MW01198899

Yamada's Textbook of Gastroenterology

Yamada's Textbook of Gastroenterology

Seventh Edition

Volume One

Edited by

Editors

Timothy C. Wang, MD

Chief, Division of Digestive and Liver Diseases
Silberberg Professor of Medicine
Department of Medicine and Irving Cancer Research Center
Columbia University Medical Center
New York, NY, USA

Michael Camilleri, MD

Atherton and Winifred W. Bean Professor
Professor of Medicine, Pharmacology and Physiology
Distinguished Investigator
Division of Gastroenterology and Hepatology
Mayo Clinic
Rochester, MN, USA

Associate Editors

Benjamin Lebwohl, MD

Associate Professor of Clinical Medicine and Epidemiology
Columbia University Medical Center
New York, NY, USA

Anna S. Lok, MD

Alice Lohrman Andrews Research Professor of Hepatology
Division of Gastroenterology and Hepatology
University of Michigan
Ann Arbor, MI, USA

William J. Sandborn, MD

Professor of Medicine
University of California
San Diego, CA, USA

Kenneth K. Wang, MD

Russell G. and Kathleen M. Van Cleve Professor of Medicine
Division of Gastroenterology and Hepatology
Mayo Clinic, Rochester, MN, USA

Gary D. Wu, MD

Ferdinand G. Weisbrod Professor in Gastroenterology
Division of Gastroenterology and Hepatology
Perelman School of Medicine
University of Pennsylvania
Philadelphia, PA, USA

WILEY Blackwell

This seventh edition first published 2022

Edition History
John Wiley & Sons Ltd (6e, 2016); Blackwell Publishing Ltd (5e, 2009)

Registered Offices
John Wiley & Sons, Inc., 111 River Street, Hoboken, NJ 07030, USA
John Wiley & Sons Ltd, The Atrium, Southern Gate, Chichester, West Sussex, PO19 8SQ, UK

Editorial Office
9600 Garsington Road, Oxford, OX4 2DQ, UK

For details of our global editorial offices, customer services, and more information about Wiley products visit us at www.wiley.com.

Wiley also publishes its books in a variety of electronic formats and by print-on-demand. Some content that appears in standard print versions of this book may not be available in other formats.

Library of Congress Cataloging-in-Publication Data

Names: Wang, Timothy C., editor. | Camilleri, Michael, editor.
Title: Yamada's textbook of gastroenterology / edited by Timothy C. Wang, Michael Camilleri ; associate editors, Benjamin Lebwohl, Anna S. Lok, William J. Sandborn, Kenneth K. Wang, Gary D. Wu.
Other titles: Textbook of gastroenterology (Yamada) | Textbook of gastroenterology
Description: Seventh edition. | Hoboken, NJ : Wiley, 2022. | Includes bibliographical references and index.
Identifiers: LCCN 2021060154 (print) | LCCN 2021060155 (ebook) | ISBN 9781119600169 (cloth) | ISBN 9781119600183 (adobe pdf) | ISBN 9781119600176 (epub)
Subjects: MESH: Digestive System Diseases | Digestive System–anatomy & histology | Digestive System Physiological Phenomena | Nutrition Disorders | Gastrointestinal Microbiome
Classification: LCC RC801 (print) | LCC RC801 (ebook) | NLM WI 140 | DDC 616.3/3–dc23/eng/20220106
LC record available at https://lccn.loc.gov/2021060154
LC ebook record available at https://lccn.loc.gov/2021060155

Cover Design: Wiley
Cover Images: Courtesy Dr. Rosa Miquel; Courtesy of Iain Kirkpatrick; Courtesy of Dr. Richard A. Kozarek; Courtesy of Dr. Krish Ragunath and Dr. Jon White; Courtesy of Dr. Martin L. Freeman; Courtesy of Dr. Martin L. Freeman

Set in 9.5/12 pt MinionPro-Regular by Straive, Pondicherry, India

Printed in Singapore
M000523W_140323

Contents

VOLUME ONE

PART 1 General principles

VOLUME TWO

VOLUME THREE

Contributors

Dwight Aberle, MD
Resident, Radiology
Columbia University Irving Medical Center, New York, NY, USA

Chathur Acharya, MD
Internist
Virginia Commonwealth University and McGuire VA Medical Center, Richmond, VA, USA

Andres Acosta, MD, PhD
Consultant
Mayo Clinic, Rochester, MN, USA

Paul C. Adams, MD, FRCP
Professor
Western University, London, ON, Canada

Joseph Ahn, MD, MS, FAASLD, FACG, AGAF
Section Chief
Oregon Health and Science University, Portland, OR, USA

David Armstrong, MA, MBChir
Professor
Department of Medicine, McMaster University, Hamilton, Ontario, Canada

Fred Askari, MD, PhD
Clinical Associate Professor
Hepatology Clinic, University of Michigan, Ann Arbor, MI, USA

Mary Raina Angeli Abad, MD
Research Fellow
Digestive Diseases Center, Showa University Koto Toyosu Hospital, Tokyo, Japan

Badr Al-Bawardy, MD
Assistant Professor of Medicine
Yale University, New Haven, CT, USA

Ahmad H. Ali, MD, FACE
Endocrinologist
Division of Gastroenterology and Hepatology, College of Medicine, Mayo Clinic, Rochester, MN, USA

Ashwin N. Ananthakrishnan, MBBS, MPH
Gastroenterologist
Massachusetts General Hospital, Boston, MA, USA

Yumi Ando, MD
Gastroenterologist
Oregon Health and Science University, Portland, OR, USA

Juan Pablo Arab, MD
Assistant Professor of Medicine
Department of Gastroenterology and Hepatology,
Medicine School, Pontifical Catholic University of Chile, Santiago, Chile

Amanda K. Arrington, MD, MHM, FACS
Associate Professor
Department of Surgery, University of Arizona, Banner University Medical Center, Tucson, AZ, USA

Stephen R. Atkinson, PhD
Visiting Research Scholar
The University of Pittsburgh, Pittsburgh, Pennsylvania, PA, USA;
Department of Hepatology, Department of Metabolism
Digestion and Reproduction, Imperial College London
London, UK

Jasmohan S. Bajaj, MD
Professor
Virginia Commonwealth University and McGuire VA Medical Center, Richmond, VA, USA

Veroushka Ballester, MD
Assistant Professor
Columbia University Irving Medical Center, New York, NY, USA

Sarah Ballou, PhD
Assistant Professor of Medicine
Beth Israel Deaconess Medical Center, Boston, MA, USA

Giorgos Bamias MD, PhD
Associate Professor
National and Kapodistrian University of Athens, Sotiria Hospital, Athens, Greece

Todd H. Baron, MD
Director of Advanced Therapeutic Endoscopy
University of North Carolina, Chapel Hill, NC, USA

Kim E. Barrett, PhD
Distinguished Professor of Medicine
Division of Gastroenterology, Department of Medicine and Program in Biomedical Sciences, University of California, San Diego, School of Medicine, La Jolla, CA, USA

Sina Bartfeld, MD
Group Leader
Research Center for Infectious Diseases, Würzburg, Germany

Adam J. Bass, MD, MSc
Associate Professor
Dana-Farber Cancer Institute and Harvard Medical School, Boston, MA, USA

Ramon Bataller, MD, PhD
Chief of Hepatology
Center for Liver Diseases, Division of Gastroenterology, Hepatology, and Nutrition, Department of Medicine, Pittsburgh Liver Research Center, University of Pittsburgh, Pittsburgh, PA, USA

Luo Xiao Bei, MD
Gastroenterologist
Department of Gastroenterology, Nanfang Hospital, Southern Medical University, Guangzhou, China.

Daniel P. Beiting, PhD
Assistant Professor
University of Pennsylvania, School of Veterinary Medicine, Philadelphia, PA, USA

Stuart Bentley-Hibbert, MD, PhD
Division Chief, Body Imaging
Columbia University Irving Medical Center, New York, NY, USA

Matthew Berger, MD
Gastroenterology Fellow
Department of Medicine, University of Rochester Medical Center, Rochester, NY, USA

Diane Bergin, MD, BCh, BAO
Consultant Radiologist
University Hospital Galway, Galway, Ireland

Adil E. Bharucha MBBS, MD
Gastroenterologist
Division of Gastroenterology and Hepatology, Mayo Clinic College of Medicine, Rochester, MN, USA

Jacob Bilhartz, MD
Professor
Department of Pediatrics, University of Michigan, Ann Arbor, MI, USA

Shrinivas Bishu, MD
Assistant Professor
Department of Medicine, Division of Gastroenterology and Hepatology, Crohn's and Colitis Center University of Michigan, Ann Arbor, MI, USA

Maurizio Bonacini, MD
Clinical Associate Professor
University of California San Francisco, San Francisco, CA, USA

Michael J. Bourke, MBBS, FRACP
Director of Endoscopy
Westmead Hospital, Westmead Clinical School University of Sydney, Sydney New South Wales, Australia;
Department of Medicine, University of British Columbia Vancouver, British Columbia, Canada

Albert J. Bredenoord, MD, PhD
Consultant Gastroenterologist
Academic Medical Center, Amsterdam, The Netherlands

Sidney Z. Brejt, MD
Assistant Professor of Radiology
Columbia University Irving Medical Center, New York, NY, USA

Robert S. Brown Jr., MD, MPH
Professor of Medicine
New York Presbyterian Weill Cornell Medical Center, Department of Gastroenterology and Hepatology, New York, USA

James Buxbaum, MD
Assistant Professor of Clinical Medicine
University of Southern California, Los Angeles, CA, USA

Michael Camilleri, MD
Atherton and Winifred W. Bean Professor
Professor of Medicine, Pharmacology and Physiology, Distinguished Investigator, Division of Gastroenterology and Hepatology, Mayo Clinic, Rochester, MN, USA

E. Ramsay Camp, MD, FACS
Professor and Chief
Division of Surgical Oncology, Baylor College of Medicine, Houston, TX, USA

David Cangemi, MD
Gastroenterologist
Mayo Clinic, Jacksonville, FL, USA

Peter Capucilli, MD
Fellow
Children's Hospital of Philadelphia, Perelman School of Medicine at University of Pennsylvania, Philadelphia, PA, USA

Lizmar Cerezo, MD
Resident
University of Puerto Rico Medical Sciences Campus, San Juan, Puerto Rico

John A. Chabot, MD, FACS
Chief, Division of GI/Endocrine Surgery
Columbia University Irving Medical Center, Herbert Irving Comprehensive Cancer Center, New York, NY, USA

Andrew T. Chan, MD, MPH
Professor
Massachusetts General Hospital and Harvard Medical School, Boston, MA, USA

Sandra D. Chanez-Paredes, PhD
Research Fellow in Pathology
Laboratory of Mucosal Barrier Pathobiology, Department of Pathology, Brigham and Women's Hospital and Harvard Medical School, Boston, MA, USA

Lin Chang, MD
Professor of Medicine
David Geffen School of Medicine at UCLA, Los Angeles, CA, USA

Julius Chapiro, MD
Assistant Professor
Yale School of Medicine, New Haven, CT, USA;
Johns Hopkins University School of Medicine Baltimore, MD, USA

Suresh T. Chari, MD
Professor
Department of Gastroenterology, Hepatology and Nutrition, Division of Internal Medicine, The University of Texas MD Anderson Cancer Center, Houston, TX, USA

Kyung Jae Cho, MD, FSIR
Professor Emeritus
Radiology, Department of Radiology, Division of Vascular and Interventional Radiology, Michigan Medicine, Ann Arbor, MI, USA;
University of Michigan Frankel Cardiovascular Center, Ann Arbor, MI, USA

George Cholankeril, MD
Assistant Professor of Medicine
Division of Gastroenterology and Hepatology, Stanford University School of Medicine, Stanford, CA, USA

Daniel C. Chung, MD
Associate Professor
Massachusetts General Hospital, Boston, MA, USA

Robert R. Cima, MD
Colon and Rectal Surgeon
Division of Colorectal Surgery, Mayo Clinic College of Medicine, Rochester, MN, USA

John O. Clarke, MD
Clinical Professor
Division of Gastroenterology and Hepatology, Stanford University School of Medicine, Redwood City, CA, USA

Hans Clevers, MD, PhD
Group Leader
Hubrecht Institute for Developmental Biology and Stem Cell Research, Oncode Institute and University Medical Centre Utrecht, Utrecht, the Netherlands; The Netherlands Princess Maxima Center for Pediatric Oncology, Utrecht, the Netherlands

Mitchell B. Cohen, MD
Chair
Department of Pediatrics, University of Alabama at Birmingham, Birmingham, AL, USA

Darwin L. Conwell, MD
Physician
Division of Gastroenterology, Hepatology, and Nutrition, The Ohio State University Wexner Medical Center, Columbus, OH, USA

Emmanuel Coronel, MD
Gastroenterologist and Advanced Therapeutic Endoscopist
University of Texas, MD Anderson Cancer Center, Houston, TX, USA

Marcia Cruz-Correa, MD, PhD
Professor
University of Puerto Rico Medical Sciences Campus and Comprehensive Cancer Center, San Juan, Puerto Rico

Zobeida Cruz-Monserrate, PhD
Assistant Professor
Department of Internal Medicine, Division of Gastroenterology, Hepatology, and Nutrition; and The James Comprehensive Cancer Center, The Ohio State University Wexner Medical Center, Columbus, OH, USA

Sushila R. Dalal, MD
Assistant Professor of Medicine
University of Chicago Medicine, Chicago, IL, USA

Rafael U. deAzevedo, MD
Research Fellow
Department of Surgery, Mayo Clinic, Rochester MN, USA

Laurie D. DeLeve, MD, PhD
Professor of Medicine
USC Keck School of Medicine, USC Research Center for Liver Diseases and Division of Gastrointestinal and Liver Diseases, Los Angeles, CA, USA

Evan S. Dellon, MD, MPH
Professor
Department of Medicine, Division of Gastroenterology and Hepatology, School of Medicine, University of North Carolina, Chapel Hill, NC, USA

Melinda Dennis, MS, RD, LDN
Nutrition Coordinator
Beth Israel Deaconess Medical Center, Boston, MA, USA

John K. Dibaise, MD
Professor of Medicine
Mayo Clinic in Arizona, Scottsdale, AZ, USA

Raymond N. DuBois, MD, PhD
Dean, College of Medicine
Medical University of South Carolina· Charleston, SC, USA

Parambir S. Dulai, MBBS
Assistant Professor of Medicine
Division of Gastroenterology, University of California San Diego health, La Jolla, California, USA

Rafael Duran, MD, PD, MER
Radiologist
Department of Radiology and Interventional Radiology, Lausanne University Hospital and University of Lausanne, Lausanne, Switzerland

Lars Eckmann, MD
Professor of Medicine
University of California, San Diego, La Jolla, CA, USA

Eric C. Ehman, MD
Assistant Professor
Mayo Clinic, Rochester, MN, USA

Xiaowen Fan, MD
Nutrition Fellow
Department of Medicine, Columbia University Irving Medical Center, New York, NY, USA

Emad M. El-Omar, BSC (HONS), MB CHB, MD (HONS)
Professor of Medicine
Microbiome Research Center, St George and Sutherland Clinical School, University of New South Wales, Sydney, Australia

Paul T. Fanta, MD
Clinical Professor of Medicine
Moores Cancer Center, University of California San Diego, La Jolla, CA, USA

David R. Farley, MD
Professor of Surgery
Mayo Clinic, Rochester MN, USA

James J. Farrell, MBChB
Director
Yale Center for Pancreatic Diseases and Advanced Endoscopy, Yale School of Medicine, New Haven, CT, USA

Andrew P. Feranchak, MD
Director
Division of Pediatric Gastroenterology, Hepatology and Nutrition, University of Pittsburgh Medical Center, Pittsburgh, PA, USA

M. Rosario Ferreira, MD
Assistant Professor
Medicine (Gastroenterology and Hepatology), Northwestern University Feinberg School of Medicine, Chicago, IL, USA

José Ferrusquía-Acosta, MD
Hepatologist
Hepatic Hemodynamic Laboratory, Liver Unit, Institute of Gastrointestinal and Metabolic Diseases, Hospital Clínic Barcelona, Institute of Biomedical Research August Pi i Sunyer (IDIBAPS), Barcelona, Spain

Elliot K. Fishman, MD
Professor of Radiology and Radiological Science
Johns Hopkins University, Baltimore, MD, USA

Mary Flanagan, MD
Specialist Registrar
Paediatric Gastroenterology, Children's Health Ireland at Crumlin, University College Dublin, Dublin;
Royal College of Surgeons in Ireland, Dublin, Ireland

Robert J. Fontana, MD
Professor
Division of Gastroenterology, University of Michigan, Ann Arbor, MI, USA

Linda J. Fothergill, PhD
Research Fellow
Florey Institute of Neuroscience and Mental Health, Parkville, VIC, Australia

Alyson N. Fox, MD
Medical Director
Living Donor Liver Team, Center for Liver Disease and Transplantation, New York Presbyterian Columbia University Medical Center, Department of Gastroenterology and Hepatology, New York, USA

John B. Furness, PhD, FAA, FAHMS
Professor
Florey Institute of Neuroscience and Mental Health, Parkville, VIC, Australia.

John J. Garber, MD
Associate Medical Director
Translational Medicine at Vertex Pharmaceuticals Boston, MA, USA;
Massachusetts General Hospital, Instructor, Harvard Medical School Boston, MA, USA

Denise I. Garcia, MD
Professor
Department of Surgery, Hollings Cancer Center, Medical University of South Carolina, and Ralph H. Johnson VA Medical Center, Charleston, SC, USA

Guadalupe García-Tsao, MD
Professor of Medicine
Yale University School of Medicine New Haven, and VA-CT Healthcare System, West Haven, CT, USA

Timothy B. Gardner, MD, MS
Associate Professor of Medicine
Dartmouth-Hitchcock Medical Center, Lebanon, NH, USA

Ishan Garg, MD
Professor
Department of Radiology, Mayo Clinic College of Medicine, Mayo Clinic, Rochester, MN, USA

Sushil Kumar Garg, MBBS
Assistant Professor of Medicine
Mayo Clinic Health System, Eau Claire, WI, USA

John Geibel, DSc, MD, AGAF, MS, FRS
Professor
Department of Surgery and Department of Cellular and Molecular Physiology, Yale University School of Medicine, New Haven, CT, USA

Jean-Francois Henri Geschwind, MD
Professor
Johns Hopkins University School of Medicine, Baltimore, MD, USA

Janna R. Gewirtz O'Brien, MD, FAAP
Fellow
Department of Pediatrics, University of Minnesota, MN, USA

Omar M. Ghanem, MD
Bariatric Surgeon
Department of Surgery, Mayo Clinic, Rochester, Rochester, MN, USA

Marc G. Ghany, MD
Gastroenterologist
National Institute of Diabetes, Digestive and Kidney Diseases, National Institutes of Health, Bethesda, MD, USA

Kevin A. Ghassemi, MD
Assistant Professor
David Geffen School of Medicine UCLA, Los Angeles, CA, USA

Victoria Gómez, MD
Associate Professor of Medicine
Mayo Clinic, Jacksonville, FL, USA

Tamas A. Gonda, MD
Gastroenterologist
Chief of Endoscopy, Department of Medicine, Tisch Hospital, and Pancreas Disease Program, New York University, New York, NY, USA

Yuna Gong, MD
Assistant Professor of Clinical Pathology
USC Keck School of Medicine, Los Angeles, CA, USA

Nirmala Gonsalves, MD
Professor of Medicine (Gastroenterology and Hepatology)
Feinberg School of Medicine, Northwestern University Rochester, MN, USA

Sugantha Govindarajan, MD
Professor of Pathology
USC Keck School of Medicine, Los Angeles, CA, USA

Chandan Guha, MBBS, PhD
Professor
Department of Radiation Oncology, Albert Einstein College of Medicine, Montefiore Medical Center, New York, NY, USA

Kristyn Gumpper, PhD
Postdoctoral Researcher in Cachexia and Pancreatic Cancer
The James Comprehensive Cancer Center; Department of Internal Medicine, Division of Gastroenterology, Hepatology, and Nutrition, The Ohio State University Wexner Medical Center, Columbus, OH, USA

Christina Ha, MD
Clinical Associate Professor
F. Widjaja Foundation Inflammatory Bowel and Immunobiology Research Institute, Cedars-Sinai Medical Center, Los Angeles, CA, USA;
David Geffen School of Medicine at UCLA, Los Angeles, CA, USA

Yuri Hanada, MD
Gastroenterologist
Mayo Clinic, Rochester, MN, USA

Phil A. Hart, MD
Program Director
Pancreas Fellowship, The Ohio State University Wexner Medical Center, Columbus, OH, USA

Gail A. Hecht, MD
Professor
Division Director, Gastroenterology and Nutrition
Department of Medicine, Loyola University Medical Centre
Maywood, IL, USA

Yasmin G. Hernandez-Barco, MD
Gastroenterologist
Massachusetts General Hospital, Boston, MA, USA

Melissa Hershman, MD
Assistant Professor
Department of Medicine, University of Rochester Medical Center, Rochester, NY, USA

Luke Higgins, MD, PhD
Medical Resident
Johns Hopkins University School of Medicine, Baltimore, MD, USA

Ikuo Hirano, MD
Professor of Medicine (Gastroenterology and Hepatology)
Northwestern University Feinberg School of Medicine, Chicago, IL, USA

Stefan D. Holubar, MD, MS
Colon and Rectal Surgeon
Colorectal Surgery, Digestive Disease Surgery Institute, Cleveland Clinic, Cleveland, OH, USA

Brian D. Hosfield, MD
Resident
Indiana University School of Medicine, Department of Surgery, Indianapolis, IN, USA

Jonathan O'B. Hourihane, MD
Professor
Paediatrics and Child Health, Royal College of Surgeons in Ireland, Dublin, Ireland

Séamus Hussey, MD
Consultant Gastroenterologist
Children's Health Ireland at Crumlin, University College Dublin, Dublin; Royal College of Surgeons in Ireland, Dublin, Ireland

Haruo Ikeda, PhD
Professor
Digestive Diseases Center, Showa University Koto Toyosu Hospital, Tokyo, Japan

John M. Inadomi, MD
Professor
Department of Internal Medicine, University of Utah School of Medicine, Salt Lake City, UT, USA

Haruhino Inoue, MD, PhD, FASGE
Professor and Chairman
Digestive Diseases Center, Showa University Koto Toyosu Hospital, Tokyo, Japan

Shayan Irani, MD
Gastroenterologist
Digestive Disease Institute, Virginia Mason Medical Center, Seattle, WA, USA

Edward N. Janoff, MD
Clinical Professor
University of Colorado Health Sciences Center Denver, Aurora, CO, USA; Veterans Affairs Medical Center, Denver, CO, USA

Dennis M. Jensen, MD
Professor of Medicine
David Geffen School of Medicine UCLA, Los Angeles, CA, USA; CURE Digestive Diseases Research Center, and VA Greater Los Angeles Healthcare System, Los Angeles, CA, USA

Robert T. Jensen, MD
Section Chief
Gastrointestinal Cell Biology Section, Digestive Disease Branch, National Institute of Diabetes and Digestive and Kidney Diseases, National Institutes of Health, Bethesda, MD, USA

Amanda M. Johnson, MD
Gastroenterologist
Division of Gastroenterology and Hepatology, Mayo Clinic College of Medicine, Rochester, MN, USA

Stella Joyce, MB, Bch, BAO, MRCPI, MRCP(UK)
Radiology Specialist Registrar
Department of Radiology, University College Cork, Cork University Hospital, Cork, Ireland

Barbara Jung, MD
Professor of Medicine
University of Washington, Seattle, WA, USA

Anthony N. Kalloo, MD
Professor Emeritus
Division of Gastroenterology and Hepatology, Johns Hopkins University School of Medicine, Baltimore, MD, USA

Margaret G. Keane, MD
Advanced Endoscopy Fellow
Johns Hopkins Hospital, Baltimore, MD, USA

Mouen A. Khashab, MD
Associate Professor
Division of Gastroenterology and Hepatology, Johns Hopkins Hospital, Baltimore, MD, USA

Peter J. Kahrilas, MD
Professor of Medicine (Gastroenterology and Hepatology)
Feinberg School of Medicine, Northwestern University, Chicago, IL, USA

Patrick S. Kamath, MD
Professor of Medicine
Mayo Clinic College of Medicine and Science, Rochester, MN, USA

Amrit K. Kamboj, MD
Gastroenterologist
Division of Gastroenterology and Hepatology, Mayo Clinic, Rochester, MN, USA

John Y. Kao, MD
Professor
Department of Internal Medicine, Division of Gastroenterology, Michigan Medicine, University of Michigan, Ann Arbor, MI, USA

Alyson J. Kaplan, MD
Fellow
New York Presbyterian Weill Cornell Medical Center, Department of Gastroenterology and Hepatology, New York, USA

Fay Kastrinos, MD
Associate Professor
Columbia University Irving Medical Center, New York, NY, USA

Jesse Katon, MD
Professor
Cancer Research Institute, Beth Israel Deaconess Medical Center, Boston, MA, USA

David A. Katzka, MD
Professor of Medicine
Department of Gastroenterology and Hepatology, Mayo Clinic, Rochester, MN, USA

Stephen J. Keely, MD
Assistant Director
Department of Molecular Medicine, Royal College of Surgeons in Ireland, Dublin, Ireland

Todd A. Kellogg, MD
General Surgeon
Department of Surgery, Mayo Clinic, Rochester, MN, USA

Samuel Kesseli, MD
Resident
Duke University Medical Center, Durham, NC, USA

Dong Wook Kim, MD
Assistance Professor
Department of Medicine, Boston University School of Medicine, Boston, MA, USA

Sun A. Kim, MD, MS, PhD
Assistant Professor of Pathology
The George Washington University, Washington, DC, USA

Ravi Pokala Kiran, MD
Chief and Program Director, Division of Colorectal Surgery
Director, Center for Innovation and Outcomes Research
Columbia University Irving Medical Center,
Department of Surgery, New York, USA

Richard A. Kozarek, MD
Executive Director
Digestive Disease Institute, Virginia Mason Medical Center, Seattle, WA, USA

Abraham Krikhely, MD, FACS
Assistant Professor of Surgery
Columbia University Irving Medical Center, New York, NY, USA

Shilpa Kulkarni, PhD
Research Assistant Professor
Department of Radiation Oncology, Albert Einstein College of Medicine, Montefiore Medical Center, New York, NY, USA

Sonia S. Kupfer, MD
Associate Professor of Medicine
The University of Chicago Medicine, Chicago, IL, USA

Brian E. Lacy, MD, PhD
Gastroenterologist
Mayo Clinic, Jacksonville, FL, USA

Uri Ladabaum, MD
Professor of Medicine
Division of Gastroenterology and Hepatology, Stanford University School of Medicine, Stanford, CA, USA

Laura Lamps, MD
Director
Department of Gastrointestinal Pathology, University of Michigan, Ann Arbor, MI, USA

Luis F. Lara, MD
Associate Professor
Department of Internal Medicine, Division of Gastroenterology, Hepatology, and Nutrition, The Ohio State University Wexner Medical Center, Columbus, OH, USA

Ryan J. Law, DO
Gastroenterologist
Mayo Clinic, Rochester, MN, USA

Konstantinos N. Lazaridis, MD
Professor of Medicine
Division of Gastroenterology and Hepatology, College of Medicine, Mayo Clinic, Rochester, MN, USA

Jocelyn Lebow, PhD, LP
Assistant Professor of Psychology
Mayo Clinic, Rochester, Minnesota, USA

Anne Marie Lennon, MD, PhD
Director
Division of Gastroenterology and Hepatology, Johns Hopkins Hospital, Baltimore, MD, USA

Allen A. Lee, MD
Clinical Lecturer
Department of Internal Medicine, Division of Gastroenterology, Michigan Medicine, University of Michigan, Ann Arbor, MI, USA

William Lee, MD
Professor
Department of Internal Medicine, University of Texas Southwestern Medical Center, Dallas, TX, USA

Daniel A. Leffler, MD
Gastroenterologist
Beth Israel Deaconess Medical Center, Boston, MA, USA

Jonathan A. Leighton, MD
Internist
Division of Gastroenterology and Hepatology, Mayo Clinic, Scottsdale, AZ, USA

Anthony Lembo, MD
Gastroenterologist
Beth Israel Deaconess Medical Center, Boston, MA, USA

John Leung, MD
Director
Division of Gastroenterology and Hepatology, Department of Internal Medicine, Tufts Medical Center, Boston, MA, USA

Joseph W. Leung, MD
Professor Emeritus
Sacramento VA Medical Center, VA Northern California Health Care System, Mather, CA, USA;
University of California Davis School of Medicine, Sacramento, CA, USA

Marc S. Levin, MD, AGAF
Professor of Medicine
VA St. Louis Health Care System and Washington University School of Medicine in St. Louis, St. Louis, MO, USA

Marc S. Levine, MD, FACR
Emeritus Professor CE of Radiology
Hospital of the University of Pennsylvania, Philadelphia, PA, USA

Andrew A. Li, MD
Fellow
Division of Gastroenterology and Hepatology, Stanford University School of Medicine, Stanford, CA, USA

T. Jake Liang, MD
Chief
Liver Diseases Branch, National Institute of Diabetes, Digestive and Kidney Diseases, National Institutes of Health, Bethesda, MD, USA

Amy L. Lightner, MD
Colon and Rectal Surgeon
Colorectal Surgery, Digestive Disease Surgery Institute, Cleveland Clinic, Cleveland, OH, USA

Berkeley N. Limketkai, MD, PhD
Associate Clinical Professor
UCLA School of Medicine, Los Angeles, CA, USA

Simon K. Lo, MD
Gastroenterologist
Cedars-Sinai Medical Center, Los Angeles, CA, USA

Benjamin Lebwohl, MD
Associate Professor of Clinical Medicine and Epidemiology
Columbia University Medical Center, New York, NY, USA

Edward V. Loftus Jr., MD
Professor of Medicine
Division of Gastroenterology and Hepatology, Mayo Clinic College of Medicine, Rochester, MN, USA

Anna S. Lok, MD
Professor
Division of Gastroenterology and Hepatology, Department of Internal Medicine, University of Michigan, Ann Arbor, MI, USA

Val J. Lowe, MD
Professor
Department of Radiology, Mayo Clinic College of Medicine, Mayo Clinic, Rochester, MN, USA

Andrew M. Lowy, MD, FACS
Chief
Division of Surgical Oncology, Moores Cancer Center, University of California San Diego, La Jolla, CA, USA

Shelly C. Lu, MD
Gastroenterologist
Cedars-Sinai Medical Center, Los Angeles, CA, USA

Jay Luther, MD
Director
Massachusetts General Hospital and Harvard Medical School, Boston, MA, USA

Michael M. Maher, MD
Professor
Department of Radiology, University College Cork, Cork University Hospital, Cork, Ireland

Carolina Malagelada, MD
Digestive System Specialist
Hospital Universitari Vall d'Hebron, Autonomous University of Barcelona, Barcelona, Spain

Juan-R. Malagelada, MD
Researcher
Digestive System Research Unit, Hospital General Universitari Vall d'Hebron, Autonomous University of Barcelona, Barcelona, Spain

Harmeet Malhi, MBBS
Associate Professor of Physiology
Mayo Clinic, Rochester, MN, USA

Michael P. Manns, MD
President
Hannover Medical School, Hannover, Germany

Troy A. Markel, MD
Associate Professor of Surgery
Indiana University School of Medicine, Department of Surgery, Indianapolis, IN, USA

Jorge A. Marrero, MD
Medical Director
Liver Transplantation, Division of Digestive and Liver Disease, University of Texas Southwestern Medical Center, Dallas, TX, USA

Laura E. Matarese, MD
Professor of Medicine
Gastroenterology, Hepatology and Nutrition, East Carolina University, Greenville, NC, USA

Marlyn J. Mayo, MD
Professor of Internal Medicine
University of Texas Southwestern Medical Center, Dallas, TX, USA

Thomas R. McCarty, MD
Research Fellow
Division of Gastroenterology, Hepatology and Endoscopy, Brigham and Women's Hospital, Boston, MA, USA;
Harvard Medical School, Boston, MA, USA

Stephen A. McClave, MD
Professor
University of Louisville, Louisville, KY, USA

Dermot McGovern, MD, PhD
Director of Translational Medicine
David Geffen School of Medicine at UCLA, Los Angeles, CA, USA;
F. Widjaja Foundation Inflammatory Bowel and Immunobiology Research Institute, Cedars-Sinai Medical Center, Los Angeles, CA, USA

Rachel M. McQuade, MD
Post Doctoral Research Fellow
Florey Institute of Neuroscience and Mental Health, Parkville, VIC, Australia;
University of Melbourne, Parkville, VIC, Australia

Kenneth McQuaid, MD
Professor & Vice Chair
Department of Medicine, Division of Gastroenterology, University of California, San Francisco, San Francisco, CA, USA

Gil Y. Melmed, MD, MS
Assistant Clinical Professor of Medicine
David Geffen School of Medicine at UCLA, Los Angeles, CA, USA;
F. Widjaja Foundation Inflammatory Bowel and Immunobiology Research Institute, Cedars-Sinai Medical Center, Los Angeles, CA, USA

Stacy Menees, MD
Clinical Associate Professor
Gastroenterology, Internal Medicine, Michigan Medicine, Ann Arbor, MI, USA

David C. Metz, MBBCh
Professor of Medicine
Perelman School of Medicine, University of Pennsylvania, Philadelphia, PA, USA

Donald G. Mitchell, MD
Professor
Department of Radiology, Thomas Jefferson University, Philadelphia, PA, USA

Ann M. Moyer, MD, PhD
Associate Professor
Laboratory Medicine And Pathology, Mayo Clinic College of Medicine and Science, Rochester, MN, USA

Gerard E. Mullin, MD, MS
Associate Professor of Medicine
Gastroenterology, Johns Hopkins University School of Medicine, Baltimore, MD, USA

Kevin P. Murphy, MD
Consultant Radiologist
Mercy University Hospital, Cork, Ireland;
Department of Radiology, University College Cork, Cork University Hospital, Cork, Ireland

Haresh Naringrekar, MD
Clinical Assistant Professor
Diagnostic Radiology, Thomas Jefferson University Hospital, Philadelphia, PA, USA

Owen O'Connor, MD
Senior Lecturer and Consultant Radiologist
Department of Radiology, University College Cork, Cork University Hospital, Cork, Ireland

Audrey R. Odom John, MD, PhD
Chief
Children's Hospital of Philadelphia, Division of Pediatric Infectious Diseases, Philadelphia, PA, USA

Paula O'Leary, MD
Professor
Department of Medicine Roinn na Sláinte, University College Cork, Cork, Ireland

Manabu Onimaru, MD, PhD
Professor
Digestive Diseases Center, Showa University Koto Toyosu Hospital, Tokyo, Japan

Amy S. Oxentenko, MD
Professor of Medicine
Division of Gastroenterology and Hepatology, Mayo Clinic, Rochester, MN, USA

Lucian Panait, MD, FACS
Bariatric Surgeon
Geisinger Commonwealth School of Medicine, AtlantiCare, Atlantic City, NJ, USA

John E. Pandolfino, MD
Chief
Gastroenterology and Hepatology, Northwestern University Medical School, Chicago, IL, USA

Darrell S. Pardi, MD
Gastroenterologist
Division of Gastroenterology and Hepatology, Mayo Clinic College of Medicine, Rochester, MN, USA

Henry P. Parkman, MD
Professor
Department of Medicine, Lewis Katz School of Medicine at Temple University, Philadelphia, PA, USA

Shabana F. Pasha, MD
Gastroenterologist
Division of Gastroenterology and Hepatology, Mayo Clinic, Scottsdale, AZ, USA

Tushar Patel, MB, ChB
Professor of Medicine
Mayo Clinic, Jacksonville, FL, USA

Richard M. Peek Jr., MD
Director
Division of Gastroenterology, Vanderbilt University Medical Center, Nashville, TN, USA

Roman Perri, MD
Assistant Professor of Medicine
Vanderbilt University Medical Center, Nashville, TN, USA

Brian A. Perrino, PhD
Associate Professor
Department of Physiology and Cell Biology, University of Nevada, Reno School of Medicine, Reno, NV, USA

Bret T. Petersen, MD
Internist
Division of Gastroenterology and Hepatology, Mayo Clinic, Rochester, MN, USA

Daniel K. Podolsky, MD
Professor
Internal Medicine, University of Texas Southwestern Medical Center, Dallas, TX, USA

Piero Portincasa, MD, PhD
Professor (Associate)
University of Bari Medical School, Bari, Italy

David O. Prichard, MB, BCh, PhD
Gastroenterologist
Mayo Clinic College of Medicine, Rochester, MN, USA

Deborah D. Proctor, MD
Professor of Medicine (Digestive Diseases)
Yale University, New Haven, CT, USA

Ruslan V. Pustovit, PhD
Postdoctoral Research Fellow
Florey Institute of Neuroscience and Mental Health, and University of Melbourne, Parkville, VIC, Australia

Jianwen Que, MD, PhD
Associate Professor of Medicine
Columbia University Medical Center, New York, NY, USA

Eamonn M. M. Quigley, MD
Professor of Medicine
Houston Methodist Hospital and Weill Cornell Medical College, Houston, TX, USA;
University College Cork, Cork, Ireland

David S. Raiford, MD
Chief, Medical Staff
Vanderbilt University Medical Center, Nashville, TN, USA

Aashish Rajesh, MD
General Surgery Resident
University of Texas Health Science Center, San Antonio, TX, USA

Mitchell L. Ramsey, MD
Fellow
Division of Gastroenterology, Hepatology, and Nutrition, The Ohio State University Wexner Medical Center, Columbus, OH, USA

Satish S.C. Rao, MD, PHD, FRCP, FACG, AGAF
Professor
Division of Neurogastroenterology & Motility, Department of Medicine, Augusta University, Augusta, GA, USA

Jean-Pierre Raufman, MD
Division Head
Gastroenterology & Hepatology, University of Maryland School of Medicine and Veterans Affairs Maryland Health Care System, Baltimore, MD, USA

Craig C. Reed, MD, MSCR
Assistant Professor of Medicine
Department of Medicine, Division of Gastroenterology and Hepatology, School of Medicine, University of North Carolina, Chapel Hill, NC, USA

Joel M. Reid, PhD
Associate Professor
Pharmacology, Mayo Clinic College of Medicine and Science, Rochester, MN, USA

Anupam Rej, MD
Professor
Royal Hallamshire Hospital, Sheffield Teaching Hospitals, Sheffield, UK

Douglas K. Rex, MD
Distinguished Professor Emeritus
Division of Gastroenterology and Hepatology, Indiana University School of Medicine, Indianapolis, IN, USA

Mona Rezapour, MD, MHS
Gastroenterologist
University of California Los Angeles, Los Angeles, CA, USA

Nicole E. Rich, MD
Assistant Professor
Internal Medicine, Division of Digestive and Liver Disease, University of Texas Southwestern Medical Center, Dallas, TX, USA

Don C. Rockey, MD
Professor
Digestive Disease Research Center, Department of Internal Medicine, Medical University of South Carolina, Charleston, SC, USA

Sabine Roman, MD, PhD
Associate Professor
Digestive Physiology, Lyon I University, Lyon, France

Stephen E. Rubesin, MD
Emeritus Professor CE of Radiology
Hospital of the University of Pennsylvania, Philadelphia, PA, USA

Deborah C. Rubin, MD, AGAF
Professor
Washington University School of Medicine, Saint Louis, MO, USA

Rebecca Rudel, MPH, RD, CNSC
Graduate Teaching Fellow
Boston University School of Public Health, Boston, MA, USA

Anil K. Rustgi, MD
Professor of Medicine
Herbert Irving Comprehensive Cancer Center, Columbia University, Irving Medical Center, New York, NY, USA

David S. Sanders, MB, ChB, MD, FRCP, FACG
Honorary Professor of Gastroenterology
Department of Infection, Immunity and Cardiovascular Disease, Royal Hallamshire Hospital, The Sheffield Teaching Hospitals, Sheffield, UK

William J. Sandborn, MD
Professor of Medicine
University of California
San Diego, CA, USA

Kenton M. Sanders, PhD
Professor & Chair
Department of Physiology and Cell Biology, University of Nevada, Reno School of Medicine, Reno, NV, USA

Arun J. Sanyal, MD
Professor
Department of Internal Medicine, Division of Gastroenterology, Hepatology & Nutrition, Virginia Commonwealth University, Richmond, VA, USA

Todd R. Schlachter, MD
Radiologist
Johns Hopkins University School of Medicine, Baltimore, MD, USA

Carol E. Semrad, MD
Professor of Medicine
University of Chicago Medicine, Chicago, IL, USA

Antonia R. Sepulveda, MD, PhD
Professor of Pathology
The George Washington University, Washington, DC, USA

David S. Seres, MD, ScM, PNS
Associate professor
Institute of Human Nutrition and Department of Medicine, Columbia University Irving Medical Center, New York, NY, USA

Nicholas J. Shaheen, MD, MPH
Chief
Department of Medicine, Division of Gastroenterology and Hepatology, School of Medicine, University of North Carolina, Chapel Hill, NC, USA

Neal Shahidi, MD
Gastroenterologist
Department of Medicine, St. Paul's Hospital, University of British Columbia, Vancouver, British Columbia, Canada;
Department of Gastroenterology and Hepatology, Westmead Hospital, Sydney, New South Wales, Australia

Nizamuddin Shaikh, MD
General Surgeon
Department of Surgery, Mayo Clinic, Rochester MN, USA

Anisa Shaker, MD
Assistant Professor of Medicine
Keck School of Medicine of the University of Southern California, Los Angeles, CA, USA

Bo Shen, MD
Professor of Medicine
Columbia University Irving Medical Center, New York Presbyterian Hospital, New York, NY, USA

Nicole T. Shen, MD
Fellow
New York Presbyterian Weill Cornell Medical Center, Department of Gastroenterology and Hepatology, New York, USA

Courtney B. Sherman, MD
Hepatologist
Department of Medicine, Division of Gastroenterology, University of California, San Francisco, CA, USA

Yuto Shimamura, MD
Assistant Professor
Digestive Diseases Center, Showa University Koto Toyosu Hospital, Tokyo, Japan

M. Shadab Siddiqui, MD
Associate Professor
Department of Internal Medicine, Division of Gastroenterology, Hepatology & Nutrition, Virginia Commonwealth University, Richmond, VA, USA

Leslie Sim, PhD, LP
Psychologist
Department of Pediatrics, Mayo Clinic, Minneapolis, MN, USA

Magnus Simrén, MD, PhD
Professor of Gastroenterology
University of Gothenburg, Gothenburg, Sweden

Siddharth Singh, MD
Assistant Professor of Medicine
Division of Gastroenterology, University of California San Diego, La Jolla, CA, USA

Phillip D. Smith, MD
Professor of Medicine
Division of Gastroenterology and Hepatology, University of Alabama at Birmingham, AL, USA

Sergei A. Sobolevsky, MD, MBA
Managing Physician
Modern Vascular Hospital, Mesa, Arizona, AZ, USA

Rhonda F. Souza, MD
Co-Director
Baylor University Medical Center and Baylor Scott & White Center for Esophageal Diseases, Dallas, TX, USA

Stuart Jon Spechler, MD
Gastroenterologist
Baylor University Medical Center and Baylor Scott & White Center for Esophageal Diseases, Dallas, TX, USA

Jonathan M. Spergel, MD, PhD
Professor of Pediatrics
Children's Hospital of Philadelphia, Perelman School of Medicine at University of Pennsylvania, Philadelphia, PA, USA

James E. Squires, MD, MS
Assistant Professor
Department of Pediatrics, School of Medicine, University of Pittsburgh, Pittsburgh, PA, USA

Martin J. Stebbing, BSc (Hons), PhD
Senior Research Fellow
Florey Institute of Neuroscience and Mental Health, and University of Melbourne, Parkville, VIC, Australia

Neil Stollman, MD, FACP, FACG, AGAF
Associate Clinical Professor
Alta Bates Summit Medical Center, East Bay Center for Digestive Health, Oakland, CA, USA

Sarah Streett, MD
Clinical Associate Professor
Division of Gastroenterology and Hepatology, Stanford University School of Medicine, Stanford, CA, USA

Grace L. Su, MD
Professor
Gastroenterology, Michigan Medicine, University of Michigan, Ann Arbor, MI, USA;
Veterans Administration, Ann Arbor Healthcare System, Ann Arbor, MI, USA

Debra Sudan, MD
Professor of Surgery
Duke University Medical Center, Durham, NC, USA

Kazuki N. Sugahara, MD, PhD
Assistant Professor
Surgical Sciences, Columbia University Irving Medical Center, New York, NY, USA

Kazuki Sumiyama, MD, PhD
Professor
Department of Endoscopy, The Jikei University School of Medicine, Tokyo, Japan

Seth Sweetser, MD
Associate Professor
Division of Gastroenterology and Hepatology, Department of Medicine, Mayo Clinic College of Medicine, Rochester, MN, USA

Lawrence Szarka, MD
Gastroenterologist
Mayo Clinic College of Medicine, Rochester, MN, USA

Vania Tacher, MD
Radiologist
Greater Paris University Hospitals, Paris, France

Jan Tack, MD
Professor
Department of Gastroenterology, University of Leuven, Belgium

Andrew W. Tai, MD
Gastroenterologist
University of Michigan and VA Ann Arbor Healthcare System, Ann Arbor, MI, USA

Richard Taubert, MD
Gastroenterologist
Hannover Medical School, Hannover, Germany

Christopher C. Thompson, MD
Professor
Division of Gastroenterology, Hepatology and Endoscopy, Brigham and Women's Hospital, Boston, MA, USA; Harvard Medical School, Boston, MA, USA

Judy A. Trieu, MD
Fellow
Gastroenterology and Hepatology, Loyola University Medical Center, Maywood, IL, USA

Jerrold R. Turner, MD, PhD
Professor
Laboratory of Mucosal Barrier Pathobiology, Department of Pathology, Brigham and Women's Hospital and Harvard Medical School, Boston, MA, USA

Travis W. Vandergriff, MD
Associate Professor of Dermatology
University of Texas Southwestern Medical Center, Dallas, TX, USA

Johan H. van Es, PhD
Researcher
Hubrecht Institute for Developmental Biology and Stem Cell Research, Oncode Institute and University Medical Centre Utrecht, Utrecht, The Netherlands

Stephen J. Vanner, MSc, MD
Professor
Queen's University, Kingston, ON, Canada

Hugo E. Vargas, MD
Gastroenterologist
Mayo Clinic, Scottsdale, AZ, USA

John J. Vargo, MD, MPH
Director of Endoscopic Operations
Cleveland Clinic Foundation, Cleveland, OH, USA

Elizabeth J. Videlock, MD
Clinical Instructor
Division of Digestive Diseases, Department of Medicine, David Geffen School of Medicine at UCLA, Los Angeles, CA, USA

Kavel H. Visrodia, MD, PhD
Assistant Professor
Division of Digestive Diseases, Columbia University Irving Medical Center, New York city, NY, USA

Erik C. von Rosenvinge, MD
Associate Professor
University of Maryland School of Medicine, Baltimore, MD, USA

Vaibhav Wadhwa, MD
Gastroenterologist
Gastroenterology & Hepatology, Cleveland Clinic Foundation, Cleveland, OH, USA

David H. Wang, MD, PhD
Associate Professor
Department of Internal Medicine, The University of Texas Southwestern Medical Center, Dallas, TX, USA

David Q.-H. Wang, MD, PhD
Professor
Department of Medicine and Genetics, Albert Einstein College of Medicine, Bronx, NY, USA

Kenneth K. Wang, MD
Russell G. and Kathleen M. Van Cleve Professor of Medicine
Division of Gastroenterology and Hepatology,
Mayo Clinic, Rochester, MN, USA

Timothy C. Wang, MD
Chief, Division of Digestive and Liver Diseases
Silberberg Professor of Medicine
Department of Medicine and Irving Cancer
Research Center,
Columbia University Medical Center,
New York, NY, USA

Mary Kay Washington, MD, PhD
Professor of Pathology
Vanderbilt University Medical Center, Nashville, TN, USA

Irving Waxman, MD
Professor of Medicine and Surgery
Department of Medicine and Surgery; Division of Digestive Diseases & Nutrition; Digestive Disease Service Line for Rush University System for Health, Chicago, IL, USA

Joel V. Weinstock, MD
Professor of Medicine
Division of Gastroenterology and Hepatology, Department of Internal Medicine, Tufts Medical Center, Boston, MA, USA

Theodore H. Welling, MD
Director
Liver Tumor Program, NYU Langone Health, New York, USA

Maria Westerhoff, MD
Associate Professor
Gastrointestinal and Hepatobiliary Pathology, Department of Pathology, Michigan Medicine, University of Michigan, Ann Arbor, MI, USA

David C. Whitcomb, MD, PhD
Professor of Medicine
Giant Eagle Foundation Professor of Cancer Genetics, Department of Medicine, Cell Biology & Molecular Physiology, and Human Genetics,
Division of Gastroenterology,
Hepatology and Nutrition, University of Pittsburgh and University of Pittsburgh Medical Center, Pittsburgh, Pennsylvania, USA

C. Mel Wilcox, MD
Professor Emeritus
University of Alabama-Birmingham, Birmingham, AL, USA

Grace L.H. Wong, MD, FRCP
Professor
Institute of Digestive Disease, Department of Medicine and Therapeutics, and State Key Laboratory of Digestive Disease, The Chinese University of Hong Kong, Hong Kong Special Administrative Region, China

Louis M. Wong Kee Song, MD
Consultant
Department of Medicine, and Division of Gastroenterology and Hepatology, Mayo Clinic College of Medicine and Science, Rochester, MN, USA

Gary D. Wu, MD
Ferdinand G. Weisbrod Professor in Gastroenterology
Division of Gastroenterology and Hepatology,
Perelman School of Medicine, University of Pennsylvania,
Philadelphia, PA, USA

Ramnik J. Xavier, MD, PhD
Director
Center for the Study of Inflammatory Bowel Disease, Kurt Isselbacher Professor of Medicine, Harvard Medical School, and Massachusetts General Hospital, Boston, MA, USA

Mohammad Yaghoobi, MD
Associate Professor
Department of Medicine, McMaster University, Hamilton, Ontario, Canada

Amoah Yeboah-Korang, MD, MPH
Assistant Professor
Digestive Diseases, University of Cincinnati Medical Center,
Cincinnati, OH, USA

Andrew W. Yen, MD
Gastroenterologist
Sacramento VA Medical Center, VA Northern California Health Care System, Mather, CA, USA;
University of California Davis School of Medicine, Sacramento, CA, USA

Eugene F. Yen, MD
Gastroenterologist
University of Chicago Pritzker School of Medicine, NorthShore University Health System, Evanston, IL, USA

Howard Yim, BSc(Hons), PhD
Senior Postdoctoral Fellow
Microbiome Research Center, St George and Sutherland Clinical School, University of New South Wales, Sydney, Australia.

Vincent B. Young, MD, PhD
Professor
Department of Internal Medicine, Division of Infectious Diseases, Michigan Medical School, University of Michigan, Ann Arbor, MI, USA

Camila Zamboni, MD
Resident
Johns Hopkins University School of Medicine, Baltimore, MD, USA

Harvey A. Ziessman, MD
Professor
Division of Nuclear Medicine, Russell H. Morgan Department of Radiology and Radiological Sciences, Johns Hopkins University, Baltimore, MD, USA

Preface to the Seventh Edition

It has now been nearly 30 years since the publication of the first edition of the *Textbook of Gastroenterology*, formulated and developed by the first Editor, Dr Tadataka Yamada, a leading figure in gastroenterology. The goal at that time was to create the most comprehensive textbook and reference in the field, covering in encyclopedic fashion all of clinical gastroenterology and hepatology and, at the same time, grounding the discussion and approach in basic science. Dr Yamada brought together some of the best known thought leaders in the field to serve as Editors, and they in turn sought out luminaries in relevant areas to author cutting edge chapters that elucidated the molecular and pathologic basis of gastrointestinal diseases. This first edition was spectacular, and was followed by four subsequent editions by Dr Yamada and his colleagues, which included Drs David H. Alpers, Chung Owyang, Daniel K. Podolsky, Don H. Powell, and Fred E. Silverstein. Over the years, the textbook became firmly entrenched in the digestive community as an essential resource for students, residents, fellows, and practicing GI clinicians.

A sixth edition, published 5 years ago, was led by a different Editor-in-Chief, Dr Daniel K. Podolsky, who was in many ways the natural successor to Dr Yamada as the main Editor for this formidable textbook. Dr Podolsky assembled a brand new team of Associate Editors, which included Drs Michael Camilleri, J. Gregory Fitz, Anthony N. Kalloo, Fergus Shanahan, and Timothy C. Wang. More substantial changes were made in this sixth edition, compared to previous editions. The changes nicely updated, supplemented, and reinvigorated the textbook with web-based links, shortening the list of references to key references and moving the remainder online, and adding a new section entitled "Approaches to the patient with . . .." that provided a convenient source and framework for clinical management of common gastrointestinal problems. More emphasis was given to the ancillary fields of endoscopy, imaging, histology, and pathology. Coverage of inflammatory bowel diseases, a rapidly changing field, was expanded and reorganized as a stand-alone section, and the textbook as a whole encompassed a more global view of gastroenterology with greater attention to geographic differences.

Three years ago, leadership of this fine textbook was entrusted to two of the Editors from the last edition, Drs Michael Camilleri and Timothy Wang, who stepped forward to lead the seventh edition of the Yamada textbook. A new team of Editors was assembled, which included Benjamin Lebwohl, Anna Lok, William Sandborn, Kenneth K. Wang, and Gary D. Wu. This new team was particularly well suited to address several new initiatives and additions to the textbook. A key change has been a much greater focus on the structure and function of the human microbiome, with implications for health and disease. The textbook has also been expanded to include a section on the role of gastroenterologists in the management of obesity, which is become an increasing component of GI practice. The endoscopic offerings have been bolstered by new chapters on bariatric endoscopy and endoscope reprocessing. Finally, a greater geriatric focus has been achieved by a new chapter on the aging gastrointestinal tract. Despite these new additions, broadening and increasing the scope of the textbook, the overall number of authors and length of the textbook have not increased, with the consolidation and/or elimination of several older chapters, as well as shortening of others.

Despite the continued growth and utilization of internet-based sources of information, we strongly believe that textbooks such as this one remain a vital resource for both experienced clinicians and novices to the fields of gastroenterology and hepatology. Information found on the internet in all fields of knowledge continues to exhibit an inconsistent quality, with a lack of sufficient vetting and expert review on many internet sites. A great advantage of the Yamada textbook is that it is both comprehensive and well sourced by expert authors and editors, such that vital information on the widest spectrum of GI and liver diseases, ranging from essential clinical features to the molecular underpinnings, can be found in one convenient location. As such, a comprehensive reference such as this is still a highly dependable and valued source of knowledge.

We would like to thank the many individuals who contributed to this work. The textbook represents the efforts of the

Editors and authors, as well as our many teachers and colleagues over the years, from whom we have learned about the rewarding specialties of gastroenterology and hepatology. We would also like to thank our patients, who educated us more directly about the real meaning of GI diseases and their impact on patients' lives. Finally, we are grateful to all the previous Editors of this textbook, who set a high standard for excellence in a GI textbook. We acknowledge our many partners at Wiley, including Jennifer Seward, Ambikapathi Raja, and Pri Gibbons, for their invaluable assistance in this project.

We are hopeful that the combined work of our team has resulted in an enjoyable and useful set of volumes for our esteemed readers.

Timothy C. Wang, MD
Michael Camilleri, MD
Benjamin Lebwohl, MD
Anna S. Lok, MD
William J. Sandborn, MD
Kenneth K. Wang, MD
Gary D. Wu, MD

Foreword to the Seventh Edition

Tadataka Yamada

When the Editors of the first edition of the *Textbook of Gastroenterology* gathered together to plan the book's design and contents 35 years ago, the internet as we know it today did not exist. At that time, it was still a National Science Foundation project that permitted access only to government agencies and universities. It wasn't until 1991, the year that the first edition of the *Textbook*, was published that the internet was opened up to commercial service providers and started to become what it is today. How could we possibly have known then the manner in which students, trainees, and practitioners of gastroenterology would learn the subject a third of a century later? The growth of readily accessible information on the internet through handy devices that fit neatly and unobtrusively in our pockets has fundamentally changed the way people gain information about disease states that define our discipline of gastroenterology. In the day of tools such as *UpToDate*, why would anyone need a textbook, some might question.

Without any foresight into the age of the internet, we, the first editors, took an approach to the design of the *Textbook* that I believe has allowed it to be every bit as relevant today as it was back then. By way of explanation, permit me to return to the day I left Japan at the age of 15. My father told me then that the reason he was sending me away at such a tender age to obtain my education in the United States was the way in which Americans teach and learn. He was concerned that the Japanese system of education at that time was based on memorization of facts while the American system was based on deductive reasoning. Staying true to the educational approach championed by my father, my associate editors and I endeavored to design a textbook that contained not only the factual information about disease states but also the scientific basis behind the diseases, the way to approach patients with symptoms but without defined diseases, the tools and instruments that could be applied to learn more about a patient's problems and the images that allow us to see the organs of interest in our very visual discipline. As I wrote in the Preface to the first edition of the *Textbook*:

> "The purposes of the *Textbook of Gastroenterology*, then, are multiple: to teach the scientific basis of gastroenterology, to provide practical approaches to common gastrointestinal problems, to serve as an encyclopedic reference for gastrointestinal diseases, and to indicate the current applications and future directions of the technology of gastroenterology. Above all, the *Textbook* is planned to integrate the various demands of science, technology, expanding information, good judgment, and common sense in the diagnosis and management of gastrointestinal patients."

In other words, this textbook has been designed from the beginning not to be simply a compendium of information that can be readily accessed on the internet but a source of knowledge and information in a single place that would allow the reader to learn the discipline of gastroenterology by "deductive reasoning." As with any good textbook, each edition has been refreshed and improved with new chapters, authors and editors but the book has not wavered from its initial educational strategy.

To Dan Podolsky who served as the editor of the *Textbook* in its sixth edition, my deepest gratitude for your masterful job in enhancing the quality of the book. To the newest editors of the book, Tim Wang and Michael Camilleri, renowned leaders, educators, scientists, and practitioners of gastroenterology, I join the world of students of our discipline in looking forward to learning from the unique insights that you and your associate editors have brought to the seventh edition.

Addendum

While this edition of the *Textbook* was in production, on August 4, 2021, Dr Tadataka Yamada passed away rather suddenly and unexpectedly. Many glowing commentaries and obituaries were quickly written about Dr Yamada and his long and varied career, his many accomplishments and his tremendous impact on the field of healthcare. Born in Japan but educated at Phillips Andover Academy, Stanford University and

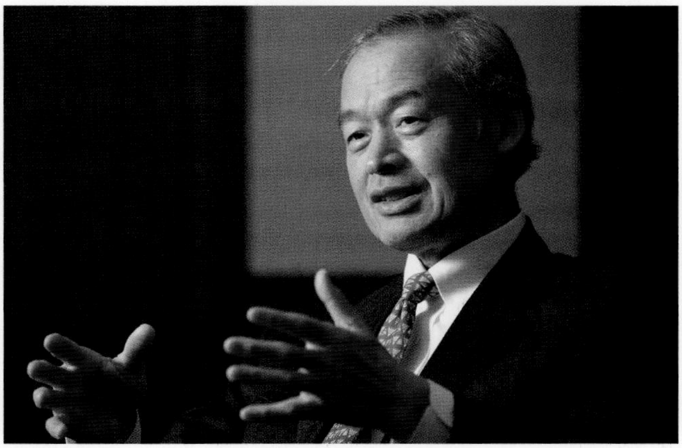

Dr Tadataka Yamada

NYU, "Tachi" initially pursued the life of a physician-scientist at the University of Michigan, but was recognized early on for his inspirational leadership qualities and quickly rose to positions of Division Chief and Chairman of Internal Medicine before leaving academic medicine to take on senior positions at GlaxoSmithKline, the Gates Foundation, Takeda, and finally Frazier Healthcare Partners. However, even during his time in industry, Dr Yamada remained loyal to his roots in medicine, and his inspirational presence continued to be felt in the field of gastroenterology and hepatology. He encouraged us to continue this textbook of gastroenterology, which he felt was one of his most treasured achievements, and we are deeply saddened by the knowledge that he will not be with us to see this latest edition. Nevertheless, this textbook is one of his many great gifts and his enduring legacy in the field of digestive diseases.

About the companion website

This book is accompanied by a companion website:

www.yamadagastro.com/textbook7e 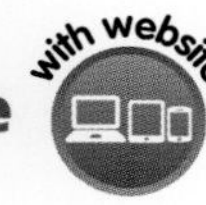

The website includes:
- Full lists of references
- Digital edition access instructions

PART 1

General principles

CHAPTER 1

Development and differentiation of the gastrointestinal system*

Jianwen Que[1] and Daniel K. Podolsky[2]

[1] Columbia University Medical Center, New York, NY, USA

[2] University of Texas Southwestern Medical Center, Dallas, TX, USA

Chapter menu

Previous studies of animal models have elucidated cellular and molecular events that are essential for building an organism. Central to the field are questions about differentiation, morphogenesis, and growth – the processes that give rise to our physical appearance, physiology, and (when perturbed) diseases. Despite many years of intensive research, our understanding of the molecular mechanisms that guide normal vertebrate development remains incomplete. Perturbations in these processes, resulting in congenital malformations or functional diseases, are difficult to study because developmental insults may occur weeks or months before a defect is detectable.

Although an understanding of how the body is formed is intrinsically important, it is also clinically relevant. Exploiting developmental processes offers the promise of creating "cell therapies" – that is, growing tissues ex vivo for use in tissue transplantation and augmentation, or coaxing cells in vivo to acquire characteristics that restore function. Fulfilling this promise will undoubtedly require a more complete delineation of developmental mechanisms.

The chapter has been divided into several sections to facilitate an appreciation for the complexity of the development of the gastrointestinal system. *Early development* outlines the basic mechanisms by which the embryo achieves a spatial "pattern," setting the stage for further developmental steps. *Organogenesis* focuses on the known molecular mechanisms that guide development of the liver, pancreas, and lumenal gastrointestinal tract. *Developmental physiology* samples important events during the functional maturation of the gastrointestinal tract. *Disorders of development*, the fourth and final section, focuses on specific diseases that highlight the relationship between molecular events and clinical consequences. The embryology of the human gastrointestinal tract involves many temporally and spatially regulated tissue interactions and the creation of many varied structures. The ensuing discussion focuses on the mechanisms of gastrointestinal development. What hurdles must be surmounted to create a gastrointestinal tract with normal form and function, and how can these processes be controlled for therapeutic benefit?

Early development

The transformation from a fertilized egg to newborn occurs in many steps marked by discrete milestones (Figure 1.1). The fertilized egg initially grows in cell number through cleavage divisions into a blastocyst – an asymmetrical collection of cells containing the precursors of both embryo and placenta – which implants in the uterine wall. After implantation, the

* This is an update of a chapter in which Dr. Ben Stanger at the University of Pennsylvania served as an author.

Yamada's Textbook of Gastroenterology, Seventh Edition. Edited by Timothy C. Wang, Michael Camilleri, Benjamin Lebwohl, Anna S. Lok, William J. Sandborn, Kenneth K. Wang, and Gary D. Wu.

Companion website: www.yamadagastro.com/textbook7e

endoderm – the cell layer from which the epithelium of all gastrointestinal organs is derived – is formed through the process of *gastrulation*. Subsequently, the endoderm is segmented (*patterned*) into domains that become *committed* to create specific organs. Finally, solid organ buds emerge from the gut tube, and organogenesis proceeds with the processes of *differentiation* and *morphogenesis*.

Many studies of gastrointestinal development have been performed in model organisms, including fruit flies (*Drosophila melanogaster*), frogs (*Xenopus laevis*), zebrafish (*Danio rerio*), and mice (*Mus musculus*). Despite differences in anatomy and timing of development (see Figure 1.1), most studies suggest that many developmental mechanisms in the mouse are comparable with those in human. Information gained from model organisms can therefore be reasonably extrapolated to humans because of evolutionary conservation of mechanism. Indeed, recent progress made in the differentiation of human pluripotent stem cells confirmed that most, if not all, signaling pathways demonstrate conserved functions in the generation of epithelial cells lining the gastrointestinal tract.

Gastrulation and tube formation

To understand gastrointestinal form and function, it is necessary to recognize the steps that precede organogenesis. The most important of these is *gastrulation*, the process by which three distinct "germ layers" – ectoderm, mesoderm, and endoderm – are formed. The embryo exists as a disc of cells called the *epiblast* after implantation in the uterus. Two structures – the node and the primitive streak – appear in the posterior half of the epiblast layer, and cells migrate caudally toward, and down through, the primitive streak, generating new layers of cells – the embryonic mesoderm and embryonic endoderm (Figure 1.2). As a consequence of gastrulation, the three axes of the embryo are also established: the anterior–posterior (or rostral–caudal) axis is defined by the location of the primitive streak (posterior), the dorsal–ventral axis is defined by the ectoderm (dorsal) and endoderm (ventral), and the left–right axis is defined by the other two axes.

How the cells that migrate through the primitive streak are instructed to become mesoderm or endoderm is incompletely understood. Phylogenetic analyses of organisms, including fish, frogs, and mice, point to a conserved pathway for endoderm development that involves the transforming growth factor-β (TGF-β)-related nodal pathway and several classes of DNA-binding transcription factors that belong to the homeobox, forkhead (winged helix), zinc finger, and high mobility group families [1].

The tubular structure of the gut arises from two ventral invaginations that form at the anterior (proximal) and posterior (distal) ends of the embryo after gastrulation (see Figure 1.2). These will eventually form the structures of the foregut and hindgut, respectively. The anterior fold, or anterior intestinal portal, and the caudal fold, or caudal intestinal portal, move toward each other and meet in the midline of the embryo at the level of the yolk sac. As a result, ventral structures close to the midline (e.g., lung, liver, and ventral pancreas) derive from endoderm that is distinct and distant from the endoderm that gives rise to dorsal structures (e.g., dorsal pancreas). This arrangement means that the dorsal and ventral portions of the pancreas are independently induced, although these tissues eventually combine to form one functioning organ.

Several genes have been identified that are required for tube formation of the gut (Table 1.1). One of these genes encodes GATA4, a zinc finger-containing, DNA-binding protein. Although endoderm is able to develop in *Gata4* mutant mice, formation of the anterior intestinal portal is faulty and results in failure to form a foregut [2–4]. Other genes that are required for tube formation or closure include those encoding the forkhead-winged helix DNA-binding transcription factor FOXA2 (previously hepatocyte nuclear factor 3B [HNF3B]), which has additional roles in foregut and midgut development, and the FURIN protease, which may be necessary to process TGF-β signals [5–7]. A critical and conserved role for two other families – the high mobility group domain-containing SOX factors and the homeodomain-containing MIX (Mesoderm Inducing Factor [MIF]-inducible homeobox) factors – has been demonstrated [8–10]. GATA4-like and FOXA-like factors are involved in gut development in organisms as distantly related to mammals as the fruit fly *Drosophila* and the nematode *Caenorhabditis elegans* [11], whereas the involvement of SOX and MIX factors

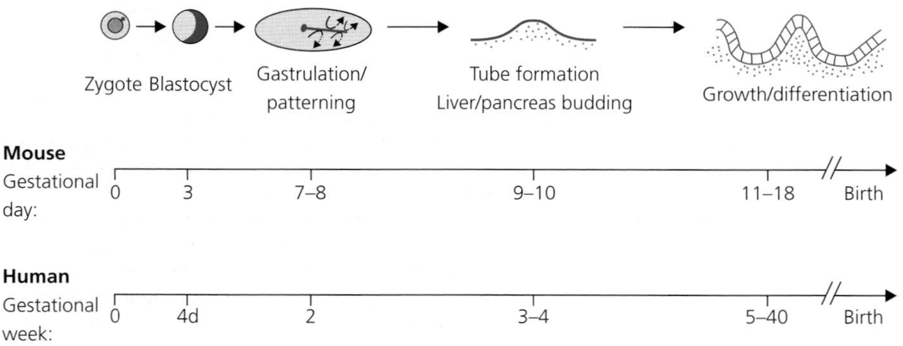

Figure 1.1 Overview of gastrointestinal development. Timelines for milestones of mouse (18-day gestation) and human (40-week gestation) embryogenesis. See text for details of individual steps.

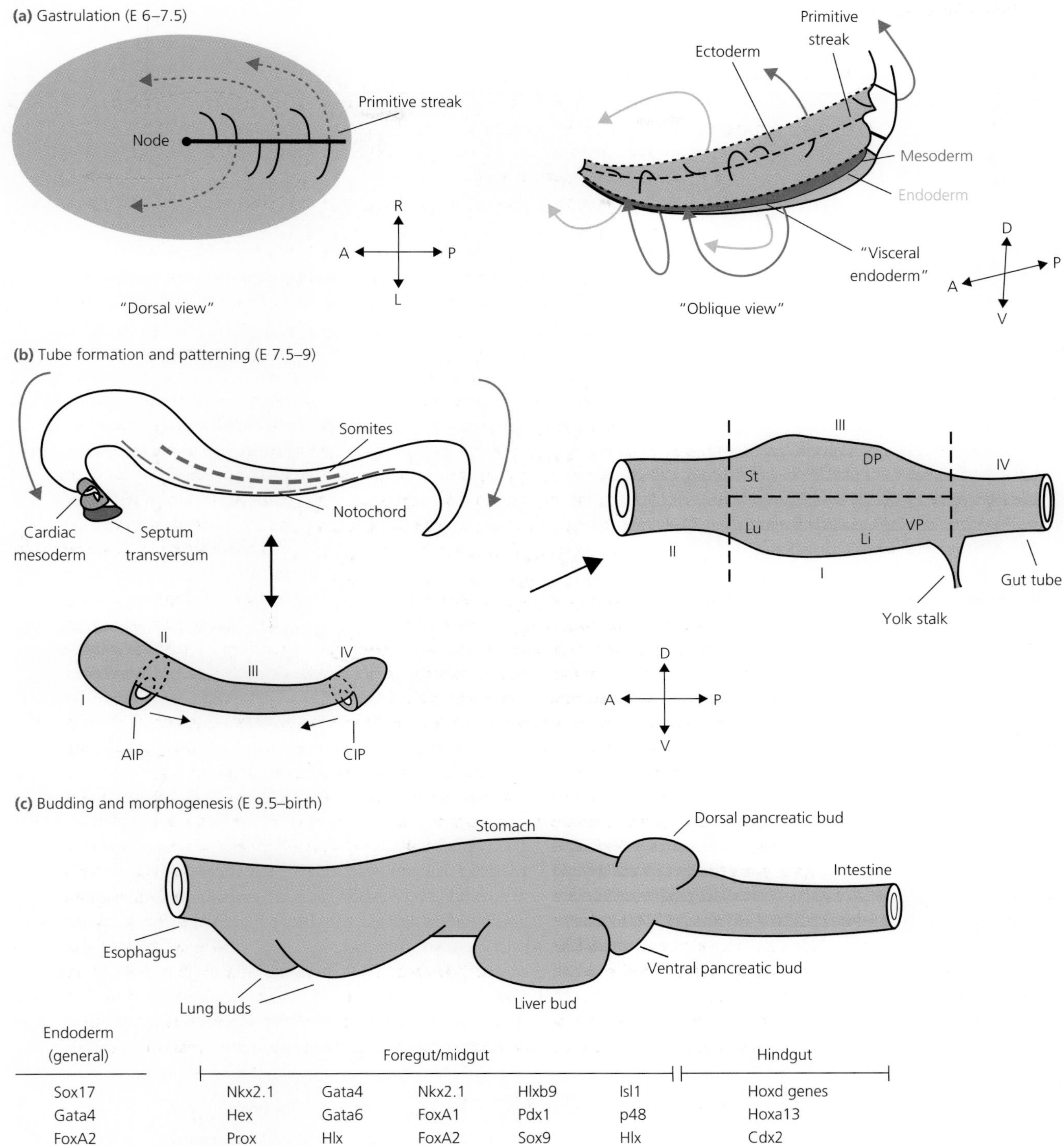

Figure 1.2 Major events in early mammalian endoderm development. **(a)** Gastrulation. **(left)** The embryonic epiblast (blue) viewed from above. Epiblast cells (solid black) migrate down through the primitive streak, becoming mesoderm (dashed red) or endoderm (dashed yellow) cells. **(right)** Oblique view of migrating epiblast cells, in which formation of the new mesoderm and endoderm is visible. **(b)** Tube formation and patterning. **(left)** The mesoderm and ectoderm have been pulled back to reveal the endoderm below. At this stage, the anterior endoderm is adjacent to the cardiac mesoderm and septum transversum (which mediate liver induction), whereas more dorsal portions of the endoderm are in contact with the notochord (which mediates pancreas induction). The folds of the anterior intestinal portal (AIP) and caudal intestinal portal (CIP) form the gut tube as they migrate toward each other at the midline. Blue arrows indicate the process of turning, by which the embryo switches from a convex to a concave shape, with the endoderm on the "inside." The roman numeral designations are derived from fate-mapping studies and indicate the prospective regions of endoderm that will give rise to later endoderm derivatives. (*right*) The relative position of endoderm domains changes with the completion of gut tube folding; the region that previously constituted the most anterior portion of endoderm (I) shifts to the ventral midline and gives rise to lung (Lu), liver (Li), and ventral pancreas (VP). **(c)** Budding and morphogenesis. Budding of endoderm derivatives begins shortly after the gut tube is formed and involves many transcription factors. A, anterior; D, dorsal; DP, dorsal pancreas; E, embryonic day; L, left; P, posterior; R, right; St, stomach; V, ventral. Source: Stanger and Melton 2003 [241]. Reproduced with permission of Oxford University Press.

Table 1.1 Transcription factors in gastrointestinal development.

Gene class	Region	Function
HMG-box genes		
SOX17	Endoderm	Formation of definitive endoderm
SOX10	Enteric nervous system	Development of neural crest derivatives
SOX9	Intestine	Formation of pyloric sphincter
SOX2	Esophagus	Formation of stratified squamous epithelium
GATA genes		
GATA4	Endoderm	Anterior intestinal portal and foregut development
GATA6	Liver	Liver bud outgrowth, regulates HNF4
FOXA genes		
FOXA1 (HNF3A)	Endoderm, liver	FOXA1/A2 cooperate to specify the liver
FOXA2 (HNF3B)	Endoderm, liver	FOXA2 required for foregut and midgut development
FOXA3 (HNF3G)	Endoderm, liver	Liver gene transcription
Onecut factors		
HNF6 (OC1)	Liver, pancreas	Bile duct, pancreatic duct, and islet development
OC2	Liver	Bile duct development
bHLH genes		
HES1	Liver, pancreas, intestine	Notch signaling; numerous roles in differentiation
NGN3, NEUROD	Pancreas, intestine	Pancreatic, gut endocrine cell specification
PTF1/p48	Pancreas	Early development of pancreas; exocrine transcription
MATH1	Intestine	Secretory vs enterocyte cell fate specification
Homeobox genes		
HEX	Liver	Growth of early liver bud
PROX1	Liver, pancreas	Growth of early liver bud, endocrine differentiation
HNF1B	Liver	Cholangiocyte formation
PDX1	Pancreas	Growth of pancreatic progenitor cells
HLXB9	Pancreas	Budding of dorsal pancreas, β-cell development
ISL1	Pancreas	Budding of dorsal pancreas, islet development
NKX2.2	Pancreas	β-Cell development
NKX6.1	Pancreas	β-Cell development
PAX4	Pancreas	β-Cell development
PAX6	Pancreas	Islet development (α cells > β cells)
ARX	Pancreas	α-Cell development
BARX1	Stomach	Patterning of the stomach
HLX	Intestine, liver	Early growth of liver and intestine
NKX2.5	Intestine	Formation of pyloric sphincter
CDX2	Intestine	Anterior–posterior patterning of intestine
HOXA/HOXD clusters	Intestine	Anterior–posterior patterning
Other		
HNF4	Liver	Terminal differentiation of hepatocyte
SMAD2	Endoderm	Endoderm development
Trp63	Esophagus	Formation of stratified squamous epithelium

bHLH, basic helix–loop–helix; HMG, high mobility group; HNF, hepatocyte nuclear factor.

appears to become important only in "higher" vertebrates, including zebrafish, *Xenopus*, and mammals.

Pattern formation

The process of "pattern formation" ensures that the esophagus and lung are positioned in the anterior or rostral part of the gastrointestinal tract, while the colon is always positioned in the posterior or caudal region. Pattern formation also enables the embryo to "know" where along the newly formed gut tube each of these organs should sprout, ensuring that new tubes (e.g., the pancreatobiliary system) form at the appropriate location.

Patterning refers to the stereotypical commitment of cells to certain *fates*, constituting in its most overarching form the establishment of the "body plan" – that is, the spatial arrangement of all tissue types in three-dimensional space. In the endoderm, patterning establishes the correct relationship of domains that will generate the respiratory tract and the gastrointestinal organs along the anterior–posterior axis. Our understanding of how embryos are patterned comes largely from classical studies in *Drosophila*, in which homeobox-containing transcription factors (*Hox* genes, in particular) were identified as the major determinants of the body pattern [12]. Subsequent studies have confirmed the critical role that *HOX* genes (and related homeobox-containing genes) also play in establishing the body plan of all higher organisms, including humans, a testament to the remarkable conservation of biological mechanisms across evolution.

HOX genes, of which there are 39 in humans, have a distinct organization in the genome. Specifically, *HOX* genes are arranged sequentially within each of four distinct "clusters" (A, B, C, and D). This chromosomal organization of the *HOX* genes within the DNA sequence mirrors their spatial expression in the embryo, so-called colinearity of expression. For example, the mouse *Hoxa* cluster consists of 12 genes; *Hoxa1* is expressed more anteriorly in the embryo than *Hoxa2*, which in turn is expressed more anteriorly than *Hoxa3*, and so forth. Loss-of-function analyses, also known as "gene knockout" studies, have shown that these carefully regulated expression boundaries dictate the *pattern* of the ectoderm and mesoderm. Mutations in *Hoxa2* therefore cause more anterior malformations that affect the head, while mutations in *Hoxa3* affect the neck and chest; this property holds true for all *Hox* clusters and genes. Conversely, ectopic expression of a *Hox* gene in a particular segment can cause it to turn into a more anterior (or posterior) segment. This respecification of fate is referred to as a *homeotic transformation*.

On the basis of the key role that *Hox* genes play in establishing the anterior–posterior pattern of the ectoderm and mesoderm, it would be logical to assume that these genes function similarly in the endoderm. Indeed, there are rare cases of homeotic transformations resulting from the misexpression of homeobox-containing proteins; for example, *Cdx2* is expressed in the early preimplantation embryo, and its expression is maintained in the endoderm throughout development [13]. Although *Cdx2*-deficient embryos die before implantation, animals heterozygous for *Cdx2* develop colonic lesions that exhibit an anterior histology [14,15]. Conversely, misexpression of *Cdx2* in the stomach causes intestinal metaplasia [16,17], a more posterior phenotype. Thus, *Cdx2* seems to pattern the endoderm by directing cells to adopt a more posterior fate. Nevertheless, *Cdx2* seems to be the exception rather than the rule, and the rarity of homeotic transformations in the endoderm suggests that homeobox-containing genes are for the most part indirectly responsible for regulating endoderm pattern. Although many *Hox* mutations result in intestinal malformations [18–21], these phenotypes are not specific to the endoderm despite the fact that boundaries of *Hox* expression in the endoderm correlate with organ boundaries [22–24].

After gastrulation, the developing gut tube is surrounded by mesoderm from the so-called lateral plate. It has long been appreciated that patterning is normally influenced by interactions between mesoderm derivatives (mesenchyme) and endoderm derivatives (epithelia). Epithelial–mesenchymal interactions can be demonstrated by transplantation experiments in which pieces of endoderm and mesoderm from different regions are recombined [25–28]. When tissues from postgastrulation embryos are recombined in this way, the fate of the endoderm is largely dependent on the type of mesoderm with which it is cultured; thus, anterior endoderm becomes "posteriorized" when recombined with posterior mesoderm, and posterior endoderm becomes "anteriorized" when recombined with anterior mesoderm [29]. Importantly, the mesoderm may be capable of providing the endoderm with a pattern because it has already been patterned by *Hox* gene activity.

Finally, other factors may participate in endoderm patterning, among them the vitamin A derivative retinoic acid. Embryos exposed to excess doses of retinoic acid exhibit congenital malformations resulting from the transformation of anterior embryonic structures to more posterior fates, a "posteriorization" phenotype that also involves the endoderm [30,31]. The mechanism by which retinoic acid influences patterning in such a global fashion remains unclear, but almost certainly involves the corruption of regulated retinoic acid-related signaling that occurs in normal development.

Fate and potential

The role of epithelial–mesenchymal crosstalk in endoderm patterning makes it clear that the fate of endodermal epithelial cells is strongly influenced by adjacent mesoderm/mesenchyme. Yet even before gastrulation, cells in the epiblast contain information about their future identity and position. This has been shown through the construction of *fate maps*, in which individual cells are marked and their progress is traced during development. Fate maps of the epiblast illustrate a stereotyped pattern of development, in which the endoderm is largely derived from cells that surround the anterior primitive streak before gastrulation [32,33]. However, assignment of cell *fate* may not be irreversible, and cells may remain capable of adopting identities other than their assigned fates. This capacity to change fate in response to environmental cues is referred to as *potential*, and it confers the cell with a certain amount of plasticity. Fate and potential represent important and complementary properties of a cell during development, and they provide the embryo with the means to correct errors that may occur in the course of embryogenesis.

It is generally accepted that a loss in potential accompanies gastrulation. The ability of cells within the very early embryo to become any cell type (*totipotency*) is therefore reduced within each germ layer to a more limited set of possibilities after gastrulation. This progressive *commitment* means that the parenchymal cells of the gastrointestinal organs are derived exclusively from endoderm, and at later stages, different organs are derived only from specific portions of the endoderm. This classical notion of progressive commitment has been challenged by studies in which cells appear to be capable of traversing germ layer boundaries, a process known as *transdifferentiation*. As discussed later, it remains unclear whether such cellular behavior contributes significantly to normal tissue homeostasis.

Attention has focused on the importance of *chromatin* in the regulation of tissue competence. Chromatin defines the structural state of DNA–protein complexes, determining whether a given DNA sequence is "open," or accessible, for transcription factors to bind. A model in which competence and commitment are achieved through sequential changes in chromatin has been suggested by studies of the regulatory region of the liver-specific albumin gene [34]. In these studies, the binding of the endodermal transcription factors GATA and FOXA to the albumin gene was assessed in several different cell types. In neural tube cells, which lack GATA and FOXA, the albumin enhancer is empty. In dorsal endoderm, the albumin enhancer is bound by GATA and FOXA, even though albumin is not transcribed in these cells, whereas in embryonic liver cells, the albumin promoter is bound by these and other factors and is transcriptionally active. This suggests that it is the chromatin state of a cell that confers a given set of potential fates. Consistent with this model, FOXA factors are themselves capable of modifying chromatin [35], and the ability to form a liver is lost in *Foxa1/Foxa2* mutant murine embryos [36].

Signaling in development

The assignment of cell fate in the endoderm is achieved through cell–cell signaling between neighboring cells or between adjacent cell layers. Such signals can be divided into two classes: *permissive* signals, which allow a tissue to progress to a fate that has already been assigned, and *instructive* or *inductive* signals, which divert a tissue to a new fate that would not otherwise have been followed. Instructive signals play an important role in regulating patterning by assigning cells that have not yet become committed (i.e., multipotent cells) to specific lineages.

Developmental signals have traditionally been identified through transplantation studies, in which different embryonic structures (e.g., epithelium and mesenchyme) are cocultured. The resulting fate (or absence thereof) indicates whether signals are present or absent, and if present, whether the signals are permissive or instructive. Several features of development complicate the study of the specific ligands that mediate this intercellular communication. Because development is a highly dynamic process, cells and cell layers are in constant movement relative to each other. Cell or tissue interactions may exist only transiently – long enough for a signal to be received, but not long enough to be easily characterized experimentally. Furthermore, signaling often occurs in a *reciprocal* manner (Figure 1.3). For example, the epithelium may respond to signal A from the mesenchyme by supplying signal B, which in turn prompts the mesenchyme to secrete signal C, and so forth. The number of secreted factors encoded in the genome is vast, further precluding straightforward analysis of epithelial–mesenchymal signaling.

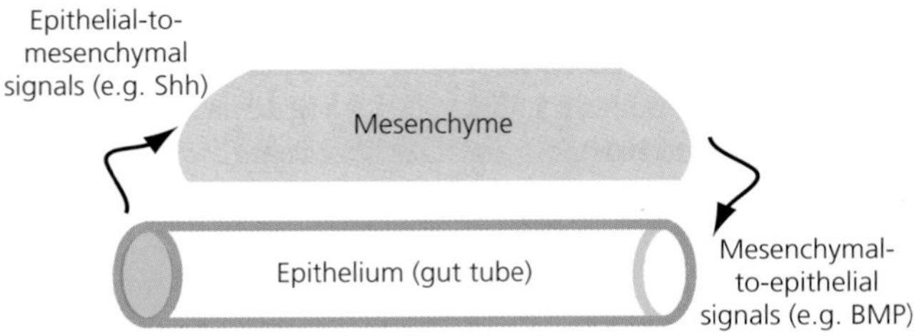

Figure 1.3 Epithelial–mesenchymal signaling. The gut tube, derived from the endoderm and composed of epithelial cells, produces soluble signals (e.g., Sonic hedgehog [Shh]) that diffuse outward to the surrounding mesoderm-derived mesenchyme. Receptors on mesenchymal cells receive this signal, causing them to produce a reciprocal signal (e.g., bone morphogenetic proteins [BMPs]), which diffuses back to the epithelial cells. This kind of epithelial–mesenchymal crosstalk is important for patterning, tissue outgrowth, and morphogenesis (and is also critical in carcinogenesis, where it takes the form of "tumor–stroma interactions").

Even though additional layers of complexity will undoubtedly be discovered, it appears that a limited repertoire of signals controls development. At least four signaling *modules*, each consisting of a family of ligands, receptors, and signal-modifying factors, are used iteratively during development: the fibroblast growth factor (FGF), hedgehog (Hh), bone morphogenetic protein (BMP), and BMP-related TGF-β families (Figure 1.4 and Table 1.2). In addition, three other classes of signaling modules – Wnt, Notch, and Hippo (Hpo) – act predominantly in regulating proliferation and differentiation within established organs. Crosstalk between signaling modules active in specific tissue layers (in particular, epithelium-derived Hh and mesenchyme-derived FGF and BMP) exemplifies the reciprocal nature of epithelial–mesenchymal signaling.

Fibroblast growth factors

The FGFs comprise a large family of ligands that are capable of binding to one of four FGF receptors. Both ligands and receptors are subject to a significant degree of regulation of splicing. Therefore, the combinatorial ligand–receptor repertoire is vast and subject to complex variability in binding specificity and

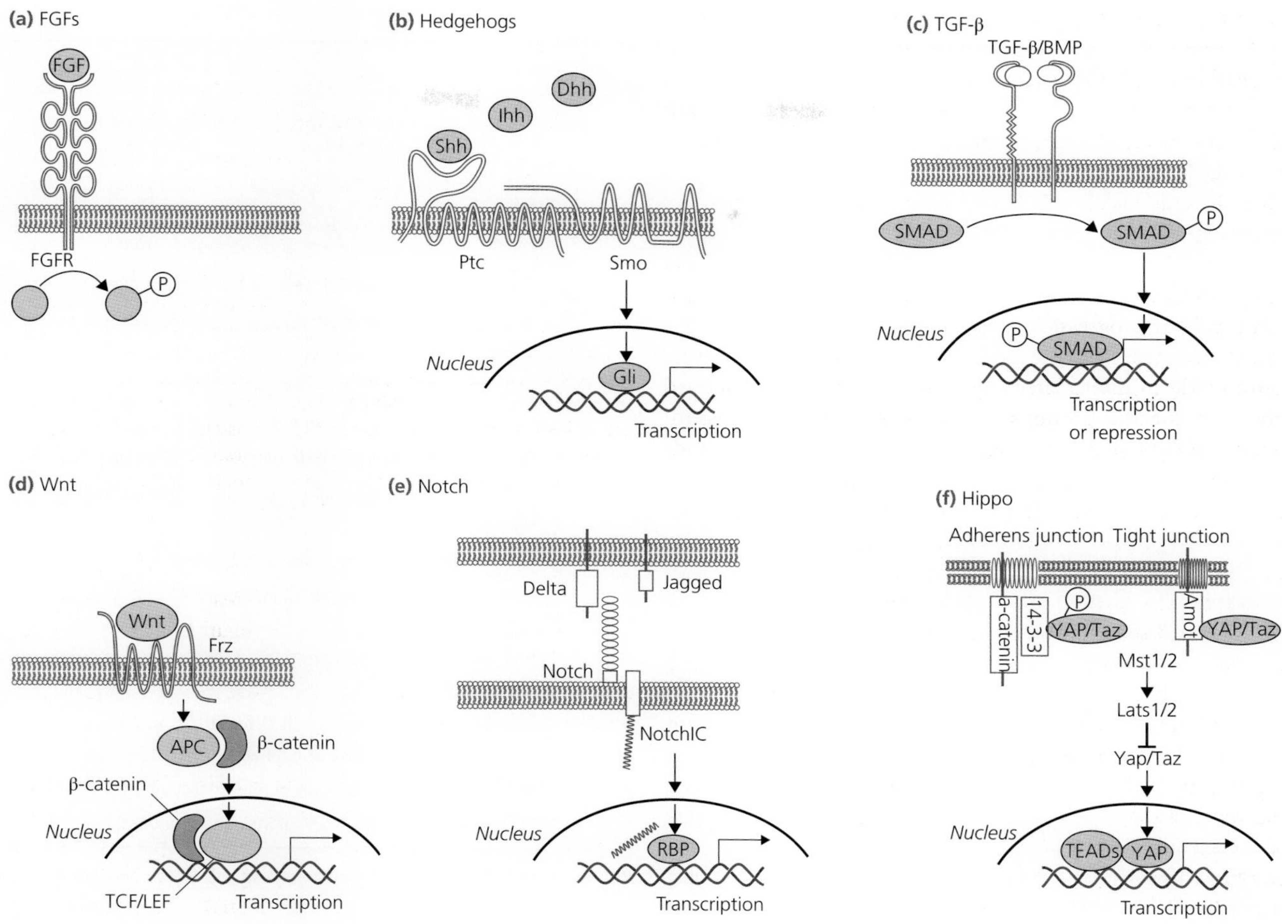

Figure 1.4 Ligand–receptor pairs in gastrointestinal development. **(a)** Fibroblast growth factor (FGF) signaling. Binding of an FGF ligand to one of four FGF receptors (FGFRs) leads to receptor dimerization and activation of FGFR tyrosine kinase activity. Phosphorylation of target proteins leads to the activation of multiple pathways, including Ras, phosphatidylinositol 3-kinase, phospholipase C, and STAT pathways. **(b)** Hedgehog signaling. All three hedgehog ligands – Sonic hedgehog (Shh), Indian hedgehog (Ihh), and Desert hedgehog (Dhh) – are capable of binding to the Patched receptor (Ptc). Ligand binding causes the membrane-bound signaling mediator Smoothened (Smo) to activate downstream transcription factors in the Gli family. These factors migrate to the nucleus and activate transcription. **(c)** Transforming growth factor (TGF)-β/bone morphogenetic protein (BMP) signaling. TGF-β family members bind to a heterodimeric membrane receptor complex consisting of a type I receptor and a type II receptor. The activated receptor complex phosphorylates SMAD transcription factors, which migrate to the nucleus, where they mediate or repress transcriptional activation. **(d)** Wnt signaling. Binding of a soluble Wnt ligand to one of the seven transmembrane Frizzled (Frz) receptors results in the activation of the canonical Wnt pathway, in which adenomatous polyposis coli (APC) dissociates from β-catenin, allowing the latter to migrate to the nucleus, where it becomes part of a transcriptionally active complex that includes T-cell factor/lymphoid enhancer factor (TCF/LEF) transcription factors. **(e)** Notch signaling. Cell–cell signaling is mediated by an interaction between one of the membrane-associated Notch ligands, Delta or Jagged, and one of the four Notch receptors on an adjacent cell. Ligand binding causes the intracellular portion of the Notch receptor (NotchIC) to migrate to the nucleus, where it activates the retinol-binding protein (RBP) transcription factor. **(f)** Hippo signaling. The kinases Mst1 and Mst2 phosphorylate Lats1 and Lats2, which in turn phosphorylate Yap and Taz. Phosphorylated Yap and Taz are sequestered in the cytoplasm through association with 14-3-3. Without Hippo activation, unphosphorylated Yap and Taz translocate to the nucleus, where Yap and Taz bind Tead1–4 and other transcription factors to initiate gene expression. Yap and Taz can also localize at cell–cell junctions through interacting with junctional proteins, including α-catenin and Amot.

tissue-specific expression. FGF receptor signaling is largely mediated by the tyrosine kinase activity of the receptor, acting through Ras and phospholipase C pathways [37]. FGFs are expressed in the primitive streak, mesodermal structures of the postgastrulation embryo, and developing organs, and they have important roles in endoderm patterning (possibly through a concentration gradient) and in organogenesis of the liver, pancreas, and intestine (see *Organogenesis*) [29,38,39].

Hedgehogs

The Hh genes were first identified through studies of *Drosophila*, and their names, like those of other developmental genes (e.g., *Notch*), arise from the Hh-like appearance of mutant flies. There are three mammalian hedgehogs – Indian, Sonic, and Desert – all of which bind to the membrane receptor Patched (Ptc). In the absence of ligand, Ptc acts as a repressor of the signaling mediator Smoothened (Smo); after Hh ligand binding to Ptc, Smo is

Table 1.2 Soluble signals in gastrointestinal development.

Tissue	Signal	Source	Function
Liver	FGF	Cardiac mesoderm	FGF1, FGF2, and/or FGF8 specify prehepatic endoderm, promote liver bud outgrowth
	BMP	Septum transversum mesenchyme	BMP4 (and other BMPs?) cooperates with FGFs in specification, outgrowth
	HGF	Septum transversum mesenchyme	Mediate hepatoblast growth and suppress apoptosis
	Unknown	Blood vessels	Expansion of liver bud into septum transversum mesenchyme
	Jagged 1	Portal mesenchyme	Specification or survival of cholangiocyte precursors (ductal plate)
Pancreas	Shh	Endoderm	Shh repression signals pancreatic specification
	FGF/activin	Notochord	Candidate mediators of Shh repression
	FGF10	Pancreatic mesenchyme	Outgrowth of pancreatic bud, pancreatic epithelium
	Delta/Jagged	Unknown	Notch-mediated inhibition of pancreatic progenitor cell differentiation
	TGF-β family	Unknown	Regulation of endocrine vs exocrine fate decisions
Intestine	Shh	Epithelium	Epithelial–mesenchymal crosstalk (Shh–BMP) regulates intestinal pattern
	BMP	Mesenchyme	Shh mediates radial pattern of gut; BMP regulates intestinal stem cell niche
	GDNF	Mesenchyme	Migration and/or survival of enteric neurons
	Endothelins	Mesenchyme	Migration and/or survival of enteric neurons
	Frizzled	Mesenchyme and Paneth cells	Receptors for Wnt regulation of intestinal stem/progenitor cells
	Delta/Jagged	Mesenchyme and Paneth cells	Ligands for Notch regulation of intestinal stem/progenitor cells

BMP, bone morphogenetic protein; FGF, fibroblast growth factor; GDNR, glial-derived neurotrophic factor; HGF, hepatocyte growth factor; Shh, Sonic hedgehog; TGF, transforming growth factor.

derepressed and activates Gli transcription factors. Importantly, cells are able to distinguish different concentrations of Hh ligand, allowing Hh to create patterns through a "gradient effect" in which cell fate depends on whether a high, intermediate, or low concentration of ligand is sensed. Shh is particularly important in gastrointestinal development. Shh is expressed in the endoderm at the time of formation of the gut tube (in the anterior and caudal intestinal portals) and participates in the specification of the pancreas and regionalization/morphogenesis of the gut.

Bone morphogenetic proteins and the TGF-β superfamily

BMPs are members of the TGF-β superfamily of secreted proteins, a family that also includes the activins. Receptors for TGF-β family members are serine–threonine kinases that modulate the activity of TGF-β-responsive transcription factors (termed SMADs) through phosphorylation. The relevance of BMPs to gut development was also first suggested by studies in *Drosophila*, which showed that the BMP ortholog *decapentaplegic* responds to Hh signaling and is necessary for midgut development. This specific example of reciprocal signaling between TGF-β and Hh family members is conserved in mammals, where Shh is expressed in the epithelium of the developing gut, and induces expression of particular BMPs in the adjacent mesenchyme.

Wnts

Wnt ligands play a critical role in the formation of differentiated cell types in the embryo, a process called *cell fate determination*. Wnts are a family of secreted factors (there are at least 19 known mammalian Wnts) that bind to "frizzled" receptors on the membrane. A complex series of events follows receptor binding. In the best characterized, or canonical, pathway, Wnt signaling leads to the release of β-catenin from the adenomatous polyposis coli (APC) protein, and the former then moves to the nucleus, where it activates T-cell factor/lymphoid enhancer factor transcription factors.

Despite the involvement of Wnt signaling in multiple developmental systems, including the intestine, developmental disorders with prominent gastrointestinal tract manifestations have not yet been associated with perturbed Wnt signaling. Rather, alterations in Wnt signaling are predominantly associated with carcinogenesis, particularly in the colon (colon adenocarcinoma), liver (hepatoblastoma), and pancreas (pancreatoblastoma) (Box 1.1).

Box 1.1 Cancer and its relationship to development: cancer stem cell hypothesis.

The observation that developmental signaling pathways are often activated in adult tumors has forged a bridge between the fields of developmental biology and cancer biology. The notion that cancer recapitulates development dates to the 19th century (reviewed by Sell [243]) and is embodied in the hypothesis that tumors arise from stem cells in adult tissues that retain an embryonic phenotype. Strong evidence for such a model exists in hematopoiesis, but it remains to be determined whether stem cells represent a target for malignant transformation in solid organs.

Further evidence for a link between development and cancer comes from the "reemergence" of signals normally prominent in development during the course of tumor initiation and progression. Wnt signaling, normally important during embryogenesis, is commonly activated in pediatric hepatoblastomas and pancreatoblastomas. Mutations in the type 1A BMP receptor (BMPR1A) or the downstream signaling element SMAD4 are common in juvenile polyposis syndrome.

Links between developmental signals and tumorigenesis are not limited to cancers that occur in children or inherited cancers. Like their heritable counterparts, most sporadic colorectal cancers exhibit activated Wnt signaling. Many adult pancreatic adenocarcinomas exhibit a reactivation of PDX1, Shh, and Notch signaling, which are either completely absent or present in only a subset of cells in the adult pancreas. Furthermore, several gastrointestinal malignancies (esophageal and gastric, in particular) are preceded by metaplasia. This replacement of one tissue type with another may reflect the emergence of more primitive cells with a greater capacity for growth.

Furthermore, tumors are composed of both mutant cancer cells and nonmutant "stromal cells" that comprise the so-called tumor microenvironment. The formation of the malignant stroma is reminiscent of the process of epithelial–mesenchymal crosstalk that occurs during normal organogenesis (see Figure 1.3), because it arises through reciprocal signaling between cancer cells and mesenchyme-derived noncancer cells.

Similarly, the concept of "cancer stem cells" – special cells within a tumor that provide the tumor with an inexhaustible supply of new cancer cells – is based on this apparent link between development and cancer. The *cancer stem cell hypothesis* posits that most cells within a tumor have a limited capacity for division and are themselves generated from cells with an unlimited capacity for division. In several tumors (breast and brain, in particular), a small subset of tumor cells has been identified and shown to be uniquely capable of reconstituting the tumor [244,245].

The cancer stem cell hypothesis has significant implications for cancer therapy. Most cancer therapies are assessed by their effect on tumor mass, the easiest assay for antitumor activity. However, if the cancer stem cell hypothesis is true, these agents would primarily target a cell population with a limited self-renewal capacity – analogous to a "transient amplifying population" – but may only inefficiently kill the cancer stem cells that are actually fueling the growth of the tumor. Stem cells that normally reside in adult tissues seem to be more resistant to chemotherapy than other cells [246], giving additional plausibility to this model. If the cancer stem cell hypothesis is correct, then it would be highly desirable to have therapies that specifically target these cells, because they might provide more durable cures and simultaneously generate less toxicity.

Notch

Like Wnt, Notch signals regulate the differentiation of cells within established tissues (Figure 1.5). Notably, a role for Notch in the formation of endoderm itself has also been postulated [40,41]. There are four mammalian Notch receptors, which are activated by two classes of ligands, Delta and Serrate/Jagged. In contrast with ligands from the other important signaling modules, including Wnts, FGFs, BMPs, and Hhs, Delta and Serrate/Jagged are transmembrane ligands. Hence Notch mediates signaling exclusively between cells that are in direct contact with each other. Ligand engagement leads to the detachment of the intracellular portion of the Notch receptor from the membrane, where it travels to the nucleus and alters the transcriptional program of the cell. Like Wnt signals, Notch signals are subject to complex regulatory inputs at all stages of the signal transduction pathway, from ligand binding to cytoplasmic and nuclear activation of downstream mediators.

Hippo

The Hpo pathway is highly conserved between insects and mammals. In *Drosophila*, Hpo signaling regulates tissue homeostasis and organ size. Genetic inactivation of the pathway components such as Hpo and Warts (Wts) leads to overgrowth of organs, such as the eye and wings. In contrast, mutation of downstream effectors Yorkie (Yki) and Scalloped (Sd) results in reduced organ size. In the midgut, Yki overexpression induces expansion of intestinal stem cells [42]. Consistently, in mice, combined deletion of Mst1 and Mst2 (mammalian Hpo orthologs) leads to increased activities of the Yki ortholog Yes-associated protein 1 (Yap) and crypt dysplasia [43]. Removal of one or both copies of Yap blocks stem cell expansion and intestinal dysplasia in Mst1/2 deletion mutants, confirming that Yap is a downstream effector of Mst1/2 [43]. Taz (also called Wwtr1 [WW domain-containing transcription regulator 1]) is another ortholog of Yki. When not phosphorylated, Yap and Taz accumulate in the nucleus and serve as transcriptional coactivators, facilitating the transcription initiated by the transcription factors TEA domain family members 1–4 (Tead1–4, orthologs of Sd). Although deletion of *Yap* seems not to impact intestinal development, possibly because of genetic compensation by Taz [44], Yap is required for bile duct development and hepatocyte survival in the liver [45]. Yap is also required for the formation of the stratified squamous epithelium in the esophagus [46], suggesting tissue-specific function of Hpo signaling in gastrointestinal organ development.

The role of these signaling modules in adult homeostasis remains to be fully defined. However, it is known that some signals are necessary for function throughout life. For example, Notch and Wnt signals maintain the proper balance of cell types in both the embryonic and the adult intestine. It is not clear how developmental specificity is achieved when signals from a single family are used repeatedly. It is likely that signals are interpreted in the context of cellular identity, thereby causing the same signal to have different effects on different tissues (i.e., pancreas versus liver versus intestine).

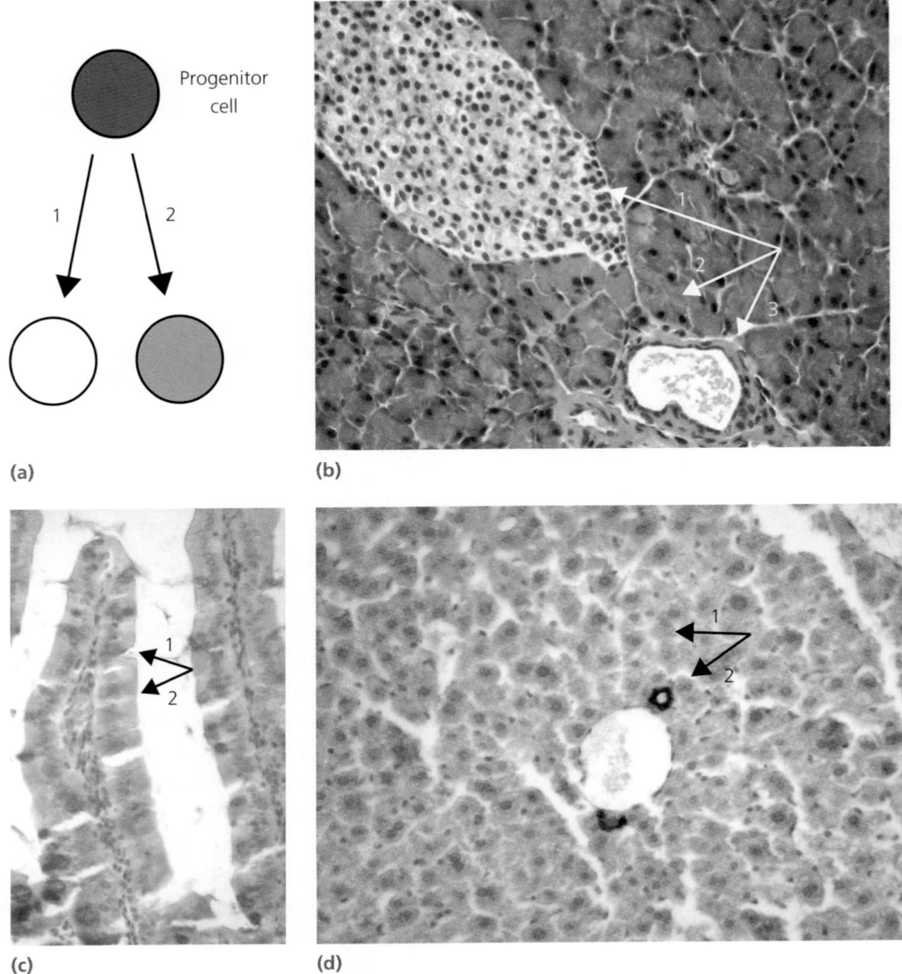

Figure 1.5 Control of gastrointestinal development by Notch. **(a)** The fate of a multipotent progenitor cell (dark blue) is influenced by whether it receives a signal from a Notch ligand (Delta or Jagged). In this example, active Notch signaling causes the cell to adopt fate 1 (white), whereas absence of signaling results in fate 2 (light blue). Evidence supports distinct roles for Notch in various gastrointestinal tissues. In the pancreas **(b)**, a Notch signal prevents the differentiation of the progenitor cell into any of the mature pancreatic cell types – islet (1), acinar (2), or ductal (3). In intestinal progenitor cells **(c)**, activation of Notch signaling promotes the formation of enterocytes (2). The formation of secretory cells (1), such as the goblet cells visualized here with Alcian blue staining, is inhibited by Notch signaling. In the liver **(d)**, Notch signaling is required for the proper formation of bile ducts (2), visualized by staining for cytokeratin 19 (CK19).

Transdifferentiation and dedifferentiation

Several studies have challenged the notion that commitment imposes a nearly absolute boundary between different lineages. Investigators have reported that certain somatic cells, particularly the cells derived from bone marrow, have the capacity to generate many different tissues in vitro and in vivo, including the cells of skin, lung, kidney, muscle, and all of the gastrointestinal organs [47]. A significant fraction of this apparent plasticity may actually reflect the effect of cell fusion between the bone marrow-derived cells and other differentiated cells, giving rise to tetraploid cells with the characteristics of hepatocytes, cardiomyocytes, and neurons [48–50]. Although it is possible that bone marrow-derived cells can transdifferentiate, albeit with low efficiency, into other somatic cells, the physiological significance of such a rare event is unclear, and the paradigms of lineage commitment established early in the 20th century remain largely intact.

A major exception to this rule of irreversible commitment from a less-differentiated state to a more-differentiated state is the finding that under experimental conditions, a terminally differentiated cell can be induced into a pluripotent stem cell capable of producing all differentiated cell types [51]. Known as *cellular reprogramming*, this process can be used to generate pluripotent cells from an individual patient that have the potential to generate cell types that are lost from injury or degenerative disease. In the future, the ability to manipulate the identity of adult cells – either through fusion or exploitation of developmental plasticity – may constitute a method for cell replacement in such disease states through an approach that is now being called *regenerative medicine*.

Conclusions

Early development of the gastrointestinal tract is characterized by gastrulation and endoderm formation, followed by midline migration of anterior and posterior invaginations (i.e., the anterior and caudal intestinal portals), resulting in a gut tube. The endoderm is patterned into organ domains along its anteroposterior axis through the activity of homeobox-containing transcription factors and epithelial–mesenchymal signaling. Cell fate remains plastic during the initial stages of development, with tissue identity depending on reciprocal signals that are refined until the commitment to a particular organ fate is made. Cells maintain their differentiated identity once commitment has occurred, although a new paradigm of cellular reprogramming may make it possible to convert cells from one identity into another (e.g., liver into pancreas).

Organogenesis

After gastrulation, the endoderm undergoes more easily recognizable changes of organogenesis. Studies delineating the development of the gastrointestinal tract were performed over the 20th century, and the timing of most key biochemical, physiological, and morphological events during human development was established at least 40 years ago [52]. Accordingly, this section will focus primarily on the mechanisms that underlie these remarkably complex and integrated events.

Importantly, the same signaling pathways described in the previous section on early development (e.g., BMPs, FGFs) are used iteratively in the specification of organ domains and the growth and differentiation of tissues. Sometimes, a single signal is involved in the development of two different organs, or one signal may mediate two different effects in the same tissue. In these instances, it is cellular *context* – the identity of the cell on which a given signal acts – that determines the signaling outcome.

Gastrointestinal organogenesis can be divided into several overlapping phases:

1. *Specification* – a direct consequence of the patterning processes previously described, results in the commitment of cells to restricted tissue fates
2. *Budding* – of liver and pancreas
3. *Morphogenesis* – the formation of a three-dimensional structure that facilitates the physiological function of the tissue (e.g., hepatic sinusoids and intestinal villi)
4. *Cell fate determination* – the restriction of specific lineages within the tissue (e.g., hepatocytes and cholangiocytes).

These components of organogenesis do not occur sequentially or independently, but rather, they occur in parallel, in a coordinated fashion. Finally, differentiation programs are implemented within those lineages, allowing the expression of physiological function (discussed further later in *Developmental physiology*).

Liver

Specification

The liver provides a good example of how a prepatterned mesenchyme can influence epithelial fate. The developing cardiac mesoderm, which gives rise to the heart, lies adjacent to the anterior endoderm fated to give rise to the liver (see Figure 1.2b). Experiments performed decades ago showed that cardiac mesoderm plays a critical role in the formation of the liver. These studies consisted of transplantation assays in which pieces of endoderm and mesenchyme were independently assembled. Such experiments demonstrated that an interaction between endoderm and cardiac mesoderm, during a critical time window, is necessary for the endoderm to activate a liver program [25]. As the cardiac mesoderm moves anteriorly, the space adjacent to the prehepatic endoderm is replaced by the septum transversum, a mesoderm derivative that later gives rise to part of the diaphragm. Other signals mediate the outgrowth of the expanding liver bud into the septum transversum mesenchyme (see also Chapter 10).

Tissue transplantation studies using molecular markers have confirmed an important role for embryonic mesenchyme in liver development. For example, ventral endoderm expresses albumin (a marker of liver specification) when it is cocultured with cardiac mesoderm. However, other studies suggest that a more complex regulatory circuit underlies the process. For example, *dorsal* endoderm expresses albumin when it is simply removed from its adjacent endoderm. This surprising result implies that the normal function of cardiac mesenchyme is permissive rather than inductive, in that it may allow the expression of a "default" liver program [53]. Such a default mechanism may also apply to the ventral pancreas, which forms from a lip of anterior endoderm that constitutes the "leading edge" of the anterior intestinal portal. This piece of endoderm exhibits "bipotential" pancreatic/hepatic properties; that is, it expresses pancreatic genes if cultured on its own, but represses the pancreatic program and expresses albumin if cocultured with signals from the cardiac mesoderm [38]. Although it is enticing to interpret these experiments as an indication that intrinsic endoderm fates are reprogrammed by specific mesenchymal elements, it is more likely that the liver, like all parts of the endoderm, is specified through a combination of early signals that provide cells with an intrinsic bias, as well as later permissive and inductive signals.

Although it is likely that a combination of FGF and BMP signals is among the specific signals involved in hepatic specification, FGFs are both sufficient and necessary for isolated anterior endoderm to activate albumin expression [54], and BMPs expressed by the septum transversum mesenchyme appear to act in concert with these FGFs [55]. The transcription factors Foxa1 and Foxa2 are critical mediators of these signals within the adjacent endoderm, because liver specification fails to occur in mice with a targeted inactivation of both of these genes [36].

Budding

After hepatic specification by the cardiac mesoderm, a bud that will grow into the liver begins to emerge. The first morphological evidence of budding is a thickening of the adjacent endoderm into a "hepatic diverticulum," which is followed by the outgrowth of liver cells into the septum transversum mesenchyme. FGFs are also necessary for this outgrowth, although their role in budding appears to be permissive, and their actions alone are not sufficient for liver bud outgrowth [56]. BMPs (specifically BMP4) are independently required for liver budding into the septum transversum, as demonstrated with the use of *Bmp4* mutant mice and the BMP antagonist noggin [55]. Furthermore, endothelial cells within the septum transversum mesenchyme are a source of growth-promoting signals, because *Flk1* mutant embryos (which are incapable of forming mature endothelial cells or blood vessels) undergo liver specification but fail to bud [56].

Many genes are required after endoderm specification for outgrowth into the septum transversum. These include three homeobox-containing transcription factors – Hex, Prox1, and Hlx – and the zinc-finger transcription factor GATA6. *Hex* is expressed during gastrulation in the first endoderm cells to pass through the primitive streak that ultimately give rise to the liver. Mice lacking *Hex* form a small hepatic diverticulum, but subsequent outgrowth and budding fails to occur [57,58]. *Hlx* and *Prox1* mutant mice also exhibit growth arrest at the bud stage, although the livers of *Prox1* mutant mice ultimately reach nearly a third of the size of a normal liver [59,60]. *Hex* and *Prox1* are expressed in the hepatic epithelium, whereas *Hlx* is normally expressed in the septum transversum mesenchyme.

As previously noted, the GATA4 zinc-finger transcription factor binds to the albumin promoter before albumin expression, suggesting a role in liver specification [34]. Another GATA family member, GATA6, also plays an important role in liver development. GATA6 regulates HNF4, an important transcriptional regulator of hepatocyte genes (described in later in *Morphogenesis and cytodifferentiation*), and liver bud outgrowth is retarded in mouse embryos lacking *GATA6* [61]. Further studies are needed to determine whether a regulatory relationship exists between *Hex*, *Hlx*, *Prox1*, and *GATA6*, given the similar phenotypes that mutations of these genes exhibit. Further studies are also required to determine the signaling hierarchy between soluble FGFs and BMPs and the activity of these transcription factors; for example, *Hex* expression can be induced by BMP signaling [62].

Morphogenesis and differentiation

After this migration into the septum transversum, epithelial cells intercalate with mesenchymal cells, eventually leading to the formation of the hepatic sinusoids that support embryonic hematopoiesis. These morphogenetic changes are accompanied by dramatic growth of the liver through the action of mesenchymal factors. The most important of these is hepatocyte growth factor (HGF), which signals through the c-met receptor. Mutation of either *Hgf* or c-*met* leads to marked liver cell apoptosis in some, but not all, analyses [63,64]. This signaling pathway also seems to modulate the response to injury in adult liver [65,66]. Mutations in several other genes, including components of the tumor necrosis factor (TNF)–nuclear factor-κB signaling pathway, lead to similar developmental apoptosis phenotypes [67–69]. Hepatocyte apoptosis in many adult liver diseases is mediated by a TNF-like "death receptor" pathway [70], suggesting that these cell death signaling mechanisms are active throughout life.

The two major parenchymal cell types of the liver – hepatocytes and bile ducts – arise from multipotent embryonic "hepatoblasts." Intrahepatic bile ducts (IHBDs) are derived from "ductal plates," precursor structures that form around branches of the portal vein. Inductive signals from the portal vein mesenchyme induce surrounding hepatoblasts to form the ductal plate, which can be recognized by the expression of distinctive CK molecules, such as CK19 (Figure 1.6). Mature IHBDs emerge after remodeling of the ductal plate, in conjunction with selective apoptosis of duct precursors. The "extrahepatic" bile ducts (EHBDs) and the gallbladder have a separate embryonic origin from the IHBDs, because these larger ductal structures arise through a process of branching from the gut tube into the liver well after budding has occurred. It remains unclear how the connection between IHBDs and EHBDs occurs.

Several signaling pathways are involved in biliary specification and morphogenesis. Among those first identified were liver-enriched HNFs. HNFs belong to several different transcription factor families and contribute to the expression of liver-specific genes. Inactivation of either HNF6 (a member of the onecut transcription factor family) or HNF1B (a homeodomain factor) perturbs biliary development [71,72]. The reduced HNF1B expression in the livers of *Hnf6* mutant mice suggests that HNF6 likely acts through HNF1B [71]. Alternatively, HNF6 and the onecut transcription factor OC2 act through activin/TGF-β family member(s) to regulate biliary fate decisions. The liver normally exhibits a gradient of TGF-β signaling activity, with high activity near the ductal plates and low activity in the remaining parenchyma. In livers lacking both HNF6 and OC2, this gradient is disrupted, resulting in high levels of activin/TGF-β signaling throughout the liver and the appearance of cells exhibiting features of both hepatocytes and cholangiocytes. Thus, onecut transcription factors may shape a gradient of activin/TGF-β signaling to allow localized induction of the bile ducts.

In addition, there is convincing evidence that Notch signaling is important for biliary development. Mutations in the Notch ligand Jagged 1 (*JAG1*) result in Alagille disease, a clinical syndrome that includes a paucity of IHBDs [73,74], and the mechanism appears to involve a failure of proper biliary differentiation [75]. The molecular pathogenesis of Alagille syndrome is discussed further later in *Disorders of remodeling*.

A cellular differentiation program is executed after the assignment of biliary or hepatocyte fate. Evidence that this program is distinct from the assignment of hepatocyte cell fate comes from the targeted inactivation of HNF4. Remarkably, this transcription factor has been reported to bind to nearly half of the actively expressed genes in the liver [76]. Among the genes whose

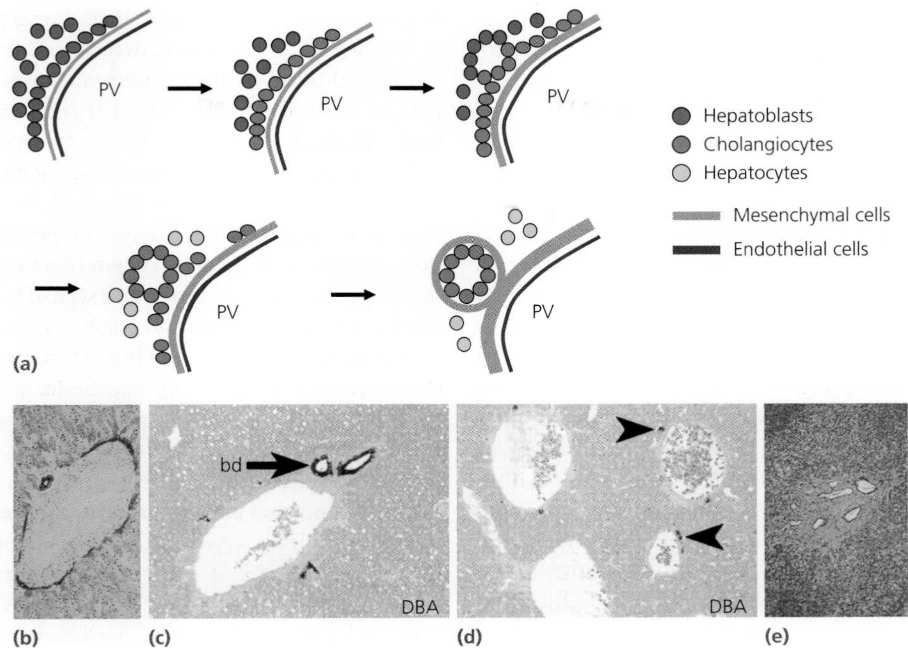

Figure 1.6 Biliary tract development. **(a, b)** Normal biliary development. **(a)** Branches of the portal vein (PV) induce embryonic hepatoblasts (red) to form the ductal plate, a ring of biliary epithelial precursor cells (green). These cells become arranged into a tube that undergoes remodeling late in embryogenesis or early in postnatal life to yield mature bile ducts. This process involves Notch and TGF-β signaling. **(b)** The ductal plate expresses cytokeratin 19, a marker of mature bile ducts. **(c, d)** Disorders of biliary development. **(c)** Normal mouse portal tract with bile duct (bd) (visualized by Dolichos biflorus agglutinin [DBA] lectin staining), hepatic artery, and portal vein branches. **(d)** Portal tract from a mouse lacking one copy of both *Jagged1* and *Notch2*, a model of human Alagille syndrome. **(e)** Periportal expansion of bile ducts in a patient with the ductal plate abnormality characteristic of congenital hepatic fibrosis. **(a)** Source: Zong and Stanger 2011 [75]. Reproduced with permission of Elsevier. **(c, d)** Source: Adapted from McCright et al. 2002 [230]. Reproduced with permission of The Company of Biologists, Ltd.

expression "defines" the hepatocyte are albumin, apolipoproteins A and B, and transferrin. Despite exhibiting normal morphogenesis, HNF4-deficient embryos exhibit reduced expression of all of these genes, demonstrating a role for this transcription factor in hepatocyte differentiation, but not liver specification and morphogenesis [77].

In summary, FGF and BMP signals from the cardiac and septum transversum mesoderm/mesenchyme induce a portion of the ventral foregut endoderm to become the liver. Budding and parenchymal growth involve homeobox-containing transcription factors and mesenchyme-derived soluble factors, such as HGF, that mediate proliferation and suppress apoptosis. Poorly understood epithelial–mesenchymal interactions mediate the morphogenesis of the hepatic sinusoids, which support hematopoiesis during fetal life. Biliary development involves the formation of perivascular ductal plates and subsequent remodeling, a process that requires Notch and TGF-β signals and the activity of several onecut transcription factors. In hepatocytes, other transcription factors, including HNF4A, are required for the full manifestation of the differentiated hepatocyte program.

Pancreas

With some important exceptions, development of the pancreas follows a paradigm that is similar to that of the liver. Specifically, signals from adjacent mesoderm specify the pancreatic endoderm, FGFs mediate pancreatic growth, and a variety of signaling components (including Notch and homeobox-containing transcription factors) regulate the differentiation of the parenchymal cell types of the pancreas – its exocrine, endocrine, and duct cells.

Specification

Unlike the liver, the pancreas forms from two distinct pieces of foregut endoderm – a dorsal pancreatic domain and a ventral pancreatic domain (see Figure 1.2c) – that later fuse into a single gland. Patches of endoderm on opposite sides of the gut tube must therefore somehow be instructed to become pancreas. Transplantation studies similar to those previously described have shown that the dorsal pancreatic region of the endoderm is specified before the 13-somite stage, a period when this endoderm is in contact with the notochord [78]. At a slightly later stage, the "prepancreatic endoderm" (the patch of endoderm fated to become pancreas) is in contact with the aorta (dorsally) and the vitelline veins (ventrally). Thus, the notochord or blood vessels could be mesenchymal sources for inductive pancreatic signals, akin to the role played by the cardiac mesoderm in the developing liver.

Indeed, evidence suggests that both the notochord and the blood vessels are important for pancreatic specification and growth. Isolated dorsal endoderm fails to show evidence of pancreatic differentiation when cultured on its own, but a pancreatic program is induced on reassociation with the notochord [79]. Similarly, coculture of dorsal endoderm with aortic cells (or other endothelial cells) induces a pancreatic program, whereas removal of aortic precursor cells from the embryo causes a failure in pancreatic development [80].

The most important consequence of mesenchymal signaling appears to be the repression of Shh expression. Shh is expressed throughout the entire gut tube, with the notable exception of the prepancreatic regions (both dorsal and ventral). The notochord is directly responsible for repressing Shh in the dorsal prepancreatic endoderm, possibly through the activity of FGF2 or activin β-B [81]. Repression of Shh alone is able to reproduce the pancreatic inductive activity of notochord [81], and blocking Shh signaling with an inhibitor (cyclopamine) causes ectopic pancreas formation [82]. Furthermore, Shh repression must be maintained throughout pancreatic development, and ectopic expression of Shh after pancreatic budding inhibits further pancreas development [83]. Shh repression is therefore both necessary and sufficient for pancreas specification. It is unclear what structure serves the function analogous to that of the notochord to repress Shh expression in the ventral prepancreatic endoderm.

Budding

The pancreatic buds form at about 3–4 weeks of embryonic development (embryonic day 9.5 in the mouse), with formation of the ventral bud lagging behind that of the dorsal bud. One of the earliest and most important genes to be expressed in these nascent buds is the homeobox transcription factor *PDX1*. All mature pancreatic cell types are derived from cells that expressed *PDX1* [84], and ectopic *PDX1* expression in the intestine is sufficient to promote the early steps of pancreas formation [85]. Although pancreatic buds form in *Pdx1*-deficient embryos, further pancreas development is arrested at this stage [86,87], a phenotype that has also been observed in humans (Box 1.2) [88,89]. In adults, PDX1 is a major transcription factor for insulin, and its loss in adult mice causes diabetes [90]. Several other transcription factors that play roles in mature differentiated pancreas cells are also expressed in the early progenitor cells of the pancreas, including p48/PTF1A, Hes1, and Nkx6.1.

As noted, specification of the dorsal and ventral pancreas occurs by different mechanisms (notochord for dorsal, unknown for ventral). This differential regulation repeats itself later, because several genes exhibit distinct activities in dorsal versus ventral pancreatic development. One of these is *Hlxb9*, which encodes a homeobox transcription factor that is required for dorsal, but not ventral, pancreatic budding in mice [68,91]. Similarly, the homeobox transcription factor Isl1 is required in the pancreatic mesenchyme to promote dorsal, but not ventral, pancreas development [92]. Mesenchymal *Isl1* expression is maintained in *Hlxb9* mutants, suggesting that *Isl1* is not downstream of *Hlxb9*. Because there are no profound functional or histological differences between the postnatal derivatives of the ventral (head and uncinate process) and dorsal (body and tail) pancreas, it is unclear why *Isl1* and *Hlxb9* mutations cause such selective phenotypes.

Once formed, the ventral pancreas rotates across the midline to meet the dorsal pancreas (Figure 1.8). The two pancreatic derivatives undergo complete functional and anatomic integration, and the ventral ductal system (duct of Wirsung) serves as the major conduit for pancreatic secretion through the major papilla. Failure of integration results in the common anatomic variant *pancreatic divisum*, which is marked by persistence of the dorsal duct of Santorini and drainage through the minor papilla.

Morphogenesis and cytodifferentiation

Mutant phenotypes demonstrate that early pancreas organogenesis occurs in two steps: an early phase of pancreatic budding (which requires ISL1) and a later phase of outgrowth and branching (which requires PDX1). Wessells and Cohen [78] suggested a two-step process after observing that the substitution of heterologous mesenchyme for pancreatic mesenchyme supported later stages of development, but not early budding.

For many years, investigators looked for "mesenchymal factors" that control pancreatic growth, branching, and differentiation [93]. FGF10 was discovered to be such a pancreatic mesenchymal factor. In the lung, FGF10 expression causes budding and branching of the pulmonary epithelium [94]. This growth is "stereotyped" – primary, secondary, and tertiary branch formation are spatially and temporally regulated to ensure a consistent branching pattern. Although branching in the pancreas does not appear to be stereotyped in the same way that it is in the lung, FGF10 has a strikingly similar function in the development of the pancreas. FGF10 is expressed in the mesenchyme and drives the proliferation of progenitor cells expressing PDX1 during branching by binding to the FGF receptor 2b on epithelial cells [95]. Consistent with this, *Fgf10* mutant mice exhibit arrested pancreas development at the bud stage [96]. An additional activity of FGF10 during pancreas growth is to keep the expanding pancreatic epithelium in an undifferentiated state. This is achieved through the activation of Notch signaling, a potent regulator of pancreatic differentiation [97–101].

Gastrointestinal tract

Specification

Although the gastrointestinal tract is composed of a single continuous tube, it is partitioned into discrete domains from anterior to posterior (esophagus, stomach, small intestine, and colon) that are demarcated by sphincters (lower esophageal sphincter, pylorus, ileocecal valve, and anal sphincter). Each domain has a distinct function and a unique architecture. Similar to the liver and the pancreas, the different functional domains of the gastrointestinal tract are patterned on the activities of multiple signaling pathways, including BMP, FGF and a

Box 1.2 Pancreatic agenesis.

PDX1 homeodomain-containing transcription factor (also known as IDX1, STF1, and IPF1) is absolutely required for development of the pancreas, because both mice and humans lacking the gene have an arrest in pancreatic development [86,88] (Figure 1.7). Heterozygous mutations in PDX1 caused maturity-onset diabetes of youth in a subset of patients, reflecting the protein's later role as the major transcriptional regulator of insulin gene expression [89].

The mature pancreas contains exocrine cells that make digestive enzymes, ducts that carry these enzymes to the gut, and hormone-producing endocrine cells. The exocrine pancreas is the largest compartment, comprising more than 80% of the pancreatic mass. The transcription of exocrine-specific genes is dependent on the PTF1A transcriptional complex, which contains the pancreas-specific transcription factor p48. Like PDX1, p48 is expressed in the early stages of development in multipotent pancreatic progenitor cells [102], and it is the major transcription factor for the expression of exocrine-specific genes [103]. p48 is required for exocrine differentiation, and *p48* null mutant mice develop an endocrine pancreas but lack exocrine cells [104]. Another transcription factor, MIST1, is required for the assembly of the exocrine secretory machinery [105].

During the growth of the pancreatic epithelium within the bud, endocrine cells arise in waves of differentiation (glucagon-producing α cells preceding insulin-producing β cells); these cells delaminate from the epithelium and reaggregate postnatally into the islets of Langerhans (which also include somatostatin-producing δ cells and pancreatic polypeptide [PP]-producing cells). The development of these different endocrine lineages is complex and regulated by multiple factors. The basic helix–loop–helix (bHLH) transcription factor Neurogenin 3 (NGN3) is both necessary and sufficient for endocrine differentiation in the pancreas [85,106,107]. NGN3, and its target gene *BETA2/NEUROD*, are regulated by Notch signals [108] and the onecut transcription factor HNF6 [109]. Additional transcription factors involved in the delineation of different endocrine lineages in appropriate numbers include NKX6.1, NKX2.2, PAX4, and PAX6 [110].

Islets are not derived from the monoclonal expansion of endocrine precursor cells, but rather from the polyclonal coalescence of distinct endocrine cells or endocrine precursors [111]. The aggressive search for putative "adult stem cells" in the pancreas has yielded ambiguous results. One laboratory that used a genetic labeling method failed to show that adult stem/progenitor cells give rise to β cells, suggesting that the adult β-cell mass is maintained principally by replication [112].

In summary, the repression of Shh signaling induces the formation of dorsal and ventral pancreatic buds from the endoderm. Signals provided by blood vessels, as well as mesenchymal FGF10, promote the outgrowth of multipotent pancreatic progenitor cells into a branched epithelium. Complex signals, including members of the Notch and TGF-β families, as well as numerous bHLH and homeodomain proteins, regulate the subsequent differentiation of pancreatic endocrine, exocrine, and ductal lineages.

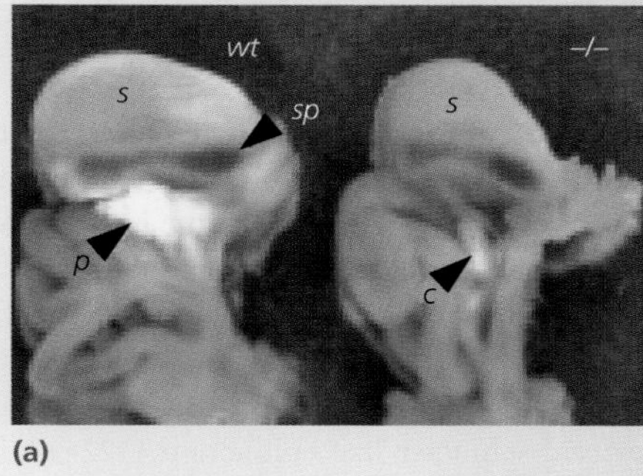

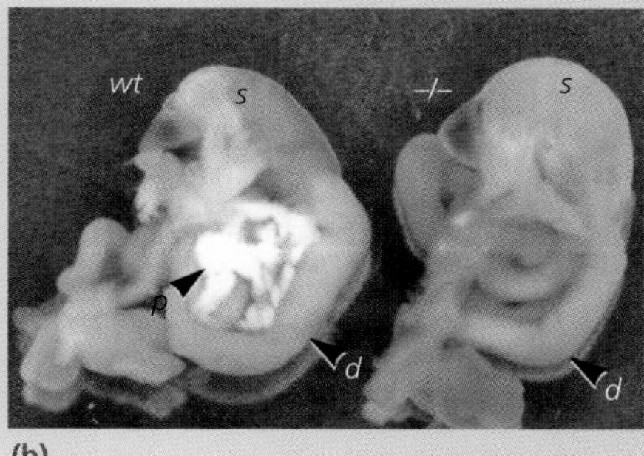

Figure 1.7 **(a, b)** Modeling pancreatic agenesis in the mouse. Images of dissected mouse stomach (s), spleen (sp), duodenum (d), and pancreas (p) from wild-type (wt) and mutant mice lacking the *Pdx1/IPF1* gene (–/–). In the absence of Pdx1/IPF1, the pancreas does not develop and is instead replaced with a cystic structure (c). Source: Offield et al. 1996 [86]. Reproduced with permission of The Company of Biologists, Ltd.

repertoire of homeobox genes. These signaling pathways and transcription factors serve as critical mediators of the epithelial–mesenchymal crosstalk.

BMP signaling molecules are expressed throughout the primitive gut and play tissue- and stage- specific roles during gastrointestinal tract development. At the proximal end, esophageal development requires both inactivation and activation of BMP signaling, depending on stages. Before trachea–esophageal separation, the BMP inhibitor Noggin is expressed transiently in the dorsal epithelium and is required for the specification of esophageal cells. Deletion of *Noggin* leads to failed trachea–esophageal separation, resulting in the birth defect esophageal atresia with or without trachea–esophageal fistula [113]. After stratification, BMP activities are required for promoting the squamous differentiation of top layers of esophageal epithelium [114]. BMP signaling is also required for the specification of gastric epithelium. Deletion of *Bmpr1a* in the mouse foregut endoderm with *Foxa3-Cre* caused an anteriorization of the stomach, with the expansion of the forestomach region, which is lined by stratified squamous epithelium in mice [115]. Although BMP signaling is important for the morphogenesis and epithelial differentiation (see later), it plays a rather minor role in the early specification of intestinal fate from the primitive gut. Instead FGF signaling seems to be critical for the early patterning of the intestine. Deletion of *Fgf10* leads to colon and duodenal atresia with failed cecal formation [116].

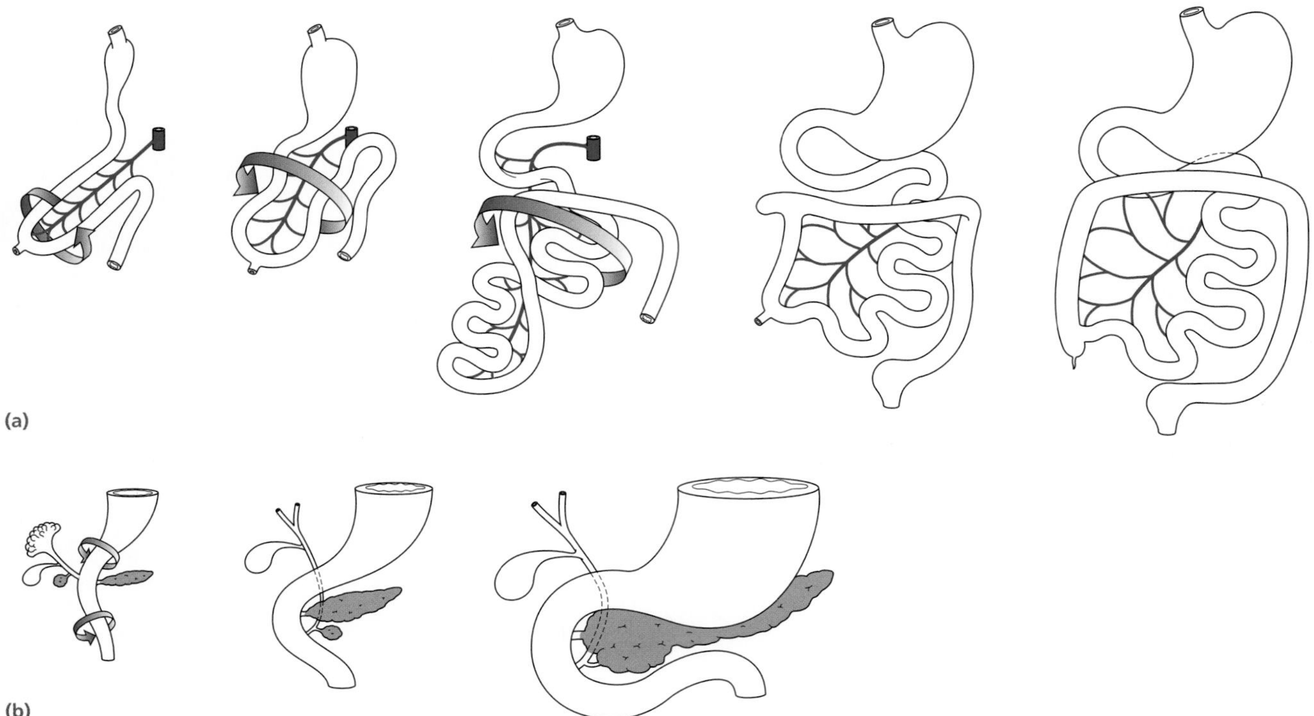

Figure 1.8 Rotation during development of the gastrointestinal tract. **(a)** Rotation of the gut. **(b)** Rotation of the pancreas.

Homeobox-containing genes are expressed in a regionalized manner in the gut epithelium and mesenchyme [14,23], and several examples of "homeotic transformations" have been observed after the dysregulated expression of homeobox genes. *Hoxa13* and *Hoxd13* are expressed in the hindgut, and ectopic expression of either of these *Hox* genes in the midgut leads to acquisition of hindgut characteristics [117,118]. Likewise, the *Hox* gene *Hoxa5* is expressed in stomach mesenchyme and is necessary for gastric fate specification [119]. Sphincters constitute a special case of endoderm patterning, and they reside at boundaries between intestinal segments. Again, *Hox* genes are important for the process of sphincter formation. *Hoxa13/Hoxd13* mutant mice have defects in anal sphincter formation, and mice with a large deletion in the *Hoxd* cluster (*Hoxd4–d13*) lack an ileocecal valve [20,21].

Epithelial–mesenchymal signaling is essential for the establishment of an intestinal pattern. In some cases, such as the murine cecum, a clear hierarchy of epithelial–mesenchymal signaling (through FGFs in cecal development) mediates organ growth [120]. In other cases, it is less clear whether transcription factors (such as homeobox-containing proteins) establish an initial pattern that is refined by further epithelial–mesenchymal signaling, or whether epithelial–mesenchymal signaling is responsible for establishing the pattern of transcription factor gene expression. An alternative possibility is that the basement membrane, an aggregate of extracellular matrix strategically placed between epithelial and mesenchymal cells, regulates crosstalk between the two tissue layers [121].

Pyloric sphincter development is a particularly instructive example of this complex process of specification. In the chicken, the pyloric sphincter forms at the junction of the gizzard (caudal stomach) and the small intestine. Two transcription factors – the homeobox factor Nkx2.5 and the HMG-box factor Sox9 – are both markers of the mesenchyme of the pyloric sphincter, and ectopic expression of either gene is sufficient to convert the gizzard into pyloric sphincter-like epithelium [122–124]. Moreover, mesenchymal BMP4 is both necessary and sufficient to induce the expression of these transcription factors [118,124,125]. This result is surprising, because BMP4 is expressed widely throughout the gut mesenchyme. The specificity of BMP4 activity to induce sphincter development likely reflects specific spatial regulation of its own expression and spatial regulation of its receptor [125,126]. Moreover, the ability of the downstream factor Nkx2.5 to induce pyloric sphincter development is spatially regulated; Nkx2.5 can induce pyloric sphincter development when it is expressed anteriorly (in the gizzard), but not posteriorly (in the duodenum) [123]. These studies provide insight into the final steps regulating the development of the pyloric sphincter, but a deeper question remains: What regulates the regulators?

Complex signals that are both intrinsic and extrinsic to the developing epithelium control tissue identity. The extent to which these or similar inductive events contribute to common congenital anomalies, including intestinal stenoses and atresias, duplications, and anorectal malformations, is unknown. However, congenital anomalies of the gastrointestinal tract are commonly associated with malformations in other organ systems or chromosomal abnormalities, including trisomy 21 (Down syndrome), suggesting that the regulatory signals involved in patterning are disrupted widely.

The clinical relevance of these regulatory networks may extend beyond putative relationships to congenital errors. For example, intestinal metaplasia, a premalignant lesion in which portions of the esophagus or stomach are replaced with intestinal mucosa, may represent reactivation of developmental programs. Studies of BARX1, a homeobox-containing transcription factor that is expressed transiently in the gastric mesenchyme, provide support for this concept. BARX1 mediates gastric specification by inhibiting Wnt signaling, and mouse embryos with a targeted disruption of the gene exhibit a homeotic transformation of stomach to intestine [127]. One interpretation of this result is that intestinal differentiation represents a "default" state for gut endoderm that must be overcome (through inhibition of Wnt signaling) to allow stomach specification. Although unproved, this model may explain why intestinal metaplasia of the stomach and esophagus is common, whereas the converse, gastric metaplasia of the midgut or hindgut, is uncommon.

Morphogenesis

The lumenal gastrointestinal tract acquires its shape through rotational changes at a gross level, and through tissue remodeling at a microscopic level. Left–right (L–R) asymmetry of the intestine is generated through the same mechanisms that regulate the L–R axis of the body plan. This process involves the clockwise movement of cilia, which promotes the asymmetric distribution of inductive signals [128]. Dysregulation of cilium function leads to randomization of L–R asymmetry and clinical phenotypes, including situs inversus.

The intestine undergoes tremendous growth during the initial embryonic period, and elongates about 1000-fold between the 5th and 40th weeks of human development [129]. The intestine exists outside the abdominal cavity for much of its early embryonic life ("physiological herniation") to accommodate a large embryonic liver. Early in development, the growing midgut and hindgut undergo a two-step rotation (see Figure 1.8) totaling 270° (counterclockwise orientation viewing the embryo en face). Both growth and looping of the intestine require the action of HLX, a homeobox transcription factor that is expressed in the midgut and hindgut mesenchyme, and that is also required for liver development (see subsection *Budding* in the *Liver* section). *Hlx* mutant mouse embryos have a shortened and single-looped gut that undergoes normal differentiation [59]. Although many congenital anomalies are related to errors in these gross movements of the intestine, most notably midgut malrotation with risk for ensuing volvulus, the mechanisms underlying normal rotation are poorly understood.

Although our understanding of this dramatic intestinal growth and rotation remains mainly descriptive and phenomenological, the mechanisms controlling the cross-sectional makeup of the intestine are better understood. The stereotyped circumferential arrangement of cells according to each intestinal segment has been referred to as the *radial axis* of the gastrointestinal tract. Starting from the lumen, the radial axis goes from innermost epithelium, lamina propria, muscularis mucosae, submucosa, outer muscular layers, out to the serosa. Each intestinal segment has a unique epithelial and mesenchymal composition – for example, the stratified squamous epithelium and thin submucosa and muscular layers of the esophagus versus the columnar epithelium and thickly muscled mesenchyme of the stomach.

Shh–BMP crosstalk appears to be important for determining the composition of the radial axis in each intestinal segment. This conclusion is based on several lines of evidence. First, Shh is expressed throughout the gut epithelium (except for the pancreas, as discussed in the subsection *Specification* in the *Pancreas section*) and is a potent activator of mesenchymal BMP expression so that the two signaling pathways regulate each other. Second, ectopic BMP expression affects the degree of muscularity of the mesenchyme along the anterior–posterior axis [116], suggesting that it regulates mesenchymal morphology. Third, Shh signaling is necessary for normal crypt–villus structure [130], and Shh regulates mesenchymal fate according to the distance from the epithelium [131]. These results are consistent with a model in which a concentration gradient of Shh (expressed by the innermost epithelium) organizes the mesenchymal rings of the gut, possibly through the activity of BMPs. According to this model, mesenchymal cells closest to the epithelium are induced to adopt a lamina propria or submucosal fate, whereas only those cells farthest from the epithelium adopt a muscle fate [131].

The gastrointestinal tract possesses both inner and outer muscle layers. (The stomach also has an extra third muscle layer.) The inner layer in the intestine is circumferentially aligned before the formation of the longitudinally aligned outer layer. During patterning of the two layers, mesenchymal cells in each layer have different proliferation rates: the inner mesenchyme shows a higher proliferation rate than the outer mesenchyme. This differential growth generates mechanical strain and aligns the inner layer circumferentially. Reduction of differential growth leads to impaired smooth muscle alignment in chicken midgut explants [132]. In addition, cyclic contractions of the inner layer orient the outer layer longitudinally. Alignment of the outer muscle layer is inhibited by prevention of circumferential muscle contraction in chicken intestinal explants [132].

Shh and Bmp signaling appear to be important for gastrointestinal smooth muscle development. Shh controls smooth muscle differentiation in the inner muscle layer through mesenchymal BMP signaling in a dosage-dependent manner. Inhibition of Hh signaling in chicken midgut explants leads to a lack of smooth muscle differentiation. However, high levels of Shh signaling activate BMP4 expression in the mesenchyme adjacent to the epithelium, which in turn inhibits smooth muscle differentiation [132]. BMP signaling also plays a role in the formation of the outer muscle layer. BMP antagonists are expressed in the inner muscle layer and neurons close to the outer layer in chick and mouse. Loss of the antagonists *Noggin* and *Gremlin1* in mesoderm and neural crest results in defective smooth muscle differentiation in mouse, suggesting that inhibition of BMP signaling activity is required for the differentiation of mesenchymal cells in the outer layer [132].

The intestinal lumen forms after 7–8 weeks of gestation (human) and arises through the processes of canalization and morphogenesis. The failure of canalization is thought to account for some cases of duodenal atresia, a partial or complete obstruction of the duodenum that occurs with a frequency of 1 in 5000 to 1 in 10 000 births, whereas morphogenesis involves polarization of the epithelium and transformation of a stratified epithelium to a columnar epithelium. As villi emerge from the stratified epithelium, they acquire a distinctive crypt–villus architecture, a process that is dependent on the cytoskeleton. One of these cytoskeletal elements is the "bridge" protein ezrin, which links membrane proteins to the actin cytoskeleton. Ezrin-deficient mice exhibit normal intestinal differentiation and polarity but abnormal villi, including nascent villus structures that are unable to break away from each other [133].

Cell proliferation and kinetics

The adult small intestinal epithelium has a rapid and regular turnover, with the average lifespan of intestinal enterocytes measured in days [134]. To support this constant need for new cells, the intestine recapitulates the embryonic processes of differentiation from stem cells throughout life (Figure 1.9). Stem cells are specialized cells that can generate multiple differentiated cell types ("multipotentiality") and also produce more stem cells ("self-renewal"). Intestinal stem cells reside near or at the bottom of the crypts and are characterized by their relatively low rate of cell division and long life [135].

Progenitor cells with a more limited potential and shorter half-life coexist with stem cells in the crypts [136]. A subset of stem cell-derived progenitor cells, known as the *transient amplifying population*, undergoes rapid cell division within a region of the crypt–villus axis known as the *proliferative zone* (see Figure 1.9). Mesenchymal factors, including the winged helix transcription factor Fkh6 [137], and several intercellular signaling pathways regulate cell division in this zone. Recent advances in coupling organoid culture and genetic manipulation uncover a series of signaling molecules and transcription factors that are critical for the self-renew and differentiation of gastrointestinal stem/progenitor cells [138–142]. Stem cell regulation in the gastrointestinal tract is discussed in detail in Chapter 2.

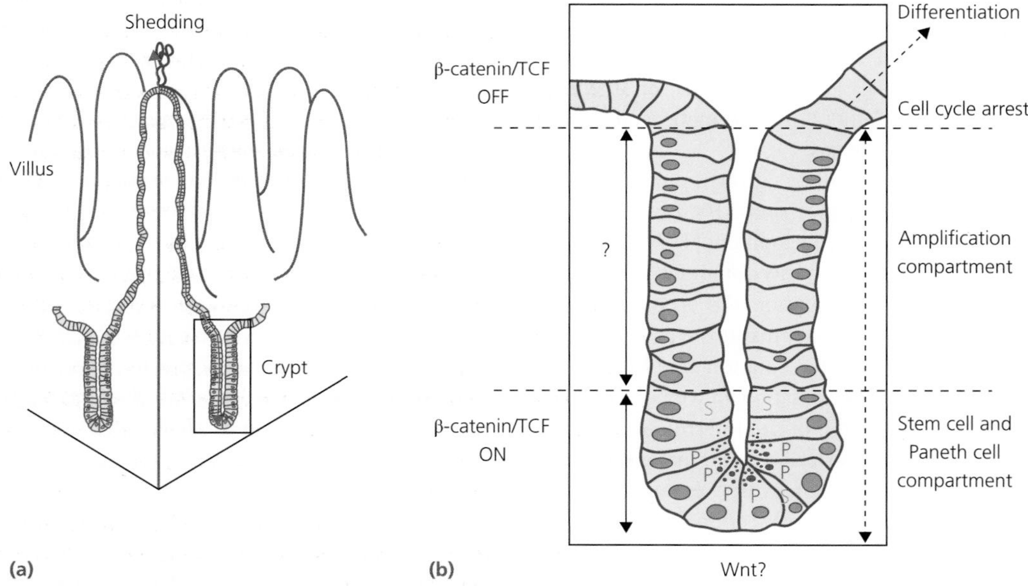

Figure 1.9 Small intestinal maturation. **(a)** Maturation of the crypt–villus axis. Stem cells near the base of the crypt give rise to a transient amplifying multipotent population of cells that reside in the middle and upper portions of the crypt. These cells give rise to mature enterocytes, enteroendocrine cells, and goblet cells, which migrate up the villus and are eventually shed into the intestinal lumen. Paneth cells are also derived from the transient amplifying population, but these cells migrate down to the crypt base, where they intermingle with stem cells. **(b)** Small-intestinal crypt. Schematic showing the crypt is divided into compartments. At the base are stem cells (S), which are thought to reside slightly above the crypt base, and Paneth cells (P). Canonical Wnt signaling is active in these cells. Above this compartment is the transient amplifying population, containing actively dividing cells. Cells withdraw from the cell cycle as they reach the crypt–villus interface and adopt an absorptive or secretory fate. Source: Sancho et al. 2003 [242]. Reproduced with permission of Elsevier.

Differentiation

The differentiated cells of the intestine (see Chapter 5) can be divided into *absorptive* and *secretory* cells on the basis of cellular function. The precise identity and relative abundance of absorptive and secretory cells vary along the anterior–posterior axis. The major secretory cells of the stomach (and their secretory products) are parietal cells (acid), chief cells (digestive enzymes), and endocrine G cells (gastrin). By contrast, the major secretory cells of the small intestine are goblet cells (mucus), Paneth cells (antimicrobial peptides), and enteroendocrine cells (myriad hormones). Nevertheless, the genetic mechanisms that regulate the development of these different cells are shared between different segments of the gastrointestinal tract.

As in the pancreas, Notch signaling plays a critical role in the regulation of intestinal cell fate by mediating the expression of several downstream bHLH proteins – NGN3, BETA2/NEUROD, HES1, and MATH1. The general conclusion from studies of mice with mutations of these proteins is that differentiation of the secretory cell lineage is triggered by repression of Notch signaling and HES1, with the resulting derepression of MATH1 [143,144]. Additional signals control the selection of different intestinal secretory cell lineages (endocrine, goblet, and Paneth). One of these signals, NGN3, is absolutely required for endocrine cells to form in the intestine, but not in the stomach; by contrast, the formation of goblet and Paneth cells is normal in *Ngn3*-deficient mice [145,146]. Other complex signals and lineage relationships underlie the development of the 10 or so different types of enteroendocrine cell [147].

There is additional evidence that Notch signals are coordinated with Wnt signals to regulate the balance between proliferation and differentiation. Either embryonic activation of Notch or inhibition of Wnt results in the loss of secretory cell lineages [148–150]. Furthermore, Wnts have a special role in ensuring proper compartmentalization of the crypt–villus axis by regulating another family of cell–cell signaling molecules known as ephrins [151].

Several studies suggest that major regulators of embryonic differentiation, Notch and Wnt, are also involved in adult intestinal homeostasis. These are discussed in Chapter 2. Notably, activation of Wnt signaling through the loss of the *APC* gene and the subsequent activation of β-catenin is known to be a key step in colorectal carcinogenesis (see Chapters 26 and 71), suggesting that intestinal stem cells or transient amplifying cells are most sensitive to the inactivation of *APC* and represent a likely target for malignant transformation.

In summary, the formation of sphincters during midgestation divides the gut tube into segments – esophagus, stomach, small intestine, and large intestine – that prefigure their distinct morphologies and functions. The mechanisms underlying sphincter formation and gut tube patterning are incompletely understood but involve significant epithelial–mesenchymal crosstalk. Similar crosstalk is involved in the morphogenesis of the different intestinal segments. Subsequently, intestinal development proceeds by differentiation from stem cells, a process that depends on Wnt and Notch signaling, among other pathways. Such signals control proliferation and differentiation in the adult intestine and are dysregulated during carcinogenesis.

Conclusions

After gastrulation, the gut tube is exposed to regional signals from adjacent nonendodermal cells. In prespecified organ domains, the epithelium responds by growing into adjacent mesoderm-derived mesenchyme, resulting in the budding of lung, liver, and pancreas. In the remaining gut epithelium, reciprocal signaling with mesenchyme results in the formation of sphincters or regionally distinct submucosal layers. Complex morphogenetic changes and differentiation events occur in each of these developing organs, giving rise to organized functional tissues. Tissue-specific gene expression begins, setting the stage for further refinement of regulated expression and function. In the adult esophagus, stomach, and intestine, differentiated cell types are generated throughout life from stem cells that reside within the basal layers (esophagus), isthmus (stomach), and crypts (intestine), an ongoing process that recapitulates many developmental events. In the liver and the pancreas, by contrast, the replication of existing cell types appears to be the major mechanism for tissue maintenance.

Developmental physiology

The development of complex anatomical structures with distinct differentiated cell lineages would be purposeless if it did not facilitate function. The functions of the gastrointestinal organs include assimilation of nutrients, detoxification and elimination of waste, maintenance of blood glucose, and synthesis of plasma proteins. In addition, the gastrointestinal tract subserves secondary roles in water and electrolyte balance and immunological defense (see Chapter 16).

The connection between form and function is reflected in an economy of mechanism. Many genes exhibit dual function and are involved in both development and physiological regulation. As previously described, FOXA2 and GATA4 bind to the albumin promoter as part of a program of endoderm commitment, and are thus involved in both patterning and the functional expression of a liver-specific gene. There are several other instances of such developmental "parsimony"; for example, the *Pdx1* and *p48* genes play important roles in pancreatic development and are also the major transcriptional regulators of insulin and of several exocrine genes, respectively [87,103]. Similarly, the *CDX2* homeobox gene product plays an important role in endoderm patterning [14,16,17,152] and also functions as a major transcription factor for the expression of brush border enzymes and intestinal carbonic anhydrase [153–155]. Such economy is not surprising because the use of a limited set of genetic tools reduces the need for additional layers of complexity during specification and differentiation. Fortuitously, this arrangement facilitates the study of developmental physiology, and identification of the genes that regulate development provides a list of candidate regulators of function, and vice versa.

Maturation of the gastrointestinal tract

After parturition, the gastrointestinal tract faces two challenges. Immediately after birth, the individual must convert from a diet that is predominantly parenteral (provided by the maternal circulation), to one that is completely enteral (consisting of colostrum and breast milk). Later, at weaning, the gastrointestinal tract must be able to assimilate nutrients from a vast array of solid foods. These adjustments occur in a hormonal milieu that is increasingly under the control of the infant. Therefore, unlike structural development, which follows a set of preprogrammed genetic events, functional development is likely to be considerably more dependent on environmental forces [117].

Gastrointestinal "maturation" refers to the progressive attainment of features of adult gastrointestinal physiology during development. Given the imprecise nature of such a definition, several surrogate markers are used to understand how the physiology of the gastrointestinal tract changes over time. These include biochemical measurements of intestinal enzyme and hormone activities, morphological grading, mutant analysis, and measurements of permeability, motility, and immune performance. It has been suggested that the human gastrointestinal tract is structurally and functionally mature at the time of parturition, whereas the rodent gastrointestinal tract is altricial, or immature, at birth. However, given the comprehensive nature of maturation, and the fact that the neonatal diet of all mammals is similar (i.e., milk), the implications of such a distinction are unclear.

Carbohydrate digestion and absorption

A focal point in the study of intestinal maturation has been the characterization of the major brush border enzymes that digest carbohydrates. Lactase–phlorizin hydrolase (LPH) cleaves lactose, the major dietary carbohydrate of breast milk. In rats, LPH is expressed at high levels early in embryogenesis, whereas peak expression in human embryos occurs during the third trimester. LPH expression declines with age in both species. The observation that LPH expression across species is highest after birth and subsequently lower likely reflects the critical requirement for lactase during nursing [156].

Sucrase–isomaltase (SI) is another well-studied brush border enzyme. In contrast with LPH, the expression of SI is discordant between humans and other mammals. In rats and pigs, SI expression is undetectable before a dramatic burst of expression in the postnatal period, corresponding to the time just before weaning when the major carbohydrate source shifts from milk to starch. By contrast, SI expression in humans begins in the first trimester and reaches its peak level just before birth [156]. The earlier expression of SI during human ontogeny is not understood, and it is unclear whether differences in enzyme expression levels reflect differences in overall functional maturation between species.

Protein digestion and absorption

The embryo has a limited capacity to digest proteins, a result of the late expression of digestive zymogens, the low-level expression of the activating enzyme enterokinase, and the insensitivity of embryonic pancreatic exocrine cells to the action of secretagogues (see *Hormonal control of gastrointestinal development*). Furthermore, gastric pH is neutral until birth, declining rapidly from 6.0 to 2.2 in the first day of life [157]. Instead, other systems handle the limited protein load delivered to the intestine prenatally and perinatally. Brush border and microvillar peptidases and dipeptidases, which complete peptide digestion, are present in the fetal small intestine at levels of activity comparable with levels in the adult small intestine. High levels of amino acid transporters in the newborn permit the uptake of free amino acids.

Macromolecular transport also plays an important role in the digestion of proteins and lipids in the fetus and the neonate [158–160]. In experimental animals, the small-intestinal epithelium is most permeable to amino acids and peptides in the immediate postnatal period. Macromolecular tracers infused into the amniotic fluid or the intestinal lumen late in gestation are absorbed into the enterocytes of humans, monkeys, guinea pigs, and rats, reflecting a high rate of pinocytosis [160]. This process is extremely active in the first 2 weeks postnatally and decreases at weaning. This mechanism accounts for the absorption of intact maternal immunoglobulins and other proteins from milk.

In parallel with pinocytosis, enterocytes exhibit high levels of lysosomal proteases, such as cathepsins and other peptidases, during the first 2 weeks postnatally. These intracellular enzymes provide a mechanism for protein digestion before the appearance of the pancreatic proteolytic enzymes. Intact proteins also are absorbed in premature and term human infants during the first few months of life. Macromolecules may continue to cross the healthy adult small intestine, but the quantity is low compared with those in the newborn. The relative permeability of the intestine during the first months of life may play an important role in conferring tolerance or sensitivity to dietary proteins during the development of immune function.

Lipid digestion and absorption

Fats and unhydrolyzed triglycerides are present in the stools of human neonates at a rate that is greater than that of adults, a phenomenon that correlates with the low activity of pancreatic lipase and the low intralumenal concentrations of bile acids. Although pancreatic lipase levels increase significantly during the third trimester, lipase activity at week 32 of gestation is only 50% of term levels, which are themselves only 10% of adult levels. Fat digestion in human neonates is aided by "preduodenal" lipases (lingual and gastric lipases) and maternal milk lipase. Lingual lipase increases to adult levels by 2 years of age [161]. Gastric lipase appears as early as 10–13 weeks into gestation and reaches adult levels by 16 weeks [162]. Gastric lipase appears to be a major determinant of lipolytic activity in gastric aspirates of premature infants. As with peptides, the newborn intestine exhibits increased permeability to both triglycerides and cholesterol [163].

The synthesis of bile acids from cholesterol and their conjugation with taurine and glycine can be demonstrated in organ culture in vitro with human liver tissue obtained from fetuses after 15 weeks of gestation. Biliary secretion is observed as early as the 22nd week of gestation. Bile acid reabsorption occurs in the neonate by passive diffusion throughout the small intestine, but active sodium-dependent ileal transport of bile acids does not occur until weaning [164]. As a result, the bile acid pool is reduced in neonates; this is of particular concern in premature infants, in whom 10%–20% of ingested fat may not be absorbed.

Dietary control of gastrointestinal development

The expression of SI, LPH, and other brush border enzymes appears to be under autonomous control, because their normal expression pattern does not change significantly with delayed or early weaning or early introduction of dietary sucrose [165]. Indeed, transplanted human fetal intestine is able to undergo normal cytodifferentiation in an immunodeficient "nude" mouse host [166]. However, other aspects of gastrointestinal development, particularly growth, are regulated by diet. Exposure of the gut lumen to nutrients begins in utero with the swallowing of amniotic fluid, which contains amino acids and carbohydrates, and which the embryo uses to meet some of its nutritional requirements.

The importance of the lumenal environment is supported by studies in which the timing, the composition, or the route of delivery of nutrition is varied. Ligation of the embryonic sheep esophagus causes reversible and specific inhibition of growth of the gastrointestinal tract [167]. Although normally absent in human amniotic fluid, galactose can nevertheless be absorbed by the embryonic jejunum. Intraamniotic infusion (and therefore increased enteral delivery) of galactose induces an increase in the mucosal transport of galactose by the rabbit intestine, as well as an overall increase in mucosal weight, suggesting that the fetal intestine is competent to respond to small changes in enteral carbohydrate composition [168]. Consistent with this, intestinal growth in the first day of life depends on the composition of milk [169]. Importantly, it is not simply the metabolic consequences of feeding that provide a signal; the intestinal mucosa itself must be exposed to these nutritional components [170]. A requirement for lumenal stimulation has long been appreciated in the "adaptation" observed after massive intestinal resection – a compensatory increase in intestinal surface area that depends on enteral feeding [171]. It is possible that this adaptation reflects a reemergence of a developmental program that regulates intestinal size and surface area. Indeed, microarray analysis of gene transcription during development and adaptation supports this hypothesis [172].

Hormonal control of gastrointestinal development

A possible regulatory role for corticosteroids and thyroid hormone in intestinal development has been extensively explored because of the dramatic increase in the level of both hormones observed in rats immediately before the spike in SI activity and coinciding with a reduction in LPH activity. Direct effects on the activity of several disaccharidases have been documented after the administration of exogenous hormones. Notably, prenatal administration of cortisone reduces the incidence of necrotizing enterocolitis in a rat model, presumably by accelerating the maturation of the mucosal barrier [173]. Conversely, intestinal maturation is slowed by treatments that reduce levels of circulating corticosteroids. Similar effects are seen with enhancement or inhibition of thyroid hormone expression, although some of these effects may be mediated through corticosteroids [156]. However, mice lacking corticotropin-releasing hormone or thyrotropin-releasing hormone do not exhibit an overt gastrointestinal phenotype [174,175]. The regulation of gastrointestinal maturation by other hormones and circulating growth factors has also been investigated through similar approaches. In particular, cholecystokinin, gastrin, insulin, and members of the insulin-like growth factor (IGF), epidermal growth factor, and TGF families have been the focus of numerous studies.

These analyses have yielded evidence for the involvement of hormones and systemic growth factors in gastrointestinal development. However, distinguishing between primary and secondary effects is challenging, and for the most part, the precise functions of these molecules in development remain to be delineated. It is worth noting that mice with a targeted inactivation of the gastrin gene exhibit a deficiency of acid-producing parietal cells [176,177], suggesting a role in cellular differentiation rather than maturation per se.

Despite lingering uncertainty over the precise role of hormones in intestinal maturation, it is clear that the responsiveness of some gastrointestinal tissues to hormones changes over the course of fetal and postnatal life. The responsiveness of the exocrine pancreas is an example of such regulation. Pancreatic digestive and lipolytic enzymes are detected in the early bud stage, and high levels of protein are detected in the acinar cells before term. Despite the abundance of these proteins, embryonic acini are insensitive to secretagogues until after birth [178]. Similarly, sensitivity to the acid-secretory action of gastrin develops during the first week of life; poor expression of the gastrin receptor in the immediate postnatal period renders newborns relatively insensitive to gastrin [179]. Finally, as a source of insulin, the pancreas is the major regulator of glucose homeostasis, and the intestine contains numerous peptides that regulate motility, ion transport, feeding, and satiety [180].

Development of the enteric nervous system

The enteric nervous system (ENS) regulates many aspects of gastrointestinal physiology, including peristalsis and smooth muscle activity, sphincter tone, glandular output, microcirculation, and possibly, inflammation [181]. Through these activities, the ENS controls the response to feeding by coordinating intestinal transit, secretion, and continence. The cells that generate the ENS migrate from the neural crest during the first trimester, induced by complex and poorly understood signals. Similar to other neural crest derivatives, the ENS is part of the peripheral nervous system, constituting its largest subdivision. Although the ENS receives input from the vagus nerve, it possesses marked independence from the central nervous system, exhibiting function even after complete dissociation from all brain and spinal inputs. On the basis of its size and autonomy, the ENS has been referred to as the "second brain" [182]. Although many disorders may be related to ENS dysfunction, only Hirschsprung disease is clearly attributable to developmental errors in ENS formation (see *Disorders of specification and formation*).

Fate mapping in the chick has shown that enteric neurons are largely derived from rostral (vagal) and caudal (sacral) precursors that migrate from the neural tube and intermingle to populate the entire gut tube [183]. Although some details remain controversial, studies in mice have confirmed the general picture of neural crest migration mapped out by studies in the chick. The ENS is composed of two types of ganglionated plexuses: the Auerbach (myenteric) plexus, which is located in the outer muscular layer and regulates gastrointestinal tract motility and function of extralumenal organs, and the Meissner (submucosal) plexus, which regulates enteral secretory activity [182]. Enteric neurons can be further subclassified according to the neurotransmitters (e.g., vasoactive intestinal polypeptide and serotonin) and enzymes (e.g., tyrosine hydroxylase and choline acetyltransferase) they express. Although details regarding the migration and terminal differentiation of neural crest precursors are still emerging, neuronal subtypes appear to arise in overlapping developmental waves [184]. The functional roles of these neuronal subtypes and specific neuropeptides in gastrointestinal physiology are described elsewhere in this textbook (see Chapter 12).

In contrast with the neural crest-derived cells of the enteric plexuses, interstitial cells of Cajal (ICCs), which serve as the "pacemakers" of the intestine, arise from intestinal mesenchyme [185,186]. The development of these cells requires the function of another receptor tyrosine kinase, c-Kit. Mice with reduced or absent c-Kit function exhibit abnormal slow-wave activity in the small intestine and develop paralytic ileus [187,188]. It has been discovered that those mesenchymal tumors known as gastrointestinal stromal tumors (GISTs) have activating mutations in *KIT* that confer constitutive kinase activity in the absence of ligand [189,190]. Ultrastructural similarities between ICCs and GISTS, and other shared features, have led investigators to propose that GISTs arise from ICCs [191] or from a common ICC–smooth muscle precursor cell [192].

A central role for the c-Ret tyrosine kinase pathway in the development of most enteric neurons has been demonstrated through targeted inactivation of pathway components (see *Hirschsprung disease* later in this chapter). Furthermore, important neural crest subpopulations have been recognized from the more limited phenotypes that results from the targeted mutation of other genes. For example, the bHLH protein MASH1 is required for the development of a subset of enteric neuronal precursors with noradrenergic features, and endothelin B signaling is required to prevent the differentiation of neuronal precursors that will enervate the distal colon [193]. The significance of these different subtypes is unclear, and the mechanisms by which they achieve regulatory integration require further study.

The ENS begins to function early in embryonic development, but its maturation continues well into postnatal life. Fetal swallowing is first detectable during the first trimester [194], and by term, the fetus swallows about 450 mL amniotic fluid (half of the total amniotic volume) per day [195]. A spectrum of neuropeptides is detectable between weeks 11 and 18 of human development [196]. Peak numbers of both neurons and ganglion cells are achieved during the second trimester and decrease during the third trimester [197]. Although the structural elements of the esophagus and stomach are largely developed by midgestation, gastroesophageal motility does not fully mature until after birth. Lower esophageal sphincter pressure increases dramatically during the last trimester and again postnatally [198], achieving adult levels by 3–6 weeks of age. Despite this, gastroesophageal reflux is common postnatally and persists in up to 10% of infants for the first year [199].

Mucosal immune system

The gastrointestinal tract, particularly the small intestine, contains a highly complex mixture of immune cell populations. The gut-associated lymphoid tissue (GALT) encompasses organized aggregates dominated by lymphocytes (Peyer's patches) and a diffuse heterogeneous population of lymphocytes, monocytes, or macrophages, and other cells, such as eosinophils and mast cells in the lamina propria. Intraepithelial lymphocytes are also scattered throughout the surface epithelium. Structures resembling Peyer's patches are evident as early as 11 weeks of human gestation; by 14 weeks, $CD4^+$ and $CD8^+$ lymphocytes can be detected. By the end of the second trimester, Peyer's patches histologically resemble the adult structure, indicating that antigen exposure or bacterial colonization are not necessary for their development; however, germinal centers do not form until after birth. Mice carrying a null mutation for TNF-α do not develop Peyer's patches or lymph nodes, and splenic organization is markedly abnormal; if the 55-kD receptor for TNF-α is disrupted, lymph nodes and splenic tissue develop normally, but Peyer's patches are still absent, suggesting that the 55-kD receptor provides specificity for Peyer's patch development. Other targeted mutations that result in the absence of Peyer's patch development in mice include knockout of the inhibitory helix–loop–helix transcription factor Id2, lymphotoxins, and the lymphotoxin-β receptor. Mice lacking Peyer's patches do not develop oral tolerance. Targeted disruption of the homeodomain containing the transcription factor gene *Nkx2.3* in mice results in significant defects in intestinal development and also smaller Peyer's patches and loss of expression of the mucosal cell adhesion molecule 1 (MadCam1), which is normally responsible for B-cell and T-cell homing to peripheral lymphoid organs. Full maturation of the immune system, and specifically Peyer's patch formation, is dependent on postnatal bacterial colonization.

Lamina propria lymphocytes are first detected after 11 weeks of gestation. Macrophages are present at 12 weeks but increase greatly in number after birth. Recruitment and maturation of mucosal lymphocytes depend on retinoic acid, presumably produced by intestinal epithelial populations. During fetal life, lymphocytes consist of increasing numbers of scattered T cells and B cells. In contrast with αβ T cells, γδ T cells, which make up 5%–15% of small-intestinal and 40% of colonic intraepithelial lymphocytes, can develop extrathymically, as well as in the thymus. The γδ T cells undergo clonal expansion soon after birth, but with further maturation they become clonally restricted and unique in each individual. Targeted deletion of γδ T cells in mice results in a lack of mucosal B cells that produce immunoglobulin A (IgA) but has no effect on αβ T-cell development, which is thought to occur within the thymus. IgA- and IgM-producing plasma cells are not found in the lamina propria until after birth and antigenic exposure. Intraepithelial lymphocytes appear at 11 and 12 weeks of gestation. Fetal lamina propria lymphocytes are mostly $CD4^+$ as in the adult lamina propria, and fetal intraepithelial lymphocytes are often $CD4^-$ $CD8^-$; $CD8^+$ cells become more predominant after birth.

As noted earlier, exposure to the luminal flora is necessary for maturation of the mucosal immune compartment. In rats, suckling and germ-free animals have fewer intestinal lymphocytes than adults, and weaning – associated with intestinal maturation and increasing bacterial colonization – is also characterized by marked development of the mucosal immune system. Cyclosporine (cyclosporin), an inhibitor of T-lymphocyte activation, retards normal lymphocyte development in the small intestine. Natural killer activity of intraepithelial and lamina propria lymphocytes is absent before birth, increasing dramatically after weaning.

Conclusions

The genes and signals that give rise to the primitive structures of the gastrointestinal tract become progressively invested with functionality during embryogenesis and postnatal life. Some features (e.g., synthesis of pancreatic hormones, neuropeptides, and certain digestive enzymes) are largely under autonomous control, whereas other features (e.g., intestinal growth and development of mucosal immunity) are highly dependent on interactions with the environment.

Disorders of development

The earlier sections have described the basic events and mechanisms that allow the normal development of the gastrointestinal tract, pancreas, and liver. Although dysgenesis may result from disturbances of any one of these steps, errors in gastrulation or endoderm formation do not present clinically because the global importance of these early steps for further development render them lethal during embryonic development. The range of observable clinical phenotypes is therefore confined to those that are compatible with advanced embryonic development. It should be emphasized that developmental disorders involving the gastrointestinal tract are most commonly observed as part of multigenic disorders. Of these, the most common is Down syndrome (trisomy 21 syndrome), which is associated with duodenal atresia, tracheoesophageal fistula, Hirschsprung disease, and imperforate anus. In the following sections, disorders have been selected to illustrate key events in organ formation and organogenesis, along with their (known) molecular underpinnings.

Disorders of specification and formation

Congenital gastrointestinal malformations may occur in the setting of Down syndrome or other syndromes, or they may occur as isolated findings. For example, anorectal malformations are common birth defects that may be found in isolation or as part of a syndrome, such as the VACTERL syndrome (vertebral, anal, cardiac, tracheal, esophageal, renal, and limb abnormalities). Clinical features of anorectal malformations are discussed in Chapters 6 and 67.

The etiology for most congenital malformations is unknown. Certain anomalies result from lesions in a single gene (e.g., see Box 1.2), whereas others may be associated with a disruption of a signaling pathway (e.g., see Box 1.3 and later *Heterotopias* section). Another class of congenital syndromes may reflect a common final pathophysiological pathway that can be disrupted by any of a number of events. Hirschsprung disease is an instructive example of this last class.

Hirschsprung disease

As already noted, neural crest cells migrate from the neural tube during midgestation to give rise to the ganglion cells of the ENS. Absence of these cells (aganglionosis) in the colon results in Hirschsprung disease, a male-predominant disorder that most commonly presents in the perinatal period. Absent peristalsis in the affected segment of colon causes constipation (or failure to pass meconium), distal obstruction, and megacolon. Hirschsprung disease always affects the rectum; more proximal segments are affected in a few patients and, rarely, the small bowel (see Chapters 6 and 67 for a detailed clinical discussion). Although Hirschsprung disease can be inherited in an autosomal or recessive fashion, most cases exhibit non-Mendelian inheritance with a genetic component. Hirschsprung disease is commonly associated with Down syndrome.

Receptor tyrosine kinase RET

Heterozygous mutations in *RET*, a transmembrane tyrosine kinase (chromosome 10q11.2), represent the most common genetic alteration resulting in Hirschsprung disease. The gene for RET is expressed in ENS precursors, whereas those for its ligands (which include GDNF and neurturin [NRTN]) are expressed in the mesenchyme of the developing gut. On binding

Box 1.3 Meckel syndrome.

Meckel diverticulum is the most common congenital malformation of the gastrointestinal tract, occurring with a frequency rate of 2% of births [247]. The disorder reflects a persistence of the vitelline duct – the embryonic structure connecting the gut to the yolk sac (Figure 1.10). Meckel diverticula are generally located near the terminal ileum, and in about 50% of patients the diverticulum contains ectopic tissue, most commonly gastric or pancreatic, but occasionally also colonic, duodenal, jejunal, hepatic, and endometrial [248]. Secretion of gastric acid (and in some cases, pancreatic bicarbonate) causes ulceration of adjacent small intestinal mucosa; the disorder commonly presents as unexplained gastrointestinal hemorrhage in a child or young adult (see Chapters 5 and 60). Note that heterotopia is distinct from metaplasia, which represents an acquired replacement of one tissue type with another over time.

What mechanism might account for the defective patterning leading to heterotopia?

Bossard and Zaret [249] observed that 3% of mouse embryos exhibit an albumin-expressing ectopic bud at the site of the vitelline duct, near the terminal ileum, which led them to propose that Meckel diverticula result from the loss of normal mesenchymal inhibitory signals at the site of the vitelline duct. According to this attractive model, heterotopic tissue forms not as a result of ectopic cells "left behind" by the nonregressed vitelline structure, but because a signal required for patterning and specification was disrupted by the error in regression (see *Heterotopias*).

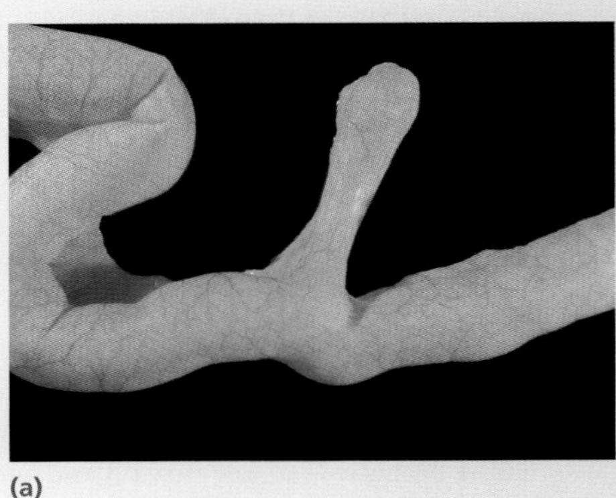

(a)

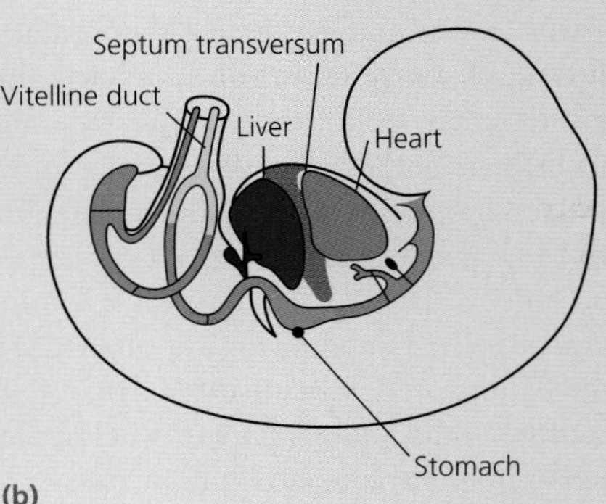

(b)

Figure 1.10 **(a)** Gross specimen showing a Meckel diverticulum in the embryo. Source: Courtesy of Beth Furth, University of Pennsylvania School of Medicine. **(b)** Embryonic vitelline duct.

to one of its cognate ligands, RET normally activates a membrane complex that includes a glycosylphosphatidylinositol-anchored signaling component (GFRA1–4) [193]. Mutations in the *RET* gene cause disease by reducing kinase function, which interferes with the proper differentiation, survival, or migration of these cells. Such mutations are present in up to 50% of patients with familial disease. Consistently, loss of *Ret* also causes Hirschsprung disease in mice through impacting multiple tissue compartments, including ENS precursors, enteric mesenchyme and epithelium [200]. A small percentage of patients with sporadic disease have inactivating RET mutations, and polymorphisms in the gene may also play a role [193,201,202]. Mutations in the RET ligand GDNF also have been found in patients with Hirschsprung disease [203,204], and mutations in the NRTN ligand may contribute to disease severity [205]. Polymorphisms in the homeobox transcription factor PHOX2B, a putative regulator of RET [206], are also associated with Hirschsprung disease [207]. Consistent with a specific role for RET in neural crest cell biology, a high frequency of activating mutations occurs in patients with multiple endocrine neoplasia type 2, who experience development of a spectrum of neural crest-derived tumors [208].

Sox10

Mutations in genes with no apparent link to RET signaling are also associated with Hirschsprung disease. One of the first models of Hirschsprung disease was Dominant megacolon (Dom), a naturally occurring mouse mutant that exhibited pigmentary defects and aganglionosis [209]. Mutations in the SRY-related transcription factor SOX10 are responsible for the Dom phenotype [210,211]. In contrast with most mouse models of Hirschsprung disease, haploinsufficiency of SOX10 is sufficient to cause colonic aganglionosis in *Sox10*$^{+/-}$ mice. *SOX10* mutations are also found in patients with Waardenburg–Shah syndrome, who exhibit Hirschsprung disease, pigmentary defects, and deafness. Thus, like RET, SOX10 also likely has a general role in the development of neural crest derivatives.

Endothelins

Mutations in endothelin 3 (*EDN3*) and its receptor (*EDNRB*) have also been found in patients with isolated Hirschsprung disease or the Waardenburg–Shah syndrome. Similar to *RET*, *EDNRB* is expressed in neural crest cells before and during migration, whereas its ligand is expressed by the gut mesenchyme; mutations in these genes account for about 10% of

Hirschsprung disease cases [212]. In addition, a mutation in an endothelin-processing enzyme (ECE1) has been found in a patient with Hirschsprung disease [213].

The final common pathology in Hirschsprung disease is aganglionosis; hence the disorder may reflect defects in the specification, migration, or survival of enteric neurons. Much work remains to be done to understand precisely how the identified genes function in normal ENS development and how mutations in these genes result in a Hirschsprung disease phenotype. Given that most patients with Hirschsprung disease lack identifiable mutations, polygenic contributions are likely to be important. Alternatively, "errors" in migration, without a genetic contribution, may play a role in some cases.

Disorders of differentiation and patterning

Clinical phenotypes caused by the developmental failure to form a particular cell type are rarely observed. It is likely that many mutations affecting critical regulatory pathways (e.g., Notch signaling) are incompatible with life. Alternatively, redundancy or plasticity may lead to adaptive compensatory changes that permit normal or nearly normal differentiation in a mutant background.

Instead, disorders that affect patterning leading to *misplacement* of differentiated tissues occur with some frequency. These conditions may be the result of an acquired (metaplasia) or congenital (heterotopia) tissue placement. Metaplasia is often the harbinger of malignant transformation, as mentioned in the *Specification* subsection of *Gastrointestinal tract* and discussed in greater detail in Chapter 26. Although the possible mechanism of heterotopia is discussed in the following section, note that the mechanism of metaplasia is entirely unknown. In particular, it is not clear whether the premalignant intestinal epithelium that replaces the normal squamous mucosa of the esophagus is a consequence of *transdifferentiation* between the two cell types or the growth and replacement of squamous cells by a quiescent stem/progenitor cell that exists within the esophagus.

Heterotopias

The presence of ectopic cell types (heterotopia) is observed in several tissue types, although in some cases the displacement is the result of faulty migration. Ectopic placement of gastric, pancreatic, and liver tissues has been described and may occur in the setting of congenital gastrointestinal duplications. Of the simple heterotopias, two types occur with relative frequency: inlet patches and pancreatic heterotopias.

Inlet patches consist of a segment of gastric mucosa within the cervical esophagus and occur with a frequency rate of up to 4.5% in autopsy studies. Inlet patches contain true gastric mucosa, and most exhibit oxyntic histology. Most cases are asymptomatic, although some may be complicated by infection with *Helicobacter pylori*, inflammation, bleeding, and malignant transformation [214]. Inlet patches are sometimes associated with intestinal metaplasia and pancreatic heterotopia.

Pancreatic heterotopias, also known as pancreatic rests, consist of ectopic pancreatic tissue, most often located within the proximal gastrointestinal tract. Autopsy studies estimate their frequency to range from 0.5% to 14%, although the true prevalence is probably on the lower end of the scale [215]. As with inlet patches, most pancreatic heterotopias are asymptomatic.

Both of these conditions are believed to be congenital, but the causes are unknown. One study shed light on a possible mechanism: the segmental absence of a developmental signal. As discussed in the *Organogenesis* section related to the pancreas, a key signal during the specification of the pancreas is the *repression* of Shh expression in the endoderm. Consistent with Hh repression being sufficient to specify pancreatic development, the exposure of mouse embryos to the drug cyclopamine, an inhibitor of Shh signaling, results in ectopic pancreas formation with an anatomic distribution that mimics that of human pancreatic heterotopia (stomach > duodenum > small intestine; Figure 1.11; see also Box 1.4 for a discussion of the related subject of annular pancreas). Thus, the failure of a patch of endoderm to receive a Hh signal could result in the specification of an ectopic patch of pancreatic tissue. Similarly, the cervical esophagus could be particularly susceptible to the absence of a normally inhibitory signal during development, creating an inlet patch. This presumptive mechanism could account for the development of ectopic tissues in other organs as well (see also the discussion of Meckel syndrome in Box 1.3).

Disorders of remodeling

Much is known about remodeling – the molding of patterned tissue through growth and development – in certain tissues, especially the developing central nervous system. By contrast, little is known about remodeling during gastrointestinal development. How are the vascular supplies of the intestine, pancreas, and liver tailored to physiological need? What mediates the integration of the ventral and dorsal pancreatic ductal systems (the failure of which causes pancreatic divisum)? How are the different endocrine cells in the pancreas guided to coalesce into the islets of Langerhans? Because the pathophysiology of some developmental disorders (e.g., Hirschsprung disease) may have a component of defective remodeling, the following discussion focuses on biliary tract remodeling as an example.

Abnormal biliary development

As discussed in *Morphogenesis and differentiation* related to the liver, the ductal plate – a ring of specialized cells surrounding branches of the portal vein – gives rise to the IHDBs. Ductal plate remodeling appears to occur in two steps: formation of discrete tubules within the ductal plate followed by elimination of remaining cells through apoptosis, attrition, or differentiation.

Developmental or neonatal biliary disorders fall into two categories: ductal plate malformations and bile duct paucity. Ductal plate malformations refer to a collection of overlapping disorders that are characterized by faulty remodeling of the IHBDs, resulting in the persistence of the embryonic ductal plate

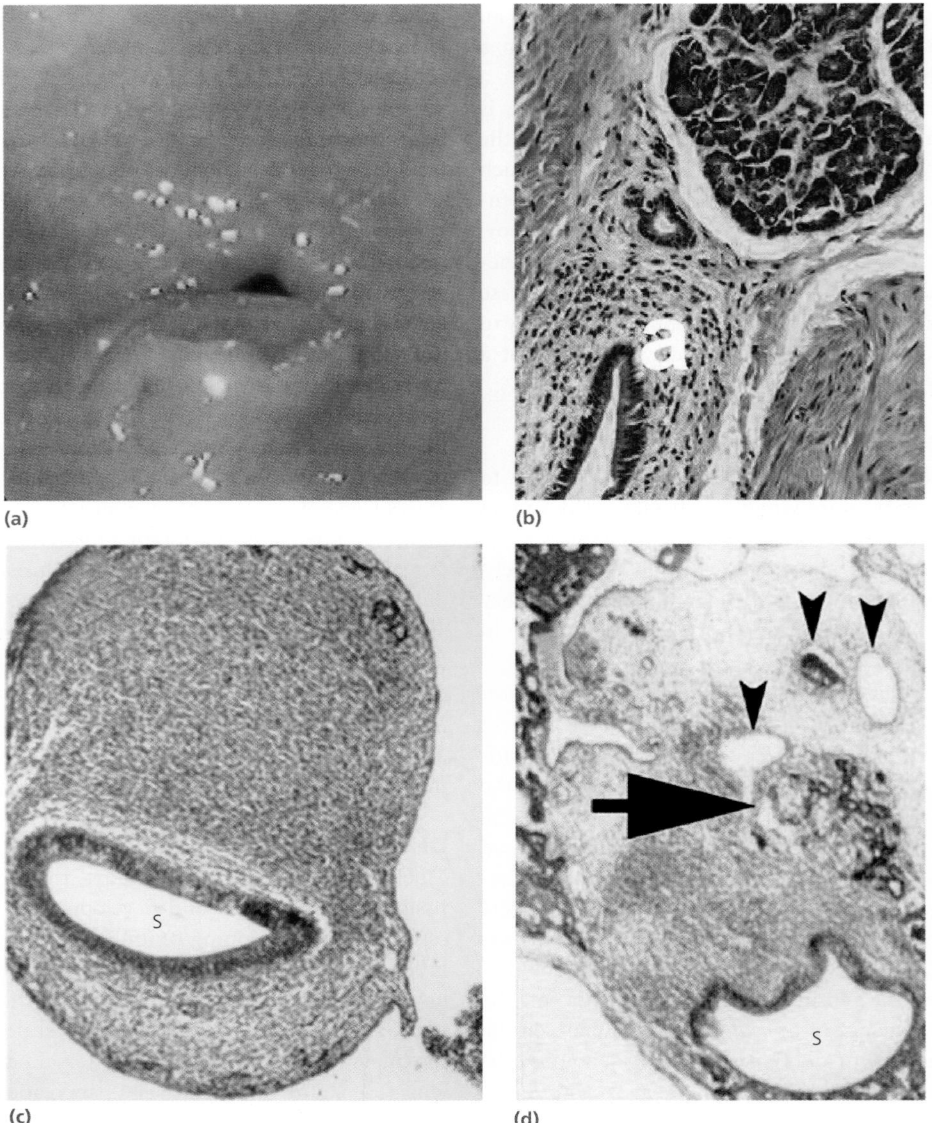

Figure 1.11 Pancreatic heterotopias (rests) in human and mouse. **(a, b)** Pancreatic heterotopia in human. **(a)** Endoscopy reveals dimpling of gastric epithelium. **(b)** Histology reveals pancreatic acini (a) adjacent to gastric mucosa. **(c, d)** Mouse model of pancreatic heterotopia. **(c)** Normal mouse stomach (S). **(d)** Mouse treated with cyclopamine exhibits pancreatic differentiation within the stomach (arrow). Arrowheads show vascular structures. **(a)** Source: Courtesy of William R. Brugge, MD, Massachusetts General Hospital. **(c, d)** Source: Kim and Melton 1998 [82]. Reproduced with permission, Copyright (1998) National Academy of Sciences, USA.

configuration (see Figure 1.5) [222]. Congenital hepatic fibrosis is an autosomal recessive disease with variable histological and clinical features in which the portal tracts and bile ducts exhibit fibrosis and a ductal plate configuration. The histopathology of congenital hepatic fibrosis is seen in association with both autosomal recessive and autosomal dominant polycystic kidney disease. A related disorder, Caroli syndrome, is characterized by the ductal dilation of Caroli disease (type IVA/type V choledochal cysts; see Chapters 9 and 82) with the superimposed fibrosis of congenital hepatic fibrosis, suggesting an overlapping pathophysiology [222]. Although the shared histopathological characteristics observed in these and similar abnormalities (e.g., von Meyenburg complexes) are intriguing, the etiology of these disorders remains completely unknown.

Insight into one potential mechanism for biliary malformation comes from studies of patients with a paucity of IHBDs, also known as Alagille syndrome. Although bile duct paucity is the sine qua non of Alagille syndrome, patients may also have several extrahepatic manifestations, including abnormalities of the great vessels and skeletal and ocular malformations, as well as characteristic facies (see Chapters 9 and 82). Two studies have shown that mutations in the Notch ligand JAG1 are responsible

Box 1.4 Annular pancreas.

The pancreas forms from two buds – a ventral bud and a dorsal bud – that only later fuse into a single integrated gland during the rotation of the abdominal viscera (at which time the ventral portion rotates *behind* the duodenum to meet the dorsal portion). Dysregulation of this process is thought to result in annular pancreas, a condition in which the duodenum is encircled by pancreatic tissue (Figure 1.12). Annular pancreas was first described in 1818 by Tiedemann [216] and is the most common congenital anomaly of the pancreas to present in childhood, although nearly half of cases are first recognized in adults [217], in whom the condition presents with early satiety, nausea, and vomiting [218,219]. In pediatric patients, the disorder is associated with other congenital anomalies, and it is more common in patients with Down syndrome.

The etiology of annular pancreas is not understood, although several theories have been proposed, including hypertrophy or failure of atrophy of the left ventral pancreatic bud, fusion of heterotopic pancreatic rests, and malrotation [217]. Others have suggested that annular pancreas is not a primary malformation at all, but instead is a secondary consequence of duodenal obstruction from other causes. A mouse model of annular pancreas was serendipitously discovered while looking at the role of Hh signaling in pancreas development. Inactivation of Indian hedgehog (Ihh) and rarely Shh results in a high frequency of an annular pancreas that encircles the duodenum [220]. This observation provides an experimental framework for determining whether rare cases of familial annular pancreas [221], or the more common annular pancreas associated with Down syndrome, are caused by disruptions in Hh signaling.

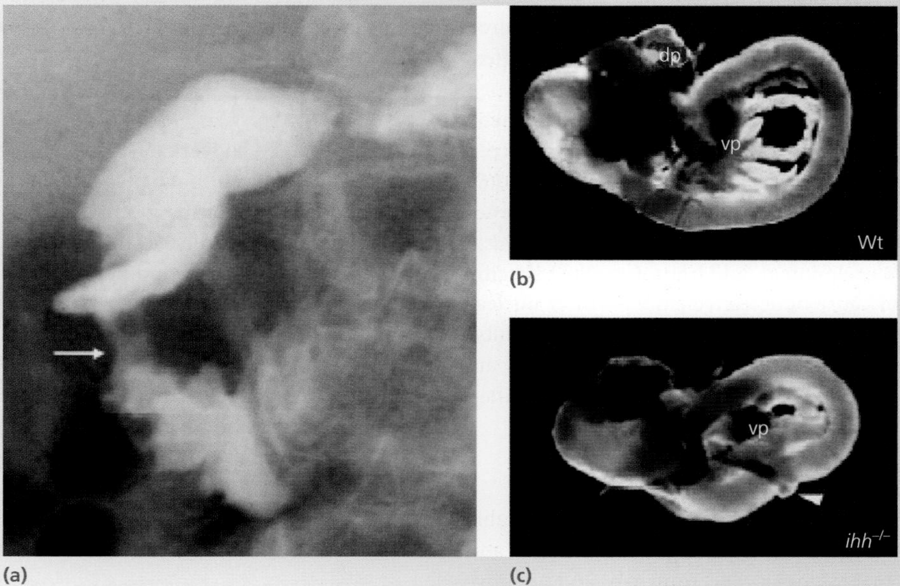

Figure 1.12 **(a)** Upper gastrointestinal radiograph showing narrowing of the duodenum in the area of a pancreatic annulus. **(b)** Foregut structures from a wild-type (Wt) mouse have been dissected out, revealing strands of ventral pancreatic tissue (vp) within the duodenal loop. **(c)** In mutant animals lacking Indian hedgehog (*Ihh*$^{-/-}$), a piece of pancreatic tissue encircles the proximal duodenum (arrowhead). dp, dorsal pancreas. Source: Hebrok et al. 2000 [220]. Copyright MDPI.

for Alagille syndrome and strengthened the link between this developmental signaling pathway and the disease [73,74]. Consistent with this notion, many patients with Alagille syndrome who lack JAG1 mutations have mutations in the NOTCH2 receptor instead [223].

An understanding of the molecular mechanisms underlying this disorder has come from mouse studies. JAG1 is expressed by portal veins and hepatic arteries [224–226], and mice with compound heterozygous *Jagged/Notch* mutations exhibit a paucity of IHBDs [227]. Furthermore, embryos deficient in the Notch target Hes1 develop ductal plates with normal appearance at the appropriate developmental time, but these ductal plates fail to form the tubular structures that precede normal duct development [228]. Finally, mutations in the Notch effector RBP-J lead to bile duct paucity, whereas activation of Notch signaling leads to bile duct excess [229]. Taken together, these studies suggest that Alagille syndrome results from the faulty specification of bile ducts in the absence of Notch signaling.

Biliary atresia, by contrast, is characterized principally by the loss of the extrahepatic bile ducts rather than IHBDs. Biliary atresia is a heterogeneous disorder that presents with two major clinical patterns: a prenatal form that presents almost immediately after birth and is associated with other congenital anomalies, and a perinatal form that presents in the first few weeks of life. Although the etiology of both forms is poorly understood, defective morphogenesis of the bile ducts may play a role in the prenatal form of the disease [230]. Congenital anomalies affecting body symmetry, such as cardiac anomalies, intestinal malrotation, and abdominal situs inversus, often accompany the prenatal form of biliary atresia [231]. Mice with a mutation of the *inversin* gene exhibit abdominal situs inversus and a defective extrahepatic biliary tree [232,233]. Furthermore, missense mutations in *JAG1* have been observed in patients with severe refractory biliary atresia, suggesting that this Notch ligand contributes to disease progression [234]. Consistent with a connection between intrahepatic and extrahepatic ductal pathology, some patients with biliary atresia exhibit the histological characteristics of ductal plate malformation observed with congenital hepatic fibrosis [222].

Disorders of growth control

Several rare disorders that affect the growth of specific parts of the body highlight another developmental phenomenon: genomic *imprinting*. In mammals, which contain sets of paired chromosomes, the maternally inherited chromosome differs from the paternally inherited chromosome both in terms of primary sequence (polymorphisms) and additional epigenetic (noninherited) differences. Epigenetic differences are conferred by DNA methylation, a process that occurs early in embryonic development and results in the differential expression of genes from maternal and paternal alleles. Imprinting is enormously important in normal development, and improper allele-specific methylation is a major cause of defective embryos after nuclear transplantation (cloning). Several human disorders that exhibit growth abnormalities and an increased cancer susceptibility are linked to abnormalities in genomic imprinting, as exemplified by Beckwith–Wiedemann syndrome.

Beckwith–Wiedemann syndrome

Beckwith–Wiedemann syndrome is characterized by variable growth defects, including generalized overgrowth (prenatal and postnatal), as well as macroglossia, visceromegaly, and hemihypertrophy (enlargement of half of the body). Patients with Beckwith–Wiedemann syndrome have an increased frequency of several tumors, including Wilm tumor, hepatoblastoma, and pancreatoblastoma. In the last decade, it has become clear that Beckwith–Wiedemann syndrome is linked to chromosome 11p15, a region containing several imprinted genes.

Two genes in this imprinted region are thought to play a causative role in Beckwith–Wiedemann syndrome: *CDKN1C* (a negative regulator of cell proliferation that acts by inhibiting cyclin-dependent kinase) and *IGF2* (a major regulator of fetal growth). Classical mutations of either of these genes affect growth. For example, mutations in *CDKN1C* have been described in patients with Beckwith–Wiedemann syndrome [235], and the overexpression of *Igf2* in mice is sufficient to cause an overgrowth syndrome [236]. However, the more common mechanism of gene activation (*IGF2*) or inactivation (*CDKN1C*) is related to abnormalities in methylation-dependent imprinting.

Under conditions of normal imprinting, *CDKN1C* is expressed from the maternal allele and *IGF2* is expressed from the paternal allele. Two different patterns of abnormal imprinting are associated with the development of Beckwith–Wiedemann syndrome. In most cases, abnormal methylation results in the loss of *CDKN1C* expression from both alleles, whereas in a few cases, abnormal methylation results in *IGF2* expression from both alleles [237]. Notably, the converse pattern of dysregulated methylation (resulting in loss of *IGF2* expression from both alleles) is associated with Silver–Russell syndrome, a congenital disorder characterized by growth retardation and asymmetry [238–240]. Although the mechanism by which dysregulation of *CDKN1C* or *IGF2* results in isolated growth phenotypes is not known, it is likely that alterations in cell proliferation underlie both the abnormal growth and the tumor propensity in patients with Beckwith–Wiedemann syndrome.

Conclusions

Despite a detailed conceptual framework for understanding the events that govern normal patterning, organogenesis, and physiological adaptation of the gastrointestinal tract, the pathogenesis of congenital disorders of the gastrointestinal tract is poorly understood, reflecting the numerous questions about gastrointestinal development that remain unanswered. To date, most insights have come from human (reverse) genetics and serendipitous similarities between animal and human phenotypes. Specific challenges to further advances include the association of many developmental disorders with complex genetic syndromes and the separation in time between a developmental lesion and its phenotypic manifestations.

References are available at www.yamadagastro.com/textbook7e

Further reading

Brookes M., Zietman A. Clinical Embryology: A Color Atlas and Text. Boca Raton, FL: CRC Press; 1998.

Johnson L.E. Physiology of the Gastrointestinal Tract. New York: Raven Press; 2006.

Larsen P., Kronenberg H., Melmed S., et al. Williams Textbook of Endocrinology, 10th edn. Philadelphia: Saunders; 2003.

Sadler T. Langman's Medical Embryology, 10th edn. Philadelphia: Lippincott Williams & Wilkins; 2006.

Sato T., Clevers H. Growing self-organizing mini-guts from a single intestinal stem cell: mechanism and applications. Science 2013;340:1190.

Zorn A.M., Wells J.M. Vertebrate endoderm development and organ formation. Annu Rev Cell Dev Biol 2009;25:221.

CHAPTER 2

Gut stem cells and tissue renewal

Johan H. van Es[1], Sina Bartfeld[2], and Hans Clevers[1,3]

[1] Hubrecht Institute for Developmental Biology and Stem Cell Research, Oncode Institute and University Medical Centre Utrecht, Utrecht, the Netherlands

[2] Research Center for Infectious Diseases, Würzburg, Germany

[3] The Netherlands Princess Maxima Center for Pediatric Oncology, Utrecht, the Netherlands

Chapter menu

The epithelium of the intestinal tract, continuously attacked by mechanical, chemical, and biological insults, is the most vigorously self-renewing tissue of mammals with a turnover rate of 5–7 days. To sustain this, new cells are continuously generated by a population of multipotent intestinal stem cells that create daughter or progenitor cells, which can subsequently differentiate into the different mature cell types. The balance between intestinal stem cells self-renewal and differentiation must be carefully regulated to maintain tissue homeostasis. This chapter summarizes the current understanding of the identity, location, and maintenance of intestinal stem cells and the tools available to study their behavior in normal and pathological conditions.

In mammals, embryonic stem (ES) cells and adult stem cells comprise two broad categories of stem cells. ES cells, present in the inner cell mass of early embryos (blastocysts), are pluripotent stem cells characterized by their ability to differentiate into derivatives of all three germ layers: ectoderm, endoderm, and mesoderm. These derivatives include each of the more than 200 cell types in the adult body. As development proceeds, ES cells gradually lose their plasticity, ultimately giving rise to adult tissues, each harboring a limited reservoir of tissue-specific adult stem cells. These adult stem cells have long-term self-renewal capacity and are multipotent; that is, they maintain their own numbers while producing all differentiated cell types of the pertinent tissue. Thus, adult stem cells are key to tissue homeostasis and regeneration upon damage.

Architecture and function of the gastrointestinal tract

The intestinal tract, comprising the small intestine and colon, is established during mid to late gestation [1]. It is a complex organ system in which a single layer of specialized epithelium performs its primary functions of digestion, absorption, protection, and excretion. The intestinal epithelium consists of different epithelial cells that secrete digestive enzymes, mucus, and antibacterial agents, absorb food particles, or produce hormones (see Chapter 1).

The epithelium of the small intestine is organized into finger-like villi and adjacent invaginations called *crypts of Lieberkühn* (Figure 2.1). Within crypts, which project deep into the underlying mucosa, new cells are produced and key cell fate decisions are made. The crypt compartment of the small intestine contains the stem cells, the progenitors, and some differentiated cells, while the villus compartment consists entirely of differentiated cells. The colon lacks villi and has a flat surface epithelium.

Pluripotent stem cells located near the crypt base give rise to transit-amplifying (TA) cells. The vigorously dividing TA cells migrate upward in a conveyor belt fashion from the crypts onto the villi. Concomitantly, the TA cells exit the cell cycle and differentiate into the different functional epithelial cell types: enterocytes (colonocytes in the colon), goblet cells,

Yamada's Textbook of Gastroenterology, Seventh Edition. Edited by Timothy C. Wang, Michael Camilleri, Benjamin Lebwohl, Anna S. Lok, William J. Sandborn, Kenneth K. Wang, and Gary D. Wu.

Companion website: www.yamadagastro.com/textbook7e

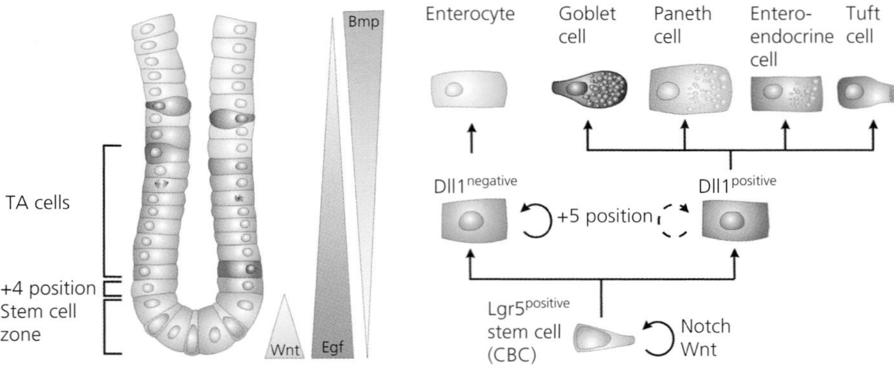

Figure 2.1 Anatomy of the adult small-intestinal epithelium. The epithelium of the adult small intestine is shaped into crypts and villi. The crypt compartment contains Lgr5^{positive} stem cells intercalated between Paneth cells, putative (quiescent) stem cells above the Paneth cells (the +4 position), and the transit-amplifying (TA) cells, while the villus compartment is made up entirely of enterocytes, goblet cells, Tuft cells, and enteroendocrine cells (left). The stem cell niche controls stem cell activity and maintenance by providing short-range molecular signals. In the intestine, various signaling pathways (Wnt, Notch, and Bmp) act in concert at the crypt base to maintain stem cell-driven epithelial renewal. If the multipotent Lgr5^{positive} stem cells leave the stem cell niche, they give rise to Dll1^{negative} and Dll1^{positive} cells, which are the precursors of the absorptive (enterocytes) or secretory lineage (Paneth cells, goblet cells, Tuft cells, and enteroendocrine cells, respectively) (right).

enteroendocrine cells, or Tuft cells. The differential cells continue their upward migration until they reach the villus tip, where they undergo apoptosis and exfoliate into the lumen of the intestine. They are rapidly replaced by advancing cells. In contrast, the Paneth cells, also derived from intestinal stem cells, migrate to the bottom of the crypt as they differentiate and mature. M cells reside exclusively over the Peyer's patches, the lymphoid follicles located in the wall of the intestine.

Enterocytes, the most abundant intestinal epithelial cells, are highly polarized with a basal nucleus and an apical brush border. These cells are responsible for absorption and transport of nutrients across the epithelium toward capillaries in the underlying mesenchyme. Goblet cells contain mucin granules, which are discharged onto the surface. The secreted mucins are required for the movement of luminal contents and provide protection against shear stress and chemical damage [2]. Enteroendocrine cells are scattered in a dispersed fashion in the epithelium. At least 10 different enteroendocrine cell types can be distinguished based on the hormones they produce [3]. The less well-characterized Tuft cells are also scattered along the crypt–villus axis and are characterized by pronounced actin bundles [4,5]. They express signaling components typical of chemosensory cell types. Paneth cells secrete antimicrobial agents, including defensins/cryptdins and lysozyme, to control the microbial content of the intestine [6–8]. Perhaps even more important, Paneth cells act to maintain stem cells via the expression of important niche signals, including Egf, Tgf-α, Wnt3, and Dll4 [9]. Paneth cells reside at the base of the crypt for up to 6 weeks before they are cleared [10]. The developmental hierarchy of the colon essentially resembles that of the small intestine, with the notable exception of the absence of the Paneth cells. Instead, the colon contains differentiated deep crypt secretory (DCS) cells, a cKit^{positive} goblet cell population, which reside between colon stem cells [11]. Of interest, DCS and Paneth cells have some markers in common. M cells, found solely in the specialized epithelium of the Peyer's patch, transport antigenic particles from the gut lumen via endocytosis or phagocytosis and deliver it to immune cells (dendritic cells and T cells) across the epithelial barrier, and thereby mediate mucosal immunity [12].

The system is highly dependent on the continuous supply of all cell types in appropriate ratios. Homeostatic self-renewal of the intestine is achieved through a complex interplay between processes involved in cell proliferation, differentiation, migration, adhesion, and cell death, coordinated by a relatively small number of highly evolutionarily conserved signaling pathways. These pathways include the bone morphogenetic protein (BMP), Notch, Hippo, and Wnt signaling pathway [13–16]. Disruption of these pathways can lead to pathological conditions, including cancer [17–19].

Role of the Wnt signaling pathway in the intestine

The highly regulated Wnt signaling cascade plays an essential role during embryonic patterning, in cell proliferation, differentiation, and cell-fate determination [20]. It is also essential in stem cell maintenance in the mature intestine [21]. The canonical Wnt pathway regulates the stability of the multifunctional protein ß-catenin, which can activate the transcription of specific Wnt target genes [22].

In the absence of Wnt signals, free cytoplasmic ß-catenin is actively targeted for degradation (Figure 2.2). This is accomplished by two scaffolding proteins (APC and Axin/Axin2) that are able to bind ß-catenin. They reside in the so-called destruction complex. Two kinases (CKI and Gsk3β) residing in the same destruction complex sequentially phosphorylate a set of highly conserved Ser and Thr residues of ß-catenin. Once phosphorylated, ß-catenin is ubiquitinated and then targeted for degradation by the proteosome. As a result, free cytoplasmic ß-catenin in the cells remains virtually undetectable. In the absence of Wnt signaling, the nuclear DNA binding proteins of the Tcf/Lef family act in the nucleus as transcriptional repressors via the recruitment of transcriptional corepressors (such as TLE/Groucho) to the target gene promoters and/or enhancers.

Secreted signaling Wnt proteins (19 family members) can induce signaling via interaction with Wnt receptors consisting of a member of the frizzled family (10 family members) and members of the low-density lipid receptor family (Lrp5 or Lrp6) and Leucine-rich repeat-containing G protein-coupled receptor 4 (Lgr4) and/or Lgr5 [20–22] (see Figure 2.2). On binding of a Wnt protein to this receptor complex, the activity of the destruction complex is inhibited. As a direct consequence, ß-catenin accumulates in the cytoplasm, enters the nucleus, and binds to a member of the Tcf/Lef family, converting these Tcf/Lef transcription factors from a transcriptional repressor into a transcriptional activator. The Tcf/ß-catenin complex, in association with other transcriptional coactivators, activates the transcription of a specific set of Wnt target genes. When the Wnt signal subsides, ß-catenin is removed from the nucleus by APC and degraded. As a result, Tcf reverts into a transcriptional repressor.

The Wnt signaling pathway is the most important force controlling epithelial physiology of the intestine [20,21,23–25]. A Wnt signaling gradient exists along the crypt–villus axis. When cells migrate from the Wnt source at the base of the crypt, they progressively lose their proliferative capacity and differentiate. Nuclear ß-catenin, the hallmark of active Wnt signaling, is observed at the bottom of the crypts in the intestine. Moreover, several Wnts and Frizzleds are expressed in the crypt of the intestine, as is the Wnt effector Tcf4 [26]. In addition, genetic studies have shown that Wnt signaling plays an essential role in regulating intestinal epithelial cell proliferation. In neonatal mice lacking Tcf4, proliferative crypts do not develop, implying that Wnt signals are required for the establishment of the stem cell compartment [27]. In adult mice, the conditional deletion of β-catenin or Tcf4 or transgenic overexpression of the diffusible Wnt inhibitor Dickkopf 1 (Dkk1) results in a complete block of cell proliferation [28–30]. By contrast, the transgenic overexpression of R-spondin-1, a Wnt agonist that acts through the Lgr4/5–Wnt receptor complex [31–33], results in a marked hyperproliferation of intestinal crypts [34].

The Wnt-driven crypt gene program, as well as the roles of individual Wnt target genes (including *Lgr4/5*, *EphB2/B3*, *Frizzled-5*, *cMyc*, *cyclin-D1*, and *Sox9*), have been studied extensively in genetically modified mouse models [32,35–40]. These studies have demonstrated that the Wnt signals near the bottom of crypts are not only crucial for the maintenance and proliferation of the undifferentiated progenitors but, unexpectedly, also for the maintenance of the postmitotic Paneth phenotype [35–37]. Moreover, the Wnt signaling gradient controls the expression of the EphB/EphrinB sorting receptors and ligands. These receptors facilitate the correct positioning of epithelial cells in conjunction with a Wnt gradient along the crypt–villus axis, as well as the positioning of Paneth cells at the bottom of the crypt [38]. The intestinal Wnt target genes *cyclin-D1* and *cMyc* are drivers of the proliferation of undifferentiated cells. Indeed, gene knockout of

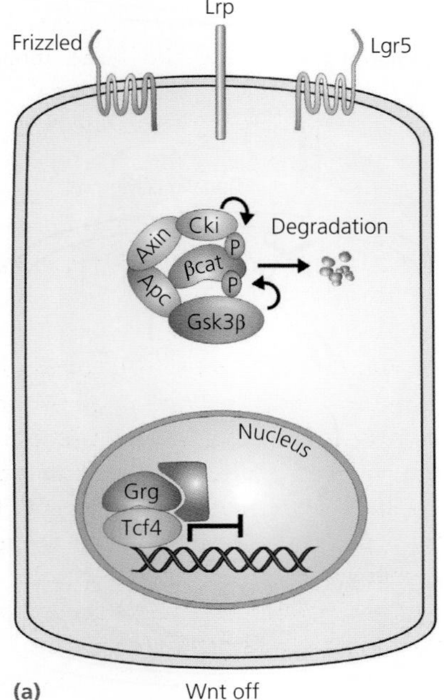

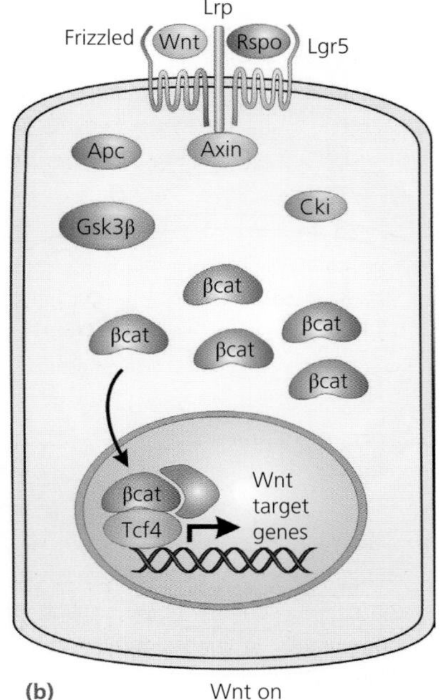

Figure 2.2 A simplified overview of the Wnt signaling pathway. In cells devoid of a Wnt signal **(a)**, β-catenin is held in a tight grip by the "destruction complex" composed of APC, Axin, CKI, and Gsk3β, ultimately resulting in the degradation of β-catenin. Tcf/Lef transcription factors associate in the nucleus with transcriptional repressor Groucho. This association blocks Wnt target gene activation. Upon binding of Wnt to the Wnt receptor complex (Frizzled, Lgr4/5, Lrp5/6) **(b)**, the destruction complex is inactivated, resulting in the accumulation of β-catenin, which subsequently enters the nucleus. In the nucleus, a transcriptionally active Tcf/β-catenin complex is formed that leads to the activation of a specific set of Wnt target genes (for a detailed description, see Gehart and Clevers [16], Bertrand et al. [17], and Brabletz et al. [18]). R-spondins (Rspo) binding to Lgr5 potentiates the Wnt signaling pathway.

cMyc gradually slows down crypt self-renewal [41]. The simultaneous deletion of the Wnt targets *Lgr4* and *Lgr5*, the receptors for R-spondins, leads to the demise of the crypts [32].

Thus, the Wnt signaling pathway controls intestinal stem cell fate and maintenance, TA proliferation and differentiation, Paneth cell maturation, as well as sorting of crypt epithelial cells along the crypt axis.

Role of the Notch signaling pathway in the intestine

The Notch signaling pathway also plays a critical role in developmental processes, typically controlling binary cell fate decisions [1,42–44]. Notch genes encode single-pass transmembrane receptors that interact with transmembrane ligands on adjacent cells. The mammalian genome encodes four receptors (Notch 1–4) and five ligands (Delta-like-1, -3, and -4 and Jagged-1 and -2) (Figure 2.3). Notch activation generates a rapid feedback amplification process that differentially regulates transcription in each cell, ensuring differences in identity. Upon ligand–receptor binding, a series of proteolytic cleavages modifies the reception. This ultimately results in cleavage of the Notch intracellular domain (NICD) of the Notch receptor. The NICD is subsequently translocated into the nucleus, where it binds to the DNA binding protein Rbp-J, activating Notch target gene transcription. The best-characterized Notch target genes are the basic helix–hoop–helix (bHLH) proteins hairy/enhancer of split (Hes). These proteins repress expression of downstream genes, including *neurogenin* (*ngn*), *Achaete-Scute*, and *Math-1*. In the absence of a Notch signal, Rbp-j associates with transcriptional corepressors, which together block target gene activation. The Notch signaling pathway is critical for maintaining cells in the undifferentiated state [44–46]. Indeed, genes of the Notch signaling pathway are also active in intestinal epithelial cells [47,48].

Different Notch genes have been implicated in intestinal homeostasis. Notably, the fetal intestine of mice lacking *Hes1*, a Notch target gene, exhibit an increase in goblet and enteroendocrine cells at the expense of enterocytes [49]. Moreover, the pharmacological inhibition of Notch signaling in the crypts activates the expression of Math1, driving the TA and stem cells into the secretory lineage [50,51]. Definitive proof of an essential role of Notch in regulating intestinal stem cell fate has been provided by studies deleting Rbp-J or the simultaneous deletion of Notch1 and Notch2 or the simultaneous deletion of Dll1 and Dll4, all of which resulted in the terminal differentiation of intestinal stem cells into the secretory lineage [50,52,53]. A complementary gain-of-function study has yielded the reciprocal phenotype. Transgenic expression of the NICD in the epithelium of the murine intestine results in a block of differentiation of secretory cells and an expansion of immature progenitor cells [54].

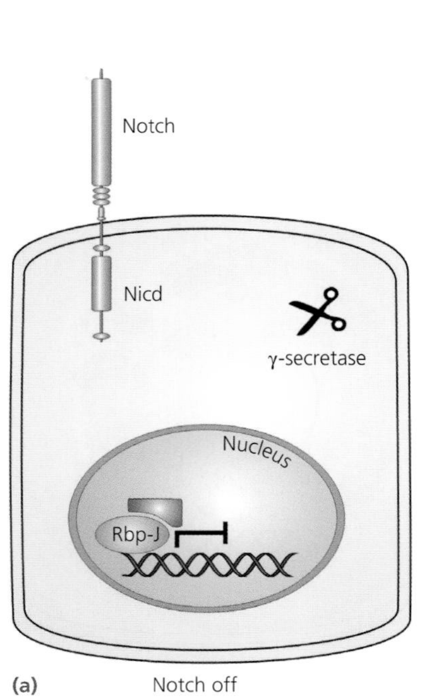

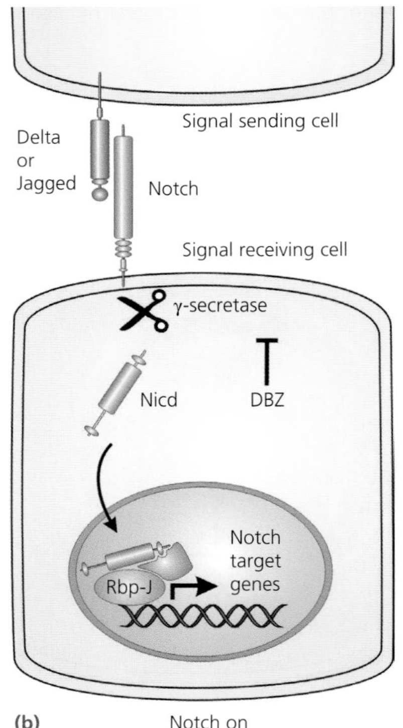

Figure 2.3 A simplified overview of the Notch signaling pathway. On binding of the receptor (Notch) with its ligand (Delta or Jagged), a series of proteolytic cleavages and posttranslational modifications occur **(b)** (for a detailed description, see Noah et al. [1]). This ultimately results in cleavage of the Notch intracellular domain (NICD) of the Notch receptor. The NICD subsequently translocates into the nucleus, where it binds to the DNA binding protein Rbp-j and several coactivators, thereby activating a specific set of Notch target genes. As a result, the downstream target genes, such as the repressor Hes, are upregulated. This results in the inhibition of various basic helix–hoop–helix transcriptional activators, including Math-1. In the absence of a Notch signal, Rbp-j associates with transcriptional corepressors, which together block target gene activation **(a)**.

Collectively, these studies show that the Notch signaling pathway controls the decision of intestinal stem cells to self-renew or differentiate into one of the secretory lineages.

Intestinal stem cells

The nature and location of the intestinal stem cell population was long uncertain [55–58]. Formal proof has been made possible by the discovery of specific marker stem cell populations.

Intestinal stem cells: "the stem cell zone"

Since the Wnt pathway was shown to be the driving force behind proliferation in the crypts, the elucidation of the transcriptional target gene program has made delineation of stem cell-specific genes possible [59]. In situ hybridization analysis of the intestine showed that most Wnt target genes were expressed throughout the crypt, reflecting the role of Wnt signaling in cell proliferation of the TA compartment and in Paneth cell differentiation at the crypt base. However, a small group of genes, including Lgr5, were expressed in a more restricted fashion in the crypt-based column (CBC) cells at the base of the crypt [60]. Every crypt contains approximately 10–14 Lgr5^{positive} proliferating CBC cells intercalated between Paneth cells. The expression of the Lgr5 receptor in the CBC cell was confirmed in genetically modified mice containing a LacZ knockin allele (Lgr5^{LacZ}) or an enhanced fluorescent GFP-expressing allele (Lgr5$^{EGFP\text{-}ires\text{-}CreERT2}$) in the Lgr5 locus [60] (Figure 2.4).

In vivo lineage tracing was performed to determine whether these Lgr5-expressing cells are actually intestinal stem cells [57]. This involves the targeted introduction of a permanent genetic mark into the candidate population, allowing the visualization of both the modified stem cell and its descendants over time. This is possible using the well-known Cre-LoxP recombination system, which allows the Cre-mediated excision of targeted LoxP sites to delete or to activate gene expression in temporal or tissue-specific fashion on induction with tamoxifen [61]. To facilitate this, investigators crossed the genetically modified mouse model Lgr5$^{EGFP\text{-}ires\text{-}CreERT2}$ with a Cre-activatable Rosa26^{LacZ} reporter mouse strain [62] (schematic representation in Figure 2.4). Activation of the Cre-enzyme by the administration of tamoxifen results in the removal of a roadblock from the Rosa locus, resulting in the irreversible activation of the LacZ reporter in Lgr5-expressing cells. This trait is inherited by their cellular offspring. One day after Cre induction, LacZ reporter gene activity was restricted to Lgr5^{positive} CBC cells at the crypt base of the small intestine (see Figure 2.4c) and the colon. At later time points, ribbons of LacZ^{positive} cells extended from the crypt base to the villus tips in the small intestine and contained cells of all intestinal lineages (see Figure 2.4d,e). Importantly, these multilineage LacZ^{positive} ribbons persisted for years.

The combined data unequivocally demonstrated that LGR5^{positive} CBC cells fulfilled both criteria of stemness: generation of multiple lineages and long-term self-renewal. Interestingly, Lgr5 not only marks intestinal stem cells in the intestine but also in many other organs, including, for example, stomach, hair follicles, liver, kidney, and mammary gland [63–66].

From isolated Lgr5^{GFP} cells, a gene expression signature has been determined, revealing additional stem cell genes [67,68]. Thus, the secreted molecule Olfm4 was found to be a robust CBC stem cell marker [69], and Ascl2, which encodes bHLH transcription factors involved in determining the cell fate, was also found to be expressed in stem cells. Conditional Ascl2 gene ablation in the mouse small-intestinal epithelium resulted in rapid ablation of the Lgr5 stem cells, whereas misexpression in nonstem cells resulted in de novo crypt formation on the villi, suggesting it is a master regulator of CBC stem cells [70].

Intestinal stem cells: the "+4 cells"

Although many studies have established the stem qualities of CBCs, other studies have suggested that the intestinal cells above the Paneth cells, also known as "+4 cells," have stem cell characteristics. These radiosensitive cells were identified as cycling but still able to retain incorporated nucleoside analogs, which are widely used as a surrogate stem cell marker [71]. Presumably, the long-term label-retaining cell (LRC) trait of +4 cells does not reflect quiescence, but rather is the result of asymmetric segregation of old (labeled) and new (unlabeled) DNA strands into stem cells and their daughters, respectively [55]. This "immortal" strand hypothesis was originally postulated to protect the stem cell genome from mutation [72] but has remained controversial [73]. Genes that mark +4 cells have been identified (e.g., Bmi1, mTert, Hopx, Lrig1), and the same lineage tracing strategy as for Lgr5 has been used to evaluate the stemness of these cells in the intestinal crypts [74–77].

Bmi1, a member of the polycomb group family, which has important roles during development and in regulating progenitor self-renewal in many tissues, was the first +4 stem cell marker investigated by lineage tracing [74]. Bmi1 was reported to mark rare, slowly cycling or quiescent cells at the +4 cell position, yet was uniquely expressed in the proximal small intestine only. In vivo lineage tracing yielded ribbons under noninjury conditions that resembled those obtained in the Lgr5 mouse model. Targeted ablation of the Bmi1^{positive} intestinal cells with diphtheria toxin also impaired epithelial renewal, consistent with loss of stem cell function [74]. Bmi1-expressing cells are dramatically increased after Lgr5 cell ablation, and thus may function as a reserve stem cell pool contributing to intestinal lineage development via an Lgr5-independent pathway [78].

Mouse telomerase reverse transcriptase (mTert)-expressing cells are distributed in a pattern along the crypt–villus axis similar to long-term LRCs and are resistant to tissue injury [75]. Expression of mTert was shown to be expressed in less than 1% of the crypts, while only a fraction of these mTert-GFP^{positive} cells were LRCs. Lineage-tracing studies demonstrate that mTert^{positive} cells give rise to Lgr5^{positive} cells and to all differentiated intestinal cell types, persist long term, and contribute to the regenerative response after injury. It appears that mTert expression may mark a radiation-resistant pool of stem cells, distinct from Lgr5^{positive} cells [79].

Homeodomain-only protein X (Hopx) encodes an atypical homeobox protein, which functions as a cofactor to modulate

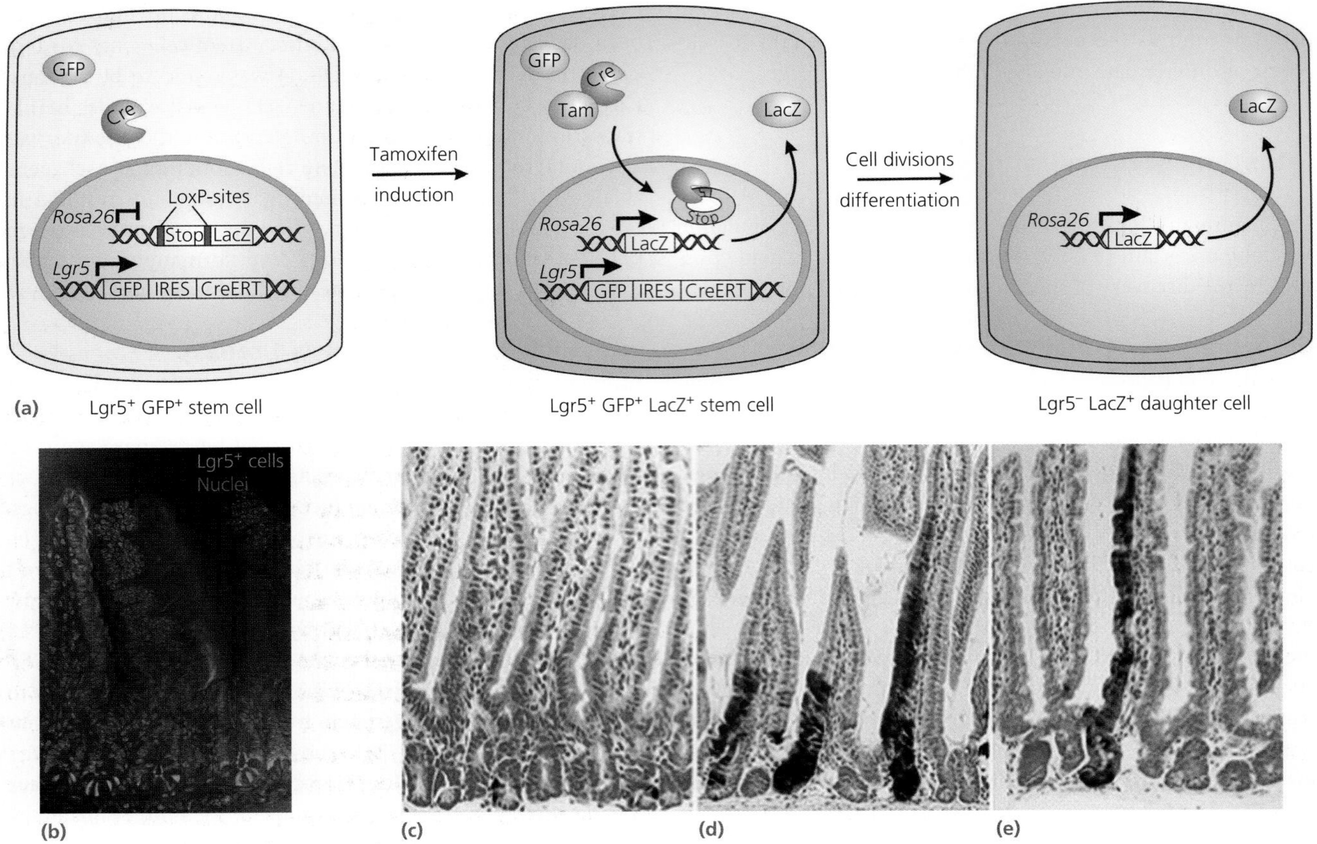

Figure 2.4 Lgr5 marks intestinal stem cells. Intestinal stem cells are defined as long-lived cells that exhibit self-renewal and have the ability to differentiate into all differentiated cell types. Stem cell activity can retrospectively be evaluated by the investigation of marked cellular descendants via in vivo; lineage tracing/gene fate mapping studies. To determine whether intestinal Lgr5^{positive} cells faithfully assessed all characteristics of intestinal stem cells, the Lgr5$^{EGFP\text{-}ires\text{-}CreERT2}$ mouse [57], which expresses the fluorescent GFP in conjunction with a tamoxifen-inducible Cre enzyme, was crossed with the Rosa26^{LacZ} reporter mouse [59]. Activation of the Cre enzyme by the administration of tamoxifen results in the removal of a roadblock from the Rosa locus, resulting in the irreversible activation of the LacZ reporter in Lgr5-expressing cells (**a**: schematic representation). This trait is inherited by their cellular offspring. One day after Cre induction, LacZ reporter gene activity (blue cells) was specifically restricted to the Lgr5^{positive}-GFP^{positive} CBC cells at the crypt base of the small intestine (**b, c**) and the colon (not shown). Telltale blue ribbons of LacZ^{positive} cells, emanated from the marked Lgr5^{positive} cells, reached the villus tips 5 days after tamoxifen induction (**d**) and persisted for at least a year (**e**). The blue ribbons contained cells of all intestinal lineages [57]. The results demonstrated that Lgr5^{postive} cells fulfill the definition of intestinal stem cells. (**a**) Source: Courtesy Dr. Hugo Snippert. Reproduced by permission. (**b**) Source: Snippert et al. 2010 [120]. Reproduced by permission of Elsevier. (**c**) Source: Barker et al. 2007 [60]. Reproduced from by permission of Nature Publishing Group. (**d, e**) Source: Courtesy Hans Clevers.

gene expression. A genetically modified mouse containing a LacZ knockin allele in the Hopx locus showed predominant expression by cells located in the LRCs at the +4 position along the entire intestinal tract [76]. Lineage tracing from the Hopx locus suggested that Hopx-expressing cells can give rise to CBCs and all mature intestinal epithelial lineages. Conversely, CBCs can give rise to +4 Hopx^{positive} cells. These findings suggest a bidirectional lineage relationship between active and quiescent stem cells in their niches. Additional evidence indicates that the Hopx^{positive} and Lgr5^{positive} populations represent slow- and fast-cycling stem cell populations that are interrelated.

Lrig1 encodes a transmembrane protein that has been shown to interact with receptor tyrosine kinases of the Egfr family, Met and Retz [80]. It is highly expressed by most proliferative crypt cells, and its removal leads to a rapid expansion of the proliferative compartment. Lineage tracing from a Lrig1^{CreERT2} allele initiated at crypt bottoms along the entire length of the intestinal tract yielded ribbons by 7 days [77]. Around 20% of the Lrig1^{positive} cells were LRCs. Comparative microarray profiling revealed that sorted Lgr5^{positive} cells display a proliferation signature, whereas the Lrig1^{positive} population showed signs of downregulation of the cell cycle. In a simultaneous study, it has been reported that approximately 30% of all crypt cells express Lrig1, with the highest levels in the Lgr5^{positive} stem cells [81].

The significance of the +4 cells remains uncertain. Comparison between the +4 populations delineated by the different markers reveals major differences between the different +4 populations, and independent studies report that the +4 markers Bmi1, mTert, Hopx, and Lrig1 are all expressed rather broadly, including in the Lgr5-expressing stem cells [67,82,83]. These findings complicate the interpretation of the lineage-tracing experiments, suggesting that non-Lgr5 cells actively function as stem cells.

Although lineage tracing experiments confirm the pattern of stem cell fate, it does not resolve the underlying molecular mechanisms that control stem cell competence. Indeed, the local niche environment is considered to be instrumental in regulating adult stem cell function in vivo. Recently, further insight into the mechanism of stem cell regulation in the small intestine has been provided by a combination of in vitro and in vivo assays.

Three-dimensional in vitro organogenesis

Current in vitro studies of the intestinal epithelium are typically performed with epithelial cell lines derived from human colon cancer cells. It was believed that it would be inherently impossible to establish long-term cultures from primary adult tissues without inducing genetic transformation.

Extensive genetics studies in mice have provided insights into the growth factor dependence of Lgr5 intestinal stem cells. This knowledge was the basis of the establishment of a unique long-term in vitro culture model in which three-dimensional (3D) intestinal organoids can be grown from a single Lgr5^{positive} stem cell in Matrigel, a 3D laminin/collagen-rich matrix that mimics the basal lamina (Figure 2.5a) [84]. However, culturing from a single stem cell is inefficient (1–2% plating efficiency), whereas stem cell/Paneth cells doublets efficiently form organoids in vitro [9]. This suggests that Paneth cells express factors important for the growth and maintenance of Lgr5^{positive} intestinal stem cells. On mechanical dissociation of the in vitro grown organoids, crypt fragments or fluorescence-activated cell sorting (FACS)-sorted Lgr5^{positive} intestinal stem cells quickly grow out into new organoids. The architecture of these 3D organotypic structures is remarkably similar to that of the normal intestinal epithelium and consists of multiple crypts containing basal Lgr5 cells and a proliferative TA population (see Figure 2.5b–d). Moreover, the central lumen-lining epithelium resembles the villus domain, harboring the same differentiated cell-type composition, that is, enterocytes (colonocytes in the colon), goblet cells, enteroendocrine cells, Paneth cells, or Tuft cells as the in vivo situation (see Figure 2.5e–h). The culture system has been adapted to grow epithelia from many different human organs, including the human small intestine and the colon.

Careful analysis of these organoids reveals the absence of nonepithelial/mesenchymal cells surrounding the organoid epithelium. Maintenance of intestinal organoids is absolutely dependent on the presence of a defined cocktail of secreted growth factors, including R-spondin1, Noggin, and Egf. R-spondin has been identified as a secreted activator of the canonical Wnt signaling pathway and as the ligand of the Lgr4/5 receptors [32,85]. Egf signals exert strong mitogenic effects on stem and TA cells. Indeed, the Ras/Raf/Mek/Erk signaling axis is active in crypt epithelium, whereas inhibition of Mek ablates intestinal stem cells [81]. Finally, Bmp signals are active in the villus compartment [84]. When Bmp signaling in the villus is inhibited by transgenic Noggin, crypt-like structures appear along the flanks of the villi, implying that Bmp inhibition creates a "crypt-permissive" environment [85]. For colon crypt culture, a Wnt ligand has to be added to maintain Lgr5^{positive} CBC cells, because the epithelium makes little, if any, Wnt.

The organoids recapitulate the epithelial stem cell differentiation hierarchy and allow in vitro study of cell fate determination. Inhibition of the Notch signaling pathway via the administration of pharmacological drugs (GSI inhibitors) in vitro phenocopies the effects of the same manipulation in vivo [50,84,86], with overproduction of goblet cells. Peyer's patch M cells are normally absent in organoid culture. However, the addition of Rankl, a member of the tumor necrosis factor (Tnf) cytokine family, which is essential for M cells in vivo, robustly induces M cell formation [87]. Malignant transformation, through the introduction of activating Wnt pathway mutations, such as loss of APC, generates organoids that are spheroid and no longer require R-spondin1 for their growth. Similarly, deletion of the Egf inhibitor Lrig1 allows the mutant organoids to grow without Egf [81].

The presence of various differentiated cells types facilitates their use as a model to study infectious diseases and host–pathogen interactions. Indeed, intestinal organoids have been used to model multiple host–pathogen interactions and represent the first reproducible in vitro cultivation system to study, for example, norovirus [88] and the life cycle of Cryptosporidium [89].

Organoids allow all laboratory methods that are applied to cell lines, such as transfection with plasmid DNA, infection with recombinant viruses imaging, in vitro throughput drug screening CRISPR/Cas9 modification, among others.

Multiple studies exploit human organoid technology, for instance, by converting normal organoids into cancer organoids by multistep CRISPR mutations [90], by determining mutational processes that lead to cancer [91], or by modeling tumor–immune interactions [92], to model metastasis and cancer stem cell behavior in CRISPR-modified cancer organoids [82] and to functionally repair disease loci in stem cells of intestinal organoids from patients with cystic fibrosis [93].

Treatment protocols and predictions of clinical drug response are currently based on pathological examination, sometimes refined by biomarker analyses. Individual patients are assigned into subclasses, for which the average response rates are known. Cancer organoids from an individual patient are currently cultured in the laboratory, exposed to a series of cancer drugs and radiation, after which the drug combination that scores best is given to the patient [94,95]. Indeed, novel studies showed that cancer organoids do have predictive value [96,97].

The 3D culture system of intestinal stem cells may contribute to new tissue-replacement therapy [98]. Indeed, in vitro expanded colon organoids derived from a single mouse Lgr5^{positive} colon stem cell have been engrafted into the colon of a dextran sodium sulphate-colitis mouse model [99] and were able to regenerate epithelial patches that were perfectly integrated into the existing but damaged epithelium. Histological analysis demonstrated the formation of normal crypts containing all differentiated cell types that persisted for a long time without changing their histological appearance, suggesting adult intestinal stem cell therapy may be possible.

It is anticipated that these (combined) technologies will be instrumental for the usage of (genetically modified) organoids in many aspects of the treatment of human disorders, such as

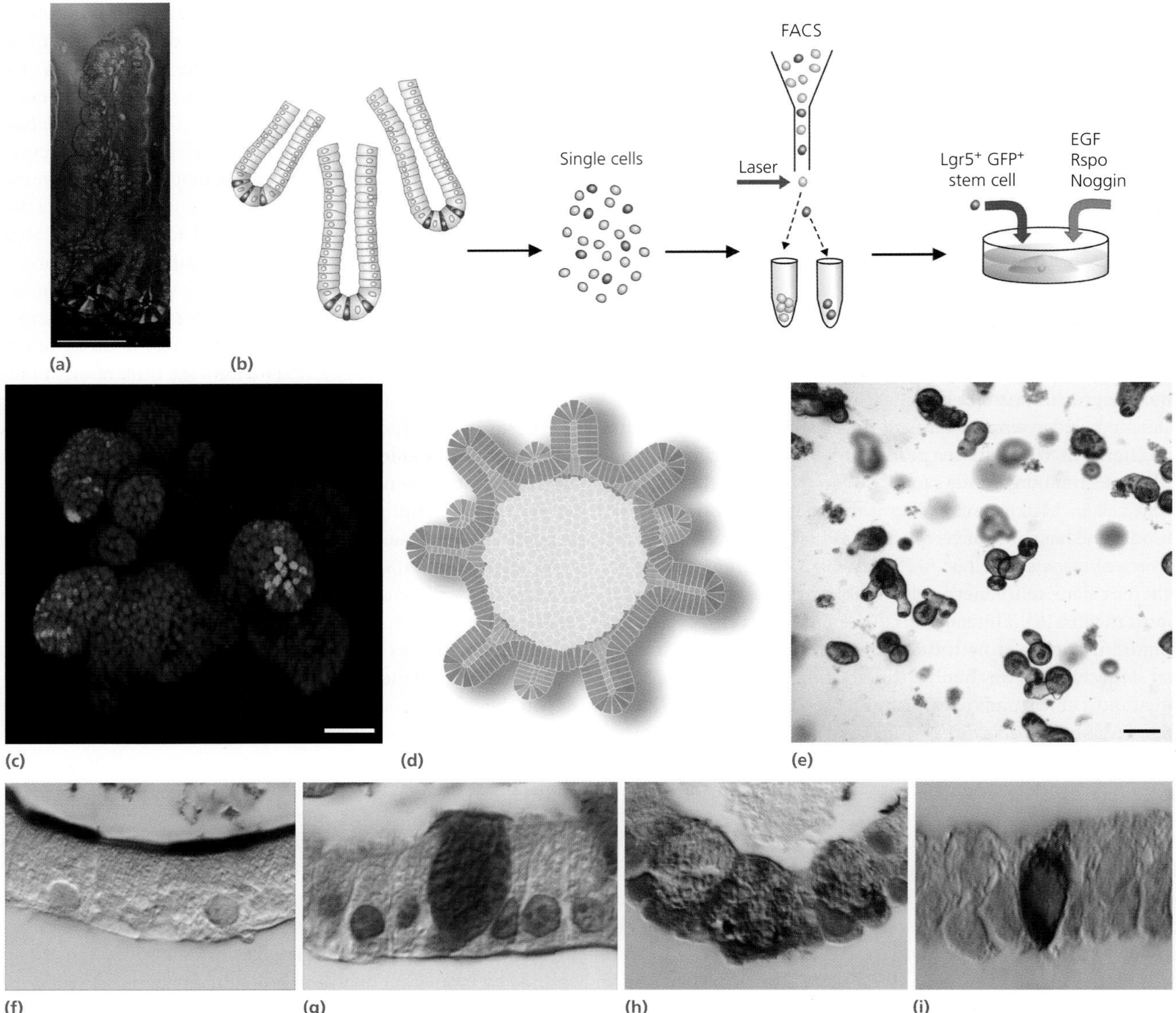

Figure 2.5 The in vivo; growth of three-dimensional intestinal organoids. Intestinal $Lgr5^{Positive}$ cells are genetically labeled by the fluorescent marker GFP **(a)**. GFP expression allows the isolation by FACS of intestinal stem cells, which can be grown in vitro;. The culture medium consists of the growth factors Egf, Noggin, and R-spondin **(b)**. A single isolated $Lgr5^{Positive}$ stem cell grows into organoids. The budding structure resembles that of the normal intestinal epithelium **(c–e)**. It consists of basal Lgr5 cells intercalated between Paneth cells and a proliferative TA population. Moreover, the central lumen-lining epithelium resembles the villus domain, harboring all differentiated cell-type composition, that is, enterocytes **(f)**, goblet cells **(g)**, Paneth cells **(h)**, and enteroendocrine cells **(i)**. Source: Courtesy Toshi Sato. Reproduced by permission. **(a)** Source: Snippert et al. 2010 [120]. Reproduced by permission of Elsevier. **(c, d, f)** Source: Sato et al. 2009 [84]. Reproduced by permission of Nature Publishing Group. **(g–i)** Source: Courtesy Hans Clevers.

drug discovery, precision medicine, regenerative medicine, and gene therapy in combination with editing technology.

Intestinal stem cell niche

The stem cell niche is defined as the microenvironment that is in close proximity to the stem cells and controls stem cell activity and maintenance by providing short-range molecular signals. In the intestine, various signaling pathways (e.g., Wnt, Notch, and BMP) act in concert at the crypt base to maintain stem cell-driven epithelial renewal [13].

The mesenchyme surrounding crypts consists of smooth muscle cells, pericytes, neural cells, fibroblasts cells, and the intestinal subepithelial myofibroblasts and has been considered to constitute the niche for the intestinal stem cells, providing the necessary repertoire of growth factors and physical interactions [100]. Indeed, the epithelium is dependent on the presence of mesenchymal cells. Diphtheria toxin-mediated ablation of a $FOXL1^{+}$ mesenchymal population in mice leads to proliferative arrest in the stem cell and TA zone because of reduced WNT signaling in the crypt, which results in intestinal failure [101]. Moreover, $GLI1^{+}$ and $CD34^{+}GP38^{+}aSMA^{-}$ mesenchymal cells act as a source of WNT2B [102] or WNT2B, RSPO1, and the BMP inhibitor Gremlin 1 [103], respectively. The extent to which the three described cell populations are overlapping or distinct is not yet clear.

The observation that crypts can be grown continuously for long periods and that even single-stem cells can be grown into organoid suggested that these nonepithelial cells were dispensable for the creation of stem cell niches in vitro. This unexpected finding was explained by the identification of a role for the post-mitotic Paneth cells as an essential epithelial component of the intestinal stem cell niche. The long-lived Paneth cells are in intimate connection with the Lgr5^{positive} stem cells at the crypt base in the small intestine, suggestive of a functional interaction in vivo. Ablation of the Paneth cell compartment in vivo leads to rapid crypt death, consistent with loss of stem cell function [9,104]. Moreover, in vitro, CD24^{high} Paneth cell/Lgr5^{positive} stem cell doublets were found to be 10-fold more efficient at generating self-renewing epithelial organoids than single Lgr5^{positive} cells [9]. Gene expression profiling of the CD24^{high} Paneth cells revealed them to be the source of many growth factors essential for maintaining Lgr5^{positive} stem cell function, including Wnt3, Egf, and Tgf-α. The combined data showed an essential role for Paneth cells in the maintenance of Lgr5^{positive} intestinal stem cells. The conditional deletion of Math1/ATOH1, a target gene of Hes1-mediated repression, resulted in the complete elimination of Paneth cells [105]. Unexpectedly, stem cells are present and do proliferate in the absence of Paneth cells. This apparent contradiction is explained by the fact that the removal of the pivotal differentiation factor Math1 also removed the dependence on Notch signals that are normally provided by Paneth cells [106]. Indeed, although Math1 deletion eliminates Paneth cells in vivo without obvious changes to stem cells, the Math1-mutant intestinal organoids did not grow in vitro. This finding implied a critical in vitro dependence of the stem cells on one of the other signals provided by Paneth cells, likely Wnt3. The genetic deletion of Wnt3 has no effect in vivo but results in the same in vitro growth inhibition of stem cells, which can be overcome by the addition of exogenous Wnt, suggesting it may be the other function provided by Paneth cells that is required by stem cells [107].

The Paneth–stem cell interaction also plays a central role in the response to the nutritional status of an organism [108–110]. Paneth cells serve as sensors for nutritional status and enhance or restrict stem cell function in response to a specific diet. These findings are among the first to assign a direct role to niche cells in controlling stem cell activity in the context of physiology in mammals.

As the key determinant of the stem cell niche, Paneth cell numbers must be tightly controlled under homeostatic conditions. This is accomplished through the action of two Wnt target genes: Rnf34 and Znrf3 [111]. Rnf34 and Znrf3, both expressed in Lgr5^{positive} stem cells, encode transmembrane E3 ligases that remove the Wnt-Frizzleds from the cell surface, constituting a negative feedback loop in the Wnt pathway. Simultaneous conditional deletion in crypt stem cells results in rapidly expanding stem cell/Paneth cell compartments and, ultimately, in large adenomas. Strong Wnt signals from Paneth cells are required for stem cell expansion. Paradoxically, strong Wnt signals are also required for Paneth cell differentiation [36]. Apparently, interruption of the Rnf43 negative feedback loop results in the exclusive production of stem cells and Paneth cells.

Classical Paneth cells are absent from the majority of the colon, but a Reg4 or CD24/cKit^{positive} goblet cell population (so-called DCS cells) have been noted at the base of the colonic crypts intermingled with Lgr5^{positive} stem cells, raising the possibility that a similar epithelial niche may also regulate colon Lgr5^{positive} stem cell function [11]. Indeed, diphtheria toxin-treated Reg4-diphtheria toxin receptor mice, which express the diphtheria toxin receptor under the control of the Reg4 promoter, showed loss of the Lgr5^{positive} colon stem cells in vivo [112].

Together, findings indicate that Paneth/DCS cells constitute (part of) the niche for Lgr5 stem cells in intestinal crypts.

Role of Lgr4/5 on intestinal stem cells

Lgr5 and its close relatives Lgr4 and Lgr6 belong to the family of Lgr receptors [113,114]. Lgr5 and Lgr6 are markers of cycling adult stem cell populations in various tissues, including the hair follicle, stomach, intestine, and skin [60,63,66,115]. In contrast, Lgr4 has a broader expression pattern [116]. Lgr4 and Lgr5 knockout mice are both neonatal lethal, indicating an essential role for Lgr4 and Lgr5 during embryogenesis [117,118]. The functions of Lgr4 (present in the entire crypt, including the stem cells) and Lgr5 (present only on intestinal stem cells) in the intestine have been elucidated in vivo and in vitro.

Intestine-specific conditional ablation of Lgr5 expression in the adult small intestine, using the Cre-LoxP system, surprisingly yielded no obvious phenotype. In contrast, the conditional ablation of *Lgr4* in the intestine caused a block in crypt proliferation and widespread crypt loss within 5 days [32]. Simultaneous conditional deletion of *Lgr5* and *Lgr4* in adult mice markedly enhanced the small-intestinal phenotype, resulting in almost complete crypt ablation within 3 days, thereby phenocopying Wnt pathway inhibition. This phenotype was confirmed with the analysis of in vitro grown organoids on deletion of Lgr4/5. The severity and accelerated onset of this phenotype showed that Lgr4 and Lgr5 have essential, yet partially redundant roles in maintaining intestinal stem cell function in vivo. This was further substantiated when gene expression of the Lgr5^{positive} intestinal stem cells, derived from intestinal crypts isolated 1 day after deletion of *Lgr4* and *Lgr5*, were analyzed. This analysis revealed the selective loss of many stem cell-enriched genes and the reduction of the typical intestinal Wnt target gene signature [32,59,67]. This is consistent with a role for Lgr4/5 receptors in mediating Wnt signaling at the crypt base. The link with the Wnt signaling pathway was further underscored when mass spectrometry analyses revealed a direct physical interaction of Lgr4 and Lgr5 with the Frizzled/Lrp Wnt receptor complex [32]. Other studies have demonstrated that members of the R-spondin family of secreted Wnt agonists are physiological ligands of Lgr4 and Lgr5 [31–33]. Lgr4 and Lgr5 act thereby as an optional Wnt coreceptor that facilitates the enhancement of local canonical Wnt signals by circulating R-spondins.

Dynamics of intestinal stem cells

The specific dynamics of stem cell homeostasis in the intestine have been investigated using an in vivo lineage-tracing approach to map the division fates of individual adult stem cells in the small intestine [103]. Short-term fate mapping of individually marked stem cells 1 day postinduction demonstrates that symmetric division predominates within the intestinal stem cell compartment. Longer-term tracing analysis of the Lgr5 stem cell population dynamics revealed a neutral drift toward clonality over time. A similar mechanism was indirectly observed by Winton and coworkers [119]. Collectively, these observations show that Lgr5 stem cells divide symmetrically every day and stochastically acquire either stem cell or TA cell fate based on the availability of contact to Paneth cells. An optimal balance for stem cell self-renewal is likely to be achieved by competition for Paneth cell surface between 10 and 14 symmetrically dividing stem cells within the space-limited niche at the crypt base [120].

Plasticity of intestinal cells

The intestine has the capacity to survive the acute loss of its active stem cell pool. This may be because of the existence of quiescent "reserve" stem cells, but could also be explained by the plasticity of (progenitor) epithelial cells present in the crypt of Lieberkühn.

Dll1 is a receptor of the Notch signaling pathway, which marks an early daughter of Lgr5^{positive} stem cells residing around position +5 [121,122]. Lineage tracing studies in genetically modified mice showed that these Dll1^{positive} cells represent short-lived progenitors that (under physiological conditions) produce small, mixed clones of exclusively secretory cells [121]. However, when Lgr5^{positive} intestinal stem cells are killed by radiation, these Dll1^{positive} secretory progenitors readily revert to Lgr5^{positive} stem cells to enable regeneration. Moreover, the examination of the potential stemness of Dll1^{positive} cells in vitro showed that, although cycling Lgr5 CBC cells grow under standard conditions, the addition of Wnt3A can force the Dll1^{positive} secretory precursor to revert into Lgr5^{positive} stem cells.

Intestinal plasticity is also seen in the analysis of mice in which Lgr5^{positive} intestinal stem cells were inducibly killed via transgenic expression of the receptor for diphtheria toxin from the Lgr5 locus [78]. On injection of diphtheria toxin, the Lgr5^{positive} cells died, yet crypts remained intact for at least a week, implying that the self-renewal process can be maintained in the absence of Lgr5^{positive} cells. After cessation of toxin injections, Lgr5^{positive} cells reappeared. These data showed that non-Lgr5-expressing cells can take over the role of the Lgr5^{positive} stem cells and/or are able to revert to Lgr5-expressing stem cells. The nature of crypt long-term LRCs has been reassessed genetically. This was conducted by briefly expressing the stable chromatin marker histone 2B yellow fluorescent protein (H2B-YFP) throughout the crypt [123]. In addition to the expected label retention by Paneth cells, non-Paneth cell LRCs remained evident in the first 2–3 weeks after the pulse. Surprisingly, these quiescent cells coexpressed Lgr5, Paneth cell markers, and +4 cell markers. It was concluded that this Lgr5-expressing LRC type represents a nondividing Paneth/enteroendocrine precursor that persists for weeks before terminal differentiation. A sophisticated strategy that directly exploits the quiescent state to genetically mark the Lgr5^{positive} LRCs was developed to test further the properties of these cells. In healthy mice, the marked Lgr5^{positive} LRCs failed to divide and disappeared over time, presumably because of their terminal differentiation. However, when crypts were damaged, the Lgr5^{positive} LRCs generated the telltale stem cell ribbons. In addition, in vitro studies, whereby organoids of the nondividing Paneth precursors were cultured, showed that they have the capacity to revert to stem cells. Although these studies focused on dedifferentiation of secretory cells, plasticity in the intestinal epithelium is not limited to the secretory lineage. Committed absorptive progenitors also have the ability to return to the stem cell state when LGR5^{+} CBC cells are depleted with diphtheria toxin [124]. Similarly, Paneth cells [125] and enteroendocrine cells [126] have been shown to possess at least some potential to restore the crypt stem cell pool after damage or loss of the endogenous intestinal stem cell population.

Thus, intestinal cells contain a high degree of plasticity depending on their location, and this plasticity allows the intestine to survive the loss of its active stem cell pool.

Lgr5^{positive} cancer stem cells

Colorectal cancer is one of the leading causes of cancer-related deaths in the world. The high frequency with which gastrointestinal malignancies occur likely in part is related to the high rate of self-renewal in the intestine. Almost invariably, intestinal tumors carry activating mutations in the Wnt pathway, leading to the formation of nuclear Tcf4/ß-catenin complexes and the subsequent uncontrolled Tcf4 target gene transcription. Indeed, allelic loss and somatic mutations of the APC tumour suppressor genes are the most frequent molecular alteration found in colorectal cancers. APC was originally cloned as the gene that is mutated in the germline of patients with familial adenomatous polyposis [127–129]. Up to 80% of sporadic colorectal tumors, as well as essentially all colorectal tumors in familial adenomatous polyposis, carry inactivating APC gene mutations. APC mutations typically delete the central domain of APC containing the binding sites for ß-catenin. Consequently, nuclear ß-catenin increases to induce transcriptional activation of target genes of Tcf4 [130]. About 2–3% of colorectal tumors carry activating mutations in the highly conserved serine/threonine residues of ß-catenin that are phosphorylated by GSK-3ß and that are required for recognition and degradation of ß-catenin [131]. As a result, mutant ß-catenin becomes stabilized. Mutations in the scaffolding protein Axin2 have also been observed in some hepatocellular tumors, as well as in colorectal cancers defective in DNA mismatch repair [132]. Inactivating Axin2 mutations prevent normal functioning of the destruction complex and, like the other mutations, lead to constitutive, high levels of nuclear ß-catenin. Rare oncogenic point mutation in Rnf43 [112], frameshift mutations or gene fusions involving Tcf4 [133], and the secreted R-spondin Wnt agonists [134] have also been observed in colon cancer.

The progression from benign adenoma to invasive and metastatic adenocarcinoma involves multiple additional genetic alterations, many of which remain to be characterized [135]. The progression of adenomas into carcinomas in situ is thought to depend on a strict sequence of events, in which mutations in the Wnt pathway are followed by mutations in KRAS, SMAD4, and finally p53. Genomic instability is one of the important characteristics of late-stage colon cancer. Additional genetic alterations that are thought to be involved in the progression of colon cancer include the loss of positional cues. In the normal epithelium, the Wnt gradient establishes a border between the crypt and villus. This gradient also controls the expression of EphB/EphrinB receptors and ligands responsible for positional migration of intestinal cells [38]. Progression of colon carcinogenesis is accompanied by EphB2 downregulation, a step required for adenomas to progress to carcinomas by freeing themselves of their positional constraints [136].

The cell of origin in cancer development remains an important question. Deletion of APC gene specifically in the Lgr5^{positive} intestinal stem cell compartment results in efficient adenoma formation in the small intestine, as well as in the colon, of the mouse [137]. In contrast, adenoma formation is greatly reduced when APC is deleted in TA cells, with most APC-deficient cells being quickly lost. Conditional expression of oncogenic β-catenin in Bmi^{positive} or Prominin1^{positive} intestinal stem cell pools was also found to promote intestinal neoplasia in mice [74,138]. Similar observations were made using CD133 as a marker of CBC cells [139]. These observations show that the normal intestinal stem cell serves as a very efficient initiator of tumorigenesis, but do not preclude the possibility that tumors can be formed from early descendants of the stem cell.

The possibility that established tumors are maintained by dedicated stem cells, the so-called cancer stem cell hypothesis, has attracted great interest but remains controversial. in vivo evidence of cancer initiation by a potential cancer stem cell was shown via xenotransplantation studies in immune-deficient mice. Only a subset of cells derived from human acute myeloid leukemia expressing the CD34 but lacking the CD38 cell surface antigen (CD34^{positive}/CD38^{negative}) was sufficient to initiate leukemic transformation in immunodeficient mice [140]. The existence of intestinal cancer stem cells was demonstrated in studies using human colorectal primary tumors in which only certain minor subsets of tumor cells were able to initiate tumor formation on transplantation into immunodeficient mice [141–143]. Other subsets of cells derived from the original human cancer were not able to initiate tumors in mice, supporting the notion that tumors are heterogeneous in cellular composition. Studies using other solid types of tumors have also yielded similar results [144–148]. However, the relevance of xenotransplantation as an experimental approach to detect cancer stem cells is uncertain [149].

Studies to identify specific markers for intestinal cancer stem cell are ongoing. The adenomas that develop after APC deletion in Lgr5^{positive} cells support the notion that these cells may act as cancer stem cells within the adenoma [137]. Human Lgr5^{positive} colorectal cancer cells serve as cancer stem cells in growing cancer tissues [150]. Indeed, "lineage retracing" studies demonstrate that Lgr5 marks a subpopulation of adenoma cells that fuel the growth of established mouse and human intestinal adenomas [150,151]. These Lgr5^{positive} tumor cells, which represent about 5–10% of the cells in the adenomas, generate additional Lgr5^{positive} cells, as well as all other adenoma cell types. Interestingly, the Lgr5^{positive} cells are intermingled with Paneth cells near the adenoma base, a pattern reminiscent of the architecture of the normal crypt niche.

In addition, FACS-based detection of human Lgr5^{positive} cells in primary colorectal tumor cells revealed the presence of a distinct subpopulation of Epcam^{positive}/Lgr5^{positive} cells [152]. Similarly, primary colorectal cancer-derived organoids contain high levels of Lgr5^{positive} cells, which decrease on in vitro differentiation of these cancer stem cells. Selection of the Lgr5^{high} colorectal cancer cells identified the clonogenic fraction in vitro, as well as the tumorigenic population in vivo. These studies provide additional evidence that Lgr5 is, in addition to being a functional intestinal stem cell marker, a selective marker for human colorectal cancer stem cells. Importantly, the tumor-initiating cells in human colorectal cancers have expression profiles similar to healthy human intestinal stem cells [59,67,153]. Collectively, these studies show that the Lgr5^{positive} intestinal stem cell is induced by uncontrolled active Wnt signaling, the cell of origin of adenomas, and that a small subpopulation of Lgr5^{positive} cells within an intestinal adenoma can both self-renew and create cells of multiple other lineages, fulfilling the characteristics proposed to define cancer stem cells.

Acknowledgments

The authors thank Drs. Nick Barker, Hugo Snippert (see Figure 2.4), and Toshi Sato (see Figure 2.5) for providing figures.

References are available at www.yamadagastro.com/textbook7e

Further reading

Barker N., van Es J.H., Kuipers J., et al. Identification of stem cells in small intestine and colon by marker gene Lgr5. Nature 2007;449:1003.

Barker N., Ridgway R.A., van Es J.H., et al. Crypt stem cells as the cells-of-origin of intestinal cancer. Nature 2009;457:608.

Beyaz S., Mana M.D., Roper J., et al. High-fat diet enhances stemness and tumorigenicity of intestinal progenitors. Nature 2016;531:53.

Drost J., van Jaarsveld R.H., Ponsioen B., et al. Sequential cancer mutations in cultured human intestinal stem cells. Nature 2015;521:43.

Ettayebi K., Crawford S.E., Murakami K., et al. Replication of human noroviruses in stem cell-derived human enteroids. Science 2016;353:1387.

Sato T., Vries R.G., Snippert H.J., et al. Single Lgr5 stem cells build crypt-villus structures in vitro; without a mesenchymal niche. Nature 2009;459:262.

Shimokawa M., Ohta Y., Nishikori S., et al. Visualization and targeting of LGR5(+) human colon cancer stem cells. Nature 2017;545:187.

Tian H., Biehs B., Warming S., et al. A reserve stem cell population in small intestine renders Lgr5-positive cells dispensable. Nature 2011;478:255.

Valenta T., Degirmenci B., Moor A.E., et al. Wnt ligands secreted by subepithelial mesenchymal cells are essential for the survival of intestinal stem cells and gut homeostasis. Cell Rep 2016;15:911.

Vlachogiannis G., Hedayat S., Vatsiou A., et al. Patient-derived organoids model treatment response of metastatic gastrointestinal cancers. Science 2018;359:920.

CHAPTER 3

Esophagus: anatomy and structural anomalies

Ikuo Hirano
Northwestern University Feinberg School of Medicine, Chicago, IL, USA

Chapter menu

The majority of developmental and structural anomalies covered in this chapter are important although infrequently encountered. In contrast, some specific entities, including esophageal heterotopic gastric mucosa (inlet patch) and Schatzki's rings, are commonly identified but only occasionally produce clinical manifestations. With the widespread use of upper endoscopy, recognition and understanding of both common and uncommon esophageal pathology are of relevance to clinical care. Embryology and normal gross anatomy and histology of the esophagus are reviewed as background pertinent to all esophageal disorders.

Embryology (see Chapter 1)

During the first 2 weeks of gestation, the human embryo forms a bilaminar disk with adjacent layers composed of ectoderm and endoderm [1–3]. In the fourth week, the tracheobronchial diverticulum forms on the ventral surface of the endodermally derived foregut adjacent to the pharyngeal gut. This diverticulum gradually separates from the dorsal foregut with formation of the esophagotracheal septum that separates the trachea and esophagus. During the sixth week of gestation, the muscularis layers form, derived from the splanchnic mesoderm. The striated muscle of the upper esophagus is derived from branchial arches 4, 5, and 6 with innervation by corresponding branches of the vagus nerve. Vagal neural crest cells derived from the ectoderm populate the foregut, forming the enteric nervous system. Unlike the mid and hindgut, axial migration of the neural crest cells is not an important factor in the development of the foregut enteric nervous system [4,5]. Complex interactions between the gut microenvironment regulated by control regulatory genes coordinate the development of the myenteric and submucosal plexi. Growth factors have a direct and indirect effect on neural crest cell migration [6].

The esophageal epithelium rapidly proliferates and almost completely occludes the lumen in the seventh and eighth weeks, leaving residual channels. A single esophageal lumen returns in the tenth week lined by a superficial layer of ciliated epithelial cells. In the fourth month, the ciliated cells are replaced by stratified squamous epithelium, a process that continues until birth. Residual islands of ciliated epithelium at the proximal and distal ends of the esophagus remain and give rise to esophageal glands.

Adult anatomy

Gross anatomy (see Chapters 4 and 5)

The proximal origin of the esophagus is at the pharyngoesophageal junction that anatomically corresponds with the anterior thyroid cartilage and physiologically with the upper esophageal sphincter (UES). The UES is identified manometrically as a

Yamada's Textbook of Gastroenterology, Seventh Edition. Edited by Timothy C. Wang, Michael Camilleri, Benjamin Lebwohl, Anna S. Lok, William J. Sandborn, Kenneth K. Wang, and Gary D. Wu.

Companion website: www.yamadagastro.com/textbook7e

2–3 cm focus of elevated resting pressure between the hypopharynx and the esophagus. The UES is primarily composed of the transversely oriented cricopharyngeus with contributions from the inferior pharyngeal constrictor and thyropharyngeous muscles [7–10]. The cricopharyngeus is a C-shaped muscle that has attachments to the lateral aspects of the cricoid cartilage at the level of the cervical 5–6 vertebral interspace. The inferior fibers of the cricopharyngeus merge with the circular muscle of the esophageal body which courses through the posterior mediastinum to end at the esophagogastric junction, corresponding with the thoracic (T) 10 vertebral level.

The esophageal lumen can distend to approximately 2 cm in anteroposterior diameter and up to 3 cm in lateral diameter in adults. Muscle tone and elastic properties of the mucosa, submucosa, and muscularis contribute to the distensibility of the esophageal lumen. Furthermore, variation of esophageal distensibility along the length of the esophagus has been demonstrated in vivo using impedance planimetry studies [11]. The resting length of the adult esophagus is variable but ranges from 18 to 26 cm [12]. Significant shortening of the esophagus occurs during both deglutition and transient lower esophageal sphincter relaxation that can axially displace the esophagogastric junction by several centimeters. The cervical esophagus extends from the pharyngoesophageal junction to the suprasternal notch and is about 4–5 cm long. At this level, the esophagus is surrounded by the trachea anteriorly, the vertebral column posteriorly, and the carotid sheaths and thyroid laterally (Figure 3.1a).

The thoracic esophagus passes just posterior to the tracheal wall and courses to the right and posterior to the aortic arch that corresponds with the T4 vertebral level and posterior to the tracheal bifurcation and left main stem bronchus (Figure 3.1b). At the T8 vertebral level, the esophagus turns left and crosses anterior to the aorta at the level of the diaphragmatic hiatus. At the T10 vertebral level, the esophagus passes through the diaphragmatic hiatus and enters into the cardia of the stomach, at an acute angle referred to as the "angle of His" which functions with the lower esophageal sphincter and diaphragmatic hiatus to prevent the reflux of gastric contents.

The abdominal portion of the esophagus varies in length from 0.5 to 2.5 cm [13]. At this level, the left lobe of the liver lies anteriorly, the caudate lobe of the liver lies to the right, the fundus of the stomach is to the left, and the right crus of the diaphragm and aorta lie posteriorly (Figure 3.1c). The intraabdominal segment of the esophagus is compressed by

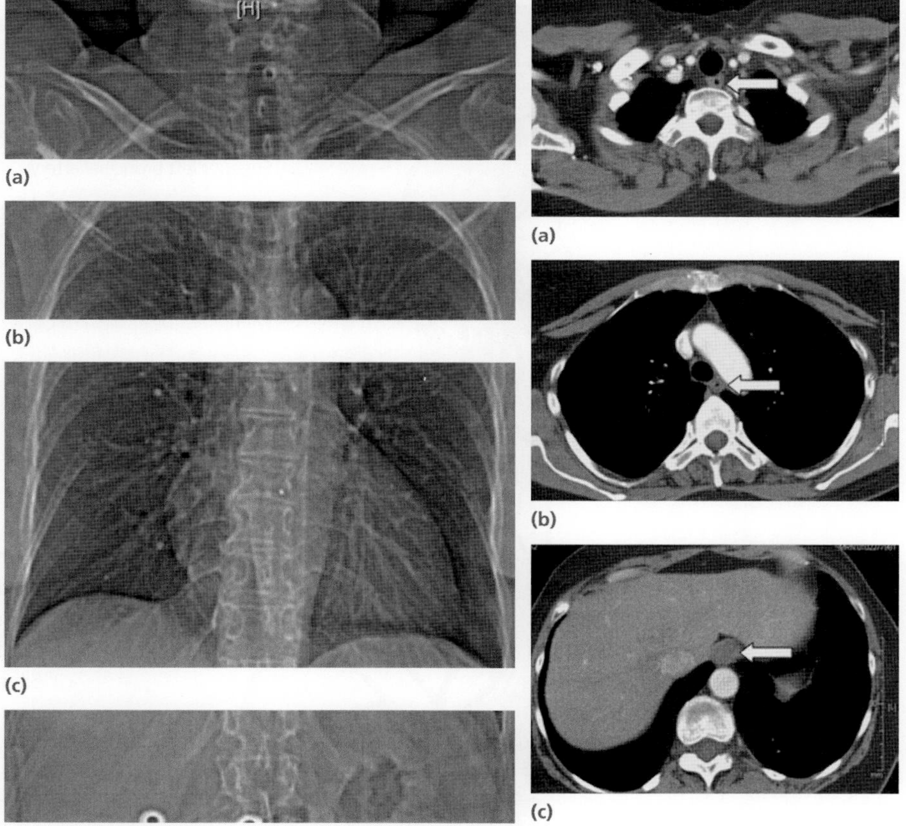

Figure 3.1 Cross-sectional CT images of the thorax demonstrating the relationships between the esophagus and adjacent structures. **(a)** Image is at the level of the cervical esophagus with the trachea anteriorly and thoracic spine posteriorly. The carotid arteries and jugular veins are situated laterally. **(b)** Image is at the level of the thoracic esophagus with the aortic arch visible anteriorly and left laterally and trachea right anterior. **(c)** Image is at the level of the abdominal segment of the esophagus with the liver anteriorly and aorta posteriorly.

physiologic events that increase intraabdominal pressure, creating resistance to esophageal reflux during such events. The borders of the esophageal hiatus are formed by the diaphragmatic crura and median arcuate ligament, if present. The crura arise from the first four lumbar vertebrae, intervertebral disks, and anterior longitudinal ligament. The fibers of the left and right crura pass upward and anteriorly to form the muscle borders of the hiatal ring and then insert into the transverse ligament of the central tendon of the diaphragm [14–16]. At the level of the diaphragm, the phrenoesophageal membrane extends from the hiatal margin to insert into the circumference of the esophagus both above and below the diaphragm [17,18]. With age, the esophagus is less firmly fixed to the hiatus and adipose tissue is incorporated into the membrane [19].The membrane is absent in patients with hiatal hernia [20].

The esophagogastric junction is represented intraluminally by the cephalic margin of the longitudinal mucosal folds in the gastric cardia [21,22].These folds are best appreciated when a hiatal hernia is present and used as an anatomic landmark for the esophagogastric junction in patients with Barrett esophagus. In patients without Barrett esophagus, the esophagogastric junction corresponds with the squamocolumnar mucosal junction or Z line which is demarcated by the abrupt disappearance of the visible vascular pattern and the color change from white-tan to the reddish orange, slightly granular appearance of gastric mucosa [21]. Manometrically, the junction is defined by the lower esophageal sphincter (LES), which has both an intrinsic, smooth muscle and extrinsic, skeletal muscle components [23]. The smooth muscle of the LES generates myogenic tone that is modulated by neurotransmitters from the enteric and autonomic nervous system. The extrinsic component of the LES represents contractions of the crural diaphragm.

Blood supply

The arterial blood supply to the esophagus is segmental, with limited vascular overlap (Figure 3.2). The cervical esophagus is

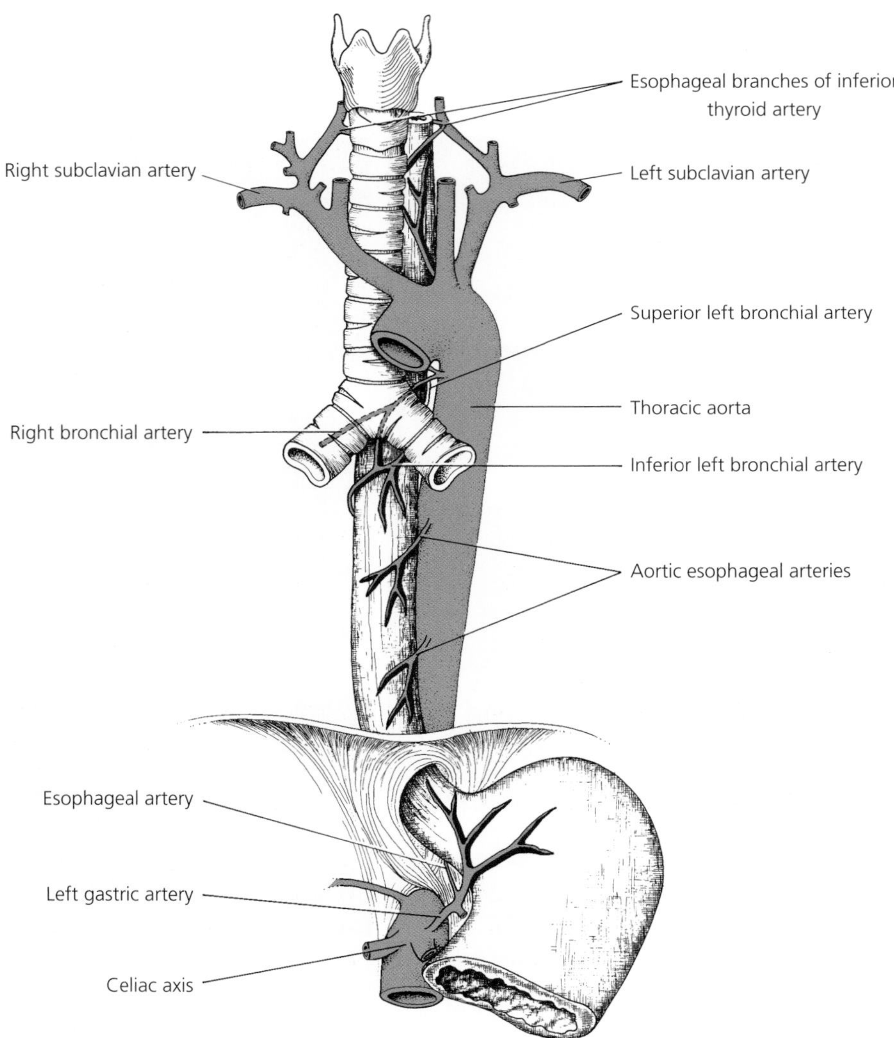

Figure 3.2 Arterial system of the esophagus.

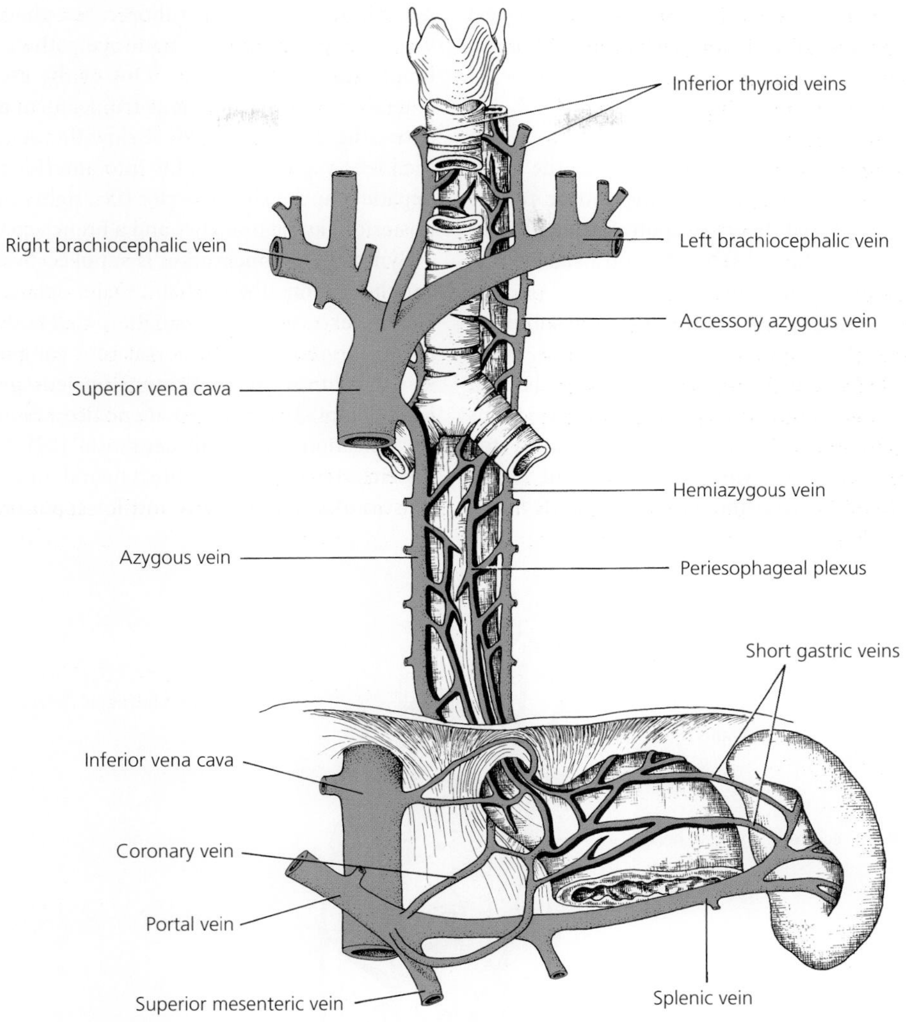

Figure 3.3 Venous drainage of the esophagus.

supplied mainly by branches of the inferior thyroid artery. Branches of other arteries, such as the common carotid, subclavian, vertebral, and ascending pharyngeal, may provide additional blood supply. The thoracic esophagus is supplied by branches of the aorta and the right intercostal and bronchial arteries. The abdominal esophagus is supplied by branches of the left gastric, short gastric, and left inferior phrenic arteries.

The venous anatomy of the esophagus is depicted in Figure 3.3. Fine intraepithelial channels drain into a subepithelial superficial venous plexus that connects with intrinsic veins in the submucosa. At the level of the gastroesophageal junction, the superficial venous plexus and deep intrinsic veins communicate with their gastric counterparts [24]. Perforating veins connect the deep intrinsic veins to adventitial veins. At the level of the cervical esophagus, the adventitial veins drain into the inferior thyroid vein, deep cervical vein, vertebral vein, and peritracheal venous plexus.

At the thoracic level, adventitial veins drain into the azygous vein on the right, the hemizygous vein on the left, and the intercostal veins when the hemizygous vein is absent. At the gastroesophageal junction, the portal systemic circulation involves venous drainage of the esophagus, stomach, pancreas, spleen, diaphragm, and retroperitoneum. Anatomic studies have suggested a high-pressure watershed region between the portal and azygous systems at the region of the gastroesophageal junction that is prone to venous dilation in portal hypertension [25]. Esophageal varices may extend up to the level of the aortic arch, the upper limit of the venous drainage of the lower esophagus by way of the azygous vein system into the superior vena cava. Varices in a location cephalic to this level have been termed "downhill" varices. The "downhill" description refers to the anatomic site of venous obstruction above the level of the varices, in either the cervical venous system or the superior vena cava. The varices then develop below the site of venous obstruction, whereas the more commonly encountered distal esophageal varices develop in a location cephalic to or above the portal venous flow.

Innervation

Motor innervation of the esophagus is dominated by the vagus nerve, which supplies parasympathetic innervation to the esophagus (Figure 3.4). Vagal fibers responsible for motor innervation of the upper esophageal sphincter and striated muscle esophagus originate from cell bodies in the nucleus ambiguus. The distal esophagus and lower esophageal sphincter derive vagal projections from the dorsal motor nucleus. Vagal afferent fibers responsive to chemical, thermal, and mechanical stimuli have cell bodies in the nodose ganglia with projections to the nucleus solitarius. The cervical esophagus is innervated by the recurrent laryngeal nerves, which arise from the vagus. Branches of the vagus nerves and the left recurrent laryngeal nerve innervate the upper thoracic esophagus. The left and right vagus nerves intertwine with sympathetic fibers to form the esophageal plexus [26,27]. Out of the esophageal plexus, the anterior and posterior vagus trunks form at a variable distance above the diaphragm [26]. Below the diaphragm, the anterior (i.e., left) vagus trunk splits into anterior gastric branches and hepatic branch. The posterior (i.e., right) vagus trunk splits into posterior gastric branches and a branch to the celiac plexus.

Sympathetic innervation is supplied by the superior cervical ganglion, sympathetic chain, major splanchnic nerve, thoracic aortic plexus, and celiac ganglion. Cell bodies for spinal afferent nerves originate in the dorsal root ganglia and project to the spinal column and brainstem nucleus gracilis and cuneatus [28]. Spinal afferents mediate nociception from both mechanical sensation and chemosensation [29]. The enteric nervous system is responsible for direct neural innervation of the smooth muscle of the esophagus and lower esophageal sphincter [5].

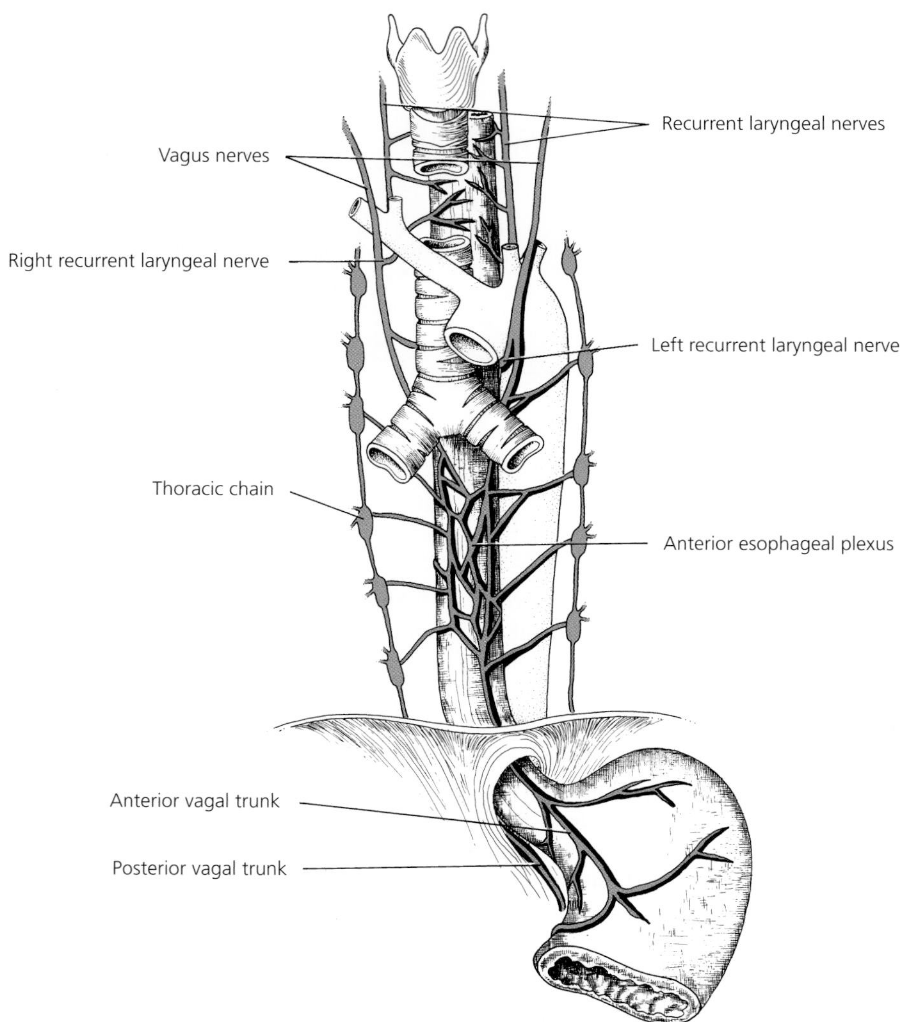

Figure 3.4 Innervation of the esophagus.

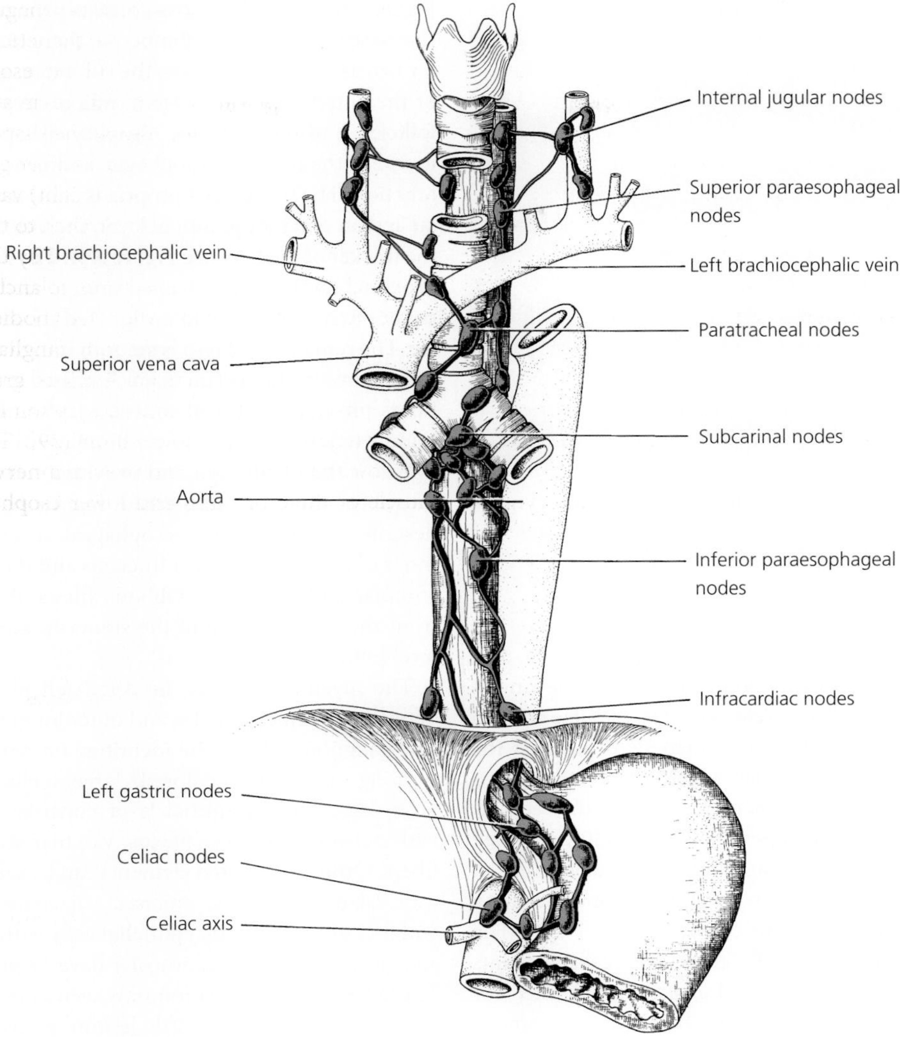

Figure 3.5 Lymphatic system of the esophagus.

Interestingly, the enteric nervous system is present within the striated portion of the esophagus but its function is unclear.

Lymphatics

Lymphatic vessels in the mucosa and submucosa of the esophageal wall extend through the muscularis propria before emptying into adventitial lymph nodes (Figure 3.5). Cervical lymph nodes drain the proximal esophagus while more inferiorly, the lymphatics drain into the paraesophageal lymph node chain. Internal jugular, tracheal, tracheobronchial, posterior mediastinal, and pericardial nodes drain adjacent esophageal segments. In contrast to the arterial supply, the lymphatic drainage of the esophagus is not segmental. Multiple interconnections exist between nodal chains. This arrangement accounts for the frequent wide intramural and mediastinal lymphatic spread of esophageal carcinoma (see Chapter 47).

Histology

Light microscopy

Similar to other regions of the digestive tract, the esophageal wall is composed of a mucosa, submucosa, and muscularis propria (Figure 3.6) [30]. The esophagus does not have a serosa but only a loose connective tissue that makes up the adventitia. The absence of a serosal layer allows esophageal perforations and malignancies to disseminate more readily and makes esophageal anastomosis and surgical repair more difficult.

The esophageal mucosa is composed of nonkeratinized, stratified squamous epithelium, connective tissue of the lamina propria, and the muscularis mucosa. The squamous epithelium resembles that of the skin and oral cavity and is composed of a basal cell layer known as the stratum basale or germinativum, the stratum intermedium or spinosum, and a superficial layer

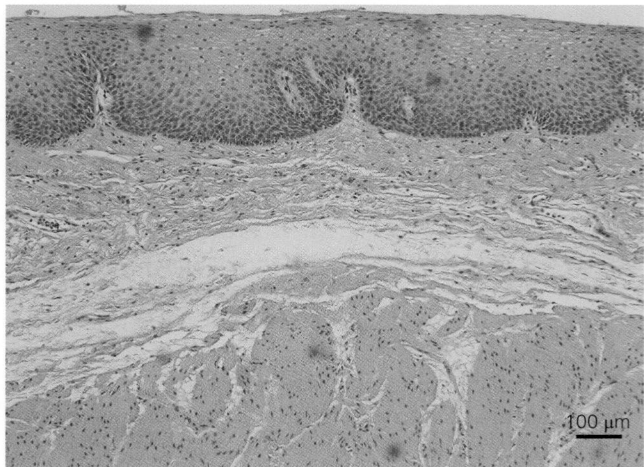

Figure 3.6 Histologic cross-section from the distal third of the esophagus demonstrating the stratified squamous epithelium, lamina propria, submucosa, and muscularis propria. Source: Courtesy of Guang-Yu Yang, MD, Chicago.

known as the stratum superficiale or corneum. The inner aspect of the epithelium undulates owing to protrusions of the lamina propria, called dermal papillae or rete pegs. The papillae contain vasculature and normally extend less than two-thirds of the overall thickness of the mucosal layer. The basal cell layer is composed of basophilic, cylindrical cells that have the capacity to divide and repopulate the superficial layers [30]. The cell turnover rate for the squamous epithelium is 5–8 days. Cells of the stratum spinosum contain glycogen and membrane-coating granules believed to play a role in cell cohesion [31,32]. The presence of glycogen in the superficial mucosal cells accounts for their brownish black staining by Lugol iodine applied for chromoendoscopy. In the stratum superficiale, the squamous epithelial cells are more flattened and oriented parallel to the surface. Tight junctions and intercellular mucin secretions form a protective seal between cells. Dilation of the intercellular spaces has been demonstrated to be significantly increased in patients with both erosive and nonerosive gastroesophageal reflux disease as well as eosinophilic esophagitis [33–35]. Acid and neutral mucosubstances are found on all layers of epithelial cells and may play a protective role [36].

The esophagus contains cells that are a part of the gut-associated lymphoid tissue. Cytotoxic T cells (i.e., intraepithelial lymphocytes) and Langerhans cells are found in the squamous epithelium. The presence of mucosal neutrophils, lymphocytes, or eosinophils is indicative of inflammatory conditions such as reflux esophagitis, lymphocytic esophagitis or eosinophilic esophagitis respectively. T helper cells and B lymphocytes are seen primarily in the lamina propria [30,37,38].

The muscular components of the esophageal wall include the muscularis mucosa and muscularis propria. The muscularis mucosa is composed of longitudinally oriented smooth muscle cells that separate the lamina propria from the submucosa (see Figure 3.6). The submucosa consists primarily of loose connective tissue. Within the submucosa, there are a vascular network known as the Heller plexus, the submucosal or Meissner plexus of the enteric nervous system, mucin-secreting glands, lymph follicles, and lymphocytes. Esophageal submucosal glands are found in the proximal esophagus and near the esophagogastric junction. The muscularis propria is composed of an inner circular and an outer longitudinal layer, the inner circular layer being the thicker of the two (see Figure 3.6). The first centimeter of the proximal esophagus is striated muscle alone, the muscle of the next 6–8 cm consists of interdigitated striated and smooth muscle. The remaining length is smooth muscle alone. In situ, longitudinal muscle fibers run in an elongated spiral. Circular muscle fibers run in an elliptical course, with some fibers leaving their bundle to join higher or lower bundles [3].

Below the diaphragm and proximal to the angle of His (i.e., the abdominal or submerged segment), an area has been described in fixed gastroesophageal specimens in which the inner circular muscle layer thickens and the fibers become semicircular and interlaced. Oblique fibers of gastric type, arising from the greater curve of the stomach, are also present at this level [39].

The myenteric plexus, or Auerbach plexus, is interspersed between the inner circular and outer longitudinal muscle coats. The ganglion cells can be identified on hematoxylin and eosin staining as lavender-colored, larger cells clustered in small groupings. The adventitial layer consists of connective tissue with networks of nerve plexus, vascular structures, and elastic fibers. Other specialized elements can be seen in the esophageal wall. Islands of gastric mucosa, sebaceous glands, taste buds, and foci of hyperplastic epithelial cells with intranuclear glycogen (i.e., glycogenic acanthosis) have been described [40–42]. The latter condition is commonly seen during esophagoscopy as scattered, focal, white, sessile lesions, a few to several millimeters in diameter. Glycogenic acanthosis is of no clinical consequence. It stains more intensely with Lugol iodine than the surrounding typical mucosa.

Developmental anomalies

Congenital tracheoesophageal fistula and esophageal atresia

Owing to a shared embryologic origin, congenital disorders affecting the esophagus often involve abnormalities of the respiratory tract. During embryogenesis, the process of elongation and separation of the trachea and esophagus can be disrupted. If fusion of the tracheoesophageal septum is incomplete, the result is a tracheoesophageal fistula (TEF). Five basic types of TEF and atresia have been described (Figure 3.7). Esophageal atresia with lower-pouch fistula is by far the most common [3,43,44]. Esophageal atresia and congenital TEF occur in 1 in 2400–5500 individuals [45,46]. Hydramnios and prematurity are common in infants with atresia or TEF [47–49]. Up to 50% of infants may

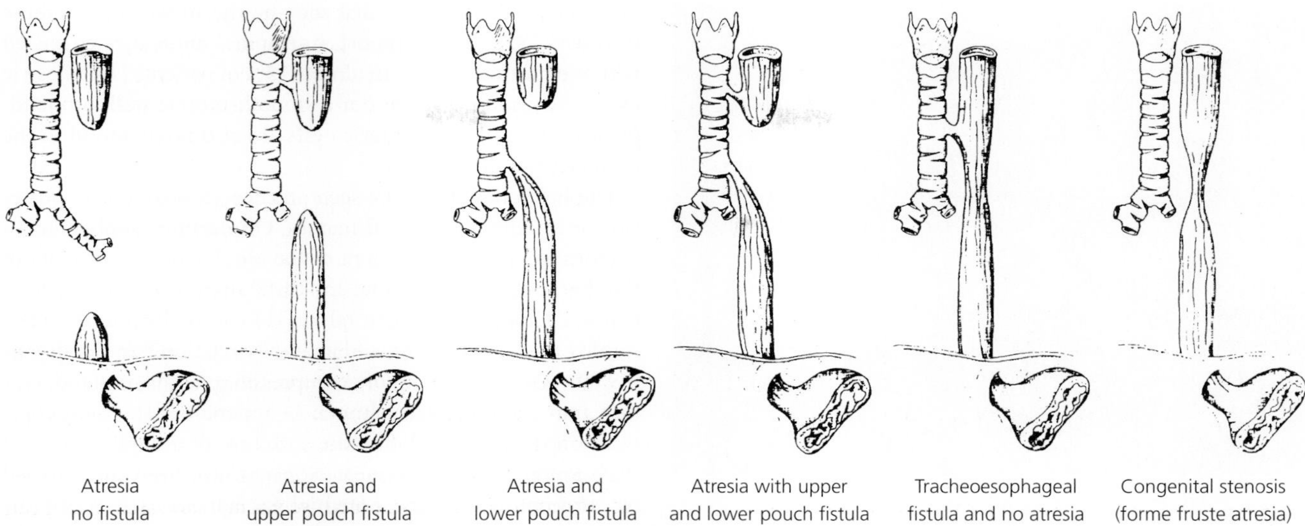

Figure 3.7 The spectrum of esophageal atresia, tracheoesophageal fistula, and congenital stenosis. Atresia with lower pouch fistula (third from left) is the most common anomaly.

have other associated congenital anomalies that include cardiac, genitourinary, gastrointestinal, skeletal, and central nervous system anomalies [45].

VACTERL is a term describing the combined occurrence of the vertebral, anal, cardiac, tracheoesophageal, renal, and limb anomalies in the same patient. Genetic defects have been identified in a subset of patients with VACTERL. Some features may be absent in VACTERL syndrome. There may be an association with the 16q24.1 FOX transcription factor gene cluster [50].

Symptoms vary with the type of tracheoesophageal anomaly. In infants with atresia alone, the diagnosis is often made after birth with signs of retention and regurgitation of saliva and feedings. Infants with proximal fistula exhibit respiratory distress during feedings. In infants with atresia and distal fistula, excessive salivation and regurgitation occur along with cyanosis and pneumonia secondary to reflux of gastric contents. The fifth type, isolated TEF or H-type fistula, leads to cough and choking with feedings, recurrent pneumonia, and intermittent abdominal distension. In rare cases, this anomaly may present in adulthood given the absence of associated esophageal atresia. In such cases, secondary causes of TEF such as infection, chronic inflammation, and cancer need to be excluded. Adult patients present with a history of recurrent aspiration pneumonia and bronchiectasis [51–54].

In most infants with esophageal atresia and TEF, a surgical repair with division of the fistula and primary esophageal anastomosis can be accomplished. In cases of atresia with wide separation of the proximal and distal esophageal remnants, esophageal lengthening procedures or interposition using small or large intestine is necessary. Gastrointestinal complications can result from the underlying congenital defect as well as surgical repair. Dysphagia is common and can result from anastomotic stricture formation as well as esophageal dysmotility and rarely from concomitant congenital esophageal stenosis [55]. Abnormalities of the myenteric plexus have been described and may account for the dysmotility [56]. Gastroesophageal reflux and delayed gastric emptying have also been reported in a high proportion of patients [55].

Congenital esophageal stenosis

Congenital esophageal stenosis is rare, estimated to occur in 1 of 25,000–50,000 live births, and is thought to result from failure of the normal embryonic separation of trachea and esophagus that is frequently associated with esophageal atresia and TEF [57,58]. Stenoses caused by tracheobronchial cartilaginous remnants, fibromuscular wall hypertrophy, and membranous web formation have been described (Figure 3.8) [58–62]. Fibromuscular wall hypertrophy is the most common type (54%) followed by tracheobronchial remnants (30%) and membranous webs (16%) [58]. Unlike atresia and TEF, congenital stenosis often is not diagnosed until later in childhood, and several cases have been reported in adults [3,63,64]. Symptoms include regurgitation, prolonged eating time, and dysphagia with recurrent food impaction. An esophagram typically demonstrates a focal stenosis in the esophagus. Membranous webs are found in the upper and middle thirds of the esophagus whereas fibromuscular hypertrophy occurs in the middle and distal thirds and tracheobronchial remnants in the distal third of the esophagus [58].

Endoscopic ultrasonography can visualize the presence of tracheobronchial remnants. Esophageal dilation has been used in children and adults with success but esophageal perforation risk exceeds that for more common benign strictures [58]. Segmental resection has been advocated for symptomatic patients, particularly those failing esophageal dilation [58,65]. Eosinophilic esophagitis can present with focal esophageal

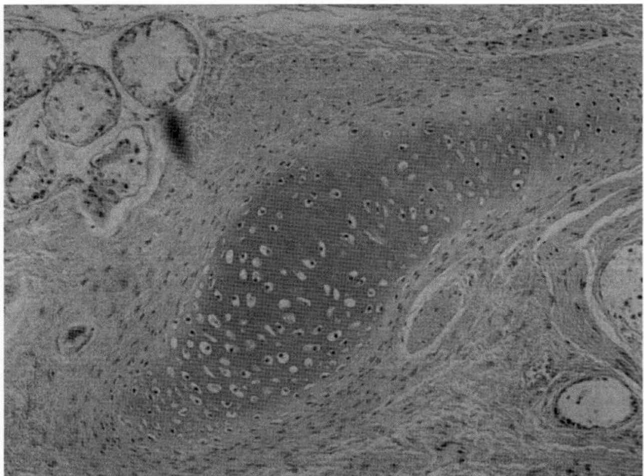

Figure 3.8 Histologic section from the esophageal wall of a resected segment of congenital esophageal stenosis with cartilagenous tracheobronchial remnant [65].

strictures as well as concentric mucosal rings in both children and adults, and is an important consideration in the evaluation of a patient with possible congenital esophageal stenosis. While the ringed appearance of eosinophilic esophagitis is sometimes referred to as "trachealization" of the esophagus, this is neither congenital nor cartilaginous in origin [66]. Several reported cases of congenital esophageal stenosis in adults were unrecognized cases of eosinophilic esophagitis.

Congenital esophageal duplication

Congenital esophageal duplications, tubular or cystic, represent about 15% of digestive duplications [67]. They develop in the third week of embryonic development due to failure of vacuoles to coalesce properly, interfering with normal recanalization of the esophageal lumen. As a result, a cyst or parallel tubular channel forms within the esophageal wall [68].

Duplications of the gastrointestinal tract have three common characteristics: they are contiguous with some segment of the gastrointestinal tract; they are lined by alimentary epithelium; and smooth muscle is present in their walls. Most patients present before 1 year of age, but as many as 25–30% of cases are first diagnosed in adults [69]. The most common presenting symptom is dysphagia, but the diagnosis is often made as an incidental finding in patients studied for other indications [70].

Congenital duplication cysts constitute less than 3% of mediastinal masses. They are the second most common benign esophageal submucosal lesion, with gastrointestinal stromal tumors being the most common [71,72]. They are lined by squamous columnar, cuboid, pseudostratified, or ciliated epithelium [73,74]. Sixty percent arise in the distal third of the esophagus, 17% in the middle third, and 23% in the upper third [67,75]. Cysts located posterior to the heart have been associated with cardiac arrhythmias [76]. Intraspinal cystic extensions can cause neurologic deficits that may be the initial sign of these disorders [77]. In one report, intraspinal anomalies coexisted with mediastinal masses in almost 25% of patients [78]. Gastric cysts, inclusion cysts without a smooth muscle wall, bronchogenic cysts, and neuroenteric cysts are also rarely found in the esophageal wall [67].

Duplication cysts can be seen on chest radiographs as posterior or middle mediastinal masses. On barium esophagram, a smooth, curved displacement of the esophagus is seen without the sharp, step-like proximal and distal margin seen with a leiomyoma. Computed tomography (CT) can be helpful in determining the location, size, and anatomic relation to other organs [79,80]. At endoscopy, a soft, compressible submucosal indentation into the esophageal lumen is apparent [81]. Endoscopic ultrasonography can define the structure of a duplication cyst [82]. Preoperative esophageal biopsies have been discouraged by surgeons due to the potential for adhesions between the esophageal mucosa and cyst wall that may make surgical resection more difficult.

Tubular duplications are rare and may be associated with other congenital cardiac, spinal, pulmonary, and extremity abnormalities [70]. Tubular duplications may communicate at both ends with the esophageal lumen or be closed at one end, but more than 80% do not communicate with the lumen [3,83–85]. Spontaneous, submucosal dissection of the esophagus has been reported and can radiographically present with a double-barrel esophagus that mimics a tubular duplication [86]. Surgical resection is usually recommended for pathologic diagnosis and definitive treatment [87–89]. Both laparoscopic and thoracoscopic resection have been reported [90,91]. Surgical incision and suturing of the edges of the cyst to create a common cavity with the esophageal lumen (marsupialization) has been used for the treatment of large cysts where surgical excision of the cyst may be undesirable [92,93]. Although rare, both adenocarcinoma and squamous cell carcinoma within tubular or cystic duplications have been reported [94–96].

Bronchopulmonary foregut malformation

The term bronchopulmonary foregut malformation was proposed by Gerle in 1968 to include pulmonary developmental abnormalities both with and without communication to the gastrointestinal tract. Since then, confusion in the terminology has occurred owing to the inclusion and exclusion of a number of gastrointestinal, pulmonary, and vascular anomalies as well as attempts to histologically, pathogenetically and anatomically classify the varying presentations described largely in case reports and small series. Bronchopulmonary foregut malformations include a focus of pulmonary parenchyma or sequestration with a patent congenital communication to the upper gastrointestinal tract [3,97–99]. They are considered distinct from TEF, which result from failure of initial foregut septation.

Bronchopulmonary foregut malformations develop when cell rests with respiratory potential arise from the foregut caudal to the lung bud or when a portion of the lung bud arises from the dorsal esophagus rather than the ventral trachea [98]. The tract within the sequestered pulmonary lobe typically involutes because of outgrowth of its blood supply; incomplete involution of the tract leads to a gastrointestinal tract communication [99]. Bronchopulmonary foregut malformations are most commonly seen in the lower lobes [3]. Up to 40% of children with communicating bronchopulmonary foregut malformations have associated congenital anomalies. The clinical presentation in infants is respiratory distress exacerbated with feedings. In older children and adults, recurrent pneumonia, bronchiectasis, hemoptysis, gastrointestinal bleeding, and dysphagia may develop. Contrast esophagram, CT scans, and angiography are used for diagnosis and surgical planning.

Aortic arch vessel abnormalities producing extrinsic compression of the esophagus (dysphagia lusoria)

It has been estimated that 3% of the population have a congenital abnormality of the aortic arch vessels, but only rarely does this result in symptomatic compression of the esophagus [100]. In the embryo, the foregut is surrounded by vascular structures of the branchial arches. Normally, portions of the branchial arches obliterate to form the great vessels and aortic arch. Abnormalities in developmental obliteration of the branchial arches may lead to vascular compression of the trachea and esophagus [101].

The term dysphagia lusoria, literally translated from the Latin lusus naturae ("trick or freak of nature"), is used to describe symptomatic esophageal compression resulting from any vascular anomaly of the aortic arch. Another term used is dysphagia arteritica. Most commonly, it results from an aberrant right subclavian artery [102]. The root of the aberrant artery often has a broad base referred to as Kommerell diverticulum. Symptoms of this anomaly may occur at the onset of semisolid feedings, later in childhood, or in adult life. With this anomaly, the right subclavian artery arises from the left side of the aortic arch and compresses the esophagus from the posterior aspect in an oblique manner (Figure 3.9a). Based on autopsy studies, an aberrant right subclavian artery occurs in 0.7 % of the general population, with only 10% of these affected individuals having symptoms related to compression [3,103]. During esophageal endosonography performed in 3334 patients, an aberrant right subclavian artery was identified in 12 (0.36%). None of the patients had symptoms of this entity [104]. While esophageal motility abnormalities have been observed, the patterns have been variable and nonspecific [105]. This vascular anomaly most typically causes symptoms later in life [106]. The reason for this is unclear but may be attributed to age-related changes to the vasculature.

Barium esophagram demonstrates an oblique filling defect just above the level of the aortic arch (Figure 3.9b). CT and magnetic resonance imaging have largely replaced the need for angiography

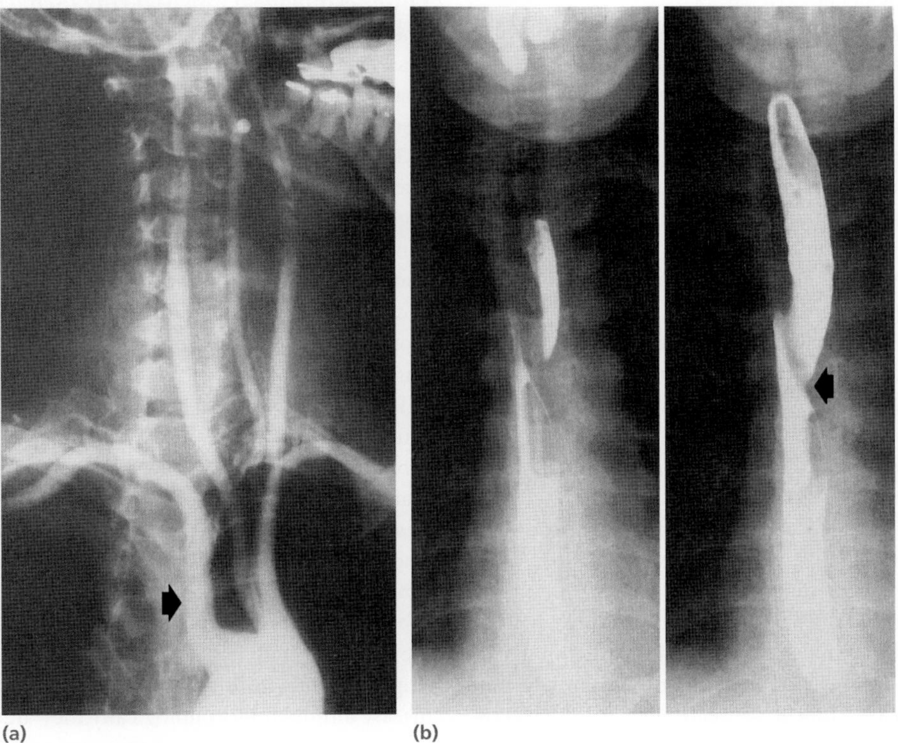

Figure 3.9 **(a)** Angiography reveals an aberrant right subclavian artery (*arrow*) arising from the aortic arch. **(b)** Barium esophagram in the same patient reveals oblique esophageal compression (*arrow*) by the aberrant right subclavian artery posterior to the esophagus.

in the diagnosis. Endoscopy may demonstrate a posterolateral pulsatile compression of the lumen of the proximal esophagus. Correction is performed in children by division and ligation of the aberrant artery. In adults, reanastomosis to the ascending aorta is performed to avoid the development of a subclavian steal syndrome, which is reversed flow of blood in the vertebral artery leading to brainstem ischemia [107]. Surgery is not always needed because many adult patients can easily tolerate minor degrees of dysphagia by simply modifying their diet.

Esophageal compression by an anomalous vertebral artery and right aortic arch with constricting left ligamentum arteriosum has been reported in adults and can be successfully repaired surgically [108,109]. Other vascular anomalies are causes of tracheoesophageal compression in infants, and these require early surgical intervention [110,111].

Heterotopic gastric mucosa (inlet patch)

Heterotopic gastric mucosa, also known as an inlet patch, is a focus of gastric epithelium most commonly located in the cervical esophagus. An autopsy series of 1000 children demonstrated a prevalence of 4.5% [112].Endoscopic studies reported a prevalence of 0.1–10% [113–116]. Most commonly, the inlet patch is situated immediately distal to the upper esophageal sphincter, making endoscopic detection difficult. Substantially higher prevalence frequencies are reported if microscopic foci of gastric tissue are included in the definition. Inlet patches have been reported to occur in 5.6% of patients with Barrett esophagus but in none with achalasia [117].

At endoscopy, these areas of gastric mucosa typically are well-circumscribed patches of reddish orange or salmon-colored mucosa that range in size from 2 mm to 4 cm [118]. The lesions can be unifocal, multifocal or circumferential. Inlet patches can be dramatically demonstrated by applying topical dilute iodine solution to stain the squamous mucosa around their margin. Histologically, the majority contain fundic type gastric mucosa that include parietal cells [113]. The inlet patch is generally considered to be a congenital abnormality that results from incomplete replacement of the early embryonic columnar epithelium with squamous epithelium. On the other hand, some investigators have reported that inlet patches share features with Barrett esophagus, suggesting that the former is an acquired condition associated with acid reflux [119–121]. *Helicobacter pylori* has been detected in mucosal biopsies of inlet patches [122,123].

Complications of heterotopic gastric mucosa include those secondary to acid production and neoplastic transformation. Acid secretion has been demonstrated in several reports [113,124–126]. While the majority of inlet patches are asymptomatic, symptoms of odynophagia, dysphagia, and globus have been reported [127]. Cervical esophageal strictures or webs and even esophagotracheal fistula have been demonstrated [128–130]. Plummer–Vinson or Paterson–Kelly syndrome is characterized by dysphagia due to a cervical esophageal web with concomitant iron deficiency anemia. The anemia and strictures may be secondary to esophageal erosions produced by acid secretion. In terms of cancer risk, 30 cases of progression of heterotopic gastric mucosa to adenocarcinoma have been reported [131,132]. Given the high prevalence of inlet patches and low prevalence of cervical esophageal adenocarcinoma, both the absolute and relative risks of malignant transformation are quite low. In light of this, biopsies of endoscopically detected inlet patches are generally not performed.

Symptomatic inlet patches should respond to proton pump inhibition through the same mechanism by which gastric acid suppression is achieved. Complications of strictures and webs are amenable to standard esophageal dilation techniques with the caveat that detection of such strictures can be more difficult given the location adjacent to the upper esophageal sphincter. Transendoscopic thermal ablation of the mucosa of the inlet patch by means of argon plasma coagulation combined with high-dose omeprazole therapy has been shown to allow replacement of the inlet patch by normal squamous mucosa, with resolution of related symptoms [133,134]. As most patients are asymptomatic and symptomatic patients should respond to acid inhibition or dilation, the role for ablation techniques is yet undefined.

Structural anomalies

Esophageal rings and webs

Lower esophageal mucosal ring (Schatzki ring)

The lower esophageal mucosal ring, or "B" ring, was initially described by Templeton in 1944 [3]. In 1953, Ingelfinger and Kramer, and Schatzki and Gary independently described the association of lower esophageal mucosal rings with dysphagia [3,135,136]. Schatzki and Gary attributed the symptoms to a fixed, mucosal stricture at the squamocolumnar junction. Ingelfinger and Kramer, on the other hand, postulated that a contractile muscular ring at the gastroesophageal junction produced the symptoms. Ring-like narrowings at the esophagogastric junction are now differentiated into two types: lower esophageal muscular ring, or A-ring, and lower esophageal mucosal ring, or B-ring.

Lower esophageal mucosal rings are located at the level of the squamocolumnar junction. These rings consist of mucosa and submucosa and are covered by squamous mucosa on the proximal aspect and either columnar mucosa or several millimeters of squamous mucosa on the distal or gastric aspect [137,138]. The lower esophageal mucosal ring is circumferential and 3 mm or less in thickness (Figure 3.10). An autopsy study of 100 subjects reported a 9% prevalence for the mucosal rings and they are detected in 4–15% of radiographic studies [139]. The rings are likely acquired and may be a manifestation of reflux disease although morphologically they are distinct from peptic strictures. The majority of patients with Schatzki rings have abnormal distal esophageal acid exposure on pH monitoring although this does not prove causation [140]. A congenital

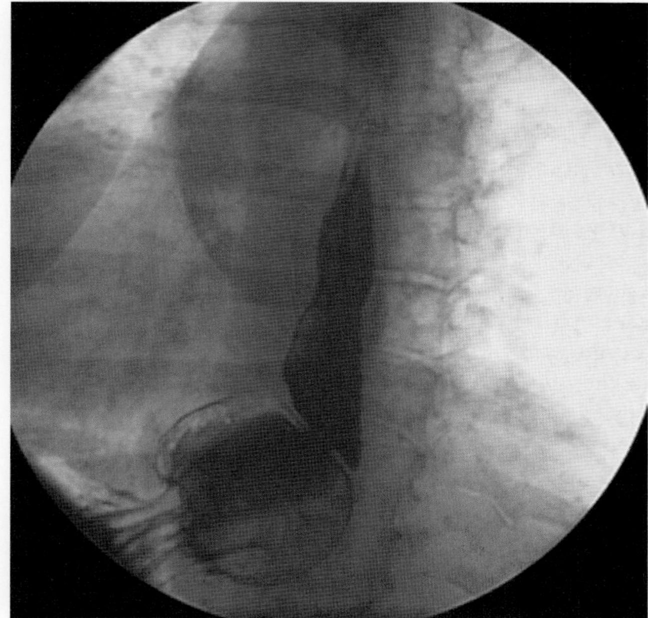

(a)

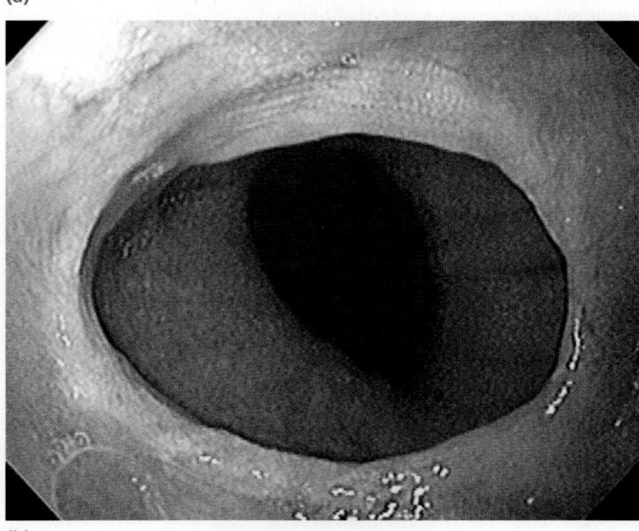

(b)

Figure 3.10 **(a)** Barium esophagram demonstrates a lower esophageal mucosal ring, also known as Schatzki or B ring, at the proximal end of a hiatal hernia pouch. Constriction of the distal end of the hernia is secondary to the diaphragmatic hiatus. The ring is appreciated with both a distended (*left*) and undistended (*right*) hiatus hernia. **(b)** Endoscopic view of a Schatzki ring with hiatal hernia immediately below. The ring margin is smooth, less than 3 mm thick, and without inflammation or evidence of fibrosis.

origin and association with esophageal shortening have also been proposed [139].

Most patients with lower esophageal mucosal rings are asymptomatic; however, they are one of the most common causes of intermittent dysphagia and food impactions, typically presenting in patients older than 40 years of age [141,142]. The severity of symptoms depends on the inner diameter of the ring. Rings larger than 20 mm in diameter usually are asymptomatic, rings 13–20 mm in diameter cause variable degrees of dysphagia depending on type and size of bolus, and rings less than 13 mm in diameter frequently cause solid food dysphagia [143,144]. Serial esophagrams have demonstrated the development and progressive narrowing of lower esophageal mucosal rings, providing evidence that these are acquired and not congenital lesions [145–147]. Misunderstanding in the literature and in practice has resulted from confusing Schatzki rings with short, annular, peptic strictures and, more recently, eosinophilic esophagitis. Lower esophageal mucosal rings identified in the setting of eosinophilic esophagitis should be considered distinct from the Schatzki ring as the former has characteristic histopathology and occurs in the setting of diffuse, endoscopically identified esophageal abnormalities [66,148,149].

On esophagram, a lower esophageal mucosal ring appears as a thin (<3.0 mm) transverse circumferential ridge above the hiatus of the diaphragm. To visualize the ring either endoscopically or radiographically, the esophagogastric junction must be adequately distended (see Figure 3.10). By definition, a hiatal hernia is invariably present although this may be related to the limited ability to visualize the ring when it is collapsed by the constriction of the diaphragmatic hiatus. Lower esophageal mucosal rings are absent in patients with long segment Barrett esophagus. Barium esophagram with a prone full-column technique is more sensitive than double-contrast radiography or endoscopy in detecting lower esophageal mucosal rings [150]. Performing a Valsalva maneuver during the esophagram is helpful in demonstrating a ring [151]. The use of a barium tablet or marshmallow bolus may further improve the sensitivity of the barium esophagram to correlate dysphagia with the ring. The standard barium tablet has a diameter of 12.8 mm and will therefore not usually detect rings in the 13–20 mm category which may still be clinically significant.

The endoscopic characteristics of lower esophageal rings and the associated findings are readily recognized (Figure 3.10b) [152]. Symptomatic lower esophageal rings can be effectively treated with single passage of a 17–20 mm (51–60 French) Maloney or Savary dilator [153]. For very tight rings, some clinicians use the standard gradual sequential dilation technique rather than passage of a single large-diameter bougie. Hydrostatic balloon dilation is also effective. Disruption of the ring using four-quadrant mucosal biopsies and needle knife incision has been described [154,155]. While most patients achieve immediate relief of dysphagia following dilation, a follow-up study noted that 32% of patients had recurrent dysphagia at 1 year and 65% at 2 years [156]. Proton pump inhibitor therapy may reduce the occurrence of recurrent dysphagia, again pointing to a possible link with reflux disease. A randomized controlled trial of omeprazole in patients with symptomatic Schatzki rings found that 7% of patients receiving the drug experienced recurrent dysphagia requiring dilation compared with 47% of patients on placebo [157].

It should be kept in mind that Schatzki rings are common and when detected in a patient with dysphagia, may be an incidental finding. For patients demonstrating a poor or short duration response to esophageal dilation of a presumed symptomatic lower esophageal mucosal ring, other etiologies should be sought, including motility disorders and eosinophilic esophagitis.

Lower esophageal muscular ring

In an autopsy series, lower esophageal muscular rings were found in 5% of an asymptomatic cohort of 100 patients [139]. The location proximal to the squamocolumnar junction makes it likely that the rings represent an exaggeration of the proximal aspect of the lower esophageal sphincter. Symptomatic muscular rings are unusual and typically present with dysphagia. Unlike the dysphagia that occurs with Schatzki rings, muscular rings present with intermittent dysphagia for both liquids and solids without food impactions. On barium esophagram, muscular rings are smooth, symmetric narrowings that are several millimeters in axial extent with a luminal aperture that varies during the course of fluoroscopic examination (Figure 3.11). Endoscopically, the appearance is that of a constriction with intact overlying squamous mucosa situated 2–3 cm above the squamocolumnar junction. Unlike achalasia, the constriction is very focal and does not encompass the distal aspect of the esophagogastric junction. Lower esophageal muscular rings have been associated with esophageal manometric abnormalities that include high-amplitude, long-duration esophageal body contractions and esophageal spasm [158]. Esophageal dilation is often attempted but provides incomplete and short-lasting relief. Several case reports have noted significant improvement in dysphagia following injection of botulinum toxin [158–160]. Surgical myotomy has been described but is necessary only in rare instances [135,161–163].

Cervical and midesophageal webs

Esophageal webs are thin (1–2 mm), transverse membranes of squamous epithelium. They most commonly occur in the cervical esophagus and usually originate on the anterior wall. They are rarely circumferential but may be multiple. Due to proximity to the upper esophageal sphincter, cervical webs are easily missed on upper endoscopy. Radiographic studies detected esophageal webs in 6–12% of patients, with the higher prevalence reported in patients with symptoms of dysphagia [164,165]. Like Schatzki rings, most webs are asymptomatic. Intermittent solid food dysphagia is the usual complaint in symptomatic patients.

Cervical esophageal webs have been reported to occur in association with heterotopic gastric mucosa and in some instances may represent a form of peptic stricture related to local acid secretion [166]. Cervical webs should be distinguished from proximal, mucosal, web-like strictures secondary to a number of other conditions producing esophageal injury, including epidermolysis bullosa, cicatricial pemphigoid, pill esophagitis, chemotherapy-induced mucositis, graft-versus-host disease, radiation, and eosinophilic esophagitis.

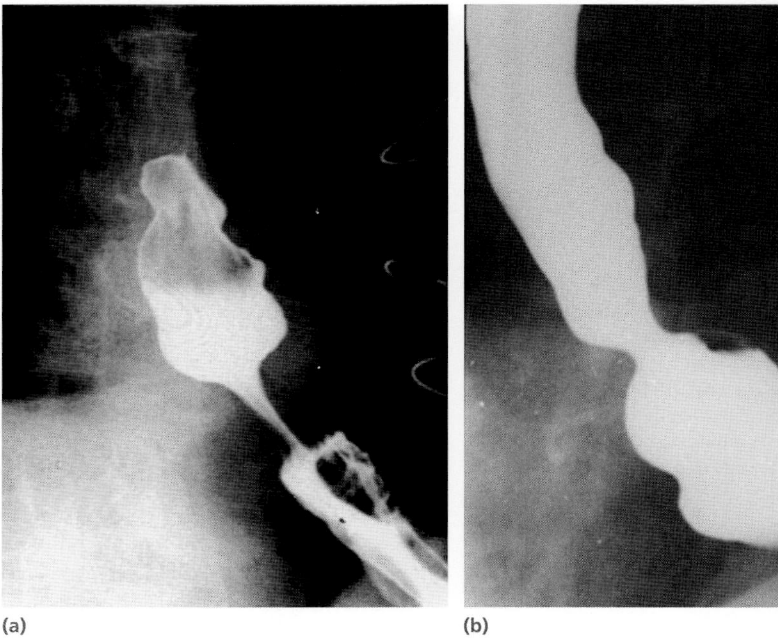

Figure 3.11 Lower esophageal muscular ring (A-ring). Two views from the same patient show marked, 3 cm long constriction in the distal esophagus proximal to a hiatal hernia (*left*). The right panel depicts partial relaxation of the A-ring with distension of the phrenic ampulla proximal to a concomitant Schatzki ring. The distended hiatal hernia is visible distal to the Schatzki ring.

The association of postcricoid webs with iron deficiency anemia (i.e., Plummer–Vinson or Patterson–Kelly syndrome) is both infrequent and controversial [3,167,168]. The existence of the syndrome is debated although some indirect evidence points to the possibility that iron deficiency could predispose to web formation. On the other hand, as discussed in a preceding section of this chapter, acid secretion from heterotopic gastric mucosa could be a cause of blood loss from esophageal erosions as well as cervical webs.

Midesophageal webs are rare and typically present with dysphagia. They may be single or multiple and are believed to be of congenital origin [168–172]. In addition to midesophageal mucosal lesions resulting from the conditions causing esophageal injury noted above, they may also be confused with congenital esophageal stenosis. If symptomatic, they are best treated with bougienage. Treatment with transendoscopic incision or surgical resection has been reported but is rarely necessary [169–171,173,174].

Cricopharyngeal bar

Cricopharyngeal (CP) bar is a common radiographic finding, reported in 5–19% of patients undergoing dynamic pharyngeal radiography [175,176]. It appears as a prominent and persistent posterior indentation at the level of the lower third of the cricoid cartilage (Figure 3.12). The majority of patients with CP bar do not experience significant dysphagia. In one report, dysphagia was not statistically more prevalent in patients with CP bar than in controls (13% vs 8%) [177]. Symptomatic CP bars most commonly present in the elderly with dysphagia for solids and occasionally liquids as well [178]. Studies have also shown histologic changes comparable with Zenker diverticulum that include muscle degeneration and fibrosis [179]. It is important to exclude other more common etiologies for dysphagia because a CP bar may be an incidental finding. Furthermore, CP bars may be secondary to neuromuscular causes, including central and peripheral nervous system abnormalities (multiple sclerosis, amyotrophic lateral sclerosis, syringomyelia, cerebral vascular disease), inflammatory myopathies, and myoneural junction disorders (myasthenia gravis, diphtheria, tetanus).

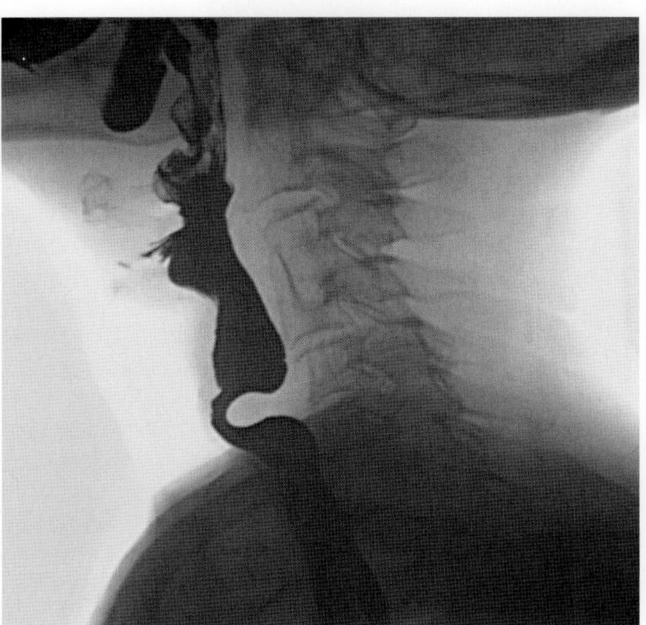

Figure 3.12 Barium swallow depicting a prominent cricopharyngeal bar in the cervical esophagus in a patient presenting with dysphagia.

Early studies attributed the pathophysiology of CP bars to failed UES relaxation, UES spasm, and basal UES hypertension. It has subsequently been recognized that the radiographic appearance of a CP bar is associated with neither high basal UES pressure nor incomplete sphincter relaxation. Moreover, one study found that neither peak pharyngeal pressure nor incoordination were predictors of outcome following cricopharyngeal disruption in a heterogeneous group of patients with oropharyngeal dysphagia [180]. Using simultaneous pharyngeal videoradiography and manometry, these investigators demonstrated that increased hypopharyngeal intrabolus pressure was a significant predictor of positive outcome following CP disruption. Similar to the studies in Zenker diverticula patients, these authors suggested that increased intrabolus pressure implies impaired sphincter opening and may be an indirect measure of sphincter compliance, all of which predict response to CP disruption. An earlier study by Dantas et al. demonstrated significant impairment of cricopharyngeal opening in patients with a CP bar when compared to control subjects without a CP bar, which further supports the concept of sphincter dysfunction in the pathogenesis of CP bars [176].

Treatment options for symptomatic CP bars include esophageal dilation and surgical myotomy. Several small case series have described significant relief of dysphagia with a 1–2-year follow-up after dilation to 17–20 mm [180–183] Esophageal dilation is an attractive alternative to surgery, especially in older patients with comorbidities.

Pharyngoesophageal and esophageal diverticula

Zenker diverticulum

Pharyngoesophageal diverticulum was first described by Ludlow in 1769 and critically reviewed a century later by the pathologists Zenker and Ziemssen [3]. Pharyngoesophageal or Zenker diverticula represent an outpouching of the posterior hypopharyngeal mucosa proximal to the esophageal inlet. The site of origin of the diverticulum between the oblique fibers of the inferior pharyngeal constrictor and the transverse fibers of the cricopharyngeus was described by Killian in 1907 and is referred to as Killian's dehiscence or the triangle of Killian.

A number of theories have been suggested to explain the pathogenesis of Zenker diverticulum [184].The observation that both symptomatic and asymptomatic Zenker diverticula occur in the elderly population supports an acquired defect that is a consequence of aging. Early studies suggested that the upper esophageal sphincter failed to relax in this condition, leading to the term cricopharyngeal achalasia. Subsequent combined manometric-fluoroscopic studies demonstrated complete UES relaxation but diminished opening [185,186]. As a result, hypopharyngeal pressures are increased and thought to lead to progressive protrusion through an area of relative mural weakness in the Killian triangle. The limitation in UES opening is most likely a myogenic rather than neurogenic phenomenon.

Histologic studies of muscle biopsies taken during the time of surgical treatment have demonstrated connective tissue replacement of skeletal muscle fibers and muscle fiber degeneration [186–188]. The cause of the muscle changes is unclear. Evidence linking gastroesophageal reflux disease with Zenker diverticula is limited. Initial reports of UES hypertension and contraction in response to distal esophageal acid exposure have not been confirmed in subsequent studies [189,190]. Others have theorized that esophageal shortening induces mural weakness, allowing for mucosal herniation in patients with Zenker diverticula [191].

The prevalence of Zenker diverticula ranges from 0.01% to 0.11%, with the majority of patients being asymptomatic [192]. The median age is approximately 70 years with a male predominance, and presentation in a patient younger than 30 is unusual. The predominant symptoms are dysphagia and regurgitation. Throat pain, cough, aspiration, halitosis, and neck gurgling or mass are also reported. The diagnosis is apparent on esophagram but the fluoroscopic field needs to visualize the hypopharynx which is not routinely included by all radiologists (Figure 3.13). For unclear reasons, the majority of diverticula deviate to the left. Complications include aspiration pneumonia, pill retention, ulceration, fistula, and bleeding. Squamous cell cancer was reported in 0.4% of 1249 patients with Zenker diverticula over a 53-year period [193]. Spindle cell carcinoma and benign tumors also have been reported to arise in pharyngoesophageal diverticula [194,195].

Endoscopy is not essential to the management of symptomatic Zenker diverticula and carries a risk of perforation. With direct visualization and awareness of the posterior location of the diverticular orifice, endoscopy is not contraindicated and may demonstrate concomitant esophageal pathology or secondary complications. Blind esophageal intubation with nasogastric tubes, manometric catheters, and transesophageal echocardiographic devices can lead to inadvertent perforation. A fluoroscopically placed guidewire and use of smaller, pediatric or transnasal endoscopes can facilitate esophageal intubation in cases with significant stenosis of the UES.

Patients with minimal or no symptoms can be followed clinically for potential progression. Symptomatic pharyngoesophageal diverticula are managed by endoscopic or surgical approaches [196]. Early surgical reports of divertulectomy alone were associated with a very high recurrence rate, leading to the current recommendation for upper esophageal sphincter myotomy in most cases. For the open surgical approach, myotomy

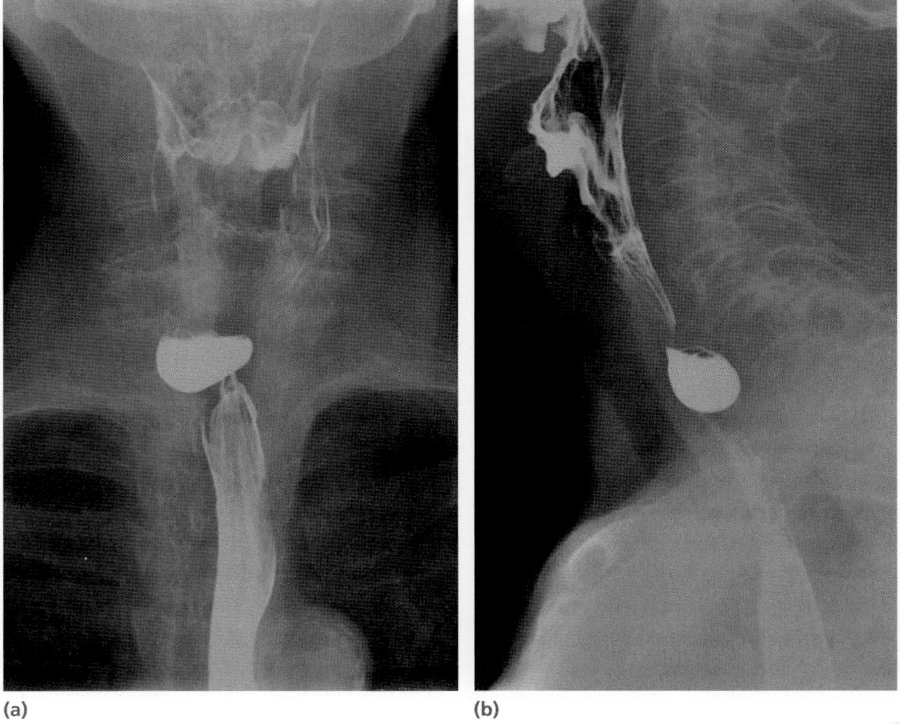

Figure 3.13 Barium swallow demonstrating a 25 mm Zenker diverticulum on anterior **(a)** and lateral **(b)** views. The opening to the pharyngeal diverticulum originates above the cricopharyngeous at the level of the sixth cervical vertebra. Unlike most Zenker diverticula, this example deviates slightly to the right of midline on the anterior view.

alone may suffice for small diverticula while a myotomy with either diverticulectomy or diverticulopexy is performed for larger diverticula. Diverticula greater than 5 cm in size are typically resected. In spite of the elderly population that is afflicted with this condition, operative mortality is less than 2% [197]. Reported morbidity is highly variable but approximates 5–10% and includes esophageal leak, bleeding, mediastinal emphysema, fistula, nerve palsy including injury to the recurrent laryngeal nerve, and mediastinitis.

The transoral, endoscopic approach to Zenker diverticula dates back to 1917 but has become increasingly popular with advances in the use of electrical or laser cautery or endoscopic stapling devices. The technique involves dividing the common septum between the diverticulum and esophagus that is largely composed of the upper esophageal sphincter. Several hundred patients have been treated by this approach in the literature with outcomes, morbidity, and recurrence rates that are similar to the open surgical approach [198]. Advantages include shorter recovery and hospital stays. Disadvantages include a remnant anatomic defect as the diverticulum is divided but not resected but the clinical significance of this defect is unclear. The transoral technique using rigid endoscopy is primarily performed by thoracic surgeons and otorhinolaryngologists. An approach utilizing flexible endoscopes has increased interest amongst gastroenterologists in the management of Zenker diverticulum [184,199,200]. Septotomy performed by means of per oral submucosal tunnel techniques has produced both technical success and clinical effectiveness [199,200]. Long-term follow-up studies comparing the safety and durability of the different surgical and endoscopic therapies for Zenker diverticulum are needed to better understand the optimal management strategy.

Killian–Jamieson diverticula

Killian–Jamieson diverticula are outpouchings arising from the proximal cervical esophagus immediately below the upper esophageal sphincter [201]. They are less common and less likely to present with dysphagia than Zenker diverticula [202]. While more commonly unilateral with a left-sided predilection, bilateral diverticula occur in 25% and may coexist with Zenker diverticula [202]. The occurrence of these anatomic lesions is important to recognize because they can be confused with Zenker diverticula (Figure 3.14). It is interesting to speculate on their pathogenesis given their location below the upper esophageal sphincter. An underlying esophageal motility disorder of the striated muscle of the cervical esophagus has neither been described nor carefully excluded in these patients. Located at the transition zone between the striated and smooth muscle segments of the esophagus, incoordination of muscular contractions might account for their origin.

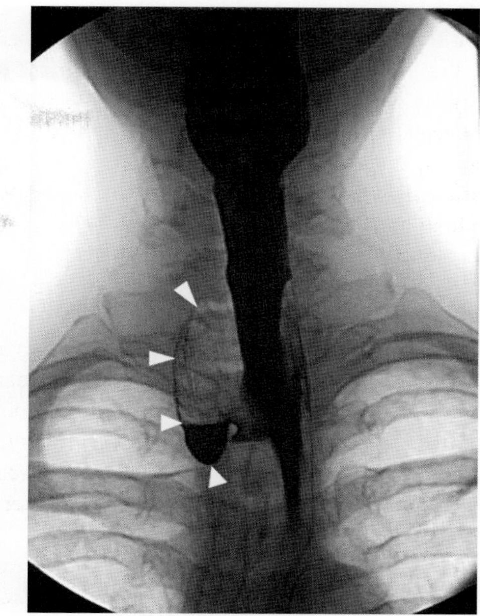

Figure 3.14 Barium swallow demonstrating a Killian–Jamieson diverticulum. In contrast to the Zenker diverticulum, Killian–Jamieson diverticula originate caudal to the cricopharyngeus muscle and are therefore true esophageal diverticula.

Midesophageal and epiphrenic diverticula

Diverticula also may occur in the mid or distal esophagus (Figure 3.15). Prevalence estimates of less than 1% are based on retrospective reviews of radiographic studies but are affected by the indications for the radiographic examination [3]. A century ago, midesophageal diverticula were described secondary to pulmonary tuberculosis. They were termed traction diverticula and felt to result from tethering on the outer aspect of the esophagus created by an inflammation of adjacent mediastinal lymph nodes. Midesophageal diverticula have also been reported in cases of anthracosis, sarcoidosis, histoplasmosis, and lymphoma, all with a presumed similar pathogenesis [203].

The majority of both midesophageal as well as epiphrenic diverticula are seen in conjunction with esophageal dysmotility [204–209]. They are typically referred to as pulsion-type diverticula, thought to be caused by increased intraluminal pressure induced by high-amplitude or uncoordinated esophageal body contractions or failed lower esophageal sphincter relaxation. Hypercontractile peristaltic contractions and esophagogastric junction outflow obstruction can be identified but a proportion of cases have normal esophageal motility [209]. Interestingly, esophageal diverticula are uncommon sequelae of achalasia. Cases of hypertensive lower esophageal sphincter, nutcracker esophagus, and nonspecific motility disorders have also been reported although the causative nature of these diagnoses in the pathogenesis of diverticula is uncertain.

A study utilizing high-frequency intraluminal ultrasonography reported temporal incoordination between circular and longitudinal muscle contractions in patients with nutcracker esophagus [210]. The investigators postulated that the asynchrony resulted in increased esophageal wall stress that could be a mechanism for diverticulum formation. Esophageal diverticula

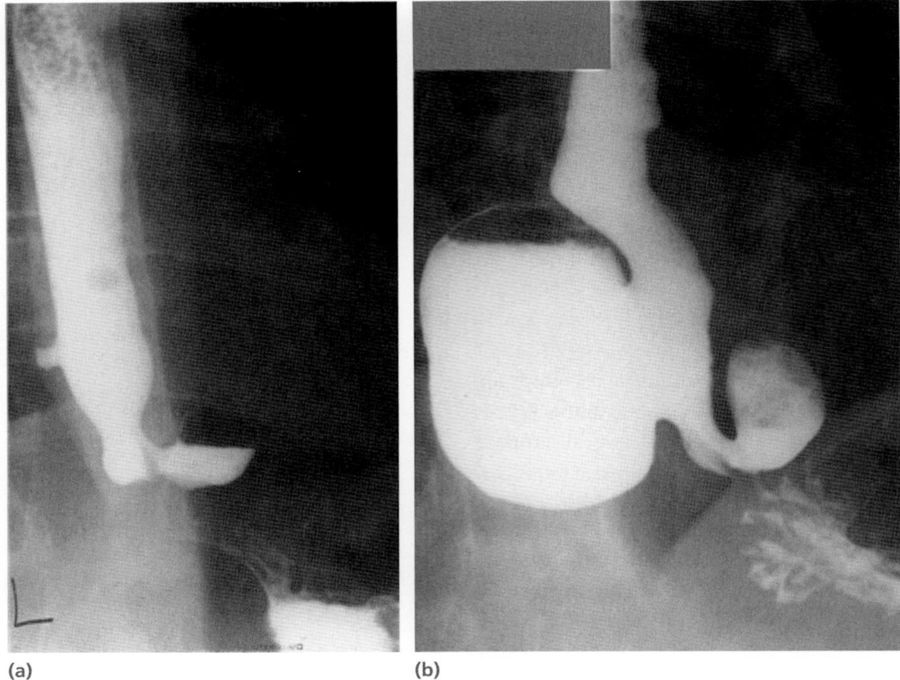

Figure 3.15 Barium radiograph depicting significant enlargement of epiphrenic diverticula in a patient on initial presentation (*left*) and 10 years later (*right*).

also may be secondary to esophageal wall anatomic weakening as in cases following Heller myotomy or per oral esophageal myotomy for achalasia [211].

Symptom presentation for esophageal diverticula closely mirrors that of the underlying esophageal motility disorders, making it difficult to discern whether a particular symptom is a direct result of the diverticulum. Dysphagia and regurgitation are the dominant presenting complaints with additional symptoms including chest pain, heartburn, weight loss, and respiratory symptoms including chronic cough [203]. In general, symptoms tend to correlate more closely with the motility disorder rather than the size of the diverticulum [203,207]. An exception to this general principle is giant diverticula that increase the retention of food and likely increase the risk of regurgitation and aspiration. Epiphrenic diverticula more commonly protrude from the right. Uncommon complications of esophageal diverticula include ulceration, hemorrhage, perforation, and fistulization. Rare cases of carcinoma arising from esophageal diverticula have been reported [212,213].

Many patients with esophageal diverticula are asymptomatic at the time of presentation with the finding incidentally noted on a radiographic or endoscopic procedure performed for another indication [203]. Natural history studies of untreated esophageal diverticula are few. In one radiologic series, enlargement of the diverticula was noted in 16% over a mean 12-year period [214]. Clinical case series have noted the development or progression of symptoms in less than 10% with a follow-up of several years [203].

Surgery remains the primary treatment for symptomatic esophageal diverticula. Botulinum toxin A injection of the lower esophageal sphincter has been effective in providing relief of dysphagia in a small series of patients with diverticula, although the moderate efficacy and durability of this approach limit its utility [215–217]. Recognizing the importance of underlying esophageal dysmotility, most surgical approaches combine a diverticulectomy with esophageal myotomy [203]. Several retrospective reports have noted a higher rate of postoperative esophageal leak and recurrent diverticula for diverticulectomy compared with diverticulectomy with myotomy. Even when combined with myotomy, esophageal leak is a major source of surgical morbidity and significantly more common than reported with myotomy alone in the treatment of achalasia without diverticula. A thorough presurgical evaluation, including barium esophagram, esophagoscopy and esophageal manometry, should be performed. Proximal extension of the myotomy into the esophageal body is considered in cases of esophageal spasm and vigorous achalasia, and can be guided by the proximal extent of the diverticula or hypercontractile manometric abnormalities. Divertulectomy, accompanied by lower esophageal sphincter myotomy plus some degree of fundoplication, has been successfully accomplished via the laparoscopic transhiatal approach [203].

Esophageal intramural pseudodiverticulosis

Esophageal intramural pseudodiverticulosis is a rare condition, detected in less than 1% of radiologic studies of the esophagus [218]. First described by Mendl and colleagues in 1960, multiple, small diverticula form in the wall of the esophagus by dilation of the excretory ducts of the submucosal esophageal glands [219–221] (Figure 3.16). The diagnosis is best appreciated on barium studies where intramural tracking of contrast can also be appreciated in 50% of studies [222]. Thickening of the esophageal wall due to chronic submucosal inflammation and fibrosis can be appreciated on CT scans as well as endoscopic ultrasonography [223,224]. Most cases present after the sixth decade with chronic dysphagia. Esophageal strictures, typically proximal, are seen in 70–90% of patients, and esophageal manometric abnormalities have been found in two-thirds of those studied [220,225,226]. Unlike the association between achalasia and esophageal spasm with esophageal diverticula, the reported abnormalities are most commonly nonspecific and may not be involved in the pathogenesis of intramural pseudodiverticulosis. Only one case of pseudodiverticulosis has been reported in achalasia [227]. A relationship between corrosive injury of the esophagus and intramural pseudodiverticulosis has been reported [228]. A report of 14 cases of this entity in 59 patients with corrosive esophageal injury noted that an esophageal stricture was a constant association. No correlation was found between the length of the stricture and the number of diverticula, and the diverticula regressed in number or disappeared altogether after the stricture was dilated.

In contrast to the surgical management of other esophageal diverticula, esophageal intramural pseudodiverticulosis is managed medically. Dilation of strictures, antireflux therapy, antifungal therapy, and calcium channel blockers have been reported to relieve symptoms [223,228]. Esophageal candidiasis has been described in up to 50% of reported cases; however, its role in the development of esophageal intramural pseudodiverticulosis is unknown and it is likely secondary to stasis. Rare complications include perforation, mediastinitis, fistula formation, and bleeding. An association between intramural pseudodiverticulosis and esophageal cancer has been reported but cause and effect has not been proven [229].

References are available at www.yamadagastro.com/textbook7e

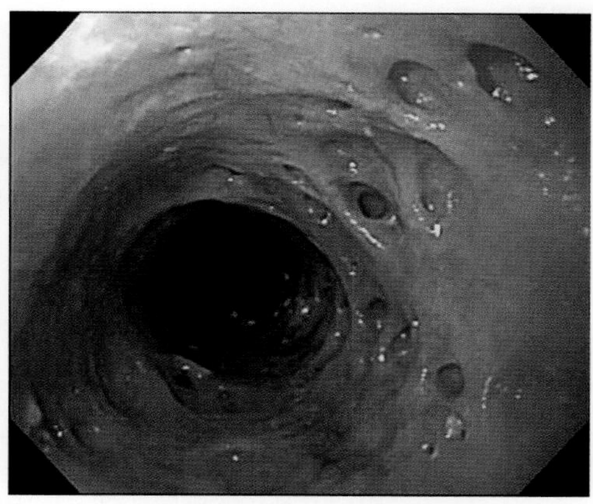

Figure 3.16 Endoscopic view of intramural pseudodiverticulosis with numerous small orifices in the esophageal mucosa. In other cases, the orifices can be punctate and may be overlooked on endoscopy. Source: Image courtesy of Prakash Gyawali MD, Washington University School of Medicine, St Louis.

Further reading

Ishaq S., Sultan H., Siau K., Kuwai T., Mulder C.J., Neumann H. New and emerging techniques for endoscopic treatment of Zenker's diverticulum: state-of-the-art review. Dig Endosc 2018;30(4):449.

Krishnan U., Mousa H., Dall'Oglio L., et al. ESPGHAN-NASPGHAN guidelines for the evaluation and treatment of gastrointestinal and nutritional complications in children with esophageal atresia-tracheoesophageal fistula. J Pediatr Gastroenterol Nutr 2016; 63(5):550.

Levitt B., Richter J.E. Dysphagia lusoria: a comprehensive review. Dis Esophagus 2007;20(6):455.

Terui K., Saito T., Mitsunaga T., Nakata M., Yoshida H. Endoscopic management for congenital esophageal stenosis: a systematic review. World J Gastrointest Endosc 2015;7(3):183.

Yang J., Novak S., Ujiki M., et al. An international study on the use of peroral endoscopic myotomy in the management of Zenker's diverticulum. Gastrointest Endosc 2020;91(1):163.

CHAPTER 4

Stomach and duodenum: anatomy and structural anomalies

Erik C. von Rosenvinge[1] and Jean-Pierre Raufman[1,2]
[1] University of Maryland School of Medicine, Baltimore, MD, USA
[2] Veterans Affairs Maryland Health Care System, Baltimore, MD, USA

Chapter menu

Embryology of the stomach and duodenum

The primitive foregut gives rise to the stomach and proximal duodenum. The duodenum distal to the ampulla of Vater derives from the cephalic end of the midgut [1,2]. About the fourth week of intrauterine development, the primitive stomach rotates 90° clockwise around its longitudinal axis, ending with the left side facing anteriorly and the right side posteriorly [3]. This accounts for the course of the left vagus along the anterior wall and the right vagus along the posterior wall. The left wall of the stomach grows faster than the right, resulting in the size difference between the curvatures. As the stomach grows and rotates, the cephalic end moves leftward and downward, forming the fundus and cardia. The caudal end moves upward and to the right, forming the antrum and pylorus. Hence, the long axis of the stomach runs from above left to below right.

The duodenum also grows rapidly, forms a C-loop projecting ventrally, rotates to the right and becomes retroperitoneal. Because of rapid epithelial proliferation during the fifth and sixth weeks of embryogenesis, the duodenal lumen is temporarily obliterated; it recanalizes over ensuing weeks as some cells degenerate.

The epithelium and glands of the stomach and duodenum derive from the embryonic endoderm. The connective tissue, muscle, and serosa derive from the mesoderm.

Gross anatomy of the stomach and duodenum

The gross and microscopic anatomy of the stomach and duodenum are intrinsically linked to their functions in mediating and regulating digestion and nutrition. Their structural organization facilitates sequential physiologic events that promote the fragmentation, enzymatic digestion, and absorption of nutrients. Also, appropriately timed autocrine, paracrine, and hormonal secretions from gastric and duodenal endocrine cells recruit other cells and organs to aid in the digestive process.

Anatomical relationships and divisions

The stomach – a large distensible sac with the largest diameter of any part of the gastrointestinal tract – is located in the epigastrium, just inferior to the diaphragm (Figure 4.1). The size and shape of the stomach vary greatly from person to person, depending on age, body habitus, posture, and interval since eating. The ability of the stomach to enlarge to accommodate meals is facilitated by its free mesentery, distensibility, and location. Although fixed proximally to the esophagus and distally to the duodenum, and by the gastrocolic and gastrophrenic ligaments, the stomach has great latitude in distension and motion. When the stomach is nearly empty, gastric volume

Yamada's Textbook of Gastroenterology, Seventh Edition. Edited by Timothy C. Wang, Michael Camilleri, Benjamin Lebwohl, Anna S. Lok, William J. Sandborn, Kenneth K. Wang, and Gary D. Wu.

Companion website: www.yamadagastro.com/textbook7e

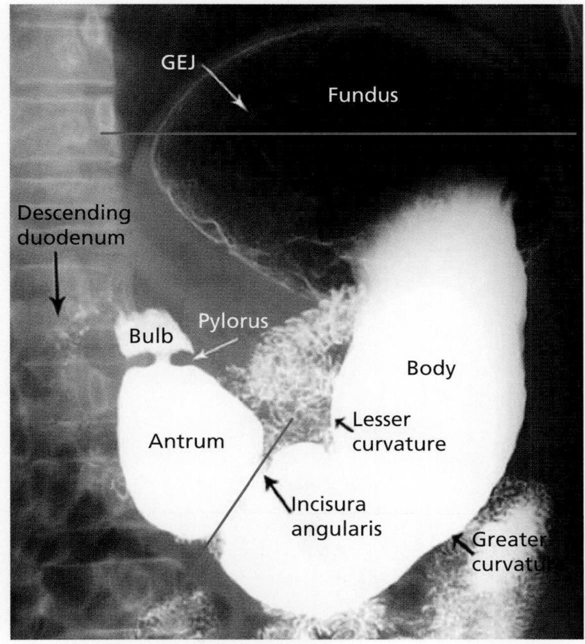

(a)

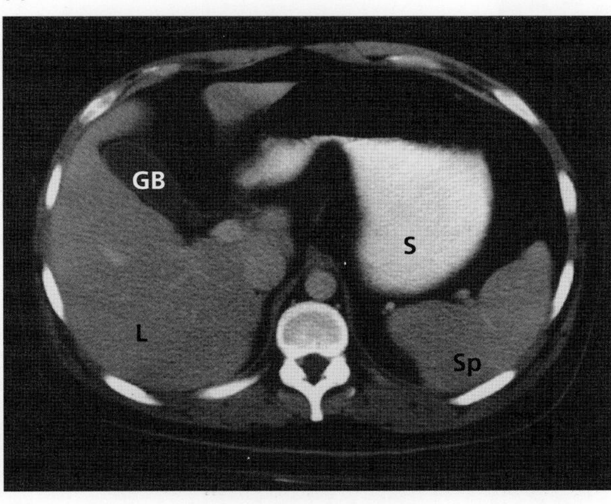

(b)

Figure 4.1 **(a)** Barium contrast radiograph of the stomach and proximal duodenum. The pyloric channel can be seen connecting the gastric antrum to the duodenal bulb. GEJ, gastroesophageal junction. Source: Brant and Helms 2012 [88]. Reproduced with permission from Lippincott, Williams & Wilkins. **(b)** A computed tomogram of the abdomen shows the stomach in relation to adjacent organs. GB, gallbladder; L, liver; S, stomach; Sp, spleen. Source: Courtesy of Drs Timothy Carter and Hemendra R. Shah, University of Arkansas for Medical Sciences, Little Rock, AR, USA.

approximates a few hundred milliliters; when distended with food, the stomach can accommodate in excess of 2 L. With full distension, the stomach may extend from the diaphragm to the pelvic brim.

As a consequence of its size and central location in the abdomen, the stomach abuts many organs. These include the diaphragm superiorly, hepatobiliary organs to the right, spleen to the left, pancreas posteriorly, and transverse colon inferiorly (Figure 4.1). The anterior surface of the stomach abuts the abdominal wall. The stomach is separated from other abdominal organs by visceral peritoneal lining. The close proximity of the stomach to other abdominal organs, such as the pancreas, permits endoluminal imaging techniques such as endoscopic ultrasonography to evaluate intraabdominal viscera. Because the anterior surface of the stomach is adjacent to the abdominal wall, percutaneous feeding tubes can be placed directly into its lumen.

By convention, the stomach is divided into the cardia, a 1–2 cm segment adjacent to the esophagogastric junction; the fundus, the superior portion of the stomach lying above and slightly posterior to the rest of the stomach; the body or corpus, the voluminous portion of the stomach below the fundus; the antrum, the distal region of the stomach; and, most distally, the pylorus or pyloric channel, a narrow (1–2 cm diameter) channel connecting the stomach with the duodenum (Figure 4.2). The shorter, right side of the stomach is the lesser curvature; the opposite, longer left side is the greater curvature. An intrusion, about two-thirds along the distal lesser curvature, near the junction of the body and antrum, is designated the angular notch or incisura angularis.

The tubular, C-shaped duodenum, surrounding the head of the pancreas, starts at the pylorus and extends to the ligament of Treitz, a landmark separating the fourth portion of the duodenum from the jejunum (Figure 4.3). The word *duodenum* derives from its length, approximately the same as the breadth of 12 fingers (about 25–30 cm). The duodenum has no mesentery and, in contrast to the stomach, is largely retroperitoneal and fixed in position.

The first, or superior, part of the duodenum is about 5 cm long, starting at the pylorus and passing posteriorly, upward and to the right. The initial 2–3 cm of the first part of the duodenum is the duodenal bulb. In contrast to the rest of the duodenum which is lined by circular folds (plicae circulares), the lining of the bulb is relatively flat. The second, or descending, part of the duodenum takes a sharp curve and descends along the head of the pancreas for 7–10 cm. The close proximity of the second portion of the duodenum to the head of the pancreas allows endoscopic ultrasonography and transduodenal biopsy of lesions in the head of the pancreas. The common bile duct and ventral pancreatic duct (Wirsung) enter the second portion of the duodenum via the posteromedially located ampulla of Vater. The accessory pancreatic duct (Santorini) enters the duodenum approximately 2 cm proximal to the ampulla of Vater. The third, or horizontal, part of the duodenum passes from right to left across the spine, inclining upward about 5–8 cm. The fourth, or ascending, part of the duodenum starts left of the spine, ascends leftward and terminates at the ligament of Treitz, where the intestine angles anteriorly and downward as the jejunum.

Circulation

Gastric and duodenal blood supply is derived from the celiac and superior mesenteric (SMA) arteries; both arise from the abdominal aorta. The short celiac artery branches to form the splenic, left gastric, and common hepatic arteries. A dense anastomotic network encircles the stomach, formed by vessels

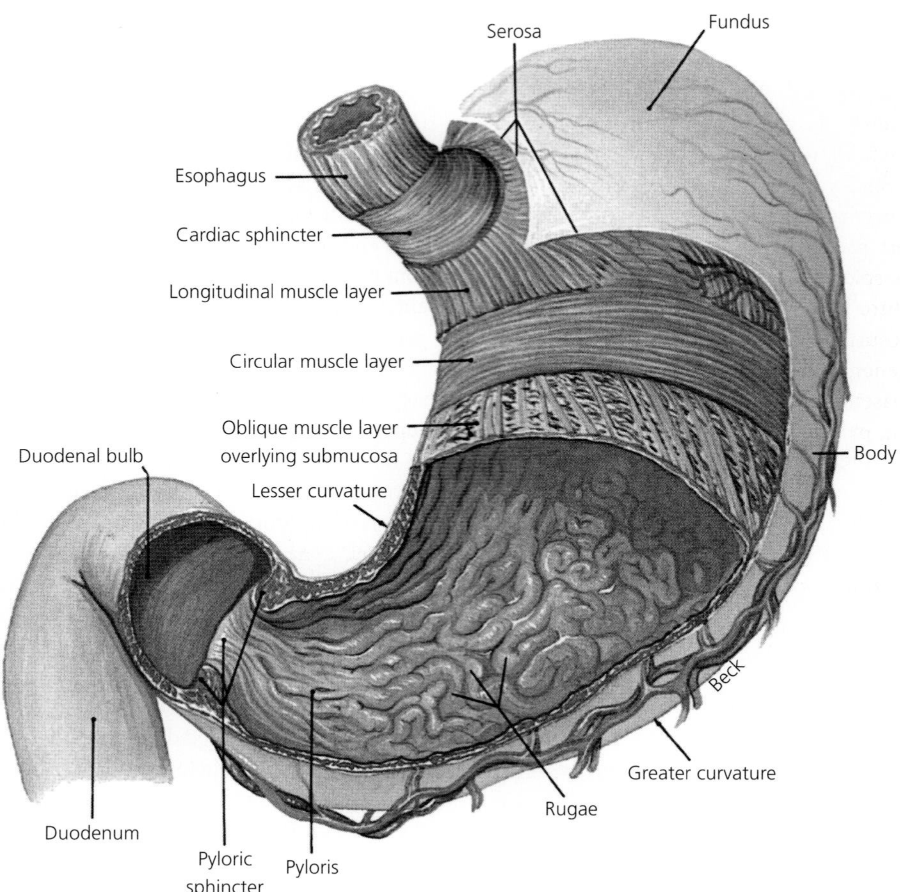

Figure 4.2 Muscle layers and rugal folds of the stomach. Source: Thibodeau and Patton 1996 [89]. Reproduced with permission of Elsevier.

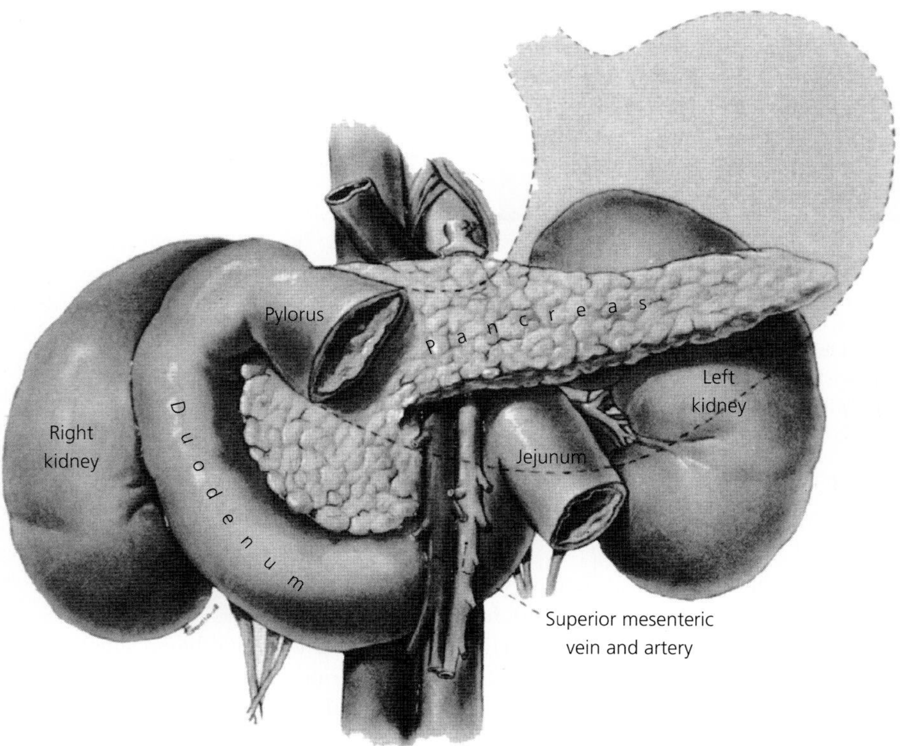

Figure 4.3 Anatomical relationships of the four parts of the duodenum to adjacent organs. The stomach is shown in outline. Source: Rosse and Gaddum-Rosse 1997 [90]. Reproduced with permission of Wolters Kluwer Health.

that branch from these major arteries. These vessels include the left gastric artery, which feeds the anterior and superior portions of the stomach; the right gastric, gastroduodenal, and right gastroepiploic arteries, which arise from the hepatic artery and feed the lower right portion of the stomach and the lower greater curvature; and the short gastric and left gastroepiploic arteries, which arise from the splenic artery to feed the fundus and the upper greater curvature (Figure 4.4). Because of the extensive anastomotic network surrounding the stomach, gastric ischemia is uncommon and generally occurs only with systemic aberrations in blood flow, gastric volvulus, or previous gastric surgery.

The distal stomach, pylorus, and duodenum are supplied by the inferior pancreaticoduodenal branch of the SMA. The duodenum is also nourished by the right gastric and superior pancreaticoduodenal arteries that arise from the hepatic artery.

Venous drainage from the stomach and duodenum leads directly or indirectly to the portal vein. From the stomach, the left and right gastric veins drain the lesser curvature, and the right and left gastroepiploic and short gastric veins drain the greater curvature. The short gastric veins and often the gastroepiploic veins drain into the portal circulation via the splenic vein. From the duodenum, the anterior inferior and superior pancreaticoduodenal veins drain into the superior mesenteric vein. The posterior superior pancreaticoduodenal vein drains directly into the portal vein. Venous drainage of the stomach becomes clinically relevant in the presence of portal hypertension or splenic vein thrombosis. With increased portal venous pressure or obstruction, venous drainage from the gastric vein is diverted to the systemic circulation via the azygous vein, resulting in the development of gastroesophageal varices. Isolated gastric varices occur as a result of splenic vein thrombosis which impairs the drainage of the short gastric and gastroepiploic veins.

Lymphatics

The pattern of lymphatic drainage of the stomach is similar to that for its vasculature, with most lymph draining ultimately into celiac nodes. Submucosal, muscular, and serosal lymphatics join to drain into four major groups from the stomach and two from the duodenum. The first group of gastric lymphatics follows the left gastric artery, receives branches from the upper stomach, and ends in the superior gastric nodes surrounding the gastroesophageal junction. The second group drains the fundus and proximal stomach, follows the short gastric and left gastroepiploic arteries, and ends in the pancreaticolienal and splenic nodes, which drain into celiac nodes. The third group drains the distal greater curvature into inferior gastric nodes connected to subpyloric nodes. The final group of gastric lymphatics drains the pyloric area into superior gastric, hepatic, and subpyloric nodes. In the duodenum, anterior and posterior lymphatics drain into a series of small pancreaticoduodenal nodes near the boundary between the pancreas and duodenum. Efferents from these lymph nodes run superiorly and inferiorly to hepatic and pancreatic nodes, respectively, and to preaortic (superior mesenteric) nodes near the origin of the SMA.

Innervation

The stomach and duodenum are innervated by sympathetic and parasympathetic neurons of the autonomic nervous system. Sympathetic neuron cell bodies are located in the gray matter of the anterior columns of spinal thoracic segments T6–T12. Neural axons exit the spinal cord by the ventral roots and unite to form the greater and lesser splanchnic nerves that synapse in the celiac ganglia. Postganglionic fibers follow the hepatic, splenic, and left gastric arteries to the stomach, where they form perivascular intramural autonomic plexuses. Gastric afferent fibers follow the

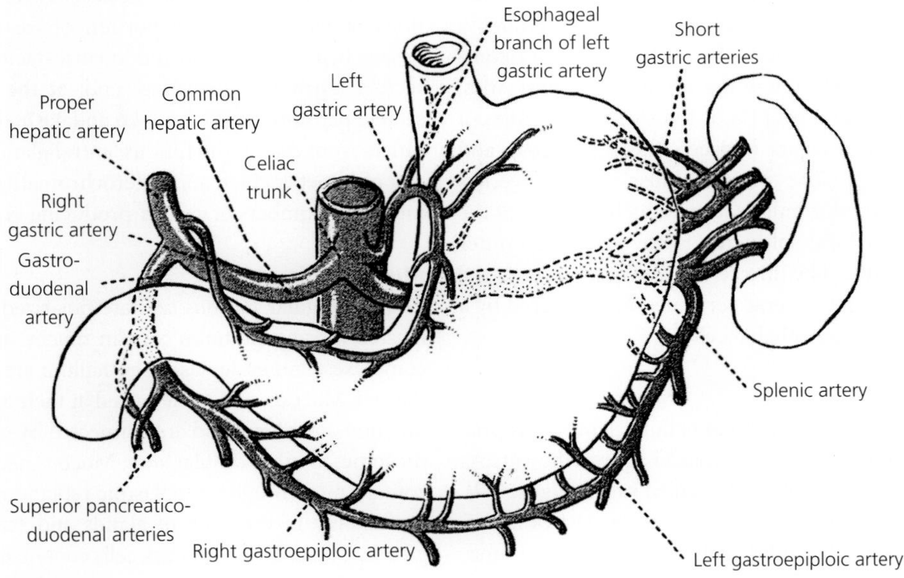

Figure 4.4 Illustration of the arterial supply of the stomach. Source: Hollinshead and Rosse C. 1985 [91]. Reproduced with permission of Wolters Kluwer Health.

same course as efferent fibers; however, they pass through the celiac ganglia without synapsing, reaching cell bodies in dorsal root ganglia of the spinal cord. Afferent fibers transmit visceral pain sensation from the stomach and duodenum.

The vagus nerve, originating in the dorsal motor nucleus in the medulla, provides parasympathetic innervation to the stomach and duodenum. Vagal fibers course along the esophagus and enter the abdomen as the posterior and anterior vagal trunks containing preganglionic efferent and visceral afferent fibers. Efferent fibers synapse with gastric cholinergic and peptidergic neurons that innervate cells directly. Although afferent vagal fibers predominate, little is known about their function.

After entering the abdomen at the esophageal hiatus of the diaphragm, the anterior vagal trunk divides almost immediately into anterior gastric and hepatic branches. The anterior branch innervates the cardia and provides a branch running to the right of the lesser curvature as the anterior nerve of Latarjet. The hepatic branch innervates the liver, gallbladder, pylorus, and proximal duodenum. The posterior vagal trunk divides into celiac and posterior gastric branches. The former innervates the pancreas and other abdominal viscera. The posterior gastric branch innervates both surfaces of the stomach and forms the posterior nerve of Latarjet. The anterior and posterior nerves of Latarjet course along the lesser curvature, give off branches to the fundus and body, and terminate in a crow's foot neural distribution to the antrum and pylorus.

Preganglionic vagal fibers synapse with ganglia in the intrinsic plexuses of the gastric wall: the myenteric (Auerbach) and submucosal (Meissner) plexuses. Postganglionic fibers innervate secretory and muscle cells. A growing body of literature suggests the nervous system plays an important role in gastric neoplasia, and is a potential therapeutic target [4,5].

Microscopic anatomy

The stomach and duodenum have four tissue layers: mucosa, submucosa, muscularis propria, and serosa. The submucosa represents a connective tissue layer beneath the mucosa composed of a loose framework containing vasculature, lymphatics, and nerves. The muscularis propria of the stomach consists of a series of three muscle layers between the submucosa and the serosa (Figure 4.2). The oblique muscle layer overlies the submucosa. The circular muscle layer, which thickens at the pylorus to form the pyloric sphincter, is covered by an outer longitudinal muscle layer. The thin serosa, the outer layer of the stomach that serves as the visceral peritoneum, is covered by a monolayer of squamous mesothelial cells.

Stomach

The gastric mucosa is divided into epithelium, lamina propria, and muscularis mucosae. When the stomach is empty, the mucosa and submucosa contract into thick folds called *rugae* (Figure 4.2). As the stomach distends, the rugae flatten. At the gastroesophageal junction, the mucosal boundary between the stratified squamous epithelium of the esophagus and the glandular columnar epithelium of the stomach can be detected as an irregular line encircling the lumen (Z-line or squamocolumnar junction [SCJ]). Cells from this region may play a role in the development of Barrett's esophagus and subsequent esophageal adenocarcinoma. Research utilizing mouse models suggests that cells making up the epithelium in Barrett's esophagus derive from a distinct population of basal progenitor cells at the SCJ [6]. The gastric cardia is predominantly composed of mucous glands and, to a lesser extent, mixed mucous/oxyntic mucosa. Pure oxyntic mucosa is rare in the cardia, but characteristic of the fundus. At birth, cardia-type mucosa is found only within 1 mm of the SCJ and, in adults, expands as a result of chronic inflammation induced by injurious agents such as acid or infection with *Helicobacter pylori*. This expansion creates a squamo-oxyntic gap; the length of this gap correlates with the degree of gastroesophageal reflux [7,8].

Gastric pits (foveolae gastricae) which serve as exit channels for underlying gastric glands stud the gastric mucosal surface. This surface epithelium is lined by a single layer of columnar epithelial cells that extends into the gastric pits and glands. Differences in the cellular makeup of glands permit histologic division of the gastric mucosa into three types that differ in structure and function: cardiac (junctional), fundic, and antral (pyloric) (Figure 4.5). The lamina propria comprises loose connective tissue containing strands of collagen and smooth muscle, lymphatics, blood vessels, nerves, and a variety of cells, including plasma cells, mast cells, fibroblasts, macrophages, and eosinophils. Very few lymphocytes are found in the normal lamina propria, but increased numbers are present with inflammation or infection with *H. pylori* or other pathogens [9]. The muscularis mucosae, a smooth muscle layer, forms the inferior margin of the mucosa and separates it from the submucosa, which contains dense connective tissue, arterioles, venules, lymphatics, and neural plexuses. Morphologically, fundic (oxyntic) mucosa is characterized by clusters of functionally distinct mucosal cells proceeding from the luminal surface epithelium towards the bases of the gastric pits: mucous cells line the luminal surface and mucous neck cells extend into the upper portions of pits; in the mid-portion of gastric pits, parietal cells secrete hydrochloric acid and intrinsic factor, and endocrine cells secrete hormonal mediators; and, at the pit bases, chief cells secrete pepsinogen (Figures 4.6 and 4.8) [10–12]. Antral mucosa differs from that in the fundus; antral glands have a relative paucity of parietal, chief, and enterochromaffin-like (ECL) cells and increased numbers of gastrin-producing G cells.

Mucous cells

The rectangular *mucous cells* are polarized (Figure 4.7); apically located mucous granules contain mucin, and the nucleus, Golgi complexes, and endoplasmic reticulum are located at the base of the cell. Mucous cells are attached at their apical margins by tight junction complexes and are connected by gap junctions and desmosomes at other cellular sites. Mucous neck cells are similar but contain more rough endoplasmic reticulum and are located predominantly in the neck of glands and scattered deeper within glands. Because mucous neck cells contain acidic mucus (glycosaminoglycan), their granules are generally less dense than those in surface mucous cells. Mucus is released by stimulated exocytosis; hence the degree of granule filling depends on the stage of digestion.

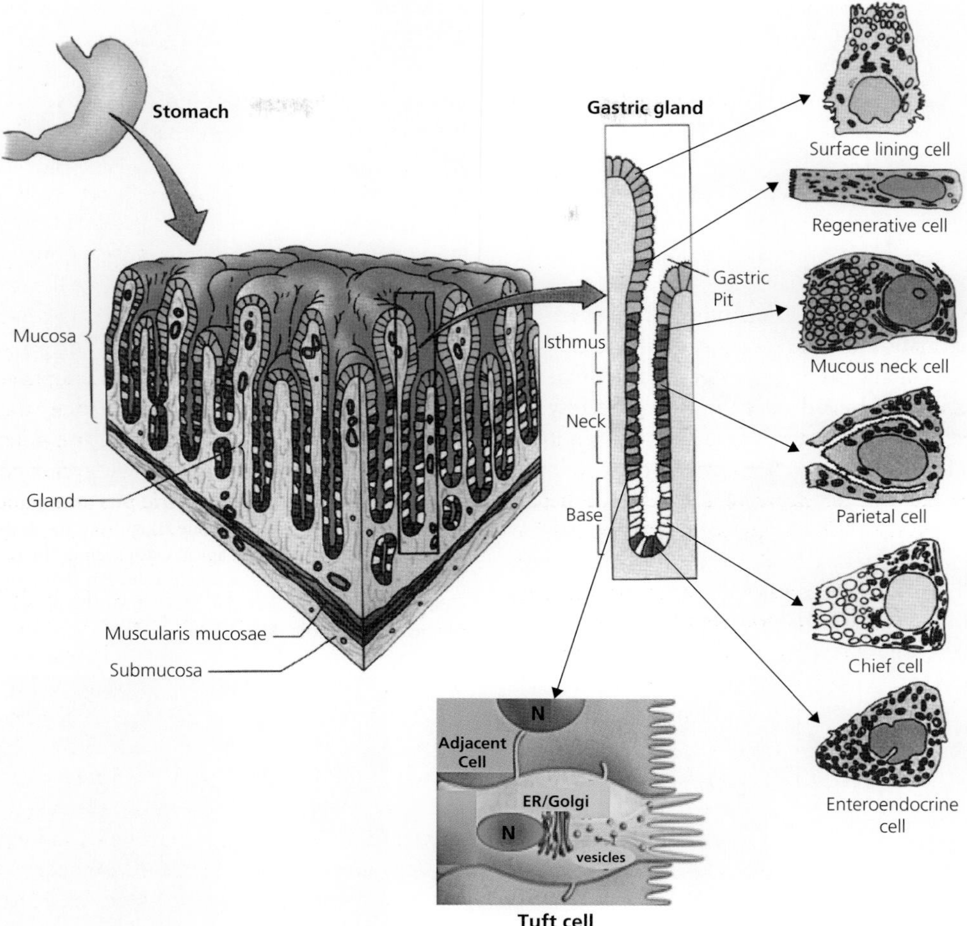

Figure 4.5 Drawing of gastric glands from fundus/body region of stomach showing approximate location within a representative gastric gland and typical histology of surface epithelial, mucous neck, parietal, chief, and enterochromaffin-like cells. Source: Gartner and Hiatt 1997 [92]. Reproduced with permission of Elsevier. Inset: Illustration of a tuft cell. N, nucleus; ER, endoplasmic reticulum. Source: Banerjee et al. 2018 [93]. Reproduced with permission of The American Society for Clinical Investigation.

It is likely that surface mucous cells, also known as pit cells, arise from different progenitor cells than mucous neck cells. This determination is based upon studies showing that mucous neck cells, but not pit cells, express trefoil factor 2 peptide (TFF2) [13].

Parietal (oxyntic) cells

Parietal cells, situated in the lower two-thirds of fundic-type glands, secrete hydrochloric acid and intrinsic factor (Figure 4.5). In glands of the fundus and body, these cells have a concentric nucleus and appear pyramidal, with the tubular apical end abutting the glandular lumen. Numerous mitochondria and tubulovesicles occupy much of the cytoplasm (Figure 4.6a). When parietal cells are stimulated, tubulovesicles expand into microvillus-lined canaliculi that course through the cytoplasm and fuse with the apical membrane to connect with the lumen of the gastric gland (Figure 4.6b) [14]. In unstimulated cells, H^+,K^+-adenosine triphosphatase (ATPase), the "proton pump" which mediates electroneutral exchange of cytoplasmic hydronium ion for potassium in the canalicular lumen, is located in tubulovesicle membranes; in stimulated cells this enzyme is relocated to canalicular membranes. Translocation of the proton pump and expansion of the canaliculi are required for the acid-secreting function of parietal cells.

Chief cells

Chief cells, a type of digestive enzyme-secreting zymogenic cell, arise from differentiation of mucous neck cells [15]. Chief cells in the lower third of gastric glands (Figure 4.5) secrete the proenzyme pepsinogen that is hydrolyzed to the acid protease pepsin at acidic pH. Chief cells maintain polarity with basally located nuclei, granular endoplasmic reticulum and prominent Golgi complexes, and apically located pepsinogen-containing secretory granules (Figure 4.8). When chief cells are stimulated, zymogen granules migrate to the apical pole, fuse with the cell membrane, and release their contents into the lumen of the gastric gland by exocytosis.

Tuft cells

Epithelial tuft cells contain a characteristic tubulovesicular system and apical bundle of microfilaments attached to a tuft of

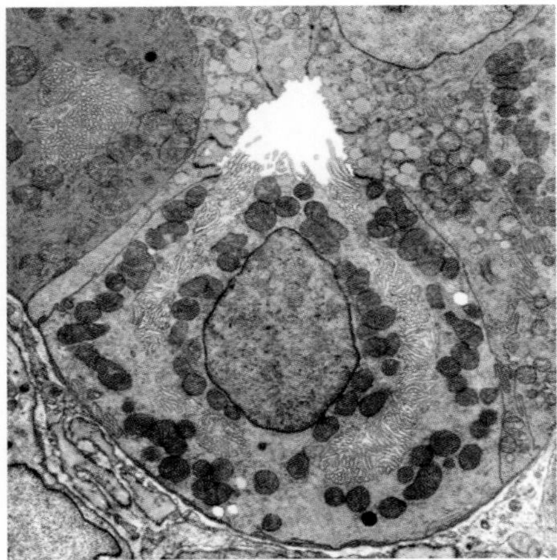

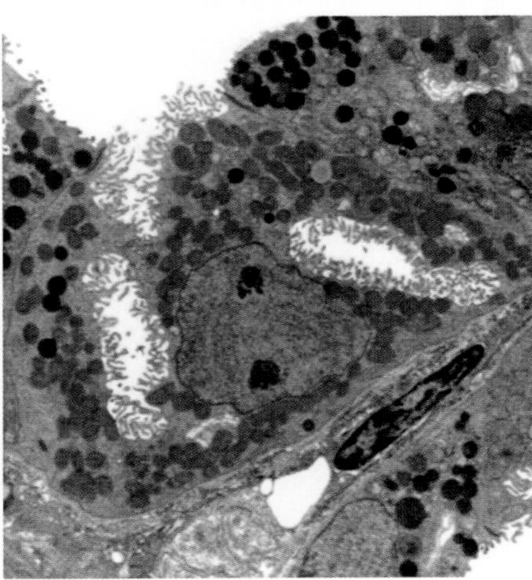

Figure 4.6 Electron micrographs of parietal cells. (Top) Resting parietal cell showing concentric nucleus (blue), abundant tubulovesicles (yellow) and mitochondria (red) within the cytoplasm (green). (Bottom) Activated parietal cell with secretory canaliculi extending from the apical surface to near the base of the cell. Nucleus (blue), mitochondria (red), Golgi apparatus (yellow), endoplasmic reticulum (cyan), lysosomes (black), and cytoplasm (green). Source: Reproduced with permission from histologyguide.com.

long, dense microvilli protruding into the lumen of the gastrointestinal tract (Figure 4.5). Tuft cell structure and signaling components suggest they play a chemosensory role, e.g., detection and immune response to intestinal parasites [16,17], and increased numbers of gastric tuft cells may be seen in gastric inflammation [18]. There is increasing evidence that tuft cells act as niche cells for gastrointestinal stem cells [19]. Indeed, tuft cells are the major site of expression of COX-1 and COX-2, and they also express choline acetyltransferase and secrete acetylcholine, thus supporting gastric stem cells [5].

Endocrine cells

Enterochromaffin-like cells (ECL) are small, irregularly shaped cells scattered near parietal cells in fundic-type gastric glands. ECL cells, which do not connect with the lumen of the glands, are packed with histamine-containing granules. Histamine release from ECL cells regulates parietal cell function [20].

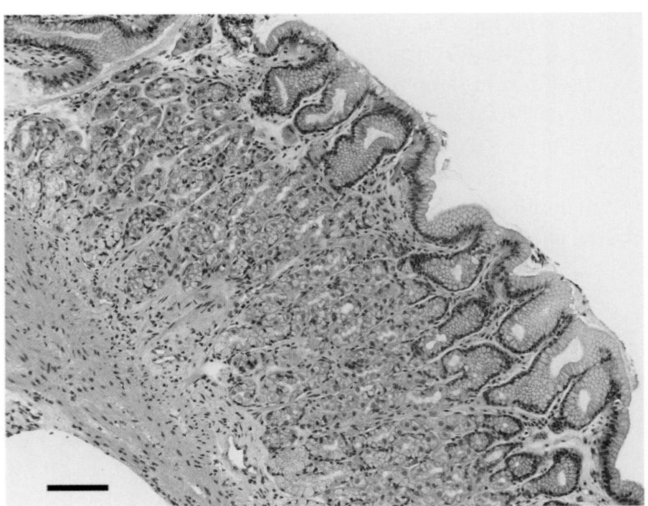

Figure 4.7 Normal gastric tissue taken from the gastric fundus. Mucus granules can be seen in the apical cytoplasm of the mucosa with nuclei located near the base of the mucus cells. Bar is 100 microns. Source: Courtesy of William Twaddel, MD, University of Maryland School of Medicine, Baltimore, MD, USA.

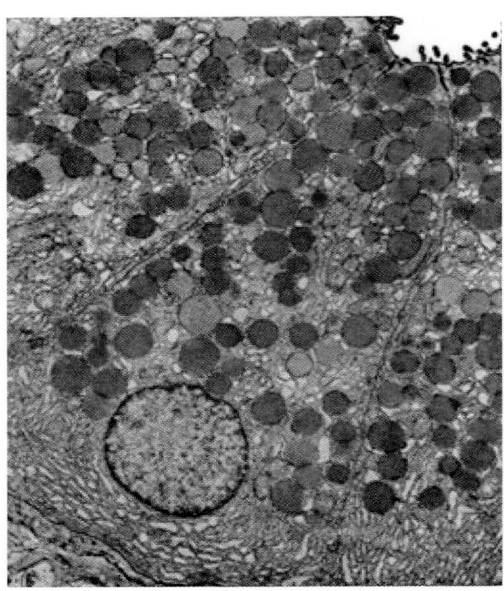

Figure 4.8 Electron micrograph of a digestive enzyme secreting chief cell. Nucleus (blue), secretory granules (purple), Golgi apparatus (yellow), mitochondria (red), rough endoplasmic reticulum (cyan), cytoplasm (green). Source: Reproduced with permission from histologyguide.com.

G cells, located in the mid-portions of antral glands and in duodenal crypts, have a broad base resting against the basement membrane that runs beneath the epithelium [21]. Dense secretory granules containing gastrin cluster near the base. A narrow apex extends to the lumen of the gland. In response to stimuli associated with eating, such as vagal stimulation, antral distension and the luminal presence of aromatic amino acids, G cells secrete the hormone gastrin into the systemic circulation.

D cells, located in fundic and antral glands, contain the inhibitory peptide somatostatin. Neuron-like extensions terminate near other gastric mucosal cells, particularly G, ECL, parietal, and chief cells. Inhibitory actions of D cells are mediated by paracrine actions of somatostatin released from these extensions [22].

P/D_1 cells are the second most abundant gastric endocrine cell, accounting for 20–30% of oxyntic gland endocrine cells [23,24]. Ghrelin and obestatin are peptide hormones secreted by P/D_1 cells. Ghrelin enhances appetite; levels are increased before and decreased after meals. Obestatin, a peptide that decreases appetite, is encoded by the same gene that produces ghrelin; cleavage of the prepropeptide gene product yields both peptides [25]. Ghrelin is produced in many organs and its receptors are found in many tissues, suggesting diverse biological functions. In the gastrointestinal tract, ghrelin has proinflammatory effects in response to oxidative stress, including promoting intestinal cell proliferation and inhibiting apoptosis [26].

Duodenum

In the pylorus, the mucosal pattern changes from pits and glands (typical of gastric mucosa) to villi and crypts (typical of intestinal mucosa) [27]. From the proximal to distal duodenum, the villi become progressively taller and thinner until they reach a villous-to-crypt ratio of 4 or 5:1, characteristic of jejunal mucosa. A monolayer of epithelial cells consisting of absorptive, mucous, Paneth, and endocrine cells covers the villi and lines the crypts. The lamina propria, composed of loose connective tissue, contains lymphatics, blood vessels, nerves, and smooth muscle fibers, as well as varying numbers of plasma and mast cells, lymphocytes, fibroblasts, macrophages, and eosinophils. The muscularis mucosa lies below and perpendicular to the crypts.

The submucosa of the duodenum provides a connective tissue framework for blood vessels, lymphatics, and nerves, and contains Brunner glands that secrete alkaline mucus. Brunner glands extend through the muscularis mucosae into the mucosa and empty into the crypts. The muscularis propria consists of a layer of inner circular fibers and outer longitudinal fibers. The myenteric plexus is located between these muscle layers.

Cellular interactions

The juxtaposition of secretory cells and neurons in the stomach and duodenum is crucial to their physiologic interactions that regulate digestion. For example, in the fundus and body, ECL cells, D cells, and cholinergic neurons must be close enough to parietal cells to allow paracrine secretory products, such as histamine, somatostatin, and acetylcholine, to diffuse through the interstitium and reach receptors on these acid-secreting cells [14]. Likewise, in the antrum, interplay between neurons containing gastrin-releasing peptide and vasoactive intestinal polypeptide, histamine-containing mast cells, somatostatin-containing D cells, and gastrin-containing G cells requires physical proximity [20].

Cellular renewal

Gastric and duodenal mucosal epithelial cells undergo continuous rapid renewal, a process involving proliferation, migration, differentiation, senescence, and loss of epithelial cells [28]. To replace surface mucous cells, nascent cells migrate upward from the base of gastric pits or duodenal crypts to the mucosal surface or villous tip. Migration of basal cells to the surface takes 2–6 days [29,30]. In contrast, parietal and chief cells are replaced by cells in the upper proliferative zone of the gastric glands, a process that takes weeks to months. Senescent gastric or duodenal mucosal cells are sloughed into the lumen.

Aspirin, indomethacin, and ethanol stimulate epithelial proliferation, perhaps by causing mild injury [31–36]. Epithelial proliferation is also stimulated by chronic inflammation, as in chronic superficial gastritis caused by *H. pylori* infection, gastric atrophy associated with pernicious anemia, and hypergastrinemic states, such as Zollinger–Ellison syndrome [37]. In these conditions, the zone of proliferating cells is expanded. In contrast, corticosteroids and physiologic stress suppress epithelial proliferation [34]. Prostaglandins appear to delay senescence and loss of epithelial cells; the resulting mucosal thickening contributes to their cytoprotective effects [38].

Gastric and intestinal epithelial stem cells

Understanding the response of gastric epithelial stem cells to inflammation is likely to advance our understanding of patterns of gastric differentiation and the development of gastric adenocarcinoma [39]. All gastric mucosal cells derive from stem cells [40,41]. Epithelial stem cells in the gastric antrum are located near the base of glands, but are located in the isthmus of the glands in oxyntic mucosa. It is likely that parietal cells influence stem cell proliferation in response to specific types of injury [39]. For example, intestinal metaplasia, a precursor of adenocarcinoma, reflects activation of stem cells in response to *H. pylori* infection, pernicious anemia, or other chronic inflammatory states.

Studies have identified markers of pluripotent gastrointestinal epithelial stem cells, including Sox2 in the antrum and corpus of the stomach, and Lgr5 in the antrum and intestine [42,43]. Stem cell markers differ between the antrum and corpus. In the antrum, Lgr5, the first marker reported [43], was followed by the discovery of several others including Axin2 [44], CCK2R [45], Mist1 (BHLHa15) [46], and a Runx1-enhancer element or eR1 [47]. In the corpus, Mist1 was the first isthmus stem cell marker used for lineage tracing in oxyntic glands [48]; $Mist1^+$ stem cells appear unique in their slowly cycling nature. In contrast, Stathmin1 (Stmn1), a recently described corpus stem cell marker, identifies an active cycling isthmus stem cell population [49]. Evidence suggests gastrointestinal epithelial stem cells are supported by vagal innervation and niche cells that provide R-spondin [4,44].

Although it was suggested that a subset of chief cells marked by the stem cell marker Troy serve as quiescent "reserve" stem cells [50], this is controversial. Lineage tracing by Mist1 may be due to isthmus stem not chief cells [48] and tracing by Troy may have resulted from haploinsufficiency of Troy-CreERT knockin mice [50]. More recent studies suggest chief cells have limited capacity to undergo dedifferentiation or lineage tracing [51].

Congenital abnormalities of the stomach

Atresia

Gastric atresia results in a blind end in the antrum or pylorus. Atresia may involve only the mucosa and submucosa or may involve the entire gastroduodenal wall. Atresia probably results from failure of the antrum and pylorus to recanalize after transient occlusion by epithelium during embryogenesis. Complete atresia is a familial disorder with autosomal recessive transmission [52].

Signs of gastric atresia in the newborn include persistent, nonbilious vomiting, upper abdominal distension, dehydration, and hypochloremic hypokalemic metabolic alkalosis. Gastric rupture may occur. Abdominal radiographs demonstrate gaseous gastric distension without intestinal gas. Initial therapy includes nasogastric suction and fluid resuscitation. Surgical treatment of a short atretic segment, involving only the mucosa, requires resection of the membrane and pyloroplasty. Extensive atretic segments require resection and gastroduodenostomy. Gastrojejunostomy should be avoided because, in the absence of vagotomy, peptic stomal ulceration may occur. Careful exploration must exclude unsuspected distal atresias.

Mucosal membranes

Congenital mucosal membranes occur in the antrum or pylorus and encircle but do not occlude the lumen. Membranes may contain squamous or columnar epithelium. Peptic ulceration can result in acquired membranes. Vomiting may occur in infancy, but symptoms usually develop in late childhood or adulthood.

Plain abdominal radiographs usually appear normal, but barium studies reveal a band-like defect in the prepyloric antrum. The antrum between the mucosal membrane and the pylorus may simulate a second duodenal bulb. Endoscopic lysis of membranes may be effective, thereby obviating the need for surgery [53].

Gastric duplication

Gastric duplications containing mucosa, submucosa, and muscle usually involve the greater curvature and share a common wall with the stomach. They may or may not communicate with the stomach. Gastric duplications vary widely in size, occur more commonly in girls, may coexist with other duplications of the digestive tract, and usually present in the first year of life. Symptoms depend on size, location, and communication with the gastrointestinal tract. Small children may present with vomiting, failure to thrive, and weight loss. In older children, epigastric pain, abdominal fullness or mass, gastrointestinal bleeding, or symptoms of gastric obstruction may occur. Rare complications include peritonitis from duplication cyst perforation, hemoptysis from fistulation to the lung, or cancer in the duplication [54]. Barium radiography, ultrasonography, computed tomography, or magnetic resonance imaging may demonstrate the anomaly. If a large part of the gastric wall is involved and complete surgical excision is not feasible, then partial excision, partial gastrectomy, and cystgastrostomy are options.

Microgastria

Microgastria is a rare congenital disorder where the stomach fails to enlarge during embryogenesis, resulting in a tubular stomach with small capacity. Infants usually present soon after birth with vomiting, diarrhea, aspiration pneumonia, malnutrition, and anemia. Microgastria is associated with developmental cardiac abnormalities, upper limb and spinal deformities, micrognathia, asplenia [55,56], and death within weeks to months. Supportive treatment requires frequent, small, high-caloric feedings and parenteral alimentation. If the child survives, surgical formation of a jejunal reservoir should be attempted, but anastomotic ulceration is common [57].

Gastric teratoma

These congenital tumors contain all three primary embryonic germ layers. They are rare in the stomach and occur almost exclusively in males. *Gastric teratomas* may present with bleeding, obstruction, or an upper abdominal mass in children, and less commonly in adults.

Imaging and endoscopic studies may demonstrate a mass sometimes containing calcified teeth or bone. Teratomas tend to be large and may require total gastrectomy and formation of a jejunal pouch [58]. Gastric teratomas are not associated with other congenital anomalies and the prognosis is good [59].

Gastric diverticula

Congenital *gastric diverticula* are rare, comprise all layers of the gastric wall, and arise primarily from the posterior gastric wall near the gastroesophageal junction. They may also occur in the antrum and pylorus, and may be associated with ectopic pancreatic tissue. Gastric diverticula may present with ulceration or bleeding, or mimic mucosal or submucosal tumors. Acquired gastric diverticula often result from the scarring and dilation that accompany peptic ulceration, outlet obstruction, cancer, or surgery.

Gastric diverticula are commonly asymptomatic and discovered incidentally on endoscopy or imaging studies [60]. They must be distinguished from acquired false diverticula, peptic ulcers, ulcerated neoplasms, and prominent folds [61]. Epigastric pain, chest pain, heartburn, and vomiting are reported. Severe symptoms or complications, such as bleeding, obstruction, and perforation, require surgical excision.

Ectopic gastric mucosa

Rests of *ectopic gastric mucosa* can be found in any part of the gastrointestinal tract and may cause ulceration, obstruction, or bleeding. In the upper esophagus, a gastric inlet patch has been observed in as many as 5% of people [62]. In the small intestine, colon, and rectum, ectopic gastric mucosa may form bleeding masses resembling polyps [63,64]. Meckel diverticula in the distal ileum may contain gastric mucosa with acid-secreting parietal cells that cause ulceration and bleeding, typically in children and young adults [65].

Hypertrophic pyloric stenosis

Neonates

Neonatal hypertrophic pyloric stenosis is a congenital condition wherein muscular hypertrophy and mucosal edema of the pylorus result in gastric outlet obstruction. This disorder is more frequent in boys than in girls – 1/150 births versus 1/750 births, respectively [66]. It has a genetic basis and is more common in Caucasians. Although the cause is unknown, lack of nitric oxide synthase in pyloric tissue may contribute to pylorospasm [67,68]. Cases cluster in families and can be associated with other disorders, including maternal myasthenia gravis, fetal rubella, phenylketonuria, Hirschsprung disease, Turner syndrome, Smith–Lemli–Opitz syndrome, Cornelia de Lange/Amsterdam dwarf syndrome, and esophageal atresia [66].

Symptoms of pyloric stenosis, including regurgitation and nonbilious projectile vomiting, typically do not occur until 3–4 weeks after birth. However, 20% of infants may develop symptoms sooner [66]. The vomitus is classically nonbilious, but it may contain blood. Despite vomiting, the infant remains hungry until malnutrition and weakness cause interest in feeding to wane. Decreased delivery of food and fluid to the intestines results in constipation, oliguria, and failure to thrive.

The baby generally appears thin, weak, and dehydrated. Abdominal examination often reveals gastric dilation, visible gastric peristalsis, and a palpable pyloric mass. Whereas gastric dilation and visible peristalsis are more evident during feeding, the olive-like pyloric mass is more likely palpable immediately after vomiting when the abdominal wall is more flaccid.

Typical upright radiographs demonstrate a large gastric air bubble with minimal intestinal air. In most cases, the detection of an "olive" on physical examination of babies with typical symptoms is sufficient for diagnosis [69]. If further testing is needed, barium studies appear to be most cost-effective [70] and may reveal a long narrow pyloric channel, giving the appearance of a double channel, and a mass effect that indents the prepyloric antrum and duodenal bulb (Figure 4.9).

Initial therapy includes replacement of fluid and electrolytes, as well as correction of alkalosis resulting from repeated vomiting. Definitive therapy is surgical. The preferred operation is Ramstedt pyloromyotomy: longitudinal division of the anterior pyloric muscle from the serosa to the submucosa. Mild vomiting may persist, but symptoms usually disappear within several days. After surgical correction of the defect, growth and development are normal, and the prognosis is excellent.

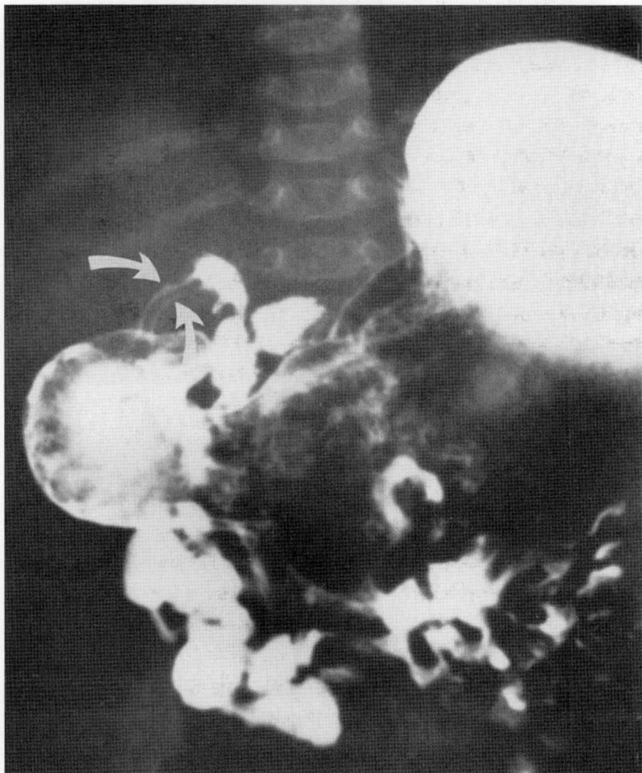

Figure 4.9 Barium contrast upper gastrointestinal series shows the long narrow double channel of the pylorus (arrows) in a patient with hypertrophic pyloric stenosis.

Adults

Most cases of pyloric stenosis in adults are acquired and result from peptic ulcer disease or cancer. While extremely uncommon, congenital pyloric stenosis can be diagnosed in adults. In these cases, there is usually a long-standing history of symptoms that began in infancy, including early satiety, nausea, vomiting, epigastric pain, and anorexia. Absence of an olive-like mass may contribute to a delay in diagnosis. Contrast imaging may reveal gastric dilation, delayed emptying, and a long narrow pyloric channel. Endoscopic dilation or surgical pyloromyotomy may be therapeutic, but to exclude a small focus of cancer, pyloric resection with gastroduodenostomy may be preferable [71].

Congenital abnormalities of the duodenum

Atresias, stenosis, and membranes

The duodenal lumen is obliterated by epithelium during the fifth to sixth weeks of development. *Duodenal atresia*, *stenosis*, and *membranes* result from subsequent failure of the lumen to recanalize. This rare cause of duodenal obstruction occurs distal to the ampulla in 80% of cases and is frequently associated with other congenital anomalies, including Down syndrome, intestinal malrotation, tracheoesophageal fistula, annular pancreas, cardiac and renal anomalies, and anorectal malformations.

In newborns with compete obstruction caused by a duodenal membrane or atresia, vomiting develops within hours to days after birth. The vomitus is nonbilious if obstruction is proximal to the ampulla and is clinically indistinguishable from pyloric stenosis. With partial obstruction, symptoms may be delayed and less severe. Rarely, duodenal membranes that persist or develop in adulthood cause upper abdominal distension, vomiting, and weight loss.

When obstruction is distal to the duodenal bulb, plain abdominal radiography or ultrasonography shows a "double bubble" caused by a distended stomach and duodenal bulb (Figure 4.10) [72]. The absence of distal intestinal gas suggests complete obstruction.

Initial treatment consists of nasogastric suction, with fluid and electrolyte repletion. Definitive treatment is surgical, with gastrojejunostomy or duodenojejunostomy, depending on the level of obstruction [73]. At surgery, other correctable anomalies should be sought as the prognosis usually depends on the outcome of associated anomalies. In adults, endoscopic obliteration of duodenal membranes may be successful [74,75].

Annular pancreas

Annular pancreas is a rare condition that may result in complete or partial obstruction of the second part of the duodenum [76]. The cause is unknown but probably involves incomplete migration of the ventral pancreatic bud during embryogenesis. This results in a

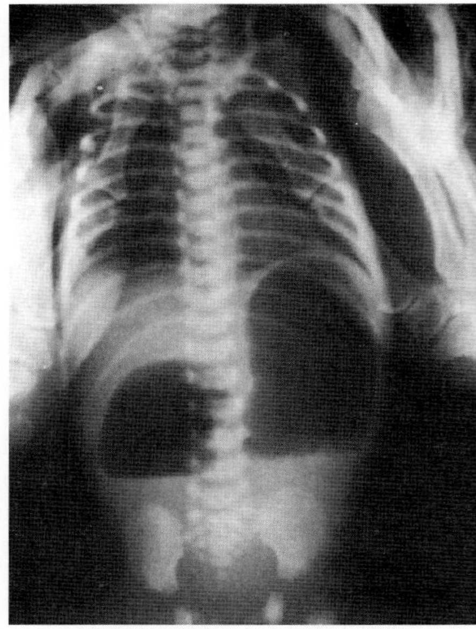

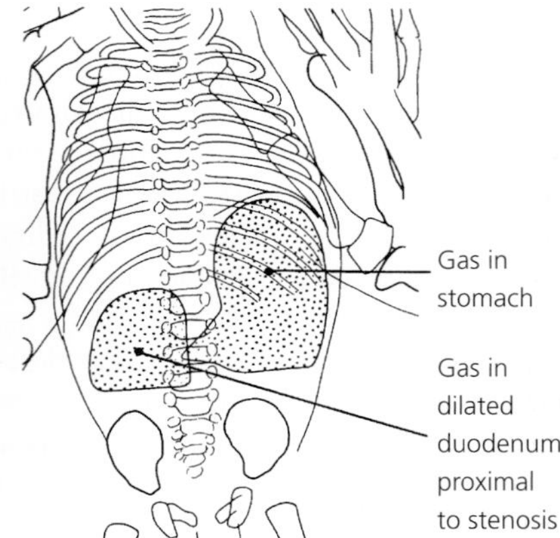

Figure 4.10 Plain abdominal radiograph in an infant with duodenal atresia shows the double-bubble sign. The stomach and the proximal duodenum are distended with air. Source: Misiewicz et al. 1994 [94]. Reproduced with permission of Elsevier.

pancreatic remnant within the duodenal wall or pancreatic encirclement of the duodenum. Annular pancreas is associated with intestinal malrotation, Down syndrome, facial cleft, imperforate anus, and cardiac and tracheoesophageal malformations [77].

Neonates present with intractable vomiting whereas children and young adults have abdominal pain and distension with less dramatic vomiting. The clinical presentation and plain abdominal radiographs are similar to those for duodenal obstruction caused by duodenal atresia, including a double-bubble sign. Imaging and endoscopy confirm the level of duodenal obstruction and may establish the diagnosis (Figure 4.11). In adults, endoscopic retrograde cholangiopancreatography can establish the diagnosis if the duct from the annular pancreas joins the main pancreatic duct. Endoscopic ultrasonography can identify bands of pancreatic tissue encircling the duodenum [78]. Impaired pancreatic ductal flow may result in acute or chronic pancreatitis.

Resection or division of the annular pancreatic segment may cause pancreatitis or fistulas and should not be performed. Definitive therapy requires duodenoduodenostomy or duodenojejunostomy. Laparoscopic gastrojejunostomy has been successful in adults [79]. Surgical results are good; long-term prognosis depends on the outcome of associated anomalies.

Duplication

Duplications are cystic or tubular malformations that contain all layers of the normal duodenum and may communicate with the main lumen. Intestinal obstruction may be secondary to compression by mass effect causing symptoms of upper abdominal distension, early satiety, and vomiting. Duodenal duplications may ulcerate, bleed, and, rarely, penetrate into the head of the pancreas, causing pancreatitis [80,81]. Diagnosis can be established by imaging. Treatment is surgical; the approach depends on the relationship of the cyst with the biliary and pancreatic ducts, as well as the vasculature. If total resection is not possible, cystenterostomy may suffice.

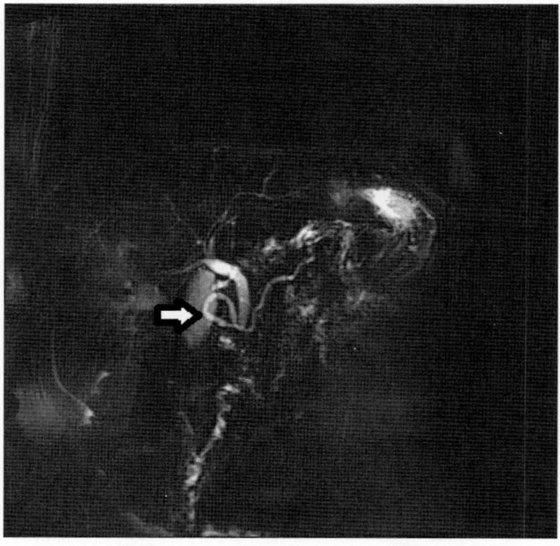

Figure 4.11 Magnetic resonance cholangiopancreatography image showing annular pancreas. The pancreatic duct is seen encircling the duodenum (arrow). Source: Courtesy of Barry Daly, MD, University of Maryland School of Medicine, Baltimore, MD, USA.

Malrotation

In children, *intestinal malrotation* is the most common cause of duodenal obstruction [82]. It results when the embryological duodenojejunal loop does not rotate normally around the SMA and the duodenum fails to complete its rotation. Consequently, the ligament of Treitz is situated to the right of midline, thereby kinking the duodenum. If the cecum fails to rotate completely into the right lower abdomen, or when the hepatic flexure lies medial to the duodenum, mesenteric bands may also compress the duodenum. Other developmental anomalies, such as duodenal atresia, annular pancreas, or Hirschsprung disease, are present in 30–60% of patients with intestinal malrotation.

Patients with malrotation typically present within the first few weeks of life with bilious vomiting and abdominal distension. Intestinal peristalsis may be visible on the abdominal wall. Occasionally, lax mesentery results in intestinal or cecal volvulus. If the vasculature becomes twisted, intestinal ischemia can ensue. Some patients with malrotation present later in life with weight loss, hypoproteinemia, chylous ascites, postprandial vomiting, and abdominal distension.

Plain films demonstrate a large gastric air bubble and distended duodenum proximal to the obstruction. An upper gastrointestinal series or computed tomography scan can confirm the obstruction and may identify the type and extent of malrotation. Ultrasonography may reveal obstruction or volvulus caused by malrotation in utero.

Treatment is surgical: division of obstructing bands, resection of infarcted bowel, and fixation of the cecum to prevent further episodes of volvulus. When extensive bowel resection is required, mortality approaches 20% and survivors may develop short bowel syndrome.

Superior mesenteric artery syndrome

Rarely, the SMA obstructs the third portion of the duodenum by compressing it against fixed retroperitoneal structures. Although *SMA syndrome* has been attributed to an acute angle between this vessel and the aorta, thereby trapping the duodenum, the exact cause is unknown. This syndrome has been associated with rapid childhood growth, profound weight loss, abdominal surgery, inflammatory diseases of the abdomen, and immobilization in a cast that increases lordosis and accentuates the angle of the SMA with the aorta [83,84]. Symptoms include episodic epigastric pain associated with vomiting, and may be acute or chronic.

In adults, plain abdominal radiographs are usually unremarkable, but in children a double-bubble sign may be seen (Figure 4.10). Upper gastrointestinal contrast studies may show dilation behind an abrupt cutoff in the third portion of the duodenum. On abdominal angiography, lateral views may show the narrowed angle of the SMA with the aorta. It is important to exclude other causes of abdominal pain.

Medical therapy includes frequent small feedings and patients may benefit from lying prone or on their left side postprandially. In some cases, weight gain or removal of a body cast improves symptoms. Laparoscopic lysis of the ligament of Treitz was beneficial in a few cases [85]. Duodenojejunostomy is required in refractory cases.

Preduodenal portal vein

A *preduodenal portal vein* is an extremely rare condition that can cause duodenal obstruction. In early embryonic life, the preduodenal vein helps to drain the primitive gut. A preduodenal portal vein occurs when this vein does not atrophy later in embryogenesis and is associated with other congenital malformations, including duodenal stenosis or atresia, annular pancreas, intestinal malrotation, and biliary tract abnormalities [86].

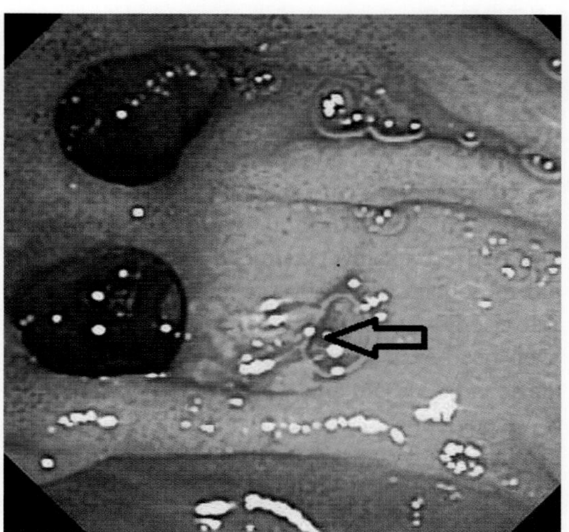

Figure 4.12 Endoscopic image of duodenal diverticula adjacent to the duodenal papilla (arrow).

Duodenal diverticula

Congenital and acquired *duodenal diverticula* usually occur within a few centimeters of the ampulla of Vater (Figure 4.12) [87]. The ampulla may lie within the diverticulum or on its rim. These diverticula are usually asymptomatic and found incidentally on imaging or endoscopy. Rarely, duodenal diverticula can bleed, perforate, or obstruct the common bile duct. Most cases of biliary obstruction associated with a duodenal diverticulum result from another cause, such as choledocholithiasis or neoplasms. Symptomatic diveticula are best treated by choledochoduodenostomy or Roux-en-Y choledochojejunostomy rather than excision of the diverticulum.

References are available at www.yamadagastro.com/textbook7e

Further reading

Bekaii-Saab T., El-Rayes B. Identifying and targeting cancer stem cells in the treatment of gastric cancer. Cancer 2017;123:1303.

Eisenberg R. Gastrointestinal Radiology: A Pattern Approach. 4th ed. Philadelphia: Lippincott, Williams and Wilkins; 2002.

Han M.E., Oh S.O. Gastric stem cells and gastric cancer stem cells. Anat Cell Biol 2013;46:8.

Amrita A., Mckinley E.T, von Moltke J., et al. Interpreting heterogeneity in intestinal tuft cell structure and function. J Clin Invest 2018; 128:1711.

Kumar R. Textbook of Human Embryology. New Delhi: I. K. International Pvt Ltd; 2008.

Morris G., Kennedy A., Cochran W. Small bowel congenital anomalies: a review and update. Curr Gastroenerol Rep 2016;18:16.

Netter F. Atlas of Human Anatomy, Professional Edition. 7th ed. Philadelphia: Elsevier; 2018.

Ovalle W., Nahirney P. Netter's Essential Histology. 2nd ed. Philadelphia: Saunders; 2013.

Schubert M.L. Stomach and duodenum. Curr Opin Gastroenterol 2019;35:507.

Sell S. Stem Cells Handbook. 2nd ed. Totowa, NJ: Humana Press; 2013.

Wani A.A., Maqsood S., Lala P., et al. Annular pancreas in adults: a report of two cases and review of literature. JOP 2013;14:277.

CHAPTER 5

Small intestine: anatomy and structural anomalies

Anisa Shaker[1] and Deborah C. Rubin[2]
[1]Keck School of Medicine of the University of Southern California, Los Angeles, CA, USA
[2]Washington University School of Medicine, Saint Louis, MO, USA

Chapter menu

Embryology and development

A brief synopsis of the major events in midgut morphogenesis is presented as a basis for understanding the congenital anomalies discussed in subsequent sections (see also Chapter 1).

The primitive human gut forms when the dorsal part of the yolk sac is incorporated into the embryo at the fourth week of development, giving rise to the foregut, midgut, and hindgut [1]. The foregut is the progenitor of the esophagus, stomach, duodenum up to the biliary duct ampulla, pharynx, respiratory tract, liver, pancreas, and biliary tract. The midgut gives rise to the duodenum distal to the common bile duct, jejunum, ileum, cecum, appendix, ascending colon, and half to two-thirds of the transverse colon. The rest of the colon and the superior anal canal are derived from the hindgut.

The gut endoderm is the precursor of the gastrointestinal tract epithelium. Its endothelium arises from the ectoderm of the stomodeum and proctodeum as well as the endoderm. The splanchnic mesenchyme supplies the muscular and connective tissue components of the gastrointestinal tract. The midgut first freely communicates with the yolk sac and then narrows to be connected by the omphalomesenteric or vitelline duct. The primitive gut forms a U-shaped loop; this grows so rapidly in comparison with the embryo that it herniates into the umbilical cord at the sixth week of gestation. The proximal limb of the loop elongates into multiple intestinal loops, whereas the distal limb simply develops into the cecal diverticulum. The first stage of rotation is 90° counterclockwise around the superior mesenteric artery axis. At 10 weeks, the intestines return into the abdominal cavity and rotate a further 180° counterclockwise in the second stage. Finally, the cecum and appendix descend from the right upper quadrant to the right lower quadrant, and the proximal part of the colon elongates to form the hepatic flexure and ascending colon (third stage of rotation). Fixation occurs as the ascending colonic mesentery fuses with the parietal peritoneum and becomes fixed retroperitoneally. The small bowel mesentery attains a broad-based attachment to the posterior abdominal wall, extending from the duodenal–jejunal junction to the ileocecal region. The end result of this process is the normal location of the small and large intestine (Figure 5.1).

Gross anatomy

The small intestine begins at the pyloric sphincter of the stomach and extends to the cecum. Approximately 600 cm long, the small bowel is composed of three major segments: the duodenum, the jejunum, and the ileum. The junction between the duodenum and the jejunum is anatomically demarcated by the ligament of Treitz. No similar landmark distinguishes the jejunum from the ileum, but the jejunum is usually defined as the proximal two-fifths of the small bowel, and the ileum as the distal three-fifths.

Yamada's Textbook of Gastroenterology, Seventh Edition. Edited by Timothy C. Wang, Michael Camilleri, Benjamin Lebwohl, Anna S. Lok, William J. Sandborn, Kenneth K. Wang, and Gary D. Wu.

Companion website: www.yamadagastro.com/textbook7e

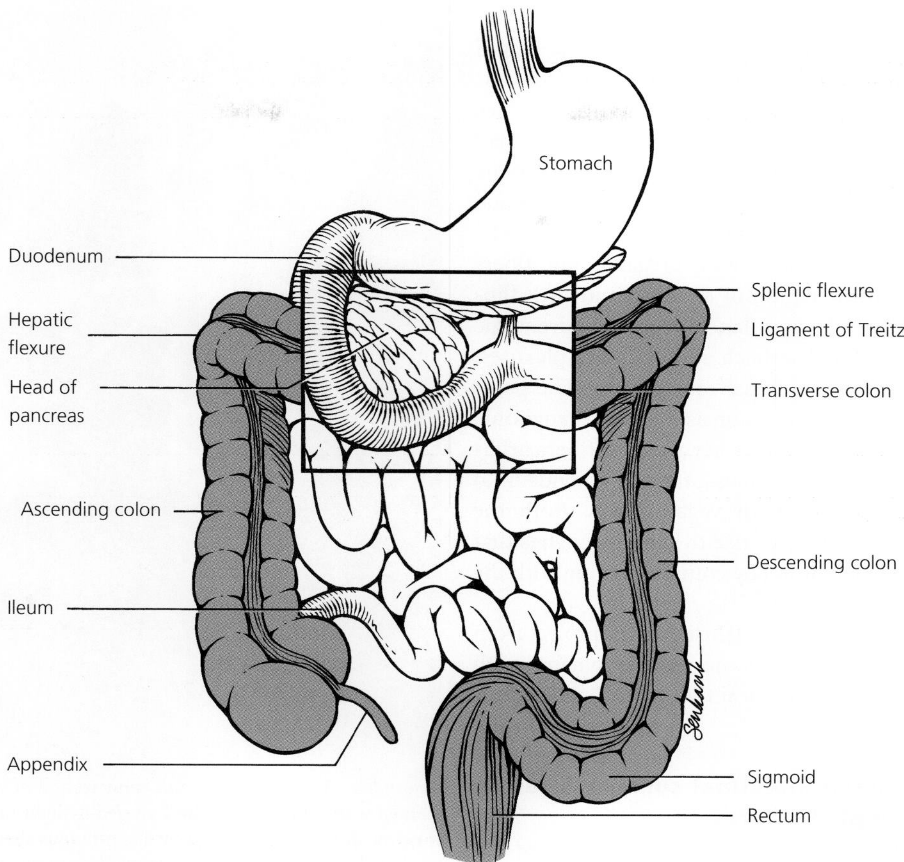

Figure 5.1 Anatomical relations of the stomach, small intestine, and large intestine. The duodenum encircles the head of the pancreas and is retroperitoneal. As the intestine reenters the peritoneal cavity at the ligament of Treitz, it becomes the jejunum. Generally, the jejunal bowel loops are located in the left and middle upper abdomen, the proximal ileum in the middle abdominal region, and the distal ileal loops in the right lower quadrant. Inset: Retroperitoneal duodenal loop and the ligament of Treitz, located behind the transverse colon.

After the appropriate rotation of the gut and its return to the abdominal cavity in fetal life, the normal position of the small bowel loops is attained. The jejunum is generally located in the mid upper and left upper quadrants, the proximal ileum in the middle abdominal region, and the distal ileum in the right lower quadrant [2].

The first part of the duodenum, the bulb, is invested with mesentery. The descending, transverse, and ascending parts of the duodenum are retroperitoneal and partially encircle the pancreatic head (see Figure 5.1). The jejunum begins at the ligament of Treitz as the small intestine reenters the peritoneal cavity. The jejunum and the ileum are invested with mesentery. The very distal ileum may occasionally be retroperitoneally located [3].

The gross appearance of the small intestine changes from the jejunum to the ileum. The wall of the jejunum generally is thicker than that of the ileum. Also, the plicae circulares, or circular folds of mucosa and submucosa that invaginate the lumen and increase the gut surface area, are prominent in the duodenum and jejunum and disappear in the middle ileum [1]. Peyer patches usually are found on the antimesenteric border of the small intestine. They are particularly prominent in childhood and atrophy with aging.

Extrinsic arterial, venous, and lymphatic supply

The arteries, veins, and lymphatics that supply the small bowel travel through the mesentery (see Chapter 11). The hepatic artery gives rise to the gastroduodenal artery, which branches into the anterior and posterior superior pancreaticoduodenal arteries. These anastomose around the duodenum and communicate with the inferior pancreaticoduodenal artery, which arises from the superior mesenteric artery. The superior mesenteric artery also supplies the jejunum and the ileum through a series of branches that form numerous arcades in the mesentery and then penetrate the intestine.

The superior mesenteric vein serves as the major venous conduit and joins the splenic vein to empty into the portal vein. Small lymph channels or villus lacteals drain into mesenteric lymph nodes located near the intestine and along the superior mesenteric and celiac arteries. These drain into the cisterna chyli and the thoracic duct.

Neural supply

The intestine contains an abundant, complex intrinsic neural supply that coordinates motor activities and consists of myenteric (Auerbach) and submucosal (Meissner) plexuses (see Chapter 12). The extrinsic autonomic innervation of the small intestine consists of components from the parasympathetic and sympathetic systems [4]. Postganglionic fibers arising from the superior mesenteric ganglion supply sympathetic motor innervation. These synapse with preganglionic fibers from the spinal cord in the region of the 10th and 11th thoracic roots and travel in the lesser splanchnic nerve. Adrenergic neurons innervate both the Auerbach and Meissner plexuses. Sensory nerves arise from the dorsal root ganglia. The parasympathetic motor innervation consists of preganglionic nerve fibers that arise from the vagus nerve. Vagal fibers originate from the dorsal motor nucleus and then divide into esophageal, anterior, and posterior vagal trunks. Both the anterior and posterior trunks give rise to celiac branches that directly innervate the small bowel by communicating with the intrinsic nervous system.

The axons of a small number of intrinsic nerves project from the intestine to travel with extrinsic nerves and synapse with sympathetic postganglionic neurons at the sympathetic prevertebral ganglia.

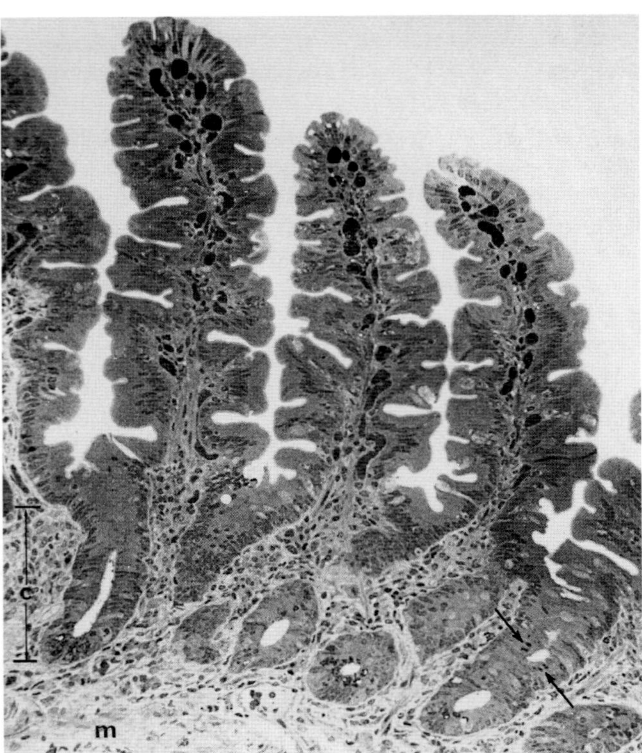

Figure 5.2 This semi thin 1 µm epon section of human jejunum, stained with toluidine blue and viewed by light microscopy, depicts the mucosa. The villi are formed by a continuous sheet of columnar epithelial cells and underlying connective tissue, the lamina propria. The epithelial sheets are composed primarily of enterocytes; mucus-secreting goblet cells are also present but are much less abundant, as are rare enteroendocrine cells and tuft cells. At the base of the villi, the epithelial cells descend into the lamina propria to form the crypts, one of which is denoted at the left (c). The crypts are lined mainly by undifferentiated crypt cells, which can be observed in mitosis (arrows). Differentiation proceeds as these cells migrate up the villus. Paneth cells at the bases of the crypts are recognized by their dark granules. The muscularis mucosae (m), a thin layer of smooth muscle, separates the mucosa from the submucosa below. Original magnification ×150. Source: Rubin 1971 [318].

Maximization of small intestinal surface area: gross and microscopic features

The surface area of the small intestine is enhanced by three features that are peculiar to the gut: the plicae circulares or valvulae conniventes, the villi, and the microvilli [2]. The plicae circulares, or circular folds, consist of visible mucosal/submucosal invaginations that are predominantly located in the duodenum and jejunum. The villi, finger-like projections that protrude into the intestinal lumen, are approximately 0.5–1.5 mm long and cover the mucosal surface. They can be viewed by close inspection of the mucosa under low-power microscopy or as tiny mucosal protrusions at endoscopy. They consist of a layer of epithelial cells overlying the lamina propria. Their microscopic appearance varies; duodenal villi are characteristically broad and leaf shaped, jejunal villi are tall and thin, and ileal villi are short and broad. At the base of the villi, the epithelium enters the lamina propria and forms the crypts of Lieberkühn (Figures 5.2 and 5.3), which extend almost to the muscularis mucosae. The microvilli are sublight microscopic tubular projections that are extensions of the apical cell membrane and compose the brush border. This complex membranous network contains the enzymes, receptors, and carriers required for terminal digestion and absorption.

Microscopic anatomy

The small intestine is composed of four concentric layers: the serosa, muscularis propria, submucosa, and mucosa.

Serosa and muscularis propria

The thin serosal lining of the small bowel consists of mesothelial cells overlying loose connective tissue. This outer layer becomes continuous with the mesentery as it joins the small bowel; many large blood vessels course through it. Those portions of the gut that are invested with mesentery are completely covered by serosa, whereas the retroperitoneal segments are invested only on the anterior surface. The muscularis propria consists of two muscle layers: an outer, longitudinally oriented layer and an inner, circumferential layer. Between the two layers lies the myenteric or Auerbach nerve plexus, composed of intrinsic ganglion cells and nerve fibers. The muscular layers of the gut are responsible for generating coordinated peristaltic movements.

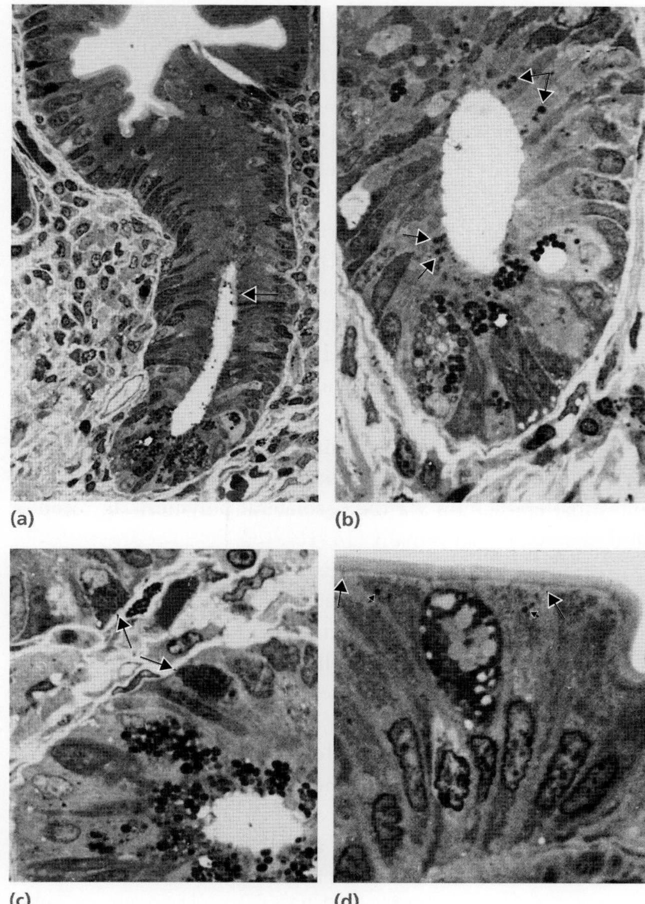

Figure 5.3 High-power views of the crypt. **(a)** A crypt is observed extending to the base of a villus. Note the prominent brush border on the differentiated cells above the villus base and the inapparent brush border on the crypt cells below. The arrow shows a short and irregular brush border on an upper crypt cell. Large, dense Paneth cell granules are evident at the crypt base; the smaller apical granules higher in the crypt are in undifferentiated crypt cells. Original magnification ×300. **(b)** The large granules in Paneth cells at the base of another crypt are located mainly in the apical cytoplasm. The scantier, lighter apical granules in cells above (arrows) are in undifferentiated crypt cells. Flask-shaped cells interspersed between the Paneth cells are crypt base stem cells. Original magnification ×700. **(c)** The large, dense apical granules in Paneth cells at another crypt base should be contrasted with the smaller, barely resolved basal infranuclear granules observed in two endocrine cells (arrows). Original magnification ×700. **(d)** Differentiated villus epithelial cells and a goblet cell. Note the tall, prominent brush border. The narrow, light zone below the brush border represents the terminal web. The numerous light structures within the cells are mitochondria. The occasional dense apical structures are lysosome derivatives (arrowheads). The apical densities between adjoining cells at the level of the terminal web (arrows) are the terminal bars. They represent the junctional complexes of electron microscopy – the tight junctions, intermediate junctions, and desmosomes; these are specialized structures that serve to bind adjoining epithelial cells at their apices. The accumulation of mucus granules within the apical cytoplasm of the goblet cell distends it into the shape of a brandy goblet. Original magnification ×1500. Source: Rubin 1971 [318].

Submucosa

The submucosa is a dense connective tissue layer containing numerous arteries as well as venous and lymphatic plexuses. Typical connective tissue cells are also present, but vascular structures predominate, consistent with the role of this portion of the gut as a conduit for absorptive and digestive products. In the duodenal bulb and descending duodenum are specialized Brunner glands that secrete mucus and bicarbonate. These are branched epithelial glandular structures that fill the submucosa and are thought to be important in neutralizing stomach acid. The submucosa also contains ganglion cells and nerve fibers, termed the Meissner plexus, a collection of autonomic nerves that communicate with the Auerbach plexus. A variety of neuroendocrine substances are produced in the Meissner plexus (see Chapter 12). These plexuses interact to produce regulated, coordinated gut peristalsis [5].

Mucosa

The mucosal layer of the gut consists of epithelial cells overlying the lamina propria, or connective tissue core, and resting on a narrow layer of smooth muscle, the muscularis mucosae (see Figure 5.2).

Lamina propria

The connective tissue core of the villus (lamina propria) contains a variety of cells and vascular structures (Figure 5.4). The immune cellular component of the lamina propria constitutes yet another line of defense between the lumen and the intestinal surface and includes lymphocytes, macrophages, granulocytes, plasma cells, and mast cells (see Chapter 14). Lying beneath the intestinal epithelium and composed of a supportive connective tissue, the lamina propria contains distinct lymphoid structures that detect and respond to antigens and microbes [6]. Most of the lamina propria lymphoid tissue is organized into aggregates of isolated lymphoid follicles or Peyer patches, clusters resembling lymph nodes [7]. Adaptive (T helper [Th], T regulatory [T_{regs}], and B regulatory cells [B_{regs}]) and innate immune intestinal lamina propria cells (dendritic cells, macrophages, intraepithelial lymphocytes, and innate lymphoid cells [ILCs]) play a role in maintaining gut homeostasis. The majority of lamina propria T lymphocytes are T helper/inducer cells that are surface antigen CD4+. There has also been identification of IL-17-producing helper T cells, Th17 cells [8]. Smaller numbers of T cytotoxic/suppressor cells (CD8+) are also present [9]. B_{reg} cells, present in the gut-associated lymphoid tissue, contribute to regulation of the adaptive immune system [8]. The lamina propria also contains subpopulations of ILCs [10], including natural killer (NK) cell subsets. ILCs are bone marrow-derived lymphocytes that react quickly to immune stimulation and lack antigen-specific receptors. Many ILC immune responses involve signals from commensal microbiota [10].

Dendritic cells initiate innate immune responses during microbial invasion and inflammation via Th1/Th17 polarization or stimulation of CD4+ and CD8+ T-cell proliferation [11].

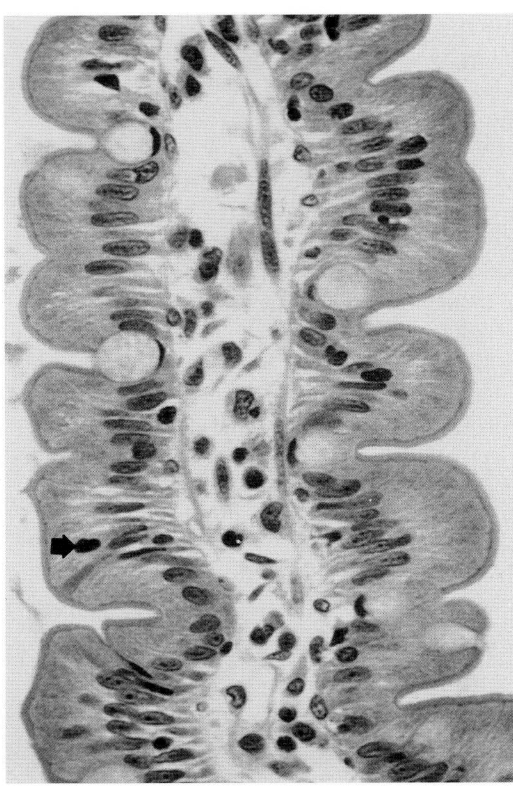

Figure 5.4 Upper villus region, with lamina propria, goblet cells, enterocytes, and intraepithelial lymphocytes (arrow). Hematoxylin and eosin stain; original magnification ×495. Source: Phillips 1989 [319]. Copyright © 1989 Elsevier.

T_{regs} and B_{regs} suppress intestinal inflammation via IL-10 production. Depending on the subtype, macrophages produce anti- and proinflammatory cytokines. CD11b+CD11c− macrophages produce IL-10, which limits inflammation through modulation of T_{regs} and inhibits myeloid cell production of IL-12 and tumor necrosis factor (TNF)-α. Finally, a subset of innate immune myeloid cells (M_{reg}) that associate with CD4+ T cells has been identified in the intestinal lamina propria. Dysfunction of these cells has been implicated in the pathogenesis of inflammatory bowel disease [8].

Intraepithelial lymphocytes (IELs) represent a heterogeneous group of T cells that reside as single cells on the basolateral side of the villus epithelial cells [12]. This specialized population of T cells is involved in barrier maintenance, reconstruction of injured gut, and host defense [8]. IELs are distinguished by an effector/memory phenotype and expression of oligoclonal repertoire of T-cell antigen receptors (TCRs) [7]. Unlike conventional T cells, antigen receptors expressed by IELs have limited diversity and do not require a priming step. In response to activation, IELs can immediately release cytokines that in turn activate and recruit innate immune cells and thereby contribute to the adaptive immune response [7]. IELs in the small intestine consist predominantly of CD8+ T cells. Classification of IELs into subtypes is based on the mechanism of their activation and antigen recognition. "Natural" or non-conventional IELs (previously known as type b) are activated in the thymus in the presence of self antigens and are permanent residents of the gut epithelium [13]. "Natural" IELs predominate in the small intestine and express T-cell receptor subtypes TCRαβ and TCRγδ. "Induced" or conventional (previously known as type a) IELs are derived from postthymically activated T cells in response to peripheral antigens. They are acquired memory T cells, similar to peripheral spleen and lymph node T cells, which migrate into the gut epithelium as well as the lamina propria and thoracic duct lymph after an encounter with antigens outside the gut [13].

The intestinal lamina propria plasma cells produce immunoglobulin, especially dimeric immunoglobulin A (IgA), which after joining with secretory component is taken up into the intestinal epithelium via the basolateral polymeric Ig receptor and secreted intraluminally [14–16].

Although the overall mechanisms underlying IgA production have not yet been fully elucidated, with ongoing debate over the relative contributions of different anatomical compartments as inductive sites, IgA plasma cells are generally thought to be derived from germinal center responses in organized gut-associated lymphoid tissue (GALT) such as Peyer patches and isolated lymphoid follicles [16–18]. IgA is the major immunoglobulin isotype in humans and its production is greater than that of all the other immunoglobulins combined [17]. IgA isotypes IgA1 and IgA2 are present in equal amounts in the small intestine [17]. A much smaller number of plasma cells produce IgM or IgG. The maturation of the B cell to an IgA-secreting plasma cell occurs during the course of a migratory journey throughout the body's vascular system. Cells exit the Peyer patches through lymph vessels, enter the mesenteric lymph nodes, thoracic duct, and peripheral blood, and then finally "home" to the lamina propria of the gut (as well as to other organs, such as the lung, genitourinary tract, and breast). T lymphocytes similarly migrate from one lymphoid organ to another and eventually home to mucosal sites, which are determined by their interactions with specific proteins expressed on lymphoid cells as well as the high endothelial venules, specialized vessels of the lymph nodes, Peyer patches, and appendix [19]. These vascular structures can also proliferate in organs affected by chronic inflammation. Macrophages and eosinophils are present in the normal human intestinal lamina propria. However, neutrophils are primarily found in inflamed rather than normal gut [16].

Mucosal immune responses are coordinated by GALT, which includes Peyer patches, the appendix, and isolated lymphoid follicles [17,18]. Isolated lymph follicles (ILFs) are small collections of lymphocytes in the mucosa and submucosa, scattered throughout the gastrointestinal tract [20]. ILF development in humans is not completely understood. While the contribution of ILFs to IgA induction in healthy individuals is not clear, evidence suggests ILFs may serve as a mechanism for IgA production once other pathways are impaired [17]. ILFs are most abundant in the distal small intestine [18].

Peyer patches are localized collections of lymphoid follicles that may be as large as 30 mm in diameter. They are most prominent in the terminal ileum mucosa and submucosa [17]. Peyer patches develop prenatally and increase in number in the gut after birth. The Peyer patch contains specialized epithelial cells, known as microfold or M cells, that overlie the lymphoid cells and allow sampling and transport of luminal antigens across the epithelial barrier [17,18,21,22]. The dome area of the Peyer patch lies above the lymph follicles and just below the M cells, and contains lymphocytes, macrophages, and an extensive dendritic cell network. The follicular or central region contains large numbers of precursor B cells that undergo active cell division. The interfollicular zone is populated predominantly by T cells. Peyer patches are also involved in the induction of mucosal immune responses [16], and are a major contributor to generation of IgA-secreting plasma cells that populate the gut lamina propria [17].

Other cellular components of the lamina propria include fibroblasts and smooth muscle cells. Arterioles, venules, and a central lacteal function to deliver nutrients into the vascular system (see Figure 5.4).

Epithelium

The villi and crypts contain a complex, rapidly proliferating, and perpetually differentiating epithelium, a continuous sheet of simple columnar cells that rests on a filamentous basal lamina or basement membrane (see Figures 5.2 and 5.3). It constitutes the major barrier between the intestinal lumen and the lamina propria and regulates flux between these two compartments. The villus enterocytes vectorially transport the products of digestion into the lamina propria, where they enter the venous capillaries or lymphatic system and are transported to other areas of the body. Tight junctions (zonula occludens) bind adjacent epithelial cells tightly together near their apices to restrict flux between adjoining cells (the paracellular route) to small ions, small molecules, and water [22,23].

The crypt and villus form the basic structural and functional unit of the small bowel (see Figures 5.2, 5.3, and 5.5). Stem cells located in the crypts of Lieberkühn are the source of the six terminally differentiated cell types: absorptive enterocytes, mucus-secreting goblet cells, enteroendocrine cells, Paneth cells, tuft cells, and M cells [24–26]. The tuft or caveolated cell is a rare but important constituent of the villus [27], and the M or microfold cell is a specialized epithelial cell that overlies the Peyer patch [28]. Cellular differentiation proceeds during a

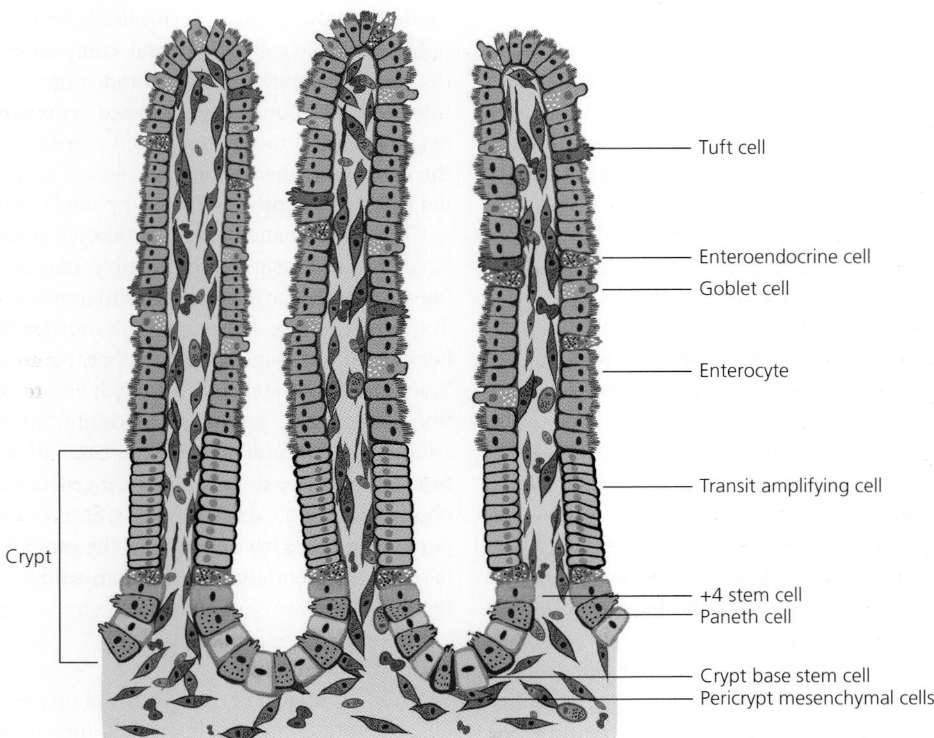

Figure 5.5 Organization of the crypt–villus axis in the small intestine. Intestinal stem cells that undergo frequent cell division are located near the crypt base next to Paneth cells. A second, longer-lived label-retaining putative stem cell population is located at position +4 above the crypt base. The stem cells divide to give rise to proliferating progenitor cells that migrate up toward the villus and differentiate into enterocytes, goblet, enteroendocrine, and tuft cells (not shown), or migrate downward to the crypt base and differentiate into Paneth cells. Pericryptal mesenchymal cells and Paneth cells provide the crypt stem cell niche. Source: Illustrated by Jessica Kion.

bidirectional migration process (Figure 5.5) [29]. Two populations of stem cells reside in the crypts: the rapidly proliferating G-protein coupled receptor LGR5+ crypt base stem cells [30] and the label-retaining injury-responsive "reserve" stem cell population located 4 cell positions ("+4 cells") from the crypt base [31–33]. Components of the stem cell niche include Paneth cells, pericryptal fibroblasts, and other mesenchymal cells [34–36]. Plasticity of the gut epithelium is a newly recognized process by which differentiated cells convert to stem-like phenotypes in response to injury [37,38].

Stem cells give rise to proliferating progenitor or transit amplifying cells, which differentiate as they migrate up the crypt onto the villus to become enterocytes, goblet cells, and enteroendocrine cells. In contrast, the Paneth cells arise as their progenitors journey to the crypt base [25,33]. Several crypts contribute cells to a single villus. The number of crypts supplying each villus varies from the duodenum to the ileum. Epithelial cell migration and differentiation occur continuously, and the process of cellular renewal and migration to the villus tip takes approximately 5 days in humans. Apoptotic cell death occurs spontaneously near the stem cell region in the crypts, presumably to regulate stem cell numbers. Effete cells are removed from the villus tip by a process known as *anoikis*, in which altered cellular adhesion results in apoptosis [39].

Cellular and topographic organization of the crypt

Knowledge of the organization of the crypt and its cellular kinetics (see Chapter 2) has increased dramatically over the past 10 years. Rapidly dividing stem cells are located near the base of the crypt [40], with a second, quiescent, label-retaining population at the +4 position, which may function as an accessory source of stem cells in gut injury states [33,40]. Also, dedifferentiation of crypt progenitors into stem cells occurs in response to injury [36,37].

The crypt base contains multiple stem cells. These give rise to proliferating progenitor cells, also known as transit amplifying cells located in the mid crypt region, above the presumptive stem cell region, which give rise to the major differentiated cell types. Wnt and bone morphogenetic (Bmp) signaling pathways are implicated in crypt formation and maintenance [41,42]. The stem cell is regulated by Wnt and Wnt ligands. Wnt signal abrogation via deletion of TCF4, an end target of Wnt signaling or mutation of β-catenin, results in stem cell depletion, crypt loss, and contraction of the proliferative compartment [43,44]. Conversely, transgenic expression of the Wnt agonist R-spondin results in an increase in crypt proliferation. Mesenchymal derived Bmp signals in turn inhibit stem cell self-renewal through modulation of Wnt activity [26]. The Bmp inhibitor protein, noggin, cross-talks to the Wnt–β-catenin pathway via PTEN/PI 3 kinase and regulates the production of transit amplifying (proliferative) cells [45] (see Figure 5.5). The sources of these signaling molecules include crypt epithelial cells, Paneth cells, myofibroblasts, and other mesenchymal cells [34,35,46].

Absorptive enterocytes

Cellular differentiation commences during migration to the upper crypt and villus base. The production of a differentiated epithelium is regulated by Notch signaling pathways. The transcription factors Hes1 and Math1 are required for the normal production of the columnar (e.g., enterocytic) versus secretory (goblet, Paneth, and enteroendocrine) cell types, respectively [47–49]. As they reach the crypt–villus junction, the cells that are fated to become the absorptive enterocytes begin to express proteins that enable the cells to digest and absorb many different nutrients. These highly polarized cells have an apical microvillus membrane and a basolateral membrane. The microvillus membrane contains brush border enzymes (disaccharidases, peptidases, and alkaline phosphatase), proteins involved in lipid absorption and trafficking (apolipoproteins and fatty acid-binding proteins), and many receptors, carriers, and transporters. Immunohistochemical and in situ hybridization analyses indicate that most major enterocyte genes and their products, such as disaccharidases, apolipoproteins, fatty acid-binding proteins, and the sodium-dependent glucose transporter, are expressed as cells emerge above the crypt–villus junction but are not found in the crypts. This precise vertical differentiation continues as cells migrate up the villus. Microvilli become more prominent, and the capacity of the cell to absorb lipids, sugars, and amino acids increases. Tight junctions are found in the apical domain and regulate permeability between epithelial cells.

Despite rapid cellular renewal, complex spatial differentiation in the gut is maintained from duodenum to colon. Many enterocyte genes are abundantly expressed in the proximal small bowel, but mRNA and protein expression levels decrease markedly in the distal gut, whereas other genes are specifically expressed in the ileum as recently confirmed by single cell analyses [50].

Cloning, sequencing, and promoter analysis of these genes have provided insight into the molecular mechanisms underlying the regulation of regional differentiation in the gut [51]. Transgenic mouse and cell culture transfection techniques have been used to map out regulatory promoter elements [52]. Transgenic mice and mice in which embryonic stem cell mutations have been generated to delete specific gene products ("knockout" or null mice) have been used to determine the function of these novel regulatory genes, including the homeobox-containing Cdx family [53]. Studies using induced pluripotent stem cells have elucidated the genes that are required for in vitro differentiation to foregut, midgut, and hindgut cell types [54,55].

Ultrastructural features

As undifferentiated crypt cells travel up the villus, they acquire longer, more numerous microvilli, measuring 0.1 μm in width and about 1 μm in height, which produce a prominent striated (brush) border by light microscopy. The development of these long microvilli, finger-like extensions of the apical cell membrane markedly increases the absorbing surface of the small intestine (Figure 5.6). The basolateral membrane is relatively smooth in comparison. As cells migrate up the villus, they acquire more mitochondria and rough endoplasmic reticulum, lose their secretory granules, and acquire large apical dense bodies, which represent lysosomal derivatives (see Figures 5.3d and 5.6). Deep apical tubules visualized by ruthenium red staining are situated between microvilli and represent areas of the apical cell surface that function in endocytic or exocytotic membrane trafficking [56]. The functional polarity of the enterocyte, with its specific apical and basolateral membrane domains, is strictly maintained, thereby ensuring the vectorial transport of a variety of nutrients and ions from the apical to the basolateral surfaces of these cells.

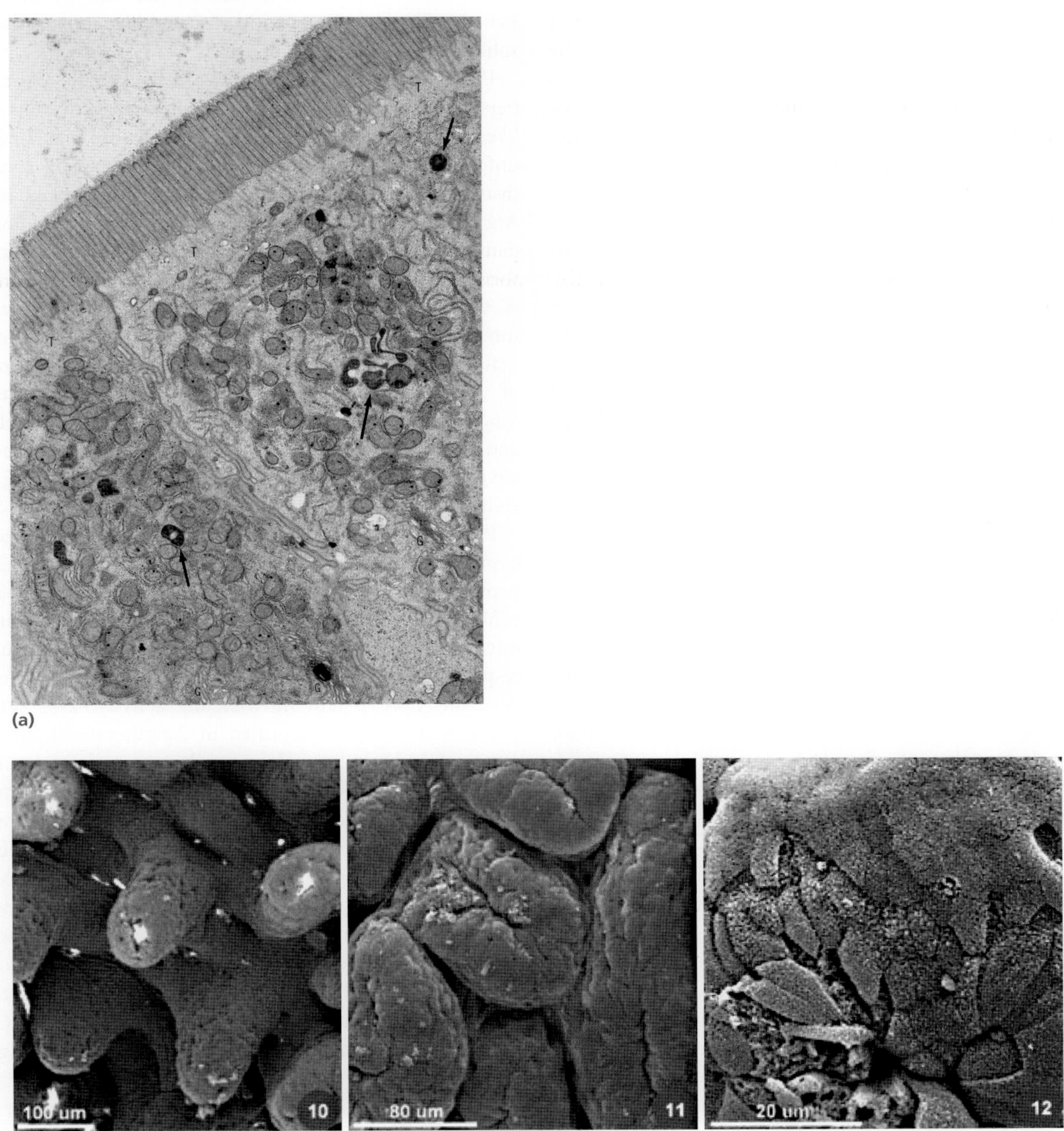

Figure 5.6 Electron microscopic images of villus epithelium. **(a)** An electron microscopic picture of the apical halves of differentiated villus epithelial cells. Note the numerous tall microvilli covered with glycocalyx and an organelle-free apical zone, the terminal web (T), just below the microvilli. There are abundant mitochondria and profiles of rough endoplasmic reticulum. The irregularly shaped dense bodies (arrows) are lysosome derivatives. The intercellular space is obliterated between the apices of adjoining cells just below the level of the microvilli by the tight junction (zonula occludens), an apparent fusion of adjoining cell membranes (best seen between the two cells on the left). Transport of substances from the lumen between cells (paracellular route) is restricted to water and small molecules and ions. Most products of digestion enter the cell by crossing the microvillar membrane. Original magnification ×15 000. Source: Rubin 1971 [318]. **(b)** Scanning electron microscopy images of intestinal villi. Source: Skrzypekh 2005 [322].

Filaments composed of actin extend from a dense plaque just beneath the cell membrane at the tip of the microvillus down the core of the microvillus into the terminal web [57,58]. The terminal web is a dense meshwork of filaments that contain actin, myosin, and other cytoskeletal proteins. The meshwork is oriented parallel to the surface and perpendicular to the microvillus filaments, and is attached to the lateral cell membrane at the intermediate junction (zonula adherens). The numerous filaments in the microvilli and terminal web, known as the cytoskeleton of the brush border, probably confer a structural rigidity to the apices of the differentiated villus cells and may provide for the movement of the microvilli. This cytoskeleton probably also affects the uptake of certain nutrients and paracellular permeability.

Short, thin, filamentous material extends from the outer leaflet of the cell membrane covering the microvilli into the intestinal lumen, producing a surface coat, the glycocalyx (or "fuzz"). The glycocalyx represents external extensions of proteins and glycoproteins in the microvillus membrane [59]. The microvillus membrane of the differentiated villus cells contains many of the enzymes, receptors, and carriers necessary for terminal digestion and absorption, such as the disaccharidases, alkaline phosphatase, peptidases, the ileal cobalamin–intrinsic factor receptor, the bile acid receptor, and the Na+-dependent glucose and amino acid transporters. The components of the microvillus membrane and glycocalyx turn over and are replenished by continuous synthesis and are transported from the rough endoplasmic reticulum via the Golgi apparatus to the microvillus membrane.

The selective vesicular transport of microvillus constituents from the Golgi apparatus to the cell apex is dependent on microtubules. Some of the microvillus enzymes are finally processed in the glycocalyx by the proteolytic activity of pancreatic enzymes, especially elastase, that are adherent to the glycocalyx.

Paneth cells

Paneth cells are pyramid-shaped secretory cells located at the base of the crypts of Lieberkühn in the small intestine. They contain large apical eosinophilic secretory granules that consist of multiple antimicrobial peptides. Although the colon is generally devoid of Paneth cells, metaplastic Paneth cells are observed under dysbiotic conditions such as inflammatory bowel disease [60]. They are much longer-lived than enterocytes, with a half-life of approximately 6–8 weeks in the mouse, longer than the original 20 days originally suggested by nucleotide incorporation studies [61,62]. The half-life of human Paneth cells is not known. There are approximately 5–12 Paneth cells per crypt in the mouse. They are removed from the bottom of the crypt by cellular fragmentation and phagocytosis from macrophages [63].

A critical role in innate immunity, host defense, and regulation of microbial density is suggested by their abundant expression of antimicrobial peptides such as lysozyme, cryptdins, and other antibiotic proteins, and by their ability to degranulate in response to live and heat-killed bacteria [64]. Wnt/β-catenin signaling and the Wnt transcriptional target SOX9 have been implicated in Paneth cell differentiation and maturation [41]. The importance of this cell type for intestinal homeostasis is supported by evidence that Paneth cells constitute part of the niche for Lgr5+ stem cells in the intestinal crypts [65] via production of secreted (Wnt, EGF) and surface bound (Notch) niche signals. Of note, recent studies in mice with depletion of Paneth cells show enteroendocrine and tuft cells as alternative sources of Notch signals [63].

Paneth cells detect microbiota and regulate antimicrobial peptide production via MyD88-dependent activation of Toll-like receptors. Paneth cell function is further regulated by the unfolded protein response (UPR) and autophagy. For example, disruption of the UPR gene Xbp1 or the autophagy gene Atg16l1 in mice leads to decreased crypt lysozyme levels and defects in Paneth cell granule content and exocytosis, respectively [66]. Crohn's disease patients homozygous for the ATG16L1 risk allele show similar Paneth cell abnormalities to those observed in Atg16l1-deficient mice [67]. Human and animal models also suggest a role for Paneth cells in pathogenesis of necrotizing enterocolitis, which afflicts premature infants [68]. Loss of murine Paneth cell function using chemical and genetic models results in an alteration of immature intestinal microbiome and mimics changes seen in necrotizing enterocolitis (NEC) [68].

Paneth cells express several of the defensins, a family of small peptides abundant in human neutrophils [64]. These 3–4 kDa peptides are also known as *cryptdins*, for crypt defensins, and exhibit microbicidal activity toward many different bacterial microorganisms in vitro. Paneth cells release defensins in response to bacteria but not to fungi or protozoa, and the defensins have potent microbicidal activity. Two enteric α-defensins have been identified in Paneth cells at the base of crypts of Lieberkühn in humans: human α-defensins (HD) 5 and 6 [69,70]. HD5 and 6 are present in a precursor form of the peptide and are processed to the mature form by the enzyme trypsin, which is colocalized in Paneth cell granules [70]. Decreased expression of HD5 and 6 has been reported in patients with ileal Crohn's disease. It is not entirely clear whether altered defensin levels are implicated in the pathogenesis of inflammatory bowel disease or are a consequence of mucosal inflammation, epithelial cell loss, and reduced Paneth cell number [66,70]. Nucleotide oligomerization domain 2 (NOD2) is expressed in Paneth cells. NOD2 activates NF-κB, which in turn regulates transcription and expression of various genes involved in both innate and adaptive immunity [70]. Defective NOD2 function has been implicated in the pathogenesis of Crohn's disease [71] and polymorphisms of CARD15 encoding NOD2 are associated with Crohn's disease [71].

Enteroendocrine cells

The intestine contains a complex enteroendocrine cell population composed of a variety of paracrine–endocrine cell types. These cells were first characterized as argentaffin or argyrophil cells, depending on their reaction to silver staining in the presence or absence of a reducing agent. These cells are classified based on their primary neuroendocrine product. For example, the D cell produces somatostatin, the L cell produces glucagon-like immunoreactivity (including glicentin, glucagon-like peptide-1 [GLP-1], and GLP-2), and the enterochromaffin cell makes serotonin. A subset of enteroendocrine cells express more than one peptide and/or amine. Taste receptors and taste signaling elements are expressed in enteroendocrine cells [72,73].

Enteroendocrine cells have two different secretory pathways, characterized by the presence of classic large, dense core vesicles, as well as a second vesicle that is smaller and synaptic-like. At least 10 different enteroendocrine cell types producing over 15 gut hormones have been identified in the small intestine [74]. These cellular subpopulations exhibit a very specific spatial distribution along the crypt-to-villus and duodenal-to-colonic axes of the gut. For example, serotonin cells are abundant throughout the gastrointestinal tract, whereas secretin and cholecystokinin cells are much more localized to the duodenum and proximal jejunum. In the mouse, secretin cells are predominantly located on the villi, whereas substance P-containing cells are found primarily in the crypts. Enteroendocrine cells may also simultaneously express more than one neuroendocrine product [75].

Enteroendocrine cells arise from common precursor cells located in the crypts [74]. The three secretory lineages (enteroendocrine, goblet, and Paneth cells) require Atoh1 for differentiation [76]. Early cell fate decisions are regulated by Notch signaling [77,78]. Inactivation of Hes1, a downstream target of Notch, results in increased enteroendocrine cell numbers. Math1 expression determines a secretory cell fate and neurogenin 3 specifies the enteroendocrine cell lineage. Neurogenin 3 cells are multipotent, and contribute to goblet and Paneth cell lineages [74]. Neurogenin 3 cells are also found near the crypt base and express stem cell markers such as Lgr5 [79]. Loss of function mutations in the neurogenin-3 gene (NEUROG3) have been identified as a cause of congenital malabsorptive diarrhea and lack of enteroendocrine cells [80]. NeuroD expression is required for secretin and cholecystokinin cell differentiation [74]. The genes that regulate the appearance of other enteroendocrine cell types are still being elucidated.

Some of the secreted products of these cells act in a paracrine manner and function locally, whereas others are true endocrine products. The peptides and amines are released postprandially [81] and variably affect bowel motility, intestinal cellular secretion, epithelial cell proliferation (e.g., GLP-2, a product of the intestinal L cell [82]) and play important roles in energy balance and glucose homeostasis [83]. In contrast to exocrine cells, which secrete apically into the lumen of an organ or the duct of a gland, endocrine cells are morphologically oriented toward the basement membrane. They exhibit an appreciable basal surface, and they narrow superiorly so that only narrow bands of apical cytoplasm reach the lumen. Their secretory granules are located predominantly in the basal cytoplasm below the nucleus, ready to be secreted by exocytosis through the basal membrane into the lamina propria (see Figure 5.3c).

Goblet cells

The mucin-secreting goblet cells are present throughout the entire gastrointestinal tract but are more numerous in the ileum than the jejunum. These cells have the shape of a brandy goblet and have apically located granules filled with mucin. They are the most abundant epithelial cell of the secretory lineage, constituting up to 15% of the small intestinal epithelium. There is evidence to suggest that goblet cells share a precursor lineage with Paneth cells. Loss of SOX9, for example, results in a decrease in both goblet and Paneth cell number [41]. Mucin is the primary secretory product of goblet cells and, as a key component of the mucosal barrier, presumably serves a cytoprotective lubricant function in the gastrointestinal tract [66,84].

In the small intestine, the epithelium is lined by a single layer of mucus that is loose, unattached, and composed of MUC2 [85]. One of the functions of the small intestinal mucus layer, therefore, is entrapment and distal transport of bacteria [85]. Biochemical differences among mucins expressed in the stomach, small intestine, and colon suggest heterogeneity among goblet cell populations. The expression of specific mucins is also developmentally regulated. Other important products include trefoil proteins, which serve both protective and reparative functions, and antibacterial proteins such as resistin-like molecule B (RELM-B) [86,87]. Goblet cells have recently been shown to form goblet cell-associated antigen passages (GAPs) that deliver luminal substances to antigen-presenting cells in the lamina propria and induce adaptive immune responses [84,88]. Goblet cells arise from the same committed stem cell as the other principal cell types. Production of a secretory cell type (including goblet, Paneth, and enteroendocrine cells) is dependent upon Math1 expression, a basic helix-loop-helix transcription factor that is a downstream component of the Notch pathway. Studies using mice lacking downstream components of Math1 have demonstrated impaired maturation of Paneth and goblet cells [89].

M cells

M cells, or microfold cells, are specialized epithelial cells with a unique cellular structure characterized by microfold ridges on their apical surface. In the gastrointestinal tract, they are most often associated with the follicle-associated epithelium of non-encapsulated mucosal lymphoid tissue such as the Peyer patch although they may also be occasionally found in the normal villi of the small intestine [22,90]. Unlike the absorptive enterocytes, they lack a typical brush border, demonstrating fewer, shorter microvilli and numerous apical endocytic vesicles. Their cytoskeleton is less rigid and the cells can be deformed by migrating lymphocytes [20]. M cells also possess a thin glycocalyx that provides better accessibility to large particulate antigens, allowing them to serve as antigen-sampling cells [91,92] and to endocytose a variety of macromolecules, viruses, and bacteria from the lumen. These molecules are then rapidly transported across the epithelium via vesicles to the basolateral surface where they are delivered to dendritic cells and then to lymphoid tissue (Peyer patches or isolated lymphoid follicles), initiating protective mucosal immune responses associated with IgA production [92].

The M cell basolateral pocket is populated by CCR6-expressing B cells and CX3CR1-expressing dendritic cells, which can extend dendrites through M cell pores to directly sample antigens overlying the dome epithelium of Peyer's patches, where they receive antigens transported from the mucosal surface by the M cells [90].

Mechanisms involved in transepithelial transport (transcytosis) of antigens across the M cell include pinocytosis and receptor-mediated endocytosis [93]. Efficient M cell transcytosis of particulate antigens and whole bacteria, including commensal organisms that are part of the normal microbiota, is facilitated by a variety of receptors, including glycoprotein, uromodulin, and annexin V, all of which bind to bacterial components [90].

M cells can be formed by culturing Peyer patch lymphocytes together with the intestinal Caco-2 cell line, or with native enterocytes [94]. B cells are required for Peyer patch development and maintenance of M cells [95]. Intestinal epithelial cells can be induced to differentiate into M cells when cocultured with intestinal lymphocytes or with Peyer patch lymphocytes that are stimulated with anti-CD3/CD28 monoclonal antibodies [96]. These and other data suggest that M cell differentiation may be immunoregulated and that lymphoepithelial cross-talk may induce M cell formation from follicle-associated epithelial cells.

The TNF superfamily member receptor activator of NF-κB ligand (RANKL) is required for initiation of differentiation of Lgr5-positive stem cells into M cells [97]. Cell-specific genetic deletion studies have demonstrated that subepithelial mesenchymal cells serve as M cell inducers or Mci [97]. These podoplanin+ subepithelial mesenchymal cells abundantly express RANKL on their cell surface and interact with follicle-associated epithelium to direct differentiation of stem cells into M cells [97]. Cross-talk between canonical and alternative NF-κB pathways may be important for augmentation of M cell differentiation. Spib is a target gene of RANKL-NIK-NF-κB signaling and is important for commitment to M cell fate. Transcriptome studies have identified several M cell-expressing genes associated with the antigen uptake process and/or transcytosis. M cell signature genes include Spib, Tnfaip2, Ccl9, Pgryrp1, and Anxa5 [97].

Two functionally different subtypes have been identified in FAE M cells based on glycoprotein 2 (GP2) expression. GP2-high M cells are mature cells that actively take up luminal microbeads, whereas GP2-negative or GP2-low M cells are immature cells that scarcely ingest them. Impaired M cell uptake and transcytosis of bacteria and toxins in the absence of GP2 suggests GP2 is an uptake receptor for a subset of commensal and pathogenic bacteria. GP2 interaction with FimH, a component of the outer membrane pilus of gram-negative enterobacilli, is necessary for efficient M cell uptake of *Escherichia coli* and *Salmonella typhimurium* [97]. Exposure of follicle-associated epithelium to *Salmonella* induces epithelial to mesenchymal transition of follicle-associated enterocytes to M cells, via a *Salmonella*-derived effector protein that induces Wnt signaling and RANKL and RANK induction [98].

Botulinum neurotoxin (BoNT), produced by *Clostridium botulinum*, is a potent metalloprotease toxin and causative agent of food-borne botulism. On its own, it is not absorbed by the intestinal epithelium. Recent work suggests that the toxicity is derived from M cell GP2-mediated translocation of botulinum toxin A as part of a large progenitor toxin complex (L-PTC) through the intestinal epithelium to neuronal cells. Mice that lack intestinal M cells due to anti-RANKL antibody treatment are less susceptible to orally administered L-PTC [97]. Similarly, cellular prion protein (PrPC) on M cells may serve as a major uptake receptor for *Brucella abortus*, which causes brucellosis during oral infection [97]. M cells are also involved in uptake of prions from the intestinal lumen [99]. Neutralization antibodies against RANKL and intestinal epithelial cell-specific RANKL-deficient mice block invasion of prion proteins into Peyer patches. Conversely, exogenous RANKL administration to mice enhances oral prion uptake and toxin absorption [97].

Finally, improved molecular understanding of M cell biology has furthered our understanding of mucosal immunity and as such, M cells have been proposed as a potential target for oral vaccines [21]. Targeting antigen delivery to M cells and regulating M cell density can lead to improvements in design of oral vaccines [97].

Tuft or caveolated/brush cells

Tuft cells are rare, secretory, chemosensory epithelial cells found in a variety of tissues, including respiratory and olfactory epithelia of the nose, trachea, and proximal airways [100]. In the gastrointestinal tract, tuft or caveolated cells are found in the stomach, small and large bowel, pancreatico-biliary system, and gallbladder [101]. They were initially identified by their unique morphology, an apical microfilament bundle connected to long, thick microvilli tufts projecting from bottle-shaped epithelial cells into the lumen [100,102]. Unlike other epithelial cells of secretory lineage, specification of tuft cells from intestinal stem cells appears to be independent of the transcription factor ATOH1. Mouse studies with intestinal epithelial-specific disruption indicate that SOX4 promotes tuft cell lineage allocation independent of ATOH1 [103].

Tuft cells are best described in the mouse, in which they constitute 0.4% of the small intestinal epithelium [104]. They are distinguished from other nonproliferative, differentiated cells of the epithelial villi by unique expression patterns of villin, fimbrin, the serine-threonine kinase 1 involved in microtubule polymerization DCLK1, growth factor independent 1b (Gfi1b) transcription factor, cytokeratin 18, acetylated tubulin, and ankyrin [102,104]. They are defined by expression of the lineage-defining transcription factor POU domain, class 2, transcription factor 3 (POU2F3) [100,102]. They facilitate chemoreception in the gut, and express proteins involved in taste transduction pathways including guanine nucleotide-binding protein G(t) subunit α3, also known as α-gustducin, and the cation channel TRPM5 [104]. Pou2f3-deficient mice lack tuft cells in the intestinal epithelium along with Pou2f3 expressing taste cells and TRMP5 expressing chemosensory cells in the nasal cavity and olfactory epithelium [102]. Tuft cells are also the major epithelial source of intestinal opioids and express components of eicosanoid biosynthetic pathways, including cyclooxygenase 1 (COX1) and COX2, and arachidonate 5-lipoxygenase (ALOX5) [27,100].

Most recently, tuft cells have been shown to be a major component of the type 2 immune response of the small intestine to parasitic helminths and protozoans by using taste chemosensory signaling pathways [100]. They are the source of epithelial IL-25 via a TRMP5-dependent mechanism and are central to type 2 immune circuits involving innate lymphoid cells (ILC2s). IL-25 activates ILC2s, promoting IL-5- and IL-13-mediated type 2 inflammation to luminal helminths [100]. TRPM5 likely acts upstream of IL-25 as TRMP5 deletion impairs the type 2 response following infection with the *Tritrichomonas muris* protozoan and TRMP5-deficient mice have impaired tuft cell expansion, reduced IL-25 expression, and a lowered frequency of lamina propria IL-17RBþ ILC2s [102].

Tuft cells input environmental signals and relay into functional outputs via G-protein coupled receptor (GPCR) signaling. Luminal succinate, a metabolic endproduct of protists, activates small intestinal tuft cells via GPCR transmembrane succinate receptor 1 (SUCNR1) followed by IL-25-dependent activation of lamina propria ILC2s [100].

Transcriptional profiling has identified tuft cell heterogeneity across and within tissues. SUCNR1 is abundantly expressed in small intestinal tuft cells but not in other gastrointestinal tuft cell populations. Transcriptomics has also identified two subtypes of tuft cells in the small intestine: tuft-1 and tuft-2 cells. Tuft-1 cells appear to be involved with neuromodulation while tuft-2 cell gene signature is associated with immunological responses [100]. Single cell RNA sequencing approaches have also demonstrated that the type 2-associated cytokine thymic stromal lymphopoietin (TSLP) is enriched in tuft cells of the small intestinal epithelium, with significantly greater expression by tuft-2 cells, suggesting differential regulation of TSLP by tuft cells unlike IL-25 which is expressed by all tuft cells [102].

Congenital anomalies

Meckel diverticulum

Description and pathophysiology

During early gestation, the omphalomesenteric or vitelline duct connects the fetal yolk sac to the primitive gut. By 7–8 weeks of gestation, this duct is normally completely obliterated. A Meckel diverticulum, the most common congenital anomaly of the gastrointestinal tract, results when this structure fails to resorb completely. The duct remnant most commonly persists as a diverticular sac; alternatively, the diverticulum may be connected to the mesentery or umbilicus by a fibrous band. Occasionally, only a thick connective tissue band remains, attaching the gut to the umbilicus. These bands may lead to volvulus or the strangulation of bowel loops. Rarely, a fistula remains patent from the ileum to the umbilicus, leading to persistent external drainage of ileal contents. Other, more unusual duct remnants include umbilical polyps and vitelline cysts.

Ultimately, proper development of the gastrointestinal tract requires balanced expression of key transcription factors involved in specification of anterior/proximal and posterior/distal domains. SOX2 is a highly conserved transcription factor important for vertebrate embryogenesis and differentiation of the gastric epithelium that is normally expressed in the proximal primitive gut. CDX2 is a homeobox transcription factor involved in establishment of anterior–posterior polarity normally expressed in the posterior gut. Aberrant expression of these transcription factors may lead to gut malformation. For example, analysis of expression pattern of these transcription factors in intestinal anomalies with gastric-type heteroplasia such as Meckel diverticulum has demonstrated SOX2 expression in gastric tissue with patches of CDX2 expression. These findings suggested that aberrant SOX2 expression rather than absence of CDX2 expression may be partially responsible for the presence of ectopic gastric tissue in the intestinal epithelium [105].

Classic presentation of Meckel diverticulum is exemplified by the "rule of twos" [106]. Large autopsy series indicate a 2–3% prevalence of Meckel diverticulum in the general population [107]. This anomaly is 2–3 times more common in males and nearly 50% of symptomatic patients present before the age of 2 years [106].

Meckel diverticula are true diverticula, containing all layers of the bowel from serosa to mucosa. Located on the antimesenteric border of the gut, they are most commonly found within 100 cm of the ileocecal valve but may also be in other regions of the small bowel. Most diverticula are between 1 and 10 cm in size; giant lesions may be as large as 100 cm in diameter. The two types of giant diverticula are the type I lesions, which are long but of the same caliber as the ileum, and the less common type II, or ovoid, lesions [108]. Heterotopic tissue is present in approximately 50% of all diverticula [109]. The most commonly found heterotopic tissue is gastric mucosa, pancreatic tissue, or a combination of the two; a recent metaanalysis showed that gastric heterotopic tissue is found in 24–70% of symptomatic Meckel diverticulum [110]. Diverticula containing colonic mucosa, Brunner glands, or jejunal or hepatobiliary tissue have also been rarely described [106]. The presence of heterotopic mucosa correlates with an increased risk for symptomatic, complicated Meckel diverticulum [110]. Diverticular gastrointestinal bleeding occurs in adults and children when acidic secretion of heterotopic gastric tissues lead to ulceration of adjacent normal ileal mucosa; almost all bleeding diverticula contain gastric mucosa [111]. Although the data are conflicting, some studies have indicated that *Helicobacter pylori* may rarely colonize the diverticular gastric mucosa and is associated with gastritis in this site [112]. Heterotopic tissue is also associated with a modestly increased risk for other complications, including small bowel obstruction and diverticular inflammation.

The risk for complications dramatically decreases with age [110], although most adults with a Meckel diverticulum remain asymptomatic and diagnosis is incidental [113–115]. Patients with Meckel diverticulum have a lifetime risk of complications of ~4–6% [115,116]. Females are less likely than males to be symptomatic [113,114]. The complications of Meckel diverticulum include bleeding, intestinal obstruction, diverticulitis, perforation, and carcinoma [117]. Obstruction is caused by intussusception of the diverticulum into adjacent bowel; volvulus around or herniation into a fibrous band; entrapment in inguinal, femoral, or umbilical hernia sacs (Littre hernia); or inflammation and scarring leading to blockage around the diverticular neck and adjacent ileum. Meckel diverticulum lithiasis can result in intestinal obstruction by movement of the stone out of the diverticulum into the distal ileum or by causing diverticular inflammation that then leads to intussusception [106].

The frequency of specific complications varies in adult and pediatric patients. The most common complications in children are gastrointestinal bleeding, occurring most often in infancy and early childhood (before 5 years of age) [118], followed by intestinal obstruction [106]. In adults, intestinal obstruction is the most frequent complication. Although earlier studies indicate that gastrointestinal bleeding is relatively uncommon, more recent series indicate that bleeding from Meckel diverticulum is also an important complication in adults [113]. Whereas adults most often describe melena, children usually present with painless, multiple, rapid, bright or dark red bowel movements. Meckel diverticulitis is more commonly seen in older adults and accounts for up to 20% of complications. It is frequently misdiagnosed as appendicitis [106].

More unusual complications in adults include the development of carcinomas such as carcinoids, sarcomas, and rarely adenocarcinomas [119,120]. Carcinoid tumors are typically small, with biological characteristics resembling those of jejunoileal rather than appendiceal carcinoids (e.g., immunohistochemical staining and metastatic potential). Patients with carcinoid of a Meckel diverticulum are generally older (in their sixth decade) and frequently asymptomatic. Other complications include enteroliths, which may become lodged in the diverticulum and cause abdominal pain, vomiting, bleeding, and obstruction.

Diagnosis

The diagnosis of Meckel diverticulum remains a challenge [110]. Sodium pertechnetate ^{99m}Tc radionuclide scanning is particularly useful in children, with a sensitivity of 80–90% and specificity of 95% [77]. The ^{99m}Tc isotope is taken up by normal stomach tissue and by ectopic gastric mucosa in the Meckel diverticulum. Surface mucus cells from the intestine as well as the stomach accumulate and secrete this anion [121,122]. To enhance the sensitivity of this test, H_2 antagonists such as cimetidine may be administered to decrease anion secretion from the gastric mucosa [123]. Pentagastrin may also be useful, enhancing anion uptake by a poorly understood mechanism [124]. The major drawback of this detection method is that heterotopic gastric mucosa must be present in the diverticulum if a true-positive result is to be obtained [125]. In children with lower gastrointestinal bleeding from a Meckel diverticulum, this test is sensitive and specific because almost all bleeding diverticula contain gastric mucosa, but in adults, the false-positive and false-negative rates of the method are high, even in patients with bleeding [126,127]. Crohn's disease and other inflammatory disorders lead to false-positive scans. In children, a scan for Meckel diverticulum is often followed by a technetium or stannous pyrophosphate red blood cell scan to localize the site of bleeding definitively.

A small bowel follow-through barium study is usually not useful because the diverticulum may not fill with barium and is also rapidly emptied. Enteroclysis examinations improve the sensitivity of barium studies because the contrast material under increased pressure better fills the diverticulum. When bleeding is present, angiography can localize the source of hemorrhage and may also demonstrate the vitelline artery and its embryonic branches. This vessel arises from a distal branch of the superior mesenteric artery and ends in a characteristic blush of tortuous small vessels. Frequently, the vitelline artery involutes, and the diverticulum is directly supplied by branches from the superior mesenteric artery. Computed tomography can detect Meckel diverticulum but is not sensitive for detecting bleeding [117]. Small bowel video capsule endoscopy has been used successfully to detect Meckel diverticulum [128,129]. Retrograde double-balloon enteroscopy may further aid in the detection of obscure GI bleeding due to Meckel diverticulum [130–132], although the diagnosis remains difficult when the lesion is far from the ileocecal valve. In these instances, MR enterography can be considered in order to localize the lesion [133].

Management

The treatment of Meckel diverticulum complicated by bleeding, obstruction, or perforation is surgical. Diverticulectomy is performed, sometimes with concurrent ileal resection if the adjacent small bowel is ulcerated, inflamed, or obstructed. These operations can be complicated, and postoperative morbidity occurs in up to 6% of all cases [116,117,134,135]. Laparoscopic removal has been reported [136–139]. Some published series recommend a search for Meckel diverticulum in appendectomy and laparotomy cases performed for acute abdomen and suggest that a diverticulectomy/resection be performed to avoid future complications [140]. However, management of Meckel diverticulum incidentally detected during an abdominal surgery remains controversial [141]. Similarly, the management of asymptomatic diverticula is controversial [142] and the data on the role of resection are sparse.

Because of the low risk for complications of Meckel diverticulum in adults, some have not recommended prophylactic removal [114,134,143,144]. However, others prefer to resect asymptomatic diverticula that are highly likely to cause complications, such as large (>2 cm) diverticula; lesions associated with an omphalomesenteric band, which are at risk for volvulus and obstruction; lesions containing a palpable mass, which may represent tumor or ectopic mucosa; or lesions in younger male patients [111,113,120].

Duplications

Duplications of the gastrointestinal tract are rare, congenital cystic anomalies attached to the intestinal mesenteric border (Figure 5.7). They may be spherical or tubular in shape. They are usually lined by gut mucosa but, like Meckel diverticula, they may contain heterotopic gastric mucosa or, less commonly, pancreatic, squamous, thyroid, or bronchial epithelium as well as lymphoid aggregates. They share a blood supply with the associated native intestine and may also communicate lumen to lumen.

Duplications may occur anywhere along the gastrointestinal tract from mouth to anus. Those of small bowel origin are most commonly found in the ileum [145]. The embryonic origin of gut duplications is unknown. Postulated mechanisms include aberrant recanalization of the gut lumen during morphogenesis, creating two attached yet distinct gut structures [105,146], intrauterine ischemic events, and aborted (partial) twinning [147]. Intestinal atresia may be associated with duplications, supporting a possible vascular etiology. Duplications are also associated with genitourinary tract anomalies [148]. Human duplications express SOX2 in ectopic gastric mucosa; CDX2 is also expressed ectopically in gastric mucosa of duplications [105]. Approximately one-third of patients with duplications have associated anomalies elsewhere [149].

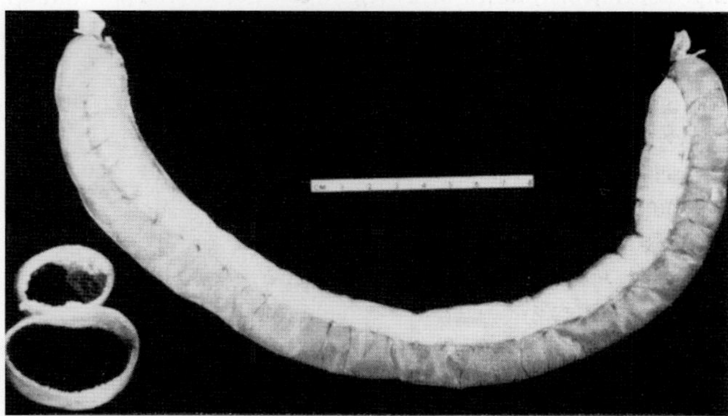

Figure 5.7 Tubular duplication of the terminal ileum in a 7-month-old boy. The duplication, lying on the mesenteric border of the bowel, was 29 cm long and communicated with the adjoining bowel near its distal end. The duplication, which is the smaller of the two cross-sections, was lined largely by gastric mucosa, and an ulcer was within it, near its point of communication with the bowel. An island of aberrant pancreas was also in its wall. Source: Arey and Valdes-Dapena 1992 [320]. Copyright © 1992 Elsevier.

Signs, symptoms, and complications

In most patients, duplications are diagnosed in infancy or early childhood, but duplications are occasionally newly discovered in an adult [150]. The frequency of symptoms varies inversely with age. Pediatric patients most commonly present with abdominal pain, obstructive symptoms (e.g., nausea, vomiting, pain), and hemorrhage. Obstruction may result from a mass effect, from volvulus produced by a large lesion, or more rarely from inflammation of the duplication. Much less frequently, these lesions are asymptomatic and are discovered incidentally. In adults, the evaluation of relatively mild abdominal complaints by computed tomography (CT) or ultrasonography may lead to detection [151], and ultrasonography has been used for prenatal detection [152]. Intussusception may be precipitated if a duplicated gut acts as a lead point and invaginates into normal intestine. Gastrointestinal hemorrhage may result from ulceration of the duplicated or surrounding mucosa; very frequently, these lesions contain ectopic gastric mucosa that secretes acid and causes ulceration.

A rare complication in adults is the development of carcinoma in the duplication and an association with autoimmune hemolytic anemia has been described [153,154]. Carcinoid tumors, adenocarcinoma arising in ectopic gastric mucosa, and squamous cell carcinoma have been reported.

Diagnosis

Small bowel duplications can be difficult to detect. Plain films may show a partially calcified wall of the duplication. Small bowel follow-through or enteroclysis barium examinations may reveal the duplication if it communicates with the gut lumen. Cysts that contain gastric mucosa may be detected by ^{99m}Tc abdominal scintigraphy [155], which specifically delineates gastric surface mucus cells (see section on Meckel diverticulum). Ultrasonography (effective for prenatal diagnosis) or CT can provide clues to the diagnosis by revealing the presence of a cystic mass, and these tests are also valuable for detecting rare carcinomas [156], which appear as solid tissue within the cyst.

Management

Duplications are treated surgically. The use of minimally invasive surgery has been reported although conversion rates are still high, particularly in infants [157]. Lesions detected antenatally can be electively resected, because the majority are asymptomatic at least for a few months after birth [158]. Resection within 6 months has been recommended [149]. If small, the lesions are easily resected with the adjacent small bowel. If the duplicated bowel is quite extensive and resection would require the removal of too much normal bowel, the duplication is opened and the mucosa removed, with the serosa and muscular layers left intact. Alternatively, the common wall can be excised. It is important to remove all mucosa because residual ectopic gastric mucosa can lead to recurrent hemorrhage [147].

Intestinal atresia and stenosis

In intestinal atresia, the lumen of a segment of the gut is completely occluded. Stenosis is a narrowing of the gut lumen that leads to partial obstruction. Atresia is one of the most common causes of bowel obstruction in neonates. Duodenal atresia and stenosis are frequently associated with Down syndrome, midgut malrotation, esophageal atresia, annular pancreas, imperforate anus (see Chapter 6), and intrauterine growth retardation. Duodenal atresia is also associated with intestinal atresia, with an incidence of 2.8% and a miss rate of 0.8% [159]. Jejunoileal atresia is much less frequently associated with other congenital anomalies. Atresias are most often single but may be multiple and can be found from esophagus to rectum. The reported incidence of small bowel atresias varies but is approximately 1 in 3000 to 1 in 5000 live births [160,161].

Several types of small intestinal atresias have been described (Figure 5.8) [162]. In type I atresia, a membranous septum or diaphragm of mucosa and submucosa obstructs the lumen, but the bowel wall and mesentery are intact. In type II, two blind bowel ends are connected by a fibrous cord, with intact mesentery in between. In type IIIa lesions, two blind bowel ends are separated by a mesenteric gap, and type IIIb is the "apple peel" atresia, characterized by proximal small bowel atresia and absence of the distal superior mesenteric artery (<5% of all atresias) [163]. In this case, the bowel distal to the atresia is foreshortened and coiled and receives a retrograde blood supply from the ileocolic, right colic, or inferior mesenteric artery. Finally, in type IV, multiple atresias are present throughout the small bowel, creating the appearance of a "string of sausages"; they may individually be of type I, II, or IIIa.

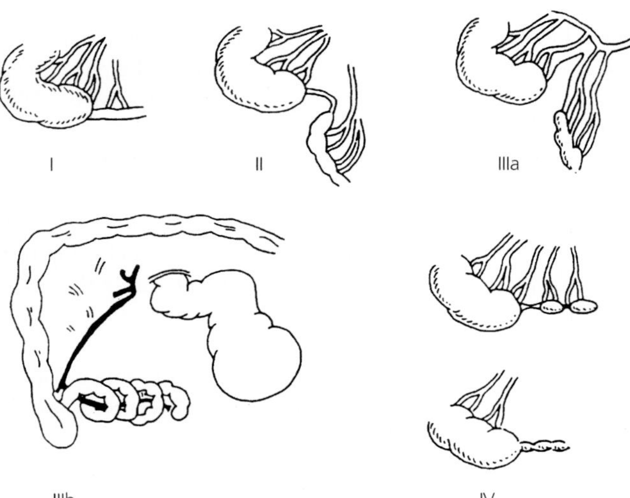

Figure 5.8 Classification of intestinal atresias. In type I, or membranous atresia, a membranous septum or diaphragm of mucosa and submucosa obstructs the lumen, but the bowel wall and mesentery are intact. In type II, two blind bowel ends are connected by a fibrous cord, with intact mesentery between them. In type IIIa, bowel lesions are separated by a mesenteric gap. Type IIIb is an "apple peel" atresia with features of proximal small bowel atresia, absence of the distal superior mesenteric artery, and coiled and foreshortened bowel. Type IV consists of multiple atresias of any type (I–IIIa). Source: Smith and Glasson 1989 [321]. Reproduced with permission of John Wiley & Sons.

Pathophysiology

The pathogenesis of atresia and stenosis is unknown. Duodenal atresia is considered separately from jejunoileal atresia. Duodenal atresia is thought to be caused by a failure of recanalization of the intestinal lumen after the solid cord stage, which takes place at 4–8 weeks of gestation [164]. Mutations in the α6- and β4integrin genes have been reported in families affected by junctional epidermolysis bullosa and duodenal or pyloric atresia [165,166]. In mice, deletion of the fibroblast growth factor (FGF) 10 receptor, FGF2Rb, results in duodenal and colonic atresia, along with other defects such as pulmonary agenesis [167].

Whole-exome sequencing of four French-Canadian families affected by hereditary multiple intestinal atresia [168–170] led to the identification of mutations in the tetratricopeptide repeat domain 7A gene (TTC7A). The precise function of this gene is unknown but is thought to be critical in maintaining intestinal homeostasis. More than 20 distinct disease mutations have been described [171], with multiple associated diseases include early-onset inflammatory bowel disease and severe combined immunodeficiency [170].

Ischemic intrauterine events such as midgut volvulus, arterial occlusion, intussusception, and localized volvulus secondary to meconium ileus or duplication have been implicated in the pathogenesis of small intestinal atresia, especially in single atresia and stenosis [172,173]. Atresia has been associated with intrauterine volvulus, gastroschisis, cardiac and other anomalies [174], and cystic fibrosis [174,175]. A retrospective review showed a more than 200-fold increased risk for cystic fibrosis in Caucasian infants with jejunoileal atresia [176], leading to a recommendation that all infants with jejunoileal atresia be screened for cystic fibrosis [177]. In a population-based study, small bowel atresia was associated with low birthweight, low gestational age, maternal age, and multiple births [161]. Analysis of a large European congenital anomaly database suggests that maternal age <20 is a risk factor for small bowel atresia [178]. To further explore the vascular ischemic hypothesis, genomic DNA from 206 small bowel atresia patients was sequenced for 32 single nucleotide polymorphisms (SNPs) in genes involved in vascular processes such as coagulation, inflammatory response, and blood pressure regulation, and compared to 573 normal infants [179]. SNPs in SERPINE 1 (plasminogen activator inhibitor 1), MMP3 (matrix metalloproteinase 3), and ADRB2 (β_2 adrenergic receptor) were associated with reduced risk, and SNPs in ITGA2 (glycoprotein 1a) and NPPA (atrial natriuretic peptide) were associated with higher risk. Meconium ileus is thought to predispose the bowel to ischemia or cause volvulus as a consequence of hyperperistalsis.

Pathological examination of atretic segments resected from neonates with multiple intestinal atresias suggests a role for either ischemia or a defect in recanalization of the gut lumen [180]. Rare familial cases of multiple intestinal atresias and apple peel (type IIIb) atresias have been reported [180–183]. An autosomal recessive inheritance pattern has been suggested [182], but variability in the types of atresia found within families and discordance in a set of monozygotic twins suggest a more complex genetic transmission [163]. Other factors implicated in the pathogenesis of atresia and stenosis are maternal ergotamine use, vasoconstrictive exposures such as pseudoephedrine and amphetamine, combined with cigarette smoking [184], fetal exposure to methylene blue, which was formerly used as a marker during amniocentesis of twin pregnancies to ensure that both sacs had been sampled [185], and toluidine blue [186]. Multiple intestinal atresias have also been reported to be associated with neonatal immunodeficiency states [187], and a syndrome in which neonatal diabetes and hypoplastic pancreas were found in association with intestinal atresia and gallbladder hypoplasia [188].

Clinical presentation

Polyhydramnios is frequently detected in proximal gastrointestinal atresia, but the amniotic fluid may be normal in distal atresia [172,173]. Neonates most commonly present with signs and symptoms of obstruction within hours to 3 days after birth. Bilious vomiting early after birth is a characteristic symptom of proximal atresia, whereas abdominal distension occasionally associated with visible bowel loops, later vomiting, and a failure to pass meconium are frequent presenting complaints of distal lesions. High atresias of the jejunum and duodenum are also associated with jaundice. The course of infants who have intestinal stenosis without atresia may be much more indolent because the obstruction is usually partial. The diagnosis may therefore be delayed.

Diagnosis

Polyhydramnios is an indication for ultrasonography, which may identify the obstructing defect [152]. Fetal echogenic bowel, enlarged stomach, and dilated loops of bowel are frequently detected [189]; the presence of fetal ascites and extraluminal calcifications may indicate aseptic perforation of the bowel, with meconium peritonitis. The intralumenal calcifications found in type IV atresias may also be seen. Ileal atresias are generally not associated with an enlarged stomach or polyhydramnios [189]. The presence of polyhydramnios and fetal bowel dilation in gastroschisis patients is associated with atresia; absence of fetal bowel dilation seems to exclude atresia [190]. After birth, routine abdominal radiography may demonstrate multiple air–fluid levels throughout the small bowel or dilated bowel proximal to the obstruction with an absence of gas distally. A double-bubble sign on abdominal radiography or ultrasonography is classic for duodenal atresia. Barium enema shows an unused microcolon. The anatomical defect should always be definitively identified by plain films and cautious contrast radiography before surgical intervention is attempted. It is also important to identify all atretic sites, with the risk for multiple atresias kept in mind.

Important in the differential diagnosis of neonatal bowel obstruction are Hirschsprung disease, malrotation, meconium ileus associated with cystic fibrosis, duplications, Meckel diverticulum, and mesenteric bands [191]. Barium enema is recommended to rule out Hirschsprung disease and malrotation with volvulus and to identify other atresias in the bowel distal to the primary obstruction.

Treatment and prognosis

Initial therapy consists of intravenous hydration, correction of electrolytes, and nasogastric suction to remove accumulated fluid and decompress the bowel. Surgical resection of atretic small intestine is the primary treatment, which may be challenging because bowel preservation is critical and dilation of the small bowel proximal to the obstruction makes anastomosis difficult.

Several different surgical procedures have been developed, including tapering enteroplasty and the creation of an ileostomy [192,193]. Patients with type IIIb and type IV atresias often require extensive resective surgery, which results in short bowel syndrome and a poor prognosis. A study has suggested that transluminal stent placement in lieu of surgical resection may be a viable approach although the outcomes of only nine patients were reported [194]. Patients with hereditary multiple intestinal atresias have particularly poor outcomes, because of the extensive involvement with multiple atresias from antrum to rectum that cannot be surgically corrected [183]. Small bowel transplantation in a patient with multiple intestinal atresias and immunodeficiency resulted in partial correction of immune defects, by recruitment of immune cells from the donor [195].

All patients after surgery are placed on total parenteral nutrition and monitored for a return of normal bowel function as the diet is slowly advanced. A central venous catheter should be placed early in the course of the disease. Intestinal atresia is a common prenatal cause of short bowel syndrome in children [196]. Patients with short bowel syndrome frequently require prolonged parenteral nutrition. Factors that hinder progress to full oral intake include meconium peritonitis, the number of anastomoses, luminal discrepancy between proximal and distal intestine, and the presence of immature ganglion cells as well as short bowel syndrome [197]. The morbidity and mortality rates in infants have dramatically decreased since the 1950s. Postoperative survival is approximately 90–95% [164,172,198]. Enhanced survival is a result of improved management of the nutritional and pulmonary status. However, overall survival has remained at approximately 84–88% [180,197]. Intestinal rehabilitation programs for patients with short bowel syndrome improve liver function and reduce TPN requirements [198].

Factors adversely affecting prognosis include the presence of other congenital anomalies (especially cardiac), chronic pulmonary disease, or pulmonary aspiration [164,166]. Prolonged disturbance in motility is common postoperatively. The development and maturation of the enteric nervous system are impaired below the atretic segment [199].

Malrotation

Description and pathophysiology

Alterations in the normal rotation and fixation of the gut during embryogenesis result in a series of anomalies with various clinical manifestations. Malrotation or incomplete rotation is the most common disorder of rotation and fixation; it occurs when the normal 270° bowel rotation is not completed. As a result, the cecum may lie in the subpyloric region or may be in a subhepatic location. The small bowel is not attached by a broad mesentery but remains suspended from a narrow vascular pedicle. Peritoneal bands (Ladd bands) may pass from the cecum across the duodenum to the right upper quadrant or may attach to the duodenum.

The two major complications of malrotation are volvulus, caused by free rotation of the midgut around the vascular pedicle, and duodenal obstruction secondary to the Ladd bands. In nonrotation, the embryonic midgut loop does not rotate and the caudal limb of the loop reenters the abdominal cavity first. Subsequently, the small intestine (jejunum and ileum) lies on the right side of the abdomen and the colon is entirely on the left. The cecum is usually located in the left iliac fossa. Frequently, the broad attachment of the small bowel mesentery does not develop, and the small bowel remains suspended by a narrow pedicle, at risk for volvulus. In reversed rotation, clockwise instead of counterclockwise rotation of the gut leads to reentry of the colon into the abdomen first. The position of the colon is then posterior to the superior mesenteric artery and the duodenum. The placement of the duodenum is anterior to the superior mesenteric artery. The small bowel mesentery passes in front of the transverse colon, so that a mesenteric tunnel forms that causes colonic compression and obstruction. Finally, failure of the cecum to descend into its normal position in the right lower quadrant may lead to mobile cecum; the cecum remains in the right upper quadrant and is unfixed posteriorly, predisposed to cecal volvulus. The ileum may similarly be unfixed and susceptible to volvulus.

The incidence of malrotation is unknown; estimates range from 1 in 200 to 1 in 6000 live births [200, 201]. Mutations in the FILAMIN A (FLNA) gene, the Coxsackie and Adenovirus Receptor Like Membrane Protein (CLMP) gene, L–R asymmetry genes, and the FOXF1 gene have been found in infants with intestinal malrotation in the context of multiorgan defects [202,203].

Clinical manifestations

In approximately 50–80% of cases of midgut malrotation, symptoms develop in infancy. Related concurrent anomalies are biliary atresia and congenital heart disease. Intestinal atresia and stenosis may result from malrotation, and omphalocele and diaphragmatic hernia may lead to malrotation secondary to abnormal placement of the bowel during rotation. In adults, malrotation is sometimes associated with absence of the superior mesenteric vein and extrahepatic biliary anomalies. The most severe complications of malrotation are small bowel obstruction and volvulus, which cause recurrent bilious vomiting, passage of bloody stools or acute onset of constipation, and bowel loop distension. In patients with Ladd bands, symptoms of duodenal obstruction may develop [204]. Patients from 1 month of age through adolescence may have symptoms that are more varied and indolent, including intermittent vomiting, failure to thrive, and recurrent abdominal pain [200]. Adults may be asymptomatic for many years [200,205] and then present with midgut volvulus causing abdominal pain, bloody stools, and distension [200,201]. Alternatively, in adult patients with a long history of recurrent abdominal pain with nausea and vomiting since childhood, the obstruction or volvulus may never have been diagnosed because it was transient and resolved before presentation [204].

Diagnosis

The diagnosis may be challenging in the older child and adult [206–208]. Plain films may reveal evidence of duodenal or small bowel obstruction. A classic double-bubble sign may be seen, indicating duodenal obstruction. However, early in the course of midgut volvulus, plain radiographs may be unrevealing, and children with bilious vomiting should undergo a contrast study to rule out volvulus [209]. Contrast radiographic studies may demonstrate anomalous small bowel, ligament of Treitz, and cecal locations. In adults with midgut volvulus, upper gastrointestinal contrast series may reveal a dilated stomach and duodenum with a typical "corkscrew" appearance of the barium in the twisted duodenum and proximal jejunum [210]. Barium enema may reveal malposition of the right colon and cecum [201,207]. CT may show reversed positions of the superior mesenteric artery and vein.

Treatment

The surgical correction of malrotation (incomplete rotation) in symptomatic patients includes relieving the obstruction caused by Ladd peritoneal bands, freeing the duodenum, reducing midgut volvulus, and broadening the mesentery to prevent recurrent rotation of the bowel around a narrow mesentery [201]. In the Ladd procedure, the bowel is placed in the position of nonrotation (small bowel on the right side of the abdomen and colon on the left). Appendectomy is performed because the cecum is incorrectly located. Variations of this operation are used to correct nonrotation and the very rare reversed rotation. Elective repair in adults with incidentally discovered malrotation or with mild gastrointestinal symptoms results in improved outcomes compared to adults who undergo surgery emergently [211].

In most patients, bowel function returns to normal. However, some children with recurrent and prolonged symptoms of nausea, vomiting, and pain preoperatively do not fare as well postoperatively, possibly because of persistent dysmotility syndromes associated with malrotation or damage to the small bowel resulting from long-standing, indolent obstruction [199].

Gastroschisis and omphalocele

Description and embryonic origin

Although gastroschisis and omphalocele both result from abdominal wall defects, these rare disorders are distinct entities (see Chapter 104). The incidence of gastroschisis has recently increased to 44.9 per 10 000 live births [212,213] and omphalocele is 1.5–3 per 10 000 births [214,215]. The incidence of gastroschisis appears to be increasing worldwide and is associated with young maternal age, drug use, smoking, and maternal infection [212,213,216–219].

In omphalocele, the abdominal viscera herniate through the umbilical ring and persist outside the body, covered by a membranous sac but not by skin. In gastroschisis, massive evisceration of the intestines occurs through a small defect in the abdominal wall, usually to the right of the closed umbilical ring. The bowel has no membranous covering, has been exposed to amniotic fluid in utero, and is often matted, thickened, foreshortened, and covered with adhesions. It has been hypothesized that omphalocele is caused by a failure of embryonic folding at the level of the lateral folds or persistence of the body stalk [214,220]. Gastroschisis may be caused by rupture of the amnion at the umbilical ring, and vascular disruption in utero, leading to failure of differentiation of the somatopleural mesenchyme [216,221] or later between the time of herniation into the umbilical cord and fixation, or by disruption of the right omphalomesenteric artery. The defect is thought to occur between the fifth and tenth weeks of gestation, but perinatal insults have also been suggested in patients in whom gastroschisis was not detected sonographically [222]. Potential teratogens include tobacco, alcohol, cocaine, and other drugs [215,223,224].

Other congenital anomalies that occur in association with omphalocele are chromosomal [225]; about one-third of individuals with omphalocele and multiple anomalies have trisomy 13, trisomy 18, or Beckwith–Wiedemann syndrome, which is characterized by macroglossia, large infant size, visceromegaly, early hypoglycemia, and increased risk of Wilms and other tumors. Gastroschisis is associated with intestinal anomalies, including atresia and malrotation, vascular disruptions, and renal and gallbladder agenesis [214].

Several mouse models of gastroschisis have been described [226–230]. In mice that are null for the bone morphogenetic protein 1 (BMP1) gene, the ALX4 gene, or the aortic carboxypeptidase-like protein gene, gastroschisis develops with early mortality. ALX4 is a homeodomain transcription factor. Both BMP1 and the aortic carboxypeptidase-like protein appear to have important functions in the extracellular matrix. The relevance of these gene defects to human disease is unclear; a mutational analysis of the BMP1 gene in human patients with gastroschisis was unrevealing [231]. Mouse models of omphalocele have also been described [226] in knockout models of insulin-like growth factor 2 (IGF-2), calreticulin, and several transcription factors. The TGF-β signaling pathway has been suggested to be important in ventral body wall closure [226].

Prenatal diagnosis

Elevated levels of maternal serum α-fetoprotein are associated with ventral abdominal wall defects. Gastroschisis is detected with greater sensitivity than omphalocele [174]. Prenatal ultrasonography is the mainstay of diagnosis [213–215,232]. One of the major advantages of prenatal diagnosis is that the obstetrician is alerted, so that at the time of delivery the mother can be taken to a tertiary care center where appropriate surgical and neonatal intensive care support is available [220], and the surgeon and others can provide early counseling and information about this condition [219]. The role of preterm delivery or early-term versus full-term delivery to minimize intestinal damage and prevent intrauterine death is still being examined, and the factors that should determine the need for this intervention are still being defined [232–238]. Vaginal delivery is becoming increasingly prevalent, although caesarean section rates remain increased due to planned deliveries and intrapartum heart rate anomalies [213,239,240].

Treatment and outcomes

Surgical closure of omphalocele and gastroschisis is attempted shortly after birth. Options include primary reduction with a sutured or sutureless immediate closure if reducible. If irreducible, delayed reduction with silo placement or sutured or sutureless delayed closure can be performed [241–243]. Primary closure may be possible with the use of retention sutures and stretching the abdominal wall. If this cannot be achieved, a silo or Silastic sac can be used with successive compression to reduce the herniation further [241–243]. Because almost all children have bowel hypomotility, total parenteral nutrition is recommended early in the course of the illness. Advances in surgical correction have greatly improved the prognosis of patients with gastroschisis, despite the fact that the bowel is usually damaged and slow to return to normal function.

The survival rate for gastroschisis and associated complications continues to improve and is more than 90% [219,244–246]. The presence of necrotizing enterocolitis and other anomalies affecting other organs or associated intestinal conditions (e.g., atresias [247], perforations, necrotic segments, and volvulus) affects mortality rates [248]. In the absence of severe associated anomalies, the immediate survival and long-term outcome of patients with omphalocele have also improved but are worse than for gastroschisis [249–251]. Survival from omphalocele is also related to the severity of the associated anomalies and medical conditions [219].

Structural anomalies

Volvulus

A volvulus is an abnormal twisting of the intestine around the axis of its own mesentery, resulting in obstruction of the more proximal bowel. Twisting of the mesentery may involve the mesenteric vessels and so make the involved loop particularly susceptible to strangulation and gangrene, with resulting perforation, peritonitis, and sepsis. In contrast to colonic volvulus, particularly of the cecum and sigmoid colon that are the most common types, small bowel volvulus is relatively rare in the United States and most of Europe [252–257]. The estimated annual incidence in the US is 1.7–5.7 cases per 100 000 [252,253]. It occurs more frequently in parts of Africa, the Middle East, and the Indian subcontinent [252,253,255]. In these countries, volvulus occurs in the absence of anatomical abnormalities and is probably related to dietary factors. It has been postulated that ingesting large amounts of bulky foods after fasting may predispose to torsion of the small bowel loops [254]. In the US, small bowel volvulus is usually caused by a preexisting defect, such as an anomaly of rotation and fixation, postoperative adhesion, or congenital bands [258]. Other causes include jejunal diverticula [259], postsphincterotomy bleeding [260], stromal tumors, pregnancy, endometriosis, internal hernias, and hematomas [261]. Small bowel volvulus is rare in adults, who typically complain of chronic symptoms compared to pediatric patients [255,262].

Clinical presentation and diagnosis

Patients present with symptoms of small bowel obstruction and an acute abdomen. Abdominal pain, nausea, and vomiting are almost always present [252,253,255]; the severity of the pain may be out of proportion to the physical findings. Signs include abdominal distension, rebound, guarding and rigidity, and occasionally a palpable abdominal mass.

Computed tomography scan or multidetector CT angiography is the imaging modality of choice [208,210]. The "whirlpool" sign, which is a whirl-like rotation of the small bowel around the axis of the superior mesenteric artery, is a sensitive indicator of volvulus [253,255]. Plain abdominal radiographs taken in supine and upright positions may demonstrate distended bowel with air– fluid levels, consistent with obstruction. Perforation may be indicated by the presence of free air. Barium studies can be useful. A typical corkscrew-like appearance of the barium in the distorted duodenum and jejunum is diagnostic. Angiography may reveal twisting of the branches of the superior mesenteric artery. A multiinstitutional study showed that point-of-care ultrasonography can be used for pediatric emergency room diagnosis of malrotation and volvulus [263,264].

Treatment and outcome

The treatment of small bowel volvulus is surgical. Ischemic or gangrenous loops of bowel should be resected, although derotation of the bowel may be sufficient therapy in itself. Vascular compromise of the small bowel with subsequent gangrene is common and leads to increased morbidity and mortality postoperatively. Rapid recognition of volvulus and prompt surgical intervention are the keys to decreasing the fatality rate associated with this condition. Long-term outcomes have improved for pediatric patients with resulting ultra-short bowel syndrome, including transplant-free enteral autonomy [265].

Intussusception

Description and pathophysiology

Intussusception occurs when a segment of bowel (the intussusceptum) invaginates, or telescopes, into adjacent distal bowel, leading to obstruction and possible ischemic injury. The incidence, causes, clinical presentation, and therapy of intestinal intussusception are different in adult and pediatric patients [263,266,267].

Intestinal intussusception is one of the most common causes of small bowel obstruction in children younger than 2 years of age [268] but it is an unusual cause of bowel obstruction in adults. Most pediatric cases occur in children younger than 5 years of age [269]. Pediatric intussusception is most often idiopathic but may be associated with a pathological lead point in 8–12% of cases [270,271], including Meckel diverticulum; a variety of benign and malignant tumors, such as polyps, leiomyomas, and lymphomas; duplications; and Henoch–Schönlein purpura, in which an intramural hematoma acts as a lead point. An association between adenovirus and rotavirus infection [272] and rotavirus vaccination and intussusception [273–275] has been described, perhaps secondary to a lead point of viral or vaccine-induced lymphoid hyperplasia. In idiopathic intussusception, an association with prominent Peyer patches and enlarged mesenteric lymph nodes has been observed [263]. In children, ileocolic intussusceptions are most common, followed by ileoileocolic, cecocolic, and, much less frequently, ileoileal involvement.

In adults in the western world, small bowel intussusception occurs rarely, accounting for approximately 5% of all cases of intestinal obstruction [276,277]. A causative factor can be identified in more than 90% of adult patients [266], whereas it cannot in children [263,266,267]. Small intestinal intussusception may result from tumors, including leiomyomas, neurofibromas, lipomas, lymphomas, small bowel adenomatous polyps, and metastatic tumors with or without peritoneal carcinomatosis. Other causes include Meckel diverticulum or other diverticular disease and celiac disease with chronically dilated flaccid bowel. Intussusception has been reported in association with *Yersinia enterocolitica* enterocolitis [278]. Postoperative intussusception may result from adhesions, or intussusception may follow trauma [279]. Small bowel intussusception may occur as a complication following Roux-en-Y gastric bypass, possibly due to altered motility of the divided small bowel [280,281]. Jejunogastric intussusception may occur after Bilroth II surgery, and bypassed bowel may become intussuscepted after jejunoileal bypass. Patients with acquired immunodeficiency syndrome and Kaposi sarcoma or diffuse enteritis are also at risk [282]. Pregnancy and the use of long intestinal or Cantor tubes are other predisposing factors.

Signs and symptoms

The typical pediatric patient is a well-nourished, previously healthy child between the ages of 5 months and 5 years. The peak presenting age is 3–11 months [283]. Classic signs and symptoms include the acute onset of intermittent abdominal pain, vomiting, and hematochezia. A palpable abdominal mass, diarrhea, and somnolence are other frequent findings [270,271]. In older children, these diagnostic signs and symptoms are often not present [269]. In adults, the clinical picture may be confusing. Abdominal pain is almost always present [284,285] but is often low-grade and chronic; patients may present after several episodes have spontaneously resolved [286,287]. A partial or complete small bowel obstruction may be present, and an abdominal mass is often palpable. Nausea and vomiting are particularly associated with small bowel compared with large bowel intussusception. Weight loss may also occur in patients with chronic, indolent symptoms.

Diagnosis and therapy

Pediatric patients

In children, ultrasonography or an air or water-soluble contrast barium enema is performed as the initial diagnostic procedure because the ileocecal region is so frequently involved. In many centers in the USA, ultrasound has become the initial diagnostic procedure of choice [268,288] with a sensitivity of 97.9% and specificity of 97.8%. In a Markov decision model that evaluated the use of ultrasound followed conditionally by contrast enema versus contrast enema alone, it was determined that the use of ultrasound decreases radiation-induced malignancy, and reduces the number of perforations and laparotomies, and thus is the more effective diagnostic algorithm [289]. Contrast enemas demonstrate the location of the intussusception and are often successful in reducing it. Air enemas are also safe and effective in reducing intussusceptions [209,290–292], and pneumatic reduction has a higher success rate [268]. The enema is usually administered with a surgeon in attendance in case of perforation or failure to reduce. In extremely ill patients with peritonitis, perforation, or shock, enema reduction is contraindicated and operative intervention must be pursued [268]. If necessary, the patient is taken to laparotomy for manual reduction. Resection is performed if ischemia or gangrene of the bowel is present. A careful search is made for a possible pathological lead point. Recurrent intussusception occurs but is rare [293].

Plain films (two view or three view) may reveal a crescent of gas capping the intussusceptum, outlining its leading edge (rim sign), or a target sign, consisting of two concentric radiolucent curvilinear lines outlining the intussusception [268,294]. A gasless area may also be identified, corresponding with the soft tissue mass of the intussusception. Plain films that show intestinal obstruction may predict a worse outcome with decreased success rate of therapeutic enema and increased rate of complicated surgical reductions and resection [295]. Ultrasonography may show a classic target, bulls-eye, or doughnut sign, characterized by multiple concentric rings of sonolucency alternating with one or two echogenic foci. The edematous outer and inner walls of the intussusception create two hypoechoic areas ringing the hyperechoic luminal mucosa [296]. CT may similarly be useful, but is usually avoided in children. Upper gastrointestinal contrast series may show proximal dilation and a "bird's beak" at the site of obstruction, but are contraindicated if perforation or peritonitis are suspected.

Adult patients

Intussusception is diagnosed and treated differently in adult patients because its location and causes are different from those in children [263,266,267,276]. Most intussusceptions in adults are in the small bowel, although they may also occur in the colon [297]. Therefore, a combination of plain film, upper gastrointestinal series, barium enema, and CT or ultrasonography is used in adult patients.

Because of the often puzzling presentation of intussusception in this age group, CT is frequently performed [276,277]. A mass of alternating high and low attenuation may be seen as a target, sausage-shaped, or bilobed lesion [287]. Mesenteric fat appears as areas of low attenuation, whereas the bowel wall itself appears as an area of high attenuation. Thickened bowel loops and an intralumenal soft tissue mass may be seen. However, this technique is not sensitive enough to determine the nature of the pathological lead point.

Because a pathological lesion is found so frequently, treatment in adults consists of surgical intervention with bowel resection. Manual reduction alone may be pursued only if it is certain that no other lesions are present [286]. With present diagnostic techniques, however, it is unlikely that a tumor or another anatomical cause can be ruled out preoperatively. Therefore, manual reduction of intussusception in adults is usually not recommended because manipulation can lead to intralumenal or intravenous tumor seeding [284]. Colonic intussusception is never treated with manual reduction because of the very high likelihood of malignancy [287].

Lymphangiectasia

Description and pathophysiology

Intestinal lymphangiectasia is characterized by the obstruction of lymph drainage from the small intestine and the dilation of lacteals and other intestinal lymphatics, such as those in the serosa and mesentery, depending on the level of obstruction. As a result of obstruction and increased pressure in the intestinal lymphatics, the absorption of chylomicrons and fat-soluble vitamins such as vitamin D is impaired, the reentry of intestinal lymphocytes into the peripheral circulation is impeded, and excessive amounts of intestinal lymph "leak" into the intestinal lumen. Lymphenteric fistulas may form, and intestinal lymph containing chylomicrons, protein, and lymphocytes drains directly into the intestinal lumen. Chylomicrons are sequestered in the lamina propria as well as in the distended lymphatics. Blockage of serosal and mesenteric lymphatics may lead to chylous ascites, and blockage of the thoracic duct to chylous pleural effusions.

Intestinal lymphangiectasia may occur as a primary congenital disorder or may be secondary to a disease that blocks the intestinal lymph drainage at some level [298]. CD55 deficiency due to loss of function mutations leads to early-onset protein-losing enteropathy [299–301].

Causes of secondary lymphangiectasia include extensive abdominal or retroperitoneal carcinoma or lymphoma, retroperitoneal fibrosis, chronic pancreatitis, mesenteric tuberculosis or sarcoidosis, Crohn's disease, Whipple disease, scleroderma, celiac disease [302], constrictive pericarditis, systemic lupus erythematosus [303], chronic congestive heart failure, and after the Fontan operation (right atrium to pulmonary artery anastomosis) [304,305]. Lymphangiectasia occurs after the Fontan procedure in up to 24% of patients [305] and is thought to be due to increased systemic venous pressure resulting in increased lymph production and decreased drainage. However, focal involvement has been reported, detectable by radionuclide studies and amenable to surgical resection [305]. Congenital intestinal lymphangiectasia (Milroy disease) results from a malformation of the lymphatics that often affects many areas of the body.

Clinical presentation

Patients present with varying degrees of steatorrhea and malabsorption, lymphocytopenia (especially of T lymphocytes), marked hypogammaglobulinemia with impaired cell-mediated immunity, and prominent manifestations of protein-losing enteropathy. They often have edema and low serum protein levels, the reduction in serum albumin usually being the most pronounced and the only one of clinical significance. Patients with congenital disease present at any time from birth to adulthood, often with asymmetrical edema of an extremity caused by peripheral lymphatic obstruction. They may also present, as do the secondary cases, with more diffuse, symmetrical edema, usually the result of marked hypoproteinemia. Despite lymphocytopenia and impaired delayed hypersensitivity reactions, opportunistic infections are not common. Gastrointestinal symptoms are usually not prominent, but some patients may have diarrhea, abdominal pain, distension, nausea and vomiting, and occasionally gastrointestinal bleeding.

Diagnosis

Protein-losing enteropathy should be suspected in any patient with unexplained hypoalbuminemia, and intestinal lymphangiectasia should be considered if lymphocytopenia and steatorrhea are also present. Asymmetrical lymphedema, especially dating from infancy or childhood, should suggest congenital (Milroy) disease.

A diagnosis of lymphangiectasia rests on peroral jejunal biopsy demonstrating dilated lymphatic lacteals. Several specimens may be required to demonstrate the diagnostic findings because the lesions are often patchy and localized [306]. Endoscopy may reveal dilated lacteals that appear as white opaque spots or white-tipped villi, and nodular lesions and xanthomatous plaques have also been noted [307,308]. These findings aid the endoscopist in selecting appropriate regions to sample. Other pathological findings include moderate villus blunting and mild to moderate inflammatory infiltration [306].

Other tests demonstrate protein-losing enteropathy by detecting excessive enteric loss of plasma proteins. The use of radiolabeled plasma proteins, such as ^{131}I-albumin, ^{51}Cr-albumin, and ^{51}Cr-chloride, has been generally replaced by the measurement of gastrointestinal clearance of α1-antitrypsin. The use of ^{99m}Tc to detect the site of protein loss appears sensitive and specific [305]. Double-contrast radiographs of the small bowel may reveal folds thickened by intestinal edema, nodular protrusions, and an absence of mucosal ulceration [308]. Magnetic resonance lymphangiography can be used to image central conducting lymphatics and helps to differentiate protein-losing enteropathy due to Fontan physiology from congenital lymphangiectasia [309,310]. If secondary lymphangiectasia is suspected, appropriate tests such as CT of the abdomen should be performed to diagnose the underlying disease. The degree of malabsorption and nutritional deficiency may be assessed by quantifying stool fat and by measuring the prothrombin time, which is nonspecific, and the serum levels of calcium and carotene. In congenital cases, if necessary, the malformed, hypoplastic lymphatics can be demonstrated by lymphangiography. Pleural effusions and ascitic fluid may be tapped for conventional diagnostic studies and examined for chylomicrons.

Treatment

The therapy for lymphangiectasia should be directed toward treating the pathophysiological consequences, and, in the case of secondary lymphangiectasia, the underlying disease (e.g., lymphoma, tuberculosis, sarcoidosis, constrictive pericarditis) should be diagnosed and treated. A low-fat diet and substituting medium-chain triglycerides for the usual long-chain triglycerides may reduce enteric protein loss, malabsorption, and diarrhea and may improve serum albumin levels [298,311–313]. Medium-chain fatty acids are more water soluble and may be more readily absorbed through portal venous channels than through the lymphatics. The concomitant reduction in dietary long-chain fat presumably reduces chylomicrons in obstructed lymphatics and thereby decreases the lymphatic pressure and rate of lymph loss. Anecdotal reports have demonstrated the efficacy of octreotide [298,311,314–317]. Peripheral edema can be minimized by postural drainage and the use of elastic stockings to reduce the risk for cellulitis and lymphangitis. Lymphangiectasia from CD55 deficiency has been successfully treated by eculizumab [301].

Celiac artery compression

The topic of celiac artery compression is covered in Chapter 55.

References are available at www.yamadagastro.com/textbook7e

Further reading

Avitzur Y., Guo C., Mastropaolo L.A., et al. Mutations in tetratricopeptide repeat domain 7A gene result in a severe form of very early onset inflammatory bowel disease. Gastroenterology 2014;146:1028.

Duerr C.U., Ganal-Vonarburg S.C. The interaction of intestinal microbiota and innate lymphoid cells in health and disease throughout life. Immunology 2020;159:39.

Gehart H., Clevers H. Tales from the crypt: new insights into intestinal stem cells. Nature Rev Gastroenterol Hepatol Rev 2019;16:19.

Gerbe F., Jay P. Intestinal tuft cells: epithelial sentinels linking luminal cues to the immune system. Mucosal Immunol 2016;9:1353.

Haber A.L., Biron M., Rogel N., et al. A single-cell survey of the small intestinal epithelium. Nature 2017;551:333.

Kimura S. Molecular insights into the mechanisms of M-cell differentiation and transcytosis in the mucosa-associated lymphoid tissues. Anat Sci Int 2018;93:23.

Marinis A., Yiallourou A., Samanides L., et al. Intussusception of the bowel in adults: a review. World J Gastroenterol 2009;15:407.

McDole J.R., Wheeler L.W., McDonald K.G., et al. Goblet cells deliver luminal antigen to CD103+ dendritic cells in the small intestine. Nature 2012;483:345.

Moens E., Veld M. Epithelial barrier biology: good fences make good neighbours. Immunology 2012;135:1.

Papadimitriou G., Marinis A., Papakonstantinou A. Primary midgut volvulus in adults: report of two cases and review of the literature. J Gastrointest Surg 2011;15:1889.

Powell D.W., Pinchuk I.V., Saada J.I., et al. Mesenchymal cells of the intestinal lamina propria. Annu Rev Physiol 2011;73:213.

Schneider S., Wright C.M., Heuckeroth R.O. Unexpected roles for the second brain: enteric nervous system as master regulator of bowel function. Ann Rev Physiol 2019;81:235.

Spencer N.J., Hu H. Enteric nervous system: sensory transduction, neural circuits and gastrointestinal motility. Nat Rev Gastroenterol Hepatol 2020;17:338.

Uppal K., Tubbs R.S., Matusz P., et al. Meckel's diverticulum: a review. Clin Anat 2011;24:416.

Vaos G., Misiakos E.P. Congenital anomalies of the gastrointestinal tract diagnosed in adulthood – diagnosis and management. J Gastrointest Surg 2010;14:916.

CHAPTER 6

Colon: anatomy and structural anomalies

Bo Shen
Columbia University Irving Medical Center, New York Presbyterian Hospital, New York, NY, USA

Chapter menu

The large bowel consists of the colon and rectum. Our current understanding of colon and rectum anatomy began with the work of Andreas Vesalius in 16th century. Although anatomy of the colon is considered as well understood, insight into the complex anatomy of the rectum and particularly the anal sphincter and pelvic floor complex continues to evolve. Our understanding of functional and anatomical relationships between the structures surrounding the rectum and anus within the confined space of the pelvis has been augmented by the availability of high-definition magnetic resonance imaging (MRI) and high-resolution ultrasound. Advances in imaging modalities, particularly computed tomography colonography and MRI, have also enabled a more detailed understanding of relationships of the colon, rectum, and anus with surrounding structures and anatomical pathways involved in tumor spread. Knowledge of the normal anatomy of the colon and rectum also provides a basis for recognition of the presence of congenital or acquired abnormalities. Appreciation of embryological development is especially important when approaching congenital conditions, such as imperforate anus, intestinal malrotation, and Hirschsprung disease. In addition to understanding the gross anatomy of the colon and rectum, detailed knowledge of their histological features and cellular components are critical in the appreciation of physiological and pathological processes of the large bowel.

Embryology

The colon, rectum, and anus are derived from the distal segment of the midgut and the hindgut. During the third week of embryological development, the human primitive intestine appears as a straight tube that is suspended along the sagittal plane by its mesentery. At this stage of development, the foregut is located in the head fold and the hindgut located in the smaller tail fold. The midgut begins to protrude into the yolk sac, where the growth of the intestine takes place. During embryological development, the intestine undergoes extensive elongation and rotation within the yolk sac before returning into the abdominal cavity [1]. The initial stage of the rotation begins between the sixth and eighth week of development, and by the eighth week counterclockwise 90° rotation from the sagittal plane into the horizontal plane occurs. A few rare anomalies originating from this stage include inverted duodenum and extroversion of the cloaca. During the second stage of the rotation, which occurs around the tenth week of the intrauterine life, the midgut returns into the abdomen from its umbilical herniation as it simultaneously rotates an additional 180° counterclockwise around the pedicle of the mesentery. The duodenal and proximal jejunal loops return to the abdomen first and as the rotation continues the duodenum becomes situated posterior to the superior mesentery artery. Abnormalities that occur during this

Yamada's Textbook of Gastroenterology, Seventh Edition. Edited by Timothy C. Wang, Michael Camilleri, Benjamin Lebwohl, Anna S. Lok, William J. Sandborn, Kenneth K. Wang, and Gary D. Wu.

Companion website: www.yamadagastro.com/textbook7e

stage of development are more common and include intestinal nonrotation, malrotation, reverse rotation, internal hernia, and omphalocele. During the third and final stage of the rotation, the sequential fixation of the colon takes place. The cecum, initially located in the right upper abdomen, descends caudally and migrates to the right lower quadrant to its typical anatomical position, as counterclockwise rotation completes the 360° turn. Once the intestine is in its proper anatomical position, fixation begins, starting with the duodenum, followed by ascending and descending colon. Anomalies during this stage are also common and include mobile cecum, subhepatic or undescended cecum, hyperdescendent cecum, and persistent colonic mesentery.

The midgut-derived portion of the intestine includes the duodenum distal to the papilla, the entire small intestine, and the ascending and proximal two-thirds of the transverse colon. The distal transverse colon, descending colon, and rectum are derived from hindgut. At the level of the dentate line, the endodermal and ectodermal tubes fuse to form the anal transition zone (ATZ). Before the fifth week of intrauterine development, the intestinal and urogenital tracts terminate as a common opening termed the *cloaca*. Between the sixth and eighth weeks of fetal life, the urorectal septum forms to divide the cloaca into an anterior urogenital plate and a posterior anal plate. During this stage of development, even a slight posterior shift in the position of the septum can reduce the size of the anal opening and potentially cause anorectal defects. The segment within the newly formed anal canal that is derived from cloaca and that bears both endodermal and ectodermal elements becomes the ATZ. The internal anal sphincter is formed between the 6th and 12th weeks of development, deriving its muscle fibers from the circular layer of the rectum [2].

Gross anatomical considerations

The colon and rectum are considered as a single organ. However, it is prudent to subdivide the colon and rectum for the purposes of anatomical discussion because there are considerable differences between the two in their anatomical features, structural relationships, and physiological aspects. The colon is a tubular structure of approximately 150 cm in length that courses through the abdomen and pelvis beginning at the right lower quadrant with the ileal cecal valve (ICV) and cecum to the rectum in the pelvis. Throughout its course, the colon has variable degrees of fixation to the retroperitoneum, as a reflection of its embryological development. The ascending and descending colon are secondarily retroperitoneal, with normally no mobility, while the cecum, transverse, and sigmoid colon are intraperitoneal, freely mobile often with a long, well-developed mesentery. The primary function of the colon is the absorption of water from the luminal contents as they advance toward the rectum, ultimately leading to formed stool.

Ileocecal valve

Various shapes of ICV (Figure 6.1a) can be visualized with colonoscopy. The terminal ileum joins the cecum at its posteromedial aspect forming the ileocecal valve. The circular sphincter muscle that comprises the ileocecal valve is derived from hypertrophied muscular layers of the terminal ileum and contributes to its typical nipple-like appearance. Although the ICV often appears incompetent on barium enema, it is known that a competent ICV can prevent decompression of a markedly distended cecum, as seen in cases of high-grade colonic obstruction. Patients with ileocolonic Crohn's disease often have stenotic ICV (see Figure 6.1b), whereas those with ulcerative colitis, backwash ileitis, and primary sclerosing cholangitis commonly presented with patulous ICV (see Figure 6.1c). The functional importance of the ileocecal valve remains speculative. Some authors contend that its primary role is the regulation of ileal emptying [3], whereas others view its principal function as the prevention of reflux of colonic contents into the terminal ileum [4]. The observation that the presence of an intact ileocecal valve in patients at risk for short bowel syndrome is associated with improved absorption and decreased transit time through the small intestine supports the conclusion that the ileocecal valve regulates ileal emptying [5]. In addition, loss of the ileocecal valve, such as ileocolonic resection with

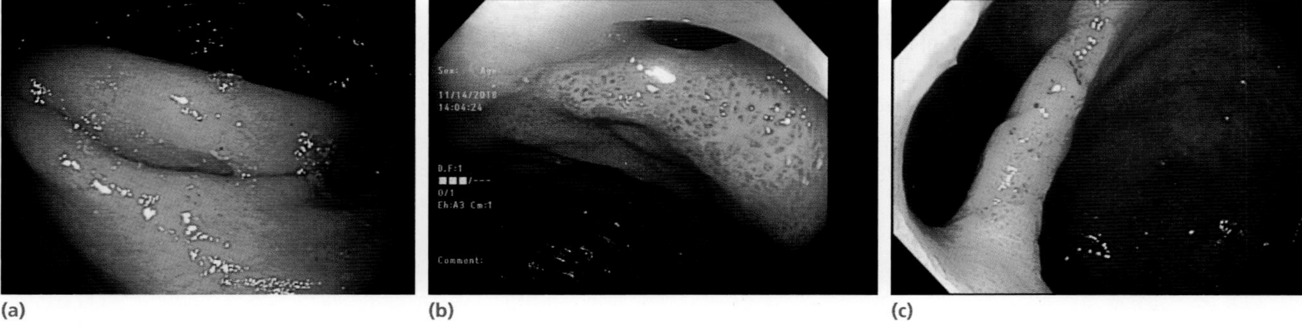

Figure 6.1 Ileocecal valve. **(a)** Ileocecal valve with the proximal and distal lips in a retroflex view on colonoscopy; **(b)** nonulcerated strictured ileocecal valve in Crohn's disease; **(c)** patulous ileocecal valve in a patient with current ulcerative colitis, backwash ileitis, and primary sclerosing cholangitis. Source: Courtesy Bo Shen.

anastomosis for cecal cancer or Crohn's disease of the terminal ileum, may put the patients at risk for small intestinal bacterial overgrowth.

Appendix

The vermiform appendix is located at the base of the cecum at the site of convergence of the three colonic taenia (Figure 6.2). The appendix usually measures 8–10 cm in length. Its location is quite variable, the most common being posteromedial and directed toward the terminal ileum [6]. Another common position for the appendix is retrocecal. Because of its variability in location, the presentation of acute appendicitis can also be quite variable. An appendix located intraperitoneally is more likely to produce symptoms associated with irritation of the parietal peritoneum earlier than one located retrocecally. The rudimentary appendage contains predominantly lymphoid tissue that serves no apparent digestive purpose. However, evidence suggests it may serve an important role in maturation of mucosal immunity. Epidemiological and clinical studies suggest that appendectomy is associated with an increased risk for Crohn's disease [7], while the surgery has been used for the treatment of ulcerative colitis [8,9].

Colon

The cecum, the most proximal part of the colon, is a blind saccular organ. The diameter of the colon at the level of the cecum is approximately 7.5–8.5 cm but can distend significantly further during certain motility or obstructive disorders, such as colonic pseudoobstruction. The bowel wall of the cecum is thinner than that in other parts of the colon. Therefore, endoscopic therapy, such as polypectomy, should be performed with extreme caution. The physiologically large lumen of the cecum makes a retroflex view of the area behind the ileocecal valve during screening or surveillance colonoscopy possible [10] (see Figure 6.1a). The colon continues from the cecum to the ascending colon, which becomes the transverse colon at the hepatic flexure (Figure 6.3). The ascending colon is usually short, approximately 15 cm length. It is secondarily retroperitoneal with its mesocolon fused to the retroperitoneum. The transverse colon is the longest segment measuring approximately 45 cm as it courses across the upper abdomen from hepatic to splenic flexure. During colonoscopy, the hepatic flexure can sometimes be identified by transluminal visualization of a bluish structure, that is, the liver (Figure 6.4). The transverse colon crosses the upper abdomen toward the spleen, where it becomes the descending colon at the splenic flexure and terminates as the sigmoid colon in the left lower quadrant. The triangular-shaped lumen is a landmark for the transverse colon (Figure 6.5). The endoscopist often uses this feature of the transverse colon to separate the descending colon from the ascending colon during colonoscopy. It usually has a well-developed mesentery that allows significant mobility so that the transverse colon can drape as low as the pelvic inlet. The greater omentum is fused to the inferior surface of the transverse colon at the *taenia mesocolica*. The splenic flexure with its watershed location of blood supply is vulnerable for the development of ischemic colitis (Figure 6.6). The descending colon, along with the ascending colon, is secondarily retroperitoneal but is somewhat longer, measuring 25 cm. It courses caudally along the left side of the

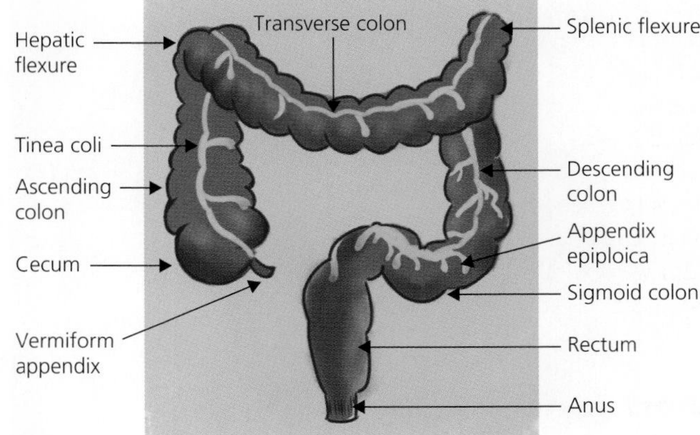

Figure 6.3 Schematic depiction of the colon and rectum and its anatomical segments.

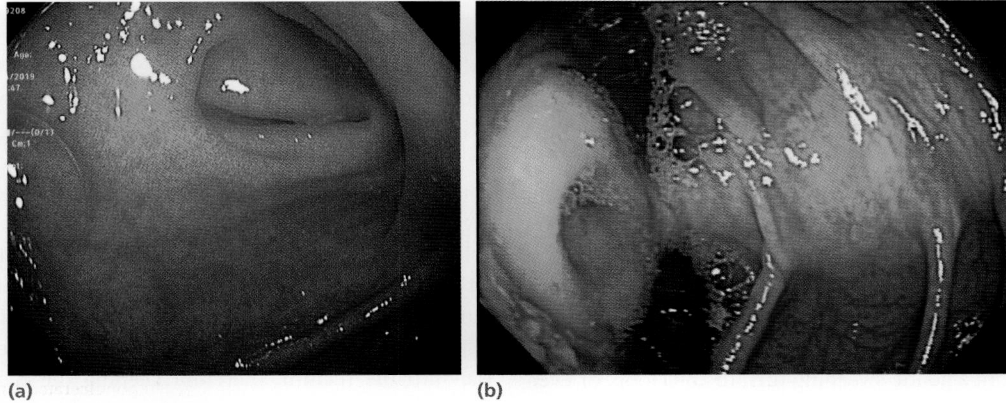

Figure 6.2 The appendiceal orifices at the cecal on colonoscopy (**a** and **b**). Source: Courtesy Bo Shen.

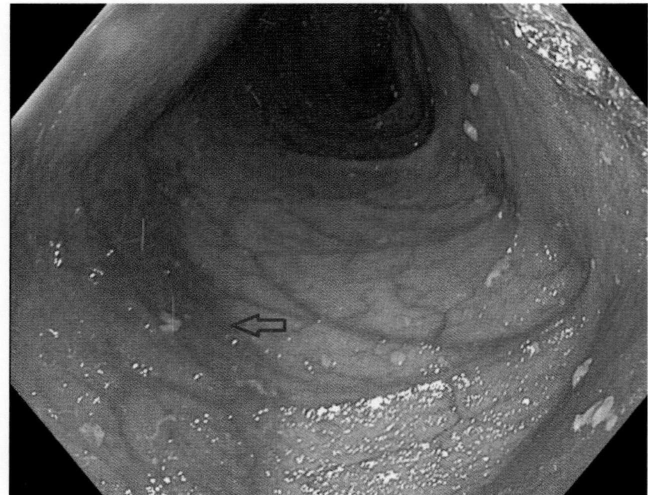

Figure 6.4 Hepatic flexure on colonoscopy. The liver is visualized transmurally as a bluish structure (blue arrow). This feature is used as a topographic marker to describe the location of pathologies in the colon. Source: Courtesy Bo Shen.

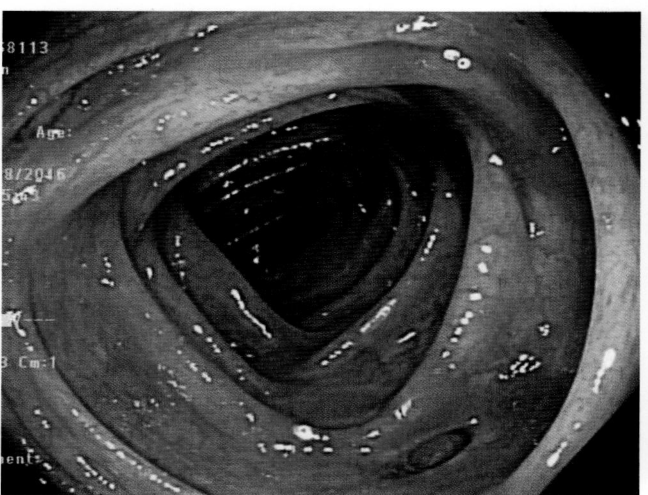

Figure 6.5 The triangular-shaped lumen is a hallmark for the transverse colon. The segment divides the left and right colon on colonoscopy. Source: Courtesy Bo Shen.

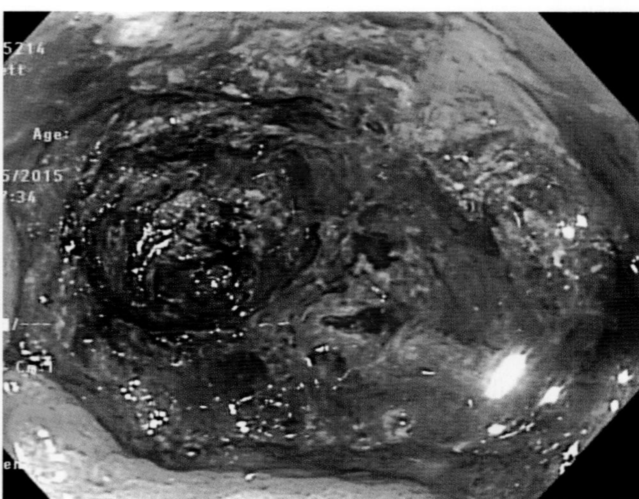

Figure 6.6 Acute ischemic colitis at the splenic flexure with edematous and erythematous mucosa and spontaneous bleeding on colonoscopy. Source: Courtesy Bo Shen.

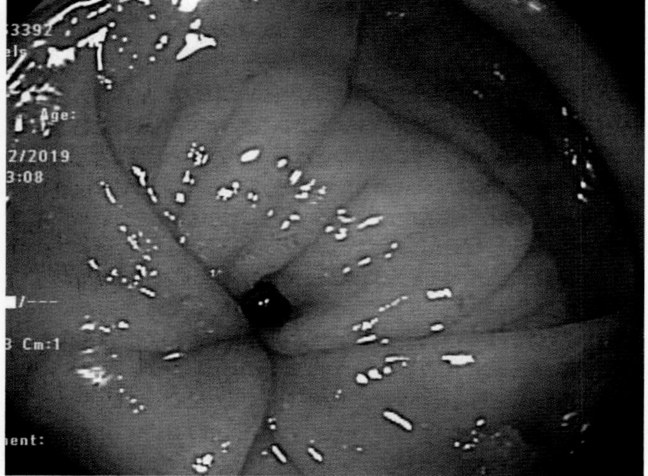

Figure 6.7 Sigmoid volvulus with luminal narrowing undergoing colonoscopic detorsion. Source: Courtesy Bo Shen.

abdomen, where it joins the sigmoid colon. The diameter progressively diminishes to approximately 2.5 cm at the level of the distal sigmoid colon.

The sigmoid colon varies greatly in length, measuring from 15 to 50 cm with a mean length of 38 cm. The sigmoid colon makes a sweeping turn in the pelvis occasionally reaching to the right side, then joining the rectum at the sacral promontory. The sigmoid colon is a mobile segment of the large intestine as it is completely invested by peritoneum. Its anatomical configuration can vary from a gentle sweeping turn to an ω loop, or even a remarkably redundant coiled appearance. This gross feature of the sigmoid colon should be taken into account during colonoscopic navigation of a markedly redundant torturous sigmoid colon. A redundant, floppy sigmoid colon may undergo axial rotation about its mesentery, resulting in sigmoid volvulus or floppy sigmoid (Figure 6.7). The rectosigmoid junction is considered by some anatomists and clinicians to be a distinct segment containing what is described in essence as a functional sphincter mechanism [11]. Although no distinct muscle fibers have been identified, the narrowed diameter of the rectosigmoid, together with its sharp angulation, does appear to provide a sphincter-like function that retards the advance of fecal material into the rectum, therefore keeping the rectum relatively empty. This functional feature is believed to be responsible for the delayed transit through the rectosigmoid junction that contributes to the increased intraluminal pressure in the sigmoid colon and predisposes to the development of sigmoid diverticulosis [12] (Figures 6.8 and 6.9).

In contrast with the small bowel, the colon is notable for its saccular or haustral appearance, resulting from the arrangement of the external muscular layer into three thick longitudinal muscular bands termed the *tenia coli*. The colon assumes its macroscopic saccular appearance because the length of the tenia is approximately one-sixth shorter than the length of the rest of the colonic wall [13]. The haustra are separated by the *plicae semilunares*, crescentic folds that give the colon its distinctive appearance (Figure 6.10), which is more pronounced when the colon is filled with air or barium contrast. Colonic *plicae semilunares* span only a portion of the bowel lumen, in distinction to *plicae circulares* of the small intestine, which extend around the luminal circumference. This difference becomes particularly useful in distinguishing the large intestine from the intestine on abdominal imaging when small bowel is distended and the colon is relatively collapsed.

It is commonly assumed that the colon lacks a complete circumferential longitudinal layer of the muscularis propria because of its consolidation as tenia. However, Fraser and colleagues [14] demonstrated that the colon in fact has a complete longitudinal muscular layer over its entire circumference, but that the external muscular layer appears to be much thicker at the taeniae. The taenia coli on the anterior aspect of the colon is

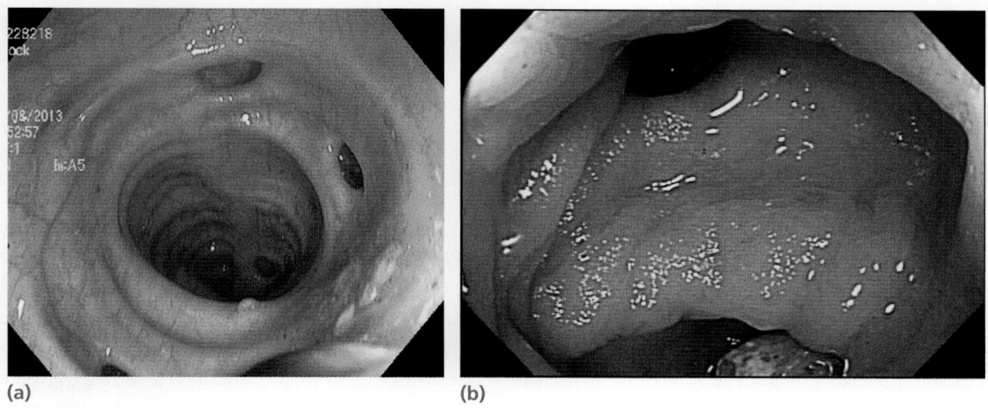

Figure 6.8 Extensive sigmoid diverticulosis on colonoscopy (a and b). Source: Courtesy Bo Shen.

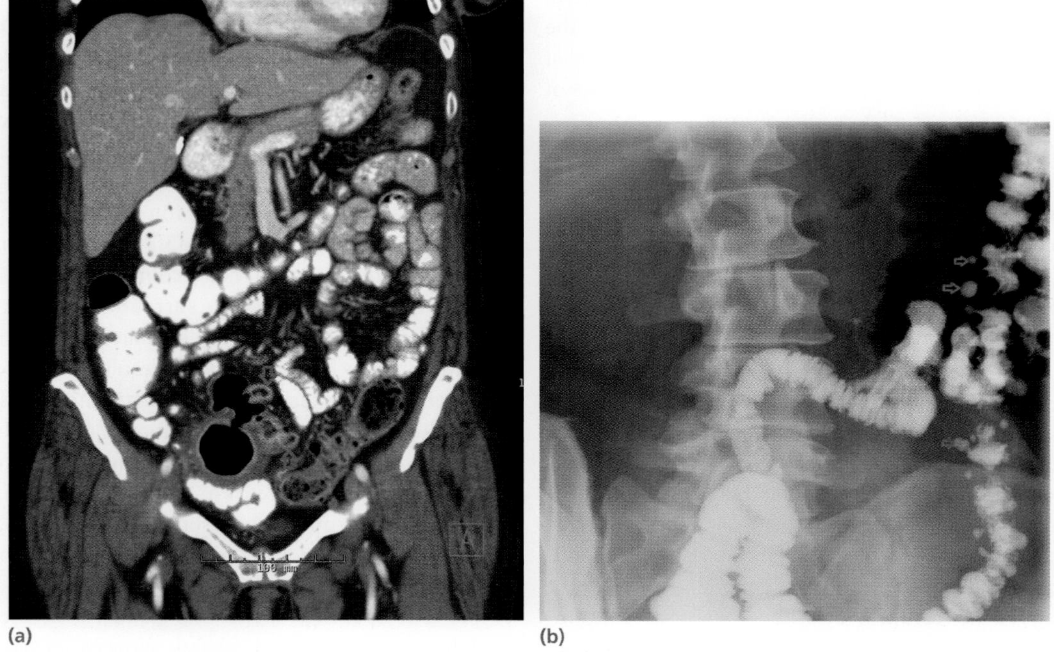

Figure 6.9 Diverticulosis on abdominal imaging. (a) Sweeping sigmoid colon on computed tomography with diverticulosis (red arrows); (b) diverticulosis in the left colon (red arrows) on colon barium enema. Source: Courtesy Bo Shen.

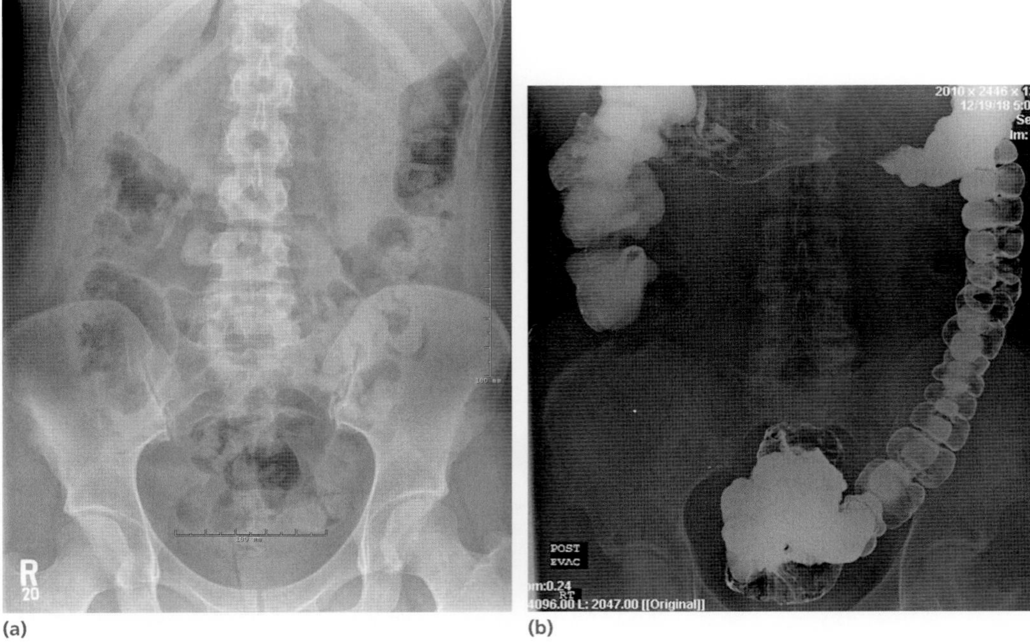

Figure 6.10 Colon haustra. (a) Colon haustra on plain abdominal radiograph; (b) crescentic folds of colon on barium enema. Source: Courtesy Bo Shen.

called *taenia libera*, with the taenia on the posteromedial and posterolateral aspects termed the *taenia mesocolica* and *taenia omentalis*, respectively. Taeniae are generally absent from the surface of the rectum. The transition between the colon and the rectum at the level of the sacral promontory is gradual, marked by splaying of the taenia coli into a confluence of the muscle fibers covering the surface of the rectum resulting in distinctive taenia-free appearance. Another feature that distinguishes the colon from the rectum or small intestine is the presence of *appendices epiploicae*, fatty appendages located at the serosa of the colon that may serve as a fat storage reserve.

Blood is supplied to the colonic wall by the *vasa recta*, which traverse the muscularis propria layer to provide blood supply to the mucosa and submucosa [15]. The sites of entry of the vasa recta leave potential weak areas in the muscularis propria that are thought to predispose to the formation of pseudodiverticula wherein colonic mucosa may progressively protrude through the muscularis propria [16] (see Figures 6.8 and 6.9).

Rectum

The rectum (from the Latin *rectum intestinum*, meaning "straight intestine") is a tubular organ that is straight in its course toward the anus and is 12–15 cm in length (Figure 6.11). The proximal extent of the rectum is somewhat arbitrary because there are no precise anatomical landmarks to differentiate it from the sigmoid colon. Surgeons generally consider the proximal extent of the rectum to be at the level of sacral promontory, whereas anatomists argue that the rectum begins more distally, at the level of third sacral vertebra. On its external surface, the rectum has three gentle curves that correspond intraluminally to the valves of Houston (Figure 6.12). The rectum is distinguished from the colon by the absence of taenia, appendices epiploicae, and a well-defined mesentery. The proximal third to half of the rectum is intraperitoneal and enveloped by visceral peritoneum. The rectum is distally supported by the mesorectum that locates mostly posteriorly, occupying the entire posterior space of the true pelvis. The mesorectum is enveloped by the fascia propria of the rectum (Figure 6.13). It is within this mesorectal envelope that lymph node metastases and direct extension of rectal cancer typically occur. It is of paramount importance during surgical removal of a rectal cancer to maintain the integrity of the mesorectal envelope to minimize the risk for local recurrence [17].

The distal rectum continues inferiorly to become the anal canal. Despite being rather short (3.2–5.3 cm in men and 3–5 cm in women), the anal canal has a complex anatomy, particularly because of its relationship to surrounding structures [18]. It opens externally as the anus, an anterior–posterior slit that remains virtually closed at rest as a result of tonic contraction of the internal sphincter muscle. Approximately in the middle of the anal canal, the distal rectal mucosa of endodermal origin transitions into lower (cutaneous) lining derived from the ectoderm. This transition occurs at the dentate line, an area notable for toothlike mucosal protrusions pointing cephalad (Figure 6.14). The folds of the distal rectal mucosa form the columns of Morgagni that in turn form pits known as anal sinus crypts. The openings of the anal glands, which secrete mucus for lubrication of the anal canal to allow easier passage of stool, are located within these crypts. Anal glands are more numerous at the posterior aspect of the anal canal and extend through the

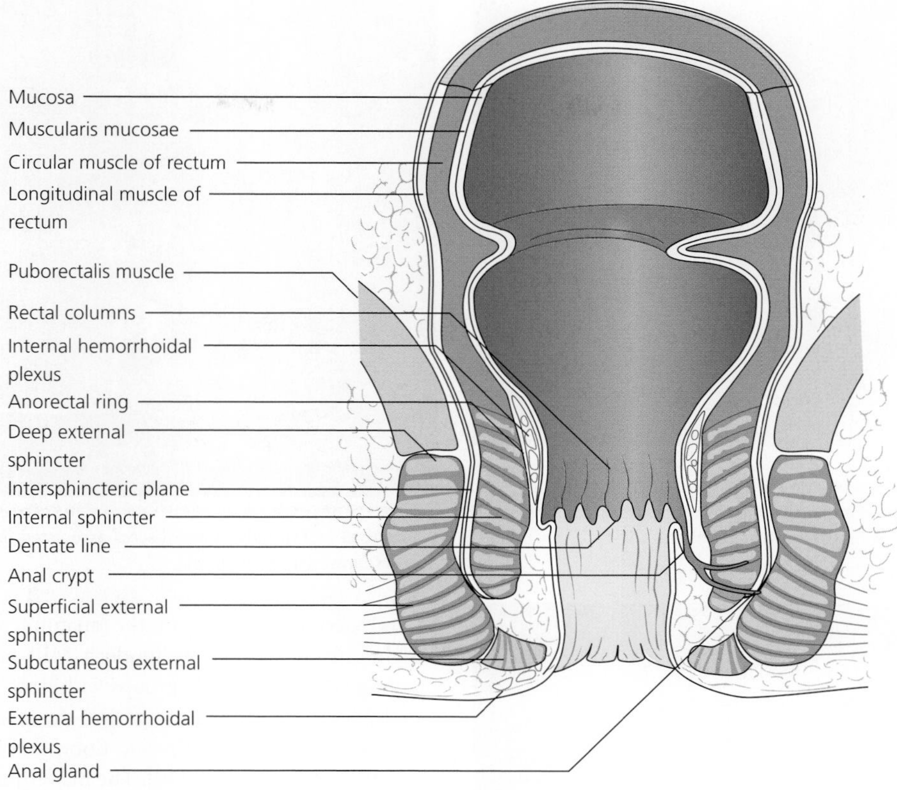

Figure 6.11 Anorectal anatomy.

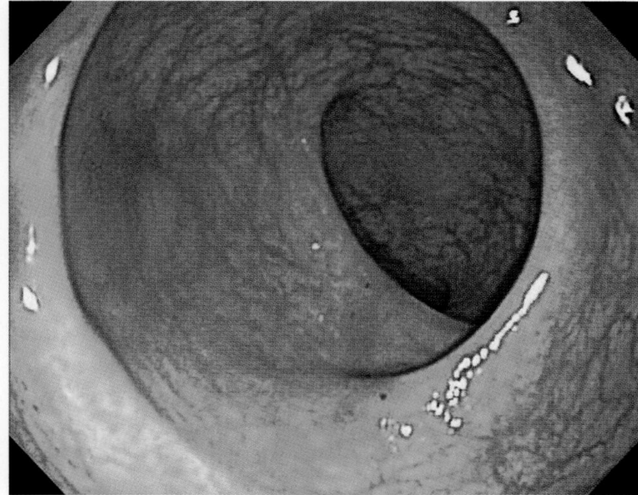

Figure 6.12 Valves of Houston as crescent-shaped folds in the lumen of the rectum. Source: Courtesy Bo Shen.

submucosa, with half of them traversing the internal sphincter muscle and terminating in the intersphincteric space. Obstruction of the glands at their opening within the anal crypts is thought to be responsible for the development of cryptoglandular abscesses and fistula-in-ano (Figure 6.15). Cryptoglandular

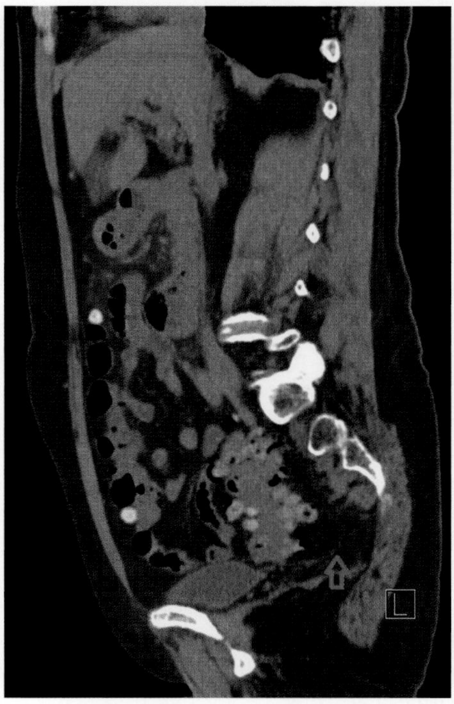

Figure 6.13 Mesorectum wrapping around the rectum (red arrow) on computed tomography. Source: Courtesy Bo Shen.

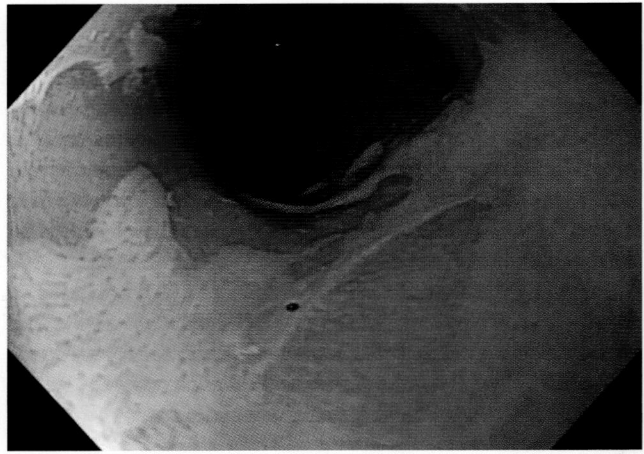

Figure 6.14 Anal transition zone on endoscopy. Notice the salmon-colored rectal columnar mucosa and white-colored anal squamous epithelia on colonoscopy. Source: Courtesy Bo Shen.

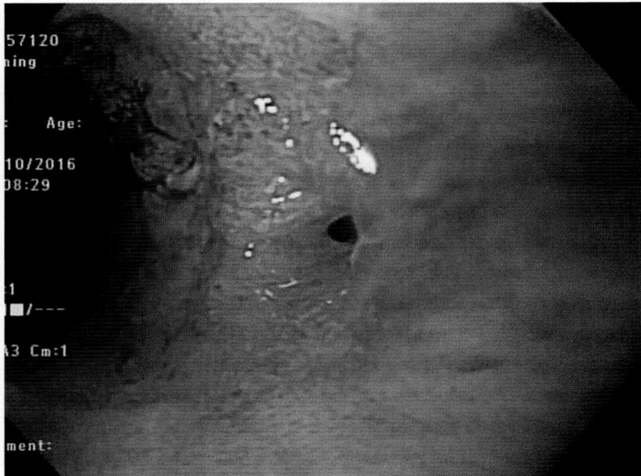

Figure 6.15 Cryptoglandular abscess and fistula. An fistular opening at the dentate line on colonoscopy. Source: Courtesy Bo Shen.

abscesses can expand through the planes of perianal and potential ischiorectal spaces, resulting in ischioanal, intersphincteric (Figure 6.16), or transsphincteric abscess. The distal aspect of the anal canal continues toward the anal opening, where the epithelium of the anal canal meets with an ectoderm-derived epithelium of the anal margin or anal verge. The anal margin is an anatomical landmark that has been used to measure and communicate the distance to the findings of interest during colonoscopy. Although some anatomists recommend using the dentate line as a reference because of its readily identified location, it is more convenient for clinical purposes to use the anal margin instead because the dentate line cannot be reliably visualized during routine endoscopy.

Our understanding of anal sphincter musculature and composition of the pelvic floor in general has evolved over the past several decades because of the anatomical and physiological insights made possible by modern MRI and ultrasonographic imaging [19]. The muscle groups within the pelvis can be subdivided into three general categories: the anal sphincter complex itself, the muscles of the pelvic floor, and the muscles located along the pelvic sidewalls [20]. The major muscle that contributes fibers to the external sphincter is the *levator ani* (Figure 6.17). This muscle derives its name from its functional characteristic of elevating the pelvic floor and anus during the act of defecation. It is a broad, thin muscle composed of skeletal muscle fibers that originate from both sides of pelvic sidewall and meeting in the middle to form anococcygeal raphe. *Levator ani* is a muscular aggregate made up by the ileococcygeus, pubococcygeus, and puborectalis muscles supplied by the roots of the sacral nerves S2–S4, as well as the perineal branch of the pudendal nerve [2,21]. The midline of the pelvic floor has several openings through which pass the lower rectum, urethra, and either the dorsal vein of the penis in the male or the vagina in the female. The puborectalis muscle has an anatomical configuration similar to a U-shaped sling that is tonically contracted at rest. This tonic contraction “kinks” the rectum, resulting in an increase in the anorectal angle and limiting movement of stool into the distal rectum [22,23]. During defecation, in a synchronized motion with the rest of the pelvic floor, the puborectalis muscle relaxes, allowing return of the rectum into a straighter position, allowing for passage of fecal material into the distal rectum (Figure 6.18). On digital rectal examination, this muscle can easily be appreciated by gently curving the examining finger posteriorly as the finger advances above the anorectal ring. The anal canal is described differently by anatomists and clinicians. Whereas anatomists define the anal canal as extending from anal verge to the dentate line, clinicians find this definition of limited clinical utility and instead consider the anal canal as extending to the top of the anorectal ring marked by the upper edge of the puborectalis

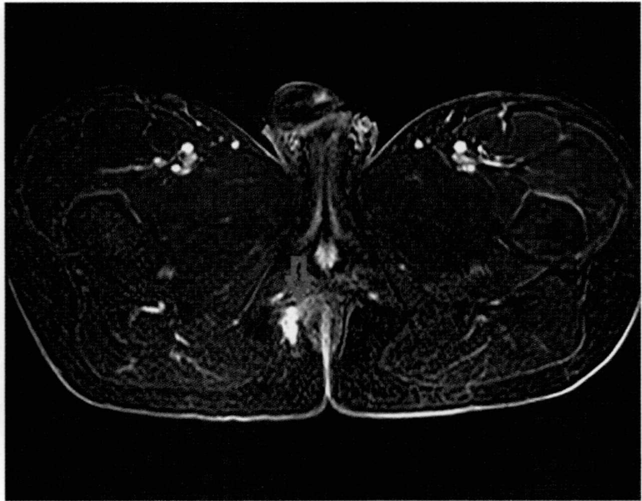

Figure 6.16 Cryptoglandular abscess-associated fistula-in-ano on magnetic resonance imaging.

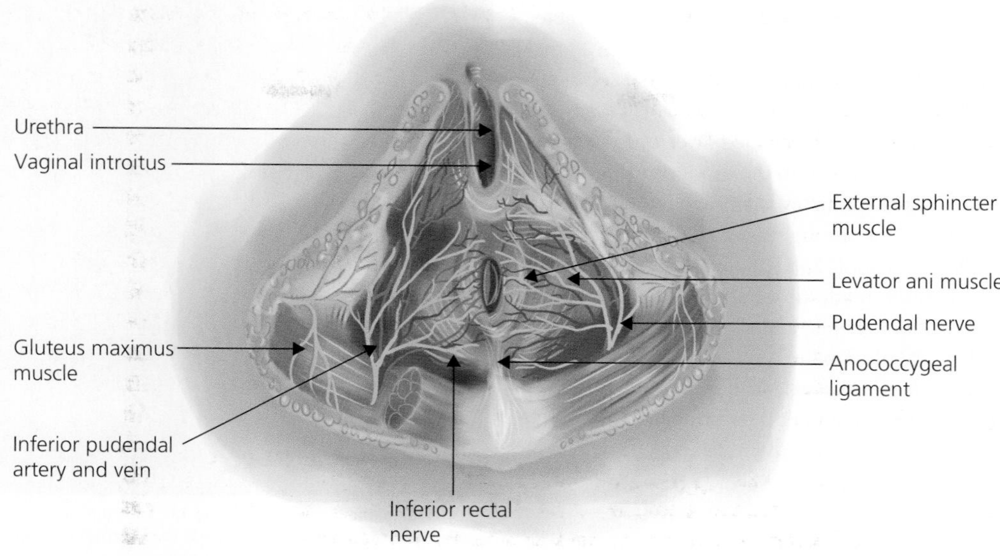

Figure 6.17 Pelvic floor (female) anatomy and anal sphincter innervation.

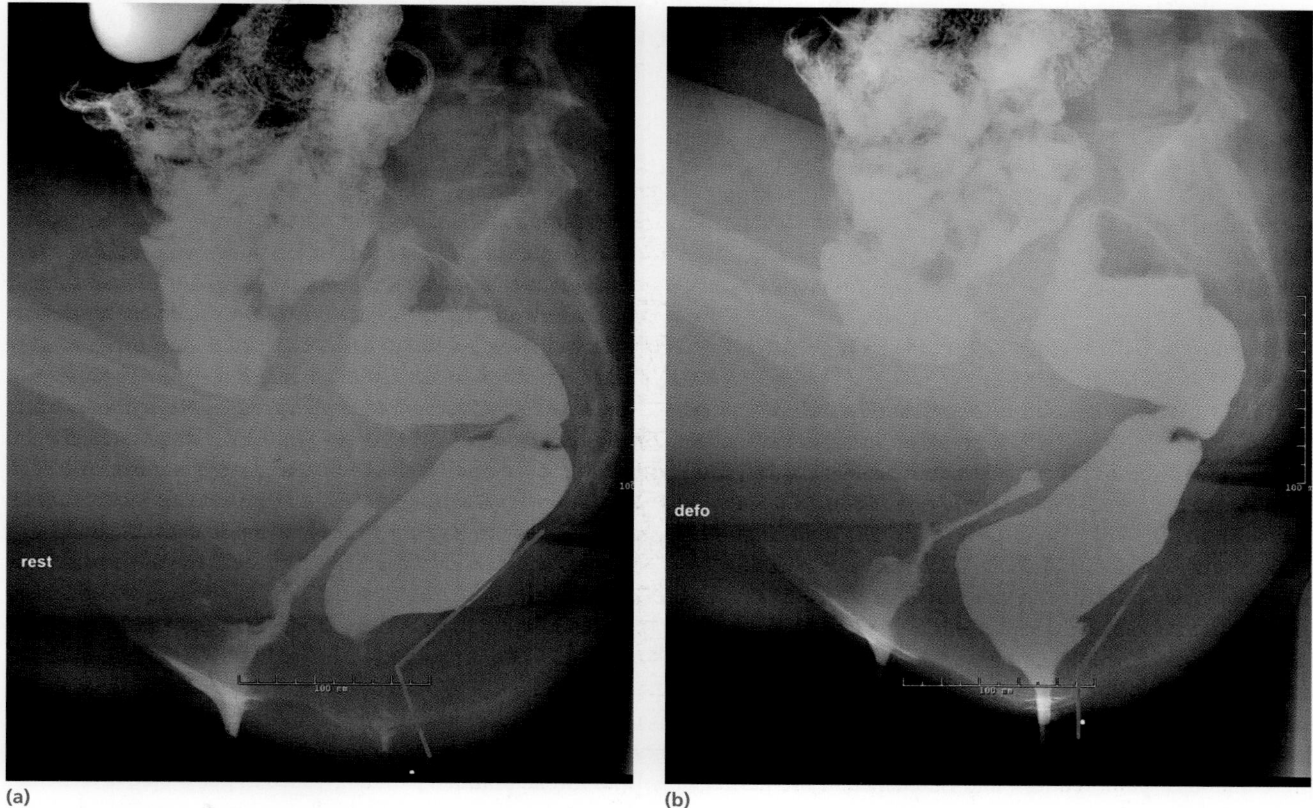

Figure 6.18 Change of anorectal axis before and during defecation on barium defecography (red lines). **(a)** The anorectal angle is about 100–110° before defecation; **(b)** the angle becomes straight (around 160°) during defecation. Source: Courtesy Bo Shen.

muscle [18]. This definition is more useful for decisions regarding surgical intervention that requires division of the anal sphincter or evaluation of the extent of pathological conditions, such as anal or distal rectal cancers [24]. In addition to the external sphincter consisting of the levator muscles, the anorectal ring is composed of the internal sphincter muscle, a thickened layer of muscularis propria of the rectum that extends from the distal rectum into the anal canal. The internal anal sphincter is an involuntary smooth muscle that is responsible for resting anal tone contributing to continence of gas and liquid stool [25]. It is tonically contracted at rest. The external sphincter, made up of striated muscle fibers, provides additional continence, particularly with physical exertion associated with a Valsalva maneuver, such as coughing or sneezing [26,27]. In contrast, the external sphincter muscle is controlled voluntarily and can augment the resting pressure of the internal sphincter when a bowel movement needs to be deferred.

Anus

The anal canal has a rich blood supply with six arteries running longitudinally within the wall of the distal rectum and anus [28]. They supply three internal hemorrhoids located on the left lateral, right posterior, and right anterior aspect of the anal canal. Internal hemorrhoids serve a physiological purpose of providing complete continence, particularly to liquid stool and gas, because the anal canal, being shaped as an anterior–posterior slit, cannot otherwise close completely to provide a water-tight and airtight seal. Internal hemorrhoids are the venous cushions located submucosally and are covered by a rather thin layer of anoderm. They can become enlarged as a result of a variety of conditions, such as constipation, frequent Valsalva maneuvers, or genetic predisposition. Internal hemorrhoids can protrude through the anal canal and could be confused with external hemorrhoids, which are small venous cushions located at the anal margin. Internal hemorrhoids that protrude through the anal canal can be differentiated from external hemorrhoids by the appearance of the overlying tissue. Whereas internal hemorrhoids are covered with mucosa of anal canal, external hemorrhoids are covered with skin of the anal margin.

Perianal and perirectal space

Surrounding the rectum and anal canal are clinically significant potential spaces within which perirectal or perianal abscesses can fester. These spaces are defined as ischiorectal, ischioanal, intersphincteric, submucosal, superficial, and deep postanal [20]. In addition, there are supralevator and retrorectal spaces. The ischiorectal fossa is a commonly affected potential space filled with a loose areolar fatty tissue located between ischial bones of the pelvis and the rectum. This space is a frequent location of cryptoglandular abscesses that originate in infected anal glands. Large abscesses in ischiorectal or ischioanal fossa can extend to the skin of the buttock resulting in classic presentation of pain, redness, and fluctuance in the perirectal region. There is also a small potential intersphincteric space between the internal and external sphincters. Abscess formation in this area can result in significant pain in the absence of external signs of infection [29]. Digital rectal examination is usually extremely painful, suggesting an abscess located between the sphincter complexes. Intersphincteric abscess can be easily identified on imaging by computed tomography or MRI (Figure 6.19). Abscesses in the supralevator region can result from intraabdominal pathology, such as perforated diverticular abscess. The postanal space is also a common site of perirectal infection and can give rise to a horseshoe-shaped extension bilaterally around the ischioanal fossae (Figure 6.20).

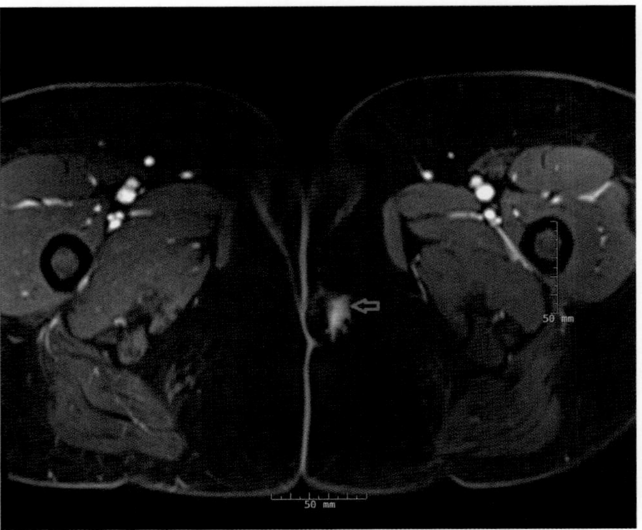

Figure 6.19 Intersphincteric fistula (red arrow) on computed tomography. Source: Courtesy Bo Shen.

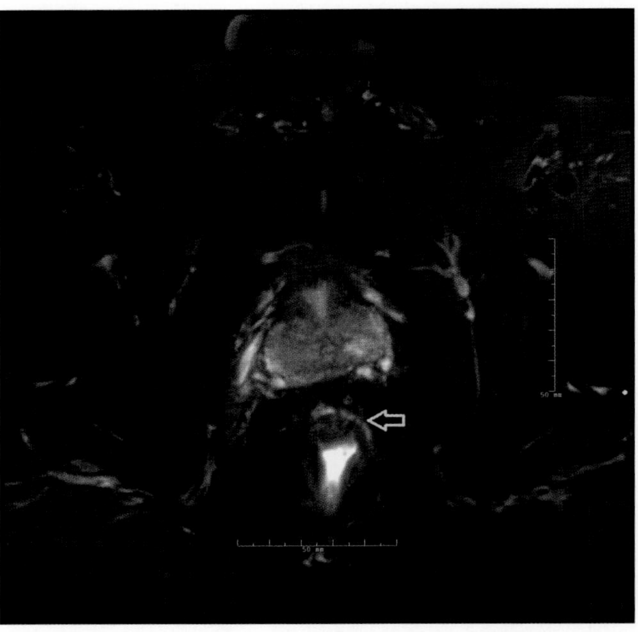

Figure 6.20 Horseshoe fistula (yellow arrow) between the rectum and prostate on magnetic resonance imaging. Source: Courtesy Bo Shen.

Histology of the colon

The wall of the colon is composed of five layers, each serving unique functions. Starting from the lumen, the colon is lined by the mucosa, which rests on the lamina propria (Figure 6.21). Beneath the mucosa are the muscle fibers of the muscularis mucosae followed by submucosa, muscularis propria, and serosa. The muscularis propria consists of circumferential and longitudinal muscles and neural plexuses.

Colon epithelia

The colonic mucosa is composed of a continuous polarized simple columnar epithelium comprising the luminal surface and lining the crypts, lamina propria, and a thin muscularis mucosa layer [30]. The colonic mucosal layer is organized as an array of crypts that appear as a row of test tubes in a rack under light microscopy (Figure 6.22). Unlike the small intestine, the colonic mucosa does not have true villous projections. Regularly spaced crypts located in parallel alignment are a hallmark feature of colonic mucosal architecture. It is present throughout the entire colon, except in proximity to mucosal lymphoid collections, in areas of transition to small intestinal mucosa (i.e., ileocecal valve), or the squamous epithelium at the anorectal junction [31]. The colonic surface epithelium is a simple columnar cuboidal epithelium that functions as a protective barrier between the host and the luminal environment and to absorb water from the colonic lumen. It is composed of absorptive and goblet cells residing on a basement membrane complex [32]. Absorptive surface epithelial cells are responsible for colonic ion and water transport. These cells project microvilli and glycocalyx as seen by transmission electron microscopy. The nuclei of absorptive cells are oval and located toward the basement membrane in parallel with the long axis of the cells, while the cytoplasm is highly eosinophilic [33,34].

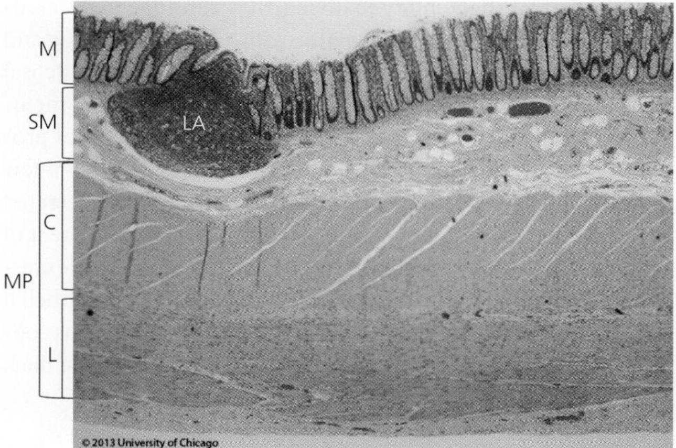

Figure 6.21 Anatomy of the colonic wall. The histological section represents all layers of the colonic wall. At the top of the figure is the colonic mucosa (M) with one lymphoid aggregate (LA) extending into the submucosa (SM). Muscularis propria (MP) consists of circular smooth muscle layer (C) and longitudinal layer (L). Source: Courtesy Dr. Shu-Yuan Xiao, Department of Pathology, University of Chicago, Chicago, IL, USA.

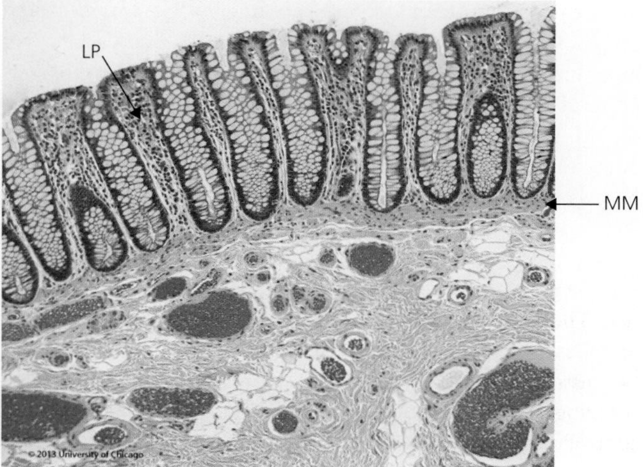

Figure 6.22 Normal colonic mucosa. Simple columnar surface epithelium at the top of the figure forms mucosal crypts arranged in parallel "row of test tubes." The lamina propria (LP) consists of the stromal elements investing the crypts and extending from the surface epithelium to the smooth muscle cells of the muscularis mucosa (MM). Prominent vascular structures (arterioles, venules, and lymphatics) are noted within the submucosa. Source: Courtesy Dr. Shu-Yuan Xiao, Department of Pathology, University of Chicago, Chicago, IL, USA.

Goblet cells (so named for their wine goblet-like appearance) synthesize, store, and secrete mucous granules by exocytosis [35]. These cells also contain luminally directed microvilli, which are small and irregular in shape and size as visualized by electron microscopy. The cytoplasm of goblet cells is almost entirely filled with mucin, which does not stain with standard hematoxylin and eosin (H&E) stain, giving its vacant appearance. Specialized mucin staining can be used to highlight their cytoplasm [36].

The cellular composition of the epithelium within the colonic crypts is different from that of the surface epithelium. In addition to absorptive and goblet cells, colonic crypts contain immature and undifferentiated precursor cells, as well as specialized endocrine, and in the right colon maybe a few Paneth cells. Endocrine cells can be distinguished from more numerous absorptive and goblet cells by their eosinophilic staining granules within the cytoplasm oriented toward the basement membrane with a nucleus residing somewhat higher toward the apex of the cell. These cells are readily visualized on an H&E-stained section (Figure 6.23). Endocrine cells can also be visualized by the special silver staining techniques because most of these cells are argyrophilic. They may be further identified immunohistochemically with varying immunoreactivity to chromogranin A, synaptophysin, neuron-specific enolase, and specific antibodies [37]. Paneth cells, normally found at the base of the crypts, are pyramidal in shape and contain large eosinophilic secretory granules (Figure 6.24). These granules contain lysozyme, epidermal growth factor, and arginine-rich basic protein, as well as glycoprotein. Paneth cells are normally found only in the midgut-derived segments of colon (cecum and right colon); their presence in other regions of the colon could indicate metaplasia

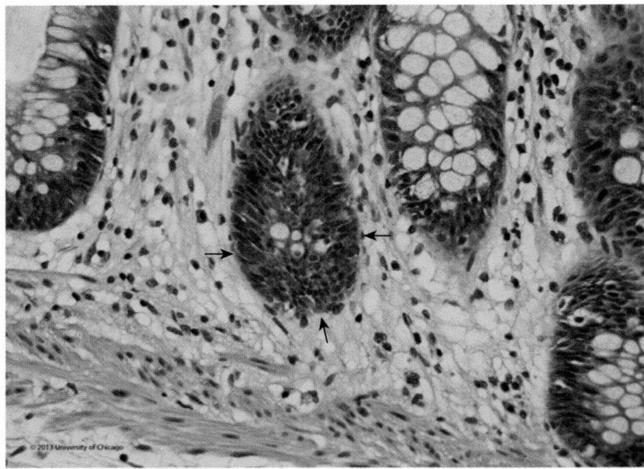

Figure 6.23 Normal colonic basal crypt epithelium. Among the absorptive cells and goblet cells are endocrine cells with basally oriented secretory granules (arrows). Source: Courtesy Dr. Shu-Yuan Xiao, Department of Pathology, University of Chicago, Chicago, IL, USA.

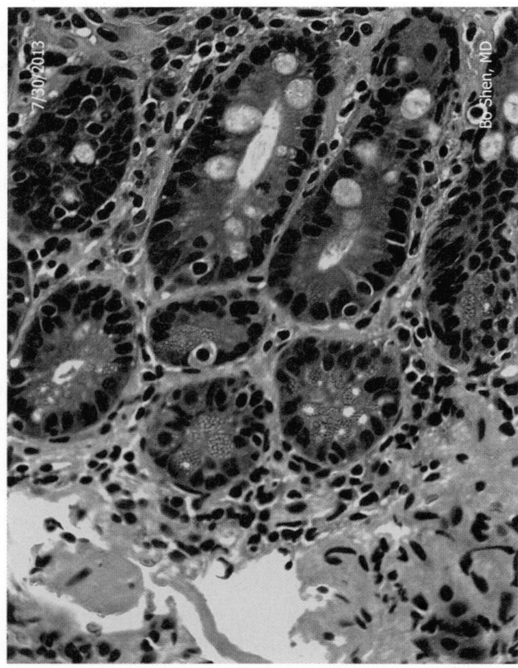

Figure 6.24 Paneth cells at the intestinal crypt with characteristic intracytoplasmic granules on hematoxylin and eosin histology.

developing in the context of chronic inflammation. Paneth cell granules and cellular components contain α-defensins, β-defensins, nucleotide-binding oligomerization domain-containing (NOD)-2, lysozyme, phospholipase A_2, secretory leukocyte inhibitor, immunoglobulin A (IgA), tumor necrosis factor-α, trypsin and trypsinogen, Fas ligand (CD95L), CD44v6, CD15, and many others [38]. The contents of the Paneth cells reflect their role in innate immunity, apoptosis, and stem cell maintenance. Membranous (M) cells are a variant of epithelial cells found in the dome of lymphoid follicles and cannot be reliably distinguished from the absorptive colonocytes under light microscopy. The M cells provide docking sites for intraepithelial B and T lymphocytes, as well as a small number of macrophages. These cells are able to sample luminal contents and transfer the antigens to the antigen-presenting cells through the specialized process of transcytosis [39]. The intramucosal lymphocytes in the small intestine are the first members of immune system to encounter dietary and bacterial antigens and are likely to play a role in oral tolerance [40,41]. Within the paracellular space, the predominant cell types are $CD3^+$, $CD8^+$, T-cell receptor $\alpha\beta^+$ suppressor T cells, and a relatively smaller number of T-cell receptor $\gamma\delta^+$ suppressor T cells [37]. T lymphocytes can be recognized by nuclei that densely stain by hematoxylin with usually only a thin rim of cytoplasm visible under light microscopy. $CD3^+$/$CD45RO^+$ activated memory T lymphocytes with smaller numbers of $CD45RA^+$ naive T cells and IgM-secreting B cells reside within the M cell-covered lymphoid aggregate. The presence of an excessively large number of intraepithelial lymphocytes is a histopathological feature of lymphocytic colitis, an autoimmune diarrheal disorder. Intraepithelial eosinophils occasionally can be seen in normal colon, but they are present in much smaller numbers than lymphocytes.

Colonic crypts serve an important function in renewing the surface epithelium. Mucosal renewal is attributable to colonic epithelial stem cells residing within the so-called mesenchymal niche (see Chapters 1 and 2). These multipotent cells slowly divide, contributing new epithelial cells that migrate toward the surface epithelium replacing those lost by continuous exfoliation into the lumen or as a result of apoptosis [42,43]. As the cells migrate toward the surface, they differentiate into one of five distinct cell types: colonocyte, goblet cell, endocrine cell, Paneth cell (see Figure 6.18), or M cell. Even though most epithelial cells lose their ability to divide, they continue to differentiate and become more functionally mature while migrating and eventually undergoing apoptosis or exfoliate from the mucosal surface. The colonic epithelium rests on a thin basement membrane complex composed of collagen and other structural proteins [44,45]. The basement membrane is normally only a few microns thick and is readily permeable to absorbed or secreted substances, including water and proteins. It allows movement of lamina propria lymphocytes into the epithelial layer. The excessively thickened collagenous band, along with intraepithelial lymphocytosis, is a histopathological feature of collagenous colitis, an autoimmune disorder of the colon causing watery diarrhea of patients.

Lamina propria

The lamina propria located beneath the columnar epithelium forms an investing stroma for the colonic mucosa and extends from the basement membrane complex to the muscularis mucosa. It contains a variety of cell types residing within loosely organized collagen fibers [46]. Most of the cells in lamina propria are responsible for immunologically mediated host defense. The majority of the cells are organized in lymphoid aggregates, while mature B lymphocytes, plasma cells T cells (helper, suppressor, and lymphokine-activated killer), eosinophils, and macrophages comprise the pool of free lamina propria inflammatory cells. The predominant cell type within the lamina propria is IgA-secreting plasma cells with a smaller proportion Ig-, IgG-, and IgE-secreting cells [47]. The remaining lymphocytes in the lamina propria are predominantly CD3$^+$ T cells with smaller numbers of CD8$^+$ T and CD20$^+$ B lymphocytes. Eosinophils can be found in the lamina propria of a normal colon; their numbers are highly variable, but they are relatively rare compared with plasma cells and lymphocytes.

Mast cells, also referred to as tissue-based basophils, are even less numerous than eosinophils. Their density appears to be increased in the ileocecal region compared with other sites in the colon [48]. Mast cells are difficult to distinguish on routine H&E stain, but these cells stain well by Giemsa or toluidine blue, and for tryptase and CD117 (c-kit) [49]. Despite the abundance of other immune cells, neutrophils normally are absent within the colonic epithelium or lamina propria. The presence of neutrophils in the colonic epithelia or the lumen of crypt is indicative of acute or active inflammation, namely, cryptitis or crypt abscess (Figure 6.25). Macrophages, representing tissue-based monocytes, are common within the lamina propria and play an important role in processing and presenting antigenic materials to other immune cells. Macrophages are not easily identified on light microscopy unless H&E-stainable apoptotic debris or pigment is present within their cytoplasm, for example, deposits from anthracene-type laxatives as seen in melanosis coli [50]. Neuroendocrine (amine precursor uptake and decarboxylation) cells are present within the lamina propria outside the basement membrane of the crypts. These cells may give rise to carcinoid and neuroendocrine tumors [51]. Lamina propria myofibroblasts form a reticular network called *subepithelial myofibroblast syncytium*. The myofibroblasts interact closely with the epithelium, lamina propria inflammatory cells, and muscularis mucosa. They play a role in water absorption, ion and mucin secretion, immune regulation, and maintenance of stem cells [52]. Vascular structures within the lamina propria are limited to small capillaries, which can be identified by the presence of erythrocytes, cells, and sometimes neutrophils within their lumen.

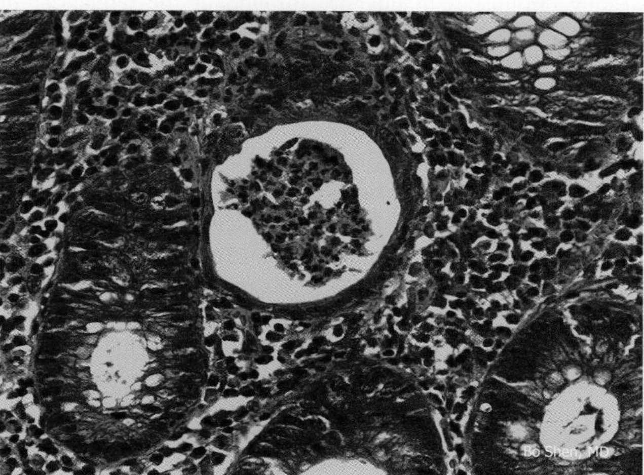

Figure 6.25 Cryptitis and crypt abscess in active colitis with infiltration of neutrophils in the colon epithelia and crypt lumen on hematoxylin and eosin histology.

Muscularis mucosae

A thin layer of muscle fibers termed *muscularis mucosa* is located deep to the lamina propria and separates the mucosa (lamina propria and epithelium) from submucosa.

Submucosa

The submucosa forms an elastic interface between the mucosa and the muscularis propria allowing mucosa to slide over relatively rigid muscularis during peristalsis. It is composed of loosely arranged smooth muscle fibers, fibroelastic and adipose tissue, a small number of inflammatory cells (lymphocytes, plasma cells, fibroblasts, and macrophages), and neural plexuses. Submucosal smooth muscle fibers are closely associated with the interstitial cells of Cajal (ICCs), which form neuroeffector junctions with the nerve fibers located in the immediate proximity. These junctions are thought to transmit central, sympathetic, and parasympathetic nervous system signals. ICCs are modified myofibroblasts as evidenced by their H&E appearance of fusiform bodies with large oval nuclei. Mutation in the *c-kit* gene of ICCs is responsible for 80%–90% of gastrointestinal stromal tumors [50]. c-kit, a tyrosine kinase receptor, is activated by binding its ligand (known as c-kit ligand, stem cell factor, steel factor, or mast cell growth factor), which results in dimerization of c-kit molecules on the cell surface [53,54]. The resulting activation of c-kit's tyrosine kinase moiety causes autophosphorylation and phosphorylation of downstream signaling molecules leading to inhibition of apoptosis and increased cell proliferation. In gastrointestinal stromal tumors, *c-kit* mutations cause transcription of a protein that is constitutively active and results in ligand-independent signaling ultimately leading to the development of cancer [53,55].

Vascular structures are more abundant in the submucosa and include arterioles, venules, and lymphatics. These submucosal vessels may appear large and tortuous even in an otherwise normal colon (see Figure 6.22). Tumors invading into the submucosa can produce distant metastases through invasion of vascular or lymphatic submucosal networks [56].

Muscularis propria

The muscularis propria of the colon includes a circular inner layer and a longitudinal outer layer [14,57]. In addition to the complete longitudinal layer of muscularis propria as noted earlier, three longitudinal bands known as taenia coli run along the length of the colon. ICCs, located within the muscularis propria, are thought to serve as pacemaker cells creating and propagating slow waves that lead to smooth muscle contraction [58]. They can be identified by immunostaining for CD117 and CD34 [59]. The segments of colon located intraperitoneally are covered by a serosal lining derived from mesothelial cells.

Serosa

Intraperitoneal segments of colon and rectum are covered by visceral peritoneum forming its serosal surface. The serosa consists of a single layer of cells.

Enteric nerve system

Meissner's neural plexuses lie immediately below the muscularis mucosae, and the deeper Henle's neural submucosal plexus is located along the inner aspect of the muscularis propria and is analogous to the myenteric plexus of Auerbach [60,61]. Between the muscle layers of muscularis propria lies the neural plexus of Auerbach. Cell bodies of neurons or ganglion cells with their characteristic appearance of round or oval nuclei containing prominent nucleolus and surrounded by generous basophilic cytoplasm can be found within the submucosa. Nerve axons and plexuses have a fibrillar appearance and seem to traverse in and out of the plane of the histological section when examined under light microscopy.

Anal transition zone

The region where distal rectal mucosa and the squamous mucosa of the anoderm gradually intersect is called the ATZ and is located approximately 1 cm above the dentate line of the anal canal. There is no visible line or landmark that can be noted on gross or clinical examination that would indicate its location. ATZ epithelium consists of four to nine cell layers, with the surface cells arranged as a columnar, cuboidal, or polygonal layer, whereas the basal cells are small with their nuclei arranged perpendicular to the basement membrane (Figure 6.26) [62]. Within the ATZ, small areas of mature squamous epithelium may be present, especially at the upper border of the anal canal (see Figure 6.14). Anal glands, responsible for secreting lubricating mucus, arise from anal sinuses in ATZ. The median number of anal glands is 6 with a range of 3–10. Whereas some glands are located within the submucosa, others extend into the internal sphincter, and a few reach the intersphincteric space or penetrate the external anal sphincter, terminating in the ischioanal space [63]. At the distal aspect of the transition zone, approximately at the level of the dentate line, the squamous epithelium becomes more uniform, indicating the beginning of the squamous zone. The squamous epithelium in this zone is unkeratinized with short or no papillae. Anal glands or skin appendages are never present within this zone. As the squamous zone transitions into the perianal skin, keratinization becomes apparent. Perianal skin contains sweat glands, hair follicles, and sebaceous glands. A characteristic finding in the perianal skin is the presence of apocrine glands within the subcutaneous tissue.

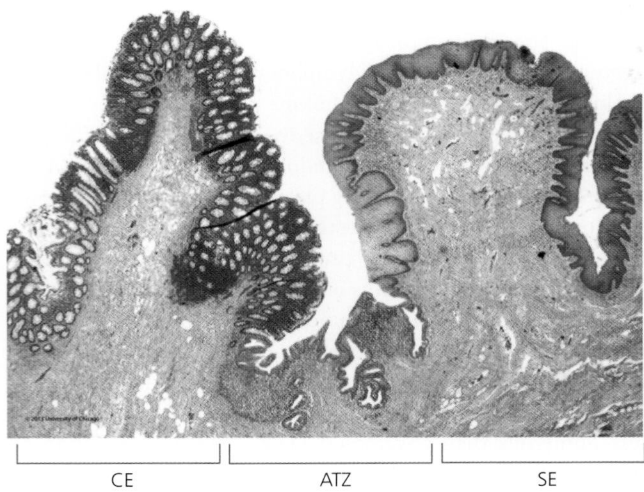

Figure 6.26 Anal canal. Transition between the colonic epithelium (CE) on the left, anal transition zone (ATZ), and squamous epithelium (SE) of the anal canal on the right. Source: Courtesy Dr. Shu-Yuan Xiao, Department of Pathology, University of Chicago, Chicago, IL, USA.

Histology of the appendix

The histology of the appendix varies from that of the colon. In contrast with the colon, where crypts line up evenly like test tubes in a rack, appendiceal crypts are more irregular in shape, length, and distribution [64]. The appendix has abundant lymphoid tissue, most of it organized in lymphoid aggregates (Figure 6.27) [65]. Although a characteristic feature of the appendix, the amount of lymphoid tissue varies in quantity with age. The appendix of a newborn contains scant or no lymphoid tissue. With age, lymphoid nodules accumulate, peaking in the first decade, then steadily diminishes in quantity throughout the remainder of life [66]. Appendices excised incidentally from middle-aged adults can still occasionally demonstrate prominent organized lymphoid components. In areas containing lymphoid tissue, crypts are typically absent. Appendiceal lymphoid aggregates can extend beneath the muscularis mucosae into the underlying submucosa. These aggregates are confluent and appear similar in composition and function to Peyer's patches of the small bowel. As in Peyer's patches, the lymphoid framework of the appendix is compartmentalized into follicles, dome, interfollicular region, and follicle-associated epithelium [67]. The follicle in most cases has a germinal center containing a polymorphic cellular population of small and large lymphocytes in various stages of maturation, occasional $CD4^+$ T-helper cells, and macrophages. Immediately surrounding the germinal center is the mantle zone containing small round B lymphocytes. Overlying the lymphoid aggregate and beneath the epithelium is the dome region composed of a heterogeneous population of cells, including B and T lymphocytes, macrophages, and occasional plasma cells.

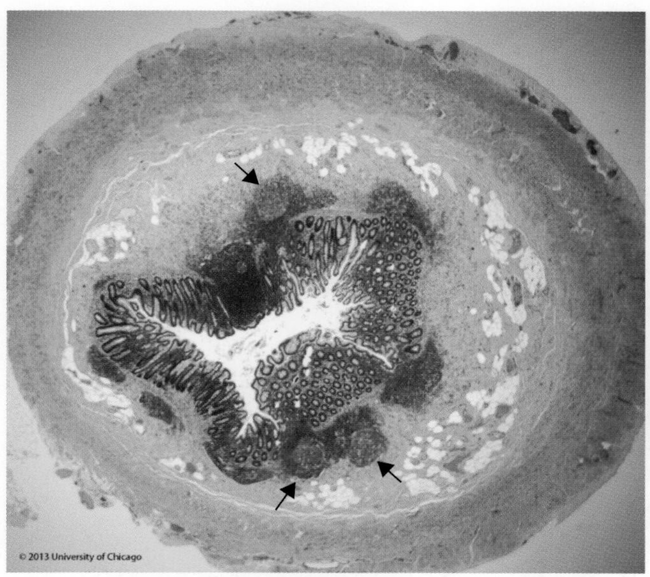

Figure 6.27 Low-magnification view of a cross section of vermiform appendix. The irregular (stellate) lumen is lined by a single layer of surface epithelium. Note the characteristic lymphoid follicles within the lamina propria that also extended to submucosa (arrows). Source: Courtesy Dr. Shu-Yuan Xiao, Department of Pathology, University of Chicago, Chicago, IL, USA. Copyright 2013, University of Chicago.

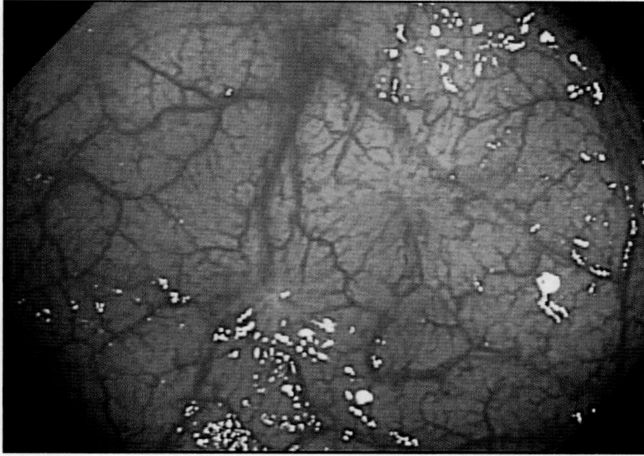

Figure 6.28 Normal vascular pattern of the colon under near-transparent epithelia on colonoscopy.

Blood supply, lymphatic drainage, and innervation

The blood supply to the colon and rectum is derived from the superior and inferior mesenteric arteries and veins [68]. The vascular pattern of the colon can clearly be visualized through mucosa (Figure 6.28). The lymphatics drain via the corresponding arterial supply.

Arterial system

The watershed area between the territory supplied by the superior mesentery artery and the inferior mesenteric artery is located between the proximal two-thirds and the distal segment of the transverse colon, which corresponds to the area where the midgut joins the hindgut. The superior mesenteric artery originates from the aorta posterior to the pancreas at the level of L1 (Figure 6.29). It courses anteriorly to the third portion of the duodenum and continues caudally and slightly to the right, traveling within the mesentery of the small bowel as it gives off 12–20 jejunal and ileal branches and continues as the ileocolic artery toward the cecum. On the right side, the superior mesenteric artery gives rise to the middle and right colic arteries. Although the ileocolic artery is quite constant, the right colic and middle colic arteries can have varying anatomy. The right colic artery originates directly from the superior mesenteric artery in approximately 20% of the individuals and in the remainder, it originates as a branch of the ileocolic artery or can be absent altogether. The ileocolic artery bifurcates into an ascending branch coursing superiorly and anastomosing with the right colic artery and a posterior branch that supplies the cecum and appendix [69]. The middle colic artery has a short common trunk and bifurcates early in its course into left and right branches. The left branch supplies the distal half of the transverse colon and splenic flexure, whereas the right branch supplies the hepatic flexure and provides collateral circulation through anastomosis with branches of the ileocolic and right colic arteries.

The inferior mesenteric artery originates from the aorta about 3–4 cm cephalad to its bifurcation at the level of L2–L3 and courses caudally and to the left toward the pelvis. Just distal to its origin from the aorta, the inferior mesenteric artery gives off the left colic artery, which bifurcates into an ascending branch, contributing to the arc of Riolan, and a descending branch that runs caudally and supplies the descending colon. As the inferior mesenteric artery continues its course into the pelvis it gives off two to six sigmoidal arteries and becomes the superior hemorrhoidal artery, also commonly referred to as the superior rectal artery. Unlike most of the colonic blood supply, which is segmental in its architecture, the sigmoidal arteries form arcades that more closely resemble the small bowel vasculature with multiple anastomoses between them.

Due to its segmental blood supply that originates from two major arterial systems, the collateral circulation within the colon plays a critical role when blood supply through one of the arteries is interrupted surgically or through disease processes. The central anastomotic artery connecting the colonic mesenteric vascular beds is the marginal artery of Drummond [70]. It provides collateral circulation between the superior and inferior mesenteric arterial systems as it runs along the mesenteric border of the entire colon. A potential watershed area between the inferior and superior mesenteric arterial systems is located at the splenic flexure and is called Griffiths' critical point [71]. Even though some authors postulate that this watershed area

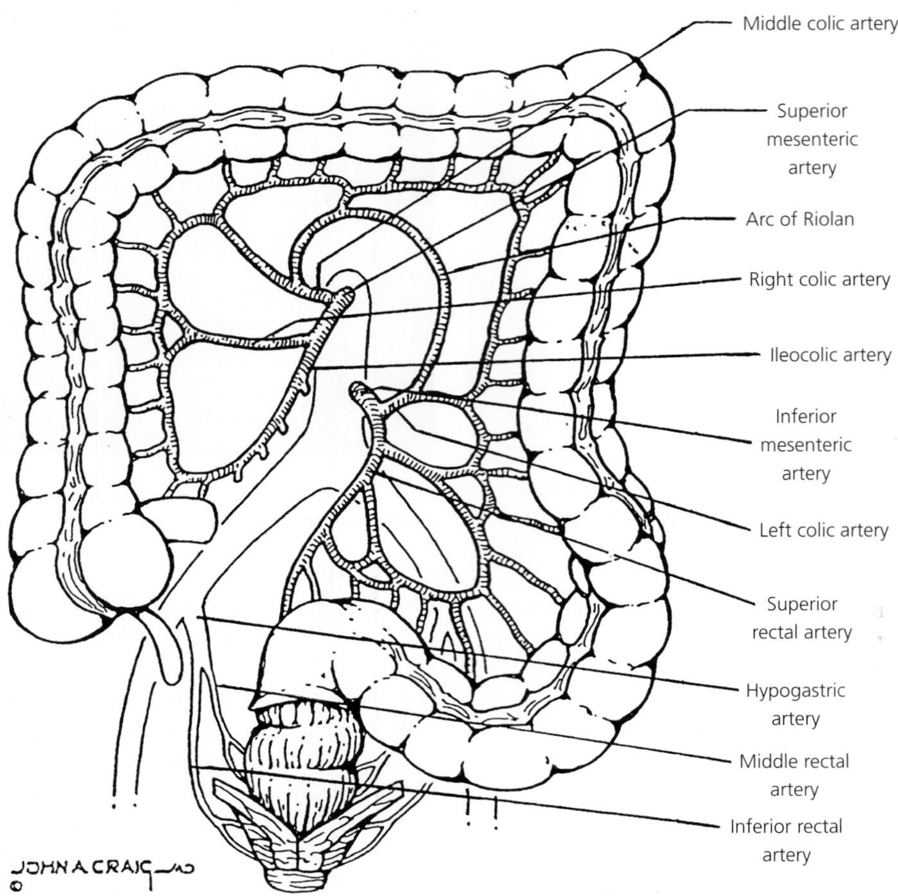

Figure 6.29 Arterial blood supply of the colon and rectum. Source: Kodner et al. 1993 [100]. Reproduced with permission of McGraw-Hill.

predisposes patients to ischemic colitis [72] (see Figure 6.6), this has not been supported by clinical evidence [73]. Another area of potentially diminished blood supply is Sudeck's point located at the watershed area between the inferior mesenteric artery and the internal iliac artery. This point is located near the rectosigmoid junction. Similar to Griffiths' point, there is no convincing clinical evidence that Sudeck's point is more prone to ischemia than any other segment of the left colon. Another communicating arc between inferior and superior mesenteric systems is the arc of Riolan, a thick torturous vessel that is often referred to as the meandering artery [74]. It tends to become more pronounced as it plays a critical role in establishing collateral circulation between the middle colic artery and the ascending branch of the left colic artery when either the superior or inferior mesenteric artery is occluded in advanced atherosclerotic disease. Correspondingly, the presence of a meandering artery with antegrade flow indicates stenosis or occlusion of the inferior mesenteric artery, whereas retrograde flow indicates occlusion of the superior mesenteric artery.

The blood supply to the colonic lumen is provided by short straight arteries, *vasa recta*, arising from the marginal artery of Drummond. These vessels divide into anterior and posterior branches and run submucosally within the colonic wall. At the level of the taenia epiploica and taenia libera they penetrate the muscularis propria and continue within the submucosa toward the antimesenteric border. At the mesenteric aspect of the colonic wall, short straight vessels, *vasa recta brevia*, course toward the submucosa by penetrating the muscularis propria in multiple locations. These sites are thought to represent potential weak areas prone to formation of colonic pseudodiverticula [75]. Clinical observation supports this notion because colonic diverticula are rarely found on the serosal surface of the colon between taenia epiploica and taenia libera as this segment of colon is not supplied by *vasa recta brevia*, but rather by continuation of submucosal vessels coursing within the colonic wall. Interestingly, linear ulceration in Crohn's disease is characteristically located along the mesentery border (Figure 6.30).

There is a dual blood supply to the rectum that combines inflow from the inferior mesenteric and internal iliac arterial systems. The superior hemorrhoidal artery coursing caudally into the pelvis gives off multiple branches within the mesorectum. These branches form multiple anastomoses with the middle and inferior rectal arteries. The middle rectal arteries in most instances arise from the internal pudendal arteries

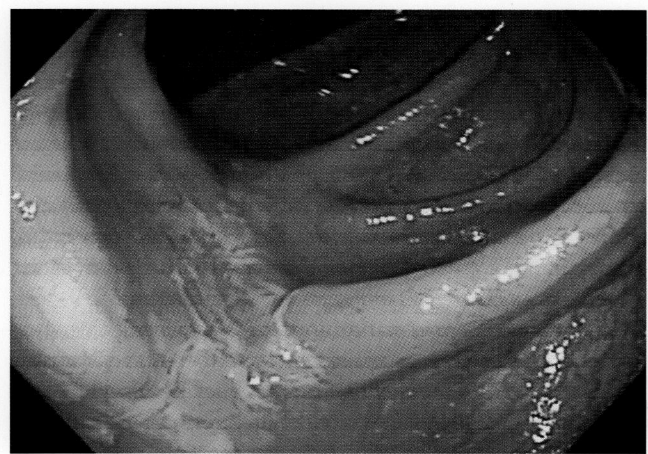

Figure 6.30 Longitudinal linear ulceration along the mesentery edge in Crohn's disease on colonoscopy. Source: Courtesy Bo Shen.

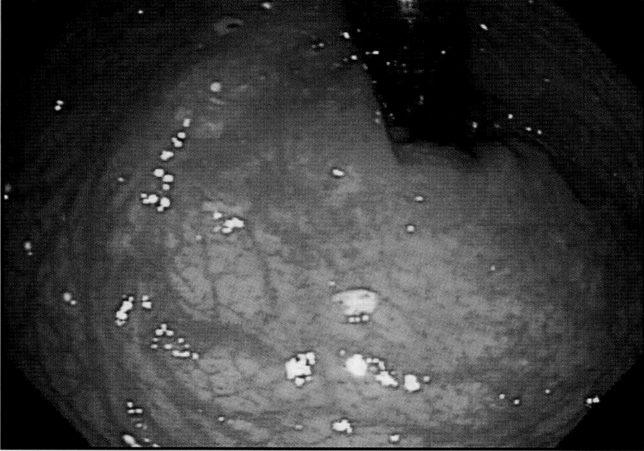

Figure 6.31 Prominent veins underneath the rectal mucosa on an endoscopic retroflex view. Source: Courtesy Bo Shen.

(approximately two-thirds of the time); in the remaining instances, they arise from the inferior gluteal or internal iliac artery. The middle rectal artery is often quite small in diameter measuring less than 1 mm; in fact, a middle rectal artery measuring 1–2 mm in diameter is present in less than 5% of population. The inferior rectal arteries originate from the pudendal arteries and supply the anal canal and external anal sphincter muscles. The anastomoses between the inferior rectal artery and the other rectal arterial systems occur primarily within the walls of the rectum and anal canal.

Venous system

The venous drainage of the colon essentially follows arterial blood supply. The vascular distribution of the superior mesenteric artery is drained by the superior mesenteric vein that joins with the splenic vein to form the portal vein. The inferior mesenteric vein drains the distribution of the inferior mesenteric artery and usually joins the splenic vein posterior to the body of the pancreas.

Rectal venous outflow follows the course of the rectal arteries. Prominent veins beneath the rectal mucosa are often visualized on endoscopy (Figure 6.31) The hemorrhoidal cushions located within the anal canal at left lateral, right anterior, and right posterior positions lack muscular wall and are considered to be sinusoids rather than veins. The subepithelial vessels and sinuses above the dentate line, which constitute the internal hemorrhoid plexus, are drained by way of the middle rectal veins to the internal iliac veins. The venous plexus and sinuses below the dentate line constituting the external hemorrhoidal plexus drain primarily via the inferior rectal veins into the pudendal veins and into internal iliac veins.

Lymphatic system

The colon has a rich and well-developed network of lymphatic vessels that follow the vascular supply. The lymphatic basins are typically divided into epiploic, paracolic, intermediate, and principal. The epiploic lymph nodes reside on the bowel wall under the peritoneal lining, as well as in the appendices epiploicae. The paracolic nodes are located along the marginal artery of Drummond and along the vascular arcades. The intermediate lymph nodes are situated along the primary named colic vessels. The principal nodes are located along the superior and inferior mesenteric vessels. The lymph from the colon drains into the cisterna chyli through a chain of lymph nodes. Pathological evaluation of lymph nodes for the presence or absence of metastases is critical in the staging of colorectal cancers. Therefore, proximal ligation and division of major blood vessels is required during colon resection to achieve removal of a segment of mesocolon with sufficient numbers of lymph nodes.

Lymphatic drainage from the upper and middle parts of the rectum proceeds along the superior hemorrhoidal artery through the inferior mesenteric lymph nodes (Figure 6.32). The caudal part of the rectum drains cephalad through superior rectal lymphatics into inferior mesenteric nodes and laterally into middle rectal lymphatics to the internal iliac nodes. Lymphatic drainage from the anal canal above the dentate line proceeds cephalad via superior rectal lymphatics through inferior mesenteric nodes and laterally along both the middle rectal vessels and inferior rectal vessels through the ischioanal fossa toward the internal iliac lymph nodes [76]. Lymph from the anal canal below the dentate line usually drains to the inguinal nodes. It can also drain to the superior rectal lymph nodes or along inferior rectal lymphatics to the ischioanal nodes if obstruction to the lymph flow occurs along the primary drainage pathway. It is therefore important to consider metastatic spread of distal cancers to the inguinal lymph nodes, which should always be meticulously examined as a part of a detailed physical examination of the patient with rectal cancer.

Innervation

Similar to the lymphatics, the innervation of the colon closely follows its blood supply. The sympathetic supply of the right colon originates from the lower thoracic segments. These nerves synapse in the celiac, preaortic, and superior mesenteric ganglia. The postganglionic fibers course along the superior mesenteric

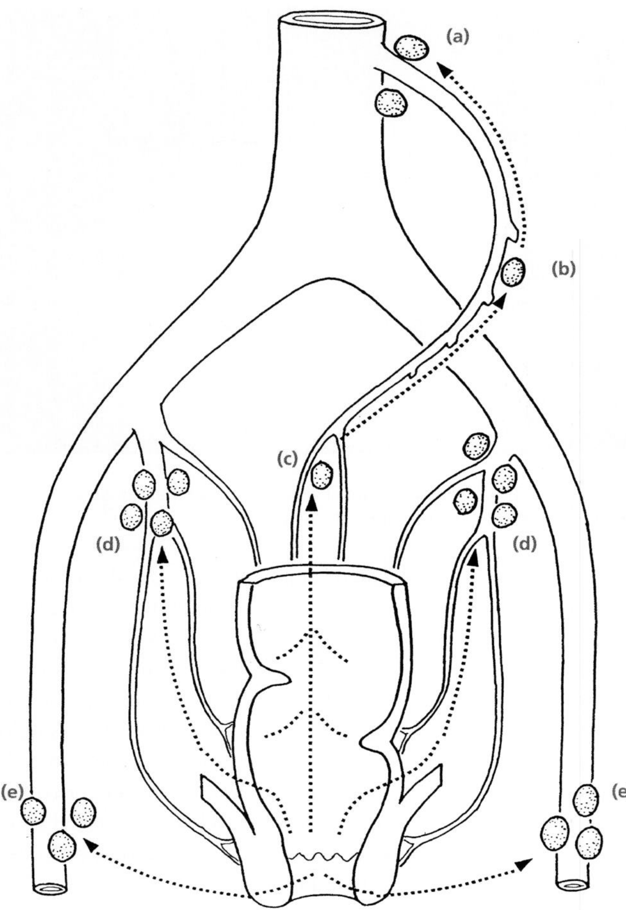

Figure 6.32 Lymphatic drainage of the rectum and anus. **(a)** Nodes at the origin of the inferior mesenteric artery; **(b)** nodes at the origin of the sigmoid branches; **(c)** sacral nodes; **(d)** internal iliac nodes; **(e)** inguinal nodes. Source: Kodner et al. 1989 [101]. Reproduced with permission of McGraw-Hill.

artery supplying the small bowel and right colon. The parasympathetic innervation is supplied by the right vagus nerve branch and the celiac plexus. The sympathetic nerves supplying the left colon and rectum arise from L1–L3. The preganglionic fibers synapse in the preaortic plexus, while postganglionic fibers continue along the superior rectal artery into the pelvis, supplying the left colon and upper rectum.

Colorectal malformations

The large bowel and anus are common organs affected by congenital malformation.

Malrotation

Malrotation can result from failed completion of a full 360° rotation around the root of the mesentery of the cecum. Most commonly, the cecum will cease rotation and become fixed in the right upper quadrant by fibrotic Ladd's bands that may lead to extrinsic compression of the duodenum [77]. An abnormal location of the cecum can also contribute to an atypical presentation of acute appendicitis with symptoms localizing to the left or right upper quadrant [78]. Reverse rotation occurs when the midgut rotates clockwise instead of counterclockwise, placing the duodenum anteriorly and the transverse colon posteriorly. Omphalocele occurs when the midgut fails to completely return to the abdominal cavity and remains covered by a thin membrane. Incomplete attachment of the cecal mesentery is relatively common. In the majority of individuals, the cecum is located intraperitoneally, fully invested by visceral peritoneum. It usually has a short mesentery that limits its mobility; however, in approximately 5% of the population, the peritoneal covering of the cecum is absent, resulting in a fully mobile cecum [79]. Such excessive mobility may predispose the individual to the development of cecal bascule or volvulus.

Colonic atresia

Among other congenital malformations is atresia of the colon, a rare cause of intestinal obstruction that comprises only 5% of all forms of intestinal atresia. It can present as partial occlusion of the colonic lumen by a membrane or web, complete occlusion with proximal and distal colonic segments that are joined by a completely obliterated cordlike remnant of the intestine, and a variant where there is complete separation of the proximal and distal segments appearing as blind pouches without any communication between them. Colonic atresia can occur at any segment of the colon and can be of varied length.

Intestinal duplication

Intestinal duplication is a rare congenital anomaly that can occur anywhere along the gastrointestinal tract. The colon and rectum account for 5–10% of all intestinal duplications [80]. In the colon, there are three general groups of congenital malformations: mesenteric cysts, diverticula, and long colonic duplication [81]. Mesenteric cysts are lined by intestinal epithelium with variable amounts of smooth muscle and located within the mesentery of the colon or behind the rectum. Diverticula arise either from the mesentery wall or the mesenteric border of the bowel. They may have heterotopic gastric mucosa or pancreatic tissue. Long colonic duplication is exceedingly rare. In this malformation, the two parts lie in parallel, sharing a common wall throughout most of the length of the colon and rectum.

Hirschsprung disease

Hirschsprung disease results from the absence of ganglion cells in the myenteric plexus of the colon and rectum. This condition is caused by an interruption of migration of neuroenteric cells from the neural crest as they advance toward the distal colon and rectum. Hirschsprung disease occurs in 1/5000 live births and has an overall 4:1 male predominance [82]. The internal anal sphincter is involved in all cases, and in most cases the colon and rectum are involved as well. The length of the aganglionic colonic

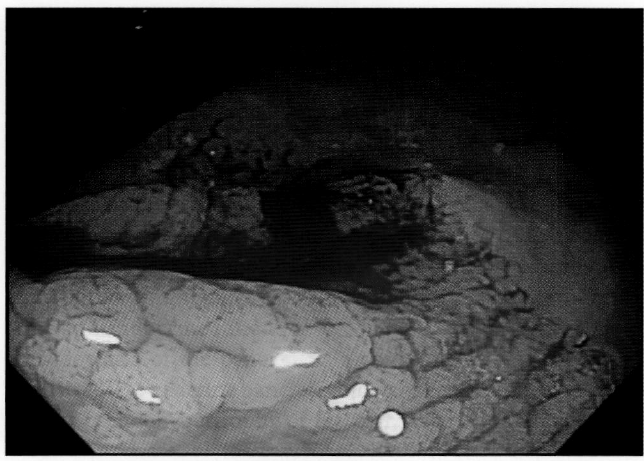

Figure 6.33 Mucosal bleeding after deep rectal biopsy for the evaluation of Hirschsprung disease.

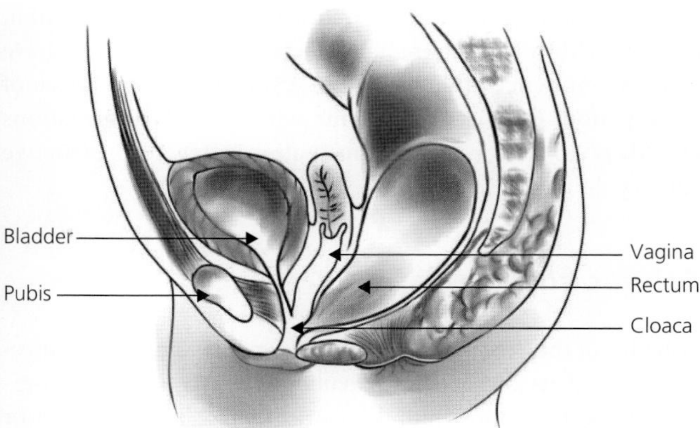

Figure 6.34 Cloaca. The rectum, vagina, and urinary tract are fused together forming a common channel. This single channel opens at a location where the urethra would be typically found in normal female individuals. Source: Courtesy Bo Shen.

segment varies. In the most common type, affecting 80–85% of patients with Hirschsprung disease, the aganglionic segment involves the rectum and most of the sigmoid colon. In 10% of patients, the aganglionic segment extends to the level of splenic flexure. Total colonic aganglionosis occurs in 3–8% of patients, sometimes affecting a segment of terminal ileum [83]. Deep rectal biopsy is helpful for the diagnosis (Figure 6.33).

In the so-called ultra-short Hirschsprung disease, the aganglionic segment is very short, extending just a few centimeters above the dentate line. Because this variant has such a short aganglionic zone, ganglion cells may be present in the biopsy [84]. Clinical presentation is characterized by sustained contraction of the aganglionic bowel segment, leading to intestinal obstruction and distension of proximal segments (megacolon). In most instances, the diagnosis of Hirschsprung disease is made before the child reaches the age of 1 year. However, in those affected by very short or ultra-short segment of distal rectum, diagnosis may not be made until they are adults.

Neuronal intestinal dysplasia

Neuronal intestinal dysplasia is an abnormality that includes hypertrophy of ganglion cells, presence of immature ganglia, hypoganglionosis, hyperplasia of the submucosal and myenteric plexus giant ganglion cells, as well as hyperplasia or aplasia of the sympathetic innervation of the myenteric plexus. This condition can occur in either a localized or a disseminated manner and can clinically resemble Hirschsprung disease. The patients with neuronal intestinal dysplasia, however, lack the typical histological features of aganglionosis found in Hirschsprung disease [85].

Anorectal malformations

Anorectal malformations are inborn defects characterized by the absence of the anal orifice (imperforate anus). The majority of patients with anorectal malformations also have an abnormal communication between the rectum and other pelvic organs or structures (e.g., vagina, bladder, or urethra) or perineum. In girls, the most common type of associated defect is rectovestibular fistula [86]. In some female patients there is a common channel between the anus and vagina called a *cloacal abnormality* (Figure 6.34) [87]. In male patients, the most common abnormality associated with imperforate anus is rectourethral fistula. The incidence of anorectal malformations is 1/5000 with slight male predominance. Ninety-five percent of patients with anal malformation have some form of fistulization. Urogenital abnormalities are quite common, comprising approximately 50% of anorectal anomalies [88]. As a result, the urological problems associated with the imperforate anus are a major source of morbidity. Sacral and spinal abnormalities are also very common and range from an entirely normal well-developed sacrum to a completely absent sacrum. The degree of sacral abnormality appears to correlate with the outcome of the corrective surgery for imperforate anus: the more the sacrum is deformed, the less likely the patient will have a satisfactory functional outcome. Twenty percent of patients with anorectal malformation will have a defect called *tethered cord* [89]. In this condition, the cord is abnormally attached to the spine. During the natural growth of the infant it is thought that the spine growth rate is faster than that of the cord, resulting in traction of the nerve fibers. Tethered cord is also associated with poor functional prognosis. Approximately 8% of patients with anorectal malformations will also have esophageal atresia. These patients are likely to have a high imperforate anus and high likelihood of associated urological abnormalities. Cardiovascular abnormalities are also commonly associated with imperforate anus, with the most frequent being patent ductus arteriosus, atrial septal defect, ventricular septal defect, and tetralogy of Fallot [89].

The main concern for the patient with anorectal malformation is whether they will have adequate bowel, urological, and sexual function. With higher levels of anorectal malformation, patients tend to have worse functional outcomes. In addition, patients with higher anorectal defects are more likely to have fecal incontinence after repair but a much smaller chance of constipation. Conversely, patients with lower malformations are likely to suffer from constipation after reconstructive surgery.

Colonic volvulus

Volvulus of the bowel refers to a twisting or torsion of the intestine around its mesentery. Volvulus of the colon most commonly affects its most mobile segments, that is, the cecum or sigmoid colon, but volvulus can occur in any other segment of the colon if it becomes sufficiently mobile (transverse colon, splenic flexure). A concurrent volvulus of both cecum and sigmoid colon can occur. In the United States, volvulus is an uncommon condition, comprising only 10–15% of all causes of colonic obstruction [90,91]. In contrast, this condition is much more prevalent worldwide, comprising up to 50% of cases of bowel obstruction in some Asian, African, and Latin American countries [90].

Cecal volvulus accounts for approximately 40–60% of colonic volvuli. The worldwide incidence is estimated at 2.8–7.1/1 000 000 people per year. Most cases occur in younger individuals with a slight predilection for female sex with a female/male ratio of 1.4:1 [92]. Cecal volvulus is an axial rotation of the cecum terminal ileum and the ascending colon about its mesentery (Figure 6.35). Cecal bascule, conversely, is a partial torsion of the cecum that does not involve a true axial twist. It is considered as a variant of volvulus because it involves folding of the cecum along its junction with ascending colon and may result in transient or more prolonged symptoms of colonic obstruction. Cecal bascule affects approximately 10% of patients who present with cecal volvulus or volvulus-type symptoms [90]. Cecal volvulus has been classified into three types: type I, the axial torsion type resulting from clockwise axial torsion or twisting of the cecum along its long axis; type II, loop type caused by a torsion or twisting of the cecum and a portion of the distal ileum; and type III, cecal bascule type with a upward folding of the cecal bascule [93].

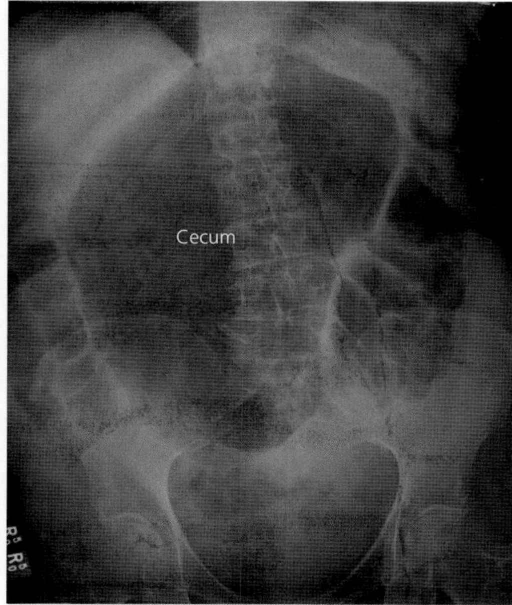

Figure 6.35 Radiograph of the cecal volvulus. Massively dilated cecum occupies most of the abdomen. Gas-filled intestinal loops result in a "coffee bean" sign. Source: Courtesy Bo Shen.

An anatomical abnormality responsible for the development cecal volvulus is thought to be a mobile cecum and descending colon, that is, a lack of fixation of the right colon that then assumes an intraabdominal position. In cadaver studies, 37% of individuals have a sufficiently mobile cecum that it is able to fold or axially rotate [90]. Despite the relatively high prevalence of individuals with mobile cecum, cecal volvulus is uncommon. Oher risk factors include a history of prior abdominal surgery with colonic mobilization, intraabdominal adhesions, distal colonic obstruction [92], pregnancy, and pelvic masses. Prior abdominal surgery appears to have a strong correlation with cecal volvulus because 30–70% of patients with cecal volvulus have previously undergone abdominal surgery. Most patients with a cecal volvulus require surgical intervention.

Sigmoid volvulus is the most common form of colonic volvulus. There is a substantial male predominance, especially in developing nations [94]. However, sigmoid volvulus is the most common cause of intestinal obstruction in pregnancy, accounting for up to 45% of intestinal obstructions in this group of women [95]. The primary reason for observed geographical differences in the incidence of sigmoid volvulus is thought to be the consumption of a high-fiber diet that results in elongation of the colon and that may lead to the development of sigmoid volvulus in relatively younger patients. A long redundant sigmoid colon with a narrow mesenteric attachment and two relatively fixed points of attachment between the descending sigmoid junction and rectosigmoid located at close proximity may put the patient at risk for the development of sigmoid volvulus [96]. This allows markedly elongated and redundant sigmoid colon to form an ω or α loop.

Colonic dysmotility is considered a risk factor for sigmoid volvulus. In the western world, the typical scenario is that sigmoid volvulus occurs in an elderly institutionalized man with a history of chronic constipation. The factors that are thought to contribute to sigmoid volvulus are laxative abuse, previous abdominal surgery, and diabetes mellitus. In other parts of the world, patients tend to be significantly younger and do not necessarily suffer from constipation. Megacolon from any cause, particularly Hirschsprung disease or Chagas disease, also predisposes to volvulus [97]. The gross anatomical features of the sigmoid colon as it becomes prone to volvulus include progressive widening and

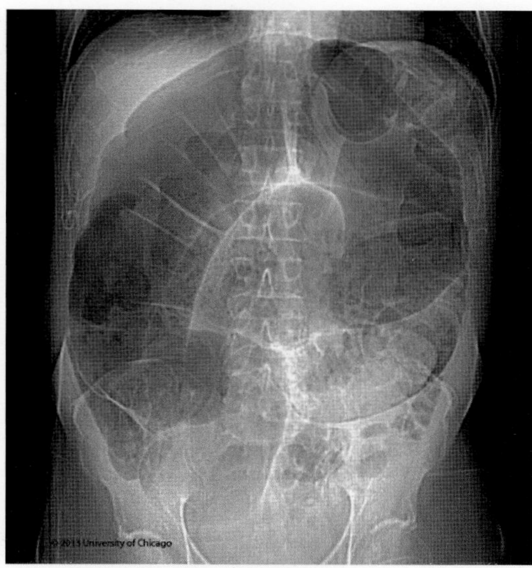

Figure 6.36 Computed tomogram of the abdomen (scout image) of a patient with sigmoid volvulus. Markedly dilated gas-filled sigmoid colon with a "bent inner tube" sign. Source: Courtesy Bo Shen.

loss of taenia coli, disappearance of appendices epiploicae, and the development of a thickened narrow fibrosed mesentery. In many instances, patients can experience repeated undiagnosed episodes of sigmoid volvulus that reduce spontaneously. These episodes are thought to result in scarring and fibrotic changes within the sigmoid mesocolon. The sigmoid colon can undergo volvulus in either direction, clockwise or counterclockwise, and on completion of the 360° turn, a closed-loop obstruction occurs within the affected segment (Figure 6.36). Obstruction of the colonic lumen and impairment of vascular perfusion occur when the degree of torsion exceeds 180° and 360°, respectively [98]. The hyperperistalsis and fluid secretion that follow further contribute to colonic distension and increased tension within the colonic wall, which in turn result in hypoperfusion, ischemia, and eventually, colonic wall necrosis. Colonic perforation can occur either at the neck of the volvulus, within the closed loop, or in the proximal descending colon or distal rectum as a result of the retrograde mesenteric thrombosis. Upstream perforation of the cecum as a consequence of sigmoid volvulus has also been described. Surgical intervention is required in patients with symptoms and signs of perforation or peritonitis. Endoscopic detorsion can be attempted in those without signs of perforation or peritonitis (see Figure 6.7).

Volvulus of the transverse colon is exceedingly rare. It is estimated to represent at most 1–4% of all forms of colonic volvulus. The risk factors for the development of transverse colon volvulus are physiological rather than congenital and are related to history of chronic constipation, previous abdominal surgery, and diets high in fibers [99]. Specific factors that may increase the risk are redundant or elongated transverse colon mesentery, a narrow distance between the flexures, and a lack of fixation of the mesentery.

References are available at www.yamadagastro.com/textbook7e

Further reading

Akinkuotu A., Samuel J.C., Msiska N., et al. The role of the anatomy of the sigmoid colon in developing sigmoid volvulus: a case-control study. Clin Anat 2011;24:634.

Ananthakrishnan A.N. Environmental risk factors for inflammatory bowel diseases: a review. Dig Dis Sci 2015;60:290.

Beck D.E., Roberts P.L., Saclarides T.J., et al. The ASCRS Textbook of Colon and Rectal Surgery. 2nd edn. New York: Springer; 2011.

Butler-Tjaden N.E., Trainor P.A. The developmental etiology and pathogenesis of Hirschsprung disease. Transl Res 2013;162:1.

Corman M.R., Nicholls J., Fazio V.W., et al. Corman's Colon and Rectal Surgery. 6th edn. Philadelphia: Lippincott Williams & Wilkins; 2012.

Dujovny N., Quiros R.M., Saclarides T.J. Anorectal anatomy and embryology. Surg Oncol Clin N Am 2004;13:277.

Gordon P.H., Nivatvongs S. Principles and Practice of Surgery for the Colon, Rectum, and Anus. 3rd edn. New York: Informa Healthcare; 2007.

Myrelid P., Landerholm K., Nordenvall C., Pinkney T.D., Andersson R.E. Appendectomy and the risk of colectomy in ulcerative colitis: a national cohort study. Am J Gastroenterol 2017;112:1311.

Mills S.E. Histology for Pathologists. 4th edn. Philadelphia: Lippincott Williams & Wilkins; 2012.

Netter F.H. Atlas of Human Anatomy. 5th edn. Philadelphia: Saunders; 2007.

Raizada V., Mittal R.K. Pelvic floor anatomy and applied physiology. Gastroenterol Clin North Am 2008;37:493.

Rex D.K. Accessing proximal aspects of folds and flexures during colonoscopy: impact of a pediatric colonoscope with a short bending section. Am J Gastroenterol 2003;98:1504.

Sahami S., Wildenberg M.E., Koens L., et al. Appendectomy for therapy-refractory ulcerative colitis results in pathological improvement of colonic inflammation: short-term results of the PASSION study. J Crohns Colitis 2019;13:165.

Walker T.G. Mesenteric vasculature and collateral pathways. Semin Intervent Radiol 2009;26:167.

CHAPTER 7

Pancreas: anatomy and structural anomalies

Kazuki N. Sugahara[1] and John A. Chabot[2]
[1] Columbia University Irving Medical Center, New York, NY, USA
[2] Columbia University Irving Medical Center, Herbert Irving Comprehensive Cancer Center, New York, NY, USA

Chapter menu

The pancreas has a complex anatomy, making it one of the most challenging abdominal organs to manipulate. It is located deep in the upper retroperitoneum posterior to the stomach and transverse colon, and anterior to the great vessels of the abdomen. The head of the pancreas is nestled in the duodenal concavity and harbors the common bile duct and the pancreatic duct. The body extends toward the left connecting to the tail, which passes anterior to the kidney and adrenal gland and terminates near the splenic hilum. The pancreas is intimately associated with vital major vessels of the epigastrium, such as the celiac axis, common hepatic artery, portal vein, superior mesenteric vein, and superior mesenteric artery. The central position of the pancreas provides for lymphatic drainage along several major routes, namely, the splenic, hepatic, and superior mesenteric nodal systems, as well as the aortocaval and other posterior abdominal wall lymphatics. Posteriorly, the pancreatic nerve plexus, which originates from the celiac plexus, innervates the pancreas to control its endocrine and exocrine functions.

Recent imaging technologies, such as computed tomography (CT) using thin-cut triple-phase pancreatic protocols and magnetic resonance imaging combined with magnetic resonance cholangiopancreatography, have greatly increased the understanding of pancreatic anatomy. As a result, a major advancement has been made in interventional gastroenterology and radiology technologies, which have significantly broadened our knowledge in the biological functions, histological features, and disease processes of the pancreas. These imaging and interventional technologies have become indispensable for the screening and control of pancreatic diseases, and for performing safe and effective surgical procedures. In this chapter, we will discuss in detail the anatomy of the pancreas in relation to some disease processes.

Development/Embryology

The pancreas develops from two primordial outpouchings, one in the ventral foregut and the second in the dorsal midgut, and is first apparent at 4 weeks of gestation (Figure 7.1a) [1]. Cells in both regions express the Pdx1 transcription factor, but only cells in the ventral foregut express the Sox17 transcription factor. Eventually, the $Pdx1^{+}/Sox17^{+}$ cells differentiate into $Pdx1^{-}/Sox17^{+}$ cells, which give rise to the extrahepatic biliary tree, and $Pdx^{+}/Sox17^{-}$ cells, which give rise to the ventral pancreas. The cells within the dorsal midgut eventually give rise to the dorsal pancreas. The dorsal pancreatic bud grows more rapidly than the ventral pancreas and by the sixth week extends into the dorsal mesentery (Figure 7.1b). The ventral pancreas remains smaller and is carried away from the duodenum by the development of the hepatic rudiment into the biliary system.

Yamada's Textbook of Gastroenterology, Seventh Edition. Edited by Timothy C. Wang, Michael Camilleri, Benjamin Lebwohl, Anna S. Lok, William J. Sandborn, Kenneth K. Wang, and Gary D. Wu.

Companion website: www.yamadagastro.com/textbook7e

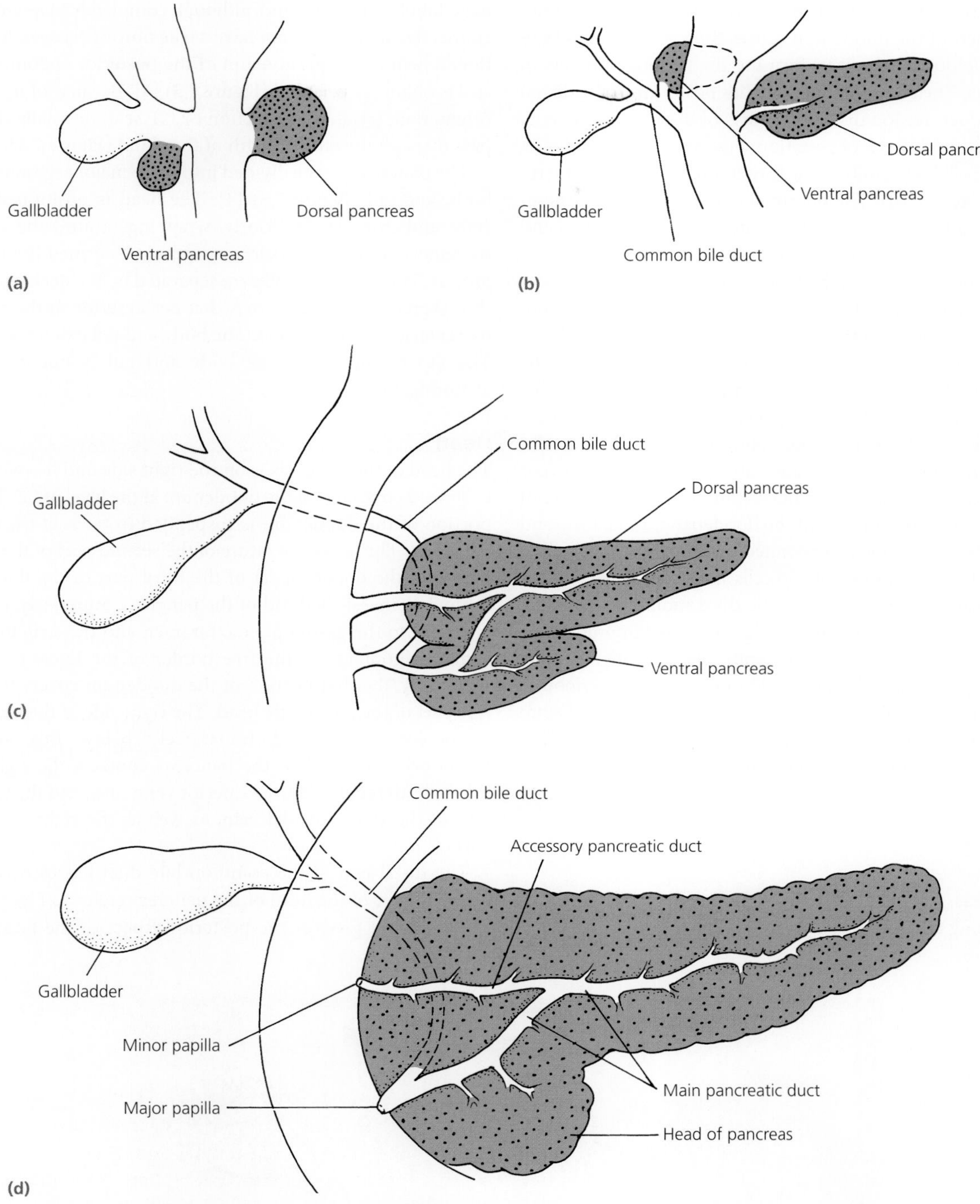

Figure 7.1 Embryological development of the pancreas. The various stages of intrauterine pancreatic growth are shown at 4 weeks **(a)**, 6 weeks **(b)**, 7 weeks **(c)**, and birth **(d)**. Source: Arey 1974 [1]. Reproduced with permission of Elsevier.

Investigations have shown that sonic hedgehog (SHH) expression in the embryonic foregut suppresses pancreatic differentiation of the stomach and duodenum. In the dorsal bud, signals from overlying notochord and dorsal aorta result in downregulation of SHH expression and development of pancreatic tissue. The ventral endoderm closer to the developing major papilla differentiates into pancreatic tissue, whereas signals from the septum transversum lead to upregulation of SHH in the nascent hepatic bud [2].

Differential growth of the duodenum and axial rotation of the gut result in the dorsal pancreas being carried to the left and the ventral pancreas being carried to the right of the duodenum

(Figure 7.1c). Migration of the distal common bile duct behind and to the left of the duodenum causes the ventral pancreas to lie below the dorsal pancreas, forming the uncinate process of the pancreas. The common bile duct lies posterior to the dorsal pancreatic duct. Fusion of the two parts of the pancreas occurs during the seventh week of gestation. Fusion of the ventral duct with the dorsal duct results in the formation of the main pancreatic duct (Figure 7.1d). The proximal end of the dorsal pancreatic duct usually does not communicate with the main duct and forms the accessory pancreatic duct.

The pancreatic acini and the first zymogen granules appear at 12 weeks of gestation. Groups of endocrine cells develop from multipotent stem cells in the ductular epithelium (nesidioblasts) at 9 weeks of gestation. Discrete islets of Langerhans cells can be identified at 12 weeks. Most of the islet cells develop within the tail of the pancreas and the dorsal pancreas. The first cells to produce granules are the α cells, soon followed by the β and δ cells. Complete maturation of the pancreatic gland does not occur until the end of gestation. The smooth muscle of the sphincter of Oddi develops independently of the duodenal musculature, and only later does it become incorporated into the duodenal wall.

Most evidence indicates that islet cells arise from stem cells that appear in pancreatic ducts during the third month of gestation. Insulin-containing granules may be demonstrated immunocytochemically by the end of the third month. Islet cells migrate away from the ducts in which they arise and move into the interlobular connective tissue. Mature islet morphology is established before birth. Refer to Chapter 1 for a detailed discussion on the development and differentiation of the gastrointestinal system.

Anatomy

The pancreas is a soft, flattened, elongated gland, which is 12–20 cm long and weighs 85–95 g in adults (Figure 7.2) [3]. It has a lobular structure and, although completely invested in fine connective tissue, does not have a true fibrous capsule. It is positioned behind the peritoneum of the posterior abdominal wall and is obliquely oriented (Figure 7.3) [4]. Because of its oblique orientation, a transverse section or CT scan normally does not pass through the entire length of the gland (Figure 7.4).

The pancreas can be divided into three major segments: head, body, and tail (Figure 7.5) [4]. The head is positioned to the right and extends posteriorly, wrapping around the superior mesenteric vein. This posterior segment is termed the *uncinate process*. The head and body are separated by the neck, which is a thin segment of the pancreas that lies anterior to the superior mesenteric artery and vein. The body and tail extend to the left. The exact junction of the body and tail is not discernible anatomically.

Head

The head of the pancreas is on the right side and lies within the C-shaped concavity of the duodenum at the level of L2. The first portion of the duodenum is suspended in front of the head of the gland. The lesser curvature of the second part of the duodenum and the upper aspect of the third part of the duodenum intimately invest the head of the pancreas. Superiorly, the head is related to the gastroepiploic foramen and the structures that form the contents of the free border of the lesser omentum. Anteriorly, the first portion of the duodenum covers the superior part of the pancreatic head. The right side of the transverse mesocolon is attached transversely below this segment. Posteriorly, the head of the pancreas contacts the right renal hilum, both renal veins, the inferior vena cava, and the termination of the right gonadal vein, as well as the right side of the aorta [5].

The distal end of the common bile duct passes behind the upper border of the head of the pancreas (refer to Figure 7.1d). The bile duct grooves the posterior aspect of the head of the

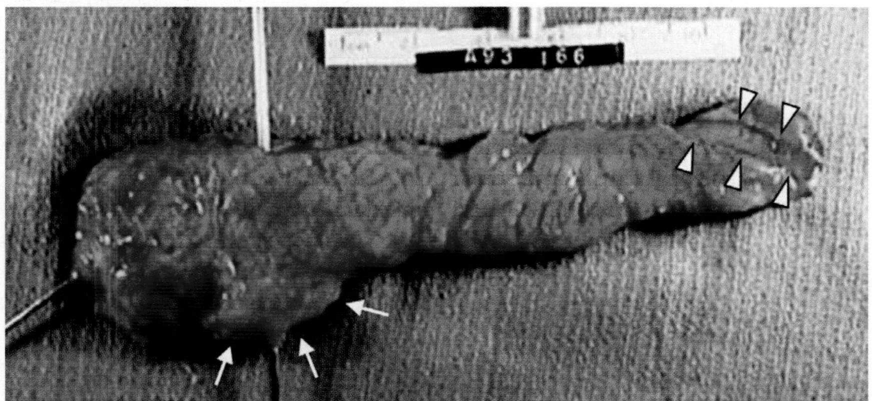

Figure 7.2 The human pancreas. A horizontal probe has been put into the main pancreatic duct, and a vertical probe is in the portal-superior mesenteric vein behind the pancreas. The diagonal groove in the tip of the tail (arrowheads) marks the course of a branch of the splenic artery or vein. The uncinate process (arrows) is fused to the remainder of the head. Source: Adapted from Longnecker 2014 [3]. Reproduced with permission of the American Pancreatic Association.

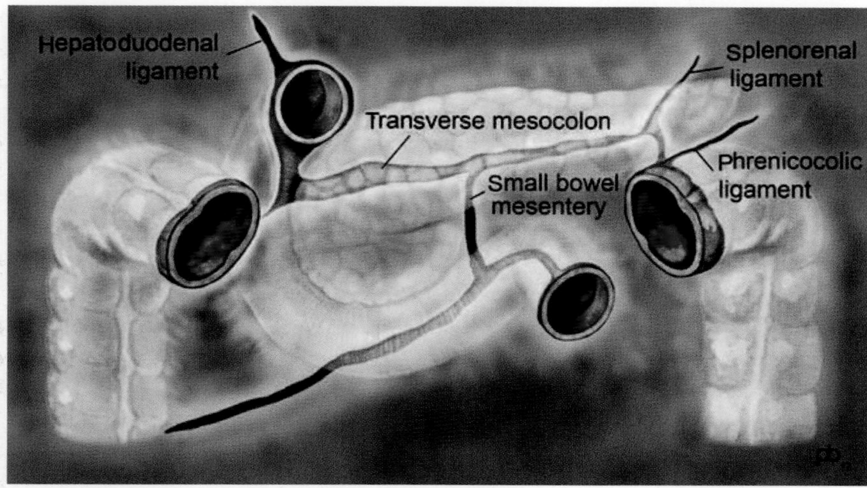

Figure 7.3 Peritoneal lining in relation to the pancreas. The entire pancreas is located retroperitoneally. Peritoneal lining of the anterior surface is lacking at the root of the transverse mesocolon and the small-bowel mesentery. The bare area of the former is contiguous with the splenorenal and phrenicocolic ligament. Source: Campbell and Verbeke 2013 [4]. Used with permission of Springer Nature.

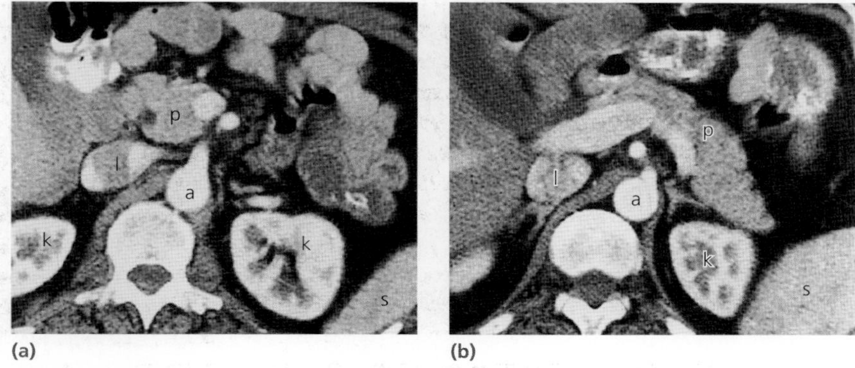

Figure 7.4 Computed tomographic scan of the abdomen demonstrates the relation of the head **(a)** and the body and tail **(b)** of the pancreas to surrounding structures. a, aorta; I, inferior vena cava; k, kidney; p, pancreas; s, spleen.

gland before passing through the substance of the head to reach the duodenal papilla of Vater. From the posterior aspect of the head, the uncinate process extends to the left to occupy the concavity formed by the third and fourth portions of the duodenum. The uncinate process lies anterior to the inferior vena cava and aorta and is covered superiorly and anteriorly by the superior mesenteric vessels as they emerge below the neck of the pancreas.

Neck

The neck of the pancreas is 3–4 cm wide and bridges the head to the body of the gland that extends to the left. The neck lies behind the posterior peritoneum of the lesser sac, and its inferior border is covered by the attachments of the transverse mesocolon and the root of the small-bowel mesentery. The splenic vein merges into the superior mesenteric vein behind the neck to form the splenic-mesenteric confluence, which is the proximal portion of the portal vein. During a Whipple procedure, the pancreas is divided at the neck, making it a critical anatomical landmark during the procedure.

Body

The body of the pancreas starts at the midline positioned anterior to the aorta. It is held securely against the aorta and the posterior parietes by the posterior peritoneum of the lesser sac and courses toward the left in the retroperitoneum. The antrum and the body of the stomach cover the body of the pancreas anteriorly. Posteriorly, the left renal vein, passing between the aorta and the pancreas, is separated by the latter from the first part of the superior mesenteric artery. At a slightly higher level, elements of the celiac and superior mesenteric plexus ramify between the pancreas and the aorta.

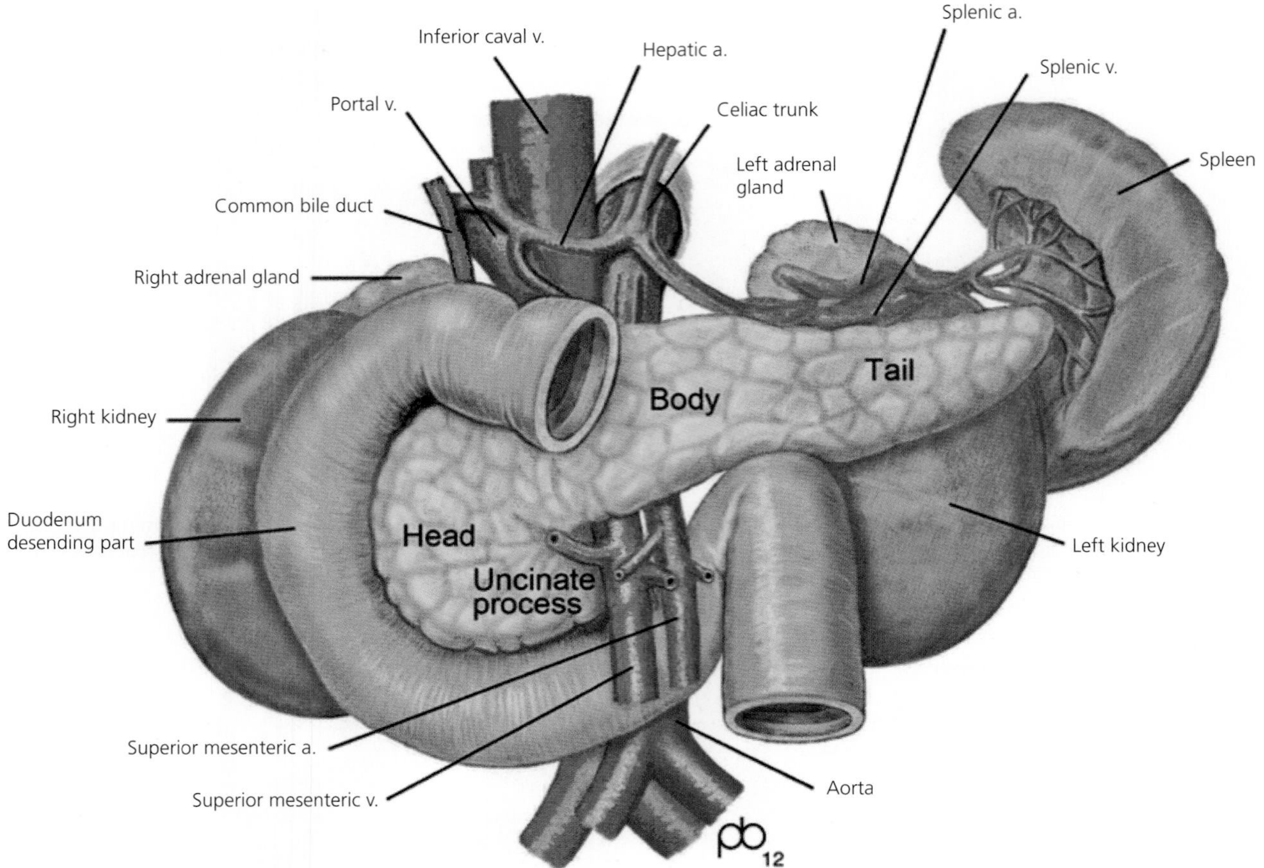

Figure 7.5 The pancreas in relation to surrounding organs and structures. The pancreas consists of the head (including the uncinate process), body, and tail. The neck is a thin segment anterior to the superior mesenteric artery and vein, which connects the head to the body (not labeled). a, artery; v, vein. Source: Campbell and Verbeke 2013 [4]. Used with permission of Springer Nature.

The midline part of the body of the pancreas is pushed anteriorly by the bodies of L1 and L2 and, therefore, lies closest to the anterior abdominal wall. Because of its prominence and fixity in this region, this area of the pancreas is most vulnerable to blunt abdominal injuries. In addition, a tumor in this region may be palpated as a mass that does not move with respiration and that strongly transmits the aortic pulsation. The celiac axis, surrounded by the celiac plexus, divides into its major branches between the superior border of the body of the pancreas and the crura of the diaphragm.

Tail

The body of the pancreas passes laterally, posteriorly, and slightly cephalad behind the posterior peritoneum of the lesser sac and merges imperceptibly with the tail of the gland. Various anatomic landmarks for the division between the body and tail of the pancreas have been proposed (e.g., left border of the aorta, one-fourth of the pancreas from the tip of the tail, sharp narrowing of the gland that exists in some individuals) [6–9]. However, none of them has been universally accepted. The posterior relationships of the body and tail of the pancreas include the posterior attachment of the left crus of the diaphragm, the left suprarenal gland, the upper pole of the left kidney, and the splenic hilum. The splenic vein above and the left renal vein below lie close to one another behind the body and tail of the gland. At the upper border of the body and tail of the pancreas, the splenic artery courses to the left from its origin at the celiac axis. The transverse mesocolon is attached to the anterior part of the lower border of the gland. The splenocolic ligament connects the splenic flexure of the colon to the hilum of the spleen and brings the colon adjacent to the tail of the pancreas.

The shape and disposition of the pancreas varies, as demonstrated by pancreatography. In 57% of people, the bulk of the head of the gland is to the right of the spinal column. In about 38% of people, it lies directly over the spine, but only rarely (5%) does the head of the pancreas lie to the left of the spine. There is a tendency in elderly people for the pancreas to be ptotic, or to show abnormal drooping. The duodenal opening of the main pancreatic duct lies at the level of L2–L4 in 92% of people, but rarely has it been described at a lower level.

Structural functions/relationships

Surgical exposure

Although the pancreas is located retroperitoneally, it is usually approached by way of an anterior laparotomy incision. The gland is usually not seen or palpated at laparotomy without dissection. In a thin patient, small areas of the head may be seen directly behind the peritoneum of the supracolic and right infracolic compartments, and the inferior border of the body and tail may be seen from the left infracolic compartment at the root of the transverse mesocolon. However, these limited views usually are obscured by omental, mesocolic, and retroperitoneal fat. The neck of the pancreas may be felt from above by a finger passed through the gastroepiploic foramen of Winslow.

The head of the pancreas may be inspected and palpated more closely by performing two maneuvers [10]. First, the hepatic flexure of the colon is mobilized downward and medially, dividing the attachments of the transverse colon to the front of the duodenum and pancreatic head as far as the origin of the middle colic vessels. In addition, the attachments of the right side of the greater omentum to the transverse colon are divided. Thus, the lesser sac can be widely exposed on the right side of the middle colic vessels. Second, the peritoneum lateral to the second part of the duodenum is incised, and the duodenum and pancreatic head may be elevated and swept to the left by blunt dissection, exposing the right renal vein, the inferior vena cava, the right gonadal vein, the origin of the left renal vein, and the retroduodenal and retropancreatic portions of the distal common bile duct. After this mobilization (Kocher maneuver), the head of the pancreas may be palpated anteroposteriorly between the thumb and fingers. The mesenteric vessels are obscured from view by the uncinate process.

Limited sight of the superior part of the body of the pancreas may be obtained by opening an avascular part of the lesser (gastrohepatic) omentum and retracting the lesser curvature of the stomach inferiorly. This maneuver also brings the celiac axis into view. A much better view of the body of the pancreas may be obtained by widely opening the lesser sac, which can be achieved by dividing the gastrocolic omentum at its attachment to the transverse colon. Extending this opening to the right into the subpyloric region allows visualization of the anterior aspect of the head and neck of the pancreas, especially if the right gastroepiploic vessels are ligated and divided. Extending the opening to the left and dividing the short gastric (gastrosplenic) vessels in the gastrosplenic ligament superiorly and the relatively vascular splenocolic ligament inferiorly will give complete visualization of the anterior surface of the body and tail of the pancreas. The spleen, splenic vessels, and tail of the pancreas may be mobilized medially and anteriorly en bloc, allowing inspection of the posterior aspect of the tail and body of the gland. All these surgical maneuvers may be carried out quickly and safely with little risk for damage to vital structures or troublesome bleeding. By this means, all except the region of the neck and uncinate process of the pancreas may be evaluated fully.

The pancreas can also be exposed using a minimally invasive approach, whether for a laparoscopic/robotic Whipple or, more frequently, for a laparoscopic/robotic distal pancreatectomy/splenectomy. Five ports can be used: a periumbilical camera port, a right flank/subcostal port, a right abdominal/midclavicular line port, a left abdominal/midclavicular port, and a left flank/subcostal port. A long, laparoscopic energy device (e.g., LigaSure, Harmonic scalpel, Enseal, or Thunderbeat) can be used. For exposure of the pancreatic head, the proximal transverse colon, hepatic flexure, and even the entire right colon all the way down toward the terminal ileum is mobilized to expose the duodenum and reflecting the right colon away from the operative field. The duodenum is Kocherized as described earlier. For exposure of the pancreatic body/tail, the greater curve of the stomach is mobilized, up to and including the short gastric vessels. The splenic flexure of the colon is then mobilized and reflected inferiorly. The distal stomach and proximal duodenum are lifted anteriorly and detached from the anterior surface of the pancreas. This dissection can be carried all the way toward the gastroduodenal artery. The inferior border of the pancreas is then dissected free from the tail toward the neck of the pancreas until the middle colic vein is seen emptying into the superior mesenteric vein, which courses underneath the neck of the pancreas. The splenic vein can be dissected free under the pancreas. The splenic artery can be dissected along the superior border of the pancreas.

Arterial blood supply

The pancreas derives its blood supply from the celiac axis and the superior mesenteric artery (Figure 7.6). These major vessels and their branches also provide the blood supply to other vital organs adjacent to the pancreas.

Typically (in 90% of people), the celiac axis divides into the common hepatic, splenic, and left gastric arteries. The common hepatic artery passes to the right, anterior to the portal vein, to reach the free border of the lesser omentum and usually lies to the left of the common bile duct. After giving off the gastroduodenal artery, the hepatic artery turns upward toward the porta hepatis and divides into the left and right hepatic arteries. The middle hepatic artery, supplying the caudate lobe of the liver, is usually a branch of one of these two vessels. This arrangement of the hepatic arterial blood supply, however, occurs in only 55% of people. Replaced or accessory hepatic arteries are frequent, occurring in as many as 30% of people. Michels [11] identified 10 types of hepatic arterial anatomy through 200 cadaveric dissections (Table 7.1). The most frequent variation from normal is the right hepatic artery branching off from the superior mesenteric artery and coursing behind the uncinate process and the head of the pancreas to reach the free border of the lesser omentum (Michels type III) [12].

The gastroduodenal artery usually originates from the common hepatic artery. The gastroduodenal artery courses from its

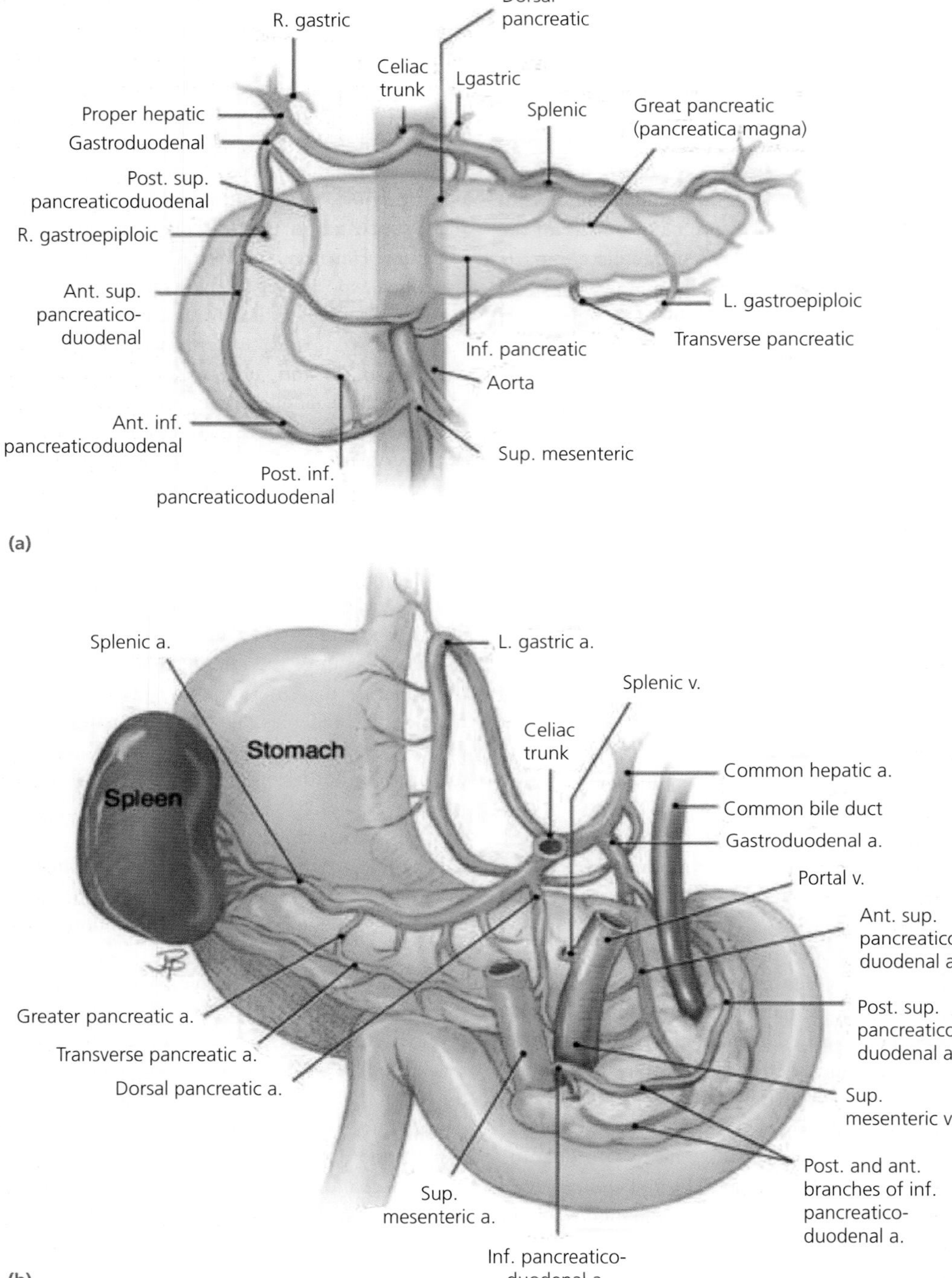

Figure 7.6 Arterial blood supply of the pancreas. **(a)** Frontal view. **(b)** Posterior view. a., artery; ant., anterior; inf., inferior; L., left; post., posterior; R., right; sup., superior; v., vein. Source: Hruban, Pitman, and Klimstra 2007 [8]. Used with permission of American Registry of Pathology.

origin behind the first part of the duodenum and, after giving off the posterior superior pancreaticoduodenal artery, lies on the anterior surface of the head of the pancreas. At the lower border of the first part of the duodenum, it branches into the right gastroepiploic artery and the anterior superior pancreaticoduodenal artery.

For the most part, the head of the pancreas and the duodenum have a common blood supply from the anterior and

Table 7.1 Anatomical variations of the hepatic artery as classified by Michels.

Michels type	Variation
I	Normal
II	Replaced LHA from the LGA
III	Replaced RHA from the SMA
IV	Replaced RHA and LHA
V	Accessory LHA
VI	Accessory RHA
VII	Accessory RHA and LHA
VIII	Replaced RHA or LHA with an additional accessory hepatic artery
IX	Hepatic trunk from the SMA
X	CHA from the LGA

CHA, common hepatic artery; LGA, left gastric artery; LHA, left hepatic artery; RHA, right hepatic artery; SMA, superior mesenteric artery.
Source: Based on data from Michels 1966 [11].

posterior pancreaticoduodenal arcades. The anterior arcade gives off the only arteries that enter the head of the gland from its anterior aspect. This arcade is formed by the anastomosis of the anterior superior pancreaticoduodenal artery, which is a terminal branch of the gastroduodenal artery, and the anterior inferior pancreaticoduodenal artery, which is usually a branch of a common inferior pancreaticoduodenal artery, arising from the superior mesenteric artery.

The posterior pancreaticoduodenal arcade is formed by the anastomosis of the posterior superior pancreaticoduodenal artery, usually a branch of the gastroduodenal artery, and the posterior inferior pancreaticoduodenal artery, which arises in a way analogous to the anterior pancreaticoduodenal artery. Of surgical importance is the relation of the posterior superior pancreaticoduodenal artery to the common bile duct. Typically, this vessel arises from the gastroduodenal artery and passes to the right, anterior to the common bile duct, contributing the major source of the structure's blood supply. The supraduodenal portion of the common bile duct may also be crossed anteriorly by the right hepatic artery, the right gastric artery, and the supraduodenal artery, making mobilization of the lower end of the common bile duct more difficult.

Because of the shared blood supply of the duodenum and pancreatic head, extensive interference with the pancreaticoduodenal arcades in the course of a 95% pancreatectomy may compromise the blood supply of the duodenum [13]. In addition, ligation of the inferior pancreaticoduodenal artery vessels may render the proximal jejunum ischemic because branches of the vessels may supply the duodenojejunal flexure and the first part of the jejunum.

The body and tail of the gland derive their blood supply chiefly from branches of the splenic artery. This vessel, the largest branch of the celiac axis (5–11 mm in diameter), courses laterally at the upper border of the pancreas; its characteristic marked tortuosity appears to be related to age. The tortuosity is often absent in infants and is most marked in the elderly. The splenic artery gives multiple side branches to supply the neck, body, and tail of the pancreas. The termination of the splenic artery passes between the layers of the lienorenal ligament, and four or five branches enter the splenic hilum separately. Refer to Chapter 11 for additional discussion on the blood flow of the gastrointestinal system.

Venous drainage

The general pattern of veins draining the pancreas is the same as that of the arterial blood supply (Figure 7.7). Blood from the pancreas drains ultimately into the portal vein, which is formed by the junction of the superior mesenteric vein and splenic vein behind the neck of the gland. The close relationship of the portal and superior mesenteric veins to the head, neck, and uncinate process of the pancreas is of vital surgical importance; in determining the resectability of a pancreatic lesion, a key step is to assess the involvement of these veins. The portal vein originates from behind the neck of the pancreas as a continuation of the superior mesenteric vein after it becomes confluent with the splenic vein. The portal vein passes upward to the right to gain access to the free border of the lesser omentum, where it lies posterior to the hepatic artery and the common bile duct. At the porta hepatis, it divides into a short, broad right branch and a longer, narrower left branch. In adults, the portal vein is about 8–10 cm long and 8–14 mm wide. Its average length is about 8.4 cm [14].

The splenic vein originates at the hilum of the spleen by the confluence of five or six tributaries draining the spleen. It receives the basal brevia (short gastric veins) and left gastroepiploic veins at the hilum. It passes through the lienorenal ligament behind the tail of the pancreas and below the splenic artery and is the large, straight vein that courses to the right in contact with the posterior surface of the pancreas. It receives many tributaries from the tail, body, and neck of the gland.

Below the pancreas, the ileocolic vein passes directly, and usually without tributaries, from the ileocecal region to join the right side of the superior mesenteric vein in the midline just above the inferior border of the third part of the duodenum. At about the same level on the left side, the superior mesenteric vein is joined by the jejunointermediate vein. The confluence of these three veins forms the lower limit of what has been termed the surgical trunk of the superior mesenteric vein. Above this point, about two-thirds of the superior mesenteric vein lies below the inferior border of the neck of the pancreas, with the remaining one-third retropancreatic. The superior jejunal vein joins the left side of the superior mesenteric vein. The middle colic vein usually joins the superior mesenteric vein immediately below the inferior border of the pancreatic neck.

The inferior mesenteric vein typically joins the splenic vein vertically behind the body of the pancreas. The latter passes

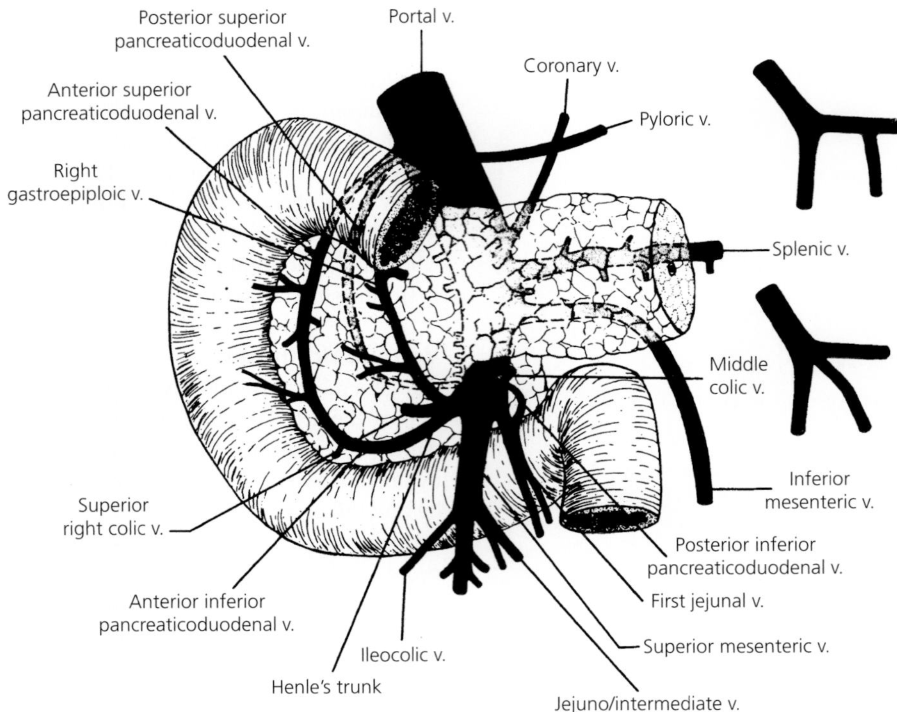

Figure 7.7 Venous drainage of the pancreas. The pancreas and duodenum are viewed from their anterior aspects. Insets: normal variations in the termination of the inferior mesenteric vein (v.).

horizontally and combines with the superior mesenteric vein at a right angle to form the portal vein, which turns obliquely to the right to pass into the free edge of the lesser omentum. Small veins draining the head of the pancreas pass directly into the portal vein. Similarly, small veins draining the uncinate process terminate in the right and posterior aspects of the retropancreatic superior mesenteric vein. The anterior aspects of the major veins are usually free from tributaries. From the left side, the coronary vein joins the retropancreatic portal vein, and the pyloric vein joins the suprapancreatic portal vein. The superior and posterior pancreaticoduodenal veins drain into the portal vein from the right side, deep to the first part of the duodenum and opposite the pyloric vein. In 60% of cases, the coronary, or left gastric, vein drains into the left side of the retropancreatic portal vein, but it may have a high termination well above the neck of the pancreas.

The close anatomical relationship of the splenic vein with the pancreas often leads to splenic vein occlusion in inflammatory or neoplastic diseases that involve the body and tail of the gland. Retrograde venous drainage toward the splenic hilum and then by way of the short gastric veins and the left gastroepiploic vein creates the syndrome of left-sided portal hypertension and gastric varices.

Lymphatic drainage

The lymphatic vessels of the pancreas conform to the general pattern of deep lymphatic drainage and accompany the arterial supply (Figure 7.8). The duodenum and head of the pancreas have a common lymphatic drainage; lymph from the foregut and midgut structures, including the pancreas, liver, stomach, spleen, small bowel, and proximal large bowel, flows eventually into the celiac and superior mesenteric groups of paraaortic nodes and into the cisterna chyli [15]. The lymphatics of the tail of the pancreas pass to the splenic nodes at the hilum of the spleen, and those of the body of the pancreas pass upward to the pancreaticosplenic nodes lying along the superior border of the gland. These nodes, along with the retropancreatic nodes, drain into the celiac nodes. Lymphatics of the upper anterior part of the head of the pancreas pass through the subpyloric nodes lying behind the first part of the duodenum. Obstruction of these pancreatic lymphatic drainage pathways by tumor may result in the shunting of lymph through local collateral channels, resulting in the involvement of nodes primarily concerned with hepatic or gastric drainage. Inferiorly, the retropancreatic and antepancreatic group of nodes drain into the superior mesenteric nodes, and lymph from the latter also may pass into nodes in the root of the transverse mesocolon. The absence of fascial or retroperitoneal coverings on the posterior aspect of the pancreas allows easy communication between lymphatics of the pancreas and those of neighboring retroperitoneal tissues and organs. The lymphatic network is so rich that a thorough lymphadenectomy en bloc with a pancreatic resection frequently produces a profuse postoperative chylous leakage [16].

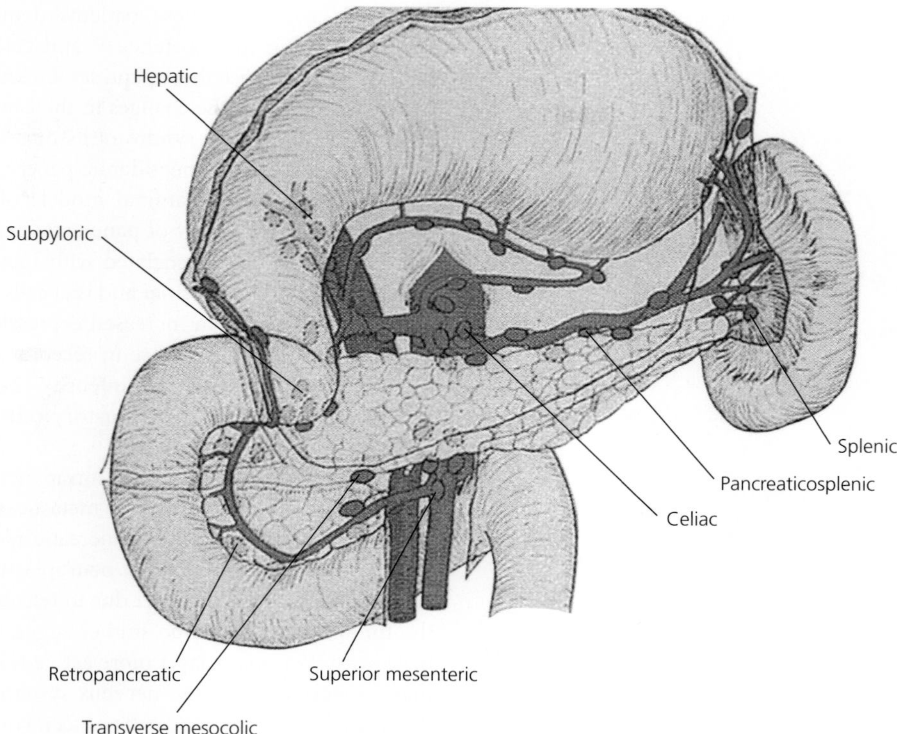

Figure 7.8 Lymphatic drainage of the pancreas. The pancreas is viewed from its anterior aspect. The gastrocolic ligament has been divided along the greater curvature of the stomach, which has been retracted anterosuperiorly. The transverse mesocolon has been detached from the peritoneum of the posterior abdominal wall. Labels indicate representative lymph nodes in the major regional nodal groups.

Nerve supply

The sympathetic efferent innervation of the pancreas is derived from the greater, lesser, and least splanchnic nerves (Figure 7.9) [17]. The bodies of the preganglionic sympathetic neurons originate in the lateral gray matter of thoracic spinal segments 5–10. After traversing the sympathetic trunks, presynaptic nerve fibers synapse with postganglionic sympathetic neurons within the celiac plexus, although there is some minor distribution to the pancreas through the hepatic and superior mesenteric plexuses. The celiac ganglion consists of two masses that lie on either side of the aorta, anterior to the crura of the diaphragm and close to the adrenal glands. The right celiac ganglion is partly covered by the inferior vena cava, and the left celiac ganglion is covered by the peritoneum of the lesser sac close to the upper border of the pancreas. The cell bodies of afferent sympathetic neurons are located in the dorsal root ganglia. Afferent fibers often cross the midline in celiac ganglia before projecting centrally so that sympathetic afferent innervation is bilateral.

The parasympathetic innervation of the pancreas is derived from the vagal nerves. The cell bodies for efferent vagal fibers are located in the medulla in the dorsal motor nucleus. Efferent fibers pass to the pancreas by way of the celiac division of the posterior vagal trunk. No synaptic connections are made within the celiac ganglia; postsynaptic neurons are located within the pancreatic parenchyma. Afferent vagal fibers also pass through the celiac ganglia; afferent cell bodies are located within the nucleus ambiguus [18].

The ultrastructure of pancreatic innervation has been studied extensively in several animal species in addition to humans. Myelinated fibers usually are not found within the parenchyma. Intrapancreatic ganglion cells are seen within the interlobular tissues, with nonmyelinated fibers passing to both exocrine and endocrine portions of the gland. The sites of nerve termination may be generally grouped as blood vessels, pancreatic acinar cells, ductal cells, and pancreatic islets. Functional correlates suggest that pancreatic nerves may modulate the function of each of these pancreatic elements. In addition to the classic cholinergic and adrenergic neurons, evidence suggests that a large number of peptide-containing neurons also exist within the pancreas. Immunocytochemical methods have demonstrated the presence of fibers or cell bodies containing vasoactive intestinal polypeptide, substance P, cholecystokinin-8, gastrin-releasing peptide, enkephalin, galanin, neuropeptide Y, and calcitonin gene-related peptide [19]. Anatomical studies suggest that modulation of release of acetylcholine and catecholamines from autonomic nerve terminals within the pancreas may be important in pancreatic function.

Pain fibers from the pancreas travel through the celiac ganglia and by way of the sympathetic splanchnic nerves and the

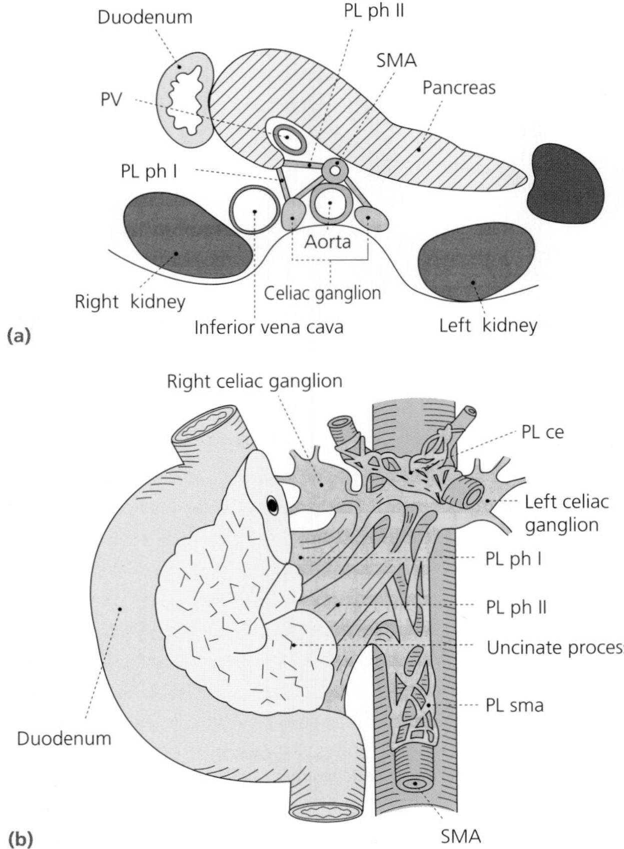

Figure 7.9 Innervation of the pancreas. **(a)** Cross-sectional diagram of pancreatic nerve plexuses. **(b)** Standard anatomical depiction of extrapancreatic nerve plexuses. PL ce, celiac plexus; PL cha, common hepatic artery plexus; PL hdl, plexus within the hepatoduodenal ligament; PL ph I, pancreatic head plexus I; PL ph II, pancreatic head plexus II; PL sma, superior mesenteric plexus; PL sp, splenic plexus; PV, portal vein; SMA, superior mesenteric artery. Source: Japan Pancreas Society 2003 [17]. Reproduced with permission of Japan Pancreas Society and Kanehara & Co. Publishers, Ltd.

thoracic sympathetic chain to reach the spinal root ganglia. Pain from the head of the pancreas tends to be broadly localized in the midepigastrium, and pain from the body and tail tends to be localized in the left upper quadrant. Visceral pain from the pancreas usually is sensed as a severe, constant discomfort in the epigastrium. Because the pancreas does not contact the somatically innervated parietal peritoneum, sharply localized pain usually does not occur. Radiation of pancreatic pain to the back in the area of the lower thoracic vertebrae is common.

Studies suggest that pancreatic innervation may be altered in chronic pancreatitis. In patients with chronic pancreatitis, the number and diameter of intralobular and interlobular nerve bundles have been reported to be increased relative to normal. Evidence of neuronal sprouting and neuritis are also evident. These changes have been strongly associated with clinical pain scores, and thus suggest they represent an important factor in the pathogenesis of pain in chronic pancreatitis [20,21]. Pancreatic nerves in these patients demonstrated increased immunostaining for substance P and calcitonin gene-related peptide [22]. Because these peptides are known to be expressed in afferent neurons, the changes in their expression levels have been linked to the pain syndrome associated with chronic pancreatitis. Alterations in peptidergic pancreatic innervation also have been reported in animal models of chronic pancreatitis [23]. The hypertrophy of pancreatic nerves seen in chronic pancreatitis has been associated with increased expression of nerve growth factor by acinar and islet cells. Expression of nerve growth factor results in increased expression of its receptor in neural tissue, and an increase in receptor expression has been shown to correlate with pain intensity [24,25]. Interactions of nerves with pancreatic inflammatory cells and glia have been proposed as a cause [26].

Perineural tumor invasion of intrapancreatic nerves, neurogenic inflammation, and tumor metastasis along extrapancreatic nerves are key features of pancreatic adenocarcinoma. It has traditionally been thought that neuroplastic changes are a consequence of pancreatic cancer due to release of substances from the tumor. However, some studies suggest that the peripheral nervous system may play a more active role in tumor development, suggesting that the nervous system may be a potential therapeutic target for pancreatic cancer. For example, in a genetically engineered mouse model system, changes in neurotropic factor expression and pancreatic innervation were found to be important not only for the subsequent development of pancreatic cancer-related pain, but also for driving disease progression from premalignant stages to cancer via sensory afferent sensitization and neurogenic inflammation [27]. More recently, catecholamines were found to drive a feed-forward loop to facilitate pancreatic cancer development: norepinephrine promoted pancreas cancer development in a β_2-adrenergic receptor-dependent manner and facilitated secretion of neurotrophins, which in turn promoted tumor innervation leading to increased norepinephrine and tumor growth [28]. Importantly, blockade of β_2-adrenergic or neurotrophin receptors improved the therapeutic effect of gemcitabine in this study, suggesting that control of the nervous system may be a critical factor in pancreatic cancer treatment. The readers are directed to Chapter 12 for additional discussion on the innervation of the gastrointestinal tract.

Ductal system

The main pancreatic duct of Wirsung extends from the tail of the pancreas to the major duodenal papilla or ampulla of Vater (Figures 7.10 and 7.11) [29]. The average diameter of the duct in the adult tapers from 4 to 2 mm, and it is widest in the head of the gland [30]. The main duct is close and almost parallel to the distal common bile duct for 2–3 mm, then combines to form a common duct channel before opening into the duodenum. The accessory pancreatic duct of Santorini, which is present in 40–70% of people, usually communicates with the main duct and passes transversely to the right in the upper part of the head of the pancreas. The duct of Santorini lies anterior to the

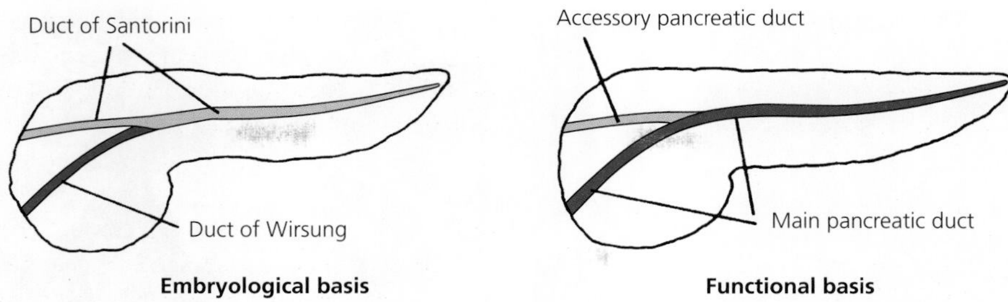

Figure 7.10 Terminology variously applied to describe the pancreatic duct system. One system indicates an understanding of ductal embryology, particularly with regard to the development of the more unusual variations (left). For clarity and practicality, however, the terms given on the right are preferred.

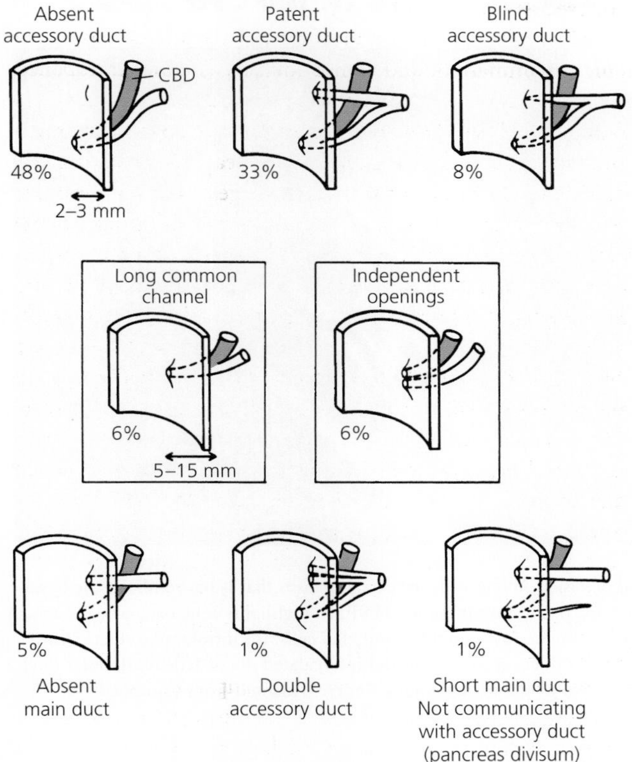

Figure 7.11 Variations of main and accessory pancreatic ducts, and their relation to the common bile duct (CBD) from a series of 143 postmortem preparations. Accessory duct variations and usual short common channel for CBD and main pancreatic duct (top); variations of CBD and main pancreatic duct terminations (middle); miscellaneous variations (bottom). Source: Berman et al. 1996 [29]. Reproduced with permission of American College of Surgeons.

intrapancreatic common bile duct and usually opens into the proximal portion of the second part of the duodenum at the minor papilla, proximal to the ampulla of Vater.

This "typical" ductal anatomy actually may be present in as few as 33% of people. Important variations include nonpatency of the accessory duct (8%), independent openings of the common bile duct and the main pancreatic duct (6%), an absent main duct (5%), and patent double accessory ducts (1%). Noncommunication between the main duct and the accessory duct, with the body and tail of the gland draining exclusively by way of the duct of Santorini, results in the anatomical variant known as *pancreas divisum*, which occurs in 2–6% of otherwise healthy individuals.

The sphincter of Oddi consists of circular smooth muscle that surrounds the common channel of the common bile duct and the main pancreatic duct at the ampulla of Vater. The muscle fibers of the sphincter of Oddi extend around the common bile duct just distal to the latter's oblique entry into the wall of the duodenum to form the choledochal sphincter. A short region of circular smooth muscle also surrounds the pancreatic duct just before its termination to form the pancreatic duct sphincter.

Histology/Cell types

The pancreas is a mixed endocrine and exocrine gland. Its glandular constituents by weight are 80% exocrine tissue, 18% ductular system, and 2% endocrine tissue. Also, the pancreas is a lobulated organ with lobular subunits composed of acini; the latter are rounded or have a short tubular form and consist of single rows of epithelial cells lying on a basal lamina (Figure 7.12). Lining the lumen of the acinus are pyramidal acinar cells and pale-staining centroacinar cells, which are unique to the pancreas. The acinar lumen connects with the intralobular ducts to form the interlobular ducts, which, in turn, coalesce to form the main pancreatic duct. Lining the ductules are columnar cells, goblet cells, and occasional argentaffin cells. The large ducts are surrounded by thick layers of connective tissue and elastic fibers.

In the resting state, the basal portion of the acinar cell contains a centrally located spherical nucleus lying within a highly basophilic cytoplasm secondary to the large number of ribosomes in the rough endoplasmic reticulum. The abundant ribosomes attest to the high protein-synthesizing capacity of the acinar cells. A clear region containing the Golgi complex separates the nucleus from numerous eosinophilic zymogen granules, each about 1 μm in diameter, lying at the apex. The acinar

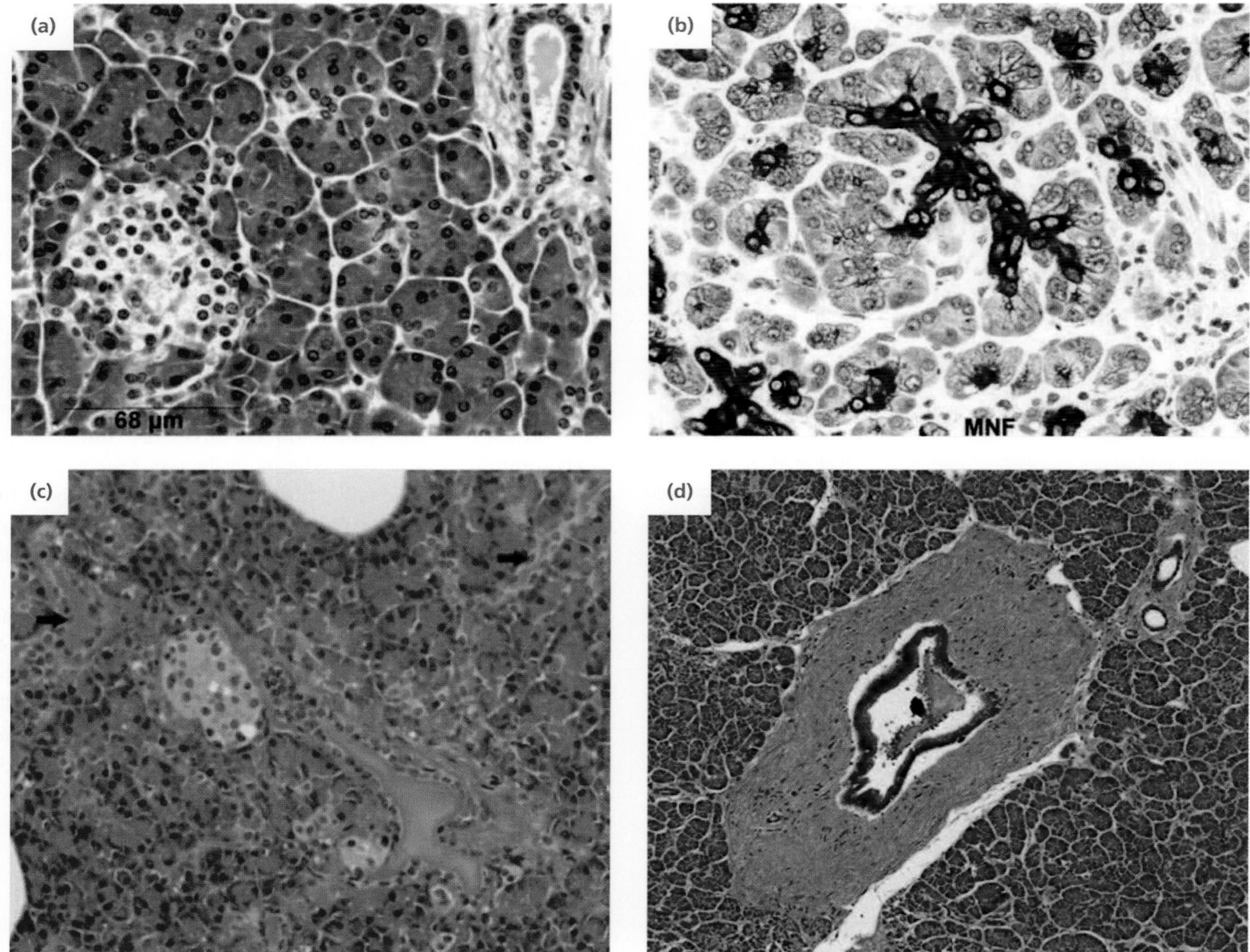

Figure 7.12 Ultrastructure of the pancreas. **(a)** Normal acini, duct, and Langerhans islet. Acinar cells have a cytoplasm that is basophilic at the basal pole and eosinophilic at the apical pole. **(b)** Intercalated ducts and centroacinar cells. Immunostaining for MNF116 highlights centroacinar cells, which are located within the acini, and intercalated ducts, which consist of a single row of similar, low-cuboidal epithelial cells. **(c)** Intralobular ducts. An intralobular duct lies within densely packed acini. Arrows represent small intralobular duct ramifications and intercalated ducts. **(d)** Interlobular duct. The duct has a larger caliber that lies within the thin fibrous septum that separates two neighboring lobules. Source: Adapted from Campbell and Verbeke 2013 [4]. Used with permission of Springer Nature.

cell has short microvilli, averaging 0.2 µm in length, which protrude into the acinar lumen. At the apical portion, the cells are held together by tight junctions, which prevent reflux of lumenal contents. Laterally, the cells are connected by gap junctions, which permit intercellular communication.

The thin basal lamina on which the acini rest is supported by collagen fibers. A rich capillary plexus surrounds the acinus in this connective tissue, and this plexus is penetrated by numerous nerve fibers, which reach the acinar cells.

The endocrine portion of the pancreas consists of about one million islets of Langerhans, which are distributed throughout the gland but are relatively concentrated in the tail of the pancreas. The islets are about 200 µm in diameter, and each is associated with a prominent capillary plexus. The islets contain several cell types. About 75–80% of islet cells are β cells (or B cells), which secrete insulin, and 10–20% are α cells (or A cells), which contain glucagon. δ cells (or D cells) constitute about 5% of the islets and contain somatostatin [31]. The β cells occupy the center of the islets, whereas the perimeter is lined by α cells. δ cells are dispersed between these groups. Other peptide-secreting cells that may be associated with the islets include enterochromaffin cells, containing 5-hydroxytryptamine, and pancreatic polypeptide cells, containing pancreatic polypeptide.

Structural congenital anomalies

Agenesis or hypoplasia of the pancreas

Agenesis of the pancreas is a rare and, in the past, was a universally fatal condition [32]. Failure of the pancreas to develop may occur as an isolated anomaly, or it may be associated with other congenital defects, such as absence of the gallbladder [33]. Although the cause is not known, pancreatic agenesis has been associated with retarded intrauterine growth, presumably resulting from failure of the endocrine pancreas to produce insulin [34]. Partial agenesis of the pancreas results from incomplete formation of either the dorsal or ventral pancreas and has a more favorable outcome than complete agenesis. Involvement of the dorsal segment appears to be more common than involvement of the ventral pancreas. These glands possess normal exocrine and endocrine function.

Hypoplasia of the pancreas is a congenital disease involving exclusively the exocrine pancreas and has been referred to as lipomatous pseudohypertrophy of the pancreas [35]. Pathologically, the gland appears enlarged and of normal shape but of a fatty consistency. The major pancreatic ducts are developed, and islets of Langerhans are present; however, secondary pancreatic ducts and acinar lobules are absent or underdeveloped, and fatty tissue replaces normal acinar cells [36]. The finding that the gland is of normal shape, but missing differentiated cellular components, led investigators to postulate that embryological development is normal in this condition. It is proposed that an intrauterine insult, such as infection, may be the cause of hypoplasia of the exocrine gland [37]. Although this disease usually is diagnosed in infants, it has been reported to occur in adults sometimes in association with malignancy [35,36,38]. It is also seen in two autosomally recessive diseases, Shwachman–Diamond syndrome and Bannayan–Riley–Ruvalcaba syndrome [39,40]. Manifestations result from severe pancreatic exocrine insufficiency.

Annular pancreas

Annular pancreas is an unusual complication of disturbed embryological development in which the head of the pancreas surrounds the duodenum, often resulting in duodenal obstruction (Figure 7.13a) [41]. Annular pancreas frequently is associated with other congenital defects, including Down syndrome, Meckel diverticulum, malrotation of the intestine, duodenal atresia and bands, intestinal webs, tracheoesophageal fistulas, imperforate anus, absence of the gallbladder, and certain types of cardiac defects [42–46]. Annular pancreas has been described in association with pancreas divisum (see *Pancreas divisum* section later in this chapter) [47]. Men appear to be affected more commonly than women. The occurrence of annular pancreas is usually sporadic, although several reports describe a familial association and apparent autosomal dominant transmission [48–51].

Typically, the annulus is a band of pancreatic tissue completely encircling the second portion of the duodenum. The ring usually lies proximal to the major papilla, and in a few cases the annulus involves the first or third portion of the duodenum. Histologically, pancreatic tissue frequently invades the muscularis layer of the duodenum [52].

The most popular etiological theory suggests that the ventral pancreatic bud becomes fixed; as the pancreas and duodenum rotate, a band of pancreatic tissue is left encircling the duodenum [53]. Supporting this theory, a high concentration of pancreatic polypeptide cells, which is characteristic of the ventral pancreas, was found in annular tissue [54]. Other theories propose that hypertrophy of the dorsal and ventral ducts or ectopic pancreatic tissue causes the annulus [55].

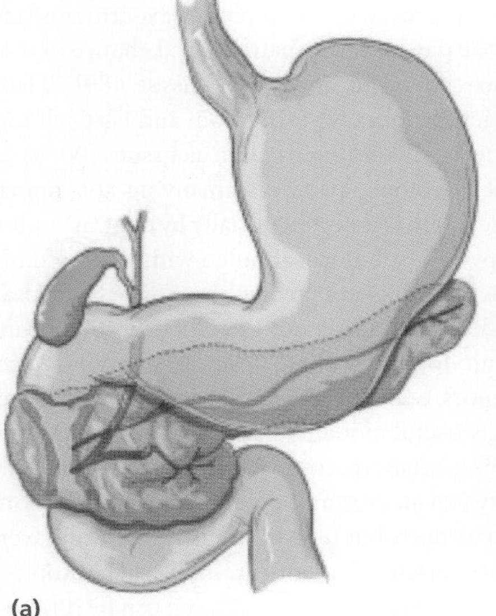

(a)

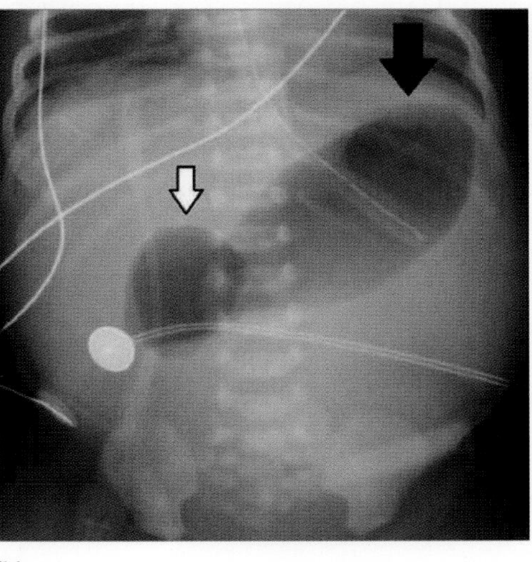

(b)

Figure 7.13 Annular pancreas. **(a)** Normal acini, duct, and Langerhans islet. Acinar cells have a cytoplasm that is basophilic at the basal pole and eosinophilic at the apical pole. Source: Zyromski et al. 2008 [41]. Used with permission of Elsevier. **(b)** Supine frontal radiograph of a neonate, with two gas-filled structures in the upper abdomen (double bubble sign). The larger bubble in the left upper abdomen (black arrow) is the gas-distended stomach. The smaller bubble in the right midabdomen represents gas in a distended proximal duodenum (white arrow). Source: Adapted from Koberlein and DiSantis 2016 [61]. Used with permission of Springer.

More than half of all cases are diagnosed in the first year of life. Severe duodenal stenosis is usually apparent within the first few days of birth. Because pancreatic tissue encircles the duodenum, causing obstruction, newborns and infants are intolerant of oral feedings and have vomiting, often of bilious material. Upper abdominal distention and visible peristalsis are often present on physical examination [56]. Although vomiting is the usual presenting symptom in children, adults often complain of postprandial colicky abdominal pain, bloating, and fullness that also may be associated with nausea and vomiting [57–60]. Upper gastrointestinal bleeding and duodenal ulcer disease occur in one-third of adults, and acute pancreatitis is a common associated finding in this disorder.

The radiographic signs of annular pancreas are those of duodenal obstruction. Plain radiographs of the abdomen often show a "double-bubble" sign resulting from dilation of the duodenum and stomach (Figure 7.13b) [61]. With high degrees of obstruction, a duodenal cut-off sign also may be seen. In infants, these findings are the only necessary radiographic tests. Radiographic findings are not specific in older children and adults, and it is usually necessary to document duodenal obstruction by upper gastrointestinal contrast studies. Constricting bands, 0.8–5 cm long, around the duodenum can be detected radiographically [62]. Other signs include dilation and reverse peristalsis of the proximal duodenum. Endoscopic evaluation of annular pancreas usually is not helpful, although endoscopic ultrasound (EUS) will occasionally reveal a circumferential bandlike structure with the same echo pattern as the pancreas surrounding the duodenum [63]. The mucosa usually is normal, and it is difficult to appreciate mild narrowing of the duodenum. In severe cases, concentric narrowing of the duodenum or stenosis and associated peptic ulcer disease are suggestive of the diagnosis. Endoscopic retrograde cholangiopancreatography (ERCP) has been used to visualize the ductal system in annular pancreas and is diagnostic of the disorder [64–67]. Magnetic resonance pancreatography is being used with increasing frequency as a noninvasive alternative to diagnostic ERCP in the evaluation of pathological conditions of the pancreas, such as annular pancreas and pancreas divisum [68]. Characteristic features can also be determined by CT [69]. In symptomatic patients, treatment of annular pancreas is surgical alleviation of the obstruction. Division of the annulus is not recommended because of the high incidence of pancreatitis and pancreatic fistulas complicating that procedure, and bypass of the obstructed intestinal segment is preferred [70].

Heterotopic pancreas

Aberrant localization of pancreatic tissue, also known as heterotopic pancreas or pancreatic rests, refers to segments of pancreatic tissue not in continuity with the main body of the pancreas. The condition is usually asymptomatic, and therefore its true incidence is difficult to determine. Heterotopic pancreas has been identified in 1 of every 500 laparotomies, and autopsy studies have reported frequency rates ranging from 0.6% to 15% [71,72]. Seventy percent of such rests are found along the upper gastrointestinal tract, with the stomach (25.5%), duodenum (27.7%), and jejunum (15.9%) representing the most frequent locations. Other intraabdominal locations include the gallbladder, liver, small intestine, colon, appendix, omentum, and Meckel diverticulum [73–75]. In the stomach, heterotopic pancreas is found primarily in the prepyloric region along the greater curvature. Extraabdominal sites include the lung and umbilicus [76–78]. Histologically, heterotopic pancreas can contain acinar tissue, islets, ducts, or any combination thereof. Seventy-five percent is located in the submucosa of the stomach or intestine and appears as firm yellow nodules, 2–4 cm in diameter, underlying the mucosa. These often have a central mucosal depression, thought to represent the presence of a vestigial duct that may be recognized endoscopically or by radiographic contrast studies. The origin of heterotopic pancreas is not known, and it is likely that several abnormalities of embryological development account for the locations in various sites. As pluripotential cells, pancreatic rests may represent abnormal differentiation of endodermal stem cells. Conversely, disturbances in migration of the pancreas as it rotates around the gut may account for some heterotopic locations [79].

Heterotopic pancreas is usually an asymptomatic condition that is an incidental finding at surgery or autopsy. Symptoms attributed to this disorder include abdominal pain, nausea, vomiting, and gastric outlet obstruction [80,81]. Peptic ulcer disease and upper gastrointestinal bleeding also have been described. Because of the varied locations of pancreatic rests, involvement of other organs can occur. Pancreatitis, biliary obstruction with jaundice, intestinal obstruction, and intussusception all have been associated with heterotopic pancreas [82–88]. As a result of the combined exocrine and endocrine function of the pancreas, any pathological change in the normal pancreas also can occur in ectopic tissue [89]. Therefore, malignant degeneration, cyst formation, and islet cell tumors also may be found in heterotopic pancreas tissues [90–96].

Heterotopic pancreas involving the upper gastrointestinal tract often is detected initially by contrast radiography or endoscopy as a submucosal bulge with central umbilication [97,98]. These lesions are covered by normal mucosa, making routine endoscopic biopsy not useful. Heterotopic pancreas may be difficult to differentiate from leiomyomas, fibromas, carcinoid tumors, or other malignant tumors. EUS has become an increasingly useful modality in the evaluation of these submucosal gastrointestinal masses. It allows one not only to distinguish between an intramural lesion and compression from an extraluminal mass but also to identify the wall layer from which the mass originates. For example, heterotopic pancreas tissue, located in the submucosal layer, can be differentiated from leiomyomas, the most commonly encountered submucosal masses, which are located in the layer of the muscularis propria [99]. In other patients in whom a definitive diagnosis cannot be made based on EUS appearance, EUS-guided fine-needle aspiration may be used to obtain a histological diagnosis [100,101].

Treatment of heterotopic pancreas is indicated only for those who have significant symptoms or complications, such as recurrent upper gastrointestinal bleeding, biliary or intestinal obstruction, or malignant degeneration. Definitive treatment is surgical removal of the ectopic tissue. Asymptomatic people with incidental discovery of heterotopic pancreas do not require further evaluation or treatment [102]. If unsuspected heterotopic pancreas is found at surgery, excision prevents the possible complication of malignant degeneration and eliminates confusion if subsequent symptoms develop [102].

Pancreas divisum

Pancreas divisum, the most common congenital anomaly of the pancreas, is caused by failure of the ducts of the dorsal and ventral anlagen to fuse during the fifth and sixth weeks of gestation. Normally, the proximal one-third of the dorsal pancreatic duct regresses as it fuses with the ventral duct, forming the main pancreatic duct. In pancreas divisum, the ventral duct of Wirsung empties into the duodenum through the major papilla but drains only a small portion of the pancreas. Secretions from the tail, body, neck, and remainder of the head of the pancreas drain into the duodenum through the minor papilla by way of a persistent duct of Santorini. In 2–3% of cases in which the ducts do not fuse, the ventral duct may not be demonstrable. Normally, drainage of the pancreas can occur by either duct, depending on fusion of the two ductal systems and the degree of patency of each. Most pancreatic drainage is through the duct of Wirsung, and although some drainage occurs through the duct of Santorini, this volume is relatively small. Occasionally, the duct of Santorini ends blindly in the duodenal wall.

Although pancreas divisum is a long-recognized entity, only with the advent of ERCP has its clinical significance become apparent. In autopsy series, pancreas divisum has an incidence rate of 5–10% [103]; as an ERCP finding, its incidence rate is 4% [104–106]. Importantly, pancreas divisum appears to be one of the causes of pancreatitis. In a series of patients with pancreatitis, however, there was a 16% incidence rate of pancreas divisum, and the incidence rate of the abnormality increased to 25% in idiopathic pancreatitis [104]. It has been postulated that pancreatitis may result from a combination of pancreas divisum and stenosis at the level of the accessory papilla, with impediment of pancreatic secretory flow. As a congenital defect, clinical manifestations of pancreas divisum may occur at any age but are uncommon in childhood. Symptoms may be mild with only occasional epigastric pain occurring postprandially, but more often episodes of severe acute pancreatitis occur. Chronic pancreatitis also may develop, with all of its associated sequelae. Changes in the pancreatic ducts characteristic of chronic pancreatitis may be detected on ERCP.

Pancreas divisum is diagnosed by pancreatography (Figure 7.14). On ERCP, the major papilla is often difficult to cannulate, but on injection with contrast fluid, the duct of Wirsung appears short and thin. There is rapid filling of small accessory ducts, and too much contrast can be injected before it is realized that the duct of Wirsung is not in communication with the main pancreatic duct. As a result, the patient may experience sudden pain, and pancreatitis of the ventral pancreas can develop. What appears as an abrupt cut-off of the duct of Wirsung must not be confused with a mass lesion, such as a malignancy or pancreatic pseudocyst. The delicate nature of the accessory ducts on the pancreatogram is a helpful indicator of pancreas divisum. If possible, the accessory papilla should be cannulated, which should reveal a duct of Santorini running the entire length of the pancreas that is not in communication with the duct of Wirsung. Although ERCP remains the gold standard for the diagnosis of pancreas divisum, magnetic resonance pancreatography is becoming more frequently used given its noninvasive nature. If stenosis of the papilla is not demonstrated radiographically, pancreatic manometry and secretin ultrasound scanning may be useful in identifying patients who may benefit from endoscopic or surgical intervention [107,108].

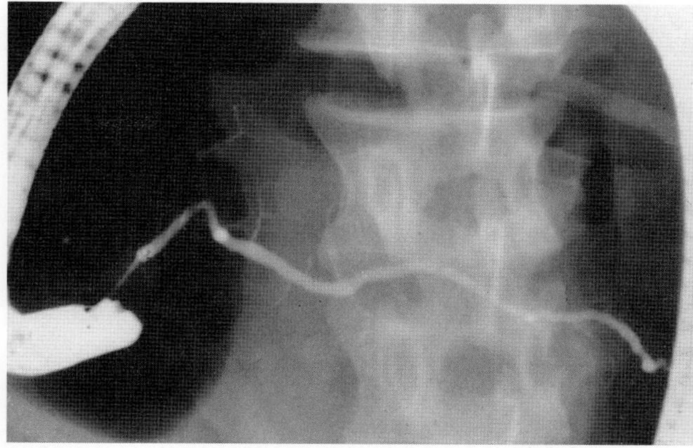

Figure 7.14 Pancreas divisum. An endoscopic retrograde pancreatogram performed through the accessory papilla shows the dorsal duct in pancreas divisum. Source: Courtesy of Peter B. Cotton, Durham, NC.

Patients with mild symptoms can be managed conservatively. Patients with recurrent episodes of acute pancreatitis or chronic pain require intervention to alleviate accessory ductal stenosis. Surgical accessory duct sphincteroplasty has been successful in treating patients, with the best results observed in patients with recurrent episodes of acute pancreatitis [109–111]. Endoscopic therapy with a combination of minor duct sphincterotomy and stenting has achieved similar rates of success; however, the follow-up period in these patients has been less than in the surgical groups [112–114], and long-term stenting of the pancreatic duct has been reported to result in chronic ductal changes [115]. Determination of which patients with acute recurrent pancreatitis would be served best by surgical or endoscopic treatment awaits further study. Patients with chronic pancreatitis have a poor response to both surgical and endoscopic treatment modalities. If sphincterotomy fails or the ductal involvement is extensive, direct ductal drainage or resection of the involved pancreas is necessary [116,117].

Cystic lesions of the pancreas

Cysts of the pancreas are distinguished from more common pseudocysts by the presence of an epithelial lining. Pseudocysts often follow bouts of acute pancreatitis, with trauma being a major precipitant. Identification of true columnar or cuboidal epithelium in cystic lesion may be difficult, and it is not always possible to distinguish a congenital or neoplastic cyst from a pancreatic pseudocyst. In cysts located in the peripancreatic space, identification of pancreatic enzymes in the cyst fluid is helpful in determining that it is of pancreatic origin; however, not all pancreatic cysts contain fluid rich in pancreatic enzymes. Solitary congenital cysts are rare [118]. They are more commonly diagnosed in early childhood but may remain asymptomatic and undetected into adulthood. Although other congenital anomalies have been reported with pancreatic cysts, these are more often isolated defects [119].

The most common presentation of a solitary pancreatic cyst is as an abdominal mass, which may be associated with abdominal pain or complications resulting from expanding size, such as gastroduodenal obstruction. Encroachment on the intrapancreatic or extrapancreatic common bile duct may cause biliary obstruction [120]. Subcutaneous fat necrosis and osteolytic lesions secondary to pancreatic enzymes leaking into the circulation from a developmental pancreatic cyst have been described [121].

The presence of a pancreatic cyst may be suggested by a plain radiograph of the abdomen or an upper gastrointestinal radiographic series demonstrating a mass displacing a portion of the stomach, duodenum, or colon. The best diagnostic test is CT, which demonstrates a fluid-filled cystic lesion in the pancreas and its relationship to surrounding structures. In considering the differential diagnosis, it is important to consider the different possible cystic lesions of the pancreas, including congenital cysts (rare), pseudocysts, and cystic neoplasms. Cystic neoplasms of the pancreas include mucinous cystic neoplasms, serous cystadenomas, solid pseudopapillary neoplasms, cystic pancreatic endocrine neoplasms, and intraductal papillary mucinous neoplasms [122] (see Chapter 77 for a detailed discussion).

Multiple cysts

Multiple congenital pancreatic cysts are rare and usually are associated with other congenital anomalies, most frequently polycystic kidney disease and cystic fibrosis. Other clinical syndromes involving multiple pancreatic cysts include von Hippel–Lindau syndrome, Ivemark syndrome, and Gruber syndrome, in which cysts of the lung, liver, and central nervous system also are found [123,124]. Many of the associated anomalies are lethal, although patients may have no symptoms referable to the pancreatic cysts. Because of the numerous cysts and the involvement of several organ systems, no treatment is necessary unless specific symptoms or a particular complication, such as infection of a cyst, dictates surgical excision or drainage. Multiple pancreatic cystic lesions can present as a manifestation of intraductal papillary mucinous neoplasms of the pancreas (see Chapter 77 for a detailed discussion on cystic neoplasms of the pancreas).

References are available at www.yamadagastro.com/textbook7e

Further reading

Bockman D.E., Buchler M., Malfertheiner P., et al. Analysis of nerves in chronic pancreatitis. Gastroenterology 1988;94:1459.

Ceyhan G.O., Bergmann F., Kadihasanoglu M., et al. Pancreatic neuropathy and neuropathic pain – a comprehensive pathomorphological study of 546 cases. Gastroenterology 2009;136:177.

Coleman S.D., Eisen G.M., Troughton A.B., et al. Endoscopic treatment of pancreas divisum. Am J Gastroenterol 1994;89:1152.

Dawson W., Langman J. An anatomical-radiological study on pancreatic duct pattern in man. Anat Rec 1961;39:59.

Farrell J.J., Fernandez-del Castillo C. Pancreatic cyst neoplasms: management and unanswered questions. Gastroenterology 2013;144:1303.

Fulcher A.S., Turner M.A. MR pancreatography: a useful tool for evaluating pancreatic disorders. Radiographics 1999;19:5.

Lloyd-Jones W., Mountain J.C., Warren K.W. Annular pancreas in the adult. Ann Surg 1972;176:163.

McLean A., Fairclough P. Endoscopic ultrasound – current applications. Clin Radiol 1996;51:83.

Silen W. Surgical anatomy of the pancreas. Surg Clin North Am 1964;44:1253.

Stopczynski R.E., Normolle D.P., Hartman D.J., et al. Neuroplastic changes occur early in the development of pancreatic ductal adenocarcinoma. Cancer Res 2014;74:1718.

CHAPTER 8

Abdominal cavity: anatomy, structural anomalies, and hernias

Stella Joyce[1], Kevin P. Murphy[1,2], Michael M. Maher[1], and Owen J. O'Connor[1]

[1] Department of Radiology, University College Cork, Cork University Hospital, Cork, Ireland

[2] Mercy University Hospital, Cork, Ireland

Chapter menu

Introduction

Awareness of the embryological development and anatomy of the abdominal cavity is key to understanding the basis for many anomalies and acquired defects that may occur both in infancy and later in life, in addition to the patterns of disease spread that may be observed in the abdominal cavity. This chapter details the salient points regarding abdominal cavity development and anatomy, developmental and childhood structural anomalies of the abdominal cavity, and adult abdominal hernias.

Abdominal cavity development and anatomy

Key components of the abdominal cavity include the peritoneum and its reflections that envelop, suspend, or form boundaries around many intraabdominal organs. The abdominal cavity is divided into intraperitoneal and retroperitoneal components by the peritoneum, a serous membrane composed of visceral and parietal layers. The visceral layer covers the surfaces of abdominal viscera, while the parietal layer lines the walls of the abdominal cavity. As a strict definition, the peritoneal cavity refers to the potential space between both layers of peritoneum; this normally contains only a small amount of fluid, and is not usually visible on imaging [1]. In broader terms, the peritoneal cavity refers to an area bounded by the diaphragm and pelvic floor superiorly and inferiorly, respectively, and by the anterior abdominal muscles and vertebrae anteriorly and posteriorly, respectively [2].

Peritoneal embryology

The embryonic abdominal cavity within the fetus, known as the coelomic cavity, has formed by the fourth week of gestation. In general embryonic terms, the intestine develops from the endodermal germ layer, while the mesentery develops from the mesodermal germ layer [3]. Though previous descriptions of mesenteric embryology included commentaries on mesenteric regression, fragmentation and discontinuity, the mesentery is now regarded as a contiguous structure [4], spanning the intestine from duodenum to rectum. As such, the accepted understanding of mesenteric embryological development has required reevaluation. Mesenteric embryology can now be defined by a number of key processes: suspension at points of vascular connectivity; differential elongation of focused areas of the intestine and mesentery with a resultant counterclockwise rotation of both; mesenteric flattening against the posterior abdominal wall; and development of Toldt's fascia and the peritoneal membrane maintaining attachments in this configuration [5].

The primitive gut tube, suspended from the posterior abdominal wall, consists of the foregut, midgut, and hindgut; each has its own arterial supply, which subsequently become the celiac,

Yamada's Textbook of Gastroenterology, Seventh Edition. Edited by Timothy C. Wang, Michael Camilleri, Benjamin Lebwohl, Anna S. Lok, William J. Sandborn, Kenneth K. Wang, and Gary D. Wu.

Companion website: www.yamadagastro.com/textbook7e

superior mesenteric, and inferior mesenteric arteries, respectively. The closing process of the primitive gut facilitates the opposition of two layers of mesothelium (peritoneum) ventrally and dorsally to the gut. These are referred to as primitive mesenteries, with the embryological process confirming the mesentery to be a peritoneal derived structure [6].

Distal to the major papilla, the second part of the duodenum forms the junction between foregut and midgut in the adult. The junction of the middle and distal thirds of the transverse colon marks the site of transition between the midgut and hindgut. The foregut undergoes a 90° clockwise rotation by the 10th week of gestation such that the left side of the stomach faces anteriorly as per normal adult configuration. The spleen moves to the left upper quadrant, the liver predominantly occupies the right upper quadrant, and the stomach bridges the gap between. The pancreas also becomes a retroperitoneal structure during the same period. Midgut development is characterized by rapid elongation, physiological herniation into the umbilical cord, and 270° of counterclockwise rotation during return to the abdominal cavity between the fifth and 11th weeks of development. As a result, the jejunum is normally located in the left upper quadrant and the cecum in the right lower quadrant (Figure 8.1). When this rotation fails to occur, malrotation of the bowel ensues, appreciable on cross-sectional imaging when the normal orientation of the superior mesenteric artery (SMA) to the superior mesenteric vein (SMV) is reversed (Figure 8.2). The normal anatomical relationship of the mesenteric vessels consists of the SMV lying to the right of the SMA. Although reversal of the normal SMA and SMV orientation should suggest the possibility of malrotation, reversal is not pathognomonic of malrotation and the intestine can be appropriately positioned even with the SMA and SMV configuration reversed [7]. Furthermore, normal configuration of the SMA and SMV does not definitively exclude intestinal malrotation; ultrasound imaging is useful as a screening tool in the diagnosis of midgut malrotation, particularly in children [8].

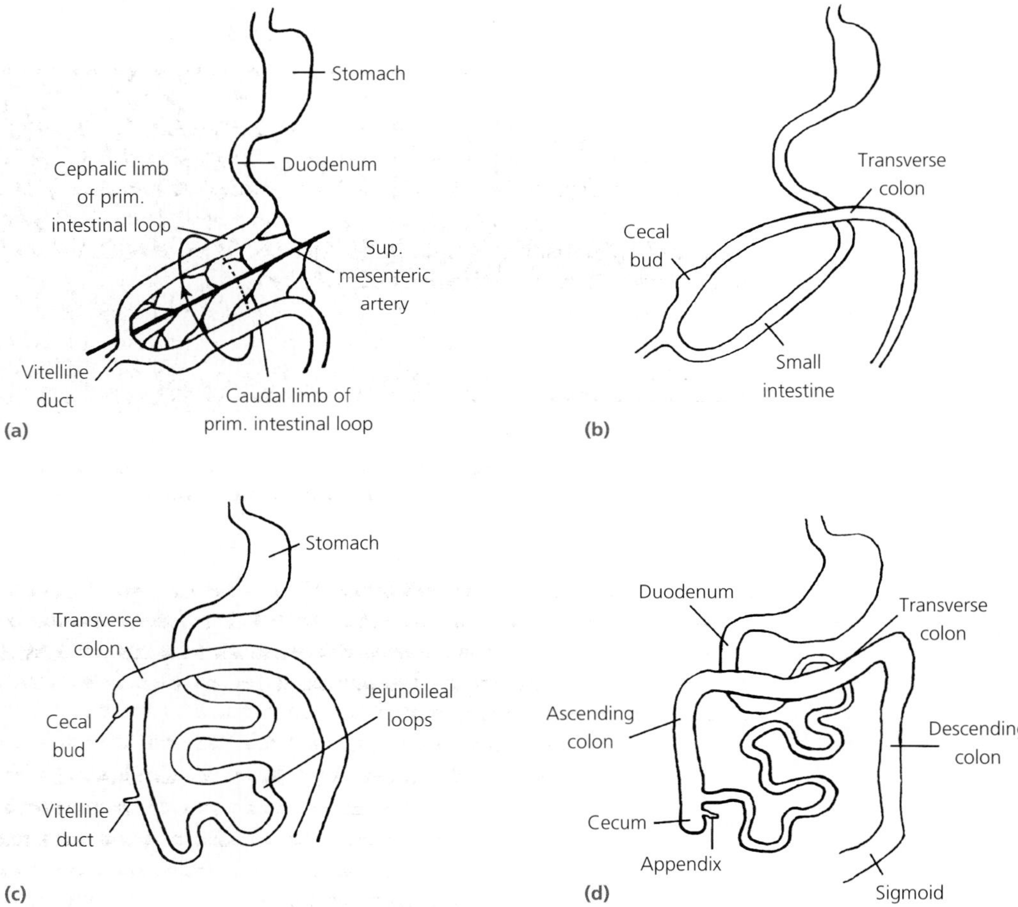

Figure 8.1 Embryonic development of the midgut. **(a)** Schematic drawing of the primary intestinal loop before rotation (lateral view). The superior mesenteric artery forms the axis of the loop, and the arrow indicates the counterclockwise rotation around this axis. **(b)** Similar views as in **(a)** showing the primary intestinal loop after 180° counterclockwise rotation. The transverse colon is shown as passing in front of the duodenum. **(c)** Anterior view of the intestinal loop after the 270° counterclockwise rotation. Note the cecal bud in the right upper quadrant. **(d)** Similar view as in **(a)** with the intestinal loops in the final position. Cecum and appendix are now in the right lower quadrant. Source: Sadler 1985 [9]. Reproduced with permission of Wolters Kluwer Health.

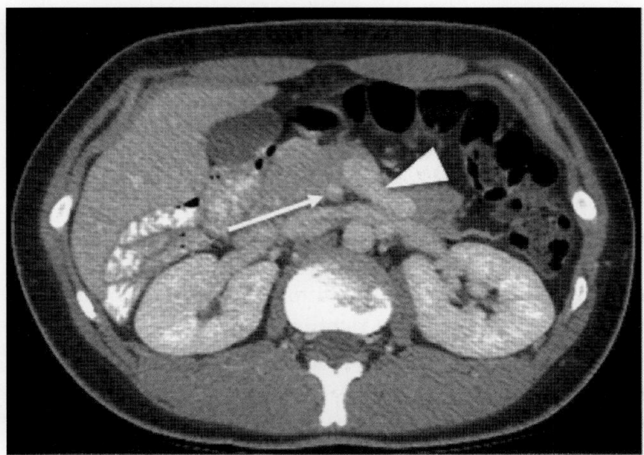

Figure 8.2 Axial computed tomography (CT) image demonstrating malrotation with reversal of the normal superior mesenteric artery and vein orientation. The superior mesenteric artery (arrow) is located to the right of the superior mesenteric vein (arrowhead).

Peritoneal reflections

The peritoneum derives from mesoderm; it assists in suspending the gut tube via ventral and dorsal mesenteries. The mesentery, which anchors the anterior and posterior abdominal wall, is an extension of the peritoneum. The ventral mesentery forms the lesser omentum, whilst the dorsal mesentery maintains function as a mesentery, and also consists of the greater omentum and gastrosplenic ligament.

The peritoneal cavity is subdivided into several spaces and recesses via peritoneal reflections. These reflections are double-layered folds of peritoneum, which are composed of remnants of the primitive ventral and dorsal mesenteries that result from the visceral rotation (Figure 8.3). They interconnect and suspend the organs, and are subdivided into ligaments, omenta, and mesenteries. The relationship of an organ to the peritoneum has surgical significance; retroperitoneal organs include the aorta, pancreas, kidneys, ureters, adrenal glands, esophagus, ascending and descending colon, and second and third parts of the duodenum.

A peritoneal ligament consists of two folds of peritoneum that enclose a structure. Peritoneal ligaments are named based

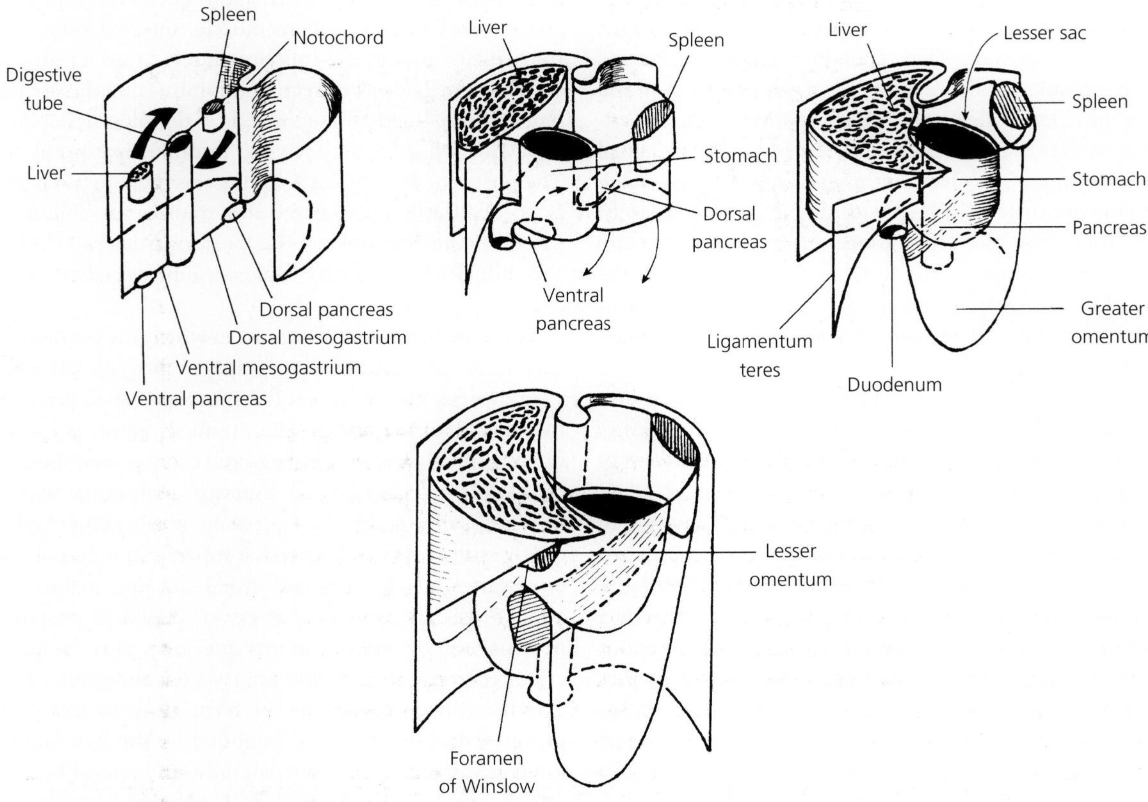

Figure 8.3 Embryological mesenteric folding. The organs of the upper gastrointestinal tract rotate 90° clockwise (when viewed from above) in a transverse plane. Originally, ventral structures like the liver are situated to the right, and posterior organs such as the spleen and dorsal pancreas and the dorsal aspect of the future stomach are positioned to the left side of the abdominal cavity. The dorsal mesogastrium elongates and folds to the left to form the greater omentum.

on the structures that they connect. Examples include the phrenicocolic, hepaticoduodenal, gastrosplenic, gastrocolic, gastrophrenic, splenorenal, and duodenocolic ligaments. The liver is connected via the triangular ligament, plus the superior and inferior coronary ligaments, to the diaphragmatic undersurface. The falciform ligament, which contains the obliterated umbilical vein, connects the liver to the anterior abdominal wall at the umbilicus.

An omentum is a subtype of ligament that joins the stomach to another organ. The greater omentum is composed of four peritoneal layers, which drape downwards to connect the greater curve of the stomach with the anterior transverse colon. The gastrocolic, gastrosplenic, and duodenocolic ligaments are components of the greater omentum. The lesser omentum encloses the hepatoduodenal and hepatogastric ligaments [10]. It connects the lesser gastric curve with the fissure for the ligamentum venosum and contains the left gastric artery, coronary vein, and lymph nodes. This ligament is a potential route of disease spread between the two organs because the ligament is contiguous with the hepatic capsule between the caudate lobe and left lobe of liver. The foramen of Winslow, a small opening at the free distal margin of the hepatoduodenal ligament, serves as the only natural communication between the lesser sac and greater peritoneal cavity [10].

Mesenteries are composed of subperitoneal tissue between two layers of visceral peritoneum [1] that connect bowel to the posterior abdominal wall. They contain mesenteric arteries, veins, and lymphatics. The mesentery has a role in attaching and supporting the colon; collectively, this component of the mesentery is referred to as the mesocolon [11]. Anatomically, the small and large bowel mesentery has a number of subsections, which take the following anatomical sequence: small intestinal mesentery, right, transverse and left mesocolon, mesosigmoid, and mesorectum [5]. Though assumed to be continuous with the mesentery of the jejunum, ileum and colon, the exact alignment of the mesogastrium and mesoduodenum is being evaluated from an embryonic perspective.

The small intestinal mesentery attaches to 15 cm of the posterior abdominal wall from the level of the duodenojejunal junction to the ileocecal junction, enveloping between 6 and 8 m of small bowel.

The transverse mesocolon divides the peritoneal cavity into supra- and inframesocolic compartments. The supramesocolic space is bounded by the transverse mesocolon and diaphragm. It contains the pancreas, liver, spleen, duodenum, and lesser sac. The inframesocolic section lies inferior to the mesocolon and is divided into the larger left inframesocolic space and smaller right space by the small bowel mesentery. The left inframesocolic space communicates freely with the pelvic peritoneal space. It contains the small intestine, left colon, and spleen. The contents of the equivalent right-sided space include part of the small intestine, a fraction of the liver, and the right colon.

Peritoneal reflections are not normally visible on cross-sectional imaging unless there is thickening of the peritoneum. There is normally a small volume of fluid in the peritoneal cavity. This measures less than 100 mL in volume and allows friction-free movement. The abdominal cavity acts as a natural pathway for disease spread, with potential routes along the mesenteries and ligaments, in addition to along ducts. Transperitoneal or transcoelomic spread describes progression of disease through the visceral peritoneum of an organ, with dissemination into the peritoneal cavity.

Fluid circulation within the abdominal cavity follows an orderly pattern; peritoneal fluid follows a caudocranial clockwise direction towards the right into the subphrenic submesothelial lymphatics that absorb peritoneal fluid. The left subdiaphragmatic space is discontinuous with the left paracolic gutter due to the phrenicocolic ligament. Fluid spread between the right and left subdiaphragmatic spaces is limited by the falciform ligament [12]. Peritoneal metastases tend to occur in regions of relative stasis or dependency, such as the subdiaphragmatic space, the paracolic gutters, pouch of Douglas, porta hepatis, and falciform ligament.

Boundaries of the abdominal cavity

The abdominopelvic cavity is bounded superiorly by the diaphragm, inferiorly by the pelvic floor, and by the abdominal wall in other directions. The layers of the anterior and lateral abdominal walls from superficial to deep are: skin, subcutaneous fascia, external oblique muscle, internal oblique muscle, transversus abdominis muscles, fascia transversalis, fat, and peritoneum. The paired rectus abdominis muscles are the dominant muscles medially separated by the bloodless plane of the linea alba which is conducive to midline laparotomy incisions. The posterior abdominal wall muscles include psoas major, iliacus, quadratus lumborum, and transversus abdominis. The osseous contributions to the posterior, lateral, and anterior abdominal walls are ribs, xiphisternum, vertebral bodies, and pelvis.

There are a number of regions in which the peritoneum must accommodate structures entering or leaving the abdominal cavity; these sites are potential sources of structural weakness in the abdominal cavity. The inguinal region is of particular interest in this regard. The inguinal canal is an oblique channel through the inferomedial anterior abdominal wall, which measures approximately 4 cm long in an adult, and extends downwards from the deep to the superficial inguinal rings. The boundaries of the inguinal canal are the external oblique aponeurosis anteriorly, the transversalis fascia posteriorly, the inguinal and lacunar ligaments inferiorly, plus the arching fibers of internal oblique and transverses abdominis superiorly. The Hesselbach triangle is the term given to that part of the posterior wall of the canal bounded by the inguinal ligament inferiorly, epigastric vessels laterally, and lateral border of the rectus muscle medially. The deep opening of the canal is the deep inguinal ring, which is an opening in the transversalis fascia. The superficial inguinal ring is a defect in the external oblique aponeurosis.

The canal transmits the spermatic cord in males (vas deferens, spermatic vessels, and cremasteric muscle), the round ligament of the uterus in females, and the ilioinguinal ligament in both sexes. The canal forms from a diverticulum of the peritoneum called the processus vaginalis, which extends through the abdominal wall layers. The processus' connection with the peritoneal cavity is normally obliterated in the neonate but more likely to be patent in premature infants leading to an increased incidence of inguinal hernia. Deep to the inguinal ligament, the arrangement of the normal femoral neurovascular structures from lateral to medial is the femoral nerve, femoral artery, femoral vein, and femoral canal. The femoral canal is approximately 13 mm in length and represents the medial compartment of the femoral sheath. The femoral ring is the superior opening into the canal. Its boundaries are the inguinal ligament anteriorly, superior pubic ramus posteriorly, femoral vein laterally, and lacunar ligament medially. The femoral canal normally contains fat, lymphatics, and a deep inguinal node (Cloquet node).

Developmental and structural anomalies of the abdominal cavity

The normal anatomy, described in the section above entitled *Abdominal cavity development and anatomy*, has a number of variations, some of which result in pathological conditions. These include disorders of bowel rotation, consequences of physiological umbilical herniation, as well as failure of membrane formation leading to development of hernias.

Disorders of bowel rotation

The peritoneum and its reflections, including the mesentery, omentum, and ligaments, are intimately related to the development of bowel structure. Any disorder of the physiological 270° rotation of the small bowel is termed malrotation. Nonrotation, a specific subtype where the duodenojejunal flexure and small bowel lie to the right of midline and the colon lies to the left of midline, is noted as an incidental finding on approximately 2 out of 1000 upper gastrointestinal contrast studies [13]. This configuration results in a short small bowel mesentery. The key concern in patients with malrotation is the propensity for midgut volvulus around the axis of this short mesentery with development of obstruction and subsequent bowel ischaemia [14–19]. The true incidence of malrotation is unclear, as rotational anomalies may be asymptomatic throughout a person's life span. Neonatal symptomatic malrotation has a reported frequency of approximately 1 in 6000 live births.

Approximately 50% of patients with malrotation present in the first month of life, with symptoms of partial or complete obstruction [14,15]. Though rarely diagnostic, radiographs are useful as a first-line imaging tool to exclude perforation. An upper gastrointestinal fluoroscopic contrast study will visualize the duodenum [18], though ultrasound, sensitive and specific for the diagnosis of volvulus [20], is an alternative imaging option in institutions with experienced pediatric radiologists. Fluoroscopy has a high sensitivity and specificity, though is equivocal in approximately 15% of cases. The key finding in cases of nonrotation is that the third part of the duodenum does not cross the midline and the duodenojejunal flexure lies to the right of midline. Furthermore, in cases of malrotation, the ligament of Treitz is typically displaced both inferiorly and to the right; upper GI contrast studies, demonstrating the abnormal position of the ligament of Treitz, are useful for confirmation of malrotation diagnosis (Figure 8.4). The duodenum may have a corkscrew appearance if a volvulus is present at the time of contrast medium ingestion (Figure 8.5), or an abrupt cut-off if obstruction exists [18]. Reversal of the normal superior mesenteric artery–vein relationship is frequently seen on cross-sectional or ultrasound imaging but this sign is not pathognomonic [21].

Patients presenting with intestinal malrotation and volvulus, or suspected volvulus, should be treated by an appropriately trained surgeon in an emergent manner [22]. Intraoperatively, volvulus, if present, is untwisted in a counterclockwise fashion. Additionally, the Ladd procedure for correction of malrotation is conducted; Ladd bands, if present, are released, viable bowel is placed in a nonrotation position, and the base of the mesentery is widened. Appendectomy is also performed. In the absence of bowel ischemia or volvulus, the Ladd procedure may be conducted laparoscopically, particularly in adults or older children [23–27].

Of the remaining 50% of patients with malrotation who do not present in the first month of life, some have chronic intermittent abdominal symptoms, but many are asymptomatic and the finding is incidentally made during adulthood [14,16].

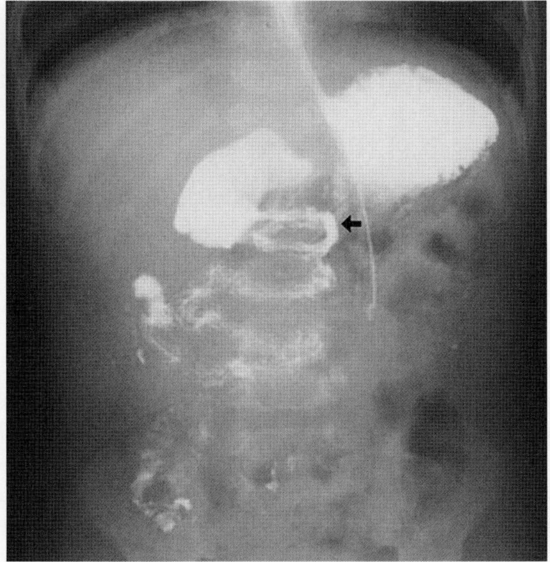

Figure 8.4 Upper gastrointestinal contrast study demonstrating malrotation. The small bowel is located to the left of midline and the ligament of Treitz (arrow) is not normally positioned.

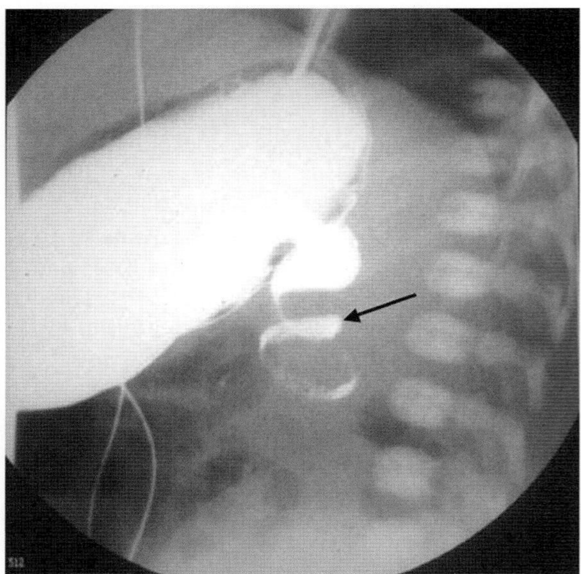

Figure 8.5 Upper gastrointestinal fluoroscopic contrast study in a neonate with vomiting due to malrotation. Lateral view shows a "corkscrew" appearance of the duodenum (arrow) that has torted around itself.

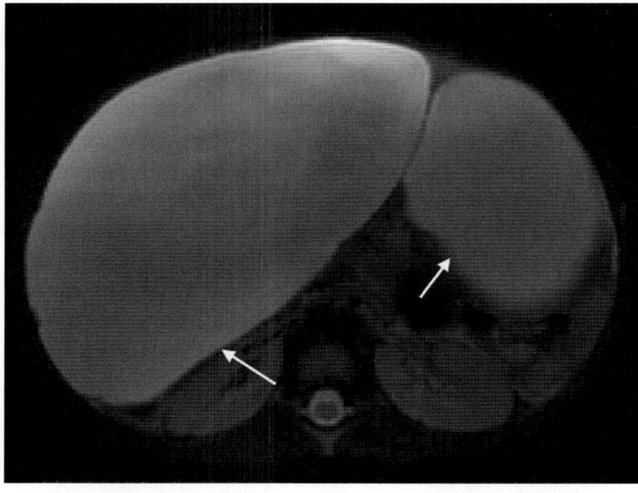

Figure 8.6 T2-weighted magnetic resonance image (MRI) in a newborn with congenital abdominal lymphangioma. There is a loculated, high-signal, thin-walled malformation anterior to the kidneys (arrows).

Congenital intraabdominal cystic lesions

Intraabdominal cystic lesions are traditionally classified on the basis of their location and histology [28]. They include lymphangiomata (Figure 8.6), mesenteric cysts, enteric cysts, and enteric duplication cysts (commonly referred to as duplication cysts) [29,30]. All of these lesions are associated with the mesentery, omentum, and small bowel. Though abdominal ultrasound is the imaging modality of choice for initial evaluation, CT or MRI are frequently required for detailed lesion characterization [31].

Lymphangiomata are congenital vascular malformations and appear as multiloculated thin-walled lesions on imaging. Mesenteric and enteric cysts are predominantly unilocular with imperceptible walls. Mesenteric cysts primarily affect the small bowel mesentery, though a small number of cases have been recognized beyond the mesocolon or retroperitoneal colon [32]. Enteric duplication cysts are chiefly unilocular with walls that mirror the small bowel wall [29,30]. Though typically located in the proximal small intestine, enteric duplication cysts may also affect the esophagus (Figure 8.7), stomach, and colon. Many of these lesions are detected antenatally and are frequently asymptomatic. Small asymptomatic intraabdominal congenital cystic abnormalities do not need any intervention and are generally monitored to ensure regression or stability [33].

Pediatric anterior abdominal wall hernias

A hernia is defined as an abnormal bulge, protrusion or projection of an organ, or part of an organ, through the wall of a cavity within which it is usually contained.

Failure of reduction of physiological small bowel herniation in the first trimester may result in exomphalos or gastroschisis. Exomphalos, also known as omphalocele, is a persistence of small bowel herniation into the base of the umbilical cord. It most commonly contains small bowel, and is covered by a three-layer membranous sac of amnion, peritoneum, and Wharton's jelly. Exomphalos has a prevalence of 1.86 per 10 000 live births in the United States [34]; in excess of 90% of cases are diagnosed prenatally. It is associated with other congenital anomalies in 54% of infants [35], and it is these anomalies that generally determine patient prognosis. Associated anomalies include chromosomal aberrations, which result in other gastrointestinal, genitourinary, cardiac, and central nervous system defects [35–37].

Gastroschisis involves an anterior abdominal wall hernia that lies lateral to the umbilicus and lacks any coverings. It has a prevalence of 4.49 per 10 000 live births in the US [34] but has a much lower incidence of associated anomalies compared with exomphalos. Both gastroschisis and exomphalos are detected antenatally in the majority of cases [36,37], and repaired in the antenatal period in an emergent fashion.

The umbilical ring normally closes spontaneously after birth, with continued growth of the rectus abdominis muscles toward one another; persistent opening of the umbilical ring results in an umbilical hernia. Pediatric umbilical hernias are common, affecting 15–23% of newborns in the US [38]. There is an increased prevalence among African-American children. They typically remain asymptomatic and resolve spontaneously. Surgical intervention is required in only a minority of cases, usually for incarcerated and symptomatic hernias [39].

Disorders involving persistence of the urachus are an uncommon congenital anomaly [40,41]. During bladder development, a patent connection exists between the cloaca and allantois. This lumen usually fibroses by birth. The connection can persist completely as a patent connection between the anterosuperior

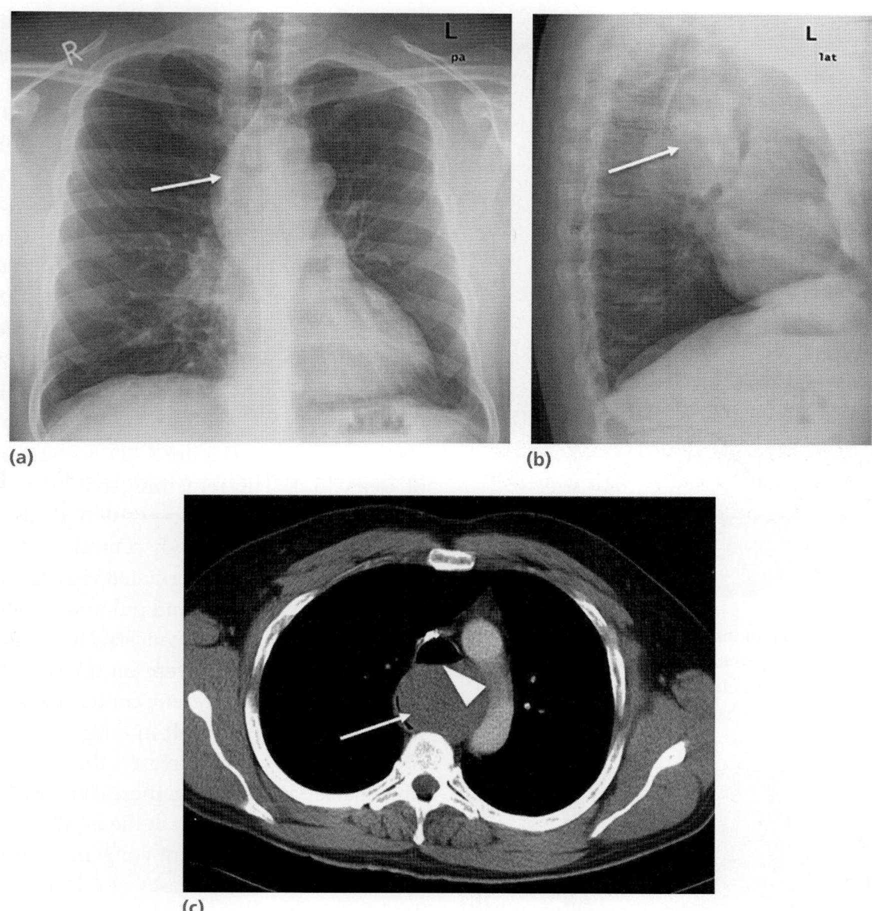

Figure 8.7 Posterior mediastinal mass in a 39-year-old male patient. Frontal **(a)** and lateral **(b)** chest radiographs demonstrate a soft tissue density lesion (arrow) adjacent to the right upper mediastinum, with right paravertebral stripe thickening. The cardiac contour is maintained, and hilar vessels remain visible, placing the mass in the posterior mediastinum. Axial computed tomography (CT) **(c)**, taken just above the level of the carina, demonstrates a cystic posterior mediastinal mass (arrow), with secondary bowing of the inferior trachea (arrowhead). Differential diagnoses would include an esophageal duplication cyst and bronchogenic cyst.

bladder and the umbilicus, or partially anywhere along the length of the connection. Four variations of urachal persistence exist: completely patent urachus, urachal cyst, urachal–umbilical sinus, and vesicourachal diverticulum. Allantoic cysts may also arise from persistence of the urachus. If a complete urachus persists then urine drains onto the anterior abdominal wall via the umbilicus. Urachal remnants can cause pain, a palpable mass, sinus discharge, or recurrent infection. An increased risk of adenocarcinoma is also seen [40–42]; this is a rare malignancy which frequently produces mucin and may contain calcification. Disorders of the vitellointestinal duct are discussed elsewhere (see Chapter 5).

Pediatric groin hernias

The vast majority of congenital groin hernias are indirect inguinal hernias as a result of incomplete closure of the processus vaginalis (Figure 8.8) (canal of Nuck in females). A number of other anomalies associated with the processus vaginalis can occur, including congenital hydrocele, communicating hydrocele, and hydrocele of the cord. Primary inguinal hernia affects 1–5% of all newborns, with an increased incidence of 9–11% among premature infants [43]. Males are affected more commonly than females, with a male to female ratio slightly in excess of 4:1 [44].

The hernial sac most frequently contains fat or small bowel. The etiology behind an acute groin swelling can usually be diagnosed on clinical evaluation, though ultrasound is the modality of choice if further assessment is necessary [45,46]. Typically, a lump is noticed by a parent when the child cries; this is usually reducible but sometimes an irreducible swelling is seen medially in the groin. Thickening of the inguinal-scrotal fold may also be detected clinically (Figure 8.9). The defect itself can often be palpated with a fingertip. Obstruction or incarceration is rare.

Surgical repair remains the definitive management option for inguinal hernia. This can be done via an open or laparoscopic route with comparable results [47–49]. Laparoscopic repair has

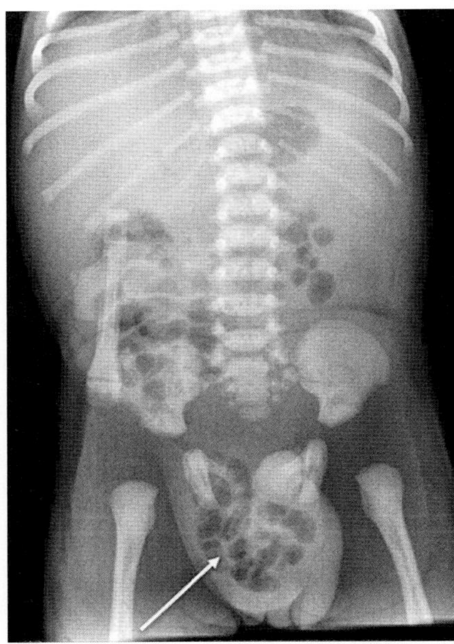

Figure 8.8 Abdominal radiograph of an infant male patient demonstrating a right-sided indirect inguinal hernia. This is secondary to a persistently patent right processus vaginalis (arrow), which contains loops of small bowel without features of obstruction.

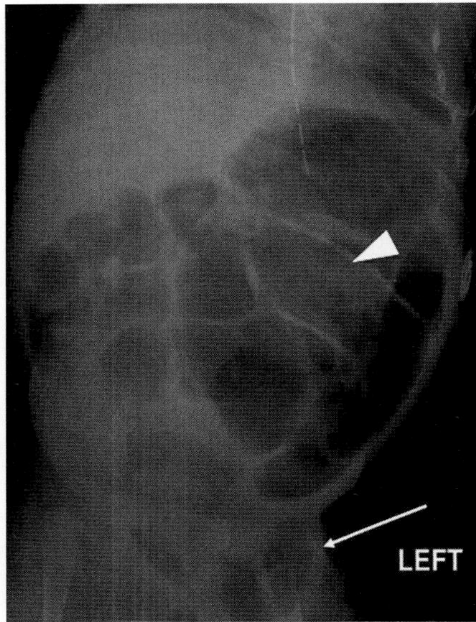

Figure 8.9 Abdominal radiograph of an infant demonstrating an incarcerated indirect left inguinal hernia, with secondary small bowel obstruction. Bowel loops are demonstrated in the hernia (arrow), with proximal small bowel dilation consistent with obstruction (arrowhead). A nasogastric tube has been sited.

the advantage of bilateral access but space is often limited due to small patient size. Additionally, the requirement for contralateral inguinal exploration is controversial [50]. Given the risk of metachronous hernia in children with a unilateral inguinal hernia is 5–12% [51–54], routine contralateral exploration is not deemed justifiable, and is now warranted only for children at particularly high risk for hernia development.

Congenital diaphragmatic hernias

Congenital diaphragmatic hernia (CDH) is a developmental defect, characterized by the presence of an orifice in the diaphragm, which allows abdominal viscera to herniate into the thoracic cavity (Figure 8.10). It is a rare condition, with a prevalence of approximately 1–4 cases per 10 000 live births [55–57].

Classic CDH presents as a diaphragmatic opening, secondary to failure of normal closure of the pleuroperitoneal folds. Complete absence of the hemidiaphragm, referred to as diaphragmatic agenesis, carries a poorer prognosis than classic CDH [58]. Bochdalek hernias, caused by a posterolateral diaphragmatic defect (Figure 8.11), account for approximately 95% of cases [57]. The remaining minority of CDH are anterior-retrosternal or anterior-peristernal defects, referred to as Morgagni hernias, or rarely central.

Compromise of the herniated viscera is not common in CDH. Pulmonary hypoplasia and pulmonary hypertension as a result of compression are key concerns in the antenatal and neonatal period. Whilst most severe on the ipsilateral side, pulmonary hypoplasia may be present contralaterally if there is sufficient mediastinal shift to result in lung compression. As the severity of lung compression increases, there is a corresponding reduction in arterial branching, increasing the likelihood of persistent pulmonary hypertension of the newborn (PPHN) [59].

Associated multisystem congenital anomalies are present in approximately 50% of cases of CDH; their presence increases

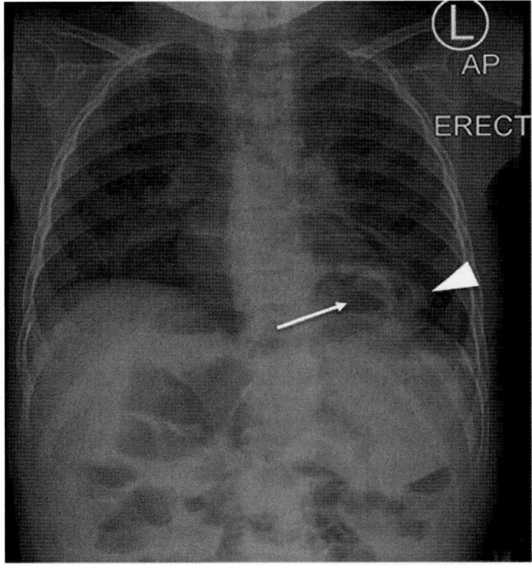

Figure 8.10 Chest radiograph of an 18-month-old pediatric patient, with a background of congenital diaphragmatic hernia repair at 8 days of age. Retrocardiac lucency is demonstrated (arrow), suggestive of recurrence of diaphragmatic hernia. Associated atelectasis of adjacent lung is also demonstrated (arrowhead).

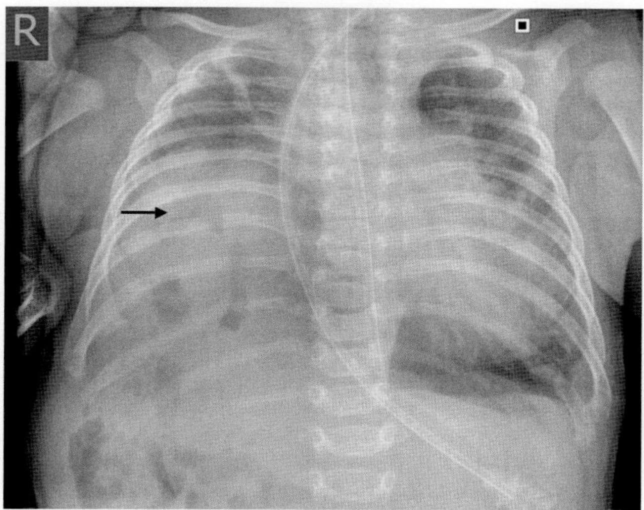

Figure 8.11 Neonatal chest radiograph with Bochdalek hernia. There is a right-sided posterior diaphragmatic defect (Bochdalek hernia) with associated bowel and abdominal content (arrow) herniation into the chest cavity.

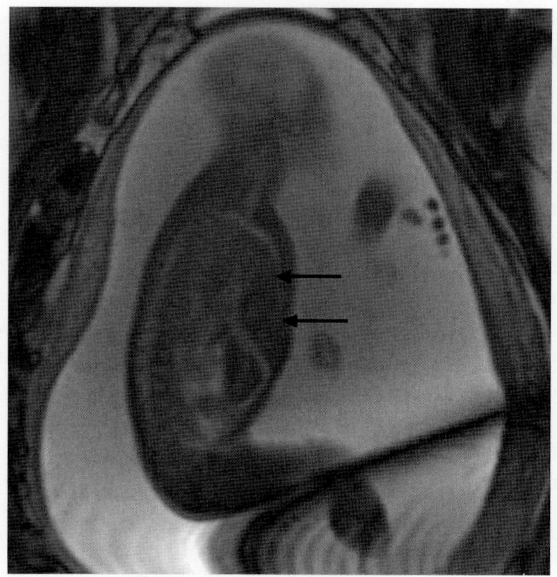

Figure 8.12 Fetal magnetic resonance image of a Morgagni hernia showing protrusion of part of the liver (arrows) through a right-sided Morgagni hernia.

the sensitivity of CDH detection [60]. The majority of clinically significant hernias are detected antenatally; in excess of 60% of cases are suspected at the classic 18–22-week fetal anatomic sonographic survey [57]. Antenatal ultrasound is the standard of care for screening, with prenatal CDH diagnosis dependent on characteristic ultrasound findings [61]. Visualization of abdominal viscera within the thoracic cavity is definitive of a diagnosis of CDH. Fetal magnetic resonance imaging (MRI) is reserved for characterization once an anomaly is suspected or detected on ultrasound (Figure 8.12). Postnatally, a chest radiograph is usually sufficient for diagnosis, demonstrating herniation of abdominal contents into the hemithorax [61]. Typically, only minimal or no aerated lung will be visible on the affected side.

Antenatal detection helps ensure that provisions are made for adequate perinatal planning in a center where the neonate can be managed appropriately. The initial priority following birth of an infant with a CDH is to adequately oxygenate and stabilize the newborn. This may require extracorporeal membrane oxygenation. Surgical repair can be done through an approach from either side of the diaphragm. Larger defects require a muscle flap or synthetic graft to prevent recurrence [62]. In utero fetal repair is feasible and has shown results comparable to open postnatal repair in carefully selected cases [63]. Despite advances in treatment, mortality remains high and is up to 40% [64].

Adult abdominal hernias

The key elements of a hernia are the hernia sac, neck, and contents [65]. The contents of an abdominal hernia most commonly consist of fat and bowel, but any solid or hollow abdominopelvic viscus can be partly or completely contained within a hernial sac.

An incarcerated hernia describes a hernia which cannot be reduced by manipulation (Figure 8.13); incarcerated hernias may or may not be strangulated. Strangulation implies vascular compromise of the incarcerated hernia contents, and may occur within just two hours of incarceration [66].

Classification and pathogenesis

Abdominal hernias can be classified based on their site of origin; abdominal wall, internal, and diaphragmatic varieties are all recognized entities. Abdominal wall hernias may be further subclassified based on location or etiology, with ventral, groin, and pelvic varieties the most common.

Any cause of increased intraabdominal pressure, which compromises mechanical integrity of the abdominal wall, will predispose to abdominal wall hernia [67]. These mechanisms include chronic cough, obesity, ascites, bladder outlet obstruction, constipation, and heavy lifting. In addition, conditions that precipitate localized or generalized weakening of the anterior abdominal wall can contribute to hernia formation. Prior surgery, congenital defects, trauma, aging, connective tissue disorders, and pregnancy are well-documented premorbid conditions. In the case of incisional hernias from prior surgery, problems with wound healing, collagen formation, and extracellular matrix formation are factors that lead to defects.

Epidemiology

Abdominal wall hernias are common, with a prevalence of 4% for individuals aged 45 years and older [68]. Across the US, inguinal hernia repair is now one of the most commonly performed general surgery operations, with rates of 28 per

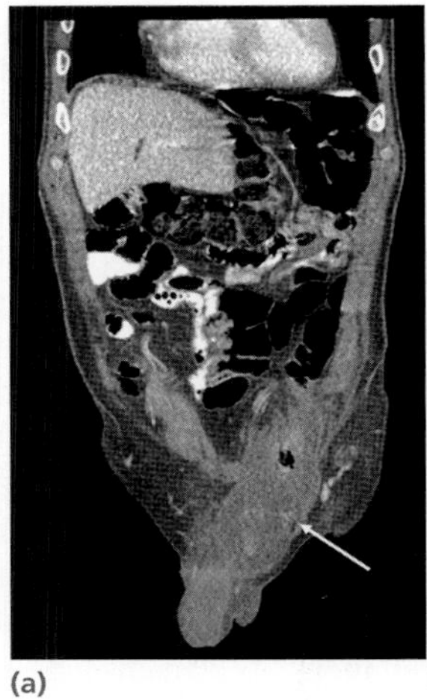

(a)

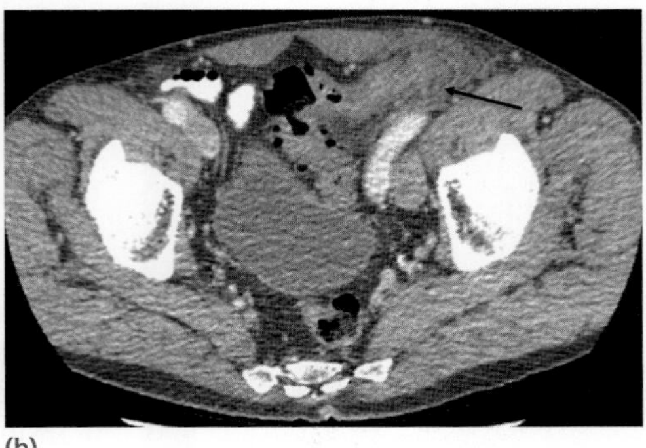

(b)

Figure 8.13 Computed tomography (CT) images demonstrating an incarcerated indirect left inguinal hernia, containing sigmoid colon (arrow). Coronal oblique **(a)** and axial **(b)** images demonstrate extensive fat stranding and mural edema in the sigmoid colon, with reduced mucosal enhancement, concerning for ischemia.

100 000 [69]. In 2006, 348 000 ventral hernia repairs were conducted in the US, costing an estimated $3.2 billion; a significant proportion of the cost burden arose from postoperative complications and emergency repairs [70].

Inguinal hernias are far more common in men than women, with an estimated lifetime risk of 27% and 3% for men and women, respectively [68]. They are bilateral in up to 10% of cases. Inguinal hernias account for approximately 75% of abdominal wall hernias, with femoral, umbilical, epigastric, and incisional hernias accounting for most other types [71]. Though femoral hernias more commonly affect females, inguinal hernias remain twice as common as femoral hernias across the female population.

Clinical findings

Abdominal wall hernias may vary in their clinical presentation depending on size and location of the hernia; small hernias may be completely asymptomatic. Typically, patients describe a lump that appears or increases in size with coughing, standing, or straining, and that reduces spontaneously on relaxation or with manual pressure. Localized pain or tenderness is more commonly present if the hernia is irreducible (incarcerated). Exquisite local tenderness and pain should raise concern for ischemia/strangulation. The risk of strangulation is inversely proportional to the size of the neck. If bowel is contained within the hernia, then symptoms associated with acute or recurrent bowel obstruction may occur; obturator and sciatic hernias are frequently first identified only once they present as bowel obstruction due to incarceration.

Clinical evaluation is sufficient for abdominal wall hernia diagnosis in the majority of patients. Clinical examination should include a complete abdominal assessment. The hernia should be evaluated for size, contents, and location, as well as for neck size and ease of reducibility. The latter two features are better appraised with the patient recumbent. A cough impulse is present when the swelling enlarges as the patient coughs.

In patients presenting with groin hernias, it is important to ascertain whether the hernia is femoral or inguinal. A femoral hernia can be palpated below and lateral to the pubic tubercle whereas an inguinal hernia may be felt above and medial to the tubercle. Differentiating between a direct and indirect inguinal hernia is not of key importance as the repair is the same [72]. Passing a gloved finger through the superficial ring into the canal by invaginating the skin can help differentiate. A direct hernia causes an impulse on the side of the examining finger, as the defect is in the posterior wall medial to the inferior epigastric vessels, whereas an indirect hernia leads to an impact on the tip of the finger on coughing, as the sac comes through the deep ring lateral to the vessels.

Whilst a clinical diagnosis will be definitive in most patients with groin or ventral hernias, hernias in obese patients, in addition to very small hernias, may require imaging studies for formal diagnosis. Additionally, the use of ultrasound, CT or MRI can be beneficial both in determining the size of the hernia defect, and for preoperative planning [73,74].

Adult groin hernia

Variants of adult groin hernia

Collectively, inguinal and femoral hernias are referred to as groin hernias. Femoral hernias (Figure 8.14) are less common than inguinal hernias, generally accounting for approximately 3% of all groin hernias [75]. However, they more frequently present with complications including incarceration and strangulation. Femoral hernias carry a female-to-male ratio of about 10:1.

Direct inguinal hernia occurs due to protrusion of contents through the posterior wall of the canal at the Hesselbach triangle medial to the epigastric vessels. The indirect type (Figure 8.15,

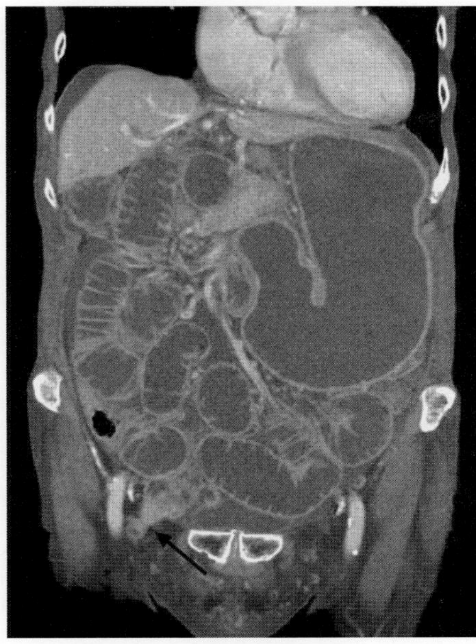

Figure 8.14 Computed tomography image of an obstructed femoral hernia. There is a right-sided femoral hernia (arrow) with proximal bowel obstruction from an incarcerated loop demonstrated on coronal reformatted CT scan.

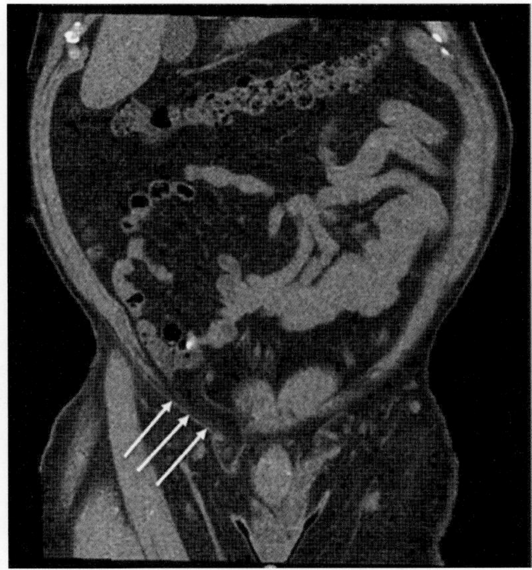

Figure 8.15 Coronal CT image demonstrating an indirect right inguinal hernia. The abdominal wall defect is located lateral to the inferior epigastric vessels, and the hernia sac contains fatty tissue.

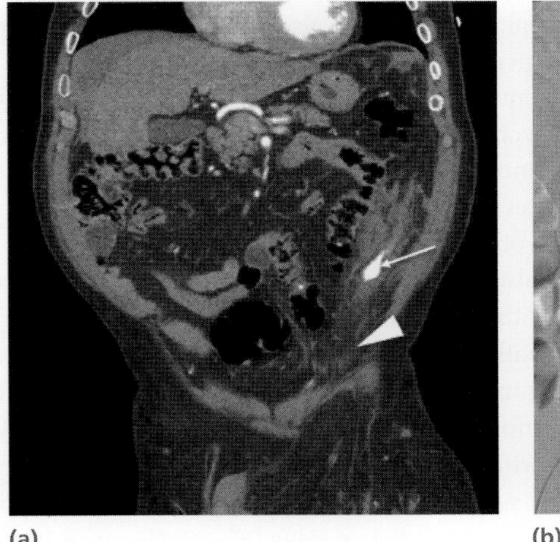

(a)

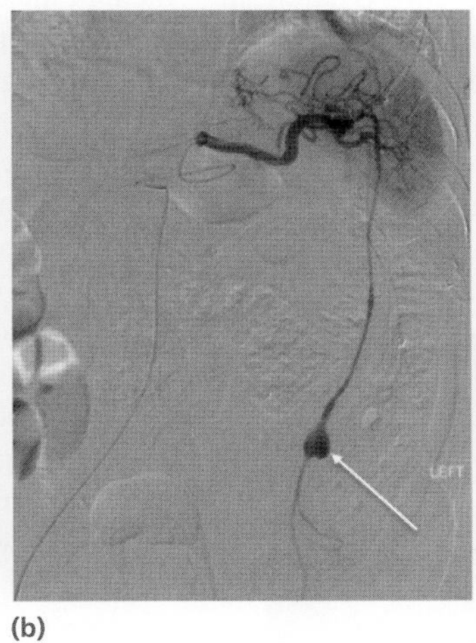

(b)

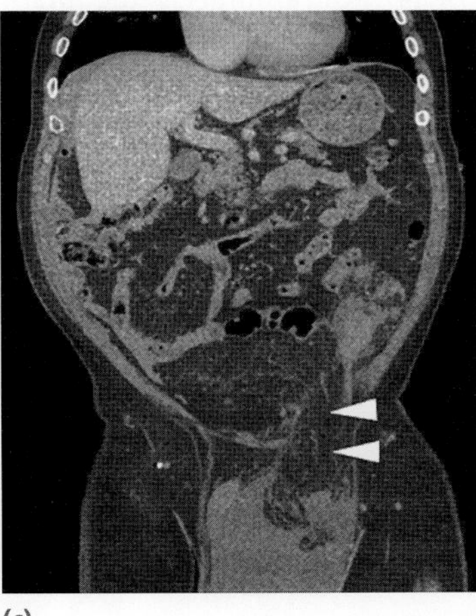

(c)

Figure 8.16 Computed tomography and fluoroscopic images of a spontaneous pseudoaneurysm of a splenic arterial supply to omentum contiguous with a large inguinal hernia. CT mesenteric angiogram, coronal slice **(a)** demonstrates a pseudoaneurysm (arrow) of the vascular pedicle supplying a large inguinal hernia containing omental fat (arrowhead). Fluoroscopic examination **(b)**, acquired during a planned embolization procedure, demonstrates a pseudoaneurysm of a splenic artery branch (arrow). Follow-up reformatted CT mesenteric angiogram, coronal slice **(c)**, demonstrates resolution of the pseudoaneurysm, with no residual filling defect. A large left indirect inguinal hernia is also evident (arrowheads), containing omentum; the extent of stranding within the hernial sac raises clinical suspicion for hernia incarceration.

Figure 8.16) leads to extension of contents through the deep ring into the canal.

A pantaloon hernia occurs when direct and indirect inguinal hernias simultaneously exist on the same side. Littré hernia describes the incarceration of a Meckel's diverticulum within an abdominal wall or internal hernia [76,77]. They are most commonly inguinal, accounting for up to 50% of cases [78]. Amyand hernia refers to the vermiform appendix, whether inflamed or not, being present within the hernia sac. Approximately 1% of all inguinal hernias are complicated by an Amyand hernia; up to 33% of these cases will be noted to have associated acute appendicitis [79].

A Richter hernia contains a single wall of bowel, usually the antimesenteric border [80]; hence, this type can strangulate without bowel obstruction. A Maydl hernia, on the other hand, contains more than one loop of bowel, meaning that this variety can result in closed loop obstruction. A sliding inguinal hernia is when part of the sac wall is formed by a retroperitoneal (or partly retroperitoneal) viscus, usually colon or bladder. A femoral hernia leads to herniation of contents into the femoral canal through the femoral ring. A femoral hernia can be palpated below and lateral to the pubic tubercle whereas an inguinal hernia can be felt above and medial to the tubercle.

A "sportsman's hernia" (Figure 8.17), synonymous with the term "sports hernia," is a common cause of chronic groin pain in athletes. The term is a misnomer as there is no true herniation of soft tissue [81]. Instead, a series of injuries to the abdominal and pelvic musculature associated with the hip joint result in a weakness of the posterior wall of the inguinal canal [82].

Other pathologies which may also present with groin swelling include inguinal adenopathy, saphena varix, femoral artery aneurysm, psoas abscess, hydrocele, varicocele, epididymal cyst, spermatic cord cyst, lipoma, and soft tissue tumor.

In most cases of inguinal or femoral hernia, the diagnosis can be made based on history and clinical examination, avoiding the requirement for further investigations [83]. Radiological investigation of a suspected groin hernia can be performed with CT, MRI, ultrasound (Figure 8.18), or fluoroscopic-guided herniography [74,84]. Ultrasound is the first-line investigation in children, and also has an excellent positive predictive value for hernia detection in adults [85], although it lacks sensitivity in the latter. CT and MRI both offer the clinician the advantage of good regional evaluation, which can identify alternative causes of groin pain. CT is optimal in the acute setting, whilst MRI is superior when the main clinical differential diagnosis is a musculoskeletal cause, as when sportsman's hernia is a consideration. CT and MRI are also excellent modalities for the assessment of the extent of a hernial defect in the nonacute setting.

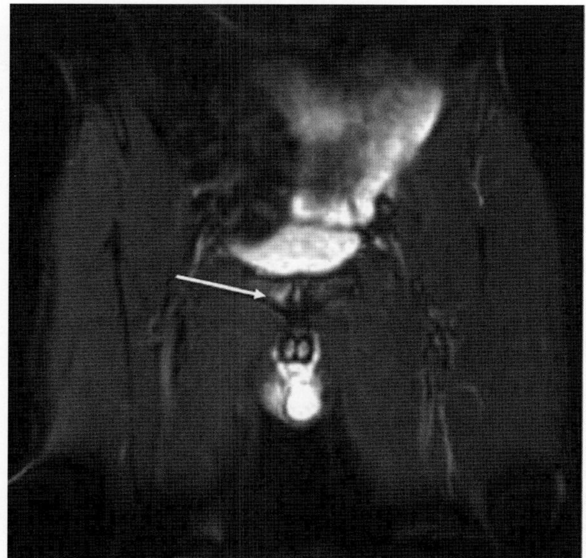

Figure 8.17 Coronal STIR MRI of a sportsman's hernia in a patient presenting with groin pain. There is increased T2 signal indicative of bone marrow edema in the right pubic body (arrow). No true hernia is present.

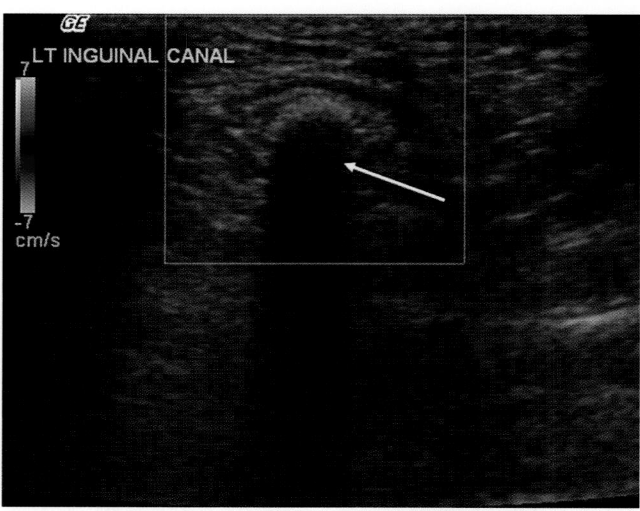

Figure 8.18 Ultrasound image of a bowel containing left inguinal hernia in a 37-year-old male patient. Ultrasound demonstrates a curvilinear echogenic band and posterior acoustic shadowing within the inguinal canal due to air within a bowel loop in the hernial sac.

Fluoroscopic herniography, also known as peritoneography, is a safe radiological investigation, in experienced hands, for assessment of patients with groin pain who clinically lack a palpable hernia. The technique involves percutaneous introduction of iodinated contrast medium into the peritoneal cavity [86]. The hernial orifices are then fluoroscopically examined with the patient in the prone, oblique or erect position at rest, and while the patient performs Valsalva maneuvers. Though slightly more accurate compared with other imaging studies, herniography is invasive and infrequently required given the availability of alternative noninvasive imaging. However, in the small cohort of patients considered for diagnostic laparoscopy to definitively identify or exclude a hernia following inconclusive imaging, herniography may avoid the need for surgical exploration. Herniography is sensitive and has a high negative predictive value [87–89] (Figure 8.19).

Treatment of adult groin hernia

Regardless of type, surgical repair is the only definitive therapy for management of hernias [90].

Surgical repair is recommended for hernias in almost all patients; in patients with uncomplicated groin hernias, repair aims to relieve symptoms and reduce the risk of future complications. The requirement for elective surgical repair is particularly applicable to patients with femoral hernias, regardless of symptoms or gender. Femoral hernias carry a higher risk of developing complications compared with inguinal hernias, with rates of strangulation at 3 and 21 months of 22% and 45% respectively [91]; timely repair avoids complications which may necessitate urgent surgery.

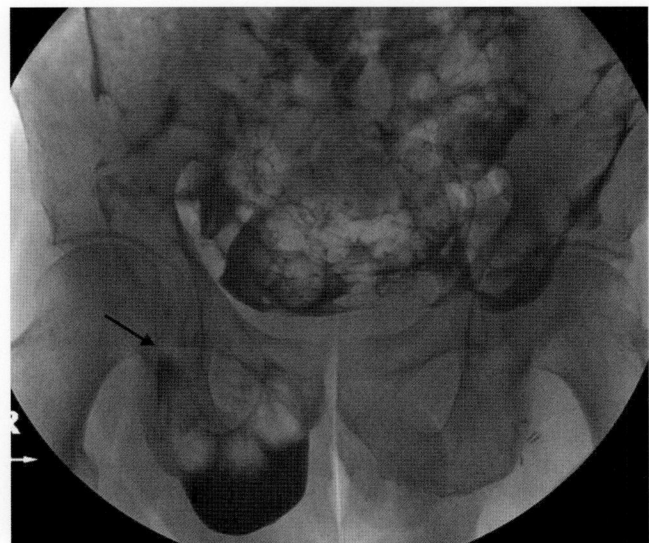

Figure 8.19 Inguinal hernia on herniogram. An indirect right inguinal hernia (arrow) is demonstrated on this frontal image from a herniogram examination.

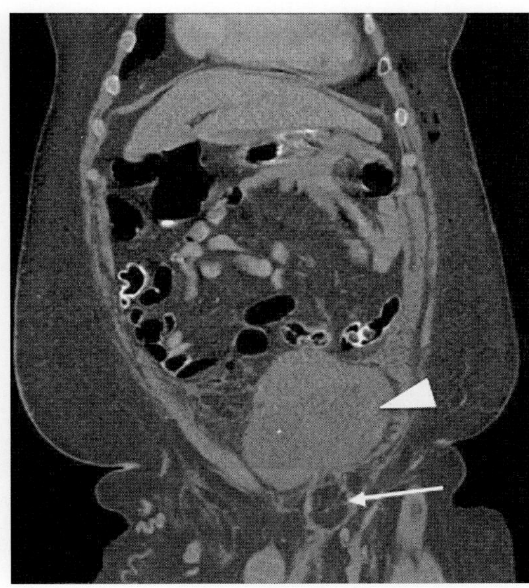

Figure 8.20 Coronal CT image with recurrent left inguinal hernia (arrow) 2 days after attempted repair. An associated postoperative hematoma is seen superiorly (arrowhead).

The European Hernia Society recommends that inguinal hernia repair be performed via the Lichtenstein open approach or total extraperitoneal laparoscopic approach [92]. The results are comparable for both types of repair, but the latter is associated with less postoperative pain and an earlier return to work [93]. Repair of femoral hernias involves emptying and excising the sac before closing the canal by suturing the pectineus fascia to the inguinal ligament. This can also be performed via open (femoral/low incision or Lotheissen/high incision) or extraperitoneal laparoscopic methods. The laparoscopic route is advantageous when it is unclear if the groin hernia is femoral or inguinal preoperatively, or if the patient has more than one hernia. A mesh plug repair is a less commonly performed alternative. This technique is an open repair that employs a mesh plug to close the defect. Proponents of this method claim that it is easier to perform, and requires a smaller incision, with less tissue dissection and fewer sutures. Recurrence rates are relatively high following mesh plug closure of an inguinal hernia but overall results are acceptable in management of a femoral hernia. The majority of authors recommend repair of the posterior wall of the inguinal or reattachment of the rectus muscle [94–96].

All groin hernia repairs can be done under local, spinal, epidural, or general anesthetic, with a single overnight stay or as a day case. Laparoscopic procedures are best performed under general anesthetic. Complications related to repair, such as recurrence, infection, and postoperative collections, occur in up to 20% of patients [74,97] (Figure 8.20).

While conservative management, including rest and antiinflammatory medication, is recommended initially for sportsman's hernia, most athletes report symptom recurrence on return to usual activity levels. Treatment options for this cohort of patients include physical therapy and surgical repair. Surgical exploration may be conducted laparoscopically or open using an anterior approach; a transabdominal preperitoneal approach has gained support [98].

Adult nongroin abdominal wall hernias

Among the most common nongroin hernias are epigastric, umbilical, paraumbilical, hypogastric, incisional, parastomal, Spigelian, and lumbar types. Epigastric, hypogastric, and umbilical/paraumbilical hernias occur in the midline below the xiphisternum and above or adjacent to the umbilicus. Umbilical hernias are the most common nongroin abdominal wall hernia [99].They have a higher association with pregnancy, obesity, and ascites than groin hernias [100]. Omental fat and small bowel typically enter the sac at the umbilicus, which presents as a protuberant mass. Umbilical rupture and bacterial peritonitis are infrequent complications in patients with umbilical hernia and ascites. The risk of strangulation from an umbilical hernia approaches 30%.

Spigelian hernias are uncommon (Figure 8.21), accounting for only 0.1–2% of all ventral hernias [101]. They are typically recognized after the age of 50, and are rarely described in children; when present in pediatric patients, they may point to an associated anomaly, including undescended testes [102,103]. Fat usually fills the sac of epigastric and hypogastric hernias. Epigastric hernias occur between the umbilicus and the xiphoid process.

Lumbar hernias, either primary (acquired) or congenital, consist of two types: superior and inferior. These may arise from one of two triangular defects within the lumbar region [104]. The superior (Grynfeltt–Lesshaft) lumbar triangle transmits

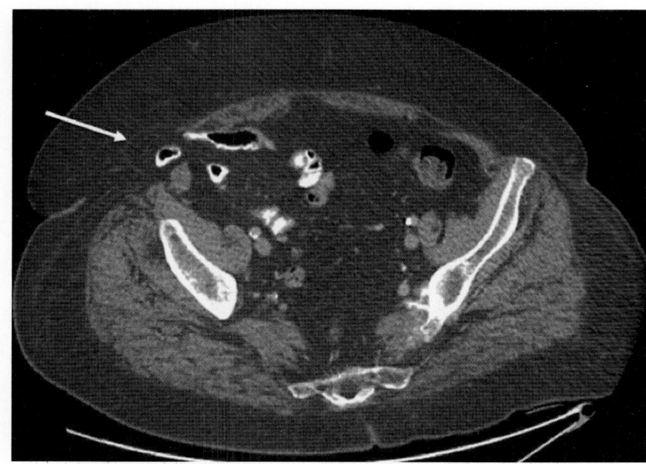

Figure 8.21 Right-sided Spigelian hernia (arrow) demonstrated on an axial CT slice. There is a defect in the anterior abdominal wall adjacent to the semilunar line.

superior lumbar hernias. The 12th rib and the internal oblique and erector spinae muscles form the borders of the superior lumbar triangle. Inferior lumbar hernias pass through a defect in the inferior (Petit) lumbar triangle bounded by the iliac crest inferiorly, the latissimus dorsi medially (posteriorly), and the external oblique muscles laterally (anteriorly). Whilst the majority of lumbar hernias are acquired, up to 20% are congenital [105]. In cases where lumbar hernias extend beyond the margins of the lumbar triangular boundaries delineated above, they are referred to as flank hernias [104].

In cases of severe obesity, the laparoscopic Roux-en-Y gastric bypass (LRGB) has become the favored surgical management option [106]. Internal hernia, resulting in secondary bowel obstruction, is a well-recognized complication of this operation, and a leading cause of late postoperative morbidity. The diagnosis is difficult, requiring a high index of suspicion in patients presenting with abdominal pain, with a history of LRGB; clinical and radiological findings can be of little assistance in diagnosis [107].

Incisional or parastomal hernias occur following 9.9% of laparotomies and 0.7% of laparoscopies [108]. Risk factors for hernia occurrence include a transverse laparotomy incision, use of absorbable sutures for fascial closure [108], large incisions, wound infection, and obesity [109–111]. Deficient collagen and extracellular matrix formation also contribute to defect occurrence [112]. The formation of a colostomy is more likely to result in a hernia than the fashioning of an ileostomy [108].

Clinical assessment of these types of anterior abdominal wall hernias is the same as for other types. The appraisal is difficult in obese patients, and those with small irreducible epigastric or umbilical forms. Differential considerations include intraperitoneal mass, lipoma, soft tissue lesion, divarication (diastasis) of the recti, or, in the case of a periumbilical lesion, a metastatic Sister Joseph nodule. CT is the modality of choice for assessing the extent of ventral abdominal defects and confirming diagnoses. Ultrasound offers a reasonable alternative for detecting small abdominal wall deficiencies and may confirm the constituent contents of the hernia sac.

Surgical repair is recommended for all these nonincisional hernias. Small defects do not require mesh insertion but mesh is almost inevitably required to close larger defects [113]. These repairs can be performed open or laparoscopically, with improved outcomes in terms of postoperative pain, length of stay, and wound infection in favor of laparoscopy [114–116]. The risk of recurrence following epigastric or umbilical hernia repair is approximately 10%; recurrence rates in excess of 20% are observed following incisional hernia repair [117,118].

Adult internal, pelvic, and diaphragmatic hernias

Internal hernias are formed by an abnormal protrusion of a viscus through a normal or abnormal peritoneal or mesenteric orifice, within the peritoneal cavity. Paraduodenal hernias (PDH), also referred to as mesocolic hernias, represent approximately 53% of all internal hernias [119], though fortunately account for less than 1% of all intestinal obstruction cases.

Other types of internal hernia in order of decreasing frequency are pericecal, transmesenteric, foramen of Winslow, supravesical, pelvic, and transomental hernias [120,121]. Internal hernias are difficult to diagnose clinically [122] and imaging is key to diagnosis. Congenital, postoperative, or posttraumatic defects are the most common underlying etiologies. The incidence of internal hernia formation is rising because of the increasing number of minimally invasive abdominal surgeries. CT assessment plays an important role in the investigation of internal hernias. Key CT findings include clusters of dilated small bowel loops in an abnormal location in the setting of bowel obstruction, with a twist in the mesenteric root. In this setting, adhesions remain the most common differential consideration.

Noninternal pelvic hernias are frequently seen in elderly females with acquired pelvic floor weakness. Contents may protrude through the obturator foramen, greater or lesser sciatic foramina, or through the perineum [74]. The former is most common. Similar to other hernia types, precipitants of raised intraabdominal pressure are usually identifiable. However, obturator hernia most commonly occurs in the context of emaciation or cachexia [123]; preperitoneal fat in the obturator canal typically provides support for the neurovascular bundle, preventing herniation.

Obturator hernias are very rare, predominantly affecting thin, elderly female patients. They may occur in conjunction with a femoral hernia, and are often confused with femoral hernias on initial clinical assessment; in cases of diagnostic uncertainty, CT, ultrasound or MRI may be performed for further evaluation.

Diaphragmatic hernia (DH) may be classified as two main types: congenital and acquired (see the section above entitled *Congenital diaphragmatic hernia*). Acquired adult DH is rare, with the majority being posttraumatic in origin [124]. The left hemidiaphragm is most frequently affected. Other causes of adult DH include delayed diagnosis of CDH and iatrogenic DH, an uncommon postoperative complication following abdominal or thoracic surgery [125,126].

Adult Bochdalek DH is rare; the majority of diagnoses are incidental findings, with asymptomatic diaphragmatic defects [127]. In symptomatic cases, patients most commonly present with pulmonary or gastrointestinal symptoms, which may relate to incarcerated bowel, intraabdominal organ dysfunction, or significant pulmonary disease [128–132].

On clinical examination, adult DH may reveal decreased or absent air entry at the involved lung base. Typically the inferior thoracic region is dull to percussion. The diagnosis is often suggested on chest radiograph when the hemidiaphragm appears elevated, bowel loops are seen in the hemithorax, or a nasogastric tube is seen to curl back into the hemithorax. CT and MRI play an important role in both confirming the diagnosis and analyzing the defect size. The main diagnostic differentials are diaphragmatic eventration or paralysis, pleural mass, or pleural effusion. Hiatus hernia is a subtype of DH and is discussed in Chapter 3.

Whilst surgical repair is recommended for the majority of internal, pelvic, and diaphragmatic hernias, asymptomatic and smaller adult Bochdalek DHs do not necessarily require definitive surgical treatment [133]. Internal hernia repair often requires laparotomy but can be safely performed laparoscopically by experienced surgeons. Despite treatment, mortality remains in excess of 50% in some series, particularly when strangulation is present [134,135]. Obturator and other pelvic hernias can be repaired via open or laparoscopic routes, with the min imally invasive method possibly having a decreased complication rate [136,137].

Diaphragmatic hernia repair can be performed through transabdominal or transthoracic routes using open or minimally invasive approaches; thoracoscopy may be preferential when treating hernias with associated significant pleural fibrosis and adhesions [138]. The aim of repair is primary closure [139]; in cases where this is not possible with nonabsorbable sutures, mesh repair provides an alternative option [140].

Conclusions

Knowledge of the normal embryology and anatomy of the abdominal cavity related to the peritoneum (ligamental, omental, and mesenteric) and abdominal margins is key to understanding the pathological processes of the abdominal wall. These include disorders of bowel rotation, pediatric or adult hernia formation, and intraabdominal disease spread. Acquired adult abdominal hernias are common. Each hernia is composed of a hernia sac, neck, and contents. Symptoms and complications are determined by hernia morphology and location, which in turn determine their natural history and treatment.

References are available at www.yamadagastro.com/textbook7e

Further reading

Aguirre D.A., Santosa A.C., Casola G., et al. Abdominal wall hernias: imaging features, complications, and diagnostic pitfalls at multidetector row CT. Radiographics 2005;25:1501.

Chiu P.P., Langer J.C. Surgical conditions of the diaphragm: posterior diaphragmatic hernias in infants. Thorac Surg Clin 2009;19:451.

Diesen D.L., Pappas T.N. Sports hernias. Adv Surg 2007;41:177.

Doyle N.M., Lally K.P. The CDH Study Group and advances in the clinical care of the patient with congenital diaphragmatic hernia. Semin Perinatol 2004;28:174.

Martin L.C., Merkle E.M., Thompson W.M. Review of internal hernias: radiographic and clinical findings. Am J Roentgenol 2006;186:703.

Nehra D., Goldstein A.M. Intestinal malrotation: varied clinical presentation from infancy through adulthood. Surgery 2011;149:386.

Pickhardt P.J., Bhalla S. Intestinal malrotation in adolescents and adults: spectrum of clinical and imaging features. Am J Roentgenol 2002;179:1429.

Simons M.P., Aufenacker T., Bay-Nielsen M., et al. European Hernia Society guidelines on the treatment of inguinal hernia in adult patients. Hernia 2009;13:343.

Slater N.J., van der Kolk M., Hendriks T., et al. Biologic grafts for ventral hernia repair: a systematic review. Am J Surg 2013;205:220.

Yiee J.H., Garcia N., Baker L.A., et al. A diagnostic algorithm for urachal anomalies. J Pediatr Urol 2007;3:500.

CHAPTER 9
Gallbladder and biliary tract: anatomy and structural anomalies

Theodore H. Welling
NYU Langone Health, New York, USA

Chapter menu

The extrahepatic biliary tract has a great number of variations, with a wide range of these variations also seen in the vasculature surrounding the extrahepatic biliary tree. Increasing use of diagnostic and interventional radiology as well as therapeutic endoscopy has made it essential for a wide variety of physicians to become familiar with the anatomy of the extrahepatic biliary tract. This review of anatomy and anomalies of the extrahepatic bilary tree will assist surgeons, gastroenterologists, and radiologists in understanding and recognizing the variations they may encounter.

Embryological development

The biliary tract develops from the primitive gastrointestinal tract, in the distal foregut, as a ventral sacculation; it is first apparent at week 5 of gestation when the embryo is 3 mm long (Figure 9.1a). This sacculation grows and extends into the ventral mesentery, dividing into two buds: the cranial bud develops into the liver and intrahepatic bile ducts and the caudal bud develops into the gallbladder and cystic duct (Figure 9.1b). The base of the diverticulum ultimately becomes the common bile duct. Another small bud develops from the proximal aspect of the caudal bud and grows inferiorly, ultimately developing into the ventral pancreas (see Figure 9.1a,b).

The cranial bud divides into two smaller buds that grow upward toward the septum transversum (future diaphragm). These eventually become the right and left lobes of the liver. The caudal bud is carried superiorly by the growth of the cranial bud and stops at the undersurface of the cranial bud to become the gallbladder and cystic duct (Figure 9.1c). Rarely, continued advancement of the caudal bud too far superiorly will result in an intrahepatic gallbladder, which is almost always embedded within the right lobe of the liver.

As the cranial and caudal buds are advancing, the ventral pancreatic bud rotates 180° from right to left, allowing it to fuse with the dorsal pancreatic bud to form the complete pancreas. Fusion of the two parts of the pancreas occurs during week 7 of gestation. Because the lower end of the common bile duct is attached to the ventral pancreatic bud, the rotation results in fusion of the junction of the common bile duct and the duodenum on the posteromedial duodenal wall, posterior to the dorsal pancreatic duct (Figure 9.1d).

The ventral sacculation from which the biliary tract arises is originally composed of a solid cord of endodermal cells and contains no lumen. Beginning at week 7 of gestation, vacuolization begins to occur and a completely open lumen is formed in the gallbladder, cystic duct, hepatic ducts, and common bile duct within 1 week. By the third month of gestation, bile flow is demonstrable through the canalized biliary tract into the duodenum [1].

Yamada's Textbook of Gastroenterology, Seventh Edition. Edited by Timothy C. Wang, Michael Camilleri, Benjamin Lebwohl, Anna S. Lok, William J. Sandborn, Kenneth K. Wang, and Gary D. Wu.

Companion website: www.yamadagastro.com/textbook7e

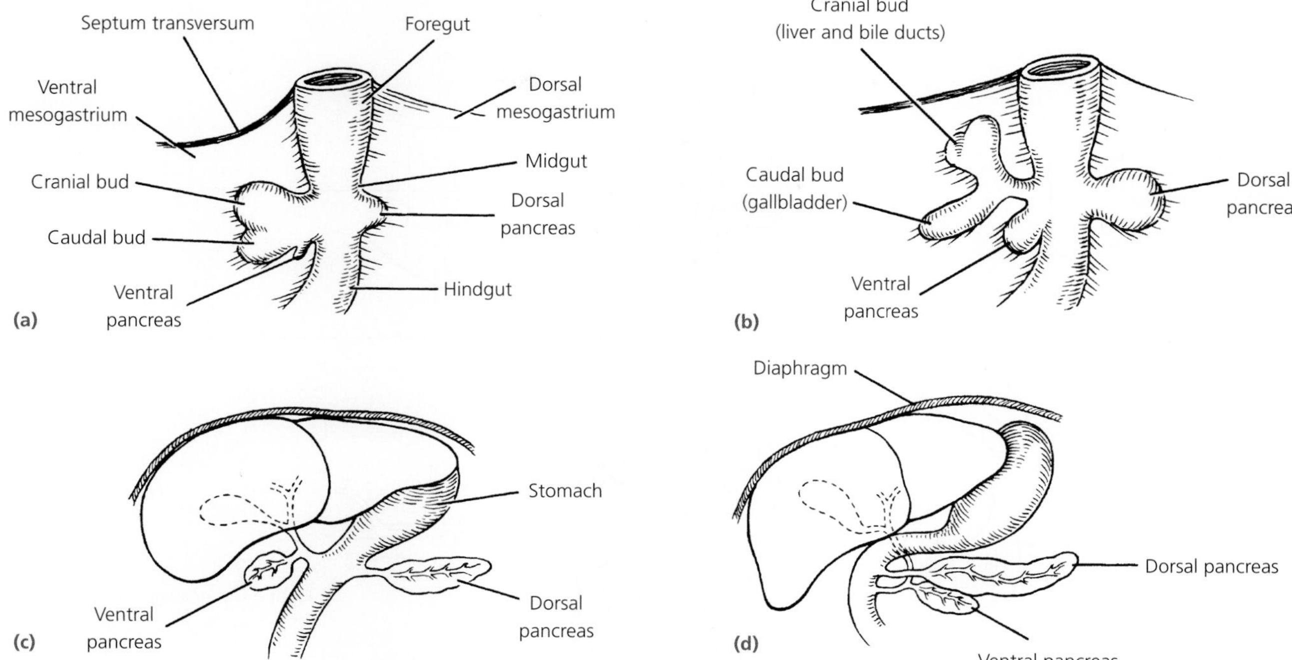

Figure 9.1 Embryology of the developing biliary tract. (a) At the 3 mm stage of the embryo, the ventral bud enters the mesogastrium and soon divides into a cranial and a caudal bud. A smaller caudad bud represents the origin of the ventral pancreas. (b) As the embryo reaches 5 mm, the cranial bud, which will form the liver and intrahepatic biliary tract, moves toward the septum transversum, pulling the caudal bud, which will form the gallbladder and extrahepatic bile ducts. (c) When the embryo reaches 7 mm, the right and left lobes of the liver occupy the position under the septum transversum. The ventral pancreas and the extrahepatic biliary tract are visible. As the ventral pancreas rotates to reach the dorsal pancreas, it pulls the lower end of the common bile duct with it. (d) At the 12 mm embryonic stage, the ventral pancreas has rotated, and the anatomic relations between the bile ducts and the gastrointestinal tract have assumed their mature forms.

Anatomy of the gallbladder

Gross anatomy

The gallbladder is a pear-shaped sac located along the inferior surface of the liver in the line of division of the anatomical left and right lobes; it lies in a depression known as the gallbladder fossa (Figure 9.2). The adult gland is typically 7–10 cm in length and has an average capacity of 30 mL. The gallbladder is intimately attached to the liver by loose connective tissue, which contains small veins and lymphatics that connect between the gallbladder and liver. Occasionally, one or more small accessory ducts from the liver traverse this connective tissue to enter the gallbladder directly. Inadequate ligation of an accessory duct may account for the occasional bile leak that occurs after cholecystectomy.

The remainder of the gallbladder not in direct contact with liver is covered by peritoneum reflected from the liver. The gallbladder is divided into four anatomical areas: fundus, body, infundibulum, and neck. The fundus is the rounded end of the gallbladder that normally extends 0.5–1 cm beyond the liver margin and is covered with peritoneum. The fundus rests on the duodenum and hepatic flexure of the colon (see Figure 9.2) and is in direct contact with the anterior abdominal wall, usually near the lateral border of the right rectus abdominis muscle at approximately the level of the ninth costal cartilage; however, its position may vary. The fundus may occasionally possess a kink, known as a phrygian cap deformity, which has no pathological significance.

The fundus merges imperceptibly into the body, which is the largest part of the gallbladder and the segment that is closely attached to the liver on one side. This intimate contact is responsible for early direct spread of gallbladder carcinoma into the liver. The infundibulum represents a transitional region between the body and neck. It is notable because occasionally a shallow diverticulum may be present on the inferior surface of the infundibulum, referred to as a Hartmann pouch. Gallstones may become impacted within the Hartmann pouch, causing cystic duct obstruction and thus acute cholecystitis.

The neck is a short (usually 5–7 mm) region that tapers into the cystic duct. The neck occupies the deepest part of the gallbladder fossa and lies in the free border of the hepatoduodenal ligament.

Arterial blood supply

The blood supply to the gallbladder is usually from a single cystic artery that arises from the right hepatic artery, traverses the triangle of Calot, and divides into two branches close to the gallbladder wall [2] (Figure 9.3a). One branch runs along the peritoneal surface of the gallbladder and the other branch in the gallbladder fossa between the gallbladder and liver. When the cystic artery arises from the right hepatic artery, its course is often parallel and medial to the cystic duct. Double or accessory cystic arteries have been reported in up to 20% of people. Variations in the site of origin and course of the cystic artery are common. The cystic artery typically arises from the right hepatic artery (95%), but also

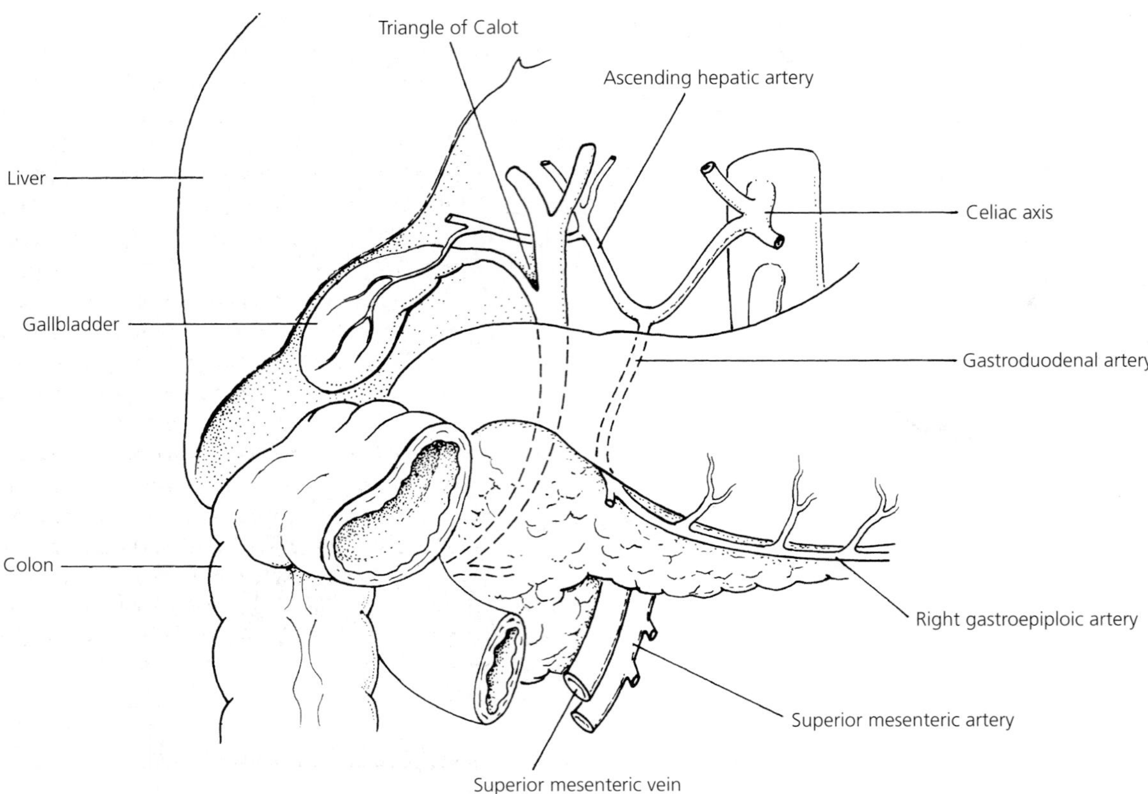

Figure 9.2 Relation of the gallbladder and the extrahepatic biliary tract to the liver, duodenum, colon, and pancreas.

may arise from the left hepatic artery, the common hepatic artery, an aberrant right hepatic artery that arises from the superior mesenteric artery, the gastroduodenal artery, the superior mesenteric artery, or celiac axis directly (see Figure 9.3). The cystic artery may be short or long, and may either pass behind the hepatic duct (84%) or cross the hepatic duct anteriorly.

The cystic artery, when it originates from the right hepatic artery, may closely parallel the right hepatic artery for a distance before reaching the gallbladder. In 5–10% of cases, the cystic artery does not arise from the right hepatic artery until just before it enters the right lobe of the liver, thus creating a very short (only a few millimeters) cystic artery. Failure to recognize this may lead to inadvertent ligation of the right hepatic artery during cholecystectomy.

Venous and lymphatic drainage

The gallbladder lacks a major cystic vein but rather drains through a network of small veins. These veins run either from the hepatic surface of the gallbladder directly to the liver or toward the cystic duct and join venous collaterals from the common bile duct before ultimately draining into the portal vein.

The lymphatic drainage of the gallbladder parallels the venous drainage pattern. Lymph flows directly from the gallbladder to the liver or may drain toward the cystic duct into a single node or group of nodes. From these lymph nodes, lymph may ultimately drain into several nodes along the surface of the portal vein and common bile duct.

Nerve supply

The gallbladder is innervated by branches of both the sympathetic and parasympathetic nervous systems, which pass through the celiac plexus. Preganglionic sympathetic nerves arise from the T8 and T9 levels. Postganglionic sympathetic nerves originate at the celiac plexus and travel along the hepatic artery and portal vein to the gallbladder. Parasympathetic nerves arise from branches of the vagal trunks. Unlike the branches of the posterior vagal trunk that pass through the celiac plexus, branches of the anterior vagal trunk reach the gallbladder by way of the gastrohepatic ligament (Figure 9.4). Visceral pain caused by gallbladder wall distension or inflammation is conducted through afferent sympathetic fibers and referred to the epigastric, right subcostal, or right scapular regions. The nerve supply to the common bile duct is the same as for the gallbladder.

Although gallbladder contractility is primarily mediated by cholecystokinin (CCK), innervation of the gallbladder also modulates gallbladder contractility. Vagal activity contributes to normal gallbladder tone and enhances the ability of subthreshold doses of CCK to promote gallbladder mobility [3]. Sympathetic fibers enhance gallbladder relaxation. In addition to the classic parasympathetic and sympathetic nervous systems, a large number of peptide-containing neurons exist within the gallbladder. The peptides identified thus far by immunocytochemical techniques include CCK [4], vasoactive intestinal polypeptide [4], gastrin-releasing peptide [5], neuropeptide

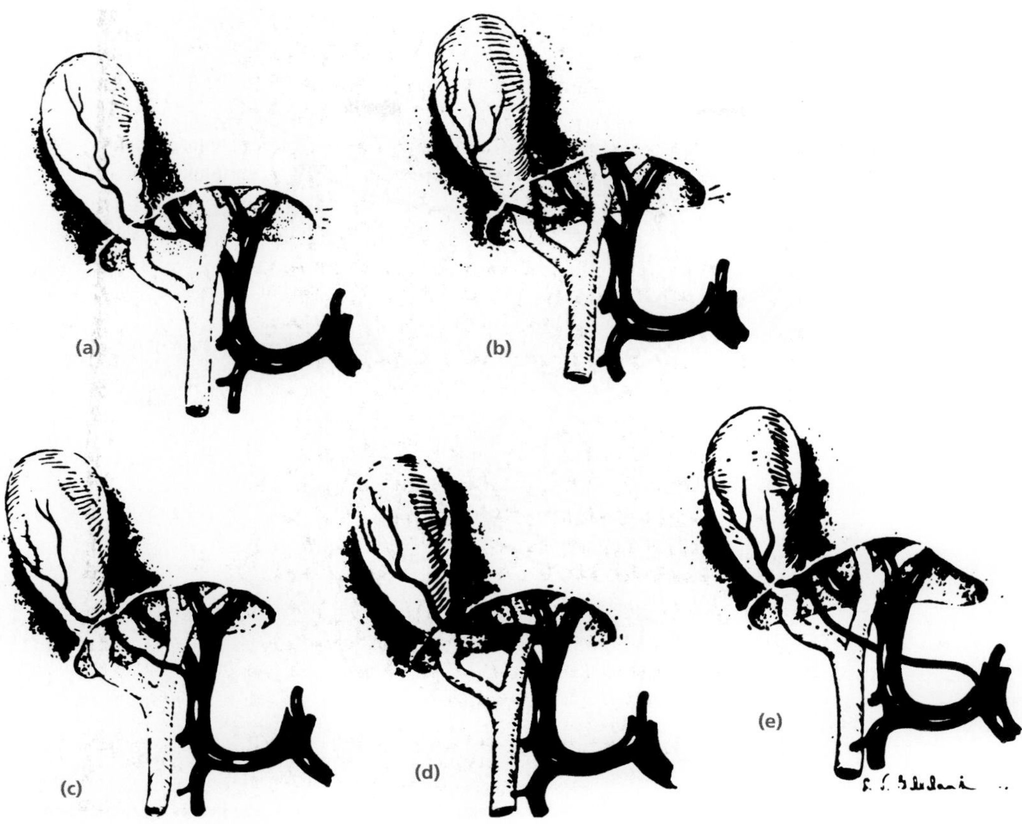

Figure 9.3 Common variations in the origin of the cystic artery. **(a)** It originates most commonly from the right hepatic artery; it traverses the triangle of Calot, and, upon reaching the gallbladder, it divides into two main branches. **(b)** Occasionally the two branches come off the right hepatic artery independently. The cystic artery may cross the hepatic duct anteriorly **(c)**, come off the left hepatic artery **(d)**, or, more rarely, come directly from the celiac axis **(e)**. Source: Lindner H. Embryology and anatomy of the biliary tree. In: Way LW, Pellegrini CA (eds). Surgery of the Gallbladder and Bile Ducts. Philadelphia: WB Saunders; 1987. Reproduced with permisison of Elsevier.

Y [6], pituitary adenylate cyclase-activating polypeptide (PACAP) [7], calcitonin gene-related peptide (CGRP) [7], and substance P [7]. The physiologcial functions of these peptidergic nerves within the gallbladder remain to be elucidated.

Histology and ultrastructure

The gallbladder has five layers: epithelium, lamina propria, muscularis, perimuscular connective tissue layer, and serosa. The mucosa, lined with a simple columnar epithelium, consists of many folds that increase the efficiency of the gallbladder in concentrating bile. The apical surface of the epithelium is covered with abundant microvilli. The basal surface of the epithelium is in contact with the lamina propria, which is rich in loose connective tissue, elastic fibers, blood vessels, and lymphatics. The muscularis is an arrangement of circular, longitudinal, and oblique fibers without any well-developed layers. Ganglia may be found between the muscle fibers of the muscularis. The subserosa contains loosely arranged collagen and elastic fibers, as well as larger blood vessels and lymphatics. This thick subserosal layer attaches the gallbladder to the liver. Dissection during cholecystectomy usually takes place between the subserosa and serosa, which in normal circumstances is an avascular plane. The serosa is absent on the surface of the gallbladder that is in direct contact with the liver. Mucus is secreted into the gallbladder from tubular alveolar glands found in the mucosa lining the infundibulum and neck of the gallbladder.

At the ultrastructural level, the gallbladder epithelium is well suited for its physiological role of concentrating bile. The columnar epithelial cells have basally located nuclei and apices covered with numerous microvilli that protrude into the gallbladder lumen. Numerous mitochondria are present within the epithelial cells, which facilitate the active process of bile concentration. Epithelial cells are joined together along their lateral membranes by tight junctions, which separate the gallbladder lumen from the intercellular spaces. During active bile concentration, the intercellular spaces become distended with water and electrolytes. Water extracted during this process passes into a rich capillary network in the lamina propria.

Anatomy of the extrahepatic biliary ducts

Hepatic ducts

The common hepatic duct is formed by the union of the right and left hepatic ducts. In 95% of cases, this union takes place

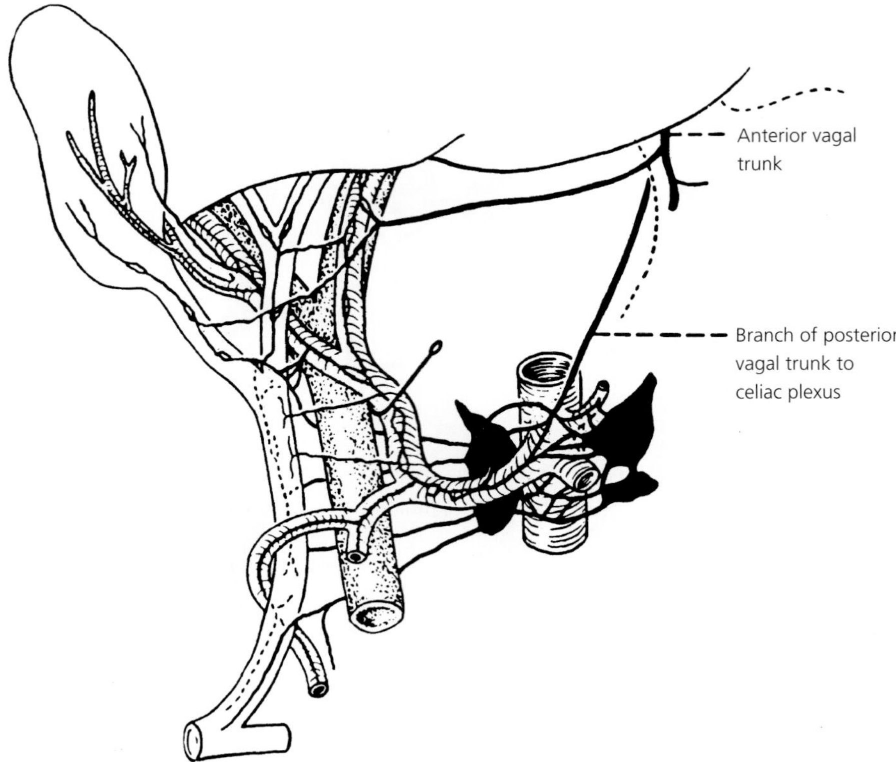

Figure 9.4 Schematic representation of the innervation of the gallbladder and extrahepatic biliary tract. The nerves originate from both vagi and from the celiac axis. They reach the biliary tract, traveling along the walls of the hepatic artery, except for the direct vagal branches of the anterior vagus, which cross through the gastrohepatic ligament.

outside the liver, just below the level of the porta hepatis. In 5% of cases, the left and right hepatic ducts join within the substance of the liver. The right and left hepatic ducts vary from 0.5 to 2.5 cm in length, with the left hepatic duct usually longer than the right. The ducts may join at a wide or acute angle, depending on their extrahepatic length; however, they usually join about 1 cm below the porta hepatis to form the common hepatic duct. The confluence of the right and left hepatic ducts lies anterior to the portal venous bifurcation, usually overlying the origin of the right branch of the portal vein. An accessory right hepatic duct is present in 10% of people.

Anatomical variations of the hepatic duct confluence most commonly involve the right hepatic duct with the right anterior and right posterior branches often taking a variable course. The right anterior and posterior branches join to form a common right hepatic duct 60–65% of the time whereas the right anterior and posterior duct branches join at the confluence approximately 12% of the time. About 20% of the time, the right anterior duct will join separately onto the common hepatic duct with the right posterior and left hepatic duct joining first to form the common hepatic duct. The common hepatic duct passes downward in the superior portion of the hepatoduodenal ligament and lies anterior to the portal vein and to the right of the hepatic artery (Figure 9.5). In cases when the cystic duct inserts on the right hepatic duct or at the junction of the union of the right and left hepatic ducts, there is no common hepatic duct. The length of the common hepatic duct varies from 2 to 6.5 cm. It joins the cystic duct to form the common bile duct.

The course of the right hepatic artery is variable in relation to the right hepatic duct and common hepatic duct. Usually, the right hepatic artery passes posterior to the common hepatic duct near the junction of the right and left hepatic ducts (64%). In 24% of people, the right hepatic artery or the cystic artery may pass anterior to the common hepatic duct. In the remaining patients (12%), the right hepatic artery arises from the superior mesenteric artery and runs parallel and to the right of the common bile duct and posterior to the cystic duct. Because of the inconstant location of the right hepatic artery and its close proximity to the cystic artery, the right hepatic artery may be mistaken for the cystic artery and is particularly vulnerable to injury during biliary tract surgery.

The triangle of Calot, originally described in 1891, is bounded superiorly by the hilum of the liver, on the right by the cystic duct, and on the left by the common hepatic duct [8] (see Figure 9.5). Dissection of the triangle of Calot during cholecystectomy must be carried out with care because many important structures run through this triangle: the right hepatic artery, the cystic artery, 90% of accessory hepatic ducts, and 95% of aberrant right hepatic arteries. In cases when there is a replaced right hepatic artery originating from the superior mesenteric artery, the vessel travels toward the liver in a position posterolateral to the common bile duct and just behind the cystic duct. Here it is vulnerable to injury. Complete dissection of the triangle of Calot, with separation of the neck of the gallbladder from the liver bed, allowing identification of the only two structures that should be emanating from the gallbladder, the cystic duct and cystic artery, is critical to avoid injury during cholecystectomy.

Cystic duct

The cystic duct arises from the neck of the gallbladder and joins the common hepatic duct. Its lumen usually measures 1–3 mm but it may occasionally be as large as 10 mm, allowing larger gallstones to enter the common bile duct. While the cystic duct typically joins the common hepatic duct directly (70%), the site of the cystic duct junction with the extrahepatic biliary tree may vary from the right hepatic duct down to the level of the ampulla (Figures 9.6 and 9.7). Thus the length of the cystic duct may vary from 0.5 to 8 cm. The cystic duct may join the right hepatic duct, may run parallel to the common hepatic duct for a distance with connective tissue ensheathing both ducts, and, in some instances, may not enter the common hepatic duct until passing behind the duodenum. Additionally, the cystic duct may spiral around the common hepatic duct, passing either dorsal or ventral to the common hepatic duct before joining it. These anatomic variations may lead to bile duct injury during cholecystectomy, especially if dissection is carried out to clearly define the union of the cystic duct and common bile duct, a practice that is unnecessary during cholecystectomy.

Within the cystic duct, the mucosa forms a series of 5–10 crescent-shaped folds, known as the spiral valves of Heister. They span the length of the cystic duct and project into the cystic duct lumen. These valves serve to prevent excessive distension or collapse of the gallbladder with changes in cystic duct pressure and may function to block passage of gallstones into the common bile duct. They may make catheterization during intraoperative cholangiogram difficult.

Common bile duct

Union of the cystic duct and common hepatic duct forms the common bile duct. Its length is approximately 7.5 cm, but can vary depending on the relative lengths of the cystic and common hepatic ducts. The mean diameter of the common bile duct is about 6 mm, but it may dilate significantly in the face of distal obstruction. The common bile duct is divided into four anatomic segments: supraduodenal, retroduodenal, pancreatic, and intraduodenal. The supraduodenal segment is usually 2.5 cm in length and is located in the right border of the hepatoduodenal ligament. It lies anterior to the portal vein and to the right of the ascending common hepatic artery. This anatomic relationship allows the surgeon to compress these three

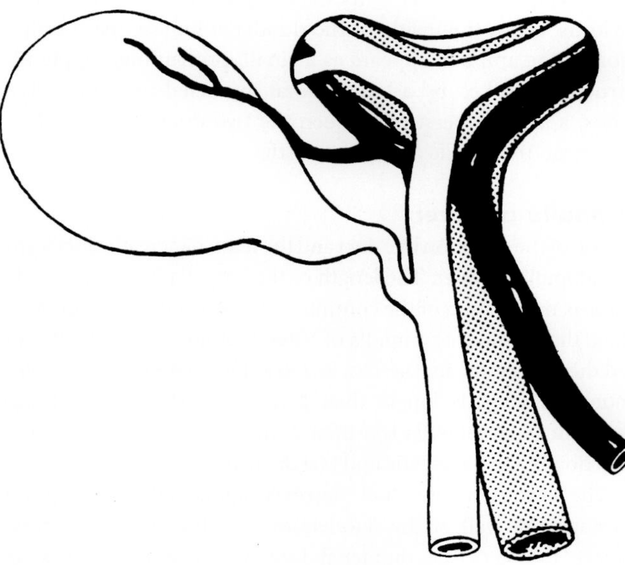

Figure 9.5 Schematic representation of the hilum of the liver. The right anterior and posterior hepatic ducts join to form the right hepatic duct. This duct and the left duct join outside the liver capsule to form the common hepatic duct. The left duct is usually longer and more superficial than the right. The triangle of Calot, with the right hepatic artery and the cystic artery, is also clearly displayed. Source: Lindner H. Embryology and anatomy of the biliary tree. In: Way LW, Pellegrini CA, eds. Surgery of the gallbladder and bile ducts. Philadelphia: WB Saunders, 1987. Reproduced with permission of Elsevier.

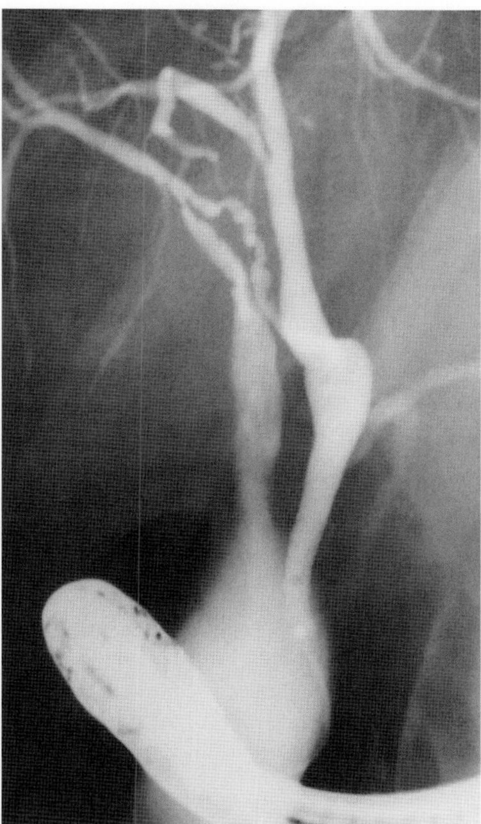

Figure 9.6 Endoscopic retrograde cholangiopancreatogram demonstrating an anomalous junction of the cystic duct with an accessory right hepatic duct.

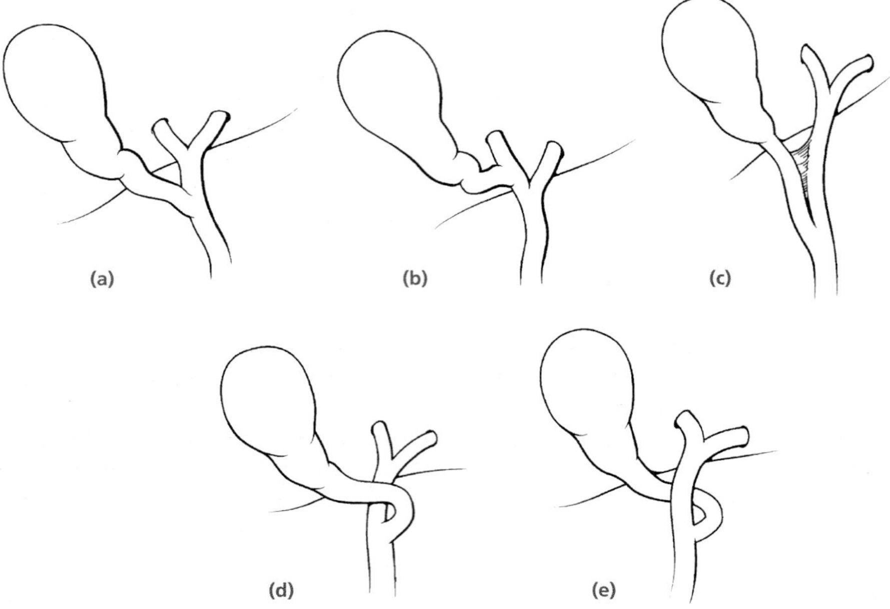

Figure 9.7 Variations in cystic duct anatomy. **(a)** Cystic duct joins common hepatic duct directly (most common). **(b)** Cystic duct joins the right hepatic duct. **(c)** Low junction of cystic duct with common hepatic duct. **(d)** Anterior spiral of cystic duct before joining common hepatic duct. **(e)** Posterior spiral of cystic duct before joining common hepatic duct.

structures between an index finger inserted through the foramen of Winslow into the lesser sac and a thumb placed anteriorly across the hepatoduodenal ligament. This maneuver is referred to as the Pringle maneuver and allows rapid occlusion of the blood supply to the liver, which is useful for controlling major liver hemorrhage.

The retroduodenal segment lies posterior to the first part of the duodenum and is about 2.5–4 cm long. As it runs to the inferior surface of the duodenum, it moves right to left, lying just to the right of the gastroduodenal artery. The retroduodenal common bile duct is loosely attached to the duodenum by a thin layer of areolar tissue. Because of the close relationship of this portion of the common bile duct and the duodenal bulb, it may occasionally be involved in the inflammatory process of a posterior penetrating duodenal ulcer and may be inadvertently injured during antrectomy.

The pancreatic segment of the common bile duct extends from the lower border of the first part of the duodenum to the posteromedial wall of the second portion of the duodenum where the duct penetrates the duodenal wall. It may be entirely retropancreatic or it may lie within the substance of the head of the pancreas. Obstruction of this segment of the common bile duct is common with cancers of the pancreatic head, which often initially present with painless jaundice.

The common bile duct then turns 90° to the right to enter the posteromedial wall of the descending duodenum. The final, or intraduodenal, segment of the common bile duct is about 2 cm long and travels obliquely through the duodenal wall with the main pancreatic duct. The common bile duct may join the main pancreatic duct outside the duodenum, or the ducts may form a common channel as they traverse through the duodenal wall, in both of these cases opening through a single ostium on the major ampulla of Vater. This site is typically 7–10 cm from the pylorus. From the inside of the duodenal lumen, the termination of the ampulla appears as a small, protruding, nipple-like structure marked by a longitudinal duodenal fold. In 29% of cases, a septum persists between the two ducts, and the ducts empty on the papilla as separate ostia.

Ampulla of Vater

Union of the common bile duct and the main pancreatic duct forms the ampulla of Vater. The length of the ampulla is variable, and if there is no junction of the common bile duct and main pancreatic duct, there is no true ampulla of Vater. Rienhoff and Pickrell studied the pancreatic duct system in 250 autopsy specimens [9]. They found an ampulla longer than 2 mm in 46% of cases (range 3–14 mm), an ampulla less than 2 mm in 32% of cases, and no junction of the pancreatic and bile ducts in 29% of cases.

The common bile duct narrows significantly as it passes through the wall of the duodenum, and the ampulla narrows before it enters the duodenal lumen. These narrowings are frequent sites for stones to lodge and cause either biliary or pancreatic obstruction. Additionally, these are potential sites of injury when instrumented during common bile duct exploration.

Sphincter of Oddi

The intraduodenal segment of the common bile duct and the ampulla is surrounded by a sheath of smooth muscle fibers referred to collectively as the sphincter of Oddi. The sphincter of Oddi is a unique group of muscle fibers that arise from the bile duct wall and manometric studies have verified that the sphincter acts independently of the duodenal musculature. The resting pressure of the sphincter of Oddi is approximately 13 mmHg above duodenal pressure [10]. Regulation of bile flow is primarily controlled by the sphincter of Oddi. Relaxation of the sphincter occurs with CCK stimulation and is facilitated by parasympathetic stimulation. Sympathetic stimulation causes increased sphincter tone.

The preampullary portion of the common bile duct is invested in a sheath of circular muscle referred to as the sphincter choledochus (sphincter of Boyden) (Figure 9.8). The distal main pancreatic duct may have a short sphincter called the sphincter pancreaticus. If present, the sphincter pancreaticus and sphincter choledochus may intertwine in a figure-of-eight manner. The smooth muscle sheath surrounding the ampulla is called the sphincter of the ampulla; if there is no ampulla, the distal sphincter is simply called the sphincter of the papilla. During endoscopic sphincterotomy, the sphincter of Oddi is divided using electrocautery to relieve common bile duct obstruction from a common duct stone.

Arterial blood supply

The arterial blood supply to the extrahepatic bile ducts is segmental. Because of the segmental nature of the blood supply, extensive mobilization of the extrahepatic bile ducts may lead to ischemic injury and development of postoperative biliary stricture and thus should be avoided [11]. The hepatic ducts and the supraduodenal portion of the common bile duct are nourished by small arterial branches from the cystic artery (Figure 9.9). The retroduodenal portion of the common bile duct is supplied by branches of the retroduodenal and posterior superior pancreaticoduodenal arteries. The pancreatic and intraduodenal segments of the common bile duct are supplied by both the anterior and posterior superior pancreaticoduodenal arteries.

Venous and lymphatic drainage

The veins of the hepatic ducts and proximal common bile duct, like those from the gallbladder and cystic duct, enter the liver directly. Veins from the lower portion of the common bile duct drain into the portal vein. The lymphatic drainage from the hepatic ducts and upper common bile duct flows superiorly

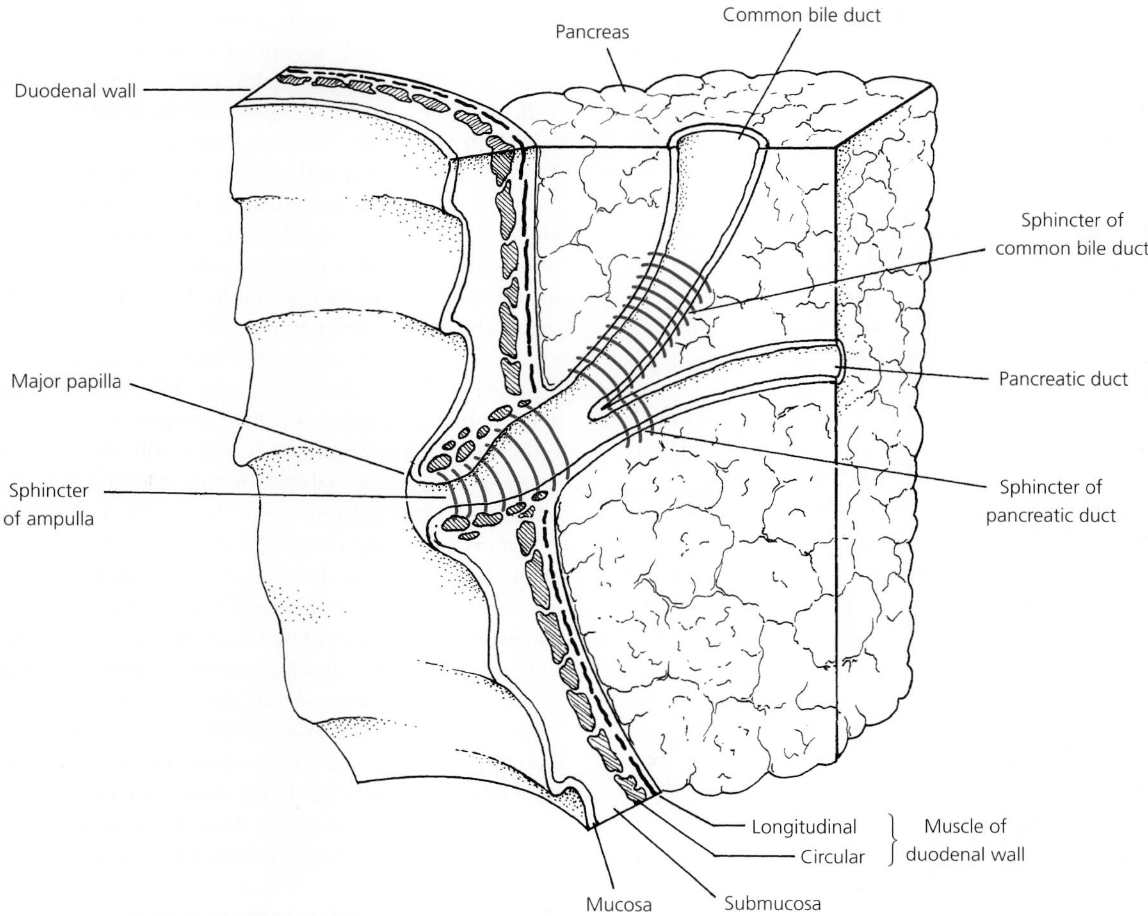

Figure 9.8 The muscular apparatus at the terminal end of the common bile duct. The bile duct is closely associated with the pancreatic duct, and they both enter the medial wall of the duodenum tangentially. Each duct has its own sphincter, which is poorly developed in the pancreatic duct.

along the course of the common bile duct to lymph nodes in the porta hepatis. Some lymphatic drainage arising from the inferior portion of the common bile duct may reach the deep pancreatic nodes near the origin of the superior mesenteric artery. All lymphatic drainage ultimately reaches the celiac lymph nodes.

Histology and ultrastructure

The mucosa of the extrahepatic bile ducts contains columnar epithelium surrounded by a layer of connective tissue. The epithelium contains many mucous glands. Muscle fibers in the hepatic ducts and proximal common bile duct are relatively few and discontinuous, and may be arranged in either a longitudinal or circular direction. As the common bile duct approaches the duodenum, it begins to develop a more substantial muscle layer, which merges into the sphincter of Oddi complex, where distinct bundles of muscle fibers are evident.

Congenital variations and malformations

Gallbladder and cystic duct

Congenital anomalies of the gallbladder may be classified into three different categories: anomalies of number, anomalies of form, and anomalies of position. Duplication of the gallbladder is thought to occur in approximately one of every 4000 human

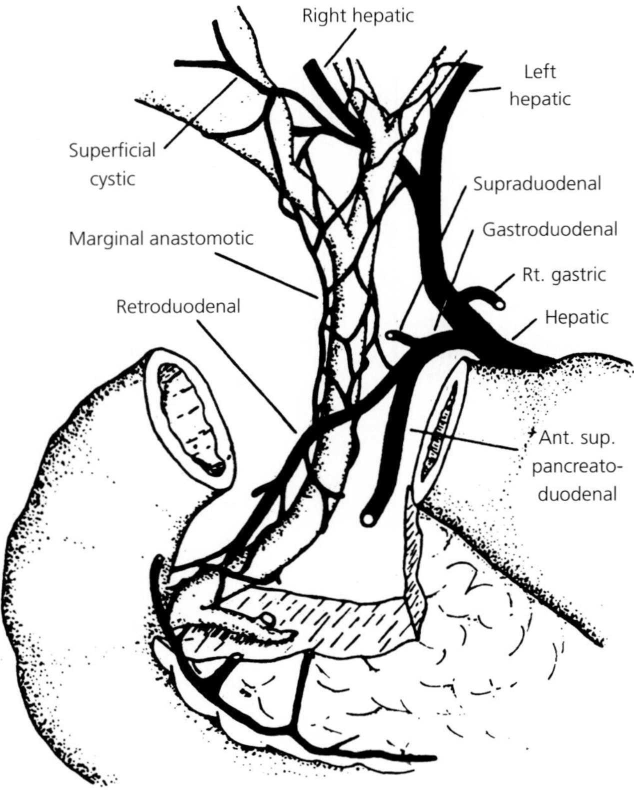

Figure 9.9 The extrahepatic biliary tract is supplied by a rich vascular net of vessels from the hepatic and gastroduodenal arteries. The relationship between the hepatic arteries and the extrahepatic biliary tree is evident.

gallbladders [12]. With complete duplication, the gallbladders are separate, and the cystic ducts may join one another before entering the common duct or each cystic duct may enter separately. Partial duplications can result in bilobed gallbladders (Figure 9.10a), in which the two gallbladder cavities are separate at the fundus but joined at the neck and drain via a common cystic duct. Gallbladders may also be septate (divided by a partial or complete septum) with septa present in either a longitudinal or transverse direction, the latter referred to as an hourglass gallbladder (Figure 9.10b). Septate gallbladders are thought to be a result of incomplete vacuolization of the solid endodermal cord during development. None of these abnormalities of the gallbladder by themselves have clinical significance unless they are involved in a pathological process.

Lack of development of the gallbladder bud results in agenesis of the gallbladder. Most cases are associated with extrahepatic biliary atresia [13]. In the absence of associated biliary atresia, an intrahepatic gallbladder or left-sided gallbladder must be ruled out before the diagnosis is made.

Abnormal migration of the caudal bud (future gallbladder and cystic duct) of the ventral diverticulum during development may cause an anomalous gallbladder position. If the caudal bud advances beyond the cranial bud (future liver), it may become buried in the liver substance, creating an intrahepatic gallbladder. These are usually identified by ultrasonography prior to cholecystectomy and may make cholecystectomy slightly more difficult. If the caudal bud lags behind the cranial bud, a floating gallbladder is created. A floating gallbladder is a gallbladder that is completely covered with peritoneum; it is usually suspended from the liver by a mesentery. A floating gallbladder is at a higher risk for torsion. Left-sided gallbladders are rare, but they have been described in the setting of situs inversus (all abdominal viscera are reversed right for left) or in the setting in which the gallbladder alone is transposed [12]. The gallbladder has also been found in other unusual locations such as the falciform ligament [14], the abdominal wall [15], and the retroperitoneum [16]. Regardless of the anomalous position of the gallbladder, it is important to realize that in almost all cases, the cystic duct will inevitably join the common bile duct in a relatively normal position.

Abnormal development of the gallbladder bud may also cause anomalies in the cystic duct. Double cystic ducts may drain a single, nonseptated gallbladder and join the biliary system at the common bile duct or right hepatic duct. There may be absence of the cystic duct, and, in this case, the neck of the gallbladder drains directly into the common bile duct. Failure to recognize this anomaly has resulted in excision of a segment of the common bile duct during cholecystectomy in which the common bile duct has been mistakenly identified as the cystic duct. Liberal use of intraoperative cholangiography has been emphasized when intraoperative anatomy is confusing or anomalies are present.

Hepatic ducts and common bile duct

True accessory hepatic ducts result from the development of an extra bud from the biliary anlage during development. Accessory ducts are much more common on the right than the left. They

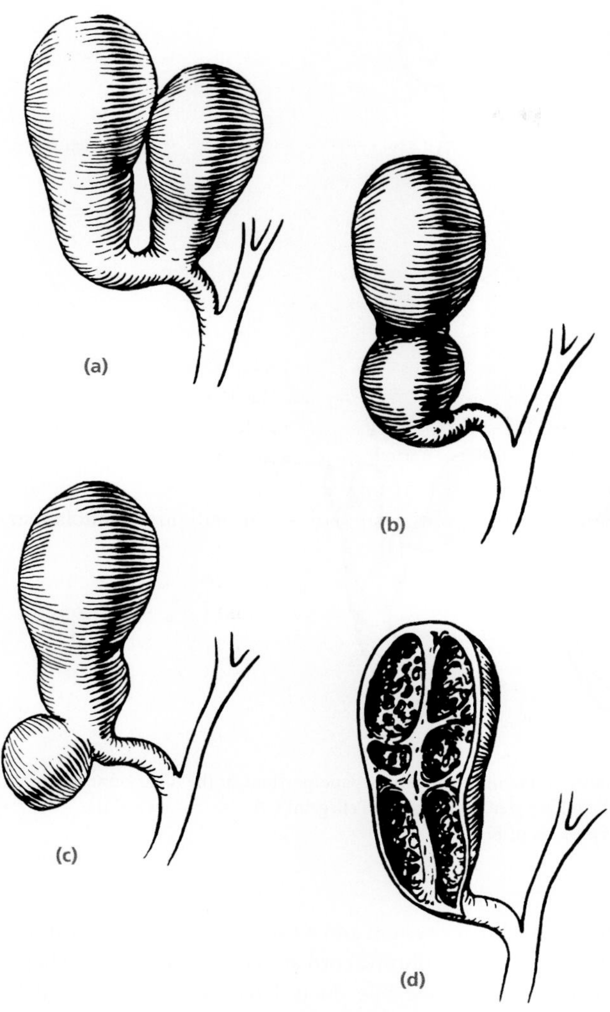

Figure 9.10 Two gallbladders **(a)**, a bilobed gallbladder **(b)**, a diverticulum at the neck **(c)**, and a septated gallbladder **(d)** are all anatomic variations that relate to the embryological development of the biliary tract. Source: Lindner H. Embryology and anatomy of the biliary tree. In: Way LW, Pellegrini CA, eds. Surgery of the gallbladder and bile ducts. Philadelphia: WB Saunders, 1987. Reproduced with permission of Elsevier.

may drain directly into the gallbladder, the right or left hepatic ducts, the cystic duct, or the common bile duct. Accessory hepatic ducts are present in about 10% of individuals. Cystohepatic ducts that drain bile directly from the liver to the gallbladder are rare. Aberrant hepatic ducts, unlike true accessory ducts, result from an extrahepatic course of a duct that is normally contained within the liver parenchyma. Accessory ducts provide a second drainage route from a region of the liver, in contrast to an aberrant duct, which represents the only drainage to a particular region of the liver, but lies in an unusual location. Almost all aberrant hepatic ducts represent the right anterior segmental duct, which joins the right posterior segmental duct outside the liver. This extrahepatic union occurs in about 10% of cases and may result in mistaken identification of the right anterior segment duct as the cystic duct during cholecystectomy, with inadvertent ligation [17]. Both aberrant and true accessory hepatic ducts are at equal risk for injury during cholecystectomy.

Anomalies in the common bile duct do exist but are quite uncommon. The common bile duct may contain two lumens but appears to be single externally. The common bile duct may be completely duplicated, with one duct draining the right lobe of the liver and one duct draining the left lobe. Duplicated ducts usually empty separately into the duodenum [18,19]. Rarely, the common bile duct may open into the gastrointestinal tract at an ectopic site. The common bile duct has been reported to drain into the stomach [20] and the duodenal bulb [21], as well as the distal duodenum [22,23].

Biliary atresia

Biliary atresia is defined as the obliteration of the extrahepatic and/or intrahepatic bile ducts, with many different variations described (Figure 9.11). The incidence of biliary atresia is 1 per 15 000 births. Ten to 15% of patients with biliary atresia have associated anomalies of the inferior vena cava (absence), portal vein (preduodenal portal vein), intestine (intestinal malrotation), and spleen (polysplenia) [24]. Most patients have a form of biliary atresia with complete obstruction of the gallbladder and extrahepatic bile ducts, whereas 10–15% of patients have obstruction of the proximal hepatic ducts with patency of the gallbladder and distal common bile duct. Only 1–2% of patients have proximal hepatic duct patency.

In biliary atresia, the bile ducts are replaced by dense fibrotic tissue containing evidence of both an acute and chronic inflammatory process [25]. Typically, there is obliteration of the entire extrahepatic biliary tract, including the gallbladder. Extrahepatic biliary atresia frequently extends into the intrahepatic bile ducts, probably as an end result of a destructive process leading to fibrosis and obliteration of the biliary tree, with development of secondary biliary cirrhosis [26]. If left untreated, the typical course is one of progressive hepatic insufficiency, with an average survival of 12–19 months [27].

The pathogenesis of biliary atresia is not known. Existing data seem to contradict the theory that failure of recanalization of the bile ducts during development is the cause. Data accumulated from the surgical experience using portoenterostomy have provided some insight into the disease process. Early establishment of bile drainage, typically before 60 days, can reverse the liver injury and is associated with long-term survival, while delay in establishing bile drainage until after 120 days is often associated with progression of cirrhosis and a poor outcome. In addition, infants who develop biliary atresia are rarely jaundiced at birth and frequently have bile-stained meconium; biliary atresia has rarely been demonstrated in autopsy studies of fetuses [28]. These observations suggest that biliary atresia is a dynamic process targeting the extrahepatic bile ducts, with progressive destruction rather than a static process. The best available data suggest that 80% of cases are secondary to infection with a cholangiotropic virus such as cytomegalovirus (CMV), reovirus, or rotavirus followed by an exhuberant immune response destructive to the ductal epithelium that may persist even after eradication of the offending agent [29–31].

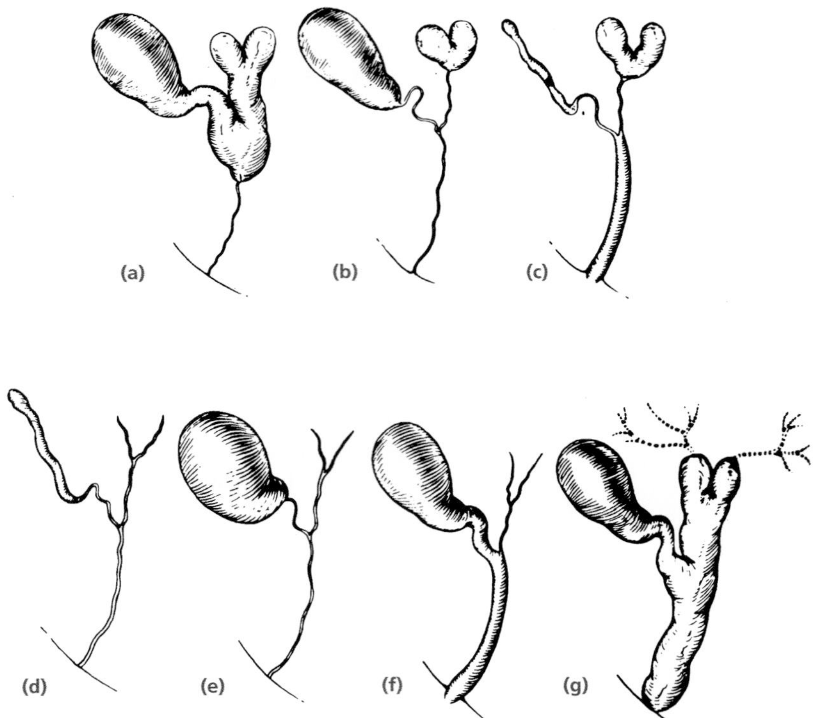

Figure 9.11 The different forms of biliary atresia. Biliary atresia may be partial, affecting the intra- or extrahepatic portions of the biliary tract, or it may be a complete process **(d)**. Source: Lindner H. Embryology and anatomy of the biliary tree. In: Way LW, Pellegrini CA, eds. Surgery of the gallbladder and bile ducts. Philadelphia: WB Saunders, 1987. Reproduced with permission of Elsevier.

The clinical presentation of biliary atresia is progressive neonatal jaundice with an onset in the first few weeks of life. Jaundice usually becomes visible in the first 2–4 weeks of life. Biliary atresia must be differentiated from neonatal physiological jaundice, as well as congenital infectious causes, such as CMV and rubella, and genetic diseases, including α1-antitrypsin deficiency.

Technetium 99m-iminoacetic acid (^{99m}Tc-IDA) hepatobiliary scanning is the imaging test of choice for biliary atresia, especially when preceded by a 5–7-day course of phenobarbital to increase bilirubin conjugation and excretion. The sensitivity of the test for biliary atresia is 100%, with a specificity of 94% [32]. An abdominal ultrasound should also be performed as a standard part of the evaluation of the jaundiced infant and is helpful to evaluate the possibility of other sources of biliary obstruction. Liver biopsy is nondiagnostic in up to 25% of patients and is often unnecessary to make a diagnosis.

Because of the near 100% mortality associated with medical management of biliary atresia, surgical therapy has become the treatment of choice. The standard operation, hepatic portoenterostomy, termed the Kasai procedure, was first described by Kasai in 1959 [33] following his original observation of residual microscopic bile channels in the fibrous tissue of the porta hepatis in patients with biliary atresia. The Kasai procedure consists of exploratory laparotomy with excision of the occluded extrahepatic biliary system and a Roux-en-Y enteric anastomosis to the transected fibrotic cord at that level of the porta hepatis where microscopic bile ducts have been documented by frozen section. Primary hepatic transplantation is reserved for patients with a delayed diagnosis and advanced cirrhosis at presentation or patients with failed Kasai procedures [34].

Most series report a 40–60% 5-year survival rate following portoenterostomy [35,36]. In general, one-third have good long-term results with minimal or no liver dysfunction and normal growth and development, one-third do poorly and are dependent on immediate liver transplantation for survival, and one-third have slow, progressive liver dysfunction over a period of months to years and subsequently need liver transplantation. Although the failure rate is fairly high, the fact that one-third of patients will do well and never require transplantation and another subset will experience normal growth for a period of years before potentially requiring transplantation, in addition to the shortage of transplantable organs, has prompted centers to use the Kasai procedure as first-line therapy for biliary atresia [37–39].

Choledochal cyst

See Chapter 83 for detailed discussion.

References are available at www.yamadagastro.com/textbook7e

CHAPTER 10

Liver: anatomy, microscopic structure, and cell types

Maria Westerhoff and Laura Lamps
University of Michigan, Ann Arbor, MI, USA

Chapter menu

The liver is a unique organ with remarkable capabilities and a vast range of functions. It filters blood from the gastrointestinal tract before it reaches the rest of the body, detoxifies foreign substances, and produces bile, albumin, and coagulation factors. Understanding the individual components of the liver both macroscopically and microscopically is crucial to truly comprehending liver diseases. It also allows for better interpretation of laboratory test results used to evaluate a patient's liver health and disease. Finally, being aware of hepatobiliary embryology not only assists in understanding pediatric liver disease, but also aids in comprehending adult liver conditions.

With these goals in mind, this chapter outlines embryological development as well as the gross, histological, and electron microscopic characteristics of the liver with a practical, patient-oriented mindset.

Embryology

The primordial liver first appears toward the end of gestational week 3, and is called the "hepatic diverticulum." It is formed by an outpouching of the distal foregut (future duodenum), and is composed of proliferating endodermal cells [1–9]. By the fourth week, these endodermal cell cords ("hepatoblast cords") of the diverticulum grow cranially into a mesodermal plate called the septum transversum. This sheet of mesoderm lies beneath the pericardial cavity; it is a major source of the connective tissue framework of the liver as well as the diaphragm.

The cranial part of the diverticulum that grows into the septum transversum eventually becomes the liver (Figure 10.1). The hepatic diverticulum also gives rise to a caudal bud, which becomes the gallbladder and cystic duct. The cranial end of the hepatic diverticulum ultimately divides to form the right and left liver lobes. The stalk of the diverticulum between the developing liver and foregut narrows, forming the extrahepatic biliary system and gallbladder. By week 5, as the hepatoblast cords extend radially from the hepatic diverticulum and into the septum transversum, capillary plexuses from the vitelline veins simultaneously grow into the septum transversum from its outer margins and penetrate between the epithelial cords. These vessels ultimately meet the growing, anastomosing epithelial sheets and are enmeshed to form the primitive hepatic sinusoids.

The septum transversum mesoderm initially surrounds the liver and is in continuity with the lesser curvature of the stomach, duodenum, and ventral body wall. The mesoderm becomes stretched between the liver and lesser curvature, forming the lesser omentum, and between the diaphragm and ventral abdominal wall, forming the falciform, coronary, and triangular ligaments. A portion also develops into the hepatic (Glisson) capsule. The developing hepatic artery and vagus nerve branches follow the mesoderm adjacent to the portal vein. The mesoderm on the liver surface is also in continuity with the

Yamada's Textbook of Gastroenterology, Seventh Edition. Edited by Timothy C. Wang, Michael Camilleri, Benjamin Lebwohl, Anna S. Lok, William J. Sandborn, Kenneth K. Wang, and Gary D. Wu.

Companion website: www.yamadagastro.com/textbook7e

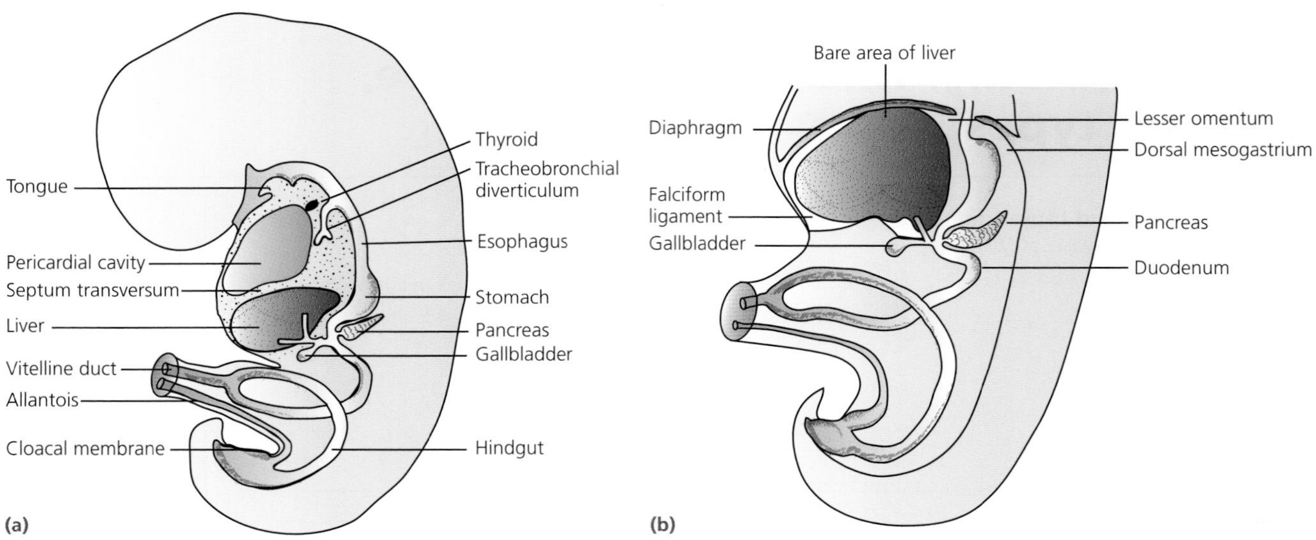

Figure 10.1 Developing embryo. **(a)** The drawing represents a 9 mm embryo, estimated at about 36 days of gestation. The liver is derived from the hepatic diverticulum (midline outgrowth stalk of the distal foregut) and projects cranially into the septum transversum and caudally into the abdominal wall. **(b)** The drawing represents an embryo that is slightly older, with the falciform ligament noted between the hepatic parenchyma and the anterior abdominal wall. Source: Langman 1969 [5]. Reproduced with permission of Wolters Kluwer Health.

peritoneum, while the portion in contact with the future diaphragm remains unperitonealized (*bare area*). Hematopoiesis begins at about 6 weeks and becomes most active during the fifth gestational month. After this, the process rapidly regresses and the bone marrow takes over. Hematopoiesis is responsible for the prominent size of the fetal liver (up to 10% body weight by week 10, with the liver occupying most of the abdominal cavity). The liver size regresses at birth and only a few islands of hematopoietic cells are left; at that point, the liver weighs about 5% of body weight. Hematopoiesis is usually absent by 3–4 weeks after birth. Initially, the enlarged fetal liver has symmetric right and left lobes; with time, however, the growth rate diminishes but affects the left lobe more than the right, causing the size difference seen at birth. The caudate and quadrate lobes develop as subdivisions of the right lobe.

The liver's vascular network is originally derived from both the vitelline and umbilical veins. It occurs at the same time as the proliferation of the hepatoblasts. The hepatoblast cords enmesh the vessels, forming the hepatic sinusoids. Initially, the sinusoidal network receives blood through the vitelline veins and drains into the sinus venosus. By the fifth gestational week, the right and left umbilical veins also supply the sinusoidal network. Most of the major vessels, including the right and left umbilical veins, the transverse portal sinus, and the ductus venosus, are also identifiable at this time. The ductus venosus shunts blood directly from the umbilical vein into the inferior vena cava to supply oxygenated blood to the heart, bypassing the liver. Around this time, the left umbilical vein becomes the main source of blood flow from the placenta to the fetus including the liver; and the right umbilical vein atrophies. The paired vitelline veins become a single portal vein, which then subdivides into the right and left branches. Ultimately, the left umbilical vein blood flow has three major branching routes: (1) the sinusoidal plexus of the left hepatic segment; (2) the sinusoidal plexus of the right hepatic segment by way of retrograde flow from communications with the left portal vein branch; and (3) the ductus venosus. At birth, the umbilical vein blood flow is eliminated and the ductus venosus closes. The closed umbilical vein becomes the ligamentum teres and the fibrotic ductus venosus becomes the ligamentum venosum.

Hepatocytes and bile duct epithelial cells (cholangiocytes) both derive from hepatoblasts, the progenitor cells. The hepatic cords' rapid growth rate allows sheets that are several cells thick. This persists until birth, after which the sheets narrow to two cell layers and, by 5 years of age, into one cell-thick trabecular cords [8,10–12].

Portal tract formation is largely determined by hepatic vascular development. The portal vein enters the liver through the porta hepatis and the mesenchyme that condenses around the intrahepatic portal venous system makes up the portal tracts. The hepatoblasts immediately adjacent to the portal mesenchyme become the ductal plates [10]. The ductal plate cells ultimately form intrahepatic bile ducts, but also provide molecular signals that drive hepatic arterial growth. The hepatic artery arises from the celiac axis and branches into the developing liver from the porta hepatis along the mesenchyme of the portal tract. Hepatic arterial development is thus elegantly harmonized with that of the intrahepatic biliary tree, which explains the 1:1 pairing of the hepatic arteries and terminal bile ducts in the terminal portal tracts.

Intrahepatic bile ducts develop from the hepatoblasts immediately adjacent to the mesenchyme of the portal tracts. At 9–10 weeks, the hepatoblasts surrounding the portal tracts near the hilum of the liver form a layer of bile duct-type cells, followed by a second layer forming a primitive duct structure called the ductal plate. By the third gestational month, a lumen is seen within the ductal plate, with formation of associated double-layered tubular structures. This process repeats itself centrifugally along the portal tracts from the hilum toward the periphery of the liver. As remodeling of the ductal plate continues, invading connective tissue separates the ductal structures from the liver parenchyma, incorporating the duct structures into the portal tract mesenchyme. The intrahepatic bile ducts are not fully developed at term [13]; immature structures may persist for up to a month. Postnatal remodeling forms the true interlobular bile ducts that link the biliary canaliculi and the extrahepatic biliary system. The biliary network is supplied by a delicate peribiliary plexus formed by the hepatic arteries. The biliary canaliculi are first seen as intercellular spaces between the hepatoblasts at the sixth gestational week. They develop from membranous infoldings between junctional complexes that form luminal channels between hepatocytes. Bile synthesis occurs by week 9, with bile secretion by week 12.

Other individual cell functions become apparent at different times, but all early in embryological development [11,14,15]. α-Fetoprotein, which is found in high amounts at birth, is present by 1-month gestation, and continues throughout fetal development. Glycogen may be seen by 2 months, with glycogen synthesis becoming most apparent by 3 months; at birth, the amount of glycogen rapidly diminishes owing to rapid and active glycogenolysis. Fatty change within the hepatocyte parallels that of glycogenesis. Hemosiderin is usually visible in early stages and becomes most marked as intrahepatic hematopoiesis decreases. It then gradually decreases but may still be seen at birth in the periportal hepatocytes. The Kupffer cells appear by the third gestational month.

Gross anatomy

Anatomically, the liver has four lobes: right, left, caudate, and quadrate. Grossly, the right lobe is divided from the left by the falciform ligament. Functional divisions of the liver follow the branching pattern of the portal structures (portal vein, hepatic artery, and bile duct). Consequently, there are eight functional segments, each with its own supportive vascular and biliary drainage [1,2,8,16–23] (Figure 10.2).

The hepatoduodenal ligament connects the liver to the superior aspect of the duodenum and supports the hilar vessels and

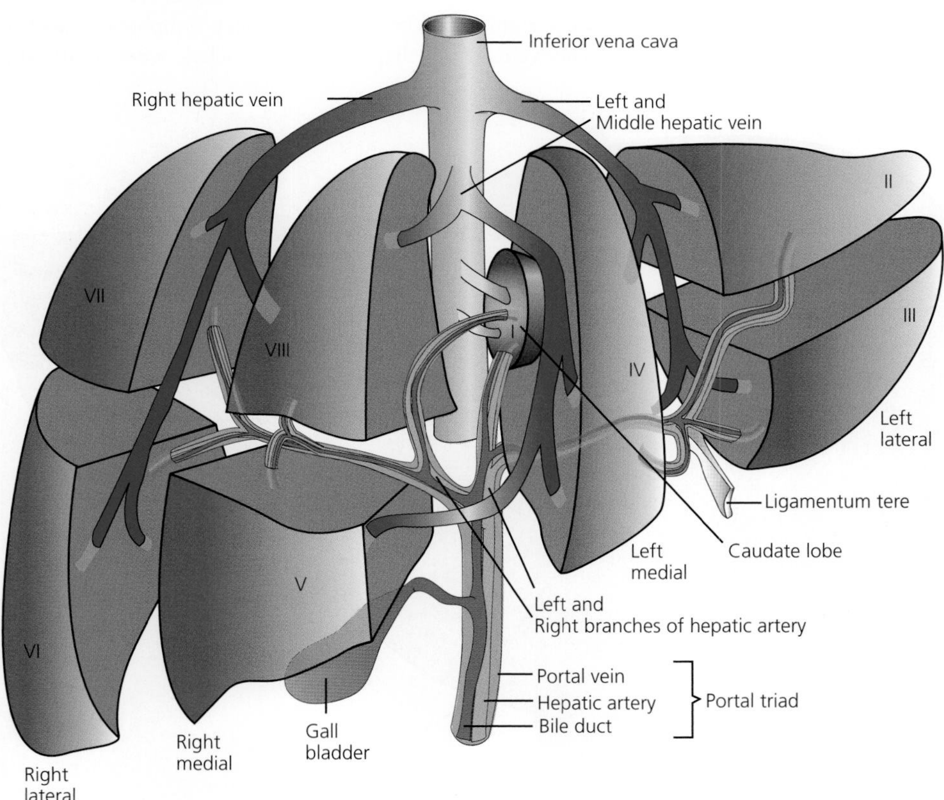

Figure 10.2 Anatomical and functional subdivisions. The liver is divided into eight functional anatomical segments, each having its own vascular flow and biliary drainage. The caudate lobe is segment I. Segments II and III are the left lobe lateral subdivisions, while segment IV is the left lobe's medial subdivision. The quadrate lobe is considered a part of segment IV, deemed IVb. The right lobe is subdivided into the lateral (segments VI and VII) and medial (segments V and VIII) divisions. Source: Moore and Dalley 1999 [70]. Reproduced with permission of Wolters Kluwer Health.

ductal structures. The transverse fissure separates the right lobe from the caudate lobe anteriorly. The umbilical fissure is located to the left of the quadrate lobe, which itself is bordered on the right by the gallbladder. The peritoneal layers forming the falciform ligament, which extends between the liver and the anterior abdominal wall, separate to form the superior layer of the coronary ligament and the left triangular ligament. The ligamentum teres is located along the lower edge of the falciform ligament.

The portal vein is the main vascular drainage of the gastrointestinal tract, and is formed by the convergence of the superior mesenteric and splenic veins. It also receives blood from the left gastric (coronary) and cystic veins. Increased portal venous pressure can result in reversed flow at these sites of portosystemic anastomoses (known as portosystemic shunts). The portal vein is located along the hepatoduodenal ligament posterior to the hepatic artery and common bile duct, and ends at the porta hepatis, dividing into its right and left main branches. The right branch divides early into anterior and posterior segments, whereas the left branch divides into the pars transversus and the pars umbilicus. The caudate lobe veins arise from both the right and left main portal vein branches (Figure 10.3). The hepatic vein is composed of three major tributaries (right, middle, and left), each having intrahepatic branches. The middle and left hepatic veins often converge to form a single outflow vessel before draining into the inferior vena cava, whereas the right hepatic vein enters through a separate ostium. The veins draining the caudate lobe enter directly into the inferior vena cava; consequently, the caudate lobe may be spared in the event of venous outflow obstruction.

The hepatic artery is a branch of the celiac artery, which ascends along the hepatoduodenal ligament and eventually divides into right and left main branches. The right hepatic artery is typically located behind the common hepatic duct after giving rise to the cystic artery; it eventually divides into the anterior and posterior segmental branches. The left hepatic artery passes obliquely upward and to the left in the porta hepatis, eventually dividing into medial and lateral segmental branches. The quadrate lobe is fed by the middle hepatic artery branch, whereas the caudate lobe is fed by both the right and left hepatic artery branches.

The right hepatic lobe biliary drainage is derived from anterior and posterior segmental duct branches that merge to form the right hepatic duct. Lateral and medial segmental branches merge, forming the left hepatic duct that drains the left lobe. The caudate lobe is drained from three duct branches directly into the right and left hepatic ducts (Figure 10.4). The intra- and extrahepatic bile duct structures are directly supplied by the hepatic artery and its anastomosing branches, which parallel the ducts as they course through the various hepatic segments.

The lymphatics of the liver are divided into deep and superficial branches. The deep lymphatic branch parallels the portal and hepatic vein branches, whereas the superficial lymphatic

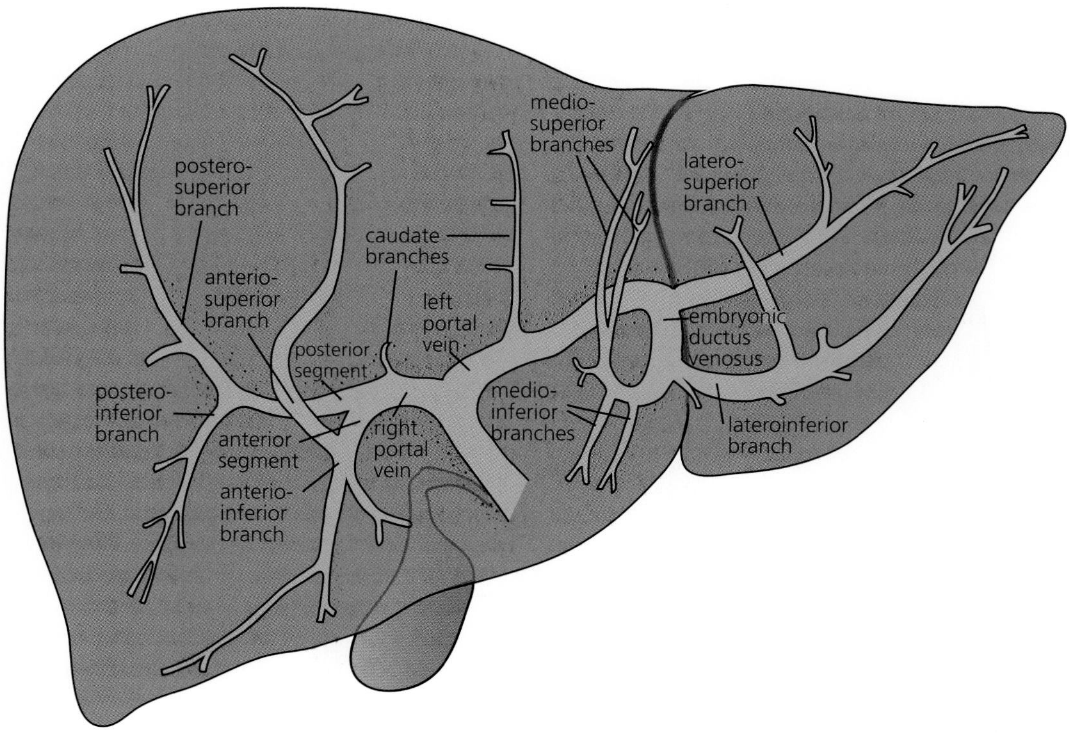

Figure 10.3 Intrahepatic branches of the portal vein. A, anterior segment; br., branch; L., left; P, posterior segment; R., right; U, embryonic ductus venosus. Source: Skandalakis et al. 1992 [71].

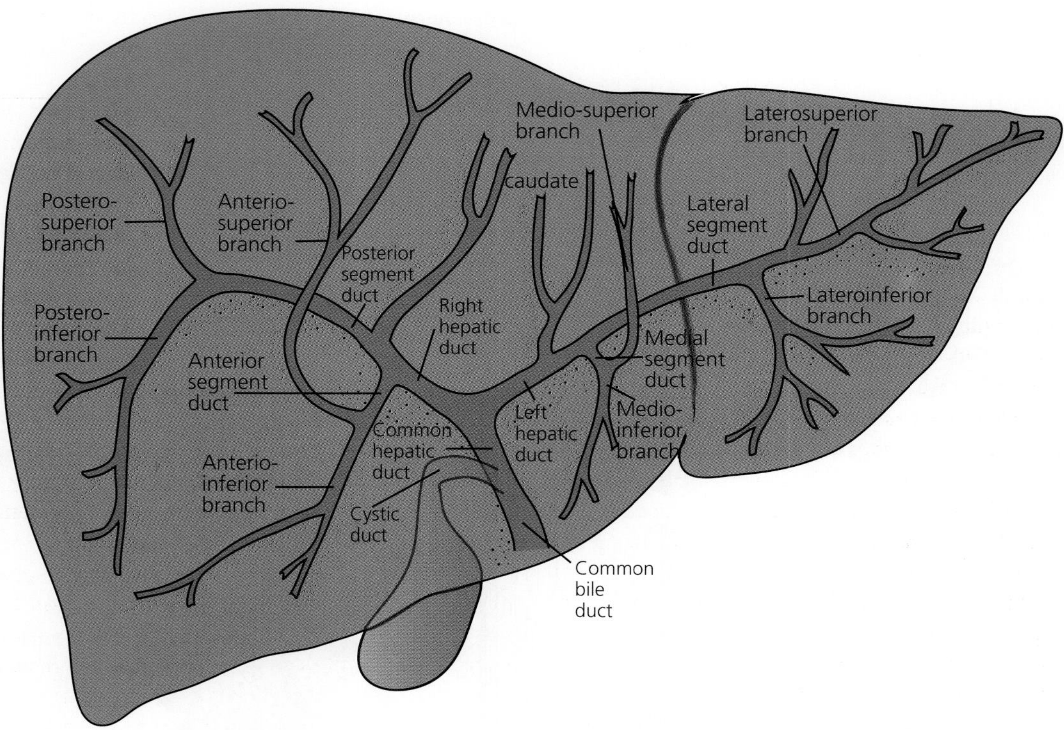

Figure 10.4 Branching segments of the intrahepatic bile ducts. br., branch; Med seg., medial segment; L., left; R., right. Source: Adapted from Skandalakis et al. 1992 [71].

structures arise from Glisson capsule and drain through the adjacent falciform ligament, diaphragm, esophagus, and hilar lymph nodes [1,2,24].

The nerve supply is divided into parasympathetic and sympathetic fibers. The former are preganglionic and derived from the vagus nerve, whereas the latter are postganglionic and receive their nerve supply from T7–T10. The nerves enter the hepatic hilum through both anterior and posterior routes, and innervate the arteries and bile ducts through sympathetic innervation. The nerve fibers branch through the main portal tracts, with smaller unmyelinated branches supplying the periportal hepatocytes. In addition, many of the nerve fibers terminate on endothelial cells lining the smallest arterioles and along Kupffer cells, stellate (fat-storing) cells, and hepatocytes [25].

Histology

Architecture

The three-dimensional architecture of the liver is fairly homogeneous throughout all lobes (Figure 10.5) [26,27]. Although the architecture may be difficult to assess when acute liver injury is present, the spatial arrangement of the various liver components may return close to baseline on recovery. On the other hand, in advanced chronic liver disease, fibrosis distorts the architecture. Even with regression of fibrosis due to treatment or removal of the agent of injury, the liver architecture does not revert to normal.

The classic Rappaport acinus concept can be appreciated under the light microscope [28]. It subdivides the parenchyma into zones 1 (periportal), 2 (between periportal and pericentral/perivenular), and 3 (area around hepatic venule), with decreasing oxygenation and increasing susceptibility to ischemia and toxic/drug-induced injury toward zone 3 (Figure 10.6). Biliary drainage runs parallel to the vascular sinusoidal circulation. The other popular model of the hepatic lobule is hexagonal; it centers on a hepatic vein branch (central vein) and is surrounded by six portal tracts. The hexagonal equivalents to the acinus zones 1, 2, and 3 are the periportal, midzonal, and centrilobular areas, respectively [29].

Portal tracts

The portal tracts (Figure 10.7) contain branches of the portal vein, interlobular bile duct, and hepatic artery (portal "triad"). The density of portal tract fibroconnective tissue varies depending on how far it is from the hepatic hilum. Portal tracts normally contains small numbers of inflammatory cells, predominantly lymphocytes with occasional histiocytes [30].

The interlobular bile ducts are usually seen immediately adjacent to the hepatic arterioles, which are responsible for their blood supply. The hepatic arteriole and bile duct are intimately associated from the time of development, which explains both

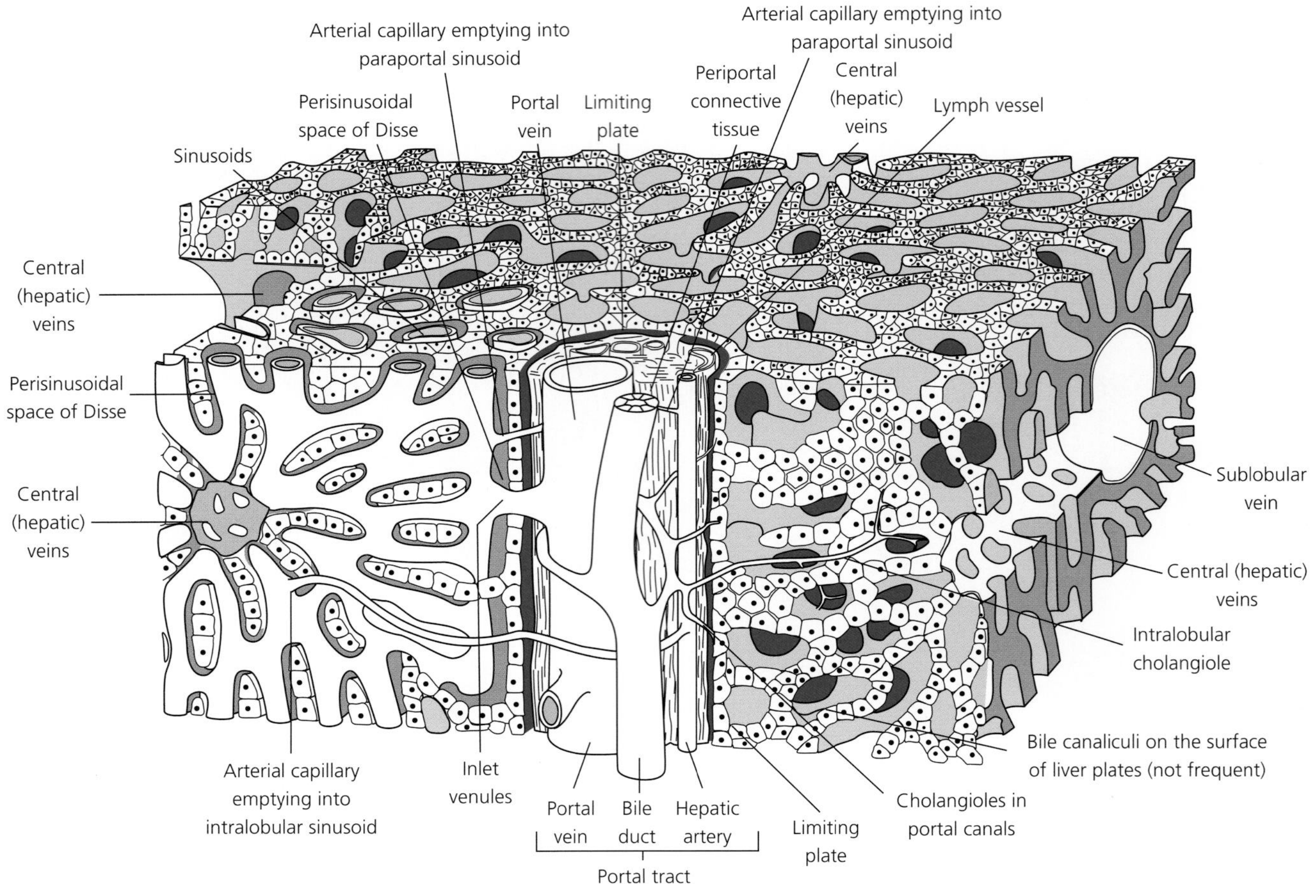

Figure 10.5 Structure of the normal liver. Source: Sherlock and Dooley 2002 [2]. Reproduced with permission from John Wiley & Sons, Ltd.

the pairing of these structures and the fact that the hepatic arteriole is approximately the same size as the bile duct. This is important diagnostically, as bile duct injury or paucity can be easily determined by looking for a hepatic arteriole and bile duct of the same caliber in each portal tract. The portal venules are about three times bigger than hepatic arteriole or bile duct lumens. A true increase in the number of portal venules is characteristic of portal hypertension, and may be seen in conjunction with portal fibrosis or cirrhosis.

Parenchyma

In adults, the hepatocytes are arranged in cords that are 1–2 cells thick. Each cord, or *trabecula*, of cells has a sinusoid on either side, exposing the hepatocyte to portal blood on two surfaces. Within the cords, the hepatocytes are adjoined via intercellular surfaces, with a groove (hemicanaliculus) surrounding each hepatocyte. The hemicanaliculi of two adjacent cells together form the bile canaliculus, which is separated from the rest of the intercellular space by tight junctions.

The perisinusoidal space (space of Disse) is located between the endothelial cells and hepatocytes, and harbors hepatic stellate cells and collagen fibers. On routine staining, the space of Disse is usually inconspicuous. However, it appears dilated in autopsy liver specimens secondary to hepatocyte shrinkage from autolysis. The sinusoids drain from the portal venule and hepatic arterioles into the terminal hepatic venules (Figure 10.8).

Parenchymal cellular components

Hepatocyte

Hepatocytes are polygonal cells with a single, central nucleus, generally measuring about 25–40 μm in diameter. Hepatocytes have three notable and distinct cell boundaries [8,11,31].

The sinusoidal (basolateral) aspect of the hepatocyte has microvilli present along the surface that extends into the perisinusoidal spaces, increasing the cell surface area. The plasma membranes immediately beneath these microvilli exhibit various membrane pits and infoldings involved in secretory and absorptive functions.

The intercellular (lateral) aspect is the interface between adjacent hepatocytes. It is divided into a number of junctional subunits [1,31], including gap junctions, which mediate

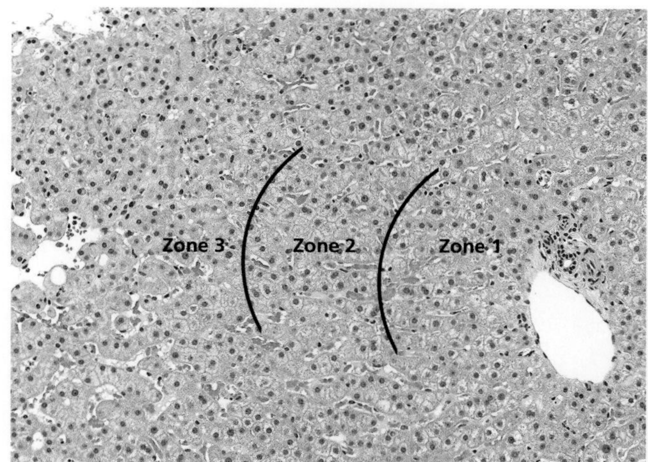

Figure 10.6 The three hepatic parenchymal zones. Zone 1 is periportal, 2 is between periportal and pericentral/perivenular zones, and 3 is the area around the hepatic venule. There is decreasing oxygenation toward zone 3.

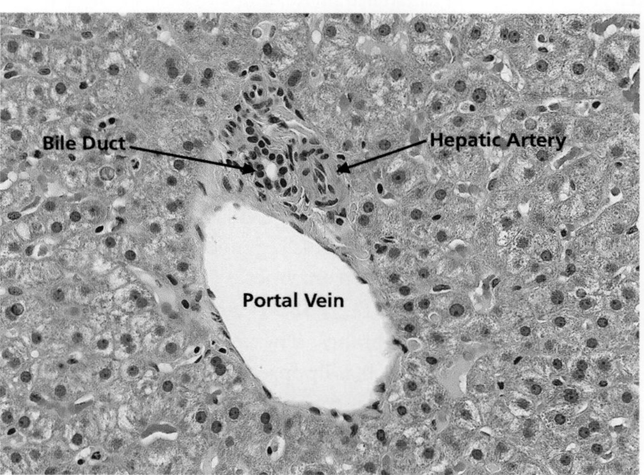

Figure 10.7 Portal tract. The major components include the hepatic arteriole, portal venule (large vessel), and bile ductule (cuboidal epithelium). There is a normal amount of collagen seen in this portal tract.

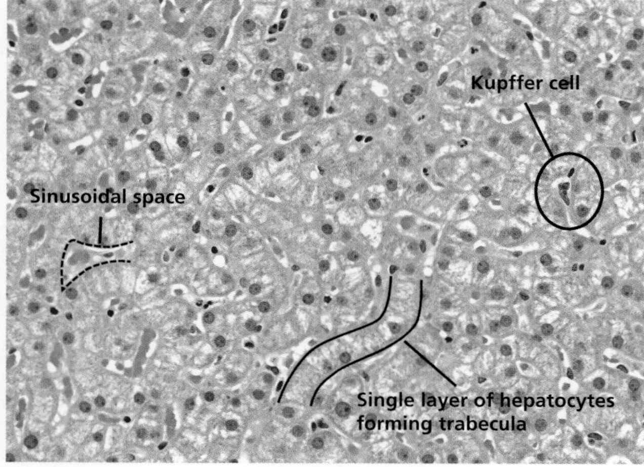

(a)

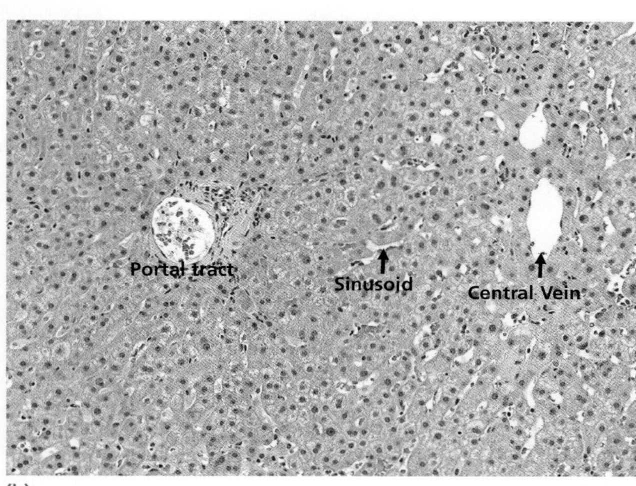

(b)

Figure 10.8 Parenchyma. **(a)** The liver cell plates are one cell thick and are composed of polyhedral hepatocytes with centrally placed nuclei. These cells are bordered by sinusoids lined by both Kupffer and endothelial cells. **(b)** The sinusoids drain directly into the terminal hepatic (central) venules.

communication between cells via transport of metabolites (bobbins); desmosomes, which are attached to intermediate filaments and promote cell membrane resilience; intermediate junctions, which are attached to various cytokeratin filaments that also aid in cellular resilience; and tight junctions, which are zones of membrane-to-membrane contact that represent a permeability barrier to macromolecules [32].

The canalicular membranes lie toward the center of the intercellular confluence of hepatocytes and are immediately adjacent to the tight junctions. As above, they represent the beginning of the biliary drainage system (Figure 10.9). The canalicular membranes are lined by microvilli and measure between 0.5 μm in diameter in the perivenular zone to 2.5 μm in the periportal zone. Various contractile microfilaments surround the canaliculi, allowing hepatocytes to move the bile forward.

Nucleus

The hepatocyte nucleus is centrally located, round, and, measures about 10 μm in diameter, with clumped chromatin and small nucleoli [28,32]. Usually hepatocytes contain only one nucleus, although binucleate forms may be seen, more often in elderly patients in the perivenular zone (zone 3 of Rappaport). Multinucleated hepatocytes can be seen in several pathologic conditions, including cholestasis when the detergent effect of retained bile salts dissolve cellular membranes, and in autoimmune hepatitis, as a regenerative feature due to increased cell proliferation without cell division.

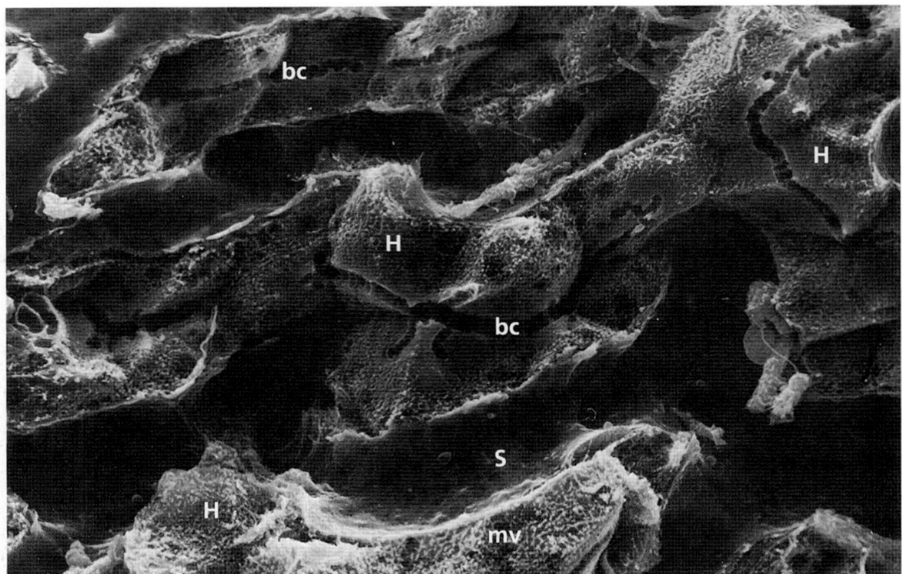

Figure 10.9 Biliary canaliculi. Using scanning electron microscopy, the liver cell plates and adjacent fenestrated sinusoids (S) are seen with the bile canalicular (bc) network located between the adjacent hepatocytes (H). Microvilli (mv) are also present. Source: Phillips et al. 1987 [31]. Reproduced with permission of Wolters Kluwer Health.

Mitotic figures are infrequent, but may be prominent during active regeneration (e.g., resolving acute hepatitis) or in carcinoma. Various nuclear inclusions may be identified in hepatocytes [31,33,34], including glycogen (frequently seen in diabetic patients), lipid, and cytoplasmic invaginations (pseudoinclusions, or nuclear membrane irregularities). Nuclear glycogen is most often seen in periportal hepatocytes as clear nuclear vacuoles on routine stain, and bright pink on periodic acid–Schiff stain.

Cytoplasm

The superstructure of the hepatocyte cytoplasm is maintained by the cytoskeleton, and includes microfilaments, microtubules, and intermediate filaments [8,11,31,35–37]. These are responsible for the overall three-dimensional framework of the hepatocytes as well as organization of the various intracellular functions.

The mitochondria are one of the most prominent intracellular organelles, and are responsible for many metabolic functions [8,11,31]. On average, there are up to 2200 mitochondria per hepatocyte. They are larger in the perivenular zone but more numerous in the periportal zone.

The endoplasmic reticulum (ER) is composed of a network of parallel cistern structures. If polyribosomes are attached to the cytoplasmic aspects of the surfaces, this constitutes rough ER. The remaining smooth ER lacks a ribosomal coat and communicates with the Golgi apparatus. The ER is responsible for various important functions such as protein synthesis and fatty acid metabolism.

The cytochrome p450 oxidative system is also located in the ER, which plays a large part in drug metabolism and toxin degradation. Perivenular hepatocytes have the highest level of cytochrome p450 activity. This degree of activity correlates with the considerable amount of smooth ER that resides in this area compared to the periportal zone, as well as with the darker hue of the hepatocyte cytoplasm in this region due to the presence of heme in the cytochrome p450 enzymes.

The Golgi apparatus [8,11,31,38,39] consists of a complex of vesicles and folded membranes. The vesicles detach, transferring secretory material such as lipoproteins into the sinusoids or biliary canaliculi. The Golgi functions also include bile secretion, carbohydrate incorporation into proteins, and membrane synthesis and repair.

Lysosomes [8,11,31,40,41] contain and store enzymes such as acid phosphatase, esterases, proteases, and lipases, and are most frequently located adjacent to the canalicular membrane. They are divided into *primary* and *secondary* lysosomes. The primary lysosomes digest intracellular degradation products (autophagocytosis), forming secondary lysosomes that secrete these vacuoles into the biliary system. Various pigments such as lipofuscin, hemosiderin, and copper also may accumulate within lysosomes over time. This accumulated residue of nondigested material or pigments forms *residual bodies.*

There are various other intracellular components readily seen by light microscopy that contribute to the function and appearance of the liver cell [26,27]. *Lipofuscin* pigment appears as fine to coarse brown granules and is derived from increase in lysosomal activity and intracellular condensation of various cellular remnants. It appears in the pericanalicular region of centrilobular hepatocytes and is most numerous in older individuals. Two other intracellular pigments that can resemble lipofuscin include *bile* and *hemosiderin*. Bile consists of clumped green to green-yellow globules. Hemosiderin pigment, representing red blood cell degradation remnants, is refractile, coarsely granular, and golden brown, and best highlighted by the Perl iron stain. Stainable iron is usually absent or in trace amounts in the adult liver. In the newborn, a slight baseline liver siderosis is normal.

Intracellular lipids appear as clear, distinct, rounded vacuoles, and are composed predominantly of neutral triglycerides. The size of the fat droplets varies. Macrovesicular steatosis refers to the presence of large, well-demarcated fat droplets in the hepatocyte cytoplasm that displaces the nucleus to the periphery. Routine histological sections of liver show these fat droplets as being optically clear cytoplasmic vacuoles because the fat washes out during tissue processing [42]. The normal liver may contain macrovesicular fat droplets in small amounts (<5% of the parenchyma). On the other hand, microvesicular steatosis represents numerous miniscule fat droplets that diffusely occupy the cytoplasm and cause a foamy or bubbly appearance to the cytoplasm without displacing the nucleus. Microvesicular steatosis can be subtle on routine staining. Practically speaking, the presence of diffuse, purely microvesicular steatosis is seen mostly in critically ill patients with liver failure and in genetic or acquired causes of mitochondrial defects (i.e., acute fatty liver of pregnancy, Reye's syndrome, toxins). Macrovesicular steatosis is commonly seen in metabolic syndrome due to nonalcoholic fatty liver disease, alcohol-related liver disease, and inherited disorders such as glycogen storage diseases and even Wilson disease. A variant of macrovesicular steatosis referred to as small droplet macrovesicular steatosis has multiple, clearly defined fat vacuoles that are smaller than half of the hepatocyte and do not displace the nucleus. The presence of small droplet fat may have some clinical outcome ramifications in the transplant setting, but is not standardly included in estimating the percentage of steatosis during donor liver evaluation for transplant use [43,44]. *Intracellular glycogen* is distributed throughout the cytoplasm but is more frequently seen adjacent to the smooth endoplasmic reticulum. Glycogen is easily demonstrated by periodic acid–Schiff (PAS) stain.

Sinusoidal lining cells

Kupffer cells

Kupffer cells are tissue macrophages that line the sinusoids of the liver. They represent more than 75% of noncirculating macrophages throughout the body [8,11,28,45–50] and can enlarge and proliferate in response to a variety of stimuli. Although originally derived from the circulation, they eventually come to rest along the sinusoidal borders. Nevertheless, they maintain the ability to divide and migrate along the sinusoidal spaces, especially into regions of liver cell damage where it is not uncommon to find hyperplastic and hypertrophic Kupffer cell clusters and aggregates. Kupffer cells measure up to 9 μm in length, have oval to elongated nuclei, and abundant pyramidal stellate cytoplasm. They express macrophage markers such as CD68 and CD163. Kupffer cells contain various lysosomes and function in phagocytosis and clearance of bacteria, endotoxins, and degenerating cellular components. Other roles include lipid synthesis and catabolism as well as clearance of immune complexes. PAS with diastase staining can highlight debris-filled Kupffer cells in areas of hepatocyte death, indicating recent hepatocyte necrosis in patients who have been biopsied soon after an acute hepatitis event.

Endothelial cells

The sinusoidal endothelial cells are fenestrated, flattened, and elongated cells [31,45,48,51–54] (Figure 10.10). They are characterized by numerous gaps (fenestrae) within the cytoplasm that function as a filtration barrier (Figure 10.11). The fenestrae vary in size: there are small clusters of fenestrae that are 0.2 μm in diameter each, as well as larger ones up to 1 μm in diameter that are more numerous at the distal end of the sinusoid. In this way, the degree of endothelial permeability differs depending on the region; permeability is higher near the hepatic venule than the periportal region. The sinusoidal endothelial cells have slightly different functions from endothelial cells seen in other

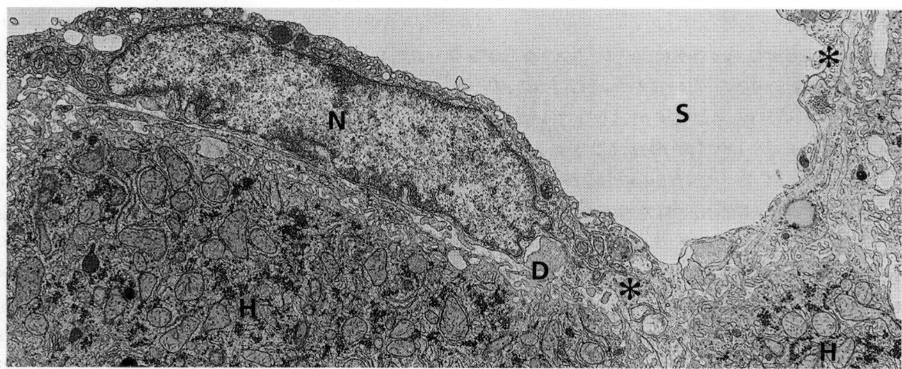

Figure 10.10 Endothelial cell. Electron microscopy of a sinusoid (S) shows an endothelial cell with an elongated nucleus (N) and scanty cytoplasm (*). The space of Disse (D) and adjacent cytoplasm of two hepatocytes (H) are noted. Source: Phillips et al. 1987 [31]. Reproduced with permission of Wolters Kluwer Health.

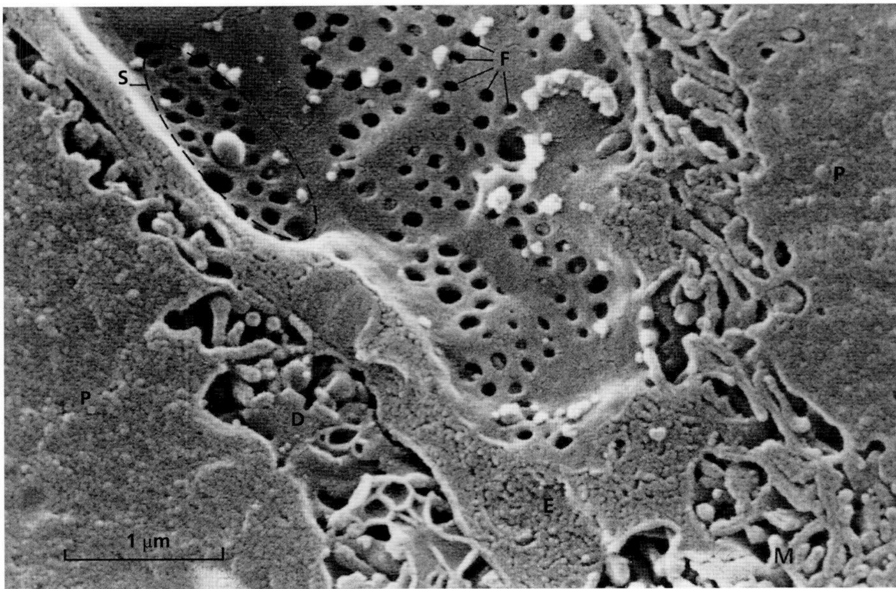

Figure 10.11 Scanning electron micrograph of the hepatic sinusoid. Numerous fenestrae (F) grouped into sieve plates (S) are demonstrated. D, space of Disse; E, endothelial cell; M, microvilli; P, parenchymal cell. Source: Sherlock and Dooley 2002 [2]. Reproduced with permission of John Wiley & Sons, Ltd.

organ systems in that they do not bind lectin or factor VIII-related antigen. In their normal state they also express very little CD31 or C34 [8], although expression of these markers is common along the hepatocyte sinusoidal endothelium of patients with chronic liver diseases and hepatocellular carcinoma.

Hepatic stellate (perisinusoidal) cells

Previously known as *fat-storing cells* or *Ito cells*, the hepatic stellate cells are located within the perisinusoidal liver cell recesses along the space of Disse [31,45,48,55–62]. Normally, hepatic stellate cells are difficult to see on routine staining. They range in diameter from 2 to 10 μm and contain small triangular-shaped nuclei without prominent nucleoli. The cytoplasm often contains variably sized lipid droplets. Besides being the major source of vitamin A storage, these cells produce hepatocyte growth factor and synthesize extracellular matrix by way of cytokine activation and resultant transformation to myofibroblasts in response to liver injury, with enhancement of protein and collagen synthesis [63,64].

Stroma (extracellular matrix)

The Glisson capsule, composed of dense hypocellular collagen, encapsulates the liver and extends at the hilum into the hepatic parenchyma, forming the tensile connective tissue structure of the portal tracts. Extension of this collagen within the sinusoids and into the space of Disse as reticulin fibers maintains the intralobular framework. For this reason, reticulin stains are useful to highlight normal liver cords and assisting in detection of pathological conditions that disrupt the normal architecture.

Five basic types of collagen are seen within the liver stroma, with types I and III representing more than 95% of the total [8]. Type I is found in mature collagen fibers, and is seen predominantly within the portal tracts but also around the terminal hepatic, sublobular, and hepatic veins. Type III characterizes new collagen fibers which, along with type IV collagen, make up the sinusoidal reticulin framework. Type IV collagen is also present in the basal lamina (membrane) around small vascular structures and ducts, and represents about 1% of the total hepatic collagen. The noncollagenous proteins are composed of numerous matrix glycoproteins including *laminin*, the major glycoprotein component within basement membranes that is responsible in part for cell adhesion and formation of capillaries within the sinusoids; *fibronectin*, synthesized by perisinusoidal cells responsible for collagen adhesion; and *elastin*, which stabilizes blood vessel walls [8]. Collagen deposition is often triggered by activation of hepatic stellate cells due to a variety of inflammatory conditions.

Biliary network

The main function of the biliary tract is to transport bile that has been synthesized in the hepatocytes into the gastrointestinal tract. It does so by way of the intra- and extrahepatic biliary network (see above). In addition, the transport proteins synthesized by biliary epithelium and located within the microvilli aid in secreting bicarbonate-rich fluid and reabsorbing various fluids and solutes that generally enhance bile flow [65].

The smallest structural components of the biliary tract [66] are the biliary canaliculi, located along the intercellular spaces between hepatocytes. The canaliculi have numerous anastomotic connections and may undergo contractions secondary to actin, myosin, and tropomyosin [67], enabling and enhancing forward bile flow.

Near the portal tract limiting plate (interface between the portal tract and the liver parenchyma), the *canals of Hering* connect the canaliculi to the *terminal bile ductules*, which then communicate with the interlobular bile ducts that lie within the portal tracts. The canals of Hering are lined by hepatocytes as well as bile duct epithelium. Although in the normal liver canals of Hering are usually inconspicuous on routine light microscopy, stem cells that reside in canals of Hering may proliferate, resulting in cells that first take on a cholangiocytic phenotype. This is most apparent in liver damage (such as hepatitis) where these ductules may extend to and involve the periportal zones. It can also be seen in biliary tract obstruction and other cholestatic processes due to the accumulation of bile acids, which trigger bile ductular reaction.

The *interlobular bile ducts* are located within small portal tracts, and range in diameter from 15 to 20 μm. They are lined by a single layer of cuboidal cells with discrete round nuclei, inconspicuous nucleoli, and scant eosinophilic cytoplasm. The duct cytoplasm has abundant intermediate cytokeratin filaments (cytokeratins 7, 19) [3]. A basement membrane is apparent and easily demonstrated on PAS stain. Although the smaller ducts have no apparent wall, the larger interlobular ducts, which measure up to 100 μm in diameter, develop a small periductal fibrous sheath.

The larger *interlobar* and *septal ducts* measure more than 100 μm in diameter, have a fibrous wall, and are lined by a single layer of cuboidal to columnar epithelium. Periductal fibrous tissue in this location is typical and should not be confused with the distinct periductal concentric "onion-skinning" fibrosis seen in long-term bile duct obstruction and primary sclerosing cholangitis. The interlobar and septal ducts lead into the *segmental ducts*, which measure up to 800 μm in diameter, and eventually form the major *hilar ducts* that measure up to 1.5 mm in diameter. The hilar ducts ultimately branch into the *main right* and *left hepatic ducts*. The hilar ducts are lined by columnar mucinous epithelium, have a distinct fibromuscular wall, and are associated with both intramural and extramural seromucinous peribiliary glands, which communicate with the bile duct lumen. The same type of peribiliary glands are also demonstrated around intrahepatic large bile ducts [68].

Vascular and lymphatic network

The major blood vessels that supply the liver are the *portal vein* and *hepatic artery*, the former supplying approximately two-thirds of the total blood flow. The portal vein sequentially divides into interlobar, segmental, and interlobular veins and preterminal branches, with the terminal portal venules present in the smaller portal tracts measuring about 20–30 μm in diameter.

The hepatic artery branches accompany the portal vein, dividing within the smaller portal tracts into two segments: the periportal plexus and peribiliary plexus. The periportal plexus branches around the portal vein and drains into the sinusoids; the peribiliary plexus provides blood to the accompanying interlobular bile ducts by way of small capillaries layered around the ducts. Various connections are seen between the small arterioles and the sinusoids, which are most prominent in the periportal zone. The sinusoids, which receive blood from both the portal vein and hepatic artery, eventually drain into the terminal hepatic venules, which have no fibrous wall. These then drain into the terminal hepatic and sublobular intercalated veins and exit the liver from the three main hepatic vein branches into the inferior vena cava.

The majority of hepatic lymph is derived from the space of Disse and ultimately exits the liver at the porta hepatis to drain into the lymph nodes that are along the hepatic artery. The space of Disse lymph is protein-rich filtrate. Approximately 10% of lymph is protein-poor filtrate from peribiliary capillary leakage [1,69]. There are lymphatic vessels within the portal tracts, but how the lymph from the space of Disse gets to the portal tract is controversial. This is because there are no channels connecting the space of Disse to the portal lymphatics. One possibility is that the lymph within the space of Disse travels into the portal tract lymphatic vessels by way of "endothelial massaging," where circulating intrasinusoidal leukocytes create a pulsatile effect that moves the lymph along to the portal tract. The terminal lymphatic branches form plexuses lined by endothelial cells; they are accentuated around the hepatic arterioles in the smaller portal structures; lymphatics are also seen near portal veins and bile ducts in larger portal tracts. Small branches can be seen along the hepatic veins as well. Finally, the Glisson capsule lymphatic plexus communicates with the intrahepatic lymphatics through anastomotic channels. Most lymphatics exit the liver at the porta hepatis. In conditions of impaired venous drainage (e.g., venous outflow obstruction or cirrhosis), lymphatic drainage is prominent through the Glisson capsule.

References are available at www.yamadagastro.com/textbook7e

Further reading

Crawford J.M., Bioulac-Sage P., Hytiroglou P. Structure, function, and responses to injury. In: Burt A., Portmann B., Ferrell L. (eds). MacSween's Pathology of the Liver, 7th ed. Edinburgh: Elsevier; 2018: 1.

Eleazar J.A., Memeo L., Jhang J.S., et al. Progenitor cell expansion: an important source of hepatocyte regeneration in chronic hepatitis. J Hepatol 2004;41:983.

Friedman S.L. The cellular basis of hepatic fibrosis. N Engl J Med 1993;328:1828.

Gaudio E., Carpino G., Cardinale V., et al. New insights into liver stem cells. Dig Liver Dis 2009;41:455.

Jungermann K., Kietzmann T. Zonation of parenchymal and nonparenchymal metabolism in liver. Annu Rev Nutr 1996;16:179.

Lamers W.H., Hilberts A., Furt E., et al. Hepatic enzymic zonation: a reevaluation of the concept of the liver acinus. Hepatology 1989;10:72.

Phillips M.J., Poucell S., Patterson J., et al. The Liver: An Atlas and Text of Ultrastructural Pathology. New York: Raven Press; 1987.

Teutsch H.F. The modular microarchitecture of human liver. Hepatology 2005;42:317.

Turner R., Lozoya O., Wang Y., et al. Human hepatic stem cell and maturational liver lineage biology. Hepatology 2011;53:1035.

Wanless I.R. Physioanatomic considerations. In: Schiff E.R., Sorrell M.F., Maddrey W.C. (eds). Schiff 's Diseases of the Liver, 9th ed. Philadelphia: Lippincott Williams & Wilkins; 2003: 17.

CHAPTER 11
Gastrointestinal blood flow

Brian D. Hosfield and Troy A. Markel
Indiana University School of Medicine, Department of Surgery, Indianapolis, IN, USA

Chapter menu

The ultimate function of the gastrointestinal (GI) tract is to assimilate nutrients and water from the external environment and make them available to cells throughout the body; in this context, the blood and lymph circulations provide the conduits for transferring absorbed nutrients and water to the entire body. The vascular supply to the GI mucosa is particularly well suited for the absorptive and secretory functions of this tissue in that it can accommodate a high rate of blood flow, has a large exchange surface area, and permits easy permeation of nutrients and water, yet largely retains proteins within the plasma compartment. This chapter summarizes current concepts regarding circulatory control and function in the GI tract during normal physiological conditions. The chapter also reviews mechanisms by which the GI and hepatic circulations interact, and summarizes information relevant to the pathophysiology of intestinal ischemia. Additionally, this chapter examines the unique differences in the intestinal circulation of the newborn.

Embryology of gastrointestinal circulation

Intestinal vasculogenesis in the developing embryo occurs by vascular endothelial precursor cells (angioblasts) migrating to the position of future vessels. These angioblasts are primarily induced by fibroblast growth factor 2 (FGF-2) [1]. They subsequently differentiate into endothelial cells and form cords, and after flow is established, form patent vessels [2]. Growth factors such as vascular endothelial growth factor (VEGF), transforming growth-factor-β (TGF-β), and platelet-derived growth factor (PDGF) promote angiogenesis which add additional capillaries and microvasculature to the developing fetal intestine [3]. Additionally, erythropoietin (EPO) has been shown to stimulate angiogenesis in the gastrointestinal endothelium in neonatal rat models [4].

The developing fetal intestine is divided into three different sections: foregut, midgut, and hindgut [5,6]. Each portion of the intestine has its own respective blood supply: the celiac artery supplies the foregut, the superior mesenteric artery supplies the midgut, and inferior mesenteric artery supplies the hindgut (Figure 11.1) [7]. Contrary to the arterial supply, the venous drainage of the developing fetal intestine is much more variable [2].

Anatomy of the gastrointestinal circulation

Extramural vessels

Arteries

After birth, the major arteries supplying the stomach and intestines are the celiac, superior mesenteric, and inferior mesenteric

Yamada's Textbook of Gastroenterology, Seventh Edition. Edited by Timothy C. Wang, Michael Camilleri, Benjamin Lebwohl, Anna S. Lok, William J. Sandborn, Kenneth K. Wang, and Gary D. Wu.

Companion website: www.yamadagastro.com/textbook7e

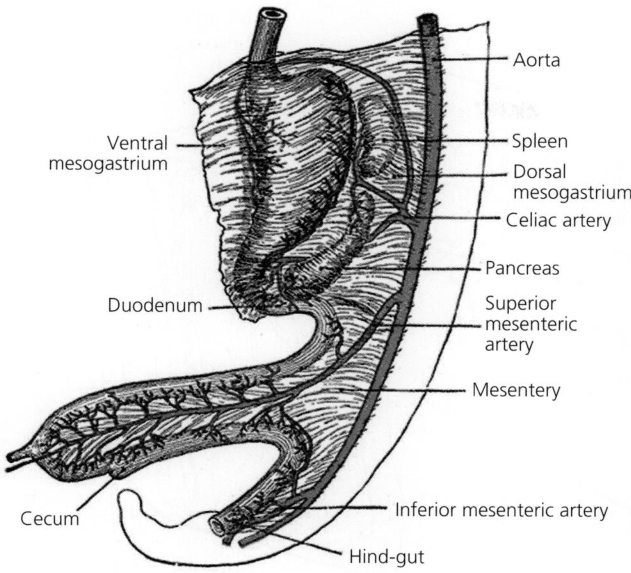

Figure 11.1 Embryologic development of blood supply to the gut, showing the celiac artery supplying the foregut, the superior mesenteric artery supplying the midgut, and the inferior mesenteric artery supplying the hindgut. Source: Based upon Gray and Lewis 1918 [7]. Public Domain.

arteries. The celiac artery supplies the stomach, the first portion of the duodenum, a portion of the pancreas, and the liver. The superior mesenteric artery supplies the remainder of the pancreas and duodenum, the jejunum, the ileum, and the colon through two thirds of the transverse segment. The inferior mesenteric artery supplies the remainder of the colon and rectum, except the distal rectum, which is supplied by rectal arteries arising from the internal iliac arteries. Along the mesenteric border of the intestine, arterial and venous branches form multiple arcades, anastomose with one another, and provide a pathway for collateral blood flow. The arcades give rise to vasa recta, which branch to encircle the intestine and ultimately pierce the circular muscle [8–10].

Veins

Blood from the stomach, pancreas, and intestines drains into the portal vein, except for that of the distal rectum, which drains into the internal iliac veins. The vessels that drain the intestines course within the mesentery, except those vessels supplying retroperitoneal portions [8–10].

Intramural vessels and microcirculation

Stomach

In the human stomach, submucosal arterioles branch into capillaries at the base of the gastric glands, pass perpendicularly through the mucosa, form a lumenal capillary network, and drain into mucosal venules only at the most lumenal level of the lamina propria (Figure 11.2). These venular branches converge on infrequent mucosal collecting venules, which then pass directly to the submucous venous plexus without receiving any direct capillary tributaries within the mucosa [11].

Small intestine

Small arteries pierce the muscularis layers and give rise to 1A submucosal arterioles that in turn generate an extensive, anastomosed series of 2A arterioles. These arterioles function as a pressure manifold for 3A arterioles that descend into the mucosa to form the villus microcirculation; as well, 4A arterioles branch from the 3A vessels and ascend into the muscularis layers. A tufted pattern of capillaries, derived from the tubular capillary plexus underlying the epithelium of the crypts, supplies the basal 70–80% of the villus and also drains into the venule high in the villus (Figure 11.3) [9,12].

Colon

The colonic mucosa is devoid of villi; therefore, the arterioles and their capillary branches pass to the basal epithelial surface between the crypts to form a network of capillary plexuses around the crypts. The colonic capillaries are much closer to the epithelial cells than are the villus capillaries in the small intestine [13].

Mechanisms of blood flow regulation

Intrinsic systems

Blood flow in the GI tract is tightly controlled within narrow limits. This is largely due to intrinsic vascular regulatory systems, or stated differently, mechanisms that originate and remain within the intestinal parenchyma and its attendant circulation. Three well-identified systems merit review: the myogenic mechanism, metabolic mechanism, and nitric oxide (NO) derived from the endothelial isoform of NO synthase (eNOS). Integration of these systems occurs at a molecular level and their relative activities are most certainly modified by other vasoactive stimuli (e.g., peptides, hormones, neural input) that arise from intrinsic or extrinsic sites.

Myogenic vascular response

The Frank–Starling law states that as the heart stretches, its force of contraction increases [14]. British physiologist William Bayliss described a similar phenomenon in 1902 known as the intrinsic myogenic response, where vascular smooth muscles in vasculature contract more forcefully as they stretch [15]. The myogenic response has been repeatedly demonstrated within the intestinal circulation, most commonly by documenting vasoconstriction in response to increased intravascular pressure [16–21]. Conversely, reduced intravascular pressure leads to myogenic dilation [22]. Though the complete mechanism of the myogenic response remains understood, there are several theories that postulate that contraction is mediated by calcium induced phosphorylation of myosin followed by activation of the actin-myosin motor unit [23,24]. Protein kinase C (PKC) also may increase the sensitivity of the actin-myosin motor unit to calcium [25].

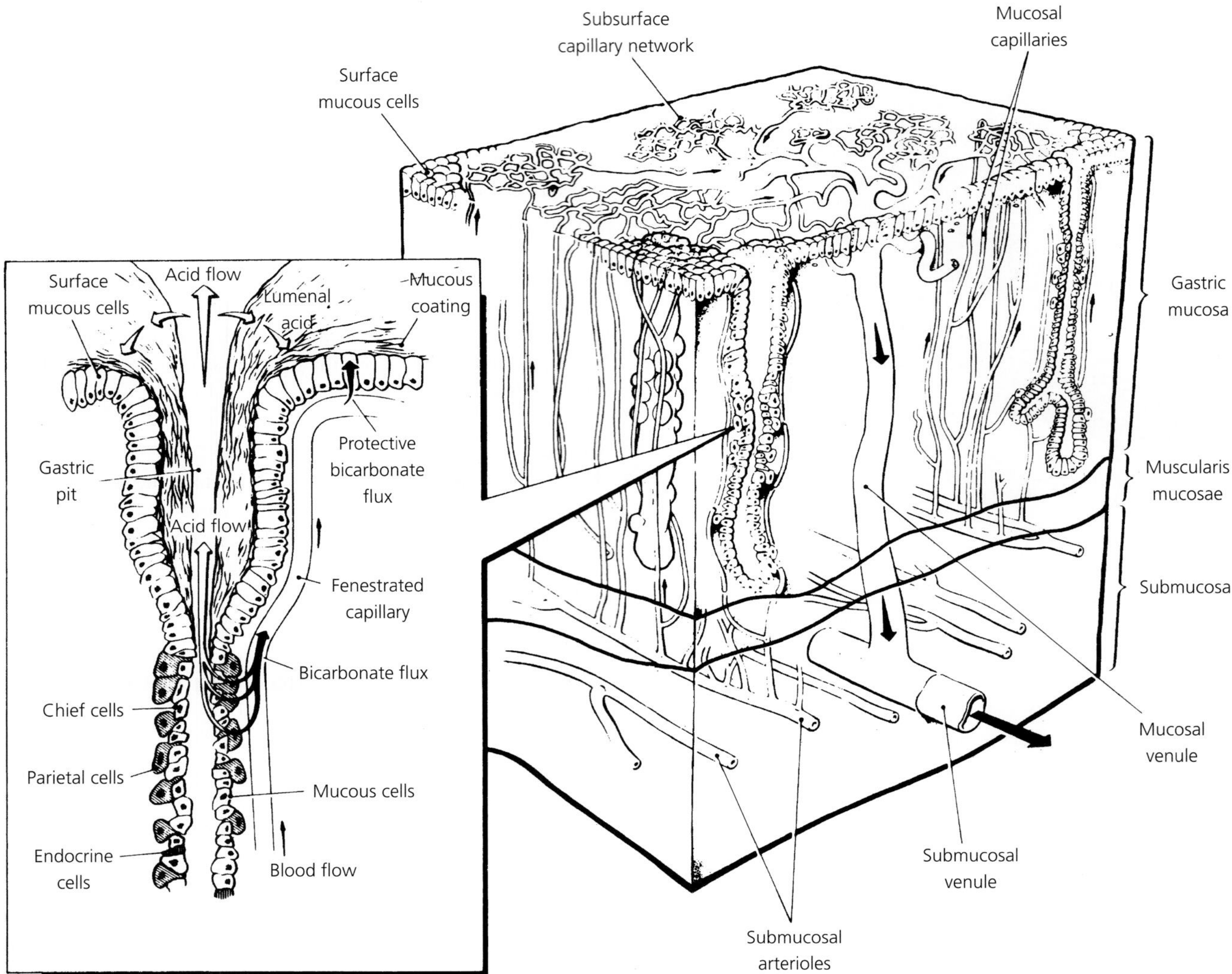

Figure 11.2 The vascular organization in gastric mucosa **(right)**. The proposed mechanism for the vascular transport of HCO_3^- is toward the surface mucous cells from deeper within the mucosa **(inset left)**. Source: Gannon et al. 1984 [11]. Reproduced with permission of Elsevier.

Intrinsic myogenicity of the intestinal vasculature has at least two physiological roles. First, it contributes to the basal vascular tone and thus participates in setting vascular resistance across the intestine; in this context, the myogenic mechanism generates vascular tone that is independent of extrinsic neural stimuli [22,26]. Second, it serves to regulate vascular wall tension and in this capacity participates in pressure–flow autoregulation [16,19,27,28] and helps preserve homeostasis of capillary filtration [17,29–32].

Metabolic vascular regulation

A consistent experimental observation is that the intensity of vasoregulation within the intestine is contingent upon its momentary rate of O_2 utilization (O_2 demand), a finding which strongly suggests that the gut parenchyma produces a factor that is indexed to tissue metabolic activity and that this factor regulates the gut circulation. This concept is the basis of the metabolic theory of local blood flow regulation, which states that tissue oxygenation, not blood flow, is the principal variable regulated by intrinsic vascular control mechanisms. The theory partitions microvascular control into two sites: resistance vessels and precapillary sphincters. The former regulate the flow of blood, and hence oxygen delivery to the capillary level, wherein O_2 delivery is defined as the product of blood flow rate and O_2 concentration. Precapillary sphincters govern perfusion of individual capillaries, and hence the surface area available for O_2 diffusion from capillary to cell. The metabolic feedback signal serves to vasodilate resistance vessels and open precapillary sphincters. Anything that reduces the O_2 delivery-to-demand ratio (e.g., hypotension, hypoxemia, or increased tissue O_2 demand during digestion) increases production of the metabolic feedback signal, an action that increases net O_2 transport to the gut parenchyma and restores O_2 homeostasis [33].

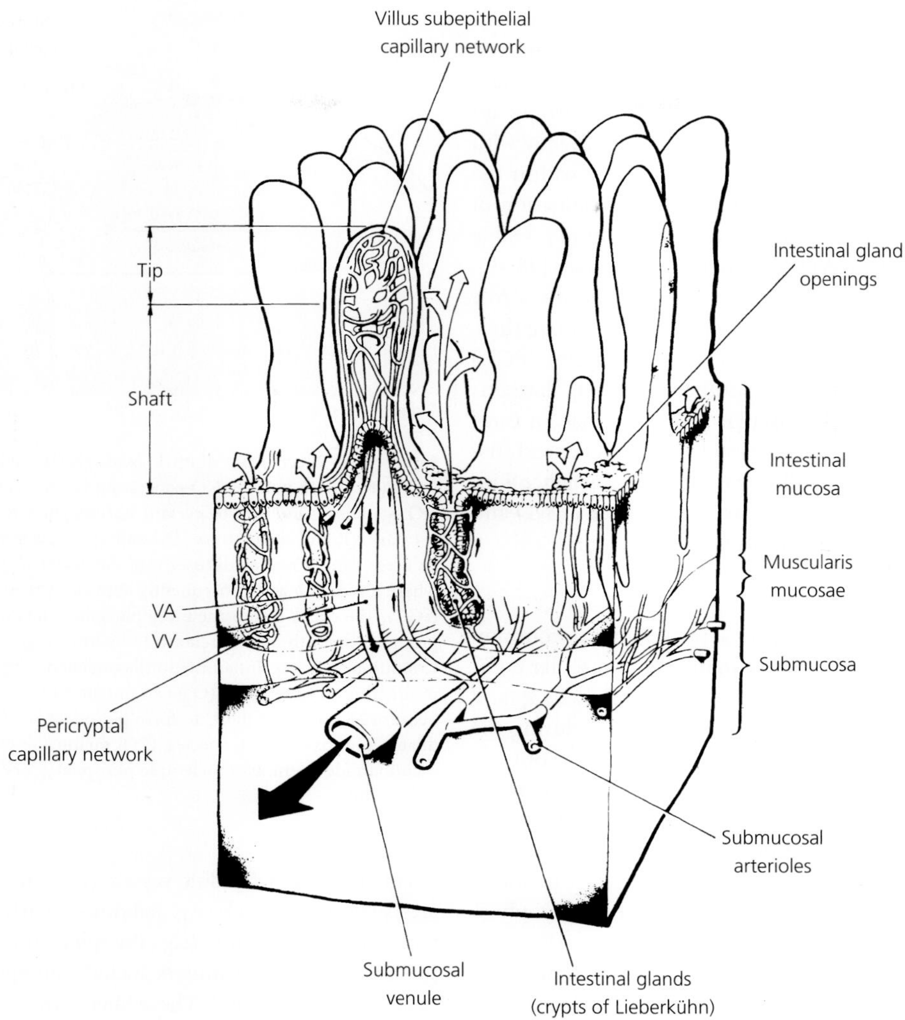

Figure 11.3 Mucosal microcirculatory patterns typical of human and rabbit small intestine. VA, villus arteriole; VV, villus venule. Source: Adapted from Frasher and Wayland 1972 [12].

An important aspect of the metabolic theory is that precapillary sphincters are more sensitive to the metabolic feedback signal than resistance vessels [33]. Hence, the first response to a reduction in the O_2 delivery-to-demand ratio is the opening of closed precapillary sphincters, an effect that has been experimentally confirmed by noting increases in the capillary filtration coefficient ($K_{f,c}$) and the arteriovenous O_2 content difference across the intestine in response to a reduction in the O_2 delivery-to-demand ratio [20,34–36]. Dilation of resistance vessels and hence augmentation of flow only occur when capillary PO_2 is no longer sufficient to drive the capillary cell O_2 diffusion process. This phenomenon may explain why the intrinsic regulation of intestinal blood flow is enhanced when the intestinal metabolic rate, and hence tissue O_2 demand is increased [18,37,38].

The precise identity of the metabolite that drives this theory is unknown, although several reports suggest adenosine as a viable candidate for this role. Adenosine is generated during metabolic utilization of adenosine triphosphate (ATP) and its accumulation in venous blood has been demonstrated under conditions where tissue oxygenation might be reduced, such as following arterial hypoxemia or occlusion, or during the active transport of nutrients. Indeed, this is the same mechanism that governs metabolic coronary vasodilation, as the accumulation of adenosine augments increased coronary blood flow [39]. There are studies to suggest that adenosine is also a powerful intestinal vasodilator [40]. The role of adenosine in local vasoregulation has been assessed using substances such as theophylline, a competitive antagonist, by the enzyme adenosine deaminase, which converts adenosine to inosine, and by dipyridamole, an inhibitor of adenosine reuptake. These agents have been shown to attenuate or completely abolish the vasodilation associated with reductions in arterial pressure, release of an arterial occlusion, hypoxemia, and absorption of nutrients [41,45].

Other studies suggest that molecular O_2 itself dictates vascular tone, either directly or via generation of endothelium-derived autacoids – biological factors that act like local hormones near the site of synthesis. Microvascular studies demonstrate an inverse relationship between villus PO_2, measured directly with O_2 sensitive electrodes, and the rate of blood flow within the submucosal and villus microvasculature [46,47]. Reduction of PO_2 within vascular smooth muscle causes relaxation, possibly due to the effects of PO_2 on ATP-dependent K^+ channels [48,49]. Alternatively, a considerable body of evidence supports a role for the vascular endothelium as an oxygen-sensing organ; thus, release of vasorelaxing autacoids such as prostacyclin (PGI_2) and NO can occur in response to endothelial hypoxia that ultimately lead to a reduction in vascular resistance that, in turn, increase bloodflow and O_2 delivery [50,51]. In this context, tissue PO_2 functions as the controlled variable (in accordance with the metabolic theory), while secondary agents such as NO and PGI_2 are the effector mechanisms (the feedback signal).

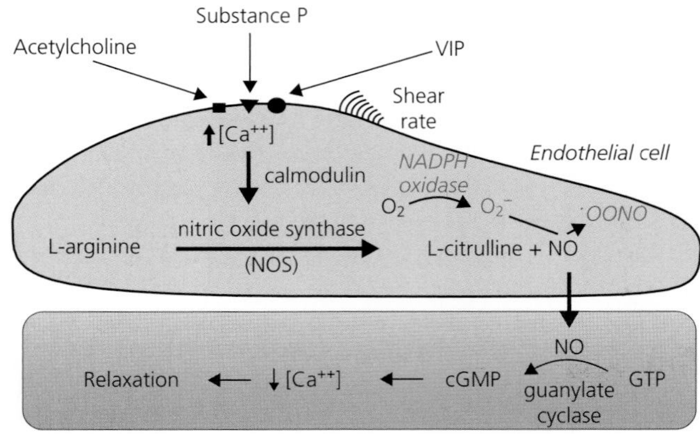

Figure 11.4 Mechanism of nitric oxide (NO)-mediated relaxation of vascular smooth muscle. NO generation by the endothelial cell enzyme NO synthase is induced by certain stimuli, such as acetylcholine, substance P, and shear stress. The endothelial cell-derived NO produced by these stimuli readily diffuses into the underlying smooth muscle cells, where it binds to and consequently activates soluble guanylate cyclase (sGC). The cyclic guanosine monophosphate (cGMP) produced by sGC promotes smooth muscle relaxation by lowering intracellular calcium. Conditions (such as inflammation) associated with an increased production of superoxide (O_2^-) can impair NO-mediated vasodilation because NO reacts with O_2^- to form peroxynitrate (·OONO), a less potent dilator and toxic radical species. GTP, guanosine triphosphate; NADPH, nicotinamide adenine dinucleotide phosphate; VIP, vasoactive intestinal polypeptide.

Nitric oxide

eNOS-derived NO has emerged as a pivotal "final common pathway" in vasodilation and its role in intestinal vascular regulation has been established by both anatomical [52,53] and physiological studies [54–57]. eNOS generates NO during the reduction of L-arginine to L-citrulline, in the presence of Ca^{2+}, calmodulin, O_2, tetrahydrobiopterin, and nicotinamideadenine-dinucleotide phosphate (NADPH). The principal mechanism of NO-based vasodilation is activation of soluble guanylate cyclase in adjacent vascular smooth muscle. This leads to a cascade of events characterized by: increased cyclic guanosine monophosphate (cGMP) production, reduced [Ca^{2+}], cell relaxation, and net increase in vessel diameter (Figure 11.4) (see [58] and [59] for reviews of eNOS biochemistry and molecular biology).

The most convincing evidence for NO-based intestinal vasoregulation comes from microvascular studies using NO-sensitive microelectrodes placed immediately adjacent to submucosal vessels. Periarteriolar NO exceeds the dissociation constant for soluble guanylate cyclase; as well, this variable exists in direct correlation with arteriolar diameter and increases in response to shear stress, hypoxemia, and nutrient absorption, perturbations that lead to arteriolar dilation [55,60,61]. Moreover, attenuation of eNOS activity with L-arginine analogs causes relative vasoconstriction of the intestine, indicating that constitutive eNOS activity (and hence NO production) participates in gut vasoregulation [54]. eNOS-derived NO also participates in flow-induced dilation within the intestine, i.e., the vascular phenomenon by which an increase in flow rate increases vessel diameter [56].

Extrinsic systems

Central nervous system

The GI tract is innervated by postganglionic (sympathetic) fibers emanating from celiac, superior mesenteric, and inferior mesenteric ganglia [63]. Both anatomical and physiological studies demonstrate sympathetic innervation in virtually all portions of the gut circulation, from conduit vessels (e.g., the superior mesenteric artery) to microvessels (e.g., submucosal arterioles) to the mesenteric venous vasculature (e.g., the splanchnic capacitance vessels). Identified neurotransmitters include norepinephrine, ATP, and neuropeptide Y [64,65]. These fibers provide the sole neurogenic vasoconstrictor stimuli to submucosal arterioles [65].

Direct stimulation of the postganglionic mesenteric nerve fibers causes brisk vasoconstriction; however, this effect is not sustained, even in the face of continued nerve stimulation. This response is termed autoregulatory escape (Figure 11.5) [62,66–68]. A similar phenomenon occurs during intraarterial infusion of the neurotransmitter norepinephrine [62]. Autoregulatory escape occurs in arteriolar smooth muscle, but not in venous smooth muscle [66]. Additionally, it is unaltered by β-receptor blockade [67] or by administration of atropine [68]. Three proposed mechanisms to explain autoregulatory escape are redistribution of blood flow from the mucosa to the submucosa, adaptation of adrenergic receptors to continued nerve stimulation, and accumulation of vasodilator metabolites during tissue hypoxia resulting from nerve-induced ischemia. The last explanation is the most widely accepted [69–72]. Consistent with this theory is experimental evidence that the propensity for blood flow to escape from sympathetic vasoconstriction is significantly greater in the metabolically active mucosa than in the more metabolically dormant muscularis [73]. Adenosine appears to play at least a partial role in autoregulatory escape [62].

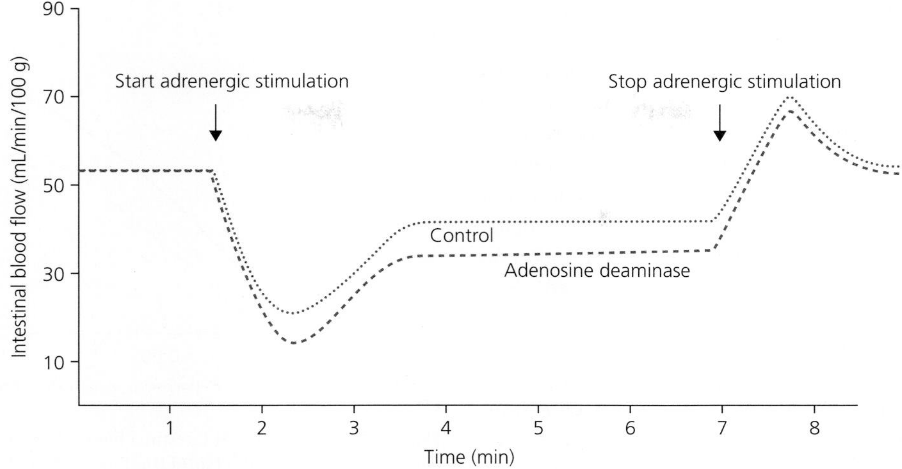

Figure 11.5 Autoregulatory escape from adrenergic stimulation in autoperfused piglet small intestine. Adenosine deaminase pretreatment reduced the steady-state escape response to norepinephrine infusion, whereas pretreatment with chlorpheniramine, a histamine H_1 blocker, had no effect. Source: Data from Crissinger et al. 1988 [62].

Extrinsic, preganglionic, afferent (sensory) fibers that arise from dorsal root ganglia also innervate the GI vasculature [65]. Substance P (SP) and calcitonin gene-related peptide (CGRP) serve as neurotransmitters for these fibers. Stimulation of extrinsic afferents with capsaicin causes vasodilation of submucosal arterioles [74–76].

The GI tract also receives extensive cholinergic parasympathetic innervation via the vagus nerve (stomach, small intestine) and pelvic nerve (colon), although the role of these fibers in regulation of gut perfusion is unclear. Early studies failed to demonstrate significant change in gut vascular tone following direct stimulation of the vagus or after vagotomy [77,78]. Subsequent work, however, has revealed vasodilation of intestinal submucosal arterioles in response to vagal stimulation [79]. For more in-depth discussion on the central nervous system's role in gastrointestinal blood flow, see Chapter 12.

Enteric nervous system

The GI tract has a complex nervous system that contains both sensory and motor neurons capable of function in the absence of extrinsic neural input [80]. Submucosal arterioles are innervated by afferent and efferent fibers that emanate from both myenteric and submucosal neurons; currently, it is believed that myenteric long fibers synapse with submucosal neurons that in turn innervate submucosal arterioles [65]. Direct stimulation of myenteric ganglia induces vasodilation of the submucosal arterioles [81] that is mediated by a variety of neurotransmitters: acetylcholine [82], SP [82], CGRP [83], and neuropeptide Y [84]. Additionally, a reflex arc connecting afferent fibers arising from the villi to submucosal and myenteric ganglia, and thence to submucosal arterioles, has been identified. Chemical and mechanical stimulation of the mucosa activates this reflex arc and induces submucosal arteriolar vasodilation [83,85]. This phenomenon suggests that the enteric nervous system may elicit vasodilation in response to mucosal events such as nutrient absorption, as well as the mucosal inflammation present in ulcerative colitis [65]. Reviews of the role of the enteric nervous system in gut vascular regulation are available [65,83].

Circulating vasoactive substances

Circulating vasoactive substances that affect GI blood flow include catecholamines, vasopressin, and angiotensin. Norepinephrine, a predominantly α-adrenergic receptor stimulant, causes intestinal vasoconstriction, a decrease in capillary density, and a reduction in oxygen uptake [69,86,87]. With continuous intraarterial infusion, the intense initial vasoconstriction is followed by the return of blood flow toward control levels despite continued norepinephrine infusion. Epinephrine can cause either α-receptor-mediated vasoconstriction at high doses or β-receptor-mediated vasodilation at low doses, as well as a variable response in oxygen uptake [69,88,89].

Both vasopressin and angiotensin II are potent physiological vasoconstrictors that increase vascular resistant and subsequently reduce blood flow in all GI organs. These agents cause generalized vasoconstriction, with a disproportionate selective reduction in mesenteric blood flow at doses that have been measured in pathophysiological states of hypotension [90]. Vasopressin causes a decrease in capillary density and a reduction in intestinal oxygen uptake, whereas angiotensin II reduces or does not affect splanchnic oxygen uptake [91]. In normal rat intestine, α-adrenergic and vasopressin activity account for most extrinsic vasoconstrictor tone. In a portal hypertension rat model, vasopressin and angiotensin II account for the majority of extrinsic vasoconstrictor tone [92]. Renin-angiotensin and vasopressin systems are also involved in the intestinal vasoconstrictor response to hemorrhage and hypovolemia, and significant attenuation of this increase in vascular resistance occurs only when both systems are blocked simultaneously [93,94], even in the presence of an intact sympathetic system.

Another key circulating vasoactive substance is hydrogen sulfide (H_2S). H_2S is an endogenous gasotransmitter that is known to have vasodilatory properties [95,96]. By donating a sulfur moiety to cysteine, H_2S can modify several proteins by replacing a -SH group on cysteine to an -SSH group (also known as a perisulfide group), a process known as persulfidation [97]. Though the exact mechanism which H_2S causes vasodilation remains unknown, there are data to suggest it may be mediated through potentiating eNOS and NO. When eNOS undergoes persulfidation by H_2S, it dimerizes [98]. Once dimerized, eNOS is able to produce NO and subsequent downstream vasodilation [58]. Mesenchymal stem cells (MSCs) have been shown to have mesenteric vasodilatory properties [99]. and these benefits are dependent upon H_2S. When H_2S producing enzyme cystathione β synthase (CBS) was knocked down with siRNA, MSCs lost their vasodilatory properties [100]. Additionally, when MSCs were given to mesenteric arteries isolated from eNOS knockout mice, vasodilation was attenuated, further suggesting a dependency on eNOS (100). However, there are other studies that have shown H_2S has NO-independent vasodilatory properties [101]. H_2S donors have been studied in animal models for attenuating intestinal injury, including NSAID-induced intestinal injury [102,103], colitis [104,105], and ischemia/reperfusion injury [96,106–108]. Aside from vasodilatory properties, H_2S has also been shown to decrease cell death and apoptosis [109].

Response of the intestinal circulation to systemic circulatory perturbations

Pressure–flow autoregulation

Pressure–flow autoregulation, or more simply autoregulation, is a physiological response designed to maintain blood flow relatively constant in the face of fluctuation in the pressure gradient across an organ or tissue. The relationship among flow, pressure, and resistance is given by the equation

$$\text{flow} = (P_A - P_V)/R$$

where P_A and P_v are arterial and venous pressures, and R is resistance. Assuming that P_V remains constant, evidence of autoregulation would include an increase in R (vasoconstriction) in the face of increased P_A (hypertension), or a reduced R (vasodilation) in response to a lowered P_A (hypotension). Autoregulation is also elicited in the stomach [110,111], small intestine [37], and colon [19,20,112] (Figure 11.6).

Autoregulation is generally ascribed to both myogenic [113] and metabolic [18,37,112,114] processes. The myogenic response would reflect the inherent tendency of the circumferential arterial vascular smooth muscle to contract or relax as a function of the prevailing intravascular pressure, insofar as that pressure affects the stretch stimulus applied to the muscle cells [22]. The metabolic response is less straightforward. For example, hypotension would initially compromise gut perfusion and reduce O_2 delivery. This circumstance reduces the O_2 delivery-to-demand ratio, producing more adenosine and subsequent vasodilation as described above [40]. However, active regulation

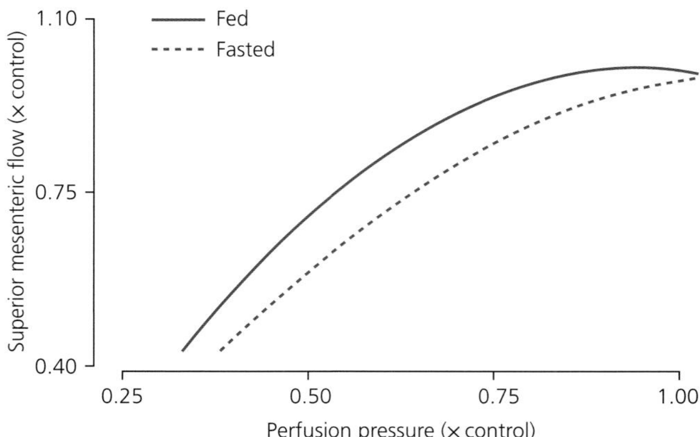

Figure 11.6 Responses of intestinal blood flow to step reductions in perfusion pressure in fed **(solid line)** versus fasted **(dashed line)** dogs demonstrate an increased intensity of autoregulation during enhanced functional activity. Source: Granger and Norris 1980 [38]. Reproduced with permission of the American Physiological Society.

of precapillary sphincters designed to enhance capillary surface area and hence the diffusive flux of O_2 from capillary to cell is the first response to hypotension. This response is evidenced by a rise in the capillary filtration coefficient, a marker of the perfused capillary density, as pressure falls [34,36,38]. Evidence of autoregulation (vasodilation) only occurs when capillary PO_2 falls below the level needed to drive O_2 diffusion to maintain tissue oxygenation, the variable controlled by the metabolic mechanism [115]. This circumstance explains why the efficacy of autoregulation is significantly enhanced when the oxidative requirements of the intestine are increased by feeding [18,37,38].

Alterations in arterial blood gas tensions (hypoxemia) and hematocrit

Alterations in arterial blood gases affect GI blood flow. Arterial hypoxemia increases the perfused capillary density and causes vasodilation, and hence increased perfusion in denervated intestinal preparations [115,116]. The vasodilation and increased perfused capillary density tend to minimize the reduction in oxygen uptake induced by the limited oxygen delivery. When blood flow is held constant, the intestine maintains oxygen consumption within 48% of control during arterial hypoxemia. When both blood flow and capillary density are free to increase, however, oxygen uptake remains within 26% of control despite the hypoxia. Similar to hypoxia, hypercapnia induces a marked relaxation of resistance vessels [116]. In contrast to hypoxia, hypercapnia causes the precapillary sphincters to constrict and the capillary density to decrease [116].

Alterations in arterial hematocrit also influence GI blood flow and oxygenation [117–120]. An inverse linear correlation exists between the intestinal blood flow and hematocrit, and a direct linear correlation between the arteriovenous oxygen difference and hematocrit in both the intestine and stomach. The relation between intestinal oxygen uptake and hematocrit is

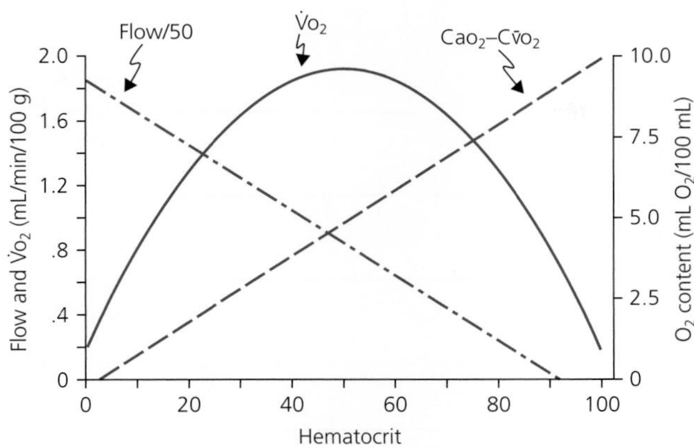

Figure 11.7 Effect of hematocrit on canine intestinal blood flow, oxygen consumption (VO_2), arterial oxygen content, and arteriovenous oxygen difference (C_AO_2 – CvO_2). Source: Shepherd and Riedel 1982 [120]. Reproduced with permission of Wolters Kluwer Health.

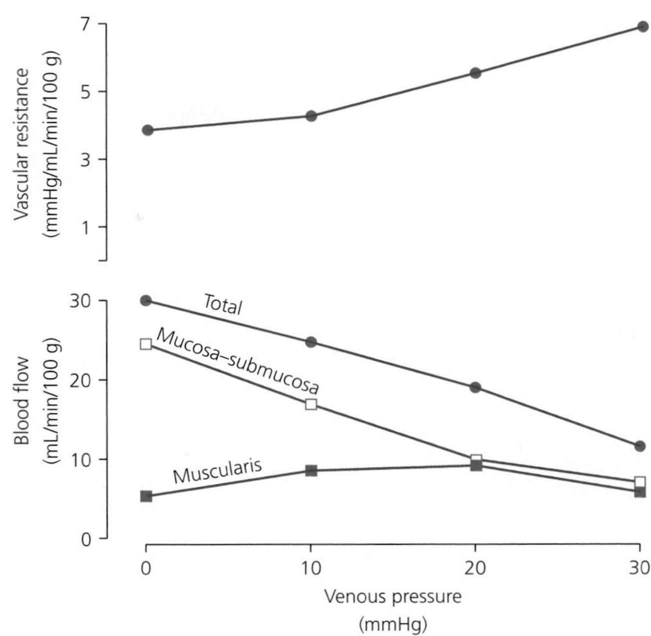

Figure 11.8 Intestinal vascular responses to acute venous hypertension in cats. The increase in vascular resistance and decrease in blood flow during acute venous pressure elevation are consistent with the myogenic theory of intrinsic vasoregulation. Source: Data from Granger et al. 1979 [29].

parabolic (Figure 11.7) [120], showing a maximal uptake at a hematocrit of 48.7% – that is, the optimal hematocrit. Intraluminal placement of nutrients increases the optimal hematocrit to 57.1%. In the stomach, the optimal hematocrit is 38.2% during resting conditions, and it increases to 45.7% during pentagastrin-stimulated acid secretion.

Venous pressure elevation

Studies of the stomach, small intestine, and colon in adult animals indicate that vascular resistance rises in response to venous pressure elevation, findings consistent with a myogenic mechanism (Figure 11.8) [16–21,27,29–31,112,121,122]. Acute venous hypertension in the adult intestine elicits vasoconstriction as a result of rising precapillary (arteriolar) resistance while postcapillary resistance falls [123]. Capillary exchange capacity decreases in the small intestine during venous hypertension [124]. Despite the intense capillary derecruitment initiated by venous hypertension in the small intestine, oxygen extraction increases disproportionately to the reduced blood flow and consequently oxygen consumption rises [31]. The elevated intestinal oxygen utilization during venous hypertension has been attributed to increased villus motility [125]. Animal studies have demonstrated conflicting reports regarding the influence of enhanced oxidative metabolism on the vascular responses to elevations in venous pressure. Some investigators have observed that increased oxygen demand significantly reduces or abolishes the rise in vascular resistance [38,121], whereas others have noted an exaggerated resistance response to venous pressure elevation [120].

Acute venous hypertension alters the distribution of blood flow within the bowel wall [29,126,127]. As venous pressure is elevated, blood flow is redirected from the mucosa and submucosa to the muscularis. These observations indicate that the constriction of arteriolar and precapillary sphincter smooth muscles elicited by venous hypertension takes place in the mucosal and submucosal layers, and that the vasculature of the muscularis dilates in response to venous hypertension (see Figure 11.8).

Oxygen uptake–blood flow relation: functional implications

Considerable attention has been devoted to the interaction between GI blood flow and oxygen uptake, and the relevance of this interaction to mucosal function and integrity. Blood flow is altered in response to oxygen uptake in a graded manner (Figure 11.9) [34]. Oxygen uptake is relatively constant and it is independent of blood flow, but becomes compromised when blood flow reaches a critically low level. Below this level, oxygen uptake is dependent on blood flow. Resting blood flow in the small intestine, stomach, and colon is usually greater than the critical blood flow at which oxygen uptake is blood flow dependent [21,128–130].

The mechanism of reduction in oxygen uptake that occurs when blood flow falls below a critical level can be explained in terms of the normal relation between mitochondrial oxygen consumption and cell PO_2. This relation predicts that oxygen uptake remains constant over a wide range of cell PO_2 levels, and uptake is reduced only when cell PO_2 falls to a low level, the critical PO_2. The resting cell PO_2 is normally well above the critical PO_2. Evidence indicates that graded reductions in blood flow produce concomitant reductions in cell PO_2 without altering oxygen uptake in the stomach [91]. At very low rates of blood

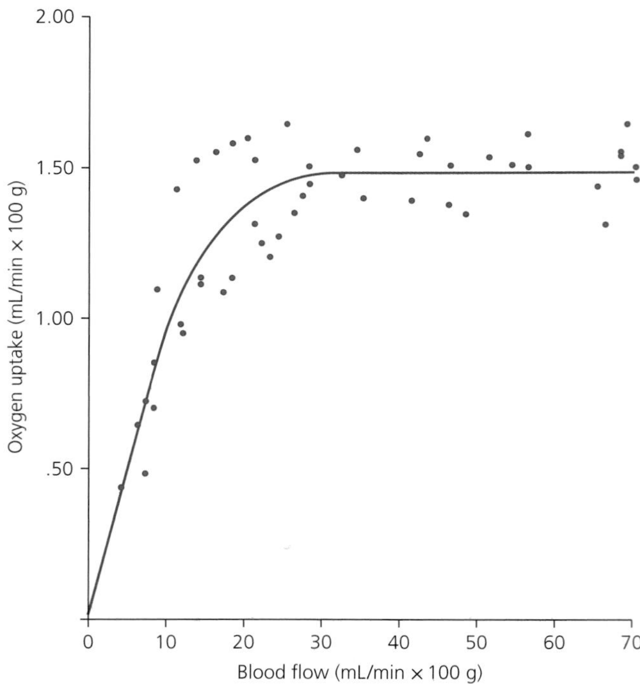

Figure 11.9 Relation between intestinal blood flow and oxygen uptake in feline jejunoileum when blood flow is altered with a pump or by graded reductions in perfusion pressure. Source: Granger et al. 1982 [34]. Reproduced with permission of the American Physiological Society.

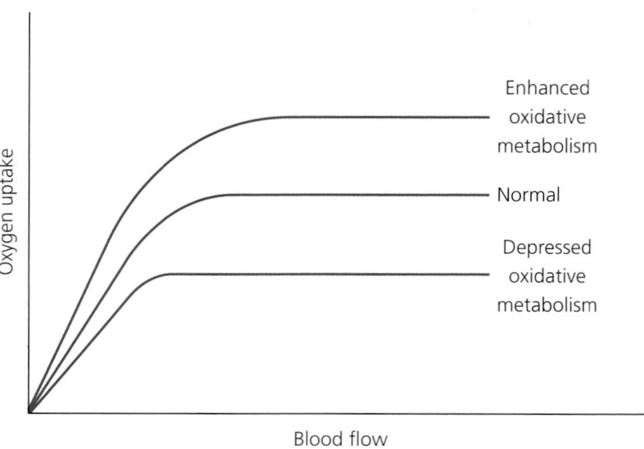

Figure 11.10 Relation between blood flow and oxygen uptake during stimulation or inhibition of oxidative metabolism. Source: Kvietys and Granger 1982 [91]. Reproduced with permission of the American Physiological Society.

flow, however, the rate of oxygen diffusion to the cells is so low that the intracellular PO_2 falls below the level required to maintain normal oxidative metabolism. This reduction in oxygen uptake observed at low blood flow may simply reflect a depression in oxidative metabolism caused by the limited oxygen availability.

Many conditions alter the relation between oxygen uptake and blood flow such that oxygen uptake is dependent on blood flow even when it is increased above the previously discussed critical low threshold. These include luminal distension [131], alterations in hematocrit [132], and devascularization [113]. All these conditions are thought to reduce tissue oxygenation severely in discrete or generalized regions of the stomach or gut. Luminal distension and devascularization reduce tissue oxygenation by compromising blood flow or redistributing it to the muscularis layer, whereas a low hematocrit limits oxygen delivery, even at high blood flows. Normal physiological conditions can also influence the relation between oxygen uptake and blood flow. Stimulation or inhibition of oxidative metabolism will shift the plateau of the blood flow–oxygen uptake curve upward or downward, respectively (Figure 11.10) [91]. Stimulation of intestinal motility or enhancement of active transport raises the plateau of the blood flow–oxygen uptake curve [36]. Conversely, decreasing the temperature of isolated bowel segments lowers the plateau. Another important aspect of the blood flow–oxygen uptake relation in the small bowel is that it can predict the influence of blood flow reductions on oxygen-requiring processes, such as absorption and secretion. For example, it has been shown that the reductions in glucose absorption produced by graded decrements in blood flow parallel the decline in oxygen uptake [133], suggesting that oxygen availability limits solute transport when cell PO_2 falls.

The relation between blood flow and oxygen uptake has also been useful in explaining some of the reported observations regarding the influence of blood flow on gastric acid secretion [134]. The production of gastric acid is an energy-consuming process that results in an increase in gastric oxygen uptake. The consistent finding that acid secretion and oxygen consumption are highly correlated raises the question of whether acid secretion in the stomach is dependent on blood flow. The answer to this question largely depends on the experimental preparation employed. In some preparations, a number of vessels supplying the stomach are occluded, and the end result is flow-dependent oxygen uptake. In this situation, an increase or decrease in blood flow is associated with a corresponding change in acid secretion. In normally perfused preparations, however, acid secretion and blood flow exhibit a relation similar to that observed between oxygen consumption and blood flow; acid secretion is dependent on blood flow at low blood flow rates and is independent at higher flow rates. This explains why vasoconstrictors tend to reduce gastric acid output and why some vasodilators (i.e., acid secretagogs) increase acid output whereas others (i.e., nonsecretagogs) do not.

Postprandial hyperemia

The term *postprandial hyperemia* is used to describe the increase in blood flow that occurs in response to a meal. The anticipatory-ingestion phase of digestion is characterized by transient increases in heart rate, cardiac output, and aortic pressure; however, GI blood flow is either unchanged or slightly increased [135–139]. These transient hemodynamic responses appear to be mediated by activation of the sympathetic nervous system, because they can be attenuated by adrenergic blocking agents [139].

In conscious animals, blood flow to the stomach and proximal bowel increases 30–90 min after ingestion of a meal [135–138]. Blood flow to the ileum increases 45–120 min postprandially. However, colonic blood flow generally does not increase postprandially [140–142]. Transient decreases in distal colon blood flow have been observed 30 min after a meal, a response attributed to tonic contractions produced by the gastrocolic reflex [142]. Blood flow in the superior mesenteric artery of conscious animals typically increases by 25–130% after ingestion of a meal [135–137,143]. The splanchnic vasodilation may last for 4–7 h, depending on the nature and quantity of the meal [144,145]. A smaller increase (10–60%) in blood flow is observed in isolated bowel segments in adult animals after intralumenal placement of digested food or nutrient solutions. This is consistent with findings in human subjects wherein intraduodenal perfusion with a test meal elicits a 35–45% increase in superior mesenteric artery flow, with no differences in postprandial splanchnic flow noted between genders [146]. While the performance of a mental task (color-word conflict test) tends to exert a vasoconstrictor influence on superior mesenteric blood flow in fasting subjects, it does not counter the vasodilatory effect of meal ingestion [146].

Constituents of chyme responsible for postprandial hyperemia

Considerable effort has been devoted to defining the lumenal stimuli responsible for postprandial hyperemia. Lumenal placement of undigested food does not elicit hyperemia, whereas digested food significantly increases blood flow [147]. The latter observation indicates that hydrolytic products of food digestion initiate the hyperemia.

Bile appears to play an important role in postprandial intestinal hyperemia. The role of bile in postprandial intestinal hyperemia is dependent upon its concentration. In canines, ten percent gallbladder bile, the steady state concentration in proximal bowel in the early postprandial period, does not increase jejunal blood flow, yet it appears to render glucose and long-chain fatty acids vasoactive [148]. Thirty-three percent gallbladder bile renders both short-chain fatty acids (e.g., caproic acid) and amino acids vasoactive and further enhances glucose-induced hyperemia. Although intralumenal placement of endogenous or synthetic bile does not have a direct vasoactive effect in the jejunum, bile more than doubles blood flow in the ileum [148,149]. Bile acids are largely responsible for bile-induced hyperemia, an assertion supported by the observation that cholestyramine abolishes the vasodilator effects of endogenous bile on ileal blood flow in canines [149].

Ingestion of protein-rich meals in humans and gastric placement of protein in conscious rats produces marked increases in splanchnic blood flow. In isolated loops of proximal small bowel, a protein-rich diet (64%) increases blood flow by the same extent as a carbohydrate-rich diet (68%) [150]. Although hydrolyzed proteins are well known to induce postprandial hyperemia, the precise hydrolytic metabolites of protein digestion that mediate the response remain unknown.

Solubilized long-chain fatty acids appear to be the most potent lumenal stimulus of postprandial intestinal hyperemia. Oleic acid (10–20 mM) solubilized in 10% gallbladder bile produces a 20–60% increase in intestinal blood flow [150–153]. Evidence suggests that this increase in blood flow may be a response to epithelial cell injury [152]. Relatively little is known about the vascular response of the gut to the lumenal placement or ingestion of other dietary lipids. Short-chain fatty acids (e.g., caproic acid) do not alter blood flow, even in the presence of 10% gallbladder bile. Although lipids produce the largest intestinal hyperemia, the vascular responses elicited by protein and carbohydrate are significant in that the three major dietary components of food – that is, fats, proteins, and carbohydrates – appear to act synergistically on blood flow when placed in the bowel lumen (Figure 11.11) [154].

Mechanisms

Numerous mechanisms of postprandial hyperemia relevant to the gut vasodilation that occur during the digestive/absorptive phase have been investigated. The current consensus is that the final vascular effect reflects integration of multiple inputs and that this orchestration is region specific, i.e., that the inputs relevant to the stomach, jejunum, and ileum are unique [155].

Tissue metabolic rate

Nutrient absorption is an energy-dependent process that increases intestinal metabolic rate; hence, tissue O_2 demand increases after feeding under in vivo conditions, as well as in in vitro gut loops. This effect reduces the O_2 delivery-to-demand ratio and activates the metabolic mechanism described previously. Mathematical modeling of the intestinal circulation predicts expansion of capillary surface area and intestinal vasodilation in response to this perturbation [156] and these predictions have been experimentally confirmed [38]. However, a metabolic mechanism alone does not account for all facets of postprandial hyperemia. For example, intraluminal placement of solubilized oleic acid induces a brisk hyperemia in the absence of any change in tissue O_2 uptake, and hence demand [157].

The putative role of tissue PO_2 as a stimulus for postprandial hyperemia has also been assessed on a microvascular level. Mucosal suffusion with isotonic glucose reduces villus PO_2 from ~17 to ~8 mmHg and simultaneously increases flow through the villus arteriole [115]. If the PO_2 of the mucosal suffusate is increased so that the glucose suffusion does not reduce villus PO_2, the villus arteriolar vasodilation is attenuated [47]. Once again, however, a metabolic mechanism cannot entirely account

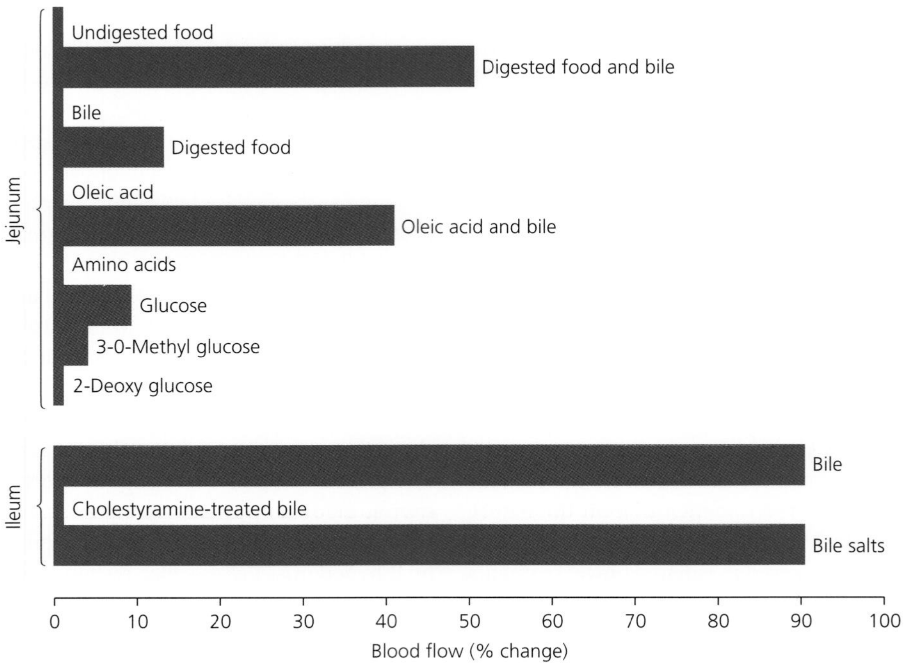

Figure 11.11 Effects of intralumenal placement of various constituents of chyme on intestinal blood flow. Source: Granger et al. 1983 [154]. Reproduced with permission of S. Karger AG.

for the villus blood flow response to glucose; vasodilation of upstream submucosal arterioles also occurs in response to glucose, despite the fact that periarteriolar PO_2 is unchanged at the submucosal level.

Adenosine

As previously discussed, adenosine has been proposed as an integral component of the metabolic mechanism, possibly functioning as a metabolic feedback signal. Adenosine is released into the venous effluent of isolated jejunal gut loops in response to intraluminal placement of a predigested meal [155]. Moreover, treatment with theophylline (adenosine receptor antagonist), dipyridamole (blocks adenosine reuptake), or adenosine deaminase attenuates food-induced vasodilation [41,158]. Other work, however, failed to demonstrate an effect of adenosine antagonism on postprandial hyperemia [37].

Sodium-induced hyperosmolarity/nitric oxide

Sodium is cotransported during the active uptake of glucose or amino acids across the villus membrane [159]. Ultimately, this process can lead to activation of eNOS and resultant NO-induced vasodilation. This process is dependent upon maintaining intracellular Na^+ homeostasis by exchanging Na^+ for Ca^{2+}, as intracellular Ca^{2+} is a potent stimulus for eNOS [160]. The perivascular concentration of Na^+ increases both within the villus and submucosal arterioles during glucose absorption [161]. Furthermore, the temporal sequence of increased perivascular Na^+ noted at the villus arterioles and thereafter at the submucosal arterioles is consistent with the timing of the vasodilation of these vessels during glucose absorption [46]. Movement of cotransported Na^+ to the submucosal space during villus glucose absorption may occur via lymphatics, as evidenced by an increase in lymph osmolarity following mucosal glucose suffusion [162]. The anatomical juxtaposition of the extensive submucosal lymphatic plexus and submucosal arterioles is ideally suited for the flux of lymphborne Na^+ to adjacent arterioles [162]. It also appears that Na^+induced eNOS activation occurs within the lymphatic with subsequent diffusion of NO to the immediately adjacent submucosal arteriole, leading to vasodilation [163,164].

eNOS-derived NO may also participate in dilation of the small arteries that lie upstream from the submucosal arteriolar plexus [163]. These vessels, the vasa recta, represent the terminal portion of the mesenteric arterial arcade and are a vital portion of the intestinal resistance vasculature [165]. The perivascular concentration of NO increases at this site during glucose infusion. Additionally, downstream blockade of the immediately adjacent venule reduced both the postglucose rise in periarteriolar NO and its subsequent vasodilation. The subsequent rise in flow rate through the arteriole would generate an additional mechanostimulus for eNOS activation, i.e., shear stress [56].

Gastrointestinal hormones

Feeding induces the production of vasoactive peptides and hormones by the gut. This effect was initially believed to contribute to postprandial hyperemia; however, subsequent work determined that postprandial concentration of these agents is below that necessary to induce a vascular effect [166]. This is best demonstrated by reviewing cholecystokinin (CCK). Intraarterial infusion of CCK induces vasodilation, but only when it is given at concentrations well above those noted after feeding [167,168]. However, the peptide neurotensin, produced by gut neuroendocrine cells in response to feeding does induce vasodilation at physiologically relevant concentrations [168,169]. Interestingly, the vascular effect of neurotensin appears to be site specific: neurotensin-induced vasodilation occurs in the ileum [169] but not in the jejunum [167].

Enteric nervous system

While it is well accepted that extrinsic nerves play no role in the digestive/absorptive phase of postprandial hyperemia, some evidence supports a role for the enteric nervous system in this process [170]. Afferent fibers from neurons of the submucosal ganglia innervate the villi and synapse with efferent fibers that reach submucosal arterioles [85]. VIP, an effective intestinal vasodilator, is one of several neurotransmitters localized to these neurons [170]. Stimulants of VIP release and subsequent vasodilation include chemical stimulation by luminal instillation of bile oleate [171] while mechanical stimulation of the mucosal surface also causes both VIP release and vasodilation [83].

Interactions between gastrointestinal and liver circulations

Blood draining the GI tract, pancreas, and spleen accounts for approximately 80% of the resting blood supply to the liver, with the remaining 20% of liver blood flow derived from the hepatic artery. This dual supply of blood to the liver reflects a combination of well-oxygenated blood from the high-pressure hepatic artery that mixes with poorly oxygenated blood from the low-pressure portal vein. Because of the higher oxygen content of arterial blood, the hepatic artery and portal vein contribute roughly equal amounts of oxygen to the liver in the fasting state.

A unique feature of the liver circulation is the role of capillary (sinusoidal) constriction in the regulation of intrahepatic vascular resistance and blood flow. This ability of sinusoids to constrict has been attributed to stellate cells that reside in the space of Disse in close contact with sinusoidal endothelial cells. Stellate cells exhibit anatomical features that are remarkably similar to smooth muscle-like pericytes that have been implicated in the sprouting and remodeling of capillaries and may represent the anatomical equivalent of the precapillary sphincter that controls perfused capillary density in other vascular beds. A variety of vasoconstrictors, including endothelin-1, angiotensin II, and vasopressin, are known to elicit stellate cell contraction that colocalizes with sinusoidal constriction. The gaseous monoxides, NO and carbon monoxide (CO), also appear to play an important role in modulating stellate cell contraction, possibly through the activation of soluble guanylyl cyclase. The interplay of NO with vasoconstrictors like endothelin-1 may be a major determinant of liver blood flow, especially following liver injury, which is often associated with stellate cell activation and an enhanced contractility. It has been proposed that exaggerated stellate cell contractility may contribute to the increased intrahepatic resistance and portal hypertension that can accompany liver injury. Through this effect on portal vein pressure, the stellate cell-mediated sinusoidal constriction may exert a significant influence on blood flow in those tissues, including the GI tract, that are drained by the portal vein [145,172–175].

Although the liver receives the majority of its resting blood flow from venous drainage of the GI tract, it appears to be relatively well protected against the deleterious consequences of GI hypoperfusion. This protection largely results from the unique hydrodynamic interaction between portal venous and hepatic arterial blood flows that has been termed the hepatic arterial buffer response (HABR). With the HABR, an increased blood flow in the portal vein leads to an increased hepatic arterial resistance, while a reduction in portal vein flow produces hepatic arterial dilation, resulting in blood flow to the liver being kept relatively constant. Adenosine washout from the space of Mall has been proposed as a major determinant of the altered hepatic arteriolar tone that accompanies changes in portal venous blood flow. The adenosine washout hypothesis predicts that adenosine levels are inversely related to portal venous blood flow and that adenosine exerts a potent dilatory effect on hepatic arterioles. Although the reciprocal relationship between hepatic arterial and portal vein blood flows tends to prevent large changes in total blood flow through the liver, hepatic arterial flow can only compensate for about 30% of the change in portal venous inflow. However, compensation relative to oxygen delivery is much greater because of the higher oxygen content of hepatic arterial blood, compared to the portal vein. For example, it has been shown that liver oxygen supply remains relatively normal during hemorrhage until the blood loss exceeds a critical threshold at 30%. The liver is more effective in maintaining constant oxygen consumption than tissues in the GI tract because the extraction of oxygen from hepatic blood is very efficient. This highly efficient oxygen extraction results from the small diffusion distances for oxygen transport between blood and hepatocytes. The combined effects of a large capacity for efficient oxygen extraction and the HABR ensures that liver can tolerate substantial reductions in GI blood flow without impairment of hepatocellular function [173,176].

Portal venous hypertension

Whereas exposure of the splanchnic circulation to an acute elevation in portal venous pressure is likely to elicit a myogenically mediated constriction of splanchnic arterioles, chronic portal hypertension tends to dilate the splanchnic vasculature. Pathogenic dilation of splanchnic vasculature is commonly seen in cirrhosis, and this is due to portal hypertension [177]. Furthermore, chronic portal hypertension has a significant impact on other regional vascular beds and on systemic hemodynamics. Blood flow to the GI tract, kidneys, and skeletal muscle is significantly elevated. This presumably results from an increase in circulating vasodilators (e.g., glucagon) and a decrease in vascular sensitivity to vasoconstrictors (e.g., norepinephrine). The widespread dilation of arterioles results in a reduction of peripheral vascular resistance and a corresponding reduction of arterial blood pressure. In addition, cardiac output is elevated as a consequence of the increased venous return associated with the splanchnic and peripheral vasodilation. The elevated portal pressure results in the opening of portosystemic shunts to divert portal blood from the liver and reduce portal pressure. These shunts generally run along the esophagus (i.e., esophageal varices). The increase in portal pressure impairs venous drainage from the spleen into the portal vein, resulting in the accumulation of blood within, and distension of, the spleen (i.e., splenomegaly) [177–180].

Organ blood flow is determined by the arterial venous pressure gradient and vascular resistance. It follows then that portal pressure is determined by portal venous inflow and portal venous resistance. The relationship between portal venous flow and portal pressure at a normal portal vascular resistance is depicted in Figure 11.12 as a solid line. In this instance, an increase in portal venous flow will produce a proportional increase in portal pressure (point A to point B on Figure 11.12; flow-induced portal hypertension). When portal vascular resistance is increased, the relationship between portal pressure and portal venous flow is shifted upward and to the left, as depicted by the dashed line. At any given portal venous inflow, an increased portal vascular resistance will result in an increase in portal pressure (point A to point C on Figure 11.12; resistance-induced portal hypertension).

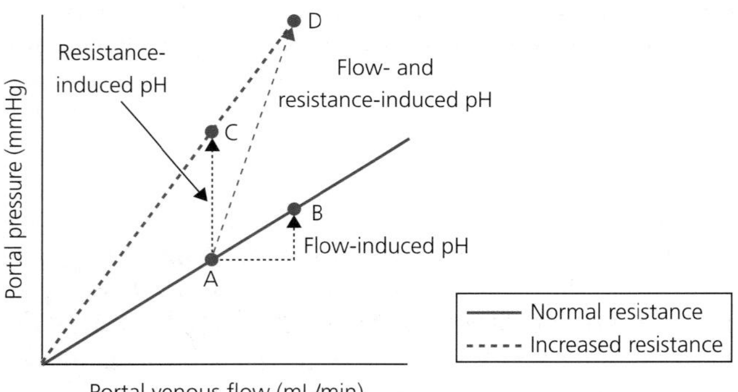

Figure 11.12 Hypothetical relationship between portal pressure and portal venous flow in the presence of a normal **(solid line)** or elevated **(broken line)** portal vascular resistance. Even when portal vascular resistance is normal, an increase in portal blood flow (from point A to point B) can result in an increase in portal pressure – that is, portal hypertension. An elevation in portal vascular resistance in the absence of increased portal blood flow (point A to point C) can also lead to portal hypertension. When both portal blood flow and vascular resistance are increased (point A to point D), the increase in portal pressure is more substantial. Source: Adapted from Premen et al. 1985 [168].

Portal pressure can be further increased by a concomitant increase in portal venous flow and portal vascular resistance (point A to point D on Figure 11.12; flow- and resistance-induced portal hypertension) [168]. Indeed, the latter situation appears to reflect the vascular changes that account for the elevated portal pressure observed in some experimental models of chronic portal hypertension, and it is likely to account for the portal hypertension associated with some forms of liver disease. With a portal vascular resistance that is 40% higher in the portal hypertensive than in the control state, it is predicted that increased portal inflow and increased portal vascular resistance account for 40% and 60% of the increase in portal pressure, respectively [181].

The portal hypertensive state leads to the development of collaterals (mostly along the esophagus; esophageal varices) to shunt blood from the congested portal vein, around the liver, to the systemic circulation (i.e., portosystemic shunting). Because a large proportion of portal venous blood bypasses the liver as a result portosystemic shunting, the hepatic degradation of different compounds, including circulating vasodilators, such as glucagon, is reduced. The diminished catabolism of circulating vasodilators increases their concentration in the plasma, allowing these agents to relax arteriolar vascular smooth muscle and reduce splanchnic vascular resistance. Another important action of some of the vasodilators that accumulate in chronic portal hypertension (e.g., glucagon) is to reduce the sensitivity of the splanchnic arterioles to vasoconstrictors such as norepinephrine, vasopressin, and angiotensin. Consequences of the direct and indirect actions of the accumulated circulating vasodilators include increased splanchnic blood flow and higher shear rates in splanchnic arterioles. The mechanical and humoral factors also exert an influence on NO generation by eNOS. The increased NO production that accompanies portal hypertension appears to result from endothelial cell responses that include increased intracellular calcium, protein kinase B (AKT) activation, and the production/mobilization of molecular chaperones. However, some studies have revealed that eNOS-deficient mice exhibit a hyperdynamic state during portal hypertension, suggesting that eNOS-derived NO is not required for the induction of this vascular response. The net result of the vasodilation induced by all of these mechanisms is perpetuation of the portal hypertensive state [178–185].

Pathophysiology of ischemia

Ischemic damage to the intestine occurs when blood flow falls to a level at which delivery of oxygen and other nutrients are insufficient to maintain oxidative metabolism and hence cell integrity. Blood flow to the GI tract may be reduced during generalized nonocclusive ischemia (e.g., circulatory shock, congestive heart failure, treatment with cardiac glycosides) and in occlusive disorders (e.g., embolism, atherothrombosis) that primarily involve the mesenteric circulation. For occlusive disorders, surgical intervention (e.g., embolectomy, intestinal resection) [186] may be used, but the mortality of this disease continues to be significant. The mortality of acute arterial mesenteric ischemia in adults has been reported at 54–77%, and acute mesenteric venous thrombosis at 32% [187], primarily because of the difficulty of making an early diagnosis before bowel infarction occurs. Fortunately incidence is low and is estimated at 0.9–2.0% of all acute admissions to emergency departments [186]. Experimental nonocclusive mesenteric ischemia in dogs has been treated successfully with intravenously administered selective mesenteric vasodilators (e.g., urotensin I, sauvagine, and corticotropin-releasing factor) [188], thereby potentially obviating the risk of an indwelling angiographic catheter, but the use of these drugs in humans remains to be investigated.

Alterations of intestinal morphology with ischemia

The response of the intestine to decreased blood flow can range from no damage to transmural necrosis [189], and a gradient of sensitivity to ischemic injury has been demonstrated from the villus tips to the muscularis [189–191]. Mesenteric ischemia is associated with characteristic mucosal lesions that progress from subepithelial edema within 30 min after total vascular occlusion, to loss of epithelial cells along the villus after 1 h of total occlusion, to total loss of villi after 2 h of occlusion [189,190]. Within 30–60 min after total mesenteric artery occlusion, changes indicative of cellular failure appear, such as mitochondrial vacuolization and decreased oxygen uptake, loss of ATP, and release of lysosomal enzymes [191].

Changes in vascular and mucosal permeability with ischemia

The permeability of intestinal capillaries to water and solutes (including albumin) is increased after ischemia [192]. The increase in permeability is largely derived from an increase in the number of large (200 Å) pores. The small-pore (50 Å) population, however, is unaffected. Transcapillary water exchange is enhanced as a result of both the increased pore size and an increased capillary surface area. Increases in mucosal permeability induced by ischemia and reperfusion have been estimated based on the clearance of solutes ranging from 700 to 70 000 Da [193,194]. The ischemia/reperfusion-induced increases in mucosal permeability are dependent on both the duration and severity of the ischemic insult (Figure 11.13) [195]. Mucosal permeability increases significantly after 1–2 h of mesenteric artery occlusion in adult animals.

Blood flow, oxygenation, and ischemic injury

Ischemic injury to the intestine occurs when blood flow is reduced to a level at which delivery of oxygen and other nutrients to the tissue is compromised. Although the correlations of tissue PO_2, mucosal blood flow, and mucosal injury have not been investigated, it has been demonstrated that reduction of blood flow to levels that do not affect oxygen uptake are not associated with any evidence of mucosal damage in adult animals [196]. Furthermore, substantial increases in mucosal albumin clearance are not seen until blood flow is reduced to produce ≥50% reduction in oxygen consumption (Figure 11.14) [196].

The importance of collateral blood flow in the prevention of intestinal ischemia is well recognized in humans and adult animals [197–199]. Intestinal collateral blood flow may occur through anastomotic connections at several levels of vessel branching, including the main arterial trunks (i.e., celiac, superior, and inferior mesenteric arteries) [198,200], extramural vessels (i.e., arterial arcades, marginal arteries) [201,202], and intramural vascular plexuses located within the intestinal wall itself [198,202]. Quantitative studies in adult animals have demonstrated that collateral channels among the major arterial trunks and between adjacent bowel segments both play a role in

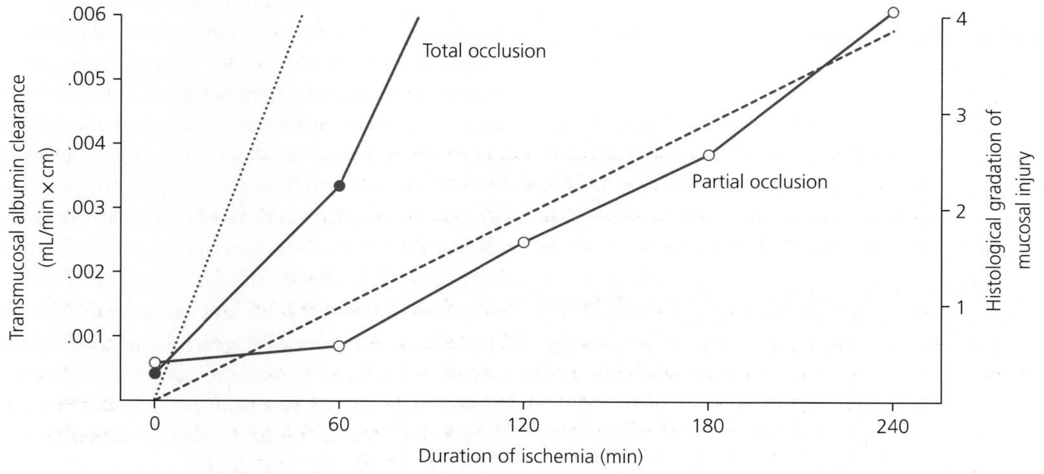

Figure 11.13 Comparison of quantitative morphological data **(dotted and broken lines)** and mucosal albumin clearance results **(solid lines)**. Source: Parks et al. 1982 [195]. Reproduced with permission of Elsevier.

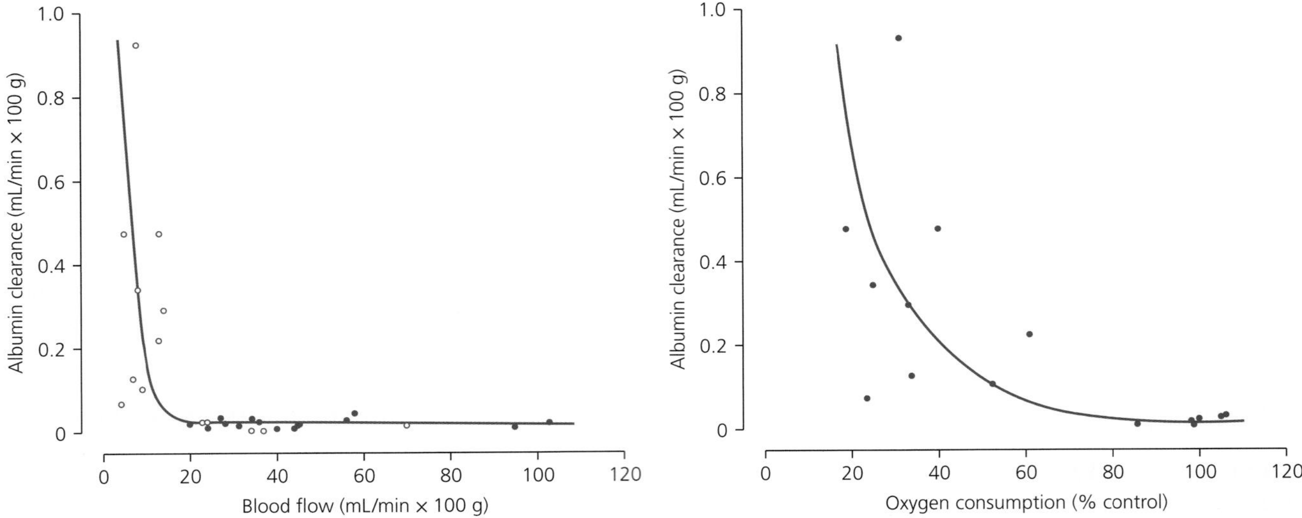

Figure 11.14 Relation between blood flow during control **(closed circles)** and ischemia **(open circles)** and mucosal albumin clearance during reperfusion of canine jejunum **(left)**. Relation between intestinal oxygen consumption during control and ischemia and mucosal albumin clearance during reperfusion of canine jejunum **(right)**. Substantial increases in albumin clearance were not seen unless blood flow was reduced to below 20 mL/min × 100 g or oxygen consumption was reduced to approximately one-half that of the control values. Source: Bulkley et al. 1985 [196]. Reproduced with permission of Elsevier.

the prevention of intestinal ischemia. In the adult cat, perfusion through collateral vessels after occlusion of the superior mesenteric artery maintained flow to the small intestine and proximal colon to within 30–65% of preocclusion flow [200]. However, the efficiency of collateral perfusion by way of the celiac and inferior mesenteric arteries is substantially lower in dogs after superior mesenteric artery occlusion [203]. In adjacent segments of canine small bowel, collateral vessels maintain blood flow in one segment at approximately 55% of its control level when the artery to that segment is totally occluded. The percentage of collateral flow attributed to extramural vessels is 67%, whereas that attributed to intramural vessels is 33% [201].

Possible mechanisms of injury or villous necrosis

Ischemic injury in the intestine appears to be related, either primarily or secondarily, to the effects of tissue hypoxia. In some species, the hypoxic stress induced by ischemia is exacerbated by the presence of a countercurrent exchange mechanism [159]. Experimental data to suggest that hypoxia plays a role is supported by the observation that intralumenal perfusion with oxygenated saline solution markedly attenuates mucosal injury during ischemia induced by hypotension [204], whereas perfusion with nitrogenated saline solution does not attenuate injury. Possible mechanisms of mucosal injury induced by tissue hypoxia include depletion of high-energy phosphates necessary to produce protective substances, such as mucus, leading to increased susceptibility to the action of intralumenal proteases [205]; accumulation of histamine, leading to increased microvascular permeability [206]; production of metabolic acidosis, leading to release of lysosomal enzymes and cellular digestion [207]; conversion of xanthine dehydrogenase to xanthine oxidase, an enzyme that can produce cytotoxic oxygen-derived free radicals during reoxygenation [208]; and attraction of circulating granulocytes into the mucosa, or activation of resident leukocytes within the mucosa, with release of neutrophilic proteases and oxidants to initiate or propagate mucosal injury [209].

Another proposed mechanism involved direct cellular damage from digestive enzymes. It has been demonstrated that changes in the intestinal mucosa induced by circulatory shock lead to an increased vulnerability to the digestive action of trypsin and chymotrypsin. Inhibition of pancreatic proteases by aprotinin [210] or previous ligation of the pancreatic ducts [211] significantly attenuates ischemic mucosal injury. In addition, an intralumenal injection of trypsin exacerbates mucosal injury [210]. The digestive action is caused by enzymes already present along the intestinal wall before shock, because removal of the pancreas has no effect if the animal is subjected to shock immediately after pancreatectomy [199]. Inhibition of pancreatic elastase and bile salts, both of which contribute to the loss of protective brush border glycoproteins [212,213], also decreases mucosal injury. Furthermore, it has been demonstrated that mesenteric ischemia leads to protease-independent mucin degradation that renders the gut mucosa more vulnerable to the digestive action of pancreatic enzymes [205]. Self digestion by pancreatic enzymes has been proposed as a major mechanism for the gut injury and multiorgan failure associated with hemorrhagic shock [214].

A role for reactive oxygen species (ROS) in the pathogenesis of injury associated with reperfusion of the ischemic bowel has received considerable attention during the past 30 years. The digestive system is particularly well endowed with the enzymatic machinery capable of generating significant quantities of ROS. For example, the intestine and liver are the richest sources of xanthine oxidase (XO) [215], an enzyme that catalyzes the production of both superoxide and hydrogen peroxide. XO activity in the small intestine is located primarily within the mucosa, with a gradient of activity from villus tip to the base [216]. In addition, the intestine contains a large, resident population of phagocytic cells, which when activated produce considerable quantities of superoxide, hydrogen peroxide, and hypochlorous acid [217]. Oxidants generated by either XO or activated phagocytes can injure cells by a variety of mechanisms, including lipid peroxidation, degradation of the extracellular matrix, protein and carbohydrate decomposition, and DNA strand breakage [218]. Cellular enzymatic defense mechanisms against ROS include superoxide dismutase, which converts the superoxide anion to hydrogen peroxide and oxygen, as well as catalase and glutathione peroxidase, which detoxify hydrogen peroxide [219]. Glutathione is another critical free radical scavenger, which serves both as a cosubstrate for the glutathione peroxidase-catalyzed decomposition of hydrogen peroxide and as a stand-alone free radical scavenger [218].

A large body of experimental data supports the hypothesis that ROS mediate the microvascular and mucosal permeability changes after reperfusion of the ischemic intestine and stomach in adult animals [209,220–224]. Superoxide dismutase (which scavenges superoxide anions), catalase (which detoxifies hydrogen peroxide), and dimethylsulfoxide (which scavenges hydroxyl radicals and decomposes hypochlorous acid) attenuate the vascular permeability changes observed after reperfusion of the ischemic intestine [218].

A role for XO in the microvascular and mucosal dysfunction induced by ischemia-reperfusion (I/R) has been proposed. Using the I/R animal model, which involves causing intestinal ischemia by clamping the superior mesenteric artery for a fixed period of time followed by subsequent reperfusion, demonstrated attenuated injury responses following treatment with XO inhibitors allopurinol or pterin aldehyde [221,225,226]; increased vascular and mucosal permeability during intraarterial infusion of hypoxanthine-XO, a superoxide anion-generating system [227]; attenuation of injury by agents that prevent the conversion of xanthine dehydrogenase to XO [223]; and a blunted I/R injury response in animals placed on a tungsten-supplemented, molybdenum-deficient diet, which inactivates XO [228].

There is also evidence to suggest that granulocytes play a role in I/R-mediated injury. Ischemia may lead to neutrophil activation, release or production of neutrophilic oxidants (e.g., superoxide, hydrogen peroxide, hypochlorous acid, *N*-chloramines) and proteases, and subsequent tissue injury [217,229–231]. A five- to sevenfold increase in mucosal myeloperoxidase (MPO) activity, which is an index of granulocyte number, occurs during ischemia, whereas reperfusion induces an 18-fold increase in MPO activity in feline intestine [222]. Both neutrophil depletion and prevention of neutrophil adherence significantly attenuate the increased intestinal microvascular permeability induced by ischemia and reperfusion in cat intestine [209], suggesting that neutrophils, which migrate into the mucosa, mediate the injury produced by I/R.

It has also been proposed that xanthine oxidase-derived oxidants may serve as chemoattractants for granulocytes in postischemic adult intestine. This is supported by the XO inhibitor allopurinol [222], superoxide dismutase (a superoxide scavenger and inhibitor of neutrophil adherence) [222], catalase (a scavenger of hydrogen peroxide) [232], deferoxamine (an iron chelator) [232], dimethylthiourea (a hydroxyl radical scavenger) [232], and IB_4 (a CD18-specific monoclonal antibody that inhibits neutrophil adherence) [233] all inhibit I/R-induced granulocyte accumulation in the small intestine.

The view that leukocyte–endothelial cell adhesion plays an important role in the pathogenesis of I/R injury, as well as in other inflammatory conditions of the GI tract [234,235], has led to an increased interest in defining the factors that modulate leukocyte adherence and emigration in postcapillary venules. Intravital microscopic techniques have been used to monitor and quantify leukocyte–endothelial cell adhesion in venules exposed to I/R [41,227–239]. During the final 10 min of a 60-min 80% reduction in mesenteric blood flow, the numbers of adherent and emigrated leukocytes increase by fourfold and threefold, respectively. At 60 min after reperfusion, sevenfold and eightfold increases in adherence and emigration are noted. Electron microscopic analyses of postischemic mesenteric venules reveal that more than 85% of the leukocytes that emigrate into the adjacent interstitial compartment are neutrophils [240]. The recruitment of adherent leukocytes after reperfusion is associated with a corresponding accumulation of adherent platelets, with each blood cell exerting an influence on the recruitment of the other. There is mounting evidence that platetet attachment to leukocytes and the products of platelet activation greatly enhance the inflammatory response to I/R [236,238,239].

Several chemical mediators produced by endothelial and/or parenchymal cells have been implicated in the leukocyte–endothelial cell adhesion elicited by mesenteric I/R. Some evidence implicates XO-derived superoxide as a major mediator in this process. A role for superoxide is supported by reports describing an attenuating influence of superoxide dismutase (a free radical scavenger), whether administered before ischemia or after reperfusion, on the number of adherent and emigrated leukocytes in mesenteric venules exposed to I/R [237,238]. Superoxide dismutase is also effective in attenuating the adherence of neutrophils to endothelial cell monolayers exposed to anoxia and reoxygenation [241]. These results have been replicated by allopurinol [232,240–242], suggesting that XO is a likely source of the superoxide produced after reperfusion. XO, rather than neutrophils, also appears to be responsible for generating the oxidants that mediate reperfusion-induced lipid peroxidation in intestinal mucosa. This contention is based on reports demonstrating that although both allopurinol and CD18-specific monoclonal antibodies prevent the reperfusion-induced increase in mucosal MPO activity, only allopurinol prevents the rise in tissue conjugated dienes, an index of membrane lipid peroxidation [243,244].

A likely explanation for the proadhesive action of superoxide is that it inactivates an antiadhesion molecule that is normally produced by endothelial cells. NO, a product of L-arginine metabolism in endothelium that is rapidly inactivated by superoxide, may be such an endogenous antiadhesion molecule. NO donors are very effective in preventing the recruitment of leukocytes, platelet–leukocyte aggregation, and tissue injury associated with I/R [245]. Additionally, inhibitors of NO production lead to a dramatic increase in the number of leukocytes adhering to and emigrating from mesenteric venules, further supporting that NO donors are effective in preventing leukocyte recruitment [246]. This adhesion response can be prevented or reversed by simultaneous exposure of venules to a NO synthase inhibitor and either L-arginine (but not D-arginine) or nitroprusside, which spontaneously generates NO. The observations that NO synthase inhibitors promote leukocyte adherence while superoxide dismutase reduces reperfusion-induced adherence are consistent with the view that the enhanced formation of superoxide by postischemic endothelial cells leads to NO inactivation and consequently results in enhanced leukocyte adhesion. Such a mechanism would explain why superoxide dismutase exerts an antiadhesive effect in postischemic tissues, because the enzyme would prevent inactivation of NO. NO also stabilizes mast cells through a mechanism that involves superoxide [247].

Catalase, another free radical scavenger, has been shown to attenuate reperfusion-induced leukocyte adherence in mesenteric venules [242]. This observation is consistent with reports that demonstrate that hydrogen peroxide is produced by endothelial cell monolayers exposed to anoxia and reoxygenation [247], and hydrogen peroxide promotes neutrophil adherence to cultured endothelial cells and in mesenteric venules [248,249]. The levels of hydrogen peroxide required to promote adherence are well within the range of the hydrogen peroxide concentration produced by activated neutrophils. Both in vivo and in vitro studies indicate that hydrogen peroxide-induced neutrophil adherence is mediated by platelet-activating factor (PAF) [248,249]. PAF receptor antagonists effectively attenuate the neutrophil adherence induced by hydrogen peroxide in feline mesenteric venules [231] and isolated canine carotid arteries [250]. The hydrogen peroxide-induced, PAF-mediated leukocyte adherence is prevented mostly by monoclonal antibodies directed against the common β-subunit of CD11/CD18.

The proposed mechanism of reactive oxygen (hydrogen peroxide, superoxide) and nitrogen (NO) species in mediating the endothelium-dependent inflammatory responses observed in the GI microcirculation after ischemia/reperfusion is summarized in Figure 11.15. I/R leads to an increased production of superoxide and hydrogen peroxide by XO, with a corresponding reduced production of NO by eNOS. The enhanced generation of ROS results in the activation and deposition of complement, and phospholipase A_2-mediated production of leukotriene B_4 and PAF. Oxidants also mediate the initial expression of P-selectin by mobilizing the leukocyte rolling receptor from its preformed pool (Weibel–Palade bodies) in endothelial cells. Firm adhesion of leukocytes, which is mediated by β_2-integrins (CD11/CD18), is induced by the engagement of activated complement, leukotriene B_4, and PAF with their receptors on rolling leukocytes. Sustained rolling and adhesion of leukocytes on endothelial cells is ensured by an oxidant-dependent synthesis of endothelial cell adhesion molecules, such as E-selectin and intracellular adhesion molecule-1 (ICAM-1). Oxidants, derived from either endothelial cells or leukocytes, elicit this biosynthetic response by activating specific nuclear transcription factors (e.g., nuclear factor-κB) that bind to the genes for these adhesion molecules. Platelets coursing through the postischemic microvasculature are activated by endothelial cell-derived mediators such as thrombin and adenosine diphosphate (ADP). The activated platelets express adhesion molecules such as P-selectin and glycoprotein IIb/IIIa (GPIIb/IIIa), which bind to counterreceptors expressed on the surface of endothelial cells (P-selectin glycoprotein ligand-1 or PSGL-1, ICAM-1 bound fibrinogen) and adherent leukocytes (PSGL-1). The adherent and activated platelets release a variety of chemicals that can amplify the inflammatory response to I/R. Further amplification occurs as a result of the activation of (and mediator release from) mast cells and macrophages that normally reside near postcapillary venules [251,252].

Ischemic preconditioning

Ischemic preconditioning (IPC) is one of the most effective and reproducible forms of protection against the tissue injury and organ dysfunction caused by intestinal ischemia. The phenomenon of IPC is observed in the intestine and other tissues that are exposed to a brief period of ischemia and subsequently exhibit resistance to the deleterious effects of prolonged ischemia followed by reperfusion. There is an early, acute phase of IPC that is manifested within minutes following the preconditioning insult. The acute phase is powerful, persists for 1–4 h, and relies on preexisting effector molecules (Figure 11.16). A late or delayed phase of IPC is also evident, emerging 24 h later and persists for 2–4 days. The late phase (also known as the "second window of protection") requires gene expression and is less powerful than the acute phase response. IPC in the intestine has been demonstrated following temporary occlusion of the superior mesenteric artery (direct) as well as after an artery not responsible for direct blood supply (remote) of the intestine (e.g., renal artery) is temporarily occluded. The protective effects of direct and remote IPC against intestinal I/R include decreases in epithelial cell apoptosis, inflammatory cell infiltration, mucosal injury, capillary permeability, and bacterial translocation, as well as an improvement in microvascular perfusion and tissue oxygenation. Local IPC has also been shown to improve the stability of

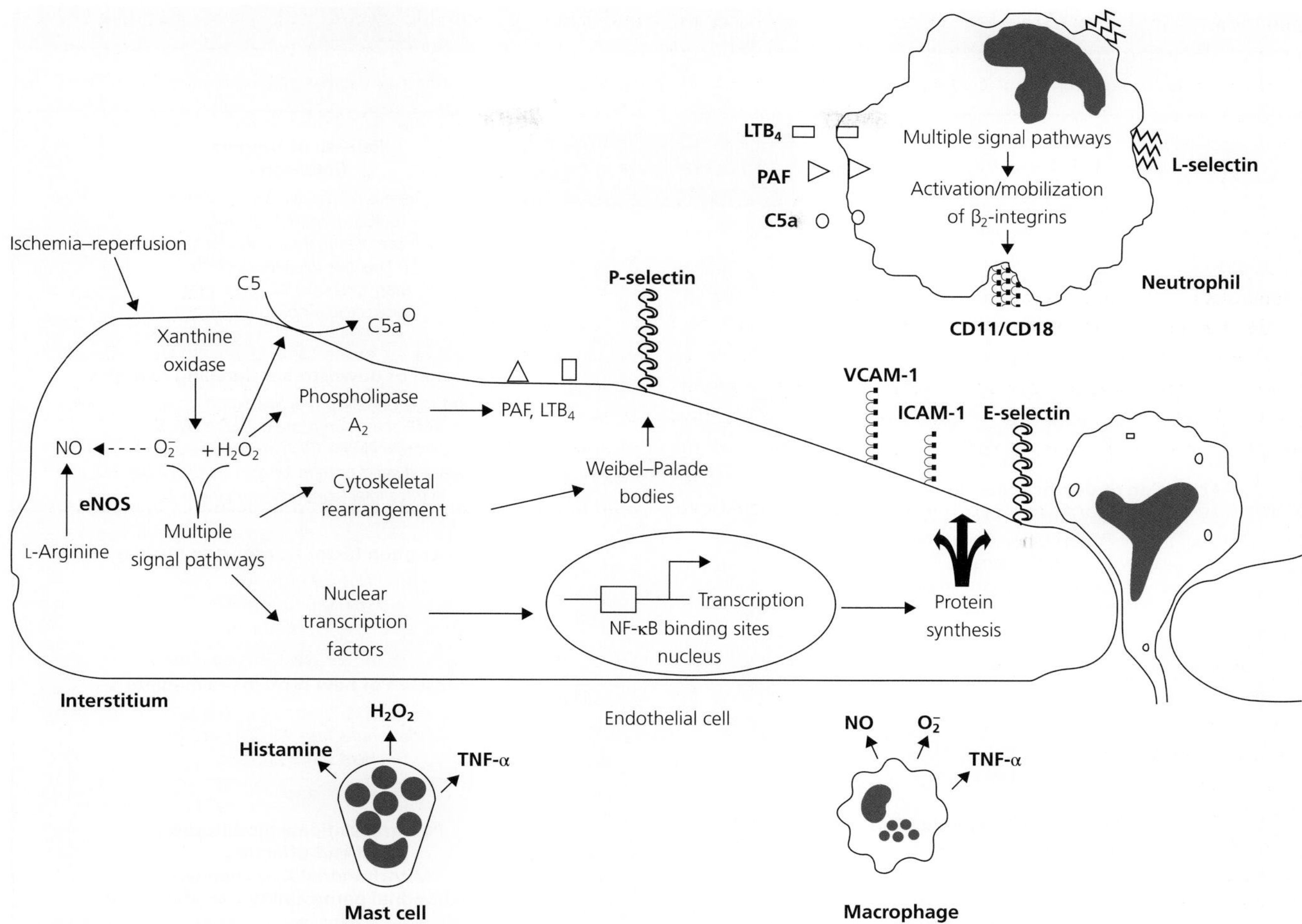

Figure 11.15 Mechanism proposed to explain the endothelium-dependent inflammatory responses observed in the postischemic microvasculature. C5a, complement 5a; CD11/CD18, leukocyte adhesion glycoprotein; eNOS, endothelial nitric oxide (NO) synthase; H_2O_2, hydrogen peroxide; I/R, ischemia–reperfusion; ICAM, intracellular adhesion molecule; LTB_4, leukotriene B_4; NF-κB, nuclear factor-κB; O^-_2, superoxide; PAF, platelet-activating factor; TNF-α, tumor necrosis factor-α; VCAM, vascular cell adhesion molecule. Source: Carden and Granger 2000 [251]. Reproduced with permission of John Wiley & Sons, Ltd.

intestinal anastomoses [252–256]. However, a randomized prospective trial utilizing remote ischemic preconditioning (RIPC) by using a blood pressure cuff on the upper extremity of patients undergoing CABG did not demonstrate that RIPC affected intestinal injury in these patients [257].

While not fully elucidated, the cellular signaling pathways and genetic responses to IPC in the intestine have been extensively characterized (see Figure 11.15). Adenosine, NO, ROS, bradykinin, opioids, and sarcolemmal K-ATP channels have been implicated as key initiators that are released in response to the brief IPC episode and serve as triggers for both the acute and late phases of IPC. These initiator molecules then activate downstream signaling cascades, some of which contribute to the acute phase IPC response (e.g., phosphatidylinositol-3-kinase/AKT/eNOS), while others (e.g., large conductance, calcium-activated potassium channels) mediate the late-phase response. Transcription factor activation and the expression of genes for new protein mediators are responses critical for the late phase response, while posttranslational modification of end-effector molecules (e.g., mitochondrial permeability transition pore) contribute to both the acute and late IPC responses. The net effect of these signaling mechanisms is the appearance of protective phenotype that resists the deleterious consequences of a prolonged ischemic insult, followed by reperfusion. A similar protective phenotype can be initiated using endotoxin, cytokines, and low to moderate alcohol ingestion as the preconditioning stimulus [252,253,256,258,259].

Angiogenesis

While capillary growth and proliferation are rarely observed in normal GI tissues in adults except during wound healing, the process of angiogenesis (the formation of new blood vessels

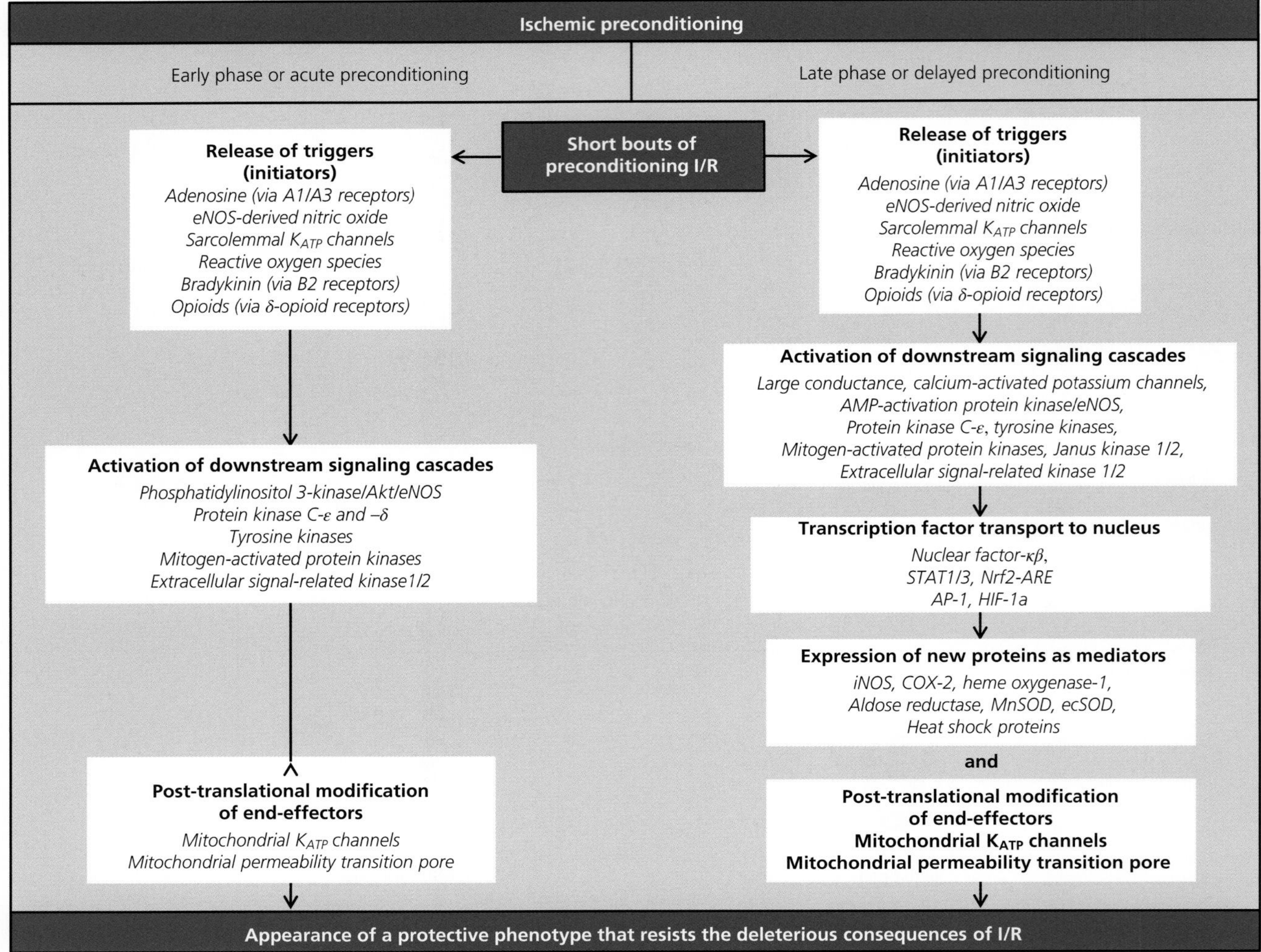

Figure 11.16 Mechanisms proposed to explain the phenomenon of ischemic preconditioning, wherein a brief period of ischemia followed by reperfusion (I/R) renders the intestine resistant to the tissue damaging effect of a subsequent ischemic insult of longer duration (which would otherwise cause severe damage). AMP, adenosine monophosphate; AP-1, activator protein-1; eNOS/iNOS, endothelial and inducible nitric oxide synthases; HIF, hypoxia inducible factor; Nrf-ARE, nuclear respiratory factor-antioxidant response element; STAT, signal transducer and activators of transcription. Source: Krenz et al. 2013 [252] Reproduced by permission of Morgan & Claypool Life Sciences.

from existing microvessels) is detected under certain pathological conditions, such as inflammation and tumorigenesis. Angiogenesis is a tightly controlled process that involves regulatory inputs from a variety of activators (proangiogenic) and inhibitors (antiangiogenic). Conditions that tip the balance in favor of proangiogenic factors result in rapid formation of new blood vessels. The process of angiogenesis consists of two phases (Figure 11.17): (1) an initial destabilization of the vasculature to facilitate sprouting of new vessels, followed by (2) a restabilization or maturation of the newly formed microvessels. The destabilization phase involves the activation of cells that generate proangiogenic molecules, such as VEGF and tumor necrosis factor (TNF)-α. For example, when macrophages sense hypoxia, VEGF is produced in response to the generation of hypoxia inducible factor (HIF). The destabilization process includes endothelial cell junction dissociation, basement membrane degradation, and the migration and proliferation of endothelial cells. A consequence of the events associated with the destabilization phase is the formation of hyperpermeable vascular sprouts, which is a characteristic feature of tumor microvessels. During the restabilization phase, the interendothelial junctions and cell–cell contacts are strengthened and stabilized, a new basement membrane is deposited, and a nonleaky tube is formed [260–262].

Angiogenesis has been implicated in the pathogenesis of inflammatory bowel diseases. A variety of proangiogenic factors (e.g., cytokines, VEGF, ROS) are produced in the inflamed bowel and there is evidence for vessel proliferation and increased capillary density in the chronically inflamed bowel. An increased angiogenic capacity of the inflamed bowel is supported by

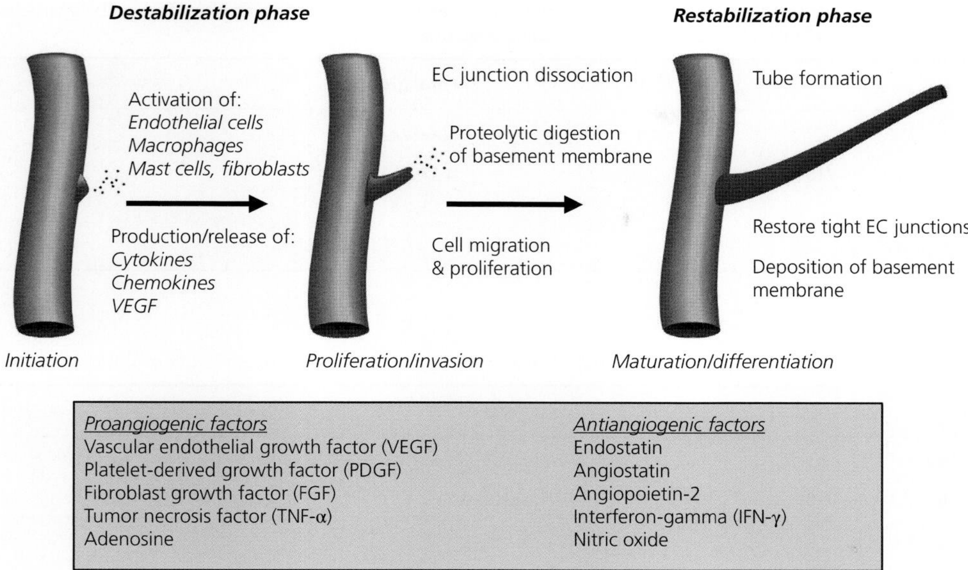

Figure 11.17 Events associated with angiogenesis. Following tissue injury or during inflammation, angiogenesis is initiated by the activation of different populations of cells that release proangiogenic factors. This leads to vessel destabilization resulting in endothelial cell (EC) junction dissociation, degradation of the basement membrane, and the proliferation and migration of endothelial cells. The final stage (restabilization) includes tube formation and the restoration of a normal vessel wall. The rate of angiogenesis is determined by the balance of pro- and antiangiogenic factors. Source: Granger and Senchenkova 2010 [268]. Reproduced by permission of Morgan & Claypool Life Sciences.

reports describing a dose-dependent enhancement of the migration rate of human microvascular endothelial cells exposed to mucosal extracts from patients with inflammatory bowel disease. In both human and animal models of inflammatory bowel disease there is a direct correlation between disease activity (e.g., tissue injury, inflammatory cell infiltrate), local expression of VEGF, and vascular density. It has been proposed that angiogenesis is both a consequence and cause of the inflammatory response associated with inflammatory bowel disease. This contention is supported by reports describing increased disease severity following VEGF treatment in experimental models of inflammatory bowel disease while antiangiogenic agents or VEGF neutralization (e.g., with soluble VEGF receptor) have the opposite effect. Based on these observations, it has been proposed that angiogenesis may be an effective therapeutic target for the treatment of inflammatory bowel disease. However, the clinical utility of such a therapeutic strategy may be limited due to the essential role that angiogenesis plays in normal wound healing [263–267].

Circulatory physiology of the newborn intestine

The physiology of gastrointestinal circulation of the newborn is unique when compared to adults. This is likely due to the functional difference of the intestine. Whereas the intestine of infants is dynamic and rapidly growing and relies solely on breastmilk or formula for enteral nutrition, the adult intestine is static and utilizes solid foods for enteral nutrition. This section will explore the unique features of the circulatory physiology of the newborn intestine.

Transition from fetal to newborn life

At birth, vascular resistance to the bowel falls significantly and blood flow subsequently increases. Consequently, oxygen extraction and oxygen uptake in the intestinal vasculature also increase. This was demonstrated by Edelstone and Holzman et al. using a lamb model, where both fetal and newborn lambs were catheterized and intestinal blood flow was calculated by radionuclide microsphere techniques (Table 11.1) [117,269]. This is unsurprising and advantageous as fetal nutrition is provided by the umbilical vein, which carries oxygenated blood rich in maternal nutrients from the placenta to the fetus [270]. The fetal intestine, in contrast, does not functionally absorb nutrition and is a relatively dormant organ, so limited blood flow and oxygen uptake are adequate to meet its metabolic needs [271]. These changes continue in the first month of life and are likely due to the rapid growth and maturation of the intestine in response to enteral feeding [272,273].

Experiments in swine demonstrate that vascular resistance continues to decline and blood flow continues to increase from 1-day-old piglets to 3-day-old piglets [271]. Both oxygen delivery and uptake also increase. As piglets continue to grow and are weaned from the sow to a cereal diet at 35 days old, vascular resistance increases and blood flow falls. Subsequently, oxygen delivery and uptake fall (Table 11.2) [274–277]. The mechanism for why vascular resistance falls after weaning has yet to be

Table 11.1 Catherization studies by Edelstone and Holzman demonstrated differences in basal gastrointestinal blood flow and oxygen extraction between fetal and newborn lambs. These data are taken from the text in the following references [117,269].

	Fetal group	Newborn group
Blood flow (mL/min/100 g)	100 +/- 21	196 +/- 50
Vascular resistance (mmHg/mL/min/100 g)	0.41 +/- 0.09	0.31 +/- 0.10
Oxygen extraction (%)	23 +/- 4	26 +/- 4
Oxygen uptake (mLO_2/min/100 g)	0.4 +/- 0.1	4.8 +/- 1.1

Table 11.2 Hemodynamic and oxygen changes in 1-, 3-, and 35-day-old pigs. These figures are taken from the text from articles [274–277].

	[tch]1 d/o	3 d/o	35 d/o
Blood flow (mL/min/100 g)	64 +/- 4	99 +/- 5	45 +/- 5
Vascular resistance (mmHg/mL/min/100 g)	0.77 +/- 0.12	0.65 +/- 0.09	1.74 +/- 0.14
Oxygen delivery (mLO_2/min/100 g)	6.5 +/- 0.4	12.5 +/- 0.9	5 +/- 0.5
Oxygen uptake (mLO_2/min/100 g)	2.24 +/- 0.13	2.97 +/- 0.13	1.88 +/- 0.15

determined. In regard to postprandial hyperemia, the newborn experiences a transient increase in gastrointestinal blood flow after feeding that is similar to adults [278,279].

Factors that affect intestinal basal vascular resistance

External neural stimuli

Basal intestinal vascular resistance in the newborn is partially mediated by external neural stimuli. This has been demonstrated in 1-day-old swine by transecting the splanchnic nerve, which decreased mesenteric vascular resistance in piglets. Additionally, newborn piglets required a larger stimulus to the splanchnic nerve to achieve an increase in vascular resistance when compared to 1-month-old piglets, suggesting that α-adrenergic mechanisms are present at birth, but relatively immature [280,281].

Intrinsic myogenic tone

The vascular myogenic tone has been shown to be an important factor in maintaining basal vascular tone in newborn mesenteric vasculature. An in situ experiment using saline-perfused rabbit mesenteric arteries demonstrated that when vessel diameter was increased passively, vessel diameter decreased below control values with increased perfusion pressure, reflecting intrinsic myogenic activity [282]. As stated above, the precise molecular mechanism for intrinsic myogenic activity remains unknown. Regardless, it is an important physiological mediator of the basal tone of the mesenteric vasculature of infants, and myogenic vasoconstriction is present to a greater extent in the newborn than adult intestine [283–285].

The more prominent role of myogenicity in the newborn in maintaining blood flow may be due to the newborn being particularly susceptible to changes in systemic blood pressure. Newborns are vulnerable to changes in blood pressure because of their inability to autoregulate in response to changes in arterial pressure [286]. Additionally, the newborn intestine cannot increase perfused capillary density in response to reduced perfusion pressure [276]. These circumstances render the newborn intestine profoundly susceptible to tissue hypoxia. Systemic hypotension also compromises intestinal perfusion in an age-specific manner, having a greater impact in the newborn [287,288].

Chemical mediators that affect vasodilation

Nitric oxide

The primary stimulus for eNOS to generate NO in the mesenteric endothelium is from a process called flow-induced dilation [289]. This key stimulus is generated by shearing forces on the wall of the endothelium, and the generated NO serves to reduce the vascular resistance and improve blood flow [290]. The newborn is better able to overcome the vascular resistance mediated by myogenic tone by constitutively producing more NO from eNOS within the postnatal endothelium. Stated otherwise, the production of NO by eNOS is age dependent, with NO production being greater in younger nonweaned infants than weanlings [26,54,291]. This may be due to increase in eNOS expression immediately postnatally [54,283]. This was demonstrated by measuring the basal rates of NO production in mesenteric arterial arcades in 3- vs 35-day-old swine, with the concentration being 43.6 vs 12.1 nmol/min respectively [291].

The ability to overcome intrinsic myogenic vasoconstriction and augment flow is more pronounced in the newborn. In an elegantly designed experiment using pressure myography, Reber et al. demonstrated that the presence of flow in mesenteric

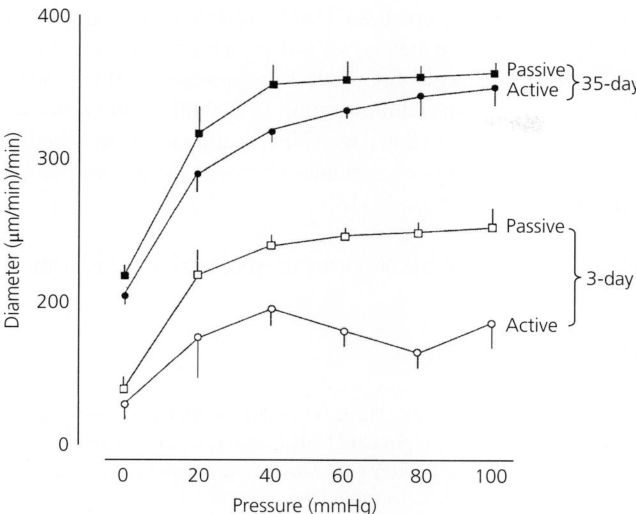

Figure 11.18 Effects of increases in intravascular pressure, delivered in absence of flow, on diameter of terminal mesenteric arteries from 3-day-old and 35-day-old swine. This figure demonstrates that the presence of flow eliminated myogenic vasoconstriction in response to increase in pressure in 3-day-old arteries, but not in 35-day-old arteries Source: Reber et al. 1998 [277].

arteries was able to overcome myogenic vasoconstriction in arteries isolated from 3-day-old piglets. When the experiment was repeated with mesenteric arteries isolated from 35-day-old swine, the presence of flow was *not* able to overcome myogenic vasoconstriction (Figure 11.18) [277]. Stated otherwise, flow-induced dilation is also age dependent [292]. As the infant matures and reaches 1 month of age, the role of NO in mediating intestinal vascular resistances declines [271].

Chemical mediators that affect vasoconstriction

Endothelin-1

Endothelin-1 (ET-1) is a 21-amino acid protein that is a potent vasoconstrictor and constitutively produced by endothelial cells [293]. ET-1-mediated vasoconstriction is done by binding G-protein coupled receptor endothelin receptor A (ET_A) [294]. ET-1 undergoes negative feedback inhibition by binding endothelin receptor B (ET_B) on endothelial cells, which produces eNOS-mediated NO production and prostacyclin synthesis with subsequent vasodilation [295]. Aside from vasoconstriction, ET-1 also mediates cell proliferation through the MAPK pathway and may be involved in tumor angiogenesis [296,297].

Endothelin-1 plays an important role in newborn intestinal physiology. It is expressed at higher levels in younger subjects and it is hypothesized that this may be due to its role in angiogenesis [271]. Production of ET-1 by endothelial cells is age specific, with greater production being performed in younger subjects [298]. Additionally, endothelin receptor population is age dependent, with both ET_A and ET_B being more highly expressed in younger piglets than older swine [299]. Ontogeny studies looking specifically at the swine superior mesenteric artery have demonstrated that both receptors are expressed at higher rates in younger pigs [300].

Platelet activating factor

Platelet activating factor (PAF) is a lipid proinflammatory molecule derived from phospholipid membranes and synthesized by numerous cell types [301]. It is known to have both vasodilator and vasoconstrictor properties [302]. When given exogenously to piglets, it causes profound mesenteric vasoconstriction without a significant rise in systemic arterial pressure, indicating that the newborn gastrointestinal tract is vulnerable to its effects [303].

Necrotizing enterocolitis

Necrotizing enterocolitis (NEC) remains a devastating disease that affects the gastrointestinal tract of the newborn [304]. Despite decades of research, the pathophysiology remains poorly understood and is thought to be multifactorial, composed of intestinal dysbiosis, aberrant immune signaling, and intestinal immaturity [305]. The incidence of NEC is estimated to be as high as 5–7% of all preterm infants [306]. Additionally, mortality is estimated at 42% for very low-birthweight infants [307].

The role of ischemia in NEC has been debated for several years. The initial hypothesis of ischemia's involvement in NEC may have come from a correlation between perinatal asphyxia and subsequent gastrointestinal perforation, thought to be due to a maladaptive "diving reflex" where shunting of bloody supply from splanchnic organs to the brain occurred in the setting of hypoxia [308]. Although this theory has been abandoned, there are several experimental studies that support NEC being an ischemic process. The histological pathology features of mucosal ulceration, vascular congestion, and coagulative necrosis seen in NEC are consistent with ischemia [309]. Immunohistochemical staining of hypoxia markers in human tissue has shown increased staining in intestinal NEC tissue versus control tissue [310]. Additionally, NEC is replicated in mouse models by ischemia-reperfusion and hypoxia [311–313]. However, hypoxia is not necessary to cause NEC in a swine model [314].

The proposed molecular mechanism for the role of ischemia in NEC involves an imbalance of vasoactive chemical mediators, with a proposed increase in vasoconstrive ET-1 and relative decrease in vasodilatory NO [315]. This is supported by several studies and is summarized nicely in a review paper by Watkins and Besner (316). Agents that augment NO have been shown to attenuate the severity of intestinal injury in NEC animal studies [317,318]. In a rat NEC model, pharmacological eNOS blockade has been shown to decrease intestinal perfusion as well [319]. Additionally, there have been two mouse studies that have shown an increase in NEC severity in eNOS knockout mice [318,320]. eNOS isolated from human intestinal vasculature from babies with NEC showed extreme dysfunction, and loss of the ability to mediate critical flow-induced dilation, as discussed earlier [321]. As discussed earlier, H_2S is another vasodilatory gasotransmitter that has been studied in NEC. Exogenous H_2S administration has reduced NEC severity in a mouse animal model [107,322]. Similarly, the benefits of umbilical stem cells (USCs) in attenuating NEC severity were eliminated when H_2S-producing enzymes were knocked down by siRNA, demonstrating that USCs' beneficial properties were dependent on the production of H_2S [323].

Exogenous ET-1 given to guinea pigs has been shown to narrow the lumen of microvessels in the submucosa of the small intestine [324]. When given exogenously to rats, ET-1 causes intestinal malperfusion and subsequent tissue damage [325]. Interestingly, the deleterious effect of exogenous ET-1 was attenuated when given with an ET_A receptor blocker, but not an ET_B receptor blocker [326]. Using an ischemia-reperfusion model in swine and rats, pretreatment with ET_A blockade reduced intestinal injury [327,328]. There have been higher levels of ET-1 found in human NEC tissue [329]. These findings have been replicated in mice and higher levels of ET-1 have been found in the ileum of mice that developed NEC [330]. Similar to ET-1, exogenous administration of PAF has also been shown to cause NEC in animal models [331]. Additionally, PAF inhibitors have been shown to attenuate the severity of NEC [332]. Lastly, PAF serum levels have been explored as a biomarker for NEC, as PAF levels have been shown to be increased in babies with NEC [333].

Clinical data has not been as conclusively supportive of the role of ischemia in NEC. One study in infants found that abnormal SMA doppler flow on ultrasound increased the risk of later developing NEC [334]. However, there is more data to suggest that abnormal doppler SMA velocity has been predictive of bowel dysmotility rather than true clinical NEC [335,336]. This is likely because the true malperfusion and endothelial dysfunction associated with NEC are at the submucosal level, rather than at the large splanchnic artery level [337]. Additionally, many other clinical variables that are known to decrease intestinal blood flow are not associated with NEC, such as the presence of a PDA, indomethacin, or caffeine administration [338–340]. While intestinal ischemia is clearly correlated with NEC in animal studies, whether it is a causative factor or a secondary factor to the disease process remains to be determined [316].

References are available at www.yamadagastro.com/textbook7e

Further reading

de Aguilar-Nascimento J.E. The role of macronutrients in gastrointestinal blood flow. Curr Opin Clin Nutr Metab Care 2005;8:552.

Ceppa E.P., Fuh K.C., Bulkley G.B. Mesenteric hemodynamic response to circulatory shock. Curr Opin Crit Care 2003;9:127.

Chaaban H., Stonestreet B.S. Intestinal hemodynamics and oxygenation in the perinatal period. Semin Perinatol 2012;36:260.

Hass D.J., Kozuch P., Brandt L.J. Pharmacologically mediated colon ischemia. Am J Gastroenterol 2007;102:1765.

Holzer P. Efferent-like roles of afferent neurons in the gut: blood flow regulation and tissue protection. Auton Neurosci 2006;125:70.

Jacob S.M. Splanchnic blood flow in low-flow states. Anesth Analg 2003;96:1129.

Kvietys P.R. The gastrointestinal circulation. In: Granger DN, Granger JP (eds). Integrated Systems Physiology: From Molecule to Function. San Rafael, CA: Morgan & Claypool Life Sciences; 2010.

Matheson P.J., Wilson M.A., Garrison R.N. Regulation of intestinal blood flow. J Surg Res 2000;93:182.

ter Steege R.W., Kolkman J.J. Review article: the pathophysiology and management of gastrointestinal symptoms during physical exercise, and the role of splanchnic blood flow. Aliment Pharmacol Ther 2012;35:516.

Treiber G., Csepregi A., Malfertheiner P. The pathophysiology of portal hypertension. Dig Dis 2005;23:6.

CHAPTER 12

The innervation of the gastrointestinal tract

John B. Furness[1,2], Ruslan V. Pustovit[1,2], Linda J. Fothergill[1], Rachel M. McQuade[1,2], and Martin J. Stebbing[1,2]
[1]Florey Institute of Neuroscience and Mental Health, Parkville, VIC, Australia
[2]University of Melbourne, Parkville, VIC, Australia

Chapter menu

Overview

The central nervous system (CNS), the enteric nervous system (ENS) and their interconnections through sympathetic ganglia (Figure 12.1) provide integrated neural control of the digestive system. Although the ENS is capable of regulating aspects of intestinal function by itself, as demonstrated by the persistence of functionally relevant motility, vasomotor and secretomotor reflexes in the intestine that is fully isolated from the CNS [1–4], it does not actually act independently of the CNS in a healthy individual.

Central nervous system control of gastrointestinal function is exerted through the vagus nerves, sympathetic pathways, and pelvic nerve connections. The vagus receives substantial sensory information from the gastrointestinal tract and the CNS has major roles in the control of esophageal and gastric movements, gastric acid secretion, secretion by the exocrine pancreas, and gallbladder emptying. ENS circuits have essential roles in the control of motility, blood flow and water and electrolyte transport in the small and large intestine, and they also influence gut immune and tissue defense system [4,5]. The sympathetic pathways have roles in regulating motility and fluid movement (particularly in relation to fluid balance in the whole body), and controlling vascular resistance and the gut immune system [6]. Major roles of the pelvic nerve connections are to receive sensory input from the distal bowel and to control distal colonic transit, defecation, and fecal continence [7]. Sensory pathways that are primarily concerned with perception of pain follow the sympathetic and pelvic nerves and enter the spinal cord through the dorsal roots.

Many CNS actions on final effectors such as the muscle and lining epithelium are exerted via the ENS. For example, the vagus nerves innervate enteric ganglia of the stomach, pancreas, and gallbladder, but not the muscle directly, sympathetic pathways innervate myenteric and submucosal ganglia, and pelvic nerves innervate the ganglia of the distal colon and rectum. However, some connections are direct, notably the vagal innervation of esophageal striated muscle, sympathetic innervation of the gastrointestinal sphincters, and, in large animals, muscle of nonsphincter regions and sympathetic innervation of gastrointestinal blood vessels.

Essential role of the ENS

It is notable that ENS, but not CNS, control of the gastrointestinal tract is essential to life. If the ENS is missing or depleted, then humans and other mammals die or suffer deficiencies in digestive function, depending on the extent of the loss of enteric neurons.

Yamada's Textbook of Gastroenterology, Seventh Edition. Edited by Timothy C. Wang, Michael Camilleri, Benjamin Lebwohl, Anna S. Lok, William J. Sandborn, Kenneth K. Wang, and Gary D. Wu.

Companion website: www.yamadagastro.com/textbook7e

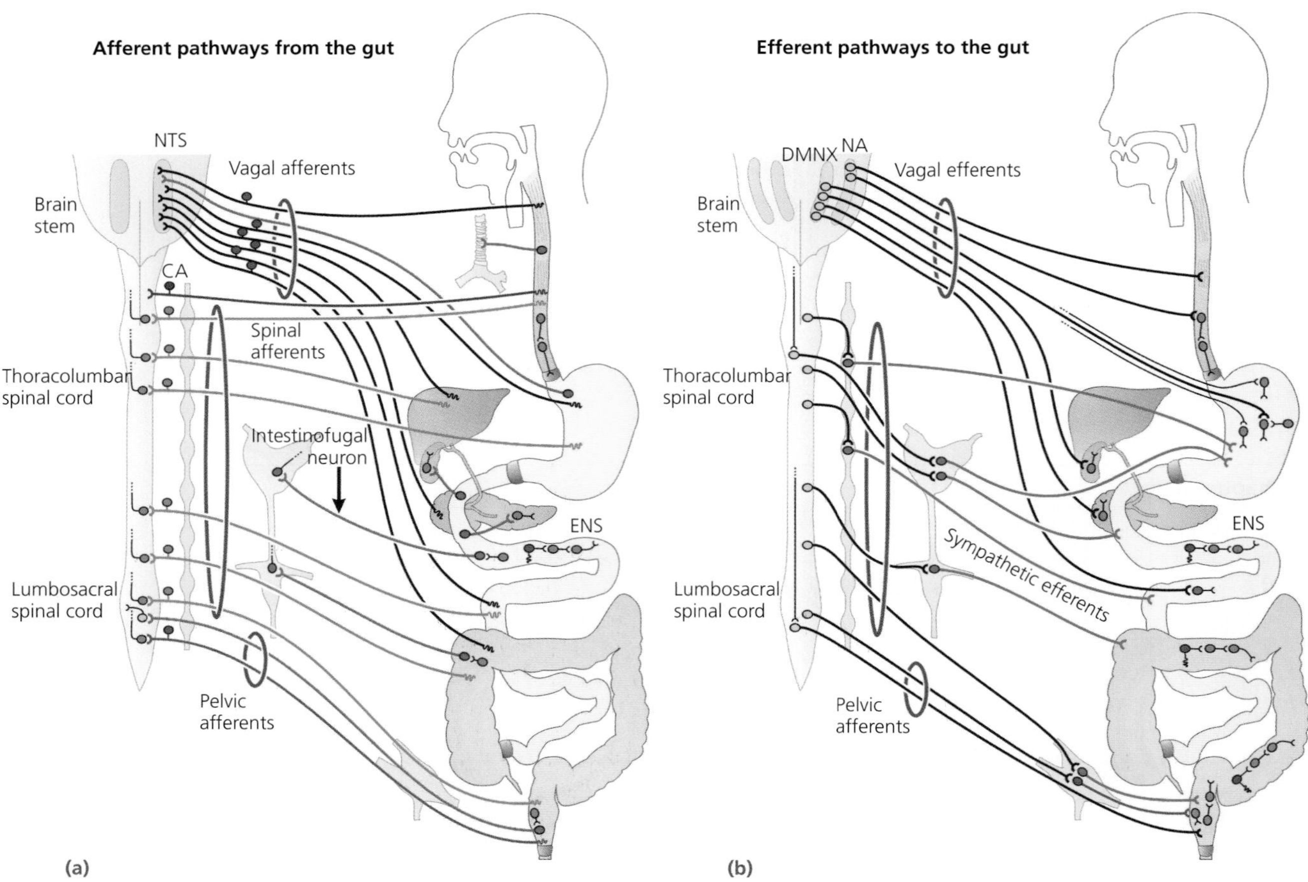

Figure 12.1 The innervation of the gastrointestinal tract. The neural connections between the central nervous system (CNS), sympathetic ganglia, enteric nervous system (ENS), and gastrointestinal effector tissues are complex. **(a)** Afferent signals travel along connections from the digestive system to other organs and the CNS. Vagal afferents end in the nucleus tractus solitarius (NTS) and spinal afferents end in the thoracolumbar spinal cord. In addition, cervical afferents (CA) connect the esophagus to the cervical spinal cord. Some afferent pathways involve intestinofugal neurons that project away from the gut to the CNS, sympathetic ganglia, gallbladder, pancreas, and trachea. Some sensory information is transferred by intrinsic sensory neurons to the ENS. **(b)** Efferent signals travel along connections from the CNS to the digestive system. Pathways from the CNS reach the ENS and gastrointestinal effector tissues through vagal, sympathetic, and pelvic pathways. The sympathetic pathways pass through sympathetic chain ganglia. The vagal efferent neurons have cell bodies in the dorsal motor nucleus of the vagus (DMNX) and nucleus ambiguus (NA). Thoracolumbar and lumbosacral efferents have cell bodies in the autonomic intermediolateral nuclei, and Onuf's nucleus (see Figure 12.10). Neurons of vagal medullary and pelvic spinal outflows synapse with enteric neurons, and many gut-projecting sympathetic neurons with cell bodies in prevertebral ganglia are also preenteric neurons. Some neurons in sympathetic prevertebral ganglia receive both CNS and ENS inputs.

An extreme outcome occurs with Hirschsprung disease, in which there is a congenital absence of enteric neurons (aganglionosis) in all, or part, of the large intestine (see Chapter 110). Hirschsprung disease patients die if the aganglionic segment is not removed. Conversely, when the aganglionic segment is removed, and the patient has an intact ENS throughout the remaining bowel, the patient returns to good health [8]. Severe dysmotility occurs when there is degeneration of the ENS, such as occurs when the ENS is targeted by the infective organism of Chagas disease, *Trypanosoma cruzi* [9]. By contrast, there is survival, with minimal pathology, after removal of CNS connections to the gut, by vagotomy [10,11] or by total sympathectomy [12]. If the pelvic nerves are severed, there is loss of voluntary control of defecation, but the animal or patient is otherwise healthy [13,14].

Although there is a structurally well-developed ganglionated myenteric plexus in the walls of the esophagus and stomach, the neural control of these organs is almost completely dependent on centers in the caudal brain stem and on vagovagal reflexes [15]. Propulsive activity of the esophagus and the activity of the lower esophageal sphincter are controlled through motor pattern generators in the brainstem and reflexes that depend on centers in the CNS [16]. Vagovagal reflexes control gastric relaxation that accommodate ingested food, contractile activity that mixes the food, gastric acid secretion, and other gastric functions [15]. The small intestine and most of the large intestine are primarily dependent on the ENS for their reflex control [5]. However, the distal part of the gut (the distal colon and rectum) is dependent on the CNS for voluntary control of defecation via the pelvic nerves [7].

Structural organization of the enteric nervous system

Nerve cell bodies, their processes and enteric glial cells that are embedded in the wall of the gut form the enteric nervous system (Figures 12.2 and 12.3). The number of enteric neurons in a human is estimated to be 200–600 million, which is about the same as the number of nerve cells in the spinal cord [5]. The nerve cell bodies are grouped in small aggregates, the enteric ganglia, which are connected by bundles of nerve cell processes to form two major ganglionated plexuses in the tubular digestive tract: the myenteric and submucosal plexuses (see Figure 12.2).

Locations of the enteric ganglia

The myenteric plexus of ganglia and connecting nerve strands lies between the longitudinal and circular layers of the *muscularis externa* and forms a continuous network around the circumference of the digestive tract from the most proximal esophagus to the internal anal sphincter. In the parts of the large intestine where the longitudinal muscle is gathered into taeniae, the myenteric plexus is prominent underneath the taeniae and is sparser over the rest of the colonic surface.

Ganglia are numerous in the submucosal plexus in the small and large intestines, but ganglia are fewer the submucosa of the stomach and are rare in the esophagus.

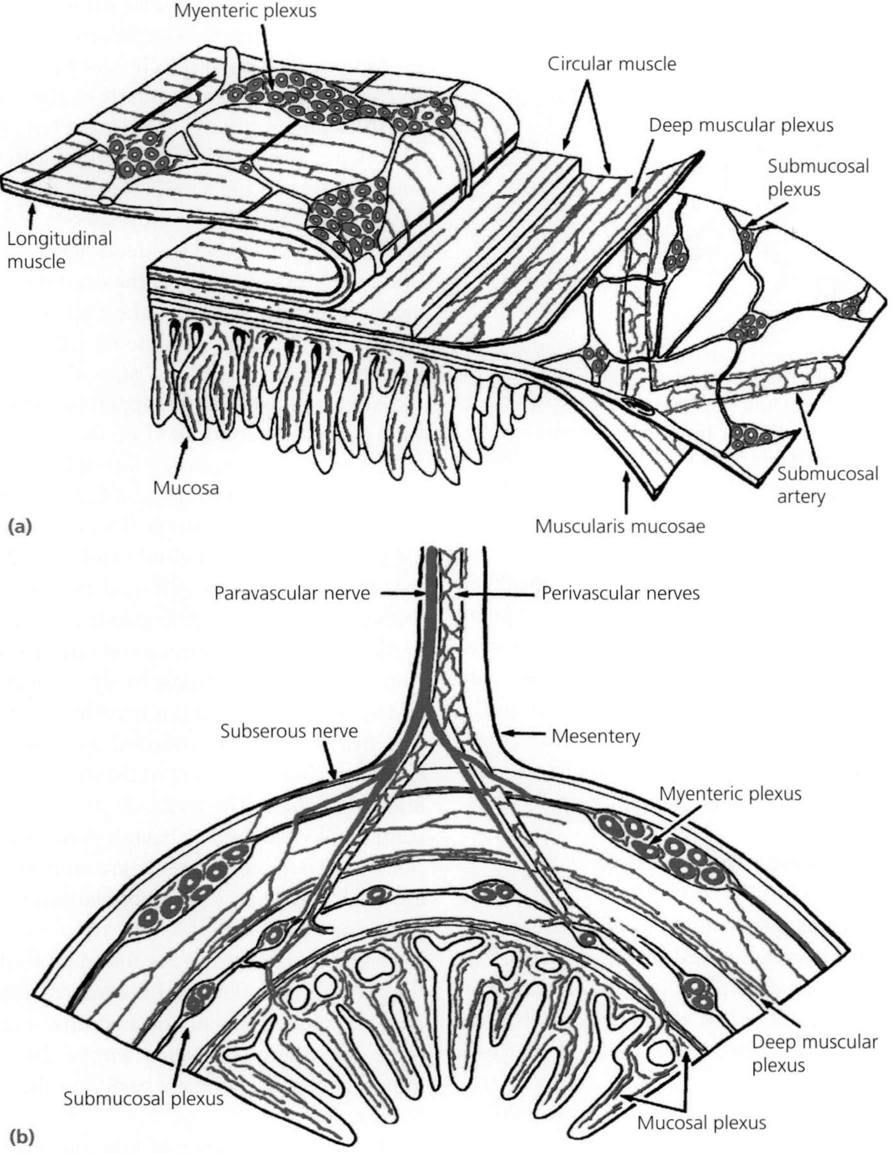

Figure 12.2 The enteric plexuses as they are seen **(a)** in wholemounts and **(b)** in transverse section of the small intestine. There are two ganglionated plexuses, the myenteric and the submucosal, in addition to plexuses of nerve fibers in the muscle and the mucosa and around the arterioles.
Source: Furness and Costa 1980 [17]. Reproduced with permission of Elsevier.

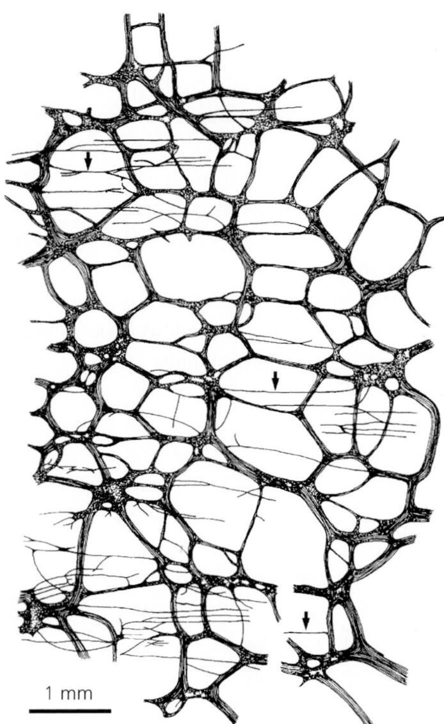

Figure 12.3 Drawing of a wholemount of the myenteric plexus of the human small intestine, prepared by Auerbach and published in *Henle's Textbook of Histology* in 1871. Republished by Furness 2006 [5]. Myenteric ganglia, internodal strands, and small nerve trunks of the secondary component of the myenteric plexus (arrows) can be seen. Source: Henle, J. (1871) Handbuch der systematischen Anatomie des Menschen. 3. Bd., 2. Abt.: Nervenlehre. Vieweg, Braunschweig. Public Domain.

Small numbers of ganglia occur in the mucosa, specifically in the connective tissue close to the *muscularis mucosae*.[5] Small ganglia are also found along the extrinsic nerves (i.e., vagus, pelvic, and mesenteric nerves) as they enter the gut. Some rare ganglia associated with the extrinsic nerves are located on the surface of the gut, particularly in the stomach and rectum; these are referred to as *subserosal ganglia*. Enteric ganglia are also present in the gallbladder, biliary ducts, and pancreas.

Nonganglionated plexuses innervating target tissues

The axons of enteric neurons mix with axons of extrinsic neurons to form a series of nonganglionated plexuses that supply effector tissues of the tubular digestive tract: the longitudinal muscle plexus, the circular muscle plexus (and its subdivisions), the plexus of the muscularis mucosae, the mucosal plexuses, and the perivascular plexuses.

The pattern of innervation of the longitudinal muscle differs according to its bulk. In humans, and in other species in which the longitudinal muscle is a thick layer throughout the intestine, the nerve fiber bundles run parallel to and within the muscle and comprise the longitudinal muscle plexus. In some species, such as the rabbit, guinea pig and mouse, the longitudinal muscle of the small intestine is less than about ten muscle cells thick. In these species, the nerve fiber bundles do not form a plexus within the longitudinal muscle, but they form the tertiary plexus, a component of the myenteric plexus, that lies against the inner surface of the longitudinal muscle [18,19]. The processes of individual tertiary plexus neurons ramify extensively on the inner surface of the longitudinal muscle [20]. There is evidence that axons in the tertiary plexus may interact with macrophages that are located at the level of the myenteric plexus [21,22].

The circular muscle plexus is formed by parallel bundles of nerve fibers throughout the thickness of this muscle layer. In some regions of the gastrointestinal tract, a dense layer of nerve fiber bundles provides additional innervation of the inner part of the circular muscle. The presence of this dense layer and its position in relation to the circular muscle differ among regions. In the mammalian small intestine, the circular muscle consists of a thick outer layer and a thin inner layer of muscle cells [23,24]. The dense plexus of nerve fibers located between these two muscle layers in the small intestine is called the *deep muscular plexus* [25]. The colon of most species lacks an inner specialized layer of circular muscle; a dense layer of nerve fibers, the *submuscular plexus*, similar to the deep muscular plexus, lies close against the inner surface of the circular muscle, adjacent to connective tissue of the submucosa [25–27]. The circular muscle plexus continues into the smooth muscle sphincters of the digestive tract without any apparent change in form. The myenteric plexus also continues into the sphincter regions.

The *muscularis mucosae* throughout the digestive tube consists of outer longitudinal and inner circular layers of smooth muscle innervated by nerve fibers running parallel to the muscle bundles. In the small intestine, muscle bundles also extend into the cores of the villi, and similar strands of muscle are found between the gastric glands [28]. In the small intestine of small animals, such as mice and rats, the muscularis mucosae is thin and barely discernible in histological sections.

The mucosal plexus is a network of fine nerve fiber bundles that lies beneath the mucosal epithelium. It is sparse in the esophagus but prominent in the stomach, small intestine, colon, and gallbladder. The mucosal plexus in the small intestine is sometimes described as having periglandular and villous components. These components are continuous with one another, although some nerve fiber populations selectively innervate the glands or villi [29,30].

Perivascular plexuses are found around the arterioles within the gut wall. The plexuses have mixed origins, from enteric neurons, extrinsic sympathetic neurons, and spinal afferent neurons. Innervation of veins within the gut wall is sparse or nonexistent and lymphatic vessels in the gut wall appear to lack innervation.

The lymphatic tissue within the gut wall, notably Peyer's patches, is innervated from intrinsic and extrinsic sources (see below). There is also innervation of the enteroendocrine (EEC) cells in the gut mucosa.

Myenteric plexus

The myenteric plexus consists of small aggregations of neurons, the myenteric ganglia, nerve fiber bundles that connect the ganglia, and nerve bundles that connect the plexus with other structures (see Figures 12.2 and 12.3). Ganglion size varies widely in the different regions of the gastrointestinal tract. For example, in the guinea pig ileum, ganglia range in size from a single cell to about 200 nerve cell bodies. The ganglia, which are flattened in the plane of the plexus, are usually 1–4 nerve cells thick, depending on the state of contraction and the size of the intestine [31].

The pattern of ganglia, determined by shape and orientation, differs among regions and species but is often readily identifiable as belonging to a particular part of the intestine [32,33]. Small bands of nerve fibers, known as *internodal strands* or *interganglionic connectives*, join the ganglia (see Figures 12.2 and 12.3).

The major targets for nerve cells of the myenteric plexus are the muscularis externa (for nonsphincter smooth muscle most of its innervation is from this source), the submucosal ganglia, and other myenteric nerve cells. Intrinsic primary afferent neurons (IPANs), with cell bodies in the myenteric plexus, and a small number of secretomotor neurons in the myenteric ganglia also innervate the mucosa in the small and large intestine. A numerically minor population of myenteric neurons is intestinofugal neurons that project to sympathetic prevertebral ganglia and other organs, notably the gallbladder and pancreas, and to the CNS (see Figure 12.1).

Submucosal plexus

A continuous network of numerous small ganglia is found in the submucosa throughout the small and large intestines. A much sparser submucosal network occurs in the stomach [34,35]. In many species, plexuses of submucosal ganglia are located in inner and outer layers, but for some regions in small animals there is only one layer [5,36]. The inner and outer plexuses contain different populations of neurons, defined by their morphological and histochemical characteristics [37,38]. Electrophysiological properties of nerve cell populations in the two plexuses also differ [39]. There is evidence that the inner plexus (closer to the mucosa) is mainly concerned with control of mucosal functions, and the outer plexus contributes to control of motility of the external muscle. Submucosal ganglia are smaller and less regularly arranged than myenteric ganglia.

The submucosal plexus harbors the cell bodies of secretomotor neurons (see below). Some neurons, notably submucosal IPANs, project from the submucosa to the myenteric plexus. Other submucosal neurons innervate the muscularis mucosae. Submucosal neurons supply a part of the innervation of the inner circular muscle in some species, including human [27,40,41]. In the stomach, which almost entirely lacks submucosal ganglia, the intrinsic innervation of the mucosa and muscularis mucosae comes from the myenteric ganglia.

Ganglia of the gallbladder, biliary ducts, and pancreas

The biliary system and pancreas develop from diverticula of the small intestine and the ganglia in their walls are part of the ENS. Plexuses of ganglia, similar to the enteric plexuses of the small intestine but differing between species in their relations to tissue layers, are found in the gallbladder, cystic duct, and common bile duct [5]. Numerous nerve fibers occur in the muscle, around blood vessels, and in the mucosa of the extrahepatic biliary tract. The intrinsic neurons of the gallbladder control motility and the flux of water and electrolytes.

Ganglia, connected to each other by small nerve trunks, are scattered through the pancreas, forming a three-dimensional plexus in this solid organ. Nerve fibers are found around the acini and the blood vessels and in the islets. In the pancreas, intrinsic neurons appear to be involved in the control of both the endocrine and exocrine components, although the most complete data exist for exocrine control [42]. Nerve fibers connect the plexuses of the biliary system and pancreas with the ganglionated plexuses of the upper small intestine [43–45]. These connections are presumed to contribute to coordination between these organs and the tubular gastrointestinal tract.

Shapes of neurons

The nerve cells of the enteric ganglia can be classified into subgroups according to their shapes [5,35,46] (Figure 12.4). The first broadly accepted classification was by Dogiel [47], who proposed that the shapes of nerve cells are related to their functions, although a similar scheme, using different nomenclature, was suggested by La Villa [48]. Dogiel defined three cell shapes: types I, II, and III. The first two are readily recognized in different species and with various staining techniques; the third type is less well defined, but bears some resemblance to a group later referred to as *filamentous neurons*. Type I neurons are generally flattened in the plane of the ganglia; they have oval cell bodies, prominent flattened (lamellar) dendrites, and a single long axon often characterized by spiny protuberances close to the cell body. Muscle motor neurons and many interneurons are type I neurons. Type II neurons have a spheroidal shape and give rise to several axons, usually 3–10, although some type II neurons are pseudounipolar [46,49]. A few type II neurons have tapering dendrites in addition to several long axon-like processes and are referred to as *dendritic type II cells* [50]. Type II neurons are IPANs (see below).

Stach [50] extended Dogiel's classification to include types IV, V, and VI and mini-neurons, based primarily on work in the pig [46]. Type IV neurons are secretomotor neurons in the guinea pig and probably in the pig. In the guinea pig small intestine, filamentous and small simple neurons (the latter being similar to the mini-neurons in the pig) have been described [49].

Enteric glia

Enteric ganglion cells and nerve fiber bundles in the gut wall are partially surrounded by glial cells that resemble astrocytes of the

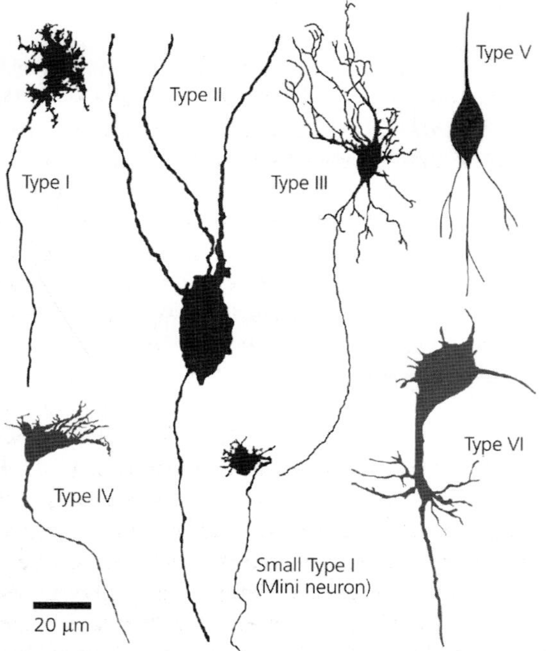

Figure 12.4 Shapes of enteric neurons. Type I neurons have short, branched, lamellar dendrites and a single axon. Most motor neurons and some interneurons have type I morphology. Type II neurons have large oval cell bodies and multiple axons that project to other neurons and to the mucosa. They interconnect with each other in networks. These are intrinsic primary afferent neurons. Type III neurons are also referred to as filamentous neurons. They have long, branched filamentous dendrites and a single axon. Some interneurons have this shape. Type IV neurons have asymmetrically arranged dendrites that often emerge opposite the single axon. Some secretomotor neurons have this shape. Type V and VI neurons are found in large mammals, notably being well documented in pig and human. Small type I neurons, also referred to as mini-neurons, are found in many species. Some of these are locally projecting muscle motor neurons. The images of type I, type II, and small type I neurons are from guinea pig small intestine; their shapes were revealed by intracellular dye injection. The type III neuron is a methylene blue-stained neuron from guinea pig large intestine. The type IV neuron was revealed by NPY immunoreactivity in a submucosal ganglion from guinea pig small intestine. Types V and VI are from pig.

CNS more than glial cells associated with peripheral nerves or other autonomic ganglia [51–53]. They can be distinguished into subtypes based on expression profiles [54]. Enteric glia are clearly not simply passive supporting cells; they interact with enteric nerves, enteroendocrine cells, and immune cells and release ATP that excites enteric neurons. For example, loss of enteric glia is associated with disordered motility and in Crohn's disease enteric glia express major histocompatibility complex (MHC) class II molecules that are normally only expressed by professional antigen-presenting cells, e.g., dendritic cells. Significant effort is currently being made to determine the roles of enteric glia in gastrointestinal physiology and in disease pathology.

Histochemical profiles and transmitter multiplicity of enteric neurons

The enteric nervous system contains more than 30 potential neurotransmitters, many being neuropeptides, that affect the activity of neurons, muscle, and epithelial cells [5,55]. Moreover, individual neurons contain several possible neurotransmitters in addition to other neuron-specific proteins (Table 12.1). The immunohistochemical localization of specific combinations of compounds in neurons provides a valuable investigative tool that allows the projections and connections of individual neurons to be determined and their functions to be deduced, even when the roles of the detected chemicals are not known. A broad range of experiments suggest that the primary transmitters are constant between species whereas differences between species occur in subsidiary transmitters or neuromodulators. In general, more than one substance contributes to the transmission process. An example is excitatory muscle motor neurons, for which acetylcholine is the primary transmitter. These neurons also release tachykinins (the main one being substance P) that contribute to postsynaptic excitation [56]. The inhibitory motor neurons to intestinal muscle also have multiple transmitters that are discussed below. The major transmitter of fast excitatory transmission between neurons is acetylcholine (Figure 12.5), that acts on postsynaptic nicotinic receptors. Gastrin-releasing peptide (GRP) is a conserved transmitter controlling gastrin release and vasoactive intestinal peptide (VIP) is consistently a transmitter of secretomotor/vasodilator neurons across species.

Physiological characteristics of enteric neurons

Electrophysiological properties of enteric neurons

Characterization of the electrophysiological properties of enteric neurons has been dominated by studies on the guinea pig small intestine. Although the types identified in this region can be recognized in other regions and species, properties of the neurons differ between regions of the digestive tract, and, even in a specific region, properties can vary depending on the circumstances of the experiment [57–59]. In the guinea pig small intestine, most neurons can be separated into two groups, AH and S, according to their electrophysiological properties (Table 12.2). These terms were introduced in 1974 [60] and the classification remains valid, although the reasons for calling them AH and S are no longer well justified.

The S neurons have properties similar to the majority of neurons in sympathetic and parasympathetic ganglia. They exhibit brief action potentials that are followed by short-duration afterhyperpolarizing potentials (AHPs) lasting 20–100 ms. These action potentials are blocked by tetrodotoxin. S neurons exhibit fast excitatory postsynaptic potentials (EPSPs), and compound fast EPSPs of sufficient amplitude to generate action potentials

Table 12.1 Major types of neurons in the enteric nervous system (ENS) and some of their defining characteristics. The numbers in brackets are the identifying numbers for the anatomical depictions of the neurons in Figure 12.6.

Functional definition	Primary transmitters	Comments
Excitatory circular muscle motor neurons (6)	ACh, cotransmitter TK. ACh receptors: muscarinic. TK receptors, NK_1, NK_2	Excitatory neurons supply all smooth muscle regions, including sphincters. Majority innervate muscle close to cell bodies, some run short distance orally to supply muscle
Inhibitory circular muscle motor neurons (7)	NO plus several cotransmitters with varying prominence: ATP-like, VIP, PACAP	Inhibitory neurons supply all smooth muscle regions, including sphincters. Majority innervate muscle close to cell bodies, some run anally to supply muscle
Excitatory longitudinal muscle motor neurons (4)	ACh, cotransmitter TK	Supply muscle adjacent to cell bodies
Inhibitory longitudinal muscle motor neurons (5)	NO plus several cotransmitters with varying prominence: ATP-like, VIP, PACAP	Supply muscle adjacent to cell bodies
Excitatory neurons to the muscularis mucosae (16)	ACh, cotransmitter TK	Similar properties to other excitatory muscle motor neurons
Inhibitory neurons to the muscularis mucosae	NO plus several cotransmitters: ATP-like, VIP, PACAP	Similar properties to other inhibitory muscle motor neurons
Myenteric ascending interneurons (1)	ACh. Nicotinic receptors postsynaptic	In the small intestine only one type. Involved in local peristaltic reflex
Myenteric descending interneurons (local reflex) (8)	ACh. ATP may be a cotransmitter	These neurons also contain NOS
Myenteric descending interneurons (secretomotor and motility reflex) (9)	ACh, 5-HT (at 5-HT_3 receptors)	This type of descending interneuron has been documented in several species. In guinea pig it is in a pathway of descending excitation
Myenteric descending interneurons (MMC) (10)	ACh	Neurons contain somatostatin. It is speculated that these neurons are involved in conducting MMC along the small intestine
Myenteric IPANs (2)	TK, CGRP, and ACh	These neurons detect distortion of their processes and intraluminal chemistry
Submucosal IPANs (11)	TK, CGRP, and ACh	Respond to intraluminal chemistry and mucosal distortion
Intestinofugal neurons (3)	ACh, cotransmitter VIP	These neurons directly or indirectly detect conditions in the gut wall and are in afferent pathways of enteroenteric reflexes
Motor neurons to gut endocrine cells	Various. Neurons innervating G cells utilize GRP	A range of endocrine cell types is innervated
Noncholinergic secretomotor/vasodilator neurons (12)	VIP. Other peptides of the VIP family may contribute	Neurons project both to the mucosa and to arterioles. The majority of these neurons are in submucosal ganglia
Cholinergic secretomotor/vasodilator neuron (13)	ACh	Dual projection, to the mucosa and to arterioles. Innervate bases of glands. The majority of these neurons are in submucosal ganglia
Cholinergic secretomotor (nonvasodilator) neurons (14)	ACh	Innervate mucosal epithelium only. The majority of these neurons are in submucosal ganglia
Submucosal uniaxonal neurons projecting to the myenteric plexus (15)	ACh (deduced). Contain VIP (NOS?)	Possibly displaced myenteric interneurons
Neurons to lymphoid tissue	ACh (deduced)	Physiology has not been directly determined

ACh, acetylcholine; ATP, adenosine triphosphate; CGRP, calcitonin gene-related peptide; GRP, gastrin-releasing peptide; 5-HT, 5-hydroxytryptamine; MMC, migrating myoelectric complex; NK, neurokinin (receptor); NO, nitric oxide; NOS, nitric oxide synthase; NPY, neuropeptide Y; PACAP, pituitary adenylyl cyclase-activating peptide; SOM, somatostatin; TK, tachykinin; VIP, vasoactive intestinal peptide.

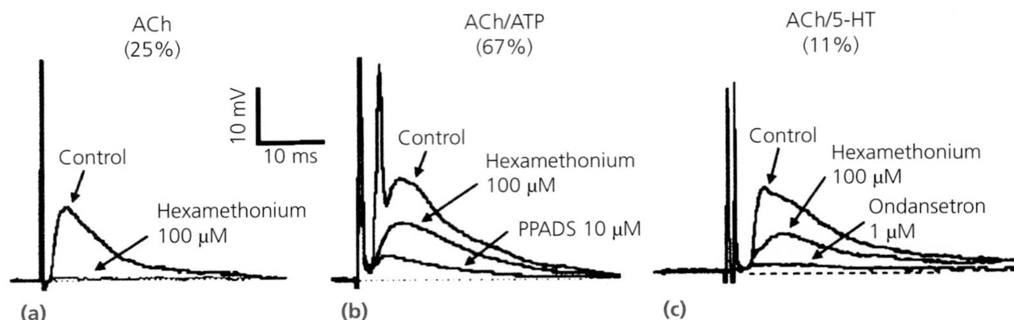

Figure 12.5 Pharmacological dissection of fast excitatory postsynaptic potentials (EPSPs) in S neurons of the myenteric plexus of the guinea pig ileum. **(a)** A fully cholinergic EPSP is blocked by the nicotinic receptor antagonist hexamethonium. **(b)** A fast EPSP is partly reduced by hexamethonium. The remaining component is largely blocked by the purinergic P_{2X} receptor antagonist pyridoxalphosphate-6-azophenyl-2′,4′-disulfonic acid (PPADS). **(c)** A fast EPSP in which the response remaining after the administration of hexamethonium is blocked by the 5-HT_3 receptor blocker ondansetron. ACh, acetylcholine; ATP, adenosine triphosphate; 5-HT, 5-hydroxytryptamine. Source: Galligan et al. 2000 [70]. Reproduced with permission of Elsevier.

Table 12.2 Comparison of properties of S and AH neurons.

	S neurons	AH neurons
Soma action potentials	Monophasic, tetrodotoxin sensitive	Hump on falling phase, tetrodotoxin insensitive
AHP following soma action potential	Brief (20–100 ms)	Brief AHP, followed by prolonged (1–2 s) AHP
Process action potentials	Tetrodotoxin sensitive	Tetrodotoxin sensitive
Fast EPSPs	Prominent, trigger action potentials	Rare, subthreshold for triggering action potentials, see text
Slow EPSPs	Observed in most S neurons	Major mode of synaptic excitation of AH neurons
Shapes	Single axon, multiple short dendrites, small and medium sized	Multiple axons, commonly without dendrites, large ovoid (type II) cell body

AHP, afterhyperpolarizing potential; EPSP, excitatory postsynaptic potentials.

can be evoked in all S neurons. These EPSPs are referred to as *compound* because they are the summed effects of transmission from several or many axons. Slow EPSPs are also recorded from S neurons. S neurons have a variety of shapes, which include the Dogiel type I and filamentous morphologies. These S neurons have a single axon.

The currents and ion channels of AH neurons in the guinea pig have been studied intensively in recent years. The degree of detail, which helps to explain how the excitability and firing patterns of these neurons are controlled, is beyond the scope of this chapter, but can be found elsewhere [61]. The soma action potentials of these neurons are carried by a combination of Na^+ and Ca^{2+} [60,62] and have an inflection (hump) on the falling phase that is contributed by the Ca^{2+} current. They are normally followed by two separate phases of hyperpolarization. An early AHP lasts 20–100 ms and is followed by the second hyperpolarization, the late AHP, that lasts 4–25 seconds. In the guinea pig small intestine, all AH neurons have Dogiel type II morphology. AH neurons in the guinea pig ileum usually do not exhibit fast EPSPs, and when they are recorded, the EPSPs have small amplitudes [58,60,63]. It is possible that the small amplitudes of fast EPSPs recorded in AH neurons are an experimental artefact. These neurons when recorded with intracellular electrodes typically have low input resistances, of the order of 100–200 MΩ, whereas whole-cell patch clamp indicates input resistance of 500 MΩ [58,64]. The leakiness that occurs when the cells are penetrated with intracellular electrodes may short out fast EPSPs. Recent studies using Ca imaging indicate that Dogiel type II/AH neurons receive hexamethonium-sensitive synaptic inputs, presumable fast EPSPs [65]. Slow EPSPS do occur in AH neurons and can trigger action potentials.

The S and AH nomenclature does not apply, or is less useful, for some other gut regions. For example, in the guinea pig rectum, some neurons that exhibit a prolonged AHP have a single axon and receive fast EPSPs [66]. In the gastric corpus, all myenteric neurons have S characteristics and do not exhibit a prolonged hyperpolarization after the action potential [67,68]. In fact, IPANs are probably absent, or very rare, in the stomach. In the absence of IPANs, most reflexes that control gastric functions pass through the CNS, notably vagovagal reflexes, such as vagovagal relaxation that increases gastric volume, vagovagal augmentation of antral contractile waves, and vagal control of acid secretion. The slow AHP is less prominent in AH neurons of the mouse intestine [69].

Synaptic transmission in the enteric nervous system

Enteric neurons receive fast and slow EPSPs and inhibitory postsynaptic potentials (IPSPs). In addition, transmitter release from terminal axons may be reduced by presynaptic inhibition. Fast EPSPs are graded in amplitude in relation to the strength of electrical stimulation, and when they are reflexly evoked, individual EPSPs of different amplitudes are observed (see below). Thus, enteric neurons receive multiple fast synaptic inputs. Fast EPSPs in S neurons have nicotinic, purinergic, and serotonergic components (see Figure 12.5). However, use of nicotinic receptor blockers, and other experimental data, show that acetylcholine (ACh) is the most prominent transmitter of fast EPSPs [70]. Some fast EPSPs are in fact completely blocked by nicotinic receptor antagonists, whereas others are reduced in amplitude (see Figure 12.5), some by as little as 20% [71–73]. In about 60–80% of neurons with a nicotinic antagonist-resistant fast EPSP, the residual EPSP is reduced in amplitude or abolished by PPADS, an antagonist of P_{2X} (purine) receptors [72,73]. In about 10% of neurons, a 5-HT_3 receptor antagonist blocks or reduces hexamethonium-resistant fast EPSPs [73,74]. Antagonists of receptors for these three transmitters, in combination, do not fully block fast EPSPs in some S neurons, which implies the existence of one or more additional transmitters of fast EPSPs.

In the guinea pig small intestine, slow EPSPs usually last between 15 and 120 s and occur in at least 75% of S neurons and in probably all AH neurons [75,76]. The slow EPSPs are evoked by short trains of stimuli, usually applied at 5–20 Hz for 1–2 s. Slow EPSPs evoked by electrical stimulation are likely to be the result of the superimposed actions of several different transmitters, each producing superficially similar synaptic potentials [75,77].

Analysis of the pharmacology of transmission and the neurochemistry of connections in the ENS indicate that acetylcholine (at muscarinic receptors), tachykinins, and 5-HT contribute to slow EPSPs [75,77–79].

Inhibitory postsynaptic potentials in myenteric neurons have been reported rarely, and then only in a low proportion of neurons in the guinea pig small intestine [80,81]. It is possible that excitatory responses may obscure IPSPs that are evoked by electrical stimulation. However, studies in which enteric reflex pathways are activated by physiological stimuli, such as distension, have also failed to evoke IPSPs in myenteric neurons. This suggests that any physiological role for this type of synaptic potential may be confined to a small group of myenteric neurons.

Electrophysiological studies of *submucosal* neurons have been performed in preparations from the small intestine, cecum, and distal colon of the guinea pig [82–87]. About 90% of all submucosal neurons exhibit fast EPSPs, and a large proportion of these also exhibit slow EPSPs, similar to those observed in myenteric neurons. The fast EPSPs are blocked by hexamethonium and are presumably mediated by ACh acting through nicotinic receptors. Pharmacological data indicate that slow transmission to secretomotor neurons in the submucosa is mediated through purine P_{2Y} receptors [88,89].

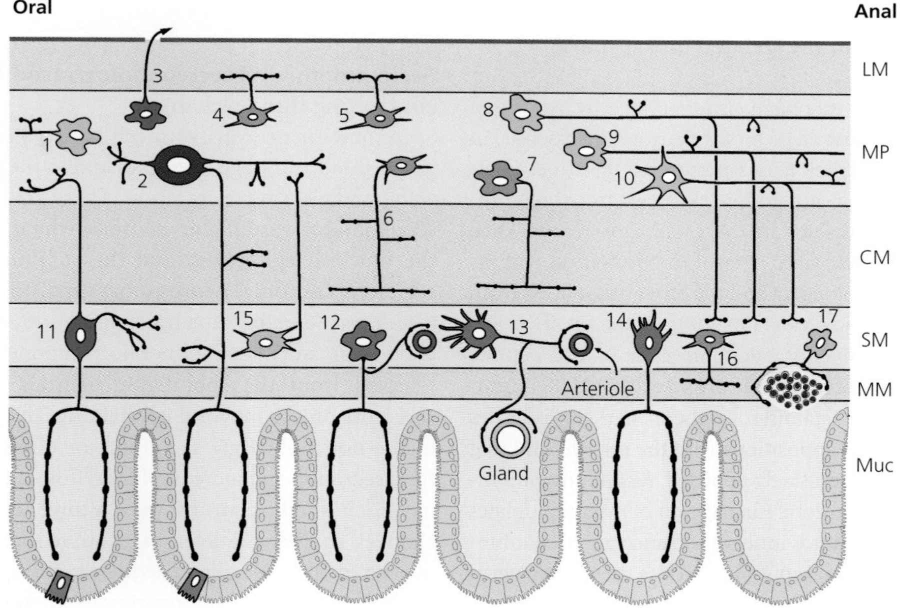

Figure 12.6 Neuron types in the ENS. The types of neurons in the small intestine, that have been defined by their functions, cell body morphologies, chemistries, key transmitters and projections to targets. LM, longitudinal muscle; MP, myenteric plexus; CM, circular muscle; SM, submucosal plexus; Muc, mucosa. Neuron types: ascending interneurons (1); myenteric intrinsic primary afferent neurons (IPANs) (2); intestinofugal neurons (3); excitatory longitudinal muscle motor neurons (4); inhibitory longitudinal muscle motor neurons (5); excitatory circular muscle motor neurons (6); inhibitory circular muscle motor neurons (7); descending interneurons (local reflex) (8); descending interneurons (secretomotor and motility reflex) (9); descending interneurons (migrating myoelectric complex) (10); submucosal IPANs (11); noncholinergic secretomotor/vasodilator neurons (12); cholinergic secretomotor/vasodilator neuron (13); cholinergic secretomotor (nonvasodilator) neurons (14); uniaxonal neurons projecting to the myenteric plexus (15); motor neuron to the muscularis mucosa (16); innervation of Peyer's patches (17). Not illustrated, motor neurons to enteroendocrine cells. Source: Furness 2006 [5]. Reproduced with permission of John Wiley & Sons, Ltd.

Although slow IPSPs are rarely observed in myenteric neurons, they are commonly seen in submucosal neurons. Substantial IPSP occur in about 50% of submucosal neurons in the guinea pig small intestine and in as many as 90% of the neurons in the cecum [82–85,90]. In the small intestine, neurons with slow IPSPs contain VIP and are noncholinergic secretomotor/vasodilator neurons [91]. Two separate contributions to IPSPs have been identified: adrenergic transmission from sympathetic neurons and nonadrenergic transmission from intrinsic neurons. The nonadrenergic transmission is contributed to by 5-HT and somatostatin [90].

Presynaptic inhibition may also have a role in the enteric nervous system. Sympathetic nerve stimulation reduces the amplitudes of fast EPSPs in both myenteric and submucosal neurons, probably by decreasing the amount of ACh released from the synapses [92,93]. It appears that the presynaptic inhibitory effect of the sympathetic transmitters is the primary mechanism by which sympathetic neurons diminish the contractile activity of the gut [5]. This inhibition is mediated through α-adrenoreceptors. ACh released from enteric nerve terminals can act presynaptically to regulate the subsequent release of ACh and possibly to modify the release of the transmitters mediating slow EPSPs.[94]

Functionally defined enteric neurons

Motor neurons

Muscle motor neurons of the striated muscle part of the esophagus

The striated muscle of the esophagus is innervated by axons that form motor endplates. These vagal motor neurons are essential to esophageal function and if their axons are severed there is esophageal paralysis [95]. Unlike motor endplates elsewhere, a high proportion of individual endplates in the esophagus receive dual innervation, one axon being from a vagal motor neuron with its cell body in the medulla oblongata and the other originating from a cell body in the myenteric plexus [96–100]. In the rat, the vagal endings are immunoreactive for calcitonin gene-related peptide (CGRP), and the endings of myenteric origin exhibit NOS immunoreactivity [100]. Double staining for these markers indicates that both fibers make close appositions with the muscle, and that the two fiber types are often closely apposed, facilitating presynaptic interaction [98]. The enteric innervation of motor endplates is presynaptic to the vagal motor innervation and causes an inhibitory modulation of the vagal input [101]. Thus the enteric nervous system seems to have a role in modulating centrally generated propulsion of content in the upper esophagus. The enteric innervation may have a greater role in young animals, because all motor endplates receive an enteric innervation at days 4–10 postnatal, after which there is partial withdrawal of innervation [102].

Muscle motor neurons of the stomach and intestines

Excitatory neurons innervate the longitudinal and circular smooth muscle and the muscularis mucosae throughout the digestive tract. They are involved in contracting the muscle during propulsive reflexes and in mixing movements. The primary transmitter of these neurons is ACh, which acts on the muscle through muscarinic receptors [5]. Tachykinins, released from the same neurons, contribute to the excitatory transmission but have a lesser role than ACh. The tachykinin component of excitatory transmission appears to be more prominent at high rates of neuron firing. These neurons are S neurons by electrophysiological classification.

Inhibitory motor neurons are involved in descending reflexes that facilitate the passage of contents along the bowel and relax regions, such as the stomach, that expand to accommodate and retain their contents. The neurotransmitters are nitric oxide (NO), ATP (or a related compound), pituitary adenylate cyclase-activating peptide (PACAP), and VIP [103–107]. Identification of the substances responsible for the "ATP" component of transmission is difficult because purines are present in all cell types, are released via numerous pathways and have overlapping pharmacologies [108]. It is likely that a major component of inhibitory transmission in the intestine is mediated by b-nicotinamide adenine dinucleotide (b-NAD+). VIP and the NO synthesizing enzyme, nitric oxide synthase (NOS), are coexpressed by the inhibitory motor neurons, and are useful immunohistochemical markers of these neurons. The primary transmitter of the neurons appears to be NO, and deficits in transmission are observed if NO synthase is knocked out [109,110]. Inhibitory motor neurons are also S neurons.

Secretomotor and secretomotor/vasodilator neurons controlling fluid exchange

Secretomotor neurons with cell bodies in submucosal ganglia in the small and large intestines and in the gallbladder enhance water and electrolyte secretion. There are two types of neuron: secretomotor/vasodilator neurons which send axons to both the mucosal epithelium and the submucosal arterioles, and secretomotor (only) neurons that supply the epithelium but not arterioles. Secretomotor transmission to the mucosa has both cholinergic and noncholinergic components [111, 112]. ACh released from the cholinergic neurons acts on muscarinic receptors on the mucosal epithelium. The primary transmitter of the noncholinergic secretomotor effect is VIP. VIP causes fluid secretion and increases blood flow [113,114]. Experiments in which single neurons were stimulated, and the resulting changes in the diameter of submucosal blood vessels were measured, provide direct evidence for the presence of both cholinergic and noncholinergic vasodilator neurons [115–117]. Immunohistochemical studies, combined with surgical denervation, confirm that both intrinsic cholinergic and noncholinergic neurons innervate submucosal arterioles [118].

Gastric vasodilator neurons

Gastric acid secretion and blood flow are enhanced when the vagus nerve is stimulated; these effects are reduced by muscarinic antagonists. In most experiments, it is not possible to determine whether vasodilation is the result of a direct vascular action of cholinergic neurons, in addition to a functional hyperemia consequent to the increased secretion [119]. However, centrally administered thyrotropin-releasing hormone stimulates a vagal pathway in the rat that caused gastric vasodilation after acid secretion is blocked by omeprazole [120]. The increased blood flow in the absence of secretory change was antagonized by atropine. There is also evidence for noncholinergic transmission from gastric vasodilator neurons that utilize VIP [121].

Gastric secretomotor neurons that stimulate acid output

Some secretomotor neurons promote gastric acid secretion. These neurons are cholinergic and act on the parietal cells through muscarinic receptors. They act with histamine and gastrin to increase acid output [122].

Motor neurons innervating enteric endocrine cells

Numerous enteroendocrine (EEC) cells reside in the mucosa of the gastrointestinal tract, and because the mucosa is densely innervated, most of these cells have nerve fibers in close proximity. It is likely that most are influenced by neurotransmitters, but there has not been a thorough investigation of neural control of gastrointestinal hormone release. The best-documented motor neurons that provide functional innervation of enteric endocrine cells are those controlling the release of gastrin from G-type EEC cells. This release is under the influence of vagal and intrinsic nerve pathways. The final neurons in both pathways are enteric neurons in the stomach wall. Transmission from the motor neurons to the G cells is mediated at least in part by gastrin-releasing peptide [122]. The basal release of motilin is reduced by atropine and tetrodotoxin and stimulated by muscarinic agonists; these findings suggest that motilin (M) cells receive an excitatory cholinergic input [123]. Stimulation of the vagus causes an atropine-sensitive release of peptide YY from L-type EEC cells of the distal small intestine [124]. Activation of a vagovagal reflex, and local nerve stimulation, both enhance glucagon-like hormone secretion from the L cells [125,126].

Innervation of lymphoid tissue (Peyer's patches)

Lymphoid aggregations of the gastrointestinal tract (Peyer's patches) have surrounding nerve fibers, some of which penetrate the capsule of the follicle to provide innervation of the suprafollicular dome region but not of the germinal centers [127–130]. Retrograde tracing from follicles reveals that they are innervated from submucosal ganglia [130]. Receptors for transmitters of enteric neurons occur on lymphocytes within the Peyer's follicles and on lymphocytes that are scattered in the connective tissue of the mucosa [131,132]. Moreover, scattered lymphocytes are close to axons; this suggests that there may be a functional innervation of isolated lymphocytes within the mucosa [128,133]. Close appositions between axons and mast cells also occur in the mucosa [134].

Neurons that influence glucose absorption

Glucose in the lumen causes the release of several gut hormones, including glucagon-like peptide 2 (GLP-2) [135–137]. In turn, there is an induction and functional activation of the sodium-glucose transporter, SGLT1 [135]. Although the induction of SGLT1 is mediated through GLP-2, the GLP-2 receptor is on submucosal neurons, not on the epithelium [138], which implies that the increased glucose transport is a nerve-mediated effect [139]. Consistent with this, GLP-2 excites submucosal neurons [140]. There is also evidence that vagovagal reflexes contribute to induction of SGLT1 in the small intestine [141]. The afferent component of the vagovagal reflex was blocked by capsaicin application to the abdominal vagus 10 days prior to infusing sugars into the duodenum [141]. The efferent pathway probably involves vagal preenteric neurons and enteric final motor neurons.

Enteric interneurons

Interneurons have been identified in all gut regions, although their characteristics may vary between regions more than those of other neuron types. For example, the ileum and colon contain the same, or very similar, motor neurons and intrinsic primary afferent neurons, but their complements of interneurons are quite different.

Within the myenteric plexus, the interneurons form chains of like neurons that run both orally and anally [142,143]. In the guinea pig small intestine, at least three classes of descending interneurons and one class of ascending interneurons exist. Detailed studies of synaptic connections indicate that the chains formed by two of the types of descending interneurons interconnect [144]. The ascending interneurons appear to be involved in local motility reflexes, as are the descending cholinergic neurons that contain NOS [5]. Another type of descending interneuron, the ACh/somatostatin interneurons, may be linked to the passage of the migrating myoelectric complexes (MMCs), which are described below. These neurons have a distinctive appearance (filamentous neurons) with numerous branching, tapering, filamentous dendrites [142]. They have very rare connections from IPANs [145,146]. The third type of descending interneuron, the ACh/5-HT interneuron, is involved in descending excitatory reflexes, and perhaps in secretomotor reflexes [147]. Interneurons also make connections between the myenteric and submucosal plexuses.

Intrinsic primary afferent neurons

About 100 years ago, it was discovered that enteric motility reflexes could be elicited in segments of intestine that had no neural connections with the CNS [1,148,149]. It was therefore assumed that primary afferent neurons were contained in the gut wall. However, it was discovered at about the same time that reflexes, notably cutaneous vasodilator reflexes, could be initiated via axon collaterals even when the axons bearing the collaterals were disconnected from their cell bodies. Thus, to demonstrate that reflexes are truly intrinsic, it is necessary to leave sufficient time for nerve endings and their collaterals to die, after the nerve has been lesioned before testing the integrity of reflexes. Such experiments applied to the small and large intestine in guinea pig, cat, and dog indicate that the motility reflexes are indeed intrinsic [2,5]. The intrinsic sensory neurons, commonly called intrinsic primary afferent neurons (IPANs), have now been identified (Figure 12.7).

Intrinsic primary afferent neurons were directly identified to be neurons with AH electrophysiological properties and Dogiel type II morphology by experiments in which activity-dependent changes were used to reveal the neurons [150,151], and by intracellular recording [152,153] in the small intestine of the guinea pig. Neurons with similar morphology, histochemistry, and projections have been found in the small and large intestines of guinea pig, mouse, rat, human, pig, and sheep. Various experiments indicate that the cell bodies of the mucosal mechanoreceptor primary afferent neurons are in the submucosal ganglia, while the cell bodies of chemoreceptor afferent neurons and stretch-responsive primary afferent neurons are in myenteric ganglia. Dogiel type II neurons are common in all gut regions except the stomach, which is consistent with neural control of the stomach being largely controlled through the CNS. In human stomach, fewer than 1% of myenteric neurons are type II [35] and gastric type II neurons are also rare in small mammals [154]. In the small and large intestines, Dogiel type II neurons generally make up 10–25% of neurons.

Intrinsic primary afferent neurons make connections with other IPANs and with inter- and motor neurons. In the colon they may make preferential connections with ascending interneurons and motor neurons [155].

Intrinsic primary afferent neurons are one of several types of afferent neuron associated with the gut (Figure 12.8; see also Figure 12.1). Others are vagal afferent neurons, spinal afferent neurons, and intestinofugal neurons. The intestinofugal neurons are probably second-order neurons in afferent pathways leading from the gut to prevertebral ganglia [156]. The extrinsic primary afferent neurons are subdivided into two groups: those with cell bodies in the vagal (nodose) ganglia and those with cell bodies in the dorsal root ganglia. The vagal afferent pathways carry information about the physiological state of the digestive organs (see below). Impulses conveying pain or discomfort are conducted through the dorsal root ganglion (spinal afferent) pathways.

Other enteric neurons that respond to mechanical stimuli

It has been assumed that the AH/ Dogiel type II neuronal subclass represents the only intrinsic sensory neurons in the gut. It is likely that these IPANs are the sole mediators of mucosally derived reflexes, as they are the only intrinsic neurons with projections to villi, and are directly activated by mechanical stimulation of the mucosa and by chemicals applied to the mucosal surface. However, recent studies provide compelling

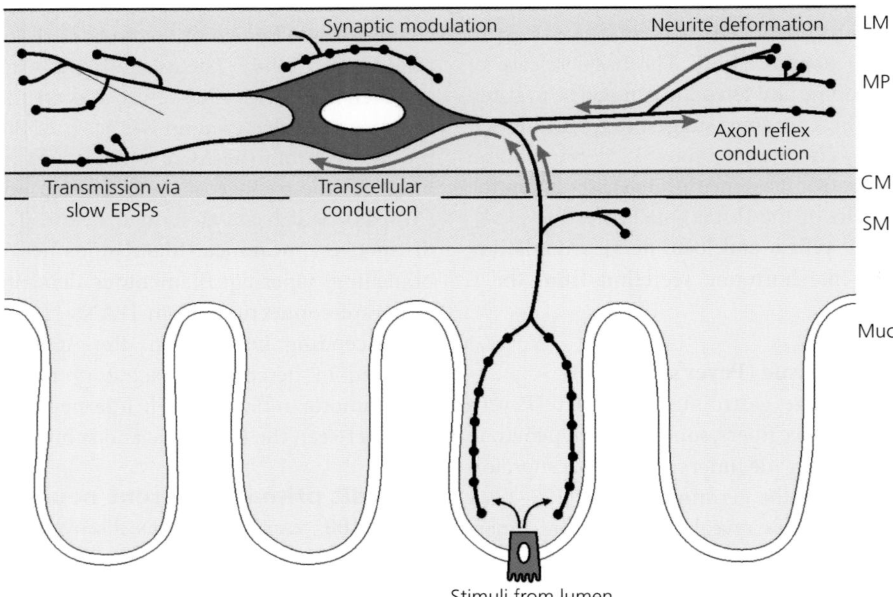

Figure 12.7 Diagram of a myenteric intrinsic primary afferent neuron (IPAN). The IPANs are multipolar type II neurons. Action potentials initiated by physiologically appropriate stimuli and by noxious stimuli can traverse the cell bodies (transcellular conduction) or can be conducted to output synapses via an axon reflex (axon reflex conduction). Conduction across the cell body is modified by the synaptic inputs that it receives. The myenteric IPANs make synaptic connections with other neurons in the myenteric and submucosal ganglia. CM, circular muscle; EPSPs, excitatory postsynaptic potentials; LM, longitudinal muscle; MP, myenteric plexus; Muc, mucosa; SM, submucosal plexus. Source: Furness 2006 [5]. Reproduced with permission of John Wiley & Sons, Ltd.

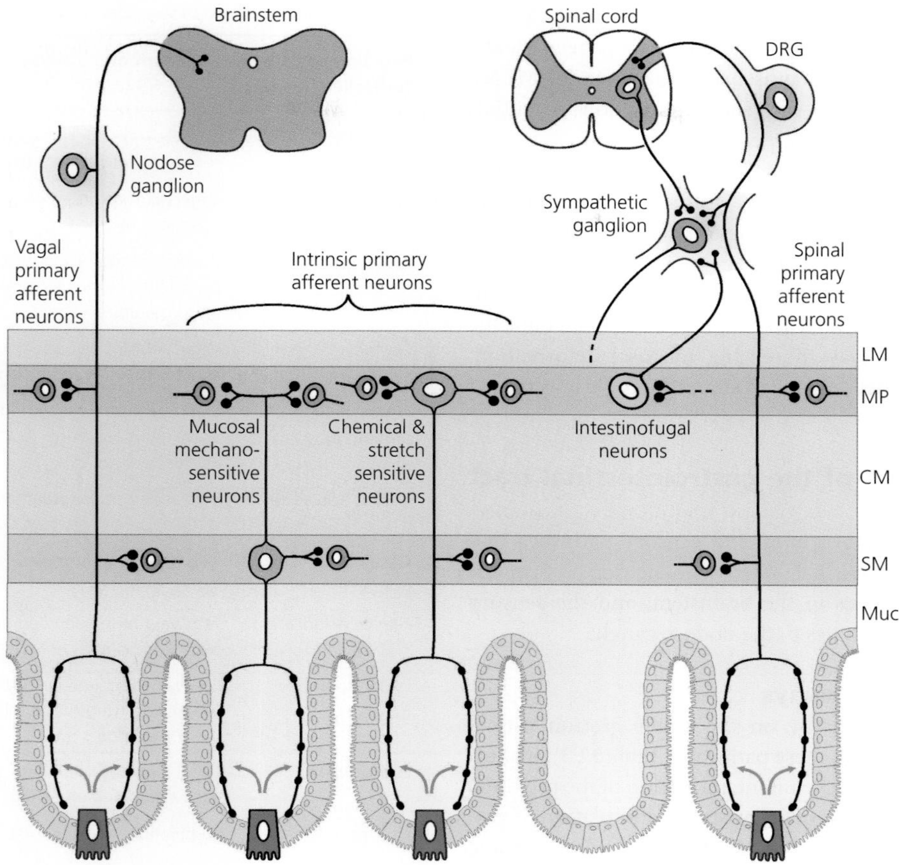

Figure 12.8 The sensory (afferent) neurons of the digestive tract. Two classes of intrinsic primary afferent neuron (IPAN) have been identified: myenteric IPANs that respond to distortion of their processes in the external muscle layers and, via processes in the mucosa, to changes in luminal chemistry, and submucosal IPANs that detect mechanical distortion of the mucosa and luminal chemistry. Extrinsic primary afferent neurons have cell bodies in dorsal root ganglia (spinal primary afferent neurons) and vagal (nodose and jugular) ganglia. Spinal primary afferent neurons supply collateral branches in prevertebral (sympathetic) ganglia and in the gut wall. Intestinofugal neurons are parts of the afferent limbs of enteroenteric reflex pathways. Nerve endings in the mucosa are activated by hormones, most prominently 5-hydroxytryptamine (5-HT), released from enteroendocrine cells (arrows). CM, circular muscle; LM, longitudinal muscle; MP, myenteric plexus; Muc, mucosa; SM, submucosa. Source: Furness 2006 [5]. Reproduced with permission of John Wiley & Sons, Ltd.

evidence supporting a role for S/Dogiel type I neurons in stretch-mediated mechanotransduction.

Spencer and Smith [157] characterized a subclass of S-type interneuron that was mechanosensitive to circumferential stretch and remained active for the duration of the stimulus period. These filamentous interneurons had dendrites located within, and parallel to, circular muscle fibers. These structures may represent sensory elements, and their presence is consistent with the requirement for connectivity between the circular muscle layer and myenteric ganglia for stretch-induced firing of these neurons. Moreover, these neurons exhibited spontaneous fast EPSPs that occurred in the muscle in time with reflexly evoked excitatory and inhibitory junction potentials. Smith et al. [158] proposed that these neurons may be analogous to the stretch-sensitive muscle spindles found in skeletal muscle, and that they are responsible for initiating stretch-sensitive, tone-independent peristaltic reflexes. Distension-evoked propagation of peristaltic contractions may be blocked by application of muscle relaxants at the site of distension, indicating that these most likely require tension-detecting IPANs [159]. Thus, it is likely that the mechanically stimulated coordinated reflex activity of the intestine is sensed and initiated by both AH and S neurons that detect muscle tension and length, respectively.

Based on motor and interneurons having sensory functions, the concept of a "multifunctional mechanosensitive neuron" with individual neurons possessing sensory, integrative, and motor functions has been proposed [160]. Experiments measuring action potential discharge in response to deformation of ganglia using fast voltage-sensitive dye imaging indicate that approximately 25% of all myenteric neurons are directly mechanosensitive [160,161]. Neurons that were morphologically and neurochemically identified as interneurons and motorneurons responded to deformation in a stimulus strength-dependent manner [160]. The authors have described these as rapidly adapting mechanosensitive enteric neurons (RAMEN). A small subset of neurons in the mouse colon has been identified as slowly adapting mechanosensitive neurons (SAMEN). These neurons are capable of generating action potentials throughout a sustained stimulus period [162].

Collectively, these studies indicate that the detection and response to sensory information within the intestine are mediated by a combination of neuron types, rather than exclusively by IPANs. There is thus evidence that the original IPAN model may be too simplistic with respect to mechanosensation. However, these reports do not discount the key roles that IPANs play in sensing mucosal deformation, chemical changes in the lumen, and smooth muscle tension.

Vagal innervation of the gastrointestinal tract

The vagus nerves contain motor and sensory pathways that innervate the gastrointestinal tract. The neurons of motor pathways have cell bodies in the brainstem, and the sensory neurons have their cell bodies in the nodose ganglia.

Motor (efferent) pathways

A variety of effects, primarily on the upper gastrointestinal tract, are mediated through these pathways (Table 12.3), including propulsion of esophageal content, relaxation of the proximal stomach, enhancement of gastric peristalsis, stimulation of gastric acid, promotion of gastrin release, stimulation of pancreatic secretion, and contraction of the gallbladder [163,164]. Except for neurons that innervate the striated muscle of the esophagus, the vagal neurons do not act directly; they are preenteric neurons that form synaptic connections with enteric neurons. Small numbers of vagal efferent neurons also project to the small intestine and proximal colon. It is interesting that Brunner's glands in the small intestine appear to be innervated directly by vagal pathways, but not by local intrinsic neurons [165].

According to the convention used for other cranial autonomic pathways, the vagal neurons of these motor pathways have been called *parasympathetic preganglionic* or *vagal preganglionic neurons.* Reference to vagal input neurons as preganglionic wrongly implies that enteric neurons are relay neurons in parasympathetic pathways. Vagal input neurons are neurons in complex circuits in which enteric reflexes of several types are integrated with signals from the central nervous system and from other parts of the gastrointestinal tract. It is preferable to refer to them as *vagal preenteric neurons.* Transmission from vagal preenteric neurons to enteric neurons is mediated principally by ACh acting on nicotinic receptors. Thus the effects of stimulating vagal motor pathways are blocked or substantially attenuated by drugs that block nicotinic receptors.

Sensory pathways

The greatest proportion of vagal sensory (afferent) fibers innervate the esophagus, stomach, proximal small intestine, liver, and pancreas. There is a less prominent vagal sensory innervation of the distal small intestine and proximal colon. The vagal afferents convey information about the physiological states of the digestive organs and their contents. The functions regulated by the vagal sensory innervation include appetite and satiety, esophageal propulsion, gastric accommodation, contractile activity and acid secretion, contraction of the gallbladder, secretion of pancreatic enzymes, and levels of inflammation of the intestines.

Table 12.3 Motor functions of vagal pathways.

Function or tissue controlled	Comment on pathway
Striated muscle esophagus,	Cell bodies in nucleus ambiguus. Respond to central pattern generators
Smooth muscle esophagus	Vagal neurons preenteric, impinging on myenteric neurons
Lower esophageal sphincter	Control through vagovagal reflexes. Vagal preenteric neurons to esophageal and gastric motor neurons
Gastric relaxation	Vagal neurons involved in vagovagal receptive relaxation and accommodation reflexes
Gastric mixing and propulsion	The rhythms are generated in the gastric muscle. Vagal input augments or inhibits contractile activity
Gastric acid secretion	Vagal neurons are preenteric. Pathways stimulate secretion from parietal cells
Gastrin secretion from EECs	Vagal pathways stimulate secretion
Gastric vasodilation	Pathways have been demonstrated, but physiological roles not clarified
Pyloric sphincter	Following vagal denervation, there is a deficit in gastric emptying that is relieved by pyloromyotomy
Gallbladder	Vagal pathways stimulate gallbladder contraction and emptying
Pancreas	Stimulation of enzyme secretion
Brunner's glands	Stimulation of vagus causes mucus secretion

EEC, enteroendocrine cell.

Three distinct types of vagal afferent ending occur in the gastrointestinal tract: intraganglionic laminar endings (IGLEs), intramuscular arrays (IMAs), and mucosal varicose nerve endings [166]. IGLEs and IMAs are mechanoreceptors, whereas the mucosal endings indirectly detect luminal chemistry and also detect mucosal distortion. IGLEs have complex branching nerve endings that give rise to flat (laminar) expansions within myenteric ganglia. In general, their frequencies of occurrence are greatest proximally in the gut and numbers decrease distally [167]. Along this gradient, regions of greater density are found in the upper esophagus, gastric corpus, and distal ileum. IGLEs in the rectum, and some of those in the distal colon, arise from pelvic nerves [168]. IGLEs respond rapidly to direct mechanical probing [169]. Firing rates diminish within the first 2–3 s, but the neurons continue to fire at a reduced rate throughout the stimulus; thus these are partially adapting mechanoreceptors. IGLEs that responded to direct probing also responded to stretching of the stomach wall, which provides direct proof that IGLEs are stretch receptors [168,169]. They almost certainly correspond to the low-threshold tension receptors that were identified in the 1950s [170,171]. IGLEs express GLP-1 receptors and, by use of a GLP-1 receptor reporter system, their mechanosensitivity has been directly demonstrated [172].

Intramuscular arrays are formed by single afferent axons that branch within the circular muscle layer to form arrays of varicose fibers that run parallel to muscle bundles [173]. They form synapse-like complexes with two types of cell, interstitial cells of Cajal (ICCs) and PDGFRα + cells that form an electrically coupled syncytium with gastric smooth muscle [174,175]. It has been suggested that IMAs, ICCs, and smooth muscle work cooperatively or synergistically to respond to stretch or muscle length information [30].

Vagal mucosal sensory nerve endings branch within the connective tissue beneath the mucosal epithelium [30,172,176]. They can therefore only react to the chemistry of the lumen indirectly. The intermediaries are chemoreceptive EEC cells that sense nutrients and also potentially noxious agents in the gut contents, and release hormones that act on vagal afferent nerve endings [177,178]. Bitter material in the lumen causes the release of the gastric hormone ghrelin from A-type EEC cells, and acidic conditions in the antrum cause somatostatin release from D-type EEC cells. It has been confirmed in humans that ghrelin signaling to hypothalamic feeding centers is via the vagus [179]. Gastric mucosal receptors are responsive to low-intensity stroking of the mucosa, but not to muscle stretch or contraction [180–182]. Solid food is triturated in the stomach into smaller particles that are able to pass through the pylorus [183]. Experiments in which the antral mucosa was separated from the underlying muscle, a procedure that abolishes vagovagal reflexes, suggest that mucosal mechanoreceptors may discriminate particles by size and regulate their passage into the duodenum [184]. The mechanosensitivity of gastric mucosal afferents is enhanced by the satiety hormone leptin, and reduced by the feeding hormone ghrelin [185,186].

Separate villus and crypt afferents innervate the mucosa of the small intestine [30]. Villus afferents have axons that project toward the villus tip, where they branch extensively. Each villus afferent fiber typically innervates a cluster of two or more neighboring villi. The villus afferents are ideally positioned to detect substances released from the epithelium, including intestinal EEC cell hormones such as cholecystokinin (CCK), 5-HT, and GLP-1 that are known to activate vagal nerve endings [172,177,178]. Fats in the proximal small intestine are detected by EEC cells that release CCK, which has three main actions: release of enzymes from the pancreas, stimulation of gallbladder contraction, and increase of satiety [187].

Pelvic nerves

The major gastrointestinal effects of the pelvic nerves are on movement, secretion, and blood flow in the distal colon and rectum. The pathways are analogous to those of the vagus; pelvic efferent neurons with cell bodies in the sacral spinal cord form synapses on enteric neurons at which ACh is an excitatory transmitter acting through nicotinic receptors. The pelvic nerves initiate defecatory reflexes [7]. Sensory axons in the pelvic nerves detect mechanical changes in the colorectum [188]. Pain signals are also conveyed through the pelvic nerves [189].

Neural control of gastrointestinal movements

Overview

The muscle layers of the gastrointestinal tract are responsible for propulsion and mixing of contents, reservoir capacity (notably in the stomach), restriction of movement between regions separated by sphincters, and expulsion of pathogens and noxious chemicals. The relative roles of extrinsic and intrinsic neurons in directing these activities differ along the digestive tract. In broad terms, the body of the esophagus is controlled through the vagus from brainstem circuits located in the medulla oblongata and the stomach is controlled through the brainstem and vagovagal reflexes. Small intestine motility is largely controlled through the ENS, as is large bowel motility, except for the essential role of the CNS in regulating defecation via the pelvic nerves. Sympathetic pathways modify the control exerted through vagal, enteric, and pelvic nerves.

The esophagus

The nerve circuits for motor programs coordinating propulsive activity in the upper, striated muscle part of the esophagus are in the medulla oblongata of the CNS. These relay through the nucleus ambiguus, which contains the cell bodies of the motor neurons that innervate the striated muscle [16,190]. Although there are numerous ganglia that form an ENS of conventional appearance in the striated muscle esophagus, the ENS has little influence on the pattern of propulsive activity, and esophageal propulsion fails and never recovers its function if the vagal innervation is severed [95]. Nevertheless, myenteric neurons supply a modulating innervation to about a majority of the end-plates (see above: *Muscle motor neurons of the striated muscle part of the esophagus*).

The nerve fibers that innervate the smooth muscle of the lower esophagus have their cell bodies in enteric ganglia. Propulsion in this region is also coordinated from the CNS. The enteric ganglia of the smooth muscle esophagus are directly innervated by preenteric neurons of the dorsal motor nucleus of the vagus, and lesion of this nucleus impairs the motility patterns of the smooth muscle esophagus [16]. The vagus is involved in relaxing the lower esophageal sphincter (LES), to allow passage of food, through a descending inhibitory reflex that relaxes the sphincter when a bolus of food enters the last part of the esophageal body and its intraluminal pressure is raised. This reflex relaxation is inhibited by cooling the vagus nerve [191]. However, sphincter relaxation still occurs in response to distension following vagal block, indicating that a local reflex can be elicited [191].

Peak intragastric pressures during gastric mixing contractions exceed resting pressures in the body of the esophagus, thus providing a gradient that would propel corrosive gastric juice into the esophagus were it not for the LES that has an important role in limiting reflux. This role is apparent when pressure in the stomach is increased and a reflex constriction of the LES is initiated [192,193]. The contraction is mediated by a vagovagal reflex pathway that passes through the brainstem. Failure of this guarding results in reflux esophagitis and esophageal mucosal damage.

Stomach

Nerve-mediated control of gastric movements is primarily exerted through vagovagal reflexes and control centers in the brainstem. The stomach has a reservoir function; it increases volume as it fills and relaxes prior to food arriving. It also has a function to mix the food with gastric juices and to push the liquefied products of gastric digestion into the duodenum. The fundus (proximal stomach) is primarily associated with the gastric reservoir function and the corpus-antrum (distal stomach) is associated with gastric mixing and antral propulsion [194]. Each antral contraction propels a small amount of liquid into the duodenum, while solid material is retained in the stomach [183].

Gastric reservoir function

The proximal stomach relaxes to accommodate meals and as a result the basal pressure in the stomach does not increase as it fills [195]. In fact, relaxation occurs even before the food arrives, a phenomenon called receptive relaxation [196]. The vagovagal reflex relaxation that occurs when the pharynx or esophagus is distended occurs even when the esophagus is severed and no food reaches the stomach [197]. Distension, for example by inflation of an intragastric balloon, relaxes the proximal stomach. This accommodation reflex is substantially reduced by vagotomy [198,199]. A vagally mediated gastrogastric reflex relaxation is also elicited when distension is confined to the antrum [200]. In addition, there appears to be a small residual component of accommodation that is due to an intrinsic reflex [201]. As the volume in the stomach reduces, the fundus contracts. This also appears to be a vagally mediated effect [199]. Thus the stomach adjusts its volume both by relaxation and contraction, primarily of the fundus, via vagovagal reflexes.

Gastric peristalsis and mixing

Gastric peristalsis, which occurs in the corpus and antrum, is not prevented when the myenteric plexus is cut through or nicotine is given in a dose that blocks peristalsis in the intestine [202,203]. Moreover, the frequency of peristalsis corresponds to the frequency of gastric slow waves in the muscle, indicating that gastric peristalsis is generated by the slow waves and, unlike peristalsis in the small intestine and colon, it does not require augmentation by the actions of excitatory neurons to be observed. However, there is augmentation of the gastric contractions, dependent on vagovagal reflexes, when the stomach is distended [204]. When the antrum, or the whole stomach, is extrinsically denervated, antral peristaltic contractions are smaller and emptying times are prolonged [204–206]. It is concluded that gastric peristalsis is a consequence of contractions that are induced in the muscle by slow waves generated by the pacemaker activity of ICCs [175]. The amplitudes of these contractions are modulated by nervous activity.

There is little evidence for an intrinsic gastric reflex that is organized like that in the small intestine. Consistent with this, IPANs, the types of neurons through which reflexes in the intestine are initiated, appear to be absent or very rare in the stomach, based on morphology, the lack of type II neurons [35,154], and electrophysiology, the lack of AH neurons [207]. Nevertheless, a number of studies indicate that there is intrinsic activity of excitatory cholinergic neurons, even in the completely isolated stomach. The isolated stomach exhibits an excitatory tone that is reduced by tetrodotoxin or by antagonists of muscarinic or nicotinic receptors, and the amplitudes, but not the frequencies of occurrence, of contractile waves are reduced when transmission from excitatory neurons to the muscle is prevented by tetrodotoxin [208–210].

The small intestine and colon

Intrinsic reflexes of the ENS are essential to the generation of motility patterns that are observed in the small and large intestines. In the small intestine, these are rapid orthograde propulsion of contents (peristalsis), mixing movements (segmentation), slow orthograde propulsion (the migrating myoelectric complex, MMC), and retropulsion (expulsion of noxious substances associated with vomiting). In the large intestine, there are mixing and propulsive movements, including the colonic MMC, typically described in small mammals, and high-amplitude peristaltic contractions (HAPC) that propel colonic contents in large mammals, including humans [188,211]. HAPCs are preceded by relaxation, and when they reach the last part of the colon, there is relaxation of the anal sphincter and defecation.

To orchestrate the movement patterns of the small intestine and colon, the state of the intestine is sensed and appropriate motor patterns are generated. The structural organization of the circuits that detect the state of the small intestine, integrate the information and direct the activities of motor neurons is known (Figure 12.9) and the colonic circuits appear to be similar [158,212] although there are some specializations of colonic circuits [155]. Although the mechanisms within the integrative circuitry through which one pattern of activity is converted to another are not known, there are some indications from computer modeling of the neuronal activities that underlie these different patterns [213,214]. Signals that trigger changes in patterns of

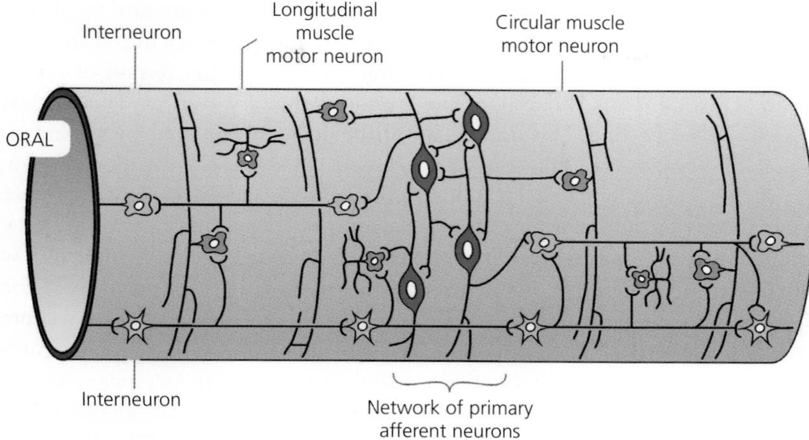

Figure 12.9 Nerve circuits for control of motility in the small intestine. This diagram is based on studies in the guinea pig small intestine. Similar component neurons have been identified in the small intestine of other species, including human, and in the large intestine. This is a simplified diagram showing the major circuit features that have been identified. Networks of interconnected intrinsic sensory neurons (IPANs) **(red)** detect mechanical distortion and luminal chemistry. These synapse with descending and ascending **(both yellow)** interneurons, and connect with excitatory muscle motor neurons and inhibitory muscle motor neurons **(both blue)** directly and via interneurons.

movement in the small intestine have been identified. For example, fatty acids added to the luminal surface convert propulsive contractile activity to mixing movements, through a neural mechanism [215]. Conversion from one pattern to another can also be achieved with drugs that target enteric neurons [216].

The circuits in the small intestine

The circuits involved in local peristaltic reflexes in the small intestine, and the projections of the component neurons, have been deduced from studies of guinea pig small intestine. Experiments in other species, including cats, dogs, and rats, suggest that the pathways are similarly organized in other mammals [5]. In all species, excitatory and inhibitory motor neurons supply the muscle; the general patterns of small intestine motility are similar, and intrinsic reflexes are evoked by the bulk and chemical nature of the luminal contents.

The movements of the intestine are a result of the contractions and relaxations of the external longitudinal and circular muscles and of the muscularis mucosae. The neural control is superimposed on an underlying rhythm of muscle activity (i.e., slow waves), which occurs at frequencies of about 3–12 per minute in humans. The major role in forming the pattern of mixing and propulsive movements appears to be taken by the circular layer of the external muscle, areas of which contract (or relax) like an annulus to decrease or increase the diameter of the lumen during both propulsive and mixing movements.

To study enteric muscle motor reflexes, investigators isolate segments of intestine to eliminate the influences of the CNS and circulating hormones. This simplifies recording from the muscle and enteric neurons. In these preparations, luminal distension, or chemical or mechanical stimulation of the mucosa, elicits reflexes whose effects on the circular muscle can be recorded with intracellular microelectrodes [217–223]. The major responses of the muscle are depolarizing potentials (i.e., excitation) in the circular layer oral to the site of the stimulus and anal hyperpolarizing potentials (i.e., inhibition). This polarization of electrical responses is analogous to that of the mechanical events seen when the intestine is distended. Longitudinal muscle motor neurons are also activated by reflex stimuli [224]. The longitudinal muscle contracts at the same time as the circular muscle, although there may be delay between the commencement of contraction in the two layers [5]. The longitudinal muscle appears to restrict the lengthening of the intestine when the circular muscle contracts. If the longitudinal muscle does lengthen, it can initiate a reflex that inhibits propulsion [225].

Neither the reflex responses to stimulation of the mucosa nor those to distension pass along the gut if the myenteric plexus is cut, but they are unaffected by interruption of the submucosal plexus [203,222,226]. Therefore, the reflex pathways excited by mucosal stimulation must pass locally from the sensory receptors in the mucosa to the myenteric plexus. Responses evoked by distention persist if the mucosa is removed [222,227–230], a finding that is consistent with some of the mechanosensitive processes of IPANs being in the external muscle. Mucosal distortion releases 5-HT from enterochromaffin cells in the epithelial lining [231] which, in turn, activates the endings of the IPANs to initiate or potentiate peristaltic reflexes [232]. However, the experiments just referred to in which the mucosa was removed or when 5-HT is absent due to genetic ablation of its synthesizing enzyme [233] indicate that there is not an essential role of mucosal 5-HT.

Enteric reflexes often extend for several centimeters along the intestine from a single point of stimulus, unlike the processes of the majority of IPANs and of motor neurons. This implies that most enteric reflex pathways include interneurons, which form interconnecting chains that run along the intestine (see above).

Most excitatory and inhibitory motor neurons supplying the circular muscle extend only 1–2 mm along the guinea pig intestine, but they run up to half the distance around its circumference, about 6–8 mm [234,235]. Thus, the response to reflex activation is spread around the intestine. This finding is consistent with the common observation that the intestine undergoes annular, not eccentric, contractions or relaxations. The reflex response probably involves a summed response to transmission from many motor neurons; each smooth muscle cell is influenced by approximately 25 inhibitory motor neurons, and a similar convergence of excitatory influence can be expected [234]. Furthermore, the electrical communication between smooth muscle cells ensures a summation of the effects of the population of motor neurons.

The intestine exhibits cyclic changes of contractile activity, which are evoked by *migrating myoelectric complexes* (MMCs). The MMCs pass along the intestine from the stomach to the terminal ileum. In humans, these cycles last about 90 minutes and are seen between digestive periods. MMCs are mediated through the intrinsic neural pathways of the small intestine [236]. Interruption of the continuity of the enteric nervous system blocks conduction of the MMC along the small intestine [237].

Control of defecation and fecal continence

Like swallowing, which introduces food into the gastrointestinal tract, control of the release of residue through defecation is under voluntary control. This is clearly demonstrated by the difficulties encountered by patients when the spinal cord is severed [238–241]. The patients are unable to voluntarily empty their bowels and the content accumulates, causing considerable discomfort. Thus, the enteric nervous system of the colorectum, in the absence of central command, will not empty the bowel. Moreover, the overfull bowel leaks through the anal sphincter, suggesting that there is a loss of voluntary control of continence. These changes involve both a loss of pelvic nerve influence on the colorectal enteric nervous system and a loss of control of the external striated muscle sphincter. The control pathways have been recently reviewed [7]. The pathways include cortical centers for voluntary control of continence and defecation, pontomedullary centers for coordination of bowel emptying and external anal sphincter relaxation, autonomic neural circuits for coordinated movement of the bowel located at the sacral level of the spine (spinal defecation center) and circuits within the ENS of the bowel wall (Figure 12.10). The somatic circuits that control the external sphincter are directed from the cortex and pons.

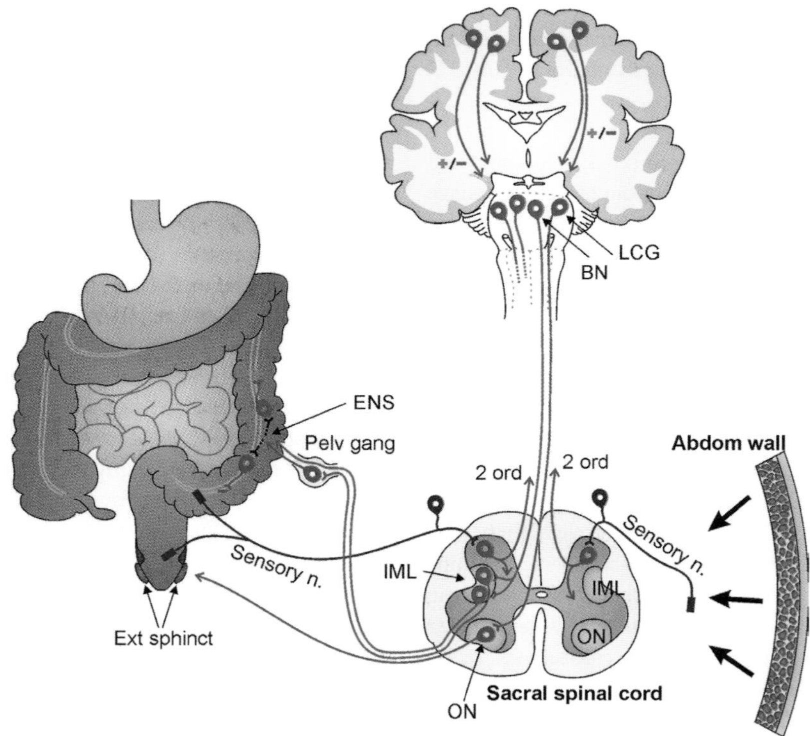

Figure 12.10 The nerve pathways for voluntary control of defecation and fecal continence. Cortical centers that govern voluntary control provide inputs that either inhibit or enhance excitability of neurons in the brainstem, a medial nucleus (Barrington's nucleus, BN) through which autonomic pathways to the distal colon and rectum are activated, and a lateral cell group (LCG) that controls the external anal sphincter. The medial group of neurons projects to the spinal defecation center in the intermediolateral column (IML) at S1 level. This in turn connects with intrinsic reflex pathways of the enteric nervous system (ENS), via the pelvic ganglia. Afferent (sensory) neurons that detect pressure and mucosal irritation in the colon contribute to urge and neurons that sense pressure in the abdominal cavity enhance defecation. These connect to second order (2 ord) neurons that make local connections in the spinal cord and provide sensory information to the pons and cortex. Descending neurons from the LCG synapse in Onuf's nucleus (ON) on motor neurons that supply the external sphincter. Source: Callaghan et al. 2018 [7]. Reproduced with permission of Springer Nature.

Neural control of secretion and mucosal blood flow

Overview

About 5–10 liters of water, derived from food and drink, salivary secretions, gastric secretion, secretions of the pancreas and biliary system, and from the intestine itself, enters the lumen of the human intestine each day. To maintain the equilibrium of fluids in the body, electrolyte that is absorbed in the gastrointestinal tract must be equalled by losses through perspiration, respiration, urination and defecation. Secretion and absorption are balanced so that the osmolarity of the fluid in the small intestine is closely matched to that in the interstitial fluid, although there are local variations from isosmolarity, for example in the lamina propria of the villi. The critical role played by regulation within the intestine itself is exemplified by the life-threatening effects of bacterial toxins, such as cholera toxin, which act on enteric neurons to cause copious secretion of fluid across the intestinal epithelium [242].

Water moves from the lumen in company with the absorption of nutrient molecules [243,244]. The major process for the absorption of nutrients, such as glucose, is cotransport with Na^+, in this case through the sodium-glucose cotransporter, SGLT1. The entry of these solute molecules draws water across the epithelium, which is one reason to add glucose to oral rehydrating fluids. Direct measurements indicate that there is cotransport of 210–260 water molecules per 1 glucose molecule [244]. It has been estimated that SGLT1 absorbs 8–9 liters of water each day from the small intestine [244]. Another way to consider the relationship between dissolved nutrient molecules and the amount of associated fluid is that 100 g of carbohydrate, if broken down to monosaccharides, would require about 1.8 L of water to be absorbed and be isotonic with blood and tissue fluids [5]. Amino acid transport is also ion coupled and in a similar way this transport involves water movement in concert with absorption. The large fluxes of water from the lumen to the fluid compartments of the body are partly balanced by intestinal secretion which is mediated by enteric secretomotor reflexes.

Enteric secretomotor and vasomotor reflexes

Distension, mechanical stimulation of the mucosa, intraluminal nutrients and the application of chemicals to the mucosa, including noxious substances, evoke secretomotor and vasodilator reflexes [245–250]. Histochemical studies in the guinea pig small intestine indicate that two of the motor neurons for secretion are also motor neurons for vasodilation; that is, these secretomotor neurons cause a physiologically appropriate vasodilation, concomitant with secretion, through collaterals to submucosal arterioles [5]. A third type of secretomotor neuron does not project to the vasculature. As indicated above, control of secretion in the small intestine contributes to the regulation of whole-body water and electrolyte status. Some of the fluid absorbed with nutrients or across the gastric mucosa can be passed back under the control of secretomotor reflexes. The source of secreted fluid in the small intestine is a mixture of serum electrolytes and locally absorbed electrolytes (Figure 12.11).

Glucose or its uptake stimulates the enteric secretomotor reflex [245]. Enteric reflexes also cause HCO_3^- secretion in response to duodenal acidification, although other acid-sensitive mechanisms, including a neurally independent stimulation of prostaglandin production, also cause secretion of HCO_3^- [251]. It is likely that the same ion channels are permeable to Cl^- and HCO_3^-, the relative amounts of Cl^- and HCO_3^- transported being dependent on the luminal pH [252]. Secretomotor reflexes can also be initiated pathologically by toxins, such as cholera toxin or enterotoxins, in the lumen (see section below: *Responses to noxious stimuli*).

The enteric secretomotor/vasodilator circuits consist of IPANs with their endings in the mucosa and an integrating circuitry that feeds back to motor neurons with cell bodies in the submucosal ganglia [5]. In some cases, the reflex pathways

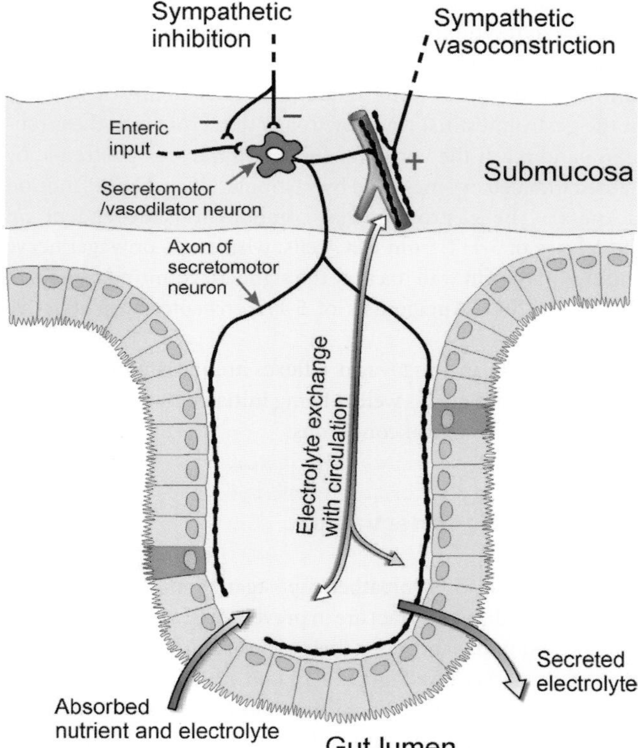

Figure 12.11 Schematic representation of the integration of enteric and sympathetic neuronal control of secretomotor and vasomotor activity in the small intestine. The circuitry provides for adjustment of the secretion of fluid and electrolyte into the intestinal lumen, according to the sources of the fluid and the needs of the whole body to maintain fluid homeostasis. The sources of fluid to supply the secretory flux are the fluid that is absorbed across the epithelium in company with nutrients and ions, and fluid from the circulation. The enteric secretomotor reflexes are under tonic inhibitory control from the sympathetic neurons that innervate secretomotor neurons and the availability of fluid from the circulation is limited by activity of sympathetic vasoconstrictor neurons. If systemic blood pressure or blood volume decreases (e.g., in hemorrhage), secretion and blood flow to the mucosa are both inhibited.

involve the myenteric ganglia (e.g., cholera toxin-induced secretion) [253] whereas reflexes initiated by mechanical stimulation of the mucosa can be mediated entirely through the submucosal plexus [112,247,254]. Pathways from the myenteric plexus also cause vasodilation [255,256].

Responses to noxious stimuli

In the small intestine and colon, protective secretory and motility responses are initiated by irritants that are included in enemas, by noxious products of bacteria, and by parasitic infestations. The intestine exhibits exaggerated secretomotor reflexes, causing diarrhea, when there are excessive levels of bacteria and bacterial toxins in the gut lumen [242,257]. Powerful propulsive reflexes are also triggered by pathogens and their products, including parasitic nematodes, the bacterial pathogen *Vibrio cholerae*, and bacterial toxins, as well as by irritants, such as ricinoleic acid, the active component of castor oil [258–260]. Vomiting, which involves retropulsive reflexes in the small intestine, is also used to eliminate undesirable contents from the gut. Vomiting is initiated by toxins or irritants in the gastrointestinal tract, by toxins that cross into the circulation and reach the vomiting centers in the area postrema, by nausea induced by smell, and by vestibular disturbance (motion sickness). The gastrointestinal component is dependent on the release of 5-HT from EEC cells, which acts on vagal nerve endings in the gut wall to carry the signal to vomiting centers in the brain [201]. Antagonists of 5-HT$_3$ receptors are effective antiemetics.

Thus enteric and vagovagal reflexes are initiated by noxious conditions in the gut, as well as being initiated by benign stimuli in normal physiological conditions.

Sympathetic innervation

The cell bodies of sympathetic postganglionic neurons that innervate the digestive tract are in prevertebral and paravertebral ganglia, and in the abdomen their axons run to the gut with the mesenteric nerves (see Figures 12.1 and 12.11). The major roles of these neurons are to regulate blood flow to the gastrointestinal tract, regulate intestinal fluid and electrolyte secretion to keep it in balance with whole body requirements, inhibit gastrointestinal motility, and reduce the intensity of inflammation. Norepinephrine is the primary transmitter of the sympathetic postganglionic neurons that supply the gastrointestinal tract.

Sympathetic effects on secretion

The sympathetic innervation of secretomotor neurons influences the net movement of water and electrolytes between the gut lumen and body fluid compartments to maintain overall fluid homeostasis. The sympathetic pathways can override the enteric secretomotor reflexes. Axons arising from the sympathetic secretomotor-inhibiting neurons in prevertebral ganglia innervate secretomotor neurons (see Figure 12.11), in which they elicit inhibitory synaptic potentials. Persuasive evidence indicates that, in day-to-day circumstances, the intrinsic secretomotor reflex activity is inhibited by tonic activity of the sympathetic secretomotor inhibitory pathways. Cutting the sympathetic pathways releases the brake on the enteric secretomotor reflex and results in what Claude Bernard, in 1859, called *paralytic secretion* [261]. Sympathetic activity is increased and water and electrolyte secretion is reduced in response to hemorrhagic hypotension, unloading of the baroreceptors, or reduction in right atrial pressure [262–265]. Bicarbonate (HCO_3^-) secretion is also inhibited by sympathetic nerves [266].

Sympathetic effects on the gastrointestinal blood supply

The sympathetic nerves to gastrointestinal supply vessels and intrinsic arterioles provide a tonic vasoconstriction that can be reduced or increased to modify the proportion of the cardiac output going to the gastrointestinal tract according to the balance of vascular need of different vascular beds. This partitioning of blood supply is centrally regulated.

Sympathetic effects on motility

The progress of contents in an oral to anal direction is restricted when sympathetic nerve activity increases. Under resting conditions, the sympathetic pathways exert little influence on motility. They come into action when protective reflexes are activated.

Sympathetic neurons slow transit by constricting the sphincters and inhibiting the contractile activity of the nonsphincter regions [267]. Sympathetic inhibition of muscle movement in the nonsphincter parts of the gastrointestinal tract is primarily through actions of the noradrenergic axons on enteric neurons, including the presynaptic inhibition of excitatory transmitter release (Figure 12.12). Sympathetic nerve fibers also have direct inhibitory actions on the nonsphincter muscle. In the sphincter regions, the sympathetic neurons contract the muscle.

Reflex pathways through which motility is inhibited are of two types. In some cases the reflexes pass via the central nervous system and then back to the intestine. Reflexes are also conducted from one part of the gastrointestinal tract to another through sympathetic prevertebral ganglia [5,268,269]. Intestinofugal neurons that synapse in the prevertebral ganglia were demonstrated by intracellular recordings from the ganglia in preparations consisting only of a segment of intestine connected to a ganglion that had been completely removed from the body [270]. Activation of intestinal tension receptors evoked fast EPSPs in many nerve cells [270–272]. The EPSPs were blocked by the application of nicotinic antagonists to the ganglia, suggesting that they are cholinergic. This conclusion has been consolidated by the observation that all intestinofugal neurons are immunoreactive for choline acetyltransferase [273]. There is also a component of slow excitatory transmission from

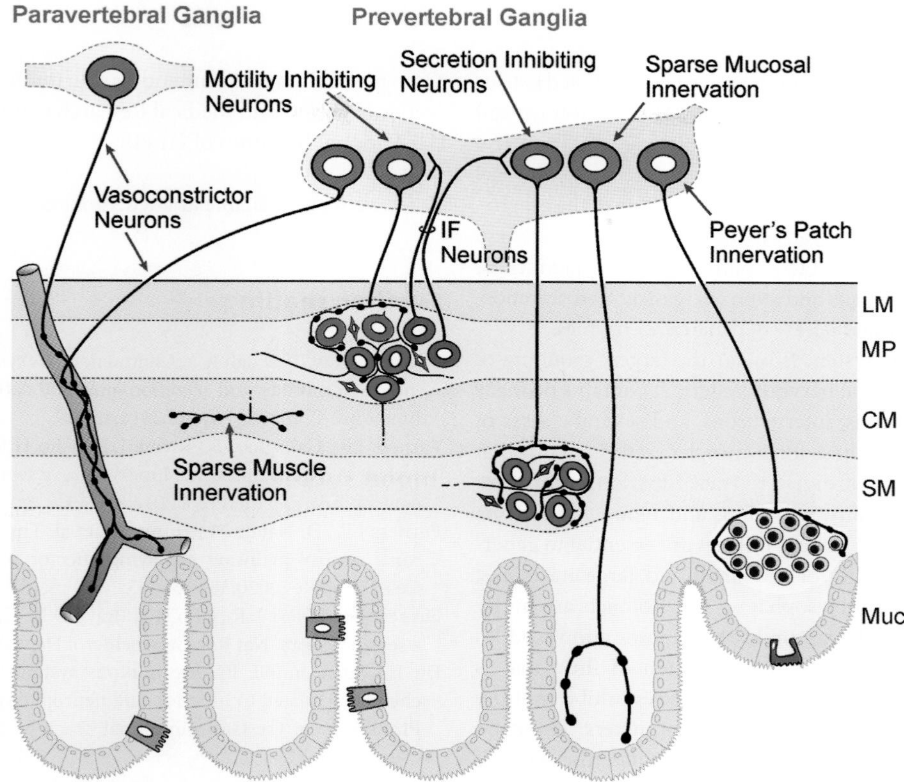

Figure 12.12 Sympathetic innervation of the gastrointestinal tract. This diagram illustrates the innervation pathways for the nonsphincter regions of the stomach, small and large intestines. The densest innervation is of the myenteric ganglia throughout these regions, the submucosal ganglia of the small and large intestines, and intramural arteries. Few sympathetic fibers innervate the muscle of nonsphincter regions, whereas the sphincter muscle is densely innervated. The postganglionic neurons that innervate gut effectors have noradrenaline as their primary transmitter. Intestinofugal neurons (IF) synapse with sympathetic neurons in prevertebral ganglia.

the intestinofugal neurons, which is a result of the release of a cotransmitter, probably VIP [269]. Most intestinofugal neurons are second-order neurons that nevertheless may also be directly activated by stretch [156].

The enteroenteric inhibitory reflexes appear to have a protective role for the gastrointestinal tract [5]. For example, in the case of enterogastric reflexes, the slowing of gastric emptying protects the duodenal mucosa from acid and osmotic stress; these reflexes are initiated by acidity or hypertonicity in the lumen of the upper small intestine. Enteroenteric inhibitory reflexes affecting other parts of the intestine can be initiated by the distension of any region. Most studies have dealt with reflexes affecting the stomach and intestine, but similar reflex pathways affect the biliary system [274]. The reflexes that pass through the CNS are commonly evoked by noxious stimuli or by pain of visceral origin. For example, biliary colic, abdominal injury, and irritation within the abdominal cavity caused by chemicals or infection activate sympathetic reflexes that inhibit gut motility.

Sympathetic modulation of inflammation

A substantial body of evidence shows that noradrenergic nerves directly control inflammation in the gut [6]. Tyrosine-hydroxylase-immunoreactive nerve endings are found near resident macrophages in the lamina propria of the mucosa, in the submucosa, around the ganglia of the myenteric plexus and innervating lymphoid follicles (see Figure 12.11). They do not, however, come in contact with the extensive network of macrophages in the muscle layers, and actions of sympathetic nerves on this subgroup of resident immune cells might be indirect via their demonstrated influences on enteric neurons some of which innervate these macrophages [22]. Macrophages express various types of adrenergic receptors. Beta-receptors mediate antiinflammatory actions on gut-derived macrophages in vitro [275] as well as in colitis models in vivo [276]. These antiinflammatory effects are distinct from the motility-modifying effects of adrenergic nerves that occur via alpha-receptors. Inflammation in experimental inflammatory bowel disease is inhibited by intermittent electrical stimulation of the sympathetic nerves to the gut, independent of inhibition of motility [277]. Consistent with a sympathetic antiinflammatory action, beta-blockers exacerbate inflammation in Crohn's disease in humans, increasing the incidence of relapse following surgery [278].

Summary

Neural control of digestive function is exerted by integrated extrinsic control through vagal, sympathetic, and pelvic pathways and intrinsic control through the enteric nervous system. The vagal control is coordinated by integrative circuitry in the brainstem. Vagal afferent neurons convey information about the state of the esophagus and upper abdominal organs to the brainstem centers and motor pathways from these centers control functions that include movements of the esophagus and stomach, gastric acid secretion, gallbladder contraction, and release of pancreatic enzymes.

The enteric nervous system is by far the largest grouping of neurons outside the central nervous system. It contains primary afferent (sensory) neurons, interneurons, and several classes of motor neuron. Together, these form complete reflex circuits that influence many aspects of digestive tract function, prominent among these being motility, secretion, and blood flow in the small and large intestines. Enteric reflexes are essential to generate the patterns of motility of the small and large intestines, whereas movements in the esophagus and stomach are under dominant vagal control. Intramural secretomotor and vasodilator reflexes control the return to the lumen of fluid that is absorbed with nutrients. Sympathetic pathways inhibit motility in nonsphincter regions and contract the sphincters. These are protective reflexes. Sympathetic pathways regulate the secretomotor reflexes to maintain secretion appropriate to whole-body fluid balance. The pelvic pathways are important in the voluntary control of defecation. Vagal, sympathetic, and enteric pathways influence inflammation in the gastrointestinal tract.

Overall, neural control of the gastrointestinal tract relies on integration of vagal, enteric, sympathetic, and pelvic influences, moderated by sensory information from digestive organs and other sources.

Acknowledgments

Our research has been and is currently supported by the National Health and Medical Research Council of Australia and the National Institutes of Health.

References are available at www.yamadagastro.com/textbook7e

Further reading

Browning K.N., Travagli R.A. Central nervous system control of gastrointestinal motility and secretion and modulation of gastrointestinal functions. Compreh Physiol 2014;4:1339.

Furness J.B., Callaghan B., Rivera L.R., Cho H.J. The enteric nervous system and gastrointestinal innervation: integrated local and central control. Adv Exp Med Biol 2014;817:39.

Furness J.B., Di Natale M., Hunne B., et al. The identification of neuronal control pathways supplying effector tissues in the stomach. Cell Tissue Res 2020;382:33–445

Furness J.B., Rivera L.R., Cho H.J., Bravo D.M.,Callaghan B. The gut as a sensory organ. Nat Rev Gastroenterol Hepatol 2013;10:729.

Hu H., Spencer N.J. Enteric nervous system structure and neurochemistry related to function and neuropathology. In: Said H. (ed.) Physiology of the Gastrointestinal Tract. St Louis, MO: Academic Press; 2018: 337.

Morarach K., Mikhailova A., Knoflach V., et al. Diversification of molecularly defined myenteric neuron classes revealed by single-cell RNA sequencing. Nat Neurosci 2021;24:34–46.

Schneider S., Wright C.M., Heuckeroth R.O. Unexpected roles for the second brain: enteric nervous system as master regulator of bowel function. Annu Rev Physiol 2019;81:235.

Sharkey K.A. Emerging roles for enteric glia in gastrointestinal disorders. J Clin Invest 2015;125:918.

CHAPTER 13

Smooth muscle and pacemakers of the gut

Kenton M. Sanders and Brian A. Perrino
Department of Physiology and Cell Biology, University of Nevada, Reno School of Medicine, Reno, NV, USA

Chapter menu

Introduction

Gastrointestinal motility is the result of complex contractile patterns of smooth muscle cells (SMCs) from the distal esophagus to the internal anal sphincter. There are many layers of regulation superimposed upon the intrinsic behaviors of SMCs, but ultimately the motor output of the gut depends upon contraction by SMCs or time-appropriate relaxation.

Years ago, regulation of motility was split into mechanisms that depended upon intrinsic smooth muscle behaviors (myogenic) and inputs from the enteric nervous system (neurogenic). While that terminology is still used, the meaning of myogenic regulation has changed. Far more is known about the complexity of smooth muscle tissues and we know, for example, that other types of cells are responsible for mechanisms previously attributed to SMCs.

At least two types of interstitial cells are electrically coupled to SMCs: interstitial cells of Cajal (ICC) and cells referred to in older literature as fibroblast-like cells, but now referred to by a biomarker, platelet-derived growth factor receptor (PDGFRα), and are thus PDGFRα$^+$ cells. Together, SMCs, ICC, and PDGFRα$^+$ cells form an electrical network called the SIP syncytium [1]. This is an important structural feature for GI motility, and it is a conserved anatomical entity through vertebrate animals and humans. Due to the electrical coupling, electrophysiological responses that develop in any of the SIP cells can affect the excitability of the entire syncytium, and we now know that the different cellular components of the SIP syncytium are responsible for various fundamental behaviors once attributed to SMCs. For example, pacemaker activity is initiated and propagated by ICC, some neural responses are transduced by ICC, and other responses are mediated by PDGFRα$^+$ cells. Recent studies have begun to delineate this division of labor between ICC and PDGFRα$^+$ cells, but the integrated responses of the SIP syncytium must now be considered the "myogenic" component of GI motility.

Although contemporary research, current therapeutic rationales, and pharmaceutical development are heavily neurocentric, many GI motility disorders have been associated with lesions in the ICC component of the SIP syncytium. It should be obvious that if myogenic mechanisms are abnormal and SMC excitability is distorted, correcting such problems by neural modulation may not be feasible. This chapter attempts to summarize important features of GI smooth muscle biology and illustrate how the SIP syncytium works to generate the basic patterns of GI motility.

Yamada's Textbook of Gastroenterology, Seventh Edition. Edited by Timothy C. Wang, Michael Camilleri, Benjamin Lebwohl, Anna S. Lok, William J. Sandborn, Kenneth K. Wang, and Gary D. Wu.

Companion website: www.yamadagastro.com/textbook7e

Anatomical organization and structure of smooth muscle cells and tissues

Gross anatomy of smooth muscle tissues in the gut

The hollow organs of the GI tract are lined with muscular coats, in most cases with bundles of smooth muscle cells (SMCs) running longitudinally along the lengths of the organs or circumferentially around the tubular structures. Between the circular and longitudinal layers is the myenteric plexus, a major organizational feature of the enteric nervous system, interstitial cells, and resident immune cells. Separating the major organs of the GI tract are thickened regions of muscle that provide sphincter functions, separating the activities of one region from the next, slowing movement of food and chyme between regions or providing protection from the acidic contents of the stomach that can damage tissues of the esophagus and duodenum. Sphincter muscles are uniquely equipped to produce tonic contraction and innervated by excitatory or inhibitory motor neurons to produce contraction or relaxation at appropriate moments. A few areas also exist in which a third muscular layer is present, such as the sling muscle in the stomach or the taenia coli, a collection of longitudinal muscle cells forming powerful cables along the wall of the colon.

Major structural features of visceral SMCs

When fully relaxed, SMCs are about 200–400 µm in length and less than 10 µm in width. For example, one study measured longitudinal SMCs in the mouse colon in situ and found cell lengths average 248 µm and widths average 8.7 µm [2]. Gut SMCs are spindle-shaped with their broadest point around the nucleus and tapering toward both ends. They have a large surface-to-volume ratio which facilitates build-up of Ca^{2+} concentration through influx to initiate contraction. SMCs lack the sarcomere structure of skeletal and cardiac muscles. This results in a lack of striations when SMCs and tissues are observed histologically. SMCs in the wall of the gut are embedded in a connective tissue matrix, consisting mainly of elastin and collagen fibrils produced by the synthetic and secretory activity of SMCs and PDGFRα^+ cells.

In spite of the lack of defined sarcomeres, smooth muscle cells possess a contractile unit analogous to other muscles and composed of actin thin filaments, myosin thick filaments, and dense plaques and dense bodies. Dense plaques and dense bodies are analogous to the Z-disks of skeletal and cardiac muscles [3]. Dense plaques are attached to the plasma membrane at adherens junctions, while dense bodies are found in the cytoplasm [4]. Dense plaques are numerous, discrete, electron-dense structures at the plasma membrane, which together account for about one-half of the total surface of cells [5]. Dense plaques form around integrins, which link the extracellular matrix to the contractile apparatus of the muscle cell, and participate in mechanosignaling processing [6].

Thin filaments are arranged obliquely in the cell, anchored at one end in opposite orientations to dense plaques or dense bodies, via a number of proteins consisting of α-actinin, paxillin, and vinculin [7]. Like Z-disks in striated muscles, the intermediate filaments, consisting mainly of desmin in visceral smooth muscle, link the dense plaques at the membrane to dense bodies in the cytoplasm and transmit the force generated by the contractile apparatus within the cell to the entire cell [8]. Adherens junctions of adjacent cells, together with collagen fibrils, transmit force from one cell to the next and couple the contractile apparatus of adjacent cells to the rest of the muscle syncytium (Figure 13.1).

Dense bodies and contractile filaments occupy about 80% of the cytoplasm of the smooth muscle cell; the remainder is occupied by organelles, including the nucleus, mitochondria, Golgi apparatus, lysosomes, and rough and smooth endoplasmic/sarcoplasmic reticulum [9]. The sarcoplasmic reticulum, occupying around 2% of the cell volume, provides sites for intracellular storage of Ca^{2+}, and well-defined processes cause dynamic uptake and release of Ca^{2+} from these sites [10]. As in other cells, mitochondria produce energy for SMCs in the form of adenosine triphosphate (ATP). There is also evidence that mitochondria also provide a low-affinity, high-capacity storage site for Ca^{2+} that can sequester large amounts of Ca^{2+} after cellular injury, when cytosolic Ca^{2+} exceeds maximal physiological levels (>1–5 µM) [11,12].

An important structure in the plasma membrane of SMCs is caveolae (Latin for "little caves"). Caveolae are 50–70 nm wide and 90–120 nm deep, regularly spaced, flask-shaped invaginations of the plasma membrane that appear in rows along the longitudinal axis of the plasma membrane, alternating with regions of dense bodies anchoring the cytoskeleton [13,14]. Caveolae constitute a substantial proportion of the smooth muscle cell membrane, and increase the surface area by up to 75% [15] (Figure 13.2). Caveolar density does not appear to change in response to physiological stretch. It is unclear whether the widening of the neck region acts as a sensor for stretch and/or volume changes [16,17]. Caveolin-1, -2, and -3 are the main structural proteins of smooth muscle caveolae [18] and are thought to act as scaffolds to facilitate signaling. The caveolin-scaffolding domain of caveolins binds several classes of signaling molecules, including G-proteins, receptor and nonreceptor tyrosine kinases, protein kinase C isoforms, small GTPases such as Rhoa, and multiple components of the dystrophin–glycoprotein complex [19]. The bases of caveolae are often in close proximity to the peripheral sarcoplasmic reticulum, the site of Ca^{2+} storage and release in smooth muscle cells. This arrangement suggests that caveolae may also be involved in the regulation of smooth muscle Ca^{2+} homeostasis [20,21].

Gap junctions facilitate communication between cells in the SIP syncytium (Figure 13.3) [22–24]. Gap junctions form channels in the plasma membranes between neighboring cells, forming low-resistance electrical coupling between cells. Gap junctions consist of junctions between connexin proteins [25]. Over 20 connexin proteins have been identified, many of which are expressed to varying degrees in SMCs, ICCs, and PDGFRα^+

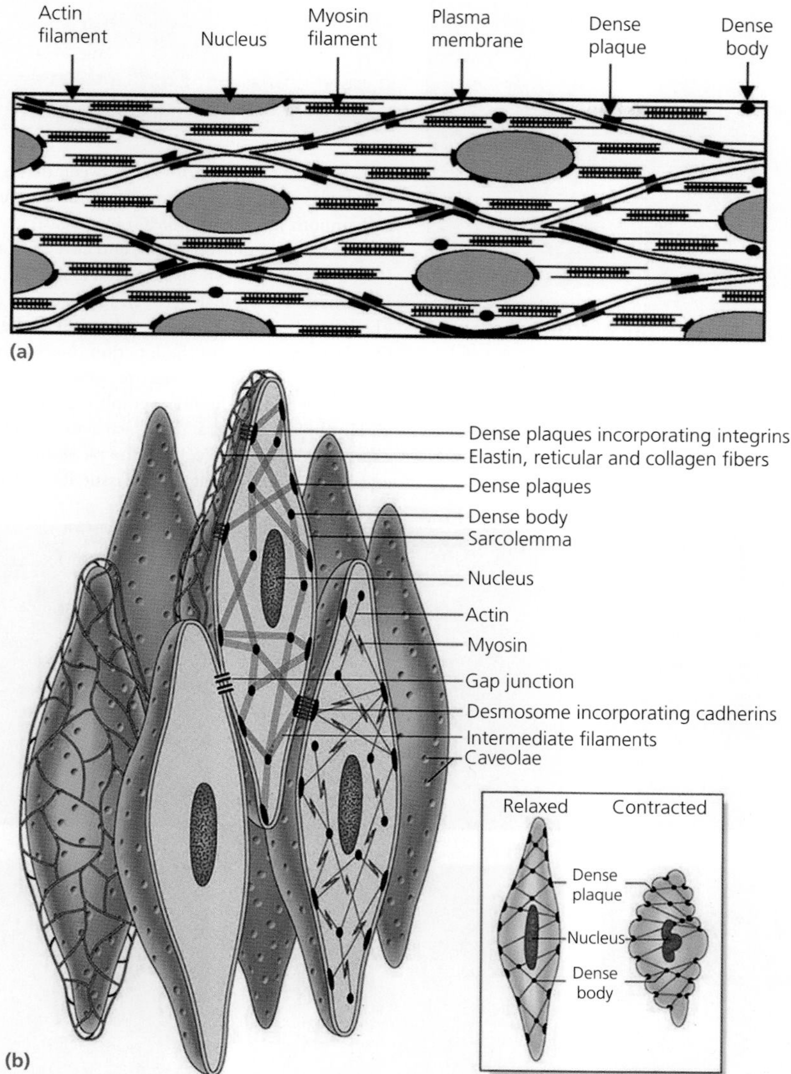

Figure 13.1 **(a)** Organization of the contractile and cytoskeletal apparatus in smooth muscle cells. Thin actin filaments are attached in opposite orientations to dense bodies in the cytoplasm and dense plaques at the plasma membrane. The other ends of the oppositely oriented actin filaments interdigitate with the thick myosin filaments. When cross-bridge cycling is activated, the actin filaments are pulled in opposite directions, contracting the cell. **(b)** Three-dimensional representation of smooth muscle cells. For clarity, some structural features have been omitted in different cells to illustrate the contributions of the different filament systems to contraction. The spindle-shaped cells interdigitate in parallel with their long axes; mechanical continuity between the cells is provided by an extracellular matrix of elastin and collagen fibers. The cytoskeletal framework consists of intermediate filament arrays (mainly longitudinal) and bundles of actin and myosin filaments (shown in separate cells) inserted into cytoplasmic dense bodies and submembraneous dense plaques to form a three-dimensional network. The sarcolemma contains anchoring desmosomes (adherens junctions), gap junctions, and caveolae. Source: Figure 6.3 from: Chapter 6 "Smooth muscle and the cardiovascular and lymphatic systems," https://basicmedicalkey.com/. Reproduced with permission of Elsevier. **(Inset)** This arrangement of the intermediate filaments and the myofilaments causes the smooth muscle cell to contract in a manner whereby the ends are pulled toward the center, causing the midsection to bulge in a corkscrew motion.

cells in different regions of the GI tract. Connexin 43 appears to be an isoform expressed dominantly by ICCs [26.27].

Concept and cells of the SIP syncytium

Smooth muscle cells do not operate independently in GI muscles. They are electrically coupled to each other, and to at least two classes of interstitial cells via gap junctions.

The first type of interstitial cell is known as interstitial cells of Cajal (Figure 13.4a–d). These cells are arranged into networks between the circular and longitudinal muscle layers in the spaces between and around myenteric ganglia. This network, known as the ICC-MY, has a pacemaker role in the GI tract [28,29]. ICC are also found within muscle bundles (Figure 13.4g). These intramuscular ICCs (ICC-IM) are closely

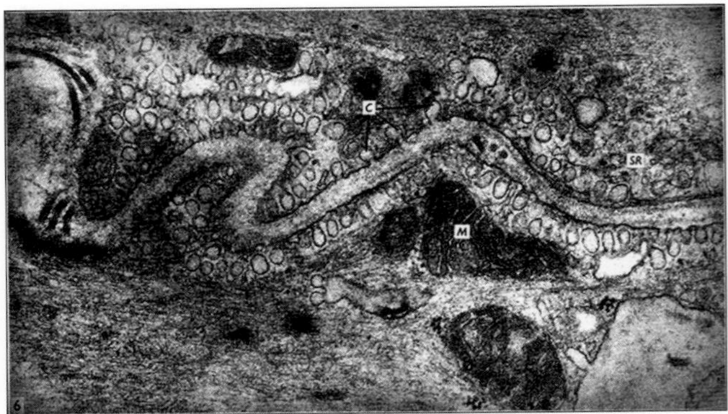

Figure 13.2 Caveolae in smooth muscle cells. Two adjacent smooth muscle cells sectioned longitudinally showing a number of caveolae (C) open to the extracellular space directly underneath the plasma membrane. A mitochondrion (M) and cisternae of the sarcoplasmic reticulum (SR) are also visible. ×43 879. Source: Riley D.A. Silver staining the caveolae intracellularis of smooth muscle. J Anat 1977;123:819.

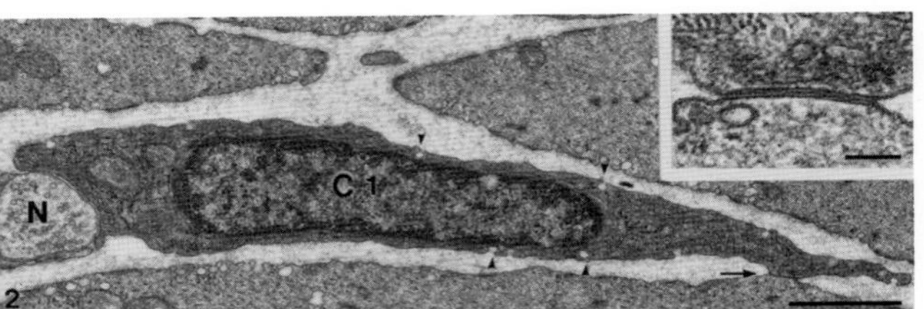

Figure 13.3 Close apposition between nerve varicosities and ICC (labeled as C1 in this micrograph), and gap junction formed between ICC and smooth muscle cell (SMC) in rat gastric antrum. Mitochondria, rough endoplasmic reticulum, and caveolae (arrow heads) are present in ICC, and caveolae can also be seen along the surface of SMCs. A distinct gap junction is present between the ICC and an adjacent SMC (arrow). The inset shows a higher magnification of the gap junction and displays the classic structure of the junction clearly. The scale bar in the inset is 0.2 μm. Close apposition occurs between a nerve varicosity (N) and the ICC. Scale bar for the micrograph is 2 μm. Source: Ishikawa K., Komuro T., Hirota S., Kitamura Y. Ultrastructural identification of the c-kit-expressing interstitial cells in the rat stomach: a comparison of control and Ws/Ws mutant rats. Cell Tissue Res 1997;289:137.

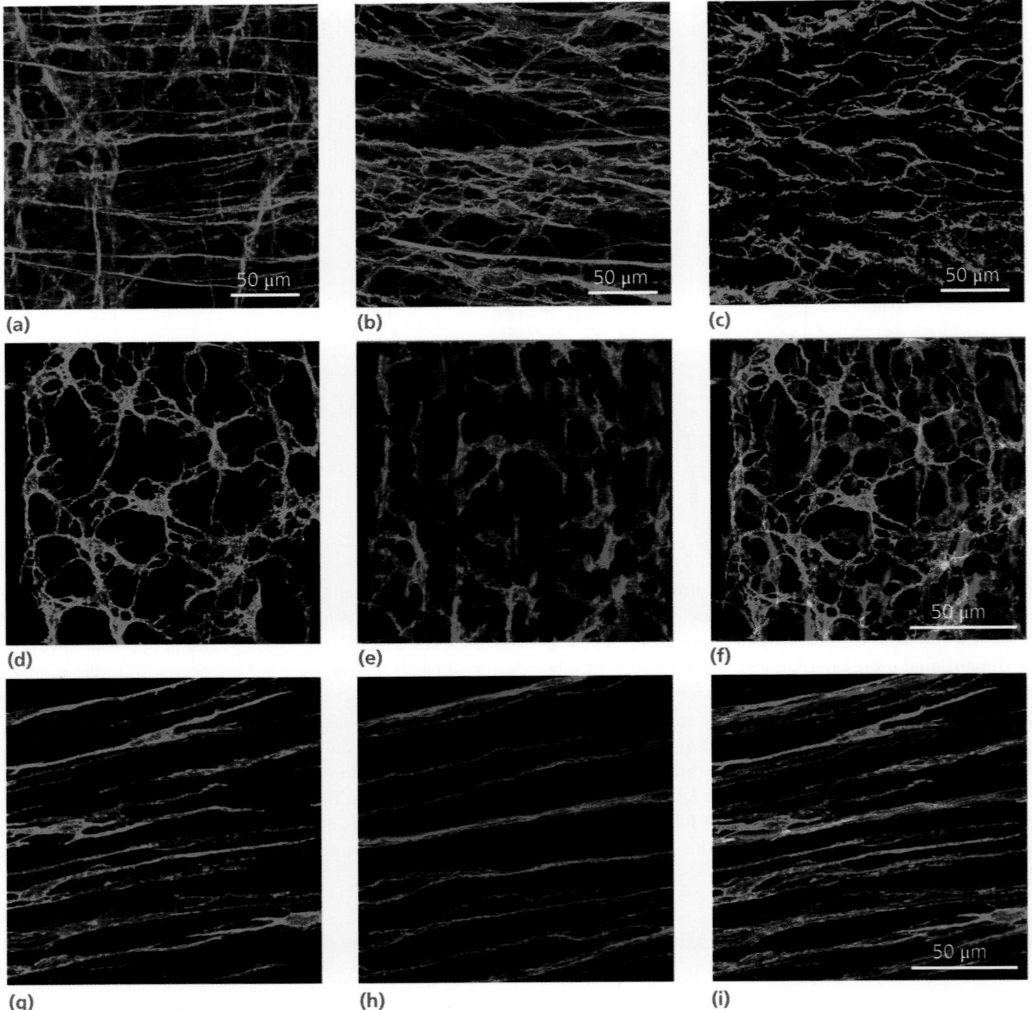

Figure 13.4 **(a–c)** c-Kit⁺ ICC-MY in mouse, monkey, and human gastric antrums, respectively. There are similarities in the structure and organization of ICC in these species. **(d-f)** c-Kit⁺ ICC-MY (d, green) and PDGFRα⁺ cells (**e**, red) in the murine colon. These are distinct populations of cells, shown by the merged image in **(f)**. **(g–i)** Intramuscular ICC (ICC-IM; g, c-Kit is labeled in green) in the monkey gastric fundus. ICC-IM are closely associated with enteric motor neurons, in this case nNOS⁺ motor neurons (**h**, labeled in red). **(i)** Merged images from **(g)** and (h). Scale bar in **(f)** applies to **(d-f)**, and scale bar in **(i)** applies to **(g–i)**. Source: Sanders K.M., Ward S.M., Koh S.D. Interstitial cells: regulators of smooth muscle function. Physiol Rev 2014;94(3):859.

associated with the varicose processes of enteric motor neurons (Figure 13.4h,i) and have a role in transduction of neural inputs [30,31]. Biomarkers for ICCs include the receptor tyrosine kinase c-Kit [29,32] and the Ca^{2+}-activated Cl^- channel, ANO1(anoctamin-1) [33,34].

A second type of interstitial cell, called "fibroblast-like" by morphologists due to the abundance of rough endoplasmic reticulum and other ultrastructural features, is also present and electrically coupled to SMCs. These cells are now labeled with and referred to as PDGFRα⁺ cells (Figure 13.4e,f) [35,36]. These cells are also closely associated with the nerve terminals of enteric motor neurons and have ultrastructure, chemical coding, and functions distinct from ICCs.

The network of SMCs, ICCs, and PDGFRα⁺ cells has become known as the SIP syncytium (Figure 13.5) [37]. This multicellular collaboration is responsible for the complex behaviors and multiple mechanisms that regulate the excitability of SMCs. Electrophysiological changes in any of the SIP cells can affect the excitability and behaviors of the other cells due to the electrical coupling between them. Classification and common naming conventions for the various types of interstitial cells that make up the SIP syncytia through the GI tract are shown in Table 13.1.

Major structural features of interstitial cells

For many years, morphologists relied on ultrastructural features to describe ICCs and PDGFRα⁺ cells and to distinguish these cells from SMCs. Mitochondria are abundant in ICCs, and these cells also display caveolae, basal lamina, rough and smooth endoplasmic reticulum (ER), and well-developed Golgi [38].

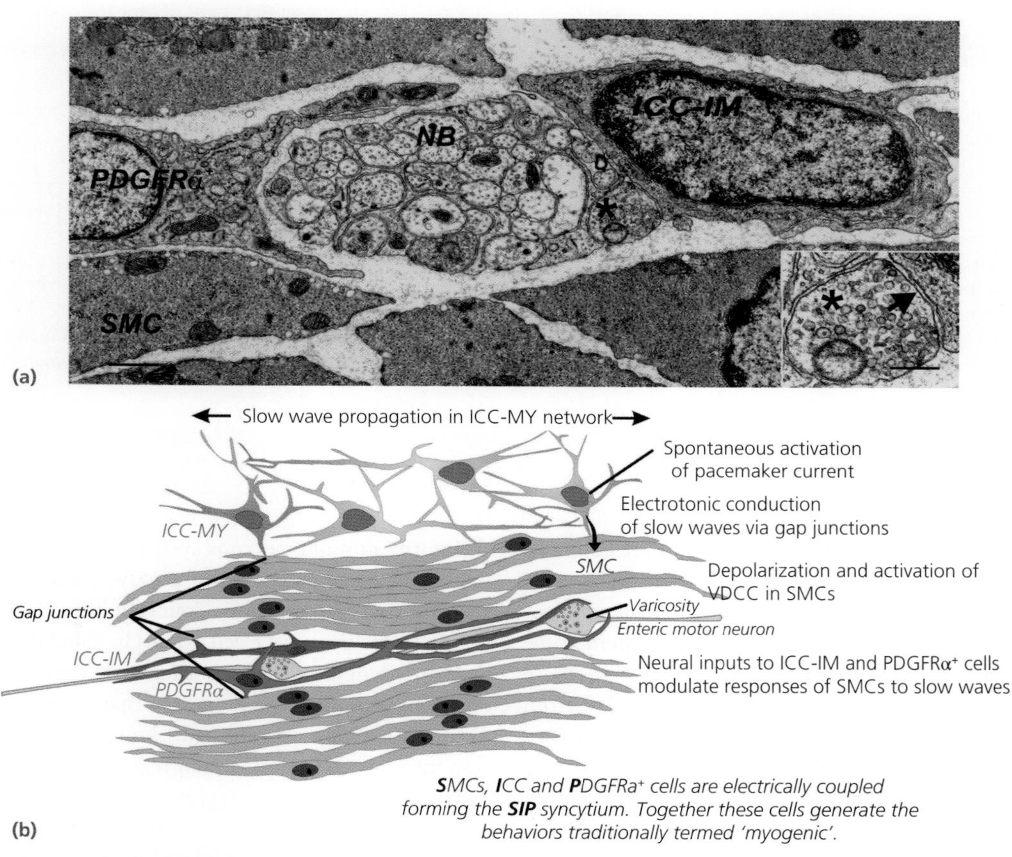

Figure 13.5 Structure and summary of functions of the SIP syncytium. **(a)** An electron micrograph, provided by Professor Terumasa Komuro, displays the cell types known as the SIP syncytium (SMC, ICC, and PDGFRα⁺ cells) in GI muscles. These cells are shown in relation to a bundle of neurons that run parallel to the long axis of the SMCs. Note varicosity at the edge of the nerve bundle (NB) labeled with *. This is shown at a higher magnification in the inset. ICC and PDGFRα⁺ cells are often closely associated with nerve bundles, and ICC make very close contacts with varicosities (<20 nm; black arrow in inset). ICC and PDGFRα⁺ cells are electrically coupled to SMCs (not shown in this image but see an example in Figure 13.3). Scale bar is 0.5 μm in main micrograph and 0.2 μm in the inset. Source: Sanders K.M., Hwang S.J., Ward S.M. Neuroeffector apparatus in gastrointestinal smooth muscle organs. J Physiol 2010;588:4621. **(b)** Depictions of SIP syncytium with addition of the network of ICC-MY that generates and propagates slow waves in the stomach and small intestine. These cells drive the phasic electrical and mechanical activities of the smooth muscle. Within smooth muscle bundles, SMCs, ICCs, and PDGFRα⁺ cells are arranged around projections of excitatory and inhibitory enteric motor neurons, as shown in the micrograph in (a). Descriptions of major functions of cellular components of the SIP syncytium are provided. VDCC is voltage-dependent Ca^{2+} channels. Source: Sanders K.M. Spontaneous electrical activity and rhythmicity in gastrointestinal smooth muscles. Adv Exp Med Biol 2019;1124:3. Reproduced with permission of Elsevier.

Table 13.1 Interstitial cells of the SIP syncytium.

Anatomical location	Common Name	Organs	Functions
Around and between myenteric ganglia between circular and longitudinal muscle layers	ICC-MY[a]	STM, SI, CLN	Pacemaker activity, innervated by motor neurons in CLN
Within muscle bundles (intramuscular); in close contact with varicosities of enteric motor neurons	ICC-IM[b]	ESG (smooth muscle portion), STM, SI, CLN and SPTRs	Express receptors for neurotransmitters released from enteric motor neurons; transduce neural inputs; mediators of responses to stretch
Intramuscular ICC concentrated in the deep muscular plexus in small intestine	ICC-DMP[c]	SI	Express receptors for neurotransmitters released by enteric motor neurons and transduce neural inputs
Submucosal border of circular muscle layer	ICC-SM	CLN, STM	Pacemaker activity in CLN; limited number of cells in STM, and function of ICC-SM in STM is unknown
Serosal surface of longitudinal muscle layer	ICC-SS	CLN (proximal)	Provide excitatory (pacemaker-like) input to longitudinal muscle layer; mediate nitrergic neural inputs
Septal spaces between muscle bundles in larger animals	ICC-SEP	STM, SI, CLN	Appear to be extensions of ICC-MY or ICC-SM networks and actively propagate slow waves into thicker GI muscles of large mammals and humans
Myenteric region	PDGFRα⁺-MY	STM, SI, CLN	Express receptors for purines and mediate purinergic and sympathetic neural responses
Distributed within muscle bundles; intramuscular spaces	PDGFRα⁺-IM	ESG (smooth muscle portion), STM, SI, CLN All SPTRs	Express receptors for purines and mediate purinergic and sympathetic neural responses

[a] Sometimes referred to as ICC-MP or ICC-AP in the literature, but this is misleading because these cells are not located within the myenteric (or Auerbach) plexus. They are disturbed around the ganglia and tertiary plexus.
[b] Some authors have broken this term down to specify in which muscle layer the cells are found (e.g., ICC-CM for cells in the circular muscle layer and ICC-LM for cells in the longitudinal muscle layer). However, to date no functional differences have been reported for ICC-IM in these different locations. Thus, ICC-IM is used in this chapter.
[c] ICC-DMP function in a manner similar to ICC-IM. They show a distinctive localization in laboratory animals and have received considerable experimental attention, so they are designated separately. Larger animals and humans have ICC-IM distributed through the circular muscle layer, as in the stomach and colon of laboratory animals.
CLN, colon; DMP, deep muscular plexus; ESG, esophagus; GI, gastrointestinal; ICC, interstitial cells of Cajal; IM, intramuscular; MY, myenteric; PDGFR, platelet-derived growth factor receptor; SEP, septal; SI, small intestine; SM, submucosa; SPTR, sphincter; SS, subserosa; STM, stomach.

Microtubules and thin and intermediate filaments are common in ICCs but myosin thick filaments are not. A prominent perinuclear region is typical and filled with mitochondria and cisternae of ER that are in close apposition to the plasma membrane, creating tiny spaces known as microdomains. Within these restricted volumes, Ca^{2+} transients, due to release of Ca^{2+} from the ER, can create relatively high local concentrations of Ca^{2+} that regulate Ca^{2+}-dependent ion channels expressed in the plasma membrane. In contrast to ICCs, caveolae and a basal lamina are lacking in PDGFRα⁺ cells. PDGFRα⁺ cells are also less electron dense than ICCs and contain an abundance of rough ER, a common feature of fibroblasts. As mentioned above, ICCs and PDGFRα⁺ cells form gap junctions with smooth muscle cells [39,40].

Nerves and glia innervating SIP syncytium

Throughout the gut, enteric neurons mediate reflexes and integration of sensory signals, and regulate motor patterns [41]. Enteric neurons have been previously regarded by Langley as the third division of the autonomic nervous system. However, they form a unique nervous system that can function independently from sympathetic and parasympathetic neurons, a fact that was first recognized by Trendelenburg.

Enteric neurons have cell bodies in ganglia distributed along the entire length of the smooth muscle portion of the GI tract. Afferent neurons have processes that sense pressures, pH or nutrient contents in the gut lumen, and organize motor responses appropriate for each region of the gut. Interneurons distribute and serve to integrate information within the enteric nervous system and help to organize large regions of SMCs to contract or relax in a coordinated manner. Motor neurons provide integrated neural information to the SIP syncytium to modulate myogenic behaviors and produce organ-level GI motility, such as the pattern of esophageal motility after a swallow, gastric accommodation during eating, efficient gastric emptying, postprandial segmentation in the small intestine, propulsive contractions in the colon, defecation reflex, and regulation of sphincters. Enteric neuron processes course through the tunica muscularis in multineuron bundles. Ganglia of enteric neurons also contain a complex network of enteric glia, the functions of which are currently a topic of active investigation [42–44]. Neural organization and regulation of motility are discussed in detail elsewhere in this text in Chapter 12.

Resident immune cells

Muscular tissues also contain resident immune cells, such as macrophages and mast cells. An extensive network of macrophages that are phenotypically different than the more commonly studied population of macrophages in the lamina propria is present in the region of the myenteric plexus between the circular and longitudinal muscle layers [45]. Some of these cells can also be found within the muscle layers and along the serosal surface of the bowel wall.

Depending upon their anatomical location, muscularis macrophages have either a stellate or bipolar morphology. The stellate morphology is characteristic of the cells within the plane of the myenteric plexus, while the bipolar cells are more typical within the muscle layers. Identification and localization of muscularis macrophages were originally performed using uptake of fluorescent dextran particles [46] but now a number of cell surface biomarkers, including CX3CR1, CD64, and F4/80, are used to identify these cells. Alternatively activated, $CD206^{+}$ (antiinflammatory, M2) macrophages provide a regulatory role and are typically present in normal tissues, but inflammatory factors can switch the phenotype toward classically activated, proinflammatory (M1) macrophages. This classic phenotypic identification, developed originally from the responses of macrophages in cell culture, is now recognized as far too simplistic, particularly in human tissues. Thus, a clear division of macrophage phenotypes, describing the range of functions of these cells in vivo;, has not yet been devised.

Significant work has been performed recently showing that bidirectional regulation occurs between enteric neurons and resident macrophages. Enteric neurons express and secrete colony stimulating factor (CSF-1) that supports survival of macrophages, and macrophages secrete bone morphogenic protein 2 (BMP2) that supports survival and normal function of enteric neurons [47]. However, macrophages are also in close contact with SIP cells, and far less is known about the impact of these cells on maintenance of myogenic mechanisms. In general, the mast cell population is sparse in mouse tissues, but these cells are present in human tunica muscularis, although to a lesser degree than macrophages.

Organization and properties of the contractile apparatus in smooth muscle cells

Smooth muscle contractile element

Three types of contractile filaments are found in SMCs: thin actin filaments (5–7 nm), thick myosin filaments (15 nm), and the intermediate desmin filaments (10 nm). Intermediate filaments link the cytoplasmic dense bodies to the dense plaques at the plasma membrane. Thin filaments consist of the 43 kD globular protein actin (G actin), which polymerizes to form the double-stranded helical thin filament. Tropomyosin lies within the groove of the actin helix and enhances caldesmon binding to actin [48]. Caldesmon functions to inhibit the ATPase activity and binding of myosin to actin [49]. When smooth muscle contraction is initiated by the influx of Ca^{2+}, Ca^{2+} binds to and activates calmodulin, which then binds to caldesmon [50]. This binding releases caldesmon from the actin filament, exposing the myosin-binding sites on the actin filament, allowing the myosin head to interact with the actin filament and cause contraction [50]. Thin filaments have a distinct polarity, and are arranged in antiparallel bundles along the long axis of the cells, with one end attached to dense plaques at the plasma membrane and the other free end surrounding and interdigitating with the thick myosin filaments [51–53]. The attachment of thin filaments to dense bodies is thus analogous to the attachment of oppositely oriented actin filaments to the Z-disks of striated muscle cells; in effect, dense bodies may be viewed as dispersed fragments of Z-disks held together and anchored to dense bands of the cell membrane by intermediate filaments.

Contractile proteins

Thick filaments are composed of myosin, a 480 kD multisubunit protein formed by the noncovalent association of six different proteins [54]. Myosin can be dissociated into one pair of myosin heavy chains and two pairs of myosin light chains (MLCs) [55]. The heavy chains are arranged in a coiled-coil to form a rigid insoluble helical core or tail, which terminates in globular head domains surrounded by two MLCs: a 20 kD regulatory chain and a 17 kD essential chain [56,57]. Each globular head contains an actin-binding domain and an actin-activated Mg^{2+}- adenosine triphosphatase (ATPase) domain. A hinge region located at the junction of the globular head and the core allows the head to rotate about the core. Another hinge in the core allows the globular heads to project laterally. The globular heads and the segments of the core between the two hinges form the cross-bridges between the myosin and actin filaments (Figure 13.6) [58,59].

The ratio of actin to myosin is higher in smooth muscle than in skeletal and cardiac muscle, averaging around 15:1, compared to the ratios of 6:1 and 4:1 in skeletal and cardiac muscles, respectively [60]. Despite the low content of myosin, smooth muscle generates as much force as striated muscle (up to 2 kg/cm^2 of cross-sectional area), and can also contract to a much shorter length than skeletal muscle [61,62]. This is partly due to the nature of the arrangement of dense bodies and dense plaques in smooth muscle cells, and the arrangement of the globular myosin heads projecting from the coiled-coli myosin tail in smooth muscles.

Myosin thick filaments in striated muscle form by antiparallel binding of the tail domains at the center of the thick filament, followed by parallel binding of the tail domains in the rest of the thick filament. Consequently, a bipolar thick filament is formed, leaving a central bare zone in the middle, with the myosin heads on either side of the bare zone arranged around the tail domains in a bipolar, helical arrangement, oriented to pull toward each

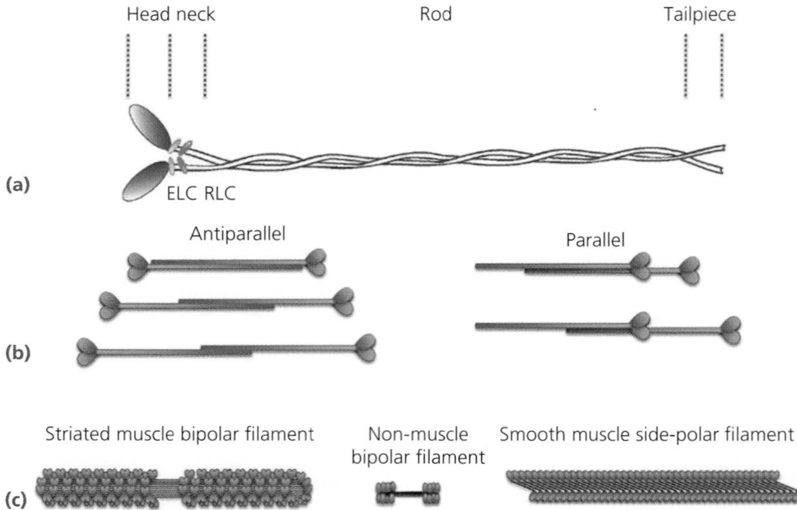

Figure 13.6 **(a)** Component proteins of the myosin molecule. A myosin protein is composed of two 230 kD heavy chains coiled around each other. Each heavy chain terminates in a globular head surrounded by two MLCs: a 20 kD regulatory chain (RLC) and a 17 kD essential chain (ELC). Cross-bridges project laterally from the main myosin core. The cross-bridge consists of a pair of myosin heads, the 17 kD and 20 kD myosin light chains, and a laterally projecting segment of the myosin core. In muscle cells, the myosin heavy chains bind in an antiparallel manner **(b)**, forming thick filaments with many projecting cross-bridges oriented oppositely to form the bipolar thick filament of striated muscle, or the side-polar thick filament of smooth muscle **(c)**. Source: Dasbiswas K., Hu S., Schnorrer F., Safran S.A., Bershadsky A.D. Ordering of myosin II filaments driven by mechanical forces: experiments and theory. Philos Trans R Soc Lond B Biol Sci 2018;26;373. Reproduced with permission of The Royal Society.

other [63]. The myosin tails in the filament backbone undergo antiparallel interactions with each other at the midpoint of the filament, where the polarity reverses (the bare zone), and parallel interactions in the remainder of each half of the filament. In this structure, the cross-bridges all have the same polarity in one half of the filament and the opposite polarity in the opposite half.

Smooth muscle myosin filaments are organized in a side polar geometry, which is distinct from the bipolar geometry of the myosin filaments in striated muscle [64]. In this thick filament structure, the myosin tails have antiparallel overlaps with each other along the entire filament length, and there is no region with pure parallel interactions. The filament has no central bare zone of polarity reversal but instead, it has asymmetrically tapered bare ends [65]. The myosin heads have a nonhelical, side-polar arrangement, and their polarity is the same along the entire length of one side of the filament, with the opposite polarity on the opposite side [66,67].

Thus, smooth muscle myosin thick filaments having cross-bridges with a single polarity along the entire length of either side allow smooth muscle to undergo extreme shortening [68]. During contraction, a thin filament can slide unimpeded along the side of a thick filament until the end of the thin filament is reached. If the thick filament were bipolar, sliding would be inhibited when the thin filament encountered cross-bridges of opposite polarity in the center of the thick filament. The side-polar mode of assembly thus confers a distinct structural advantage on a sliding filament system required to shorten by large amounts.

Electrical properties of gastrointestinal smooth muscles

Ionic conductances expressed by SMCs

Like all excitable cells, GI SMCs express a variety of ion channels in their plasma membranes. Ion channels give these cells the ability to set negative resting membrane potentials, generate action potentials, and respond to physiological stimulation. Pharmacological studies on intact organs or muscles using ion channel agonists or antagonists cannot easily determine whether responses are due to channels expressed in SMCs or in electrically coupled interstitial cells. Much has been learned about the ion channels expressed in GI SMCs from studies of isolated cells using the patch clamp technique, and common features between cells in different regions of the gut and in different species have been noted [69]. However, there are also significant variations in ion channel expression, making assumptions or extrapolations between regions or species problematic.

Ion channels responsible for inward currents in SMCs

Ionic gradients determine the directionality of transmembrane currents, and the two dominant ions carrying inward currents in GI SMCs are Ca^{2+} and Na^{+}. Membrane potentials of SMCs sit quite negative to the equilibrium potentials for both Ca^{2+} and Na^{+} so openings of channels selective for these ions will result in influx of these ions, inward currents, and depolarization.

The major type of Ca^{2+} channel expressed by SMCs is $Ca_V1.2$, an L-type, voltage-dependent and dihydropyridine-sensitive channel encoded by CACNA1C (Ca^{2+} voltage-gated channel subunit α 1C) gene [70–72]. Properties of these channels will be discussed in more detail in the section on Ca^{2+} handling mechanisms. These are key channels for excitation-contraction coupling in the GI tract. Depolarization of SMCs causes activation of this conductance, and this signaling is responsible for initiation of contraction. Regulation of $Ca_V1.2$ is typically indirect in GI muscles. Direct effects of agonists are usually directed toward other types of conductance in SMCs or in interstitial cells, and the effects of these stimuli alter membrane potential. Changes in membrane potential affect the openings of $Ca_V1.2$.

Gastrointestinal SMCs also express a variety of nonselective cation channels that show a range of selectivies for Na^+ and Ca^{2+} [73]. Activation of these channels under resting conditions tends to result in membrane potentials that sit positive to the equilibrium potential for K^+ ions (E_K). Some agonists activate nonselective cation channels in SMCs, and activation of these channels causes the depolarization associated with these compounds [74–76]. Depolarization by this mechanism is coupled to activation of $Ca_V1.2$ channels, increasing the excitability of SMCs and increasing contraction.

Ion channels responsible for outward currents in SMCs

Gastrointestinal SMCs express a variety of K^+ channels. These channels are responsible for a significant degree of the regulation of membrane potential, and therefore regulation of contraction [69]. SMCs express key voltage-dependent conductances, such as delayed rectifier K^+ channels ($K_V1.2$, $K_V1.5$, and $K_V2.1$) and large conductance Ca^{2+}-activated K^+ (BK or "big potassium" voltage-gated K^+ channels that have a large conductance) channels (also called $K_{Ca}1.1$ encoded by KCNMA1) [77,78]. BK channels are activated by depolarization and/or increased cytoplasmic Ca^{2+}. They are activated during slow waves or action potentials.

Several additional types of K^+ channels provide the dominant K^+ permeability that generates negative resting membrane potentials in SMCs. These include K_{ATP} (ATP-sensitive potassium channel), inwardly rectifying K^+ channels (K_{IR} [inward rectifier potassium channel]), and two-pore domain K^+ channels (TREK-1 and TASK-2) [69]. The varied properties of these channels add important dimensions to the regulation of membrane potential and include regulation by the metabolic state of the cells (K_{ATP}), hyperpolarization-dependent activation (K_{IR}), responsiveness to stretch (TREK-1), and regulation by pH. Several of these channels can also be regulated by agonists, particularly those coupled to the generation of cAMP or cGMP or by activation of protein kinase C.

Ionic conductances in other SIP cells

Due to the electrical connectivity between SMCs and interstitial cells of the SIP syncytium (see Figure 13.3), the openings of ion channels in interstitial cells affect the excitability state of SMCs (Figure 13.7). The complement of functional ion channels in ICC and PDGFRα$^+$ cells appears to be less complex than in SMCs, and the ion channels identified to date are encoded by highly expressed genes and are responsible for some of the primary functions of these cells in regulating motility. ICCs display very high levels of expression of ANO1 [33,34,79], and all classes of ICC from several species, including humans, express these channels exclusively in the tunica muscularis [33,34].

Due to active accumulation of Cl^- ions in ICCs [80], opening of ANO1 channels under physiological gradients results in efflux of Cl^-, which is defined electrophysiologically as inward current. Inward current causes depolarization, so ANO1 (anoctamin-1) channels in ICCs provide excitatory input to the SIP syncytium. In contrast, the dominant conductance expressed in PDGFRα$^+$ cells is SK3 (small-conductance Ca^{2+}-activated K^+) channels (encoded by KCNN3; Ca^{2+}-activated K^+channel subfamily N member 3) [36,81,82]. Under physiological gradients, opening of these channels causes efflux of K^+ ions and outward current. This tends to stabilize membrane potential or cause hyperpolarization because GI muscles have membrane potentials that lie positive to E_K. Thus, PDGFRα$^+$ cells provide an inhibitory drive or stabilizing influence on the excitability of GI muscles.

Interstitial cells express receptors to many naturally occurring, bioactive compounds [83–85], many of which have not yet been tested to determine their effects on motility. However, interesting new pathways being tested suggest these cells may mediate important signaling, such as sympathetic regulation of colonic motility [86] and responses to a variety of GI hormones.

Setting of resting potentials

The level at which the resting potentials of SMCs are set under basal conditions is an important determinant of ultimate motor responses in the GI tract. As described previously, the trigger for contraction is Ca^{2+} entry into SMCs via voltage-dependent Ca^{2+} channels. Phasic contractions, as in peristaltic or segmental contractions, occur because depolarization elicits activation L-type Ca^{2+} channels in SMCs, Ca^{2+}entry and contraction. Membrane potential normally returns to negative potentials between slow waves or action potentials, and this deactivates L-type Ca^{2+} channels and facilitates relaxation. In tonic regions of the gut, SMCs are depolarized under basal conditions, and membrane potentials lie within a voltage range, positive to -50 mV, where tonic activation of L-type Ca^{2+} channels occurs (called "window current"). This causes constant low-level Ca^{2+} entry into SMCs and tonic contraction. Responses involving SMC depolarization or hyperpolarization are superimposed upon the basal resting potential. If the basal membrane potential is set at too negative a level, excitatory stimuli may fail to reach the threshold depolarization for contraction. Under these circumstances, normal neural or hormonal excitatory inputs might fail to enhance contraction. If basal membrane potential is abnormally depolarized, then tone might develop in a region that normally generates only phasic contractions or excitatory stimuli may cause abnormally forceful contractions that might even result in sensations of cramping.

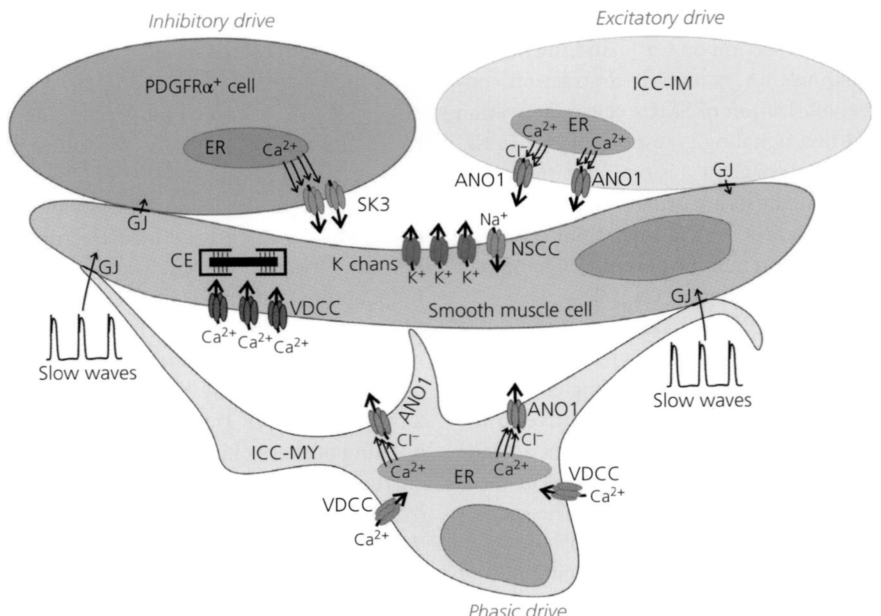

Figure 13.7 Main electrophysiological mechanisms of cells of the SIP syncytium. This figure depicts SMCs, ICC-IM, ICC-MY, and PDGFRα$^+$ cells. Gap junctions (GJ) occur between SMCs and the interstitial cells. Major ion channels in SMCs are voltage-dependent Ca^{2+} channels (VDCC) due to expression of L-type or $Ca_V1.2$ channels, a variety of K^+ channels (K chans) and nonselective cation channels (NSCC). The latter two classes of channels are involved in setting membrane potential and regulating the open probability of VDCC. Ca^{2+} entry through VDCC initiates contractions due to cross-bridge formation in the contractile element (CE). ICC-MY generate and actively propagate electrical slow waves through the activities of VDCC (in this case a T-type Ca^{2+} channel is dominant, $Ca_V3.2$) and ANO1. Ca^{2+} entry via VDCC causes Ca^{2+}-induced Ca^{2+} release into microdomains formed between the ER and the plasma membrane. Ca^{2+} release from the ER into these microdomains activates ANO1. Slow waves conduct to SMCs, causing periodic depolarization and activation of VDCC in these cells. Slow waves produce phasic excitable drive on the SIP syncytium. Membrane potential is also regulated by ICC-IM and PDGFRα$^+$ cells. In the case of ICC-IM, Ca^{2+} release from ER activates ANO1 channels. ANO1 is a Cl^- channel and efflux of Cl^- through these channels is defined by electrophysiologists as inward current. There are no VDCC in ICC-IM, so activation of ANO1 channels does not organize into slow waves. These channels exert excitatory drive through ongoing activation of spontaneous transient inward currents (STICs) in thousands of cells. Summation of STICs exerts a net depolarizing effect on the SIP syncytium. PDGFRα$^+$ cells express SK3 channels that are activated by Ca^{2+} release from ER in these cells. However, SK3 channels generate spontaneous transient outward currents (STOCs) that summate and exert a net hyperpolarizing influence and inhibitory drive on the SIP syncytium.

Setting of resting potential was thought for many years to be a function only of the ion channels and transporters present in SMCs. Now we recognize that channels active in interstitial cells of the SIP syncytium also contribute to the setting of resting membrane potentials because these cells are coupled electrically. Among the most important conductances in SMCs for regulating membrane potential are K_{ATP}, K_{IR}, TASK-2, and TREK-1 (see Figure 13.7). In some regions of the GI tract, voltage-dependent K^+ conductances may also contribute to membrane potential, depending upon the membrane potential range over which the cells function. Delayed rectifier K^+ channels may be examples of these conductances, including $K_V1.2$, $K_V1.5$, $K_V2.1$, and possibly others. It is important to mention that the complement of K^+ channels expressed by SMCs is not constant in all regions of the gut, and differences have also been noted between species.

A second class of ion channels that plays an important role in setting membrane potentials of GI muscles is nonselective cation channels (see Figure 13.7). In most instances, the presence and spontaneous activity of these channels causes membrane potentials to lie positive to the equilibrium potential for K^+ ions (E_K). Currents through nonselective cation channels are carried by monovalent (Na^+) or divalent (Ca^{2+}) ions that have equilibrium potentials positive to 0 mV. Summed activity of K^+ and nonselective cation channels causes membrane potentials of GI SMCs to lie between E_K (about -85 mV with physiological ionic gradients) and about -40 mV. Differences in the components and relative activities of channels determine the local net membrane conductance and the regional membrane potential.

Conductances in interstitial cells also contribute to the membrane potentials of SMCs. ICCs cause depolarizing trends in SMCs in two ways. ICCs generate stochastic Ca^{2+} transients (see section on Ca^{2+} handling mechanisms in SIP cells) that couple to activation of ANO1 channels and generate spontaneous transient inward currents (STICs) (see Figure 13.7) [87]. Generation of STICs in thousands of ICCs results in continuous net inward currents in the SIP syncytium, and this generates a depolarizing trend or excitatory drive. When Ca^{2+} release in ICCs (source of the Ca^{2+} transients) or ANO1 channels is blocked, the depolarizing influence of ICCs is reduced, and cells of the SIP syncytium hyperpolarize. As discussed below, ICCs also generate electrical slow waves that exert phasic depolarizations on the SIP syncytium (see Figure 13.7). PDGFRα$^+$ cells also display Ca^{2+} transients, but these cells express Ca^{2+}-activated K^+ channels (SK3). Therefore, currents activated by Ca^{2+} transients are spontaneous transient outward currents (STOCs). Summation of STOCs in thousands of PDGFRα$^+$ cells yields a hyperpolarizing trend or inhibitory drive (see Figure 13.7).

Thus, the moment-to-moment membrane potentials of SMCs result from integration of intrinsic conductances and the conductances expressed by interstitial cells. Superimposed upon resting potentials are dynamic changes in membrane potential caused by electrical slow waves, generated by ICCs, and Ca^{2+} action potentials, generated by SMCs.

Electrical slow waves

Phasic areas of the GI tract have intrinsic pacemaker activity. This activity has been referred to in the literature by a variety of names, including pacesetter potentials [88], pacemaker potentials [89], electrical control activity [90,91], basic electrical rhythm (BER) [92], slow waves [93], and action potentials [94,95]. The term in common usage now is slow waves.

Many techniques have been utilized to record slow wave activity from intact muscles and organs. Early recordings were modeled on techniques used to record cardiac or skeletal muscle electrical behaviors, and it was assumed the same approach could be used on GI muscles and organs. This technique employs the placement of metal electrodes on the surface of the abdomen or directly on the surface of organs. Signals assumed to be electrophysiological events are amplified and filtered. Unfortunately, extracellular recordings of this type are heavily contaminated by movements of the muscles and therefore do not produce valid records of the electrophysiological events occurring during slow waves or action potentials [96]. The most reliable method of recording slow waves is the use of very fine-tipped glass microelectrodes that can impale single cells and record transmembrane potentials via use of a high-impedance amplifier. Slow wave frequency, amplitude, and kinetics are obtained with this technique, and recordings of this type have been made from muscles from many species and regions of the GI tract, including from human muscles (Figure 13.8).

Slow waves consist of two major components. The first is a relatively rapid upstroke depolarization (≤1 V/s), which is quite

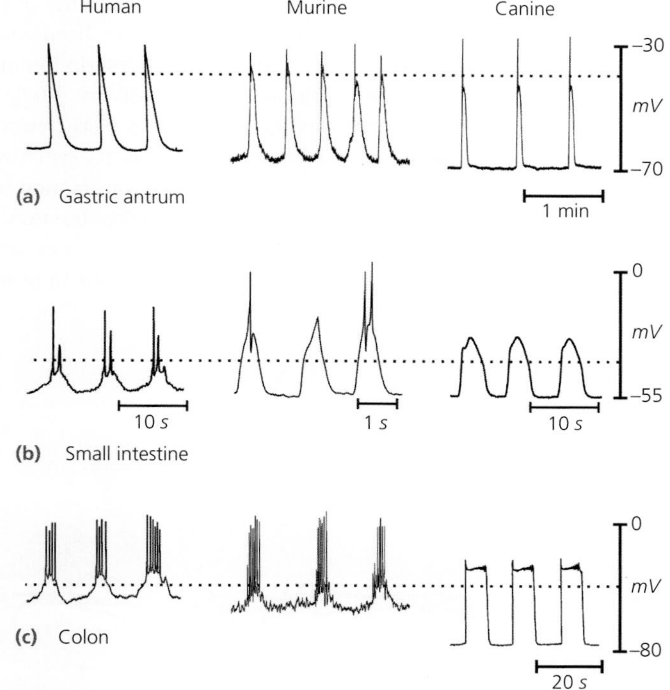

Figure 13.8 Slow waves from various regions of the GI tracts of human, mouse, and dog. Electrical slow waves were recorded from SMCs using intracellular electrical recording techniques. Slow waves consist of a fast upstroke depolarization followed by a plateau phase that persists for variable times depending upon the species and organ. Dotted lines in each series of traces show the approximate threshold potential at which L-type Ca^{2+} are activated. The slow wave upstroke and plateau depolarizations cross into voltages at which Ca^{2+} entry occurs via L-type Ca^{2+} channels. In small bowel and colon, slow wave depolarizations can elicit Ca^{2+} action potentials that are superimposed upon the slow waves. Note also the differences in resting membrane potentials (i.e., the most negative potential levels between slow waves) in different regions. Regulation of membrane potential sets the excitability of these muscles and the mechanical responses resulting from slow waves. At the most negative potentials between slow waves, the open probability of Ca^{2+} channels is very low. Therefore, slow waves cause an oscillation in Ca^{2+} channel open probability between low and higher levels of openings, and this organizes the motor outputs of these organs in phasic contractile activity. Propagation of slow waves organizes phasic contractions into peristaltic or segmental patterns of motility. Source: Sanders K.M., Koh S.D., Ward S.M. Interstitial cells of cajal as pacemakers in the gastrointestinal tract. Annu Rev Physiol 2006;68:307. Reproduced with permission of Annual Reviews Inc.

slow (≤1% of dV/dt [instantaneous rate of voltage change over time]) in comparison to cardiac and skeletal muscle action potentials. The upstroke is typically followed by a partial repolarization and then development of a plateau phase, which is a sustained depolarization that can last for seconds (see Figure 13.8) [97]. Membrane potentials of slow waves recorded from SMCs usually exceed the threshold level for activation of L-type Ca^{2+} channels, and it is during the plateau phase that excitation-contraction occurs, either by continuous Ca^{2+} entry (gastric muscles) or generation of action potentials (small bowel and colon). Slow waves occur in the absence of inputs from neurons, and have been viewed as part of the myogenic mechanisms of GI muscles. Investigators explored the origin and mechanisms of slow waves and action potentials in studies of smooth muscle tissues. When it became possible to disperse GI muscle tissues and record the electrical behaviors of SMCs directly, it became clear that SMCs display the potential to generate action potentials but do not have the ion channel apparatus necessary to generate or regenerate slow waves for the purpose of active propagation. Slow waves generated by ICC conduct passively to SMCs (Figure 13.9).

Dominant pacemaker sites usually refer to locations within organs that generate the highest frequency of electrical activity, because this drives the pacemaker activities in coupled regions, much like the SA node is the dominant pacemaker in the heart. Reasons why specific areas have higher frequency pacemaker activity and become dominant pacemakers in GI organs are presently unclear, but shifts in this dominance can negatively impact directionality and mechanical productivity of motor activities. All phasic regions of the GI tract have intrinsic pacemaker activity. Dissection experiments from specific regions of the gut have demonstrated that specific regions through the thickness of the tunica muscularis are the sources of local pacemaker activity. Muscles of the stomach displayed dominant pacemaker activity from the myenteric region between the circular and longitudinal muscle layers [98]. Small intestinal muscles showed similar dominance of pacemaker activity from the myenteric region [99]. The colon is more complex, having pacemaker zones along the submucosal surface of the circular muscle layer, as well as a second pacemaker in the myenteric region [100,101]. Morphological examination of these pacemaker regions found networks of cells known to anatomists as interstitial cells of Cajal [102–106]. ICCs within pacemaker regions were coupled electrically by gap junctions and coupled to SMCs. These morphological finding suggested the hypothesis that ICCs are the pacemakers in GI muscles. Isolated ICCs displayed rhythmic depolarizations that had properties of slow waves [107], and mutant animals (W/W^V mice) in which ICCs in the myenteric region (ICC-MY) failed to develop lacked slow wave activity (Figure 13.10) [28,29].

Summation of phasic electrical activity and the generation of tone

Sphincters have the role of restricting movements of materials from one region to another or out of the body, as with defecation. Sphincters have been referred to as purely tonic muscles [108] but this description neglects the fact that they display phasic electrical activity [109]. For example, the internal anal sphincter generates phasic electrical activity at up to 80 cycles per minute. Activity is asynchronous in sphincter muscle bundles, such that the summation of contractions in multiple bundles produces tonic contraction. The higher frequency of phasic electrical activity does not appear to leave sufficient time between depolarizations to restore intracellular Ca^{2+} to resting

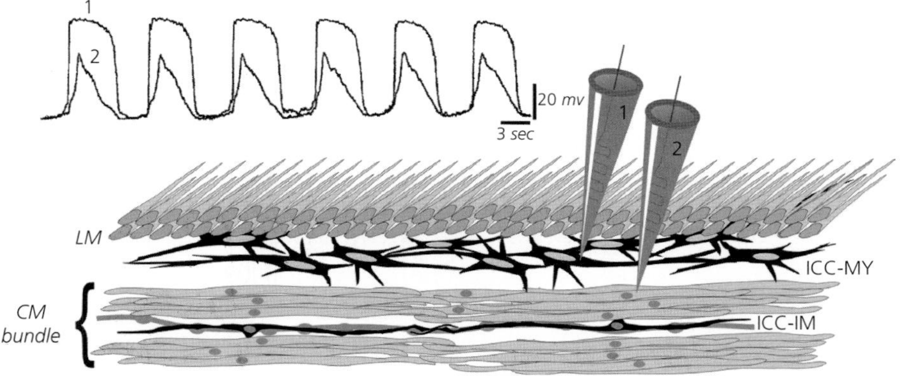

Figure 13.9 Electrical activity recorded simultaneously from ICC-MY and SMCs. Anatomical drawing depicts sites of electrical recordings for the traces shown at the top of the figure. ICC-MY between the circular (CM) and longitudinal (LM) muscle layers were impaled with microelectrodes (electrode 1). At the same time, nearby SMCs (electrode 2) were impaled. Recordings of this type showed that slow waves originate in ICC-MY (trace 1). Slow waves decay in amplitude as they conduct into electrically coupled SMCs (trace 2). Note the much larger amplitude of slow waves recorded from ICC-MY. The peak of the slow wave in ICC-MY reaches to about -10 mV (approximately the equilibrium potential for Cl^- ions) and is relatively constant for several seconds. Conductances expressed by SMCs cannot generate or regenerate slow waves, but the depolarization caused by slow waves activates voltage-dependent conductances in SMCs (e.g., L-type $Ca^{2=}$ channels and various K^+ channels). Original traces of slow waves were provided by Professor David Hirst. Source: Sanders K.M., Ward S.M., Koh S.D. Interstitial cells: regulators of smooth muscle function. Physiol Rev 2014;94(3):859. Reproduced with permission of The American Physiological Society.

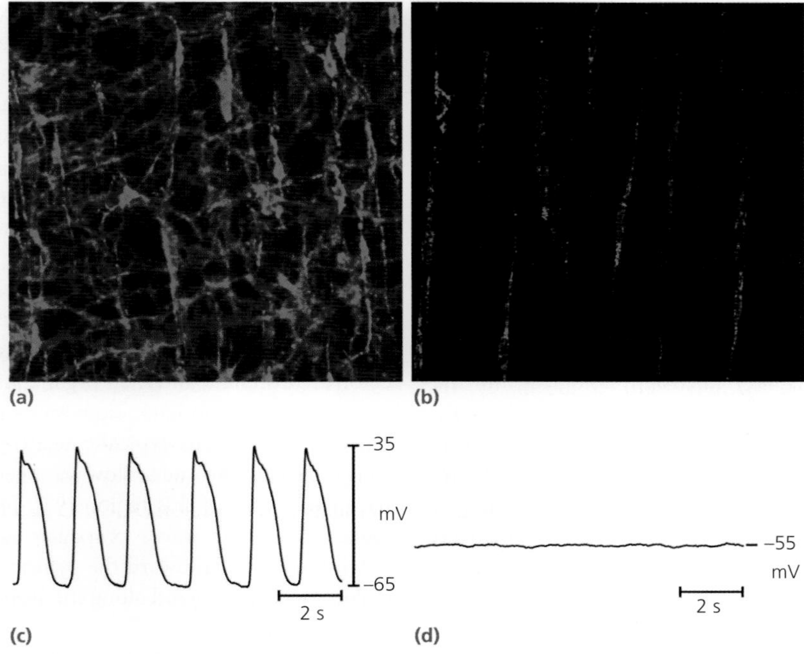

Figure 13.10 Loss of slow waves in small intestine of *W/W^V* mice. ICC-MY in the small intestine require intracellular signaling via c-Kit to develop. The *W* mutation is a loss-of-function mutation in *Kit; W^V* is also a loss-of-function mutation but less severe than *W*. The compound heterozygotes carrying this double mutation (*W/W^V*) have severely depleted ICC-MY networks in the small intestine. **(a)** The ICC-MY network in wildtype mice; **(b)** loss of these cells in *W/W^V* mice [29]. Faintly labeled cells in **(b)** are ICC-DMP that survive and still develop in *W/W^V* mice. **(c)** Normal slow waves recorded from mouse small intestine. **(d)** Loss of slow waves in *W/W^V* muscles. Source: Sanders K.M., Ward S.M., Koh S.D. Interstitial cells: regulators of smooth muscle function. Physiol Rev 2014;94(3):859. Reproduced with permission of The American Physiological Society.

levels, creating conditions of a partial tetanus. Finally, in some cases, sphincter SMCs (e.g., lower esophageal sphincter) display relatively depolarized membrane potentials [110]. Thus, these cells may experience continuous Ca^{2+} entry via L-type Ca^{2+} channels (window current), and this contributes to the development of tone.

Action potentials

Action potentials are the primary excitable events generated by SMCs in GI muscles. Action potentials are due to voltage-dependent activation of L-type Ca^{2+} channels. Openings of these channels result in Ca^{2+} influx [70,72,111,112]. Based on the upstroke velocity of Ca^{2+} action potentials, which can reach 20 V/s, Ca^{2+} current density is substantial and sufficient to increase cytoplasmic Ca^{2+} concentration and elicit contraction [113,114]. SMCs are the only cells of the SIP syncytium that produce Ca^{2+} action potentials [115].

Gastric muscles do not generate action potentials except in the most terminal antrum and pyloric sphincter [94,116]. In the small intestine, slow waves are the source of depolarization that evokes action potentials, and these events are superimposed upon the plateau phase of slow waves. When ICCs and the ability to generate slow waves are lost, such as in *W/W^V* mice, muscles are still capable of generating action potentials [117] but the pattern of action potential generation is less organized than when slow waves are present. This is an example of how the electrical activities of two cell types of the SIP syncytium are integrated to produce normal electrophysiological behaviors. Membrane potentials in colon are less negative, and very small slow wave depolarizations are capable of eliciting clusters of action potentials. Action potentials elicit strong excitation-contraction coupling. Single action potentials elicit twitch responses and multiple action potentials can elicit long-lasting contractions [118–120].

Propagation of slow waves to coordinate excitability

Action potentials do not propagate very effectively in SMCs due to the impedance properties of GI muscles, so these events alone are typically restricted to limited areas of SMCs. The inability of action potentials to organize contractions in large areas of muscle represents another important role for slow waves in motor functions. Slow waves propagate actively through networks of ICC and depolarize electrically coupled SMCs to elicit action potentials.

Smooth muscle cells do not express the molecular apparatus to support active propagation, and therefore slow waves decay in amplitude as they conduct into the syncytium of SMCs (see Figure 13.9). Thus, as observed anatomically, ICC networks extend over phasic regions of GI organs to support slow wave propagation. Slow wave propagation velocity is anisotropic; slow waves propagate more rapidly along the axis of circular muscle fibers (in one study 23 mm/s) and more slowly in the axis of the longitudinal muscle fibers (11 mm/s) [98]. In thicker smooth muscle layers of larger animals and humans, maintenance of slow wave amplitude requires regeneration, as slow waves spread from pacemaker regions into the thickness of the muscles. This appears to occur through networks of ICCs that populate the septa between muscle bundles (ICC-SEP) (see Table 13.1) [105].

Rates of slow wave propagation have been reported in studies of intact organs using extracellular recording methods. However, the interpretation of these data is controversial because the recording techniques are contaminated by mechanical artifacts and may not represent primary electrophysiological information [96]. The mechanism for slow wave propagation has also been studied using muscle strips in partitioned recording baths [121]. In such an experiment, one portion of the muscle strip is in a chamber perfused with normal physiological solution so normal slow waves can occur spontaneously or be paced electrically (Figure 13.11). Another part of the muscle can be isolated in a chamber in which test solutions can be applied. Cells in either chamber or both can be impaled for intracellular recording. Such experiments have shown that the rate of upstroke depolarization (dV/dt) of slow waves, an indication of the amount of inward current during the leading edge of advancing slow waves, is decreased in a concentration-dependent manner by reduced extracellular Ca^{2+}, reduced temperature, and antagonists of T-type Ca^{2+} channels until slow wave propagation is blocked. Propagation velocity is similarly reduced in conditions that reduce dV/dt.

Maintenance of slow wave propagation is very important for physiological behaviors such as gastric peristalsis and intestinal segmentation. Peristaltic contractions in the esophagus and colon are different, and their organization is provided by neural pathways. In the stomach, slow waves are generated in the orad portion of the corpus, typically near the greater curvature [122]. This is because the rate of slow wave generation is greatest in the pacemaker cells of this region [97]. From the dominant pacemaker area, slow waves propagate around the stomach and down the stomach toward the pyloric sphincter, causing a ring of contraction to spread along the stomach. After eating, neural

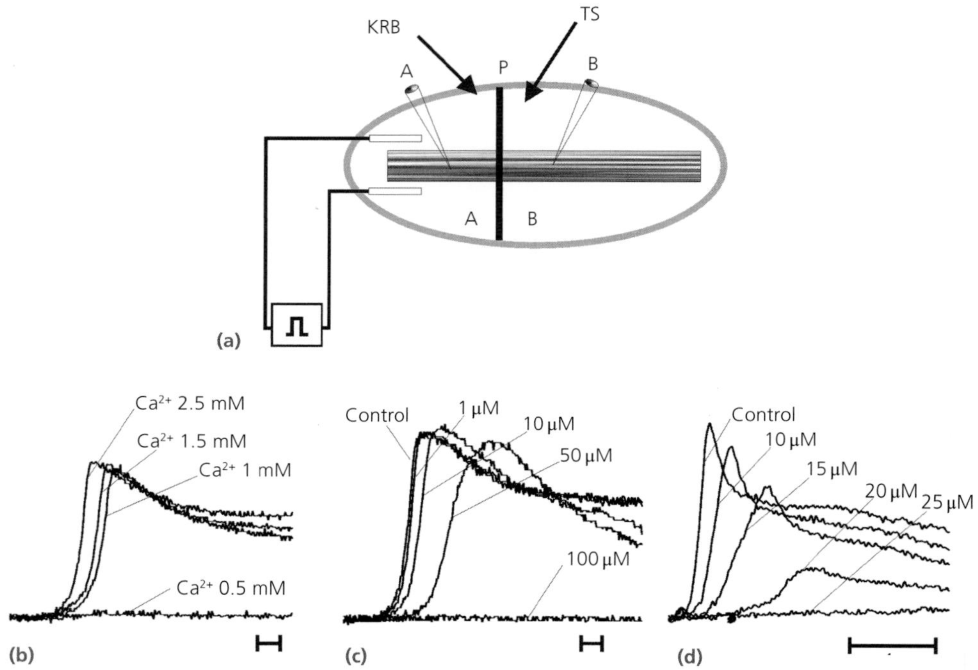

Figure 13.11 Ca^{2+} entry is required for slow wave propagation. **(a)** A partitioned bath used to study propagation of slow waves. Muscle strip is pulled through a latex partition (P) that effectively isolates the solutions perfusing the strip in the two chambers (A and B). Chamber A is perfused with normal Krebs solution (KRB) and slow waves can be generated spontaneously or as a result of pacing (current source and electrodes placed on either side of the muscle strip are shown schematically) in this chamber. Chamber B is used to perfuse Test Solutions (TS) to test conditions that sustain or do not sustain slow wave propagation. Panels **b–d** show examples of control slow waves (recorded in chamber A) and slow waves during exposure to TS containing reduced $[Ca^{2+}]_o$ **(b)**, extracellular Ni^{2+} **(c)** or mibefradil **(d)**. Concentrations resulting in each trace are shown. Sweep speeds are accelerated to emphasize the upstroke phase of slow waves. Each of the TS caused concentration-dependent decreases in the velocity (dV/dt) of the upstroke potentials, as shown by the superimposed slow waves. The TS also caused progressive decreases in propagation velocity (not shown in this example). Active propagation of slow waves was blocked by $[Ca^{2+}]_o$ (0.5 mM), Ni^{2+} (100 μM) and mibefradil, a T-type Ca^{2+} channel antagonist (25 μM), and the slow waves evoked in chamber A decayed in amplitude before reaching the cell impaled in chamber B. Time scale in **(b)** and **(c)** is 100 ms and time scale in **(d)** is 1 s. Source: Bayguinov O., Ward S.M., Kenyon J.L., Sanders K.M. Voltage-gated Ca2+ currents are necessary for slow-wave propagation in the canine gastric antrum. Am J Physiol 2007;293:C1645. Reproduced with permission of The American Physiological Society.

and hormonal inputs strengthen contractile responses to slow waves and peristaltic contractions become more powerful. As slow waves invade the terminal antrum, spread of these events into the pylorus causes contraction and closure of the sphincter. The high pressures resulting from terminal antral contraction against a closed pyloric sphincter cause retropulsion of gastric contents, and the resulting turbulence provides forces to help break apart solid food particles.

If there are breaks or uncoupling of the gastric ICC network, normal active propagation of slow waves can be compromised. Unable to regenerate in SMCs, slow waves decay rapidly within a few millimeters in areas devoid of ICCs, causing abnormal activation of muscle contractions instead of a normal coherent, unidirectional wave of excitation. Such conditions may explain delayed gastric emptying in gastroparesis in which reduced populations of gastric ICCs have been reported [123].

In spite of obvious anatomical connectivity between the musculature of the stomach and small intestine, there is separation between the electrical and mechanical behaviors of the stomach and pylorus from the duodenum. A distinct reduction in ICC networks was observed within a narrow zone in the pylorus, and this area constituted a slow wave-free zone, resulting in a block in the propagation of slow waves from the pylorus to the duodenum and facilitating independent electrical and motor behaviors in these two regions of the gut [124].

Another consequence of slow wave propagation helps explain a common behavior of the small intestine – segmentation. Like nerve action potentials, a slow wave propagating from one direction cannot pass a slow wave propagating from the opposite direction. Collisions of events block propagation due to the refractory properties of the ion channels responsible for slow waves. The network of ICCs is electrically coupled from point to point along the small intestine, but most contractions are limited to small areas of muscles in segments of intestine. The frequency of slow waves in the small intestine is about three times higher than in the stomach. A slow wave generated at any given point can propagate in both directions, but it can propagate only a short distance before colliding with slow waves generated above or below. This restricts slow wave propagation into segments of bowel and favors a segmental pattern of contraction.

Electrical pacing of the heart has been an important therapeutic tool for treating cardiac arrhythmias. The normal pacemaker tissues, the SA and AV nodes, are highly localized collections of specialized cells that can drive electrical activation of the entire organ. No such discrete area of pacemaker control exists in GI muscles, and this is why networks of ICCs, the pacemaker tissue, extend along the entire lengths of phasic regions. Pacing has also attracted interest as a means of normalizing GI motility [125]. However, differences between cardiac and GI smooth muscle tissues have made effective implementation of pacing to enhance gastric emptying or improve small intestinal function difficult. Extrinsic pacing of the gut is likely to be no more effective than intrinsic pacing if ICC networks are damaged or discontinuous, because, as discussed above, active propagation of slow waves and effective organization of electrical excitation of SMCs depend upon the integrity of ICC networks. Secondly, the relative refractory periods of slow waves are several seconds in duration. For example, pacing of dog antral muscles at 3.5 cycles per minute produced slow waves of equal wave form cycle to cycle, but increasing the rate of pacing resulted in an alternate pattern of slow waves in which every other event was compromised in amplitude and duration and therefore mechanically less productive [126].

The therapeutic purpose of pacing is to drive more effective contractile behaviors; however, the usefulness of pacing is constrained by the anatomical integrity of ICC networks and refractory properties of the slow waves.

Ca^{2+} handling mechanisms in SIP cells

Cytoplasmic Ca^{2+} ($[Ca^{2+}]_{cyt}$) is the major initiator of muscle contraction, so understanding mechanisms for Ca^{2+} handling is at the heart of understanding the GI smooth muscle function. $[Ca^{2+}]_{cyt}$ is regulated by numerous mechanisms in SMCs. Entry mechanisms include voltage-dependent and -independent ion channels, exchange proteins, store-operated proteins, and mechanosensitive ion channels. Release mechanisms include Ca^{2+} channels in the sarcoplasmic reticulum (SR) that bind inositol 1,4,5-trisphosphate or ryanodine, and Ca^{2+} homeostasis mechanisms include ion channel subunits, Ca^{2+} pumps in the plasma and SR membranes, ion exchangers, and many secondary factors that fine tune these mechanisms. Ca^{2+} handling mechanism are also of key importance to the behaviors of interstitial cells of the SIP syncytium, since the electrophysiology of these cells is mainly focused on the open probabilities of Ca^{2+}-activated ion channels.

Ca^{2+} entry mechanisms in SMCs

The primary Ca^{2+} entry mechanism in SMCs of the GI tract is a dihydropyridine-sensitive, voltage-dependent Ca^{2+} channel, commonly called L-type Ca^{2+} channel or $Ca_V1.2$. Voltage clamping of single, isolated SMCs showed this current is activated by depolarization into a threshold range of -50 to -40 mV, peaks at about 0 mV, and reverses at about +35 mV [72]. $Ca_V1.2$ channels also experience voltage-dependent inactivation, but inactivation is incomplete in the potential range of about -50 to -20 mV, creating potentials at which there is constant Ca^{2+} influx. This is known as "window current" [127] and it is an important biophysical property of GI SMCs. For example, cells in some sphincters and other regions have basal resting potentials that sit within the window current range, helping to create conditions of continuous Ca^{2+} entry and tonic contraction. The concept of window current also comes into play during slow waves, as membrane potential at the peak of the slow wave plateau often sits within the potential range for window current. This sustains Ca^{2+} entry during slow waves and allows phasic contractions to persist for several seconds.

There are highly effective agonists and antagonists for $Ca_V1.2$ channels, but the therapeutic usefulness of these drugs is minimal since the same channels are expressed in all smooth muscles in the body and in the heart. The properties and pharmacology of $Ca_V1.2$ channels are similar in these tissues. Therefore, a compound taken to enhance blood flow through coronary arteries could have negative effects on gastric emptying or cause constipation. SMCs also express receptor-operated channels that can act as a source of Ca^{2+} in response to agonist stimulation. Examples of this are P2X receptors [128] and some transient receptor potential (TRP) channels [129] that have favorable P_{Ca}/P_{Na} permeability ratios.

Ca^{2+} entry mechanisms in interstitial cells

A major difference between ICCs involved in neurotransduction and those involved in generation and propagation of pacemaker activity (slow waves) is the expression of voltage-dependent Ca^{2+} channels. Pacemaker ICCs express $Ca_V3.2$ (T-type Ca^{2+} channels), and in some cases $Ca_V1.2$ and $Ca_V1.3$ [84]. $Ca_V3.2$ channels are important for propagation of slow waves activity within networks of ICC-MY (see Figure 13.11) [121,130]. Activation of $Ca_V3.2$ channels occurs by spontaneous transient depolarizations (STDs) that are initiated by Ca^{2+} transients and transient activation of inward currents through ANO1 channels in ICCs. When the threshold is reached for activation of $Ca_V3.2$ channels, the resulting inward current causes depolarization of electrically coupled ICCs and regenerative activation of $Ca_V3.2$ channels in those cells. $Ca_V3.2$ channels are activated cell to cell within the ICC-MY networks to produce active propagation of slow waves. Ca^{2+} entry via this mechanism initiates Ca^{2+} release from intracellular stores in ICC. This mechanism is known as Ca^{2+}-induced Ca^{2+} release (CICR), and it sustains the duration of slow wave depolarizations, causing the plateau phase [130]. Voltage-dependent mechanisms for Ca^{2+} entry have not been reported in PDGFRα$^+$ cells.

Ca^{2+} release mechanisms in SIP cells

Two major mechanisms for Ca^{2+} release are expressed by SMCs in the GI tract: inositol triphosphate (IP_3) receptors, encoded mainly by ITPR1, and ryanodine receptors, encoded mainly by RYR2 and RYR3. Expression of similar Ca^{2+} release channels is found in ICCs and PDGFRα$^+$ cells [84,85]. Ca^{2+} release occurs spontaneously in each type of SIP cell [131–133] but the consequences of Ca^{2+} release vary dramatically depending upon the availability of Ca^{2+}-sensitive ion channels (see section on Ionic conductances in other SIP cells). Both types of Ca^{2+} release channels experience Ca^{2+}-induced Ca^{2+} release. In some cases, Ca^{2+} entry is coupled to Ca^{2+} release, amplifying Ca^{2+} influx. However, it should be noted that Ca^{2+} release is usually transient and directed toward the activation of Ca^{2+}-sensitive ion channels in the plasma membrane and minimally involved in the direct regulation of contraction. Ca^{2+} transients from ryanodine receptors (also called Ca^{2+} sparks) [134] are brief ($t_{1/2}$ = 50–60 ms) and highly localized (2.4 μm at half-maximal amplitude) [135]. Ca^{2+} transients from IP_3 receptors are more dynamic in nature (Ca^{2+} puffs) and can vary significantly in amplitude and duration depending upon local distribution of IP_3 receptors [136]. In some cases, regeneration of Ca^{2+} transients occurs through interactions between ryanodine and IP_3 receptors, and this can lead to generation of intracellular waves [137].

All these behaviors can be observed in SMCs and interstitial cells of the SIP syncytium spontaneously, in response to agonists or in different classes of cells. Paradoxically, Ca^{2+} release in SMCs often results in inhibitory signaling due to activation of large-conductance Ca^{2+}-activated K^+ (BK) channels rather than being directly coupled to contraction [138].

Ca^{2+} homeostasis mechanisms

Ca^{2+} entry and Ca^{2+} release must be counteracted by homeostatic mechanisms to maintain low levels of $[Ca^{2+}]_{cyt}$ between stimuli. Restoration of basal $[Ca^{2+}]_{cyt}$ occurs by sequestration of Ca^{2+} into stores and extrusion to the extracellular media. A 10^5-fold Ca^{2+} gradient exists between the lumen of the SR and the cytoplasm. Sarco/endoplasmic reticulum Ca^{2+}-ATPase (SERCA) exists to transport Ca^{2+} from the cytoplasm into the SR. SMCs express mainly two types of SERCA pumps: SERCA2b (115 kD) and SERCA3 (105 kD) [139]. SERCA uses energy from ATP hydrolysis to pump Ca^{2+} into the lumen of the SR against the significant concentration gradient [140]. Ca^{2+} is buffered in the SR lumen by proteins such as calreticulin and calsequestrin to reduce its activity [141] and this maintains a free Ca^{2+} concentration estimated to be only 10–15 mM [142].

Phospholamban, a small ER transmembrane protein, regulates the activity of SERCA pumps. Binding of phospholamban inhibits SERCA pumps, but this inhibition can be reduced by phosphorylation of phospholamban by protein kinases A or G [143,144]. Activation of SERCA pumps can shorten the duration of contractions, and this may be one of the methods by which agonists linked to production of cAMP can inhibit smooth muscle contraction. A typical means of evaluating the importance of Ca^{2+} stores in smooth muscle behaviors is to inhibit SERCA pumps with drugs, such as thapsigargin or cyclopiazonic acid [145].

Inhibition of Ca^{2+} uptake removes a major form of Ca^{2+} homeostasis and can elevate $[Ca^{2+}]_{cyt}$ and increase contractions or tone. However, experiments using inhibitors of SERCA to evaluate effects on electrophysiological or contractile behaviors of GI muscles are complicated by the fact that the behaviors of each type of SIP cell depend upon Ca^{2+} release mechanisms. Thus, treating GI muscles with SERCA pump inhibitors can produce complex, even seemingly contradictory, effects. Much of the literature on Ca^{2+} handling in GI SMCs has been performed on intact GI muscles, and conclusions from these studies have not typically considered this complexity. The plasma membrane also contains a Ca^{2+}, Mg^{2+}-ATPase (PMCA), providing an additional mechanism for removing Ca^{2+} from the cytoplasm. This enzyme differs from SERCA in that it is activated by binding of Ca^{2+}/calmodulin to an autoinhibitory domain. Thus, PMCA is activated by increased cytoplasmic Ca^{2+} concentration, serving as a negative feedback mechanism [11,146].

Low-affinity Na^+/Ca^{2+} exchangers located in the plasma membrane and the mitochondrial Ca^{2+} uniporter also aid in decreasing intracellular Ca^{2+} [147–149].

Store-operated Ca^{2+} entry

Many agonists raise intracellular Ca^{2+} through G-protein-mediated increases in IP_3 production and release of Ca^{2+} from the ER/SR stores. Loss of Ca^{2+} from stores is restored partially through the actions of SERCA, as discussed previously, but there is also net loss of Ca^{2+} to the extracellular space through the action of PMCA and Na^+/Ca^{2+} exchange. For store-dependent Ca^{2+} release mechanisms to be maintained, a regulated means of recovery must be available to refill stores without loading cells with Ca^{2+}. Such a mechanism, originally named capacitative Ca^{2+} entry (CCE), was proposed in which loss of Ca^{2+} from stores was compensated for by uptake through the plasma membrane and facilitated recovery into the ER/SR [150]. This mechanism has subsequently been renamed store-operated Ca^{2+} entry (SOCE).

Although there have been several suggestions for the mechanism of SOCE, the dominant view at this point is that two proteins are responsible. The first protein is ORAI (Ca^{2+} release-activated Ca^{2+} protein 1), a plasma membrane Ca^{2+} channel that normally has low open-probability. ORAI, of which three isoforms are expressed, is activated by an ER transmembrane, Ca^{2+}-sensing protein, stromal interacting molecule (STIM), expressed in two isoforms [151]. Store emptying leads to reconfiguration of STIMs, oligomerization, and translocation of the STIM complex within the ER/SR membrane to facilitate binding with ORAI. STIM/ORAI binding increases the open probability of ORAI channels, admitting Ca^{2+} into cells [152]. SOCE was first identified in nonexcitable cells, but now this mechanism is recognized to be available in excitable cells, such as muscle cells [153].

At present, little is known about the role of SOCE in regulation of contractions of GI SMCs; however, this mechanism plays an important role in maintaining the function of ICCs. Dynamic Ca^{2+} signaling occurs in ICC cells, as discussed previously, and a mechanism such as SOCE is required to maintain a Ca^{2+} gradient across the ER membrane to facilitate Ca^{2+} release. ICCs express multiple ORAI and STIM genes and currents attributable to SOCE were measured in isolated ICCs [154,155]. A dominant negative peptide designed to inhibit binding of STIM to ORAI blocked the current due to SOCE in ICCs and blocked the development of pacemaker currents. Pharmacological block of ORAI channels also blocked Ca^{2+} transients and the associated currents activated in ICCs. Thus, SOCE is an important factor in regulation of the pacemaker functions of ICCs.

Store-operated Ca^{2+} entry also maintains the Ca^{2+} release events in ICCs that are involved in neurotransduction. ICC-IM experience continuous, stochastic Ca^{2+} release events that elicit inward current through activation of ANO1 Cl^- channels. Enhanced Ca^{2+} release is a hallmark of excitatory neurotransduction in ICC-IM, while inhibition of Ca^{2+} release results from nitrergic, inhibitory neurotransduction [156,157]. Pharmacological block of SOCE inhibits Ca^{2+} release in ICC-IM, preventing neurotransduction by these cells [158].

Mechanosensitive ion channels/ mechanisms related to stretch

The organs of the GI tract undergo complex volume changes during the course of ingestion, digestion, and defecation. Since Ca^{2+} entry in GI SMCs occurs largely through voltage-dependent Ca^{2+} channels, mechanisms that regulate membrane potential can effectively regulate excitability. Several of the cells regulating GI motility express mechanosensitive properties that affect membrane potential, smooth muscle excitability, and contraction. Enteric neurons display mechanosensitivity and these responses are manifest upon changes in the lengths of GI muscles [159,160]. In fact, responses to stretch are likely to be integrated responses that include mechanisms present in neurons and nonneuronal, postjunctional cells.

A canonical response to stretch in many smooth muscles is the "myogenic response" [161]. However, such a response would tend to confound the reservoir function in many regions of the GI tract, such as the fundus and body of the stomach and proximal colon. In many smooth muscle tissues of the gut, stretch leads either to hyperpolarization or no change in membrane potential. Thus, a mechanism is available to stabilize excitability when muscles are stretched. Neural responses are responsible for a portion of mechanosensitive responses, with net activation of enteric inhibitory mechanisms. However, GI SMCs also express K^+ channels that have mechanosensitive properties. For example, relaxation responses to stretch in rat colon were shown to be attenuated by iberiotoxin, a sensitive and selective BK channel antagonist [162]. GI SMCs also express two-pore K^+ channels that consist of four transmembrane domains and two pore domains. Among this class of channels are mechanosensitive members, such as TREK and TRAAK (another member of the two-pore domain K^+ channel family; K2P) channels. TREK1 and TREK2 are expressed in colonic muscles, and stretching these muscles activates a K^+ conductance with properties similar to TREK channels [163]. TREK channels display interesting regulation, with cAMP-dependent phosphorylation inhibiting currents and cGMP-dependent phosphorylation enhancing current [164]. Nitric oxide (NO) donors and membrane permeable analogs of cGMP activate the TREK1-like conductance in colonic SMCs, and this conductance, via regulation by cGMP, has been suggested as a participant in nitrergic inhibition of GI muscles.

In other regions of the gut, activation of inward currents may represent dominant stretch-dependent effects. As in all GI SMCs, human jejunal muscle cells display L-type Ca^{2+} currents, and this conductance is enhanced by stretch [165]. A mechanism that included changes in membrane tension due to incorporation of lysophosphatidyl choline (LPC) was proposed for this effect [166]. LPC also altered the inactivation kinetics of L-type currents, an effect that would alter window current and might have implications for muscles that develop tone (e.g., lower esophageal sphincter). A Na^+ current, $Na_V1.5$ encoded by SCN5A (Na^+ voltage-gated channel α subunit 5), is expressed in SMCs and ICCs in the human small intestine. $Na_V1.5$ is activated by shear stress, a stimulus often employed to demonstrate mechanosensitivity (167). Slow wave frequency in intact muscles was increased by stretch, and block of $Na_V1.5$ with lidocaine or QX-314 decreased slow wave frequency. Knockdown of SCN5A by siRNA (silencing RNA) techniques caused hyperpolarization of membrane potential and reduced the amplitude and duration of slow waves [168]. A small percentage of patients with irritable bowel syndrome (IBS) display mutations in SCN5A that result in loss-of-function abnormalities in $Na_V1.5$, including aberrant voltage dependence and altered mechanosensitivity [169].

Integrated responses to stretch are also manifest in GI muscles. A study utilizing computerized application of length-ramps demonstrated how stretch can sensitize muscles to neurotransmitters [170]. Stretch-dependent hyperpolarization responses in murine colon were blocked by tetrodotoxin and a nitric oxide synthase (NOS) inhibitor, suggesting they were dependent upon release of NO from enteric inhibitory neurons. Responses to stretch were also blocked by an antagonist of TREK1 channels, and in muscles of animals pretreated with a neutralizing antibody to c-Kit that reduces the numbers of ICCs in these muscles. Apamin, a drug that blocks SK channels, also reduced stretch-dependent responses in colonic muscles. After block of inhibitory neurotransmitters, stretch elicited depolarization and excitatory responses that were blocked by neurokinin receptor antagonists. Taken together, these experiments demonstrate, in one region of the gut, the complicated nature of mechanosensitive responses and the multicellular nature of these responses. Neural pathways, SMCs, and interstitial cells may participate in stretch-dependent responses, and these responses may vary from region to region.

Other mechanosensitive mechanisms are manifest in GI muscles in addition to ion channels. In gastric antrum, computer-controlled length-ramps initiated depolarization and a positive chronotropic effect on slow waves [171]. The magnitude of these responses was tuned to the rate of muscle elongation but unaffected by neural antagonists, suggesting a myogenic origin. Responses to stretch were blocked by indomethacin, suggesting the involvement of prostaglandins. The responses were absent in W/W^V mice with severely reduced numbers of ICC-IM in the antrum. It was suggested that stretch-dependent generation of prostaglandins working on the pacemaker mechanism in ICCs is the mechanism for this response. Prostaglandin (PG) E_2 has been shown to have chronotropic effects on gastric slow waves [172,173].

The antral stretch response could have clinical significance and help to understand some of the symptoms of functional gastric disorders. Double electrode recordings from cells in the corpus and antrum showed that the chronotropic effects of stretch uncoupled the normal proximal-to-distal propagation of slow waves [171]. Thus, defective accommodation responses in the proximal stomach to food ingestion, which might be associated with early satiety, feelings of fullness and bloating, and pain, might also cause ingested food to be shuttled into the distal stomach prematurely. This alteration in the distribution of food in the stomach could lead to antral distension, chronotropic effects on antral pacemakers, disorganization of normal slow wave propagation, and delay of gastric emptying.

Mechanism and regulation of smooth muscle contraction and relaxation

Smooth muscle contraction

Like every other muscle, GI smooth muscle contraction is dependent on Ca^{2+} influx into the cytoplasm. The opening of voltage-dependent Ca^{2+} channels by membrane potential depolarization, brought on by the firing of action potentials or slow waves, the binding of neurotransmitters, hormones, and other mediators to their respective receptors, or stretch-dependent activation of ion channels in the plasma membrane, can trigger Ca^{2+} influx and contraction. As the intracellular concentration of Ca^{2+} increases, Ca^{2+} binds to calmodulin. Ca^{2+}/calmodulin binds to caldesmon to release caldesmon from the actin filament and expose the myosin-binding sites, and also binds to and activates myosin light chain kinase (MLCK) to phosphorylate MLC. For contraction to occur, MLCK must phosphorylate the 20 kD MLC of myosin to enable the molecular interaction of myosin with actin (Figure 13.12) [174].

Phosphorylation of MLC causes a conformational change to occur in the myosin head, which increases myosin ATPase activity and promotes the interaction between the myosin head and actin [175]. Myosin ATPase activity is much lower in smooth muscle than in skeletal muscle [49,176]. This factor leads to the slower cycling speed of smooth muscle, but the longer period of contraction allows smooth muscle to achieve potentially greater contractile force [177]. The energy released from ATP by myosin ATPase activity results in the cycling of the myosin cross-bridges with actin for contraction. Cross-bridge cycling, in which the myosin heads pull on the actin filaments, then occurs, generating force. There is a positive relationship between $[Ca^{2+}]_{cyt}$, MLC phosphorylation, and the generation of force.

Because most GI smooth muscles function for long periods of time without rest, their power output is comparatively low, and contractions can continue without expenditure of large amounts of energy. Contractions are sustained until ATP-dependent Ca^{2+} pumps (SERCA and PMCA) transport Ca^{2+} ions back into the SR or out of the cell. However, a low, constitutive, concentration of Ca^{2+} remains in the sarcoplasm in muscles that maintain tone [178,179]. This constitutive Ca^{2+} maintains the phosphorylation of MLC at a low level in the absence of external stimuli and generates tone. Thus, contractile activity in GI smooth muscle is determined primarily by the phosphorylation state of MLC, which can be maintained with very little energy expenditure.

Relaxation of smooth muscles

Phosphorylation of MLC promotes its binding to actin and allows cross-bridge cycling. Phosphorylation is a covalent modification, and MLC will stay bound to actin until it is dephosphorylated [180]. This creates a potential difficulty in that reducing $[Ca^{2+}]_{cyt}$ alone does not produce relaxation [181]. Dephosphorylation of MLC is required to terminate smooth muscle contraction. Myosin light chain phosphatase (MLCP), which opposes the action of MLCK, is responsible for the

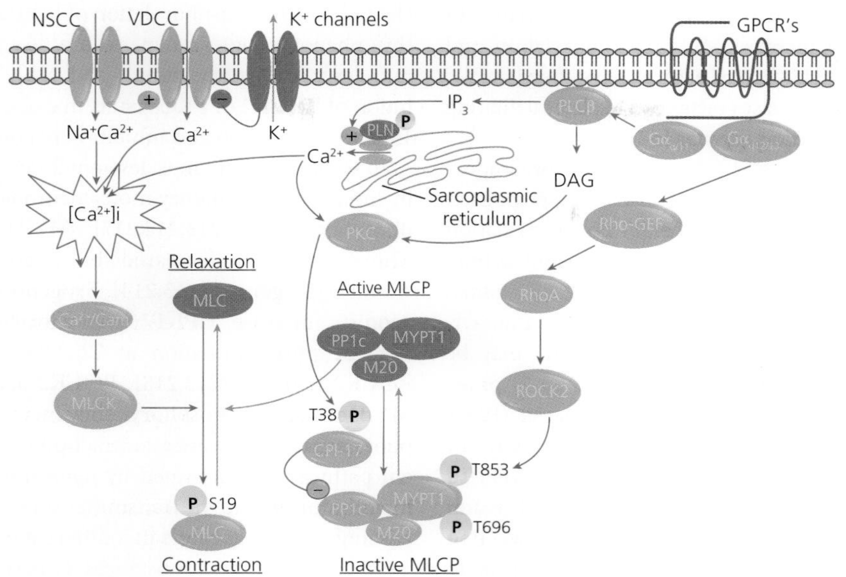

Figure 13.12 Regulation of contraction in SMCs showing Ca^{2+} mobilization and activation and deactivation of contractile proteins. Mechanisms leading to contraction are depicted in red, and mechanisms leading to reduced contraction are in blue. Ca^{2+} required for initiation of excitation–contraction coupling enters cells through voltage-dependent Ca^{2+} channels (VDCC) and can be enhanced by activation of nonselective cation channels (NSCC). The open probability of VDCC is enhanced (circle with + sign) by depolarization caused by opening of NSCC and the influx of Na^+ or Ca^{2+}. Openings of VDCC are decreased by a variety of K^+ channels expressed by SMCs; many inhibitory agonists reduce Ca^{2+} influx by activating K^+ channels. Ca^{2+} entry can be supplemented by release of Ca^{2+} from IP_3-gated Ca^{2+} channels in the sarcoplasmic reticulum membrane. Ca^{2+} release from the sarcoplasmic reticulum can also occur through ryanodine receptors (not shown). IP_3 is synthesized by PLCβ in response to agonist binding to G-protein-coupled receptors (GPCR) and coupling through G_{q11}. $[Ca^{2+}]_{cyt}$ binds to calmodulin and activates myosin light chain kinase (MLCK), which phosphorylates MLC to facilitate cross-bridge formation. Phosphorylation of MLC is balanced by the action of myosin light chain phosphatase (MLCP). Dephosphorylation of MLC reduces cross-bridge cycling and leads to muscle relaxation. Factors that lead to inhibition of MLCP increase contraction and, in effect, enhance the Ca^{2+} sensitivity of the contractile apparatus. A pathway that increases Ca^{2+} sensitization (and therefore increases contraction) occurs through binding of G-protein-coupled ($G_{12/13}$) receptors and regulation of GDP-GTP exchange factors (Rho-GEF), RhoA, and activation of Rho kinase (ROCK2). ROCK2 can phosphorylate the regulatory subunit of MLCP (MYPT1) at T853 and T696. Phosphorylation of MYPT1 decreases the activity of MLCP, preserving the phosphorylation of MLC. Protein kinase C (PKC) can phosphorylate CPI-17 (at T38), a protein that when phosphorylated inhibits the catalytic subunit of MLCP (PPlc; circle with negative sign), thus also preserving the phosphorylation of MLC.

dephosphorylation of MLC (see Figure 13.12). Relaxation results after cessation of a contractile stimulus or by the direct action of inhibitory neurotransmitters [182,183], and requires a decrease in $[Ca^{2+}]_{cyt}$ and increased MLCP activity [184–186]. Mechanisms that decrease $[Ca^{2+}]_{cyt}$ and/or enhance MLCP activity may become altered by disease, contributing to abnormal motility responses [187–189]. Removal of $[Ca^{2+}]_{cyt}$ was discussed previously in the section on Ca^{2+} homeostasis mechanisms.

Regulation of myofilament Ca^{2+}sensitivity

Excitatory neurotransmitters induce smooth muscle contractions by raising membrane potential above the threshold to activate L-type Ca^{2+} channels, trigger Ca^{2+} influx, activate MLC phosphorylation and increase the affinity of myosin for actin to form cross-bridges [97,190,191]. Termination of excitatory signals leads to decreased $[Ca^{2+}]_{cyt}$ and MLCK inactivation [192], and muscle relaxation occurs when MLC is dephosphorylated by MLCP [174,193]. Thus, the contractile force, initiated by Ca^{2+} influx, is directly correlated with the level of MLC phosphorylation, which is regulated by the relative activities of MLCK and MLCP.

The activities of MLCK and MLCP are regulated by different mechanisms. MLCK activity is increased by Ca^{2+}. The regulation of MLCP activity is more complex. MLCP is a heterotrimer of a constitutively active type 1 protein phosphatase (PP1Cδ) or (PPP1) catalytic subunit, the regulatory MYPT1 subunit, and the M20 subunit of unknown function [194,195]. The phosphatase activity of MLCP is regulated by phosphorylation. Phosphorylation of MYPT1 at Thr 696 or Thr 853 (human amino acid sequence numbering) inhibits MLCP phosphatase activity [19,196,197]. Phosphorylation of a separate regulatory protein, CPl-17, also inhibits the phosphatase activity of the catalytic subunit. When CPI-17 is phosphorylated at Thr 38, it binds to the active site of the catalytic subunit, resulting in a pseudo-substrate inhibition of MLCP [198,199]. Similarly, phosphorylation of MYPT1 at Thr 696 inhibits MLCP as a pseudo-substrate, but it is unclear how the phosphorylation of Thr 853 inhibits MLCP phosphatase activity [200,201]. There is always some level of constitutive MLCP activity because MLCP activity is never completely inhibited by MYPT1 and CPl-17 phosphorylation [202]. This gives rise to a requirement for constitutive phosphorylation of MYPT1 and CPl-17 to keep MLCP activity low, allowing Ca^{2+} to increase MLCK activity relative to the activity of MLCP to increase MLC phosphorylation and accomplish contraction [184,203,204]. Conversely, when $[Ca^{2+}]_{cyt}$ decreases, MLCK activity decreases relative to MLCP, facilitating dephosphorylation of MLC and relaxation [184,204].

Phosphorylation of MYPT1 and CPl-17 are therefore important regulators of smooth muscle contractile responses. Increasing or decreasing MYPT1 and CPl-17 phosphorylation can increase or decrease the force of contraction, respectively [174,187,205–207]. Regulation of MYPT1 phosphorylation at Thr 696 is still unclear, although zipper-interacting kinase (ZIPK) and integrin-linked kinase (ILK) may be involved [208–210]. Rho-associated kinase 2 (ROCK2) phosphorylates MYPT1 at Thr 853 and protein kinase C (PKC) phosphorylates CPl-17 at Thr 38 [196,211]. When ROCK2 or PKC is activated, MLCP is inhibited by the increased MYPT1 and CPl-17 phosphorylation, shifting the balance toward greater MLC phosphorylation [212]. ROCK2 activity and MYPT1 phosphorylation are increased by agonist-mediated G-protein coupled receptor (GPCR) activation, while PKC activity and CPl-17 phosphorylation are increased by voltage-dependent Ca^{2+} influx [200,213,214]. When MYPT1 or CPl-17 phosphorylation is increased before or during agonist stimulation, greater force is generated at equivalent levels of $[Ca^{2+}]_{cyt}$ [202,215]. This is shown as a shift to the left of the force vs $[Ca^{2+}]_{cyt}$ curve (Figure 13.13). Phosphorylation of MYPT1 and CPl-17 underlie this phenomenon, known as "Ca^{2+} sensitization" of smooth muscles to excitatory stimuli [192,216]. Pharmacological inhibition of ROCK2 or PKC results in decreased levels of MLC Ser 19 phosphorylation and inhibition of contraction [187,203].

In visceral smooth muscles, membrane depolarization evoked by inputs from excitatory motor neurons increases only CPI-17 phosphorylation [213,214,217]. MYPT1 phosphorylation at Thr 696 is not increased by endogenous or exogenous cholinergic agonists [213,214]. Exogenously applied cholinergic agonists increase CPI-17 phosphorylation and also cause MYPT1 phosphorylation at Thr 853, by recruiting of the ROCK2 pathway [213,218]. ROCK2 activation and increased MYPT1 Thr853 phosphorylation increase MLC Ser 19 phosphorylation and enhance contraction [200]. The fact that different pathways are activated by neurotransmitter released from motor neurons and the transmitter substance added to solutions bathing muscles suggests that different populations of receptors are activated by these substances. Experiments have shown that acetylcholine (ACh) released from motor neurons mainly binds to muscarinic (m3) receptors expressed by ICCs whereas receptors expressed by SMCs are also bound by muscarinic agonists added to bathing solutions [213].

Visceral smooth muscles are characterized by basal or constitutive MYPT1, CPl-17, and MLC phosphorylation [200,202,213,217,218].

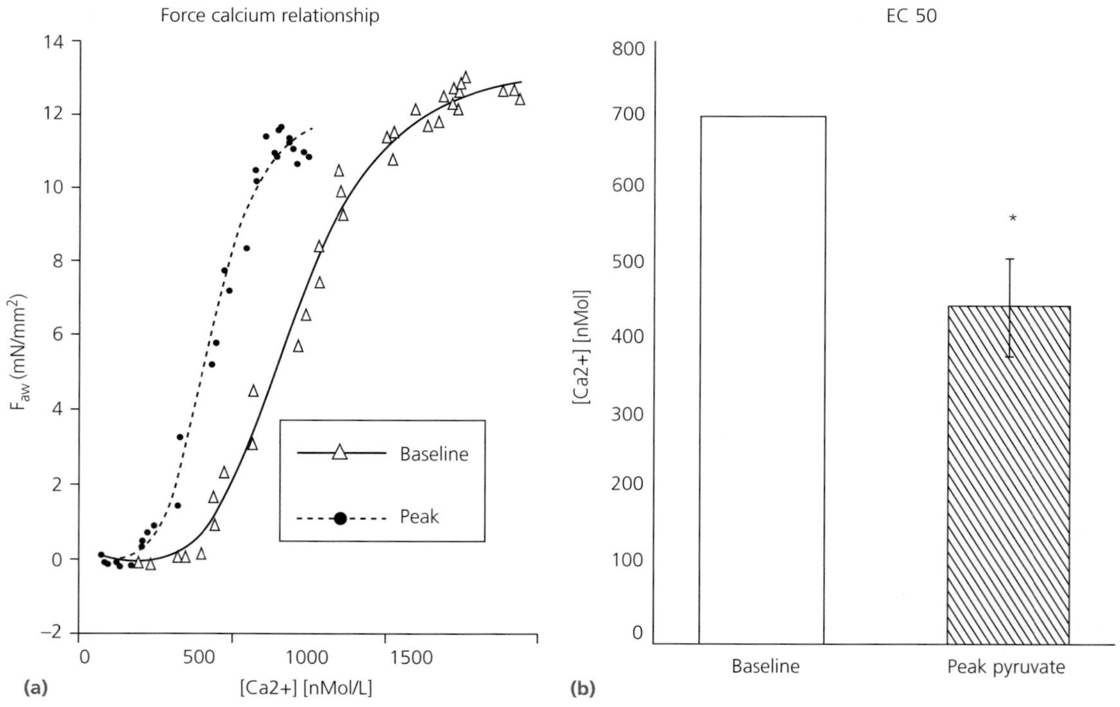

Figure 13.13 **(a)** Myofilament force-Ca^{2+} curve. The force-Ca^{2+} curve shifts noticeably to the left denoting an increase in Ca^{2+} sensitivity caused by pyruvate infusion (peak force development). Data points collected at baseline and at 20 minutes after the addition of 10 mM pyruvate, 37 °C. **(b)** Myofilament calcium sensitivity, expressed as EC_{50} for $[Ca^{2+}]_{cyt}$ at baseline and after 20 minutes exposure to 10 mM pyruvate (peak force development) demonstrates the Ca^{2+} sensitizing effects of pyruvate on the myofilaments ($p<0.01$, $n = 6$). Source: Torres C.A., Varian K.D., Canan C.H., Davis J.P., Janssen P.M. The positive inotropic effect of pyruvate involves an increase in myofilament calcium sensitivity. PLoS One 2013;8(5):e63608. Licensed under CC BY 4.0.

The basal levels of MLC phosphorylation are regulated by ongoing, low-level activities of MLCK and MLCP [184,192,202,219]. The basal levels of MYPT1 and CPI-17 phosphorylation also contribute to smooth muscle Ca^{2+} sensitization. Ongoing, low-level kinase activities that maintain constitutive MYPT1 and CPI-17 phosphorylation are responsible for regulating the ongoing low level of MLCP activity [202,213,218]. Constitutive phosphorylation of MYPT1 and CPI-17 inhibits MLCP to maintain MLC phosphorylation at a set level even when $[Ca^{2+}]_{cyt}$ is low. There is a threshold for MLC phosphorylation to trigger contraction [220]. Depending on the level of constitutive MYPT1 and CPI-17 phosphorylation, the level of MLC phosphorylation may be close to or far from the threshold required to trigger contraction. Consequently, agonist-induced force can be high or low, depending on the constitutive level of MLC phosphorylation [187,201,203,206,207,209,213,215,221].

Signal transduction mechanisms in gastrointestinal muscles

The major signal transduction pathways in GI smooth muscle cells consist of G-protein-coupled receptors (GPCRs), the heterotrimeric GTP-binding proteins that couple to the receptor, and the effector enzymes that generate the cascades of intracellular regulatory signals (Figure 13.14). A large variety of receptors and receptor subtypes are expressed by SIP cells. Among these are receptors for peptides (e.g., tachykinins, vasoactive intestinal polypeptide [VIP], pituitary adenylate cyclase-activating polypeptide (PACAP) and endothelin), amines (histamine, 5-hydroxytryptamine), pyrimidines/purines (UTP and ATP), and lipids (S1P [sphingosine-1-phosphate], LPA [lipoprotein A]) [166,222–228].

The heterotrimeric G proteins in GI smooth muscles are grouped into four main families, $G_{i/o}$, G_s, G_{q11}, and $G_{12/13}$, with each family consisting of different isotypes [229]. The different heterotrimeric G protein families interact with different receptors and effectors [230]. In general, G_s activates adenylyl cyclase, causing an increase in intracellular cAMP, while $G_{i/o}$ inhibits adenylyl cyclase, causing a decrease in cAMP. $G_{12/13}$ stimulates RhoA guanine nucleotide exchange factors (RhoGEFs), causing activation of RhoA by GTP binding and activation of downstream RhoA-dependent effector enzymes [231]. G_{q11} activates phospholipase Cβ, which hydrolyzes phosphatidylinositol-4,5-bisphosphate (PIP_2) in the plasma membrane into diacylglycerol (DAG) and IP_3.

Muscarinic receptors, a major excitatory pathway activated by ACh released from motor neurons, are coupled to G-proteins. SIP cells express m2 and m3 receptors. In general, m3 receptors couple to G_{q11}, activating PLCβ and hydrolyzing membrane-bound PIP_2 to DAG and IP_3 [232]. Increasing IP_3 increases $[Ca^{2+}]_{cyt}$ by binding to and opening IP_3 receptors in SR/ER membranes, causing the release of Ca^{2+} from intracellular stores [233]. The increase in cytoplasmic Ca^{2+} and DAG activates the conventional family of protein kinase C enzymes (PKCα, βI, βII, γ) [234]. The m2 receptors are coupled to $G_{i/o}$, inhibiting adenylyl cyclase and maintaining low levels of cAMP [232]. Muscarinic receptors on SMCs also couple through $G_{12/13}$, although the relative proportion is not clear [231]. $G_{12/13}$

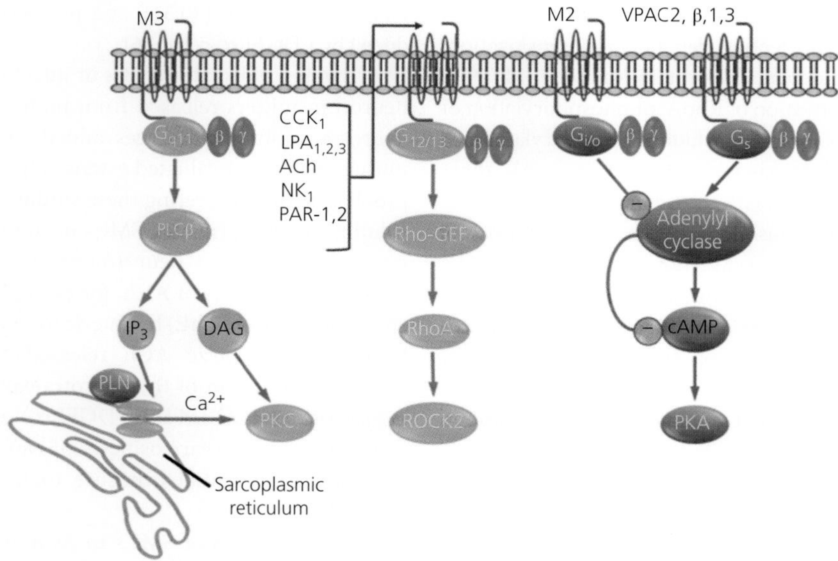

Figure 13.14 G-protein-coupled receptor signal transduction in SIP cells. Four main families of G proteins are found in GI smooth muscles: G_{q11}, $G_{12/13}$, $G_{i/o}$, and G_s. Activation of G_{q11} by m3 receptors stimulates PLCβ, generating IP_3 and DAG, leading to Ca^{2+} mobilization and PKC activation. Several excitatory neurotransmitters and peptides bind to receptors coupled to $G_{12/13}$, stimulating Rho-GEFs and activating the RhoA/ROCK2 pathway. Agonist binding to m2 receptors activates $G_{i/o}$, leading to inhibition of adenylyl cyclase, decreased levels of cAMP and PKA activity, and promotion of increased sensitivity to excitatory stimuli. Activation of G_s by the binding of the inhibitory neuropeptide VIP to VPAC2 receptors or catecholamine binding to β1 or β3 receptors stimulates adenylyl cyclase activity, which increase cAMP levels and PKA activity, leading to relaxation.

activates RhoA and its downstream effectors, including ROCK2. Activation of RhoA by $G_{12/13}$ is mediated by various Rho-specific guanine nucleotide exchange factors (RhoGEFs), which promote the exchange of GDP for GTP [235]. The RhoGEF family of proteins includes p115RhoGEF, PDZ-RhoGEF, and LARG (*l*eukemia-*a*ssociated *R*hoGEF) [236]. In the GTP-bound conformation, RhoA interacts with and stimulates the activity of downstream effectors including ROCK2 and actin cytoskeleton binding proteins [237,238].

The inhibitory enteric neurotransmitter peptide VIP binds to $VPAC_2$ receptors, which are coupled to Gs, stimulating adenylyl cyclase activity, cAMP formation, and relaxation [239]. β3 adrenoceptors are also expressed by SMCs in the GI tract, with the exception of the esophagus, where β1 receptors are expressed. The specific consequences of β receptors in motility are not fully understood [240].

Muscarinic m2 receptors are also coupled to a diverse set of downstream signaling pathways, including activation of Src family tyrosine kinases, PI 3-kinases, members of the MAPK superfamily, and PAK1, which generally function to facilitate GI smooth muscle contractile responses [241]. Src-family tyrosine kinases are membrane-associated nonreceptor protein tyrosine kinases which are expressed in most cell types, including SMCs. Src family members phosphorylate multiple substrates and participate in a wide range of cellular functions. In SMCs, Src activates voltage-dependent Ca^{2+} channels and nonselective cation channels, inactivates Ca^{2+}-activated K^+ channels, and stimulates phospholipase C activity [242].

Because m2 receptor activation inhibits adenylate cyclase in GI SMCs, it is important to note that cAMP and cGMP both desensitize the contractile process. Several mechanisms have been proposed to explain cyclic nucleotide-dependent desensitization: direct binding of cGMP-dependent protein kinase to MYPT1, phosphorylation and inactivation of RhoA, or phosphorylation of MYPT1 at Ser-695, a site that excludes phosphorylation of MYPT1 by Rho-dependent kinases [209,243,244]. All three mechanisms would activate MLCP, promote dephosphorylation of MLC, and relax smooth muscle. Therefore, activation of m2 receptors might contribute to contraction by reducing cAMP, which would favor increased or sustained MLC phosphorylation and cross-bridge cycling. The net effect of muscarinic receptor activation on contraction depends on complex interactions of cytoplasmic Ca^{2+} levels, cyclic nucleotide levels, and metabolic coupling to multiple protein kinase cascades that simultaneously regulate the relative activities of MLCK and MLCP.

Signaling by G-protein-coupled receptors is rapidly attenuated or terminated by mechanisms that target receptors or G-proteins. Agonist-occupied receptors are phosphorylated by specific G-protein-coupled receptor kinases (GRKs), the effects of which may be enhanced via feedback phosphorylation of GRK2 by second messenger-activated kinases such as PKA [245,246]. Binding of phosphorylated receptors to β-arrestin initiates receptor internalization via clathrin-coated pits, and acts as a scaffold for various mitogen-activated protein (MAP) kinases [247–249]. Src also binds to β-arrestin and phosphorylates the GTPase dynamin, promoting its ability to cleave clathrin-coated vesicles from the membrane. These eventually fuse with endosomes and the receptors are either degraded or recycled to the cell surface [250].

Two mechanisms that target the G-proteins participating in desensitization of responses involve regulator of G-protein signaling (RGS) proteins and caveolin-3. Spontaneous deactivation of Gα-subunits via their intrinsic GTPase activity is accelerated by RGS proteins [251]. Activated G-proteins can also bind to caveolin, which hinders reassociation of Gα- and Gβγ-subunits and can impede subsequent responses mediated by receptors that couple to the same G-proteins [252,253].

Neural regulation of smooth muscle contraction and motility

Organ-level and organ-specific motility behaviors are regulated by inputs from the enteric nervous system. Both excitatory and inhibitory enteric neurons innervate the tunica muscularis. With cell bodies in the myenteric plexus, neural processes innervate the circular and longitudinal muscle layers, with varicose fibers coursing along the major axes of the SMCs. Excitatory neurons release ACh and neurokinins, and inhibitory neurons release NO, purine neurotransmitters and peptides, such as VIP and PACAP [41]. While SMCs express receptors and transduction mechanisms for major neurotransmitters, neural inputs are not transduced exclusively by SMCs in GI muscles. ICCs and PDGFRα$^+$ cells have major neurotransduction roles in GI muscles. Mutant animals lacking ICCs display reduced neural responses to the two major neurotransmitters, NO and ACh [30,31], and purinergic responses are transduced by PDGFRα$^+$ cells [36].

Activation of isolated SMCs or intact muscle strips by enteric neurotransmitters released from motor neurons or exogenous neurotransmitter substances added to the solutions bathing muscles has been evaluated extensively over the past 50 years. A problem with interpreting these studies is that drugs applied to solutions bathing isolated SMCs or muscle strips may not recapitulate exposure to neurotransmitters released from motor neurons. In the case of ACh, for example, expression of acetylcholine esterase (AChE) by enteric motor neurons [254] appears to rapidly hydrolyze ACh released from nerve terminals, restricting diffusion of the neurotransmitter to sites very close to varicosities. ICC-IM and PDGFRα$^+$ cells are arranged in close proximity to nerve varicosities [255] and, as a result, these cells may have preferential exposure to higher concentrations of neurotransmitters.

Direct responses of SMCs to ACh and neurokinins include activation of nonselective cation currents [74,75,256] and enhanced Ca^{2+} sensitization of the contractile apparatus, as discussed previously. Responses to exogenous ACh and ACh released from neurons differ in that the exogenous compound causes depolarization, chronotropic effects on slow waves, and reduced slow wave amplitude in the stomach, whereas nerve stimulation evokes chronotropic effects but causes little or no depolarization [257]. Postjunctional effects were also evaluated by characterizing which proteins in the Ca^{2+} sensitization pathway, discussed previously, were phosphorylated by ACh applied in the bath [213]. Phosphorylation of MYPT1 and CPI-17 occurred in response to exogenous ACh, but only CPI-17 was phosphorylated by ACh released from neurons. Inhibitors of AChE caused activation of secondary postjunctional responses that included a second phase of junction potential, depolarization, and recruitment of MYPT1 phosphorylation [213,257].

Together, these observations suggest that ACh released from neurons may reach only a limited population of receptors, possibly those expressed by ICCs, but inhibition of AChE may increase the types of cells stimulated by ACh released from neurons and include activation of receptors expressed by SMCs. ACh activates nonselective channels in SMCs, but ACh activates Cl^- channels in ICCs. In mice with genetic deactivation of ANO1, the Cl^- channels expressed exclusively by ICCs in the SIP syncytium, stimulation of cholinergic neurons failed to activate excitatory junction potentials (EJPs) [258]. Antagonists of ANO1 also blocked postjunctional responses. These data provide direct evidence that SMCs are not the primary cells innervated by cholinergic neurons.

The role of ICCs in neurotransduction was originally demonstrated using W/W^V mutants that have greatly reduced numbers of ICC-IM in some regions of the GI tract, such as the gastric fundus, lower esophageal sphincter, and pyloric sphincter. Postjunctional nitrergic and cholinergic electrophysiological responses (junction potentials) were reduced significantly in muscles of W/W^V mutants (Figure 13.15) [30,31,259]. Postjunctional responses mediated by stimulating vagal efferent neurons were also reduced in W/W^V mice [260]. Responses to exogenous NO were also reduced in W/W^V mice, but defects in innervation by nitrergic neurons were not detected. These observations suggest involvement of ICCs in transduction of NO released from enteric inhibitory neurons. Others have argued that ICCs are not important in mediating neural responses, as contractile responses are retained in W/W^V muscles [261]. However, some of the studies summarized in that review are difficult to interpret because experiments were performed on regions of muscle in W/W^V mice with incomplete loss of ICCs. Nevertheless, the role of ICCs in neurotransmission, particularly in nonrodent species, is still debated.

Nitric oxide released from enteric inhibitory motor neurons binds to soluble guanylate cyclase (sGC) in postjunctional cells to generate cGMP [262]. The increase in cGMP in response to NO is linked to several effectors, including cGMP-dependent protein kinase (PKG1), cGMP-dependent phosphodiesterase, and cyclic nucleotide-gated ion channels. Evidence from cell-specific knockout of sGCβ1 suggests that nitrergic responses are integrated, with contributions from both ICCs and SMCs, and PKG1 serves as the major effector for cGMP in both cell types [263,264].

The actual mechanisms of nitrergic inhibitory junction potentials (IJPs) and relaxation are still controversial, with possible contributions from activation of K^+ channels (TREK1), suppression of activation of Cl^- channels (ANO1), reduced open probability of Ca^{2+} channels ($Ca_V1.2$), and Ca^{2+} desensitization of the contractile apparatus in SMCs [264–267]. NO-dependent desensitization of the contractile apparatus to Ca^{2+} can occur by PKG1-dependent phosphorylation of RhoA, preventing its activation of Rho-kinase, and by PKG1 phosphorylation of MYPT1 at Ser695, preventing the inhibition of MLCP activity by MYPT1 phosphorylation at Thr696 [192,209,268,269]. The relative contributions of these mechanisms may change from region to region in the GI tract. However, the ubiquitous expression of $Ca_V1.2$ in SMCs and ANO1 expression in ICCs throughout the gut suggest these may be common mediators of nitrergic inhibitory effects.

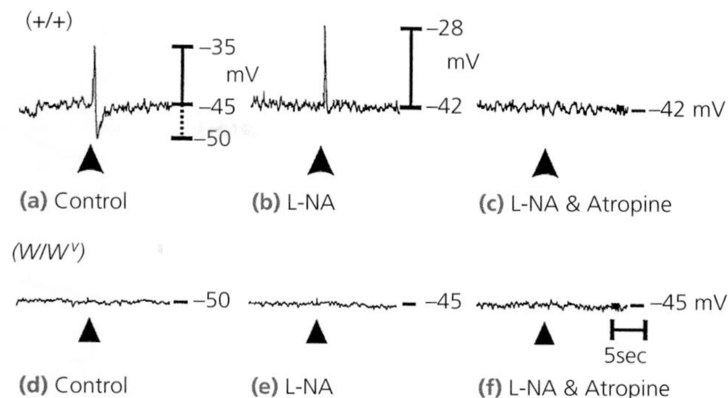

Figure 13.15 Responses to electrical field stimulation (EFS) of intrinsic motor neurons in fundus muscles of wild-type and W/W^v mice. **(a)** EFS (arrowhead; 0.5 ms duration) caused biphasic electrical responses in wild-type muscles. The responses were characterized by a rapid depolarization (excitatory junction potential; EJP) followed by a slower hyperpolarization (inhibitory junction potential; IJP). **(b)** L-NA (100 µm) inhibited IJPs and increased EJPs. **(c)** Atropine (1 µm), in the continued presence of L-NA, blocked the EJPs. These data show that muscarinic receptors mediate EJPs and IJPs are mediated by NO. **(d)** EJPs and IJPs were greatly attenuated in fundus muscles of W/W^v mice. **(e,f)** L-NA and atropine had little effect on responses to EFS in fundus muscles of W/W^v mice. Source: Ward S.M., Beckett E.A., Wang X., Baker F., Khoyi M., Sanders K.M. Interstitial cells of Cajal mediate cholinergic neurotransmission from enteric motor neurons. J Neurosci 2000;20(4):1393.

PDGFRα^+ cells also have an important role in neurotransmission. IJPs have a fast and a slow phase. The fast phase is due to release of a purine substance and the slow phase is due to release of NO (Figure 13.16) [270,271]. The purine neurotransmitter has long been thought to be ATP, but more recent evidence suggests that β-NAD better matches the postjunctional effects of the purine neurotransmitter [272]. Postjunctional responses are mediated through binding of P2Y1 receptors [273–275] and activation of small conductance Ca^{2+}-activated (SK) channels [276]. PDGFRα^+ cells, closely associated with inhibitory nerve varicosities, express both of these proteins (see Figure 13.16) [36,81]. Isolated PDGFRα^+ cells respond to P2Y1 agonists and generate significant hyperpolarization responses that are blocked by P2Y1 antagonists or SK channel antagonists (Figure 13.17). SMCs isolated from the same muscles displayed

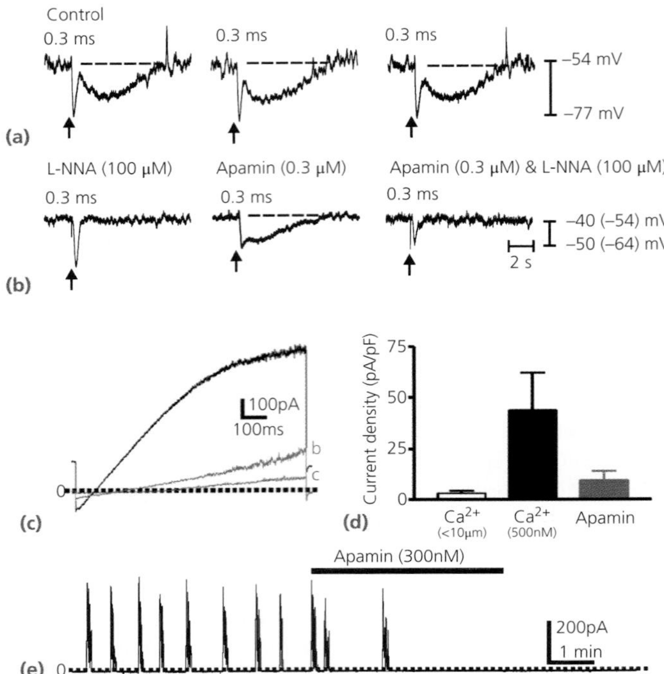

Figure 13.16 Inhibitory junction potentials (IJPs) in murine colonic muscles and the source of the apamin-sensitive component of the IJP. IJPs in the colon consist of two phases: a rapid hyperpolarization that reaches a peak and partially repolarizes followed by a more sustained period of hyperpolarization. Panel **(a)** shows these compound IJPs evoked by repetitive single pulses of EFS (0.3 ms duration). **(b)** The first trace shows that the second component of the IJP is nitrergic and blocked by L-NNA (100 μm). Apamin (0.3 μm) reduced the first component of the IJP, suggesting it was primarily due to activation of SK channels (second trace in b). Combined apamin and L-NNA (third trace in b) blocked most of the IJP. Traces in (b) were aligned for display purposes, but treatment with L-NNA in fact causes depolarization. The membrane potentials in brackets refer to the first and third traces, and the scale not in brackets refers only to the second trace. **(c)** A voltage-clamp experiment in which an isolated PDGFRα⁺ cell was ramped from -80 to + 80 mV. Current responses are displayed. Under control conditions with 500 nM Ca^{2+} in the patch pipet, a large outward current was generated (black trace). When Ca^{2+} was low in the pipet (<10 nM), very little current was evoked during the ramp (blue trace). Apamin inhibited the current elicited with 500 nM Ca^{2+}, suggesting it was due to an SK conductance (red trace). Panel **(d)** summarizes these experiments on six cells. Some PDGFRα⁺ cells generated spontaneous transient outward currents **(e)** and these currents were blocked by apamin (300 nM). These experiments show that the fast IJP in colonic muscles is due to an apamin-sensitive conductance and that conductance is expressed in PDGFRα⁺ cells. Source: Data in (a,b) from: Hwang S.J., O'Kane N., Singer C., Ward S.M., Sanders K.M., Koh S.D. Block of inhibitory junction potentials and TREK-1 channels in murine colon by Ca2+ store-active drugs. J Physiol 2008;586(4):1169; data in (c–e) from Kurahashi M., Zheng H., Dwyer L., Ward S.M., Koh S.D., Sanders K.M. A functional role for the 'fibroblast-like cells' in gastrointestinal smooth muscles. J Physiol 2011;589(Pt 3):697. Reproduced with permission of John Wiley & Sons.

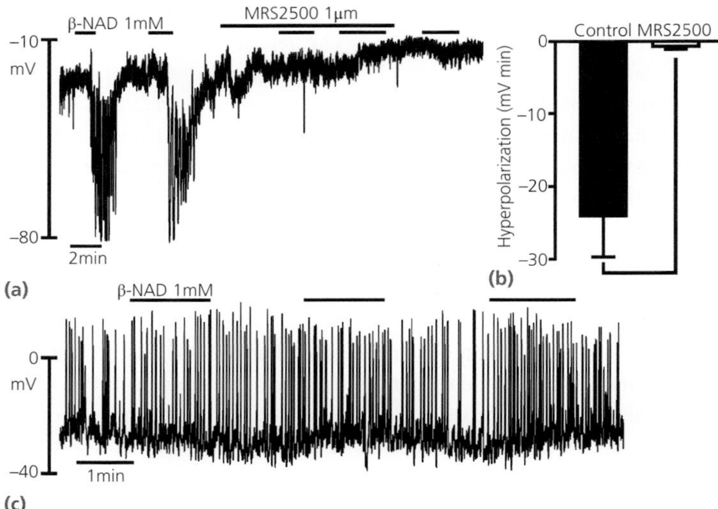

Figure 13.17 β-NAD elicits hyperpolarization in PDGFRα⁺ cells but not in SMCs. **(a)** Current-clamp recordings from an isolated PDGFRα⁺ cell in the dialyzed, whole cell configuration ($I = 0$). β-NAD (1 mM) caused transient hyperpolarizations down to about −80 mV. The hyperpolarization responses were blocked by MRS 2500 (1 μM), a selective P2Y1 receptor antagonist. **(b)** A summary of the hyperpolarization responses caused by β-NAD in five cells and the effects of MRS2500. **(c)** SMCs isolated from the same animal and muscle failed to show hyperpolarization responses to β-NAD (1 mM) and other P2Y1 agonists (not shown) under the same recording conditions. These data demonstrate that the purinergic, fast IJPs elicited in colonic muscles are due to hyperpolarization responses transduced by PDGFRα⁺ cells and not by SMCs. Source: Kurahashi M., Mutafova-Yambolieva V., Koh S.D., Sanders K.M. Platelet-derived growth factor receptor α positive cells and not smooth cells mediate purinergic hyperpolarization in murine colonic muscles. Am J Physiol Cell Physiol 2014;307(6):C561. Reproduced with permission of John Wiley & Sons.

little or no response to purine agonists [277]. Studies of the transcribed genes in both ICCs and W/W^V mice suggest that other neurotransmitter responses may be mediated by interstitial cells in the SIP syncytium [84,278], and a recent study using that information found that part of the sympathetic regulation of colonic motility is mediated by PDGFRα⁺ cells [86].

Responses to enteric motor neurons are examples of how regulation of GI motility is the product of integrated responses of the cells of the SIP syncytium (Figure 13.18). Loss or damage to ICCs has been reported in muscles from human patients with various motility disorders [279]. Loss of interstitial cells would be functionally equivalent to denervation of SMCs in GI organs, and would lead to abnormal motility responses.

More research is necessary to fully appreciate the importance of pathologies involving cells of the SIP syncytium in motility disorders.

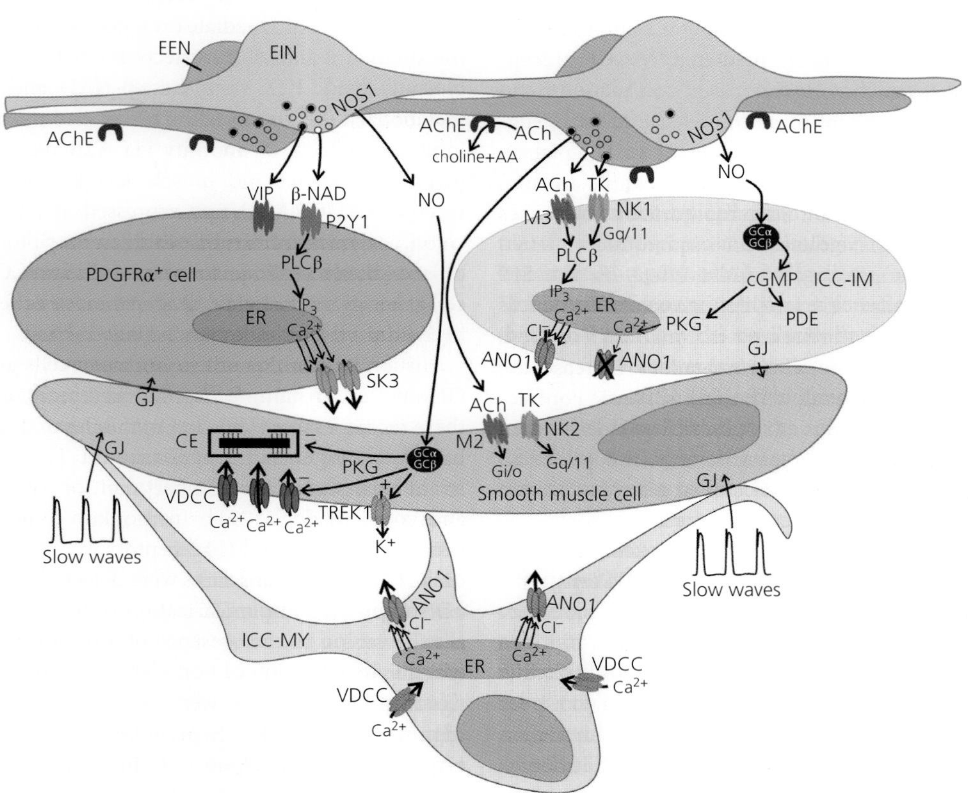

Figure 13.18 Regulation of the SIP syncytium by enteric motor neurons. This figure uses the same format as Figure 13.7, but some of the information in that figure has been removed to make room for the additional pathways displayed here. The SIP syncytium, composed of SMCs, ICCs, and PDGFRα⁺ cells, is innervated by enteric excitatory motor neurons (EEN) and enteric inhibitory motor neurons (EIN). EEN release ACh and tachykinins (TK). Predominant receptors for these transmitters include M3 muscarinic receptors and neurokinin type 1 (NK1) receptors expressed by ICC-IM in GI muscles. Motor neurons express acetylcholine esterase (AChE), and this impressive enzyme rapidly metabolizes ACh (i.e., to choline and acetic acid; AA) released into the narrow cleft between nerve varicosities and ICCs. However, under some circumstances ACh, and more than likely TK, may also reach and bind to M2 muscarinic receptors and NK2 receptors expressed by SMCs. TK activates nonselective cation channels in SMCs and can cause depolarization [256]. The role of M2 receptor activation in the SIP syncytium is poorly understood. M3 and NK1 receptors couple through Gq/11 to activate phospholipase Cβ (PLCβ) and generate IP_3. IP_3 binds to IP_3 receptors in the ER membrane and increases release of Ca^{2+} from stores. Ca^{2+} release activates ANO1 channels in the plasma membrane of ICCs, generating an inward current that conducts to SMCs through gap junctions (GJ) and exerts a depolarizing or excitable influence on the SIP syncytium. NO released from EIN diffuses to ICCs and SMCs. The receptor for NO is soluble guanylate cyclase, made up of two subunits, GCα and GCβ. Binding of NO to sGC enhances production of cGMP and this activates protein kinase G (PKG). PKG has multiple effects, including inhibition of Ca^{2+} release and ANO1 currents in ICCs, Ca^{2+} desensitization of the contractile element (CE) in SMCs, reducing openings of VDCC in SMCs and activation of TREK1 channels in SMCs. Summation of these effects reduces the excitability and contractions of SMCs. cGMP is metabolized to terminate inhibitory influences of NO by phosphodiesterases (PDE). Receptors for neurotransmitters are also expressed by PDGFRα⁺ cells. The primary receptor mediating inhibitory purinergic responses in the GI tract is P2Y1 that binds β-NAD and couples through PLCβ to generate IP_3 and activate Ca^{2+} release. Ca^{2+} release in PDGFRα⁺ cells activates SK3 channels, a K^+ conductance. SK3 channels generate outward current that conducts to SMCs through GJ, causes hyperpolarization and reduces the excitability and contractions of SMCs. Vasoactive intestinal polypeptide (VIP), another inhibitory neurotransmitter released by EIN, may also have effects transduced by PDGFRα⁺ cells. Pathways responsible for the inhibitory effects of VIP are not yet understood.

Hormonal regulation of smooth muscle contraction and motility

Many digestive hormones affect motor functions in the GI tract. Many have effects through enteric neurons, but some have direct effects on SIP cells. Comments about representative mechanisms of the latter are provided here.

Ingestion of a meal leads to release of cholecystokinin (CCK) that enhances gallbladder contractions, relaxes the sphincter of Oddi, and affects gastric motility. Some of the effects of CCK are mediated by cholinergic neurons, but relaxation of the sphincter of Oddi occurs through activation of inhibitory neurons [280]. The effects of CCK are mediated by CCK_A receptors. In the canine stomach, CCK increased contractions, and these effects were independent of neural release of ACh, suggesting direct effects on the SIP syncytium [281]. The plateau phase of slow waves was increased by CCK in canine antrum. CCK also increased the duration and amplitude of slow waves in the canine colon [282]. Neither effect was blocked by tetrodotoxin or atropine, suggesting a direct effect on the SIP syncytium.

Gastrin, another hormone released after ingestion of food, also enhances gastric motility. Gastrin analogs increase the amplitudes and frequencies of slow waves and phasic contractions in the antrum and corpus [283–285]. Atropine blocked part of the ionotropic effect of gastrin, and indomethacin blocked the chronotropic effects [286].

Humoral mediators as regulators of the SIP syncytium

In addition to neural and hormonal regulation of motility, many humoral mediators are synthesized and released in muscular tissues. These substances include, at a minimum, histamine, serotonin, ATP, adenosine and other metabolites of ATP, eicosanoids (e.g., prostaglandins, thromboxanes, and leukotrienes), proteases, and cytokines. Receptors for these substances have been reported to exist on smooth muscle cells [287]. However, genes for many of these agents are expressed preferentially by ICCs and PDGFRα$^+$ cells [84,85]. Responses to some of these agents are due to activation of intrinsic neurons [41].

Understanding cell-specific effects of humoral agents from studies of whole-muscle responses is questionable, and understanding the full range of tissue or organ effects from studies of a single cell type is also inadequate. In some cases, humoral substances are released in response to other agonists added to solutions bathing muscles (e.g., prostaglandins), so pharmacological studies investigating concentration–response relationships may include contaminating effects from humoral factors. Descriptions of several representative smooth muscle responses to paracrine substances are provided below. Responses mediated secondarily by activation of enteric motor neurons or glial cells are not addressed here.

Adenosine triphosphate was thought to be the purinergic neurotransmitter for many years [288] but more recent analysis of the enteric inhibitory neurotransmitter that activates IJPs in GI muscles suggests that β-NAD, or a metabolite, is a better match for the enteric neurotransmitter [272]. Nevertheless, there may be nonneural sources of ATP in GI muscles. The most prominent receptor for β-NAD and ATP is P2Y1, and this receptor mediates the fast IJP in GI muscles and the purinergic inhibitory response [274,289]. Genes encoding P2X1, 2, 4, 6, and 7 are expressed variably in SIP cells in murine colon [83,84,278]. These receptors encode nonselective cation channels that could mediate excitatory effects in GI muscles, but the dominant inhibitory effects mediated by P2Y1 receptors typically mask P2X responses. β-NAD and ATP are rapidly metabolized to adenosine in tissues, and this metabolite exerts inhibitory effects on motility via A2B receptors expressed in myenteric ganglia and muscle layers [290[. This adenosine receptor (ADORA2B) was expressed at low levels in murine colon, as detected in a cell-specific transcriptome analysis of SIP cells; however, ADORA1 is expressed in ICCs and PDGFRα$^+$ cells [83,84,278]. Effects of adenosine on these cells have not been characterized.

Histamine is secreted by both mast cells and eosinophils in GI muscles. Histamine has four receptors, and expression of these receptors is variable in GI muscles of different species and in different regions of the GI tract. H1, H3, and H4 were found in the smooth muscle compartment of stomach, small bowel, and colon in dogs [291]. In monkey colonic muscles, genes encoding H1, H2, and H4 receptors were expressed equally, but only H2 receptor transcripts were detected in mouse colon [76]. Histamine evoked depolarization of SMCs and contraction in monkey colon in the presence of tetrodotoxin. Depolarization was due to activation of nonselective cation channels in SMCs. Contrasting responses were noted in murine colon where histamine caused hyperpolarization and relaxation. Hyperpolarization responses to histamine in muscle strips and isolated SMCs were inhibited by antagonists of K_{ATP} channels.

Serotonin (aka 5-hydroxytryptamine, 5-HT) is an important neurotransmitter in the enteric nervous system, but it does not appear to be expressed by motor neurons. Serotonin is also released by immune cells [292]. It is unclear whether serotonin released from enteric neurons directly affects SIP cells, but these cells express receptors for this substance. 5-HT_{2A} receptors mediate contractile responses to serotonin in canine colonic longitudinal muscles [293]. However, transcriptome studies in mice have indicated that the major expression of 5-HT receptors is 5-HT_{2B}, and this gene is expressed primarily by ICCs [83,84,278]. Contractions of human colon elicited by serotonin have been attributed to 5-HT_{2B} receptors [294]. Low expression of 5-HT_{3A} receptors was also observed in SIP cells, but the relatively higher expression observed in unsorted cells is likely to be neural [295]. Nonneural effects of serotonin in GI muscles are typically contractions. 5-HT_{2B} receptors are coupled through G_{q11}, so binding of these receptors is likely to increase

Ca^{2+} release in cells that express the receptors [296]. Release of Ca^{2+} in ICCs couples to activation of ANO1 channels, producing an inward current that has a depolarizing influence on SMCs and activates L-type Ca^{2+} channels.

Another role for 5-HT_{2B} receptors in ICCs is to regulate cell proliferation [297]. Exogenous serotonin increased ICC numbers in cell cultures, and antagonism of the 5-HT_{2B} receptors by ritanserin or SB204741 blocked this effect. ICC proliferation was also inhibited by antagonists of protein kinase C (PKC) and by xestospongin C, an antagonist of IP_3 receptors [298]. ICC from PKC$\gamma^{-/-}$ mice were not affected by 5-HT_{2B} agonists.

Matrix metalloproteinase 9 (MMP-9) mediates inflammatory responses, including breakdown in the extracellular matrix and leukocyte migration [299]. Recruitment of leukocytes (neutrophils, monocytes, and mast cells) is a major factor in the development of postoperative ileus (see section on Impact of inflammation on the SIP syncytium). Resident and recruited leukocytes release a variety of cytokines, reactive oxygen species, paracrine mediators, and proteases in response to laparotomy and gut manipulation. Time-dependent increases in gene and protein expression of MMP-9 and a tissue inhibitor of metalloproteases (TIMP-1) were observed in small bowel and colon muscles after tissue manipulation (a model of postoperative ileus), and these responses were dependent upon expression and activity of inducible nitric oxide synthase [300]. Genetic deactivation of MMP-9 reduced the severity of postoperative ileus, and inhibition of MMP-9 and MMP-2 improved contractile responses to agonists after tissue manipulation.

Protease-activated receptors (PARs) are G-protein-coupled receptors that are activated by serine proteases through proteolytic cleavage of a peptide from their N termini. The cleaved peptides represent the natural ligands for the receptors [301]. Four PAR subtypes exist, and PAR1 (*F2R*) and PAR2 (*F2RL1*) are expressed in SIP cells, mainly in ICCs and PDGFRα^+ cells [302]. These receptors are coupled through G_{q11} to enhance IP_3 production and increase Ca^{2+} release [303]. Responses to these receptors are excellent examples of how each type of SIP cell contributes to integrated responses in GI muscles.

Activation of PAR1 and PAR2 via thrombin, trypsin or activating peptides causes a biphasic response characterized by transient inhibition of contractions of colonic and small intestinal muscles and followed by a more sustained increase in contractions [304]. In vivo activation of PAR1 and PAR2 increased the rate of intestinal transit [305]. The initial inhibitory response is mediated by apamin-sensitive SK channels in PDGFRα^+ cells, and the secondary excitatory component is mediated mainly by activation of ANO1 channels in ICCs; however, nonselective cation channels are also activated in SMCs [302]. The excitatory phase of the response was blocked by an antagonist of ANO1, suggesting that the tissue-level contribution of SMCs was minor. Infection with *Nippostrongylus brasiliensis* induced a potent Th2 cytokine response that increased contractions of small intestinal muscles and expression and effects of PAR1 [304]. Activation of PAR1 and PAR2 also caused relaxation in the lower esophageal sphincter; however, these responses were not blocked by apamin and were reduced by a NOS antagonist, suggesting mediation of responses by nitrergic neural inputs [306]. Other studies demonstrated indirect effects on PAR2 activation in the small intestine and showed trypsin-evoked contractions were reduced by NK1 or NK2 antagonists [307].

A biphasic pattern of responses to thrombin and trypsin was observed in the primate colon: a transient inhibitory phase was followed by a more prolonged increase in contractions [308]. As in mice, the initial inhibitory phase in primate colon was blocked by apamin, suggesting activation of SK channels in PDGFRα^+ cells. However, in contrast to the mouse colon, the excitatory phase occurred without depolarization, suggesting an alternative mechanism to activation of ANO1 channels. The excitatory phase was blocked by ROCK antagonists, suggesting it was mediated by a Ca^{2+} sensitization mechanism. This was confirmed by showing that PAR activation caused phosphorylation of CPI-17 and MYPT1, the regulatory subunit of MLCP (see section on Regulation of myofilament Ca^{2+} sensitivity). These observations suggest the more dominant response to PAR activation occurs in SMCs in the primate colon.

Prostaglandin synthetic enzymes and receptors are widely distributed in SIP cells. PGE_2, PGI_2, and $PGF_{2\alpha}$ are synthesized from arachidonic acid in smooth muscle tissues from all regions of the GI tract [309]. In cell-specific transcriptome studies of SIP cells of the mouse colon, for example, genes for PGE_2 synthesis, *Ptgs1* and 2 and *Ptges3*, are expressed, and the four PGE_2 receptors (*Ptger1–4*) are all expressed at variable levels by different SIP cells, with the highest expression of *Ptger3* in ICCs [84]. *Ptgs1* displays dominant expression in SMCs, perhaps indicating local communication between SMCs and ICCs via PGE_2. Constitutive expression of *Ptgs2* was observed in gastric and colonic muscles of the mouse [310,311]. The synthetic enzyme for prostacyclin (*Ptgis*) is also present with highest expression of the synthetic apparatus and receptor in PDGFRα^+ cells. *Akr1bB1*, encoding the synthetic mechanism for $PGF_{2\alpha}$, is expressed by all SIP cells, but receptors (*Ptgfr*) show marginal expression only in SMCs. The dominant effect of endogenous prostaglandins is to impose an inhibitory drive on circular muscles in most regions of the gut, except the proximal stomach [173,312]. Lower expression of $PGF_{2\alpha}$ receptors may explain this observation. It should also be noted that responses to PGE_2 vary in circular and longitudinal muscle and in the proximal and distal portions of the stomach [313]. PGE_2 inhibits phasic contractions in the distal stomach and increases tone in the proximal stomach [173].

Synthesis of PGE_2 suppressed small intestinal motility, and excitatory stimulation with ACh increased PGE_2 levels, suggesting this eicosanoid provides negative feedback to excitable stimuli [314]. The same response occurs in muscle strips in vitro, but the degree of this regulation in vivo; is unclear, as surgical manipulation, necessary for the experiments performed, may have induced expression of *Ptgs2* [315]. Inhibiting prostaglandin synthesis with indomethacin increased slow wave amplitude and contractions and increased electrical and mechanical responses to pentagastrin in canine gastric antrum [286]. PGE_2 has positive chronotropic effects in the distal stomach and is responsible for the chronotropic effects of pentagastrin. Chronotropic effects are mediated by EP3 receptors (*Ptger3*) expressed by ICCs [84]. Gastric peristalsis requires propagation of slow waves from the dominant pacemaker in the corpus to the pyloric sphincter. The chronotropic effects of PGE_2 resulted in functional uncoupling of gastric slow waves, such that ectopic sites of origin developed and collisions of peristaltic waves were observed in video images of contractile patterns in gastric muscle sheets [172]. Chronotropic effects are also evoked by stretch in the antrum through prostaglandin synthesis by ICCs, as discussed in the section on Mechanosensitive ion channels/mechanisms related to stretch.

Abnormal, rapid-frequency slow waves and patterns of motility were observed in the gastric antrums of *Lep^ob^* mice, a model of type 2 diabetes. This activity was similar to PGE_2 responses in wild-type mice [316]. Components of the prostaglandin signaling pathway were upregulated significantly in gastric muscles of diabetic mice, including *Ptgs2*, *Ptges*, *Ptger1–3*, *Ptgir*, and *Ptgfr*. An inhibitor of prostaglandin-endoperoxide synthase 2, valdecoxib, normalized slow wave activity, contractions, and motor patterns in diabetic muscles. This study suggested that abnormally high activity of the prostaglandin signaling pathway could be a contributing factor to the abnormal motility patterns in diabetic gastroparesis. Blocking this pathway could be a means of treating functional motility disorders associated with diabetes.

Impact of inflammation on the SIP syncytium

Initially, inflammatory events affect the mucosal compartment of the GI tract. However, events occurring in the mucosa can set off responses in the smooth muscle layers through the activation of resident immune cells, recruitment of immune cells from the circulation, such as neutrophils and macrophages, and remodeling of enteric neurons.

Transition from an innate immune response to an adaptive response depends upon antigen-presenting cells, such as macrophages and dendritic cells. Cytokines can affect the functions of SMCs and may further affect these cells through the activation of immune or nonimmune cells. Activation of immune responses leads typically to reduced contractility of SMCs [317,318], abnormal GI motility and increased transit times. In experimental models of colitis, L-type Ca^{2+} currents were suppressed, and K^+ currents via K_{ATP} were increased in SMCs from inflamed colonic muscles [319]. Both of these changes could contribute to reduced contractility. SMCs have been reported to have direct effects on mediators such as tumor necrosis factor TNF-α, interleukin IL-1β, and interferon IFN-γ [320]. For example, TNF-α has been shown to decrease the expression of CPI-17, a protein that regulates MLC phosphorylation and contractile force [321]. It should also be recognized that many studies involving the effects of inflammatory mediators on SMCs have been performed on cultured cells, and the phenotype of SMCs is unstable in culture. It is also possible that cells other than SMCs grow in these cultures and express cytokine receptors or even dominate responses to inflammatory mediators. Evaluation of transcriptomes of cells of the SIP syncytium showed expression of receptors for multiple cytokines [83,84,278].

Thorough understanding of the sites of receptor expression and cell-specific responses to inflammatory mediators in intact tissues is still needed.

While resident macrophages normally express a tolerogenic phenotype, loss of this function is associated with GI disorders, such as postoperative and septic ileus, gastroparesis, and ischemia-reperfusion injury [47]. Postoperative ileus has been linked to an inflammatory response [322] that initiates a cascade of inflammatory mediators and includes induction of expression of inducible nitric oxide synthase (iNOS) and cyclooxygenase 2 (COX2) and production of NO and prostaglandins [315,323]. SMCs and ICCs both have receptors for these substances, and are likely to be involved in prolonged inhibition of muscle contraction that occurs in postoperative ileus. Normally, gastric macrophages display an M2-like phenotype and express CD206 and heme oxygenase I [324]. However, under oxidative stress experienced in diabetes, the tolerogenic phenotype shifts to an M1-like phenotype, and this, possibly through release of TNF-α, leads to loss of ICCs, reduced nNOS expression by enteric neurons and delayed gastric emptying [325,326]. Ischemia-reperfusion injury also flips macrophages from a tolerogenic to a proinflammatory phenotype [327], causing release of cytokines and NO that impair motility [328].

Inflammatory conditions also affect the interstitial cell component of the SIP syncytium. ICC are reported to be adversely affected in Crohn's disease, ulcerative colitis, and chronic intestinal pseudoobstruction [329,330]. Animal models of inflammation, such as trinitrobenzene sulfonic acid-induced colitis or partial obstruction of the intestine, have also been associated with disrupted ICC networks [331–333]. Treatment of cell clusters containing active ICCs from the murine small intestine with IFN-γ and LPS caused impairment of ICC rhythmicity, as measured by Ca^{2+} oscillations [334]. IFN-γ and LPS induced expression of iNOS, and generation of NO was the factor inhibiting ICC rhythmicity. The inflammatory response initiated by intestinal manipulation may also include a component involving ICCs. Networks of ICCs were significantly disrupted, as assessed by immunohistochemistry and electron microscopy 24 hours after intestinal manipulation [335]. An inhibitor of iNOS, aminoguanidine, reduced disruption of ICC networks.

These findings demonstrate the susceptibility of ICCs to inflammatory damage and make the link to NO as the primary agent causing damage to ICCs. Little is known at this time about the role of PDGFRα⁺ cells in inflammation, but these cells should be investigated specifically because of the expression of cytokine receptors and genes likely to be involved in inflammatory responses.

Summary

Smooth muscle cells provide the motors for GI motility. SMCs are arranged in bundles and form the muscular layers within the walls of GI organs. Much has been learned about the contractile proteins and mechanisms regulating smooth muscle contraction. Ca^{2+} entry through voltage-dependent Ca^{2+} channels initiates SMC contraction, but regulation of the Ca^{2+} sensitivity of the myofilaments is an important mechanism that tunes mechanical responses of GI muscles. SMCs do not function in isolation in GI muscles. At least two types of interstitial cells, ICCs and $PDGFR\alpha^+$ cells, are electrically coupled to SMCs, forming a network known as the SIP syncytium. "Myogenic" regulation of GI motility is a function of the integrated responses of all SIP cells. Ca^{2+} handling mechanisms are complex and fundamental to the behaviors of all SIP cells. Ca^{2+} entry and release regulate contractile responses in SMCs, and Ca^{2+} entry and release regulate ion channels in ICCs and $PDGFR\alpha^+$ cells that affect the excitability of SMCs. ICCs generate and propagate electrical slow waves that generate the phasic contractions necessary for gastric peristalsis and intestinal segmentation. ICCs and $PDGFR\alpha^+$ cells also transduce signals from enteric motor neurons: ICCs mediate responses to ACh and NO, at a minimum, and $PDGFR\alpha^+$ cells mediate responses to purines and NE. Electrical responses that develop in ICCs and $PDGFR\alpha^+$ cells conduct to SMCs via gap junctions.

References are available at www.yamadagastro.com/textbook7e

Further reading

Berridge M.J. Smooth muscle cell calcium activation mechanisms. J Physiol 2008;586:5047.

Berridge M.J. The inositol trisphosphate/calcium signaling pathway in health and disease. Physiolog Rev 2016;96:1261.

Keef K., Cobine C. Generation of spontaneous tone by gastrointestinal sphincters. Adv Exper Med Biol 2019;1124:47.

Koh S.D., Ward S.M., Sanders K.M. Ionic conductances regulating the excitability of colonic smooth muscles. Neurogastroenterol Motil 2012;24:705.

Neshatian L., Gibbons S.J., Farrugia G. Macrophages in diabetic gastroparesis – the missing link? Neurogastroenterol Motil 2015;27:7.

Sanders K.M., Koh S.D., Ro S., Ward S.M. Regulation of gastrointestinal motility – insights from smooth muscle biology. Nat Rev Gastroenterol Hepatol 2012;9:633.

Sanders K.M., Ward S.M., Koh S.D. Interstitial cells: regulators of smooth muscle function. Physiol Rev 2014;94:859.

Somlyo A.P., Somlyo A.V. Ca^{2+} sensitivity of smooth muscle and non-muscle myosin II: modulated by G proteins, kinases, and myosin phosphatase. Physiol Rev 2003;83:1325.

Sweeney H.L., Hammers D.W. Muscle contraction. Cold Spring Harbor Perspect Biol 2018;10.

Tack J., Camilleri M. New developments in the treatment of gastroparesis and functional dyspepsia. Curr Opin Pharmacol 2018;43:111.

CHAPTER 14

Mucosal immune system

Lars Eckmann[1] and Giorgos Bamias[2]

[1] University of California, San Diego, La Jolla, CA, USA

[2] National and Kapodistrian University of Athens, Sotiria Hospital, Athens, Greece

Chapter menu

The gastrointestinal mucosal immune system is one of the largest immunological compartments in the body. It is composed of multiple cells and structures, most prominently lymphoid cells, myeloid cells, and epithelial cells, and is charged with the daunting task of maintaining a delicate homeostatic balance – defending against the many pathogenic organisms and toxins that can penetrate the epithelial barrier and cause intestinal injury, while ignoring the multitude of commensal organisms and dietary compounds present in the gut that are of no threat to the host. Of all the organ systems, only the gastrointestinal tract and a few other epithelial organs, most notably the skin and lungs, are challenged to distinguish between foreign (non-self) molecules and self-molecules in such a dramatic fashion. This chapter summarizes basic concepts and components of general and mucosal immunology and how these cooperate in maintaining homeostasis in the gastrointestinal tract.

General concepts of immunology

The immune system functions to limit host invasion and damage by live microbes and abiotic foreign compounds larger than approximately 2000 daltons (whereas smaller foreign molecules are inactivated and cleared by chemical defense systems, particularly cytochrome P450 enzymes). The system is commonly divided into two types: innate (natural) immunity and adaptive (acquired) immunity, depending on the number of foreign structures (antigens) that can be recognized, the speed with which recognition occurs, the memory it leaves for future encounters, and the primary host cells and molecules involved. Innate immunity recognizes a limited repertoire of structures (fewer than a hundred) and is rapidly activated (hours), but forms no memory. By comparison, adaptive immunity can detect a vast array (millions) of structures and develop memory to specific structures, but it is mobilized more slowly (days to weeks).

In general, adaptive immunity amplifies the initial protection provided by innate immunity in a focused, antigen-specific manner, in part through the further mobilization of the natural immune components. Immune and nonimmune cells participate in innate immunity. Innate recognition of a limited set of molecules associated with microbes occurs through specific receptors expressed on the cell surface or within specific intracellular compartments. In the adaptive immune system, lymphocytes detect antigens through receptors on their cell surface that are specific for that antigen.

The innate and adaptive immune systems are tightly linked in mammals. For example, cells within the innate immune system, such as dendritic cells, internalize, process, and present peptides to T lymphocytes. When a specific antigen is presented to a

Yamada's Textbook of Gastroenterology, Seventh Edition. Edited by Timothy C. Wang, Michael Camilleri, Benjamin Lebwohl, Anna S. Lok, William J. Sandborn, Kenneth K. Wang, and Gary D. Wu.

Companion website: www.yamadagastro.com/textbook7e

T lymphocyte that possesses a receptor capable of recognizing it, that lymphocyte undergoes clonal expansion to produce progeny cells that express the same receptor. In addition to increasing the number of cells that can fight an acute infection, the adaptive immune response also results in the expansion of long-lived memory cells, which are the progeny of the original responsive antigen-specific B- or T-cell clones. Upon reexposure to the specific offending antigen, these cells respond on a larger and more selective scale, thereby constituting the memory characteristic of adaptive immunity. Unlike adaptive immunity, innate immunity does not respond in an enhanced or more rapid fashion to repeat exposure to foreign molecules and thus does not acquire memory.

Innate immune system

Innate intestinal defenses can be conceptually divided into two major groups: nonimmunological and immunological. The mucosal surface of the gastrointestinal tract expresses a variety of nonimmunological, physiochemical barriers to exclude, inactivate, or clear pathogenic substances and organisms after ingestion. These barriers include saliva, gastric acid, intestinal mucus, digestive enzymes, bile acids, antimicrobial peptides and lysozymes, peristalsis, indigenous microbiota, and the epithelial barrier, whose intact tight junctions are usually relatively impenetrable to molecules other than water and selected small solutes. Genetic defects or pharmacological interference with one or more of these factors may increase susceptibility to ingested pathogens. As an example, blockade of gastric acid production increases susceptibility to gastrointestinal infections [1,2].

The other major group of innate intestinal defenses is composed of immunological factors, which include both cellular and soluble elements. Many types of intestinal cells participate in innate immunity, including dendritic cells, innate-like lymphoid cells, phagocytes, mast cells, and epithelial cells. These cells either engulf and kill microorganisms or secrete soluble substances that inactivate microbes, recruit and arm other cell types against microbial invasion, remove host cells altered by infection, or amplify immune responses. Many of these responses are initiated by interactions between dedicated host receptors and a limited set of highly conserved structures present in microorganisms. These "signature" microbial molecules share certain attributes: 1) they are not produced by the host; 2) they are required for microbial survival; and 3) they are found in a broad group of microbes, including many pathogens (which led to the term *pathogen-associated molecular patterns* [PAMPs], although harmless bacteria often possess the same molecules). In addition, selected host molecules, such as heat shock proteins, can be detected by innate immune receptors as proxy markers of cell injury and death [3]. These endogenous ligands, also termed *damage-associated molecular patterns*, are indicative of host cell stress and death secondary to microbial or other injuries [4].

The host receptors of the innate immune system – the pattern recognition receptors – include two prominent classes, Toll-like receptors (TLRs) and nucleotide-binding oligomerization domain (NOD)-like receptors (NLRs), which collectively recognize a distinct set of conserved bacterial, viral, and parasitic PAMPs in different extracellular and intracellular compartments. Humans possess 10 TLRs (TLR1–10) that recognize bacterial peptidoglycans, lipopolysaccharide, lipopeptides, lipoteichoic acids, and flagellin, as well as viral single- and double-stranded RNA and unmethylated bacterial DNA [5]. TLRs are membrane-bound receptors with distinct locations that allow surveillance of the extracellular space (e.g., TLR4 and TLR5) or intracellular compartments (e.g., TLR3 and TLR9). In contrast, the second major class of pattern recognition receptors, NLRs, is found in the cytosol of host cells and therefore plays a primary role in detecting microorganisms that have entered that cell compartment [6]. Humans are currently known to have 22 NLRs that recognize distinct motifs of bacterial peptidoglycan and specific bacterial proteins, such as flagellin and high-molecular-weight toxins [7]. One member of the NLR receptor family, NOD2, was the first susceptibility gene identified for Crohn's disease, underling the importance of intact innate immunity in maintaining intestinal homeostasis [8].

Pattern recognition receptors are expressed uniformly on large numbers of cells of a given class, particularly dendritic cells, monocytes/macrophages, and B cells in the gastrointestinal tract, although some are also produced by intestinal epithelial cells [9,10]. On activation, TLRs initiate a signaling cascade that results in the rapid induction of an array of genes involved in the innate immune response to infection, including cytokines and chemokines, as well as molecules involved in antigen presentation and costimulatory molecules [11]. Their widespread expression, contrary to the key receptors of the adaptive immune system where a given T cell receptor (TCR) is expressed by only a small number of T cells, places TLRs and NLRs at the front line of rapid host defense against a wide variety of microorganisms. The innate immune system is therefore much more capable than the adaptive immune system of limiting acute infections caused by pathogens new to the host.

Adaptive immune system

Adaptive immunity conceptually can be divided into humoral and cellular immunity, although both arms of the system have close interactions with each other. Humoral immunity is mediated by antibodies derived from B lymphocytes and defends against extracellular microorganisms, toxins, and other foreign molecules. Cellular immunity is derived from T lymphocytes and provides protection from deleterious intracellular microorganisms that are not amenable to the effects of antibodies. Both types of adaptive immunity possess several properties that differentiate them from innate immunity. A large number of clonally distinct lymphocytes specific for particular determinants or epitopes on a molecule are maintained to respond to a wide variety of potential antigens to which humans may be exposed during a lifetime.

The molecular basis for this clonotypic specificity is determined by a cell surface receptor unique to each cell or clone, that is, immunoglobulins expressed on the cell surface of B cells or specific receptors on T cells. Each cell or clone expressing its unique or clonotypic receptor is selected to differentiate self-antigens from foreign (non-self) antigens. This process, primarily the result of *positive selection* (i.e., selection of cells with receptors that are weakly active against self, thereby allowing productive interactions with cells that process and present antigens) and *negative selection* (i.e., deletion of cells bearing receptors that strongly recognize self, thereby avoiding autoimmunity) of B cells in the bone marrow and T cells in the thymus during lymphocyte development, results in the production of an army of lymphocytes that are tolerant or unresponsive to self [12–14].

The intestine, liver, and peritoneum may participate in extrathymic pathways of T- and B-cell development, and self-reactive lymphocytes that escape from the normal selection processes may reside within these organs. In most individuals, peripheral mechanisms in the intestine prevent the activation of potentially self-pathogenic clones. These peripheral mechanisms include the presence and/or induction of T cells and B cells that are actively involved in the suppression of other innate and adaptive immune cells. Such cells are called *regulatory T (Treg) cells* or *B cells*.

Cellular constituents of the intestinal immune system

Although multiple cell types, including most prominently epithelial cells and a range of lamina propria cells, have long been identified in the intestinal tract, advances in high-throughput sequencing and multidimensional cytometry of single-cell preparations have only recently begun to reveal the true cellular complexity of the organ [15]. Such studies have revealed more than 50 distinct epithelial, immune, and stromal (mesenchymal) cell subsets. Of these, approximately half are immune cells, including 12 subsets of T cells, 4 subsets of B cells, and 7 subsets of myeloid cells in the colon [16]. The epithelium of colon and small intestine can be divided into at least 15 subpopulations, including stem cells, transit-amplifying cells, early and late enterocyte progenitors, immature and mature proximal and distal enterocytes, enteroendocrine cells, Tuft cells, Goblet cells, and Paneth cells [17]. Such fine-mapping of cell populations has opened the door toward identifying novel cell lineages and interaction patterns in healthy and diseased conditions, a development that will undoubtedly lead to new pathophysiologic insights. The major intestinal cell lineages and their immune functions are discussed in the following sections.

T lymphocytes

T lymphocytes are a critical component of the gut mucosal immune system and make up almost a quarter of all cell types in the intestine. They must maintain tight regulation of innate and adaptive immune responses against infectious agents in an environment that is rich with benign non-self antigens. As important regulators and effectors, T cells both recognize and eliminate infectious agents and orchestrate a coordinated immune defense through their regulatory effects on other cell populations.

T cell ontogeny

Hematopoietic stem cells in the bone marrow develop into lymphoid progenitors, which differentiate into T cells (Figure 14.1). Once formed in the bone marrow, they migrate to the thymus, where they mature and develop full functionality. Self-antigens that are normally found elsewhere in the body (e.g., proteins expressed in parietal cells of the stomach) are expressed in the thymus, where they serve as a means to properly "educate" the nascent, developing T cells. A genetic loss of the ability to express these extrathymic antigens present in other organs can lead to improper cell selection and autoimmunity. Self-tolerant T cells then migrate to secondary lymphoid tissues throughout the body, including Peyer's patches of the small intestine. Such T cells are naive in that they have not been exposed to an antigen outside of the thymus. Naive T cells populate the Peyer's patches and await sensitization by luminal antigens, which are transported to the Peyer's patch follicles from specialized follicle-associated epithelial cells. A specific mucosal immune response is initiated by this interaction and directs the naive T cell to a functional, activated phenotype. The activated T cells migrate out of the intestinal tract to the afferent lymphatics that drain into the mesenteric lymph nodes, enter the efferent lymphatics of the mesenteric lymph nodes, and pass through the thoracic duct into the peripheral blood [18]. Circulating activated T lymphocytes home to the original sites of antigenic stimulation in the gut mucosa, where they provide protective immunity within the lamina propria.

Antigen recognition

During antigen encounters, most T cells recognize peptides of antigen fragments in association with components of the major histocompatibility complex (MHC), a complex of membrane proteins on the surface of antigen-presenting cells (APCs) [19] (Figure 14.2). The antigen-specific or clonotypic receptor on the surface of T cells – the TCR – is responsible for antigen recognition and is composed of immunoglobulin-like heterodimeric glycoproteins formed primarily as αβ or γδ heterodimers. Most circulating mature T cells express the TCR-αβ heterodimer, whereas only 5% express the TCR-γδ heterodimer, and rarely, the TCR exists on the cell surface as a ββ homodimer. However, among intraepithelial lymphocytes (IELs) throughout the gastrointestinal mucosa, γδ T cells are highly enriched. Indeed, their proximity to the epithelium means that γδ T cells are ideally positioned to contribute to the initial stages of mucosal immunity, as well as assist in healing of the intestinal epithelial cell barrier [20].

Although it is firmly established that the TCR-αβ heterodimer recognizes antigen in association with an MHC molecule on an apposing APC [21], the mechanisms by which γδ T cells recognize

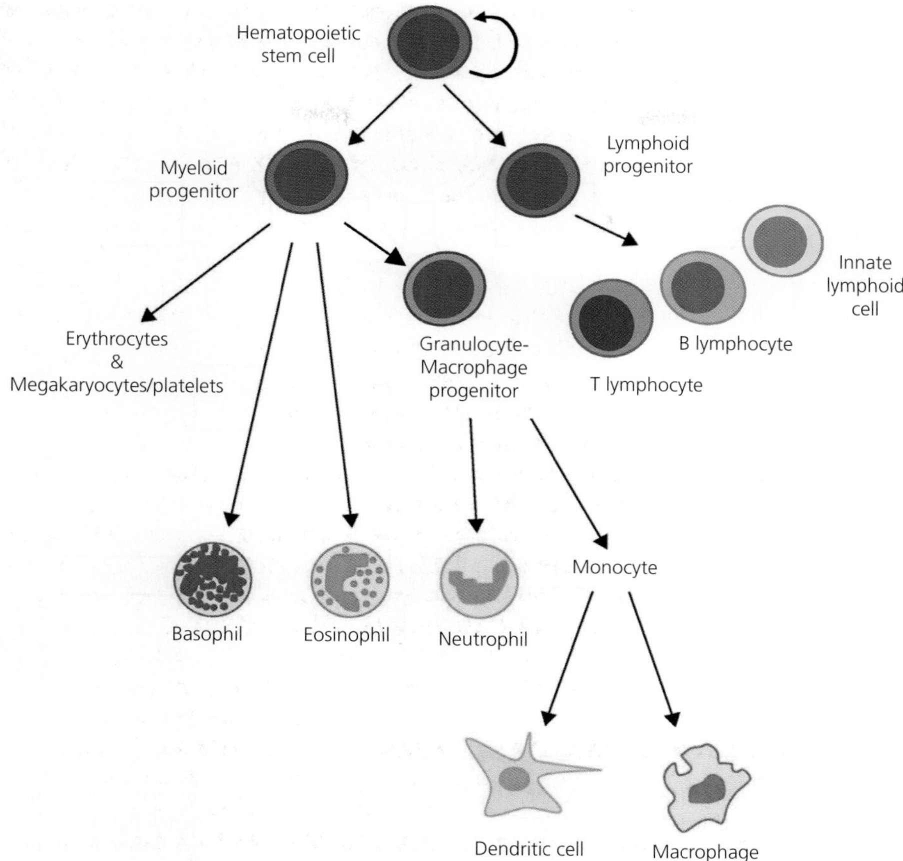

Figure 14.1 Development of lymphoid and myelomonocytic cells. Hematopoietic stem cells give rise to distinct myeloid and lymphoid progenitors in the bone marrow. The myeloid progenitors develop under the influence of various cytokines and colony-stimulating factors into erythrocytes, megakaryocytes/platelets, basophils, eosinophils, and a common precursor for polymorphonuclear leukocytes (granulocytes) and monocytes and their progeny (macrophages and dendritic cells).

antigens are not as clearly defined. Most γδ T cells recognize ligands that are fundamentally different from the short peptides that αβ T cells see in the context of MHC molecules [22]. Subsets of γδ T cells can recognize small bacterial phosphoantigens, alkylamines, and synthetic aminobisphosphonates, as well as stress-inducible MHC-related molecules (MHC class I chain-related A or B [MICA/B]) expressed on infected parenchymal cells [23]. Recognition of MICA/B is not mediated by the TCR but rather other surface receptors on the T cells.

TCR structure

The TCR is composed of a leader peptide, a long extracellular domain, a transmembrane region, and a short cytoplasmic tail [24]. These protein segments are organized into variable (V), joining (J), constant (C), and for the β- and γ-chains, diversity (D) regions (Figure 14.3a). These regions are each encoded by gene clusters on chromosomes 7 (β- and γ-chains) and 14 (α- and δ-chains), and recombine during T-cell development in the thymus. Several mechanisms contribute to the antigen-recognizing capacity of the TCR: 1) multiple V, J, and D region genes; 2) recombination of the D region in multiple reading frames; 3) addition of nucleotides not included in the germline configuration at the V–D and D–J junctions (nongermline or N region additions); and 4) different combinations of either the α- and β- or the γ- and δ-chains [24]. As a result, most of the variability of the TCR is concentrated in the V–D–J region, otherwise known as the complementarity determining region 3 (CDR3). This hypervariable region represents the clonotypic determinant of the receptor, whereas sequences closer to the amino-terminal region (CDR1 and CDR2) are more involved in interactions with MHC molecules. Simultaneous crystallization of the TCR αβ heterodimer and the MHC class I molecule has shown that the CDR3 region of the TCR is a major contact site for antigenic peptide [21]. Through these mechanisms, the T cell is able to generate enormous diversity, which allows for the recognition of a myriad of antigens.

TCR accessory proteins

The TCR is associated on the T-cell surface with functionally important accessory proteins (see Figure 14.3b). At least four

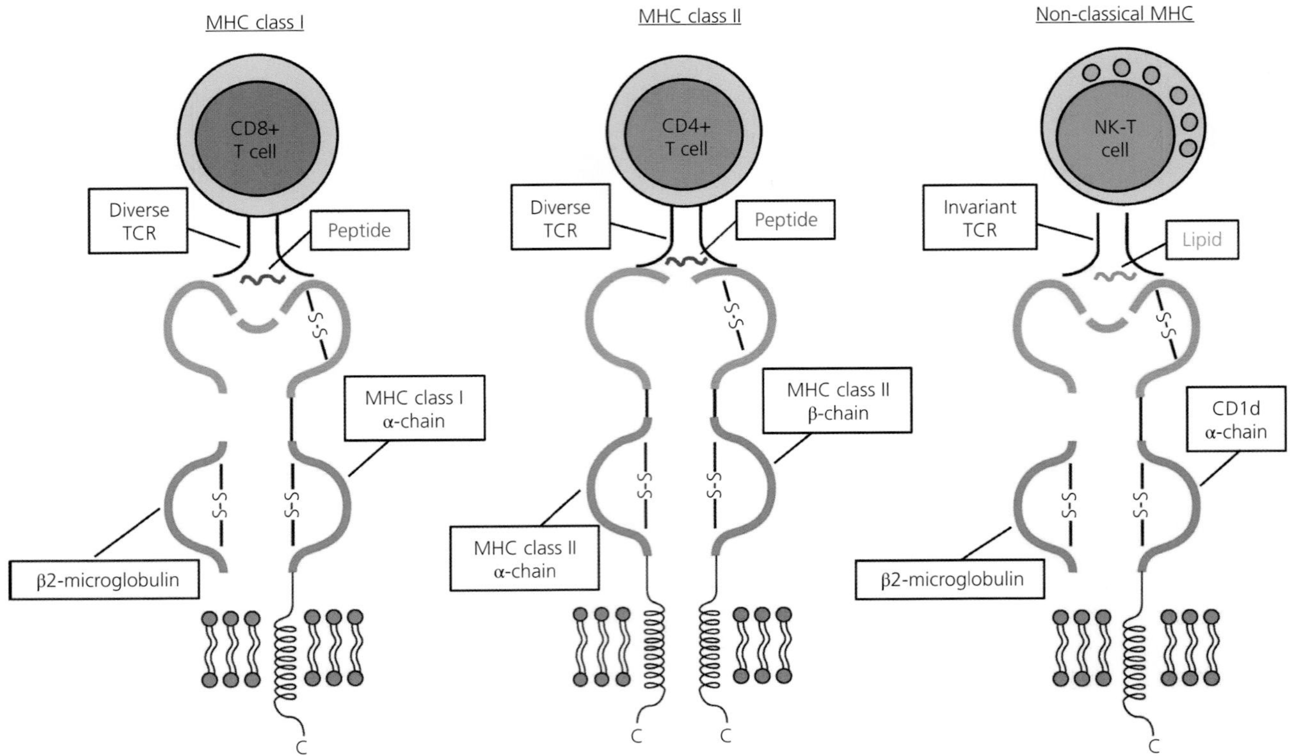

Figure 14.2 Structure of antigen-presenting molecules. Peptide and selected lipid antigens are presented for recognition by specific receptors on T and B cells by two groups of dedicated membrane molecules, major histocompatibility complex (MHC) proteins and nonclassical MHC-like molecules. MHC molecules exist in two classes, I and II. Each MHC class I protein consists of a dimer composed of two noncovalently linked polypeptide chains: the heavy (or α-) chain and an associated non-MHC-encoded nonglycosylated protein called β_2-microglobulin. The MHC class I molecule interacts with a CD8$^+$ T cell during the presentation of peptide antigen. Class II molecules are nondisulfide-linked heterodimeric glycoproteins consisting of an α-chain and a β-chain and interact with CD4$^+$ T cells. CD1d is a nonclassical MHC, related to MHC class I, involved in the presentation of lipid antigen to natural killer T (NK T) cells. TCR, T-cell receptor. Source: Based on Weiss 1990 [19].

proteins (γ, δ, ε, and ζ) of the cluster of differentiation-3 (CD3) complex form noncovalent associations with the αβ- and γδ-chains of the TCRs. The CD3 complex is invariant and therefore does not contribute to the antigen specificity of the TCR, but the CD3 proteins are involved in the assembly and transport of the TCR to the cell surface and in signal transduction after the TCR binds antigen in the context of the MHC. Together, the TCR and the associated CD3 complex are responsible for cognate, or antigen-specific, interactions of T cells with APCs.

Noncognate proteins

Several molecules play important roles in noncognate, or antigen nonspecific, interactions between a T cell and an APC. T cells are classified into distinct functional subsets according to the combinations of these molecules displayed on their cell surface and the transcription factors they express. T cells that express the 60-kD glycoprotein CD4 help coordinate immune responses and recognize antigenic peptides in the context of class II MHC molecules, whereas T cells that express the 32-kD glycoprotein CD8 recognize antigenic peptides in the context of class I MHC molecules and are either cytotoxic or secrete cytokines that influence immune response networks [25]. The interactions between CD4 and class II MHC molecules and between CD8 and class I MHC molecules provide a stabilizing environment for the cognate interactions between TCRs and antigenic peptides. CD4 and CD8 also play important roles in signal transduction through intracellular interactions with non-receptor ligands. In addition, the host contains T cells that lack CD4 or CD8 (so-called double-negative cells), which often possess TCRs that recognize CD1.

Before activation, T cells must adhere to the local connective tissue matrix and APCs. Two intracellular signals activate the T cell: an antigen-specific signal through the TCR and the CD3 complex (i.e., a cognate signal); and an antigen-independent signal through accessory molecules on the T cell, such as CD28, and their ligand counterparts on the APC, such as CD80 or CD86 (i.e., a noncognate or costimulatory signal) [26]. An intracellular signaling cascade is then initiated that leads to the expression of new cell surface antigens, cell proliferation, and expression of effector molecules.

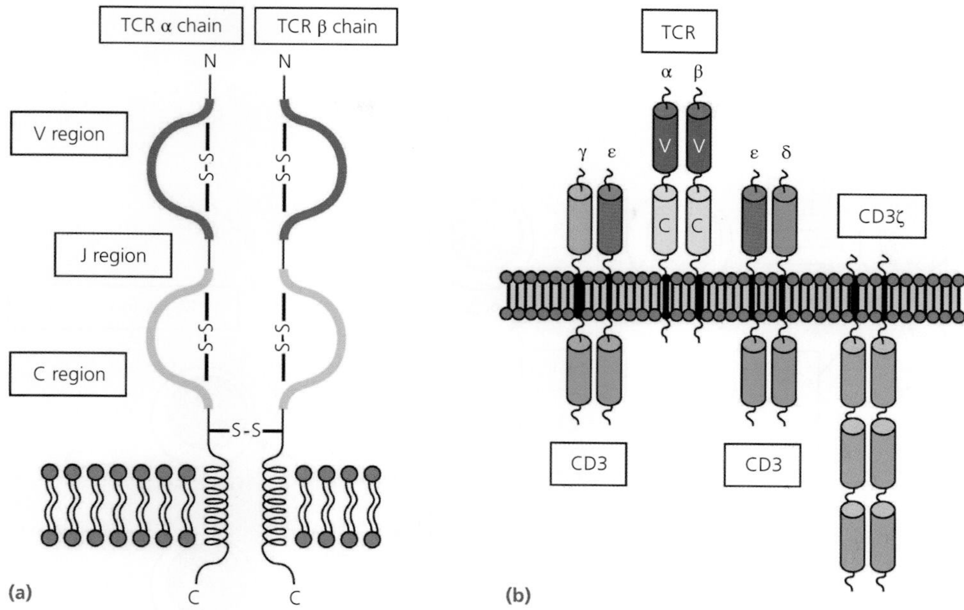

Figure 14.3 Structure of the T-cell receptor (TCR). **(a)** The TCR comprises αβ and γδ heterodimers and is responsible for antigen recognition. Its structure consists of a leader peptide, a long extracellular domain, a transmembrane region, and a short cytoplasmic tail, and it is organized into variable (V), joining (J), constant (C), and, for the β- and γ-chains, diversity (D) regions. **(b)** The cluster of differentiation-3 (CD3) complex, which forms noncovalent associations with the αβ- and γδ-chains of the TCR, is composed of at least four proteins: γ-, δ-, ε-, and ζ-chains. The TCR and associated CD3 complex together are responsible for antigen-specific interactions with antigen-presenting cells.

T-cell lineages

After antigenic stimulation, undifferentiated T cells (type 0 T helper [Th0]) develop along several different lineages that are associated with the secretion of distinct arrays of cytokines (Figure 14.4). This differentiation depends on the cognate and noncognate signals described earlier, as well as cytokines from APCs that are induced by innate immune signals. By this mechanism, the innate immune system helps shape the adaptive immune system. Th1 cells participate in the early events of T- and B-cell development (immunoglobulin G1 [IgG1] production) and cell-mediated immunity (delayed hypersensitivity). Differentiation of Th1 cells is regulated by polarizing cytokines, such as interleukin (IL)-12, IL-18, and IL-27, and transcription factors, such as T-bet, STAT1, and STAT4 [27]. Th1 cells express a characteristic profile of Th1 cytokines, including interferon-γ (IFN-γ), IL-2, and lymphotoxin, which mediate inflammatory immune responses within the gastrointestinal mucosa. In contrast, Th2 cells provide help for B cells and are involved in antibody-mediated immunity (humoral immunity). Th2 differentiation is mediated by IL-4 and the transcription factors STAT6 and GATA3. Cytokines secreted by Th2 cells include IL-4, IL-5, and IL-13 [28].

Although the Th1/Th2 paradigm was the first to be established in Th differentiation, it is now understood that other Th subsets exist. Of particular relevance to intestinal immunity, Th17 cells produce the signature proinflammatory cytokine IL-17, as well as IL-22, which has anti-inflammatory properties and promotes the secretion of antimicrobial peptides by the intestinal epithelium [29] (see Figure 14.4). Th17 may also inhibit IFN-γ release from Th1 cells. The development of the Th17 lineage depends on IL-6, IL-23, and the pleiotropic cytokine, transforming growth factor-β (TGF-β), which is also required for the development of regulatory T cells, establishing an important link between Th17 and Treg cell development [30,31]. Collectively, the Th17 subset of CD4$^+$ T cells functions to regulate the mucosal immune and inflammatory responses.

Treg cells, also known as suppressor cells, suppress the activation of other T cells at sites of inflammation and minimize collateral tissue damage. Treg cells include two distinct subsets of CD4$^+$ T cells (see Figure 14.4): 1) natural Treg (nTreg) cells, which mature in the thymus, are self-antigen specific and express CD25, glucose inducible T-cell receptor, CTLA4, and the lineage-specific transcription factor FOXP3 [32,33]; and 2) inducible Treg (iTreg) cells, which develop when mature T cells are activated under particular conditions of suboptimal antigen exposure or costimulation (e.g., when the TCR of a naive T cell is stimulated in the absence of CD28 activation). Different subsets of iTreg cells produce immunosuppressive cytokines, such as TGF-β (Th3 subset), IL-10 (Tr1), and IL-35 [34]. Treg cells may be particularly important in the prevention of autoimmune gastritis and inflammatory bowel disease (IBD) [35,36]. Treg cells suppress the activation of T cells (primarily Th1 cells) using a contact-dependent mechanism through surface expression of the T-cell inhibitory receptor, CTLA4, which, like CD28, binds CD80 and CD86 but inhibits the T cell, in the

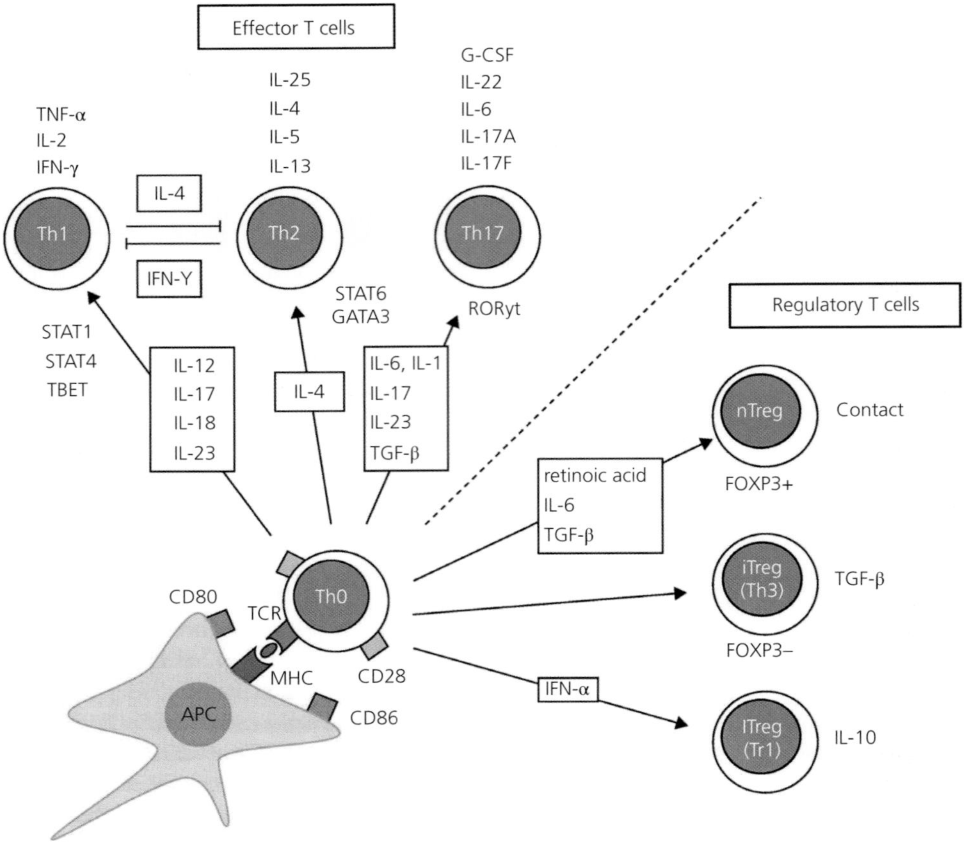

Figure 14.4 Differentiation of T lymphocytes into distinct functional phenotypes. Immature T cells (type 0 T helper [Th0]) differentiate into one of several lineages under the influence of distinct sets of cytokines and other factors. Th1 cells are regulated by polarizing cytokines, such as interleukin (IL)-12, IL-18, IL-23, and IL-27, and transcription factors, including STAT1, STAT4, and TBET. Th1 cells produce specific cytokines, such as IL-2, tumor necrosis factor-α (TNF-α), and interferon-γ (IFN-γ). Th2 cells are regulated by IL-4 and the transcription factors STAT6 and GATA3. Cytokines produced by Th2 cells include IL-4, IL-5, IL-13, and IL-25. IL-4 and IFN-γ serve as negative regulators of Th1 and Th2 polarization, respectively. Th17 cells are generated by transforming growth factor-β (TGF-β) and are also dependent on other cytokines, including IL-6 and IL-23. Th17 cells produce a distinct profile of cytokines, including IL-6, IL-22, IL-17A, and IL-17F. Regulatory T (Treg) cells include two distinct subsets of $CD4^+$ T cells: natural Treg (nTreg) cells, which are regulated by IL-6, TGF-β, and retinoic acid, express the specific transcription factor FOXP3 and suppress effector T cells by contact; and inducible Treg (iTreg), Tr1, and Th3 cells, which are $FOXP3^-$ and produce immunosuppressive cytokines such as TGF-β and IL-10, respectively. APC, antigen-presenting cell; MHC, major histocompatibility complex; TCR, T-cell receptor.

presence of TGF-β [37]. Adoptive transfer experiments have shown that nTreg cells maintain homeostasis in the healthy gastrointestinal tract by acting as primary regulators of the immune response to commensal bacteria [38,39].

Consistent with these various Th phenotypes, T cells are often considered to be either effector cells (i.e., Th1, Th2, or Th17) or regulatory cells (i.e., Treg) [40]. The balance between effector and Treg cells is vital, as demonstrated by intestinal inflammation observed in patients with cancer treated with an antibody that blocks CLTA4 normally expressed on the cell surface of activated T cells [41] and by the autoimmune enteropathy that results from a mutation of FOXP3 as one component of the immune dysregulation, polyendocrinopathy autoimmune enteropathy X-linked syndrome [42].

Natural killer T cells

Natural killer (NK) T cells are specialized T cells that carry out both innate and adaptive immune functions [43]. They express TCRs to recognize foreign and self-lipid-antigen in the context of CD1d, a nonpolymorphic antigen-presenting molecule (see Figure 14.2). The function of NK T cells is innate-like in that they react to various danger signals or inflammatory cytokines to carry out immediate effector responses, as well as stimulatory self-lipids (e.g., certain types of lysolipids) or lipid antigens from microbes. The pathogenesis of experimental intestinal inflammation and human ulcerative colitis may be partly related to aberrant responses of NK T cells through the production of IL-13 and the resulting deleterious effect on the epithelial barrier [44].

B lymphocytes

B cells mediate humoral immunity – the production of antibodies in response to an antigen – which is an integral part of the adaptive immune system. B cells are produced from hematopoietic stem cells in the bone marrow (see Figure 14.1), but unlike T cells, they also mature in the bone marrow.

B-cell immunoglobulins

Each B cell expresses a unique immunoglobulin molecule, the B-cell antigen receptor (BCR), that contains variable regions conferring its antigen specificity. B cells express two forms of immunoglobulin, a membrane form and a secreted form, that share the same antigen-binding regions but differ at their C-terminal terminus and associations with accessory proteins. The surface form consists of a covalently linked heterodimeric immunoglobulin composed of two identical light chains linked by disulfide bridges to two identical heavy chains that carry transmembrane regions at their C-terminal end. It forms the antigen-recognition component of the BCR. Associated with the immunoglobulin are two heterodimeric accessory proteins, Ig-α and Ig-β, which function in BCR signaling by linking the surface immunoglobulin with cytoplasmic protein kinases [45]. The cellular response depends on the specific signaling cascade that is activated, as well as on signal strength and duration, and modulation of the signal by coreceptor molecules (i.e., the CD19/CD21 complex, CD22, and CD72) [46,47].

The secreted form of immunoglobulin also consists of two identical light chains linked by disulfide bridges to two identical heavy chains with a shortened C-terminal end lacking a transmembrane region. Each of the five classes of immunoglobulins are defined by differences in effector function and a unique heavy chain isotype, designated α (IgA), δ (IgD), ε (IgE), γ (IgG), and μ (IgM). These five heavy chain isotypes associate with light chains of two isotypes, κ and λ. In humans, there are four different IgG subclasses (IgG1, IgG2, IgG3, and IgG4) and two different IgA subclasses (IgA1 and IgA2). Although some of the immunoglobulin heterogeneity can be attributed to the different classes and subclasses, most derives from the variable regions located on the amino terminals of the heavy and light chains and encoded by V, D, and J region gene segments that lead to structural and binding diversity in a combinatorial fashion similar to the TCR.

B-cell activation and differentiation

After binding their cognate antigens, the surface immunoglobulins of mature B cells initiate a cascade of signaling events that activate the cell, leading to clonal expansion and the generation of the secreted form of the antigen-specific immunoglobulin of that cell (Figure 14.5). Some of the clonally expanded B cells differentiate into memory B cells. Under the influence of antigen-specific T cells, B cells switch to different isotypes (usually to IgG isotypes in the periphery and IgA in the gastrointestinal-associated lymphoid tissues) and differentiate into plasma cells, which secrete high levels of immunoglobulin. The overall process results in the production of antibodies that travel throughout tissue fluids and are secreted into the lumen of the intestine and bile, where they can detect and bind to the antigenic molecules that first triggered their production [48].

Like T cells, subsets of B cells can be identified on the basis of phenotypic markers other than the membrane immunoglobulins. For example, CD5 is expressed on 5–10% of the B-cell lineage. $CD5^+$ cells, or B1 cells, are capable of producing autoantibodies in autoimmune disease. They are generated most often from fetal and neonatal splenic B-cell populations and transferred fetal precursors, and rarely from adult bone marrow [49]. Most B cells do not express CD5 and are known as B2 or common B cells.

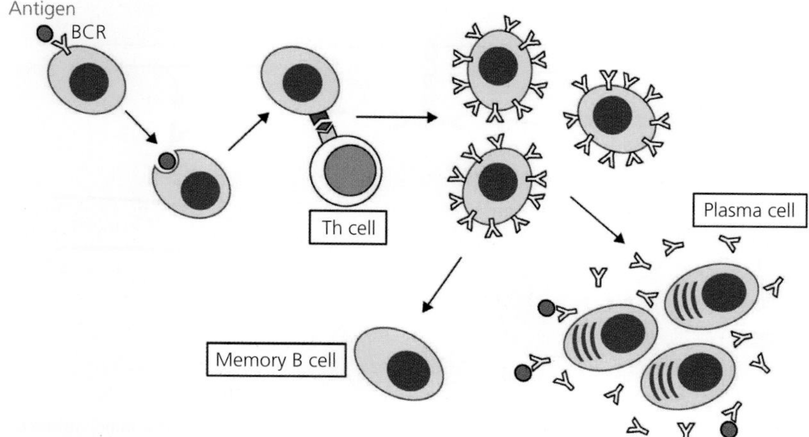

Figure 14.5 B-cell development. B cells mediate humoral immunity and the production of antibodies after interaction between specific antigens and the B-cell antigen receptor (BCR). B cells are produced and mature in the bone marrow, and first bind antigen through the surface-bound BCR, which activates the cells and leads to clonal expansion and differentiation with the help of T helper (Th) cells. After terminal differentiation into plasma cells, the cells produce high levels of secreted antigen-specific immunoglobulins. Some of the clonally expanded B cells differentiate into memory B cells that can be more rapidly activated and expanded upon reencountering the respective antigen.

IgA: the mucosal immunoglobulin

The synthesis and secretion of dimeric IgA is a major protective mechanism of the intestinal tract, which contains more than 70% of all immunoglobulin-producing cells in the body. Plasma cells produce dimeric IgA – two IgA monomers linked by a polypeptide J-chain (Figure 14.6). The J-chain participates in the transport of IgA and IgM molecules across the intestinal epithelium through interaction with the polymeric immunoglobulin receptor (pIgR) on the basal surface of epithelial cells [50]. IgA bound to a portion of the pIgR that is known as the secretory component is then secreted into the intestinal lumen. This secretory component may protect secretory IgA from proteolytic degradation in the hostile luminal environment and stabilize the structure of the polymeric IgA complex (see Figure 14.6).

IgA is also translocated across hepatocytes or bile duct epithelium into the bile and carried to the duodenum [51,52]. The presence of secretory IgA in bile provides passive immunity and protects the biliary tract and the proximal parts of the small intestine. A second implication of the hepatobiliary secretion of IgA is that complexes of IgA and antigen can be transported into the bile from the circulation. Hepatic removal of IgA–antigen complexes may protect against harmful absorbed substances, including dietary antigens and bacterial products [53].

The major function of secretory IgA in host defense is protection against bacteria, viruses, protozoa, and luminal antigens [54]. Secretory IgA provides passive immunity by inhibiting adherence of microbes to epithelial cells and preventing their effective colonization and proliferation. Secretory IgA neutralizes bacterial toxins, thereby preventing their action on intestinal epithelial cells, and can even neutralize pathogens in intracellular locations [55]. Secretory IgA also blocks the absorption of antigens from the gut and may be particularly important in disease states in which the mucosal barrier is broken. Unlike other immunoglobulins, such as IgG, which can be secreted by intestinal B cells, IgA does not activate complement.

Intestinal transport of other isotypes

Transcellular pathways for the transport of IgE and IgG also exist in intestinal epithelial cells. IgE transport is mediated by the expression of CD23 (FcεR1 or IgE receptor) on epithelial cells and may be important in intestinal allergic responses and parasitic infections [56]. IgG transport is mediated by the MHC

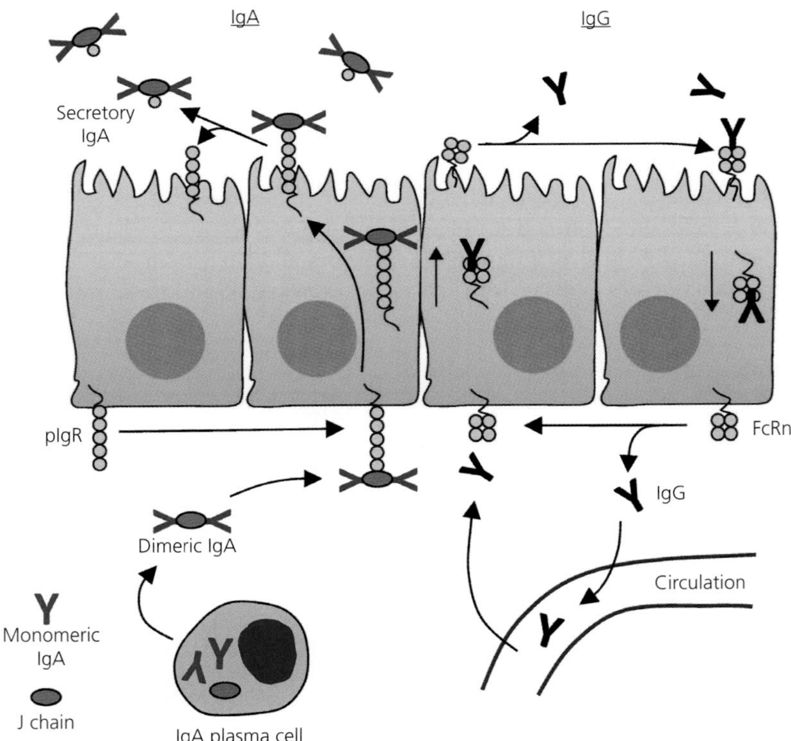

Figure 14.6 Intestinal immunoglobulin secretion. Synthesis and secretion of immunoglobulin A (IgA) is a major protective mechanism for the intestinal mucosa. Dimeric IgA is produced by plasma cells in the lamina propria by connecting two monomeric IgA molecules with a joining (J) chain. On secretion, dimeric IgA can bind to the polymeric immunoglobulin receptor (pIgR) on the basolateral side of intestinal epithelial cells and is transported across the epithelium to the apical side. After proteolytic cleavage, the dimeric IgA, along with a small fragment of the pIgR known as secretory component, is secreted into the intestinal lumen as secretory IgA. Transport of IgG across the epithelium is mediated by the major histocompatibility complex class I-related molecule, neonatal Fc receptor for IgG (FcRn). IgG transport is bidirectional, unlike that for IgA, so antigens bound in the lumen to IgG can be transported across to the lamina propria by this mechanism.

class I–related molecule FcRn (neonatal Fc receptor for IgG) [57] (see Figure 14.6). Unlike the basal-to-apical transport of IgA and IgE, IgG transport is bidirectional (i.e., both basal-to-apical and apical-to-basal) and is involved in antibody-mediated retrieval of antigens from the lumen that, when transported into the lamina propria as immune complexes, can be taken up, processed, and presented by dendritic cells, thereby contributing to host protection from mucosal infections [58].

Innate lymphoid cells

Innate lymphoid cells (ILCs) are morphologically similar to lymphocytes but do not express the characteristic cognate receptors that carry out acquired immunity, that is, TCR or BCR. These immune cells arise from common hematopoietic precursors [59] (see Figure 14.1). Through the transcriptional repressor inhibitor of DNA binding 2 and cytokine signals, ILCs differentiate into distinct populations, of which NK cells are the best studied [60] (Figure 14.7). NK cells can recognize pathogen-derived ligands through TLR surface receptors and have several cytotoxic effector functions, suggesting that NK cells provide a nonspecific first line of defense through their ability to kill pathogen-infected cells. NK cells can be divided into subsets based on surface markers, mainly CD56 and CD16 [61]. These subsets have different functional roles, such as production of IFN-γ or primarily cytotoxic activities. During innate immune responses, the NK cell recognizes target cells that lack surface expression of class I MHC molecules. Because many viruses, as well as intestinal cancers, downregulate class I MHC molecules to evade adaptive immune responses, this mechanism of recognition is important not only for antimicrobial defense but also for tumor surveillance. On contact with a target cell, NK cells release pore-forming proteins called *perforins* and proteolytic enzymes called *granzymes* into the target cell, which leads to destruction of cytoskeletal proteins, chromosomal degradation, and cell death [62]. NK cells may also function in adaptive immunity through interactions with dendritic cells [63].

In general, ILCs comprise three distinct groups (see Figure 14.7): 1) group 1 (ILC1), which is T-bet$^+$ (NK cells are also included in this group); 2) group 2 (ILC2), which is GATA3$^+$; and 3) group 3 (ILC3), which expresses the transcription factor RORγt [64]. ILC1 cells secrete IFN-γ in response to IL-15, IL-12, and IL-18. ILC2 cells respond to IL-25, IL-33, and thymic stromal lymphopoietin, which are typically secreted by epithelial cells, and secrete IL-5 and IL-13. Arylhydrocarbon receptor (AhR) ligands, IL-1β, and IL-23 stimulate ILC3 cells to secrete IL-17 and IL-22. Lymphoid tissue inducer (LTi) cells are a subset of group 3 ILCs that are involved in the process of lymph node and Peyer's patch development [65]. LTi cells are thought to play a role in inflammation by producing IL-17A and IL-22, which are important in the innate immune response to

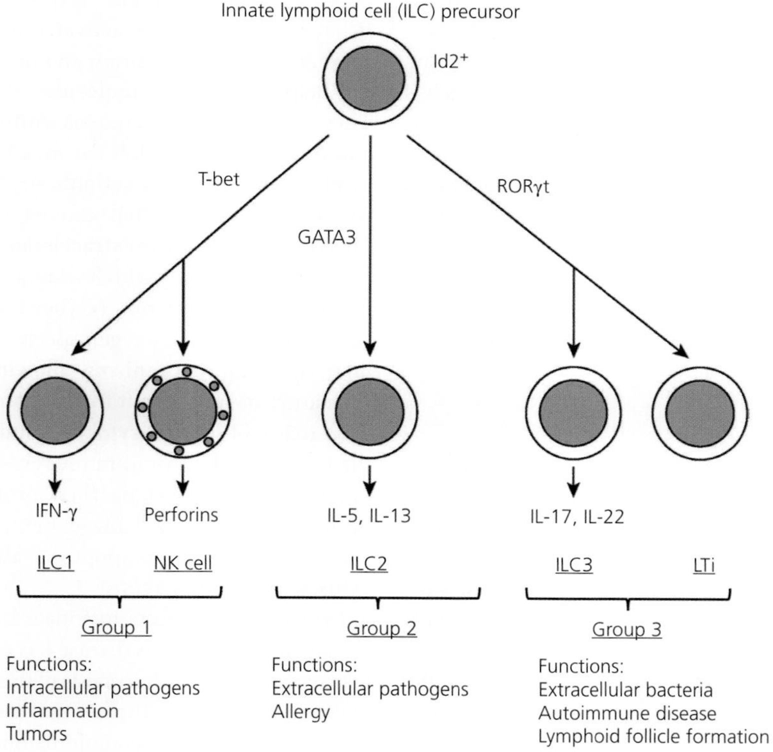

Figure 14.7 Phenotypes of innate-like lymphoid cells. Under the influence of various transcription factors, ILCs develop from an innate lymphoid precursor into three distinct groups. The individual types of ILCs within each group and the representative functions are shown. Id2, inhibitor of DNA binding 2; ILC, innate lymphoid cell; LTi, lymphoid tissue inducer cell; NK, natural killer. Source: Based on Poggi et al. 2019 [60].

microbial infection. The production of IL-22 by group 3 ILC cells may be critical in the response to infection as observed in experimental *Citrobacter rodentium* infection, a model of enteropathogenic *Escherichia coli* [66]. The development and effector function of ILCs that secrete IL-22 is largely shaped by interactions with the intestinal microbiota [67].

Myelomonocytic cells and neutrophils

Cells of the myelomonocytic lineage include monocytes and their progeny (macrophages and dendritic cells) and polymorphonuclear leukocytes (neutrophils, basophils, and eosinophils). They evolve from a common myeloid progenitor cell in the bone marrow (see Figure 14.1) in response to several lineage-specific growth factors, such as macrophage and granulocyte colony-stimulating factors (GM-CSFs).

Macrophages

Monocytes, mononuclear phagocytes that mature into macrophages when residing within tissues, and dendritic cells play central roles in both innate and adaptive immunity. In innate immunity, their phagocytic function and inflammatory cytokine secretion are important for the accumulation of inflammatory cells and the destruction of invading pathogens, whereas in adaptive immunity, they mainly exert their effects through the ability to endocytose, process, and present foreign antigens to T cells [68]. Peripheral blood monocytes almost uniformly express the CD14 marker, which they shed on entering tissues during inflammatory responses, such as infiltration into the lamina propria during IBD. These recruited monocytes evolve into tissue macrophages that have active phagocytic functions, which is important not only for the eradication of invading microorganisms but also as the essential first step in initiating antigen processing and presentation for MHC class II pathways, a prerequisite for activating $CD4^+$ T cells that orchestrate further immune responses. Macrophages promote inflammation by secreting IL-12 and IL-23, which drive $CD4^+$ T cells to the Th1 phenotype, leading to secretion of IFN-γ and subsequent activation of the phagocytic and antigen presentation functions of the macrophage.

Dendritic cells

Dendritic cells are the most potent APCs in the body and are found in Peyer's patches, lamina propria, and epithelium of the gastrointestinal mucosa [69]. Within tertiary lymphoid tissues, such as the lamina propria, dendritic cells are considered to be immature, exhibiting active phagocytic functions but poor antigen presentation functions. When exposed to microbial products – specifically, phylogenetically conserved PAMPs – dendritic cells mature and migrate to secondary lymphoid organs, including the mesenteric lymph nodes. Here they mature further, upregulate their antigen presentation functions through the expression of costimulatory molecules, such as CD80 and CD86, and activate naive T lymphocytes. It is now clear that multiple dendritic cell lineages exist, and that each contributes in a specific way to innate and adaptive immune responses within the gastrointestinal tract. A network of dendritic cells in the lamina propria of the ileum, colon, and the dome region of the Peyer's patches expresses membrane-bound CX3CR1 (fractalkine) and appears to play a unique role in luminal antigen sampling. These $CX3CR1^+$ cells can extend their dendrites through the epithelium to directly sample microbial products, in addition to the more conventional phagocytic mechanism for recognizing bacteria delivered via M cells and intestinal epithelial cells [70,71]. $CX3CR1^+CD11c^+CD11b^+$ cells are the predominant dendritic cell subset observed in the terminal ileum of mice, while expression of the integrin α-chain CD103 (αE) is characteristic of dendritic cells in the lamina propria of small intestine and colon [72,73]. Such $CD103^+$ dendritic cells possess regulatory functions that are important in maintaining tolerance against luminal antigens. The regulatory functions of such dendritic cells are determined by factors secreted by the intestinal epithelium, such as thymic stromal lymphopoietin and vitamin A, which is metabolized by the dendritic cell to retinoic acid [74].

Neutrophils

Neutrophilic polymorphonuclear leukocytes (often shortened to neutrophils) are an essential component of innate immunity and function as the first responders to infection [75]. They are continuously produced in the bone marrow and circulate through the peripheral blood, where they remain acutely posed for activation and response to invading pathogens. When infection occurs, activated neutrophils rapidly extravasate across the endothelium and into the affected mucosa with the help of adhesion molecules expressed on their surface. They infiltrate infected tissues within hours of the initial insult and phagocytose and kill the invading pathogen. Neutrophils produce antimicrobial cationic peptides, proteases, and reactive oxygen species that can be secreted directly into the phagosome or into the extracellular spaces to form neutrophil extracellular traps, which degrade virulence factors and microbes that have not yet been ingested [76]. Neutrophil secretion of reactive oxygen species can also regulate intracellular signaling mechanisms, allowing neutrophils to mediate the nature of subsequent inflammatory responses through the production of specific cytokines and chemokines that polarize the resulting adaptive immune response toward a unique phenotype [77]. To mediate their proinflammatory effects and limit collateral tissue damage, neutrophils are short-lived and constitutively undergo apoptosis, after which they are phagocytosed by macrophages.

Evidence that defects in innate immunity contribute to the pathogenesis of Crohn's disease has cast new light on the role of neutrophils in the pathogenesis of this condition [78]. In support of this theory, genetic diseases that compromise neutrophil functions, such as chronic granulomatous disease, glycogen storage disease type IB, or Turner syndrome, manifest intestinal abnormalities similar to those seen in Crohn's disease [79]. Impaired migration, decreased bactericidal and phagocytic functions, and lower superoxide production characterize neutrophils in patients with Crohn's disease [80]. Moreover, mice with a cell-type-specific disruption of the *Stat3* gene in neutrophils and macrophages develop spontaneous enterocolitis, consistent with the notion that these cell types are indeed involved in intestinal inflammation [81].

Neutrophils also contribute to acute liver damage associated with hepatic ischemia/reperfusion injury and alcoholic hepatitis [82]. In response to signals from proinflammatory cytokines, chemokines, and complement factors, neutrophils are primed and accumulate in the sinusoids, postsinusoidal venules, and portal venules of the hepatic vasculature. When a chemotactic signal is received, the neutrophils extravasate across the endothelium into the liver parenchyma, where they adhere to hepatocytes and are activated to produce reactive oxygen species and proteases, similar to their function in the intestine. Protease secretion is associated with the promotion of subsequent inflammatory responses through the production of proinflammatory cytokines and chemokines; secretion of reactive oxygen species leads to oxidative stress and neutrophil-mediated necrosis of liver cells.

Mast cells

Mast cells are granulated immune cells strategically positioned at the interfaces between the internal and the external environment to perform their numerous immunoprotective functions. In the healthy gastrointestinal tract, mast cells are located in the lamina propria, submucosa, and muscle layers, as well as on the serosal surface. Increased numbers of activated mast cells have been observed in the gastrointestinal mucosa of patients with helminth infections, ulcerative colitis, Crohn's disease, gastritis, and celiac disease.

Mast cells may be induced to degranulate through interactions of IgG complexes with specific surface immunoglobulin receptors, FcγRIIa and FcγRIIIa, and of complement with the complement C3a and C5a receptors. Expression of numerous other cell surface receptors allows for selective, nonanaphylactic activation of mast cells. Once activated, mast cells release mediators of inflammation stored in specialized granules (e.g., histamine, 5-hydroxytryptamine [5-HT, or serotonin], and proteases), as well as newly formed nongranule-associated mediators (e.g., nitric oxide, prostaglandin D_2, platelet-activating factor, and leukotrienes) and numerous chemokines and cytokines. Significant plasticity exists in the development of each mast cell. Depending on the tissue location, phenotype (such as protease expression in the granules), and external stimuli, mast cells may play diverse roles in intestinal mucosal immunology, including maintaining homeostasis at the epithelial barrier, immune defense against helminths and bacterial infection, and exacerbating inflammation in experimental colitis [83–86].

Mast cell activation caused by cross-linking of IgE and binding to the high-affinity IgE receptor is central in the pathogenesis of allergic disorders such as food allergy. However, mast cells are thought to have been conserved through evolution because of their immunoprotective function, so their role in food allergy likely represents an inappropriate inflammatory response that has the primary function of combatting intestinal parasites.

The complex of symptoms that leads to irritable bowel syndrome (IBS) likely involves interactions between the mucosal immune system and enteric nerves. Mediators that are released on mast cell activation are thought to be central in the genesis of visceral pain in this disorder [87]. Mast cells and nerves display bidirectional interactions, because neurotransmitters, particularly substance P, cause mast cell degranulation, and mast cells in turn release vasoactive intestinal peptide, which can act as a neurotransmitter. The release of various mediators on mast cell activation may link the sequence of events that have been observed in experimental IBS: changes in membrane permeability lead to low-grade mucosal inflammation and finally to activation of enteric nerves.

Intestinal epithelial cells

The intestinal epithelium serves foremost as a physical barrier that separates luminal compounds from immune cells in the lamina propria, thus preventing activation of those cells by antigens and PAMPs [88]. The integrity of the single columnar monolayer is facilitated by the continuous renewal and differentiation of epithelial cells and rapid restitution after transitory breaches. Mucus secreted by goblet cells further contributes to the physical separation of intraluminal bacteria from the subepithelial lamina propria. Mucus in the stomach and colon forms two layers, with a thick inner component being firmly attached to the epithelium and maintained bacterial-free under normal conditions. In contrast, the small intestine has only one layer of mucus. Mucin-containing mucous formation is one of the oldest protective mechanisms during evolution, as gel-forming mucins are already present in early metazoans [89].

Although generally tight, the epithelial barrier is not impenetrable and has sophisticated mechanisms to regulate the trafficking of macromolecules between the environment and the host, primarily through paracellular pathways that are controlled by tight junctions [90,91] (Figure 14.8). Tight junctions were originally believed to be impermeable but are now recognized to be composed of several tight junctional proteins (e.g., occludin, members of the claudin family, the junctional adhesion molecule [JAM], zonula occludens [ZO]-1, ZO-2, and ZO-3) that function together as a complex that controls selective epithelial permeability. Barrier disruption is important in several gastrointestinal disorders; for example, atrophic gastritis spontaneously occurs in transgenic mice deficient in claudin-18 as a result of inappropriate permeation of H^+ ions across the gastric epithelial barrier [92]. During inflammation, increased production of proinflammatory cytokines, including tumor necrosis factor-α (TNF-α) and IFN-γ, causes reorganization of several tight junctional proteins, including ZO-1, JAM-1, occludin, claudin-1, and claudin 4, and results in increased

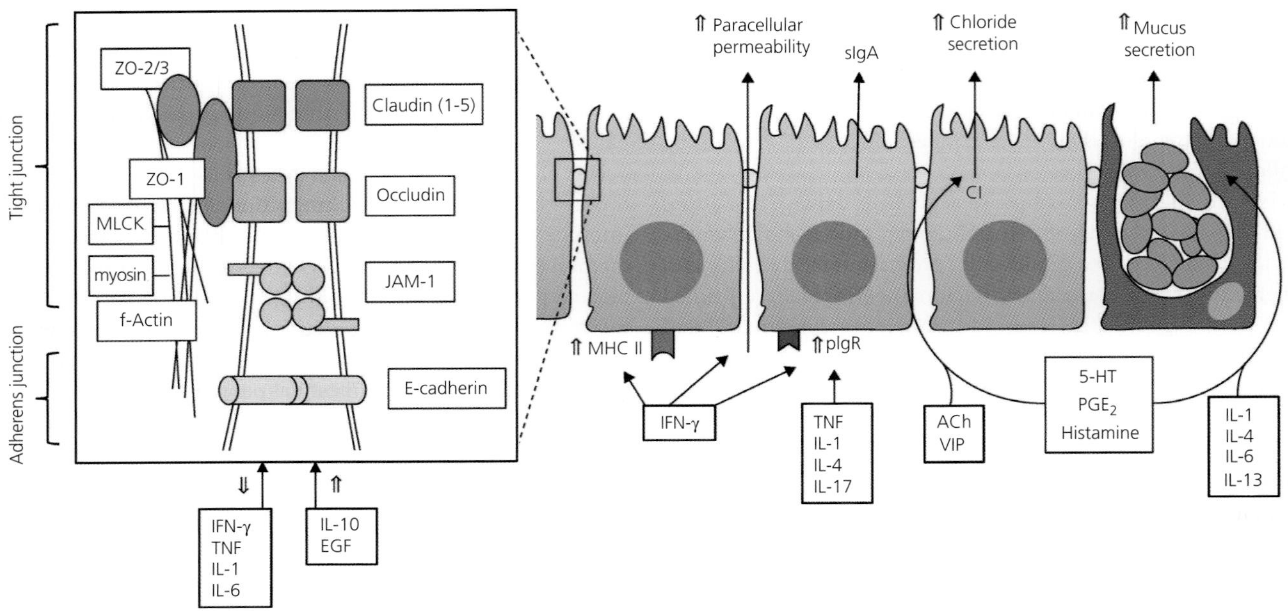

Figure 14.8 Epithelial barrier structure and function. The intestinal epithelium serves as a barrier that separates luminal antigens from immune cells of the lamina propria. The epithelial barrier is held together by adherens junctions, primarily composed of E-cadherin, and tight junctions that control paracellular pathways between adjacent epithelial cells (inset). Tight junctions are composed of several proteins, including occludin, members of the claudin family, the junctional adhesion molecule (JAM)-1, and zonula occludens (ZO) proteins. Tight and adherens junctions are anchored to complexes of actin and myosin, as well as myosin light chain kinase (MLCK), which regulate selective intestinal permeability in response to various cytokines. Epithelial cells can function as antigen-presenting cells through induction of MHC class II proteins. Transepithelial transport of IgA by the polymeric immunoglobulin receptor (pIgR) and luminal release of secretory IgA (sIgA) provides immune protection against luminal threats. Expression of pIgR is induced by a number of inflammatory cytokines. Secretion of electrolytes and water by epithelial cells is an important component of the gastrointestinal response to inflammation. Histamine, prostaglandin E_2 (PGE_2), and serotonin (5-HT) are important inflammatory mediators that induce epithelial cell chloride secretion, resulting in diarrhea when excessive. Neurotransmitters, such as vasoactive intestinal polypeptide (VIP) and acetylcholine (ACh), can also directly stimulate epithelial ion secretion, or indirectly induce mast cell activation with release of histamine and serotonin. Secretion of mucus by goblet cells provides an additional physicochemical barrier against luminal microbes. A number of inflammatory mediators and cytokines stimulate mucous expression and secretion. EGF, epidermal growth factor; IL, interleukin. Source: Fasano and Shea-Donohue 2005 [90].

permeability, or a "leaky gut" [93]. Intestinal barrier dysfunction has been proposed to be a major mechanism of disease pathogenesis in IBD and may possibly even represent a primary defect [94].

In addition to serving as a passive physical barrier, epithelial cells provide an active defense against microorganisms and foreign antigens (see Figure 14.8). The epithelium generates an adjacent luminal milieu that confers strong antimicrobial activity against microorganisms that may reach the epithelial surface. Specialized Paneth cells secrete natural antimicrobial peptides of several classes and with diverse specificities against various microorganisms [95]. Epithelial cells also actively transport secretory IgA into the gut lumen, which helps to control luminal bacteria.

Beyond barrier formation, epithelial cells are the first host cells to come into contact with intraluminal antigens and can transport them to the rich immunological system that lies beneath. This function is particularly developed in specialized, flattened epithelial cells (termed M cells) present in the epithelium overlying Peyer's patches. Antigen transport is tightly regulated via constant communication between the epithelium and gut-resident stromal and immune cells, a dialogue that is largely mediated by cytokines and growth factors. Bacterial sensing via TLRs, NOD2, and other innate immune receptors in intestinal epithelial cells and phagocytes is important for the preservation of a healthy gut mucosa. Experimental proof for this concept was obtained by use of the dextran sulfate sodium–colitis mouse model, which involves chemical destruction of the colon, followed by acute inflammation and spontaneous recovery. When innate immune receptor signaling was rendered deficient by genetic elimination of genes encoding for TLRs or their common adaptor protein myeloid differentiation primary response 88 (MyD88), or NOD1 and NOD2, the respective knockout mice had more severe colitis and compromised mucosal restitution [96]. Therefore, it appears that intact innate epithelial recognition of PAMPs is required for intestinal homeostasis. Nevertheless, the context of innate receptor activation is of paramount importance because only low-level tonic signals lead to homeostasis, whereas persistent high-level activation can cause chronic inflammation [97].

Intestinal epithelial cells can also function as APCs. Epithelial cells of the small intestine constitutively express MHC class II molecules, possibly as a consequence of IFN-γ secretion by adjacent T cells [98]. Colonic epithelial cells do not normally express measurable levels of MHC class II molecules, except in the setting of inflammation, presumably in response to local cytokine production [99]. Both in vitro and in vivo studies have shown that intestinal epithelial cells are capable of taking up, processing, and presenting soluble antigens to CD4$^+$ T cells in the context of MHC class II molecules [100]. Although soluble antigens can be taken up apically and basolaterally, MHC class II molecules primarily segregate in the basolateral region, where antigen presentation to antigen-specific, MHC class II-restricted T cells occurs. Thus, intestinal epithelial cells may augment or modify afferent immune stimulation that normally results from antigenic events within Peyer's patches. Despite in vivo evidence for functional class II MHC expression, intestinal epithelial cells seem to preferentially engage and stimulate CD8$^+$ cells that exhibit suppressor activity, which contributes to the suppressor tone of the intestine [101].

Secretion of electrolytes and water by epithelial cells is an important part of the gastrointestinal response to inflammation (see Figure 14.8). Histamine, prostaglandin E_2 (PGE_2), serotonin (5-HT), and leukotriene B_4 (LTB_4) are examples of inflammatory mediators that induce epithelial Cl^- secretion. Neural mechanisms also affect epithelial Cl^- secretion directly or indirectly through inflammatory cells. The neurotransmitter acetylcholine induces Cl^- secretion in epithelial cells [102]. Neuropeptides, such as substance P, vasoactive intestinal polypeptide, and neuropeptide Y, induce mast cell activation, resulting in the release of histamine and 5-HT, and thus the activation of epithelial cell Cl^- secretion [103]. Cl^- secretion is accompanied by Na^+ secretion and, consequently, by the passage of water across the epithelium into the intestinal lumen. Diarrhea is the clinical manifestation of the enhanced enterocyte Cl^- secretion induced by these mediators. These same inflammatory mediators induce the secretion of mucus by goblet cells in the gastrointestinal tract. Diarrhea protects the host from infectious agents and their toxins by speeding their passage through the gastrointestinal tract and out of the body. Mucous secretion protects the host from infectious agents in the gastrointestinal tract by preventing the binding of the infectious agents and their toxins to intestinal epithelial cells.

Nonimmune parenchymal cells

Intestinal cells that are not of epithelial or hematopoietic origin are collectively referred to as nonimmune parenchymal (stromal) cells. They include fibroblasts, endothelial cells, and smooth muscle cells and play instrumental roles in innate immunity, immune regulation, and epithelial barrier maintenance. These cell types, unlike dendritic cells or macrophages, likely do not initiate specific immune responses through the education of naive lymphocytes but rather integrate and enhance ongoing immune responses and contribute to the immunopathology in disease states [104]. Fibroblasts in the colon are composed of at least four subsets and myofibroblasts, while the endothelial cell cluster is made up of conventional endothelial cells, microvascular and postcapillary endothelial cells, and pericytes [16,105]. Fibroblasts, through the expression of cell surface molecules, connective tissue components, and cytokines, regulate local lymphocyte survival and function and contribute to TGF-β-mediated fibrosis associated with chronic inflammation [106]. Smooth muscle cells can present antigens in an MHC class II-restricted fashion in the context of inflammation and respond to inflammatory cytokines, such as IL-4, thereby altering intestinal motility and contributing to peristalsis and elimination of lumen-dwelling pathogens. Endothelial cells play a key role in regulating tissue inflammation by both directing the recruitment of leukocytes and myeloid cells and secreting a variety of soluble mediators that enhance inflammation [107].

Organization of the intestinal immune system

The intestinal mucosal immune system, also known as the gut-associated lymphoid tissue (GALT), is part of a larger system of the mucosa-associated lymphoid tissue, which also encompasses the mucosal surfaces of the lungs and genitourinary tract, as well as mammary glands and salivary glands. The GALT can be divided into several functionally and anatomically contained compartments: 1) the loosely organized effector sites (lamina propria and intestinal epithelium), 2) the macroscopic intestinal lymphoid structures (Peyer's patches and mesenteric lymph nodes), and 3) the microscopic intestinal lymphoid structures (cryptopatches and isolated lymphoid follicles). Peyer's patches, which are rounded lymphoid follicles in the mucosa and submucosa of the small intestine, constitute an afferent limb of the GALT. It recognizes antigens through specialized sampling mechanisms in M cells of the follicle-associated epithelium adjacent to the Peyer's patches and dendritic cells that extend their dendrites through open tight junctions in the epithelial barrier [18]. Detection of luminal antigens that cross the epithelial barrier by way of M cells results in the education and dissemination of B and T lymphoblasts to other tissues linked to the mucosa-associated lymphoid tissues and the loosely affiliated compartments of the lamina propria. The lamina propria represents an efferent or effector limb of the intestinal mucosal immune system; it is populated with lymphoid effector cells, such as B cells, plasma cells, T cells, NK T cells, NK cells and other ILCs, mononuclear and polymorphonuclear phagocytes, and mast cells. Plasma cells in the lamina propria secrete IgA, which provides protection against bacteria, viruses, and luminal antigens. The immune compartment within the epithelium consists of a unique resident population of T cells, known as IELs, which, unlike peripheral T cells, are enriched in cells that express the γδ TCR and help to maintain barrier functions.

Nonorganized lamina propria

The lamina propria lies beneath the intestinal epithelium and serves as a loosely affiliated effector compartment of T and B cells, plasma cells, NK cells, macrophages, dendritic cells, and mast cells. Virtually all T cells within the lamina propria express the $\alpha\beta$ TCR, as well as the CD45 surface marker, which indicates that these are memory cells that have had previous encounters with antigens, presumably in the Peyer's patches [108]. The $CD4^+$ T cells in the lamina propria exert an important helper–inducer function for immunoglobulin production and respond to antigens by producing cytokines rather than by proliferating [109]. $CD8^+$ cytotoxic T effector precursor cells in the intestine participate in host mucosal defense mechanisms when necessary but do not damage the surrounding tissue when they are not needed. Lamina propria lymphocytes can be induced to mediate cell-mediated cytotoxicity by incubation with IL-2, IFNs, lectins, and monoclonal antibodies directed against the TCR. This is typical of antigen-primed effector cells and is consistent with the CD45RO memory phenotype [110–112]. Although cytotoxic effector cells are present, the lymphocytes in the intestinal lamina propria are poor mediators of cell-mediated cytotoxicity, antibody-dependent cellular cytotoxicity, and cell-mediated cytolysis [113]. Activated cytotoxic $CD4^+$ and $CD8^+$ lymphocytes are more abundant in the lamina propria of patients with IBD [114].

Most mucosal T lymphocytes are also $CD95L^+$ and $CD69^+$ and exhibit elevated levels of cytoplasmic Ca^{++}, consistent with an activated phenotype [115]. Controlled activation of the intestinal immune system is important in regulating effector cell function. This includes cytotoxic functions, which may be directed at the lymphocytes themselves to dampen immune responses and regulate the level of cytotoxic function within the various compartments of the bowel wall [116]. For example, administration of anti-TNF-α therapeutics, which are used to treat human IBD, can attenuate murine ileitis through a mechanism that involves attenuation of intestinal epithelial cell apoptosis and simultaneous induction of apoptosis of lamina propria lymphocytes [117]. In this way, the gut may be said to be in a state of physiological inflammation, poised for intervention when necessary but generally held in abeyance.

About 40% of the lymphoid cells in the lamina propria are B cells derived primarily from precursors in Peyer's patches [118]. These B cells and their progeny plasma cells predominantly synthesize IgA, rather than IgM, IgG, or IgE. Lamina propria B cells are induced to differentiate terminally into IgA-secreting cells under the local influence of T-cell-derived cytokines, indicating the importance of this isotype to mucosal protection [54,119–121]. In IBD, the numbers of lamina propria B cells and plasma cells that produce IgG are markedly increased [122], and in allergy and parasitic infestations, those that produce IgE are elevated.

Intraepithelial lymphocytes

The human intestinal epithelium contains a unique population of lymphoid cells, the IELs, which reside between intestinal epithelial cells along their basolateral surfaces [123]. About 10 IELs normally exist per 100 epithelial cells in the small intestine. Given the vast surface area of the intestinal epithelium, IELs represent a significant proportion of all T cells in the human body [124]. The composition of IEL subsets differs substantially from that of the circulating T-cell subsets. IEL populations are dominated by $CD8^+$ T cells (>70% in the small intestine) and largely express the CD8$\alpha\alpha$ homodimer, which is uncommon among circulating T cells [125]. T cells lacking both CD8 and CD4 ($CD8^-CD4^-$), or double-negative cells, comprise more than 10% of murine small-intestinal IELs, as well as the majority of IELs found in other compartments, but they are rarely found among circulating lymphocytes [126]. $CD4\alpha\beta^+$ T cells, which are common in the systemic circulation and lamina propria, are underrepresented among IELs and mostly exist as double-positive cells that also express CD8$\alpha\alpha$. Lastly, IELs contain an increased proportion of cells expressing the $\gamma\delta$ TCR compared with systemic and lamina propria T cells.

The $\alpha\beta$ TCR is expressed on all of the IELs in the colon and on about half of the IELs in the small intestine, and they are mostly $CD8\alpha\beta^+$, indicating that they respond to MHC class I or class I-like molecules. IELs that express the $\alpha\beta$ TCR are cytolytic in function and secrete Th1 cytokines [123]. It has been hypothesized that these cells are primed to antigen in the Peyer's patches, enter the circulation through the mesenteric lymph nodes and the thoracic duct, and home to the lamina propria and intestinal epithelium of the small intestine and colon [127].

IELs that express the $\gamma\delta$ TCR, as well as those that express the $\alpha\beta$ TCR in conjunction with the CD8$\alpha\alpha$ homodimer, comprise the remaining half of the small-intestinal IEL population [123]. Unlike the $TCR\alpha\beta^+$ $CD8\alpha\beta^+$ IELs in the colon, these IEL subsets do not circulate through the lymphatics and blood and do not appear to be memory driven. Because they do not recognize antigen presented by MHC class I and class I-like molecules, it has been proposed that these $\gamma\delta$ IELs may be primed in situ by the epithelial cells, possibly through an autoantigen that is induced in response to infection or transformation events [128]. However, the identity and nature of this autoantigen remains unclear. A unique feature of $TCR\gamma\delta^+$ IELs is that, unlike $TCR\alpha\beta^+$ IELs, they can develop independently of the thymus, most likely within the intestinal cryptopatches [129].

Despite their proximity to the gut lumen, potential exposure to a variety of antigens, and the expectation that T cells normally express a diverse, polyclonal array of $\alpha\beta$ and $\gamma\delta$ TCRs, IELs within the small intestine and colon are oligoclonal and express only a small number of distinct $\alpha\beta$ and $\gamma\delta$ TCRs, based on an analysis of CDR3 regions [130,131]. A limited variety of T-cell clones is widely disseminated throughout the intestinal epithelium. The expression of CD8 by $\gamma\delta$ IELs suggests that they function biologically as cytolytic effectors in response to a limited number of antigens. Consistent with that, isolated IELs exhibit a high level of cytolytic activity in a variety of in vitro systems, especially after activation, and it is likely that they also do so in disease states in vivo. On activation, IELs may acquire cytolytic machinery that can contribute to epithelial cell death through apoptosis. Another biological function of $\gamma\delta$ IELs in health is the secretion of cytokines (e.g., IFN-γ and keratinocyte growth factor), which regulate epithelial cell function and possibly responses to luminal antigens [132]. Together, the cytolytic capabilities, large number, and extremely limited γδ TCR repertoire suggest that γδ IELs are a regionally specific population of cells involved in immunosurveillance against abnormal epithelial cells and maintenance of a normal epithelial barrier. IELs may be the first line of defense against deleterious epithelial events [133]. Their numbers are markedly increased in intestinal graft-versus-host disease, gluten-sensitive enteropathy, and protozoal infections of the epithelium, such as those caused by *Giardia*, *Cryptosporidium*, and *Isospora* species, underlining that IELs play a role in processes that disrupt the intestinal epithelium.

Organized lymphoid structures

Peyer's patches in the small intestine are the most clearly defined of the organized lymphoid structures in the gastrointestinal immune system. Of the ~100 developmentally determined Peyer's patches in humans, about half are located in the terminal ileum. They are located in mucosa and submucosa and are covered by the follicle-associated epithelium, which contains specialized M cells. These cells play an important role in mucosal immune surveillance by delivering luminal antigens to the organized mucosal lymphoid tissues. M cells are derived directly from undifferentiated, immature epithelial stem cells in the crypts. Their differentiation to mature follicle-associated epithelial M cells may be influenced by subjacent B cells within the lamina propria [134]. M cells have fewer, shorter, and wider microvilli than absorptive epithelial cells. Similar to the M cell antigen-sampling mechanism, dendritic cells found adjacent to intestinal epithelial cells can also directly sample luminal antigens across the epithelium by opening tight junctions and extending their dendrites into the lumen [71]. Although M cell antigen transport is important for induction of mucosal immune responses, this portal system also provides a means for pathogenic bacteria and viruses to enter the intestinal mucosa [135]. Among the many infectious agents known to undergo endocytosis and transport by way of M cells are the human immunodeficiency virus, rotavirus, reoviruses, *Salmonella*, and mycobacteria. M cells also transport commensal bacteria into the Peyer's patches, thereby initiating IgA antibody immune responses and tolerance.

Intestinal cryptopatches and isolated lymphoid follicles are two other organized lymphoid structures within the mucosal immune system. It is hypothesized that they, together with Peyer's patches, form a primary lymphoid organ. Cryptopatches are aggregates of immature T-cell precursors found adjacent to the crypts in mouse small intestine, are under the control of group 3 ILCs, and may be a site of extrathymic development of T lymphocytes [136]. The T-cell precursors residing in cryptopatches can differentiate into mature IELs expressing either the αβ TCR or the γδ TCR [137]. Isolated lymphoid follicles are organized lymphoid structures that are found in the small intestine and colon. Similar to Peyer's patches, they are covered by a follicle-associated epithelium containing M cells and are composed primarily of mature B2 B cells and $CD4^+$ T cells. Isolated lymphoid follicles are not developmentally fixed but can arise de novo in response to luminal stimulation under the influence of lymphotoxin and TNF-α signaling, as well as microbial signals that are delivered by NLRs including NOD1 [138].

Intestinal microbiota

The responsiveness and functions of the mucosal immune responses are determined by an interplay of host immune and nonimmune cells and the microorganisms that normally colonize the intestinal tract, making the microbiota a key nonhost cellular component in mucosal immunity. This section provides a brief overview of this topic as relevant to intestinal immune functions, whereas a more comprehensive discussion can be found in other chapters.

Intestinal microbiota is a collective term for the totality of bacteria, fungi, viruses, and other types of microorganisms that reside within the gut lumen. The intestinal microbiota has coevolved with the host mucosal immune system to form a symbiotic ecosystem, which is based on a close reciprocal interaction between the two. Although commensal microorganisms provide a plethora of antigens that could potentially stimulate cells of the GALT, the immune system has been trained to control its response via tolerogenic mechanisms. The microbiota provide signals that are necessary for proper development, education, and epigenetic regulation of many immune cells [139]. This is clearly demonstrated by comparing the gastrointestinal histology of rodents raised in germ-free conditions with those raised in conventional conditions. The villi in germ-free rodents are thinner and the crypts are shallower. Epithelial proliferation is diminished, and the time required for epithelial cells to migrate from the crypt to the villus tip is doubled. Germ-free rodents have fewer lymphocytes and macrophages in the intestinal mucosa, smaller Peyer's patches with fewer germinal centers, decreased numbers of IgA-producing plasma cells, and compromised isotype switching from IgM to IgA [140]. The induction of oral tolerance is also deficient in germ-free mice [141]. These abnormalities are restored by intestinal colonization of the mice with normal microbiota ("conventionalization") [142,143].

Although studies in germ-free animals consider intestinal microbiota as a single "organ," work based on monoassociation experiments shows that selected components of mucosal immunity may be regulated by individual strains of microorganisms. Both tolerogenic/regulatory and effector/inflammatory response are highly influenced by the predominant commensal species [144]. In particular, development of Treg cells is highly induced by noninvasive symbionts. For example, *Bacteroides fragilis* produces polysaccharide A, which induces conversion of $CD4^+$ T cells into $Foxp3^+$ Treg cells that produce IL-10, suppress IL-17, and protect against numerous inflammatory signals [145]. Similarly, *Clostridia* clusters IV and XIVa can enhance TGF-β1 production, leading to generation of IL-10-expressing $Foxp3^+$

Treg cells [146]. These effects may be associated with the ability of *Clostridia* to produce metabolically active substances such as short-chain fatty acids and tryptophan, which can induce Treg differentiation when sensed by their respective receptors, G-protein-coupled receptors and AhRs on T cells or dendritic cells. A similar increase in short-chain fatty acids via an intermediate step of lactic acid production was proposed as an explanation for the anti-inflammatory role of the genus *Lactobacillus* [147]. Another type of microbiota input on mucosa immunity is the Th17 polarization induced by segmented filamentous bacteria [148]. These bacteria localize in close apposition to the epithelium without deep invasion. Using serum amyloid A as an intermediate signal, they can induce secretion of TGF-β, IL-12, and IL-23 from local CD11c$^+$ DCs. This cytokine milieu upregulates RORγt expression by T cells and induces Th17 polarization. Although nominally proinflammatory, the effect is overall host protective by conferring resistance to enteric pathogens such as *C. rodentium*.

Regulators of gastrointestinal immunity

Immune responses in the gastrointestinal tract and systemic sites are highly regulated and tightly coordinated between different cell types. Although direct cell–cell contact occurs and plays a role in immune regulation, the major mediators of immune regulation are secreted cell products that influence other cells at various distances from the producer cells. Most prominent of these regulators is the group of cytokines, which are small proteins with specific receptor-mediated effects on multiple cell functions. A subset of cytokines is the interleukins, whose production and functions were thought to be restricted to leukocytes, but many of which are now recognized to be more broadly expressed and have functions beyond leukocytes. Another cytokine subset is chemokines that have primary functions in chemoattraction of target cells but also mediate other activities.

Cellular sources of cytokines include immune (e.g., lymphocytes and macrophages) and nonimmune cells (e.g., endothelium, epithelium, fibroblasts, and smooth muscle cells). These regulatory proteins have autocrine, paracrine, and endocrine functions and mediate a plethora of host responses, including those critical for immunity, inflammation, and hematopoiesis. Cytokines are produced de novo in response to immune stimulation. They generally act in a temporally and spatially limited manner at very low concentrations. Cytokines have a high level of redundancy in their effector functions, which include regulating the expression of membrane-bound proteins (including cytokine receptors) and the secretion of effector molecules [149], as well as cell proliferation and differentiation of target cells. This redundancy creates complex networks of cytokines that are difficult to classify. Cytokine function is largely context dependent, with the same cytokine exerting dichotomous effects when the local conditions change [150]. This is of particular importance in mucosal immunity because several cytokines have been shown to participate both in the preservation of homeostasis and in the induction or perpetuation of inflammation. In fact, the type and duration of antigenic stimulation, the cellular sources of the individual cytokine and its receptor, and the global immunological milieu wherein the immunological response takes place are all decisive factors for cytokine function and dictate the final outcome.

Classification schemes for cytokines have focused on their functional roles (e.g., effector vs regulatory molecules) and on the cells that produce them (e.g., Th1, Th2, Th17, and Treg for cytokines secreted by lymphocytes). For example, Th1 cells predominantly secrete IFN-γ and IL-2 and are associated with cell-mediated immunity; Th2 cells predominantly secrete IL-4, IL-5, and IL-13 and are associated with humoral and anti-helminthic immunity; Th17 cells predominantly secrete IL-17 and IL-22 and are associated with autoimmunity and extracellular bacterial responses; and Treg cells predominantly secrete IL-10 and TGF-β and are associated with suppression [151]. Despite the appeal of defining cytokines and T-cell clones in this manner, the pleiotropism and redundancy of cytokine action makes such classification problematic. For example, Th17 cells can switch from predominant IL-17 production to production of IFN-γ, a prototypic Th1 cytokine [152]. Moreover, besides T lymphocytes, the same cytokines may also be produced by other cell types, most importantly by ILCs, which follow a similar nomenclature (ILC1-3) based on the production of type 1, type 2, or type 17 cytokines. These issues are important considering the increased evidence that certain immune diseases, such as IBD, and inappropriate immune responses to certain infectious pathogens may be associated with distinct cytokine profiles.

The redundancy in cytokine effects is partly related to redundancy in their receptors, many of which are composed of common subunits shared between receptors. Cytokine receptors are grouped into families and exert their effects by activating intracellular signaling pathways within a target cell. The hematopoietic cytokine receptor (R) family includes many of the interleukin receptors. A common feature of these receptors is that they function as multimers with each other and other nonhematopoietic cytokine receptor family members, such as IL-2αR or IL-15αR. The IFN receptor family includes the receptors for type I (IFN-α and IFN-β) and type II IFN (IFN-γ); they share extracellular fibronectin-like domains with the hematopoietic cytokine receptors. Furthermore, some cytokines have more than one cognate receptor. For example, TNF-α has two receptors, tumor necrosis factor receptor p55 (TNFR1) and p75 (TNFR2), with mediate differential functions. Chemokine receptors are seven-membrane-spanning G-protein-linked receptors that are coupled to cell activation through calcium mobilization.

Homeostatic/anti-inflammatory cytokines

Several cytokines participate in maintaining homeostasis in the healthy gut by enhancing the epithelial barrier and/or regulating immunological responses against commensal microbiota and dietary antigens. Furthermore, cytokines also provide critical signals for the resolution of injury that follows acute insults and restitution of barrier integrity.

IL-10

The cytokine IL-10 is a prototypical regulatory cytokine with a prominent anti-inflammatory role. Its importance is clearly demonstrated by the development of early-onset intestinal inflammation in patients bearing mutations in the IL-10 gene, *IL10*, or the IL-10 receptor genes, *IL10RA* or *IL10RB* [153], as well as the development of spontaneous colitis in mice that lack *Il10* or *Il10r* [154]. IL-10 is primarily produced by $CD4^+$ T cells, in particular the main Treg cell populations, $Foxp3^-$ Tr1 and $Foxp3^+$ [155]. The regulatory function of IL-10 is exerted via suppression of effector T-cell responses and induction of an anti-inflammatory macrophage phenotype [156]. Subepithelial mononuclear phagocytes are also capable of IL-10 secretion when stimulated by signals from commensals, thus promoting intestinal tolerance [145].

IL-22

The IL-10 family member IL-22 has protective functions in the intestinal mucosa [157]. Main cellular sources of IL-22 are Th17 cells, ILC3s, and $\gamma\delta$ T cells. During intestinal inflammation, however, additional cell populations may become avid IL-22 producers, such as neutrophils, which were shown to be the main $IL\text{-}22^+$ population in a mouse model of infectious colitis [158]. Production of IL-22 is strongly induced by IL-23. Signals from the commensal microbiota, including those mediated via the AhR, upregulate IL-22 expression. Patients with Crohn's disease have significantly decreased intestinal expression of AhR, which might compromise IL-22 induction [159]. It was further shown that Th17 cells and IL-22 production can be stimulated by subsets of commensal bacteria (segmented filamentous bacteria) [148]. Similarly, commensal bacteria induce the production of IL-22 from ILC3s. Once upregulated, IL-22 acts downstream to confer epithelial protection by maintaining the epithelial tight junctions, strengthening the epithelial barrier via STAT3-mediated signaling in epithelial cells and stimulating the secretion of antimicrobial peptides [160].

TGF-β1

TGF-β1, an abundant cytokine, has a major role in controlling regulatory responses in the intestinal mucosa. It is produced by and acts on many cell types. TGF-β1 signaling in T cells is pivotal for the peripheral induction of $Foxp3^+$ Treg cells and development of tolerance [161]. Similar to IL-10, mutations in the *Tgfb1* gene lead to IBD-like intestinal inflammation in mice. Patients with Crohn's disease display high intestinal expression of TGF-β1, although this is paradoxically combined with defective TGF-β1 signaling because of increased levels of the inhibitory protein, Smad7, which blocks the phosphorylation of TGF-β1 transcriptional proteins Smad2 and Smad3 [162]. Nevertheless, restoring of the transcriptional deregulation via an antisense SMAD7 blocker failed to provide sustained clinical benefit in patients with Crohn's disease [163]. It should be noted that the broad functional spectrum of TGF-β1, which also includes a strong profibrotic effect, greatly impedes its clinical utility in treating inflammatory conditions.

IL-2

IL-2 is a classical T cell-produced cytokine that is required for the expansion and activation of T cells in an autocrine and paracrine fashion. This observation led to the initial hope that blockade might attenuate intestinal inflammation. However, targeting of IL-2 signaling with a biologic, daclizumab, has shown no efficacy in IBD, and loss of IL-2 in gene-targeted mice leads to spontaneous colitis [164,165]. The inflammation-suppressing functions of the cytokine are likely to be related to the ability of IL-2 to promote the development and function of $Foxp3^+$ Treg cells, which highly express the IL-2 receptor α (CD25) [166].

IFN-α/β

Although long recognized for their importance in antiviral defense, IFN-β and the different isoforms of IFN-α, collectively termed type I IFNs, have also been shown to exert protective properties at the intestinal mucosa [167,168]. IFN-α and IFN-β are produced by mononuclear phagocytes and confer protection via two separate pathways. On the one hand, acting through STAT1 and STAT2, they inhibit epithelial cell apoptosis; on the other hand, they induce secretion of anti-inflammatory cytokines and enhance Treg cell functions. Polymorphisms in the type I IFN receptor gene, *IFNAR1*, have been described in patients with IBD [169].

IL-35

IL-35 belongs to the IL-12 family of cytokines and is a heterodimer of the p35 subunit of IL-12 and the Epstein–Barr virus-induced gene 3 subunit (EBI3), which is also known as IL-27b [170]. IL-35 binds to its receptor consisting of IL-12Rβ2 and gp130 chains. The anti-inflammatory function of IL-35 is related to its close association with Treg cell populations, which appear to be its only source. In fact, nTreg cells produce IL-35, which, in turn, enhances their suppressive ability [171]. Furthermore, IL-35 signaling suppresses effector T-cell responses and induces the formation of a specific IL-35-dependent Treg cell population that also expresses Foxp3, IL-10, and TGF-β. In line with these inhibitory properties, $Foxp3^+$ Treg cells lacking IL-35 were unable to suppress adoptively transferred colitis in mice [171]. Thus, IL-35 may provide a potential therapeutic option for diseases that are characterized by exaggerated proinflammatory responses, including IBD.

Proinflammatory cytokines

Microbial attack or genetic defects can lead to a breach in the epithelial barrier, which causes an influx of an enormous number of foreign antigens into the mucosa. Immune cells respond to this challenge with a counterattack aiming to clear the triggering factors and reestablish homeostasis. Proinflammatory cytokines participate in every phase of this process. Only when the process is compromised, either because of defective clearance or persistence of the external insult, may chronic inflammation ensue that results in continuous injury to the gut and persistent disease.

TNF-α

The prototypic proinflammatory cytokine, TNF-α, was the first to be exploited for therapeutic purposes in patients with IBD with chronic intestinal inflammation. It is a pleiotropic cytokine that is produced by many cell types and signals to a variety of cellular targets that bear its receptors, TNFR1 and TNFR2. Its proinflammatory potential is indisputably proved by the development of chronic inflammation in mice with TNF overproduction as a result of compromised posttranscriptional regulation of TNF-α ($TNF^{\Delta ARE}$ mice) [172]. Signaling via TNFR2 on $CD4^+$ T cells after binding to membrane-bound TNF-α on $CD14^+$ cells promotes survival of proinflammatory T cells by preventing apoptosis [173]. At the same time, TNF induces apoptosis of epithelial cells, thus exerting a deleterious effect on barrier integrity [174]. Unsurprisingly, monoclonal antibodies against TNF have been a classic example of cytokine-targeted therapies in gastroenterological immune-mediated diseases. Several anti-TNF antibodies (infliximab, adalimumab, golimumab, and certolizumab pegol) are routinely used for patients with active Crohn's disease and ulcerative colitis [175–177]. The therapeutic success of these agents underscores the importance of proinflammatory cytokines as mediators of gastrointestinal inflammation.

Other TNF superfamily members

Although TNF and its receptor are the prototypical proteins of the TNF/TNFR superfamilies of cytokines, other members of these groups, such as the TL1A/DR3 cytokine/receptor pair, are also of relevance for mucosal immunity [178]. Expression of TL1A is inducible under inflammatory conditions. Its expression by APCs allows for interaction with DR3, which is primarily expressed on activated lymphocytes, providing costimulatory signals under low-level basal stimulation [179]. Thus, these proteins may be of importance during the chronic phase of inflammatory responses. Of particular importance, TL1A is preferentially expressed at mucosal tissues, and its overexpression leads to chronic intestinal inflammation. Furthermore, genetic variants of *TNFSF15*, the gene that encodes for the TL1A protein, have been associated with various intestinal diseases, including IBD, diverticulitis, and IBS, further underscoring the importance of the TL1A/DR3 system in mucosal immune regulation [178].

IL-1/IL-18/IL-33

The IL-1 family of cytokines consists of 11 members (IL-1α, IL-1β, IL-1Ra, IL-18, IL-33, IL-36α, IL-36β, IL-36γ, IL-36RA, IL-37, and IL-38), which signal via heterodimeric receptors. IL-1 binds to IL-1RI, IL-33 to T1/ST2, and IL-36 to IL-1Rrp2, and all recruit the same coreceptor, IL-1R accessory protein (IL-1RAcP). IL-18 signals through a heterodimer consisting of the IL-18Rα and the coreceptor IL-18Rβ. The biological effects of IL-1 are tightly regulated by naturally produced inhibitors, such as the receptor antagonist, IL-1Ra, which specifically inhibits the proinflammatory actions of IL-1 by competitively binding to IL-1Rs on target cells without exerting agonistic effects. Further attenuation of IL-1 activity occurs through the decoy receptor, IL-1R type II (IL-1RII), and the inhibitory receptors SIGIRR and IL-1RacPb [180]. Downstream signaling by IL-1 involves nuclear factor κ-light-chain-enhancer of activated B cells and MyD88, and leads to induction of other cytokines, thus amplifying the proinflammatory action during intestinal inflammation. Mucosal expression and production of IL-1 by lamina propria mononuclear cells is elevated in active IBD and correlates with the severity of inflammation. Interestingly, a marked decrease in the mucosal IL-1Ra/IL-1 ratio was found in both Crohn's disease and ulcerative colitis, suggesting an insufficiency of inhibitory signals during chronic inflammation [181]. Although the proinflammatory role of cytokines of the IL-1 family is well established, a critical characteristic of these proteins appears to be a dichotomous function that highly depends on the specific conditions and the stage of the inflammatory process [182].

IL-33 provides a typical example when studying its effects in acute chemical colitis. During the colitis induction stage, IL-33 acts in a proinflammatory fashion, because blockade of its signaling suppresses inflammation [183]. In contrast, during the resolution/restitution phase, IL-33 is necessary for effective tissue repair. Furthermore, an anti-inflammatory role of IL-33 has also been proposed via its positive effect on $Foxp3^+$ Treg cells. A two-phasic function has also been attributed to IL-18. During the acute phase of inflammation, epithelial cell-derived IL-18 acts in an autocrine manner to produce IL-11, which promotes epithelial barrier integrity. As inflammation progresses, however, IL-18 acts on IL-18R-bearing immune cells and synergizes with IL-2 and IL-12, to induce production of IFN-γ and proinflammatory Th1 responses. Similar to IL-1, the proinflammatory activity of IL-18 is tightly controlled by a soluble cytokine receptor, IL-18 binding protein (IL-18BP), which is produced by macrophages and endothelial cells under inflammatory conditions and competitively binds and neutralizes secreted IL-18 [184].

IFN-γ

IFN-γ is the only known type II IFN and the prototype cytokine of the Th1 lineage. It plays a critical role in host immunity against pathogenic intracellular microorganisms. IFN-γ is produced by T lymphocytes and NK/ILC1 cells, although production by macrophages has also been suggested. IFN-γ acts on macrophages, inducing their activation and polarization toward a proinflammatory (M1) phenotype. It also induces the expression of class II MHC molecules on APCs. Besides its indisputable role in infection immunity, increased IFN-γ activity has also been implicated in the pathogenesis of chronic inflammatory states of the gastrointestinal tract. In particular, IFN-γ and Th1 immunity are believed to have a prominent role in Crohn's disease [185]. Lamina propria T cells from patients with Crohn's disease secrete increased amounts of IFN-γ, which is paralleled by elevated mucosal expression of the Th1-related, IL-12/IFN-γ-inducible factors, STAT 4, T-bet, and IL-12Rβ2 [186]. Interestingly, the secretion of IFN-γ from CD4+ T cells isolated from the mesenteric lymph nodes of patients with Crohn's disease was 40-fold higher than the secretion of IL-17 [187], emphasizing the critical proinflammatory role of IFN-γ in the disease. Nonetheless, Th17 cells also contribute to the production of mucosal IFN-γ by upregulating expression of T-bet in T cells, thus becoming Th1/Th17 or Th1 ex-Th17 cells [188].

IL-4/IL-5/IL-13

The Th2 cytokines, IL-4, IL-5 and IL-13, have evolved as a protective mechanism against intestinal infection by multicellular metazoan parasites of mammals, also known as helminths. Their principal functions include induction of smooth muscle hypercontractility, enhanced mucous secretion, and induction of intestinal mastocytosis, all of which contribute to worm killing and expulsion. In parallel, these Th2 mediators are also involved in postinjury repair. However, when Th2 immunity becomes dysregulated, it may lead to deleterious consequences, such as unrelenting inflammation and/or excessive collagen deposition and fibrosis [189]. Abnormal Th2 responses are considered central to the pathogenesis of ulcerative colitis, with IL-13-producing NK T cells being pivotal mediators of the inflammatory process [190]. Furthermore, an exaggerated, allergic Th2-mediated immune response may underlie the pathogenesis of eosinophilic esophagitis. This disease is characterized by accumulation of eosinophils, mast cells, and T cells in the esophageal mucosa [191–193], accompanied by elevated production of several Th2 mediators of inflammation, including IL-5, IL-13, and IL-15, eotaxin, TGF-β, and fibroblast growth factor [194–196]. The role of eotaxin-3 in disease pathogenesis was discovered in genome-wide microarray studies that identified a remarkably conserved eosinophilic esophagitis transcriptome across sex, age, and allergic or nonallergic phenotypes [197]. The prominent Th2 responses that take place in eosinophilic esophagitis have led to efforts to exploit them therapeutically. Several monoclonal antibodies that target the Th2 effectors, IL-5 and IL-13, have been tested in clinical trials and resulted in amelioration of histological lesions, although without demonstrating a clear clinical benefit [198].

IL-17/IL-23

Cytokines of the Th17 axis have proinflammatory functions, with IL-17 isoforms and IL-23 being the main representatives. The discovery of IL-23 was a major breakthrough in immunology, because it was realized that experimental models of chronic inflammation that were initially considered IL-12 dependent were in fact mediated by IL-23 signaling. Because IL-12 (p40/p35) and IL-23 (p40/p19) share one common chain, antibodies against p40 simultaneously block both cytokines, making it difficult to dissect Th1- and Th17-mediated pathways. When individual cytokines are eliminated, it appears that IL-23 is the major force for experimental intestinal inflammation [199]. In later studies, however, it was shown that Th17 cells are characterized by plasticity, being capable of changing their transcriptomic program to adopt mixed Th1/Th17 or even Th1-predominant phenotypes with high production of IFN-γ [200]. The translational significance of these experimental observations is reflected in the shift from IL-12/23 blockade (with anti-p40 monoclonal antibodies such as ustekinumab) to specific anti-IL23/anti-p19 blockade for the treatment of immune-mediated disease, including IBD [201]. Contrary to the undisputable proinflammatory function of IL-23, IL-17 appears to have a more complicated role in intestinal inflammation, because anti-IL17 blockade has failed to exert beneficial effects in patients with Crohn's disease [202]. These observations indicate that the function of IL-17 is highly context and tissue dependent and may involve both proinflammatory and anti-inflammatory actions.

Chemokines

The term *chemokine* was derived from the words "chemoattractant" and "cytokine" to define members of a superfamily of cytokines, whose primary function is the regulation of cellular movement in different locations and environments. There are currently 48 identified chemokine ligands (indicated by an "L" suffix at the end) that signal through 19 G-protein-coupled chemokine receptors (indicated by an "R" suffix) [203]. Movement to a specific location is accomplished when cells that express a specific chemokine receptor migrate along a chemokine gradient that occurs in that location. When a certain chemokine concentration is reached, the process is slowed down and eventually terminated either via downregulation of the receptor or desensitization. At this point other chemokine ligand/receptor pairs may take over to complete the movement of the particular cell [204,205].

The molecular structure of chemokines includes four conserved cysteine residues that form two disulfide bonds, which pair the first with the third and the second with the fourth cysteine. Based on the arrangement of the two N-terminal cysteine residues, chemokine ligands are classified into four groups [206]. In CC chemokines, the first two cysteines are adjacent; in CXC chemokines, they are separated by one amino acid; XC chemokines lack the first and third cysteines; finally, in the only described CX3C chemokine, CX3CL1 (also termed fractalkine), three amino acids separate the two first N-terminal cysteines. The subfamily of the chemokine also dictates the nomenclature of the chemokine receptors, which are grouped into four subfamilies [207]. Although interactions between chemokines and their receptors generally follow their subclassification patterns (i.e., CXCL chemokines activate only CXCR receptors and CCLs usually activate CCRs), significant promiscuity exists [208]. Indeed, some chemokines can bind and activate more than one receptor. Similarly, one chemokine receptor may be activated by binding to multiple ligands. The high homology between members of the family may be one explanation for this promiscuity. However, from the evolutionary perspective this may be an immunological redundancy to ensure effective leukocyte response to inflammatory insults. Ligand sharing may not always be agonistic but can also lead to competitive inhibition. More recently, a subgroup of four "atypical" chemokine receptors was described that does not mediate strong chemotactic effects [209]. These receptors may act as decoys either by scavenging and removing excess chemokines or by attenuating binding affinity to other chemokine receptors by forming heterodimers.

Chemokines are further classified into "homeostatic" and "inflammatory" subcategories, although overlapping, "dual-function" chemokines exist. The homeostatic chemokines are constitutively expressed and via binding to their receptors secure a consistent and dynamic leukocyte composition in the various tissues. They navigate leukocytes during hematopoiesis in the bone marrow and thymus, during initiation of adaptive immune responses in secondary lymphoid organs, and in immune surveillance of healthy peripheral tissues. Tissue-specific expression also occurs for homeostatic chemokines, allowing for trafficking of leukocytes to specific locations [210]. Relevant examples include CCL27-CCR10 interactions for skin homing, CXCL12-CXCR421 for the brain, CCL25-CCR9 for the small intestine, and CXCL12-CXCR4 for the bone marrow. The inflammatory chemokines are inducible under inflammatory conditions and control the recruitment of effector leukocytes in infection, inflammation, tissue injury, and tumors. Highly diverse host- or pathogen-associated stimuli, which include various cytokines and TLR-mediated signals, have been shown to induce the expression of proinflammatory chemokines [211].

The molecular evolution of each subclass of chemokines appears to be different. Genes that encode for inflammatory cytokines are clustered in specific genome locations, with the CC "inflammatory" chemokines located in a human chromosome 17 cluster and the CXC "inflammatory" chemokines on chromosome 4 [203]. In contrast, genes encoding homeostatic cytokines are located in distinct genetic locations away from the clusters. This may indicate that the evolution of inflammatory chemokines was much more dynamic, because they were selected to provide evolutionary advantages critical for the protection against infectious threats [206]. As species diverted from each other, such "infectious experience" became different, and this may explain why inflammatory chemokines are not well preserved between species.

Four chemokines, namely, CCL25, CCL28, CXCL14, and CXCL17, are considered "mucosal" chemokines based on their intestinal expression pattern and importance for homeostatic leukocyte trafficking to mucosal sites [212]. In particular, CCL25 is preferentially expressed in the small intestine and involved in trafficking of T lymphoblasts that have been imprinted in mesenteric lymph nodes and bear the gut-homing molecules CCR9 and integrin $\alpha4\beta7$. CCL28 is expressed in the human colon and mediates the trafficking of IgA^+ plasmablasts, which bear the receptor CCR10.

GM-CSF

Development of specific subsets of hematopoietic cells in the bone marrow is controlled by several growth factors (historically named "colony-stimulating factors" [CSF] because of their ability to induce clonal colonies from single precursor cells in soft agar; the target cells are abbreviated as a prefix, such as G for granulocytes and M for macrophages). Among these factors, GM-CSF is relatively unique because it also affects the function of mature leukocytes, thus acting as a cytokine. Its role during intestinal inflammation remains elusive, although both protective and inflammatory effects have been described, depending on the specific conditions. In IL-23-dependent colitis, hematopoiesis and accumulation of granulocyte-monocyte progenitors is dysregulated. Neutralization of GM-CSF prevents these changes and ameliorates colitis [213]. This effect was subsequently shown to be associated with blockade of the stimulatory effect of GM-CSF on eosinophils [214]. Thus, IL-23-induced GM-CSF production by Th17 lymphocytes and ILC3s appears to be an important proinflammatory component of experimental colitis by activating recruitment of inflammatory monocytes and dendritic cells to the intestine [215]. A protective role, however, has also been proposed for GM-CSF, particularly in the context of Crohn's disease, in which a primary deficiency of innate immunity may exist. In such a scenario, administration of exogenous GM-CSF may stimulate innate immune responses and provide therapeutic effects. In fact, this has been used therapeutically for patients with rare human immunodeficiencies of innate cell function [216]. Furthermore, in patients with sporadic Crohn's disease, autoantibodies against GM-CSF have been detected and shown to correlate with disease severity [217]. These observations have led to the clinical testing of the safety and effectiveness of recombinant human GM-CSF in patients with Crohn's disease. So far, results from these studies have been inconclusive.

Lipid mediators of inflammation

Prostaglandins, leukotrienes, and platelet-activating factor are referred to collectively as lipid mediators of inflammation. These mediators are produced under many circumstances by the same cell types in response to similar stimuli. Although the lipid mediators are structurally distinct, they have many overlapping biological effects. Prostaglandins and leukotrienes are the products of arachidonic acid metabolism and are referred to as eicosanoids [218,219]. Prostaglandins are produced through the cyclooxygenase (COX) pathway, whereas leukotrienes are produced through the 5-lipoxygenase pathway. Two distinct

COXs are involved in prostaglandin synthesis. COX-1 is a constitutive enzyme found in most mammalian cell types. In the gastrointestinal tract, COX-1 is expressed in lamina propria mononuclear cells, fibroblasts, muscle cells, epithelial cells, and vascular endothelial cells. COX-2 is expressed in macrophages, fibroblasts, epithelial cells, and other cell types in response to various stimuli, including IL-1, TNF-α, and other proinflammatory cytokines.

Under most circumstances, the rate-limiting step in the synthesis of prostaglandins is the availability of arachidonic acid. Under basal conditions, cells have almost no free arachidonic acid. The activation of phospholipases (particularly phospholipase A_2) makes arachidonate available by releasing it from membrane phospholipids. A wide variety of stimuli can activate phospholipase A_2, resulting in the release of arachidonate. For example, phagocytosis in macrophages stimulates phospholipase A_2, as do receptor-mediated events, such as the binding of bradykinin to its receptor. Activation of phospholipase typically results in the rapid release of arachidonate and the production of prostaglandins within a few seconds up to 1–2 minutes. Synthesis of prostaglandins can also be increased by the infiltration of prostaglandin-producing cells into the gastrointestinal tract. For example, the large increase in prostaglandin levels in IBD may reflect the trafficking of prostaglandin-producing monocytes and macrophages into the lamina propria. A third mechanism for the regulation of prostaglandin production is increased synthesis of COX enzymes. COX-2 can be induced by proinflammatory cytokines (e.g., IL-1, TNF-α) and phorbol esters and occurs over several hours. Thus, the regulation of prostaglandin production by induction of COX-2 occurs over a longer time frame than the regulation of prostaglandin production by phospholipase activation.

Prostaglandins

Among the products of arachidonic acid metabolism through the COX pathway are PGE_2, thromboxane A_2, and prostacyclin. PGE_2 is made by macrophages, epithelial cells, and fibroblasts, and has several biological functions that suggest a role in inflammation and tumor growth. The binding of PGE_2 to its receptors, EP1–4, initiates a signaling cascade that controls cell proliferation and migration, apoptosis, and angiogenesis. PGE_2 is also capable of stimulating tumor metastasis and inhibiting tumor surveillance through the downregulation of cytokine production and NK cell activity. Epidemiological studies of colorectal cancer have demonstrated that the use of nonsteroidal anti-inflammatory drugs (NSAIDs), which block COX activity and PGE_2 production, are associated with a lower incidence of colorectal adenomas and cancer [220,221]. These studies point to a link between chronic inflammation and the subsequent development of malignancy and have resulted in the use of NSAIDs as chemopreventive agents for patients who are at high risk for development of colorectal cancer, including patients with ulcerative colitis, familial adenomatous polyposis, or hereditary nonpolyposis colon cancer [222].

Elevated PGE_2 levels in ulcerative colitis are associated with enhanced COX-2 expression in epithelial cells [223]. In many inflammatory diseases, NSAIDs diminish inflammation and relieve clinical symptoms; however, in ulcerative colitis, NSAIDs can exacerbate clinical activity, pointing to an important protective role of prostaglandins in the intestinal tract. Newer NSAIDs (e.g., celecoxib, rofecoxib) selectively block COX-2 production and were hypothesized to have better safety profiles than the original inhibitors, which block both COX-1 and COX-2; however, large clinical trials of both drugs have shown that long-term use of both groups of drugs is associated with an increased risk for cardiovascular events [224].

Leukotrienes

Production of leukotrienes is dependent on the 5-lipoxygenase pathway. The cellular distribution of 5-lipoxygenase is much more limited than that of COX-1 and COX-2. LTB_4, a potent neutrophil chemoattractant, is produced by neutrophils, macrophages, and mast cells. The peptidyl-leukotrienes (LTC_4, LTD_4, and LTE_4) are made in macrophages, mast cells, and eosinophils. They increase vascular permeability and induce vasoconstriction and smooth muscle contraction, and they may induce epithelial Cl^- secretion. Inflamed mucosa from patients with Crohn's disease and ulcerative colitis contains markedly elevated levels of LTB_4 [225], and analysis of neutrophil chemotaxis in ulcerative colitis showed that LTB_4 is a major neutrophil chemoattractant; however, randomized controlled trials in which 5-lipoxygenase inhibitors were used as single therapeutic agents have not shown benefits in treating ulcerative colitis [226].

Platelet-activating factor

Platelet-activating factor (PAF) is a phosphatidylcholine with an ether-linked alcohol fatty acid on the first carbon and an acyl-linked acetyl group on the second carbon. No intracellular stores exist for PAF, so its synthesis must be initiated by the remodeling of phosphatidylcholine through the activation of phospholipase A_2. PAF is made by neutrophils, macrophages, mast cells, and eosinophils, and it is often produced in parallel with prostaglandins and leukotrienes. The biological effects of PAF include enhanced vascular permeability, vasoconstriction, platelet aggregation, neutrophil chemotaxis, smooth muscle contraction, and epithelial Cl^- secretion. Many of these biological effects overlap with those of prostaglandins and leukotrienes. PAF is rapidly degraded to the inactive metabolite, lyso-PAF, by the enzyme acetylhydrolase, which is produced in both intracellular and secreted forms. Intestinal epithelial cells secrete acetylhydrolase, which may be an important mechanism for the defense of the gastrointestinal tract against excessive PAF actions [227].

Resolvins

Another, less well-characterized class of lipid mediators are the resolvins (short for resolution phase interaction products), which have an important role in resolution of inflammatory processes. Failure to restore homeostasis after an inflammatory insult may result in fibrosis and scarring and persistence of inflammation. In the context of experimental colitis, omega-3 polyunsaturated fatty acids, including eicosapentaenoic acid and docosahexaenoic acid, lead to the production of the lipid mediator resolvins. The resolvins have been shown to halt the influx of neutrophils [228] and macrophages [229] and to downregulate inflammatory pathways and the production of proinflammatory cytokines and chemokines [230]. Resolvin-E1 is derived from eicosapentaenoic acid and has been shown to decrease inflammation in 2,4,6-trinitrobenzene sulfonic acid-induced colitis [231].

Nitric oxide

Nitric oxide is a small (30-Da) biologically active compound formed when nitric oxide synthase (NOS) oxidizes the guanidine nitrogen of arginine. The biological effects of nitric oxide include actions as a vasodilator, a neurotransmitter, and an important component of the inflammatory response [232,233]. The three distinct isoforms of NOS differ in their cofactor requirements, tissue distribution, transcriptional regulation, and posttranscriptional modification.

Neuronal NOS (nNOS, NOS1)

The NOS isoform neuronal NOS (nNOS) is constitutively expressed in neuronal tissue. The nitric oxide produced by nNOS is the principal nonadrenergic noncholinergic neurotransmitter in the gastrointestinal tract. nNOS is found in enteric nerves in the myenteric plexus and circular muscle, and it is present in neurons containing vasoactive intestinal polypeptide [234]. Nitric oxide produced by nNOS participates in the control of peristalsis and sphincter function in the gut. Impaired nitric oxide production through nNOS may contribute to several disorders of bowel motility, including achalasia, functional dyspepsia, diabetic gastroparesis, infantile hypertrophic pyloric stenosis, and intestinal pseudoobstruction [235]. Loss of nNOS in animal models compromises intestinal defenses against lumen-dwelling pathogens that require intestinal hypermotility for clearance [236].

Endothelial NOS (eNOS, NOS3)

The isoform endothelial NOS (eNOS) is also constitutively expressed and was originally found in endothelial cells, although it is also present in epithelial cells, smooth muscle cells, platelets, and T cells. Nitric oxide produced by endothelial cells relaxes vascular smooth muscle cells and dilates the vasculature. Inhibition of eNOS in vivo; causes an increase in blood pressure, so hypertension is the major adverse effect of nonspecific NOS inhibitors. Both eNOS and nNOS synthesize nitric oxide in relatively small quantities.

Inducible NOS (iNOS, NOS2)

Unlike nNOS and eNOS, which are constitutively expressed, the third NOS isoform, iNOS, can be induced by proinflammatory cytokines (e.g., IL-1, TNF-α, IFN-γ), bacterial lipopolysaccharide, and invasive bacteria in macrophages and epithelial cells [237,238]. iNOS is produced in nanomolar concentrations compared with nNOS and eNOS, which are produced in picomolar concentrations. Therefore, iNOS produces nitric oxide in quantities that greatly exceed those required for its physiological function as a vasodilator or neurotransmitter. In addition, nitric oxide production by iNOS is delayed for several hours after stimulation but remains active for up to 5 days. In macrophages, the large quantity of nitric oxide produced by iNOS is used for killing bacteria and tumor cells. Nitric oxide works in conjunction with reactive oxygen species (i.e., hydroxyl radical, superoxide, and hydrogen peroxide) generated within phagosomes to kill phagocytosed bacteria.

Despite its clear association with inflammatory states, it remains unclear whether nitric oxide plays a pathogenic or protective role during intestinal inflammation [233]. Many studies have demonstrated that the biological effects of nitric oxide are organ specific and vary depending on the amount, the timing of production, and the particular inflammatory state. Administration of nitric oxide donors is protective to the intestinal mucosa and results in maintenance of blood flow, inhibition of platelets and leukocyte adhesion, downregulation of mast cell reactivity, and reduction of superoxide-induced damage. However, increased production of iNOS-induced nitric oxide by intestinal epithelial cells is associated with prolonged colonic inflammation. Studies using animal models of colitis have generated interesting hypotheses regarding the complex role of nitric oxide in intestinal inflammation. Models of chemically induced colitis that used NOS inhibitors to block nitric oxide production produced conflicting results: nitric oxide either improved or exacerbated the colitis [239–241]. Time-dependent studies of endotoxin-induced vascular damage have shown that early administration of NOS inhibitors results in increased tissue damage, whereas late administration results in a dose-dependent reduction in damage [242]. The specific NOS isoform has also been proposed to be a factor influencing the beneficial or pathogenic effects of nitric oxide in intestinal inflammation. However, studies using mice that lack specific NOS isoforms have produced conflicting results [243,244]. A possible explanation may be that iNOS-induced nitric oxide is protective during the early phases of acute inflammation, but that continuous high-level production during chronic inflammation contributes to inflammation.

Control of mucosal homeostasis and inflammation

The human gastrointestinal tract is the largest immunological compartment of the host that lies in close proximity to an enormous number of intraluminal non-self antigens, arising from commensal microorganisms, diet constituents, and other environmental inputs. Thus, from the immunological perspective, the gut mucosa can be considered a "danger zone" within which immune reactivity and inflammatory responses are a constant possibility. To avoid such unfavorable outcomes while maintaining its critical functions, the intestine is remarkably equipped with multifaceted and overlapping control mechanisms. These are responsible for inducing active tolerance against microbiota and food components, whereas, at the same time, maintaining the ability for defense against pathogens. These properties underlie the state of intestinal *mucosal homeostasis*, which, contrary to other tissues, refers to controlled immune responsiveness, rather than the complete absence of it. Maintenance of mucosal homeostasis requires the sequential and coordinated application of checkpoint mechanisms that regulate the interaction between the GALT and the plethora of bacterial and food material that resides within the intestinal lumen and may reach the bowel wall. The distinctive characteristics of intestinal homeostasis are reflected in the concept of "physiological inflammation" that has been long recognized as typical of healthy intestinal tissue. This term refers to the presence of significant numbers of activated immunocytes within the intestinal lamina propria in the absence of overt clinicopathological inflammation or its consequences.

General outline of mucosal immune responses

To achieve the controlled state of immune activation characteristic of the healthy small intestine and colon, antigen encounters and uptake, and the consequent activation and migration of immune cells, are highly choreographed (Figure 14.9). Generally, the process begins by transportation of antigens and microorganisms from the lumen by M cells and other epithelial cells into the lamina propria, where they come into contact with lymphocytes, macrophages, and dendritic cells in lymphoid aggregates or Peyer's patches below the M cells. Some of these immune cells enter the intraepithelial pocket, a large invaginated subdomain on the basolateral surface of the M cell that forms a docking site for specific populations of lymphocytes and occasionally dendritic cells, and that effectively shortens the distance that antigen-containing transcytotic vesicles must travel to cross the epithelial barrier [245]. Antigens that have crossed the epithelium are captured by a vast network of immature dendritic cells that exists in the subepithelial regions, particularly in the dome or apical portion of the lymphoid follicles immediately below the follicle-associated epithelium. The dendritic cells process the antigens and present them to naive lymphocytes either in the intestinal lymphoid follicles or, upon migration, in the mesenteric lymph nodes. A specific mucosal immune response is initiated by these interactions, which may preferentially direct naive T cells to a specific Th phenotype [246]. The particular Th lineage commitment is a consequence of the properties of the dendritic cells within the lamina propria and Peyer's patches and plays an important role under homeostatic conditions in generating mucosal tolerance as opposed to an aggressive immune response.

On activation in the lamina propria, lymphocytes begin a maturational journey from intestinal lymphoid follicles to afferent lymphatics that drain into the mesenteric lymph nodes [247,248] (see Figure 14.9). During this process, the lymphocytes mature into T and B lymphoblasts enriched in IgA-bearing B cells. The B lymphocytes become surface IgA-bearing lymphoblasts after being induced to switch their immunoglobulin isotype by regulatory (i.e., "switch") T cells within the Peyer's patches [249,250]. Lymphocytes then enter the efferent lymphatics of the mesenteric lymph nodes and pass through the thoracic duct into the peripheral blood. These lymphocytes subsequently reenter the gastrointestinal tract through interactions with flat endothelial cells of the postcapillary venules and home to the lamina propria. B lymphoblasts mature into IgA-secreting plasma cells under the control of antigen-activated T cells that have completed a similar maturational journey. Lymphoblasts that have homed to the gastrointestinal mucosa and matured into effector cells provide protective immunity within the lamina propria. Recirculating lymphocytes can also seed other mucosal sites and organs beyond those of the initial antigen encounter, which confers antigen-specific immune capabilities to all these sites and provides the basis for the concept of the common mucosal immune system [251].

In addition to the recirculation of lymphocyte, other leukocyte subsets, particularly neutrophils and monocytes, are recruited de novo from the systemic circulation to the mucosa, where they fulfill dedicated effector functions in host defense and subsequently either die or are shed in the lumen. This cell influx is particularly prominent in states of heightened immune and inflammatory activation.

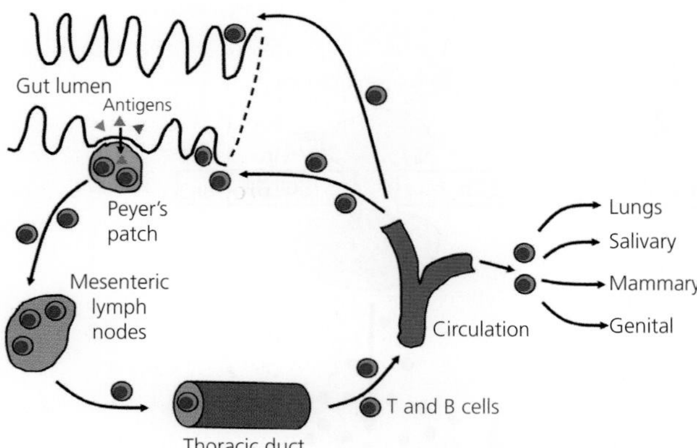

Figure 14.9 Leukocyte recirculation and the common mucosal immune system. Antigen is transported across the epithelium, particularly M cells overlying Peyer's patches, and taken up by dendritic cells, which migrate to lymphoid follicles in the Peyer's patches or the mesenteric lymph nodes and locally activate immature B and T cells. On activation, the B and T cells migrate through the mesenteric lymph nodes and into the draining thoracic duct and the systemic circulation. Specific surface adhesion molecules induced during initial activation allow targeting of the mature, effector B and T cells from the circulation to mucosal sites, including the intestinal lamina propria, as well as other mucosal organs. Sources: Dunkley and Husband 1987 [248] and Farstad et al. 1997 [247].

Immune cell trafficking

Central to the function of the mucosal immune system is the extensive and highly controlled migration of different subsets of leukocytes between the intestinal mucosa and various systemic way station. Multiple factors are involved in facilitating such movements, including chemokines (discussed earlier) that form chemotactic gradients and adhesion molecules on leukocytes and endothelial cells that allow precise tissue targeting.

Cell adhesion molecules

The adhesion molecules that participate in the binding of immune cells to the vascular endothelium fall into three groups: selectins, integrins, and the immunoglobulin superfamily of adhesion molecules (Figure 14.10).

The initial adherence of leukocytes to the endothelium is mediated by selectins expressed on the surface of both the circulating leukocytes and the endothelial cells. The three members of the selectin family are L-selectin (leukocyte adhesion molecule-1 [LAM-1]), E-selectin (endothelial leukocyte adhesion molecule-1 [ELAM-1]), and P-selectin [252]. The natural ligands for all three selectins are sialylated Lewis X oligosaccharides, which are found on almost all cell types. Among the molecules with sialylated Lewis X moieties are the selectins themselves, so that L-selectin on neutrophils can bind to E-selectin or P-selectin on endothelial cells. Selectin bonds are responsible for leukocyte rolling. Because only weak selectin bonds form between circulating leukocytes and endothelial cells, leukocytes can roll along the surface of the endothelium by making and breaking selectin-mediated bonds. Rolling reduces leukocyte velocity before the formation of stronger adhesion bonds that fully immobilize leukocytes on the surface of the endothelium. These stronger bonds are formed between members of the two other families of adhesion molecules, integrins, which are expressed on the surface of the leukocytes, and members of the immunoglobulin superfamily of adhesion molecules (e.g., intracellular adhesion molecule-1 [ICAM-1], vascular cell adhesion molecule 1 [VCAM-1], and mucosal addressin cell adhesion molecule-1 [MAdCAM-1]), which are expressed on endothelial cells.

The integrins form a large group of adhesion molecules, each of which is a heterodimer that consists of noncovalently associated α and β subunits [253]. Integrins are divided into subfamilies based on common β subunits, with the β_1 and β_2 subunits being the most important for inflammation. Neutrophils predominantly express β_2-integrins, while monocytes express both β_1- and β_2-integrins, and lymphocytes express β_1-, β_2-, and β_7-integrins (the $\alpha_4\beta_7$ heterodimer mediates lymphocyte homing specifically to the intestinal endothelium). The β_2-integrins CD11a/CD18 (lymphocyte function-associated antigen-1 [LFA-1] or $\alpha_L\beta_2$) and CD11b/CD18 (macrophage-1 antigen

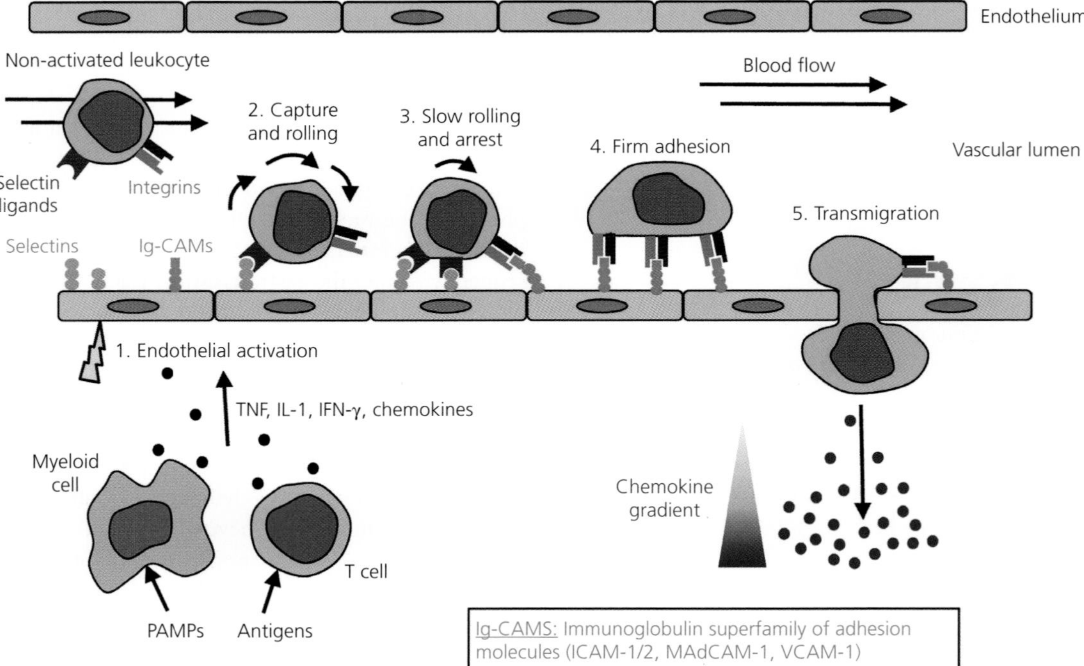

Figure 14.10 Adhesion and transmigration of leukocytes during intestinal inflammation. Leukocytes adhere to the vascular endothelium through cellular adhesion molecules. The processes of rolling and activation are dependent on selectins on the endothelial cells and leukocytes and their ligands, whereas firm adhesion and transmigration are dependent on leukocyte integrins that bind to immunoglobulin superfamily of adhesion molecules (Ig-CAMs) on endothelial cells. In the gut, the Ig-CAMs that mediate these processes include mucosal intracellular adhesion molecules (ICAM)-1 and -2, mucosal addressin cell adhesion molecule-1 (MAdCAM-1), with its natural ligand on leukocytes being integrin $\alpha4\beta7$, and vascular cell adhesion molecule 1 (VCAM-1). IFN, interferon; IL, interleukin; PAMP, pathogen-associated molecular pattern; TNF, tumor necrosis factor.

[Mac-1] or $\alpha_M\beta_2$) bind to ICAM-1 on endothelial cells. CD11a/CD18 also binds to ICAM-2 and is expressed on neutrophils in their basal state.

The most prominent members of the immunoglobulin superfamily of adhesion molecules are ICAM-1 and ICAM-2, which are expressed on endothelial cells under basal conditions. They bind to β_2-integrins expressed on the surface of adhering leukocytes [254]. ICAM-2 is expressed at higher levels than ICAM-1 under resting conditions, but ICAM-1 expression can be increased by IL-1, TNF-α, and IFN-γ stimulation, whereas ICAM-2 expression is not elevated by cytokine stimulation. Thus, the relative importance of ICAM-1 increases in conditions of inflammation.

The final step in leukocyte trafficking in intestinal inflammation is the passage of leukocytes between epithelial cells and out into the lumen [255,256]. Leukocytes that have passed into the lumen can be found in the stool, which is a clinical sign of inflammation of the gastrointestinal tract. Adhesion molecules, including ICAM-1, and neutrophil chemotactic factors are expressed on epithelial cells in the presence of inflammation. Chemotactic factors have also been identified in the colonic lumen and provide an additional driving force for neutrophil transmigration across the epithelium.

Neutrophil and monocyte trafficking

Neutrophils represent the first wave of the intestinal innate immune response and migrate within minutes to affected areas of the intestine in response to macrophage-derived chemoattractants. Th17 cells also influence neutrophil recruitment, both directly through production of CXCL8 and indirectly through IL-17-induced production of chemokines from macrophages, fibroblasts, and epithelial cells. Migrating neutrophils extravasate into the gastrointestinal mucosa by binding to adhesion molecules on the endothelium of postcapillary venules. After the neutrophil has passed between the endothelial cells, it migrates to the site of bacterial invasion or other injury by chemotaxis. The cell also acquires the ability to produce reactive oxygen species in maximal amounts through priming and activation [257]. Priming enhances the ability of neutrophils to produce reactive oxygen species, whereas activation stimulates maximal production. These processes are mediated by interaction of the cell with particulate stimuli (e.g., bacteria) or by stimulation with soluble factors, such as certain cytokines, inflammatory mediators, and bacterial products (e.g., endotoxins). Neutrophils also mediate recruitment of monocytes via production of monocyte chemoattractant proteins, thereby initiating a macrophage phase of the innate immune response, which can last several days [75]. After 1–2 days in the gastrointestinal mucosa, neutrophils either die in situ and are removed by macrophage phagocytosis or pass between epithelial cells into the intestinal lumen, where they are expelled in the stool. The migration of neutrophils across the epithelium and into the lumen is a characteristic event of the active phase of several inflammatory diseases of the gastrointestinal and hepatobiliary tracts, including *Helicobacter pylori*-induced gastritis, ulcerative colitis, Crohn's disease, bacterial enterocolitis, cholangitis, and acute cholecystitis. Because neutrophils are terminal and incapable of proliferation, elevated numbers of neutrophils in the inflamed mucosa reflect increased trafficking out of the bloodstream and into the gastrointestinal tissues.

Gastrointestinal macrophages are derived from circulating monocytes produced in the bone marrow. Monocytes enter the circulation and, like neutrophils, bind to adhesion molecules expressed on endothelial cells in the postcapillary venules of the intestine. Bound monocytes pass between endothelial cells and enter the mucosa, where they begin to differentiate into mature macrophages. As a monocyte differentiates, it acquires capacities for phagocytosis, proliferation, and bacterial killing. This process is controlled by cytokines and other soluble factors present in the lamina propria, and different combinations of cytokines and mediators result in macrophages with different phenotypes. Receptors on the surface of macrophages determine the stimuli to which the macrophage can respond, as well as the macrophage phenotype. As with neutrophils, the large increase in the number of macrophages during clinically apparent gastrointestinal inflammation reflects increased migration of monocytes out of the bloodstream, rather than proliferation of macrophages already in the lamina propria [258].

For the most part, neutrophil and monocyte trafficking in the gastrointestinal tract is similar to that in other organ systems; however, the number of leukocytes passing through the gastrointestinal tract greatly exceeds that in other organs. Because the surface area of the gastrointestinal tract is large, even the modest degree of inflammation seen in the healthy small intestine and colon involves the trafficking of a substantial number of monocytes and neutrophils. In diffuse inflammatory diseases of the gastrointestinal tract, such as ulcerative colitis, the trafficking of leukocytes through the inflamed mucosa expands to the point that most leukocytes produced in the bone marrow travel through the gastrointestinal mucosa into the lumen [259].

Lymphocyte trafficking

Lymphocyte trafficking to the GALT and intraepithelial and lamina propria intestinal compartments is tightly regulated by the expression of receptors and counterreceptors on lymphocytes and endothelial cells [260]. Lymphocyte trafficking shares many similarities with neutrophil and monocyte migration; differences, however, also exist and reflect the fact that neutrophils traffic only in the event of acute inflammation, whereas lymphocytes enter the mucosa both inducibly during inflammation and continuously in the healthy state as part of their normal recirculation. Accordingly, distinction exists between homeostatic and inflammatory adhesion molecules and chemoattractants. Added levels of variation occur in the ability of particular ligand–receptor pairs to provide regional specificity both in relation to intestinal versus extraintestinal tissues and regarding specific gut segments. Finally, different chemokine/chemokine receptor requirements characterize the various developmental stages of naive, effector, or memory lymphocytes.

Naive lymphocytes leave the primary lymphoid organs (bone marrow and thymus) and circulate through secondary lymphoid tissues, which include the peripheral lymph nodes, spleen, as well as GALT. Migration in those sites takes place through high endothelial venules. Once inside the GALT, naive lymphocytes encounter APCs, mainly dendritic cells and macrophages, which carry captured antigen. Dendritic cells enter into mesenteric lymph nodes by upregulation of CCR7, which follows antigen detention. When intestinal CD103$^+$ dendritic cells present their antigens to naive lymphocytes, the latter become activated and undergo a transcriptional modification that is called *imprinting*. This signifies the upregulation of gut-specific trafficking molecules, in particular integrin α4β7 and CCR9, which renders the lymphocytes capable of recruitment to the small-intestinal lamina propria [261,262]. Tissue specialization is accomplished via the expression of the receptors for integrin α4β7 (MadCAM-1) and CCR9 (CCL25) in the small intestine. In particular, MAdCAM-1, a member of the immunoglobulin superfamily, is selectively expressed on the high endothelial venules in lamina propria, thus attracting $\alpha_4\beta_7$ lymphocytes to the intestine. Similarly, CCR9$^+$ lymphocytes bind to a single chemokine ligand CCL25, which is specifically expressed in the small intestine. In addition to those trafficking pathways, lymphocytic homing also involves binding of the β_2-integrin lymphocyte function–associated antigen-1 (LFA-1, CD11α/CD18) to its receptor, ICAM-1 [263]. Recirculation of plasmablasts to the small intestine follows the same pattern of trafficking molecules. Entry of lymphocytes to the colon involves both common and distinct modules in comparison with the small intestine. Although MadCAM-1 is expressed in the colon, this is not the case for CCL25, hence lymphocyte blasts use alternative chemokines and chemokine receptors for large-intestinal recirculation. Besides, α4β7/MadCAM-1 binding, T-cell colon migration is supported by GPR15, an orphan G protein-linked receptor with homology to chemokine receptors [264]. Plasmablasts, in contrast, use CCR10 to migrate to the colon, via binding to intestinal CCL28.

Although the earlier interactions ensure gut trafficking during homeostasis, additional pathways may be upregulated during inflammation. For example, lymphocytes that bear the integrin α4β1 usually are excluded from the gut, because of the preferential expression of the receptor VCAM-1 in the skin, lungs, and inflamed central nervous system. Nevertheless, intestinal inflammation may lead to VCAM-1 expression in the gut, which allows for inflammatory T-cell recruitment [265]. Similarly, CCL20 is a chemokine with inducible expression during inflammation, hence it attracts T cells that bear its receptor, CCR6 [266]. This chemokine receptor is typically expressed by Th17 cells, hence CCR6/CCL20 interactions may induce the recruitment of such cells to the large and small intestine during active inflammation. Finally, Treg cells use the receptor CCR5 to enter the chronically inflamed distal small intestine [267].

Lymphoblasts recirculate or home to the sites of the original antigenic stimulation but also to other mucosal secretory sites. After antigenic stimulation in the gastrointestinal tract, IgA lymphoblasts circulate to the mucosal secretory sites of the breast, lung, and eye, where antigen-specific antibodies are secreted [268]. For example, a breastfeeding mother can passively transfer secretory IgA in her breast milk to her nursing child. The secretory IgA in breast milk protects the infant against bacteria or viruses in the mother's gastrointestinal tract. The intestinal immune system thus has the capacity to selectively sample antigens from the gut and subsequently induce immune responses that provide protection for the gastrointestinal tract and other mucosal surfaces of the host and the nursing offspring.

Immunological tolerance in the intestinal tract

Although the epithelial barrier is capable of preventing the great bulk of intraluminal antigens from reaching the lamina propria, occasional intrusions do happen and, most probably, are necessary to attain continuous education of the gut-associated, innate, and adaptive immune systems. A remarkable characteristic of the GALT is that it successfully accomplishes this task without inducing overt inflammation that could inflict bystander injury to intestinal tissues. This phenomenon of *immunological tolerance* distinguishes mucosal from systemic immunity and is exerted via specialized cellular immune populations, which also incorporate information from the overlaying epithelium and anti-inflammatory molecular modules. Accordingly, the gastrointestinal tract exhibits a fascinating example of specific tolerance to orally ingested antigens, called *oral tolerance* [269,270]. The oral administration of antigens can lead to systemic antigen-specific unresponsiveness, which results in the lack of specific T- and B-cell responsiveness to those antigens. Concurrently, local specific secretory immunity can develop, resulting in lymphoblasts capable of specific IgA production [271]. This dichotomy between systemic and mucosal compartments appears to reflect a solution to the need for excluding the specific antigen during future encounters and avoiding inappropriate systemic responsiveness. If this were not the case, numerous bacterial and viral antigens and food components could lead to frequent cross-reactive immunological stimulatory events and result in a high frequency of intestinal immune disorders, and many foods would cause diverse and uncontrollable allergic reactions.

Several cellular and molecular modules contribute to the development of intestinal immunological tolerance. In the healthy human gut, local macrophages retain the ability for phagocytosis, without, unlike macrophages in other organs, secreting proinflammatory cytokines after stimulation [272]. On the contrary, they produce anti-inflammatory molecules, such as IL-10, induce the differentiation of naive T cells into Treg cells, and suppress proinflammatory Th1 and Th17 immunity [273]. Taken together, these data show that under homeostatic conditions, lamina propria macrophages are capable of eliminating evading pathogens, while at the same time restraining excess immune responses. Intestinal dendritic cells also show phenotypic variability, which translates to functional diversity. In the healthy gut, CD103+ dendritic cells prevail and play a crucial role for the preservation of homeostasis by promoting Treg cell differentiation through a TGF-β1- and retinoic acid-dependent mechanism [274]. This homeostatic role of CD103+ dendritic cells may be dependent on the ubiquitin editing enzyme, A20, encoded in humans by the *TNFAIP3* gene, because dendritic cell-specific *Tnfaip3* deletion in mice results in spontaneous colitis [275]. Additional properties of homeostatic intestinal dendritic cells include induction of T-cell-independent IgA secretion by naive B cells and imprinting of gut-homing receptors CCR9 and α4β7 integrin on activated B and T cells [276].

Basal pathways of adaptive immunity are also enriched for anti-inflammatory responses in the human intestine. Intestinal lamina propria plasma cells secrete mainly IgA, which is delivered to the lumen as secretory IgA. This isotype protects the host by creating a barrier against microbes and by inhibiting their attachment and penetration of the epithelium; nevertheless, it does so without invoking inflammatory responses. Although commensal specific IgA is found in the normal intestine, resident flora have evolved to coexist with secreted IgA [277]. An additional tolerogenic effect may be related to the inability of IgA to activate complement and by its interference with complement activation by IgM and IgG antibodies [278]. T-cell responses are also primed for tolerance under basic conditions, most probably because of input provided by APCs. Compared with peripheral blood T cells, lamina propria T cells demonstrate weak proliferation and decreased sensitivity to IL-2 when stimulated via the TCR/CD3 complex, although retaining the ability to produce cytokines [279]. Interestingly, human lamina propria T cells do not respond to antigens derived from autologous intestinal microbiota, although they proliferate vigorously in the presence of heterologous antigens. This indicates that the tolerogenic behavior of intestinal T cells is specific for autologous gut microbial antigens [280]. Finally, antigen-specific Treg cells play a pivotal role in the generation and maintenance of tolerance to orally administered antigens and commensal microbiota. Peyer's patches appear to be the priming site for at least a component of such tolerogenic responses. Indeed, T cells in that site exhibit a memory and activated phenotype and preferentially secrete anti-inflammatory IL-10, over IFN-γ or IL-4, when activated through the TCR/CD3 complex [281].

Gastrointestinal inflammation

The development of clinically apparent inflammation suggests that the immune system has been overwhelmed by an abnormally large or invasive antigen load, by an antigen in a location inaccessible to the immune response (e.g., osteomyelitis), or by an antigen that is resistant to the immune response (e.g., tuberculosis). The inflammatory response likely evolved when our ancestors were confronted with unsanitary environments and infectious agents in contaminated food and water. Ingestion of viral, bacterial, and parasitic agents led to gastrointestinal tract infections, and the inflammatory response evolved to deal with them. Many of the inflammatory diseases of the gastrointestinal tract today reflect the activation of defense mechanisms that evolved in response to infectious agents but which have been adapted (or maladapted) to defend against noninfectious insults. Some chronic inflammatory diseases, such as IBD, may result from dysregulation of the immune response, resulting in an inappropriately prolonged and inappropriately amplified immune activation.

Gastrointestinal inflammation is remarkable in that diverse initiating events, such as infections, ischemia, radiation, and chemical toxins, all induce inflammatory responses that are clinically, endoscopically, and histologically similar. For example, the colonoscopic and histological appearances of ulcerative colitis, radiation proctitis, shigellosis, and ischemic colitis are similar. The commonality of the inflammatory responses is explained partly by the similarity between the proinflammatory cytokines, the patterns of leukocyte migration, and the inflammatory mediators induced by these initiating events. Moreover, in each of these diseases, the inflammatory response is partly caused by the normal intestinal microbiota that has activated the immune cells of the lamina propria as a result of the loss of epithelial integrity.

Inflammation in the gut is also distinguished by the organ-level physiological responses, primarily increased motility and secretion [282]. The gastrointestinal tract responds to enteric infections by attempting to wash out the offending microbes with increased electrolyte and water secretion and increased motility, resulting in cramps and diarrhea. The increases in secretion and motility are mediated by the inflammatory response. Regardless of the initiating event, the gastrointestinal tract mounts a stereotypical inflammatory response. Therefore, the same increases in secretion and motility (and resultant diarrhea and cramping) are the responses to noninfectious inflammatory events (e.g., radiation enterocolitis and IBD) for which there are no pathogenic organisms to wash out. Consequently, both infectious and noninfectious gastrointestinal inflammatory disorders manifest similar clinical symptoms.

In acute inflammation in response to infectious agents, neutrophil infiltration into the intestinal mucosa typically occurs within a few hours and monocyte infiltration occurs later, suggesting that factors promoting neutrophil chemotaxis appear earlier in the development of inflammation than those promoting monocyte chemotaxis. The process begins by adhesion of neutrophils and later monocytes to endothelial cells, followed by their migration across the endothelium to the site of microbial infiltration and tissue injury. The regulation of these events is coordinated by locally secreted cytokines, chemokines, and inflammatory mediators. A single biological event, such as the phagocytosis of bacteria by a macrophage, results in the production of proinflammatory factors (e.g., IL-1) that induce the expression of adhesion molecules and other agents (e.g., CXCL-8 and LTB_4), leading to neutrophil chemotaxis. Some soluble mediators, such as eosinophil chemotactic factor, are chemotactic for only one cell type, whereas others act on multiple cell types. Thus, the mediators that induce the expression of adhesion molecules and leukocyte chemotaxis constitute a complex and highly redundant network. In chronic inflammatory diseases, multiple agents that induce leukocyte adhesion and chemotaxis act in parallel. The complexity of the network of chemotactic agents raises the question of whether all of these factors operate in every gastrointestinal inflammatory event, or whether some factors are prominent in certain inflammatory events, but not in others. The composition of the inflammatory infiltrate may yield some insight. For example, a large number of eosinophils, such as seen in eosinophilic esophagitis, suggest the presence of eosinophil chemotactic factors. In most inflammatory states, it is likely that more than one chemotactic factor is operative, and that different factors are more or less prominent as the inflammatory response develops. This redundancy suggests that therapeutic agents aimed at one specific element in this complex network may not successfully block the overall inflammatory response.

The abundance of adhesion strategies used by immunocytes for recycling and entry into the inflamed intestine has led to therapeutic strategies that aim to block such pathways in chronic inflammatory disorders of the gastrointestinal tract. This concept has been validated in animal models of intestinal inflammation [283,284] and is now routinely used in IBD therapy. Monoclonal antibodies against α_4-integrin block the interaction between $\alpha_4\beta_7$ on T and B cells and the endothelial adhesion molecule, MAdCAM-1, which is significantly upregulated in the intestine during inflammation. Natalizumab, an anti-α4 monoclonal antibody therapy, was the first of these drugs to be approved for the treatment of Crohn's disease, but its use was subsequently associated with the rare occurrence of progressive multifocal leukoencephalopathy. This may be because natalizumab is an anti-α4 monoclonal antibody and thus neutralizes both α4β7 and α4β1. However, based on its clinical efficacy, natalizumab continues to be available to patients under highly regulated and monitored conditions [285]. Vedolizumab, a second humanized antibody that more specifically targets the entire $\alpha_4\beta_7$-integrin heterodimer (as opposed to α_4 alone), has been approved for use in both ulcerative colitis and Crohn's disease [286,287]. Not only has vedolizumab proved to be an effective treatment for IBD, but its selectivity for the gut-specific α4β7/MadCAM-1 pathway confers minimal systemic toxicity and an excellent safety profile. Currently, anti-MadCAM-1 monoclonal antibodies are also being investigated in patients with active IBD [288]. Etrolizumab is another monoclonal antibody that has shown promising results in early clinical trials. It uses a different approach by targeting the β7-chain, leading to concomitant blockade of α4β7/MadCAM-1 and αE/E-cadherin binding [289]. The theoretical advantage of this approach is the inhibition of recirculation of both α4β7 lymphocytes into the lamina propria and of αE^+ lymphocytes into the intraepithelial compartment. These novel therapeutic approaches represent an evolving class of drugs for IBD that targets immune cell trafficking to inflamed tissues of the intestine and may also apply to other immune-mediated diseases of the gastrointestinal and hepatobiliary systems [290].

References are available at www.yamadagastro.com/textbook7e

Further reading

Chen K., Magri G., Grasset E.K., Cerutti A. Rethinking mucosal antibody responses: IgM, IgG and IgD join IgA. Nat Rev Immunol 2020;20:427.

Eisenbarth S.C. Dendritic cell subsets in T cell programming: location dictates function. Nat Rev Immunol 2019;19:89.

Mowat A.M. To respond or not to respond – a personal perspective of intestinal tolerance. Nat Rev Immunol 2018;18:405.

Neurath M.F. Targeting immune cell circuits and trafficking in inflammatory bowel disease. Nat Immunol 2019;20:970.

Rankin L.C., Artis D. Beyond host defense: emerging functions of the immune system in regulating complex tissue physiology. Cell 2018;173:554.

Sonnenberg G.F., Hepworth M.R. Functional interactions between innate lymphoid cells and adaptive immunity. Nat Rev Immunol 2019;19:599.

CHAPTER 15
Epithelia and gastrointestinal function

Sandra D. Chanez-Paredes and Jerrold R. Turner
Laboratory of Mucosal Barrier Pathobiology, Department of Pathology, Brigham and Women's Hospital and Harvard Medical School, Boston, MA, USA

Chapter menu

All viscera within the alimentary tract, from the small ducts and acini of the pancreas to the gastrointestinal lumen, are lined by sheets of polarized epithelial cells. The protein and lipid components of the apical (lumenal) and basolateral surfaces of these cells are distinct, which allows them to respond differentially to each environment; this property is termed *epithelial polarity*. These epithelia form selective barriers that separate tissues from lumenal contents. Most epithelia are also able to direct vectorial (directed) transport of solutes and solvents. These essential functions are based on the structural polarity of individual cells, the complex organization of membranes, cell–cell and cell–substrate interactions, and interactions with other cell types. This chapter reviews intestinal wall structure, how the gut organization supports mucosal functions, the biological properties of the epithelial barrier and transepithelial transport, and consequences of the epithelial barrier dysregulation.

Organization of the intestinal wall

The small intestine and colon, or large intestine, share key structural features. As exemplified by the small intestine (Figure 15.1), the wall of the tubular gastrointestinal tract is composed of four principal layers: the mucosa, submucosa, muscularis propria, and serosa or adventitia. The mucosal layer, which interfaces with lumenal materials, consists of the epithelium, an underlying layer of loose connective tissue carrying nerves and vessels termed the lamina propria, and the muscularis mucosae, a thin layer of smooth muscle. The mucosa also contains an array of mononuclear cells, including lymphocytes, mast cells, plasma cells, and macrophages. Polymorphonuclear leukocytes are also present, primarily in the context of disease. In addition to their roles in host defense, these immune cells are capable of modulating epithelial function.

A layer of fibroconnective tissue, the submucosa, containing nerves, vessels, and lymphatics, lies beneath the mucosa. Recently, the submucosa has been shown to include a network of fluid-filled spaces supported by a complex array of thick collagen bundles [1]. This endows the submucosa with fluid-like, viscoelastic properties that allow it to act as a shock absorber to protect the mucosa from peristaltic contractions and other forces. The fluid within this network drains to lymph nodes and is an important route of tumor metastasis.

The submucosa rests on the muscularis propria, which is composed of two layers (three in the stomach) of smooth muscle, between which lies the myenteric plexus (see Chapters 1, 12,

Yamada's Textbook of Gastroenterology, Seventh Edition. Edited by Timothy C. Wang, Michael Camilleri, Benjamin Lebwohl, Anna S. Lok, William J. Sandborn, Kenneth K. Wang, and Gary D. Wu.

Companion website: www.yamadagastro.com/textbook7e

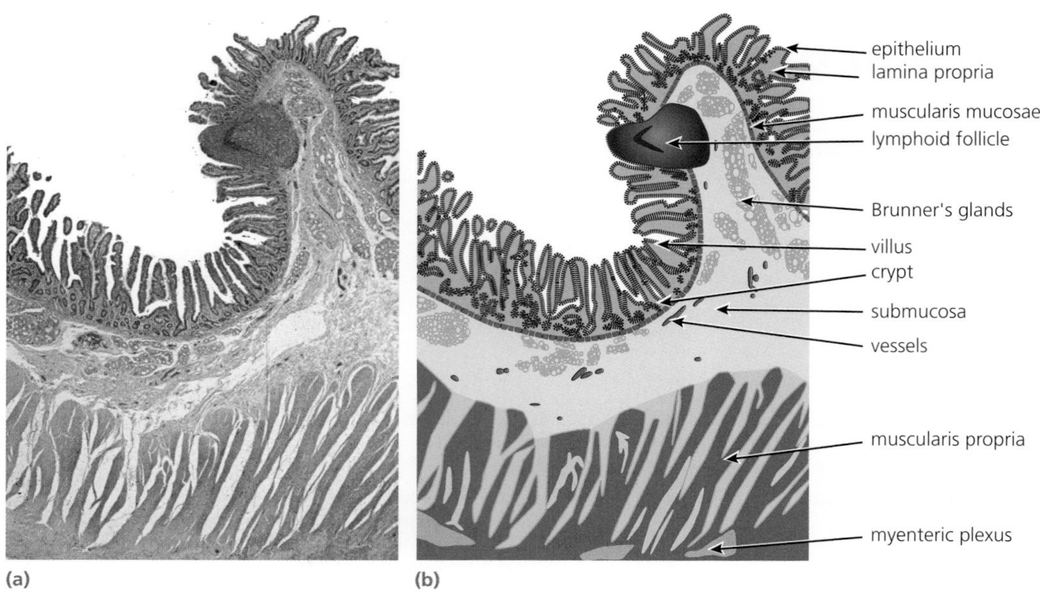

Figure 15.1 Organization of the intestinal wall. **(a)** This transmural section of normal human duodenum exemplifies many of the structural features that are common throughout the gastrointestinal tract. **(b)** The corresponding diagram delineates specific structures.

and 13). In most instances, gastrointestinal organs are encased by a delicate outermost layer of fibrofatty tissue, the serosa, encircled by a continuous layer of mesothelial cells. In areas where no serosa exists, as in portions of the esophagus and the rectum (below the peritoneal reflection), soft tissues interface with the external (longitudinal) portion of the muscularis propria. These organs are said to have an adventitial, rather than a serosal, encasement.

Mucosal organization varies throughout the gastrointestinal tract. A simple columnar epithelium lines the stomach, small intestine, and colon, as well as the pancreatobiliary ducts. In contrast, the oral cavity, esophagus, and anus are lined by a nonkeratinized, stratified squamous epithelium that is capable of withstanding the mechanical stresses of swallowing and defecation but plays no role in transepithelial transport. Mucosal structure also varies through the length of the gastrointestinal tract, e.g., villi characterize the small intestine (see Figure 15.1) while submucosal mucus salivary and Brunner glands are present in the esophagus and duodenum, respectively. Despite these complexities of regional specialization, common structural features critical to epithelial functions are present throughout the gastrointestinal tract.

Intestinal epithelial cell types

Most of the cells within the villous epithelium of the small intestine are enterocytes and are primarily charged with absorption. Enteroendocrine cells, mucin-secreting goblet cells, antigen-sampling M (or microfold) cells, and chemosensory-tuft cells are also present within villous epithelia [2,3]. The crypts contain several intestinal epithelial stem cell populations, Paneth cells, which secrete growth factors and antimicrobials, and enteroendocrine cells. Crypt-based columnar cells generate daughter cells that continue to proliferate as they migrate from crypt to villus (surface in the colon) and differentiate. This is critical, as most epithelial cells have lifespans of only 3–5 days and must therefore be replaced continuously (Chapter 2).

The development of single-cell RNA sequencing tools has allowed further subcategorization of recognized intestinal epithelial cell types and discovery of new cell types. These approaches have been applied to mouse small intestinal epithelial cells and are now being used to define epithelial reprogramming in the context of human and rodent disease. Moreover, single cell transcriptomics-based spatial reconstruction of microdissected villus segments is beginning to shed light on the gene expression profiles of crypt, transit amplifying, and villus tip cells as well as subepithelial cell types within mouse and human intestine [4–8].

Integration of epithelial cells into functional units

To work as a unit, epithelial cells must assemble into a multicellular sheet. This complex task requires individual cells to establish uniform polarity, establish intercellular junctions, and develop stable interactions with the basement membrane.

A central function of many gastrointestinal epithelia is the vectorial transport of solutes and solvents. For example, parietal cells are polarized to effect secretion of acid into the lumen (see Chapter 17). Theoretically, defective polarization of these cells could result in acid secretion into the interstitium and severe tissue damage. Absorptive villous enterocytes of the small intestine are specialized to accomplish vectorial transport of ions, nutrients, and water from the lumen to the interstitium by expressing specific transporters within the apical (lumenal), but not basolateral, membrane domain (Figure 15.2) [9,10]. These transporters often rely on a lumenal Na^+ concentration that is much higher than the intracellular Na^+; this concentration gradient is required for cotransport of sugars, amino acids, ions, and bile salts. Similarly, cAMP-induced Cl^- secretion, such as that induced by cholera toxin, requires basolateral $Na^+/K^{+}/2Cl^-$ cotransporter 1 (NKCC1) [11,12]. This creates a Cl^- gradient that results in vectorial Cl^- secretion into the lumen via the cystic fibrosis transmembrane conductance regulator (CFTR). Both NKCC1 and CFTR are activated by cAMP. Importantly, coordinated transepithelial transport requires that the entire epithelial sheet must be uniformly polarized, i.e., with all cells polarized in the same orientation, as a population of cells with apical and basolateral transport proteins misdirected to the opposite plasma membrane domain would result in vectorial

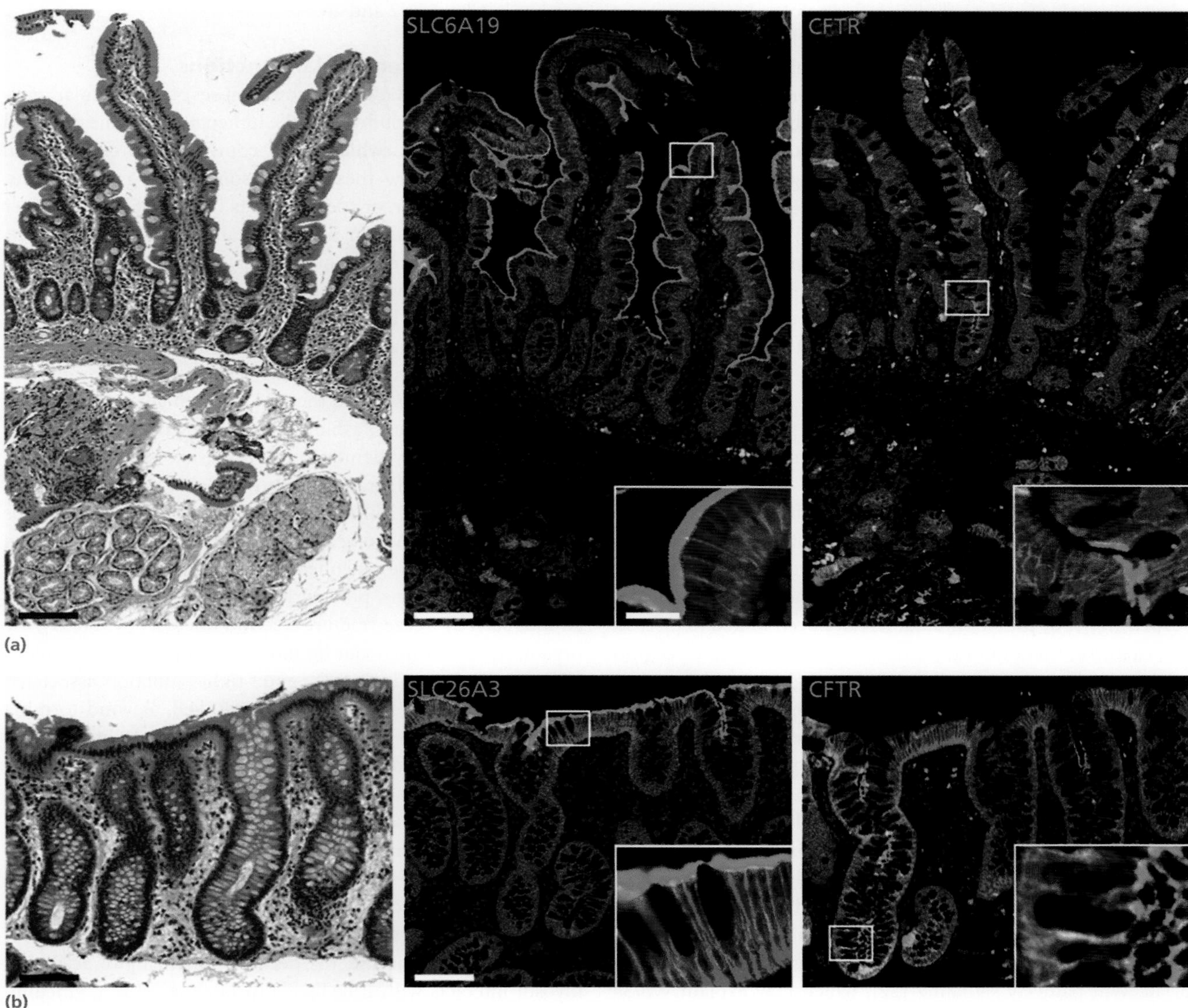

Figure 15.2 Differential transporter expression along the intestinal longitudinal (duodenum–rectum) and vertical (crypt–villus/surface) axes. **(a)** Human duodenal biopsy. Expression of the neutral amino acid transporter SLC6A19 (B^0AT1) is restricted to cells within the villus. In contrast, CFTR expression is greatest in crypt epithelia. Both are localized to the apical brush border membrane. CFTR, but not SLC6A19, is expressed in the submucosal Brunner's glands. **(b)** Human colon biopsy. Expression of the apical Cl^-/HCO_3^- transporter SLC26A3 (DRA) is restricted to surface epithelial cells. In contrast, CFTR is primarily expressed in the crypts. Both are localized to the apical brush border membrane. SLC6A19 and SLC26A3 are primarily expressed in the duodenum and colon, respectively, while CFTR is expressed throughout the length of the intestines. Bars = 50 μm and 10 μm (inset).

transport in the opposite direction and, potentially, no net transport or even net transport in the wrong direction. Thankfully, the fidelity of biological systems prevents this.

Initiation of epithelial polarization

The spatial cues that induce and maintain polarization have generally been thought to require contact with the extracellular matrix and adjacent epithelial cells. For example, the interaction between the extracellular domains of the epithelial Ca^{2+}-dependent adherens junction protein E-cadherin on adjacent cells is a critical trigger for polarization. This is followed by reorganization of the perijunctional ring of actin and myosin filaments that are linked to E-cadherin through cytoplasmic linker proteins, e.g., α-actinin and α-catenin (see Figure 15.2) [15]. The cytoskeleton then orchestrates assembly of E-cadherin clusters in the plasma membrane that join adjacent cells through membrane protrusions. Myosin II further integrates homophilic E-cadherin clustering and stabilization to reinforce the epithelial barrier [14]. These intercellular interactions synergize with integrin-dependent cellular binding to matrix components and other polarity cues that induce and maintain polarization and, ultimately, differentiation [15]. The latter include polarity proteins that define epithelial apical and basolateral plasma membrane domains [16]. These processes also play critical roles during tissue repair, including preservation of cell polarity and tissue architecture. Regulators of tissue repair include the transmembrane polarity proteins Fat (Ft) and Crumbs (Crb), which coordinate with actin-driven processes to support tissue integrity [17].

The discovery of polarity genes encoding Par proteins in *Caenorhabditis elegans* and *Drosophila* facilitated the identification of mammalian homologs which functionally define epithelial apical and basolateral plasma membrane domains (18). Not surprisingly, Par protein mutations have been linked to disease. For example, mutation of LKB1, an ortholog of the *C. elegans* protein Par-4, is associated with Peutz–Jeghers syndrome (see Chapter 70). STE20-related kinase adapter protein alpha (STRAD), that activates LKB1, can also be mutated in Peutz–Jeghers syndrome [19]. Activation of this pathway can initiate epithelial polarization in vitro, even in the absence of cell–cell and cell–matrix interactions [20]. While the mechanisms responsible for this incomplete polarization have not yet been defined, one potential mediator may be adenosine monophosphate (AMP)-activated protein kinase, which is activated by LKB1 and plays an important role in maintaining cellular energy balance [21]. Loss of LKB1 function may also facilitate inappropriate Wnt pathway signaling [22], which may explain Wnt5a upregulation in both $Lkb1^{+/-}$ mice and polyps from Peutz–Jeghers patients [23]. These data together and the ability of Wnt5a to promote crypt fission [24] may explain the complex, arborizing architecture of Peutz–Jeghers polyps.

Consistent with the idea that aberrant epithelial polarization may contribute to neoplasia, mutations of the E-cadherin and adenomatous polyposis coli (APC) binding partner β-catenin result in Wnt pathway activation and are common in human colorectal cancers [25,26]. Transcriptional repression of E-cadherin during the epithelial–mesenchymal transition accompanies invasive cancer [27]. Notably, E-cadherin loss correlates with signet ring cell features and single cell infiltration in colorectal and gastric cancers [28,29]. Moreover, germline E-cadherin mutations are associated with familial, signet ring cell (diffuse) gastric cancer, thereby providing further support for the linkage between polarity defects and neoplasia [30,31]. The underlying mechanisms by which E-cadherin, APC, and β-catenin mutations contribute to carcinogenesis are discussed further in Chapters 2 and 26.

Structure of intercellular junctions

All polarized epithelia share a common set of intercellular junctions [32]. These include, from the lumenal aspect, the tight and adherens junctions, which form continuous circumferential contacts, and, below these, desmosomes and gap junctions, which form macular, or spot, contacts (Figure 15.3a). Together these junctions maintain polarity, seal the paracellular space, provide intercellular communication, and stabilize the monolayer to preserve overall epithelial integrity.

When examined by transmission electron microscopy, tight junctions appear as zones that are 100–300 nm deep, where the plasma membranes of adjacent cells are closely apposed (Figure 15.3b). These form the seal between adjacent cells and are arrayed in a linear fashion around the cell. Freeze-fracture electron microscopy demonstrates a net-like series of anastomosing grooves and strands (Figure 15.3c). Specific tight junction proteins are differentially expressed across various epithelia [33–36]. Among the most divergent are the claudin proteins, which are encoded by 27 different mammalian genes [37]. Claudins polymerize to form the characteristic strands seen by freeze-fracture electron microscopy [38,39], the organization of which can be modulated by zonula occludens (ZO-1, ZO-2, and ZO-3) and tight junction-associated MARVEL protein (TAMP) families [40–45]. Beyond forming gates that selectively seal the paracellular space, tight junctions have been suggested to have a "fence" function that prevents mixing of transmembrane proteins and outer leaflet membrane lipids to maintain the boundary between apical and basolateral membrane domains [46]. Although supported by some data [47–50], this idea deserves further study [51].

The adherens junctions (see Figure 15.3a,b) lie directly below the tight junction, within the lateral membranes of adjacent cells [52–54]. At this site, the perijunctional ring of actin and myosin interacts with E-cadherin through α-actinin, vinculin, and α- and β-catenin [55–57]. This perijunctional actomyosin ring is also essential to the maintenance of the tight junction [49,58–60].

Directly below the adherens junctions are the desmosomes (see Figure 15.3a,b), which provide tensile strength to epithelial surfaces. These are formed by cadherin family proteins, desmogelins and desmocollins, which mediate extracellular

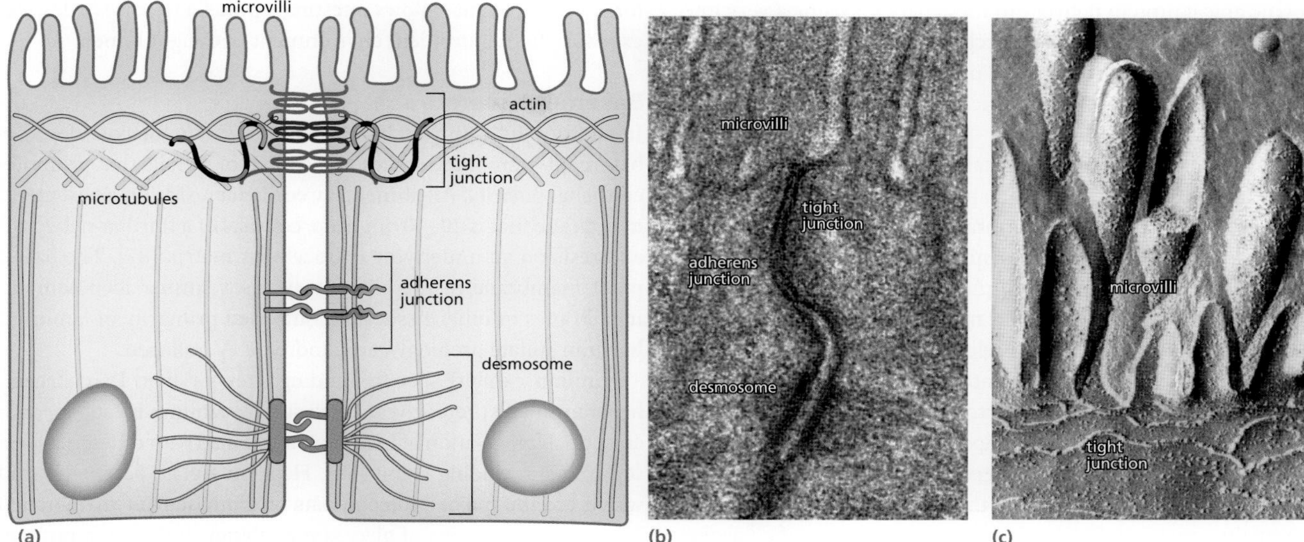

Figure 15.3 Organization of a typical gastrointestinal columnar epithelial cell. (a) The precisely orchestrated architecture of polarized epithelia includes cytoskeletal structures and intercellular junctions. (b) Electron microscopic appearance of the apical junctional complex region of a small intestinal absorptive epithelial cell. Source: Turner 2009 [145]. (c) Freeze-fracture electron microscopy demonstrates the dense interconnecting network of strands that define the tight junction. Source: Shen L., Weber C., Raleigh D., et al. Annu Rev Physiol 2011;73:283–309.

intercellular interactions [61–65]. On their cytoplasmic aspects, desmosomal proteins associate with intermediate filaments to anchor the cytokeratin-based cytoskeleton and provide resistance to mechanical stress. The spontaneous chronic colitis that develops in mice lacking keratin-8, the principal intestinal epithelial keratin, emphasizes the importance of keratin proteins in epithelial function [66,67]. Keratin-8 and keratin-18 mutations have also been identified in some patients with inflammatory bowel disease, although their significance remains to be defined [67,68].

Polarized protein delivery

Plasma membrane and secreted proteins pass through a series of distinct vesicular compartments as they are sorted to apical or basolateral surfaces. These proteins share a common site of synthesis on ribosomes bound to the rough endoplasmic reticulum and undergo posttranslational modification (e.g., glycosylation) in the Golgi apparatus. Once they reach the trans-Golgi network, proteins are sorted for polarized delivery. In most cells, proteins destined for the basolateral surface are delivered directly from the Golgi or they are transported via endosomes to that domain. Studies using live cell imaging have suggested that basolateral delivery may even be targeted to specific sites along the lateral membrane [69]. Detailed analysis of basolaterally targeted proteins has shown that specific amino acid sequences located within the cytoplasmic tail are sufficient to direct basolateral delivery [70,71]. These sequences commonly include tyrosine-based, dileucine, or monoleucine motifs [72], and several of these sequences are sorted by the epithelial adapter protein AP-1B [73]. This protein selects cargo destined for the basolateral membrane and coordinates the assembly of the exocytic machinery necessary for fusion of transport vesicles with the plasma membrane. The exocytic machinery, which is also involved in endocytic recycling of apical and basolateral membrane proteins, includes members of the Rab family of small guanosine triphosphate (GTP)-binding proteins and SNARE proteins that target delivery of transport vesicles to specific membrane domains [74].

In contrast to basolateral proteins, apically targeted proteins are transported by both direct and indirect pathways [75]. Proteins that traffic directly to the apical membrane include those that associate with glycolipid- and cholesterol-rich membrane domains, such as the brush border hydrolase sucrose-isomaltase, as well as proteins that are targeted independently of these membrane domains, such as lactase-phlorizin hydrolase. Dependence on actin also differentiates these two direct transport pathways, as transport of sucrose-isomaltase occurs along actin tracks and is inhibited by actin depolymerization, whereas lactase-phlorizin hydrolase transport is actin independent. Ectodomain glycosylation sites and transmembrane protein domains, including those that allow association with glycolipid- and cholesterol-rich membranes, have been implicated in apical targeting [76]; other apical sorting signals include glycosylphosphatidylinositol-anchored proteins (GPI-AP), N-glycans, O-glycans, and transmembrane domain sequences [72]. Direct trafficking as well as endosomal recirculation of apical membrane proteins both appear to be affected in microvillus inclusion disease (MVID), a fatal, autosomal recessive disorder of brush border development caused by myosin Vb mutations [77–79]. Recent data suggest that it may be possible to rescue apical protein delivery in these patients using a very low-fat diet [80] but neither the mechanisms of this effect nor its potential clinical utility are well understood at present. It may, however, relate to the asymmetrical lipid trafficking that parallels protein sorting.

As an alternative to direct apical trafficking, some membrane proteins are transported to the apical surface only after initial delivery to the basolateral membrane. For example, the polyimmunoglobulin (IgA) receptor is initially delivered to the basolateral surface where it binds two IgA molecules [81]. The complex is then transcytosed to the apical membrane, where the receptor undergoes proteolysis and is released, as a molecule termed secretory component, into the intestinal lumen along with two IgA molecules [82]. In addition to specific targeting sequences that direct basolateral and then apical delivery, transcytosis also requires microtubules, which serve as tracks and motors, i.e., kinesins and dyneins, that carry transcellular transport vesicles. It remains unclear why some proteins without specific basolateral functions take this indirect pathway to the apical surface. However, this mechanism is useful for the redistribution of apical proteins mistakenly targeted to the basolateral membrane, as well as for sorting of membrane proteins during the initial stages of epithelial polarization.

Organization of the cytoskeleton

The cytoskeletal organization of columnar epithelia cells exhibits only relatively minor differences among sites within the gastrointestinal tract. The stabilization of epithelial cell structure first requires support for the tall columnar shape; in the absence of the cytoskeleton, a sphere would have the most thermodynamically favorable properties. Maintenance of cell shape is primarily a function of the actin microfilaments that form a network beneath the entire plasma membrane (see Figure 15.3a). Bundles of 20–30 actin filaments also form the submembranous cores responsible for microvillous architecture [77]. Within these cores, individual microfilaments are cross-linked to each other by actin-bundling proteins and to the microvillous membrane by a member of the myosin family, myosin IA [83]. The microvillous actin bundles protrude into the apical pole of the cell and associate with a terminal web composed of actin and type II myosin that interfaces with the apical junctional complex. The contractile status of this perijunctional actomyosin ring can be adjusted in response to physiological and pathophysiological stimuli, allowing modulation of epithelial barrier function.

Microtubules also form a unique array in polarized epithelial cells. In contrast to nonpolarized cells in which microtubules radiate from a single microtubule organizing center adjacent to the nucleus, microtubules in polarized epithelia are aligned apicobasally and in a subapical network (see Figure 15.3a) [84,85].

Cables composed of intermediate filaments course through the cells and function as support structural cables. As noted above, these tonofilaments associate with desmosomes [86] to form a network that allows intestinal epithelia to survive despite exposure to the turbulent environment of the gut lumen.

Basement membrane

In addition to its important structural and supportive roles, the basement membrane serves as a source of signals that promote epithelial polarity. All alimentary epithelia reside on a basement membrane that is 20–40 nm deep, consists of a fibrillar network, and rests on an underlying extracellular matrix [87]. The basement membrane in the alimentary tract, similar to basement membranes in other tissues, is composed primarily of laminin, heparan sulfate proteoglycans, and type IV collagen.

Laminin exhibits specific binding sites for type IV collagen, heparan sulfate proteoglycans, cell surface laminin receptors, and entactin. Upregulation of laminin is associated with different types of tumors, including colon [88]. Heparan sulfate proteoglycans, which are the major proteoglycans of the basement membrane, consist of long chains of glycosaminoglycans linked to a protein core. The structure of these massive molecules, which is often likened to a test-tube brush with the glycosaminoglycan extensions representing the bristles, allows proteoglycans to hydrate this environment by binding water, and possibly imparting solute-sieving characteristics under conditions of bulk water flow. Although a controversial concept, the thickened basement membrane present in patients with collagenous colitis may result in impaired water and electrolyte absorption and the resulting watery diarrhea that is a hallmark of this condition [89].

Type IV collagen is a triple-stranded helical molecule which, unlike other collagens, does not have its propeptides removed after deposition in the extracellular space and does not cross-link into dense fibrils; instead, it assumes a loose, net-like structure by associating with other collagen IV molecules. This mesh-like organization establishes the fundamental structure of the basement membrane [87].

Basement membrane components can exert significant effects on epithelia, including modulation of proliferation, adhesion, migration, differentiation, and even barrier function. In the intestine, type IV collagen is produced primarily by mesenchymal cells, heparan sulfate proteoglycans by epithelial cells, and laminin by both mesenchymal and epithelial cells. Many basement membrane components bind to integrins, a family of epithelial cell surface molecules that are connected to the actin cytoskeleton through linker proteins. Through such associations, structural elements within the cell are able to connect with, and potentially be modulated by, events occurring within the basement membrane and even more deeply within the extracellular matrix [90].

Mucosal barriers

The mucosa interfaces with the gut lumen and is exposed to a variety of chemical and physical stressors such as gastric acid, pancreatic chyme, bile acids, and shear forces. Homeostasis

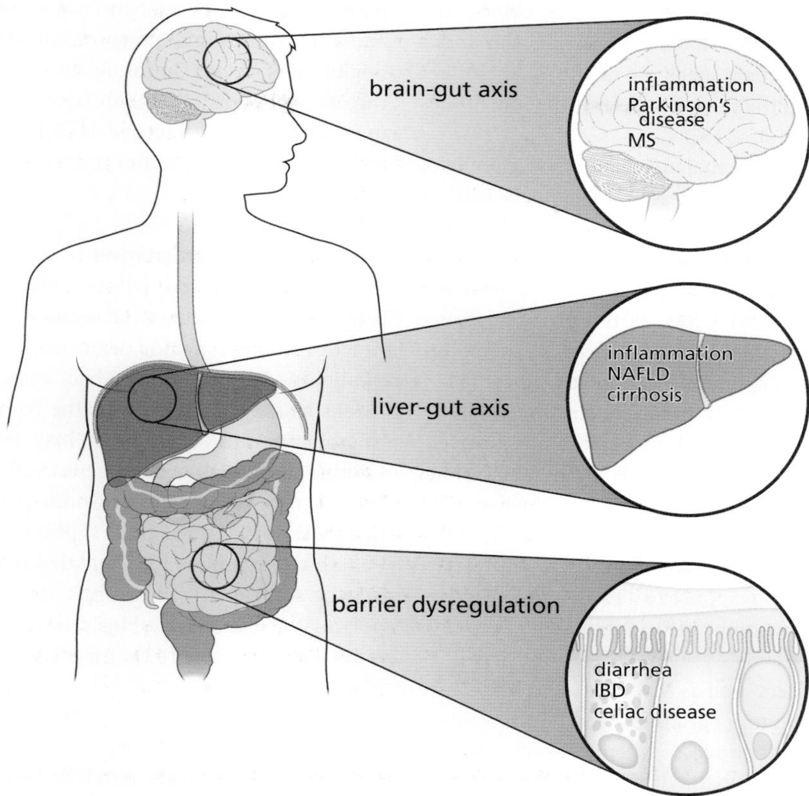

Figure 15.4 The brain–gut axis and liver–gut axis. As a result of a dysregulated epithelial barrier, microbial products and other lumenal materials gain access to the lamina propria as well as blood and lymphatic vessels. This can allow development of immune cell populations and systemic circulation of materials that cause disease in the central nervous system, liver, and other organs. MS, multiple sclerosis; NAFLD, nonalcoholic fatty liver disease; IBD, inflammatory bowel disease. See text for details.

requires that the mucosa integrate partially opposing functions, e.g., keeping the microbiota confined to the lumen while facilitating beneficial microbial interactions with gut immune cells and supporting transepithelial solute and fluid transport. It is not surprising, therefore, that the epithelial barrier is central to mucosal function. Barriers may be conceptually divided into two major categories: those that are extrinsic to the epithelium (although, in some instances, produced by the epithelium) and those provided by the physical presence of the epithelium, which we describe as intrinsic barriers. Examples of the former include goblet and Paneth cells that synthesize mucin and antimicrobial peptides, respectively.

Until recently, intestinal epithelial barrier function has been primarily associated with intestinal disease. This perspective is changing with the recognition that systemic signals can affect distant organs including the liver and brain, i.e., the liver–gut and brain–gut axes (Figure 15.4). Besides its pathophysiological role in infectious and immune-mediated intestinal diseases, e.g., inflammatory bowel disease [91–94], HIV infection [95], celiac disease [96], and Whipple's disease [97], a dysfunctional epithelial barrier may also contribute to systemic and extraintestinal diseases, such as graft versus host disease and nonalcoholic fatty liver disease (NAFLD), respectively [98–103]. This is not a unidirectional relationship, as it has been shown that, for example, microbial metabolites influence hepatic metabolism and vice versa. Increased intestinal permeability has also been linked to diseases like obesity [104], type 1 [105] and type 2 diabetes [106], rheumatoid arthritis [107], autism [108], and Parkinson's disease [109]. In the light of rising numbers of these diseases worldwide, it is important to understand that the intestinal epithelial barrier is essential to the function of the gut and other organs.

Extrinsic barriers

Mucus

The mucous layer covers the epithelium and separates lumenal content from epithelial cells and immune cells. Small intestinal mucus is organized as a loose gel. In contrast, colonic mucus includes a loose outer layer and an attached inner layer. In health, colonic microbiota are restricted to the outer layer, where they contribute to barrier function by outcompeting pathogenic organisms [110]. In the context of infectious and immune-mediated colitis, e.g., active ulcerative colitis, the mucus thins and bacteria are able to penetrate the inner layer [111,112]. As a result, pathogens are able to make direct contact with the colonic epithelium which, in turn, contributes to mucosal immune activation [113].

Mucus is composed of mucins that are encoded by a family of 22 genes. Mucins are mainly expressed by goblet cells or epithelial cells. These complex structures are synthesized and secreted by foveolar mucus cells in the stomach and goblet cells in the intestines; the specific mucins produced vary with cell type and site. For example, MUC5AC is the primary gastric mucin [114–116] but is not typically expressed in the colon. MUC5AC can, however, be expressed in colorectal cancer [117]. MUC17 and MUC12 are transmembrane mucins that are tethered to the small intestinal or colonic epithelium, respectively [114]. MUC2 is the principal secreted mucin in both small intestine and colon; its importance is demonstrated by the spontaneous colitis that develops in *Muc2* knockout mice [118]. Specialized sentinel goblet cells located at crypt openings are triggered to release MUC2 in response to TLR-mediated activation of the NLRP6 inflammasome [119]. This is thought to promote pathogen clearance.

Secreted mucin monomers such as MUC5AC and MUC2 are densely packed into secretory granules and unfold upon secretion. This finely tuned process, which is supported by bicarbonate secretion, is accompanied by mucin hydration to form a gel [120]. When CFTR function is compromised, reduced Cl^- secretion diminishes the Cl^- gradient that drives Cl^-/HCO_3^- exchange by the exchanger protein solute carrier family 26 member 3 (SLC26A3, also called downregulated in adenoma, DRA). As a result, intestinal mucus of patients with cystic fibrosis is poorly hydrated [121]. The viscous nature of this mucus occasionally manifests as meconium ileus in newborns [122] or distal intestinal obstruction syndrome in adults [123].

Unstirred layer

Peristalsis creates a turbulent environment in the gastrointestinal lumen. The epithelium is protected from lumenal convective forces by a 300–800 µm thick, unstirred aqueous layer. As noted below, the unstirred layer may contribute significantly to nutrient absorption by retaining monomers, e.g., sugars or amino acids, generated by brush border hydrolases until the monomers can be transported across the epithelium. Similarly, unstirred water layer influences drug uptake. For example, absorption of lipophilic drugs correlates inversely with the thickness of the unstirred layer [124,125].

Secreted immunoglobulins

The most abundant secreted immunoglobulin in the mucosa is immunoglobulin A (IgA) which, as discussed above, is dimerized by secretory component. IgG is transcytosed by the neonatal Fc receptor (FcRN), which can function in both basolateral-to-apical as well as apical-to-basolateral directions [126]. The latter allows FcRN, which is expressed well beyond the neonatal period, to mediate absorption of antibodies by nursing infants and also to allow IgG transport into the lumen. Secreted immunoglobulins act as immune barriers by binding to lumenal threats, including pathogenic bacteria and toxins [127,128], and may coat lumenal bacteria [129,130]. This adaptive immune barrier is highly specific and dependent on prior antigenic sensitization.

Antimicrobial peptides

Paneth cells, located within small intestinal and proximal colonic crypts, produce and secrete peptides with antimicrobial functions. These include defensins, lysozyme, and type II phospholipase A2 [131–133]. The bactericidal activity of most defensins may actually shape the composition of the intestinal microbiome [134]. This fact may link observations that the Crohn's disease-associated gene *NOD2* is required for expression of some defensins, that some Crohn's disease patients with disease-associated *ATG16L1* polymorphisms have abnormal Paneth cell granules [135], and that reduced defensin expression may be associated with Crohn's disease [136,137], thereby supporting the idea that dysbiosis, i.e., perturbation of the microbiome (see Chapter 142), may contribute to Crohn's disease pathogenesis [138].

Intrinsic barriers and transepithelial transport

The intrinsic barrier is created by polarized epithelial cells. This cannot, however, be an absolute barrier but must be selectively permeable. The tight junction defines the permeability of this seal and can be modulated in response to physiological and pathophysiological stimuli. Thus, in addition to active transcellular processes, transepithelial transport can occur via passive paracellular flux.

Transcellular transport

To traverse an epithelial cell via the transcellular route, an ion or other solute must cross the apical membrane, the cytosol, and the basolateral membrane (Figure 15.5). The two plasma membranes serve as barriers that restrict passive flux of water and hydrophilic solutes. In addition to protection, this allows maintenance of the transmembrane electrochemical gradients that provide the driving force for transport proteins. As discussed above, net vectorial transport relies on the fidelity of polarized transporter delivery to apical and basolateral membranes as well as the uniform orientation of this polarity by the entire epithelium. As an example, small intestinal glucose absorption will be considered here (Figure 15.5a). Detailed discussions of other absorptive and secretory processes are available in Chapters 16–19.

Glucose is actively transported across the apical plasma membrane by the Na^+/glucose cotransporter SLC5A1 (SGLT1) [139]. The absence of this critical transporter results in glucose–galactose

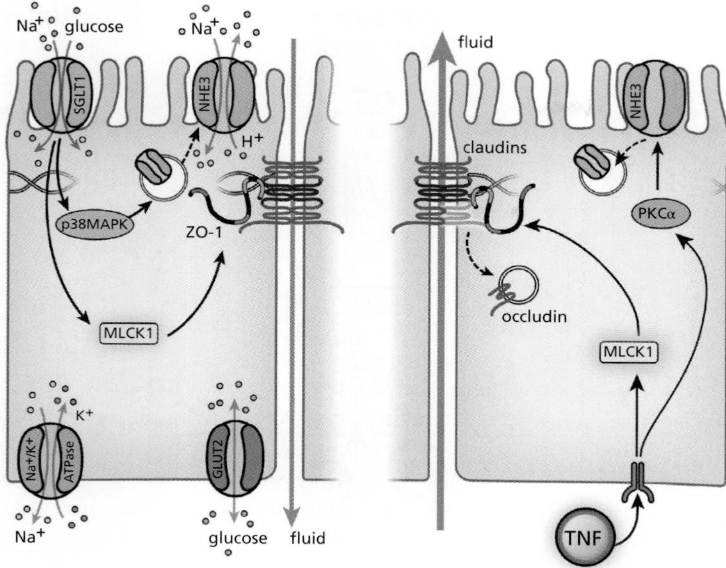

Figure 15.5 Coordination of transcellular and paracellular transport in absorption and diarrheal disease. (Left) The polarized delivery of SGLT1, GLUT2, and Na^+/K^+-adenosine triphosphatase (ATPase) to the appropriate apical (SGLT1) and basolateral (GLUT2 and Na^+/K^+-ATPase) membranes is essential for efficient vectorial glucose absorption. SGLT1 activation also activates p38 MAP kinase (p38 MAPK) to trigger insertion of apical Na^+/H^+ exchangers (NHE3) from a cytoplasmic pool. This enhances apical Na^+ transport beyond that mediated by SGLT1, thereby linking these absorptive processes. Incompletely defined downstream signaling events subsequently activate long myosin light chain kinase 1 (MLCK1) which, in turn, phosphorylates MLC and increases paracellular permeability to small molecules to augment paracellular nutrient and fluid absorption. Overall, this coordinated process drives transcellular and paracellular absorption of fluid, nutrients, and ions. (Right) Tumor necrosis factor-α (TNF) induces net fluid and solute secretion by disrupting both transcellular and paracellular transport. In contrast to SGLT1, TNF induces PKCα-dependent removal of NHE3 from the apical membrane, thereby removing the primary driving force for paracellular fluid absorption. In parallel, TNF activates MLCK1 which, in turn, triggers occludin endocytosis to increase paracellular macromolecular permeability. The combination of increased paracellular permeability and loss of the Na^+ gradient that normally promotes fluid absorption allows paracellular efflux of fluid, ions, and macromolecular solutes.

malabsorption, an autosomal recessive disease characterized by the failure to absorb these carbohydrates from the diet [140]. Affected children present with severe diarrhea, dehydration, and failure to thrive. The disease is generally fatal unless glucose and galactose are eliminated from the diet. The energy source that allows efficient uptake of lumenal glucose by SGLT1 is the steep extracellular to intracellular Na^+ gradient; two Na^+ ions are absorbed along with each glucose molecule (Figure 15.5a). The apical positioning of SGLT1 ensures that glucose is never secreted into the lumen, as the Na^+ gradient makes this thermodynamically unfavorable and also allows glucose to be absorbed against its own concentration gradient. Once within the cytosol, Na^+ and glucose diffuse to the basolateral membrane, where Na^+ ions are pumped out of the cell by the Na^+/K^+-ATPase and glucose molecules are passively transported by the facilitated transporter SLC2A2 (GLUT2). In the absence of lumenal nutrients, GLUT2 can operate in the reverse direction, bringing glucose into the epithelial cell from the subepithelial interstitium. SGLT1 and GLUT2 are specific transporters for glucose; other transporters with similar properties manage the transport of amino acids and other nutrients. One exception is the fructose transport protein SLC2A5 (GLUT5), which mediates fructose uptake across the apical brush border membrane [141].

Paracellular permeability

The paracellular pathway is a major route of passive solute flux. Although plasma membranes are highly impermeant to ions and water, intestinal epithelia have low net resistances, i.e., they are relatively permeable, due to paracellular flux. Paracellular permeability is defined by the tight junction, which is the rate-limiting step that determines passive paracellular flux. Detailed molecular and biophysical analyses, in vitro and in vivo, have shown that flux across the tight junction can be mediated by two routes; the size- (up to ~8 Å diameter) and charge-selective, high-conductance pore pathway and the relatively nonselective, low-conductance leak pathway that is permeable to macromolecules up to ~125 Å in diameter (Figure 15.6) [91,142–144]. Because they are incapable of active transport, tight junction flux pathways are necessarily symmetrical, i.e., apical-to-basal permeability is identical to basal-to-apical permeability; net paracellular transport is dictated solely by transepithelial electrochemical gradients. Preservation of barrier function is sufficiently critical that tight junctions reorganize during single cell shedding, due to either anoikis or apoptosis, in order to prevent permeability increases [145–148]. Nevertheless, complete epithelial barrier loss, termed the unrestricted pathway, occurs when there is

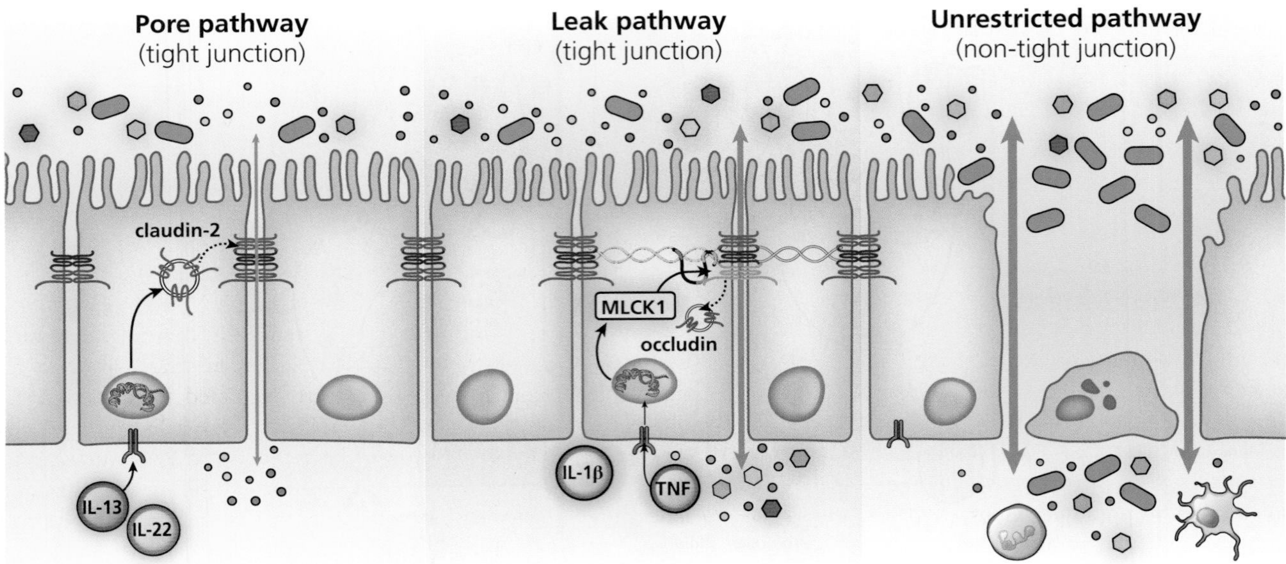

Figure 15.6 The intestinal barrier. The paracellular space between epithelial cells is sealed by selectively permeable tight junctions. Two distinct pathways for trans-tight junction flux have been characterized. The pore pathway (left) is a size- and charge-selective, high-conductance pathway whose permeability can be increased by upregulation of claudin-2, which forms paracellular channels. Both IL-13 and IL-22 have been shown to induce claudin-2 upregulation. The leak pathway (center) is a charge-nonselective, low-capacity macromolecular flux route whose permeability is regulated by long myosin light chain kinase 1 (MLCK1). TNF and IL-1β both increase MLCK1 transcription, enzymatic activity, and recruitment to the perijunctional actomyosin ring which, in turn, induce endocytic removal of occludin from the tight junction and increase leak pathway permeability. A potential third route, the unrestricted pathway (right panel), is opened as a result of epithelial damage. The unrestricted pathway is not regulated by tight junctions.

epithelial damage. This flux route is tight junction independent and is neither size nor charge selective (see Figure 15.6).

The permeability of tight junctions to ions and solutes varies between tissues (e.g., gut and renal tubule), between sites within tissues (e.g., crypt vs villus), and in response to physiological and pathophysiological stimuli [36,145,149–159]. Tight junction ion selectivity is largely defined by the ensemble of claudin protein family members expressed [150,151,156,160–162]. Claudins 1, 2, 3, 4, 5, 7, 8, 12, and 15 are expressed within intestinal epithelia [34]. Differential expression occurs across the longitudinal (duodenum–rectum) and vertical (crypt–villus) axes [34]. Regional variations in claudin expression partially explain differences in paracellular permeability at different sites within the gastrointestinal tract and nephron [34,36,149,157–159]. Expression of some claudins also varies during postnatal development [34]. For example, intestinal claudin-2 expression is highest shortly after birth but markedly downregulated by weaning [34,163–166]. Conversely, claudin-15 expression increases markedly after weaning. Despite this reciprocal developmental regulation, claudins 2 and 15 both form cation- and water-selective channels. The observations that claudin-2 knockout mice are healthy without apparent intestinal defects [166,167] while claudin-15 knockout mice develop marked intestinal hypertrophy may provide a clue to the physiology that depends on this developmental switch [166,168]. As discussed below, claudin-2 expression can be activated in the adult intestine in response to inflammatory stimuli [144,156,169].

Water transport

Despite the obvious importance of fluid transport across gastrointestinal epithelia, controversy remains about the relative importance of the transcellular vs paracellular routes. Potential mechanisms of transcellular water movement include passage through transmembrane channels created by members of the aquaporin protein family [170]. Water transport of the aquaporin protein family is well studied in tissues specialized for regulated water and salt transport, such as the collecting duct of the kidney, the parotid gland, and osmoregulatory organs of saltwater animals [171–174]. Although the aquaporins expressed vary along the length of the small intestine and colon [170], it is likely that these channels facilitate transport of other small molecules, e.g., the H_2O_2 that is released by epithelial cells as a means of defense [175,176].

Available data indicate that, unlike the renal collecting duct and parotid gland, intestinal transepithelial water transport is primarily paracellular and occurs via channels formed by claudins, e.g., claudin-2 and -15 [177–179]. Nevertheless, transcellular ion and solute transporters, e.g., Na^+-nutrient cotransporters and NHE3, direct the osmotic gradients that drive paracellular water flux [155,180–184]. Remarkably, continued activity of this transcellular Na^+ transport relies on paracellular Na^+ flux mediated by claudins-2 and-15; mice lacking both of these claudins die in the perinatal period due to inadequate transcellular nutrient absorption [166,185]. This can be understood when one recognizes that the demands of

Na^+-dependent transcellular transport exceed dietary Na^+. Na^+ flux across tight junctions from the basal interstitium back to into the lumen is necessary so that it can provide the driving force for continued Na^+-dependent transcellular transport. Failure to recycle Na^+ for this purpose explains defects in glucose, amino acid, and fat absorption in mice lacking claudins 2 and 15 [166,185].

Physiological barrier regulation

Intestinal permeability is regulated by physiological processes. For example, it is well documented that Na^+/nutrient cotransport increases tight junction permeability to small molecules [152,155,184,186–188]. These increases in permeability may represent an increase in the number or open probability of small pores in the upper villus [184], i.e., the site of nutrient transport. In contrast, flux across lower villus and crypt paracellular pathways that allow larger molecules to cross the tight junction is not affected by Na^+/nutrient cotransport [184]. Thus, the localized and size-selective tight junction permeability increases that follow Na^+/nutrient cotransport do not result in greater paracellular flux of larger molecules, such as bacterial products [189]. Na^+/glucose cotransport also activates NHE3 trafficking to the apical, brush border membrane [190,191], which results in further increases in transcellular Na^+ absorption (see Figure 15.5). This transcellular nutrient, e.g., glucose, and Na^+ absorption creates a transepithelial osmotic gradient that drives water absorption across the unstirred layer.

As noted above, the unstirred layer lies just above the brush border membranes and is enriched in small nutrients during digestion. This absorbed fluid therefore acts as a solvent that carries small nutrients through tight junction pores. This mechanism, termed "solvent drag," is most active at high lumenal nutrient concentrations, where the impact of paracellular absorption may approach that of transcellular absorption [192]. Thus, transcellular transport activates processes that enhance paracellular absorption [193]. In this manner, paracellular absorption amplifies transcellular absorption. This series of events explains the enhanced efficacy of oral rehydration solutions that include Na^+, glucose, and starches that release glucose [194,195].

Physiological tight junction regulation initiated by Na^+/glucose cotransport requires activation of myosin-light chain kinase (MLCK) [152,155]. The signal transduction mechanisms that link Na^+/glucose cotransport to MLCK activation are incompletely defined, but they result in phosphorylation of myosin II regulatory light chain (MLC). This initiates contraction of the perijunctional actomyosin ring and induces subtle morphological changes, such as perijunctional actomyosin condensation [186] and undulation of tight junction profiles [196] that increase tight junction permeability [155,196,197]. At a molecular level, MLCK activation enhances ATP- and actin-dependent cycling of the tight junction scaffolding protein ZO-1 between tight junction and cytoplasmic pools [197]. This depends, in part, on physical interactions between the ZO-1 actin-binding region (ABR) and F-actin [197] that may induce ZO-1 phase separation [49,50].

Regulation and repair of epithelial barriers in disease

Epithelial renewal

Intestinal epithelial renewal is a continuous process that depends on the capacity of intestinal stem cells (see Chapter 2). The most prominent cycling stem cells, crypt base columnar cells, express leucine-rich repeat-containing G-protein coupled receptor (LGR5) and are regulated by Wnt signaling. Because they are actively dividing, these cells are radiosensitive. They can, however, be replenished by proliferation of quiescent stem cells and dedifferentiation of specialized epithelial cells, e.g., Paneth cells. In health, coordinated proliferation within the intestinal stem cell niche and transit-amplifying zone is essential for mucosal homeostasis as the intestinal epithelium is renewed every 3–5 days. Remarkably, the barrier remains intact throughout this process, including sites where older epithelial cells are extruded into the lumen [146,198–201].

Stem cell proliferation can be upregulated in response to, and is a sensitive indicator of, epithelial damage. This, however, requires time. For rapid repair, normally columnar epithelial cells flatten and spread to resurface exposed basement membrane. This process, termed epithelial restitution, can restore the barrier within minutes to hours, well before new epithelial cells can be generated [202–212].

Tight junction regulation

Despite an intact epithelium, tight junction permeability is enhanced in many inflammatory, infectious, ischemic, and immune-mediated intestinal diseases [43,143,213–215]. For example, intestinal permeability defects that are dependent on increased tight junction permeability and occur in both graft-versus-host disease [99] and human immunodeficiency virus infection are associated with lipopolysaccharide absorption from the gut lumen [216–223].

Intestinal barrier defects are present in a subset of healthy first-degree relatives of patients with Crohn's disease [224–227]. This increased permeability in healthy first-degree subjects has been linked to specific Crohn's disease-associated *NOD2* polymorphisms [226]. Although more study is needed, emerging data indicate that healthy relatives with increased permeability may be at greater risk of developing Crohn's disease than healthy relatives without increased permeability [224]. Moreover, in Crohn's disease patients, increased intestinal permeability during remission can be a marker of impending disease reactivation [228,229]. These data have led to speculation that a primary defect in tight junction barrier function may contribute to the pathogenesis of Crohn's disease [226,230,231]. Consistent with this, experimental colitis severity is enhanced in mice with genetically encoded barrier defects [232–234]. Notably, these mice are healthy, despite barrier loss, in the absence of additional insults. Together, these human and mouse data indicate that intestinal barrier defects can contribute to the pathogenesis of colitis but, in isolation, are insufficient to cause disease.

Inflammation, including that in Crohn's disease, can also cause increased permeability. For example, treatment of patients with Crohn's disease with antitumor necrosis factor-α (TNF) antibodies both reduces inflammatory activity and restores barrier function [235]. Both in vitro and in vivo experimental models have shown that TNF-induced increases in leak pathway permeability require TNF-induced upregulation of long (epithelial) MLCK expression and enzymatic activity [236–238]. These are not, however, sufficient to cause diarrhea, which also requires inhibition of transcellular Na^+ absorption (see Figure 15.5) [239].

In mouse models, acute, TNF-induced barrier loss and diarrhea can be blocked by inhibiting MLCK expression or enzymatic activity [154]. Although enzymatic MLCK inhibitors cannot be safely given systemically [240], genetic knockout of epithelial MLCK also effectively attenuates disease and improves survival in an immune-mediated mouse model of chronic inflammatory bowel disease [241]. In addition to transcriptional and enzymatic MLCK activation, TNF triggers recruitment of the long MLCK splice variant MLCK1 to the perijunctional actomyosin ring [91]. Pharmacological blockade of this MLCK1 recruitment is as effective as either anti-TNF or long MLCK knockout in preventing acute, TNF-induced barrier loss and diarrhea as well as chronic, immune-mediated experimental IBD [91,154].

In contrast to TNF, interleukin (IL)-13 selectively increases pore pathway permeability [156]. This reflects transcriptional activation of claudin-2, which, as noted above, creates cation- and size-selective paracellular pores [156,169]. IL-6 and IL-22 also upregulate claudin-2 expression [144,242,243].

In IBD patients, MLCK expression and enzymatic activity [244] as well as claudin-2 expression are increased [169,245]. Thus, the permeability of both pore and leak pathways is increased in IBD. Nevertheless, the divergent and highly selective effects of IL-6/IL-13/IL-22 and TNF/IL-1β/LIGHT (lymphotoxin-like inducible protein that competes with glycoprotein D for herpesvirus entry on T cells) on barrier function demonstrate that the immune system can differentially target the pore pathway and leak pathways. In turn, barrier regulation can regulate mucosal immunity, as even modest increases in intestinal paracellular permeability induce complex immune responses in vivo [156,232,246]. When considered as a single system, these observations support a model where impaired mucosal barrier function can lead to immune activation, cytokine release, and further loss of barrier function that result is a self-amplifying cycle of barrier dysfunction and inappropriate immune activation [143,145]. Thus, compromised barrier function may be a critical event in disease pathogenesis. Alternatively, mucosal immune activation and cytokine release can initiate this vicious cycle. Similar mechanisms contribute to graft versus host disease [98,99,101] and have been proposed in a range of other disorders including environmental enteric dysfunction [247,248].

Conclusions

Gut epithelial function may be modulated by a host of influences from nonepithelial sources, including growth factors, cytokines and chemokines, and neural mediators. Together, these signaling and regulatory networks interact to maintain gastrointestinal mucosal homeostasis. This includes balancing barrier function with the need for transepithelial movement of ions, nutrients, and antigens; rapid repair of mucosal defects; and management of interactions between mucosal immune cells and the microbiome. The precise integration of these properties centers on the epithelium. Maintenance of the epithelial barrier is critical to these functions and requires integrity of cellular plasma membranes and intercellular tight junctions. Based on the examples provided in this chapter, as well as other chapters in this textbook, it is evident that dysregulation of any of these functions can result in diseases with overlapping clinical presentations.

Acknowledgments

We are indebted to Ms Tiffany S. Davanzo, CMI, for her outstanding illustrations. We also thank Dr. Peter Steinhagen for his contributions to development of this chapter and previous group members who have graciously allowed their data to be reformatted and presented here. Finally, we acknowledge the outstanding contributions of others in this field and apologize to those whose work we were unable to cite.

Support

This work was supported by NIH grants R01DK61931 (JRT), R01DK68271 (JRT), R24DK099803 (JRT), the Harvard Digestive Disease Center (P30DK034854), and the Department of Defense CDMRP PR181271 (JRT).

Conflict of interest

JRT is a founder of Thelium Therapeutics, Inc.

References are available at www.yamadagastro.com/textbook7e

Further reading

Choi W., Yeruva S., Turner J.R. Contributions of intestinal epithelial barriers to health and disease. Exp Cell Res 2017;358(1):71.

Quiros M., Nusrat A. Contribution of wound-associated cells and mediators in orchestrating gastrointestinal mucosal wound repair. Annu Rev Physiol 2019;81:189.

Riga A., Castiglioni V.G., Boxem M. New insights into apical-basal polarization in epithelia. Curr Opin Cell Biol 2019;62:1.

Tsukita S., Tanaka H., Tamura A. The claudins: from tight junctions to biological systems. Trends Biochem Sci 2019;44:141.

van Leen E.V., di Pietro F., Bellaiche Y. Oriented cell divisions in epithelia: from force generation to force anisotropy by tension, shape and vertices. Curr Opin Cell Biol 2019;62:9.

CHAPTER 16

Electrolyte secretion and absorption in the small intestine and colon

Kim E. Barrett[1] **and Stephen J. Keely**[2]

[1]Division of Gastroenterology, Department of Medicine and Program in Biomedical Sciences, University of California San Diego, School of Medicine, La Jolla, CA, USA

[2]Department of Molecular Medicine, Royal College of Surgeons in Ireland, Dublin, Ireland

Chapter menu

Introduction

The gastrointestinal tract deals with large volumes of fluid on a daily basis in fulfilling its physiological imperative to digest and absorb nutrients. The aqueous environment of the lumen represents a milieu where the meal is mixed with digestive secretions and within which the largely hydrophilic chemical processes of digesting the components of a meal can take place. Conversely, the end-products of digestion require a predominantly aqueous environment through which they can diffuse to the intestinal epithelium, across which they are taken up into the body. On average, the small intestine receives about 8–9 liters of fluid per day, composed of oral intake (around 1 L, depending on the types of food and beverages ingested), various digestive juices arising from the stomach as well as organs that drain into the intestine, and from the intestine itself (Figure 16.1). Of this total, the vast majority is reabsorbed, leaving only 100–200 mL to be lost to the stool in health. The balance between absorption and secretion, where absorption markedly predominates, must therefore be closely regulated. Both the small intestine and colon also have a reserve capacity for absorption, but if this is exceeded, or if absorption is inhibited and/or secretion is stimulated excessively, diarrheal symptoms will result.

Fluid movement into and out of the intestinal lumen depends, in turn, on the active secretion and absorption of electrolytes. In the small intestine, where the products of digestion are prevalent postprandially, water is reclaimed by the osmotic forces generated by active nutrient uptake, often in combination with electrolytes such as sodium ions or protons. In the colon, absorptive processes center on the active absorption of sodium and chloride ions, although uptake of products formed when intestinal bacteria ferment otherwise indigestible food substances (such as dietary fiber to form short-chain fatty acids) may also contribute appreciably. On the secretory side of the equation, fluid accumulation in the lumen is driven predominantly by the active secretion of chloride ions, although secretion of bicarbonate and potassium ions also contributes. Furthermore, even though absorption predominates overall, secretion is ongoing throughout the small intestine and colon as local conditions dictate, to maintain appropriate levels of fluidity such that the meal or its residues can be propelled along the length of the intestine, and perhaps also as a contributor to host defense, particularly to protect the vulnerable stem cell niche at the base of the crypts.

The past 25 years have seen an explosion in our knowledge of the molecular machinery that both comprises and regulates

Yamada's Textbook of Gastroenterology, Seventh Edition. Edited by Timothy C. Wang, Michael Camilleri, Benjamin Lebwohl, Anna S. Lok, William J. Sandborn, Kenneth K. Wang, and Gary D. Wu.

Companion website: www.yamadagastro.com/textbook7e

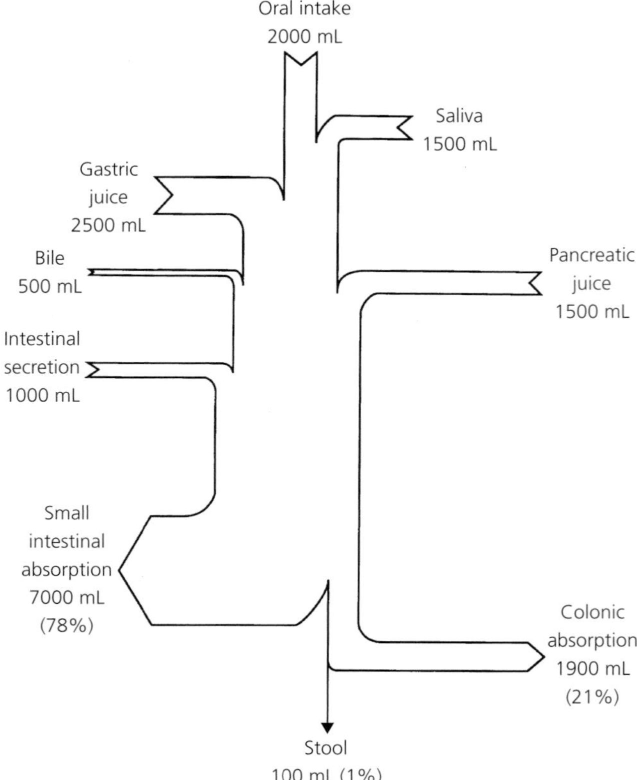

Figure 16.1 Daily water balance in the healthy human gastrointestinal tract. The amount of oral intake will vary between individuals depending on the types of meals taken. Note that even in health there is a significant secretory flux of fluid from the intestine (1000 mL). The small intestine is responsible for absorbing almost 80% of the daily fluid load, largely in association with nutrient uptake. The colon absorbs the majority of the remaining fluid, with an efficiency of approximately 95%, leaving only about 1% of the daily fluid load to be lost to the stool. Source: Reprinted with permission from Barrett K.E., Dharmsathaphorn K. Transport of water and electrolytes in the gastrointestinal tract: physiological mechanisms, regulation and methods for study. In: Maxwell and Kleeman's Clinical Disorders of Fluid and Electrolyte Metabolism, Fifth Edition, R.G. Narins, Editor, pp 493–519, McGraw-Hill, Inc., New York, 1994.

electrolyte transport mechanisms in the gut. We now enjoy a detailed understanding of the specific membrane transport proteins that mediate transepithelial transfer of ions and other solutes into and out of the lumen, the distribution of these proteins along the length of the intestine and the crypt–villus axis, the signaling mechanisms that regulate these transporters and their interactions, and the interplay of neural, endocrine, and immune effectors that establish fluid homeostasis in the healthy gut. This information has allowed the development of rational therapies for disease states where homeostasis breaks down, such as the aforementioned diarrheal diseases as well as their opposites, such as constipation and cystic fibrosis. The goal of this chapter, therefore, is to identify the components and regulation of intestinal transport mechanisms and then use these as a basis for understanding specific intestinal diseases. It is notable that diarrheal diseases, in particular, remain a scourge of humanity and a leading cause of impaired development and even mortality in infants, especially in developing countries, as well as imposing a substantial financial burden even in developed countries.

The intestinal epithelium

The intestinal epithelium is a single layer of cells that lines the entire surface of the gut lumen. Its primary functions are to act as a barrier that prevents the uptake of harmful substances from the intestinal contents, and to transport fluids, nutrients, and electrolytes into and out of the gut. Along the length of the intestine, epithelial cells must have the capacity to perform these functions under dramatically different circumstances. Moreover, they must also be able to respond rapidly to changes in the luminal environment, whether they are due to physiological or pathophysiological stimuli. To cope with this, the epithelium has evolved as a dynamic multicellular system that is in a constant state of differentiation and renewal. Despite the dramatic differences in their function along the intestinal tract, epithelial cells have common properties that enable them to perform their basic functions, most notably their capacity to undergo functional polarization and to form tight junctions with one another.

Functional polarity

In order to transport substances vectorially across the intestinal wall, epithelial cells form a selectively permeable barrier that expresses different transport proteins on its apical and basolateral sides. This feature, referred to as functional polarity, is achieved primarily through the development of intercellular tight junctions. These complex structures encircle epithelial cells towards their apical pole and perform two important functions: they act as a physical fence that separates the apical and basolateral compartments, and their components interact with partner proteins on neighboring cells to form porous seals. Development of functional polarity is important not only for the appropriate distribution of transport proteins on intestinal epithelial cells, but also for the receptors and signaling molecules that regulate their function.

When grown in single-cell suspensions, epithelial cells display no features of polarity. However, when these cells make contact with each other, the process of polarization is initiated. Firstly, E-cadherin is rapidly recruited to points of cell-to-cell contact, creating a focal point in the cell membrane around which the machinery for the development of cell polarity is assembled [1,2]. The clustering of cadherin in the membrane leads to recruitment of catenins that, in turn, leads to changes in the actin cytoskeleton at the site of cell adhesion. The membrane cytoskeleton is formed, into which is recruited a scaffold of proteins, such as fodrin, ankyrin, the atypical protein kinase C (aPKC)–PAR-6 complex, and SNAREs, that functions to direct proteins to the appropriate domain of the cell. At the same time, tight junction proteins are recruited and assembled to form a physical fence that maintains separation between the nascent apical and basolateral domains.

The signals that direct the sorting of newly synthesized proteins to the appropriate domain of the cell are complex but becoming increasingly understood. Most membrane proteins are sorted within the trans-Golgi network into vesicles destined for the apical or basolateral domain. Signals directing proteins to the basolateral side of the cell are typically contained in their cytoplasmic domains, often containing a tyrosine residue within highly conserved amino acid sequences. Such signals induce a certain conformation of the protein that targets them to vesicles bound for the basolateral pole [3]. Signals directing proteins to the apical side of the cell are generally found within their transmembrane or extracellular domains. One such signal is the glycosylphosphatidylinositol (GPI) anchor, which serves to cluster proteins into glycolipid- and cholesterol-rich rafts [4]. These rafts eventually fuse and bud off from the Golgi network, from where they travel to the cell surface. N- and O-linked glycans have also been identified as important apical sorting signals [5]. Posttranslational modification of proteins by the addition of glycan side chains is determined by the relative expression and specificities of the glycosyltransferases and glycosidases within each cell which are, in turn, dependent on cell type and differentiation state. Thus, glycosylation offers great potential for diversification of protein-sorting signals in cells from different organs and at different stages of differentiation.

Once proteins have been sorted into vesicles, they are trafficked along the cytoskeleton to the site of cell-to-cell adhesion, from where they are directed to either the apical or basolateral side of the cell. Transport vesicles express v-SNAREs on their surface, which recognize t-SNAREs in the target membrane. Different types of t-SNAREs then direct the vesicles to either the apical or basolateral membranes. For example, syntaxin 3 directs vesicles to the apical membrane, whereas syntaxin 4 sorts them to the basolateral domain [6–8]. Another important protein complex involved in directing transport vesicles to the basolateral domain is the Sec6/8 or *exocyst* complex [2]. Finally, once they have been targeted to the appropriate membrane, proteins are retained there by anchoring to the cytoskeleton and by the physical barrier posed by the tight junctions.

However, it is important to note that once polarity is established, the complement of transport proteins expressed on the apical and basolateral surfaces is not static. Indeed, their trafficking to and from the membrane is dynamically regulated by many endogenous and exogenous factors, enabling the intestinal epithelium to alter its capacity for fluid and electrolyte transport in response to changing physiological or pathophysiological circumstances. For example, under conditions of bacterial infection, perturbed sorting of proteins to the apical and basolateral domains is thought to underlie disruption of tight junctions, loss of barrier function, and dysregulated epithelial transport [9].

Tight junctions

Tight junctions, formed during the generation of cell polarity, are found towards the luminal pole of the cell and, along with adherens junctions, comprise the apical junction complex (AJC), a hallmark feature of columnar epithelial cells. At the ultrastructural level, tight junctions appear as a dense network of protein strands, the number of which is directly related to the junction's barrier properties [10,11]. Tight junction permeability is not constant along the length of the intestinal tract and tends to decrease aborally.

The structural components of tight junctions are transmembrane proteins, including a large family of proteins known as claudins, a smaller group of proteins known as TAMPs (tight junction-associated marvel domain-containing proteins), and junctional adhesion molecule (JAM) [12,13] (see also Chapter 15). These proteins interact with their counterparts on neighboring cells to form the paracellular pore through which substances can pass passively from the lumen into the body. Claudins are differentially expressed along both the jejunocolonic and crypt–villus axes and are apparently the most important of the tight junction proteins in regulating permeability [14]. Claudins have two extracellular loops that project into the lateral space and interact with partners on neighboring cells. To date, 27 claudins have been identified and the differential expression of these proteins within tight junctions dictates the size and ionic selectivity of the paracellular pore. For example, claudin 3 serves to seal the paracellular pore to ions and solutes, claudins 2 and 10a are more permeable to cations, and claudins 10b and 15 display anionic selectivity. Such ionic selectivity within the paracellular space is determined by electrostatic interactions dictated by charged amino acids in the claudin extracellular domains [15].

The role of JAM in regulating tight junctions is not as well defined as it is for claudins, but it has been proposed to play a more important role in signaling than it does in constituting part of the tight junction architecture [16]. Similarly, the TAMP proteins, which include occludin and tricellulin, are integral components of tight junctions that play important roles in the signaling pathways that regulate epithelial permeability [12,17].

Just as the membrane expression of transport proteins is coordinated with fluid homeostasis and nutritional requirements, tight junctions are also dynamic and their permeability is regulated by a wide range of endogenous and exogenous stimuli [18]. The transduction of regulatory signals occurs through a network of signaling proteins that ultimately regulate tight junction permeability either by altering the phosphorylation and/or membrane expression of their structural proteins, or by altering the perijunctional actin cytoskeleton [19,20]. Signals that induce actin polymerization physically dissociate tight junctions, while those that cause actin depolymerization, or severing, allow tight junctions to close.

Of the tight junction signaling proteins, perhaps the most studied are the zonula occludens (ZO) proteins, which belong to a class of proteins called membrane-associated guanylate kinase homologues (MAGUKs). These proteins contain several protein–protein interaction motifs and serve as important scaffolds that link structural proteins of tight junctions with intracellular signaling molecules and the cytoskeleton [21]. Interestingly, ZO proteins also contain nuclear sorting signals, implying a role for these proteins in coordinating epithelial barrier function with cell growth and differentiation [22]. Another critical regulator of tight junction permeability is myosin light chain kinase (MLCK) [19]. When activated by diverse stimuli, MLCK phosphorylates myosin light chain (MLC) and alters ZO-1 association with tight junction proteins [19].

Regulation of tight junction permeability is closely coordinated with transport function, allowing optimal synchronization of water and solute transport. Thus, increases in Na^+-nutrient coupled transport leads to an MLCK-mediated opening of tight junctions and a concomitant increase in fluid absorption [23]. Indeed, several transport proteins have been shown to regulate tight junction permeability, including sodium-hydrogen exchangers and Na^+/K^+ ATPase pumps [24–27]. Of particular interest is ClC-2, a Cl^- channel that is expressed within tight junctions and is closely associated with tight junction signaling proteins. ClC-2 has been shown to regulate occludin trafficking to the membrane and it appears to play a role in maintaining barrier function in animal models of intestinal injury [28,29].

Many extracellular factors, including nutrients, cytokines, growth factors, bile acids, and neurotransmitters, can influence intestinal fluid and electrolyte transport by altering tight junction permeability [18,30–33]. Importantly, luminal viruses, bacteria, and their toxins also have the capacity to regulate epithelial permeability. This can be achieved through direct alterations in the expression and function of tight junction structural proteins, alterations in the cellular cytoskeleton, induction of signaling cascades, or production of inflammatory cytokines [34–41]. Whatever the mechanism, tight junction opening in response to colonization of the gut by pathogens leads to an increase in paracellular permeability with concomitant fluid loss and the onset of diarrhea [9,42–44]. Conversely, numerous commensal probiotic bacteria (see Chapter 143) have been shown to have the capacity to restore normal epithelial transport and barrier function, suggesting they may have a role in treating intestinal disease [45–47].

In summary, tight junctions are essential for maintaining cell polarity, intestinal epithelial barrier function, and the osmotic gradients necessary for water transport to occur. Consequently, the opening of tight junctions, whether in response to physiological or pathophysiological stimuli, can have significant consequences, since as the paracellular pathway becomes more permeable, the barrier to nutrient, electrolyte, and water movement is diminished.

Epithelial organization and diversity

Although all epithelial cells display common characteristics of functional polarity and the ability to generate tight junctions, they are required to function under dramatically different conditions along the length of the intestine. Thus, there is a great diversity in epithelial cell type and function not only along the jejunocolonic axis, but also among the cells that constitute individual crypt and villus units (the crypt–villus axis).

Jejunocolonic axis

Since the contents of the lumen change along the length of the intestine, epithelial cells in different segments have marked differences in their capacity for absorption and secretion of fluid and electrolytes [48,49]. For example, although anion secretion occurs along the entire intestinal tract, there is an aboral gradient of the ratio between HCO_3^- to Cl^- secretion, with HCO_3^- secretion being highest in the proximal small intestine in order to neutralize gastric acid entering from the stomach. Similarly, mechanisms of Na^+ absorption differ along the intestine. In the proximal small intestine, where digestion primarily occurs, Na^+ absorption is mediated mainly by nutrient-coupled pathways, whereas in the distal colon electrogenic Na^+ absorption through the epithelial sodium channel (ENaC) predominates. Electroneutral Na^+ absorption occurs throughout the intestine and is the predominant pathway mediating fluid absorption between meals [50,51]. Interestingly, there appears to be reciprocal regulation between different absorptive pathways in the small intestine, which likely determines the extent to which each pathway contributes to the overall process of fluid and electrolyte absorption [52]. Furthermore, the epithelium displays regional heterogeneity not only in terms of electrolyte transport, but also in the transport of nutrients, vitamins, minerals, bile acids, and drugs. Accordingly, epithelial cells in different intestinal segments express distinct repertoires of transport proteins on their surface [49,53–55].

The establishment and maintenance of an epithelial phenotype is thought to be due to both location-specific intrinsic programming of stem cells and the influence of several transcription factors, notably the GATA family, which are themselves differentially expressed along the jejunocolonic axis [56,57]. Interestingly, regional differences in the expression of structural components of tight junctions also occur along the length of the intestine and this likely underlies differences in transepithelial permeability that are observed in different regions [12].

Crypt–villus axis

The mucosa of the small intestine is organized into villi, which are finger-like projections that extend into the lumen, and which surround deep invaginations into the mucosa, termed the crypts of Lieberkühn. There are four major types of epithelial cell found along the crypt–villus axis: transporting enterocytes, goblet cells, enteroendocrine cells, and Paneth cells. Tuft cells are also present, which transmit luminal information to the enteric nervous and immune systems [58]. Each of these cell types is derived from common LGR5-expressing stem cells, which are found towards the base of the crypts in the stem cell niche. Stem cells are continuously dividing to produce a population of transit-amplifying cells that migrate upwards and differentiate into the various epithelial cell types [59,60]. Enterocytes, as well as goblet, tuft, and enteroendocrine cells, continue to migrate upwards towards the villus, while Paneth cells migrate downwards to the crypt base.

Enterocytes are the most numerous of the epithelial cells along the crypt–villus axis and it is across these cells that electrolytes are either absorbed or secreted. However, the other cells of the epithelium play important roles in augmenting and regulating enterocyte transport and barrier function. For example, Paneth cells contribute to host defense by secreting antimicrobial peptides, such as lysozyme and defensins [61,62]. Furthermore, certain antimicrobial peptides produced by Paneth cells, known as cryptdins, can also directly modulate epithelial transport by forming ion channels in the apical membrane of enterocytes [63]. Goblet cells secrete mucus, which serves to lubricate and protect the epithelial surface [64,65]. Goblet cells express a similar complement of cell surface receptors as enterocytes, which ensures that mucus and fluid secretion is coordinated [66].

Enteroendocrine cells are found interspersed between enterocytes of the small intestine and colon. Many different populations of enteroendocrine cells exist, distinguished by their chemical content, with the 5-hydroxytryptamine (5-HT)-containing enterochromaffin cells being the most prominent [67,68]. The primary function of enteroendocrine cells is to sense or "taste" the luminal environment to detect changes in intraluminal nutrient contents, pH, and/or distension and to transduce these cues to sensory afferents of the enteric nervous system as well as enterocytes, thereby eliciting appropriate changes in transport function [69].

As they migrate upwards towards the villus, enterocytes differentiate from a secretory to an absorptive phenotype. For many years, it was thought that there was a strict spatial segregation of transport functions along the crypt–villus axis, with secretion occurring only in the crypts and absorption occurring only across villus cells (or surface cells of the colon). However, it is now known that the separation of absorptive and secretory function along the crypt–villus axis is not so clearly defined and can vary under different conditions [70,71]. Nevertheless, as enterocytes migrate, they develop a more absorptive phenotype. When they reach the villus tip, they are shed into the lumen by a tightly regulated form of apoptosis, known as anoikis [72].

Factors that regulate the morphogenesis of the crypt–villus axis and the differentiation of cells along its length are increasingly understood. A critical signal controlling proliferation is Wnt, a protein secreted by Paneth cells at the crypt base [61,73]. Wnt activates members of the Frizzled family of surface receptors to bring about cytosolic accumulation and nuclear translocation of β-catenin. In turn, β-catenin regulates the expression of several downstream Wnt effectors. One important downstream action of Wnt signaling is increased expression of LGR5 on stem cells. LGR5 is activated by ligands known as R-spondins and this, in turn, leads to increased abundance of Wnt receptors by preventing their degradation. Thus, regulation of this Wnt/β-catenin/LGR5-induced feedback loop is a critical factor in determining self-renewal and morphogenesis. Another important signaling pathway is that mediated by Notch receptors [73,74]. These are expressed on stem cells and cells within the transit-amplifying compartment and are activated in response to ligands, notably Dll1 and Dll4, produced by Paneth and transit-amplifying cells. Notch signaling determines cell fate and biases differentiation into enterocytes versus cells of the secretory lineage, including goblet, neuroendocrine, and Paneth cells.

Principles of epithelial transport

Transepithelial transport

Substances may traverse the intestinal epithelium by multiple routes. *Transcellular* processes require entry of electrolytes across one membrane barrier, transit through the cell cytosol, and exit across the opposite membrane. As discussed earlier, the functional polarity of epithelial cells is the basis for this net (vectorial) movement of electrolytes. *Paracellular* transport refers to the passive flux of electrolytes and water across tight junctions. Paracellular flux occurs entirely extracellularly, and can only produce vectorial transport in dissipating transepithelial chemical and electrical gradients established by active transcellular transport.

Types of transmembrane transport

Charged species, such as ions, cannot traverse the lipid core of the plasma membrane to any appreciable degree. This is vital to life, because cellular biochemistry depends on the tight control of intracellular ionic composition. Therefore, specialized proteins are inserted into the plasma membrane to mediate and regulate ion movement. Ions can cross the membrane via these proteins with either the consumption of cellular energy (active transport) or by flowing down existing electrical and/or chemical gradients (passive transport).

Transepithelial transport involves a combination of both *active* and *passive* transport pathways. Ultimately, all the net transepithelial transport mechanisms discussed in this chapter require at least one active transport step to drive vectorial transport. An additional distinction concerns transporters referred to as *secondary active* transport proteins. These are transporters that are passive, in and of themselves, in that their activity and direction of transport are dependent on existing gradients. However, they are referred to as secondary active transporters if they specifically take advantage of a gradient set up by an active transporter to move at least one of their substrates "uphill." An example would be the ability of the Na^+-glucose cotransporter, SGLT1, to move glucose into the cytosol from the intestinal lumen against its concentration gradient by coupling transport of the sugar to that of Na^+, which responds to the low intracellular Na^+ concentration established by the active transporter, Na^+,K^+-ATPase.

In addition to the distinction of active versus passive transport across a membrane, all transport reactions can be grouped into one of two classes: electrogenic or electroneutral. *Electrogenic* transport moves net charge across the membrane either via the flux of single ions (e.g., ion channels) or combinations of transport substrates whose charge is unequal (e.g., Na^+/glucose cotransporter). *Electroneutral* transporters also mediate a net flux of ions, but do so without moving net charge across the membrane during a transport cycle. Electroneutral transporters may mediate an exchange of equal charges across the membrane (e.g., Na^+/H^+ exchanger), or a cotransport of equal and opposite charges (e.g., $Na^+/K^+/2Cl^-$ cotransporter). Importantly, the electrical gradient across the membrane is not a driving force affecting electroneutral carriers, and so their rate and direction of transport are determined solely by the respective transmembrane chemical gradients of the transported ions. As discussed later (see section on Transepithelial electrolyte transport), combinations of different transport proteins can also result in overall transepithelial transport that is either electrogenic or electroneutral. Since no aqueous solution can have unequal numbers of cations and anions, transepithelial electrogenic transport requires compensatory fluxes to maintain electrical neutrality. Electrical neutrality is usually maintained by paracellular transport of an oppositely charged ion through the tight junctions. Both electrogenic and electroneutral transepithelial transport mechanisms, on the other hand, drive an accompanying flux of water in response to the osmotic gradients that they generate.

Fluid transport

Physiology of water flux

Water is crucial for physiological processes and the amount of water in the intestinal lumen is closely regulated. In healthy humans, 65–80% of secreted or ingested water is absorbed in association with nutrient and electrolyte absorption in the small intestine, so that only 1500–2000 mL enters the colon (see Figure 16.1). The colon absorbs most of this remaining fluid with high efficiency, so that normally only about 100 mL is excreted in the stool.

Molecular mechanisms of water transport

Researchers are still developing a full understanding of how water crosses the intestinal epithelium. One general principle, however, is that water always flows across membranes in response to electrolyte and/or osmolyte fluxes. In most cases, water molecules are moved into and out of the lumen by passive processes requiring no further input of cellular energy beyond that required to cause electrolyte transport.

There are multiple routes for passive water diffusion across epithelia. If the actively transported electrolyte accumulates in the small extracellular spaces between adjacent epithelial cells (during absorption) or in the gut lumen (during secretion), there is an osmotic driving force for water to equilibrate via the tight junctions. This is believed to be the mechanism for fluid absorption in the proximal small intestine. Conversely, if the electrolyte accumulates intracellularly, there is a driving force for water to equilibrate across the cell membrane, which provides a transcellular route for water transport. The transcellular route is predicted to be more important in tight epithelia (e.g., the distal colon), because flow through the tight junctions is restricted in this setting.

Like ions, water has difficulty crossing lipid membranes so membrane proteins must enhance water transport across these barriers. Attention has focused on two classes of proteins that increase water permeability across intestinal membranes: aquaporins and Na^+-dependent solute transporters. Aquaporins are members of a gene family that function as water channels in the plasma membrane. Since their initial discovery [75], eight aquaporin (AQP) isoforms have been reported in the intestine (AQP1, 3, 4, 7, 8, 9, 10, and 11) [76,77]. However, there may be significant variations between species, and certain aquaporins are apparently expressed not in epithelial cells but rather in subepithelial cell types that presumably rule out a role in transepithelial fluid movement. AQP3 has been shown to be abundant in the surface/villus cells of the colon, jejunum, and ileum, although there is controversy over whether AQP3 is apical [78] or basolateral [79]. In contrast, AQP4 is a basolateral protein in the small intestine and colon [79,80]. AQP7 and 8 have been found in surface/villus cells of the jejunum and colon of rats, although AQP8 may be absent from the small intestine in humans [76,80].

At present, only limited functional evidence links specific aquaporin isoform(s) to intestinal water transport. AQP4 knockout mice had a modest (30–40%) decrease in water absorption by the proximal colon [80], whereas AQP8 knockout mice did not [81]. On the other hand, the trichohepatoenteric syndrome, which is associated with severe childhood diarrhea, is associated with downregulation of AQP7 as well as other apical transport proteins in the gut [82]. The variable results likely highlight redundant pathways for intestinal water flux [76]. Nevertheless, alterations in aquaporin activity and/or localization may contribute to some forms of infectious diarrhea [77,83]. Moreover, there is evidence that expression of a number of aquaporins is downregulated in celiac disease (and restored when gluten is removed from the diet), which could contribute to the diarrhea exhibited by some patients [76,84].

Another potential route for transcellular water flux is via Na^+-dependent solute transporters. Some authors have argued that SGLT1 can move water molecules across the membrane each time it transports two Na^+ ions and a single glucose molecule into the cell, possibly in the form of molecules that hydrate the cotransporter glucose-binding site, or SGLT1 may even act as a water channel [85–87]. Water may be a transport substrate of SGLT1 even under isotonic conditions [88]. Results suggest that other cotransporters also enhance water fluxes [89]. On the other hand, others have argued that the relationship between the expression of SGLT1 or other cotransporters and fluid permeability is largely, if not entirely, accounted for by the ability of the transporters to establish microscopic osmotic gradients driving conventional passive water diffusion rather than water cotransport per se [90,91]. Independent of the precise model, it has been estimated that the absorption of up to 5 L of water per day could be mediated by SGLT1 alone [86].

Indeed, intestinal water transport is clearly regulated indirectly by the regulation of electrolyte transport. When electrolytes and osmolytes remain in the intestinal lumen (e.g., luminal lactose in lactase-deficient subjects), luminal hyperosmolarity decreases water absorption. The opposite is also true: when molecules are absorbed and leave the lumen, they increase water absorption. Use of this osmotic driving force constitutes the basis for oral rehydration solutions, in which a low-osmolarity substrate (e.g., starch) in the lumen is digested (e.g., to glucose) and the products avidly absorbed (e.g., by SGLT1), thus stimulating water absorption. The water transport that occurs under these circumstances is likely mediated not only by aquaporins and cotransporters, as discussed, but also via cation and water-permeable pores that are generated in intercellular tight junctions by specific claudin molecules (e.g., claudins 2 and 15) [92,93].

Electrolyte transport proteins

This section describes the building blocks of epithelial transport: individual membrane transport proteins. Different combinations of these transport molecules are expressed in individual cells to perform specific electrolyte transport events. Electrolyte transport proteins in the epithelia of the small intestine and colon and their participation in transepithelial electrolyte transport are summarized in Table 16.1.

Table 16.1 Key transport proteins and their participation in transepithelial electrolyte transport in the intestines.

TRANSPORT PROTEIN	POLARITY	GENES	TRANSEPITHELIAL FUNCTION	NOTES
ATPase pumps				
Na^+,K^+-ATPase	Basolateral	α1 subunit:ATP1A1 β1 subunit:ATP1B1	All active transport	α1β1 dimer is the only intestinal epithelial isoform
H^+,K^+-ATPase	Apical	α subunit: ATP12A	Colonic K^+ and SCFA absorption	β subunit needed for function
Exchangers and cotransporters				
Na^+/glucose cotransporter	Apical	SLC5A1 (SGLT1)	Solute-coupled Na^+ uptake	Example of Na^+-coupled cotransporter
Na^+/bile acid cotransporter	Apical	SLC10A2 (ASBT)	Bile acid reabsorption	Restricted to terminal ileum
H^+/peptide cotransporter	Apical	SLC15A1 (PEPT1)	Proton-coupled osmolyte absorption	Example of proton-coupled cotransporter
H^+/monocarboxylate cotransporter	Apical and basolateral	SLC16A1 (MCT1)	SCFA absorption?	SCFA transporter
$Na^+/K^+/2Cl^-$ cotransporter	Basolateral	SLC12A2 (NKCC1)	Cl^- and K^+ secretion	
Na^+/bicarbonate cotransporter	Basolateral	SLC4A4 (NBC1)	Bicarbonate secretion	
Na^+/H^+ exchangers	Apical	SLC9A3 (NHE3)	Small intestinal and proximal colonic electroneutral Na^+ absorption	
	Apical	SLC9A2 (NHE2)	(Electroneutral Na^+ absorption?); HCO_3^- secretion	
	Basolateral	SLC9A1 (NHE1)	HCO_3^- secretion	Ubiquitously expressed, cellular pH regulator
Cl^-/HCO_3^- exchangers	Apical	SLC26A3(DRA) SLC26A6 (PAT1)	Electroneutral Cl^- and K^+ absorption, HCO_3^- secretion	
Na^+/Cl^- cotransporter	Apical	SLC12A3 (NCC)	(Calcium absorption?)	Interacts with voltage-sensitive Ca^{++} channel
K^+/Cl^- cotransporter	Unproven	SLC12A4 (KCC1)	Electroneutral K^+ or Cl^- absorption	Presumed basolateral route for KCl exit
Channels				
Na^+ channel (ENaC)	Apical	α subunit:SCNN1A β subunit:SCNN1B γ subunit:SCNN1G	Electrogenic Na^+ absorption	Amiloride-sensitive channel
Cl^- channels	Apical	CFTR	Cl^- secretion	cAMP-activated; also conducts bicarbonate
	Apical	TMEM16A	Cl^- secretion	Calcium-activated
	Basolateral	CLCN2 (ClC-2)	Cl^- secretion?	Outwardly rectifying: volume sensitive
K^+ channels	Apical	KCNMA1	K^+ secretion	
	Basolateral	KCNN4 KCNQ1 (with its regulatory subunit, KCNE3)	Cl^- secretion, electrogenic and solute-coupled Na^+ absorption	

SCFA, short-chain fatty acid.

ATPase pumps

A transport ATPase provides the necessary driving force for net transepithelial ion transport to occur in mammalian cells. Among the known transport ATPases, Na^+,K^+-ATPase and H^+,K^+-ATPase have well-established roles in intestinal electrolyte transport. These proteins have related sequences (60–70% homology), and are both members of the P-type ATPase multigene family, so named because all members of this family become phosphorylated during part of the transport cycle.

Na^+,K^+-ATPase

In the presence of Mg^{++}, Na^+,K^+-ATPase (the sodium pump) catalyzes efflux of three Na^+ ions from the cell and uptake of two K^+ ions while hydrolyzing one ATP molecule per cycle [94]. Because more cation is pumped out than is replaced, the sodium pump is electrogenic and generates a negative intracellular electrical potential. Na^+,K^+-ATPase is localized basolaterally in all intestinal epithelial cells. It acts to maintain low and high intracellular concentrations of Na^+ and K^+, respectively. The sodium electrochemical gradient is then used as a driving force for Na^+ influx via Na^+ channels or through the many secondary active cotransporters and exchangers for which Na^+ is required (Figures 16.2–16.7). Inactivation of Na^+,K^+-ATPase with cardiac glycosides, such as ouabain, inhibits all of these transport mechanisms in the intestine.

The sodium pump exists in the membrane as a heterodimer of α and β subunits, and the α1/β1 isoforms of these subunits predominate in the intestine [95]. The α subunit has at least eight transmembrane segments, and contains the ouabain binding site and all ion binding and catalytic sites. The β subunit is essential for chaperoning the heterodimer through correct assembly and membrane targeting [96]. A variety of FXYD proteins also interact tightly with the sodium pump in a tissue-specific manner to increase its activity by increasing affinity for Na^+ [97].

H^+,K^+-ATPase

In several species, the apical membrane of cells in the distal colon contains H^+,K^+-ATPase activity. Similar to the gastric H^+,K^+-ATPase, to which it is related, the colonic form mediates cellular efflux of H^+ into the gut lumen in exchange for K^+ uptake, with hydrolysis of ATP providing energy [98]. Activity of this pump is variably inhibited by the Na^+,K^+-ATPase inhibitor ouabain, suggesting that an ouabain-insensitive K^+-ATPase may exist in different species, although it is believed that the colonic enzyme is largely insensitive to omeprazole and related inhibitors of the gastric H^+,K^+ ATPase [99–102].

Unlike Na^+,K^+-ATPase, the colonic H^+,K^+-ATPase does not play a dominant role in regulating intracellular levels of its transported ions. Although cytosolic pH can be measurably affected by the activity of H^+,K^+-ATPase, other transporters (e.g., Na^+/H^+ exchangers) are likely to have greater impact on control of resting cytosolic pH [103]. In distal colon of the guinea pig, protons secreted by the colonic H^+,K^+-ATPase are important for stimulating uptake of luminal short-chain fatty acids (SCFAs), facilitating absorption of SCFAs in their nonionized (i.e., protonated) form [104]. The colonic H^+,K^+-ATPase is also important for K^+ absorption, especially in infant animals who need to retain more K^+ than adults to avoid growth retardation [105]. Upregulation of colonic H^+,K^+-ATPase also contributes to the potassium retention in late pregnancy that is important for fetal development [106].

The colonic H^+,K^+-ATPase consists of α and β subunits [107,108]. Coexpression of the α subunit with either HKβ or a heterologous β subunit (either from gastric H^+,K^+-ATPase or Na^+,K^+-ATPase) is sufficient to reconstitute observable H^+,K^+-ATPase activity in the plasma membrane [109]. Evidence suggests that the β subunit of the Na^+,K^+-ATPase may serve this role physiologically, as it is found with the HKα subunit in the apical membrane of colonocytes [110].

Exchangers and cotransporters

Despite the limited number of ATPase pumps, an abundant assortment of electrolytes and solutes are actively transported across the intestinal epithelium. This is possible because a large number of different carrier proteins convert the energy of sodium or proton gradients into net transport of other electrolytes and solutes.

Na^+-solute cotransporters

Many food-derived products, including glucose, amino acids and vitamins, as well as endogenous luminal solutes such as bile acids, are taken up by specific Na^+-coupled cotransport proteins in the apical membrane of enterocytes. These cotransporters are the predominant route by which these diverse substances enter the body, and are also responsible for driving the majority of sodium and water absorption following a meal. Most of these cotransporters are found in the small intestine.

The intestinal Na^+/glucose cotransporter (SGLT1) has been studied the most extensively [85,111,112]. Each transport cycle results in uptake of two sodium ions and one glucose molecule, and this stoichiometry contributes importantly to absorption of glucose against its concentration gradient [85]. SGLT1 (Slc5a1) is a member of the SLC5 family of solute carriers, which also includes the renal Na^+-glucose cotransporter (SGLT2/Slc5a2), the thyroid Na^+/iodide cotransporter (NIS/Slc5a5), and the Na^+/multivitamin transporter (SMVT/Slc5a6), amongst others [113]. SGLT1 is a single polypeptide chain with 14 transmembrane segments. Studies of chimeras between SGLT1 and SGLT2 revealed that the SGLT1 C-terminal contains the sugar-binding site [114]. Further, a C-terminal mutation (Q457R) in SGLT1 resulted in glucose-galactose malabsorption by altering sugar affinity without an effect on sodium affinity, whereas mutations in other regions interrupt trafficking to the plasma membrane [85,115].

Intestinal Na^+/bile acid, Na^+/amino acid, and Na^+/vitamin cotransporters [116] are also predicted to contribute to water and sodium absorption in the intestine, but they are discussed in more detail in the chapters on bile secretion, nutrient absorption, and vitamins, respectively (see Chapters 19, 21, and 22).

Na^+-bicarbonate cotransporters

A family of basolateral cotransporters that couple uptake of bicarbonate with that of Na^+, known as NBCs, are found throughout the intestine, but particularly in those segments highly concerned with bicarbonate secretion (namely the duodenum and colon) [117]. They are members of the SLC4 gene family that also includes the AE subtypes of chloride/bicarbonate exchangers [118]. Both electrogenic and electroneutral isoforms have been described, based on their stoichiometry [118,119]. In the intestine, various splice variants of NBCe1 (Slc4a4) and NBCn1 (Slc4a7) predominate. Mice lacking NBCe1 exhibit a variety of defects including intestinal obstruction and metabolic acidosis; this gene has also been proposed as a protective modifier for the meconium ileus phenotype observed in cystic fibrosis [120,121], likely because bicarbonate secretion is required for proper mucus expansion [122,123]. NBCn1 is expressed in the duodenum and proximal colon and likewise appears to play an important role in bicarbonate secretion, pH homeostasis, and the integrity of the colonic mucus layer [124–126].

H^+-solute cotransporters

The intestinal proton-coupled peptide cotransporter (PEPT1/Slc15a1) is expressed in the apical membrane of small intestinal cells and can transport a wide variety of dipeptides and tripeptides [127]. The transporter is electrogenic, but the stoichiometry of proton:dipeptide transport depends on the net charge of the peptide substrate [127,128]. From the standpoint of fluid and electrolyte absorption, the major contribution of PEPT1 is to stimulate water transport, in cooperation with the sodium-hydrogen exchanger NHE3, which supplies protons [129]. PEPT1 remains an enigma for transport physiologists due to the extremely broad range of peptide substrates that it can accommodate. The molecular basis of this promiscuity is not fully understood and awaits determination of the crystal structure [127].

A proton-coupled monocarboxylate cotransporter (MCT1/Slc16a1) has been identified in the membranes of both small and large intestinal epithelial cells [130]. MCT1 reproduces nonionic diffusion, through coupling flux of monocarboxylate anions and protons [131]. The transporter is inhibited by α-cyano-hydroxycinnamates, and lactate is a favored substrate [131]. Evidence suggests a physiological role for colonic MCT1 as a route for basolateral SCFA flux from cells as part of transcellular SCFA absorption [132]. In this regard, MCT1 may be most important physiologically to transport monocarboxylates that are too hydrophilic for efficient flux by nonionic diffusion through the lipid bilayer. Transport of butyrate through MCT1, as well as possibly MCT4 (Slc16a3) and MCT5 (Slc16a4), has also recently been reported to regulate the secretion of K^+ via apical KCNQ-type channels in the rat colon [133].

$Na^+/K^+/2Cl^-$ cotransporters

$Na^+/K^+/2Cl^-$ cotransport is present in the basolateral membrane of certain intestinal epithelial cells, and participates in electrolyte secretion. This cotransport is electroneutral because each transport cycle moves equal numbers of cations (1 Na^+ plus 1 K^+) and anions (2 Cl^-) into the cell. The $Na^+/K^+/2Cl^-$ cotransporter plays a key role in Cl^- secretion as the predominant route for basolateral Cl^- uptake [134], and also participates in K^+ secretion by providing a second route of basolateral K^+ uptake in addition to the activity of Na^+,K^+-ATPase [135].

The NKCC1 (Slc12a2) cotransporter isoform is expressed in the basolateral membrane of human intestinal epithelial cells [136]. NKCC1 functions as a single polypeptide chain, and has 12 putative transmembrane segments. The cotransporter is inhibited by bumetanide and furosemide, which affect anion binding to the transporter [137]. Its activity is conversely promoted by phosphorylation by a kinase cascade composed of WNK4 and SPAK/OSR, which is activated upstream by a fall in intracellular chloride [138]. The abundance of colonic NKCC1 is also controlled by the ubiquitin ligase Nedd4-2, which promotes its degradation [139]. A related yet distinct thiazide-sensitive Na^+/Cl^- cotransporter (NCC/Slc12a3) has been proposed to exist in the apical membrane of enterocytes [140,141], and is implicated in the control of calcium absorption secondary to interaction with a voltage-dependent Ca^{2+} channel [142]. NCC is also found in the distal convoluted tubule of the kidney, where it participates in sodium reabsorption and is regulated by phosphorylation and trafficking. In this site, it plays a pivotal role in fine-tuning sodium homeostasis and is inhibited by an increase in dietary sodium intake [141]. It is not yet known whether similar factors regulate this transporter in the intestine.

Na^+/H^+ exchangers

Na^+/H^+ exchange activity is present in all segments of the small intestine and colon. It is defined as the tightly coupled uptake of one Na^+ ion in exchange for efflux of a proton [143]. This electroneutral exchange reaction is important for intracellular pH regulation, as well as transepithelial sodium absorption. Na^+/H^+ exchange is observed in both apical and basolateral membranes of epithelial cells from small intestine and colon [144,145].

Na^+/H^+ exchange is mediated by members of the SLC9 gene family, of which six members (NHE1–5 and NHE8, in some tissues) have been identified as plasma membrane transporters [146]. Several of these have been detected in gastrointestinal epithelia. Of the isoforms considered important for epithelial ion transport, NHE1 (Slc9a1) is present in virtually all cells of the body and is believed to be responsible for cellular pH regulation [147]. NHE1 is found in the basolateral membrane of intestinal epithelial cells [148]. NHE2 (Slc9a2) and NHE3 (Slc9a3) are predominantly epithelial isoforms of the exchanger that are expressed apically [149]. Each epithelial NHE isoform has a distinct distribution of mRNA abundance along the small and large intestines, which varies among species [150]. There are also gradients of NHE isoforms and Na^+/H^+ exchange function along the crypt-to-villus and crypt-to-surface axes. Based on immunoreactivity, NHE1 is expressed at all sites along these axes [148], but NHE2 and 3 are expressed preferentially on the villus in the small intestine and on the surface and in the upper third of the crypts in the colon [147,151]. Apical NHE activity is also regulated by so-called NHERF proteins (for NHE regulatory factors) that scaffold the transporters together with kinases that regulate their function and trafficking into the plasma membrane. Multiple NHERF isoforms provide for differing NHE regulation in different intestinal segments [152,153].

All NHE isoforms have 10–12 predicted transmembrane segments with cytoplasmic C- and N-termini [149]. Overall, NHE isoforms are 50–60% homologous within a species, with the C-terminal cytoplasmic tail having the most sequence divergence. The C-terminal portion is important for second messenger regulation of NHE isoforms, and several portions of this domain have been identified as crucial for mediating effects of calcium, calmodulin, cAMP, activation by intracellular protons, and growth factors [149,154,155]. As demonstrated by kinetic studies, all isoforms have different affinities for Na^+ and inhibition constants for amiloride and other inhibitors, reflecting their different primary structures [149].

The relative roles of NHE2 and NHE3 in electroneutral Na^+ absorption in the intestine are still debated [156]. Of note, NHE3, but not NHE2, is regulated in response to changes in extracellular sodium by insertion and removal from the plasma membrane [157]. Moreover, mineralocorticoids increase the rate of ileal brush border Na^+/H^+ exchange, correlated with an increase in the abundance of NHE3 mRNA without an effect on mRNA for NHE1 or NHE2 [158]. Further, the dose-dependency for inhibition of sodium and water absorption in dogs by dimethylamiloride is most consistent with NHE3 inhibition [159]. Finally, the patterns of second messenger regulation of sodium absorption and NHE3 are closely matched (i.e., inhibition by calcium and stimulation by phorbol esters), but differ from responses of NHE2 [149]. On the other hand, the relative importance of NHE2 may be species dependent [147], particularly under basal conditions [160,161]. Nevertheless, NHE3 knockout mice have obvious diarrheal disease whereas NHE2 knockout mice do not [162,163], and NHE3/NHE2 double knockouts have an intestinal phenotype that is indistinguishable from that produced by knockout of NHE3 alone [147].

Cl^-/HCO_3^- exchangers

Cl^-/HCO_3^- exchange in the apical membrane acts in concert with Na^+/H^+ exchange to mediate electroneutral NaCl uptake in colonocytes and small intestinal cells [164]. Unlike the apical membrane Na^+/H^+ exchanger, which is expressed predominantly in villus cells of the small intestine, Cl^-/HCO_3^- exchange appears to be equally prevalent in the apical membranes of both crypt and villus cells, suggesting it contributes to other transport mechanisms in addition to NaCl absorption. In the colon, apical Cl^-/HCO_3^- exchange is observed predominantly in the surface cells, although Cl^-/OH^- exchange remains relatively active in crypt membranes [165]. This and other kinetic evidence suggests that apical Cl^-/HCO_3^- and Cl^-/OH^- exchange may not be mediated by the same protein in either the small intestine or colon [165,166].

Clear roles in intestinal chloride absorption and/or bicarbonate secretion have been assigned to members of the SLC26 family of anion exchangers. One such transporter, DRA (for Down-Regulated in Adenoma, Slc26a3), plays a key role since mutations in this transporter are responsible for *congenital chloride diarrhea* [167], a disease characterized by a chloride-rich, acidic stool (see section on Disorders of electrolyte transport at the end of this chapter). The protein is expressed in the apical membrane of epithelial cells in the small intestine and colon [168,169]. DRA is a chloride, bicarbonate and divalent anion transporter [170,171], and mutations found in patients with congenital chloride diarrhea lead to defective anion transport function [171]. Recent work suggests that DRA activity and cell surface localization can be stimulated by cAMP, at least in cells where it is coexpressed with CFTR [172]. This may be relevant for participation of the transporter in bicarbonate secretion [173]. In addition, PAT1 (for Putative Anion Transporter 1, Slc26a6) has been characterized as a major contributor to anion exchange in the apical membranes of intestinal epithelial cells on the basis of studies in knockout mice [174]. Current thinking suggests that both DRA and PAT1 play distinct yet complementary roles in intestinal Cl^-, HCO_3^- and fluid absorption as well as enterocyte acid–base balance, since each is activated differentially by specific ionic gradients as well as extracellular pH [169]. However, DRA is linked to the activity of NHE3 because both bind to NHERF1 – this implicates DRA specifically as a major contributor to electroneutral NaCl absorption.

Multiple isoforms of the anion exchanger (AE) gene family (also known as SLC4) are expressed in the small and large intestine. Among three known AE2 (Slc4a2) transcripts (AE2a, AE2b, AE2c1), the AE2a and AE2b transcripts are most abundant in the intestine, with a basolateral localization [175,176]. In keeping with this, and rather than contributing to NaCl absorption, studies in AE2 knockout mice have revealed that this exchanger may contribute to the basolateral chloride uptake that supports stimulated anion secretion, by working in concert with either NBC or NHE1 [177]. Results have also suggested the presence of an apical AE1 isoform and a basolateral AE3 isoform in the intestines, but the presence of both of these has been controversial [176,178]. Finally, AE4 has been characterized for its involvement in bicarbonate secretion in both the stomach and duodenum, although more recent studies revealed no significant functional defects in AE4 knockout mice [179,180].

Other cotransporters

In addition to those described above, other intestinal electrolyte cotransporters include Na^+/PO_4^- (NaPi-IIb/Slc34a2) and Na^+/SO_4^- (NaS1/Slc13a1) cotransporters [174,181–183]. For phosphate, NaPi-IIb participates in a homeostatic axis linking bone, kidney, and intestinal transport processes to ensure appropriate levels of the circulating cation [184]. Mice lacking NaS1 have a 90% reduction in uptake of sulfate from the intestine and this, coupled with reduced reabsorption from the renal tubule, results in marked hyposulfatemia, which may have additional physiological consequences [183]. However, neither the absorption of phosphate nor sulfate from the intestinal lumen is likely to be quantitatively significant for fluid absorption, which is also true for uptake driven by other cotransporters, such as those for vitamins and bile acids as discussed above. The intestinal K^+/Cl^- cotransporter KCC1 [185] is a logical mechanism for electroneutral basolateral exit of K^+ and Cl^- from intestinal epithelial cells that absorb K^+ and/or Cl^- in an electroneutral fashion. Its expression increases during dietary potassium depletion [186] and its activity is increased by ligation of the zinc-sensing receptor, ZnR/GPR39, perhaps accounting for the efficacy of zinc as an antidiarrheal therapy [187].

Ion channels

An ion channel acts as a gated pore that is selective for certain ions. Open channels are passive pathways for electrolyte movement. *Gating* controls the amount of time that the pore spends in an open versus closed configuration, whereas a single open channel permits rapid flux of ions across the membrane with a characteristic *unitary conductance*. The conductance of a given channel is an intrinsic biophysical signature, whereas gating is regulated by second messengers and resulting posttranslational modifications, such as phosphorylation.

Na^+ channels

Apical Na^+ channels contribute to electrogenic sodium absorption in many distal colonic epithelia. Epithelial Na^+ channels (ENaC) are selective for sodium (>10:1 versus K^+) and are *inwardly rectifying* (i.e., they mediate cation influx more efficiently than cation efflux) [188]. Epithelial Na^+ channels are inhibited by nanomolar concentrations of phenamil and amiloride analogs, but the profile of inhibitor sensitivity is distinct from that of Na^+/H^+ exchangers [189].

ENaC is composed of three subunits: α, β, and γ. Each subunit is an integral membrane protein predicted to span the membrane twice, and the subunits share 35% homology [190]. Expression of the β and γ subunits is required to efficiently target the channel to the plasma membrane [190]. This is consistent with the observation that certain activating mutations in the β or γ subunits (see section on Disorders of electrolyte transport/Liddle's syndrome, below) cause increased numbers of sodium channels in the membrane as well as an increased activity of the expressed channels [191,192]. In contrast, a glycine near the N-terminal of the α subunit is involved in channel gating [193].

In the kidney and lung, ENaC is downregulated in response to a rise in intracellular sodium concentrations. This is thought to result from the stimulated association of the ubiquitin ligase Nedd4-2 (also referred to as Nedd4L) with the β and γ subunits of the channel, leading to ubiquitination of the channel and its resulting internalization and degradation [139,194,195]. Conversely, phosphorylation of Nedd4-2 by the serum and glucocorticoid-regulated kinase sgk1, or by protein kinase A, disrupts its association with ENaC and prolongs the channel's residence on the cell surface; sgk1 also increases channel open probability by phosphorylating the α subunit [196–198]. Thus, various growth factors, insulin, or agents that elevate cAMP can increase ENaC activity, although the extent to which this paradigm also applies to the distal colon has not yet been fully assessed [195,199]. There is even one report suggesting that sgk1 is not required for baseline or upregulated ENaC activity in the colon [200]. ENaC in this segment is, however, chronically induced by aldosterone, providing a mechanism to coordinate sodium conservation by colon and kidneys in subjects consuming a low-salt diet [201,202].

Cl^- channels

Apical chloride channels are essential components of chloride secretion. Chloride secretion in all parts of the intestine and colon is controlled predominantly by the ability of specific second messengers to regulate channel gating and localization. However, multiple chloride channel types are observed in intestinal epithelial cells, making it difficult in some cases to assign a functional role to individual proteins.

A cAMP-activated channel in the apical membrane is known to participate in hormone-stimulated Cl^- secretion, and is encoded by the gene (CFTR) that is responsible for *cystic fibrosis* (see below) [203]. The normal CFTR channel is selective for Cl >Br >I and is *nonrectifying* or *linear* (i.e., it conducts ions with equal efficiency in either an inward or outward direction). CFTR also mediates the conductance of other ions (notably HCO_3) [204], participates in a subset of cAMP-regulated apical membrane endocytosis and exocytosis events [205], and regulates the activity of other chloride and sodium channels [206,207]. The CFTR channel is a single polypeptide with 12 membrane-spanning domains, two cytoplasmic nucleotide-binding domains (NBDs), and a regulatory (R-) domain that contains the majority of phosphorylation sites. CFTR chloride channel gating is complex, involving coordinated phosphorylation of multiple R-domain serine residues and ATP hydrolysis at, and interaction between, the two NBDs [208].

In normal intestine, agonists acting via cAMP or calcium stimulate Cl^- secretion. However, in cystic fibrosis patients, neither cAMP nor calcium is able to elicit Cl^- secretion [209]. This is in contrast to airway epithelia of cystic fibrosis patients, where a Ca^{++}-activated Cl^- channel (CaCC) functions to partially restore secretory function in the absence of normal CFTR [210]. The reasons underlying the failure to detect CaCC activity in the intestine of cystic fibrosis patients are not yet understood at a molecular level, but could involve a defect in the ability of CFTR to regulate another anion channel and/or the existence of negative regulatory mechanisms in the intestinal epithelium (see section on Regulation of fluid and electrolyte transport).

CaCCs are thought to be a key target whereby NSP4 of rotavirus causes diarrheal symptoms [211,212], and both murine ileum and cultured T84 colonic epithelial cells functionally express CaCCs [211]. A candidate for this CaCC is the protein TMEM16A, also known as anoctamin 1, which encodes a calcium-activated chloride conductance in a variety of tissues. Mice lacking TMEM16A display defects in intestinal calcium-activated chloride secretion [213–215]. However, the identity of TMEM16A as a CaCC remains controversial, and it may be expressed in the basolateral rather than apical membrane where it regulates epithelial calcium signaling and thus the activity of Ca^{2+}-dependent SK4 K^+ channels required for calcium-dependent chloride secretion [216,217].

There are other candidate Cl^- channels in the gut. ClC2 and ClC5 are Cl^- channels expressed in the intestine [218–220]. ClC5 is particularly intriguing because it is expressed only in kidney and colon, has a permselectivity of I>Cl, is outwardly rectifying, but is not activated by cAMP [218]. However, many consider ClC5 to be a chloride/proton exchanger rather than a channel per se [221]. Nevertheless, since ClC5 is located in endosomes of intestinal epithelial cells [219], it may possibly be inserted into the plasma membrane upon appropriate regulatory signals. It has also been shown to be required for trafficking of NHE3, at least in the kidney [222]. ClC2 is also expressed in intestinal epithelial cells, and was originally thought to contribute to chloride secretion [223]. ClC channels are activated by cell swelling and, at a minimum, probably participate in the ion efflux necessary for cell volume regulation. However, ClC2 has been identified as a basolateral protein in distal colonic epithelial cells that is required for electroneutral NaCl and KCl absorption [224]. The ClC2 channel also attracted considerable attention as the presumed target of a channel-opening drug known as lubiprostone, which is marketed for the treatment of constipation [225–227]. However, it now seems more likely that lubiprostone acts via prostanoid receptors to stimulate CFTR rather than ClC2 [228].

Finally, an Slc26 family member, Slc26a9, is an intestinal (and airway) chloride channel (rather than a chloride/bicarbonate exchanger as seen for other family members). It is emerging as an important modifier gene for cystic fibrosis severity, and mice lacking both CFTR and Slc26a9 had significantly worsened meconium ileus than those lacking CFTR alone [229,230].

K^+ channels

Potassium channels in the apical membrane of epithelial cells are involved in K^+ secretion, and K^+ channels in the basolateral membrane are involved in Cl^- secretion [231]. K^+ channels are also involved in electrogenic Na^+ absorption and Na^+-coupled solute absorption, but the polarity of K^+ channels involved in these processes is less certain. Of note, the colon also participates in active absorption of K^+ from the lumen if whole-body potassium is depleted, but this appears to be underpinned by the apical H^+,K^+-ATPase discussed earlier rather than by a potassium channel [231].

The presence of apical K^+ channels was originally inferred indirectly by adding luminal K^+ channel blockers (e.g., barium and tetraethylammonium [TEA]) and monitoring effects on global electrical properties of the rat colonic mucosa [232]. Treatment with aldosterone increases apical K^+ conductance, suggesting an increase in K^+ channel activity or number [233]. Subsequent studies have implicated BK (KCNMA1 or $K_{Ca}1.1$) channels as mediating apical K^+ secretion, and mice lacking this channel had reduced concentrations of K^+ in their feces [231,234,235]. These channels are activated by Ca^{2+}, cAMP, and dietary K^+ loading [236]. Calcium-dependent KCNQ channels are likely also important for colonic K^+ secretion, at least in the rat [133].

Basolateral K^+ channels have been studied more extensively. Patch clamping identified a basolateral channel in human and rat colonic crypts that was selective for K^+ (49:1 vs Na^+) [237]. The open probability of this channel was increased 4–10-fold by cAMP or micromolar calcium, and the channel was blocked by quinidine and diphenylamine carboxylate (DPC) but not TEA [237,238]. The second messenger sensitivity of this channel suggests that it contributes predominantly to cAMP-stimulated Cl^- secretion. A second electrophysiologically distinct K^+ channel has also been observed in human colonic crypts. This channel has a distinct inhibitor profile: it is inhibited by TEA and quinidine but not DPC, and is highly K^+ selective (190:1 K:Na) [238]. KCNN4 and KCNQ1 (with its regulatory subunit, KCNE3), and perhaps others, are candidates for these basolateral K^+ channels in the colon that respond to Ca^{++} and cAMP, respectively, to underpin active chloride secretion [239–245].

Transepithelial electrolyte transport

The preceding section reviewed the *transmembrane* transport proteins that serve as basic building blocks for transport of the major electrolytes that drive fluid absorption and secretion in the gut, including Na^+, K^+, Cl^- and HCO_3^-. This section discusses how these proteins are combined to produce the major *transepithelial* electrolyte transport events observed in the intact intestine.

In general, net transepithelial transport requires the participation of at least two transport proteins to mediate (i) ion uptake across one plasma membrane domain, and (ii) exit of ions across the plasma membrane domain at the opposite pole of the cell. By definition, active transepithelial transport also requires involvement of a primary active transporter to provide the energy for net absorption or secretion of the ion. When the pump also serves as an uptake or exit step for the ion in question, only two transport proteins are required. Net transepithelial electrolyte transport across the epithelium can be either electrogenic or electroneutral. However, transepithelial transport mechanisms can only be electrogenic when both the apical and basolateral membranes mediate electrogenic ion fluxes as part of the mechanism, or when transcellular fluxes drive electrogenic paracellular fluxes. For instance, the electrogenic Na,K-ATPase is involved in both electroneutral and electrogenic sodium absorption depending on the accessory sodium transport events.

The voltage clamp and Ussing chamber are used in combination to define the presence of active electrolyte transport between the luminal and serosal surfaces of a tissue. The *Ussing chamber* permits mounting of intestinal tissue (or a cultured cell monolayer) between two compartments to measure transport between the luminal and serosal reservoirs. If tissue in an Ussing chamber is *voltage clamped*, where the driving force for transepithelial ion movement has been eliminated (i.e., transepithelial voltage is clamped to zero), the magnitude of the current required to offset the potential difference (termed *short circuit current* or I_{sc}) will reflect active, net electrogenic ion transport. In the same configuration, measurement of net transepithelial ion fluxes with isotopes can be used to detect transport of specific ions that is either electrogenic or electroneutral. In recent years, use of the Ussing chamber has been extended to studies of monolayers of epithelial cells derived from intestinal enteroids, which may more faithfully recapitulate the cell types and regulatory mechanisms of the native epithelium [246,247]. Studies are also revealing new information about how transport properties of the gut epithelium evolve as cells migrate and mature along the crypt–villus axis [173]. Such studies have again forced reconsideration of the dogma that secretory and absorptive processes are carefully segregated to the crypt and villus (or surface) compartments, respectively [248].

Classically, absorptive and secretory functions of the intestine are considered to be independent, and absorptive function may remain intact during periods when the secretory function is excessively stimulated. This is clinically important because some antidiarrheal strategies (e.g., oral rehydration solutions) rely on stimulating absorption in the presence of abundant secretion. However, more recent evidence suggests that there are functional, and potentially molecular, linkages between absorptive and secretory mechanisms. For example, although they are thought to be present in different cells, expression of the CFTR chloride channel affects activity of the epithelial Na^+ channel, providing an explanation for the observation that cystic fibrosis patients have increased electrogenic sodium absorption [249]. Thus, regulation of chloride secretion and sodium absorption can be intertwined.

Electrolyte absorptive mechanisms

The small intestine performs electroneutral NaCl absorption and Na^+-coupled nutrient absorption, and is responsible for most of the absorption of nutrients and water by the intestine as a whole. Sodium absorptive mechanisms in the colon vary strongly as a function of both species and segment but in most species, including humans, the large intestine absorbs Na^+ avidly through both an electrogenic mechanism involving apical Na^+ channels and an electroneutral NaCl absorptive mechanism similar to that in the small intestine. The colon is also responsible for SCFA absorption and some K^+ absorption, and is essential for conservation of fluid and electrolytes.

Electroneutral NaCl Absorption

A significant fraction of the sodium and chloride absorbed by the intestine is electroneutral and mutually dependent on the alternate ion (i.e., electroneutral Na^+ absorption requires the presence of Cl^- and vice versa) [250]. Postprandially, after absorption of nutrients has been completed, or in the fasting state, electroneutral NaCl absorption is the major route for Na^+ absorption in the small intestine [159]. This NaCl absorptive mechanism is also the principal route for Na^+ absorption in the proximal colon, with less prominence in the distal colon. The relative importance of electroneutral versus electrogenic sodium absorption in the colon also varies as a function of mineralocorticoid status. To explain its coupled fluxes, the combined action of Na^+/H^+ (NHE3 and perhaps NHE2) and Cl^-/HCO_3^- exchangers (DRA and PAT1) is the most widely accepted model for human NaCl absorption, with Na^+,K^+-ATPase in the basolateral membrane serving as the exit step for sodium (see Figure 16.2) [251]. The intestine expresses the thiazide-sensitive Na^+-Cl^- cotransporter NCC (Slc12a3) that is also present in the kidney, which theoretically could substitute for the paired exchangers. However, this protein is present at low levels and, as discussed above, may have a more important physiological role in regulating intestinal calcium absorption [141,142].

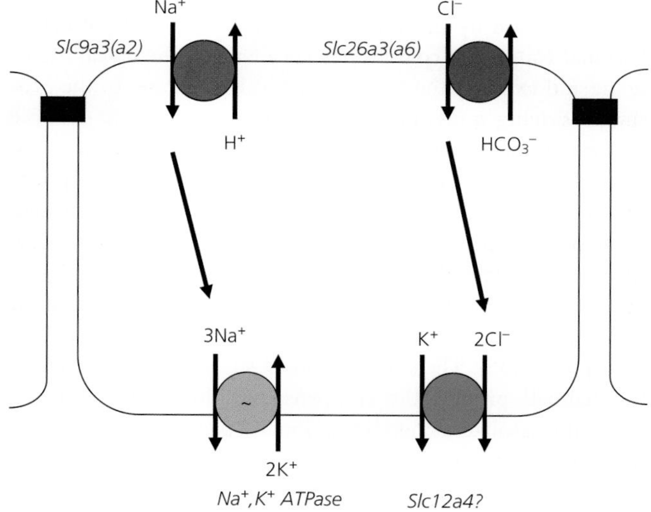

Figure 16.2 Electroneutral NaCl absorption in the small intestine and colon. As described in the text, apical NaCl entry via Na^+/H^+ and Cl^-/HCO_3^- exchange is the most strongly supported model in mammalian intestine, although directly coupled NaCl cotransport remains a possibility. In both models, Na^+ exits the cell via the basolateral Na^+,K^+-ATPase, but the route of Cl^- efflux is more speculative. Details of the model are in the text.

In the paired exchanger model, coupling of the exchangers occurs via changes in intracellular pH. For example, the Na^+ gradient drives Na^+ uptake and H^+ efflux via Na^+/H^+ exchange, which alkalinizes the cytoplasm and increases activity of the Cl^-/HCO_3^- exchanger. The action of carbonic anhydrase produces HCO_3^- which then leaves the cell in exchange for uptake of luminal Cl^-. The net reaction is Na^+ and Cl^- uptake in exchange for H^+ and HCO_3^- efflux. Once in the cell, Na^+ is pumped out by Na^+,K^+-ATPase, and Cl^- follows by way of either an electroneutral transport protein, likely to be a K^+/Cl^- cotransporter [185], or perhaps via ClC2 chloride channels [224].

Electrogenic Na^+ absorption

In humans, electrogenic amiloride-sensitive Na^+ absorption accounts for approximately 50% of the Na^+ reabsorbed in the distal colon. There is a decreasing gradient of activity through the transverse colon and only minimal levels in the proximal colon [252, 53]. Aldosterone, a mineralocorticoid well known for its Na^+-retaining and K^+-wasting effects on the distal nephron, also exerts profound effects on the distal colon. Induction of secondary hyperaldosteronism by the feeding of a low-Na^+ diet or administration of exogenous aldosterone converts the rat distal colon from electroneutral NaCl absorption to amiloride-sensitive, electrogenic Na^+ absorption [254]. Conversely, reduced electrogenic absorption of sodium and/or ENaC expression has been described in inflammatory bowel disease patients and in animal models of colitis and infectious diarrhea [199,255,256]. This may contribute to diarrheal symptoms, underscoring the importance of sodium and water salvage in the distal colon.

Figure 16.3 shows the proposed mechanism of electrogenic Na^+ absorption by the surface epithelium of the distal colon. Luminal Na^+ enters colonocytes via ENaC in the apical membrane and exits via the basolateral Na^+,K^+-ATPase. In the process of driving transepithelial Na^+ absorption, Na^+,K^+-ATPase also catalyzes K^+ uptake and creates a charge imbalance, and both effects must be compensated to sustain Na^+ absorption. The compensatory ion flux is probably achieved by electrogenic efflux of K^+ via K^+ channels. There is controversy about whether apical or basolateral K^+ channels perform this function. It is likely that the apical K^+ conductance is predominantly involved in K^+ secretion, a crypt cell function that is not linked to Na^+ absorption [135]. The simplest model suggests that basolateral K^+ channels provide the compensatory flux and recycle K^+ across the basolateral membrane. Finally, paracellular flux of Cl^- is driven by sodium movement to restore electroneutrality between luminal and serosal compartments.

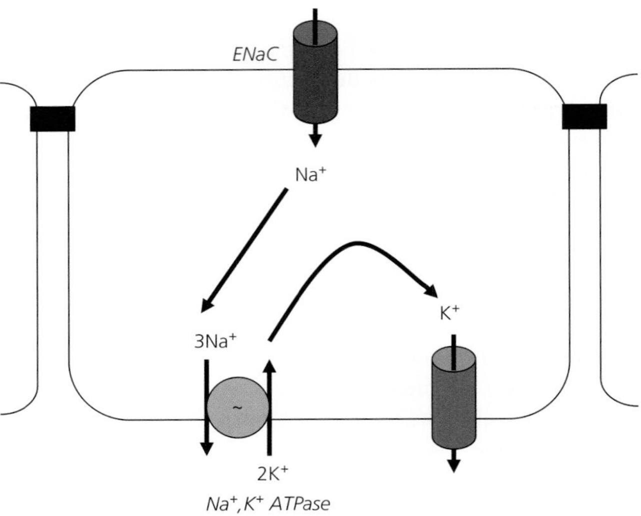

Figure 16.3 Electrogenic Na+ absorption in the distal colon. Na^+ enters cells at the apical membrane through ENaC Na^+ channels and leaves cells at the basolateral membrane through the Na^+,K^+-ATPase. The details of the model are described in the text.

Solute-coupled Na^+ absorption

The absorption of many nutrients, and also of bile acids (in the terminal ileum), is mediated by Na^+-coupled cotransporters in the small intestine. The combined action of these transporters contributes significantly to sodium and water absorption [257]. A common cellular mechanism (shown in Figure 16.4) is believed to mediate all solute-coupled Na^+ absorption, predominantly in villus cells. Luminal Na^+ enters via apical Na^+-coupled cotransporters and exits via the basolateral Na^+,K^+-ATPase. The Na^+-solute cotransporter utilizes the energy of the electrochemical gradient for Na^+ to drive intracellular accumulation of the cotransported solute above its equilibrium value. When two Na^+ ions are coupled to uptake of a single solute molecule (e.g., in

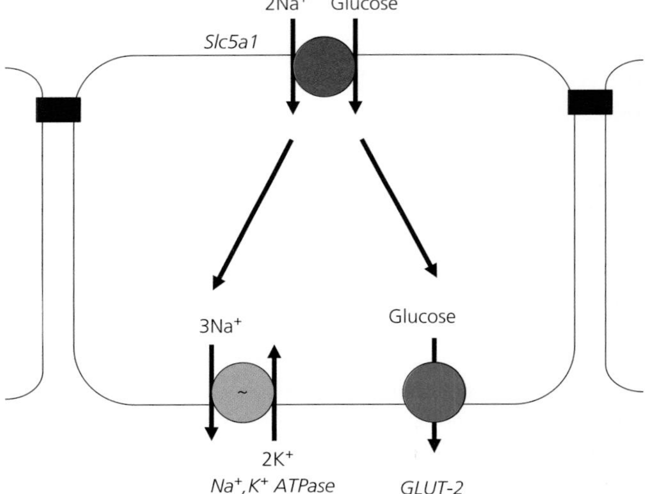

Figure 16.4 Solute-coupled Na^+ absorption in the small intestine. The model presents the mechanism for glucose as a generic solute, and is representative of Na^+-coupled absorption of glucose, many amino acids, certain B vitamins, and bile acids. Details of the model will vary among solutes due to differences in the charge of the different solute and the stoichiometry with transported Na^+ ions. Details of the model are discussed in the text.

SGLT1), the intracellular accumulation of solute can be nearly 100-fold [258]. Efflux of solute down its steep concentration gradient across the basolateral membrane is then efficiently mediated by facilitated diffusive carriers, which are passive in nature. For example, the GLUT2 passive glucose transporter performs this function for glucose absorption [112]. Electrogenic Na^+ absorption stimulates absorption of a compensatory Cl^- anion via the paracellular route, and recycling of K^+ via basolateral K^+ channels assures cellular electroneutrality.

SCFA absorption and SCFA-stimulated Na^+ absorption

Short-chain fatty acids are produced in the colon by bacterial catabolism of unabsorbed carbohydrate and protein. The combined concentration of the predominant luminal SCFAs (acetate, propionate, and butyrate) is 100–150 mM, so they are the major anions and osmolytes in the colonic lumen [259]. Absorbed SCFAs account for 7–10% of ingested calories, and serve as an important energy source for colonic epithelial cells [260]. SCFAs also stimulate electroneutral Na^+ absorption, up to fivefold in humans [261].

Short-chain fatty acids stimulate Na^+ absorption via activation of apical Na^+/H^+ exchange, which leads to subsequent exit of Na^+ via the basolateral Na^+,K^+-ATPase. Evidence suggests that luminal SCFA uptake causes intracellular acidification and luminal alkalinization, which are both known activators of Na^+/H^+ exchangers [262]. The mechanisms of SCFA uptake that lead to pH change are controversial, but it appears that both nonionic diffusion (uptake of the protonated form of these weak acids without intervention of a transport protein) and carrier-mediated transport (via either a SCFA/HCO_3^- exchanger, Slc9a3, or the proton-coupled monocarboxylate transporter, MCT1 [Slc16a1]) play a role [49,263–268]. An apical SCFA/Cl^- exchanger likely also contributes to amplifying the effect of SCFA absorption on overall Na^+ uptake [267]. The ability of SCFA-induced acidification to stimulate apical but not basolateral Na^+/H^+ exchangers of colonocytes has been perplexing. The regulation of extracellular pH in microenvironments directly adjacent to colonocyte membranes may partially explain this [269]. Physiological SCFA gradients cause alkalinization of the luminal surface and acidification of the basolateral surface [262], which preferentially activates apical but not basolateral Na^+/H^+ exchange.

Finally, there are several candidate mechanisms for SCFA efflux across the basolateral membrane, including nonionic diffusion, SCFA/HCO_3^- exchange, or SCFA/H^+ cotransport via MCT1 or MCT4 (Slc16a3) [131,270,271].

K^+ absorption

In human metabolic balance studies, ~85% of ingested K^+ is absorbed in the small intestine, with passive absorption driven by prevailing electrochemical gradients being sufficient to explain this uptake [272]. In contrast, active electroneutral K^+ absorption occurs in the distal colon [98], and is believed to mediate absorption of 5–7% of K^+ ingested daily [272], leaving 3–5% to be lost in fecal water. The absolute magnitude of colonic K^+ fluxes is underestimated by these values because colonic K^+ secretion also occurs.

An apical H^+,K^+-ATPase promotes uptake of K^+ from the lumen [273], and K^+ likely leaves the cell via the K^+/Cl^- cotransporter KCC1 [274]. The Cl^- dependent portion of K^+ absorption probably utilizes apical Cl^-/HCO_3^- exchange to neutralize protons extruded by the H^+,K^+-ATPase, providing a source of intracellular Cl^- to drive the basolateral K^+/Cl^- cotransporter. However, since not all K^+ absorption is Cl^- dependent, alternative routes for basolateral K^+ efflux, such as via KCNN4 or KCNQ1/KCNE3 K^+ channels, are likely [236].

Electrolyte secretory mechanisms

Secretory mechanisms throughout the gastrointestinal tract center around the Cl^- anion. HCl is the major secretory product of the stomach. In other intestinal segments, the predominant secreted ion is either Cl^- or HCO_3^- [275,276]. However, HCO_3^- secretion may be related to, or require, active Cl^- secretion.

Electrogenic Cl^- secretion

Electrogenic Cl^- secretion (see Figure 16.5) is found in all segments of the GI tract from the duodenum to the distal colon. Presumably, this reflects the common need for a mechanism to maintain hydration of the luminal contents. Uptake of Cl^- across the basolateral membrane is via the electroneutral $Na^+/K^+/2Cl^-$ cotransporter, NKCC1 [134]. A key function of this cotransporter is to use the energy of the Na^+ gradient to accumulate Cl^- intracellularly above its electrochemical equilibrium. Under these conditions, Cl^- will exit the cell across the apical membrane when Cl^- channels are opened. Na^+,K^+-ATPase provides energy for this overall mechanism and recycles Na^+ across the basolateral membrane. Potassium channels

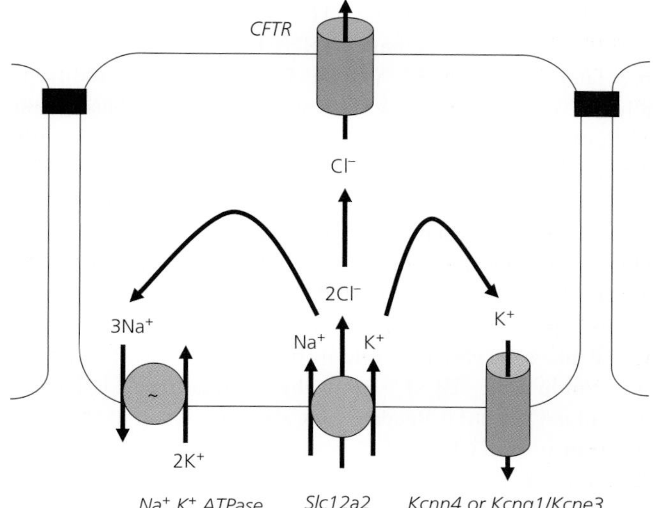

Figure 16.5 Cl^- secretion in small intestine and colon. Cl^- enters cells at the basolateral membrane through $Na^+/K^+/2Cl^-$ cotransport and leaves cells at the apical membrane through Cl^- channels. Details of the model are described in the text.

in the basolateral membrane allow for K^+ recycling, maintain cellular electroneutrality by compensating for Cl^- efflux, and keep the cell hyperpolarized (i.e., negative intracellular voltage compared to outside the cell) so that Cl^- efflux across the apical membrane can be sustained [277]. It is believed that Na^+ follows passively by paracellular flux through tight junctions to maintain electroneutrality between luminal and serosal compartments. The predominant Cl^- channel in the apical membrane involved in this mechanism is CFTR, but the TMEM16a channel may also be important, as well as others (see above).

HCO_3^- secretion

Bicarbonate secreted by the duodenal epithelium contributes to the mucus-bicarbonate layer that overlies duodenal epithelial cells, and thus may be an important protective factor that defends against duodenal ulceration [276]. Although the duodenum secretes large amounts of HCO_3^-, luminal HCO_3^- concentrations in the upper small intestine are relatively low because of neutralization by gastric acid. Bicarbonate secretion also takes place in ileum and colon, where it appears to play a critical role in determining the rheological properties of secreted mucus, establishing the surface microclimate pH, and shaping the microbiota and host defense [49,122,275]. Apical Cl^-/HCO_3^- exchange in the colon mediated by DRA also acts to conserve Cl^- at the expense of HCO_3^-. Conversely, since congenital chloride diarrhea causes systemic alkalosis, the lower GI tract may play a significant role in acid/base homeostasis.

More than one mechanism likely exists for duodenal HCO_3^- secretion. In the two mechanisms depicted in Figure 16.6, a common source of secreted HCO_3^- anion is carbonic anhydrase, which hydrates CO_2 to produce intracellular HCO_3^- and a proton. The proton is eliminated by basolateral Na^+/H^+ exchange (NHE1), and Na^+ is recycled basolaterally by Na^+,K^+-ATPase. Bicarbonate can additionally be derived from the bloodstream via a basolateral sodium-bicarbonate cotransporter, predominantly NBCe1 [278]. The models diverge in describing how HCO_3^- exits across the apical membrane. In an electroneutral mechanism, HCO_3^- is exchanged for intraluminal Cl^- [279]. The electrogenic mechanism involves HCO_3^- secretion through apical channels such as CFTR [204]. Evidence from cystic fibrosis patients and CFTR knockout mice suggests that CFTR plays an essential role in bicarbonate secretion, both by conducting HCO_3^- and by regulating Cl^-/HCO_3^- exchange [280,281]. Recent work also suggests that the relative transport of Cl^- and HCO_3^- through CFTR differs as cells differentiate along the crypt–villus axis, at least as modeled by enteroid studies. Forskolin-stimulated secretion of HCO_3^- is more prominent than that of Cl^- as the epithelium becomes more differentiated, perhaps secondary to a shift in the expression of basolateral transporters required to support the transport of each anion [173].

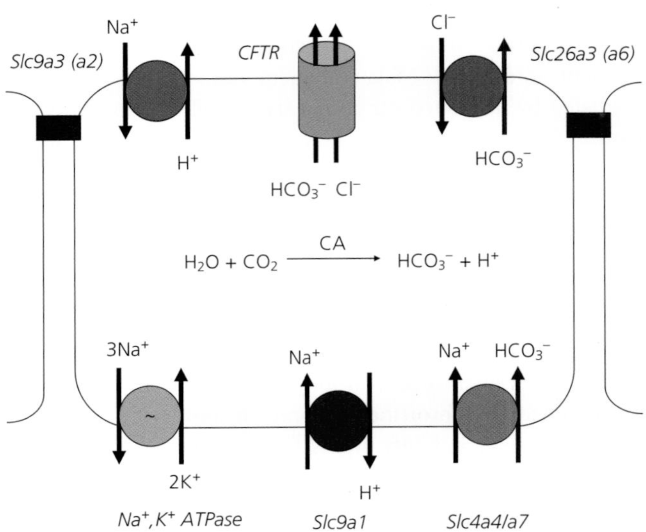

Figure 16.6 HCO_3^- secretion in duodenum. CFTR provides apical chloride to drive the activity of an apical anion exchanger, or itself serves as the pathway for HCO_3^- exit at the apical membrane. As described in the text, both mechanisms may be important in mammalian duodenum. In both models, HCO_3^- is produced by carbonic anhydrase (CA), which requires compensatory efflux of a proton by Na^+/H^+ exchange, or is taken up across the basolateral membrane by a sodium-coupled cotransporter, NBC1. Details of the model are described in the text.

In the proximal colon, bicarbonate secretion is stimulated by SCFAs [117,282], and may occur by a distinct mechanism. SCFA uptake causes alkalinization of the colonic lumen, either following nonionic uptake of protonated SCFA or via the SCFA/bicarbonate exchanger, either of which removes acid equivalents from the lumen [117,263]. The resulting transepithelial pH gradient will cause a vectorial titration of other weak acids (e.g., CO_2) across the epithelium and result in luminal accumulation of the basic form (i.e., HCO_3^-). In support of this model, transepithelial CO_2/HCO_3^- gradients drive luminal pH changes consistent with transepithelial nonionic diffusion of CO_2 [263]. More distally, on the other hand, bicarbonate secretion appears to utilize predominantly apical Cl^-/HCO_3^- exchange (via DRA) as described above [117]. In the mid colon, this is coupled with NHE3 activity whereas in the distal colon, NHE3 is absent and ENaC provides for Na^+ uptake [117,283,284].

K^+ secretion

All portions of the mammalian colon can perform active K^+ secretion. K^+ secretion is enhanced by a low-sodium diet, which leads to increased plasma levels of aldosterone, and by acute K^+ loading [135,285,286]. K^+ secretion can also be stimulated by cAMP-dependent secretagogs and occurs concurrently with Cl^- secretion, albeit from distinct cell populations [287,288]. Moreover, unlike Cl^- secretion, which is diminished in colitis, K^+ secretion is increased [289]. In health, colonic K^+ secretion may be dispensable, but it may assume an important role for

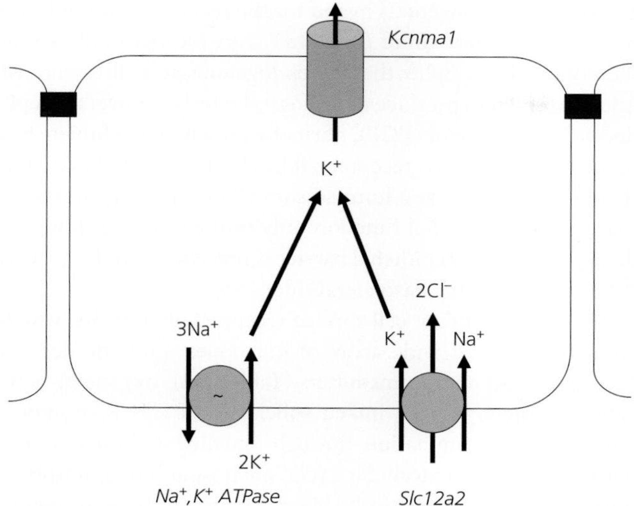

Figure 16.7 K^+ secretion in colon. K^+ uptake at the basolateral membrane is mediated by either Na^+,K^+-ATPase or $Na^+/K^+/2Cl^-$ cotransport, depending on species and segment. K^+ efflux at the apical membrane is via K+ channels. Details of the model are described in the text.

homeostasis in the setting of renal failure. In keeping with this, a patient undergoing hemodialysis who also required a temporary ileostomy following a bout of ischemic colitis developed severe hyperkalemia, which was reversed when bowel continuity was restored [290]. This has led some to advocate the exploitation of colonic K^+ secretion as an adjunctive therapy for patients with kidney failure [291].

The model of active K^+ secretion (see Figure 16.7) closely parallels that of Cl^- secretion. Since NKCC1 inhibitors block K^+ secretion, at least in some tissues (e.g., rat and guinea pig colon), the cotransporter may be an important route for basolateral K^+ uptake [292]. Potassium secretion is also ultimately dependent on the Na^+,K^+-ATPase pump to establish driving gradients, and in some tissues (e.g., rabbit proximal colon) the ATPase may supply the secreted K^+ instead of the $Na^+/K^+/2Cl^-$ cotransporter. In contrast to Cl^- secretion, active K^+ secretion is sensitive to inhibition by K^+ channel blockers applied luminally (e.g., iberiotoxin, paxilline, barium, and TEA) consistent with involvement of BK (KCNMA1) channels [288,293,294]. The entire process is electrogenic, producing a current opposite to that produced by Cl^- secretion or Na^+ absorption. Of note, mice lacking KCNMA1 expression in the colon fail to display either basal or stimulated K^+ secretion [235].

Regulation of fluid and electrolyte transport

Under normal circumstances, the absorptive and secretory processes described above act in a concerted and finely tuned manner to control the fluidity of the intestinal contents and conserve the large amounts of fluid that enter the intestine each day. However, the extent of fluid absorption and secretion is not constant, and epithelial cells must adapt to both physiological and pathophysiological cues with appropriate responses. Such dynamic regulation of epithelial transport occurs through a complex interplay of cell-to-cell interactions, intercellular mediators, and intracellular signal transduction cascades that ultimately target transport proteins to modulate their function in the short or long term.

Intracellular regulatory mechanisms

In general, epithelial cells "sense" changes in their extracellular environment through receptors expressed on their surface (Figure 16.8). Activation of these receptors, whether in response to physiological or pathophysiological stimuli, recruits complex signaling pathways that can modulate the activity and expression of transport proteins. Such changes can occur either rapidly through posttranslational modifications or altered membrane trafficking of the transporters, or over more prolonged periods of time through alterations in the rate of their synthesis or degradation. The following sections provide an overview of the intracellular signaling mechanisms that regulate epithelial transport in the gut.

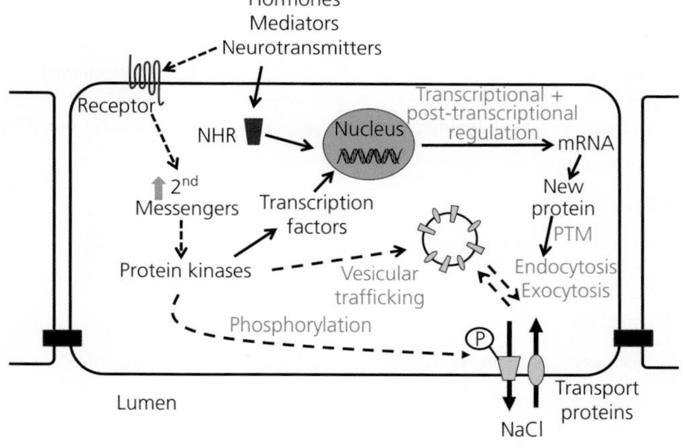

Figure 16.8 Regulation of epithelial transport. Hormones, neurotransmitters, and immune cell mediators typically exert their effects by binding to cell surface or nuclear receptors. Receptor activation, in turn, evokes acute (dashed lines) or long-term (solid lines) changes in transport function. Receptor-induced elevations in intracellular second messengers activate various proteins kinases. These signaling cascades and others as shown, in turn regulate epithelial transport in several ways: (1) via covalent modification of the transport proteins, e.g., by phosphorylation, which can activate or deactivate the transport protein; (2) trafficking of transport proteins stored in vesicles and their fusion with the cell membrane, thereby increasing the number of transport proteins expressed at the cell surface (or conversely, vesicular retrieval of transporters from the cell membrane); (3) de novo transcription either in response to kinase-induced activation of transcription factors or mediated by nuclear hormone receptors (NHR); (4) posttranscriptional fine-tuning of levels of transcribed mRNA, such as via microRNAs. Newly synthesized transport proteins can also undergo multiple posttranslational modifications (PTMs) and are then packaged into vesicles for transfer to the cell surface.

Receptor activation

In order to be able to detect changes in the huge range of endogenous and exogenous stimuli to which they are exposed, intestinal epithelial cells express many different types of receptors. Receptors at the cell surface, including G-protein-coupled receptors (GPCRs), receptor tyrosine kinases (RTKs), and tyrosine kinase-linked receptors, bind to soluble ligands, such as those released from nerves and immune cells. Nuclear receptors (NRs), on the other hand, are found in the cytosol and are activated by lipid-soluble agonists that can traverse the cell membrane, such as steroid hormones.

Most cell surface receptors are preferentially localized to the basolateral membrane, in close proximity to the regulatory cells that produce their ligands. However, some receptors are expressed apically, where they are activated by luminal stimuli, such as bacterial toxins [295]. There are, however, well-recognized exceptions to this polarization. For example, receptors for endogenous purinergic agonists are found on both sides of the epithelium [296]. This may reflect, in part, the fact that these agonists (or precursors thereof) are products of inflammatory cells that can traverse the epithelium and release mediators into the luminal compartment [297]. Similarly, receptors for guanylin, the endogenous ligand for the receptor that binds the heat stable enterotoxin of *E. coli* (ST_a), are located in the apical membrane. This implies that this endogenous peptide is secreted into the lumen to produce its biological effects. Conversely, epidermal growth factor (EGF), normally present in the lumen, has basolaterally localized receptors. It has been suggested that EGF therefore functions as a luminal surveillance peptide, in that it may regulate epithelial function only in the setting of mucosal damage, where the epithelial barrier is breeched and the growth factor can access the basolateral side [298].

The most abundant cell surface receptors are GPCRs, which are activated by a wide array of hormones, immune-derived mediators, and neurotransmitters (Table 16.2). In general, activation of the G_s- or G_q-linked subclasses of GPCR promotes luminal fluid accumulation, through signaling pathways involving increases in intracellular cyclic adenosine monophosphate (cAMP) or Ca^{2+}, respectively. Many agonists of these receptors are capable of simultaneously inhibiting absorptive processes and promoting secretion. This reciprocity in regulation of Cl^- secretion versus NaCl absorption ensures that the transport functions of different epithelial cells do not work at cross-purposes. A third subclass of GPCR expressed in intestinal

Table 16.2 Endogenous and exogenous regulators of intestinal chloride secretion.

Substance	Second messenger	Notes
Endogenous stimuli (hormones, neurotransmitters, and immune/inflammatory mediators)		
Acetylcholine	Calcium	Acts through m_3 muscarinic receptor on epithelial cells
Histamine	Calcium	H_1 histamine receptor on epithelium; indirect effects also possible[a]
5-hydroxytryptamine	Calcium, cAMP	Indirect effects also possible[a]
Prostaglandins	cAMP	E-series prostaglandins particularly potent
Bradykinin	Calcium	Bilateral BK2 receptors; indirect effects also possible[a]
Reactive oxygen species, H_2O_2	Calcium, cAMP	Effects likely to be largely indirect[a]
Platelet-activating factor	cAMP	Indirect effects[a]
Vasoactive intestinal polypeptide	cAMP	Direct effect via basolateral receptors
Guanylin, uroguanylin	cGMP	Apical receptor
Adenosine, 5′AMP	cAMP	Bilateral adenosine A2b receptors on epithelium
Lipoxygenase metabolites of arachidonic acid	Unknown	Effects largely indirect
Exogenous stimuli (bacterial products and luminally active agents)		
Cholera toxin	cAMP	
E. coli heat labile toxin	cAMP	
E. coli heat stable toxin (ST_a)	cGMP	Binds to apical guanylin receptor
C. difficile toxins A and B	Calcium, other effectors?	Indirect effects and effects on paracellular pathway likely important
Bile acids	Calcium, cAMP?	Indirect effects likely also contribute
Pharmaceutical agents (e.g., laxatives)	cAMP, cGMP	For example, lubiprostone, linaclotide

[a] Indicates agonists that may mediate at least a portion of their effects via stimulation of mucosal prostaglandin production, or activation of enteric nerves, which in turn can alter epithelial cAMP or calcium levels.
cAMP, cyclic adenosine monophosphate.

epithelial cells is coupled to inhibitory G_i proteins, of which the somatostatin receptor, $SSTR_1$, has been most studied. Activation of $SSTR_1$ inhibits accumulation of cAMP in response to agonists of G_sPCRs, thereby dampening fluid secretion [299]. This likely underlies the clinical efficacy of somatostatin analogs in cases of severe secretory diarrhea.

In addition to GPCRs, epithelial cells also express RTKs and tyrosine kinase-associated receptors. These receptors are typically activated by peptide hormones and growth factors, such as EGF and insulin. As their names suggest, they induce cellular responses through activation of tyrosine kinase-dependent signaling pathways and, similar to agonists of G_iPCRs, they can exert antisecretory and proabsorptive actions, albeit by distinct mechanisms of action [300–306].

Finally, several nuclear receptors play important roles in regulation of intestinal transport. Many bind steroid hormones and upon activation, translocate from the cytosol into the nucleus where they exert their actions by regulating gene transcription. Transcriptional regulation of epithelial transport can involve either direct effects on the genes that encode transport proteins themselves, or indirect effects involving alterations in expression of regulatory proteins. Since they involve genomic actions, the effects of nuclear receptor agonists are typically slow in onset, occurring over hours to days. Perhaps the best studied of the steroid hormones with respect to regulation of intestinal transport is aldosterone, a mineralocorticoid that regulates whole-body Na^+ homeostasis and blood pressure. In response to increased levels of serum K^+, aldosterone is released from the adrenal cortex and targets both the kidney and the colon to promote Na^+ absorption, largely via upregulation of ENaC and Na^+,K^+ ATPase expression [307]. However, other nuclear receptors, including those for glucocorticoids, estrogen, progesterone, and bile acids, exert antisecretory actions on colonic epithelial cells [254,308–312]. Furthermore, the effects of nuclear receptors on intestinal transport are not always mediated by genomic actions, since some of these receptors can also activate nongenomic signaling pathways that rapidly downregulate epithelial Cl^- secretory function [313].

Epithelial signal transduction pathways

The classic second messengers recognized for their involvement in intestinal transport regulation are cAMP, cGMP, and free cytosolic calcium. However, additional signals that can amplify, antagonize, or modify the effects of these messengers have also been identified.

Cyclic nucleotides

cAMP and cGMP have long been recognized to play important roles in the control of intestinal transport. Increases in the levels of either of these cyclic nucleotides stimulate Cl^- secretion and inhibit electroneutral NaCl absorption, via activation of PKA or PKG, respectively [314–317]. Cyclic nucleotides also regulate sodium-glucose cotransport, duodenal HCO_3^- secretion, and electrogenic sodium absorption [318–321].

Several key endogenous regulators of ion transport, including prostaglandins and vasoactive intestinal polypeptide (VIP), act via G_sPCRs and increases in cAMP production. Other agonists of intestinal ion transport may act not by stimulating increases in cAMP themselves but by relocating protein kinase A that is already active [322]. Exogenous substances may also activate the cAMP pathway. The classic example is cholera toxin, which causes irreversible activation of the G_S protein by ADP-ribosylation, leading to prolonged adenylyl cyclase activation and elevation of cAMP [323]. Similarly, the apical receptor for *E. coli* heat-stable enterotoxin (ST_a) is a membrane-bound guanylyl cyclase. Binding of toxin to this receptor thereby increases intracellular cGMP and produces a chloride secretory response as well as inhibition of NaCl absorption [316,324, 25]. The existence of a receptor for ST_a implied an endogenous ligand for this system, subsequently identified and named guanylin [326], a peptide that has been proposed to play an important role in normal intestinal water and electrolyte homeostasis [327,328].

While the effects of cAMP and cGMP on epithelial transport are primarily mediated by PKA and PKG, respectively, it is clear that there is also significant overlap in the mechanisms involved [329–331]. While most of the actions of cyclic nucleotides on epithelial transport are mediated through kinase-dependent signaling pathways, there are reports of cation channels that can be directly gated by cAMP and cGMP, and which may contribute to Na^+ absorption [332].

Intracellular Ca^{2+}

Similar to the effects of cyclic nucleotides described above, increases in intracellular Ca^{2+} stimulate both Cl^- and HCO_3^- secretion, while inhibiting electroneutral and electrogenic Na^+ absorption. Also similar to cyclic nucleotides, many of the effects of intracellular Ca^{2+} on epithelial transport are mediated by downstream protein kinases. However, in some cases, such as regulation of KCNN4 K^+ channels or TMEM16A Cl^- channels, direct interactions between Ca^{2+} or the Ca^{2+} binding protein, calmodulin, and the transport protein are involved [333–335].

The effects of agents that exert their actions through Ca^{2+} appear to be more complex than those described for cyclic nucleotides. Thus, there is a relatively poor correlation between the magnitude and duration of agonist-induced increases in intracellular Ca^{2+} and the consequent ion transport responses [336]. In general, whereas ion transport responses mediated by cyclic nucleotides are prolonged, those evoked by Ca^{2+} are transient, and terminate even if the Ca^{2+} signal persists [337]. While Ca^{2+} alone appears to be sufficient to induce epithelial Cl^- secretion, the overall effects of this messenger can be modified by other signals. For example, products of phospholipid turnover, including diacylglycerol, inositol (3,4,5,6) tetrakisphosphate ($InsP_4$), or 3-phosphorylated inositol phospholipids produced by the enzyme phosphatidylinositol 3-kinase, may downregulate Ca^{2+}-dependent responses [338,339]. In some cases, these auxiliary messengers have been shown to have reciprocal effects on secretory and absorptive processes, for example inhibiting calcium-dependent Cl^- secretion while stimulating electroneutral NaCl absorption [338,340].

Downstream targets of epithelial signaling pathways

The signaling pathways activated downstream of intracellular second messengers that bring about alterations in cell function (see Figure 16.8) can be broadly divided into two classes: (i) those mediated by posttranslational modifications (PTMs) of transport and/or regulatory proteins, and (ii) those that are transcriptionally mediated.

Posttranslational modifications

The rapid downstream effects of cyclic nucleotides and calcium in regulating epithelial transport are largely mediated by PTMs of the transport proteins involved. Such PTMs are very important in the fine-tuning of epithelial fluid and electrolyte transport, and our understanding of how they regulate the stability, activity, and membrane trafficking of transport proteins is constantly growing. PTMs of transport proteins most often involve alterations in phosphorylation, brought about by kinases and phosphatases. However, other mechanisms are also involved, including the recruitment of regulatory proteins that bind to the transporters and form complex signaling scaffolds, or through the actions of enzymes that conjugate other molecules to the transporters, such as ubiquitin. Ultimately, through the use of different PTMs, signals generated by hormones and neuroimmune mediators can either upregulate or downregulate intestinal fluid movement via coordinated regulation of multiple transporters.

A good example of how different PTMs can alter transport protein function is provided by NHE3. The contribution of electroneutral Na^+ absorption to intestinal fluid absorption varies considerably with feeding. Upon ingestion of a meal, the presence of luminal nutrients drives the activity of nutrient-coupled transporters, such as SGLT1, and the electroneutral pathway is less relevant. However, between meals, the activity of nutrient-coupled transporters decreases, with electroneutral Na^+ absorption becoming more important. A number of PTMs enable plasticity of NHE3 function, which in turn allows for rapid alterations in absorptive function [51,156,341]. First, various kinases alter NHE3 activity by phosphorylating specific residues within the protein. Perhaps the best studied is PKA, which phosphorylates the protein to inhibit its activity [342,343]. Phosphorylation of NHE3 by PKA requires the concomitant binding of other regulatory factors, including members of the NHERF (for NHE regulatory factor) family [153]. The C terminus of NHE3 is responsible for binding NHERF family members and ezrin, and in turn, the catalytic subunit of PKA. This multiprotein complex establishes a spatial relationship between PKA and the transporter residues that it phosphorylates and also regulates trafficking of NHE3 into and out of the apical membrane [156,344,345].

NHE3 activity can also be downregulated by agonists that cause elevations in cytoplasmic calcium [153,346]. In this case, protein kinase C (PKC) rather than PKA appears to be the predominant kinase effector, with the PKC-α isoform being identified as mediating inhibitory effects of effectors such as 5-hydroxytryptamine or acetylcholine [347,348]. NHERF-dependent binding of calmodulin to the transporter is also an important regulatory mechanism [349]. Indeed, the effects of agonists on NHE3 function depend on the particular isoform of NHERF that is recruited to the transporter, with NHERF2 mediating inhibition and NHERF4 (also known as IKEPP) having stimulatory effects. In turn, the particular NHERF isoform recruited is determined by the location of the transporter in membrane microdomains [350]. Clearly, the relative expression of different NHERF isoforms under different conditions has important implications for intestinal absorptive function. In addition to NHERF isoforms, many other proteins are known to be involved in the formation of the multiprotein scaffold complex that regulates NHE3 phosphorylation and trafficking, including synaptotagmin 1, AP2, α-actinin-4, and clathrin [51,156,341].

In addition to mechanisms activated by cAMP and Ca^{2+}, many other intracellular effectors are involved in regulating the activity of NHE3. For example, agents that elevate cytosolic levels of cGMP, such as *E. coli* ST_a, can inhibit NHE3 activity by a mechanism involving both NHERF2 and NHERF3 [351,352]. On the other hand, electroneutral NaCl absorption can be upregulated by signals generated coincident with meal intake. When sodium and glucose are absorbed via SGLT-1, there is concomitant upregulation of NHE3 activity that is mediated by translocation of the transporter to the apical membrane. This process involves sequential activation of p38 mitogen-activated protein kinase, MAP-KAPK-2, Akt-2, NHERF2, and ezrin [353–355]. Similarly, growth factors, such as EGF and basic fibroblast growth factor, activate NHE3 activity and membrane insertion via mechanisms involving sequential activation of PI 3-kinase and Akt [305,356].

The effects of second messengers on intestinal secretory responses are also mediated by a variety of PTMs. For example, similar to its actions on NHE3, PKA phosphorylates the regulatory domain of CFTR at multiple sites, resulting in channel opening and trafficking to the apical membrane [357]. The efficiency of this process is enhanced by clustering of PKA and CFTR into a signaling complex, with the participation of scaffolding proteins, such as AKAPs [358], and adaptor proteins, including NHERF2 [152,359], that assemble the signaling complex via interactions with PDZ domains. Similarly, guanylin and ST_a activate Cl^- secretion by a pathway involving type II cGMP-dependent protein kinase (PKG) [317,325,351]. However, it appears that this kinase does not directly phosphorylate or activate CFTR, and at least in some segments of the intestine, its effects are mediated by cross-activation of PKA [325].

Other transport proteins that constitute the Cl^- secretory pathway can also be modified by phosphorylation. For example, NKCC1 is phosphorylated and activated by PKA, with activation balanced by phosphatase activity [360]. In native colonic crypts, elevations in cAMP result in prolonged retention of

NKCC1 in the basolateral membrane, an effect that likely contributes to prolonged secretory responses observed in response to cAMP-dependent agonists [361]. Furthermore, elevated intracellular concentrations of Cl^- regulate cotransporter activity by impeding its PKA-dependent phosphorylation [360]. In this way, intracellular Cl^- levels can self-govern the rate of anion entry into epithelial cells. Recent studies suggest that direct interactions of regulatory proteins, such as AMPK, with NKCC1 are also important in controlling its activity [362].

While the prosecretory effects of agonists that elevate intracellular Ca^{2+} are thought to be mediated predominantly through calmodulin binding to KCNN4 K^+ channels [335,363,364], protein kinases, including Ca^{2+}-calmodulin-dependent (CaM) kinase and various isoforms of PKC, are also involved. The roles of PKC in regulating electrolyte transport are isoform dependent. In some systems, PKC isoforms stimulate active Cl^- secretion, an effect that may be mediated, at least in part, by phosphorylation of one, or more, of the nine PKC consensus sites within the regulatory domain of CFTR [365]. However, whether PKC exerts stimulatory or inhibitory effects on CFTR activity depends on the particular sites that are phosphorylated [366,367]. Indeed, although PKC is capable of inducing modest secretory responses, it appears more prominently to play an antisecretory role in regulating responses to both cAMP and Ca^{2+}-mobilizing agonists [368]. This appears to reflect not only effects of PKC on CFTR phosphorylation, but also the ability of specific PKC isoforms to regulate vesicular trafficking of basolateral transport proteins, including KCNN4 and NKCC1 [361,369–371].

In addition to serine/threonine kinases, tyrosine kinase-dependent signaling pathways also play important roles in regulating intestinal transport. For example, receptor tyrosine kinases (RTK), such as the EGF receptor (EGFr), stimulate electroneutral NaCl absorption in the small intestine and colon [304]. Furthermore, this proabsorptive action appears to be coupled to inhibition of Ca^{2+}-dependent Cl^- secretion [302]. Such effects of RTK activation are typically mediated by signaling cascades that lead to the activation of serine/threonine kinases, including mitogen-activated protein kinases or Akt, which ultimately alter the activity and/or surface expression of the transport protein [338,339,356,372]. However, direct phosphorylation of tyrosine residues in transport proteins by cytosolic tyrosine kinases is also important in regulating their activity. For example, Src family kinases phosphorylate a specific tyrosine residue in CFTR that, in turn, facilitates phosphorylation of a serine residue necessary for CFTR activation [373,374].

Another type of PTM that is important in regulation of intestinal transport is ubiquitination, a mechanism best studied in the regulation of electrogenic sodium absorption via ENaC. Although most findings reflect studies in renal cells [375], they are likely also representative of regulation of this channel in the distal colon. ENaC dynamically associates with a ubiquitin ligase, Nedd4-2, in response to increases in the intracellular concentration of sodium [376]. In turn, the modification of ENaC subunits by covalent association of ubiquitin targets the channel for internalization and degradation in the proteasome [377]. This provides a mechanism whereby sodium absorption is reduced if cytoplasmic sodium levels rise. This regulatory machinery also provides for upregulation of electrogenic sodium absorption in response to agonists that increase levels of cAMP. cAMP activates PKA, which in turn phosphorylates Nedd4-2, reducing its association with ENaC. Thus, by relieving an inhibitory influence on ENaC membrane abundance, cAMP can increase overall levels of sodium absorption [198,378]. Similarly, acute effects of aldosterone on sodium absorption may at least in part reflect the insertion of additional sodium channels and/or active Na^+,K^+-ATPase pumps into the appropriate membrane of the epithelial cell [379]. These effects of aldosterone, and similar effects of glucocorticoids, are mediated by acute activation of the serum and glucocorticoid-regulated kinase, sgk1. This kinase, like PKA, increases phosphorylation of Nedd4-2, thereby reducing its ability to ubiqutinate ENaC [380].

Studies from various systems suggest that ubiquitination is important in regulating not only ENaC levels but also those of other transporters, including CFTR [381,382], K^+ channels [370], Na^+/K^+ ATPase pumps [383], and NKCC1 [139]. Furthermore, not only are transporters themselves regulated by the ubiquitination/proteasome pathway but also their regulatory proteins, such as WNK [384]. Finally, an added level of complexity derives from the ability of regulatory proteins, such as NHERF, to compete with the ubiquitin ligase, Nedd4-2, for binding to its target proteins [385]. In this way, one PTM (i.e., the recruitment of an adapter protein) can prevent another type of PTM (i.e., ubiquitination) from occurring, ultimately stabilizing particular transport proteins within the cell.

Transcriptional regulation

In addition to rapidly acting PTMs, signaling cascades regulate epithelial fluid and electrolyte transport over more prolonged periods of time via alterations in transport protein expression. As discussed above, such chronic regulation of transport function classically occurs in response to several steroid hormones. For example, aldosterone upregulates ENaC expression in intestinal epithelia to promote Na^+ absorption [386], while activation of the nuclear bile acid receptor, FXR, can downregulate CFTR expression [308]. Hormones can also act by modulating the expression of regulatory proteins. An example is CHIF, a protein that is upregulated in response to aldosterone and which increases Na^+/K^+ ATPase activity by increasing its affinity for Na^+ [387]. Further, not only can nuclear receptor agonists regulate the expression of transport proteins, but so too can agonists that act at GPCRs or RTKs. For example, IL-1β can upregulate CFTR expression in cultured colonic epithelial cells [388], while EGF can promote expression of NKCC1 and TMEM16A [389,390]. In many cases, the signaling cascades activated by such agonists lead to the phosphorylation and translocation of transcription factors to the nucleus, including NFκB, AP-1, Egr, SP-1, HNF1α, and HIF1-α, among others [388,391–393], where they upregulate or downregulate transport protein gene expression.

Finally, it should be noted that extracellular factors other than receptor ligands have roles to play in transcriptional regulation of epithelial transport. For example, alterations in blood flow to the intestine can result in reduced O_2 supply to the mucosa, leading to tissue hypoxia. Under these conditions, the ability of the epithelium to generate ATP is compromised and cellular energy becomes depleted [394]. However, when hypoxia occurs, the epithelium displays an adaptive response dependent on the transcription factor, hypoxia-inducible factor (HIF). HIF induces a program of gene expression that enables epithelial cells to adapt to changes in O_2 availability, including repressing expression of CFTR and NKCC1 [391,395]. Such responses may have developed as part of a process that redirects cellular energy from costly epithelial transport processes to those that are more essential for cell survival.

When considering how alterations in gene expression are important in regulating epithelial fluid and electrolyte transport, one must also consider the role of epigenetic factors. DNA methylation and histone modifications are considered crucial in regulating gene transcription. While studies from a variety of systems have shown that expression of various epithelial transport proteins is under the control of epigenetic factors [396–400], there is still little known of their roles in regulating intestinal fluid and electrolyte transport.

Another area of epithelial biology that is poorly understood is how posttranscriptional regulatory mechanisms contribute to intestinal transport function. Posttranscriptional mechanisms are those that act on mRNAs to regulate their translation into protein. The best characterized posttranscriptional regulatory mechanisms are those mediated by microRNAs (miRNAs). miRNAs are short (~22 nucleotides) endogenously produced sequences of RNA that bind to the 3'UTR of mRNAs to either induce their degradation or repress their translation into protein. While it is now clear that miRNAs play many important roles in regulating intestinal physiology [401,402], our knowledge of how they regulate intestinal fluid and electrolyte transport is still in its infancy. However, studies from other systems do suggest that CFTR, K^+ channels, DRA, aquaporins, and Na^+/K^+ ATPase can all be regulated in this manner [403–407]. Similarly, as this complex area of research progresses it is likely to be found that other types of noncoding RNA will also emerge as important regulators of transport protein expression and activity in the intestine. For example, long noncoding RNAs (lncRNAs) are differentially expressed in conditions of intestinal disease and have been shown to modulate transport protein expression in other tissues [403,408–410].

Interactions among second messengers

The signaling pathways induced by receptor activation in intestinal epithelia rarely act independently of one another, but rather significant cross-talk takes place. In this way, interactions between second messengers can have either positive or negative effects on transport function. For example, while elevations in either intracellular Ca^{2+} or cAMP stimulate intestinal Cl^- secretion, simultaneous increases in these second messengers lead to greater than additive responses [411]. The underlying basis of such synergistic interactions appears to depend, at least in part, on the distinct set of transport proteins activated by each messenger. Thus, Cl^- secretion induced by cAMP is regulated primarily by the opening of CFTR Cl^- channels, whereas Ca^{2+} acts predominantly by opening basolateral K^+ channels. When both second messengers are elevated simultaneously, the rate-limiting step for each type of secretion is removed and synergistic responses occur [411]. The physiological implication of this phenomenon is that greater effects on ion transport can be achieved for a given level of agonist, while the pathophysiological implication is that the simultaneous release of numerous neuroimmune mediators could result in profound secretory diarrhea. Cross-talk between signaling pathways can also occur at the level of second messenger generation, since both Ca^{2+} and cAMP can influence one another's levels within epithelial cells. For example, cAMP activates a protein known as exchange protein directly activated by cAMP (Epac) that elevates intracellular Ca^{2+}, thereby activating a Ca^{2+}-dependent Cl^- conductance [412]. Conversely, a Ca^{2+}-dependent adenylyl cyclase has been identified that can associate with CFTR [413]. With these discoveries, the traditionally held idea that Ca^{2+} and cAMP-dependent transport responses in the intestine occur by distinct mechanisms can no longer be considered valid.

Agonists that act at GPCRs can also recruit signaling pathways normally associated with RTKs to regulate intestinal transport responses. For example, elevation of intracellular Ca^{2+} by G_qPCR agonists brings about transactivation of EGFr and subsequent activation of MAPKs. This constitutes an antisecretory signaling mechanism that serves to limit secretory responses to such agonists [301,414,415]. G_sPCR agonists can also transactivate EGFr. However, in this case, the EGFr-dependent signaling pathway leads to stimulation of PI3-K, which appears to be involved in mediating the full expression of secretory responses to agonists of this receptor type [416]. Further studies in native colonic crypts have shown that longer-term effects of cholinergic stimulation on epithelial transport can also be mediated by recruitment of EGFr-dependent signaling pathways. In this case, EGFr-dependent internalization of NKCC1 chronically inhibits fluid loss in response to Ca^{2+}-dependent secretagogs, unless offset by the simultaneous presence of an agonist that elevates cAMP [361].

In summary, a complex network of intracellular signals and targets underlies both acute and chronic regulation of intestinal fluid and electrolyte transport in the intestine. At any given time, the extent of absorption and secretion across the epithelium depends on intracellular levels of second messengers, rates of transport protein transcription in the nucleus, and the extent of transporter trafficking to and from the cell surface. In turn, activation of these signaling pathways depends on the pattern of receptor expression on the epithelial cells and the extracellular factors to which they are exposed.

Intercellular regulatory mechanisms

The basal tone of fluid and electrolyte transport in the intestinal tract is set by a number of factors, such as the availability of O_2 or circadian rhythms [417,418]. However, transport function is also upregulated or downregulated by a wide array of extracellular stimuli, which include luminal factors as well as blood-borne hormones, neuronal and immunological mediators. Histological examination of the lamina propria reveals various immune cell types (the mucosal immune system), an extensive neuronal network (the enteric nervous system), and enteroendocrine cells that are interspersed among the cells of the epithelial layer. The epithelium is also closely associated with an underlying layer of specialized mesenchymal cells, called myofibroblasts. Ultimately, it is the integrated effects of the many mediators released from these regulatory cells that determine the absorptive and secretory capacity of the intestine at any given time.

Luminal factors

The intestinal lumen is an ever-changing environment to which epithelial cells must rapidly adapt. For example, the intermittent presence of nutrients in the lumen induces upregulation of the surface expression of nutrient-coupled cotransporters, thereby coupling fluid to nutrient absorption. As digestion proceeds, the movement of a food bolus through the intestine also exerts physical forces on the epithelium to induce fluid secretion, thereby lubricating the epithelium and protecting it from abrasion. Such responses are mediated by enteroendocrine cells, which release mediators that act in a paracrine fashion to activate neuronal secretomotor reflexes [419].

In addition to food and digested nutrients, there are many other factors present in the lumen that can alter transport function. For example, bile acids are required for the efficient digestion and absorption of fats in the small intestine. Normally, most bile acids are reabsorbed in the ileum through Na^+-dependent apical bile salt transporters (ASBT), but small quantities enter the colon where they exert antisecretory actions, thereby promoting absorptive function [420]. In certain pathological conditions, malabsorption in the small intestine results in increased delivery of bile acids to the colon where they exert prosecretory effects and the onset of diarrhea [421]. Bile acids can also be metabolized by the colonic flora, which alters their secretory activities [422,423]. Colonic bacteria also metabolize dietary fiber to produce SCFAs, such as butyrate. SCFAs induce differentiation of epithelial cells and upregulate both electroneutral and electrogenic Na^+ absorption while downregulating secretory capacity [424,425]. In this manner, SCFAs serve to promote normal colonic absorptive function.

In addition to fermented fiber, other dietary constituents are also likely to be important in modulating intestinal fluid and electrolyte transport. In this regard, flavonoids such as genistein and quercetin, found in many types of dietary plant, have been shown to stimulate intestinal Cl^- secretion [426–429]. Other phytochemicals reported to modulate intestinal transport function include stilbenes (e.g., resveratrol) [430] and gallotannins (e.g., tannic acid) [431].

The ingestion of pathogens can also have profound effects on epithelial transport. Bacterial toxins, such as cholera toxin and *E. coli* ST_a, promote the generation of cyclic nucleotides in epithelial cells, thereby upregulating secretion and causing diarrhea [432]. Other pathogenic bacteria, for example Salmonellae, do not produce enterotoxins but can induce gastroenteritis and diarrhea through direct manipulation of host cell signaling pathways that regulate transport proteins and tight junctions [256,433]. In addition to their direct actions on epithelial cells, many bacteria can also exert prosecretory actions in the intestine by indirect means through activation of the enteric nervous or mucosal immune systems [434–436]. In addition to bacteria, other ingested pathogens, including viruses and protozoans [437,438], can induce diarrhea through alterations in epithelial transport.

Endocrine and paracrine regulation

Both endocrine (i.e., regulation by blood-borne hormones from distant sites) and paracrine (i.e., local) factors are of critical importance in the regulation of epithelial transport. Enteroendocrine cells located within the epithelium sense the nature and composition of luminal contents and also mediate responses to extraintestinal signals, such as those from neural inputs. The hormones released by these cells can then act upon epithelial receptors to alter ion transport. Table 16.2 presents a partial listing of some of the neurohumoral agents identified as potential physiological regulators of intestinal ion transport, and their presumed mechanism of action.

Hormonal regulation

The intestine is a highly vascularized organ receiving a rich blood supply through the splanchnic circulation. In addition to oxygen and nutrients, the blood supply also carries hormones that can have profound effects on epithelial transport function. Several gastrointestinal peptide hormones, such as gastrin, cholecystokinin, and secretin, are released in response to ingestion of a meal and can alter electrolyte and fluid absorption and secretion. These hormones are dealt with in more detail in Chapter 49.

However, there are also many hormones delivered via the blood to the intestine from distant organs. Interorgan signaling in this way enables intestinal electrolyte transport to be integrated and synchronized with the requirements of other systems, thereby contributing to whole-body fluid homeostasis. As discussed above, aldosterone, a mineralocorticoid produced by the adrenal cortex, is probably the best studied of hormones with respect to its chronic effects on intestinal transport. Other hormones that can induce chronic alterations in intestinal transport function include glucocorticoids, estrogen, natriuretic peptides, IGF-1, and thyroid hormone [254,310,439]. In recent years, bile acids have emerged as a new family of "enterocrine hormones." In addition to their classic roles in facilitating digestion and absorption of lipids, bile acids regulate many aspects of intestinal epithelial physiology, including fluid and electrolyte transport. These hormonal roles for bile acids are primarily mediated by two receptors: TGR5, expressed at the cell surface, and FXR, which is a nuclear receptor for bile acids [308,440–442].

While hormones have long been known to alter epithelial function through activation of nuclear receptors and induction of transport protein gene transcription, it is now known that a number of hormones also exert rapid, nongenomic effects through activation of various signaling pathways. For example, in addition to promoting ENaC expression in the colon, aldosterone rapidly activates Na^+/H^+ exchange and inhibits K^+ channel activity [443,444]. Sex steroids, such as estrogen, also exert rapid antisecretory effects in the colon, which might contribute to retention of body fluid during states of high circulating estrogen [310,370]. Other hormones that have been demonstrated to exert rapid, nongenomic effects on intestinal transport include corticosteroids, prolactin, and growth hormone [445–447].

Immune regulation

Not surprisingly, considering its continuous exposure to bacterial, viral, and dietary antigens, the gastrointestinal tract is extremely rich in immune effector cells. Intestinal immune cells are contained primarily within the lamina propria and consist of lymphocytes, plasma cells, mast cells, and phagocytes. Classically, the mucosal immune system is broadly divided on a functional basis into afferent and efferent components. The afferent component consists of lymphocyte-mediated antigen recognition and presentation as well as cytokine production which, in turn, recruits the efferent component consisting of mast cells, phagocytes, and their mediators. However, as our understanding of intestinal mucosal immunology develops, the division between the afferent and efferent arms of the MIS has become blurred as it becomes apparent that practically all cells within the intestinal mucosa are involved in both initiation and propagation of mucosal immune responses. Much has been learned of how cells and mediators of the mucosal immune system regulate ion transport, and this knowledge is increasing our understanding of how intestinal transport becomes dysfunctional in disease states [448–451].

Mast cells are the primary effector cells involved in gut allergic reactions and have also been implicated in the pathogenesis of inflammatory bowel disease and irritable bowel syndrome [452–454]. In animal models, immunological (IgE-dependent) activation of resident mast cells stimulates Cl^- secretion [455]. Treatment of human small and large intestinal tissue segments with anti-IgE antibodies also induces Cl^- secretory responses that involve many different mediators, including histamine, 5-hydroxytryptamine, adenosine, platelet-activating factor, leukotrienes, and prostaglandins. These mediators exert their prosecretory effects either by direct actions on epithelial cells or by indirect actions, involving recruitment of the enteric nervous system [456–459]. The functional association of mast cells and nerves in controlling intestinal transport is mirrored by their morphological association [460,461]. In addition to activation of the enteric nervous system, mast cells may also recruit other mucosal cell types to regulate epithelial transport. For example, mast cells produce various chemotactic factors that attract additional inflammatory cells, such as neutrophils and monocytes, to the mucosa. Furthermore, mediators released from these cell types can induce prosecretory prostaglandins from the myofibroblastic sheath that underlies the epithelium [462,463]. Thus, through recruiting multiple cell types, epithelial transport responses to activated mast cells are amplified, leading to the onset of diarrhea [464].

It should be noted that while mast cells are clearly important in the pathogenesis of diarrhea associated with allergic and inflammatory diseases, it seems that their role is even broader than this. This is illustrated in an experimental model where mice are genetically deficient in tissue mast cells. Such mice not only display defective antigen-induced transport responses, but also have reduced secretory responses to nonimmunological stimuli, such as electrical field stimulation, bile acids, or bacterial toxins [465–467].

Neutrophils are another innate immune cell type found in large numbers in the intestinal mucosa. Activation of neutrophils in colonic and ileal tissues from animals and humans by the bacterial chemotactic peptide, fMet-Leu-Phe, induces Cl^- secretory responses that, similar to mast cell activation, are due to both direct actions on the epithelium and indirect actions, mediated by enteric nerves and eicosanoids [457,468,469]. Several mediators released from activated neutrophils are thought to contribute to secretory responses, including neutrophil-derived oxidants and 5′AMP [470,471]. This latter mediator is interesting in that it is only active apically, reflecting a requirement for an apically localized 5′ ectonucleotidase that cleaves 5′AMP to its final active mediator, adenosine. This particular mediator may be an important stimulus of intestinal Cl^- secretion following migration of neutrophils into the intestinal lumen, as occurs in a crypt abscess [472].

Other inflammatory cells have not yet been examined as extensively as mast cells or neutrophils for their ability to regulate epithelial ion transport functions. However, it seems likely that such cells, including eosinophils, lymphocytes, dendritic cells, and monocyte/macrophages, also participate in the control of electrolyte transport, because they can all synthesize potent mediators that have either direct or indirect effects on the epithelium [451,473]. Such cells may also cooperate to influence the transport and barrier properties of the epithelium. For example, activation of T cells with consequent synthesis of interferon-γ and TNF-α leads to downregulation of Na^+/K^+ ATPase activity, a loss of epithelial barrier function, and reduced absorptive capacity [474,475]. Lymphocytes can also induce other mucosal immune cell populations to produce mediators that downregulate epithelial transport and barrier function [476]. In fact, it is now widely accepted that mucosal inflammation is generally associated with a more "leaky" epithelial barrier and a reduced capacity for fluid and electrolyte absorption [475,477–480].

Another highly specialized type of lymphocyte found in the intestine is the intraepithelial lymphocyte (IEL) [481,482]. These cells are found within the epithelial layer where they play an important role in surveillance and presentation of intestinal antigens. Although activated IELs have been demonstrated to produce mediators that increase epithelial permeability, they are also important in helping to maintain barrier function during microbial infection. This protective role of IELs may be due to their ability to express tight junction proteins, such as occludin, and thereby physically contribute to epithelial barrier function in times of inflammatory stress [482,483].

Another important component of the innate mucosal immune system is Paneth cells [61,484]. These cells are localized at the base of intestinal crypts in the small intestine where they synthesize a variety of antimicrobial peptides, including defensins, cathelicidins, and cryptdins. Interestingly, in addition to their bactericidal effects, cryptdins have been shown to directly interact with the apical membrane of epithelial cells to form anion channels, promote Cl^- secretion, and induce IL-8 production [485,486]. Such activities of Paneth cell-derived mediators make these cells another important mode of immune-epithelial interaction in modulation of epithelial barrier and transport function [484].

Epithelial cells themselves are now also widely considered to be important components of the mucosal immune system [487]. Enterocytes can express MHC class I and II molecules and directly participate in antigen presentation to immune cells, thereby playing an important role in induction of tolerance to food antigens or in propagation of inflammatory responses [488,489]. IELs and dendritic cells cooperate with this immune accessory function of epithelial cells [490,491]. Activated epithelial cells can also promote mucosal inflammatory responses by producing cytokines, other chemotactic substances, and antimicrobial peptides, which recruit inflammatory cells to the mucosa [492–495].

Mesenchymal cells

Immune cells may also interact with structural elements of the mucosa to control the function of the epithelium. Thus, the myofibroblastic sheath underlying the epithelium is thought to act as a regulatory site, whereby signals from lamina propria elements, including immune cells, can be amplified, suppressed, translated, and/or spatially restricted [496]. An example of such regulation is found in the observation that coculture of epithelial cells with myofibroblasts upregulates the secretory responses of the epithelial cells to both mast cell and neutrophil products. This effect may be attributable, at least in part, to the ability of the myofibroblasts to synthesize prostaglandin E_2. In turn, the capacity of the myofibroblast layer to synthesize this mediator may be selectively enhanced in the setting of local inflammation, via the induction of cyclooxygenase-2 [463]. Endothelial cells, which line the blood vessels within the mucosal layer, may act in a fashion similar to myofibroblasts in that they produce prostaglandins in response to inflammatory stimuli [497].

Neural regulation

Another key regulatory mechanism for intestinal ion and fluid transport is that provided by the enteric nervous system [498,499]. Many studies on isolated intestinal tissues have shown that electrolyte transport can be induced through direct activation of resident nerves by electrical field stimulation, or can be inhibited by pharmacological or functional denervation of the tissue. Histological studies show that effector nerve fibers from the submucosal plexus form synapses with the epithelium at the neuroepithelial junction. Neurotransmitters released by enteric nerve endings can directly bind to basolateral receptors on enterocytes and affect their function in much the same way as described above for immune mediators.

Enteric neurotransmitters identified to alter intestinal ion transport are included in Table 16.2. Many of these neurotransmitters not only act directly on epithelial cells, but also have indirect actions through their ability to recruit other lamina propria cells, such as mast cells and myofibroblasts [500,501]. Neural regulation, particularly through cholinergic pathways, appears to play an important role in maintaining the basal tone of fluid and electrolyte absorption and secretion in the intestine. Moreover, the enteric nervous system (ENS) mediates changes in epithelial transport function in response to many diverse stimuli, including endogenous hormones and immune-derived mediators or luminal factors, such as nutrients, bile acids, and bacterial toxins [499,502,503].

Activation of the ENS has various consequences depending on the segment of the intestine involved, and effects can be stimulatory or inhibitory depending on the neurotransmitters released [504,505]. Most effector neurons release several neurotransmitters simultaneously, with the net effect on transport representing the sum of their actions [506]. In the duodenum, nerve stimulation evokes HCO_3^- secretory responses [507], while in the jejunum, ileum, and distal colon, the most prominent effects are stimulation of electrogenic Cl^- secretion and inhibition of electroneutral NaCl absorption [508–510]. It should be noted that it is not just the neurons of the ENS that have important roles in regulation of epithelial transport and barrier function but also the glial cells that support and nourish them [511]. Recent studies in transgenic mice models show that activation of glial cells in the colon upregulates epithelial transport function, as measured by changes in short circuit current in Ussing chambers. These effects appear to be mediated by both stimulation of enteric nerves and direct actions of glial-derived mediators on the epithelium [511,512].

Sensory enteroendocrine cells interspersed among the transporting enterocytes are also closely associated with nerve fibers from the submuscosal plexus. These cells play a critical role in sensing, or "tasting," the luminal environment. When activated, for example, by nutrients, bile acids, or passage of a food bolus, they release messengers, most notably 5-hydroxytryptamine, that activate reflex arcs within the intestinal wall to appropriately modify epithelial secretory and absorptive processes [513,514]. Such intrinsic reflex arcs also coordinate epithelial transport function with intestinal motility through nerve fibers that run between the submucosal and myenteric plexuses. This neuronally mediated connection between epithelial and muscle cells enables integrated responses to luminal stimuli. For example, the presence of a food bolus in the lumen activates a neural reflux that increases both peristalsis and fluid secretion, thereby effectively moving the bolus along the intestinal tract [515]. Such reflexes can also be activated by luminal irritants, such as bile acids or bacterial toxins. In such cases, it is thought that increased peristalsis and fluid secretion lead to diarrhea, thereby flushing the lumen of the causative agent [516–518].

Finally, while the ENS can function in a fashion that is largely independent of the CNS, intestinal fluid and electrolyte transport can be influenced by the brain in both physiological and pathophysiological settings. The mere anticipation of a meal can activate transport processes necessary for digestion to occur when bidirectional communication between the brain and the enteric nervous system regulates fluid and electrolyte transport in the lower intestine [519]. On the other hand, psychological factors also affect intestinal transport function, as demonstrated by experiments in which rats subjected to a period of acute systemic stress had significantly increased baseline intestinal secretion and permeability [520]. Indeed, stress is widely thought to play an important role in the pathogenesis of some diarrheal diseases, most notably IBS and IBD [521,522].

Interactions between intercellular regulatory mechanisms

As discussed above, the epithelium can respond to signals from a variety of regulatory systems, including those from the endocrine, neurocrine, and immune systems, and there is substantial interplay between the mediators produced. As noted previously, mediators exert their effects on ion transport through different intracellular signaling mechanisms, displaying synergistic interactions when released at the epithelium in combination. Further, because neural input provides a basal tone to epithelial cells, they can respond more readily to increased levels of other hormones or inflammatory mediators. Evidence of the importance of this neurally defined tone is provided by the observation that the secretory responses of intestinal tissues to a wide variety of substances are reduced by blockers of neurotransmission, such as tetrodotoxin or atropine [523]. Thus, even for hormones and immune mediators that are known to have direct effects on the epithelium, the degree of neural input appears to be of paramount importance in setting the sensitivity of the system [524].

Interest in the concept of "neuroimmunophysiological" regulation of epithelial transport arose in part as a consequence of morphological studies demonstrating intimate spatial relationships between nerves, immunocytes, and the epithelium [525,526]. These spatial relationships appear to have functional correlates in that epithelial transport responses stimulated by electrical field stimulation can be reduced by antagonists of inflammatory mediators, while stimulation of immune cells, such as mast cells, induces activation of enteric nerves [456]. The idea that neuroimmune communication is likely to be an important factor in disease is underlined by observations that interactions between these systems are highly plastic and can undergo extensive remodeling in pathological states [521,527–529]. Furthermore, recent studies have shown that, just as the epithelium can be considered an active component of the mucosal immune system, it also appears to play functional roles in the enteric nervous system. For example, through release of cytokines, such as TNF-α, epithelial cells can prime enteric nerves in order to enhance their activation by mast cell mediators [530]. Furthermore, intestinal epithelial cells are now known to express enzymes involved in the synthesis and transport of acetylcholine, a predominant intestinal neurotransmitter [531–533]. These intriguing findings underline the complexity and plasticity of the multicellular interactions that regulate intestinal transport function.

Finally, when considering how interactions among extracellular signals regulate intestinal transport function, one must also consider the impact of the microbiota. Whether it is via direct bacterial–epithelial interactions or through the production of soluble mediators, the bacterial flora within the colonic lumen regulates practically all aspects of epithelial physiology, including transporter activity and expression, tight junction permeability, development of polarity, synthesis and release of inflammatory mediators, wound healing, and cell survival and differentiation [9,534–537]. For example, a variety of commensal and/or probiotic strains have been shown to increase expression of absorptive transporters DRA and NHE3, whereas pathogens suppress it [256,538,539]. On the other hand, an early effect of colonization of germ-free rats with *E. coli*, but not *Enterococcus faecalis*, *Lactobacillus intestinalis* or *Clostridium innocuum*, was to increase epithelial proliferation and suppress DRA expression [540]. Probiotics may also reverse the adverse effects of pathogens or inflammation on ion transport and barrier function and prevent diarrhea in mouse models [47,539,541–544].

Enteric bacteria not only exert their effects by acting directly on the epithelium but can also act indirectly through activation of nerves and immune cells within the lamina propria, or by metabolizing nutrients, which regulates the function and/or expression of several transporters [535,536,545,546]. Conversely, changes in ion transport can shape the microbiota. For example, mice lacking NHE3 also showed a reduction in microbial diversity that was associated with colitis [547]. Changes in the balance between commensal and pathogenic bacterial populations within the intestinal lumen have clear implications for the pathogenesis of disease, and there is growing evidence for the use of probiotics and prebiotics to induce beneficial changes in the microbiota as disease treatments [548–550]. Our understanding of the role of microbial–epithelial interactions in health and disease is rapidly developing as it becomes clear that such interactions have important implications not only for intestinal diseases, such as inflammation, diarrhea, and cancer [551–553], but also for extraintestinal disorders, including cardiovascular diseases [554], obesity [555], diabetes [556], and even, through interactions with the brain–gut axis, psychological disorders [557–559].

Disorders of electrolyte transport

The foregoing discussion should allow the reader to predict that significant morbidity should be associated with defects in the various transport pathways described and/or their regulatory mechanisms. Indeed, a number of naturally occurring genetic mutations in various transporters and channels have been instructive as to the precise physiological roles of these proteins, particularly when coupled with studies in knockout mice and/or in reductionist systems [560]. Increasingly, additional previously unexplained familial diarrheal syndromes are succumbing to high-throughput approaches to identify the responsible gene(s). Likewise, molecular information about transporters and their regulation has provided insights into the diarrheal symptoms that accompany more complex, not strictly genetic disorders, such as inflammatory bowel diseases and enteric infections. The growing understanding of the mechanisms that comprise and regulate intestinal ion transport is also allowing the more rationale design of drugs to treat conditions where transport is abnormal [561].

Genetic defects in electrolyte absorptive processes

Defects in NaCl absorption

Congenital chloride diarrhea produces profound Cl^--rich, acidic diarrhea commencing at birth, resulting in systemic hypochloremic and hypokalemic acidosis with volume depletion. First described in 1945, the disease has since been identified in more than 140 children [562]. The histology of the intestinal mucosa is normal on routine examination. Intubation studies have revealed that the transport defect is limited to the ileum and colon [563]. Na^+ absorption against a chemical gradient remains intact and is accompanied by H^+ secretion [564,565].

Mutations in DRA are now known to cause congenital chloride diarrhea, and DRA knockout in mice causes similar symptoms [167,284]. Although the disease can be accounted for by a defective Cl^-/HCO_3^- exchanger, the defect may be more subtle than a total lack of anion exchange. Indeed, increases in luminal HCO_3^- concentrations increase Cl^- secretion in these patients, suggesting that residual Cl^-/HCO_3^- exchange may still occur [563,564]. It is unclear if this is due to an alternative anion exchange protein in the apical membrane (such as PAT1) or residual DRA function. A large number of DRA mutations have been described in the disease, and some may result in a partially active protein and/or one that can be rescued, at least in part, by treatment with butyrate [566].

Congenital sodium diarrhea is an even rarer disorder. In its nonsyndromic form, this disease produces a Na^+-rich, alkaline stool and results in systemic acidosis, but without intestinal structural abnormalities. Intubation studies have revealed that the usual inverse relation between Na^+ and H^+ fluxes does not hold, suggesting a defect in Na^+/H^+ exchange [567]. This defect has been confirmed in studies demonstrating a clear lack of proton-driven Na^+ uptake in jejunal vesicles, and implicating an NHE isoform as a possible cause of the disease [568]. One genetic study failed to find an association with mutations in NHE1, -2, -3 or -5 [569] although more recent work has established that mutations in NHE-3 can be rare causes of the disease [570]. Others have reasoned that a normal developmental shift from expression of NHE8 to NHE3 in early life, along with the knowledge that some cases of congenital sodium diarrhea remit when patients reach 1 year, might suggest that mutations in NHE8 might be causative [571,572]. However, this was not borne out in a small series of five patients [573].

Thus, the major cause of classic congenital sodium diarrhea remains elusive, although mutations in genes encoding for any of the many NHE regulatory factors are obviously attractive targets. Activating mutations in guanylyl cyclase C, which would be expected to reduce electroneutral NaCl absorption and cause chloride secretion, have also been identified as causative in a subset of patients with this disease [574].

Defects in electrogenic Na^+ absorption

Liddle syndrome is an autosomal dominant disorder leading to salt-sensitive hypertension. It has been shown to be caused by mutations in ENaC [575]. The disorder leads to increased expression and activity of Na^+ channels because the normal mechanisms that internalize and degrade the channel are impaired [191,192]. No disorders of intestinal electrolyte absorption have been reported in Liddle syndrome despite severe defects in renal function. This might be predicted if ENaC, expressed only distally, plays a predominantly salvage role in colonic fluid absorption. On the other hand, in an animal model of the disease, aldosterone further enhanced the already amplified expression of electrogenic sodium absorption in the distal colon. This implies that colonic sodium salvage might be pathophysiologically significant if patients with Liddle syndrome ingest a high-salt diet [576]. It is possible, moreover, that diarrhea might be ameliorated in diseases, such as ulcerative colitis, where the diarrhea has been attributed to defective ENaC function (at least in part, see below) if the patients suffer additionally from Liddle syndrome. However, to the best of the authors' knowledge, this has not been described.

A subset of type 1 pseudohypoaldosteronism (the autosomal recessive version) is also caused by mutations in ENaC. In contrast to the gain-of-function mutants seen in Liddle syndrome, the mutations in type 1 pseudohypoaldosteronism diminish channel function and cause salt wasting. Intestinal malfunction has been noted in this disease, including elevated Na^+ in the stool [577] and a lack of colonic responsiveness to mineralocorticoids [578]. The disorder can be caused by frameshift, premature termination, and missense mutations in the α, β, or γ subunits of the channel [579].

Cystic fibrosis is associated with an increase in electrogenic Na^+ absorption, although the disease primarily reflects defects in Cl^- and HCO_3^- secretory function caused by CFTR malfunction (see below). However, CFTR is normally thought to limit ENaC activity, and lack of CFTR (or presence of mutant CFTR) therefore removes an inhibitory influence on this channel [207,249]. There is evidence in some tissues that CFTR physically associates with ENaC to limit its function, but this is controversial and may not apply in the colon where ENaC and CFTR are believed predominantly to localize to surface and crypt cells, respectively [580–583]. Nevertheless, hyperabsorption of sodium could conceivably contribute to the intestinal obstruction that is common in cystic fibrosis [249].

Defects in nutrient-coupled Na^+ absorption

Glucose-galactose malabsorption is a rare, autosomal recessive disorder in which Na^+-coupled uptake of glucose and galactose is defective [116]. Food ingestion leads to osmotic diarrhea, which can be treated by eliminating glucose and galactose from the diet. Children with this disorder can maintain normal Na^+ balance without glucose or galactose in their diets, illustrating the reserve capacity of the distal small intestine and colon for water and sodium absorption. Multiple mutations in SGLT1 that lead to glucose-galactose malabsorption have been described; these result in transport defects due to impaired trafficking of SGLT1 to the plasma membrane and/or defects in glucose transport kinetics [85,115].

Genetic defects in electrolyte secretory mechanisms

Defects in Cl^- and HCO_3^- secretion

Cystic fibrosis is an autosomal recessive disease causing defective epithelial transport in numerous organs. It is the most common genetic disease of ion transport, with one of every 20 Caucasian individuals being a heterozygous carrier and harboring a mutant CFTR allele. Almost 2000 naturally occurring missense, frameshift, and truncation mutations in CFTR cause defective Cl^- secretion by either diminishing the amount of CFTR protein in the membrane (defective trafficking or synthesis) or decreasing appropriate Cl^- channel opening (defective ATP gating, cAMP activation, or ion conductance) [584,585]. Mutations occur in all portions of the CFTR molecule, but with highest frequency in the first nucleotide binding domain, which controls channel gating. The most common mutation, found in 70% of all mutant CFTR alleles, is a triplet deletion that removes a phenylalanine (ΔF508) and results predominantly in defective trafficking of CFTR to the plasma membrane.

Cystic fibrosis is associated with meconium ileus in newborns and intestinal obstruction in older patients, which appear to result from the inability to maintain appropriate fluidity of luminal contents. Intestine from cystic fibrotic patients also fails to exhibit normal secretory responses in vitro [209,586]. While pathology in the disease has largely been attributed to defective Cl^- secretion, more recently it has been appreciated that the accompanying failure to secrete HCO_3^- that is required for appropriate mucus expansion may in fact play a more important role [587]. A meconimum ileus phenotype has also been reported in patients harboring inactivating mutations in guanylyl cyclase C, the guanylin receptor [588]. It has also been suggested that one reason for the prevalence of cystic fibrosis is a heterozygote advantage of partial protection from the severe, life-threatening consequences of infectious secretory diarrheas such as cholera. While this is an attractive possibility, others have disputed this hypothesis [589–591]. Another relevant finding is that the ability of *Salmonella typhi* to invade intestinal epithelial cells is significantly impaired in cells carrying one mutant allele of CFTR, which might confer some resistance to typhoid fever [592,593].

Other relevant genetic disorders

Microvillous inclusion disease is a rare, hereditary disease that commences in the first few days of life with the appearance of severe diarrhea that can be fatal if left untreated. The histological appearance of the intestinal epithelium is abnormal and is characterized by inclusions of brush border membranes as vesicular structures within the cytoplasm of villus cells, and a corresponding absence of apical microvilli [594]. Cytoplasmic transport of Golgi-derived vesicles destined to fuse with the apical membrane is defective in microvillous inclusion disease due to mutations in the motor protein, myosin 5B [595–598]. Endoscopic biopsies from patients with this disorder show markedly reduced levels of several apical transport proteins, with those transporters instead residing diffusely in the apical cytoplasm. Basolateral transporters, in contrast, were normal. Interestingly, a recent study has shown that CFTR continues to reside apically in both patients and in models of microvillous inclusion disease, suggesting symptoms are likely worsened by the occurrence of chloride secretion that is unopposed by electrolyte absorption [599].

A second neonatal enteropathy that causes severe diarrhea, usually arising in the context of consanguineous unions, is known as congenital tufting enteropathy, or intestinal epithelial dysplasia [600]. In this condition, the enterocytes on the villus pile up to generate characteristic "tufts" and patients are typically dependent on parenteral nutrition. The disease has been attributed to loss-of-function or deletion mutations in the cellular adhesion molecule, EpCAM [601]. Diarrhea is likely attributable to an epithelial barrier defect, and localization of the tight junction protein, claudin 7, is disrupted in models of the disease, although the precise mechanisms remain under investigation [602]. There is also a syndromic form of tufting enteropathy, associated with keratitis, in which mutations in the serine protease inhibitor, SPINT2, are causal, apparently by allowing excessive activity of the protease matriptase that results in EpCAM degradation and epithelial injury [603–605].

Finally, trichohepatoenteric syndrome, which presents with intractable diarrhea, facial dysmorphisms, immune system defects, and wooly hair, has been attributed to mutations in TTC37 (thespin) or SKIV2L. Both proteins are involved in formation of the exosome complex, which appears to be required to traffic absorptive transporters such as NHE3 to the enterocyte apical membrane. [82,606]. Thus, diarrhea in this condition likely arises from electrolyte malabsorption. Conversely, congenital bile acid diarrhea, which is caused by a defect in Slc10A2 that normally reclaims conjugated bile acids in the terminal ileum, is likely attributable to the direct prosecretory effect of high concentrations of bile acids when present in the colonic lumen [607,608]. The relevance of CFTR activation in this condition is revealed by the demonstration that inhibitors of the channel are efficacious in a rat model of the disease [609].

Mechanisms underlying other conditions associated with defective fluid and electrolyte transport

While genetic diseases associated with specific alterations in transport proteins have provided unique insights into the underlying molecular physiology of electrolyte transport, the most common diseases of fluid and electrolyte absorption are not related to transporter or regulatory protein mutations. This section serves to briefly introduce other disorders of intestinal fluid and electrolyte transport, most of which are far more common than the diseases discussed above. The reader is referred to later chapters in this text that provide more detailed descriptions of the pathogenesis of these disorders.

Infectious diarrhea

Diarrhea caused by infectious agents is usually only an inconvenience in the developed world but is a major killer in nonindustrialized nations, currently responsible for approximately 1.4 million deaths per year worldwide [610]. Many infectious diarrheas result from infections with microorganisms capable of producing classic enterotoxins. Cholera is the prototype, where a multimer toxin binds to receptors on the apical surface of intestinal epithelial cells and thereby simulates a sustained increase in intracellular cAMP [611]. In turn, this inhibits electroneutral NaCl absorption and evokes profound chloride secretion. Cholera toxin may also disrupt trafficking of tight junctional components [612]. Other bacterial toxins may subvert different cellular signaling mechanisms, such as the ability of the heat stable toxin of *E. coli* to evoke large increases in cGMP by binding to guanylyl cyclase C [613–615]. Both cholera and other enterotoxins may also activate subepithelial cell types to evoke secretion. Viral pathogens may also activate intestinal secretory mechanisms, such as the ability of rotavirus nonstructural protein 4 to induce calcium-dependent chloride secretion [212].

Information is also emerging regarding the mechanisms by which nontoxigenic pathogens, such as invasive bacteria, evoke diarrhea. Such organisms, including *Salmonella enterica* and enteropathogenic *E. coli*, may evoke a program of gene expression in intestinal epithelial cells that predisposes them to diminished absorptive function, as well as compromised barrier function. In particular, these and related pathogens have been shown to reduce expression and/or function of DRA, NHE3, subunits of ENaC, and NHERF, as well as triggering the production of chemokines that may amplify epithelial transport and barrier dysfunction secondary to the recruitment of inflammatory cell types to the mucosa [256,616–619]. Many such pathogens also impair epithelial barrier function, allowing for enhanced fluid loss via the "leak-flux" mechanism [620]. More complete information on these topics is discussed in Chapter 144.

Disaccharide intolerance

Disaccharide intolerance encompasses a variety of conditions characterized by genetic variability in the ability to conduct brush border digestion of carbohydrates, such as reduced levels of lactase in adulthood or sucrase-isomaltase deficiency. Such conditions cause osmotic diarrhea due to a reduced rate of brush border hydrolysis of specific disaccharides. Diarrhea results because only monosaccharides and not disaccharides can be absorbed by villus enterocytes. The undigested disaccharides thus remain in the lumen [621]. This should be contrasted with specific peptidase deficiencies, which do not usually result in fluid and electrolyte transport abnormalities because the intestinal epithelium has the ability to absorb both free amino acids and small oligopeptides.

Celiac disease

Celiac disease is a systemic immune-mediated disorder in genetically susceptible individuals triggered by dietary gluten, a water-insoluble protein found in certain cereal grains, notably wheat. The disease results in diarrhea and nonspecific nutrient malabsorption that can rapidly be reversed by elimination of offending substances from the diet. Celiac disease causes characteristic and striking morphological changes in the small intestine that include loss of villi, damage to remaining epithelial cells, and crypt hyperplasia. Disease pathogenesis appears to involve defective digestion of gluten and/or an inappropriate immune response to normal or improperly processed gluten molecules or peptides from these molecules that have been cross-linked to host proteins via the activity of tissue transglutaminase [622]. The accompanying diarrhea may have both osmotic and secretory components, with the latter likely being mediated, at least in part, by inflammatory mediators released by activated immune cells in the lamina propria as well as the release of acetylcholine from enteric nerves that produces a hypersecretory state (at least as observed in a mouse model) [623]. There is also emerging evidence that the active constituent of gluten in the disease, gliadin, may trigger the inappropriate release of an endogenous factor known as zonulin (now identified as prehaptoglobin-2) that impairs epithelial barrier properties [624–626].

Celiac disease is discussed in more detail in Chapter 56.

Inflammatory bowel diseases

Patients with inflammatory bowel diseases frequently present with diarrhea, although constipation is also observed. It is widely believed that the observed disorders of fluid and electrolyte absorption in inflammatory bowel disease patients are due to elevated levels of cytokines and other mediators in the inflamed bowel, although disruption of genes involved in maintaining the epithelial barrier and/or overexpression of pore-forming claudins, such as claudin-2, may also play a role [627–629]. Indeed, there is evidence for altered barrier function as a predisposing factor in inflammatory bowel disease, particularly as derived from mice lacking the multidrug resistance protein 1a [630]. This protein, expressed in the epithelium, may be responsible for effluxing toxic substances inappropriately absorbed from the gut lumen, and may also regulate the expression and function of other transport proteins, such as CFTR [631]. Likewise, there is disruption of electrolyte absorption, including Na^+-nutrient cotransport, electrogenic sodium absorption, and electroneutral NaCl absorption, as well as associated regulatory molecules, in both animal models of intestinal inflammation and human patients with inflammatory bowel disease [199,632–635].

Paradoxically, chloride secretion may also be inhibited in the setting of colitis, which is due in part to the ability of specific inflammatory mediators to downregulate expression of key components of the chloride secretory mechanism, including adenylyl cyclase 6 that predominantly contributes to agonist-stimulated increases in cAMP [199,636,637]. This suggests that reduced absorption, rather than increased secretion, may be the predominant contributor to inflammatory diarrhea, and perhaps that normal levels of secretion from the crypts are needed to maintain relative crypt sterility to protect the stem cell niche, and thus the integrity of the epithelium.

Constipation

Even more common than diarrheal disorders, the condition of constipation is associated with decreased fluidity of the colonic luminal contents, and thus challenges to their transit. Constipation is also becoming a growing clinical problem as the population ages and/or more individuals are prescribed opiates for chronic pain, and can be remarkably resistant to standard laxatives.

For a long time, constipation was predominantly attributed to defects in intestinal motility and/or a relative paucity of bulk-forming fiber in the diet, resulting in increased residence times for the colonic contents and thus a greater opportunity for their ongoing dehydration. However, the efficacy of some recently introduced therapies for chronic constipation and/or constipation-predominant irritable bowel syndrome implies, at a minimum, that the capacity of the colonic epithelium for active secretion can be exploited to ameliorate the condition. Thus, lubiprostone and linaclotide, both drugs that induce active chloride secretion (via the EP1 prostaglandin receptor or guanylyl cyclase-C dependent activation of CFTR, respectively), have been shown to be effective in increasing spontaneous bowel movements in clinical trials with little evidence of adverse effects other than mild diarrheal symptoms [228,638–641]. A small molecule activator of CFTR and a DRA inhibitor are also being studied as possible treatments for constipation [642,643]. In a similar vein, others have shown efficacy in chronic constipation with a minimally absorbed, luminally active drug that inhibits the ileal reabsorption of bile acids [644]. These clinical observations, taken collectively, imply that constipation may, in part, be a disease state where there is no longer an appropriate balance between intestinal absorption and secretion of fluid and electrolytes.

Conclusions

The ability of the intestine to control the fluidity of intestinal contents is clearly of key importance for many digestive functions. Both absorption and secretion of electrolytes, as well as other solutes, regulate this fluidity. Over the last few years, an explosion of molecular information regarding the precise structure and function of the transport proteins involved in these transport mechanisms, as well as their regulatory factors, has provided unprecedented insights into the basis of transport and its regulation. Moreover, the identification of various genetic disorders where epithelial transport function is compromised has provided a deeper understanding of molecular physiology and pathophysiology. The classic disease of intestinal transport is secretory diarrhea. However, it is also apparent that many other disease states can result when transport function is either compromised or overexpressed. In the long term, the molecular insights described in this chapter will form the basis for continuing advances in the treatment of patients with such conditions.

Acknowledgments

Related studies from the authors' laboratories have been supported by grants from the NIH and an unrestricted gift from the Estratest/ShapeUp Settlement Fund (KEB) and grants from Science Foundation Ireland (SJK).

References are available at www.yamadagastro.com/textbook7e

Further reading

Barrett K.E., Keely S.J. Chloride secretion by the intestinal epithelium: molecular basis and regulatory aspects. Annu Rev Physiol 2000;62:535.

Donowitz M., Cha B., Zachos N.C., et al. NHERF family and NHE3 regulation. J Physiol 2005;567(Pt 1):3.

Kato A., Romero M.F. Regulation of electroneutral NaCl absorption by the small intestine. Annu Rev Physiol 011;73:261.

Keating N., Keely S.J. Bile acids in regulation of intestinal physiology. Curr Gastroenterol Rep 2009;11(5):375.

Kopic S., Geibel J.P. Toxin mediated diarrhea in the 21 century: the pathophysiology of intestinal ion transport in the course of ETEC, V. cholerae and rotavirus infection. Toxins 2010;2(8):2132.

Kunzelmann K., Mall M. Electrolyte transport in the mammalian colon: mechanisms and implications for disease. Physiol Rev 2002;82(1):245.

Raybould H.E. Nutrient sensing in the gastrointestinal tract: possible role for nutrient transporters. J Physiol Biochem 2008;64(4):349.

Rowe S.M., Verkman A.S. Cystic fibrosis transmembrane regulator correctors and potentiators. Cold Spring Harbor Perspect Med 2013;3(7):a009761.

Turner J.R. Intestinal mucosal barrier function in health and disease. Nat Rev Immunol 2009;9(11):799.

Wright E.M., Loo D.D., Hirayama B.A. Biology of human sodium glucose transporters. Physiol Rev 2011;91(2):733.

CHAPTER 17

Gastric secretions

John Geibel[1,2]

[1] Department of Surgery, Yale University School of Medicine, New Haven, CT, USA

[2] Department of Cellular and Molecular Physiology, Yale University School of Medicine, New Haven, CT, USA

Chapter menu

Acid secretion plays an important role in the normal physiology and pathophysiology of the body. The stomach secretes concentrated hydrochloric acid (HCl) to aid in the digestion of foodstuffs and as a means to sterilize both fluids and liquids that enter the stomach during the digestive process and before their exit to the intestine. In this chapter, the anatomy of the stomach will be reviewed with a focus on the functional anatomy of the stomach. There are detailed reviews of the innervation and blood supply and the anatomy of the various cell types that are involved in the secretion of acid and the feedback circuit that modulates the acid. Following these discussions is a detailed review of the transport proteins that are associated with acid secretion and the peptides that act as direct or indirect modulators of the secretory process. Included in the discussion are recent findings on novel transport proteins that have been identified since the previous publication of this chapter in 2016.

Functional anatomy of the stomach

The human stomach is a specialized organ within the digestive system, situated between the esophagus and small intestine. Among its functions, the stomach serves to store and process food for absorption within the small intestine. A hallmark feature of the stomach is its ability to secrete HCl, the zymogen pepsinogen, and other important proteins and chemical messengers that play a major role in food digestion and vitamin B_{12} absorption. Absorption itself does not constitute a major function of the stomach, although some fat- and water-soluble substances are absorbed quickly and efficiently through the gastric mucosa [1].

The stomach is primarily considered a secretory organ; however, nonglandular gastric epithelium serves other important functions, such as storage mentioned earlier and additional information can also be found in Chapter 4. The human stomach is a single-chambered organ that is composed of two functional areas, the pyloric and oxyntic gland areas (Figure 17.1) [2]. The pyloric region comprises 15–25% of the stomach and consists of the pylorus and antrum. The latter region includes the "antral pump," which consists of smooth muscle in the gastric wall that serves to mix ingested food and control gastric emptying, thereby regulating the release of food products from the stomach into the small intestine for enzymatic digestion and subsequent absorption. In addition to this motor function, the pyloric region also plays an important secretory role. The oxyntic gland area of the stomach comprises 75–80% of the organ and consists of the cardia, fundus, and corpus (see Figure 17.1) [2]. As its name implies, this area contains

Yamada's Textbook of Gastroenterology, Seventh Edition. Edited by Timothy C. Wang, Michael Camilleri, Benjamin Lebwohl, Anna S. Lok, William J. Sandborn, Kenneth K. Wang, and Gary D. Wu.

Companion website: www.yamadagastro.com/textbook7e

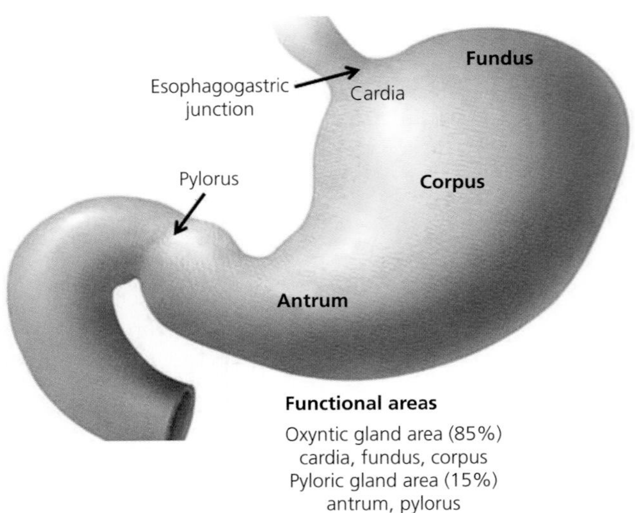

Figure 17.1 Functional, and corresponding anatomical, areas of the human stomach. Source: Based on Busque et al. 2005 [19].

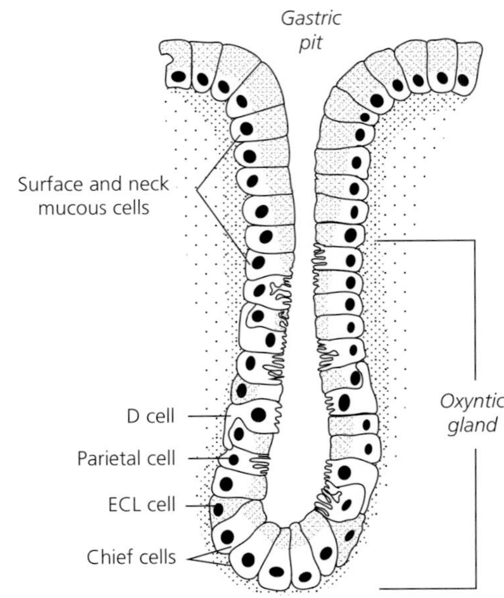

Figure 17.2 Schematic diagram of a gastric pit in the gastric corpus with an oxyntic gland at the base. D cell, somatostatin-producing cell; ECL, enterochromaffin-like.

oxyntic (parietal) glands, the principal secretory unit of the gastric mucosa (Figure 17.2).

The gastric glandular epithelium contains distinct and specialized cells, and the entire surface of the glandular stomach is lined by columnar epithelium, which includes surface mucous cells [3]. The surface epithelium is also lined with numerous gastric pits or crypts. These are tubular invaginations (see Figure 17.2), each of which opens into four or five gastric glands. The human gastric mucosa contains three distinct types of gastric glands: cardiac, oxyntic or parietal, and pyloric. The cardiac glands are located in the zone adjacent to the esophagogastric junction and consist of simple columnar cells, which are distinct from the stratified squamous epithelium of the lower esophagus. Similar to oxyntic glands, cardiac glands contain mucous, endocrine, and undifferentiated cells. However, cardiac glands can be distinguished from oxyntic glands by the absence of parietal and chief cells [1].

As noted earlier, the oxyntic portion of the stomach occupies the fundus and corpus, as well as the cardia, and is often considered the distinguishing feature of the human stomach. In addition to the presence of abundant mucous-secreting cells, the characteristic features of this region of the stomach are parietal cells, which secrete HCl, as well as intrinsic factor (IF), and chief cells, which secrete pepsinogen. These two cell types account for approximately 50% of the cells found within the corpus mucosa. Finally, endocrine cells that secrete various regulatory peptides and other chemical messengers are found in abundance in the oxyntic portion of the stomach [1].

The pyloric gland region comprises 15–25% of the gastric mucosal surface area, as eluded to earlier. The pyloric glands contain mucous-secreting cells like those found throughout the remainder of the stomach. Unlike other species, the human pyloric gland area does not include pepsinogen-secreting chief cells [4]. However, this region includes cells that secrete many hormones and other gastrointestinal regulatory peptides, the principal one being gastrin, which is secreted by gastrin cells (G cells) located in the epithelium [5].

Innervation of the stomach

The stomach is innervated by both parasympathetic and sympathetic neurons of the autonomic nervous system (see also Chapter 12). Parasympathetic innervation is provided via the vagus nerve [6]; branches of the vagi descend from the dorsal motor nucleus of the vagus in the brainstem, near the fourth ventricle, and branch extensively in the mediastinum to form an esophageal nerve plexus, which then re-forms into left (anterior) and right (posterior) vagal trunks that cross the diaphragm and innervate the stomach. Parasympathetic efferents from the vagus nerve synapse on intramural nerves in both the Meissner submucosal and Auerbach myenteric plexuses of the stomach. Vagal stimulation broadly increases the secretory and motor function of the stomach; the effect of vagal stimulation on gastric secretion is discussed in detail later. The vagus nerve also mediates sensory inputs from the stomach, and nearly three-quarters of the gastric vagal nerve endings emanate from afferent neurons, with cell bodies in the nodose ganglion, which transmit signals to the nucleus solitarius tractus in the brainstem. The nucleus tractus solitarius is adjacent to, and connects extensively with, the dorsal motor nucleus of the vagus, which generates efferent signals to the gastrointestinal tract [7]. Acetylcholine is the major parasympathetic neurotransmitter at the junction of the vagal neurons and gastric cells. However, afferent signaling also involves several other neurotransmitters, including glutamate, serotonin, and pituitary adenylate cyclase activating polypeptide [8,9].

Sympathetic innervation of the stomach is derived from the T5–T9 spinal nerves, which contribute to the greater splanchnic nerve and the celiac ganglion. These fibers primarily innervate the vasculature and nerve plexuses of the stomach, and generally act to inhibit motility, decrease secretion, and constrict the vasculature of the stomach. Norepinephrine is the primary neurotransmitter released at sympathetic nerve endings. Approximately 80% of the innervation of the stomach is derived from parasympathetic nerves, and only 20% is carried via the sympathetic system [10,11]. Additional details on recently identified neurotransmitters can be found later in the *Cephalic phase of acid secretion* section.

Blood supply to the stomach

The stomach possesses a rich vascular supply derived from branches of the celiac artery (see also Chapter 11). The left gastric artery arises directly from the celiac trunk and anastomoses with the right gastric artery (a branch of the hepatic artery) to form an arcade along the lesser curvature of the stomach. The left gastroepiploic artery arises from the splenic artery and joins the right gastroepiploic artery, which derives from the gastroduodenal artery, along the greater curvature. Additional vascular supply is provided by the short gastric arteries, which are branches of the splenic artery that supply the fundus and proximal stomach [12]. The presence of numerous feeding vessels to the stomach renders it less susceptible to ischemic injury than the small bowel and colon. The venous drainage of the stomach is of clinical importance, because the left gastric vein (also called the coronary vein) and right gastric vein drain into the portal vein. In patients with portal hypertension, it is the retrograde flow through these veins that leads to the formation of gastric and esophageal varices. The right gastroepiploic vein drains into the superior mesenteric vein, and the left gastroepiploic vein drains into the splenic vein. In cases of splenic vein thrombosis (often caused by pancreatic inflammation or neoplasm), isolated gastric varices may form as a result of pressure transmitted through the gastroepiploic vessels.

At the microvascular level, these large arteries branch to form submucosal arterioles, some of which ascend to form capillary beds surrounding the gastric glands of the mucosa (70–80% of gastric blood flow), whereas others anastomose with venules in the muscle layers of the stomach (20–30% of gastric blood flow) [13]. The mucosal capillaries then anastomose with venules at the surface and drain into submucosal venous plexuses [14]. The microvascular arrangement has important functional ramifications. As discussed later, when acid is secreted from parietal cells in the middle region of the gastric pits, the resulting intracellular bicarbonate is secreted into the surrounding capillaries and is carried to the surface of the stomach, where it can be used to buffer any acid that diffuses back to the mucosa through the protective mucous layer. The resulting "alkaline tide" that occurs after acid secretion is thereby recycled to protect the mucosal surface from the harmful effects of the secreted acid [14].

In addition, the presence of separate mucosal and submucosal arteriolar beds allows for the tight regulation of mucosal blood flow while flow to the muscle layers remains relatively constant. Sympathetic efferent neurons synapse on arterioles and induce varying degrees of vasoconstriction via the release of norepinephrine to regulate blood flow to the gastric mucosa and submucosa. In times of high sympathetic tone, blood flow to the stomach and other gastrointestinal organs is significantly decreased, shunting the energy for secretion and gastric motility to somatic muscles that can affect a fight-or-flight response. In addition to vasoconstriction, active vasodilation of gastric vessels occurs in response to the presence of acid or other damaging factors that penetrate the mucous layer and reach the mucosal surface. In response to stimulation by the secretion of gastric acid, sensory afferents present in the mucosa can release calcitonin gene-related peptide (CGRP) locally to induce vasodilation (via nitric oxide [NO] production) and provide increased blood flow to buffer and remove excess acidity. As discussed later, CGRP may also mediate the release of antral somatostatin, and thus suppression of gastrin, in response to a decrease in intragastric pH [15,16]. Finally, similar to CGRP, prostaglandins can induce vasodilation as an important part of their function in mucosal protection.

Gastric cells

Because of the cellular heterogeneity of the gastrointestinal mucosa, a thorough definition of the cellular aspects of the complex gastric physiology was not feasible until the development of an in vitro; methodology that permitted the direct assessment of the cellular mechanisms involved in regulating gastric acid secretion. These methods include the isolation and dispersion of parietal and other cells and oxyntic glands from the fundic and corpus mucosa using collagenase digestion and elutriation centrifugation to separate isolated cells according to their size or density [17]. Use of these techniques has yielded extensive information on the parietal cells receptors, as well as receptors on other cells in the fundic mucosa. Because parietal cells lose their polar orientation after dispersion, hydrogen ion (H^+ ion) secretion could not be measured directly, but rather indirect measurement was made possible using methods that measure the intracellular accumulation of the weak base aminopyrine into the acidic tubulovesicular structures described later, or by the measurement of oxygen or glucose consumption [17,18]. More recently, studies have been conducted on microdissected gastric glands from both animal and human models [19–31]. In these studies, it has been possible to examine in greater detail both the apical and basolateral transport proteins. This preparation has also allowed for studies to examine the endocrine interactions of the gland, because the receptors remain active in this preparation [21,22,24–26,28–39]. These technologies have yielded new insights into acid secretion and have led to the identification of an additional acid secretory pathway that uses the H^+ adenosine triphosphatase (H^+-ATPase) [25,26,28] (see Chapter 4).

Mucous cells

Mucous neck cells are located immediately below the isthmus, in the neck region of oxyntic glands (see Figure 17.2). A transition zone from mucous neck cells to surface mucous cells appears near the junction of gastric glands and gastric pits; this region, designated the "isthmus," represents the gastric stem cell zone. The mucous neck cells, located just below the isthmus, are progenitors for the zymogenic or chief lineage [40,41]. Mucous neck cells differ in appearance from surface mucous cells. All mucous cells synthesize large amounts of mucin in prominent Golgi stacks, and these glycoproteins are transported by vesicles to large apical mucous granules. Mucous neck cells contain acidic glycoproteins, indicating sulfated forms, and express MUC6 and trefoil factor 2 (TFF2), whereas surface mucous cells contain a neutral mucosubstance and express MUC5AC and TFF1 [42,43]. Mucous granules are larger and often paranuclear in mucous neck cells compared with surface mucous cells. Mucous neck cells possess abundant ribosomes and moderate amounts of rough endoplasmic reticulum. Their function as secretory cells and mucosal progenitor cells is different from the presumed function of surface mucous cells involved in mucosal defense. They migrate upward from the gastric pits and are replaced every 1–3 days [44]. They are thought to protect the stomach from injury by acid, pepsin, ingested materials, and pathogens by secreting mucus and HCO_3 to form a protective gel. The apical portion of the surface mucous cell is packed with secretory granules. Short microvilli extend from the apical membrane and are covered by a glycocalyx. The secretion of granular mucus appears to occur by exocytosis, apical expulsion, and cell exfoliation [45].

Parietal cells

As already noted, the distinguishing feature of the mammalian stomach is its ability to secrete large quantities of concentrated (160 mmol, pH ~0.8) HCl [17]. The normal human stomach contains approximately 1 billion parietal cells, which secrete H^+ ions into the gastric lumen in response to various physiological stimuli. Acid secretion involves an active transport process that requires significant amounts of energy, and parietal cells are notable by abundant mitochondria necessary for the generation of energy required for H^+ ion secretion and by tubulovesicular and canalicular structures [1,46–49]. The latter structures are derived from the smooth endoplasmic reticulum and contain the gastric enzyme H^+,K^+ adenosine triphosphatase (H^+,K^+-ATPase), which exchanges H^+ for K^+ ions across the apical membrane [50–54].

In the nonsecretory state, the parietal cell cytoplasm is filled with the tubulovesicular structures [55]. After stimulation, the tubulovesicles coalesce into expanded canaliculi, which become filled with elongated microvilli. With this dramatic transformation, the membrane area of the canaliculi draining to the apical surface of the parietal cell is greatly expanded, allowing access of H^+,K^+-ATPase to the gastric lumen, thereby preparing the cell for the ensuing high rates of gastric acid secretion [55]. These changes in parietal cell architecture occur within minutes of stimulation and persist throughout the duration of the stimulus. As the stimulation is withdrawn, the canaliculi collapse, the microvilli recede, and cytoplasmic tubulovesicular structures again become prominent as the cell returns to a resting state [17].

In addition to their well-established role in the production of gastric acid, parietal cells exert important biological actions in the regulation of gastric mucosal homeostasis. Parietal cells are the major site for the production of growth factors and morphogens in the gastric epithelium. These growth factors include transforming growth factor-α (TGF-α) [56] and morphogens, such as sonic hedgehog (Shh), a peptide that contributes to the regulation of complex programs of cellular growth and differentiation in the stomach [57,58]. Interestingly, loss of mature parietal cells, achieved by genetic, pharmacological, or immunological methods, appears to be associated with an increase in the number of pit cells and abrogation of the differentiation program of the zymogenic and endocrine lineages, leading to the accumulation of pre-neck cells and the depletion of their mature zymogenic and endocrine cell progenies [59,60]. Thus, Canfield et al. [59] targeted herpes simplex virus 1 thymidine kinase to parietal cells within the gastric mucosa of transgenic mice, and parietal cells were ablated by treatment of animals with ganciclovir. The drug produced the ablation of parietal cells, the dissolution of gastric glands, and the loss of chief and mucous-producing cells. Termination of ganciclovir treatment led to the reemergence of all major gastric epithelial cell types and restoration of glandular architecture, indicating the existence of a multipotent stem cell for the gastric mucosa [59].

To further examine this notion, Li et al. [61] created a transgenic mouse model to specifically define the functional interrelationships among the proliferation, differentiation, and death programs of lineages of gastric cells, including parietal cells, mucous-producing pit cells, and pepsinogen-producing zymogenic cells. Portions of the noncatalytic β-subunit gene of mouse H^+,K^+-ATPase were used to direct expression of an attenuated diphtheria toxin A subunit in the parietal cell lineage. Complete ablation of differentiated parietal cells was detected and accompanied a fivefold increase in the number of undifferentiated granule-free cells located in the proliferative compartment of gastric units. This amplified population of granule-free cells included the multipotent stem cell, as well as committed precursors of the pit and zymogenic lineages. These studies indicate that epithelial homeostasis within the stomach is maintained by interactions among different cell lineages. Unlike pit and zymogenic cells, parietal cells complete their differentiation in the proliferative compartment of the gastric epithelium before undergoing bipolar migration along gastric pits. Finally, the mature parietal cell appears to play an important role in influencing decision-making among gastric epithelial cell precursors and in modulating migration-associated terminal differentiation programs of the pit and zymogenic lineages [61]. These studies [59,61] provide strong evidence that parietal cells, possibly through their ability to produce and secrete TGF-α and Shh, are necessary for the normal differentiation and development of multiple cell lineages throughout the stomach [62,63].

Histamine-producing cells

Histamine is a primary gastric chemical messenger, which binds to H_2-specific basolateral receptors on parietal cells to stimulate the generation of H^+ ions. The primary cell containing mucosal histamine in the dog stomach is the mast cell [64], and histamine-containing mast cells also occur in the human stomach. Mast cells from canine fundic mucosa have been enriched by elutriation centrifugation and shown to contain characteristic dense granules that stain metachromatically [64]. In some species, including the rat and human, histamine is also present in endocrine cells that contain large granules and have the characteristic appearance of enterochromaffin-like (ECL) cells [65]. The relative proportion of these two histamine cell types in humans is unknown. Although in situ morphological studies have not been definitive, ECL cells are likely the principal source of histamine in humans, and it appears that these cells exist in the lamina propria in close proximity to the glandular cells.

Chief cells

The chief cell is a pepsinogen-secreting exocrine cell found in the base or fundus of oxyntic glands [17,66] (see Figure 17.2). Zymogen granules containing proenzymes are located in the apical cytoplasm and release their contents by exocytosis. The apical membrane has a few short microvilli covered by a thin coating of glycoprotein or glycocalyx. An abundant rough endoplasmic reticulum extends upward from the basal cytoplasm toward the apical granules. As H^+ ions are secreted and the intragastric pH decreases to less than 3.5, the conversion of the zymogen pepsinogen to the active proteolytic pepsin enzymes is facilitated [67]. Chief cells are relatively long-lived (~60–90 days) compared with other fundic cell types [40], and recent studies have also shown that a subpopulation of chief cells may also serve as quiescent "reserve" stem cells [68]. This point remains controversial and currently has not been resolved [62,63].

Other endocrine cells

Many different types of endocrine cell are scattered throughout the gastric mucosa. Immunohistochemical techniques have enabled a thorough characterization of these cells based on their secretory granule contents [69,70]. Their secretory products have important endocrine and paracrine effects on acid secretion. Gastric endocrine cells secrete gastrin and somatostatin, as well as ghrelin. Other morphologically distinct gastric endocrine cells may contain additional candidate hormones, but they await further characterization.

Gastric endocrine cells can be classified as open cells that have apical membranes in contact with the glandular lumen, or closed cells, which are located near the epithelial basement membrane and do not border on the lumen of the gland. The prototypical open endocrine cell is the G cell. The basilar portion of the cell is packed with secretory granules [69] from which gastrin is released, consistent with the rapid postprandial appearance of the hormone in the bloodstream. The apical portion of the cell narrows until only a small microvillous border opens on the glandular lumen. The apical membrane may contain luminal receptors that detect amino acids or their amine derivatives, which are thought to stimulate G cells during feeding [71,72]. The model of a closed gastric endocrine cell is the fundic somatostatin cell (D cell), and immunohistochemical staining of these cells reveals long, slender processes that terminate on or near parietal and chief cells [73,74]. These processes presumably help facilitate the paracrine effect of somatostatin.

Gastric acid secretion

From early recorded antiquity, acid has been considered to be present in the human stomach [75]. More than 2300 years ago, Greek scholars commented on epigastric pain, heartburn, and "sour eruptions" as maladies potentially caused by problems with the stomach. Celsus, a second-century Greek philosopher, concluded that some foods were acidic, and he recommended that "if the stomach is infested with an ulcer. . .acid is to be avoided." Scientific evidence that HCl accounted for the acidic milieu within the stomach awaited documentation by William Prout [76] in his elegant presentation before the Royal Society in London in 1823, which was published the following year in a manuscript entitled "On the Nature of the Acid and Saline Matters Usually Existing in the Stomach of Animals" [75,76].

Although it is generally assumed that gastric acid and the proteolytic enzyme pepsin are required to initiate digestion, achlorhydric individuals generally do not experience malabsorption unless small-bowel bacterial overgrowth is present [17]. It is likely that the ability of the stomach to secrete acid evolved primarily from a need to sustain a relatively sterile intragastric milieu. Animals that possessed the capacity to kill ingested pathogenic bacteria and other harmful microbes were able to avoid the development of enteric colonization and thereby ensure both the efficient absorption of nutrients and the prevention of systemic infections [67]. The discovery that *Helicobacter pylori* was adapted to survive in the acidic gastric environment overturned the dogma that the stomach is sterile. In fact, all mammals appear to possess a "normal," albeit restricted, gastric microbiome [77]. In *H. pylori*-negative individuals, gastric microbiota diversity is high, and most of the prominent gastric phylotypes (*Streptococcus*, *Actinomyces*, *Prevotella*, *Gemella*) are also abundant in the oropharynx of these individuals. These observations indicate that either many constituents are swallowed from more proximal sites, including the saliva, or that close relatives of the oral microbiota colonize more distally [77].

When present, gastric acid plays a significant role in protein hydrolysis and other aspects of the digestive process, and under various conditions, acid may play an etiological role in producing various forms of discomfort and inciting esophageal and gastroduodenal mucosal injury. Rates of gastric acid secretion generally reach adult levels during the late teens and are maintained at this rate throughout adulthood. Although a decline in the rates of acid secretion had been noted in the past near age

60 years, this decrease likely occurred as a result of a higher prevalence of chronic atrophic gastritis associated with long-standing *H. pylori* infection. Because the prevalence of infection with *H. pylori* has diminished significantly over the past few decades, atrophic gastritis is less frequently encountered.

Pathways involved in acid secretion

The generation of H^+ ions by gastric parietal cells is mediated by three pathways: neurocrine, paracrine, and endocrine [17] (Figure 17.3). The principal neurocrine transmitter is acetylcholine, which is released by vagal postganglionic neurons and appears to stimulate H^+ ion generation directly via a parietal cell muscarinic M_3 receptor. Histamine is the primary paracrine transmitter that binds to H_2-specific receptors on parietal cells. Adenylate cyclase is then activated, leading to an increase in intracellular cyclic adenosine monophosphate (cAMP) levels and the subsequent generation of H^+ ions [78,79]. The secretion of gastrin from antral G cells comprises the endocrine pathway and stimulates H^+ ion generation both directly and indirectly, the latter by stimulating histamine secretion from ECL cells of the corpus and fundus. Interactions among neurocrine, paracrine, and endocrine pathways are coordinated to promote or inhibit H^+ ion generation. Histamine appears to represent the dominant route because gastrin stimulates acid secretion principally by promoting histamine release from ECL cells [80,81]. Thus, ECL cells are often referred to as "controller" cells in the process of gastric acid secretion [67].

Parietal cell transport of hydronium ions

H^+ or hydronium (H_3O^+) ions are generated within the parietal cell from water (Figure 17.4) and are transported out of parietal cells into the gastric lumen against a substantial ionic gradient [67]. Carbonic anhydrase catalyzes the reaction that combines OH^- ions with cytoplasmic CO_2 to create bicarbonate (HCO_3^-) ions [82]. HCO_3^- ions are exchanged for Cl^- ions at the parietal cell basolateral membrane, and Cl^- ions are then transported into the secretory canaliculus along with K^+ ions via conductance pathways closely associated with H^+,K^+-ATPase and are thereby secreted. H_3O^+ ions are simultaneously exchanged at the parietal cell apical membrane for K^+ ions via an electroneutral process that is catalyzed by H^+,K^+-ATPase (see Figure 17.4) [83]. Whereas K^+ ions are primarily recycled, H_3O^+ ions are secreted at a concentration of 160 mmol (pH ~0.8). For each H_3O^+ ion secreted into the gastric lumen, a HCO_3^- ion is released from the basal side of the epithelium into the circulation, a process that has been named the "alkaline tide." The alkaline tide appears to play a pivotal role in the regulation of acid–base balance [84].

Central nervous involvement in gastric acid secretion

The important role of the nervous system in regulating gastric acid secretion has long been recognized, with prior studies demonstrating that the vagus was the sole responsible gastroacephalic neural link [85,86]. The components of the central nervous system (CNS) involved in modulating gastric secretion include the dorsal motor nucleus of the vagus, the nucleus tractus solitarius,

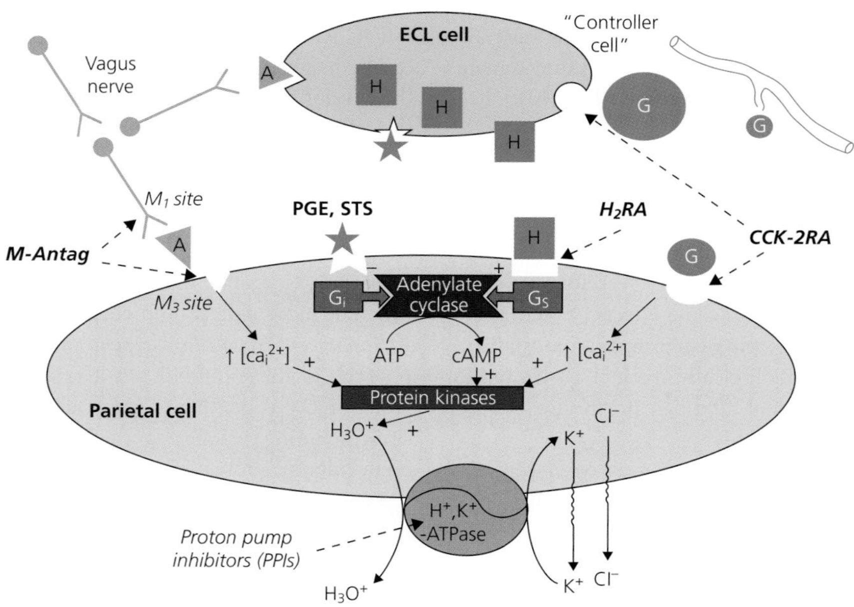

Figure 17.3 Schematic representation of the parietal cell, depicting the various pathways (solid arrows) involved in the generation and secretion of gastric acid. Also shown (dashed arrows) are the sites of action of inhibitors of acid secretion and (italicized) antisecretory agents. A, acetylcholine; ATP, adenosine triphosphate; cAMP, cyclic adenosine monophosphate; *CCK-2RA*, cholecystokinin-2 (or gastrin) receptor antagonists; ECL, enterochromaffin-like; G, gastrin; G_i and G_s, inhibitory and stimulatory catalytic subunits, respectively; H, histamine; *H_2RA*, histamine 2-receptor antagonists; *M-antag*, antimuscarinics; PGE, E series prostaglandins; STS, somatostatin.

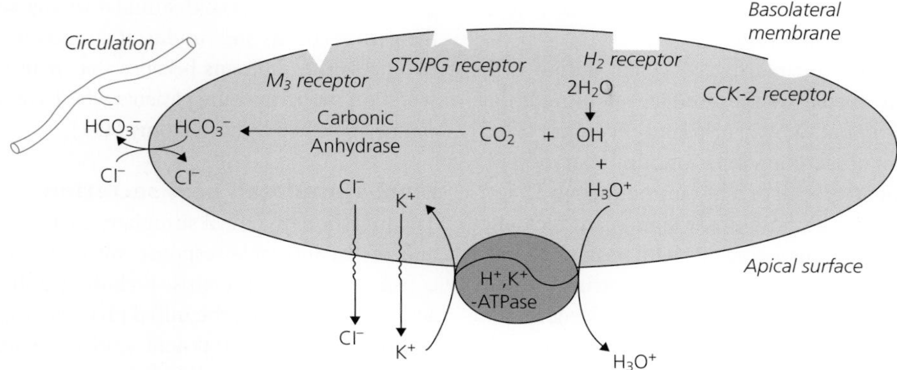

Figure 17.4 Schematic representation of the various chemical pathways involved in the generation and secretion of gastric acid. H^+,K^+-ATPase promotes the active transport of hydronium (H_3O^+) or H^+ ions in exchange for K^+ ions against a 3 000 000 : 1 ionic gradient at the apical surface of the parietal cell. A conductance pathway for K^+ and Cl^- is closely associated with H^+,K^+-ATPase. Cl^- ions are largely secreted with H_3O^+ ions, whereas K^+ ions are mostly recycled. Cl^- ions are exchanged for HCO_3 ions at the basolateral membrane, which is generated from the conversion of CO_2 and OH^- via a carbonic anhydrase pathway. HCO_3 ions are secreted into the surrounding capillaries, creating the so-called alkaline tide. CCK-2RA, cholecystokinin-2 (or gastrin); H_2, histamine subtype 2; M_3, muscarinic subtype 3; PG, prostaglandin; STS, somatostatin.

and the hypothalamus. The dorsal motor nucleus supplies stimulatory efferent fibers to the stomach through the vagus nerve [87,88]. Stimulation of the dorsal motor nucleus thereby increases gastric secretion [6,89], whereas ablation of this nucleus abolishes the secretory process [90]. The dorsal motor nucleus does not appear to initiate secretion [91], but rather integrates CNS input from the hypothalamus and visceral input from the nucleus tractus solitarius. Regions of the hypothalamus that are important for regulating gastric secretion include the ventromedial hypothalamus, which appears to provide tonic inhibition [92,93], the lateral hypothalamus, and the adjacent medial forebrain bundle; these mediate secretion in response to hypoglycemia [94]. Visceral afferents and taste fibers provide input into the nucleus tractus solitarius, demonstrating its potential involvement in stimulating gastric secretion in response to taste.

Vagal stimulation of the parietal cell appears to involve several mechanisms [17]. In addition to direct stimulation of H^+ ion generation and secretion via an M_3-muscarinic receptor, vagal stimulation also enhances the release of antral gastrin in part by the inhibition of antral somatostatin expression. The increase in circulating gastrin, in turn, contributes to stimulation of the parietal cell. Somatostatin appears to exert a continuous restraint on the antral G cell [95], an effect that occurs at both the pretranslational and the posttranslational levels [96,97]. Because vagal stimulation inhibits somatostatin, this restraint is diminished, and the expression of gastrin is enhanced. The vagal stimulation of gastrin release may also involve gastrin-releasing peptide (GRP), the mammalian homolog of bombesin, and it has been suggested that this mechanism may use noncholinergic pathways [98]. Finally, the vagal stimulation of corpus and fundic gastric mucosa lowers the threshold for gastrin stimulation [17].

Measurement of gastric acid secretion

Although no longer performed routinely, measurement of gastric acid output can provide useful information. It must be stressed that the mere determination of intragastric luminal pH, which reflects only the concentration of secreted acid, generally provides insufficient information. Because H^+ ions are secreted at a concentration of 160 mmol (pH ~0.8), intragastric pH will be nearly identical in diverse conditions, including in normal individuals, as well as in patients with duodenal ulcer caused by *H. pylori* infection and those with ulcers associated with gastrin-secreting tumors (Zollinger–Ellison syndrome).

Gastric acid output is most reliably measured by placing a tube (most commonly nasogastric) into the stomach and positioning the distal tip containing the aspiration ports in the most dependent portion of the stomach. With the person in the supine position, successful localization of the radiopaque tube in the distal stomach is generally achieved as the tube tip approaches the vertebral bodies confirmed by fluoroscopy. Initial gastric contents that are aspirated should be discarded before beginning measurements of acid output. Optimal aspiration can be achieved by placing the subject in an infusion chair, with the patient reclining to approximately 45°. Despite careful placement of the tube and positioning the subject optimally, gastric acid output can be underestimated because of three factors: back-diffusion of H^+ ions across the gastric mucosa, neutralization of H^+ ions by duodenal HCO_3^- ions, and emptying of gastric contents into the duodenum. Nevertheless, the measurement of gastric acid output using this fundamental aspiration method has proved reliable over the years.

After gastric contents are aspirated, the H^+ ion concentration can be determined by first measuring the volume over a period of time and then titrating aliquots with NaOH. A reference pH, usually 7.0, is used, and the number of millimoles (mmol) of NaOH needed to titrate to the reference pH will be equal to the acidity present in the sample. After factoring the volume, acid output is calculated and then generally expressed as either mEq or mmol per hour. Acid secretion is usually measured either under basal conditions or after stimulation by collecting acid for four to six 15-minute periods and then measuring the amount of acid generated in each aliquot [99].

Basal acid output (BAO) or interdigestive acid output is the secretion of acid that occurs in the absence of intraluminal stimuli. Maximal acid output (MAO) or peak acid output (PAO) refers to the assessment of secretion after the administration of a secretagogue such as pentagastrin or a histamine analog. The latter is rarely used at present because of the significant incidence and severity of adverse reactions associated with its use. After the determination of BAO, subjects are administered pentagastrin by subcutaneous injection at a dose of 6 μg/kg bodyweight, after which gastric contents are once again aspirated for four to six 15-minute periods. The MAO represents the sum of four collections, whereas the PAO is the sum of the two greatest consecutive 15-minute collections, which are then multiplied by 2 and expressed as mEq or mmol of H^+ secreted per hour.

The measurement of meal-stimulated acid secretion involves a far more cumbersome method that is generally reserved for the research setting [99,100]. A high-protein meal (e.g., steak and milkshake) is pureed and infused through a nasogastric tube. Gastric contents are then aspirated periodically, typically every 30 seconds to every 2–3 minutes, across a pH electrode. A reference pH, usually 4.0, is selected, and $NaHCO_3$ is infused into the stomach to keep the pH constant at the preselected value. After the meal has emptied, the total volume of $NaHCO_3$ needed to titrate the intragastric meal is measured and then regarded as the amount of acid secreted in response to the infused meal. Similar to BAO, MAO, and PAO, meal-stimulated acid output is expressed as mEq or mmol of H^+ secreted per hour.

Basal acid secretion

BAO varies widely among animal species; dogs have low BAO that is generally <1% of stimulated rates of acid secretion [101]. In contrast, in the rat and human, BAO is approximately 30% and 10%, respectively, of maximal capacity [102,103]. In addition to interspecies variations, BAO not only varies significantly among individuals but is also variable during different times of the day. The upper limit of normal BAO is less than 10 mmol/h, and BAO is generally higher in men than women, likely reflecting a larger parietal cell mass in men. BAO in humans has a circadian rhythm characterized by high rates of acid secretion in the evening, with low rates in the morning [104]. The etiology of this circadian rhythm is unknown, but the rhythmic cycle does not appear to be related to circulating gastrin concentrations [104]. Because it is abolished by atropine or vagotomy, it is likely that neurocrine pathways play a dominant role during the interdigestive phase of acid secretion [17]. BAO can be affected by external factors such as smoking and the emotional state of an individual [105–109].

Cholinergic innervation appears to play a major role in BAO because denervation of the antral pouch in dogs markedly reduces BAO from the main innervated stomach and from the denervated fundic pouch without changing plasma gastrin levels [110]. This observation suggests the presence of a local interneuronal reflex arc innervated by the vagus, which is independent of circulating gastrin and transmits acid-stimulatory signals from the antrum to the gastric corpus and fundus. It appears that these pathways are also present in humans because the small amount of basal acid secretion found in some patients who have undergone vagotomy can be abolished by antrectomy [111].

Meal-stimulated acid secretion

The ingestion of a meal stimulates gastric acid secretion rapidly, and the quantitative response varies according to the nutrient consumed [112]. Proteins, including polypeptides and amino acids derived during the initial phases of digestion, are generally considered the most potent nutrient stimuli for acid secretion [113]. In contrast with proteins, carbohydrates and lipids appear to inhibit acid secretion, which may occur as a result of the stimulation and release of intestinal regulatory peptides, such as cholecystokinin (CCK), secretin, and gastric inhibitory polypeptide (GIP), into the circulation [114]. These peptides may function as "enterogastrones," which are intestinal hormones that were postulated to function in a negative feedback capacity to inhibit acid secretion following a meal [99,114,115]. Other food substances have been shown to stimulate gastric acid secretion. Both caffeinated and, to a lesser extent, decaffeinated coffee stimulate acid secretion, whereas tea and other caffeinated beverages stimulate acid output to a lesser degree [116]. Some alcoholic beverages, such as wine and beer, stimulate acid secretion, and milk, by virtue of its alkaline pH and protein and calcium content, is a very potent stimulus for the secretion of acid [117].

Cephalic phase of acid secretion

Gastric acid secretion in response to food ingestion consists of three phases – cephalic, gastric, and intestinal – which often occur simultaneously (Figure 17.5) [17]. The cephalic phase is initiated by the release of acetylcholine from the postganglionic neurons of the vagus nerve upon the sight, smell, taste, and most importantly, thoughts of food. This phase accounts for approximately 30–40% of the total acid output in response to a meal and also accounts for basal and nocturnal acid secretion [17]. The existence of the cephalic phase of acid secretion was initially emphasized by Pavlov in the early 1900s, when he demonstrated that the anticipation of feeding, as well as visualization or smell of food, were powerful stimulants for acid secretion [118]. Despite differences observed in studies involving various species, considerable experimental and clinical evidence supports the importance of the CNS and the hypothalamus, in particular, during the cephalic phase of gastric acid secretion [119–121]. In addition to the lateral hypothalamus, electrical stimulation of the amygdala increases acid output [119,122].

Animal studies indicate that the stimulation of acid secretion during the cephalic phase is unrelated to changes in circulating gastrin [104]. Nevertheless, the mechanisms by which the initiators of the cephalic phase activate the vagal centers have not been clearly elucidated. It is widely recognized that vagotomy abolishes the response to cephalic phase stimuli [111]. In contrast, the muscarinic antagonist atropine markedly attenuates, but does not abolish, sham feeding in humans, which may

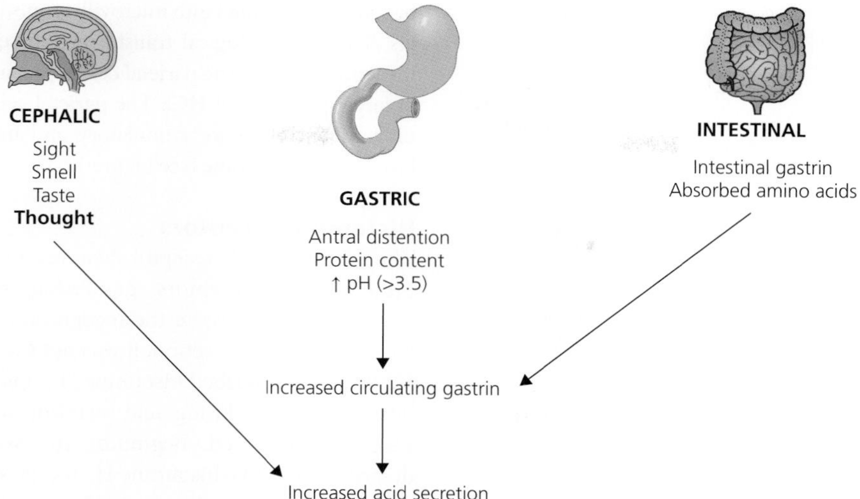

Figure 17.5 The three phases of gastric acid secretion in response to food ingestion. These phases – cephalic, gastric, and intestinal – generally occur simultaneously. More than 90% of the gastric phase occurs as a result of increases in circulating gastrin.

indicate that mediators other than acetylcholine are involved in the cephalic phase of gastric acid secretion [123]. Studies by Goto et al. [124,125] have suggested that GABAergic (γ-aminobutyric acid) neural pathways are involved in vagal efferent stimulation. Other neuropeptides, such as enkephalins, thyrotropin-releasing hormone, corticotropin-releasing factor, GRP, neurotensin, interleukin-1 (IL-1), and CGRP may also affect acid secretion via vagal stimulation [9,126–132].

Gastric phase of acid secretion

Gastric acid secretion in response to a meal increases rapidly, although the intragastric pH actually increases initially because of the buffered capacity of most meals. With time the quantity of acid secreted by parietal cells overwhelms the buffering capacity of the meal, and the intragastric pH begins to decrease. The gastric phase accounts for approximately 50–60% of meal-stimulated acid secretion, with antral distention stimulating the initial release of the polypeptide hormone gastrin [133,134]. As small amounts of food or liquid enter the stomach, the secretion of acid is increased. Studies in dogs have shown that as little as 50 mL of 0.9% NaCl stimulated acid secretion [113]. However, physiological stimulation by gastric distention postprandially is transient and involves not only gastrin release, but also vagovagal and intragastric reflexes, such as those involving GRP.

Eysselein et al. [135] demonstrated that approximately 92% of the gastric phase of acid secretion in humans could be attributed to increases in circulating gastrin. The principal stimuli for the release of gastrin during the gastric phase are the pH and protein content of the ingested meal [17]. Proteins are generally considered the most potent nutrient stimuli for acid secretion. Amino acids derived from dietary proteins undergo luminal decarboxylation to amines, which directly stimulate G cells to release gastrin into the circulation, enhancing acid secretion [69,136,137]. The aromatic amino acids phenylalanine and tryptophan are the most potent stimuli of gastrin release and gastric acid secretion in vivo; [137]. Amino acids also appear to stimulate acid secretion after systemic absorption.

Intestinal phase of acid secretion

The intestinal phase accounts for <10% of meal-stimulated acid secretion and consists primarily of digested peptides that enter into the circulation and, to a lesser extent, gastrin released from the small-intestinal mucosa. In general, agents that effectively stimulate acid secretion during the gastric phase are also stimulatory during the intestinal phase. In addition, a hypothetical regulatory peptide, which has been designated "enterooxyntin" [138,139] and appears to be distinct from gastrin, has been isolated from the small-intestinal mucosa and may possess acid-stimulatory properties.

Feedback inhibition of acid secretion

A negative feedback loop governs both gastrin release and the return of acid secretion to basal levels (Figure 17.6) [17,93,140,141]. This autoregulatory mechanism prevents postprandial acid hypersecretion. After the ingestion of a meal, gastrin release stimulates the secretion of gastric acid. Initially, the buffering capacity of ingested meals maintains the intragastric pH at >4.0. With time, however, the intraluminal pH begins to decrease, and when it reaches <3.5–3.0, somatostatin release from antral D cells is stimulated, possibly through the activation of CGRP neurons [15,17,67]. Somatostatin then appears to act via a paracrine mechanism to inhibit the further release of gastrin from G cells [73,95]. In addition to its effects on gastrin secretion from antral G cells, studies in dogs have shown that somatostatin inhibits gastrin expression at the pretranslational level [96]. Despite inhibiting gastrin gene transcription, its predominant effect

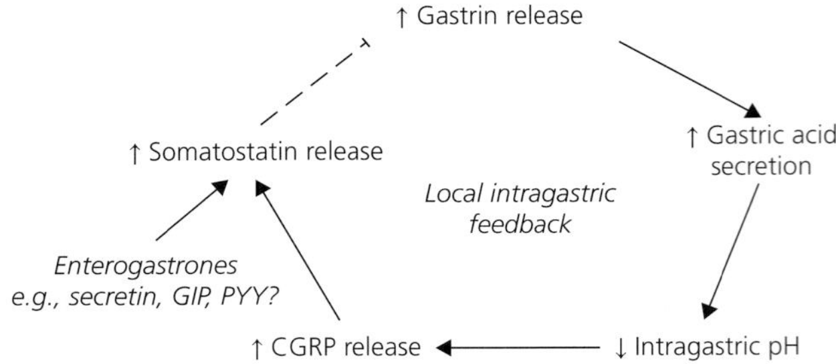

Figure 17.6 Negative feedback inhibition of gastrin release and gastric acid secretion involving both local intragastric inhibitory pathways and intestinal hormones (enterogastrones). The former appears to occur primarily as a result somatostatin inhibition of the gastrin cell. Somatostatin may also directly inhibit the enterochromaffin-like (ECL) and parietal cells (not shown). CGRP, calcitonin gene-related peptide; GIP, gastric inhibitory polypeptide; PYY, peptide YY.

on gene expression appears to occur at the posttranscriptional level by increasing the turnover of gastrin mRNA [97].

Somatostatin produced by D cells in the gastric corpus and fundus may also directly inhibit acid secretion from parietal cells and suppress histamine release from ECL cells (see Figure 17.3) [141,142]. Other observations indicate that several other neurotransmitters, including vasoactive intestinal peptide, galanin, and pituitary adenylate cyclase activating polypeptide, may play important roles in regulating gastric acid secretion, both directly and indirectly, under physiological conditions [67].

In addition to the local feedback inhibition of gastric acid secretion, it has long been recognized that various regulatory peptides emanating from the small-intestinal mucosa play a pivotal role in inhibiting postprandial acid secretion. As already noted, peptides such as CCK, secretin, GIP, peptide YY, and others have been designated as "enterogastrones," and some of these peptides function physiologically in such a negative feedback capacity [114]. Secretin and GIP function in this capacity by stimulating the release of antral somatostatin, which, in turn, inhibits gastrin release into the circulation [114,143]. These enterogastrones thereby appear to indirectly inhibit acid secretion. Whether these peptides function independently or act synergistically remains to be determined.

Pharmacology of parietal cell receptors

The parietal cell possesses a unique morphology that differs markedly between the resting and stimulated states [17,67]. Mitochondria occupy 34% of its cell volume, indicative of the importance of ATP synthesis as an energy source required for the active transport of H_3O^+ ions out of the cell against a 3 000 000 : 1 ionic gradient [67]. A large percentage of resting cell volume is also occupied by tubulovesicles, which are elongated tubes with smooth surface membranes, and by the secretory canaliculus, a small invaginated area of the apical membrane. On stimulation, which generally occurs in response to meal ingestion, the tubulovesicles decrease in number and become transformed into microvilli around the secretory canaliculus. This morphological transformation serves to greatly expand the surface area of the parietal cell in preparation for the secretion of large quantities of HCl. The parietal cell also possesses several different receptors for stimulatory and inhibitory ligands on its basolateral membrane (see Figure 17.3).

Histamine receptors

The histamine H_2-receptor belongs to a large family of G protein-linked receptors possessing seven transmembrane domains [144]. Despite the recognition that histamine stimulates gastric acid secretion, it was not until 1966, when Ash and Schild [145] described histamine H_1- and H_2-receptors, that the possibility of inhibiting acid secretion with histamine antagonists was proposed. Beginning in 1968, Black et al. [146] described selective histamine H_2-receptor inhibition, leading to the release of cimetidine in 1977, and within the next 10 years three additional H_2-receptor antagonists: ranitidine, famotidine, and nizatidine. All four drugs suppress basal and meal-stimulated acid secretion, albeit to a lesser degree than proton pump inhibitors (PPIs).

In 1991, Gantz et al. [144] successfully cloned the gene encoding the histamine H_2-receptor, which enabled the identification of the structural components of the receptor that conferred H_2 selectivity, including key areas of homology in the structures of the histamine H_2-receptor and β_2-adrenergic receptor, which suggested specific transmembrane amino acids that could be important for histamine binding. Using site-directed mutations, Gantz et al. [147] determined that an aspartic acid residue (Asp98) in the third transmembrane domain is essential for histamine binding and action, while an aspartic acid (Asp186) in the fifth transmembrane domain defines H_2 selectivity. A third amino acid residue, threonine (Thr190), located in the fifth transmembrane domain, appears to be important in establishing the kinetics of histamine binding but was not deemed essential for H_2 selectivity.

Although H_3-receptors are expressed on ECL cells, where they play a role in the autocrine regulation of histamine release, their presence on parietal cells is less well established. The H_3-receptor agonist methylhistamine is a potent stimulant of aminopyrine uptake in isolated cultured rabbit parietal cells [148]. However, this stimulatory effect can be abrogated by the H_2-receptor antagonist ranitidine, which leaves uncertainty about the selectivity of methylhistamine, as well as the physiological significance of the H_3-receptor in the regulation of H^+ ion secretion from parietal cells.

Muscarinic receptor and its antagonists

As discussed earlier, the CNS, particularly via the vagus nerve, plays a dominant role in regulating basal acid secretion, as well as the cephalic phase of meal-stimulated acid secretion [67]. Cell bodies located primarily within the Meissner plexus in the submucosa are innervated by preganglionic vagal fibers, as well as by other enteric neurons that participate in local intragastric reflexes. Acetylcholine is the principal neurotransmitter released from both short postsynaptic cholinergic neurons and postganglionic nerves emanating from the above submucosal cell bodies. Extracts of belladonna have been used to treat dyspepsia since the time of the Roman Empire, and in the recent past, nonspecific antimuscarinic agents, such as atropine and propantheline bromide, were used as inhibitors of gastric acid secretion [67]. These drugs were associated with many adverse effects, including drowsiness, dry mouth, blurry vision, and urinary retention, and as a result are rarely used today.

Five muscarinic receptors have been subtyped and cloned, and although all are G protein coupled, they signal different intracellular pathways. In vitro characterization of gastric acid secretion indicates that parietal cells normally expresses the M_3 subtype [149]. Clinically, the M_1 antagonists pirenzepine and telenzepine are effective inhibitors of acid secretion and probably exert their effect by interaction with a postsynaptic neuronal M_1 receptor [17]. Although these two agents are available in other countries for the treatment of duodenal ulcer, they have not been approved for use in the United States.

Gastrin receptor and its antagonists

As stated earlier, gastrin stimulates acid secretion via an endocrine pathway and induces H^+ ion generation both directly and indirectly. The precise location and density of the gastrin receptor has been the subject of debate and may be somewhat species dependent. Several studies in rats and other rodents have suggested that gastrin stimulates acid secretion by enhancing the release of histamine from ECL cells [150,151]. Conversely, receptors for gastrin receptors have been demonstrated on canine parietal cells [152,153]. Single-cell video imaging has provided direct evidence for a functional gastrin receptor on the parietal cells of rats and rabbits [154].

The gastrin receptor belongs to the seven-transmembrane G protein-linked receptor family [153]. It is closely related to the receptor for CCK (CCK-A or CCK-1) and is often referred to as the CCK-B or CCK-2 receptor. Gastrin-specific receptor antagonists have been developed, which include L365,260, YM022, and YF476 (netazepide) [155–159]. The former is a benzodiazepine derivative obtained from the fungus *Aspergillus alliaceus* and has been demonstrated to effectively antagonize gastrin-stimulated gastric acid secretion. Netazepide is currently in clinical trials and has shown beneficial effects in antagonizing the trophic properties of gastrin in patients with gastric neuroendocrine tumors [159]. Despite their potential benefit, these antagonists have not been used clinically as pure inhibitors of acid secretion. In addition to their benefit in neuroendocrine tumors, they may ultimately prove useful in the treatment of panic and anxiety disorders by virtue of binding to gastrin receptors in the brain [160].

Miscellaneous receptors on the parietal cell

Other receptors on the parietal cell basolateral membrane have been suggested by the ability of various agents to inhibit gastric acid secretion (see Figure 17.3). Both somatostatin and prostaglandins inhibit H^+ ion generation by binding to their respective G protein-linked receptors on the parietal cell, leading to inhibition of adenylate cyclase and a decrease in intracellular cAMP generation [161].

Five subtypes of somatostatin receptors have been cloned and characterized, each possessing distinct pharmacological properties and tissue distribution [162]. The five somatostatin receptor subtypes are expressed in all layers of the gastric mucosa [162]. Development of highly specific and selective agonists [163] has led to more precise functional characterization of these different somatostatin receptors. Although all five somatostatin receptors are expressed in the stomach, somatostatin receptor subtype 2 ($SSTR_2$) appears to be the receptor subtype most involved in regulating the gastric secretory process. It directly mediates the inhibition of gastric acid secretion in human parietal cells, as well as in rats and dogs [163–165]. Prinz et al. [166] reported that $SSTR_2$ is the predominant receptor subtype mediating inhibition of histamine release from rat ECL cells.

Specific binding sites for prostaglandin E_2 (PGE_2) have been identified in the subcellular membrane fractions of porcine fundic mucosa, suggesting localization to the plasma membrane [167–169]. Prostaglandins can displace bound $[^3H]PGE_2$ and inhibit histamine-stimulated aminopyrine uptake in isolated rabbit parietal cells [168], providing conclusive evidence for the presence of prostaglandin receptors on parietal cells. Although PGE_2 and prostaglandin I_2 (PGI_2) have no effect on parietal cell aminopyrine uptake induced by gastrin, carbachol, or dibutyryl cAMP, both prostaglandins inhibit histamine-stimulated aminopyrine accumulation and cAMP generation in enriched canine parietal cells [170]. Ding et al. [169] documented expression of the prostaglandin receptor subtypes EP3 and EP4 genes on rat gastric parietal cells.

Previous studies [128,171] have suggested that parietal cells express receptors for cytokines, such as tumor necrosis factor-α and IL-1β. In isolated rabbit and canine gastric parietal cells, these two cytokines were shown to inhibit the accumulation of the aminopyrine in the basal state and after stimulation with histamine, gastrin, and carbachol [128,171]. More recently, Howlett et al. [172] reported that IL-11 expression, which occurs in both mice and human fundic mucosa, is enhanced in parietal cells after *H. pylori* infection. They reported that this cytokine inhibits gastric acid secretion, likely by reducing the expression of the CCK-2 and histamine H_2-receptors [172]. In contrast, Yakabi et al. [173] reported that IL-8 enhanced gastrin-stimulated gastric acid secretion in rats. Thus, cytokines appear to have complex regulatory effects on gastric acid secretion, which may be mediated, at least in part, by a direct action of these agents on gastric parietal cells.

A calcium-sensing receptor has been identified on rat and human parietal cells, as well as antral G cells. The activation of this receptor by Ca^{2+} and l-amino acids appears to increase intracellular Ca^{2+} concentrations and stimulate H^+,K^+-ATPase activity and gastrin release [19,32,174]. Parietal cells also express the receptor for epidermal growth factor (EGF), which binds both EGF and TGF-α [61,175]. TGF-α is secreted by parietal cells and may thus function as an autocrine regulatory factor. Both growth factors inhibit parietal cell function in a similar fashion [176–180]. The presence of secretin, glucagon, or opioid receptors on parietal cells remains to be established.

Signaling pathways involved in gastric acid secretion

Calcium-, cAMP-, and protein kinase C-mediated stimulation of gastric acid secretion

Regardless of the initiating stimulus, after binding of an agonist to a specific receptor, a series of intracellular events are initiated that ultimately lead to H^+ ion generation. As shown in Figure 17.3, histamine, but not acetylcholine or gastrin, stimulates parietal cells by increasing the generation of cAMP, which activates specific cAMP-dependent kinases [17]. In contrast with histamine, cholinergic agonists and gastrin stimulate parietal cells through specific receptors by increasing cytosolic calcium [181]. Parietal cell stimulation by these two stimuli is abrogated by the removal of extracellular calcium with a chelating agent or by the addition of lanthanum, a trivalent cation that antagonizes calcium fluxes across the plasma membrane [17]. Some controversy remains concerning the precise source of calcium, although it is likely that it is derived from extracellular sources, as well as from the mobilization of intracellular stores [32,182–184].

Histamine stimulates a subunit of adenylate cyclase, which catalyzes the generation of cAMP from adenosine triphosphate [17] (see Figure 17.3). This catalytic subunit is linked to the receptor by G_s, a protein that binds guanosine triphosphate (GTP). G_s is the target of histamine, which induces the transfer of an adenosine diphosphate-ribose moiety to G_s, locking it into the "on" position. A mirror image of the stimulatory limb of adenylate cyclase mediates the inhibitory effects on cell function by several agents, including somatostatin and prostaglandins. This inhibitory limb contains a second GTP-binding protein, G_i, which inhibits the catalytic subunit of adenylate cyclase.

Although activation of cAMP-dependent kinases by histamine and calcium-dependent signaling pathways by cholinergic agonists is a generally recognized mechanism for increasing parietal cell HCl secretion, the role of protein kinase C (PKC) in this process is less clear. Most studies have found that direct activation of parietal cells by PKC using phorbol esters enhances gastric acid secretion [185], and that inhibition of PKC, using specific inhibitors, inhibits carbachol-stimulated [^{14}C]aminopyrine accumulation [186]. However, Chiba et al. [185] reported that the pretreatment of canine parietal cells with the phorbol ester 12-*O*-tetradecanoylphorbol-13-acetate and the synthetic diacylglycerol 1-oleoyl-2-acetyl-*sn*-glycerol inhibited both [^{14}C] aminopyrine uptake and membrane inositol phospholipid turnover in parietal cells induced by carbachol and gastrin. Moreover, Chew et al. [187] demonstrated that the PKC inhibitor Ro 31-8220 potentiated [^{14}C]aminopyrine uptake from isolated rabbit gastric glands stimulated by both carbachol and histamine. These disparate observations are likely a result of the heterogeneity among PKC isoforms, which comprise a large family of proteins with different biochemical and functional properties [188], as well as species-specific differences in both the function and the cellular localization of PKC isoforms [187]. In addition, protein kinase D is also induced by phorbol esters [189,190]. Although the presence of protein kinase D or other related protein kinases in gastric cells has not been determined, it is possible that protein kinases other than PKC mediate the effects of phorbol esters on gastric acid secretion.

Shh signal transduction pathway

Shh is a morphogen expressed in gastric glands. It appears to play an important role in the regulation of gastric epithelial cell maturation and in differentiation in the mammalian stomach [57,191–194]. Exposure to either gastrin or histamine leads to Shh gene expression [33], and this Shh gene expression has also been linked to stimulated H,K-ATPase gene expression [19]. The gastric epithelium of Shh-deficient mice exhibits intestinal transformation [195,196], and the mucosa of patients with gastric atrophy and intestinal metaplasia is characterized by the loss of Shh expression [192]. Inhibition of Shh signaling in the gastric mucosa leads to enhanced cellular proliferation [57]. The functional significance of the Shh signal transduction pathway in the stomach was initially characterized in isolated canine parietal cells [57]. These studies demonstrated that these cells express Shh and its receptor "patched" (Ptc). Incubation of the cells with EGF induces both the release and the expression of Shh.

H^+ ion secretion is required for the expression and processing of Shh [197] (Figure 17.7). Autocrine or paracrine signaling by Shh is required for full functional differentiation of the parietal cell, as well as gastric acid secretion [58]. The loss of Shh results in loss of acidity, diminished expression of somatostatin, and a resulting increase in serum gastrin levels. IL-1β has known inhibitory effects on acid secretion and stimulatory effects on gastrin secretion. However, it has also been shown to downregulate Shh, which may contribute to the loss of the parietal cells' capacity to secrete gastric acid [197]. The use of PPIs decreases Shh expression, which may explain why these agents enhance the development of gastric atrophy in patients infected with *H. pylori* [58]. Schumacher et al. [198] found that Shh secreted from gastric parietal cells after *H. pylori* infection led to recruitment of SLFN4$^+$GLI$^+$myelinoid cells [20].

Parietal cell H^+,K^+-ATPase

Various ATPase molecules regulate the transport of cations across biological membranes. Ion-motive ATPases can be classified into single or double subunit and multisubunit types, with P ATPases representing the former and F_1F_0 and V ATPases the

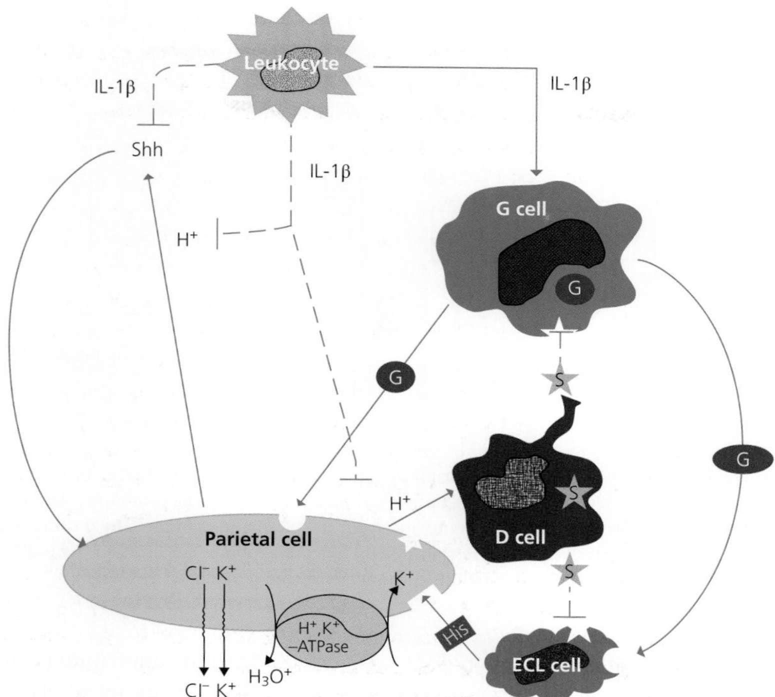

Figure 17.7 Sonic hedgehog (Shh) involvement and cytokine regulation of gastrin release and gastric acid secretion. H^+ secretion is required for expression and processing of Shh, a morphogen shown to be expressed in gastric glands. Autocrine or paracrine signaling by Shh is, in turn, required for full functional differentiation and acid secretion by the parietal cell. The loss of Shh results in loss of acidity, diminished production of somatostatin, and a resulting increase in serum gastrin levels. The cytokine interleukin-1β (IL-1β) released from inflammatory cells has demonstrable negative effects on acid secretion and positive effects on gastrin secretion. The former appears to be mediated through the downregulation of Shh, which may also contribute to the loss of the parietal cells' capacity to secrete gastric acid. The use of proton pump inhibitors (PPIs) also decreases Shh expression, which may explain why these agents may enhance the development of gastric atrophy in patients infected with *H. pylori*. Solid arrows indicate stimulatory pathways; dashed lines represent inhibitory effects. ATPase, adenosine triphosphatase; D cell, somatostatin cell; ECL, enterochromaffin-like; G, gastrin; His, histamine; S, somatostatin.

latter [67,199,200]. All ATPases possess cytoplasmic domains that bind ATP and transduce energy from the hydrolysis of ATP into conformational changes that enable binding of the ion from the cytoplasmic membrane and release of the ion from the extracytoplasmic portion of the membrane. In general, F_1F_0 ATPases are found in mitochondria and bacteria, while V-type ATPases are found in the brain and kidney [67,200].

H^+,K^+-ATPase is a member of the family of ion-motive P ATPases, which is further divided conveniently into P_1 or P_2 types, either based on the number of transmembrane segments (8 in the case of the P_1 and 10 in the case of the P_2 catalytic subunits) or based on transport of transition metals (P_1) or small cations (P_2) [67,201]. Within the P_2 family, the gastric H^+,K^+ and Na^+,K^+-ATPase isoforms are coexpressed tightly bound to a β subunit that is smaller than the catalytic or α subunit, has most of its sequence presented outside, and is glycosylated to different extents depending on the isoform [202,203]. These latter two enzymes are unique as a class in that they both serve as drug targets, digoxin for congestive heart failure in the case of the Na^+,K^+-ATPase and substituted pyridylmethylsulfinyl benzimidazoles (PPIs) for acid-related disorders in the case of the H^+,K^+-ATPase [65]. H^+,K^+-ATPase is a heterodimeric member of the eukaryotic alkali-cation P-type ion-motive ATPase family that consists of eight transmembrane segments for the catalytic α subunit and one transmembrane segment for the β subunit (Figure 17.8) [204,205]. The α subunit is composed of 1033 amino acids and the β subunit of 291 amino acids, with six or seven potential N-linked glycosylation sites [206]. The heavily glycosylated β subunit protects the enzyme from degradation and is necessary for trafficking to and from the plasma membrane [207]. The α subunit carries out the catalytic and transport functions of the enzyme, and it also contains sequences responsible for apical membrane localization [208]. Finally, the α subunit of H^+,K^+-ATPase constitutes the target of PPIs.

The H^+,K^+-ATPase enzyme of the gastric parietal cell is generally regarded as the most critical component of the ion transport system mediating acid secretion. Although mice lacking the H^+,K^+-ATPase α subunit appear healthy and exhibit normal systemic electrolyte and acid–base status, they are, as would be expected, achlorhydric and hypergastrinemic [209]. Immunocytochemical, histological, and ultrastructural analyses of these α-subunit-deficient stomachs demonstrate the presence

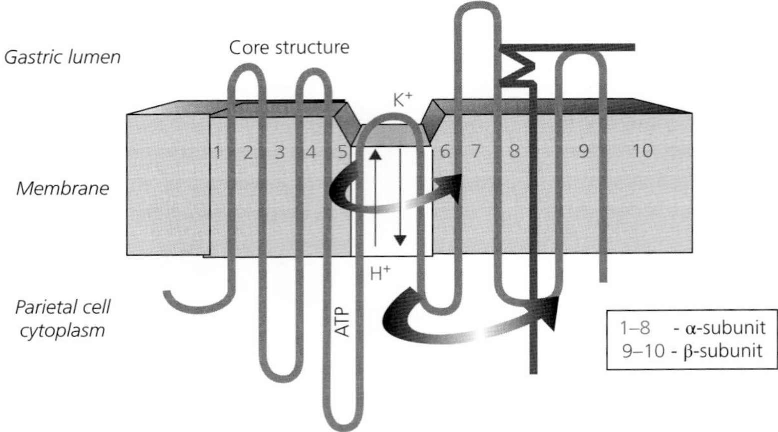

Figure 17.8 Schematic two-dimensional model of H^+,K^+ adenosine triphosphatase (H^+,K^+-ATPase), including its α and β subunits. The enzyme consists of eight transmembrane segments for the catalytic α subunit and one transmembrane segment for the β subunit. The latter heavily glycosylated subunit protects the enzyme from degradation and is necessary for trafficking to and from the plasma membrane. The α subunit carries out the catalytic and transport functions of the enzyme, and it also contains sequences responsible for apical membrane localization. As indicated, the active transport of H^+ ions in exchange for K^+ ions occurs between the fifth (M5) and sixth (M6) transmembrane domain.

of chief cells, indicating that the absence of acid secretion does not interfere with cellular differentiation. Parietal cells are also present in normal numbers and despite the absence of H^+,K^+-ATPase α-subunit mRNA and protein, the β subunit is expressed. However, the parietal cells possess dilated canaliculi and lack typical canalicular microvilli and tubulovesicles, and subsets of the cells contain abnormal mitochondria, massive glycogen stores, or both. The stomachs of adult α-subunit-deficient mice exhibit metaplasia, including the presence of ciliated cells [208]. The presence of achlorhydria and other abnormalities in these mice provides conclusive evidence regarding the vital role played by the H^+,K^+-ATPase enzyme in the process of gastric acid secretion.

The turnover of H^+,K^+-ATPase represents an important determinant of the rate of gastric acid secretion during both basal and stimulated states and in response to pharmacological inhibition. Using measurements of the loss of incorporated [^{35}S]-methionine, Gedda et al. [209] determined the turnover of the α subunit of H^+,K^+-ATPase in rats under control conditions and in response to the inhibition of K^+-stimulated ATPase activity in omeprazole- and ranitidine-treated animals. The T_2 of the α subunit under control conditions was 54 hours. Although omeprazole had no significant effect on the turnover of the gastric ATPase α subunit (15 hours), turnover was prolonged by ranitidine, with the T_2 increasing to 125 hours. The effect of ranitidine suggests that the resting H^+,K^+-ATPase enzyme in the parietal cell tubulovesicle turns over more slowly than the stimulated enzyme in secretory canaliculi. The rapid recovery of ATPase activity compared with turnover after omeprazole appears to occur as a result of both H^+,K^+-ATPase synthesis and loss of covalently bound drug [209].

In the resting nonsecretory state, H^+,K^+-ATPase activity is contained predominantly within cytoplasmic tubulovesicles (Figure 17.9a). On stimulation of the parietal cell, these tubulovesicles fuse with the apical plasma membrane, resulting in the development of a richly interdigitating intracellular canalicular system with an extensive network of microvilli and with a concomitant loss of cytoplasmic tubulovesicles (see Figure 17.9b) [210,211]. The microvilli have a central cytoskeletal core of actin filaments stabilized by other proteins [212], and these filaments appear to mediate the fusion of tubulovesicles with the canalicular system. Actin is often regarded as a "housekeeping" gene because its expression tends to remain constant. However, in the case of the parietal cell, actin plays a crucial role in the acid secretory process. With this dramatic transformation, the apical cell membrane area of the canaliculi draining to the apical surface of the parietal cell increases 5- to 10-fold, enabling the ensuing high rates of gastric acid secretion [67]. On cessation of secretion, the H^+,K^+-ATPase is retrieved from the apical membrane, and the tubulovesicular compartment is reestablished.

The precise mechanisms responsible for regulating these dramatic alterations in parietal cell morphology have not been elucidated, but in addition to actin-based microfilaments, they appear to involve small GTPases, docking/fusion proteins, cytoskeletal linkers, ezrin [213], and clathrin [214–216]. In particular, ezrin, an 80-kD membrane protein found in several cell types, is associated with the actin filaments in the microvilli of stimulated parietal cells and is phosphorylated during cAMP-mediated stimulation. In addition, other cytoskeletal proteins, such as spectrin and ankyrin, copurify with the H^+,K^+-ATPase from parietal cell microsomal membranes and cosegregate with H^+,K^+-ATPase in resting and secreting parietal cells [216]. Ankyrin may mediate the interaction of H^+,K^+-ATPase with both actin and spectrin and may thereby function to maintain the polarized distribution of the enzyme to the apical portion of

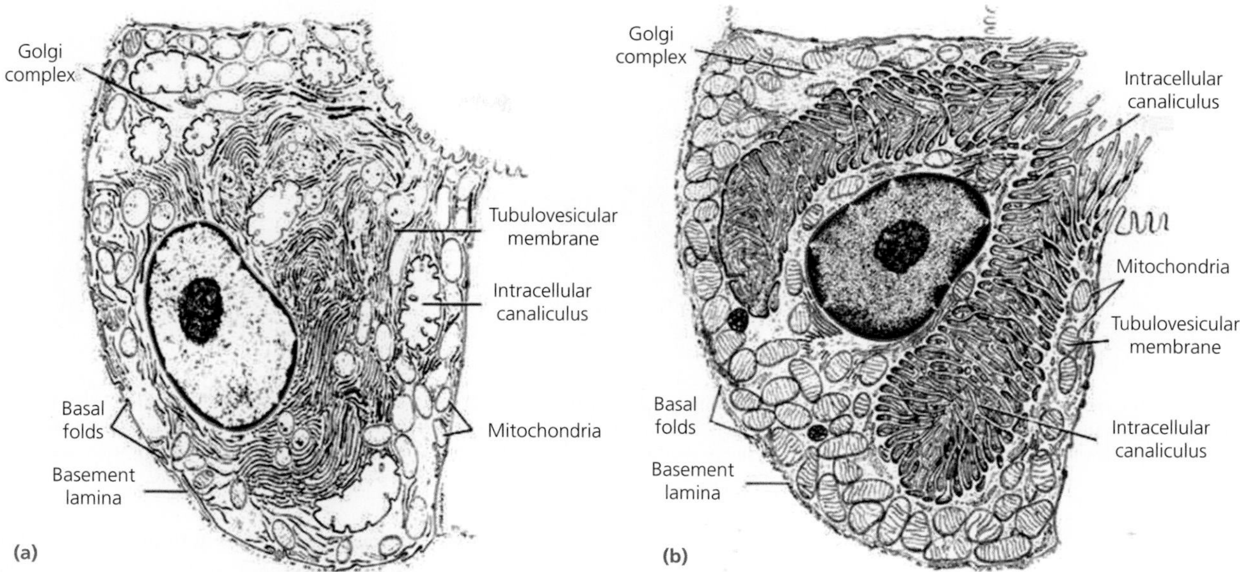

Figure 17.9 **(a)** Electron photomicrograph of the parietal cell in the resting (unstimulated) state, demonstrating abundant cytoplasmic tubovesicular membranes to which the H^+,K^+-ATPase enzyme is inserted. **(b)** Electron photomicrograph of a stimulated parietal cell, demonstrating translocation of the tubovesicular membranes containing acid activated H^+,K^+-ATPase to the intracellular secretory canalicular membranes, thereby facilitating proton pump exposure to the highly acidic secretory canalicular lumen. Source: Adapted from Ito 1987 [1]. Reproduced with permission of the author.

the parietal cell [217]. Festy et al. [218] demonstrated that rabbit H^+,K^+-ATPase binds through its N-terminal end to the spectrin-binding domain of ankyrin III. The two proteins bind directly to one another, constituting an important anchoring system for the H^+,K^+-ATPase to the plasma membrane [218].

Muraoka et al. [219] have demonstrated that basal transcriptional activity of the H^+,K^+-ATPase gene is mediated through binding of the nuclear transcriptional factor SP1 to the 5′-GCTCCGCCTC-3′ nucleotide sequence residing between bases −47 and −38 relative to the putative cap site [219]. Tamura et al. [220] identified regions within the promoters of both the α- and β subunits of the H^+,K^+-ATPase gene that are recognized by gastric-specific nuclear proteins. Maeda [221] further reported that GATA transcription factors 1 and 2 play an important role in H^+,K^+-ATPase expression. As discussed earlier, >90% of the gastric phase of acid secretion in humans occurs as a result of increases in circulating gastrin [135]. The expression levels of the H^+,K^+-ATPase α and β subunits, as well as other genes involved in the regulation of gastric acid secretion, such as the aquaporin-4 water channel, creatinine kinase B, and *KCNE2*, are diminished in the parietal cells of the gastrin-deficient mice [222]. Both the *KCNE2* gene, which encodes single-transmembrane domain subunits that regulate the function of voltage-gated K^+ channels [21], and the cystic fibrosis transmembrane conductance regulator, a cAMP-regulated Cl^- channel present in parietal cells [22], are coupled with H^+,K^+-ATPase in promoting H^+ ion secretion.

The recognition that the ATPase was the final step of acid secretion has resulted in the development of the PPIs, which are targeted toward this enzyme. All PPIs share a common structural motif (Figure 17.10), a substituted pyridylmethylsulfinyl benzimidazole, but vary in terms of their substitutions. They also share common inhibitory mechanisms and are weak protonatable pyridines, with a pKa of ~4.0 for omeprazole/esomeprazole, lansoprazole/dexlansoprazole, and pantoprazole, and ~5.0 for rabeprazole. As a result, they accumulate selectively in the acid space of the secreting parietal cell. Within that space or on the surface of the enzyme, they undergo an acid-catalyzed conversion to a reactive species, thiophilic sulfenamide or sulfenic acid, which are permanent cations (see Figure 17.10). The rate of conversion varies among the compounds and is a function of their pKa and other structural features: rabeprazole > omeprazole = lansoprazole > pantoprazole [67,223,224]. The reactive species (thiophilic sulfenamide) reacts with cysteine residues available from the external surface of the H^+,K^+-ATPase enzyme that faces the lumen of the secretory space of the parietal cell, resulting in covalent inhibition of the enzyme by disulfide bond formation. The cysteine residue that is critical for inhibition is Cys813 in the α subunit of the H^+,K^+-ATPase, strategically located in the M5/M6 sector of the enzyme, which is intimately involved in the transport process (Figure 17.11) [67]. Pantoprazole also forms a disulfide bond with Cys822 [224], located on transmembrane segment 6 deep in the α subunit, approximately 2.5 α-helical turns from the luminal surface. Pantoprazole reversal of acid inhibition may be exclusively a result of enzyme synthesis because of binding to Cys822 at a location within the ion transport pathway deep within the membrane domain of H^+,K^+-ATPase (see Figure 17.11), rendering it less accessible to reducing

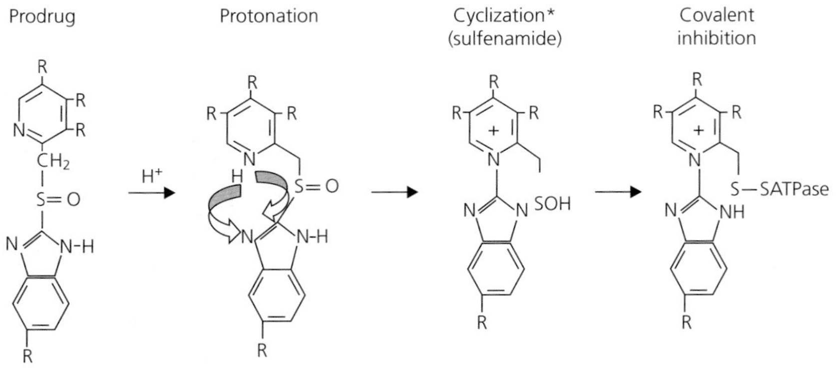

Figure 17.10 The chemical reaction involved in proton pump inhibitor (PPI) activation via protonation of the prodrug to form the activated moiety, the thiophilic sulfenamide. PPIs are concentrated in the secretory canaliculus of the parietal cell, undergo acid-catalyzed conversion to the active sulfenamide, and then form covalent disulfide bonds with cysteine residues accessible in the luminal domain of H^+,K^+-ATPase. *Activation. ATPase, adenosine triphosphatase.

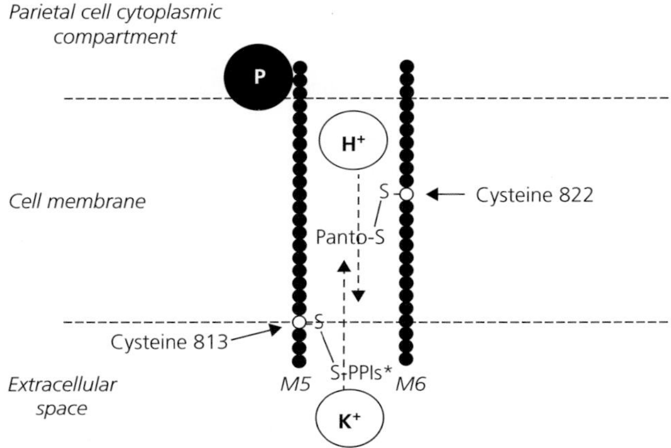

Figure 17.11 Schematic depicting the site of the active transport of H^+ (H_3O^+) ions in exchange for K^+ ions between the fifth (M5) and sixth (M6) transmembrane domain of H^+,K^+-ATPase. After stimulation of the parietal cell via receptors located on the parietal cell basolateral membrane, resulting in the generation of protein kinases (see Figure 17.3), H^+,K^+-ATPase is phosphorylated (P), resulting in the opening of the M5/M6 channel, and H^+ ions are transported from the parietal cytoplasmic compartment to the gastric lumen. After dephosphorylation of the enzyme, K^+ ions are actively exchanged and transported into the parietal cell cytoplasm. As depicted, on acid-catalyzed conversion to their respective active sulfonamide, all proton pump inhibitors (PPIs) form a covalent disulfide bond with cysteine residue 813. Pantoprazole (Panto) also forms a disulfide bond with cysteine 822, an additional reaction that has not been demonstrated to be clinically relevant. *After activation to thiophilic sulfenamide.

agents [224,225]. These differences in the reversal of acid inhibition have not been shown to be clinically relevant.

Other secretory products

Mucus

The gastric mucosal surface is covered by a layer of mucus that is approximately 0.2–0.6 mm thick [226,227]. This layer serves to protect the gastric mucosa from the actions of acid and pepsin, as well as to lubricate the mucosal surface. The mucous layer is composed primarily of water (95%) and mucins (5%). Mucins are tetrameric glycoproteins with a molecular weight of approximately 2000 kD; their protein cores are rich in serine, threonine, and proline residues, and they are heavily glycosylated. The major sugar residues in mucins include galactose, fucose, *N*-acetylgalactosamine, *N*-acetylglucosamine, and sialic acids. These carbohydrate chains attach to serine and threonine residues and are approximately 15 sugars in length. The high carbohydrate concentration is responsible for the viscoelastic properties of mucin when it is hydrated within the mucous layer [228].

Mucins are secreted by the mucous cells of the gastric pits: cells secreting both acidic and neutral mucins, while neck cells secrete primarily neutral mucin proteins. The primary gastric mucin, MUC6, is a neutral mucin synthesized in the rough endoplasmic reticulum of mucous neck cells, transported to the Golgi apparatus for final glycosylation and for intraprotein bonding via cysteine bridges, forming the mucin tetramer. The glycoproteins are then packaged in granules that rest at the apical surface of the mucous cells until they are released. In addition to these mucin glycoproteins, gastric mucus contains small amounts of fatty acids, phospholipids, trefoil factors (TFF1 and TFF2), and growth factors, including EGF and TGF-α.

Mucous secretion is stimulated by acetylcholine released by vagal efferents [229,230]. The mucosal protective effect of prostaglandins is due in a large part to their stimulation of gastric mucous production, and the decrease in mucin production seen with the use of cyclooxygenase (COX) inhibitors is an important contributor to nonsteroidal antiinflammatory drugs (NSAID)-induced mucosal damage. Histamine and gastrin also stimulate mucous secretion [231,232], helping to balance the damaging effects of increased acid and pepsin release with an increased production of mucosal defensive factors.

Within the mucous layer, the surface mucins interact with luminal pepsin and *N*-acetylcysteine, breaking the sulfide bonds that hold the tetramers together. The resulting mucin monomers form a soluble surface layer that lubricates the mucosal surface, and monomeric mucins may be washed off into the gastric juice. The deeper, tetrameric mucins form an adherent and viscous layer that binds to the mucosal surface. In addition to lubricating the mucosal surface, mucins protect the gastric cells by preventing contact between acid, pepsin, and the mucosal surface. Parietal cells secrete acid through the mucous layer in the form of finger-like projections, or "jets" of acid [233]; once the acid reaches the surface and enters the lumen, the mucous layer (along with secreted bicarbonate) prevents back-diffusion of acid [234]. This permits the luminal pH to reach 1.5–2, whereas the gastric surface maintains a pH close to 7 [235]. In addition, the phospholipid content of gastric mucus creates a hydrophobic barrier to other water-soluble molecules.

Gastric mucins also play a role in the pathogenesis of *H. pylori* infection. The bacterium appears to decrease mucin synthesis, which assists the organism in penetrating the mucous layer and reaching the gastric mucosal surface [236]. *H. pylori* also binds to Lewis blood group antigens present on mucins to facilitate surface colonization [237]. However, MUC6 mucin has an antibacterial property that is active against *H. pylori* and may inhibit bacterial proliferation [238].

Bicarbonate

Bicarbonate is secreted from the surface cells of the gastric mucosa and, in combination with gastric mucus, protects the mucosal surface from the damaging effects of gastric acid and pepsin. The surface cells are rich in carbonic anhydrase and are poised to produce large amounts of bicarbonate ion, which is secreted through a neutral HCO_3^-/Cl^- transporter on the apical surface of these cells [239]. Studies in animals have identified the anion transporter DRA (downregulated in adenoma) that, coupled with a membrane Na^+/H^+ transporter, may have a role in mediating gastric bicarbonate secretion [240]. Bicarbonate secretion is stimulated by the presence of luminal acid and by vagal acetylcholine release during the cephalic phase of gastric secretion. Gastric prostaglandins have also been shown to induce bicarbonate secretion.

Bicarbonate secretion may be coupled with acid secretion by parietal cells; when acid is secreted, bicarbonate is released into the gastric capillaries from the basolateral surface of parietal cells, the so-called alkaline tide. The bicarbonate-rich blood then travels to the mucosal surface, where sodium bicarbonate cotransporters on the surface cells take up bicarbonate for later secretion [241].

Pepsinogen

Pepsinogens are a group of proteins produced by the chief cells of the oxyntic mucosa; gastric mucous cells also secrete small quantities of these proenzymes. The protein is stored in cytoplasmic granules within the chief cell and secreted via exocytosis in response to stimulatory signals. Pepsinogen is present in two forms; pepsinogen I (PGI), which is actually a group of five isoenzymes, is secreted nearly exclusively by the chief cells and accounts for 80% of gastric pepsin production. The remaining 20% of pepsin is derived from pepsinogen II (PGII; also called pepsinogen C or progastricsin), which is secreted by cells of the gastric antrum and pylorus, as well as by the duodenal Brunner glands [242]. The various pepsinogen molecules are biochemically similar, sharing 50% of their amino acid sequence [243].

In the presence of acid, pepsinogen undergoes a conformational change that exposes its enzymatic active site. This allows pepsinogen to autocatalyze its conversion to pepsin, an aspartate protease that is enzymatically active in the digestion of animal proteins, including collagens. Pepsin is well-suited to the acidic milieu of the gastric lumen, being most active at pH 1.8–3.5 and inactivated at pH >5. When gastric pH is greater than 7, the pepsin molecule is irreversibly denatured. Pepsin cleaves peptides at sites that contain the aromatic amino acids tyrosine, phenylalanine, and tryptophan; these amino acids and their amine metabolites stimulate gastrin secretion from antral G cells [72]. The action of acid on ingested protein assists pepsin by denaturing peptides, making cleavage sites more accessible to pepsin activity.

Pepsinogen secretion is stimulated by acetylcholine from vagal efferents [243] acting at muscarinic receptors present on gastric mucosal cells. GRP also stimulates pepsinogen secretion via a vagal mechanism [244], with intracellular calcium and inositol 1,4,5-triphosphate acting as second messengers. Gastrin itself weakly stimulates pepsinogen secretion, but CCK [245] is a much more potent pepsinogen secretagogue. Secretin has also been shown to induce pepsinogen release through interaction with surface receptors on chief cells, leading to an increase in intracellular cAMP levels [246]; prostaglandins and vasoactive intestinal peptide stimulate pepsinogen release via a similar second messenger system. Several peptides have been shown to inhibit pepsinogen release, including somatostatin, peptide YY, and neuropeptide Y [246].

Pepsinogen is detectable in serum and urine [247], and it has been studied as a biomarker to predict risk for atrophic gastritis and gastric cancer in parts of the world with a high incidence of these conditions. Because PGI is produced in the oxyntic mucosa, it is markedly reduced in atrophic gastritis, whereas PGII is relatively preserved as a result of production in the antrum, pylorus, and duodenum. Thus, a low serum PGI level and a low serum PGI/PGII ratio have been used as a noninvasive predictor of gastric atrophy in areas of high prevalence [248].

Histamine

Histamine, 2-(4-imidazolyl)ethylamine, is a hydrophilic molecule composed of an imidazole ring and an amino group connected by two methylene groups [249]. The precise relationship of histamine to acid secretion was firmly established by Kay [250] during development of the augmented histamine test. Despite the central role of histamine as a potent stimulant of the generation and secretion of H^+ ions, the precise identity of the fundic cells that store histamine and regulate its release were largely unknown until recently. It appears that histamine is derived from both mast and ECL cells [251]. Although mast cells appear to account fully for the histamine content of dispersed gastric cells in the dog, in other species, including humans, it appears that the ECL cell, although comprising <1% of cells of the oxyntic mucosa, is the principal source of histamine [67,252,253]. The extent to which the stimulation of acid secretion by gastrin and acetylcholine reflects their effect on histamine release appears to vary among species. In humans, it is likely that gastrin and acetylcholine, as well as CCK, stimulate histamine release by increasing the concentration of cytosolic Ca^{2+}, whereas somatostatin appears to directly inhibit histamine release targeting the adenylate cyclase after binding to its $SSTR_2$ receptor subtype [17].

Histamine production in ECL cells occurs as a result of the decarboxylation of L-histidine by histidine decarboxylase [253], which is transcriptionally regulated by both gastrin and acetylcholine. Gastrin stimulates histidine decarboxylase transcription through PKC- and mitogen-activated protein kinase-dependent pathways [254–256]. Both in vivo and in vitro studies have demonstrated that gastrin possesses direct proliferative effects on these cells, supporting the concept that hypergastrinemia resulting from potent acid suppression, principally by the use of PPIs, represents the mechanism responsible for ECL cell proliferation [257–259].

Histamine stimulates the parietal cell directly by binding to H_2 receptors coupled to the activation of adenylate cyclase and generation of cAMP (see Figure 17.3) [78]. In addition to direct stimulation, histamine augments acid secretion indirectly by binding to H_3 receptors coupled to inhibition of somatostatin and thereby stimulation of histamine and acid secretion [260,261]. Histamine appears to regulate its own release through other H_3 receptors located on ECL cells, thus creating an autocrine feedback loop [151]. Peptide YY has also been observed to inhibit histamine release through a Y_1 receptor subtype [262].

Intrinsic factor

IF is a 50-kD glycoprotein secreted by gastric parietal cells, with a minor component of secretion from chief and endocrine cells; it has an integral role in the metabolism of cobalamin (CBL), first described by William Castle in 1929. IF is secreted in the gastric fundus and corpus but exerts its major action in the intestine. As depicted in Figure 17.12, ingested CBL is released from dietary protein by the action of gastric pepsin and then binds to R-factor, a protein present in saliva, gastric juice, and bile [263]. Although IF is present in gastric juice, at acidic pH, CBL binds with greater affinity to R-factor. In the higher pH of the small bowel, the R-CBL complex is cleaved by trypsin, allowing IF to bind the free CBL. The IF-CBL complex is resistant to proteolysis and is transported to the terminal ileum, where the CBL receptor, cubilin, promotes endocytosis of the IF-CBL complex into the ileal enterocytes, where CBL is released from IF and bound to transcobalamin II for transport in the bloodstream [264]. IF production is stimulated and inhibited by the same factors that regulate acid secretion; however, IF secretion is not dependent on the presence of gastric acid, and PPIs have not been shown to significantly inhibit IF secretion [265]. Hypochlorhydria may decrease vitamin B_{12} absorption not by affecting IF, but by inactivating pepsin and preventing release of CBL from dietary protein.

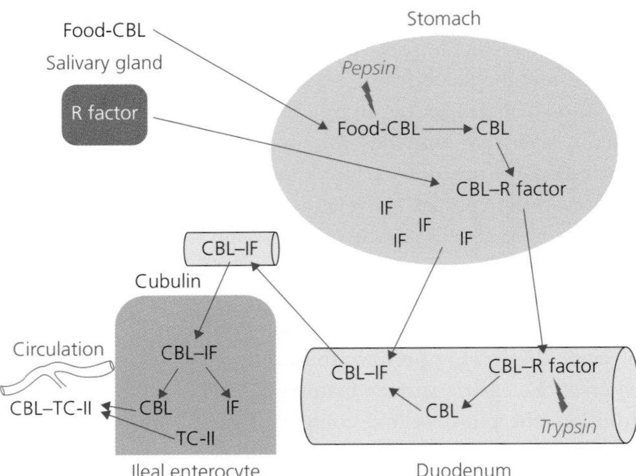

Figure 17.12 Schematic depiction of the various mechanisms involved in cobalamin (CBL) absorption. CBL (vitamin B_{12}) bound to ingested food is released in the stomach via the action of pepsin, where it binds salivary R-factor and is then transferred to the duodenum. Intrinsic factor (IF), although expressed and released into the gastric lumen, does not bind CBL until it reaches the duodenum, where pancreatic trypsin cleaves R-factor, thereby enabling IF-CBL binding. The IF-CBL complex is transported to the terminal ileum, where the surface molecule cubilin mediates the endocytosis of the IF-CBL complex. Within the ileal enterocyte, CBL is cleaved from IF and binds transcobalamin II (TC II) for transport into the bloodstream.

Pernicious anemia is an autoimmune disorder characterized by the presence of antibodies to both IF and parietal cells that leads to hypochlorhydria and IF deficiency, resulting in CBL malabsorption [266]. In the modern era, this disease is diagnosed via the detection of circulating anti-IF and anti-parietal cell antibodies. However, the Schilling test is a well-established method of diagnosing pernicious anemia that closely reflects the physiology of digestion and absorption of vitamin B_{12}. During the performance of this test, tissue receptors for CBL are first saturated by the administration of a dose of parenteral vitamin B_{12}, ensuring that any oral vitamin B_{12} that is subsequently absorbed will not bind to tissues, but rather will be excreted into the urine. Oral CBL, radiolabeled with ^{57}Co, is then administered, and urine is collected. The absence of labeled vitamin B_{12} in the urine confirms that CBL is not being absorbed. The second phase of the test is then performed to assess the role of IF deficiency in CBL malabsorption. In this phase, oral radiolabeled CBL and IF are administered together; if the urine then contains radiolabeled CBL, it indicates that IF deficiency is the cause of the vitamin B_{12} malabsorption. If CBL absorption is still deficient despite IF coadministration, then another cause of CBL malabsorption must be sought. The latter includes small-intestinal bacterial overgrowth (in which bacteria ingest dietary CBL), pancreatic insufficiency (in which trypsin deficiency prevents cleavage of the R-CBL complex), ileal diseases that prevent IF-CBL absorption, and, rarely, receptor defects in the ileum, for example, Imerslund–Gräsbeck syndrome, in which a mutation in the cubilin gene renders the receptor inactive [267].

Prostaglandins

Prostaglandins are 20-carbon fatty acid derivatives of arachidonic acid, which originate from cell-membrane phospholipids through the action of phospholipase A_2 [268]. The metabolism of arachidonic acid to prostaglandins and leukotrienes is catalyzed by the COX pathway and the 5-lipoxygenase pathway, respectively (Figure 17.13) [67,269,270]. COX rapidly metabolizes free arachidonic acid to cyclic endoperoxides, which are then converted to various prostaglandin subtypes by tissue-specific processing enzymes. PGE_2 and PGI_2 appear to be the predominant subtypes that are synthesized and secreted by the gastric mucosa in various animal species.

Mammalian cells express two related but unique isoforms of COX, designated COX-1 and COX-2 [271,272]. Despite their structural similarities, they are encoded by distinct genes that differ in their distribution and expression in tissues (Figure 17.14); the *COX1* gene is primarily expressed constitutively, whereas the *COX2* gene is inducible [268]. COX-1 appears to function as a "housekeeping" enzyme in most tissues, including the gastric mucosa, as well as the kidneys and platelets, whereas the expression of *COX2* can be induced by inflammatory stimuli and mitogens in many different cell types, including macrophages and synovial cells [273]. The important role of COX-1 in protecting the gastric mucosa is supported by studies showing that the greatest degree of gastric mucosal injury is generally caused by

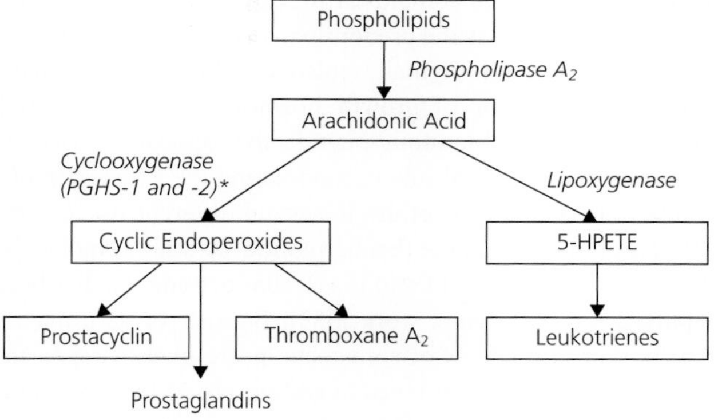

Figure 17.13 Biosynthesis of prostaglandins and leukotrienes via the cyclooxygenase (COX) and lipoxygenase pathways, respectively. The immediate precursor, arachidonic acid, is derived from membrane phospholipids by action of the enzyme phospholipase A_2. *Also designated COX-1 and COX-2. HPETE, an intermediate product in the degradation of arachidonic acid; PGHS, prostaglandin-H synthase.

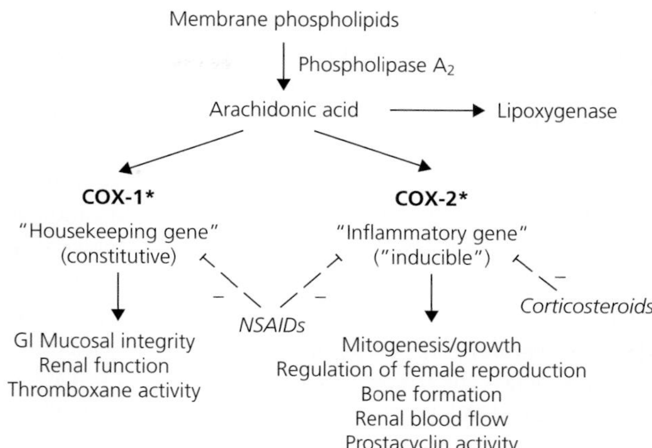

Figure 17.14 Pathways depicting the biosynthesis of prostaglandins via the cyclooxygenase (COX) pathways (also referred to as prostaglandin H synthase [PGHS]). The immediate precursor, arachidonic acid, is derived from membrane phospholipids and is catalyzed by the two COX isoenzymes, COX-1 and COX-2. The *COX1* gene is expressed constitutively and maintains normal organ homeostasis, including gastric mucosal integrity, as well as effects on gastric secretion (see Figure 17.3). In contrast, the *COX2* or "inflammatory" gene is inducible. Although both pathways can be inhibited to various degrees by different nonsteroidal antiinflammatory drugs (NSAIDs), only the *COX2* gene contains a corticosteroid-responsive repressor element in its promoter. *Also designated PGHS1 and PGHS2. GI, gastrointestinal.

NSAIDs that preferentially inhibit COX-1, such as naproxen, piroxicam, sulindac, and indomethacin [274].

Endogenously expressed prostaglandins exert mucosal protective effects by several mechanisms, including stimulating epithelial mucous and bicarbonate secretion, increasing phospholipid secretion, reducing mucosal H^+ ion back-diffusion, enhancing mucosal blood flow, and promoting epithelial cell proliferation, which all increase resistance to the development of mucosal injury [268,275]. In addition to these important physiological protective properties, as already noted, prostaglandins (primarily PGE_2) inhibit H^+ ion generation by binding to its G protein-linked receptors on the parietal cell, leading to the inhibition of adenylate cyclase and thereby a decrease in intracellular cAMP generation (see Figure 17.3) [161,276].

Nitric oxide

NO is a signaling molecule that controls a variety of biological processes, including blood flow, leukocyte and platelet adhesion, and neurotransmission [268]. NO plays a critical role in maintaining gastroduodenal mucosal integrity, exerting many of the same effects of endogenous prostaglandins [277–279]. It has been suggested that NO and prostaglandins act synergistically to mediate mucosal protective effects, including maintenance of gastric mucosal blood flow and prevention of neutrophil adherence to the vascular endothelium [268,269]. Salvemini et al. [280] demonstrated that NO stimulates expression of COX enzymes. Such redundancy in preserving normal physiological function is not unique, and it constitutes the rationale for the development of NO-NSAIDs in which NO released from such compounds compensates for the suppression of mucosal prostaglandins. The intracellular actions of NO are mediated by soluble guanylyl cyclase [281]. NO binds to guanylyl cyclase, leading to its conformational modification and activation. Active guanylyl cyclase is responsible for the conversion of GTP into cGMP, the main transducer of the biological actions of NO. The ability of NO to stimulate cGMP generation appears to mediate NO inhibition of gastric acid secretion in isolated parietal cells [25,36,281,282]. As discussed in detail in Chapter 4, the development of hypertrophic pyloric stenosis is examined and correlated with a lack of NO synthase in pyloric tissue.

Regulatory peptide secretion in the stomach

The entire stomach, and the pyloric gland area in particular, includes many different types of endocrine cells that secrete gastrointestinal regulatory peptides, the principal one being gastrin, which are secreted from G cells located in the epithelium. These endocrine cells are scattered throughout the gastric mucosa, and their secretory products possess important physiological properties.

Gastrin

The existence of a humoral substance involved in the simulation of gastric acid secretion was first postulated in 1906 by Edkins [283], who characterized an antral mucosal extract that he termed "gastrin." For many years, the activity of this substance was confused with histamine, casting doubt on the existence of an antral hormone. The studies of Komarov [284] in 1938 verified gastrin as a hormone distinct from histamine. However, it was not until 1964 that Gregory and Tracy [285] successfully isolated two gastrin peptides from porcine antral mucosa and identified their amino acid composition in sequence. These gastrins were each 17 amino acids in length (G-17) and differed only in the absence or presence of a sulfated ester on the tyrosine residue at position 12. With the introduction of gastrin radioimmunoassay by McGuigan [286,287], a larger and more basic form of the peptide was discovered by Yalow and Berson [288] in 1970. This peptide was subsequently shown to contain 34 amino acids, including the hepta-decapeptide covalently linked to a structurally distinct 17-amino acid sequence. Both the larger (G-34) and smaller (G-17) forms of gastrin share the same carboxyl-terminal pentapeptide contained in CCK [74]. Similar to the smaller form, the 34-amino acid form exists naturally in both sulfated and nonsulfated forms, each of equal potency with regard to their acid-stimulatory effects [289]. In the human gastric antral mucosa, G-17 is the predominant molecular species, with G-34 accounting for only approximately 5% of the gastrin found [290]. However, likely as a result of its far longer half-life, G-34 comprises approximately two-thirds of circulating gastrin [291]. Other circulating forms of gastrin have been described; these occur only in very low concentrations or do not increase postprandially, or both [289,292]. Rehfeld [292] has demonstrated at least 20 other different immunoreactive gastrin forms circulating in very small quantities in normal human serum.

The human gastrin gene (*GAS*) contains two introns, is located on the long arm of chromosome 17, and covers approximately 4100 bp of DNA [293,294]. Similar to other gastrointestinal regulatory peptides, gastrin mRNA encodes a preprogastrin peptide, which is directed to the endoplasmic reticulum by its hydrophobic signal sequence. The signal peptide is then cleaved and degraded, and progastrin is transported to the Golgi apparatus for further posttranslational processing by various tissue-specific enzymes, including endoproteases, tyrosyl-protein sulfonyl transferase, and carboxypeptidase [295–298]. Some progastrin remains unprocessed and secreted into the circulation, where it acts as a growth factor, particularly for the colon [299]. Gly-extended gastrin precursors, including principally G-34-Gly and G-17-Gly, both of which possess trophic properties in colorectal cancer and other gastrointestinal malignancies [300], are processed within immature cytoplasmic granules. They subsequently undergo dibasic cleavage of the glycine-extended molecule within immature granules to yield biologically active α-amidated gastrins [301]. As mentioned earlier, G-34 and G-17 are equipotent with regard to their acid-stimulatory properties, which they exert by binding to their CCK-B (or CCK-2) receptor located on ECL cells and possibly on parietal cells (see Figure 17.3).

Somatostatin

The somatostatin gene encodes a preprosomatostatin peptide, which is initially cleaved to prosomatostatin [302], then subsequently processed to a 28-amino acid peptide (S-28), and finally to its 14-amino acid form (S-14) [303]. The latter form comprises the majority of somatostatin expressed in D cells in the stomach, while S-28 is the predominant form in the small intestine [304]. Although originally isolated in the ovine hypothalamus as an inhibitor of growth hormone release [305,306], somatostatin is a ubiquitous peptide that appears to play an important physiological role in modulating the expression of a number of regulatory peptides in several different tissues [95–97]. It is of interest to note that octreotide has similar molecular characteristics as the S-14 and is a similar peptide that has been deployed for therapeutic work [303]. Because of its universal distribution, the effects of somatostatin are likely vital to the biology of most organ systems. In addition to its location in the stomach and other digestive organs, somatostatin-containing cells have been demonstrated in many organs, including the endocrine pancreas, retina, cardiac vagus, and glomerulus of the kidney [307].

Antral somatostatin exerts inhibitory effects on G cells via paracrine pathways, through release of the peptide from D cells into the immediate interstitial environment of antral G cells [73,95]. In addition to indirectly inhibiting secretion by its effect on gastrin expression, somatostatin released from D cells in the fundus and corpus directly inhibits H^+ ion generation [142] by binding to its $SSTR_2$ receptor subtype on the parietal cell membrane [164,165]. Antral D cells can be stimulated by intraluminal acid (pH <3.5–3.0), possibly through the activation of CGRP neurons [15,139], and by gastrin released from nearby G cells. D cells can be inhibited by cholinergic neurons, thereby leading to the indirect stimulation of gastrin release and acid secretion, and by histamine through its H_3 receptor. Finally, somatostatin appears to exert in autocrine inhibitory effect on D cells [95].

In addition to its inhibitory effects on the release of several peptides, such as gastrin, growth hormone adrenocorticotropin, thyroid-stimulating hormone, insulin, and glucagon, somatostatin inhibits antral G cells by pretranslational mechanisms, including a decrease in gastrin gene transcription and by increasing the turnover of gastrin mRNA [96,97]. In fact, the latter mechanism, which includes the augmentation of mRNA degradation, appears to play a dominant role in the regulation of antral gastrin biosynthesis by somatostatin.

Gastrin-releasing peptide

In addition to its role in a number of physiological and pathophysiological processes, including malignancies of the lung, colon, stomach, pancreas, breast, and prostate [308,309], GRP is a widely distributed 27-amino acid neuropeptide that stimulates gastric acid secretion both directly and through the release of gastrin from antral G cells [310]. The peptide is the mammalian homolog of bombesin, a 14-amino acid peptide originally isolated from the European fire-bellied toad, *Bombina bombina* [311]. The GRP gene encodes a 148-amino acid prepropeptide [312,313]; following cleavage of a signal peptide, the propeptide is further processed to produce either GRP or the 10-amino acid neuromedin C, also referred to as GRP-10 [314]. GRP is released from peptidergic postganglionic parasympathetic fibers and neurons of the gastric mucosa [315]. Immunoneutralization of gastrin in dogs blocks bombesin-stimulated gastric acid secretion, indicating that gastrin release is stimulated by GRP, and bombesin receptor antagonists attenuate gastric acid secretion in response to sham feeding, indicating that GRP released from postganglionic vagal fibers plays a major role during the cephalic phase of acid secretion [316].

Ghrelin

Ghrelin is a 28-amino acid peptide that is expressed mainly by P/D1 cells lining the gastric fundus, as well as in pancreatic islet α-cells [317]. Along with obestatin, ghrelin is the product of the *GHRL* gene, whose mRNA encodes the 117-amino acid ghrelin/obestatin preproghrelin, containing four exons [318]. The signaling peptide molecule of this larger precursor is cleaved to produce proghrelin, which is further processed to produce the 28-amino acid peptide ghrelin (unacylated) and C-ghrelin, from which obestatin is presumed to be a cleaved form [319]. Ghrelin is expressed in a wide variety of tissues, including the pituitary, stomach, intestine, pancreas, thymus, gonads, thyroid, and heart [320]. It binds to its G protein-coupled GHSR1 splice-variant receptor, which is present in high density in afferent cell bodies and vagal afferents throughout the gastrointestinal tract, as well as in the hypothalamus [319,321].

Ghrelin has been linked to inducing appetite and feeding behaviors [322,323]. Circulating ghrelin levels are highest right before a meal and the lowest right after [324,325]. Ghrelin administered intravenously to both humans and rats have been shown to increase food intake in a dose-dependent manner [326]. Masuda et al. [327] also demonstrated that ghrelin administered to rats increased both gastric acid secretion and gastric motility in a dose-dependent manner. The maximum response in gastric acid secretion was almost equipotent to histamine, and the stimulatory effects were abolished by pretreatment with either atropine or bilateral cervical vagotomy [327]. These observations suggest that ghrelin may play a physiological role in the vagal control of gastric function in rats.

References are available at www.yamadagastro.com/textbook7e

Further reading

Black J.W., Duncan W.A., Durant C.J., et al. Definition and antagonism of histamine H2-receptors. Nature 1972;236:385.

Fourmy D., Gigoux V., Reubi J.C. Gastrin in gastrointestinal diseases. Gastroenterology 2011;141:814.

Gantz I., Schaffer M., DelValle J., et al. Molecular cloning of a gene encoding the histamine H2 receptor. Proc Natl Acad Sci U S A 1991;88:429.

Kopik S., Murek M., Geibel J.P. Revisiting the parietal cell. Am J Physiol Cell Physiol 2010;298:C1.

Kozyraki R., Cases O. Vitamin B12 absorption: mammalian physiology and acquired and inherited disorders. Biochimie 2013;95:1002.

Kitay A.M., Ferstl F.S., Link A., Geibel J.P. Induction of secretagogue independent gastric acid secretion via a novel aspirin-activated pathway. Front Physiol 2019;10:1264.

Kopic S., Geibel J.P. Gastric acid, calcium absorption, and their impact on bone health. Physiol Rev 2013;93:189–268.

Mills J.C., Shivdasani R.A. Gastric epithelial stem cells. Gastroenterology 2011;140:412.

Schubert M.L., Peura D.A. Control of gastric acid secretion in health and disease. Gastroenterology 2008;134:1842.

Stewart B., Wallmark B., Sachs G. The interaction of H+ and K+ with the partial reactions of gastric (H+ + K+)-ATPase. J Biol Chem 1981;256:2682.

Waisbren S.J., Geibel J.P., Modlin I.M., and Boron W.F. Unusual permeability properties of gastric gland cells. Nature 1994;368:332–335.

Wolfe M.M., Sachs G. Acid suppression: optimizing therapy for gastroduodenal ulcer healing, gastroesophageal reflux disease, and stress-related erosive syndrome. Gastroenterology 2000;118(Suppl 1):S9.

Wolfe M.M., Soll A.H. The physiology of gastric acid secretion. N Engl J Med 1988;319:1707.

CHAPTER 18

Pancreatic secretion

Kristyn Gumpper[1,2], Luis F. Lara[1], Zobeida Cruz-Monserrate[1,2], and Darwin L. Conwell[1]

[1] Department of Internal Medicine, Division of Gastroenterology, Hepatology, and Nutrition, The Ohio State University Wexner Medical Center, Columbus, OH, USA

[2] The James Comprehensive Cancer Center, The Ohio State University Wexner Medical Center, Columbus, OH, USA

Chapter menu

The secretions of the exocrine pancreas, which include digestive enzymes and bicarbonate, affect the digestion and absorption of nutrients. These digestive enzymes are essential to the complete breakdown of chyme into building blocks and energy components usable by cells. In addition, bicarbonate secretion from the pancreas is crucial for neutralizing the acidic chyme coming from the stomach to optimize pancreatic enzyme function. The endocrine pancreas releases hormones that regulate glucose and fat metabolism and the disposition of the breakdown products of food within the body. The combined exocrine and endocrine functions make the pancreas one of the most important and complex organs involved in the assimilation of food.

The exocrine pancreas consists of clusters of acini that form lobules separated by loose connective tissue. Each acinus is a sphere composed of 20–50 polar, pyramidal cells arranged with their broad bases around the circumference of the acini and their apices pointed toward a central lumen. Each acinus is drained by a ductule with centroacinar cells extending from the ductule to the lumen of the acinus. The ductules drain through a series of ducts of increasing caliber until the main ducts of the pancreas are reached.

The islets of Langerhans contain the cells of the endocrine pancreas and are distributed within the pancreas. These islets consist of approximately 1–2% of the total pancreatic tissue but require approximately 10-fold more blood flow than the rest of the pancreatic tissue [1]. Morphological studies have revealed cell-to-cell contact between the exocrine and endocrine tissue, and direct connections between the capillaries of the islets and the acini [2]. These morphological arrangements may reflect the regulatory influences of the islet hormones on the function of the exocrine pancreas and vice versa. Of the pancreatic hormones, glucagon, somatostatin, and pancreatic polypeptide (PP) inhibit pancreatic exocrine secretion [3–6]. In contrast, insulin potentiates the stimulatory effect of cholecystokinin (CCK) on pancreatic exocrine secretion [7]. In addition, exocrine pancreatic secretion can influence pancreatic hormone release. The control of both endocrine and exocrine pancreatic function is complex and is highly regulated by both neural and hormonal factors.

Formation and composition of exocrine pancreatic secretion

The human pancreas secretes about 1 L of fluid daily, consisting mostly of water, ions, and digestive enzymes. The morphological appearance of the different cells of the exocrine pancreas and the results of micropuncture experiments, as well as studies from isolated acini and duct cells, suggest that the acinar cells mainly secrete digestive enzymes, while the ductal cells are mainly responsible for ion secretion [8].

Yamada's Textbook of Gastroenterology, Seventh Edition. Edited by Timothy C. Wang, Michael Camilleri, Benjamin Lebwohl, Anna S. Lok, William J. Sandborn, Kenneth K. Wang, and Gary D. Wu.

Companion website: www.yamadagastro.com/textbook7e

Water secretion

Pancreatic ions are secreted in a clear, alkaline fluid that is isosmotic with extracellular fluid. Water enters the ducts passively along osmotic gradients established by the active secretion of ions and other solutes. This water flow involves paracellular movement through junctional complexes and transcellular flow mediated by multiple aquaporin (AQP) water channels. In acinar cells, AQP12 allows for intracellular water movement between the cytosol and the zymogen granules [9,10]. Meanwhile AQP8 allows water to flow though the cell's apical membrane [11,12]. Likewise, AQP1 and AQP5 allow water to flow through the pancreatic duct cells from the basolateral side to the luminal side, respectively [13,14]. This flow of water into the duct allows for the isosmotic movement of ions as part of the pancreatic secretion.

Ion secretion

Na^+ and K^+ comprise the major cations of pancreatic secretion with trace amounts of Ca^{2+}, Mg^{2+}, and Zn^{2+}. Both N^+ and K^+ are secreted at concentrations near plasma concentrations and have constant secretory rates independent of the flow of water and other ions (Figure 18.1). HCO_3^- and Cl^- are the major anions in pancreatic secretions, along with trace amounts of HPO_4^{2-} and SO_4^{2-}, whose concentrations depend on the flow rates of water secretion. As the flow rate increases, the HCO_3^- concentration increases asymptotically, approaching a plateau value in humans of approximately 150 mM. At the same time, Cl^- secretion decreases asymptotically, reaching a plateau around 20 mM (Figure 18.1). Because HCO_3^- is vital for pH buffering in pancreatic secretions, the focus of research on exocrine pancreatic secretions has been on the mechanism of HCO_3^- secretion.

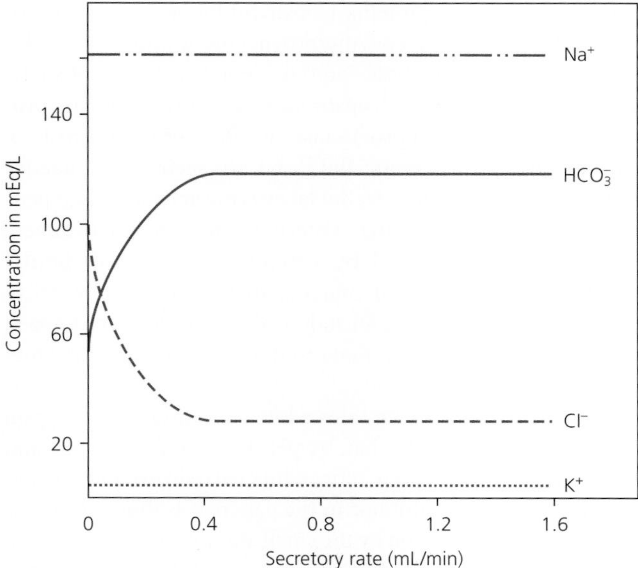

Figure 18.1 Relation of the secretory rate to the electrolyte composition of pancreatic juice.

Originally, HCO_3^- was believed to be solely derived within ductal cells by carbonic anhydrase catalyzing the interconversion between $H_2O + CO_2$ and $HCO_3^- + H^+$ [15]. However, inhibiting carbonic anhydrase decreases HCO_3^- secretion by only approximately 50% [16,17]. Rather, the remaining HCO_3^- ions are absorbed from blood through the pancreatic Na^+/HCO_3^- cotransporter 1 (pNBC1) [18]. In addition to the well-characterized secretion of HCO_3^- from ductal cells, recent evidence points to HCO_3^- efflux from the anoctamin-1/transmembrane member 16A (ANO1/TMEM16A) chloride channel in both acinar and ductal cells [19–21].

Experimental evidence and mathematical models indicate that energy input is necessary to obtain secretion of 140 mM HCO_3^- into the pancreatic ducts. Therefore, secretion of HCO_3^- into the pancreatic duct necessitates the concerted movement of several other ions to establish electrochemical gradients.

On the basolateral membrane of the duct cells, a Na^+ gradient is established by a Na^+/K^+-adenosine triphosphatase (ATPase) pump, K^+ outward channel, Na^+/H^+-ATPase, epithelial sodium channel, and pNBC1 [21]. This strong sodium gradient allows a pH neutral loading of HCO_3^- into the cell. The pNCB1 channel transports two HCO_3^- for each Na^+ and is responsible for 75% of the stimulated secretion of HCO_3^- [22–24]. In addition to pNBC1, anion exchange protein 2 is also present on the basolateral membrane, most likely as a way of supplying the apical cells with Cl^- [25]. Basolateral Na^+/H^+ exchanger 1 and luminal Na^+/H^+ exchanger 3 serve to aid in establishing the Na^+ gradient in the cell using adenosine triphosphate (ATP) hydrolysis as the energy source. This Na^+ gradient and resulting HCO_3^- gradient generate a negative membrane potential to promote HCO_3^- efflux through Cl^-/HCO_3^- exchangers in the solute-like carrier 26A (SLC26A) family and the cystic fibrosis transmembrane conductance regulator (CFTR) [26,27].

The SLC26A Cl^-/HCO_3^- exchangers are considered the major pathway for secreting HCO_3^- into the pancreatic ducts. Indeed, two isoforms of the SLC26 family reside on the apical membrane of pancreatic duct cells, SLC26A3 and SLC26A6. Interestingly, these two transporters have differing stoichiometry SLC26A3 exchanges of two Cl^- into the cell for one HCO_3^- out of the cell, whereas SLC26A6 transports two HCO_3^- ions into the duct for each Cl^- ion absorbed [28], resulting in a net recycling of Cl^- and overall secretion of HCO_3^- [29,30]. In the small ducts adjacent to the acinus, CFTR functions as a Cl^- channel, allowing Cl^- to maintain a relatively large concentration in the duct. This gives the SLC26A exchangers the fodder needed for HCO_3^- in conjunction with the Cl^- secreted from the acinar cells.

CFTR can also secrete HCO_3^- into the duct lumen. The CFTR channel has a limited permeability to HCO_3^- under basal conditions. It mainly functions as a Cl^- channel at concentrations greater than 10 mM, as is found in the small intralobar ducts [31]. However, when luminal Cl^- is greatly reduced, such as in the medium intralobar ducts (Figure 18.2) [26,32], the channel widens to become another major pathway for HCO_3^- exit into the lumen [20,33]. In addition to a decline in luminal

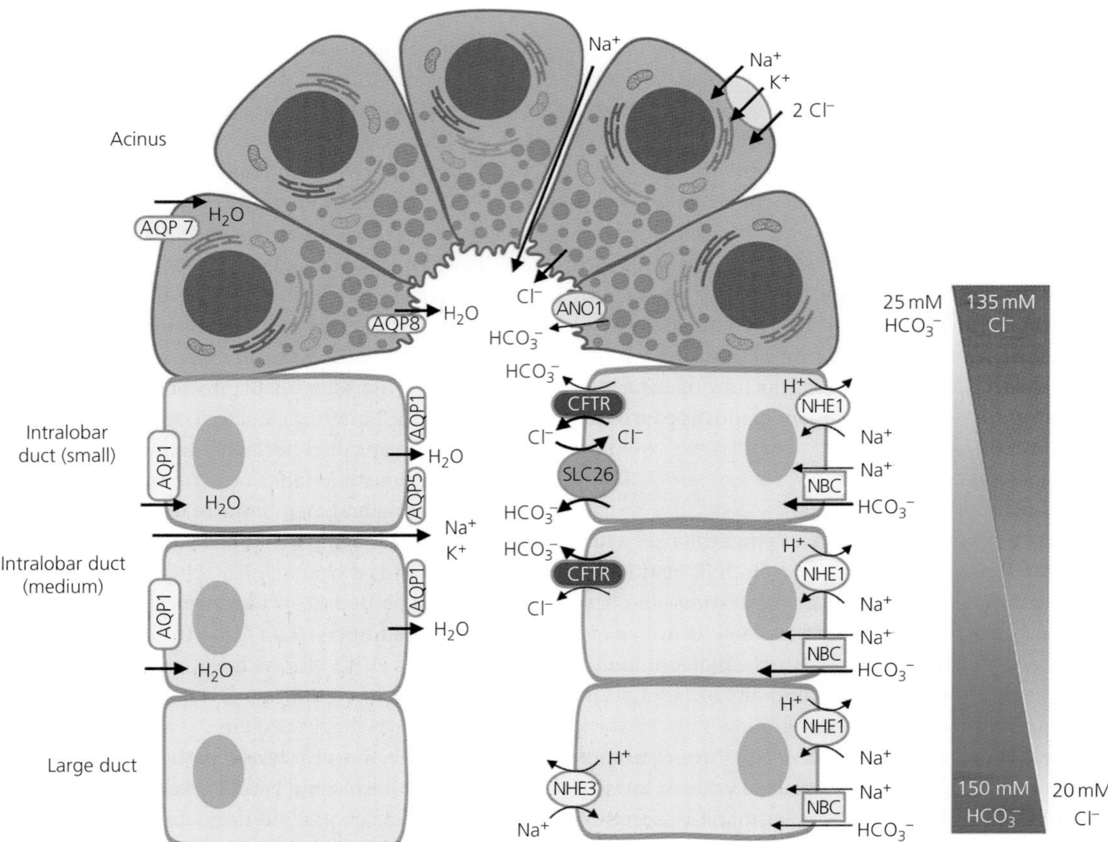

Figure 18.2 Secretion of water and ions in the exocrine pancreas. The major ion exchangers, channels, or pumps and their general localization are indicated. Some of the secreted HCO_3^- is exchanged with Cl^- in the distal ducts (not shown); however, overall an overall net gain of HCO_3^- and reabsorption of Cl^- is achieved by the time the pancreatic fluid reaches the large ducts of the pancreas. AQP, aquaporin; CFTR, cystic fibrosis transmembrane conductance regulator; NBC, Na^+/HCO_3^- cotransporter; NHE, Na^+/H^+ exchanger. Modified from Lee et al. 2012 [26] and Ishiguro et al. 2012 [32].

Cl^- concentration, CFTR increases HCO_3^- uptake by the pNBC exchanger. The transcellular secretion of anions sets up an electronegative potential across the luminal membrane of the duct cells, enabling cations such as Na^+ and K^+ to reach the pancreatic juice by moving passively through the paracellular pathway [34]. A cellular model depicting these events and in the pancreatic ductal cells is shown in Figure 18.3.

It is important to note that most of our current knowledge in pancreatic ion secretion comes from model organisms, such as guinea pigs, rats, cats, dogs, and mice. Current work in the pancreatic field is shifting toward establishing human organoid models to verify and update our current understanding of the pancreatic function in humans [35]. Indeed, even in a mouse organoid model of a pancreas, new Cl^- and Na^+ channels are being identified [21], highlighting the complexity and importance of pancreatic ion secretion.

Enzyme secretion

Human pancreatic fluid is composed of approximately 0.7–10% protein, depending on the food load. Most of these proteins are enzymes and proenzymes, with the remaining proteins consisting of plasma proteins, trypsin inhibitors, and mucoproteins. The four major enzyme/proenzyme groups are amylolytic, lipolytic, proteolytic, and nucleolytic. The proteolytic enzymes, which include trypsinogen, chymotrypsinogen, procarboxypeptidase, and proelastase, account for the majority of enzymes in the pancreatic fluid and are secreted as inactive proenzymes to prevent intraductal enzyme activation and pancreas autodigestion. After entering the intestinal lumen, trypsinogen is converted by enterokinase, a brush border enzyme on the duodenal mucosa, to the biologically active trypsin. Trypsin then autocatalytically activates trypsinogen and converts chymotrypsinogen and other proteolytic enzymes into their active forms.

Pancreatic fluid also contains a low concentration of trypsin inhibitor, a polypeptide that, at pH 3–7, combines with and inactivates trypsin in a 1:1 ratio, while partially inhibiting chymotrypsin. Trypsin inhibitor in the pancreas is thought to protect against autodigestion by the small amounts of active trypsin within the pancreas duct. Because trypsin inhibitor is present in minute quantities, the proteolytic activity of fully activated pancreatic juice in the intestinal lumen is not inhibited.

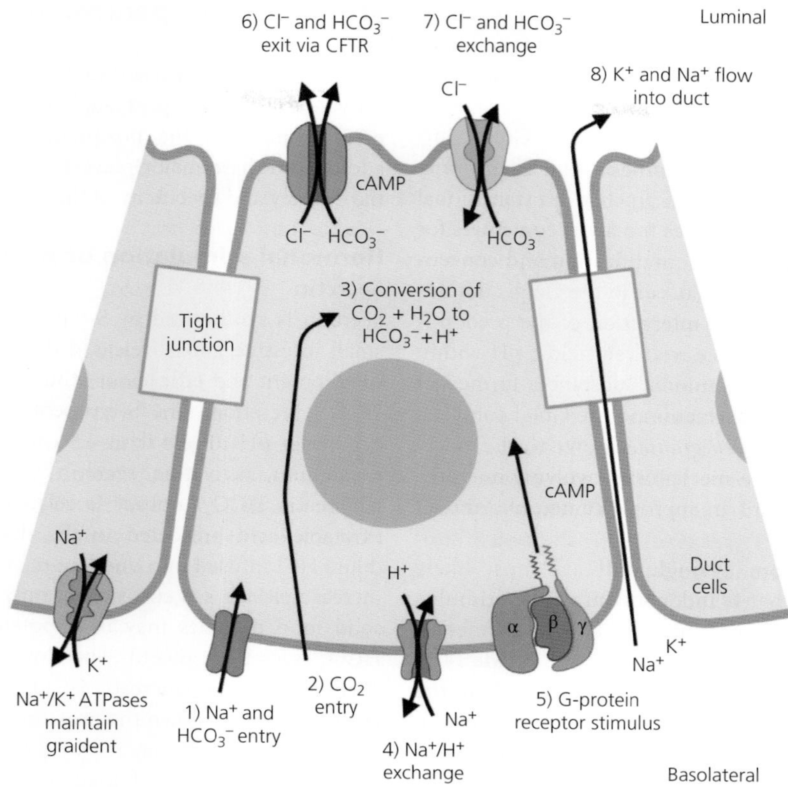

Figure 18.3 Cellular model of ion transport events in the pancreatic duct cells that cause the primary secretion of pancreatic juice. Beginning in the lower left corner of the diagram: 1) HCO_3^- enters the cell by means of the Na^+–HCO_3^- cotransporter on the basolateral membrane; 2) CO_2 enters the cell to be 3) hydrolyzed with H_2O by carbonic anhydrase to HCO_3^- and H^+; 4) H^+ moves out of the cell by the Na^+/H^+ exchanger or the vascular H^+-ATPase, contributing to the provision of intracellular HCO_3^-; 5) the secretin-activated G protein receptor signals production of cyclic adenosine monophosphate (cAMP); 6) the apical membrane contains the cystic fibrosis transmembrane conductance regulator (CFTR) anion channel; 7) a Cl^-/HCO_3^- exchanger (SLC26A6), which together secrete HCO^-_3; and 8) the transcellular electrical gradient between blood and luminal fluid drives the secretion of Na^+ and K^+. Meanwhile, the Na^+/K^+-ATPase maintains the electrochemical gradient required for Na^+–HCO_3^- cotransport at the basolateral membrane.

Unlike the proteolytic enzymes, the enzymes amylase, lipase, and ribonuclease are secreted by the acinar cells in their active forms. In addition to the enzyme lipase, pancreatic fluid also contains a peptide called colipase, which is essential for optimal lipolysis [36–38]. It facilitates lipase action by binding with bile salt/lipid surfaces to increase the interaction of lipase with triglycerides [38]. In the presence of bile salts, colipase reduces the optimal pH of lipase from 8.5 to 6.5, which is the approximate average pH in the proximal intestine.

Pancreatic enzymes are synthesized within acinar cells and packaged into zymogen granules [8,39]. The entire process, from synthesis to the point at which the enzymes are ready to be secreted into the lumen, takes about 50 minutes. According to the classical model by Palade [39], amino acids are actively transported into the acinar cells and translocated to the ribosomes for protein synthesis. Pancreatic enzymes and a variety of other exportable proteins are synthesized with an amino acid terminal peptide extension called the signal peptide [40,41]. Translation is temporarily halted when the signal peptide emerges from the ribosomal subunit and interacts with the signal recognition particle, which is associated with the large ribosomal subunit. The protein–RNA complexes then interact with another protein on the endoplasmic reticulum (ER) membrane known as the docking protein [41]. Interaction between the signal recognition particle and the docking protein permits the completion of translocation of the nascent polypeptide into the rough ER lumen, after which the ribosomal subunits, signal recognition particle, and RNA dissociate from the ER. Meanwhile the protein crosses the ER membrane into the cisternae. This process ensures that potentially destructive proteins, such as proteinases, cannot gain access to the cytosolic compartment. It also provides a mechanism for sorting the proteins not destined for export from those that must be processed by the ER–Golgi pathway and packaged for later secretion [42]. Inside the cisternae of the ER, pancreatic secretory proteins interact with chaperones and undergo conformational changes, assuming tertiary and, in some cases, quaternary structures. Abnormalities in this process result in the ER stress response, which includes translational attenuation, increased expression and function of chaperones and foldases, and activation of ER-associated protein degradation [43–45].

The transfer of pancreatic enzyme proteins to the Golgi complex occurs within 20–30 minutes of synthesis [46]. Their transfer is mediated by vesicles arising from pinched-off transitional elements of the rough ER, which act as transport containers for the secretory proteins [46]. Further modification and concentration of the proteins and peptides occur in the Golgi complex and may result partially from the interaction of the predominantly basic secretory proteins, the relatively acidic pH within the Golgi complex, and the polyanionic substances formed in the Golgi complex [47]. After formation in the Golgi complex, secretory vesicles called *zymogen granules* move to the apical portions of the acinar cell by a mechanism involving microtubules, where they remain until an appropriate neurohormonal stimulus triggers exocytosis.

Pancreatic enzymes from a single cell are most likely secreted in a fixed ratio that is independent of the stimulus but is determined at the time of synthesis. This phenomenon may be explained by the model by Scheele and Palade [48], which proposes that secretory proteins are mixed in the zymogen granule and discharged in parallel. Under certain experimental conditions, nonparallel secretion of different pancreatic enzymes may occur. In humans, increasing the doses of CCK infusion results in pancreatic secretion characterized by a greater concentration of lipase than chymotrypsin, both of which are higher than the amylase concentration [49]. Similar nonparallel enzyme secretion was reported by Dagorn and colleagues [50–52] in both rats and humans. Enzyme content and the ratio of amylase to chymotrypsin vary widely among granules taken from the same animal. Together, this supports the hypothesis that populations of acinar cells have differing mixtures of enzyme content, and that nonparallel secretion is the result of exocytosis from these heterogeneous cell populations within the pancreas [53,54].

Although controversy exists regarding short-term deviations from parallel secretion, there is little doubt that long-term adaptation of enzymes to diet occurs in animals. Adaptation has been observed in rats fed diets that contain a preponderance of carbohydrate, protein, or fat, as indicated by increases in the pancreatic content, mRNA levels, and rates of synthesis and secretion of the appropriate class of hydrolytic enzymes by the pancreas [55,56]. Moreover, the dietary effects are thought to be mediated by specific hormones. For example, insulin mediates the expression and release of amylase [57], whereas CCK released by the presence of protein in the duodenum increases the synthesis of proteases [58]. Although such adaptive changes have not been reported in humans [59], preferential secretion of lipase occurs in the chronic renal failure associated with increased plasma CCK levels, which is consistent with adaptive changes found in animals chronically given CCK [60].

Stimulation of pancreatic secretion

The hormones secretin and CCK and the vagovagal reflexes that activate cholinergic postganglionic neurons in the pancreas mediate most of the postprandial pancreatic secretion. In addition to these major players, additional hormones mediate the efficacy and specificity of the major stimulatory pathways.

Hormonal stimulation of pancreatic secretion

Secretin

Secretin is synthesized by S-type enteroendocrine cells in the small intestine and is released during a meal. Secretin is the most potent and efficacious stimulant of pancreatic fluid and HCO_3^- secretion. The S-type enteroendocrine cells detect a decline in pH to less than 4.5 caused by chyme entering the duodenum, activating secretin secretion [61]. At pH <4.5, pancreatic HCO_3^- output is related to the total amount of titratable acid presented to the duodenum. Experimentally, dilute HCl infused into duodenum at a rate of 2–4 mmol/h can increase plasma secretin significantly [62–64]. Acids bound to solid food particles may be a potent stimulus of pancreatic HCO_3^- secretion [65,66]. The slow diffusion of H^+ from the chyme stimulates pancreatic HCO_3^- secretion by triggering H^+ receptors further down the proximal small intestine. Studies of rats indicate that H^+ may release a secretin-releasing factor into the upper intestinal lumen to stimulate the release of secretin [65–67]. In addition, secretin-producing cells have acid-sensing ion channels belonging to the transient receptor potential channel family [68]. Therefore, luminal acid likely stimulates the release of secretin by more than one mechanism.

Other factors may play a role in the postprandial release of secretin. Among the major components of a mixed meal, fatty acids such as oleic acid and other digestive products of fat can increase plasma secretin levels and pancreatic HCO_3^- secretion [69,70]. Bile in the upper small intestine can also stimulate the release of secretin [71]. Some question the physiological importance of nongastric acid factors instigating the release of secretin. However, it is likely that these factors, like fatty acids, stimulate secretin release of HCO_3^- to buffer the pH for ideal function of amylase and lipase. Indeed, postprandial plasma secretin does not increase in subjects with achlorhydria or in healthy subjects in whom meal-induced acid secretion is neutralized with $NaHCO_3$. In addition, injection of anti-secretin antibodies in rats reduces HCO_3^- and enzyme pancreatic secretion [72], lending credence to this hypothesis.

Secretin given in a dose that mimics postprandial plasma secretin levels can stimulate pancreatic secretion of water, enzymes, and HCO_3^- [73,74]. With the use of radiolabeled ligand ^{125}I-labeled secretin and autoradiography, a secretin-binding site was demonstrated on pancreatic acini and duct cells of dogs [75]. In clinical practice, exogenous administration of physiological doses of secretin is often used to measure exocrine pancreatic function by measuring pancreatic juice bicarbonate concentration via the endoscopic pancreatic function test [76,77].

Physiological doses of secretin on exocrine pancreatic secretion are highly sensitive to atropine. In fact, vagal afferent pathways can mediate the effect of secretin on pancreatic exocrine secretion, gastric acid secretion, and motility [78,79]. This highlights the close interplay between endocrine and neurological stimulation of the exocrine pancreas, which will be discussed later in this chapter.

Cholecystokinin

CCK is another gastrointestinal hormone that has an important role in pancreatic secretion. It is synthesized in the I-type enteroendocrine cell and released by hydrolytic products of digestion, such as amino acids and fatty acids [80]. Undigested fat is ineffective at stimulating I cells, but products of lipolysis, such as fatty acids, are potent stimulants of CCK release [75]. Factors that influence the CCK response to fatty acids include their chain length, degree of saturation, concentration, and total load [81].

Several mechanisms drive nutrient stimulation of CCK secretion. In species such as the rat, in which feedback inhibition of pancreatic enzyme secretion occurs, CCK release may be mediated by a trypsin-sensitive CCK-releasing peptide [82]. Peptone (a mixture of large peptides produced by peptic digestion of protein) in the duodenum stimulates serotonin (5-hydroxytryptamine [5-HT]) release from the intestinal enterochromaffin cells. The serotonin released into the submucosa activates the sensory substance P neurons. Signals are then transmitted to cholinergic interneurons and to epithelial CCK-releasing peptide-containing cells by way of cholinergic secretomotor neurons [82]. In this manner, CCK release may be controlled by the level of active proteases in the duodenum [83–85]. Proteins, the major food stimulants of CCK secretion in rats, may bind or inhibit intraluminal endopeptidases, which would otherwise inactivate the CCK-releasing peptide [86]. This process was replicated in humans through intraduodenal infusion of bovine trypsin, which inhibited secretion of CCK and, consequently, pancreatic enzymes [87]. Recent work validating the stimulants needed for the secretion of CCK have focused on CCK secretion from purified CCK-producing cells. In these cells, amino acids stimulated CCK release by binding to a Ca^{2+}-sensing receptor, [88] while fatty acids bound to specific G protein-coupled fatty acid receptors to release CCK [89].

Under fasting conditions, the plasma CCK levels are low, averaging about 1 pmol/L in humans [87,90,91]. After the ingestion of a meal rich in protein and fat, CCK concentrations increase to 6–8 pmol/L within 10–30 minutes, followed by a gradual decline to basal levels over the following 3 hours [87,91]. Several molecular forms of CCK appear to be released into the circulation postprandially, including CCK-8, CCK-12, CCK-22, CCK-33, and CCK-58 [92]. Their relative contributions to the CCK activity of plasma in basal and stimulated states are species dependent. CCK-58 is the predominant form in dogs and humans and is the most potent isoform of CCK in the pancreatic feedback reflex [93–95].

CCK plays an important role in the stimulation of pancreatic enzyme secretion during the postprandial state. Infusing physiological doses of CCK produces the same levels of pancreatic enzyme secretion as during the postprandial state [96]. Furthermore, the administration of the potent CCK antagonists lorglumide or MK-329 produces a 50–60% inhibition of meal-stimulated pancreatic secretion in humans [97].

CCK can also stimulate fluid and HCO_3^- secretion [98]. The direct effect on HCO_3^- secretion is weak, but the interaction is physiologically relevant because CCK potentiates the action of secretin on the pancreas [99]. However, secretin does not potentiate CCK-stimulated pancreatic enzyme secretion [96,100,101].

CCK acts on the pancreas both indirectly, through a cholinergic neuron-mediated mechanism, and directly on the acinar cells themselves. *In vivo* studies of humans and dogs have shown that pancreatic secretion stimulated by CCK can be blocked by atropine, implying the involvement of cholinergic pathways [102–104]. Furthermore, enzyme output in response to low doses of CCK is reduced in patients after vagotomy compared with normal controls [105] (Figure 18.4). Intestinal CCK-containing I cells have pseudopod-like processes that extend from the basal surface and penetrate the basal lamina to reach the subepithelial enteric neuron [106]. This provides an enteroendocrine–neuronal connection, allowing CCK to act like a neurotransmitter.

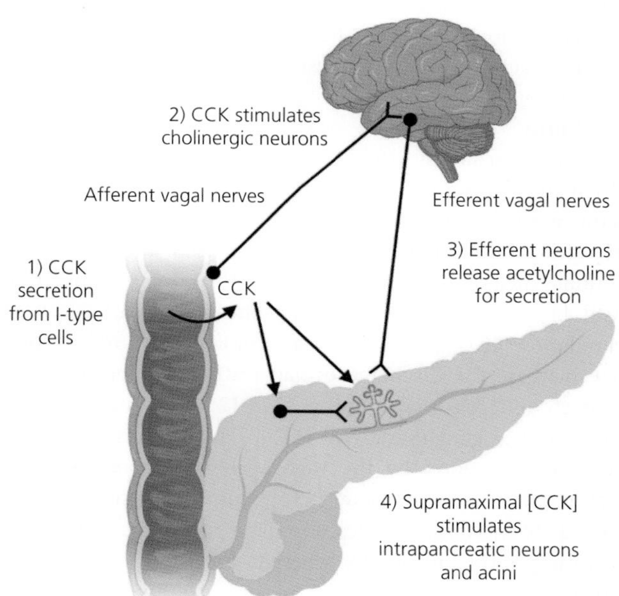

Figure 18.4 Sites and mechanisms of action of cholecystokinin (CCK) to stimulate pancreatic enzyme secretion. 1) Chyme entering the duodenum stimulates secretion of CCK from I-type enteroendocrine cells. 2) CCK stimulates afferent vagal nerves innervating intestinal wall. 3) Subsequent stimulation of efferent vagal nerves causes release of acetylcholine onto muscarinic receptors on acini to stimulate secretion. 4) Supramaximal concentrations of CCK stimulate intrapancreatic neurons, as well as directly stimulate acinar cells for secretion.

In both pancreatic acini and vagal nerves, CCK receptors exist in both high-affinity and low-affinity states [107–109]. Under physiological conditions, CCK appears to act on the pancreas through high-affinity vagal CCK_1 receptors, formerly known as CCK-A receptors, to mediate pancreatic enzyme secretion [108,110]. Both M_1 and M_3 muscarinic receptors on the pancreatic acini appear to mediate these responses [110,111].

Research has begun to reveal the mechanisms by which hormones, especially CCK and insulin, regulate protein synthesis at a translational level and account for the stimulation of pancreatic digestive enzyme synthesis with each meal. CCK and insulin can stimulate acinar protein synthesis in vitro without changes in mRNA [112]. These actions appear primarily at the initiation step in translation and involve the rate-limiting initiation factor eIF4E. Acinar secretagogues and insulin, through a series of steps most likely involving phosphatidylinositol 3-kinase (PI3K) and the mammalian target of rapamycin (mTOR), lead to the phosphorylation of the binding protein for eIF4E, and thereby the release of eIF4E, which becomes incorporated into a complex that binds the mRNA 5′ cap [113,114]. Through a separate pathway, CCK also activates the phosphorylation of eIF4E, which increases its affinity for the mRNA cap, the modified guanine nucleotide added to the 5′ end of messenger RNA shortly after the start of transcription. In addition, mTOR activates ribosomal S6 kinase ($p70^{S6K}$), thereby phosphorylating S6, which increases the translation of messages with terminal polypyrimidine tracts [115]. The importance of the mTOR pathway is shown by the fact that rapamycin can block the stimulation of acinar protein synthesis in vitro; [113].

Serotonin

Intestinal serotonin (5-HT) also mediates postprandial pancreatic secretion [116–119]. The major source of serotonin in the intestine is the gastrointestinal mucosal enterochromaffin cells [120]. Serotonin is released in response to a wide variety of stimuli, including acidification of the duodenum [120], instillation of hypertonic sugar solutions [116,121], vagal stimulation [122], and mechanical stimulation [123]. Serotonin may increase the discharge of vagal afferent fibers from the stomach and proximal intestine [124,125] and may stimulate vagal nodose ganglia activity [117]. This in turn stimulates pancreatic secretion by the vagovagal reflex mediated by a cholinergic efferent pathway [116]. Luminal factors, such as osmolarity and disaccharides, stimulate pancreatic secretion by activating $5\text{-}HT_3$ receptors, whereas mechanical stimulation activates both $5\text{-}HT_3$ and $5\text{-}HT_2$ receptors on mucosal afferent fibers in the intestine to induce pancreatic secretion [116].

Pharmacological depletion of serotonin stores using *p*-chlorophenylalanine, an inhibitor of serotonin synthesis, abolishes neuronal responses stimulated by luminal factors [117]. In contrast, pretreatment with 5,7-dihydroxytryptamine, a specific neurotoxin that destroys neurons that contain serotonin without affecting mucosal cells that contain serotonin, does not affect these responses [117]. Therefore, the vagal responses to luminal osmolarity and the digestion products of carbohydrates depend on the release of endogenous serotonin from the mucosal enterochromaffin cells, which acts on $5\text{-}HT_3$ receptors on vagal afferent fibers. In this manner, serotonin acts as a paracrine substance to stimulate pancreatic secretion by a vagal cholinergic pathway. These primary vagal afferent neurons contain mainly glutamate and substance P [126], which, on release, stimulate the nuclear tractus solitarius for sensory stimulation and, subsequently, the dorsal motor nucleus of the vagus in the brainstem to mediate postprandial enzyme secretion. An example of this would be CCK neurohormonal activation of pancreatic secretion.

There is synergistic interaction between vagal CCK and serotonin receptors in mediating pancreatic secretion [119]. Infusion of a subthreshold dose of CCK potentiates vagovagal reflex-mediated pancreatic secretion stimulated by luminal serotonin-dependent factors. Discharge recordings of single vagal primary afferent neurons innervating the duodenum reveal distinct groups of nodose ganglia neurons that possess only high- or low-affinity CCK receptors or $5\text{-}HT_3$ receptors [127]. In one group of nodose neurons, previous exposure to luminal serotonin enhanced the subsequent response to a subthreshold dose of CCK. This synergistic interaction shows how a small increase in the plasma CCK level is enough to produce robust postprandial pancreatic secretion.

Pancreatic HCO_3^- secretion and secretin release in response to duodenal acidification are inhibited by the $5\text{-}HT_3$ antagonist ondansetron and the $5\text{-}HT_2$ antagonist ketanserin [128]. In addition, pancreatic fluid and HCO^-_3 secretion stimulated by exogenous secretin are also inhibited by these serotonin antagonists. Thus, serotonin appears to regulate acid-stimulated exocrine pancreatic secretion by modulating both the release and action of secretin through two serotonin receptor subtypes.

Insulin

Insulin modulates exocrine pancreatic secretion through the acini-islet-acinar axis [7,129]. Insulin amplifies the pancreatic secretory response to secretin and CCK [130]. Ouabain, an inhibitor of Na^+,K^+-ATPase activity, abolishes the stimulatory action of insulin [131]. Pancreatic secretion of water, HCO_3^-, and enzymes stimulated by a meal or by a combined intravenous administration of physiological doses of secretin and CCK-8 is markedly reduced when the circulating insulin is neutralized with an anti-insulin antibody [132].

Pancreatic enzyme secretion is often reduced in patients with diabetes who have no overt pancreatic disease [133]. However, the mechanism responsible for this abnormality is not clear. Insulin has a trophic action on the pancreatic acinar cells and plays an important role in protein synthesis. This may account for the reduced pancreatic enzyme secretion in subjects with diabetes. Due to the close proximity of β-islet cells and acinar cells, insulin most likely enhances the release of amylase from acinar cells to facilitate sugar digestion and absorption [129].

Ghrelin

Ghrelin is a mediator of appetite and has been shown to stimulate pancreatic secretion [134]. It acts as an endogenous ligand for the growth hormone secretagogue receptor [135–140], which is found throughout the body, including pancreatic islet cells. Growth hormone secretagogue receptor is expressed in rat pancreas and in the exocrine pancreatic-derived cell line, AR42J [141]. Administration of ghrelin causes a dose-dependent increase in intracellular Ca^{2+} by binding to this receptor [142]. In acute pancreatitis, ghrelin becomes expressed in acinar cells, leading to an overload of intracellular Ca^{2+} [143] and blocking restoration of intracellular Ca^{2+} for exocytosis, as discussed later.

In vivo rat studies indicate that ghrelin also stimulates pancreatic secretion by acting centrally through the vagal cholinergic pathways [134]. Pretreatment with atropine or hexamethonium or acute vagotomy, but not perivagal application of capsaicin, abolishes pancreatic secretion in response to intravenous administration of ghrelin. Furthermore, selective ablation of the area postrema blocks the pancreatic response to ghrelin. These observations suggest that circulating ghrelin gains access to the brainstem vagal circuitry by way of the area postrema in the medulla oblongata of the brainstem, which represents the primary target on which peripheral ghrelin may act as an endocrine substance to stimulate pancreatic secretion; however, this has not yet been proved. Physiologically, ghrelin most likely acts on the pancreas to prepare it for secretion in advance of the postprandial state.

Nitric oxide

Nitric oxide (NO), a ubiquitous substance that is present in neurons and vascular endothelium [144], also appears to play a significant role in regulating pancreatic secretion. In rats, inhibition of NO production with N^G-nitro-l-arginine methyl ester (L-NAME) reduces basal amylase secretion by 60% [145,146]. A nitric oxide synthase (NOS) inhibitor also inhibits pancreatic enzyme secretion in response to a meal, duodenal infusion of acid, or intravenous infusion of physiological doses of secretin or CCK in rats [145]. In humans, L-NAME dose-dependently reduced pancreatic enzyme secretion stimulated by secretin and cerulein [147]. Because NOS inhibition has no effect on amylase release nor on the changes in intracellular Ca^{2+} concentration in rat pancreatic acini stimulated by carbachol and CCK-8 [148], the effect of NO on exocrine pancreatic secretion is likely to be indirectly mediated pancreatic secretion by nervous stimulation.

Administration of L-NAME reduces CCK-stimulated pancreatic microvascular blood flow and at the same time decreases pancreatic fluid and protein output in cats [149]. This observation may have clinical importance, because inadequate blood flow has been associated with pancreatitis. Administration of a NOS inhibitor in rats with edematous pancreatitis causes a decrease in pancreatic blood flow and exacerbates cerulein-induced pancreatitis [150].

Bombesin

Bombesin, also known as gastrin-releasing peptide (GRP), may stimulate pancreatic secretions that contain small amounts of HCO_3^- and high concentrations of enzymes in humans [151,152]. Bombesin can act directly on the pancreas through specific receptors identified on pancreatic acinar cells [153]. In rat pancreatic lobules, bombesin stimulates amylase release through the release of acetylcholine (ACh) from intralobular nerves [154,155]. However, the stimulatory action of bombesin on pancreatic secretion in humans is not affected by the CCK receptor antagonist loxiglumide [156]. The physiological importance of bombesin in pancreatic secretion is uncertain because bombesin receptor antagonists do not influence postprandial enzyme secretion in intact rats [157].

Neural stimulation of pancreatic secretion

Parasympathetic nervous system

The pancreas is innervated by parasympathetic and sympathetic nerve fibers (see also Chapter 7). The parasympathetic fibers pass to the pancreas directly through the vagus nerves and indirectly through the celiac ganglion, the splanchnic nerves, and through the intramural plexus of the duodenum.

The functional effect of vagal stimulation of the pancreas varies greatly by species and experimental conditions [119,158]. In humans, the vagus nerve appears to mediate pancreatic secretion. Insulin-induced hypoglycemia, which is presumed to stimulate the vagus centrally, augments secretin-stimulated pancreatic protein output and HCO_3^- output [159,160]. Vagotomy reduces the HCO_3^- secretory response to exogenous hormones. Maximal enzyme secretion is not significantly affected by vagotomy, but the sensitivity of the pancreas to submaximal doses of CCK is decreased [105]. As such, vagotomy reduces pancreatic enzyme responses to intestinal stimulants and food [105,161].

Baroreceptors and osmoreceptors reside in the human duodenum. Stimulation of these receptors by distention or administration of a hyperosmolar solution elicits a pancreatic enzyme response mediated by cholinergic neurons [162,163]. Increased firing rates in peripheral afferent vagal neurons and in central sites have been recorded after gastric distention and intestinal perfusion with amino acids and HCl [164–166].

Neurotransmitters and hormones in the central nervous system are likely involved in the regulation of pancreatic secretion. Microinjection of a thyrotropin-releasing hormone analog in the dorsal vagal complex of rats stimulates pancreatic juice flow and enzyme output in a dose-dependent manner [167]. Vagotomy and atropine eliminate this stimulatory effect, indicating that thyrotropin-releasing hormone modulates pancreatic exocrine secretion through the dorsal vagal complex. This highlights the role of the hypothalamus in mediating pancreatic secretions to coordinate pancreatic function with multiple other metabolic processes regulated by endocrine secretions.

Hypothalamic regulation

Although pancreatic secretion is mediated mainly by vagovagal reflexes located within the brainstem, these reflexes are modulated by input from higher centers, such as the hypothalamus and amygdala [168–170]. After chronic decerebration, which interrupts the entire descending neural input to the brainstem, there is a 35% reduction in basal pancreatic protein output and a 40% decrease in pancreatic protein secretion stimulated by luminal perfusion of peptone [138]. This suggests that the forebrain plays a significant role in modulating the vagovagal reflex in the brainstem.

The hypothalamus receives a wide variety of convergent afferent inputs from the viscera and regulates autonomic activities by modulating neuronal input to the autonomic preganglionic neurons. Cholinergic pathways in the hypothalamus play a major role in the stimulation of pancreatic secretion. Microinjection of methscopolamine, a blood–brain barrier-impermeant cholinergic muscarinic receptor antagonist, into the lateral hypothalamic nucleus or paraventricular nucleus produces inhibitory effects like those observed after surgical decerebration [138]. In contrast, microinjection of ACh into the lateral hypothalamic nucleus and the paraventricular nucleus evokes 46% and 40% increases in pancreatic secretion over baseline, respectively [138]. Selective lesions of the lateral septal cholinergic neurons or lateral parabrachial nucleus produce significant inhibition of peptone-induced pancreatic secretion [138]. Hence cholinergic inputs from the lateral septal cholinergic neurons and the parabrachial nucleus to the hypothalamus can modulate vagal pancreatic efferent nerve activities and pancreatic secretion evoked by the vagovagal reflex.

Enteropancreatic neural reflex

Functional and anatomic enteropancreatic neural connections have been demonstrated with neurons in the ganglia of the myenteric plexuses of the stomach and the duodenum projecting directly to the pancreas [139]. Activation of the myenteric neurons in the duodenum can influence the exocrine and endocrine pancreatic functions. These enteropancreatic neural pathways have cholinergic and serotonergic components [139,140,171]. The cholinergic nerves from the duodenum stimulate intrapancreatic neurons through nicotinic synapses. Abundant enteropancreatic serotonergic axons may inhibit pancreatic secretion through presynaptic 5-HT_{1P} receptors on cholinergic nerves [139]. More recently, studies on the enteropancreatic neural reflex have established regulation of glucose metabolism through this pathway [172]. Further studies are needed to define the physiological role of the serotonergic enteropancreatic neural pathways.

Peptidergic nervous system

Immunocytochemical studies have revealed several peptides in the nerve cell bodies and fibers of the pancreas. Among these, nerve fibers and cell bodies that contain vasoactive intestinal polypeptide (VIP) are the most abundant [173]. The fibers that contain VIP appear to surround the cell bodies of intrapancreatic ganglia and innervate duct cells.

In pigs, VIP is the neurotransmitter that mediates much of the HCO_3^- secretory response by electrical stimulation to the vagus nerve [174]. However, the importance of intrapancreatic neuronal VIP as a regulator of pancreatic secretion may be species specific. VIP is a weak partial agonist in humans [174]. In some species, VIP may also induce pancreatic vasodilation and increase blood flow in response to the activation of the exocrine pancreas, providing the nutrients needed to maintain HCO_3^- secretion and enzyme formation.

Other peptidergic neurotransmitters identified in the pancreas include the carboxyl-terminal tetrapeptide of gastrin/CCK [175,176], GRP [177], substance P [175,176], peptide histidine isoleucine [178], neurotensin [179], neuropeptide Y [178], enkephalin [175,176], and calcitonin gene-related peptide (CGRP) [180]. Pharmacological studies have found that CCK, gastrin, substance P, GRP, peptide histidine isoleucine, neurotensin, and CGRP stimulate, whereas enkephalin and neuropeptide Y inhibit, exocrine pancreatic secretion. The physiological relevance of these peptides in mediating pancreatic exocrine secretion remains unknown.

Intracellular control of pancreatic secretion

Receptors

Most of the hormones and neurotransmitters that stimulate pancreatic secretion do so by directly regulating acinar and duct cells, but some may regulate indirectly by their actions on nerves or blood vessels. By using amylase secretion as the criterion for functional response, studies on the effects of agonists and antagonists on secretion have identified the presence of specific receptors for hormones and neurotransmitters on acinar cells. Electron microscopic autoradiography and confocal fluorescence microscopy have localized most ligand binding to receptors at the basolateral membrane domain, although some bound ligands are internalized by an energy-dependent process [181,182]. Acinar cells from a variety of species, including humans, have receptors for CCK, ACh, VIP, and secretin. Duct cells bear the same receptors as acinar cells with the addition of receptors for ATP and substance P. Although acinar cells and duct cells express similar receptors, acinar cells are more responsive to ACh and CCK, whereas duct cells are more responsive to secretin and VIP.

Receptors for major pancreatic secretagogues belong to the G protein receptor family. This family is characterized structurally by seven hydrophobic transmembrane domains and functionally by their interaction with guanine nucleotide binding [183]. Structure–function studies with site-directed mutagenesis and chimeric receptors have established some general principles of function for the G protein-coupled receptor family [183–185]. In brief, the transmembrane segments form a pocket for the binding of small molecules, such as ACh, while the extracellular amino-terminal end and loops may be important in the interactions with peptide molecules. The third cytoplasmic loop, projecting between the fifth and sixth transmembrane domains, is thought to interact with the appropriate G protein. The serine and threonine residues in the cytoplasmic carboxyl-terminal end may be involved with regulatory mechanisms, such as desensitization and downregulation by phosphorylation.

Transmembrane signaling

Although all membrane receptors are integral proteins spanning the lipid bilayer, the pancreatic secretagogue receptors convey information by interacting with G proteins. These G proteins are heterotrimeric proteins with unique α subunits and a smaller number of shared $\beta\gamma$ subunits [186]. Acinar cells possess α_s and α_i subunits, which respectively stimulate and inhibit adenylate cyclase. Acinar cells also possess α_q and α_{11} subunits that activate phospholipase C [187] and $\alpha_{12/13}$ subunits that activate RhoA [188]. The full complement of α and $\beta\gamma$ subunits expressed in acinar and duct cells and their functions are still being determined.

The membrane-bound G proteins work together with effector enzymes to generate intracellular messengers. There are two major effector enzymes in acinar cell membranes: polyphosphoinositide-specific phospholipase C, which cleaves phosphatidylinositol 4,5-bisphosphate, producing the intracellular signaling molecules inositol-1,4,5-trisphosphate (IP_3) and 1,2-diacylglycerol (DAG); and adenylyl cyclase, which converts ATP to cAMP [189]. There are multiple forms of phospholipase C expressed in mammalian cells. The β_1 and β_3 forms specifically are differentially activated in rat acini by CCK, carbachol, and bombesin [190,191]; however, the physiological relevance of this differential activation is still unclear.

Adenylyl cyclase is another integral membrane protein with multiple membrane-spanning domains with an intracellular catalytic site [192]. Multiple isoforms of adenylyl cyclase exist, some of which are also regulated by G protein $\beta\gamma$ subunits, Ca^{2+}, and protein kinases. In particular, the AC6 isoform in both acini and ducts is important for the formation of intracellular messenger cAMP and activation of protein kinase A [193].

Other membrane effectors in the pancreas may include CD38, the mammalian ADP–ribosyl cyclase that synthesizes cyclic ADP ribose and nicotinic acid adenine dinucleotide phosphate (NAADP) [194], phosphatidylcholine-specific phospholipase C [195] and phospholipase D [196], Na^+/H^+ ion exchanger, and various ion channels. However, these may be regulated by intracellular messengers rather than directly by G proteins.

Intracellular messengers

The major intracellular messengers involved in the regulation of pancreatic secretion are IP_3, Ca^{2+}, DAG, and cAMP [189,197]. IP_3, Ca^{2+}, and DAG are predominant in the acinar cell. Their concentration in the cell increases after the activation of phosphoinositide-specific phospholipase C by CCK and ACh. cAMP is the predominant messenger in duct cells, where it is produced in response to secretin and VIP.

When acinar cells are stimulated with ACh or CCK, phosphatidylinositol 4,5-bisphosphate and PIP levels decline rapidly as the activated phospholipase C converts them to IP_3 and DAG. IP_3 binds to its receptor on intracellular Ca^{2+} storage sites to trigger the release of Ca^{2+} into the cytoplasm. The IP_3 receptors are large 260-kD molecules that form tetramers, which function as ligand-gated ion channels. The sensitivity of the IP_3 receptors to IP_3 is regulated by phosphorylation of the IP_3 receptor [198], G protein $\beta\gamma$ subunits, Ca^{2+}, and thiol-reactive reagents, as well as ingested compounds such as caffeine [199]. Modulation of IP_3 sensitivity may explain how certain agonists can release Ca^{2+} without a measurable increase in IP_3 levels. Modulation of Ca^{2+} release by IP_3 has been directly correlated with secretion in both acinar and interlobular ducts [199].

Another homologous-gated intracellular Ca^{2+} channel, the ryanodine receptor [RyR], well known as the Ca^{2+} release channel in muscle, is also present in acinar cells. RyRs open in response to Ca^{2+} to allow for a Ca^{2+}-induced Ca^{2+} release. IP_3 receptors are present primarily in the apical pole of the cell just under the luminal membrane and partially overlapping the submembranous network of actin filaments [200,201], whereas RyRs have a more diffuse distribution and are found throughout the acinar cells.

The ER functions as the Ca^{2+} storage organelle within the acinar cells [202,203]. However, some investigators have suggested the existence of multiple populations of vesicles with different Ca^{2+} transport or release characteristics [204]. For example, CCK receptors, but not muscarinic receptors, release Ca^{2+} from a lysosome-related (acidic) organelle through the action of NAADP [205]. The mechanism of NAADP production and the receptor on which NAADP acts remain poorly understood.

High concentrations of CCK, bombesin, and cholinergic analogs cause a rapid 5-fold to 10-fold increase of $[Ca^{2+}]_i$, which declines over 2–5 minutes to a level slightly above the basal level (Figure 18.5). This initial large increase is essentially independent of extracellular Ca^{2+}. However, a small, sustained plateau increase in $[Ca^{2+}]_i$ depends on extracellular Ca^{2+}. The initial increase shows a similar time course and dependence on secretagogue concentrations, as does the rapid increase in IP_3, and is presumed to depend on IP_3-stimulated or NAADP-stimulated release of intracellular Ca^{2+}. Much of this released Ca^{2+} is extruded from the cell [197,206]. All three of the major phospholipase C-activating secretagogues (i.e., CCK, ACh, and bombesin) access the same intracellular pool of Ca^{2+}, and after maximal stimulation by one agonist, the addition of another has no augmenting effect. After removal of the agonist, the IP_3-releasable intracellular pool refills over 2–10 minutes as Ca^{2+} is taken up from the medium and resequestered. Emptying calcium from the cells likely creates a refractory period to allow the acinar cells to generate more digestive enzymes for subsequent secretion stimulation.

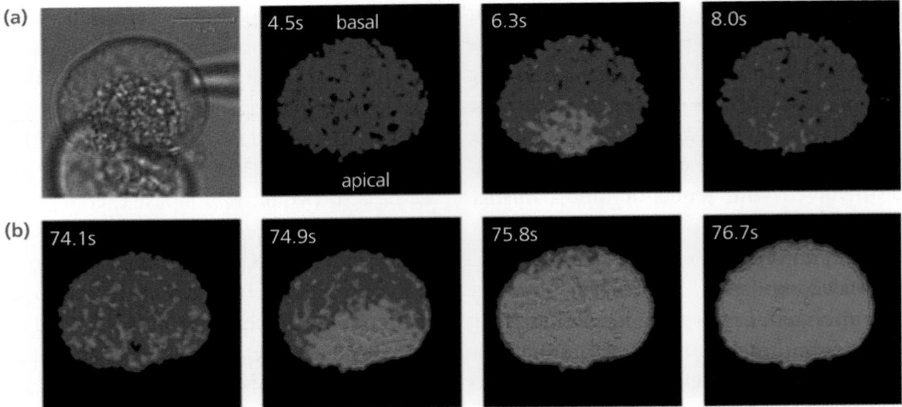

Figure 18.5 Secretagogue-induced increase in intracellular Ca^{2+} in a pancreatic acinar cell. The cell is loaded with Fluo3, a fluorescent Ca^{2+} probe, and the intensity of fluorescence is color coded so that low resting Ca^{2+} is blue and as Ca^{2+} increases the increased fluorescence shifts to warmer color, with red being the highest. **(a)** The cell was stimulated with a low dose of acetylcholine, and the Ca^{2+} increase was localized to the apical pole. **(b)** A higher concentration of acetylcholine led to a global increase but still was initiated in the apical pole. *Source:* Ashby and Tepikin 2002 [211]. Reproduced with permission of the American Physiological Society.

The sustained increase in $[Ca^{2+}]_i$ and the refilling of the intracellular Ca^{2+} pool involve activation of a Ca^{2+} entry mechanism mediated by phospholipase C. Recordings of the $[Ca^{2+}]_i$ of individual cells of rat and mouse acini have revealed that low physiological concentrations of CCK, ACh, and bombesin induce a different pattern of Ca^{2+} increase characterized by oscillations in $[Ca^{2+}]_i$ increases [207–209]. Superimposed on any steady increase are phasic increases in $[Ca^{2+}]$ of up to 250 nmol/L (see Figure 18.5). These oscillations, which occur between one and four times per minute, are relatively independent of extracellular Ca^{2+} and involve the release and reuptake from the intracellular Ca^{2+} stores. That $[Ca^{2+}]$ oscillations can drive secretion is shown by the fact that the CCK analog JMV-180 induces Ca^{2+} oscillations and can stimulate maximal amylase release [210].

Confocal digital imaging of Ca^{2+} in acinar cells has shown that the $[Ca^{2+}]_i$ increase is initiated in the apical pole of the cell and then spreads basally (Figure 18.5b) [211–213]. The response to lower agonist concentrations is a series of local increases in Ca^{2+} in the apical pole of the cell [214]. Improved imaging techniques have shown that local Ca^{2+} spikes are the result of pacemaker hotspots of Ca^{2+} release that entrain the surrounding region [215,216]. Interestingly, in the same cell, different agonists (i.e., carbachol, CCK, and bombesin) initiate $[Ca^{2+}]$ increases in distinct apical areas, indicating compartmentalization of signaling [217,218]. Further complicating the process, phosphorylation of IP_3 receptors by protein kinase A can modulate the pattern of Ca^{2+} increase [219].

Besides the apical-to-basal spread of Ca^{2+} in intact acini, Ca^{2+} waves appear to spread from cell to cell around an acinus. Gap junction coupling remains open as these Ca^{2+} waves spread but closes in response to supramaximal stimulation [220]. This cell-to-cell spread [220] increases the cellular sensitivity, allowing acinar activation and subsequent enzyme secretion to be triggered by the most sensitive cell.

Mediators of intracellular messengers

The intracellular messengers active in pancreatic acinar cells have been identified and characterized, but much less is known about the mechanisms by which they act to induce granule exocytosis, fluid secretion, protein synthesis, and gene expression. Although other mechanisms may exist, all of the intracellular messengers activate protein kinases and phosphatases, and thereby regulate the state of protein phosphorylation.

More than 25 phosphoproteins (not all identified) that are regulated by pancreatic secretagogues have been visualized by two-dimensional electrophoresis in pancreatic acini [221,222]. Some are uniquely regulated by Ca^{2+}, phorbol esters, or cAMP, whereas others are regulated by multiple second messengers.

Several Ca^{2+}-activated kinases have been identified in pancreatic acinar cells, including Ca^{2+}/calmodulin-activated type II kinase (CaMKII), CaMKIII, and myosin light chain kinase [197]. Although some kinases are highly substrate specific, CaMKII is a multifunctional kinase that phosphorylates multiple proteins in intracellular signaling pathways. Although typically stimulated by an influx of extracellular Ca^{2+} through bombesin or carbachol stimulation, CaMKII is also activated by CCK in a Ca^{2+}-independent fashion [223]. Protein kinase C, originally described as a Ca^{2+}-, phospholipid-, and DAG-dependent kinase [224], is also present in acinar cells to mediate intracellular signaling.

In addition to Ca^{2+} and cAMP-activated kinases, acinar cells contain the major classes of serine/threonine protein phosphatases (i.e., PP1, PP2A, and PP2B) [225,226]. Whereas some of these phosphatases are constitutively active and are involved in reversing phosphorylation induced by kinases, PP2B, or calcineurin, is specifically activated by Ca^{2+} through calmodulin. Calcineurin, which is activated by pancreatic secretagogues such as CCK, is essential for digestive enzyme synthesis in acinar cells, particularly at the complex formation and elongation steps of protein synthesis [227].

Stimulation of secretion normally involves synergistic interactions among intracellular messengers. In the case of ACh and CCK, this includes interactions between Ca^{2+}-activated and DAG-activated pathways. Agents such as VIP and secretin, which increase cAMP, interact at the postintracellular messenger level. Proteins localized on the granule and luminal plasma membrane and several soluble and cytoskeletal proteins may be involved in exocytosis. In pancreatic duct cells, the same intracellular messengers and kinases may regulate ion pumps, carriers, and channels involved in fluid and electrolyte secretion. The role of intracellular messengers and effectors in pancreatic enzyme secretion is summarized in Figure 18.6.

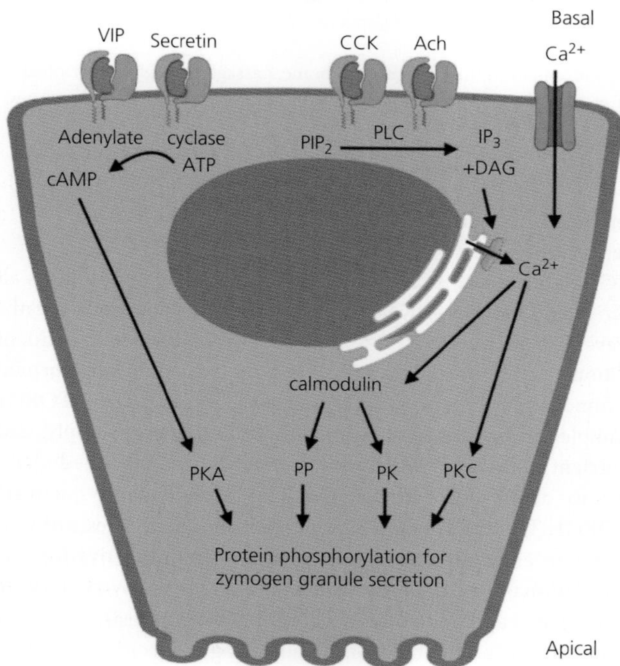

Figure 18.6 Stimulus–secretion coupling of pancreatic acinar cell protein secretion followed two major pathways. In one pathway, receptors for vasoactive intestinal polypeptide (VIP) and secretin couple through a G protein (G_s) to activate adenylate cyclase to produce cyclic adenosine monophosphate (cAMP), which subsequently activates protein kinase A (PKA). In the other and quantitatively more important pathway, receptors for cholecystokinin (CCK) and acetylcholine (ACh) couple through G proteins of the G_q family to activate phospholipase C (PLC). This enzyme hydrolyzes phosphatidylinositol 4,5-bisphosphate (PIP_2) to produce inositol 1,4,5-trisphosphate (IP_3) and diacylglycerol (DAG). IP_3 releases Ca^{2+} from intracellular stores in the endoplasmic reticulum, activating Ca^{2+} influx across the plasma membrane. Ca^{2+} binds to calmodulin to activate several protein kinases (PKs) and one protein phosphatase (PP). DAG with Ca^{2+} activates several species of protein kinase C (PKC). This battery of protein kinases and phosphatases, by altering the phosphorylation of diverse proteins, brings about the secretion of digestive enzymes and other cellular effects on growth and metabolism. ATP, adenosine triphosphate.

Zymogen granules and exocytosis

The final steps in secretion from acinar cells involve fusion of the zymogen granules with the apical membrane of the acinar cell. This fusion event shares basic mechanisms with other membrane fusion events from yeast to neurons to gastric parietal cells. Two types of proteins, SNARE proteins and small G proteins of the Rab family, play prominent roles (Figure 18.7). There are more than 35 mammalian SNARE proteins that share a homologous SNARE motif. In the SNARE paradigm, transport vesicles destined to fuse with another membrane possess a set of proteins, termed v-SNARE, that interact with proteins on the target membrane, termed t-SNARE, and with soluble attachment factors [228,229]. SNARE proteins associate into a complex of four helical bundles with SNAP25. Assembly of the SNARE protein complex is completed by zipper-like mechanism that may provide the energy for membrane fusion [230]. Modulatory proteins, such as Munc18 and Munc13, regulate the assembly of SNARE complexes, while synaptotagmin 1 provides the Ca^{2+} sensitivity to regulate this process [231].

Synaptobrevins/VAMP2, VAMP3, and VAMP8, which act as v-SNAREs on synaptic vesicles, are present on zymogen granules [232,233]. The t-SNAREs on the plasma membrane of neurons include SNAP25 and syntaxin. Multiple isoforms of syntaxin in acini have been identified and are differentially localized throughout the cell. Syntaxin 2 is present on the apical plasma membrane, while other syntaxins are present on the basolateral membranes and zymogen granules [234]. v-SNAREs VAMP2 and VAMP8 are essential to the secretion of enzymes such as amylase and trypsin. VAMP2 mediates the first 2 minutes of enzyme secretion, whereas VAMP8 is responsible for extended secretion of digestive enzymes [235,236]. In addition, syntaxin 2 is required for Ca^{2+}-stimulated secretion. A complex of VAMP2 and syntaxin 2 was involved in primary granule fusion. Meanwhile, a complex of VAMP8 and syntaxin3 is involved in compound exocytosis, a process where a zymogen granule in the cell fuses with the membrane that has undergone primary fusion with the plasma membrane [237]. VAMP-8-mediated secretion can be inhibited by supramaximal CCK stimulation, resulting in accumulation of activated trypsin in acinar cells, leading to pancreatitis [236].

Munc18, a regulatory protein for exocytosis, has isoforms that are compartmentalized in acinar cells. Munc18b is present on the apical membrane and participates in primary and compound exocytosis [237]. Conversely, Munc18c is present on the basolateral membrane and forms a complex with syntaxin 4 for basolateral exocytosis, which is increased in experimental pancreatitis in response to high concentrations of CCK and is enhanced by ethanol [238,239].

Several Rab proteins have been identified on zymogen granules by immunocytochemistry and mass spectrometry [240]. Rab3 was found on zymogen granules in pancreas [241,242], and overexpression of Rab3D in acinar cells of transgenic mice enhanced a component of amylase secretion [243], indicating that Rab3D activation may be rate limiting for secretion. Rab27B

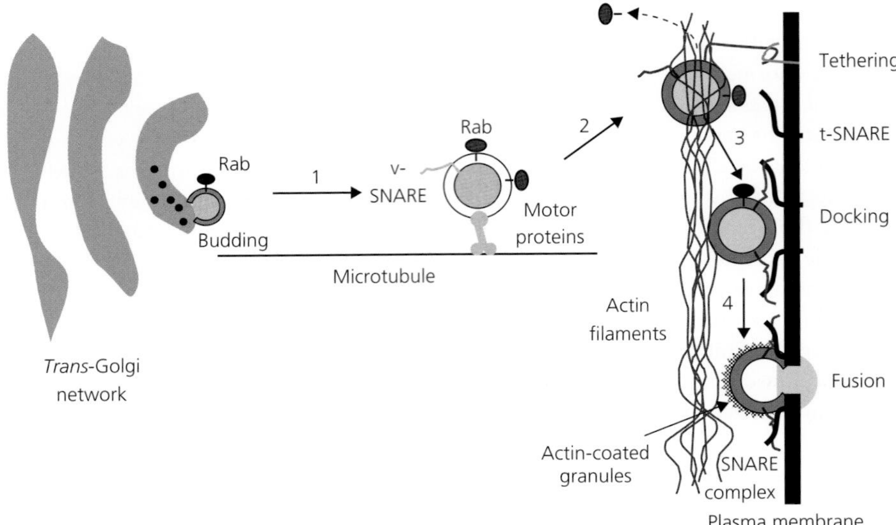

Figure 18.7 Model of the steps in the exocytosis of zymogen granules, including movement to the lumenal membrane, passage through the terminal web of actin filaments, tethering, docking, and fusion. Note, for simplicity, that not all of the SNARE complex proteins are shown. *Source:* Williams and Yule 2012 [197]. Reproduced with permission of Elsevier.

has been related to secretion in acini and in other cells [240]. RAP1, another small G protein present on the zymogen granules, is also involved in secretion by mediating movement of the zymogen granules [244]. It belongs to the RAS family and is activated by secretagogues [244].

In addition to SNARE, VAMP, and Rab proteins, the exocyst complex family of proteins is essential to targeting vesicles to docking sites on the plasma membrane. In particular, EXOC3, also known as Sec6, expression in acinar cells is essential for the transportation and docking of zymogen granules [245]. Recently, decreased expression of this protein has been associated with poor prognosis in patients with pancreatic cancer, in addition to several other proteins that regulate endocrine secretion [246]. Further investigation into this complex, as well as other zymogen granule transportation and docking proteins, is a promising field to understanding the development of pancreatic diseases, such as pancreatitis, cancer, and diabetes mellitus.

A current area of investigation is the identity of the effector proteins activated by small G proteins on zymogen granules. These include synaptotagmin-like proteins and Noc2 [247]. The actin cytoskeleton is also believed to be involved in exocytosis as a barrier, preventing premature secretion, as well as providing the scaffold for movement of zymogen granules to the cell surface. The former role may be mediated by an actin network under the plasma membrane [248]. Filamentous actin has been shown to form a coating on fused granules and may serve to promote the exit of granule contents after fusion occurs [249]. The small G proteins RhoA and Rac1 have been shown to be activated by secretagogues and to regulate secretion, presumably through effects on actin polymerization for vesicle exocytosis [250].

Intracellular pathways leading to growth and gene regulation

CCK, muscarinic ACh, insulin, and growth factor receptors all activate the PI3K–AKT–mTOR (target of rapamycin) pathway [113]. Although PI3K and AKT may have independent actions, the central pathway consists of two complexes formed around mTOR, namely, TORC1 and TORC2. The TORC1 complex integrates signals from receptors, energy supply, and nutrient sufficiency. Amino acids, especially branched-chain amino acids, such as leucine, can independently activate TORC1. TORC1 kinase activity promotes the synthesis of new digestive enzymes on a meal-to-meal basis by activating the translational machinery and in the longer term by promoting ribosome and membrane lipid biosynthesis, cellular hypertrophy, and inhibition of autophagy. Specific molecular targets of TORC1 include p70S6K, which phosphorylates ribosomal protein S6, initiation factor 4E binding protein, and elongation factor 2 kinase to activate elongation factor 2 [251].

The second pathway is the activation of focal adhesion kinase, or $p125^{FAK}$, and its downstream target, paxillin. Both molecules are associated with the cytoskeleton and, in other cells, are activated by growth factors and integrins. CCK stimulates the increase of the tyrosine phosphorylation of $p125^{FAK}$ and paxillin in rat acini [252]. This effect is probably mediated by the small G protein Rho. Adaptive growth of the pancreas can occur in response to nutrients and hormones to synthesize more digestive enzymes and prevent malabsorption. Both a high-protein diet and hyperphagia induced by pregnancy, lactation, or cold exposure can induce pancreatic growth. Much of this growth is mediated by CCK and can be modeled by adding trypsin inhibitor to increase endogenous CCK release.

Information has emerged on the intracellular signaling pathways responsible for this growth (Figure 18.6). CCK, in addition to increasing intracellular Ca^{2+}, activates three MAPK pathways and the PI3K–AKT–mTOR pathway. Most of these can be activated *in vivo* by adding trypsin inhibitor [189]. Ca^{2+}-activated phosphatase, calcineurin, is key for growth. These growth pathways are important regulators of mRNA transcription and translation. Calcineurin-mediated dephosphorylation of the transcription factor NFAT (nuclear factor of activated T cells) is associated with adaptive growth in cardiac and skeletal muscle. CCK leads to NFAT activation in pancreatic acini, which may have similar function. High levels of protein can also stimulate pancreatic growth and can do so without CCK [253]. This effect was mediated by direct activation of the mTOR pathway by amino acids. Conversely, the absence of dietary protein shuts down TORC1 in acinar cells and leads to acinar cell atrophy and a decrease in digestive enzyme synthesis [254].

Inhibition of pancreatic secretion

The regulation of pancreatic secretion depends on a balance between inhibitory and stimulatory influences on the gland, which are exerted through hormones and the autonomic nervous system.

Inhibitory phase of pancreatic secretion

Postprandial pancreatic enzyme secretion is under both hormonal and neural control. Distention of the duodenum and administration of hyperosmolar solutions into the duodenum each elicit pancreatic enzyme secretion without raising plasma CCK levels; however, addition of trypsin significantly decreases plasma CCK [163]. This stimulatory effect is inhibited by atropine, suggesting that it is cholinergically mediated. In contrast with amino acid-stimulated pancreatic enzyme secretion, pancreatic responses to stimulation by volume or osmolality in the duodenum are not suppressed by trypsin [163]. This indicates that feedback regulation of pancreatic secretion by trypsin is stimulus specific and is mediated by inhibiting CCK release.

Hormonal inhibition of pancreatic secretion

Somatostatin

Somatostatin acts as both a paracrine factor and a true hormone in inhibiting pancreatic secretion. D cells in the pancreas, as well as cells in the upper gastrointestinal tract and the central nervous system, secrete somatostatin to inhibit secretion. Somatostatin interacts with a variety of receptors on acinar cells, dorsal root ganglia, and islets of Langerhans, and on the nerves of the peripheral and central nervous systems. In humans, pharmacological doses of somatostatin cause marked inhibition of CCK-stimulated pancreatic enzyme secretion and modest inhibition of secretin-stimulated HCO_3^- secretion [5,255,256]. Studies in rats show that somatostatin inhibits 2-deoxy-D-glucose- and CCK-evoked pancreatic enzyme secretion through a vagal pathway [257]. Somatostatin does not act on peripheral vagal afferent or efferent pathways, or directly on pancreatic acinar cells. Rather, it exerts its inhibitory action at a central vagal site [257]. Indeed, somatostatin injected into the dorsal vagal complex significantly inhibits pancreatic secretion evoked by intravenous administration of CCK-8 or 2-deoxy-D-glucose. This suggests that somatostatin probably acts through the dorsal vagal complex in the brainstem to inhibit pancreatic secretion. Studies in the perfused canine pancreas have demonstrated that somatostatin is released from the pancreas during perfusion with high concentrations of amino acids or glucose [258], suggesting a paracrine negative feedback effect on the exocrine pancreas as well (Figure 18.8).

Six somatostatin receptor (SSTR) subtypes are expressed from five genes differentially throughout the body. Activation of SSTR2 inhibits exocrine pancreatic secretion, whereas SSTR5 inhibits insulin release. Injection of the SSRT2 agonist seglitide into the dorsal vagal complex inhibits CCK-8/2-deoxy-D-glucose-induced pancreatic protein secretion, indicating that the central action of somatostatin is mediated by SSTR2 on the dorsal vagal complex [259]. In addition, SSTR2A has been localized to acinar cells and to glucagon and PP immunoreactive islet cells [260]. Although somatostatin is one

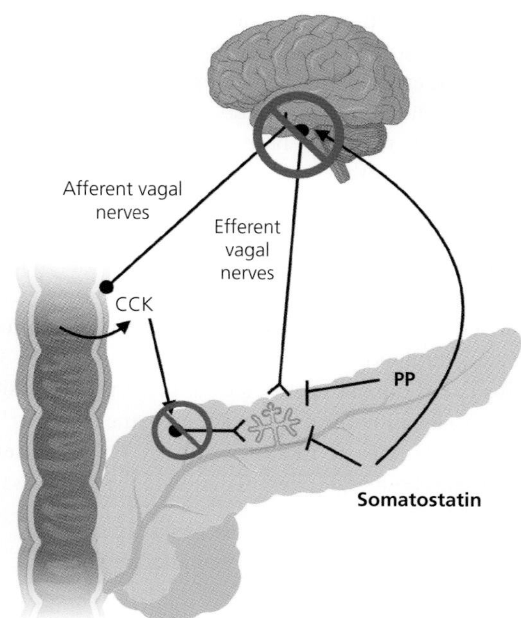

Figure 18.8 Inhibition of pancreatic secretion. An influx of amino acids and fatty acids in the blood stimulates the secretion of somatostatin and pancreatic polypeptide (PP) from the pancreas. Somatostatin moves through the bloodstream to inhibit cholecystokinin (CCK) signaling in the dorsal vagal complex in the brain, as well as the intrapancreatic nerves within the pancreas. In addition, somatostatin directly inhibits secretion from acinar cells. PP acts directly on the acinar cells to inhibit secretion.

of the few peptides to inhibit pancreatic secretion in an isolated pancreas, the role of the acinar cell SSTR may be to modulate the nonparallel secretion of digestive enzymes [261] rather than to inhibit secretion.

Pancreatic polypeptide

PP, a peptide closely related to peptide YY, is another hormone that may play an important role in inhibiting pancreatic exocrine secretion. PP is found in the islets of Langerhans and between the acinar cells of the exocrine pancreas [262]. Secretion of PP is governed mainly by a cholinergic mechanism [263]. Postprandial release of PP is mediated by a long vagovagal reflex and short local cholinergic pathways [263]. Vagal cholinergic activity is the most powerful stimulant of PP release, and it is also key to most other stimulations of the PP cell [263].

Infusion of physiological concentrations of PP inhibits basal and stimulated pancreatic secretion [6,264]. In vivo, PP appears to act preferentially by inhibiting vagal stimulation [265]. In vitro, PP inhibits pancreatic enzyme secretion by the presynaptic modulation of ACh release [266]. Because its secretion is under cholinergic control and it acts by interfering with cholinergic transmission, PP is an ideal candidate to modulate pancreatic secretion stimulated by the cholinergic enteropancreatic reflex. After ingestion of a meal, the enteropancreatic reflex is activated to stimulate pancreatic enzyme secretion and PP release. PP inhibits cholinergic transmission and reduces pancreatic enzyme secretion. Therefore, PP may participate in the negative feedback regulation of pancreatic enzyme secretion activated by the enteropancreatic reflex.

The primary target of PP appears to be the central nervous system [267]. PP receptors have been identified in discrete locations in the hypothalamus, limbic system, brainstem, and other central locations with the use of receptor autoradiography [268]. In contrast, mRNA for PP is almost undetectable [269], suggesting that peripheral PP modulates central neural function at sites that have an incomplete blood–brain barrier. Microinjection of PP into the dorsal motor nucleus of the vagus inhibits pancreatic secretion stimulated by CCK, suggesting that the dorsal motor nucleus of the vagus is a site for neural feedback inhibition of pancreatic exocrine secretion [270]. Hence PP likely acts at multiple sites in the brainstem to modulate vagal cholinergic efferent output to the pancreas [271].

Antisecretory factor

Antisecretory factor (AF) was originally described as an antidiarrheal factor by mediating intestinal fluid hypersecretion [272,273]. Recently, Nawrot-Porabka et al. [274] showed that treating rats with AF drastically reduced amylase and fluid output from the pancreas. AF's inhibition of pancreatic secretion was blocked in rats with capsaicin-deactivated sensory nerves. Although this study was performed in rats, it is likely that this protein functions similarly in humans because it is known to inhibit secretion in the intestinal tract.

Enteroglucagon

Intrajejunal perfusion of hypertonic glucose produces dose-related inhibition of secretin-stimulated pancreatic fluid and HCO_3^- secretion in humans [275,276]. This may be mediated by the release of enteroglucagon by the intestinal tract [277]. Infusion of oxyntomodulin, a 37-amino acid, glucagon-containing peptide isolated from porcine lower intestine, inhibits basal and cerulein-stimulated pancreatic secretion of HCO_3^- and enzymes [277]. This intestinal glucagon is 10 times more potent than pancreatic glucagon at inhibiting exocrine secretion.

Substance P

Substance P inhibits pancreatic HCO_3^- secretion evoked by secretin. This is mediated by neurokinin 2 and 3 receptors, which are expressed in pancreatic duct cells [278]. The receptor of substance P contributes to blocking the cAMP generation stimulated by VIP or secretin [279]. This prevents the Cl^-/HCO_3^- exchanger on the apical membrane from functioning to secrete HCO_3^- into the duct lumen.

Ileocolonic hormones

In humans, nutrients such as lipids in the colon inhibit CCK-stimulated pancreatic enzyme and HCO_3^- output [280]. These late postprandial events may function as physiological signals to reduce exocrine pancreatic secretion after the digestion and absorption of nutrients are complete. The inhibitory effect of nutrients in the distal gut on pancreatic secretion appears to be independent of the vagus and splanchnic nerves [281]. Cross-circulation studies in the rat have shown that a humoral factor mediates the inhibition of pancreatic enzyme secretion.

Harper and colleagues [281] used the term *pancreotone* to describe an inhibitory substance extracted from the colonic mucosa. The function of pancreotone is abolished when the extract is preincubated with trypsin, demonstrating it is a peptide. Peptide YY, a 36-amino acid peptide named for its amino- and carboxyl-terminal tyrosines, is ubiquitous in the distal small intestine, colon, and rectum [282]. This peptide is released by fat and, to a lesser degree, protein in the distal small intestine or colon. The infusion of this peptide in dogs significantly inhibits both basal and meal-stimulated pancreatic HCO_3^- and enzyme secretion [283]. Physiological experiments demonstrate that intraileal, but not colonic, carbohydrate increases plasma peptide YY levels and decreases amylase secretion in dogs [284].

In humans, ileal perfusion of carbohydrates inhibits exocrine pancreatic secretion. Glucagon-like peptide 1 (GLP-1), another ileal hormone, is elevated in the circulation during ileal infusion of carbohydrates. GLP-1 does not appear to act directly on the pancreas to inhibit exocrine secretion. Rather, GLP-1 acts on the dorsal vagal complex to inhibit pancreatic enzyme secretion [285].

Similarly, oxyntomodulin, which is released after ileal administration of nutrients, also inhibits pancreatic secretion by a vagal-dependent central mechanism [286]. Because oxyntomodulin does not interact with the receptor for glucagon or truncated GLP-1, its effects appear to involve an oxyntomodulin-specific receptor. Although the mediators of ileal carbohydrate-induced inhibition of exocrine pancreatic secretion have not been firmly identified, it appears that the action of these potential mediators is dependent on central neural pathways.

Other peptides

Although the list of peptides known to inhibit exocrine pancreatic secretion has expanded, little is known about how these other hormones or neurotransmitters inhibit pancreatic enzyme secretion. For example, glucagon is secreted from the endocrine pancreas after a meal and can inhibit secretin or CCK stimulation of the exocrine pancreas [3,287,288]; however, how it elicits this inhibition is not clear [289]. Many peptides suppress pancreatic enzyme secretion *in vivo* but do not act directly on the acinar cell to suppress enzyme release. Animal studies suggest that peptides such as CGRP, enkephalin, and pancreastatin inhibit pancreatic enzyme secretion by modulating cholinergic transmission, and most, if not all, act through a central vagal site [259,265,266,290–293]. Intraventricular administration of CGRP inhibitors stimulates basal pancreatic secretion in conscious rats, and this appears to be mediated by sympathetic noradrenergic efferents through the α-adrenergic receptor [294]. In contrast, CGRP in the central nervous system inhibits pancreatic enzyme secretion stimulated by 2-deoxy-d-glucose and CCK by modulating vagal parasympathetic outflow [286].

Neuronal inhibition of pancreatic secretion

Adrenergic innervation of the pancreas occurs mainly through the splanchnic nerves. Activation of the splanchnic nerves usually inhibits exocrine and endocrine pancreatic secretion; stimulation of the splanchnic nerves decreases and splanchnicectomy increases pancreatic secretion in response to pancreatic stimulants [99,175]. The pancreatic inhibitory effect of splanchnic nerve stimulation appears to be synchronous with, and dependent on, the intense vasoconstriction that is caused by stimulation of the α-adrenergic receptors on blood vessels. In isolated guinea pig pancreatic acini, norepinephrine alone has no effect on the response to submaximal concentrations of CCK-8 [295]. Meanwhile, epinephrine produces a modest stimulation of enzyme output in mouse and rat pancreas in vitro, and the stimulatory effect is inhibited by α-adrenergic receptor antagonists [296]. No clear pattern emerges from the many studies of regulation of exocrine pancreatic secretion by the sympathetic nervous system. The major role for the adrenergic mechanism appears to be the inhibition of fluid and HCO_3^- secretion, which is mediated partially by vasoconstriction.

Patterns of secretion

Basal secretion

Basal secretion rates of enzymes and HCO_3^- are about 10% and 2% of maximal levels, respectively, although there is considerable species variation. Basal pancreatic secretion appears to be driven by cholinergic tone because it is blocked by atropine but unaffected by CCK receptor antagonists. A pattern of cyclic change in basal pancreatic secretion has been demonstrated [297], and this is characterized by brief increases in HCO_3^- and enzyme secretion, which recur every 60–120 minutes during the interdigestive period. These bursts of pancreatic secretory activity are temporarily associated with periods of increased motor activity in the stomach and proximal intestine known as the interdigestive migrating motor complexes (IMMCs) [297,298].

Brief increases in gastric acid and biliary secretions are associated with the bursts of pancreatic secretion [297]. Plasma motilin and PP levels also fluctuate in phase with the interdigestive migrating motor complex [297,299]. The concentrations of pancreatic enzymes and bile acids during the transient surge of pancreaticobiliary secretion are similar to maximal postprandial outputs, although the concentrations diminish rapidly with the onset of type III duodenal motor activity [297,299]. It has been postulated that the cyclic secretion of pancreatic and biliary juice may be important in the digestion of residual food particles or cellular debris in the gastrointestinal tract during the interdigestive period.

The mechanism of control of the cyclic patterns of pancreatic secretion is unclear. Bursts of increased acid secretion are unlikely to be the principal mediators for the cyclic changes in pancreatic secretion, because removal of gastric acid by aspiration or through a fistula does not affect the pattern of interdigestive pancreatic secretion [297,299]. Infusion of motilin prematurely initiates cyclic pancreatic secretion and shortens the periodicity between peaks [300]. Administration of motilin antiserum abolishes the cyclic pattern of pancreatic secretion [301]. Cholinergic blockade with atropine also markedly decreases trypsin output and abolishes interdigestive motor activity or administration of ganglionic blockers. These observations suggest that motilin and the autonomic nervous system are responsible for the initiation of the cyclic pancreatic secretion that occurs during fasting.

Prandial and postprandial secretion

After the ingestion of a meal, the exocrine pancreas is stimulated to secrete enzymes and HCO_3^-. Total postprandial pancreatic output is about 60–70% of the output attained in response to maximal stimulation with intravenous infusion of CCK [96]. The stimulatory effect of a meal can be described by separating its components into cephalic, gastric, and intestinal phases (Table 18.1).

Table 18.1 Three phases of postprandial pancreatic secretion.

Phases	Maximal pancreatic response	Stimulants	Mediators
Cephalic	50%	Sight, smell, taste, eating	Vagal innervation
Gastric	10%? (not recorded in humans)	Distention	Vagal–cholinergic pathways
Intestinal	50–75%	Amino acids Fatty acids Ca^{2+}, H^+ Distention	Cholecystokinin, secretin Enteropancreatic reflexes Other hormones (?)

Cephalic phase

Pancreatic secretions rich in enzymes are stimulated by the sight, smell, and taste of appetizing food [302]. The contribution of the cephalic phase to the postprandial pancreatic enzyme secretion amounts to 50% of the maximal responses induced by exogenous secretin and CCK [303]. Meanwhile, the pancreatic response to sham feeding that activated gustatory receptors in the mouth lasts for only the duration of sham feeding [303]. This stimulation follows the vagus nerve as cholinergic stimulation of pancreatic secretion [304]. The CNS pathways mediating the cephalic phase of pancreatic secretion are not well defined but likely involve the dorsal and ventral anterior hypothalamus.

Gastric phase

Gastric distention increases the rate of pancreatic enzyme secretion [305–307]. Although the actual contribution of the gastric phase to the total postprandial pancreatic secretion has not been determined in humans, the magnitude of the distention-induced pancreatic response in dogs is about 10–20% of the maximal CCK response [305]. Vagotomy and atropine reduce or abolish the pancreatic response to gastric distention, suggesting that it is mainly mediated by vagal cholinergic pathways [306,307]. The mechanoreceptors in the body of the stomach sense distention and signal for stimulation of pancreatic secretion [307]. These observations suggest that the gastric phase is mediated mainly by gastropancreatic reflexes.

Gastric emptying helps determine the rate of delivery of acid and nutrients into the duodenum, thereby determining the pattern and magnitude of the intestinal phase of pancreatic secretion. Postprandial pancreatic enzyme secretion is often reduced in patients after gastric surgery because of a decrease in gastric emptying and acid production [161].

Intestinal phase

The intestinal phase is the most important phase of postprandial pancreatic secretion. The delivery of food into the small intestine stimulates pancreatic enzyme secretion to about 70% of the maximal level [161]. As discussed earlier, the major hormonal mediators of the intestinal phase of pancreatic secretion are secretin and CCK. Intestinal serotonin mediates postprandial pancreatic secretion through the vagal cholinergic pathway [116]. The intestinal mucosa has receptors for important vagal cholinergic reflexes that regulate pancreatic HCO_3^- and enzyme secretion.

The proximal intestine plays an important role in the stimulation of pancreatic HCO_3^- secretion, primarily by the release of secretin. As discussed earlier, although duodenal pH is the major regulator for the release of secretin, nonacid factors. such as fatty acids and bile. may also participate in the stimulation of pancreatic secretion.

Among the hydrolytic products of digestion, amino acids and fatty acids are potent stimulants of enzyme secretion but have only a weak effect on water and HCO_3^- secretion. Amino acid mixtures are more potent than fatty acids. Among the amino acids, only phenylalanine, valine, and methionine stimulate enzyme secretion in humans [308]. The pancreatic response to intestinal perfusion with amino acids above a concentration of 8 mmol/L depends on the total load administered [80]. In humans, the mechanisms responsible for the pancreatic response to amino acids are confined to the duodenum and jejunum because amino acid perfusion into the ileum elicits no response. Peptides that contain phenylalanine and tryptophan are effective stimulants of pancreatic secretion. These peptides generated by pepsin digestion of proteins may be more physiologically relevant because they are more abundant than individual amino acids in the lumen of the intestine after a meal.

Undigested fats are ineffective in stimulating pancreatic secretion, but fatty acids are potent pancreatic stimulants when present in micellar form [69]. Monoglycerols, the other product of lipolysis, also stimulates pancreatic secretion [69,75]. The chain length of fatty acids (indicated by the number of carbon [C] atoms in the chain) influences their potency in stimulating pancreatic secretion. In humans, the order of potency is C18 > C12 > C8 [81]. Other factors that influence the pancreatic response to fatty acids include the degree of saturation (that is, the number of double bonds between the individual carbon atoms of the fatty acid chain), the concentration, and the total load, as well as the concentration of bile salts relative to fatty acids [309]. In humans, intestinal perfusion of monoolein (10 mM) produces a pancreatic enzyme output greater than that stimulated by intestinal amino acids and almost equal to the maximal response to exogenous CCK [310].

The release of CCK and intestinal serotonin by nutrients and mechanical factors (as discussed in earlier parts of this chapter) also mediates the intestinal phase of pancreatic enzyme secretion. Plasma CCK levels increase after oral or intraduodenal administration of fat and protein or amino acids [87,90,91]. Administration of proglumide, a CCK receptor antagonist, partially inhibits pancreatic secretory responses to intestinally perfused amino acids and fat emulsions. In contrast, a wide variety of non-CCK-dependent stimuli, such as acid, carbohydrates, and mechanical factors, stimulate pancreatic secretion through intestinal serotonin [116,119]. Serotonin, in turn, stimulates submucosal vagal afferent fibers to evoke pancreatic exocrine secretion through a vagal cholinergic pathway. Increased firing rates in peripheral afferent neurons and in central sites have been recorded during intestinal perfusion with amino acids [165,311]. This finding, coupled with the observation that truncal vagotomy or administration of atropine markedly increases the latency of the pancreatic secretory response to intestinal nutrients, but not to CCK, indicates the participation of vagovagal cholinergic reflexes in the intestinal phase [311].

The human duodenum contains receptors for volume and osmolality that mediate pancreatic enzyme secretion. Volume distention or hyperosmolar solutions in the duodenum elicit pancreatic enzyme secretion by way of intestinal serotonin without increasing the plasma CCK levels [116,163]. This enzyme secretion is inhibited by atropine, suggesting mediation by cholinergic pathways [233]. The volumes of saline required to induce pancreatic secretion are as low as 1–5 mL/min, within the range observed postprandially in the duodenum. The degree of stimulation by volume receptor or osmoreceptor activation is 15–20% of the maximal enzyme response to CCK [162]. Therefore, both CCK- and non-CCK-dependent stimuli act in concert to mediate the intestinal phase of pancreatic secretion.

References are available at www.yamadagastro.com/textbook7e

Further reading

Argent B., Gray M., Steward M., et al. Cell physiology of pancreatic ducts. In: Johnson L. (ed.). Physiology of the Gastrointestinal Tract, 5th edn. San Diego, CA: Elsevier Academic Press, 2012: 1399.

Crozier S.J., D'Alecy L.G., Ernst S.A., et al. Molecular mechanisms of pancreatic dysfunction induced by protein malnutrition. Gastroenterology 2009;137:1093.

Chandra R., Liddle R.A. Neurohormonal regulation of pancreatic secretion. Curr Opin Gastroenterol 2012;28(5):483.

Lee M.G., Ohana E., Park H.W., et al. Molecular mechanism of pancreatic and salivary gland fluid and HCO3 secretion. Physiol Rev 2012;92:39.

Liddle R.A. Regulation of pancreatic secretion. In: Johnson L (ed.). Physiology of the Gastrointestinal Tract, 5th edn. San Diego, CA: Elsevier Academic Press, 2012: 1425.

Pierzynowski, S.G, Gregory, P.C., Filip, R., et al. Glucose homeostasis dependency on acini-islet-acinar (AIA) axis communication: a new possible pathophysiological hypothesis regarding diabetes mellitus. Nutr Diabetes 2018;8:55.

Williams J.A., Yule D. Stimulus-secretion coupling in pancreatic acinar cells. In: Johnson L. (ed.). Physiology of the Gastrointestinal Tract, 5th edn. San Diego: Elsevier Academic Press, 2012: 1361.

CHAPTER 19

Bile secretion and cholestasis

James E. Squires and Andrew P. Feranchak
University of Pittsburgh Medical Center, Children's Hospital of Pittsburgh, Pittsburgh, PA, USA

Chapter menu

Introduction

The importance of bile to human life has long been recognized. In fact, over 2000 years ago the Greek physician Hippocrates (460–370 SC) developed a medical theory based on four fundamental body fluids he termed "humors," consisting of phlegm, blood, "black bile," and "yellow bile" [1]. Over the last decade, utilizing complementary and sophisticated approaches in molecular biology, biochemistry, and electrophysiology, scientists have achieved profound insights into the basic mechanisms of hepatobiliary transport and bile formation. Furthermore, the recent identification of the genes and proteins involved has provided a molecular basis for our understanding of bile formation and, simultaneously, has afforded insight into the pathogenesis of many cholestatic liver diseases in which these proteins are defective or absent. Through this work, most of the major membrane transport proteins and channels responsible for the transport of organic solutes, such as bile acids, phospholipids, bilirubin, and the inorganic solutes, into bile have been identified. Importantly, these liver transporters and channels may serve as targets for the development of new therapies to augment and modify bile formation for the treatment of cholestatic liver disease.

This chapter will outline the cellular and molecular basis for bile production by the liver and highlight several specific disease entities due to defects in hepatobiliary transport, which lead directly to impaired bile formation.

Bile composition

Made continuously by the liver, bile is a complex biochemical mixture with a broad range of functions, including lipid digestion and absorption, excretion of endobiotics (bilirubin, steroids, heavy metals) and xenobiotics (drugs, environmental toxins, carcinogens), cholesterol elimination, regulation of gene transcription, and mucosal immunity. Approximately 700–800 mL/day of bile flows through the bile ducts of the liver and empties into the small intestine. Bile is mostly water, though it contains a complex composition of inorganic and organic solutes [2] (Figure 19.1). Organic solutes include bile acids, phospholipids, cholesterol, proteins, and bilirubin, while inorganic solutes are composed mostly of electrolytes [2,3].

Bile acids

Bile acids are the most abundant organic solute in bile and are synthesized from cholesterol through a series of complex chemical reactions catalyzed by specific hepatic enzymes [4]. The first enzymatic reaction introduces a hydroxyl group at position C-7 of the cholesterol ring, catalyzed by the enzyme cholesterol 7α-hydroxylase, which represents the rate-limiting step in bile acid synthesis. This initial step characterizes the classical or neutral pathway, while an initial 27-hydroxylation of cholesterol results in an alternate pathway known as the acidic pathway. Following a coordinated series of steps

Yamada's Textbook of Gastroenterology, Seventh Edition. Edited by Timothy C. Wang, Michael Camilleri, Benjamin Lebwohl, Anna S. Lok, William J. Sandborn, Kenneth K. Wang, and Gary D. Wu.

Companion website: www.yamadagastro.com/textbook7e

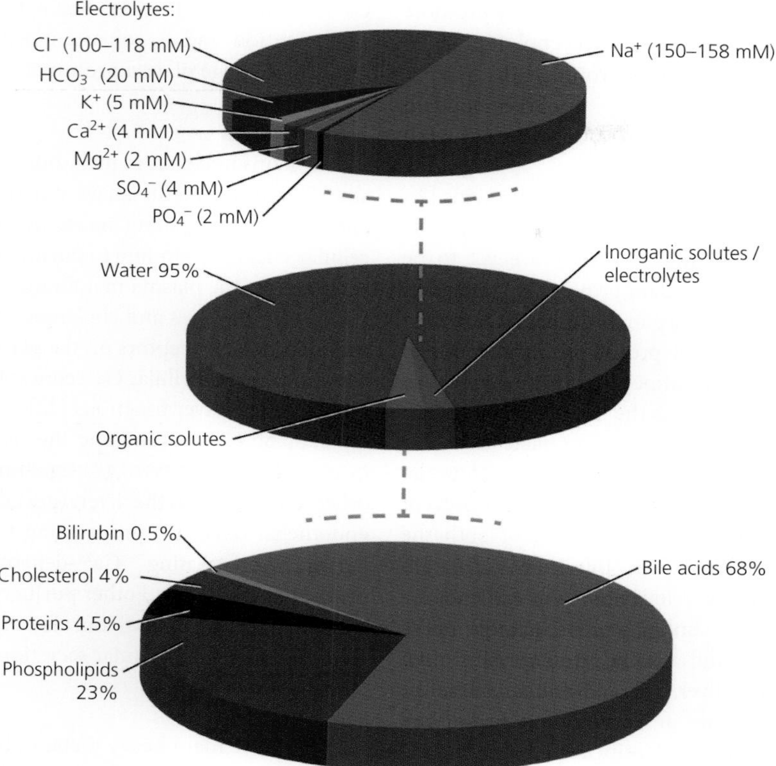

Figure 19.1 Bile composition. Composition of human bile during basal conditions. (Top) Electrolyte composition. (Bottom) Organic solutes. Data from [2,9].

involving side chain modification and hydroxylation, two primary bile acids are formed: cholic acid, a trihydroxy bile acid, and chenodeoxycholic acid, a dihydroxy bile acid [4]. In humans, cholic acid derivatives make up ~70% of bile acids, while chenodeoxycholic acid derivatives make up ~30% of the bile acid pool [5]. These primary bile acids are subsequently conjugated to the amino acids glycine and taurine by a two-step reaction involving specific ligase and transferase enzymes found predominantly in the hepatocyte peroxisome. In adult humans, glycine conjugates predominate, with a ratio of glycine to taurine of 3:1 [6]. During fetal development and infancy, the opposite is true, with taurine conjugates making up 80% of the biliary bile acids [7]. Conjugation alters the properties of the bile acids by making them more polar, limits their passive reabsorption, and minimizes the potential membrane-damaging effect of the unconjugated, more hydrophobic, bile acid species. The two primary bile acids are transported into bile by the action of specific canalicular membrane transporters, which represents the rate-limiting step for transport of bile acids into bile.

In bile, the majority of conjugated bile acids exist as mixed micelles (in combination with phospholipids and cholesterol). The formation of micelles helps maintain cholesterol in solution and also lowers the free bile acid concentration, which decreases the bile acid detergent activity and thereby prevents potential toxicity to the lipid membrane of "downstream" cholangiocytes.

In the intestine, bacteria produce the secondary bile acids by converting cholic acid to deoxycholic acid and chenodeoxycholic acid to lithocholic acid. These reactions have the potential to produce 12 major conjugated primary and secondary bile acid species, though the primary bile acids are the predominant species in humans [8].

Phospholipids and cholesterol

By volume, phospholipids and cholesterol are the next most plentiful solutes in bile. Several phospholipids exist in the hepatocyte canalicular membrane, including phosphatidylcholine, phosphatidylserine, phosphatidyletholamine, and sphingomyelin, though phosphatidylcholine is the predominant species in bile under physiological conditions [10]. While phosphatidylcholine is the predominant phospholipid in bile, cholesterol is the predominant sterol, with concentrations reaching ~300 mg/dL. It should be noted that cholesterol excretion into bile is the most important route for cholesterol elimination from the body. Approximately 1 g of cholesterol is eliminated in the feces per day, approximately one-third in the form of bile acids and approximately two-thirds in the form of steroids and steroid hormones. Importantly, the canalicular secretion of phospholipids is tightly linked with the transport of bile acids. This insures the proper ratio of phospholipids, cholesterol, and bile acids to promote micelle formation and optimum bile solubility. Disruptions in this process may alter the balance of biliary phospholipid and cholesterol concentrations and may promote gallstone formation. The biliary excretion of cholesterol and phospholipids therefore plays an important role in systemic lipid homeostasis [11].

Proteins

Bile also contains many enzymes, amino acids, and proteins [2]; in fact, proteomic studies have revealed over 2000 specific proteins in human bile [12,13]. Most of these are yet to be characterized, though the most abundant proteins include albumin and immunoglobulins which play an important role in promoting epithelial cell integrity and preventing infection. For example, secretory IgA plays an important role in mucosal immunity of the biliary tract as well as the intestine. By binding and aggregating bacteria, secretory IgA prevents bacterial motility, adherence to epithelial cells, and translocation [14]. Thus, the secretion of IgA into bile represents a mechanism to prevent colonization, overgrowth, and bacterial infection of both the small intestine and the biliary tract [15]. Bile also contains an array of other immunologically relevant substances such as human β-defensins, cytokines, and chemokines which are secreted by the cholangiocyte and act to regulate the immune system within the biliary tree, liver, and intestine [15]. Recent explorations of the bile proteome in health and disease have uncovered promising potential for identification of malignancies [16] as well as identification of disease-specific alterations which may be used to elucidate pathogenesis and define therapeutic targets [17,18].

Bilirubin

The major bile pigment in bile is bilirubin, which is responsible for the distinctive color of bile, for example "yellow bile" as noted by Hippocrates over 2000 years ago [1]. Bilirubin, the product of hemoglobin breakdown, is taken up at the hepatocyte sinusoidal membrane, conjugated via uridine 5′-diphosphate (UDP)-glucuronyl transferase in the microsome, and then secreted across the canalicular membrane into bile as glucuronide conjugates [19]. The conjugation of bilirubin is important for its excretion in bile as unconjugated bilirubin is water insoluble.

Electrolytes

The inorganic solute composition of bile is mostly made up of electrolytes, the concentration of which resembles that of plasma. The primary cation is Na^+ (141–165 mEq/L), while the primary anions include Cl^- (77–117 mEq/L) and HCO_3^- (12–55 mEq/L). Bile also contains the divalent cations Ca^{2+} (2.5–6.4 mEq/L) and Mg^{2+} (1.5–3 mEq/L) in concentrations at or above those observed in plasma [2]. An important and consistent finding is the reciprocal relationship between biliary Cl^- and HCO_3^- concentrations. Stimuli that increase net bile flow are accompanied by increases in HCO_3^- [20]. For example, after exposure to the hormone secretin, biliary HCO_3^- concentration increases from basal values of 25 mM to values as high as 60 mM, accompanied by a corresponding decrease in ductal Cl^- concentration [20,21]. The net result is an increase in bile alkalinization and is consistent with a model in which Cl^-/HCO_3^- exchange plays a prominent role at the cellular level.

Nucleotides

Bile contains nucleotides including ATP, ADP, AMP, and adenosine. These nucleotides have emerged as important autocrine and paracrine signaling molecules within the liver and exert cellular effects by binding to purinergic (P2) and adenosine (P1) receptors on the plasma membrane of target cells [22]. Released by both hepatocytes and cholangiocytes into bile, ATP can bind purinergic (P2) receptors on the plasma membrane, resulting in increases in intracellular Ca^{2+} concentration and modulation of a broad range of liver functions [23]. Thus, purinergic signaling is a means of: (1) coordinating the separate functions of hepatocytes and cholangiocytes; (2) signaling between hepatocytes and other cell types of the liver (portal fibroblasts, Kupffer cells, endothelial cells); (3) propagating Ca^{2+} waves within the liver; and (4) regulating Ca^{2+}-dependent processes [24–26]. Furthermore, ATP and other purinergic analogs, by binding apical membrane receptors on cholangiocytes, have emerged as potent agonists for ductular secretion [27–30].

Heavy metals

Copper is the main heavy metal in bile, though Mn^{2+}, Fe^{2+}, and Zn^{2+} are also present. Biliary excretion of copper is the main excretion pathway for this metal in humans. Abnormalities in the biliary excretion of copper result in Wilson disease associated with very high levels of hepatic copper [31].

Other

Bile also contains vitamins, porphyrins, exogenous drugs, xenobiotics, and environmental toxins. Vitamin D, for example, is 25-hydroxylated in the liver, excreted into bile, absorbed in the intestine, and then hydroxylated again in the kidney to form 1,25-dihydroxy vitamin D. Approximately 25% of 1,25-vitamin D undergoes enterohepatic circulation daily [32]. This enterohepatic pathway is important as vitamin D has important roles in the intestine, including promoting intestinal growth and development, and modulating Ca^{2+} homeostasis.

Anatomy and physiology of the bile secretory unit

Bile production requires the regulated function of both hepatocytes and the intrahepatic biliary epithelial cells known as cholangiocytes. While bile formation is initiated at the canalicular membrane of the hepatocyte, bile is subsequently modified by the regulated secretion and absorption of electrolytes and water by cholangiocytes as it traverses the intrahepatic ducts. Thus, these two cell types (hepatocytes and cholangiocytes) make up a functional unit responsible for bile formation. The contributions and regulation of each will be described in the following sections.

Hepatocyte

In the human liver, hepatocytes are arranged in parallel plates, the thickness of a single cell, extending approximately 20 cell lengths from the periportal to the pericentral zone. These rows of single cells are exposed to sinusoidal blood on both sides (Figure 19.2). Each hepatocyte is a specialized epithelial cell with a polygonal shape and distinct basal, lateral, and canalicular membranes [33]. The basal, or sinusoidal, membrane, which is in contact with the sinusoidal space, makes up 70% of the cell surface area; the lateral membrane, which involves the intracellular portion where adjoining hepatocytes abut, makes up 15%; and, lastly, the apical or canalicular membrane constitutes approximately 15% of the cell surface area [34]. The small canalicular space formed by the opposing canalicular membrane domains of two hepatocytes is approximately 1 μm in diameter [35]. The canalicular membrane contains numerous microvilli, increasing the surface area. Associated with, and surrounding, the canalicular membrane is a dense ring of actin and myosin filaments, which allow contraction of the canalicular membrane and promote canalicular peristalsis [36].

The movement of canalicular contents is enhanced by phasic contractions of this network, most prominent in the zone 1 hepatocytes [37]. In disease processes such as obstructive cholestasis, actomyosin contractility exerts a protective effect, inducing the formation of bile-regurgitative vesicles which serve as an early homeostatic mechanism against increased biliary pressure [36].

The canalicular space is separated from the sinusoidal space by intercellular junctions forming a permeability barrier. These cell-to-cell complexes are made up of tight junctions known as the zonula occludens [38]. The zonula occludens is composed of globular proteins known as occludens and claudins, which are connected to cytoskeletal proteins such as ZO-1 and ZO-2 [39]. These tight junctions are negatively charged, facilitating the paracellular movement of cations but preventing the movement of anions. This barrier function is critical for bile formation because it permits the concentration of organic solutes within the canalicular space and prevents the back diffusion of solutes to the sinusoidal space [40]. It should be highlighted that this is the only physical barrier between the blood and the canalicular lumen, representing an anatomical and physiological separation of these spaces.

Importantly, during cholestasis and other chronic liver diseases, the loss of tight junctions results in a physical disruption of the blood–bile barrier, resulting in "back" diffusion of canalicular contents (i.e., bile acids) into the sinusoidal space [41]. This disruption of the tight junction complexes also abolishes the normal sinusoidal-to-canalicular gradients for solutes upon which bile formation depends.

As nutrient-rich blood from the portal vein returns to the liver, it joins the oxygen-rich blood from the hepatic artery and flows into the sinusoidal space. The sinusoid is lined by endothelial cells, which contain fenestrations between adjacent cells. The fenestrations are large enough to facilitate the diffusion of nutrients and macromolecules, including albumin. The space between the endothelial cells and the basal hepatocyte membrane is known as the space of Disse and is a zone approximately 10 μm wide. Transport of substances from the sinusoidal space to the canalicular space involves movement either through (transcellular) or around (paracellular) hepatocytes [42,43]. Most solutes are transported via a transcellular route and in a regulated, precise manner due to a specific array of transporters on the plasma membrane and intracellular carrier proteins. Interestingly, hepatocytes exhibit functional differences based on their location within the lobule. The cells in the periportal region are exposed to portal blood first entering the sinusoid, which has the highest concentration of nutrients and solutes. As blood moves toward the pericentral zone, nutrients and solutes

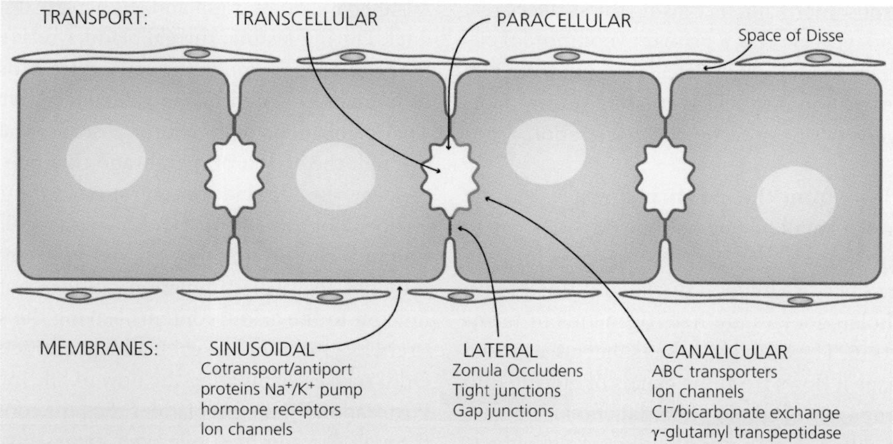

Figure 19.2 Anatomical and structural domains of the hepatocyte. Hepatocytes are polarized epithelial cells, with a basal, or sinusoidal, membrane facing the blood-filled sinusoidal space, a lateral membrane between adjacent cells, and an apical, or canalicular, membrane. Secretion of organic and inorganic solutes involves both active transport across cells (transcellular) and passive diffusion through cation-selective junctional complexes (paracellular) into the canalicular space. Source: Modified from Fitz 1996 [9].

are removed by the hepatocytes, so that the pericentral hepatocytes are exposed to significantly lower concentration of solutes. Thus, a portal-to-pericentral gradient for solutes, including bile acids, exists [44]. Furthermore, the rate of both bile acid uptake and canalicular bile acid excretion is highest in the periportal hepatocytes (zone 1). As bile acids are removed by the hepatocyte, there is a progressive decrease in the concentrations of bile acids as blood moves toward the pericentral zone (zone 3). Thus, periportal hepatocytes appear to contribute to bile acid-dependent bile flow to a greater extent than do the pericentral hepatocytes.

Bile acids are secreted at the canalicular membrane by the action of specific transporters in a process that requires energy in the form of ATP hydrolysis. Canalicular concentrations of bile acids reach concentrations of 2–45 mM, representing a >100-fold concentration above that in the portal vein [45]. Bile entering the canalicular space flows toward the portal region and enters the canals of Hering, which are small, terminal bile ductules lined by both cholangiocytes and hepatocytes, comprising a "transition" zone. Finally, bile flows into the proximal small intrahepatic bile ducts, which are formed entirely by biliary epithelial cells, or cholangiocytes.

Cholangiocyte

Cholangiocytes, the epithelial cells that line the bile ducts, represent an important component of the bile secretory unit. While bile formation is initiated at the hepatocyte canalicular membrane, cholangiocytes subsequently modify the volume and composition of bile through regulated ion and water secretion throughout the network of intrahepatic bile ducts [9]. Cholangiocytes are a polarized epithelium with distinct apical and basolateral membranes [46]. Tight junctional complexes exist between cholangiocytes of extremely high resistance (greater than 1000 ohms/cm^2), creating distinct apical and basolateral regions which are functionally isolated. The apical membrane contains numerous microvilli, increasing the surface area. Additionally, cholangiocytes express a primary (nonmotile) cilium from the apical membrane, which detects stimuli from bile and transmits the information into cells regulating several signaling pathways involved in secretion, proliferation, and apoptosis [47].

In humans, bile flows from the canalicular space, via the canals of Hering, into the small bile ducts (bile ductules, interlobular ducts, and septal ducts), which then converge into the larger bile ducts (area ducts, segmental ducts) and finally into the hepatic ducts. Cholangiocytes are heterogeneous in terms of structure and function. The initial bile ducts that are exposed to the canalicular bile as it flows from the canals of Hering into the bile ducts are composed of small, cuboidal cholangiocytes (~6 μm in diameter) with 4–5 cells per bile duct. As bile ducts become larger, cholangiocytes become progressively larger and more columnar in shape [46]. Small-sized ducts (<15 μm) and interlobular ducts (diameter 15–100 μm) are composed of small cholangiocytes (6–10 μm), while larger septal ducts (diameter 100–300 μm), area ducts (diameter 300–400 μm), and segmental ducts (diameter 400–800 μm) are composed of large, columnar cholangiocytes (12–16 μm) [48,49].

As it traverses the extensive network of intrahepatic ducts, bile becomes progressively more alkaline and dilute as a result of Cl^-, HCO_3^-, and water secretion [49]. Although duct cells only make up 3–5% of the nuclear mass of the liver, it is estimated that the combined ductular length is approximately 2 km in humans [49]. Thus, bile is exposed to a large surface area composed of the apical membrane of cholangiocytes before reaching the common bile duct. It is estimated that ductular secretion contributes approximately 40% of the total bile volume in humans [50]. Thus, cholangiocytes exhibit a prodigious secretory capacity that per cell is 50-fold greater than that exhibited by hepatocytes [9].

The predominant ion responsible for cholangiocyte secretion is Cl^- for which a gradient exists across the apical membrane. This gradient is made possible by distinct transporters and channels on the apical and basolateral membranes. Furthermore, similar to the functional differences between periportal and pericentral hepatocytes, cholangiocytes also exhibit functional differences based on their anatomical location. Notably, the larger ducts exhibit secretin-stimulated fluid and HCO_3^- secretion [51,52], whereas the smaller ducts do not. Conversely, small ducts respond to histamine with increases in Ca^{2+} and exhibit robust Ca^{2+}-dependent secretion [53]. In mice, both small and large cholangiocytes, forming the small and large bile ducts respectively, express purinergic P2 receptors on the plasma membrane and exhibit Ca^{2+}-activated Cl^- secretion in response to extracellular nucleotides [54].

Gallbladder

The chief function of the gallbladder is to provide regular, rhythmic release of concentrated bile acids into the duodenum in response to the ingestion of food [55]. Bile flows through the intrahepatic ducts, right and left hepatic ducts, into the common duct. During fasting, the gallbladder relaxes and bile flows into the gallbladder through the cystic duct. Most of the bile acid pool in humans is stored in the gallbladder during the fasting state. The gallbladder epithelium absorbs water and electrolytes through the action of membrane channels and transporters. In this way, the bile acid concentration in the gallbladder can rise to values as high as 300 mM. Following a meal, the hormones secretin and cholecystokinin are released by the duodenum in response to vagal stimulation and/or contact of the duodenal mucosa to the acidic contents leaving the stomach. In response to cholecystokinin, the gallbladder contracts and the sphincter of Oddi relaxes, facilitating the flow of bile into the small intestine. Postprandially, the gallbladder remains contracted and bile flows through the common bile duct, bypassing the gallbladder, into the intestine. The bicarbonate-rich bile optimizes the pH of the intestinal lumen for the functioning of the pancreatic enzymes.

Bile acids are necessary for fat emulsification, allowing the pancreatic enzymes lipase and colipase to break down triglycerides into monoglycerides and free fatty acids. In the intestine, bile acids again form micelles, which are taken up by the apical (luminal) membrane of enterocytes. Functionally, the gallbladder has long been regarded as a reservoir for hepatic bile awaiting secretion into the intestine; however, emerging evidence suggests a role in metabolic homeostasis regulation [55].

Enterohepatic circulation

Enterohepatic circulation describes the process by which compounds and solutes excreted into bile are reabsorbed in the intestine, travel back to the liver, and are resecreted into bile. Many solutes in bile undergo enterohepatic circulation, including bile acids, bilirubin, hormones, and drugs. This process serves to conserve the solute and is an efficient process to maintain the bile composition. Bile acids, for example, undergo 6–10 cycles/day of enterohepatic circulation. The intestinal reabsorption of bile acids is very efficient. For example, from the total bile acid pool excreted into the intestine (approximately 20–40 g), only 0.2–0.6 g/day of bile acids are lost in the feces [56]. This amount is replaced by de novo synthesis by the liver.

In the intestine, a small amount of unconjugated bile acids is absorbed in the proximal small bowel, but the majority of bile acids, including all conjugated bile acids, are absorbed in the terminal ileum. This absorption is due to the function of the apical ASBT/SLC10A2 protein, which transports bile acids into the enterocyte. After uptake by the enterocyte, bile acids bind to the carrier protein ileal bile acid-binding protein (ILBAP) [57], which transports the bile acid through the cytosol to the basolateral membrane where a heterodimer protein complex composed of Ostα and Ostβ transports the bile acids into the portal circulation [58]. The bile acids are then returned to the liver via the portal vein. Upon return to the liver, the bile acids are efficiently extracted (approximately 98% via the first pass) [58]. The bile acids that escape the first-pass clearance by the liver are filtered by the kidney glomerulus and reabsorbed by transporters in the proximal convoluted tubule and only a very small amount of bile acid is lost in the urine. However, during cholestasis associated with elevated serum levels of bile acids, urinary excretion of bile acids may increase dramatically.

Cholehepatic shunt

Bile acids in bile may also undergo recirculation before they enter the intestine This process, in which cholangiocytes take up bile acids across the apical membrane, is known as cholehepatic shunting [59]. Unconjugated bile acids are taken up passively after protonation, while conjugated bile acids are transported across the apical cholangiocyte membrane by ASBT/SLC10A2, the same protein found on the apical membrane of intestinal enterocytes [60]. Interestingly, ASBT/SLC10A2 is present on large cholangiocytes, forming the large intrahepatic ducts, but is not found on small cholangiocytes [61].

Once transported across the apical cholangiocyte membrane, bile acids are transported through the cytosol by intracellular binding proteins and transported across the basal membrane by the Ostα and OSTβ protein complex [62], as well as a truncated form of ASBT (t-ASBT) [63]. Bile acids then enter the peribiliary plexus and return to the sinusoidal space where they are again taken up by the hepatocyte. Thus, this pathway represents a structural arrangement that provides cholehepatic recirculation.

The cholehepatic shunt pathway hypothetically may serve several functions. First, the uptake of bile acids at the apical cholangiocyte membrane has been associated with increases in Ca^{2+}-activated Cl^- secretion, HCO_3^- secretion, and fluid secretion [64]. Thus, the cholehepatic shunt pathway serves to increase biliary electrolyte and fluid secretion [59]. For example, the bile acid Nor-ursodeoxycholic acid undergoes significant cholehepatic circulation, which is thought to contribute to the hypercholeresis observed with this bile acid [59]. Second, during cholestasis or bile duct obstruction, both associated with bile stasis, cholehepatic shunting may serve as a mechanism for the removal of bile acids from the bile duct lumen, thus preventing membrane damage due to the accumulation of toxic bile acids in the intrahepatic ducts [65]. Lastly, the cholehepatic shunt may also represent a hepatobiliary coupling mechanism by which hepatocytes signal to downstream cholangiocytes to coordinate a broad range of liver functions, including secretion, proliferation, and changes in the expression and/or regulation of membrane transporters and channels, as described below [64].

Mechanisms of bile formation

Bile, unlike urine, is not formed by hydrostatic filtration; rather, bile secretion is an osmotic process driven by the active secretion of organic solutes coupled to passive, or paracellular, movement of water and inorganic solutes [66,67]. Thus, the active secretion of organic and inorganic anions into the hepatocyte canalicular space is the principal driving force for bile formation. The final osmolality of bile, however, is nearly isotonic with that of plasma, suggesting that the secretory products of hepatocytes are modified by movement of water and electrolytes before it reaches the common bile duct. Thus, complementary processes exist including: (1) osmotic movement of water into the canalicular space due to concentrative bile acid transport; and (2) channel-mediated electrolyte and water transport. These complementary processes permit classification of bile formation at the canalicular membrane into two categories: *bile acid-dependent* and *bile acid-independent* bile formation [2] (Figure 19.3).

Bile acid-dependent bile formation is driven by the osmotic effects of bile acids and occurs through the transport of bile acids across the canalicular membrane [68,69]. Bile acid-independent bile formation occurs through the secretion of glutathione, inorganic solutes, and electrolytes [70,71]. Bile formation can also be categorized as "canalicular" and "ductular," describing the anatomical sites and cell types (hepatocyte versus cholangiocyte) contributing to the volume and composition

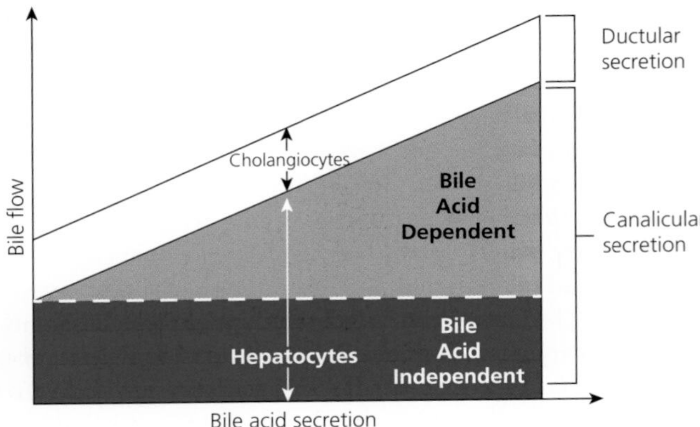

Figure 19.3 Determinants of bile flow. Canalicular bile flow and ductular bile flow both contribute to bile formation. Canalicular bile flow is composed of bile acid-dependent and bile acid-independent components. While canalicular bile flow is mediated by hepatocytes, cholangiocytes mediate ductular secretion. Source: Modified from Boyer 2002 [72].

of bile [49]. These classification systems, "bile acid-dependent" versus "bile acid-independent" and "canalicular" versus "ductular," are useful descriptive terms, but these mechanisms do not operate independently and there is substantial overlap between them. For example, bile acid-dependent bile flow, initiated by hepatocyte transport of bile acids at the canalicular membrane, is accompanied by significant increases in glutathione, electrolyte, and water transport, thus increasing bile acid-independent bile flow. Furthermore, increased canalicular transport of bile acids, resulting in an increase in the ductular concentration of bile acids, is accompanied by cholangiocyte electrolyte and water transport, thus increasing ductular secretion significantly. For example, for each 1 μmol of taurocholate secretion, there is an increase in biliary Cl^- secretion and HCO_3^- secretion resulting in an increase in bile flow of approximately 8 μL [69]. These results indicate that bile acids have intrinsic choleretic activity, though this activity is not equal among different bile acid species, as discussed further below. The general cellular principles of membrane transport, which underlie bile formation, are described below.

Principles of membrane solute and ion transport

Hepatocytes possess a variety of membrane channel proteins, which are not randomly distributed but rather restricted to specific membrane domains (canalicular versus sinusoidal). These membrane channels and transporters work in concert to establish gradients across the plasma membrane to promote the vectorial passage of ions, solutes, and water. Two primary cellular mechanisms responsible for bile formation at the hepatocyte level and ductular level include Na^+-coupled transport and transepithelial Cl^- secretion, respectively.

Coupled transport

Most organic solutes are present in the portal blood in very low concentrations. For example, while the concentration of bile acids in the portal blood is ~150 μM and that of amino acids is 1–2 mM, these solutes are concentrated intracellularly by >50-fold [73]. Passive diffusion alone cannot account for these high intracellular concentrations.

In order to achieve this high intracellular concentration, the basolateral membrane of hepatocytes contains transport proteins that facilitate solute uptake. These proteins couple the transport of the solute to movement of other ions down their thermodynamic gradient. For the uptake and intracellular concentration of bile acids, for example, hepatocytes utilize a mechanism known as Na^+-coupled transport, which uses energy derived from the Na^+ electrochemical gradient. Uptake of solutes is driven by the influx of Na^+ from an extracellular to intracellular location where concentrations are 10-fold lower [74]. At the basolateral membrane, the large out-to-in concentration gradient for Na^+ is due to the action of the Na^+/K^+ ATPase [75]. The protein is a pump that is powered by ATP hydrolysis and transports three molecules of Na^+ out and two molecules of K^+ into the cell each cycle, thus generating low Na^+ and high K^+ intracellular concentrations [76]. The Na^+/K^+ ATPase, in conjunction with membrane ion channels, also forms the basis for the electrical potential differences across the basolateral membrane, which provides the driving force for electrogenic transport systems [77]. The potential difference of the hepatocyte membrane is approximately −35 millivolts (interior negative) but is regulated over a broad range in response to changing physiological conditions [78–80]. The interior negative potential difference is due in part to the high density of K^+ channels in the basolateral membrane, resulting in a high permeability to K^+ as compared to Na^+ or Cl^-.

Thus, the pump establishes two driving forces critical for hepatic uptake mechanism: (1) an inwardly directed chemical gradient for Na^+ ions; and (2) an intracellular electrical gradient of −35 to −40 mV. The electrogenic Na^+-coupled solute transport allows for solutes to be concentrated to values approximately 40-fold or greater than concentrations in the extracellular space [80].

Na^+-coupled transport plays a critical role in bile formation and highlights the underlying importance of the Na^+/K^+ ATPase. Na^+/K^+ ATPase activity must be finely regulated, able to undergo minute-to-minute changes in activity, in order to establish proper Na^+ gradients to meet physiological needs. For example, increases in either the number or activity of Na^+/K^+ ATP pumps must accompany changes between fed and fast states in order to efficiently transport the increased load of bile acids into the hepatocyte [81].

Transepithelial Cl^- secretion

Biliary duct cells, or cholangiocytes, also express a host of transporters and channels that create gradients necessary for fluid secretion. Net fluid secretion or absorption across epithelial cells requires active transport of ions and other solutes to create osmotic gradients necessary for water movement. Cholangiocyte secretion is associated with a net flux of Cl^- and HCO_3^- into the lumen and generation of a lumen negative potential [82]. This model is consistent with a role for electrogenic Cl^- secretion. Unlike hepatocytes, which generate a gradient for cations such as Na^+ to drive cotransport of solutes, ductular secretion is driven by a gradient for Cl^- across the apical membrane [49]. Underlying this Cl^- gradient is the $Na^+/K^+/2\ Cl^-$ transporter located on the basolateral membrane, which transports two Cl^- ions into the cell along with one Na^+ and one K^+ ion. This transporter works in concert with the Na^+/K^+ ATPase, as well as membrane K^+ channels, to load Cl^- into the cell [49,83]. Under basal conditions, the apical cholangiocyte membrane is relatively impermeable to Cl^-, allowing for intracellular Cl^- concentrations to increase to values above the electrochemical equilibrium, thus creating a large gradient for Cl^- across the membrane. In response to prosecretory stimuli, Cl^- channels open in the apical membrane with efflux of Cl^- into the duct lumen [84–86]. The increase in the ductal concentration of Cl^- is thought to drive Cl^-/HCO_3^- exchange and water efflux, thus leading to alkalinization and dilution of bile [49,87].

Overall, these membrane channels and transporters in both hepatocytes and cholangiocytes underlie the basic mechanism of secretion and bile formation and highlight two important and complementary mechanisms: (1) hepatocyte membrane transporters, which create a gradient for Na^+ and use Na^+-coupled transport to move solutes from sinusoid to canaliculus; and (2) cholangiocyte membrane channels, which create a gradient for Cl^- and use channel-mediated Cl^- efflux to drive Cl^-/HCO_3^- exchange and water movement into the duct lumen.

Ion transport and cell volume regulation

While membrane ion channels underlie the electrochemical gradient necessary for coupled transport and ion and fluid movement, they also provide a critical function maintaining the volume of individual hepatocytes. Hepatocytes are exposed to large changes in the concentrations of bile acids, amino acids, and other organic solutes between fed and fasted states. Concentration of these solutes intracellularly creates large osmolar gradients sufficient to induce significant transmembrane water movement and increases in cell volume of up to 5–10% [88]. However, compensatory mechanisms are in place and activation of membrane ion channels results in rapid efflux of Cl^-, K^+, and water with restoration of hepatocyte cell volume toward basal levels [89]. This process is finely regulated by a mechanism involving ATP release and purinergic signaling [90]. In this process, increases in cell volume stimulate ATP release from hepatocytes, autocrine or paracrine stimulation of purinergic receptors on the cell membrane, activation of membrane Cl^- and K^+ channels, and water efflux, culminating in the restoration of cell volume toward basal levels [90–92]. The increase in membrane ion permeability and water efflux in response to hepatocyte volume changes contributes to the volume and dilution of bile [93]. Furthermore, volume-dependent release of ATP into the lumen allows access to purinergic receptors on downstream cholangiocytes and thereby serves as a stimulus for biliary secretion.

Thus, volume-dependent changes in membrane ion permeability and water efflux represent a potent stimulus for bile formation and this has led to the important concept that changes in cell volume per se are a mechanism for regulating bile formation and liver functions [94]. In general, increases in cell volume represent an anabolic signal, and stimulate protein and glycogen synthesis, exocytosis, and bile flow, while decreases in cell volume have opposite effects [95–97].

Bile acid-dependent bile formation

It has long been recognized that a linear relationship exists between bile acid secretion and bile flow (see Figure 19.3). As the canalicular excretion of bile acids increases, bile volume also increases proportionally [20]. Thus, bile acids represent a major driving force for bile formation. Bile acids are concentrated in bile 1000-fold compared to the sinusoidal space. Classic experiments in dogs with a duodenal fistula demonstrated that bile flow decreased as the bile acid pool was depleted and was restored when the bile acid pool was repleted [20]. Further experiments in dogs revealed that infusion of taurocholate led to an increase in bile flow of 8 μL for each 1 μmol of taurocholate infused [69]. Interestingly, infusion with unconjugated bile acids increases bile flow greater than conjugated bile acids, increasing bile flow by 20–25 μL for each μmol of conjugated bile acid infused [68]. Thus, not all bile acids have the same choleretic ability; for example, norchenodeoxycholate increases bile flow 10-fold greater than taurocholate [98,99] and norursodeoxycholic acid has the highest choleretic ability for any bile acid measured to date [100]. Bile acid secretion is also associated with simultaneous release of phospholipids, of up to 3.31 meq/L [45,68,101], and unconjugated bile acids induce a greater increase in phospholipid secretion compared to their conjugated counterparts [68]. Moreover, once in bile, bile acids that do not form micelles exhibit increased choleretic activity. Definition of the cellular mechanisms involved in bile acid-induced choleresis is of great interest because several bile acids have been introduced as therapeutic agents for cholestatic liver disease [102].

Together, these studies demonstrate the importance of bile acid transport for overall bile formation. Vectorial movement of bile acids from the sinusoidal space into the canalicular space is mediated by the coordinated activity of specific membrane transport proteins, including uptake at the sinusoidal membrane, intracellular transport, and excretion across the canalicular membrane. In general, transport across the canalicular membrane is rate limiting and represents the anatomical site for many causes of intrahepatic cholestasis. A detailed description of the transport activities at each of these membrane sites is described below.

Sinusoidal membrane uptake

The major bile acids are carried in the portal circulation bound to albumin. As portal blood enters the sinusoidal space, the bile acid–albumin complex disassociates and free bile acids are taken up into hepatocytes at the sinusoidal membrane. The rate of bile acid uptake is highest in the periportal hepatocytes of zone 1 [44], and close to 90% of bile acids are extracted from the portal blood on a single passage through the liver [103]. This efficient process occurs via a high-affinity mechanism involving several polypeptide transport proteins. Different transport systems on the sinusoidal membrane exist for uptake of conjugated and unconjugated bile acids. The majority of bile acids that return to the hepatocyte at the sinusoidal membrane are in conjugated form and are taken up by the sodium taurocholate cotransporting polypeptide, NTCP/SLC10A1 [104,105] (Figure 19.4). NTCP/SLC10A1 was the first hepatocyte transporter identified and is exclusively expressed on the sinusoidal membrane of hepatocytes and is not found in other tissues or organs [103,106,107]. It is a 349 amino acid, 50 kD protein that transports bile acids into the hepatocyte coupled to Na^+ transport [106], deriving energy for the process from the Na^+ gradient maintained by the Na^+/K^+ ATPase. While the stoichiometry has been controversial, the best evidence suggests that transport is electrogenic, with two Na^+ ions transported with each bile acid [108]. As described above, this net increase in positive charge with each transport cycle greatly increases the ability to concentrate bile acids intracellularly [109]. Thus, the Na^+ concentration gradient and the membrane potential difference work in concert to modulate the uptake of bile acids by NTCP/SLC10A1. Interestingly, NTCP has now been identified to be the entry receptor for the hepatitis B virus [110]. This explains the hepatotropism of this virus and also explains why HBV does not infect nonprimate animals as significant species-specific forms of NTCP exist. Further, in cell and liver-humanized mice, downregulation of NTCP prevents HBV infection [111].

Sodium-coupled bile acid transport accounts for greater than 80% of bile acid transport at the sinusoidal membrane. In contrast, Na^+-independent pathways are responsible for most unconjugated bile acid uptake and account for less than 20% of total bile acid transport. A family of nonspecific anion transporters, known as OATPs/SLC21A, mediates most of this Na^+-independent bile acid uptake. OATPs are predicted to have 12 transmembrane-spanning domains and, unlike NTCP/SLC10A1, are found in other tissues including kidney, intestine, and neuronal tissues [103]. In contrast to the specific, high-affinity Na^+-coupled bile acid transport by NTCP/SLC10A1, OATPs transport both conjugated and unconjugated bile acids as well as bilirubin, steroids, and xenobiotics (see Figure 19.4). This occurs through a process involving exchange of anions, primarily GSH and HCO_3^- and is nonspecific [112,113]. The sinusoidal membrane also contains transport systems for organic anions (OATs) and organic cations (OCTs), each predicted to have 12 transmembrane-spanning domains which are widely expressed, and function as electroneutral exchangers [114,115]. In general, these function as bidirectional passive facilitated diffusion of endogenous organic cations or anions, respectively.

In addition to uptake systems, the sinusoidal membrane also contains efflux systems. The OATPs, for example, have been shown to operate as bidirectional exchangers and may "back" transport solutes from the hepatocyte into the sinusoidal space (see Figure 19.4). The heterodimer protein complex composed of OSTα and OSTβ is also located in the sinusoidal membrane and may export bile acids from the hepatocyte [116]. Other sinusoidal membrane "back" transporters include MRP3/ABCC3, MRP4/ABCC4, and MRP1/ABCC1, all of which may transport solutes, including bile acids, from the hepatocyte into the sinusoid [117–119]. While the expression of these transporters is low under normal conditions, expression increases significantly during cholestasis [120]. Thus, when canalicular transport of bile acids is impaired, these pathways represent an alternative way to export bile acids from the hepatocyte. Notably, human functional studies using positron emission tomography have shown that cholestasis reduces both the uptake and secretion of conjugated bile acids and increases backflux into the sinusoidal space [121].

Intracellular transport

Once taken up at the sinusoidal membrane, bile acids and other organic solutes move rapidly through the hepatocyte cytosol prior to excretion from the canalicular membrane. Three general processes for this translocation have been identified: (1) binding to cytosolic carrier proteins, (2) diffusion within intracellular membranes, and (3) microtubule-dependent vesicular transport [122]. Which pathway a solute may take depends on its hydrophobicity, with more hydrophobic solutes taking the pathway associated with intracellular membranes and vesicular transport. For bile acids, the predominant translocation pathway occurs via binding to specific intracellular bile acid-binding proteins, followed by rapid diffusion to the canalicular membrane along the sinusoidal-to-canalicular concentration gradient [123].

The binding of bile acids to bile acid-binding proteins is therefore important for two main reasons. First, it reduces the effective diffusion constant and therefore prevents bile acids from backdiffusing into the sinusoidal space or partitioning into hepatocyte membranes and organelles. Second, it potentially prevents cellular toxicity, which could result from the detergent activity of free bile acids in the cytosol.

Several bile acid-binding proteins have been identified, including 3α-hydroxysterol dehydrogenase and GSH s-transferase [124,125]. While the majority of bile acids appear to undergo this transcellular route by binding to intracellular binding proteins, it has been suggested that increased loads of hydrophobic bile acids, as occurs during cholestasis, may be transported intracellularly via microtubule-dependent vesicular transport [126,127]. Unconjugated bile acids entering the hepatocyte are transported into peroxisomes where they undergo taurine conjugation via bile acid-CoA:amino acid N-acyltransferase (BAAT) prior to exiting the peroxisome and resecretion into the canalicular space [128]. Transport proteins also exist for other

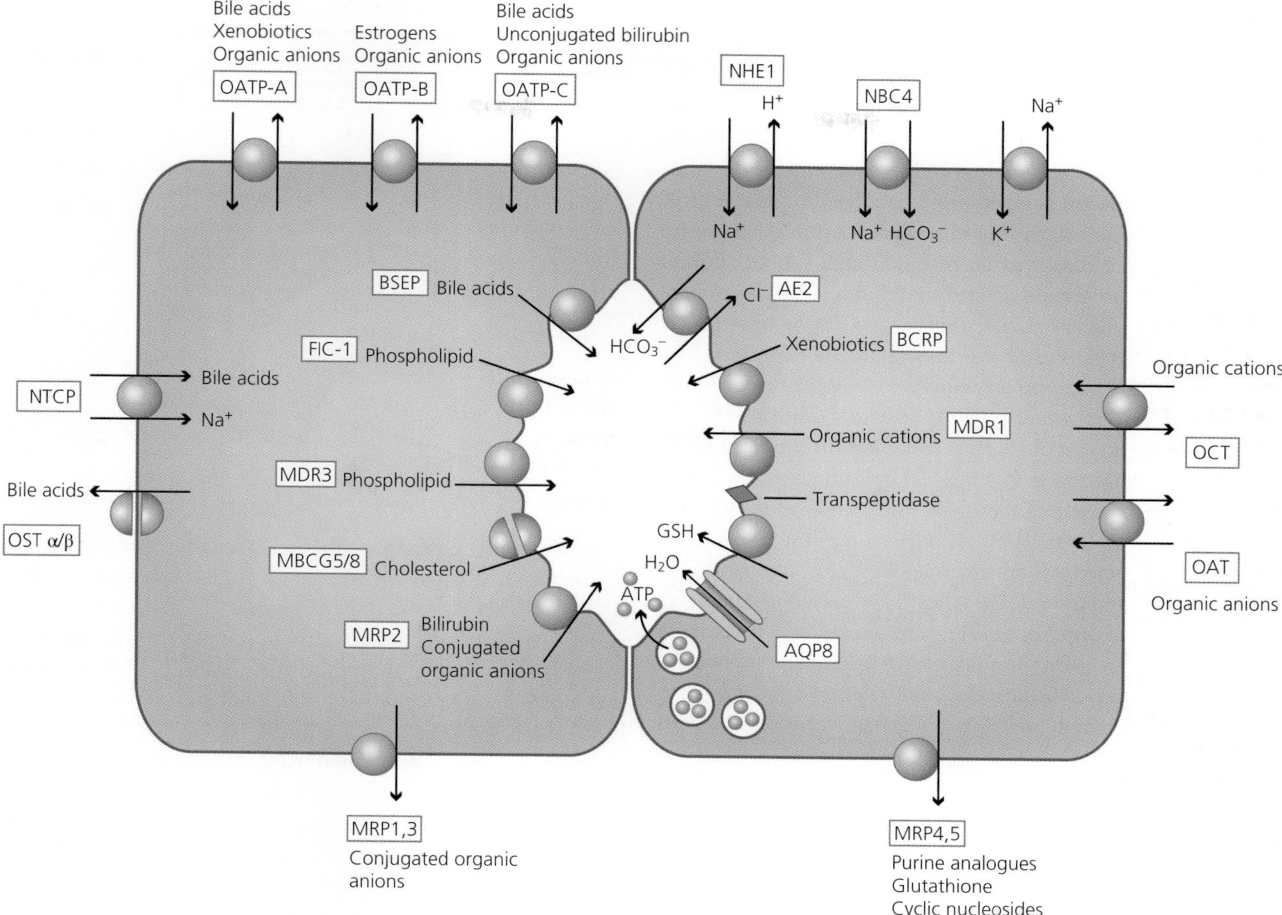

Figure 19.4 Hepatocyte transporters. Uptake of bile acids and organic solutes at the sinusoidal membrane is mediated by NTCP/SLC10A1 and three families of organic ion exchangers: OATP-A, -B, and -C, the organic anion transporter protein family; OCT, the organic cation transporter family; and OAT, the organic anion transporter family. The Na^+/H^+ exchanger, NHE1, and the Na^+/HCO_3^- cotransporter, NBC4, are located on the basolateral membrane and contribute to cellular pH regulation. Export from the hepatocyte into the canalicular space is due to the ATP-dependent transport proteins BSEP, FIC-1, MDR3, ABCG5/G8, MRP2, MDR1, and BCRP. ATP-dependent transport out of the hepatocyte into the sinusoidal space is mediated by MRP1, MRP3, MRP4, and MRP5. Inorganic secretion across the canalicular membrane is mediated by $HCO3^-$ exchange through AE2, GSH excretion, and water efflux through AQP8. ATP release into the canaliculus may contribute to hepatocyte, and downstream cholangiocyte, secretion through interaction with membrane purinergic (P2) receptors. See text for details.

organic solutes and lipids. For example, free fatty acids are bound to the liver fatty acid-binding protein (L-FABP) and bilirubin is bound to glutathione-*S*-transferase [103].

In contrast, proteins such as secretory IgA and transferrin undergo microtubule-dependent transcytotic vesicular transport. In this process, proteins bind specific receptors in the sinusoidal membrane, undergo endocytosis, transcellular trafficking, and then exocytosis at the canalicular membrane. Hepatocytes have a high rate of both constitutive and stimulated exo- and endocytosis. In fact, in in vitro models, hepatocytes have been shown to undergo endocytosis at rates capable of replacing the entire plasma membrane surface area five or more times every hour [127]. This high rate of membrane turnover suggests that vesicular trafficking is functionally important for transport activity but also highlights a potential mechanism by which hepatocytes can rapidly alter the membrane composition to meet changing transport needs.

Canalicular membrane transport

Excretion of bile acids and other organic solutes from the canalicular membrane is the major determinant of bile composition and represents the rate-limiting step in bile formation. As described above, bile is a complex mixture of solutes including bile acids, phospholipids, cholesterol, bilirubin, and other organic solutes and specific canalicular transporters exist for each of these solutes. The majority of these transporters are members of the ATP-binding cassette (ABC) protein family and use the energy of ATP hydrolysis to transport the solute into the canalicular space against large concentration gradients. Specific proteins exist for the transport of each solute, which will be described below (Table 19.1).

Table 19.1 Hepatocyte canalicular transporters.

Functional protein name	Gene symbol	Human gene locus	Predominant substrates	Tissue expression	Disease association
BSEP	*ABCB11*	2q24	Bile acids	Liver	PFIC-2, BRIC-2, ICP
FIC-1	*ATP8B1*	18q21	Aminophospholipids	Liver, intestine	PFIC-1, BRIC-1
MDR3	*ABCB4*	7q21.1	Phosphatidylcholine	Liver	PFIC-3, ICP, gallstone disease
Cholesterol 1/2 transporters	*ABCG5, ABCG8*	2p21	Cholesterol, plant sterols	Liver, intestine	β-Sitosterolemia
MRP2	*ABCC2*	10q24	Conjugated bilirubin, organic anions, glutathione conjugates	Liver, kidney, intestine	Dubin–Johnson syndrome
MDR1	*ABCB11*	7q21	Xenobiotics, organic cations	Liver, kidney	
BCRP	*ABCG2*	4q22	Xenobiotics, drugs	Liver, placenta	

BRIC, benign recurrent intrahepatic cholestasis; ICP intrahepatic cholestasis of pregnancy; PFIC, progressive familial intrahepatic cholestasis.

Bile acids

The canalicular protein responsible for transporting the majority of bile acids across the canalicular membrane into bile is the bile salt export pump, BSEP/ABCB11 [129,130]. This protein, located in the hepatocyte canalicular membrane, is a 1321 amino acid, 140–170 kD protein with four potential glycosylation sites [130,131]. It is predicted to have two transmembrane-spanning domains, each composed of six transmembrane-spanning regions, and utilizes ATP hydrolysis to transport bile acids from the hepatocyte into the canalicular space [129,132]. Both uptake of bile acids at the sinusoidal membrane and transport across the canalicular membrane, therefore, require energy in the form of ATP hydrolysis [133]. The majority of monovalent bile acids are transported by this mechanism. As BSEP/ABCB11 is the predominant pathway for bile acid excretion across the canalicular membrane, and is the rate-limiting step in this process, it therefore is a critical step for bile acid-dependent bile flow. Interestingly, BSEP/ABCB11 is expressed in the fetal liver, but is markedly below adult expression levels at birth, which may contribute to the transient elevation of serum bile acids observed in neonates [134].

Phospholipids

Phospholipid excretion across the canalicular membrane is directly related to bile acid output. As the output of bile acids increases, so does phospholipid excretion. This serves to maintain the solubility ratios between bile acids and phospholipids in bile. This transport is mediated by several pathways. Phosphatidylcholine, the phospholipid with the highest concentration in bile, is transported through the action of the canalicular protein, MDR3/ABCB4 [135,136]. MDR3/ABCB4 is a 170 kD protein that works as a "floppase", to move phosphatidylcholine from the inner to the outer leaflet of the plasma membrane in an ATP-dependent manner [101,137]. Once in the outer leaflet, phosphatidylcholine is removed and appears in the canaliculus in the form of small vesicles or incorporated into micelles. MDR3/ABCB4 activity is the rate-limiting step in this process.

Additionally, aminophospholipids may also be transported across the canalicular membrane through the actions of FIC-1/ATP8B1. The FIC-1/ATP8B1 protein is an ATPase, rather than an ABC transporter, and is found in the hepatocyte canalicular membrane as well as the apical membrane of cholangiocytes, intestinal epithelial cells, pancreas, lung, and cochlear hair cells of the ear [146]. The function of FIC-1/ATP8B1 is not entirely clear. It has been postulated to function as a flippase for aminophospholipids and thus balances the lipid asymmetry established by MDR3/ABCB4 [138–140]. Other mechanisms have also been proposed including: (1) regulation of the canalicular lipid membrane fluidity through alterations in the membrane composition of specific phospholipids and cholesterol [138–140]; (2) indirect effects on the expression or function of other canalicular transporters through a mechanism involving nuclear transcription factors such as FXR [141]; or (3) regulating the formation of microvilli in polarized epithelial cells [142]. Its location in many epithelial cells suggests an important and more general role in epithelial function beyond its role in bile formation.

Cholesterol

Cholesterol is excreted from the hepatocyte canalicular membrane through the activity of two half-transporters, ABCG5 and ABCG8, also known as sterolin-1 and -2 [143]. These ABC proteins function together as a heterodimer, each containing only one functional domain individually and, hence, each is individually termed a "half transporter" [144]. ABCG5 and ABCG8 are found in intestine and liver epithelium, and function in the elimination of not only cholesterol but also plant sterols [143,145]. Defects in either of these proteins result in a disease known as β-sitosterolemia associated with a decreased transport of sterols into bile with accumulation in the liver [143].

Organic cations and drugs

Organic cations and drugs are transported across the canalicular membrane by MDR1/ABCB1. MDR1/ABCB1 is a 1280 amino acid, 170 kD protein and is responsible for efflux of drugs and chemotherapeutic agents across the canalicular membrane [146,147]. MDR1/ABCB1, originally called p-glycoprotein, was the first ABC transporter to be localized to the hepatocyte canalicular membrane [148]. While it is overexpressed in some forms of cancer and is responsible for chemotherapy resistance in some neoplasms [146], the endogenous substrates for this transporter are still unknown. Additionally, no human disease has been identified due to mutations in the gene encoding this protein. However, MDR1/ABCB1 appears capable of transporting bile acids, but at a fivefold lower affinity compared to BSEP/ABCB11 [149]. In mouse models of cholestasis, MDR1/ABCB1 is upregulated. Together, these findings suggest that MDR1/ABCB1 may be important as an alternate bile acid transporter during cholestasis.

Sulfated conjugates and hormones

Conjugates of sulfate and hormones are transported across the canalicular membrane by the actions of BCRP/ABCG2 [150]. BCRP is found on the apical membrane of numerous types of cells and serves to protect the cell from toxic compounds. The protein derived its name from a finding that it was overexpressed in breast cancer [150,151].

Bilirubin and organic anions

Bilirubin is taken up into the hepatocyte at the sinusoidal membrane, conjugated by glucuronyl transferase, and transported across the canalicular membrane by the action of MRP2/ABCC2 [152]. MRP2/ABCC2 is a 1545 amino acid protein with three transmembrane-spanning domains and utilizes the energy of ATP hydrolysis to transport conjugated bilirubin as well as glutathione and other conjugated organic anions across the canalicular membrane [152]. The protein, which was also called the canalicular multiorganic anion transporter (cMOAT), is also located on the apical membrane of other polarized epithelial cells, including the proximal tubule cells of the kidney, small intestine, colon, gallbladder, bronchi, and placenta.

Bile acid-independent bile flow

It has been shown in the isolated perfused rat liver that even in the complete absence of bile acids, there is still significant bile flow, of ~0.8–1.25 μL/min/g of liver, accounting for close to one half of total bile output [153]. Moreover, hormones that increase cAMP are associated with increases in canalicular bile flow even without changes in bile acid output [154]. These findings support the concept that a portion of bile formation is independent of bile acids. Since movement of water into the canalicular space requires the generation of a concentration gradient for solutes as described above, the driving force for bile acid-independent bile formation must come from the transport of inorganic ions. Furthermore, while ductular secretion relies on transepithelial secretion of Cl^- to provide the driving force for secretion, there is no net driving force for Cl^- secretion across the hepatocyte canalicular membrane. However, two solutes that have been shown to contribute to bile acid independent bile formation are glutathione (GSH) and bicarbonate (HCO_3^-) [130].

Glutathione

A direct correlation exists between GSH secretion and bile acid-independent bile formation. GSH secretion is ~4–9 mM/min/g of liver, which correlates with the rate of bile acid-independent bile formation as demonstrated in the isolated perfused rat liver model [112]. GSH is transported across the canalicular membrane by the action of MRP2/ABCC2 and is found in bile in concentrations of 1–4 μM [112,155,156]. Once in bile, each molecule of GSH can be broken down by biliary transpeptidases into individual amino acids, resulting in the generation of 3 mOsm for each molecule of GSH, thus increasing its choleretic potency.

Bicarbonate

HCO3⁻ is the other important solute for bile acid-independent bile flow at the hepatocyte canalicular membrane. Removal of HCO_3^- decreases bile formation by the perfused liver by approximately 50% [157]. Bicarbonate is loaded into the hepatocytes by the combined activity of the Na^+/H^+ exchanger [158] and the Na^+/HCO_3^- cotransporter [159,160] across the basolateral membrane. Intracellular HCO_3^- concentrations may reach levels of 15 mM, a value greater than predicted for passive distribution alone. This high intracellular concentration provides a large electrochemical gradient favoring movement of HCO_3^- out of the cell. In response to hormones and stimuli that increase cGMP, efflux of HCO_3^- across the canalicular membrane occurs predominantly through Cl^-/HCO_3^- exchange [161,162]. The Cl^-/HCO_3^- exchanger works in concert with canalicular Cl^- channels, and outwardly rectifying Cl^- channels have been identified, including CLC-2 [163] and CLC-3 [164]. Both Cl^- efflux and Cl^-/HCO_3^- exchange are functionally linked to water efflux across the canalicular membrane, and the water channel, aquaporin 8 (AQP8), is localized to the canalicular membrane as well as to submembrane vesicles [165,166]. In response to secretory agonists (e.g., cAMP), AQP8 is rapidly inserted into the membrane, thus providing a means to coordinate secretion of solutes to water efflux and bile formation [165,167,168]. While this process may be important for the local or canalicular alkalization of bile, ductular HCO_3^- secretion, through the Cl^-/HCO_3^- exchange activity of cholangiocyte AE2/SLC4A2, is the predominant pathway for bile alkalosis.

The overall contribution of canalicular bicarbonate secretion to bile formation is unknown. In addition to the Cl^-/HCO_3^- exchanger, the hepatocyte membrane also contains several other anion exchangers [161,169]. These anion exchangers are transport proteins that couple movement of solutes to the movement of anions such as Cl^-, SO_4^-, or HCO_3^- and which contribute importantly to bile acid-dependent and independent bile formation [162,165,169,170].

Ductular bile formation

Once bile is formed at the canalicular membrane, it travels through an extensive network of intrahepatic bile ducts formed by cholangiocytes, increasing in volume and becoming progressively more dilute and alkaline. Cholangiocytes are a polarized epithelium and specific apical and basolateral membrane channels and transporters are responsible (Figure 19.5). Under basal conditions, the bumetadine-sensitive $Na^+/K^+/2Cl^-$ cotransporter loads Cl^- into the cell above its electrochemical equilibrium because the apical membrane is relatively impermeable to Cl^-. Upon stimulation, Cl^- channels in the apical membrane open and increase Cl^- flux into the lumen [84,85] and drive the Cl^-/HCO_3^- exchanger, AE2/SLC4A2, thus increasing alkalinization [170,171]. Moreover, the efflux of Cl^- generates a lumen-negative potential, which favors movement of Na^+ into the bile duct lumen through a paracellular pathway and water via aquaporin water channels [172,173]. AQP1 and 4 are the predominant aquaporins in cholangiocytes [173,174]. AQP1 is present on the apical membrane [173,174], while AQP4 is present on the basolateral membrane [172], and together they account for the high transcellular movement of water, which is 10-fold greater in cholangiocytes than hepatocytes [166,175]. Additionally, K^+ channels have been identified in cholangiocytes and play a role in maintaining the membrane potential difference necessary for continued transepithelial Cl^- secretion [176,177].

Overall, this model is similar to other secretory epithelium that use transepithelial Cl^- movement to drive Cl^-/HCO_3^- exchange and water movement into the lumen [178]. The transepithelial transport of Cl^- therefore represents the primary driving force for cholangiocyte secretion and Cl^- channels in the apical membrane represent a key site for regulation of bile formation [179].

Chloride channels

Several membrane Cl^- channels have been identified in cholangiocytes based on biophysical and pharmacological properties, including a cAMP-activated Cl^- channel, a Ca^{2+}-activated Cl^- channel [27], a volume-activated (or osmo-sensitive) Cl^- channel [180,181], and a G-protein regulated Cl^- channel [182] (Table 19.2). To date, only two Cl^- channels have been identified definitively on a molecular basis: (1) the cystic fibrosis transmembrane conductance regulator (CFTR/ABCC7), a cAMP-activated Cl^- channel [182]; and (2) TMEM16A (also known as anoctamin), a Ca^{2+}-activated Cl^- channel [183,184]. The best studied of these is CFTR/ABCC7, a member of the ABC family of proteins, which is activated by increases in cAMP- and PKA-dependent phosphorylation [185].

In this model, stimulation of cholangiocyte basolateral receptors by the hormone secretin results in increased intracellular concentration of cAMP [186], PKA-dependent phosphorylation and opening of CFTR Cl^- channel [52], and stimulation of Cl^-/HCO_3^- exchange [187]. Thus, secretin-mediated choleresis is thought to be primarily due to the action of CFTR on the apical cholangiocyte membrane. The CFTR is only found on the apical membrane of cholangiocytes, not on the hepatocytes, or other cell types of the liver [188,189]. In contrast, TMEM16A, a 114 kD protein with eight transmembrane-spanning domains, is found in both small and large mouse cholangiocytes [184], is activated by increases in intracellular Ca^{2+}, not cAMP, and appears to be the predominant mechanism responsible for the increase in Cl^- secretion in response to ATP and purinergic receptor stimulation [183,184]. Thus, these two Cl^- channels, CFTR and TMEM16A, are activated by different secondary messengers, cAMP and PKA for CFTR versus Ca^{2+} and PKC for TMEM16A, and by agonists acting at different membrane domains, secretin acting at the basolateral membrane for CFTR versus ATP (and other purine analogs) acting at the apical membrane for TMEM16A. Recently, a protein known as leucine repeat containing protein 8, subunit A (LRRC8A) has been identified as a component of the osmosensitive Cl^- channel in other epithelia, but further confirmation is required in cholangiocytes.

The relative contributions of these Cl^- channels to overall ductular secretion under physiological conditions are unknown. While CFTR has been shown to mediate the classical secretory pathway mediated by secretin, several observations challenge the conventional model in which CFTR represents the predominant Cl^- channel driving secretion in bile duct epithelium. First, only 15–20% of patients with cystic fibrosis, and hence absent or nonfunctional CFTR channels in biliary epithelium, develop clinically significant liver disease. This is true even in patients with identical gene mutations [190–192]. This observation suggests that in the bile ducts, other Cl^- channels unrelated to CFTR are able to compensate for the Cl^- secretory defect associated with cystic fibrosis. In fact, in animal models of cystic fibrosis, expression of alternate Cl^- channels is a determinant of organ-level disease [193]. Second, the finding that in mouse and rat cholangiocyte models, pharmacological inhibition of CFTR or knockdown of CFTR expression does not affect Ca^{2+}-activated secretion supports the notion that these alternate secretory pathways are functionally important. Furthermore, in polarized cholangiocyte preparations and isolated rat and mouse cholangiocytes, the short-circuit current response (a measure of transepithelial secretion) and the density of whole-cell Cl^- currents are two- to fourfold greater than cAMP-stimulated Cl^- secretion, respectively [27,184]. Lastly, studies in isolated cells and bile duct segments reveal that cAMP-stimulated secretion requires luminal ATP and intact Ca^{2+}-mediated pathways [194,195].

Together, these studies challenge the premise that cAMP-dependent activation of CFTR is the driving force for ductular secretion. Rather, alternate Ca^{2+}-activated Cl^- channels may represent the predominant or final common pathway contributing to ductular bile formation [25]. However, the majority of these studies have been performed in cell and epithelial models and corroborating studies in human models are lacking.

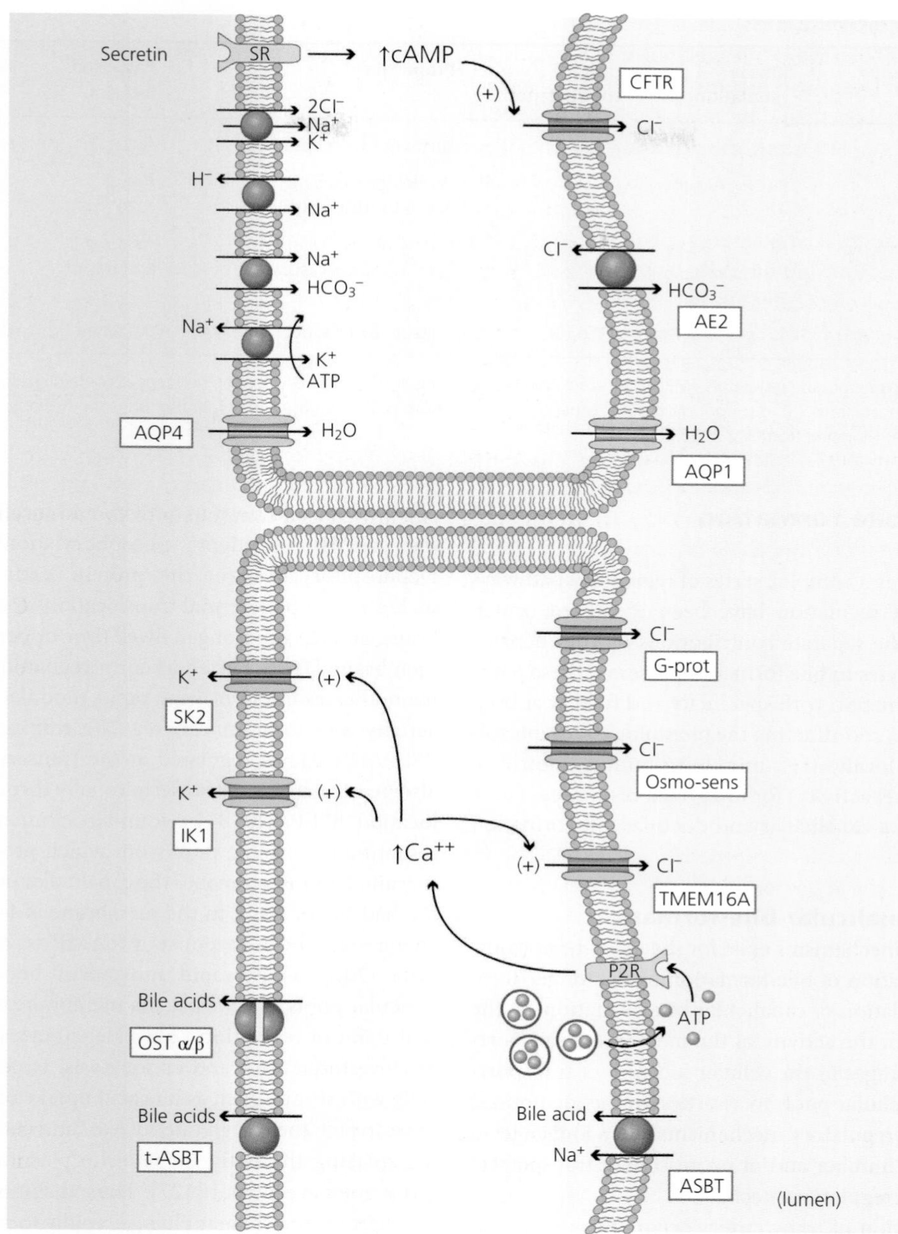

Figure 19.5 Cholangiocyte channels and transporters. Stimulation of basolateral receptors by the hormone secretin results in increases in cAMP- and PKA-dependent stimulation of Cl^- efflux through the cystic fibrosis transmembrane regulator (CFTR). The transmembrane Cl^- gradient drives Cl^-/HCO_3^- exchange through AE2. Transepithelial water flux occurs through aquaporin 4 (AQP4) on the basolateral membrane and AQP1 on the apical membrane. The increase in HCO_3^- and water secretion leads to alkalinization and dilution of bile. Other Cl^- channels have been identified, including a G-protein regulated Cl^- channel, a volume-stimulated (or osmo-sensitive) Cl^- channel, and TMEM16A, a Ca^{2+}-activated Cl^- channel. Note that cAMP- and Ca^{2+}-activated pathways represent two distinct but complementary pathways. Lumenal ATP and bile acids may also stimulate Cl^- efflux through interaction with apical membrane receptors. An apical transporter for bile acids, ASBT, has been identified. Bile acids are transported across the basolateral membrane by Ostα, Ostβ, and tASBT. On the basolateral membrane, Na^+/H^+ exchange, Na^+-dependent Cl^-/HCO_3^- exchange, and Na^+/HCO_3^- symport help to maintain intracellular pH and HCO_3^- concentrations. Cl^- uptake is mediated by a $Na^+/K^+/2Cl^-$ cotransporter. Ca^{2+}-activated K^+ channels have been identified, including SK2 and IK1, and work in parallel with apical Cl^- channels to hyperpolarize the membrane and provide the driving force for continued secretion. Note that channels and transporters are shown in two different cells for convenience only. This model represents receptors and channels in medium to large-sized cholangiocytes. Small cholangiocytes do not express secretin receptor, CFTR, AE2, or ASBT. P2R, purinergic receptor; SR, secretin receptor. See text for details.

Table 19.2 Cholangiocyte chloride channels.

Molecular origin	Stimulus	Kinase regulation	Unitary conductance	Properties	Proposed location	Function
CFTR	cAMP	PKA	~8 pS	Linear IV $Cl^- > I$ DIDS-resistant	Apical	Secretion bile formation
TMEM16A	Ca^{2+}	PKCα CAMKII	~15 pS	Outwardly rectifying IV $I^- > Cl^-$ DIDS-sensitive	Apical	Secretion bile formation
LRRC8A	Cell volume	PKCα PI3-kinase PKD	~10–50 pS	Outwardly rectifying IV $I^- > Cl^-$ DIDS-resistant	Apical and basolateral	Cell volume recovery from swelling
?	Gαi	?	~350 pS	Voltage-dependent closure	Basolateral	?

CFTR, cystic fibrosis transmembrane regulator; TMEM16A, transmembrane member 16A; LRRC8A, leucine rich repeat containing 8 protein subunit A; DIDS, 4,4′-diisothiocyanostilbene-2,2′-disulfonic acid; PKA, protein kinase A; PKCα, protein kinase Cα; PI3-kinase, phosphoinositide 3-kinase; PKD, protein kinase D.Source: Modified from Fitz 2002 [217].

Regulation of bile formation

Bile formation requires a complex series of regulatory pathways and several levels of regulation have been identified, which serve to coordinate the separate contributions of both hepatocytes and cholangiocytes to bile formation. Overall, these pathways control bile formation with specificity and fidelity at both the systemic level (i.e., coordinating the physiological events following a meal) and locally (i.e., minute-to-minute control of membrane ion channel activity) for integrated responses. These signals that coordinate canalicular and ductular bile formation are described below.

Regulation of canalicular bile formation

Different regulatory mechanisms exist for the short-term (minute-to-minute) regulation of bile formation or the longer-term (hours-to-days) regulation of canalicular bile formation. In the short term, changes in the activity of the membrane transporters themselves or changes in the cellular location of transporters, that is from subcellular pools to insertion in the membrane, account for the main regulatory mechanisms. On a longer-term basis, changes in the number and/or expression of transporters account for the main regulatory mechanism.

Short-term regulation of transporters occurs through direct changes in transporter activity via changes in the electrochemical gradients or through phosphorylation and dephosphorylation by the action of kinases and phosphatases. For example, an overall key regulatory step in the production of bile is the uptake of bile acids by NTCP/SLC10A1 on the hepatocyte sinusoidal membrane. As mentioned, the activity of NTCP/SLC10A1 is dependent on generation of an electrochemical gradient for Na^+. Thus, the activity of NTCP/SLC10A1 is regulated minute to minute by changes in the intracellular concentration of Na^+ or in the potential difference. This dependence on the potential difference is important physiologically, but also during pathological conditions. For example, during cholestasis the potential difference may change, leading to alterations in transport activity [196–198]. Additionally, NTCP/SLC10A1 is a serine/threonine phosphatide and both its activity and location are regulated by the cAMP-dependent phosphorylation state [199,200]. Dephosphorylation of the protein leads to several effects, including (1) preferential translocation to the sinusoidal membrane, and (2) a prolonged dwell time or persistence in the basal membrane [199]. The short-term regulation of BSEP/ABCB11 is another example of how rapid modulation of both protein activity and location can regulate transport function. While BSEP/ABCB11 is regulated at the transcriptional level, it can also be regulated posttranscriptionally through rapid changes in location. BSEP/ABCB11 is found in submembrane vesicles, representing a recycling pool from which proteins can be rapidly recruited for insertion into the canalicular membrane. Normally, the half-life of BSEP in the membrane is 4–6 days, but this can change rapidly in response to cAMP or other secretory agonists [201]. Thus, rapid movement between submembrane vesicular pools and the plasma membrane represents an important point of regulation [202]. Hepatocytes undergo high rates of constitutive exo- and endocytosis, which increase dramatically with stimuli such as bile acid uptake or changes in cell volume. In fact, these high rates of exo- and endocytosis are capable of replacing the entire hepatocyte plasma membrane five or more times every hour [127]. Thus, the number, type, and location of transporters may change rapidly to meet changing physiological conditions.

Over the long term, bile formation is regulated by changes in the expression of specific transporters on the sinusoidal and canalicular membranes through transcriptional regulation [203]. The transcription of these transporters is regulated by ligand-activated nuclear receptors [204]. Nuclear receptors are cytosolic receptors which bind ligands, translocate to the nucleus, and regulate transcription of target genes. Nuclear receptors have been identified for most of the solute constituents of bile, including bile acids, lipids, oxysterols, bilirubin, and xenobiotics [205–207] (Table 19.3). Binding of the ligand to the receptor results in the regulation of specific genes, and these genes are involved in the reciprocal regulation of the metabolism or transport of the ligand itself. In some cases, this may entail positive regulation and in others, negative regulation, thus representing a feedforward and feedback regulatory network.

One of the initial nuclear receptors for bile acids identified was FXR/NR1H4 [208] (see Table 19.3). FXR is a cytosolic transcription factor that preferentially binds chenodeoxycholic acid and cholic acid [209]. Upon binding by bile acids, it dimerizes with RXR and activates a number of genes involved in both the synthesis and transport of bile acids, including the genes coding for BSEP, MRP2, and FIC-1 [210]. Additionally, FXR/NR1H4 regulates expression of SHP, a transcriptional repressor, which decreases the expression of the sinusoidal NTCP/SLC10A1 [211] and 7α-hydroxylase (CYP7A1), the first step in synthesis of bile acids from cholesterol. Overall, the effect is to regulate the intracellular concentration of bile acids. In this way, increases in the intracellular concentration of bile acids decrease their own synthesis and uptake while enhancing their canalicular excretion [212].

Other important nuclear receptors include PXR, the pregnane X receptor, which binds lithocholic acid and ursodeoxycholic acid [213], VDR the vitamin D receptor (NR1I1), which binds lithocholic acid and other hydrophobic bile acids [214], and the constitutive androstane receptor (CAR/NR1I3), which binds bilirubin [213]. All of these receptors are class II nuclear receptors that heterodimerize with the retinoid X receptor α (RXRα/NR2B1) and then bind to the target region of specific gene promoters [204]. Lipids also interact with specific nuclear receptors. LXR and PPARα regulate lipid and cholesterol metabolism by binding specific ligands, including oxysterol cholesterol derivatives and fatty acids, respectively [215]. LXR regulates the expression of ABCG5 and ABCG8, the canalicular cholesterol half-transporters [215], while PPARα regulates the expression of MDR3/ABCB4, the canalicular phospholipid transporter [216]. Thus, both LXR and PPARα coordinate phospholipid and cholesterol excretion across the canalicular membrane. Together, regulation of bile formation by ligand nuclear receptors represents a powerful mechanism for regulating bile formation by coordinating the number and type of transporters on the membrane in order to match precisely the intracellular concentrations of solutes.

Regulation of ductular secretion

Biliary secretion is regulated by a variety of hormones, peptides, and small molecules acting at both the apical and basolateral membranes (Table 19.4). While the classical secretory pathway highlights the importance of the hormone secretin acting on basolateral cholangiocyte receptors, studies have demonstrated an important role for substances in bile regulating secretion directly through interaction with receptors on the apical membrane [217]. Through this mechanism, molecules secreted across the hepatocyte canalicular membrane, that is bile acids, ATP, etc., can act on downstream cholangiocytes to regulate secretion in a process known as hepatobiliary coupling.

Regulation at the basolateral membrane

The basolateral membrane of cholangiocytes contains many receptors for hormones, nucleotides, and small molecules. The best studied of these is the secretin receptor, which is found on medium and large, but not small, cholangiocytes in the mouse [51]. Secretin receptors are coupled to G-proteins and, upon binding, activate adenyl cyclase to generate cAMP. The increase in cAMP results in several steps including: (1) an increase in the rate of exocytosis with recruitment of specific vesicular pools containing CFTR, AE2/SLC4A2, and AQP1 to the apical membrane [218]; (2) direct PKA-dependent phosphorylation of CFTR with subsequent channel opening and Cl^- efflux [185]; (3) increases in AE2/SLC4A2 activity resulting in an increase in biliary HCO_3^- concentration [187]; and (4) increases in water flux through AQP1 [219]. In contrast, other hormones, including somatostatin, gastrin, and endothelin-1, counter the effects of secretin and decrease cAMP levels and inhibit secretin-stimulated secretion [220–222]. Bombesin and VIP, two neuropeptides, activate Cl^-/HCO_3^- exchange activity and increase biliary fluid secretion directly [223,224]. Cholangiocytes also express M3 acetylcholine receptors which, when bound by acetylcholine, increase biliary fluid and HCO_3^- secretion through Ca^{2+}-dependent pathways [225]. Endothelin-1 appears to have opposite effects by decreasing Ca^{2+}-dependent secretion through effects on IP3 receptors [222]. The basolateral cholangiocyte membrane also contains multiple purinergic receptors (P2 receptors), including both P2Y and P2X receptors as well as P1 receptors for adenosine [226,227].

Regulation at the apical membrane

Interestingly, constituents of bile, including bile acids and nucleotides such as ATP, have been shown to modulate cholangiocyte secretion in isolated cells and intrahepatic bile duct segments in culture through interaction with specific membrane receptors [85,228]. This mechanism, termed hepatobiliary coupling, represents a unique form of regulation where factors released by hepatocytes into bile can modulate downstream cholangiocyte functions and thereby serve as signals coordinating the separate hepatic and biliary components of secretion. Two solutes that have been shown to exert direct effects on duct cells when acting at the apical membrane are bile acids and the nucleotide ATP.

Bile acids

Cholangiocytes express transporters for bile acids on the apical membrane [229] (see Figure 19.5), including Na^+-dependent bile acid transporters (ASBT), which are capable of transporting conjugated bile acids [229]. Once taken up at the apical membrane, bile acids are shuttled through the cytosol and excreted from the basolateral cholangiocyte membrane by the proteins Ostα and Ostβ [230] and a truncated form of ASBT, t-ASBT [63]. Additionally, bile acid uptake stimulates ATP release [29,195] and increases intracellular $[Ca^{2+}]$ and Cl^-

Table 19.3 Nuclear receptors/transcription factors regulating hepatic transport protein expression.

Nuclear receptor	Alternative name	Ligands	Genes activated	Genes inactivated	Major functions
FXR	NR1H4	Bile acids, especially CDCA, DCA, CA, LCA	*BSEP, SHP, MRP2, OATP1B3, ABCB4, PXR, OSTα/β, CYP3A4, UCT2B4, UGT2B7*	*NTCP, CYP7A1*	Major bile acid sensor Increases detoxification and excretion Decreases bile acid synthesis and uptake
SHP	NR0B2			*CYP7A1, CYP8B1, NTCP, ASBT, HNF4α*	Induced by FXR Inhibits bile acid synthesis and uptake via effects on HNF4α and HNF1α
PXR	SXR, NR1I2	Numerous xenobiotics, rifampicin, statins, LCA, dexamethasone, UDCA	*CVP3A4, CYP2B6, MDR1, MRP2, GSTA2, UGT1A1*	*CYP7A1*	Induction of drug metabolism and excretion pathways Considerable overlap with CAR
CAR	NR1I3	Bilirubin, phenobarbital, xenobiotics	*CYP3A, CYP2B6, CYP2A6, OATP1B1, MRP2, UGT1A1*		Induction of drug metabolism and excretion pathways Considerable overlap with PXR Activated by bilirubin Phenobarbital promotes nuclear translocation
LXRα	NR1H3	Oxysterols, 6α-hydroxy bile acids	*ABCG5/8, ABCA1, CYP7A, CYP8B, CYP3A4, SHP*		Regulator of cholesterol metabolism and elimination
RXR	NR2B1	9-*cis*-retinoic acid	Required for function of *FXR, PXR, LXR*, and *CAR*		Heterodimerization partner for FXR, PXR, CAR, LXR, RAR Activity inhibited by cytokines
RARα	NR1B4	All-*trans*-retinoic acid	*NTCP, MRP2, ASBT*		
VDR	NR1I1	1α,25-dihydroxyvitamin D3, LCA	*CYP3A, SULTs*		Induction of bile acid hydroxylation, sulfation, and export
HNF4α	NR2A1		*CYP7A1, CYP8B1, NTCP, HNF1α*		Activity reduced by bile acids, which reduces HNF1α expression and downregulates bile acid synthesis
HNF1α	MODY3, TCF1		*OATP1B1, NTCP, CYP7A*		Major regulator of glucose homeostasis Reduced activity contributes to decreased bile acid uptake and synthesis
PPARα	NR1C1	Fatty acids, fibrates, statins, NSAIDs	*ASBT, ABCB4, UGT2B4*	*CYP7A1*	Increases β-oxidation, biliary phospholipid secretion Downregulates bile acid synthesis

CA, cholic acid; CAR, constitutive androstane receptor: CDCA, chenodeoxycholic acid; DCA, deoxycholic acid; FXR, farnesoid X receptor; LCA, lithocholic acid; NSAID, nonsteroidal antiinflammatory drug; UDCA, ursodeoxycholic acid.

Table 19.4 Regulation of cholangiocyte secretion and ductular bile formation.

Hormone/mediator	Second messenger	Effect
Ligands acting at apical receptors		
Bile acids	↑Ca^{2+}, ↑PKCα	Activation of membrane Cl^- channels
		Stimulation of Cl^- excretion and Cl^-/HCO_3^- exchange
ATP/purinergic analogues	↑Ca^{2+}	Activation of CaCC Cl^- channels
Ligands acting at basolateral receptors		
Secretin	↑cAMP, ↑PKA	Stimulation of bicarbonate-rich flow
Somatostatin	↓ cAMP	Inhibition of basal and secretin-induced bile flow
Gastrin	↓cAMP, ↑IP_3, ↑Ca^{2+}, ↑PKC	No effect on basal bile flow and bicarbonate excretion, but inhibition of secretin-induced choleresis
Bombesin	Unknown (independent of cAMP, cGMP and Ca^{2+})	Induction of a bicarbonate-rich bile flow
VIP	Unknown (cAMP independent)	Induction of a bicarbonate-rich bile flow
Acetylcholine	↑IP3, ↑Ca^{2+}	Induction of a bicarbonate-rich bile flow
Endothelin-1	↓Secretin-induced cAMP ↑IP3, ↑Ca^{2+}	Inhibition of secretin-induced choleresis

ATP, adenosine triphosphate; CaCC, Ca^{2+}-activated Cl^- channel; PKC, protein kinase C; PKA, protein kinase A; IP3, inositol triphosphate; VIP, vasoactive intestinal polypeptide.

secretion in isolated cells [228], suggesting a mechanism by which lumenal bile acids may modulate ductular secretion. This provides further evidence for the cholehepatic shunt hypothesis [100], and may help to explain the hypercholeresis, out of proportion to bile acid pool enrichment alone, observed with bile acid therapy [99]. Additionally, bile acids may interact with receptors on the cholangiocyte membrane such as TGR5 [231], a G-protein-linked receptor for bile acids found on the apical membrane and primary cilium [232,233]. Binding of bile acids to TGR5 leads to an increase in intracellular cAMP concentration and cholangiocyte Cl^- secretion [231]. Therefore, TGR5 signaling represents another mechanism by which the lumenal concentration of bile acids is coupled to ductal biliary secretion.

Nucleotides

Extracellular ATP is an important autocrine/paracrine signal that regulates diverse cellular processes by binding to one or more purinergic receptors in the plasma membrane of target cells (Figure 19.6).

Several lines of evidence provide support for ATP as a signaling molecule involved in hepatobiliary coupling and regulation of biliary secretion. First, ATP is released by primary human hepatocytes [90], and model liver and biliary cell lines [181], and is present in mammalian bile in concentrations (>100 nM) sufficient to activate purinergic receptors [234]. Second, cholangiocytes express a repertoire of purinergic (P2) receptors, including both P2Y and P2X receptors on the apical membrane [226,227]. Third, receptor binding increases Cl^- efflux rates of isolated cholangiocytes [181]. Fourth, studies in isolated cells and bile duct segments reveal that even cAMP-stimulated secretion requires lumenal ATP [194,195]. These studies challenge the premise that cAMP-dependent activation of CFTR is the driving force for ductular secretion. Rather, in the lumen of intrahepatic ducts, release of ATP and stimulation of purinergic P2 receptors may represent the final common pathway contributing to local control of ductular bile formation as well as a means of coupling hepatocyte transport to cholangiocyte electrolyte and water secretion [25]. The cellular mechanism(s) regulating ATP release into bile has not been fully elucidated. Potentially, ATP release could be mediated by two pathways: a channel-mediated pathway versus a pathway mediated by exocytosis of ATP-enriched vesicles.

Studies of CFTR and other ABC proteins in cholangiocytes and hepatocytes, respectively, suggest that while they may regulate ATP release, they are not ATP-permeable channels themselves and no other ATP channel has been identified mediating physiological ATP release in these cells [89,234,235]. Conversely, studies suggest that exocytosis of ATP-enriched vesicles may be a predominant pathway for ATP release into bile. First, stimuli that increase exocytosis in hepatocytes and cholangiocytes (e.g., cAMP, cell volume) are associated with parallel increases in ATP release and both processes require intact PKC and PI3-kinase signaling [180,181,236], key regulatory signals in vesicular trafficking. Second, both hepatocytes and cholangiocytes contain a population of ATP-enriched vesicles, which undergo regulated exocytosis and release of ATP into the extracellular space upon stimulation [237,238]. Lastly, the vesicular nucleotide transporter, SLC17A9, responsible for loading ATP into synaptic vesicles, has been identified in cholangiocytes and contributes to the formation of ATP-enriched vesicles [237].

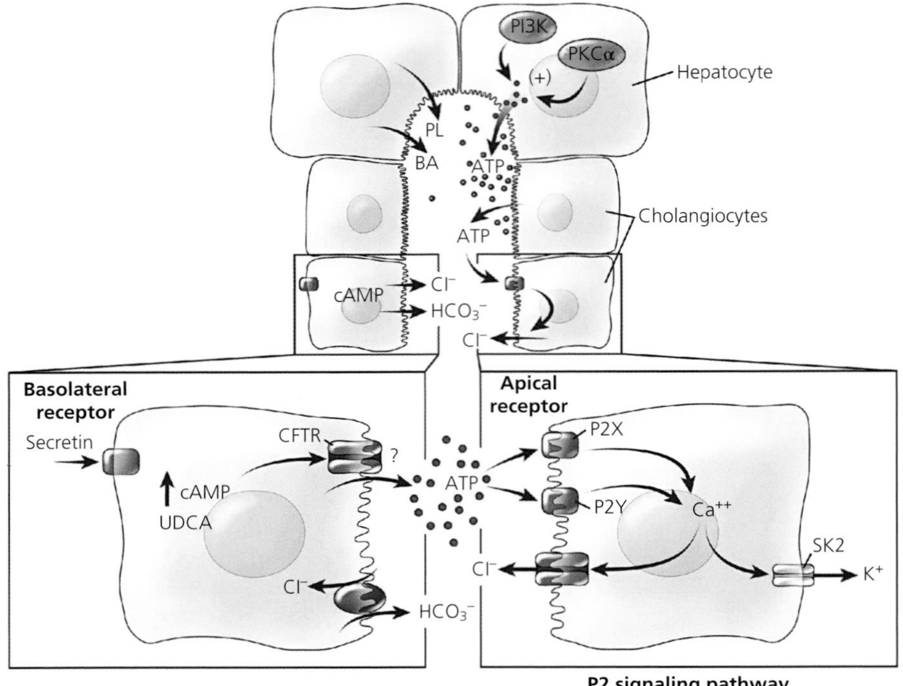

Figure 19.6 Purinergic signaling in bile formation. Proposed model for regulation of biliary secretion via extracellular ATP. Bile formation begins via transport of bile acids, phospholipids, and ATP from the hepatocyte canalicular membrane. Hepatocyte ATP release is positively regulated by PI3-kinase and PKC. Secretin stimulates increases in cholangiocyte cAMP levels via stimulation of basolateral receptors, resulting in Cl^- efflux through cystic fibrosis transmembrane conductance regulator (CFTR) and an increase in $Cl^-/HCO3^-$ exchange. Increases in cAMP, as well as exposure to the bile acid ursodeoxycholic acid (UDCA), may also increase ATP release through a CFTR-dependent mechanism. BA, bile acids; PL, phospholipids; SK2, $Ca2^+$-activated K^+ channel;. Source: Feranchak and Fitz 2007 [25]. Reproduced with permission of Elsevier.

Exosomes

The discovery that bile contains exosomes provides another potential regulatory pathway, which may coordinate the separate hepatocyte and cholangiocyte functions [239]. Exosomes are small (30–100 nm in diameter) extracellular membrane-enclosed vesicles, which contain proteins, nucleotides, and mRNAs [240] and can deliver biological information between cells and thereby regulate a host of cellular functions in target cells [241]. Exosomes can be released by both hepatocytes and cholangiocytes into bile and target downstream cholangiocytes, where they have been shown to interact with the cholangiocyte primary cilium on the apical membrane [239,242]. The uptake of specific cargo proteins and mRNAs may affect cholangiocyte functions, though the role of exosomes in the control of bile formation is not known [242].

Mechanosensitive regulation

Fluid flow or sheer stress at the cholangiocyte apical membrane has been shown to be a potent stimulus for the regulation of biliary secretion in mouse and rat models [243,244]. Increases in sheer force or increases in flow rate at the apical membrane have been shown to directly stimulate increases in ATP release, intracellular Ca^{2+} concentration, and Cl^- channel activity in polarized rat and mouse cholangiocyte preparations [183,243,244]. In this way, a rise in the shear force at the apical cholangiocyte membrane, through increases in flow rate or bile viscosity, may stimulate ATP release and, hence, result in changes in bile composition. If this model is relevant to in vivo; conditions, it may represent an attractive mechanism to increase biliary secretion and, hence, dilute bile in response to bile acid-dependent increases in bile flow or viscosity. Therefore, this would represent a "feed forward" pathway and may help to explain the hypercholeresis, out of proportion to bile acid-induced bile flow alone, observed with bile acid replacement therapy [245].

The mechanism by which the mechanical effects of flow are translated into intracellular signals is unknown. However, cholangiocytes express an apical monocilium, which mediate intracellular Ca^{2+} signals when deflected [246,247]. Additionally, the primary cilia may respond to changes in bile tonicity and express a number of receptors and proteins, such as TRPV4, PC1, and PC2, which may be mechanosensitive proteins [246,248,249].

Mechanisms of cholestasis

Cholestatic liver disease

Cholestasis is defined as absent or reduced bile flow associated with a pathological condition. The decrease in bile flow may be secondary to abnormal production, transport, or metabolism of a key constituent of bile such as bile acids or phospholipids. Cholestatic disorders may be broadly classified as genetic or acquired. In many diseases, both components exist, that is a genetic predisposition to disease development which is then initiated or propagated by acquired or environmental factors. Diseases can also be classified by the site or target of injury, such as hepatopathies, affecting primarily hepatocytes, or cholangiopathies, affecting cholangiocytes. While disorders targeting hepatocytes may lead to hepatitis and cholestasis, those targeting cholangiocytes are almost always cholestatic in nature.

This section outlines several of the genetic causes of cholestasis that are associated with alterations in the activity of the transporters and channels described in the earlier sections. Mutations in the genes for the transporters or channels at both the canalicular and ductular membranes are associated with absent or decreased function of these proteins and subsequent liver injury. For example, mutations in the genes for the canalicular proteins responsible for the transport of bile acids and phospholipids are broadly known as the progressive familial intrahepatic cholestatic (PFIC) syndromes, while mutations in the gene for the ductular Cl^- channel, CFTR, result in liver disease in some patients with cystic fibrosis. Disorders associated with abnormal production of bile acids, known as bile acid synthesis defects, are also associated with cholestasis. Lastly, defects in the development of the bile ducts are associated with disorders such as biliary atresia or Alagille syndrome. All these disorders will be discussed in more detail below, while other disorders that result in cholestasis, such as immune-mediated injury to cholangiocytes, primary biliary cholangitis (PBC), or primary sclerosing cholangitis (PSC), are discussed in Chapters 92 and 82, respectively.

General cellular mechanism of cholestasis

Insights into the cellular mechanism(s) by which cholestasis leads to liver injury are expanding. It is clear that the process is complex, with multiple steps converging on a final common pathway leading to cirrhosis [250]. As described earlier, bile acids are the major driving force for bile formation, so when bile flow decreases, bile acids accumulate in the canaliculus and in the intrahepatic bile ducts. These bile acids may be transported into hepatocytes and cholangiocytes, leading to high intracellular concentrations. The high intracellular and extracellular concentrations of bile acids may lead to direct cellular injury as bile acids are detergents capable of cellular membrane injury. The cellular injury initiates an inflammatory response with elaboration of cytokines, interleukins, and activation of Kupffer cells. This in turn leads to a cascade of signaling events converging on the activation of stellate cells and ultimately resulting in collagen deposition, fibrosis, and cirrhosis [250,251].

It should be noted that marked changes in the transcriptional regulation of canalicular and sinusoidal transporters occur during cholestasis in response to the increased concentration of intracellular bile acids [206]. Compensatory mechanisms occur involving an increased expression of sinusoidal transporters for the backtransport of bile acids from the hepatocyte into the sinusoid. This may contribute to the increase in circulating bile acids associated with most forms of cholestasis. For example, elevated levels of bile acids exert effects on the nuclear receptors FXR, PXR, and CAR [252]. Overall, this results in significant changes to the transport properties of hepatocytes with a decrease in uptake at the sinusoidal membrane, a decrease in canalicular excretion, and an increase in excretion from the hepatocyte to the sinusoid. These changes may be an attempt to limit high concentrations of canalicular and intracellular bile acids where they may contribute to cellular injury. These effects again highlight the important regulatory role of these nuclear receptors on overall bile formation during both health and disease.

Hereditary cholestasis syndromes

Progressive familial intrahepatic cholestasis (PFIC) refers to a heterogeneous group of autosomal recessive disorders that are linked by the inability to appropriately form and excrete bile from hepatocytes, resulting in a hepatocellular form of cholestasis. While the diagnosis of such disorders had historically been based on pattern recognition of unremitting cholestasis without other identified molecular or anatomic cause, recent scientific advancements have uncovered multiple specific responsible proteins. The variety of identified defects has resulted in an ever-broadening phenotypic spectrum, ranging from traditional benign recurrent jaundice to progressive cholestasis and end-stage liver disease [253].

FIC1 deficiency (PFIC-1, Byler disease)

The first reported PFIC, progressive familial intraheptatic cholestasis type 1, also called Byler disease, was described in 1969 in seven Amish children (from the original Byler kindred in western Pennsylvania) as a progressive cholestatic disease with associated extrahepatic symptoms [254]. The causative *ATP8B1* gene and corresponding FIC1 protein were identified from studies in the initial Amish cohort as well as patients from northern Europe with benign recurrent intrahepatic cholestasis type 1 (BRIC1) [255]. Deficient or defective FIC1 results in a low γ-glutamyl (GGT) cholestasis that often presents in the neonatal period, though milder forms with transient jaundice may present later in life [256–258]. Affected individuals have hyperbilirubinemia, mildly elevated aminotransferases, and elevated serum bile acids. Infants often present jaundiced, with pruritus and hepatosplenomegaly developing over the first months of life. Severe disease manifests with persistent, progressive cholestasis and the development of portal hypertension often in early childhood. Extrahepatic disease is also notable due to the broad distribution of FIC1, which can clinically distinguish FIC1 deficiency from other forms of intrahepatic cholestasis. Affected children frequently exhibit profound diarrhea, poor growth, short stature, pancreatic insufficiency, elevated sweat chloride, and sensorineural deafness [258,259]. Histopathology demonstrates canalicular cholestasis with biliary plugs, giant cell transformation, ductular paucity, and lobular disarray [260]. Visualized bile is termed as "bland" granular (Byler's) bile [256,261].

Definitive FIC1 function remains ambiguous. Current understanding of its action as an aminophospholipid translocase which transports phospholipids from outside to inside the canalicular membrane is based on studies in ATP8b1-deficient mice [262]. Additional modifiers of disease phenotype, such as mutation-specific effects on FIC1 trafficking from the endoplasmic reticulum to the canalicular membrane, have been proposed [263]. Mechanistically, disease is thought to result from inappropriate concentrations of intracellular phospholipids with resultant intracellular bile acid accumulation which are cytotoxic to the hepatocyte due to their detergent nature [256].

Treatment for FIC1 deficiency, as with all PFIC diseases, is challenging, with no definitive medical therapies available. Supportive measures are focused on improving nutritional deficiencies and managing complications of endstage liver disease. Patients should be treated with caloric, fat, and vitamin supplementation, with the majority of fat being medium chain triglycerides [256]. Ursodeoxycholic acid (UDCA) can improve pruritus and biochemical markers of cholestasis [256]. Other antipruritic agents such as rifampin and cholestyramine may also be utilized, but are often less helpful in FIC1 deficiency [256,258]. Certain CFTR folding correctors have been shown to improve defective trafficking of FIC1 in cell culture [264]; however, studies in human subjects are lacking.

When medical therapy is insufficient, surgical intervention may be considered with the goal of bypassing the enterohepatic circulation and/or decreasing reabsorption of bile salts. Procedures including partial external biliary diversion, partial internal biliary diversion, and ileal exclusion have generally, though not uniformly, resulted in sustained clinical improvement in PFIC patients [265–267]. Liver transplant is indicated in those with a refractory course and in those who develop endstage disease. Importantly, patients should be counseled that the diarrhea associated with FIC1 deficiency may persist, or even worsen, following transplant. This phenomenon has been reported concomitant with the development of both allograft steatosis and fibrosis, which can progress, requiring retransplantation [256,268]. In order to prevent damaging steatosis in the graft, ileal diversion at the time of transplant has sometimes been utilized [269].

BSEP deficiency (PFIC-2)

BSEP deficiency, PFIC-2, results from defects or deficiency in the bile salt export pump encoded by *ABCB11*. This defect results in a severe hepatobiliary phenotype and affected infants initially present jaundiced, with pruritus developing around 4–5 months of age and often progressing to the development of portal hypertension within the first year of life [256,270 271]. Scleral icterus, hepatomegaly, excoriation of skin, and poor growth due to fat malabsorption and fat-soluble vitamin deficiency may also be apparent due to cholestasis [256,259]. Laboratory findings demonstrate a low GGT cholestasis with aminotransferases typically more than twice the upper limit of normal [271]. Pathology typically demonstrates canalicular cholestasis, hepatocellular disarray, and lobular and portal fibrosis [256]. Importantly, there is up to 15% rate of malignancy (hepatocellular carcinoma and cholangiocarcinoma) that has been described in children as young as 13 months [272]. Therefore, patients with PFIC-2 should be screened for malignancy with an α-fetoprotein (AFP) level and abdominal imaging [256].

Similar to FIC1 deficiency, treatment is primarily supportive and focuses on nutritional supplementation and antipruritic agents. Zebrafish models of BSEP deficiency suggest a potential role for therapies aimed at promoting alternative transporters to excrete bile [273] while reports in human subjects using cell surface BSEP-enhancer molecules (i.e., 4-phenylbutyrate) alone [274] or as part of a cocktail of medications [275] have shown promise. Both approaches require more complete investigation, which may be facilitated through new disease models using patient-specific induced pluripotent stem cell-derived hepatocyte-like cells [276]. Surgical interruption of the enterohepatic circulation may improve pruritus but may not change the course of disease [267]. Notably, the response to diversion has been shown to be dependent on the gene defect, with those who retain some residual protein function having better outcomes than those with mutations resulting in severely dysfunctional or absent protein [277,278]. Liver transplant has been successfully used to treat severe BSEP disease and in those who develop tumor. While organ replacement has historically been considered a "cure," patients can develop alloreactive antibodies specific to the extracellular loop of the BSEP protein resulting in an immune-mediated recurrence of their BSEP disease in the allograft [279–281].

Benign recurrent intrahepatic cholestasis

Defects in both FIC1 and BSEP have been identified in individuals with benign recurrent intrahepatic cholestasis (BRIC). Patients typically experience intermittent, self-limiting but recurrent episodes of cholestasis associated with jaundice and pruritus and occasionally diarrhea. The liver disease is generally considered nonprogressive and overall the disease is thought to be benign. Laboratory evaluation reveals a low or normal GGT associated with bilirubin elevations, similar to PFIC, with biochemical resolution of cholestasis between episodes. Thus, BRIC may be thought of as a continuum, BRIC being a mild clinical phenotype with residual protein activity and PFIC a severe clinical phenotype with absent or severely deficient protein activity. Treatment of BRIC is directed at symptomatic management. Biliary drainage has been effective in relieving symptoms and this usually involves a temporary endoscopic placement of a nasal biliary drain during episodes.

MDR3 deficiency (PFIC-3)

Also described as a cholangiopathy, PFIC-3 is secondary to defects in the multidrug resistance class 3 (MDR3) glycoprotein, encoded by *ABCB4* [282]. As with other PFIC diseases, there is a spectrum of disease that can be explained by the extent to which MDR3 is impaired by a particular genetic mutation, with phenotypes ranging from transient neonatal cholestasis to more severe, progressive hepatobiliary disease [283,284]. While presentation in the first months of life is reported, MDR3 deficiency more often presents in late adolescence or even adulthood [19]. Histology typically demonstrates portal fibrosis and bile duct proliferation with mild giant cell hepatitis at disease onset with occasional intraductal cholelithiasis [256]. MDR3 immunohistochemical staining will be absent, decreased, or potentially normal if there are functional protein defects [256]. Carcinogenesis and the development of both cholangiocarcinoma and hepatocellular carcinoma have been reported [256,285,286].

Medical treatment should be initiated early in the disease course. Care is supportive, including nutrition supplementation and antipruritic agents, though it is not clear if these therapies alter the disease course [259,283]. in vitro studies have suggested that disease-associated mutations resulting in impaired ABCB4 trafficking may be functionally rescued by chemical chaperones such as phenylbutyrate and curcumin [284]. Temporizing surgical interventions as described above are rarely successful due to the severity of disease when diagnosed and liver transplant remains the only definitive therapy [19,259].

Expanded PFICs and adult disease

Progressive familial intrahepatic cholestasis has historically been used to describe the three classic genetic-based cholestatic diseases described above. Recent advances in how genetic defects in proteins affect bile acid homeostasis have led both to an expanded list of syndromes categorized in the PFIC category and a growing understanding of how adults can be affected.

Tight junction protein 2 (TJP2)

Tight junction protein 2 is one of the intracellular anchors for tight junctions that seal canaliculi and prevent damage from cytotoxic detergent bile salts [19,259]. Defects in TJP2 result in a phenotypic pattern that is similar to "classic" PFIC disease, mainly cholestasis presenting in the neonatal period. The mechanism of injury is thought to relate to TJP2's function in maintaining junction integrity, the disturbance of which enables toxic molecules to reflux into the paracellular space; however, this is not certain [287]. Though few samples are available, pathology demonstrates intracellular cholestasis and giant cell transformation, with absence of TJP2 protein staining [259]. Hepatocellular carcinoma has been described at presentation in infants [288,289] and liver transplant has been performed; however, optimal management strategies are unknown owing to the rarity of the disease.

NR1H4 (FXR)

Progressive familial intrahepatic cholestasis phenotype can also result from mutations in the *NR1H4* (nuclear receptor subfamily 1, group H, member 4) gene which encodes the farnesoid X receptor (FXR), the nuclear receptor transcription factor which regulates BSEP expression via negative feedback loop and induces FGF19 to repress bile acid synthesis [259,290]. Without appropriate regulation of BSEP, patients with this defect have presented in the neonatal period with normal GGT cholestasis, normal amino transferases, elevated serum bile acids, and extremely elevated AFP, and rapidly progressed to endstage liver disease with vitamin K-independent coagulopathy and hyperammonemia [291,292]. Patients with these defects are extremely rare, with only five reported in the literature [291,292].

MYO5B

Defects in the *MYO5B* gene result in abnormal myosin-Vb protein which BSEP requires in order to localize to the canalicular hepatocellular membrane. This usually results in microvillus inclusion disease and diarrhea, but also may result in isolated liver disease [259]. Without appropriate BSEP localization, secretion of bile acids is impaired and causes hepatocellular toxicity [293]. This results in a clinical picture of low GGT cholestasis, hepatomegaly, normal or mildly elevated aminotransferases. Patients have preserved hepatic synthetic function but struggle with pruritus and present around 1 year of age, similar to FIC1 and BSEP disease [293].

The traditional understanding of the PFIC-associated genes contributing to morbidity in adults mainly encompasses the phenotypes of BRIC and intrahepatic cholestasis of pregnancy (ICP). ICP is a common condition affecting about 1% of all pregnancies [294]. It manifests during pregnancy with pruritus, hepatic impairment, and cholestasis which usually resolves completely after delivery. While generally considered benign for the mother, adverse perinatal outcomes for the child, such as fetal distress, premature birth, and stillbirth, can occur [294].

More recently, investigators have begun looking more broadly at the contributions that these genes may have on morbidity in adult populations. Mutations in *ATP8B1*, *ABCB11*, *ABCB4*, and *TJP2* have been reported in adults with cryptogenic cirrhosis [295] while *ABCB4* defects have been linked to the development of sclerosing cholangitis, biliary cirrhosis, and low-phospholipid cholelithiasis [296,297]. Genetic sequencing of large cholestatic populations has revealed disease-causing mutations in up to a third of patients, with common variants detected in a high number of those without known disease-causing defects suggesting that they still may have a contributing role in the development of cholestasis.

Dubin–Johnson syndrome

Dubin–Johnson syndrome results from mutations in the *MRP2/ABCC2* gene [298]. MRP2/ABCC2 is an ABC protein located on the hepatocyte canalicular membrane and is responsible for transport of conjugated bilirubin and other organic anions into bile. MRP2/ABCC2 is also responsible for elimination of drugs and endogenous compounds. Patients with Dubin–Johnson syndrome have a persistently elevated direct (conjugated) bilirubin, but normal serum bile acids and GGT. It is considered to be a benign disorder but case reports of an increased risk of hepatocellular carcinoma exist. The absence of canalicular MRP2 function may be partly offset by increased expression of MRP3/ABCC3 at the sinusoidal membrane.

Bile acid synthesis defects

As bile acids are the driving force for bile formation, it is not surprising that genetic disorders associated with a decrease in bile acid production are accompanied by cholestasis. These rare disorders result from defects in the genes for the enzymes involved in the synthesis of bile acids from cholesterol [4]. Clinical manifestations are quite variable depending on the specific enzyme defect, and defects have been reported in many of the enzymes in the bile acid synthesis pathway. Cholestasis may occur due to the lack of primary bile acids that are essential for bile formation. Additionally, these defects may result in overproduction of potentially hepatotoxic, atypical bile acids proximal to the enzyme defect. Some defects are severe with accumulation of toxic hydrophobic bile acids with resultant progressive liver injury. Liver histology often reveals cholestasis with giant cell transformation. Laboratory evaluation reveals normal or low GGT, probably reflecting the lack of bile acids in bile and therefore an absence of direct biliary epithelial toxicity. Serum total bile acids may be abnormally low for the degree of cholestasis and this is a helpful clue to the diagnosis. The diagnosis can be confirmed by analysis of blood, urine, and bile (if available) for bile acid metabolites by GC mass spectrometry. Many of these disorders can be treated by administration of the primary bile acid cholic acid [299].

Defects of ductular transport

Genetic defects have been associated with absence of or abnormal ductular transport or with developmental abnormalities of the ducts themselves. These include absence of Cl^- secretion, associated with cystic fibrosis, or developmental abnormalities of the bile ducts associated with Alagille syndrome (see below) or biliary atresia.

Cystic fibrosis

Cystic fibrosis is an autosomal recessive disease characterized by abnormal electrolyte transport in the epithelial cells of many organs. The disease is due to a mutation in the *CFTR/ABCC7* gene encoding a membrane protein that functions as a Cl^- channel in the apical membrane of many epithelial cells. In the liver, CFTR/ABCC7 protein is found on the apical membrane of cholangiocytes [185]. It is not found in hepatocytes or other cells of the liver [53]. Defects in the CFTR protein lead to a wide spectrum of hepatobiliary conditions collectively referred to as CF-associated liver disease (CFLD) [300].

The mechanism of liver disease in cystic fibrosis is complex. The pathognomonic lesion of CF, focal biliary cirrhosis (FBC), presumably involves loss of biliary Cl^- and HCO_3^- secretion, bile duct plugging, and toxic injury to cholangiocytes and hepatocytes [300]. More recent findings of CFTR as a regulator of epithelial innate immunity and the possible influence of the intestinal disease with an altered microbiota on the liver complication have opened new mechanistic insights and areas of future research [301,302]. Modifiers for disease development have been sought, identifying the SERPINA1 Z allele as a potential contributor to CFLD [303]. Interestingly, most patients with cystic fibrosis (even with the most common mutation, e.g., ΔF508) do not develop clinically significant liver disease [304]. Thus, it is likely that other secretory pathways are functional and can overcome the Cl^- secretory defect associated with cystic fibrosis. As described in the previous section, cholangiocytes express several non-CFTR Cl^- channels, including the Ca^{2+}-activated Cl^- channel TMEM16A, which may serve as therapeutic targets for future treatments [183].

Currently, the treatment for cystic fibrosis liver disease is UDCA, which is associated with improvements in liver enzymes, but long-term outcome studies demonstrating improvement in morbidity and mortality are lacking [305]. The role of newly developed CFTR modulators, which target the underlying genetic defect and improve the production or trafficking of CFTR, in the progression of liver disease is unknown.

Disorders of bile duct development

Alagille syndrome

Alagille syndrome is a complex, autosomal dominant, multisystem disorder characterized by abnormal development of intrahepatic bile ducts. The liver phenotype is characterized by ductopenia, though the disorder is also associated with developmental abnormalities of the heart, kidney, face, eyes, and vertebra [306]. Therefore, the disease is often termed "syndromic bile duct paucity." Clinical presentation is quite variable though the typical liver manifestations include cholestasis during infancy or early childhood marked by jaundice, pruritus, and xanthoma formation [307]. Liver histology reveals bile duct paucity defined as a bile duct to portal region ratio of <0.9 (normal bile duct:portal region ratio is 0.9–1.8) in full-term infants or young children. Laboratory evaluation reveals blood and serum elevations of substances usually excreted in bile, including bile acids, bilirubin, and cholesterol. Cardiac, vascular, and hepatic disease account for most of the mortality associated with the disease, which is quite variable [308].

The disease is caused by abnormalities in the Jagged-1/Notch-2 signaling pathway, which is a cell fate pathway in early development. Most patients with Alagille syndrome have a mutation in the gene for Jagged-1, though a small percentage of patients have been identified with mutations in Notch-2 [309]. In liver development, Notch-2 signaling is involved in the ability of hepatoblasts to differentiate into cholangiocytes. Jagged-1 is expressed on periportal mesenchymal cells and interacts with Notch-2 expressed by hepatoblasts, determining their differentiation into ductal plate cells [304]. Abnormalities in this Jagged-1–Notch-2 interaction lead to defective peripheral branching of the biliary tree and ductopenia. As noted, the expression of disease severity is highly variable, and it is not possible to predict outcome based on specific genetic mutations. Treatment focuses on the affected organs.

Biliary atresia

Biliary atresia is the most common cause of neonatal cholestasis that causes progressive liver injury and endstage liver disease [310]. It is also the most common indication for liver transplantation in children. Biliary atresia causes a progressive fibrotic obliteration of the intra- and extrahepatic ducts. Clinically, infants present with jaundice within weeks of birth. Stools are often pale or acholic. Laboratory evaluation reveals a direct (conjugated) hyperbilirubinemia and elevated GGT. Ultrasound may reveal absence of the extrahepatic biliary ducts or gallbladder. Liver histology reveals proliferation and plugging of bile ducts, canalicular bile stasis, and portal or perilobular fibrosis.

The etiology and pathogenesis of biliary atresia are not completely understood, though two forms have been described: (1) an embryonic form and (2) the more common acquired form [311]. The embryonic form is associated with other developmental anomalies including polysplenia, asplenia, malrotation, situs inversus, portal vein abnormalities, or cardiovascular defects. This embryonic or fetal form of the disease occurs in 10–30% of patients with biliary atresia. While the associated anomalies suggest a genetic cause, few specific gene mutations have been identified. Recent identification of the potential role for the polycystic kidney disease 1 like 1 (PKD1L1) gene, associated with ciliary calcium signaling and embryonic laterality, suggests a biologically plausible, cholangiocyte-expressed candidate gene for biliary atresia associated with splenic malformations [312]. In contrast, the acquired form of the disease occurs in 70–90% of patients with biliary atresia and is characterized by a progressive obliteration of the bile ducts, suggesting an ongoing immune or inflammatory injury to the bile ducts. This has led to the hypothesis that etiology may be multifactorial, with elements of genetic predisposition, environmental trigger, and autoimmunity all contributing to disease pathogenesis [313].

Treatment involves a timely hepatoportoenterostomy (HPE), or Kasai procedure, ideally performed in the first weeks of life. If done within the first 45 days of life, HPE is associated with 65.5% survival with the native liver at 2 years of age and 40.5% at 15 years [314].

Summary

Advances in electrophysiology, molecular biology, and genetics have provided sophisticated tools to elucidate the pathways responsible for bile formation. These cellular pathways are critical for human life as evidenced by the serious diseases outlined above. We have progressed from the original ideas of Hypocrites and Galen and moved from a "humoral" understanding, in which an excess of "yellow bile" leads to a disease-causing imbalance in the "humors," to a sophisticated understanding of the genes and proteins that regulate each step of bile formation. The ongoing challenge now, and for the future, is to translate these basic mechanistic observations into new and effective treatments for cholestatic liver diseases.

References are available at www.yamadagastro.com/textbook7e

Further reading

Boyer J.L. Bile formation and secretion. Compr Physiol 2013;3:1035.

Feranchak A.P., Fitz J.G. Purinergic receptors and hepatobiliary function. In: Schwiebert E.M. (ed). Current Topics in Membranes, 54th edn. San Diego, CA: Academic Press, Elsevier Science; 2003: 395.

Fitz J.G. Cellular mechanisms of bile secretion. In: Zakim D., Boyer T.D. (eds). Hepatology, 3rd edn. Philadelphia: W.B. Saunders Company; 1996: 362.

Hofmann A.F., Hagey L.R. Bile acids: chemistry, pathochemistry, biology, pathobiology, and therapeutics. Cell Mol Life Sci 2008;65:2461.

Jansen P.L., Sturm E. Genetic cholestasis, causes and consequences for hepatobiliary transport. Liver Int 2003;23:315.

Karpen S.J. Nuclear receptor regulation of hepatic function. J Hepatol 2002;36:832.

Meier P.J. Molecular mechanisms of hepatic bile salt transport from sinusoidal blood into bile. Am J Physiol 1995;269:G801.

Trauner M., Boyer J.L. Bile salt transporters: molecular characterization, function, and regulation. Physiol Rev 2003;83:633.

Wheeler H.O., Ramos O.L. Determinants of the flow and composition of bile in the unanesthetized dog during constant infusions of sodium taurocholate. J Clin Invest 1960;39:161.

CHAPTER 20

General nutritional principles

Xiaowen Fan[1], Rebecca Rudel[2], Matthew Berger[3], Melissa Hershman[3], and David S. Seres[4]

[1]Department of Medicine, Columbia University Irving Medical Center, New York, NY, USA
[2]Boston University School of Public Health, Boston, MA, USA
[3]Department of Medicine, University of Rochester Medical Center, Rochester, NY, USA
[4]Institute of Human Nutrition and Department of Medicine, Columbia University Irving Medical Center, New York, NY, USA

Chapter menu

Introduction

Clinical nutrition is an active multidisciplinary specialty, comprising dietitians, physicians, pharmacists, and others. Gastroenterologists should have an extensive familiarity with nutrition, and be able to identify nutritional issues, provide basic advice, and then refer patients to nutrition specialists, with whom they should have a strong collaborative relationship.

In this chapter, we provide a review of important nutritional concepts, and a detailed review of nutrients, the disease states leading to risk of deficiency, and some of the approaches to addressing these.

Altered nutrition states

Deficiency

The true deficiency state requires a lack of a substance or nutrient that results in a pathological condition, and which is preventable or reversible by supplementation. This is distinguished from altered nutrient levels due to underlying disease, which may reflect disease epiphenomena for which supplementation will have no effect, rather than true deficiencies. For example, it is well accepted that low calcium levels resulting from a decrement in albumin levels do not by themselves constitute a calcium deficiency. Similarly, a low albumin level, itself, does not constitute a protein deficiency [1–3]. This is further exemplified by the attention that vitamin D has received for its potential role in prevention of numerous illnesses, and in the setting of critical illness and COVID-19. This is discussed in greater depth in the final section of this chapter.

Malnutrition

The current diagnostic criteria for malnutrition include loss of mass and poor nutritional intake [4], and are highly predictive of poor outcomes [5]. Wasting, however, may result from starvation, systemic inflammation, or both. Thus, the terms *malnutrition* and *malnourished* should not be used interchangeably. Starvation is responsive to nourishment, and these patients may be referred to as being malnourished. Metaanalyses of nutrition

Yamada's Textbook of Gastroenterology, Seventh Edition. Edited by Timothy C. Wang, Michael Camilleri, Benjamin Lebwohl, Anna S. Lok, William J. Sandborn, Kenneth K. Wang, and Gary D. Wu.

Companion website: www.yamadagastro.com/textbook7e

intervention studies of hospitalized patients with malnutrition have, in the aggregate, shown some benefit [6]. However, it has also been shown that patients with severe inflammation do not respond to nutrition interventions [7]. Thus, patients with disease-related malnutrition may or may not be malnourished, unless they are concurrently starving. Current diagnostic criteria also include phenomena, such as edema and hypoalbuminemia, which are reflective of systemic inflammation, are not responsive to supplementation, and should not be considered indications for nutritional interventions. This is reviewed in more detail in Chapter 23.

Cachexia and catabolism

Cachexia refers to muscle and fat wasting resulting from a chronic state of systemic inflammation. Definitions for cachexia vary, and include severe weight loss (more than 10% of the premorbid bodyweight with correction for fluid retention), and loss of muscle mass and strength, with or without fat loss [8,9]. However, the cause of wasting determines the treatment. Anorexia, insulin resistance, and/or biochemical alterations (anemia, elevated inflammatory markers, and low albumin) are often included [9]. Cachexia is often used to include those with wasting due to starvation. The inflammatory state, called catabolism, is characterized by accelerated muscle wasting, hypoalbuminemia, and immune dysfunction. Descriptions of catabolism as a "hypermetabolic state" are inaccurate, in that caloric consumption is not different. Nor do nutritional interventions reverse cachexia, or alter the loss of lean mass and hypoalbuminemia due to catabolism [3,10].

Cachexia is often described in the setting of cancer and in other advanced chronic illnesses including AIDS, heart failure, chronic kidney disease, and chronic obstructive pulmonary disease [11–15]. Prevalence of cachexia is as high as 85% in cancer, in particular pancreatic, gastric and lung cancer [12–14]. The prevalence of cachexia in HIV-infected patients in the United States has reduced significantly with the advent of antiviral therapy, though it still remains around 30% [16]. All patients with the above conditions should be screened for weight loss, changes in body habitus, and alterations in dietary intake.

The pathogenesis of cachexia is still somewhat poorly understood. It has been attributed mainly to release of cytokines and polypeptides by immune cells during prolonged inflammatory states. Proinflammatory cytokines such as interleukin (IL)-6, tumor necrosis factor (TNF) α, and IL-1 all elicit anorexia, lipolysis, and muscle breakdown. Other proposed factors that may contribute to cachexia include increased lipid mobilization, activation of the JAK/STAT pathway, cancer treatment (i.e., androgen deprivation therapy and antivascular endothelial growth factor therapy), reduced dietary intake, and malabsorption [17–19]. Elevated inflammatory markers are inversely related to albumin and transthyretin (prealbumin) levels, neither of which reflects adequacy of nutrient intake [1]. High levels of acute phase reactants and interleukins are associated with low albumin levels and low body mass index [20].

Patient assessment

The nutritional assessment begins with a first impression, and proceeds through a step-wise review of systems, physical assessment and review of laboratory and radiological findings. Important components for the screening of patients at risk from gastrointestinal disease are reviewed briefly here. Nutrient deficiencies may cause specific physical signs and symptoms. These are discussed in Chapter 23 and outlined in Table 23.1 of that chapter.

Review of systems

Questions related to weight change, and alterations in dietary intake and vigor are most helpful as general screening questions. However, these symptoms are often later manifestations, and are insufficient to discover early symptoms that place the patient at risk for development of nutrition deficiencies. In addition to a targeted GI review of systems, patients with any systemic disease, but gastrointestinal disease in particular, should undergo a somewhat more thorough review to discover barriers to intake. These include symptoms such as altered taste, lessened appetite, altered swallowing, changes in food preferences, and alterations of mood. This assessment should also include attention to socioeconomic factors such as affordability and access to healthy food, food purchasing and preparation patterns (e.g., grocery store and cooking vs fast food), physical self-sufficiency, and importantly isolation which has a profound impact on state of nourishment.

The review of systems should include the usual gastrointestinal symptom review. In addition, a survey of skin, vision, and neurological systems may uncover deficiencies. Drying of skin is nonspecific but may alert the practitioner to nutritional risk. Overt skin flaking may signal fat-soluble vitamin deficiencies or essential fatty acid deficiency. Lessening of vision in dim light or dry eyes may signal vitamin A deficiency. Sensory neuropathy is a symptom of many deficiencies, including most B vitamins and most fat-soluble vitamins.

Physical examination

Muscle loss

Several muscle groups, including the temporalis muscle, pectoralis, deltoids, trapezius, quadriceps and gastrocnemius, should be included in an evaluation for muscle mass. A low mass in one group may not reflect the overall muscle mass of the patient. For example, concave temples may be seen in patients with prominent brow and/or zygoma in the absence of wasting. The temples are evaluated by standing directly in front of the patient and asking them to turn their head left and right. A slight depression over the temples may be consistent with mild-to-moderate malnutrition, and a hollowing, scooping depression is consistent with severe malnutrition. The clavicular bone area assesses the deltoid, pectoralis major, and trapezius muscles based on the degree of protrusion of the clavicle. A protruding and prominent clavicle is consistent with severe malnutrition. Biceps mass can be easily evaluated with elbow flexion against resistance. Significant deltoid muscle atrophy may be present if the shoulder to arm joint appears squared. Other signs consistent with muscle loss include sharp and prominent scapular spine, bony humeral head, depressed areas between the thumb and forefinger, prominent patellar bones with limited muscle around the knee, depression line on the thigh when the patient has legs propped up in a sitting position, and limited definition of the calf muscles [21,22].

Subcutaneous fat

The loss of subcutaneous fat can be best assessed at the orbital fat pads, below the triceps muscles, and in the intercostal spaces. Orbital fat pads should be viewed while standing directly in front of the patient and palpating just above the cheekbone. A mild to moderately malnourished patient may have dark circles and a somewhat hollowed look. In severe malnutrition, the orbits will appear hollowed with depressions. The triceps should be evaluated with the arms bent and rolling skin on the back of the patient's arm between the clinician's fingers. The degree of malnutrition is defined by the thickness of the skinfold. The fat around the intercostal spaces is evaluated with the patient pressing against a solid object or wall. Small and large depressions between ribs may be consistent with mild-to-moderate and severe malnutrition, respectively [21,22].

Edema

Edema is included in the nutritional physical examination, even though the cause is not malnourishment, because it is also associated with poor outcomes. This demonstrates the ongoing confusion about malnutrition (i.e., what is due to deficiency, and what is due to disease?). While edema has long been attributed to hypoproteinemia and resultant decreased oncotic pressure, it is now known that, universally, edema is caused by capillary leak due to systemic inflammation. Moreover, oncotic pressure of hypoalbuminemic serum has, to our knowledge, never been tested. It is at least theoretically plausible that serum oncotic pressure is unchanged in the presence of edema. The decrement in oncotic proteins like albumin might be replaced by the outpouring of acute phase reactants, cytokines, and antibodies into the bloodstream during systemic inflammation. Finally, the more likely scenario is that albumin is low due to redistribution of serum proteins into the third space, rather than hypoalbuminemia being a primary cause of edema.

When assessing the extremities, the bony surfaces over the posterior ankles and anterior shins are optimal sites for examining for pitting edema. The depth of pitting or indentation of the skin correlates with the severity of the edematous state and degree of malnutrition. Ascites is associated with abdominal distension, shifting dullness and a fluid wave on percussion of the abdomen. It is important to note that weight loss is often masked by generalized fluid retention [21,23].

Muscle strength

Muscle strength is included in the nutrition-related examination, but weakness is often multifactorial and may be due to systemic inflammation. While often not predictive of nutritional deficiency, it is highly prognostic of outcomes overall.

Several methods are available to assess strength and function. Handgrip dynamometry which measures upper extremity grip strength is a preferred method due to its simplicity and standardization. Grip strength should be measured in a seated position with shoulders abducted, elbows flexed at 90° and forearms in neutral position. The grip strength is based on the mean value of the three maximum grip efforts of both dominant and non-dominant hands. A weak grip strength has been defined as strength 2.5 standard deviations below the gender-specific peak mean. Variation in measurements can occur secondary to psychological factors including motivation, depression or disease affecting the hands and nerves and muscles of the upper extremities. Muscle strength may also be tested by knee extensor strength when there are limitations to testing the upper extremities. This method of testing can be difficult, costly, and time-intensive [24].

Simple functional performance tests include walking/gait speed, stair-climb test and timed up and go. Walking gait/speed is often used and of interest as it can be predictive of poor health outcomes, including hospitalization and falling. It is measured as an individual's walking pace over a 4-meter distance. Speed <0.6 m/s is diagnostic for dysmobility [24].

Nutrition deficiencies by anatomical location

Stomach

In addition to its function in initiating food breakdown, the stomach is responsible for reduction of iron into its soluble form, and release of transporter proteins that assist with vitamin B_{12} absorption. Injury or loss of gastric tissue can lead to iron and B_{12} deficiency. Moreover, the deficiency of several vitamins and micronutrients, such as vitamin C, vitamin D, folic acid and calcium, has also been described due to alterations in gastric anatomy and physiology [25].

Chronic atrophic gastritis is caused by either autoimmune disease, with antibodies directed towards the parietal cells and/or intrinsic factor of the gastric body and fundus, or environmental factors, mainly *Helicobacter pylori* which results in loss of parietal cells and zymogenic chief cells. Chief cells are responsible for release of pepsinogen, which hydrolyzes protein-bound vitamin B_{12} to allow binding with transcobalamin. Parietal cells are responsible for the production and release of intrinsic factor, which binds vitamin B_{12} in the small intestine and facilitates its absorption in the terminal ileum [26]. Unlike the environmental metaplasia of *H. pylori*, those with autoimmune pernicious anemia or surgically altered gastric anatomy typically require lifelong and parenteral supplementation of B_{12}, though systematic reviews suggest that high-dose oral B_{12} repletion may be sufficient [27].

Parietal cells also produce hydrochloric acid. When there is significant atrophy or loss of parietal cells, achlorhydria ensues. Iron deficiency is the most common micronutrient deficiency in an achlorhydric state due to the lack of reduction of ferric iron to the more soluble ferrous iron, which is absorbed in the duodenum [25]. Iron deficiency has also been shown due to similar mechanisms in patients with chronic proton pump inhibitor (PPI) therapy [28]. Achlorhydria may also lead to poor absorption or deactivation of calcium and ascorbic acid [29–31].

Similar nutrient deficiencies are found in postbariatric or postgastrectomy patients, depending on the location and amount of stomach removed. The proximal stomach, mainly the gastric body, secretes acid, pepsinogens, and intrinsic factor. The distal stomach, mainly the antrum, secretes gastrin and somatostatin. Sleeve gastrectomy (SG) involves division of the stomach vertically with reduction in size by 75%, with preservation of the pyloric valve. By comparison, the Roux-en-Y gastric bypass (RYGB) involves a subtotal gastrectomy, leaving only a small gastric pouch [32]. The biliopancreatic diversion (BPD) also involves creation of a sleeve gastrectomy, though also reanatomizes the proximal duodenum to the distal 250 cm of small intestine. In BPD, the excluded small intestine is connected 50 cm proximal to the ileocecal valve, thus leaving little surface area for absorption of nutrients and mixing with biliopancreatic juices.

Anemia and osteoporosis often complicate bariatric surgery in the long term. Iron deficiency occurs in more than 30% of patients who have undergone SG and RYGB after 5 years [33]. Vitamin B_{12} deficiency occurs in 19–35% of patients with RYGB and BPD after 5 years [34]. Folic acid deficiency has also been described after bariatric surgeries and is felt to be secondary to reduced food intake and decreased conversion to its active form which requires B_{12} as a coenzyme [35]. The incidence of calcium deficiency approaches 10% in postsurgical patients, though is more prevalent in RYGB and BPD [32]. The American Society for Metabolic and Bariatric Surgery (ASMBS) has thus provided preventive guidance for the postoperative patient [36] (Table 20.1).

Table 20.1 Recommended supplementation after bariatric surgery [36].

Micronutrient	Recommended supplement to prevent deficiency
Vitamin B_1 (thiamine)	Minimum 12 mg daily; prefer 50–100 mg daily dose from B-complex supplement or multivitamin
Vitamin B_{12} (cobalamin)	Oral: 350–500 µg daily Nasal: as directed by manufacturer Parenteral: 1000 µg monthly
Folate (folic acid)	All: 400–800 µg daily from multivitamin Women of childbearing age: 800–100 µg daily
Iron	Low-risk males; nonanemic: 18 mg daily from multivitamin Menstruating females; all SG, RYGB, BPD, DS: 45–60 mg total elemental iron daily
Calcium	BPD, DS: 1800–2400 mg/day in divided doses LAGB, SG, RYGB: 1200–1500 mg/day in divided doses
Vitamin D	3000 IU/day vitamin D_3 until serum 25(OH)D greater than 30 ng/mL
Vitamin A	LAGB: 5000 IU/day RYGB, SG: 5000–10 000 IU/day DS: 10 000 IU/day
Vitamin E	15 mg/day
Vitamin K	LAGB, RYGB, SG: 90–120 µg/day DS: 300 µg/day
Zinc	BPD, DS: 200% of the RDA (16–22 mg/day) RYGB: 100–200% of the RDA (8–22 mg/day) SG, LAGB: 100% of the RDA (8–11 mg/day) All in multivitamin form with ratio of 8–15 mg supplemental zinc per 1 mg of copper to minimize the risk of copper deficiency
Copper	BPD, DS, RYGB: 200% of the RDA (2 mg/day) SG, LAGB: 100% of the RDA (1 mg/day)

BPD, biliopancreatic diversion; DS, duodenal switch; IU, international units; LAGB, laparoscopic adjustable gastric banding; RDA, recommended daily amount; RYGB, Roux-en-Y gastric bypass; SG, sleeve gastrectomy.

Pancreas, bile ducts, liver

Disorders of the pancreas, bile ducts, and liver result in maldigestion of proteins and fats and destruction of transport pathways for the absorption of fats and fat-soluble vitamins.

Severe pancreatic parenchymal loss caused by chronic pancreatitis, cystic fibrosis, pancreatic cancer, and pancreatic resection results in exocrine pancreatic insufficiency (EPI). In EPI, maldigestion results from the poor generation and secretion of digestive enzymes [37]. This leads to steatorrhea, fat-soluble vitamin loss (A, D, E, and K), loss of different proteins including apolipoproteins and high-density lipoproteins, and micronutrients including magnesium and selenium [38,39]. Despite the need for pancreatic proteases to hydrolyze the bond between vitamin B_{12} and transcobalamin, vitamin B_{12} deficiency is rare in EPI [40]. In addition, significant loss of pancreatic β cells may lead to pancreatogenic diabetes, also called type 3c diabetes mellitus [37].

In patients who undergo pancreatoduodenectomy (PD) or Whipple procedure, similar nutrient deficiencies are found, though these patients are at further risk for additional mineral deficiencies due to resection of the duodenum; these include iron, calcium, copper, and zinc [41–43]. Zinc deficiency has been reported in up to 68% of patients who undergo PD [41]. These patients are also susceptible to bacterial overgrowth which can further result in vitamin B_{12} and fat-soluble vitamin deficiency [44].

Bile is produced by the liver and is necessary to mediate the absorption of long-chain fatty acids and fat-soluble vitamins. Deficiencies in these nutrients ensue when there is a chronic disturbance in the flow of bile as seen in cholestatic liver diseases or bacterial overgrowth in patients having undergone RYGB. For example, in primary sclerosing cholangitis, extra- and intrahepatic bile duct obstruction occurs secondary to stricture formation. Cholestasis can also occur due to infiltrative processes or direct destruction of the bile ducts which is seen in primary biliary cirrhosis (PBC), IgG4 cholangiopathy, HIV cholangiopathy, sarcoidosis or malignancy-related cholestasis [45]. In patients with jaundice, vitamin A, D, E or K deficiencies are variable, ranging from 8% to 33%, with vitamin A being the most common [46]. The American Association for the Study of Liver Diseases (AASLD) specifically recommends annual monitoring of fat-soluble vitamins in patients with PBC and jaundice, as well as bone mineral density assessment every 2 years [47]. Because of similar risks of hepatic osteodystrophy in PSC, the AASLD also recommends periodic measurement of serum calcium, magnesium, phosphorus, 25-hydroxyvitamin D, and parathyroid hormone levels in pediatric PSC with cholestasis (in addition to vitamin A and E), as well as baseline osteopenia screening followed every 2–3 years in adult populations [48].

The liver plays a major role in the metabolism of vitamin D synthesis. The enzyme 25-hydroxylase is mainly expressed in the liver and is responsible for the conversion of vitamin D_2 and D_3 to 25-hydroxyvitamin D, a necessary process for the vitamin's activation [49]. Vitamin D deficiency is present in liver disease and correlates with degree of fibrosis [50]. This contributes to the development of osteoporosis and pathological bone fractures in patients with cirrhosis [51].

Small bowel and colon

The small bowel is responsible for the digestion and absorption of all micro- and macronutrients. The location and extent of the disturbance, global, partial, or compensated, determines to what degree each nutrient is inadequately absorbed and to what degree deficiency is likely [52]. There are multiple diseases that affect the small bowel surfaces including autoimmune diseases such as celiac disease, Crohn's disease, autoimmune enteropathy, common variable immunodeficiency, and eosinophilic gastroenteritis; infectious diseases including Whipple disease and tropical sprue; and other causes such as intestinal lymphangiectasias, radiation enteritis, bacterial overgrowth, and AIDS enteropathy [52,53].

In celiac disease, small intestinal absorptive surfaces are greatly reduced as a result of architectural distortion by an adaptive immune response to ingested gluten peptides [54]. While iron is the most well-known micronutrient deficiency, malabsorption of various other vitamins and minerals has been observed [55]. A Dutch study measured multiple micronutrients at diagnosis of celiac disease prior to starting a gluten-free diet and found deficiencies in folic acid, vitamin B_{12}, B_6, A, D, zinc, and iron. Zinc was the most common deficiency, found in up to 67% of patients [56]. Follow-up testing 3–6 months and 1 year post diagnosis might therefore include complete blood count, alanine aminotransferase, vitamins (A, D, E, B_{12}), copper, zinc, carotene, folic acid, ferritin, and iron. Consultation with a registered dietitian may help to monitor these deficiencies, and is recommended when unintentional gluten contamination is suspected [57].

In inflammatory bowel disease (IBD), the key nutrient deficiencies include calcium, folate, zinc, vitamin B_{12}, and vitamin D. Folate deficiency occurs in the setting of poor oral intake and interaction with certain IBD medications, including sulfasalazine and methotrexate [58–60]. Iron deficiency may occur due to chronic blood loss and iron sequestration in chronic disease [61,62]. Ileal resections >30 cm as a consequence of Crohn's disease are associated with vitamin B_{12} deficiency [63,64].

Short bowel syndrome (SBS) results in loss of all macronutrients, micronutrients, electrolytes, and water. SBS may be congenital or post surgical from trauma, vascular insult, Crohn's disease or tumors. Furthermore, it may result from functional loss. Examples include refractory celiac disease and radiation enteritis [65]. However, certain losses may be greater than others based on the degree of anatomical and functional intestinal losses. Ileal resections >100 cm disrupt enterohepatic circulation, resulting in bile salt deficiency and fat malabsorption. Calcium oxalate nephrolithiasis occurs when unbound oxalate freely absorbs. Oxalate is normally bound to calcium which prevents absorption but calcium will preferentially bind to fatty acids when they are unabsorbed. Sodium losses are significant due to excessive gastrointestinal secretions and losses that cannot be reabsorbed. Zinc and magnesium are often deficient due to rapid bowel transit [65,66].

Small intestinal bacterial overgrowth (SIBO) can arise in a variety of conditions, including reduced gastric acid secretion, altered small bowel motility, altered intestinal anatomy, such as bariatric gastric bypass, and impaired systemic and local immunity. Steatorrhea and fat-soluble vitamin deficiency occur secondary to deconjugation of bile acids by intraluminal bacteria, resulting in inadequate micelle formation. Carbohydrate malabsorption may result from degradation of sugars by the bacteria and impaired activity of intestinal brush border enzymes due to toxins produced by the bacteria. Enteric microbes consume vitamin B_{12} before it can be absorbed. In contrast, serum folic acid and vitamin K may be elevated due to bacterial synthesis. In rare cases, SIBO may lead to protein-losing enteropathy [44]. We have observed numerous cases of SIBO presenting in patients years after RYGB as hypoalbuminemia and multiple nutrient deficiencies. Normal treatment with nonabsorbable antibiotics does not reach the nonalimentary limb, and systemic antibiotics, usually metronidazole, are required.

The causes of protein-losing enteropathy (PLE) can be grouped into disorders of the mucosa and disorders of lymphatic flow. Conditions that disrupt the mucosa include a few of the conditions mentioned above which lead to nutrient deficiencies due to loss of absorptive surfaces. Mesenteric venous thrombosis, sclerosing mesenteritis, constrictive pericarditis, and primary intestinal lymphangiectasia are a group of disorders that cause PLE by obstructing lymphatic flow [67]. In the intestinal epithelial cell, long-chain fatty acids are esterified to triglycerides which combine with proteins to form chylomicrons to enter the lymphatic system. Increased ingestion of long-chain fatty acids increases the pressure of the lymphatic ducts in PLE. This causes leakage of proteins and poor movement of long-chain fatty acids. These patients are at risk for essential fatty acid deficiency, fat-soluble vitamin deficiency, and protein loss [68].

Body composition

The human body consists of 35 components that are organized into five levels of increasing complexity: atomic (e.g., nitrogen, potassium), molecular (e.g., water, protein), cellular (e.g., body cell mass, intra- and extracellular fluid), tissue (e.g., skeletal muscle, adipose tissue), and whole body (e.g., weight, height). A healthy, lean man is composed of 55–60% water, 15–20% fat, 15–20% protein (one-half in skeletal muscle), 1% glycogen (four-fifths in muscle, one-fifth in liver), and 4% minerals [69]. Although sophisticated techniques are available to measure each body component, the definitions of some commonly used terms can be confusing. *Fat mass* represents all body triglycerides, which are present in adipose tissue, muscle, and liver. *Adipose tissue* is about 83% fat (e.g., triglyceride), 15% water, and 2% protein. *Fat-free mass* refers to total body mass minus total fat mass. *Lean body mass* is defined as total body mass minus adipose tissue. The body also can be divided into cellular and extracellular mass. *Body cell mass* is defined as the cellular components of all tissues (35–45% of the bodyweight in healthy men, 30–40% in women) and can be measured by total exchangeable potassium [70]. *Extracellular mass* is defined as the heterogeneous group of tissues and fluids supporting the body cell mass.

Diet for healthy people

While there are certain physical states where a specific and tailored diet may improve health, for the general US population, traditional basic nutrition principles can maintain health and prevent disease. The 2015–2020 Dietary Guidelines for Americans succinctly summarize these principles into five overarching guidelines.

- Follow a healthy eating pattern across the lifespan.
- Focus on variety, nutrient density, and amount.
- Limit calories from added sugars and saturated fats and reduce sodium intake.
- Shift to healthier food and beverage choices.
- Support healthy eating patterns for all.

Clinicians can help their patients achieve better nutrition by focusing on eating patterns, rather than prescribing specific foods and nutrients to avoid or consume, remaining mindful of cultural practices and dietary requirements. The MyPlate planner, available on the USDA website (www.choosemyplate.gov), is part of an overall food guidance system designed as a reminder to help consumers make healthier food choices. Five basic food groups are emphasized: fruits, vegetables, grains, protein foods, and dairy. The concept assumes that meals are built on a basis of whole grains, fruits, and vegetables, and supplemented with low-fat dairy products and other protein sources from lean meat, fish, poultry, eggs, and plant foods such as nuts, seeds, and beans. MyPlate comes with a warning about foods with empty calories (calories from solid fats and/or added sugars) and advocates a sensible balance between food and physical activity. Simple nutrition guidance can include making 50% of the plate nonstarchy vegetables, 25% whole grains, and 25% lean proteins. Small, incremental dietary improvements are more likely to lead to sustainable change than overly restrictive diets and quick fixes. Encouraging individuals to focus on larger dietary patterns, with focus on small, attainable goals can lead to more sustainable changes.

Overweight and obesity

The prevalence of overweight and obesity continues to increase in the US and worldwide. Approximately two-thirds of US adults are overweight [71]. Body mass index (BMI) (Table 20.2) is used as a screening tool for underweight, overweight, and obesity, but it is imprecise. The calculation for BMI is:

$$\text{Weight (kilograms) / Height (meters)}^2$$

However, BMI does not account for differences in lean body mass. Waist circumference and waist-to-hip ratio can be used to supplement BMI in measurement of overweight and obesity. Waist circumference ≥35 inches for femailes, ≥40 inches in males, and a waist-to-hip ratio >8.5 in women, >9 in men, are associated with increased risk of metabolic disease.

Table 20.2 Disease risk associated with body mass index (BMI).

	Obesity class	BMI (kg/m²)	Disease risk
Underweight		<18.5	Increased
Normal		18.5–24.9	Normal
Overweight		25.0–29.9	Increased
Obesity	I	30.0–34.9	High
	II	35.0–39.9	Very high
Extreme obesity	III	≥40.0	Extremely high

Additional risks: (1) waist circumference >100 cm (40 in) in men and >90 cm (35 in) in women; and (2) poor aerobic fitness.
Source: Adapted from National Institutes of Health, National Heart, Lung, and Blood Institute [72].

Estimated energy requirements can provide caloric targets for weight gain, loss, or maintenance. The fall in resting energy expenditure (REE) during fasting or very low caloric intake varies due to differences in bodyweight, with the change in muscle mass being the most significant factor. Weight loss during starvation is not the same as on a low-calorie diet for treatment of obesity; in the latter, weight loss of fat is greater relative to fat-free mass. To calculate the estimated weight loss on a controlled diet, one must allow for the slowing of weight loss with time due to gradually decreasing body mass with a fixed caloric intake. Thus, the universal "rule of thumb" that a decrease of 500 kcal from the diet daily will result in 1 pound of weight loss each week is incorrect. To achieve consistent weight loss, individuals need to decrease caloric goals over time to account for decreasing mass. Mathematical models estimating dynamic energy balance are available [73]; calculations for individuals can be found at http://bwsimulator.niddk.nih.gov. However, individuals lack knowledge about caloric goals and intake; fewer than one-third can accurately report how many calories they should consume per day [74]. It is important to recognize that dieters struggle with calorie counting, and instead prefer assistance with motivation and goal setting [75].

Weight loss and maintenance are notoriously difficult; referral to a comprehensive weight management program, with an interdisciplinary team of physicians certified by the American Board of Obesity Medicine, mental health providers, and registered dietitians, may be useful.

Glycemic index

The glycemic index has been recommended as an alternate way to define carbohydrate-containing foods. The glycemic index of a food represents the relative increase in blood glucose that occurs over 2 hours after consuming that food, compared with either glucose or white bread [76]. In general, the factors that affect the glycemic response (index and/or load) include the amount of carbohydrate, the structure of the starch (e.g., amylose, amylopectin), the monosaccharides involved, the method of food processing, and the nondigestible/fiber content.

Most grains and potatoes have a high glycemic index, as they are rapidly hydrolyzed, while nonstarchy vegetables, fruits, and nuts, as well as poorly hydrolyzed starchy legumes, have a low index. Diets of foods with a low glycemic index and low glycemic load have been proposed to improve glycemic control in diabetes and enhance weight loss in obesity. Glycemic control is better in subjects who have type 2 diabetes if a portion of carbohydrate intake is replaced by fat [77]. A study of overweight adolescents showed that altering dietary glycemic load by reducing both total carbohydrate content (45–50% of energy intake) and consuming foods with a low glycemic index resulted in greater weight loss compared with a conventional low-fat (25–30%) diet [78]. The glycemic index concept fits well with the Dietary Guidelines for Americans 2015–2020 and MyPlate, but the clinical usefulness is still controversial, and the index has not been accepted as part of standard treatment for prevention or treatment of chronic illness. The American Diabetes Association questions the utility of using glycemic index or load in the clinical treatment of prediabetes and diabetes [79].

Nutritional chemoprevention of gastrointestinal cancers

One of the special applications of dietary recommendations for healthy people is to prevent gastrointestinal cancers. The general recommendations for such diets are similar to those that support health in the entire population. Estimates of cancers related to suboptimal lifestyle and diet vary. The World Cancer Research Fund estimates that 18% of cancers are related to excess body fat, alcohol consumption, poor nutrition, and physical inactivity [80]. Although epidemiological data have suggested associations between overall diets or environment and the risk for cancer incidence or mortality, it has proved difficult to identify the dietary components that might influence such risks.

Table 20.3 summarizes many of the data associating risks for gastrointestinal cancer with dietary components, as reported by the American Institute for Cancer Research. Few of the reported associations have been convincing. When dietary components have been identified and tested prospectively, the data, in general, are negative [81]. Data from the Nurses' Health Study and Health Professionals Follow-up Study suggest that proinflammatory diets, consisting of processed meat and refined grains, are associated with increased risk of colorectal cancer development [82]. Excess bodyweight and obesity continue to be independent risk factors for gastrointestinal (and other) cancers [83].

Table 20.3 Epidemiological evidence for associations between diet, lifestyle, and gastrointestinal cancer prevention.

Level of evidence	Decreases risk	Increases risk
Convincing	Physical activity (colorectal)	Body fatness (esophagus, colorectal, liver, pancreas)
		Alcohol (oral cavity, esophagus, liver, colorectal)
		Aflatoxin (liver)
		Tobacco (oropharynx, esophagus)
		Processed meat (colorectal)
Probable	Coffee (liver)	Red meat (colorectal)
		Alcohol (cardia)
	Whole grains, and other foods containing dietary fiber (colorectal)	Foods preserved by salting (stomach)
	Dairy products (colorectal)	Alcoholic drinks (stomach)
	Calcium supplements (colorectal)	

Source: Data from American Institute for Cancer Research 2018.

The World Cancer Research Fund/American Institute for Cancer Research (WCRF/AICR) published dietary and lifestyle recommendations to decrease risk of cancer. These recommendations include maintaining a healthy weight; participating in physical activity; consuming a diet high in whole grains, fruits, vegetables, and beans; limiting consumption of fast food, processed foods, red and processed meat; sugar-sweetened beverages, alcohol; and relying on foods rather than supplements to meet micronutrient needs [84]. A prospective cohort study of 41 543 French adults found that consuming a diet closely in line with these recommendations was significantly associated with a decreased risk of breast and prostate cancer, and a slight decrease in risk of colorectal cancer (CRC), but this finding was not statistically significant [85].

Analyses from the Women's Health prospective cohort found a modest association between fiber intake and decreased risk of CRC [86]. Analyses from the Nurses' Health Study and Health Professional Follow-up Study found that increased fiber intake after stage I–III CRC diagnosis was associated with decreased CRC mortality [87]. The impact of dietary and supplemental folate and risk of colorectal cancer has been studied at length, but evidence remains conflicted [88].

Given the inherent limitations in data collection and the necessary follow-up time, nutritional epidemiology provides lackluster evidence. Because the data supporting dietary intervention for cancer prevention are either negative or inconclusive, general recommendations should be to achieve and maintain a healthy weight throughout life, to adopt a physically active lifestyle, to consume a healthy diet with an emphasis on plant food, and to limit consumption of alcoholic beverages.

Energy metabolism

The human body continuously consumes energy for the maintenance of ionic and osmotic gradients, cell transport, nerve conduction, intermediary metabolism, biosynthesis, heat generation, and the performance of involuntary and voluntary mechanical work. Energy is provided largely by the mitochondrial production of high-energy phosphate bonds generated by the oxidation of fat, carbohydrate, and protein. After the hydrolysis of carbohydrates to simple sugars, fats to fatty acids and glycerol, and proteins to amino acids, most of these small molecules are converted to the acetyl unit of acetyl-coenzyme A (CoA), generating a small amount of ATP in the process. Acetyl-CoA is a common breakdown product of the three macronutrients. Acetyl-CoA, carrying most of the chemical energy of the original macronutrients, enters the citric acid cycle and undergoes oxidative phosphorylation, the final common pathways in the oxidation of food molecules (Figure 20.1). Many amino acids enter the citric acid cycle as α-ketoglutarate or oxaloacetate rather than as acetyl-CoA.

A portion of the energy released during substrate oxidation is not used to perform work and is dissipated as heat.

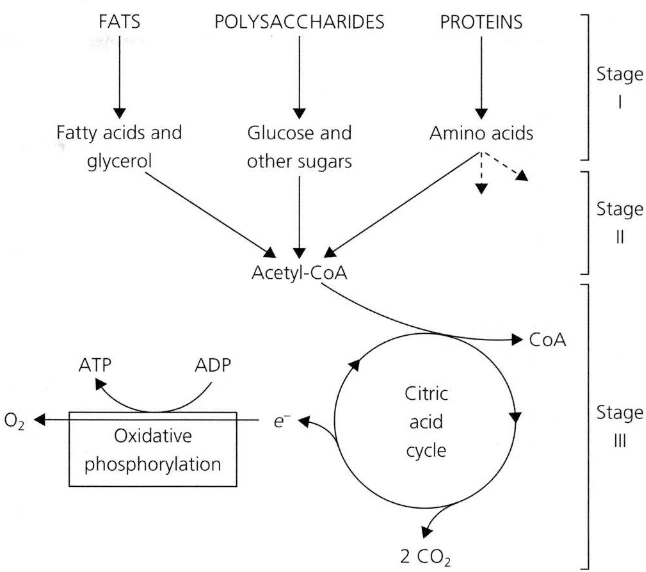

Figure 20.1 Stages in the extraction of energy from foodstuffs. CoA, coenzyme A. Source: Stryer 1988 [91]. Copyright © 1988, W.H. Freeman/Macmillan Publishers.

Therefore, energy production is traditionally measured in terms of heat production. One kilocalorie (kcal), equal to 4.184 kilojoules (kJ), is the amount of heat required to raise the temperature of 1 kg of water by 1 °C. Normally, body temperature is carefully maintained within narrow limits so that heat production equals heat loss. Energy production can be determined directly (direct calorimetry) by measuring the transfer of heat from the body to water circulating in specially designed chambers or suits. Energy production also can be measured indirectly (indirect calorimetry) by measuring carbon dioxide (CO_2) production and oxygen (O_2) consumption, because the amount of heat produced during substrate oxidation is proportional to the amount of CO_2 produced and O_2 consumed [89]. The relationship between CO_2 production and O_2 consumption can be used to estimate the relative oxidation of different substrates [90].

Dietary carbohydrates, fats, and proteins can be used as fuel soon after their ingestion, or can be stored by the body for subsequent oxidation. Endogenous energy stores (Table 20.4), which are continuously being mobilized and oxidized, become a critical source of fuel during postabsorptive conditions and when energy intake is inadequate to meet energy demands. The largest source of endogenous energy is triglyceride in adipose tissue, which is uniquely designed to store fuel. Triglycerides have a high energy density and release 39.3 kJ/g (9.4 kcal/g) when oxidized. Adipose tissue is composed almost entirely of triglycerides, which constitute 85% of adipocyte weight. In comparison, glycogen, the other major source of endogenous fuel, generates only 17.2 kJ/g (4.1 kcal/g) on oxidation.

Glycogen takes up a considerable amount of space because it is stored in liver and muscle tissue as a gel containing 2–4 g of

Table 20.4 Body energy stores.

Tissue	Fuel	Energy
Adipose tissue	Triglyceride	585 000 kJ (140 000 kcal)
Muscle	Glycogen	8400 kJ (2000 kcal)
	Triglyceride	12 500 kJ (3000 kcal)
Liver	Glycogen	1250 kJ (300 kcal)
	Triglyceride	2100 kJ (500 kcal)

water for every gram of glycogen [92]. The mobilization of adipose tissue yields 25–33 kJ/g (6–8 kcal/g), whereas the mobilization of glycogen yields only 4–8 kJ/g (1–2 kcal/g). The energy stored in the adipose tissue of a lean man can provide enough fuel for him to survive 2 months of total energy restriction [93], whereas the energy present as liver glycogen is consumed within 24 h of fasting. Certain cells and tissues, such as the brain, prefer glucose as a fuel, and others, such as bone marrow, erythrocytes, leukocytes, renal medulla, eye tissues, and peripheral nerve tissue, require glucose because they cannot oxidize fatty acids.

None of the macronutrients is completely absorbed; some are excreted in the feces. Based on the average digestibility of fat (95%) and carbohydrate (97%), the digestible energy derived from fat is 37.6 kJ/g (9.0 kcal/g), and that from carbohydrate is 16.7 kJ/g (4.0 kcal/g).

Components of energy expenditure

Total energy requirements include the sum of REE, the thermic effect of physical activity (TEPA), the thermic effect of feeding (TEF), and adaptive thermogenesis (AT). The REE is the energy consumed while lying quietly awake in the postabsorptive state. Normally, REE accounts for about 70% of total daily energy expenditure. However, energy requirements of different tissues and organs are heterogeneous. Energy consumption by the body's most metabolically active organs – the brain, liver, kidney, and heart – accounts for 60% of REE; these constitute only 5% of total body mass. By contrast, adipose tissue, which accounts for about 20% and 30% of bodyweight in lean men and women respectively, consumes less than 5% of REE.

Across mammalian species, REE is related to bodyweight; REE is proportional to the three-fourths power of bodyweight (weight$^{0.75}$) [94]. Several equations have been used to estimate resting energy requirements in humans based on measurements of REE in healthy subjects [95–98].These equations generate values that are usually within 10% of measured values in healthy volunteers but are less accurate in persons who are at the extremes of weight (i.e., extremely lean or obese) or who are ill. Starvation and severe hypocaloric feeding decrease the resting metabolic rate to values some 15–20% below that expected for actual body size, whereas illness and injury can increase energy requirements.

Physical activity usually accounts for 15–20% of total energy expenditure. The precise contribution of the TEPA to total energy expenditure depends on the intensity and duration of activities. At rest, skeletal muscle accounts for 20% of total energy requirements. However, during moderate- to high-intensity aerobic exercise, energy consumed by working muscles can increase more than 50-fold, causing a 15-fold increase in total energy expenditure.

The TEF represents the energy costs of digestion, absorption, transport, metabolism, and storage of nutrients, and it also may involve AT. Eating or infusing nutrients increases the metabolic rate by about 5–10% of the ingested or infused calories and depends on the specific foods consumed. Normally, 12–20% of the energy in ingested protein, 6–12% of carbohydrate energy, and 2–3% of fat energy is expended.

Carbohydrate metabolism

Carbohydrates, which constitute most of the earth's organic matter, are important sources of metabolic fuel. In the United States, carbohydrates normally account for about 50% of ingested calories; about 60% is complex carbohydrate, primarily starch, and most of the remainder is sucrose and lactose [99]. About 10–20 g of indigestible carbohydrate (i.e., soluble and insoluble fibers) are consumed daily. They all undergo hydrolysis in the colon to yield glucose, other simple sugars, and short-chain fatty acids. Some cells and tissues, such as erythrocytes, leukocytes, renal medulla, eye tissues, and peripheral nerve tissue, do not have the capacity for citric acid cycle activity and require glucose as a fuel for anaerobic glycolysis. The brain prefers glucose as a fuel. Daily glucose requirements include 40 g/day for anaerobic tissues and 140 g/day for the brain [100].

Absorbed glucose that is not directly oxidized can be stored as energy in the form of glycogen or fat, which require about 5% and 25%, respectively, of the original substrate oxidative energy potential. Glycogen is a branching, long-chain polymer of glucose molecules that has water and electrolytes between the chains. It is found in most tissues, but significant amounts are stored only in the liver and skeletal muscle. The primary function of hepatic glycogen, amounting to about 100 g in a healthy adult, is to maintain blood glucose levels. Plasma glucose is an essential fuel for glucose-dependent tissues. Glycogen in skeletal muscle serves to supply glucose only to the muscle itself during physical activity.

Glycolysis

The conversion of glucose to pyruvate in the cytosol of cells is known as glycolysis, a process that results in the generation of ATP but does not require oxygen. Pyruvate represents a major metabolic junction; it can be reduced to lactate, transaminated to form alanine, or enter the mitochondria and undergo carboxylation to oxaloacetate or oxidative decarboxylation to acetyl-CoA (Figure 20.2).

Citric acid cycle and oxidative phosphorylation

The citric acid cycle (i.e., tricarboxylic acid cycle, or Krebs cycle) represents a series of reactions that occur in mitochondria. Carbohydrates, lipids, and amino acids enter the cycle after

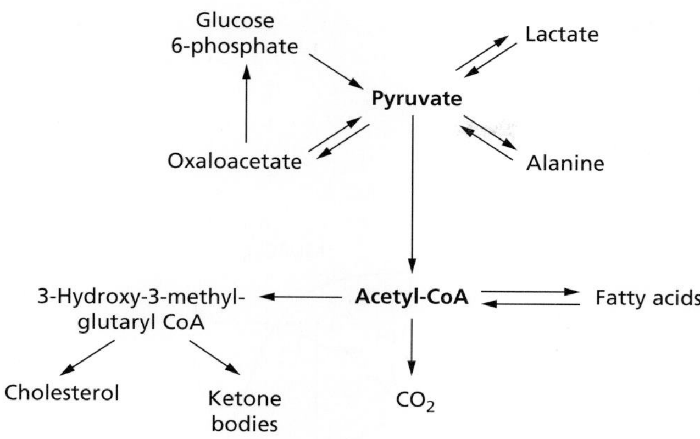

Figure 20.2 Major metabolic end-products of pyruvate and acetyl-coenzyme A in mammals. Source: Stryer 1988 [91]. Copyright © 1988, W.H. Freeman/Macmillan Publishers.

being metabolized to acetyl-CoA, and are completely oxidized to CO_2 and water. Vital biosynthetic intermediates are produced by the cycle, which plays a major role in gluconeogenesis, lipogenesis, and amino acid transamination and deamination. As acetyl-CoA is oxidized, reduced nicotinamide adenine dinucleotide (NADH) and reduced flavin adenine dinucleotide ($FADH_2$) are formed, which transfer the electrons to the respiratory chain in the inner mitochondrial membrane. In the mitochondria, the transfer of high-energy electrons from NADH or $FADH_2$ down the electron transport chain is coupled to the generation of ATP, a process known as *oxidative phosphorylation*. Glycolysis (i.e., anaerobic respiration) yields a net of only two ATPs per molecule of glucose, whereas aerobic metabolism (i.e., citric acid cycle and oxidative phosphorylation) yields 36 ATPs for each molecule of glucose oxidized.

Glucose production

Hepatic glycogenolysis is responsible for most of the glucose produced endogenously in the fed and postabsorptive states. Other mechanisms for glucose production are active and become critically important when hepatic glycogen is depleted, such as during prolonged starvation and endurance exercise. Gluconeogenesis is the process by which glucose is synthesized from noncarbohydrate precursors, lactate, glycerol, and most amino acids (principally alanine). Gluconeogenesis occurs primarily in the liver, but the kidneys also produce glucose, especially during prolonged fasting.

The Cori and glucose–alanine cycles provide mechanisms for generating plasma glucose for glucose-dependent tissues from 3-carbon intermediates released from peripheral tissues [101]. The *Cori cycle* (or lactic acid cycle) resynthesizes glucose that has been partially metabolized to lactate by peripheral tissues. Lactate produced principally by muscle, erythrocytes, and adipose tissue is transported to the liver and kidneys, where it is converted to glucose (gluconeogenesis) and released into the bloodstream. The *glucose–alanine cycle* shuttles glucose from the liver to muscle and alanine from muscle to liver. In this cycle, pyruvate is transaminated to alanine, which is transported to the liver and converted to glucose, which is then returned to muscle through the bloodstream.

Protein metabolism

Body proteins are in a state of constant flux, with protein synthesis and breakdown occurring simultaneously. Normal daily protein turnover is 1–2% of total body protein and results largely from the degradation of muscle and hepatic proteins. Protein degradation involves the enzymatic hydrolysis of protein to its constituent amino acids. More than 75% of the amino acids released by protein breakdown are reused for the synthesis of new proteins; the remaining amino acids are oxidized. Proteases within cell lysosomes are responsible for most protein degradation [102–106]. However, proteases are also found in plasma membranes and in the cytosol. The carbon skeletons of amino acids can be oxidized for energy or used for the synthesis of glucose, ketone bodies, and fatty acids [107]. Nitrogen can be released as ammonia into the bloodstream and delivered to the liver, where it is converted to urea.

The metabolism of amino acids involves the transfer of nitrogen between organs from the periphery to the liver (Figure 20.3). The liver is a workhorse for amino acid metabolism and is the site of synthesis for urea and plasma proteins. It is the main site of catabolism for the essential amino acids, with the exception of the branched-chain amino acids leucine, isoleucine, and valine, which are degraded in muscle and kidney.

Skeletal muscle preferentially takes up the branched chain amino acids after each meal and is the primary site of metabolism for these amino acids. Although leucine, isoleucine, and valine constitute only 8% of dietary amino acids, they make up 60% of the amino acids in the systemic circulation [108,109]. When muscle proteins are catabolized, the branched-chain amino acids undergo transamination, yielding alanine, glutamine, and branched-chain keto acids. The keto acids are used by the muscle as fuel, and alanine and glutamine are exported and taken up predominantly by the liver and intestine, respectively [108]. These two amino acids account for more than 50% of the total amino acid nitrogen released from muscle [109,110]. The kidneys also take up glutamine, which is the major substrate for renal ammonia production [111].

Lipid metabolism

The use of fat as a fuel requires the hydrolysis of triglyceride to free fatty acid and glycerol and the tissue uptake of free fatty acids for subsequent oxidation. Hormone-sensitive lipase within adipocytes hydrolyzes adipose tissue triglycerides and releases free fatty acids into the bloodstream, where they are bound to plasma proteins and delivered to other tissues. Lipoprotein lipase at the luminal surface of the capillary endothelium hydrolyzes plasma

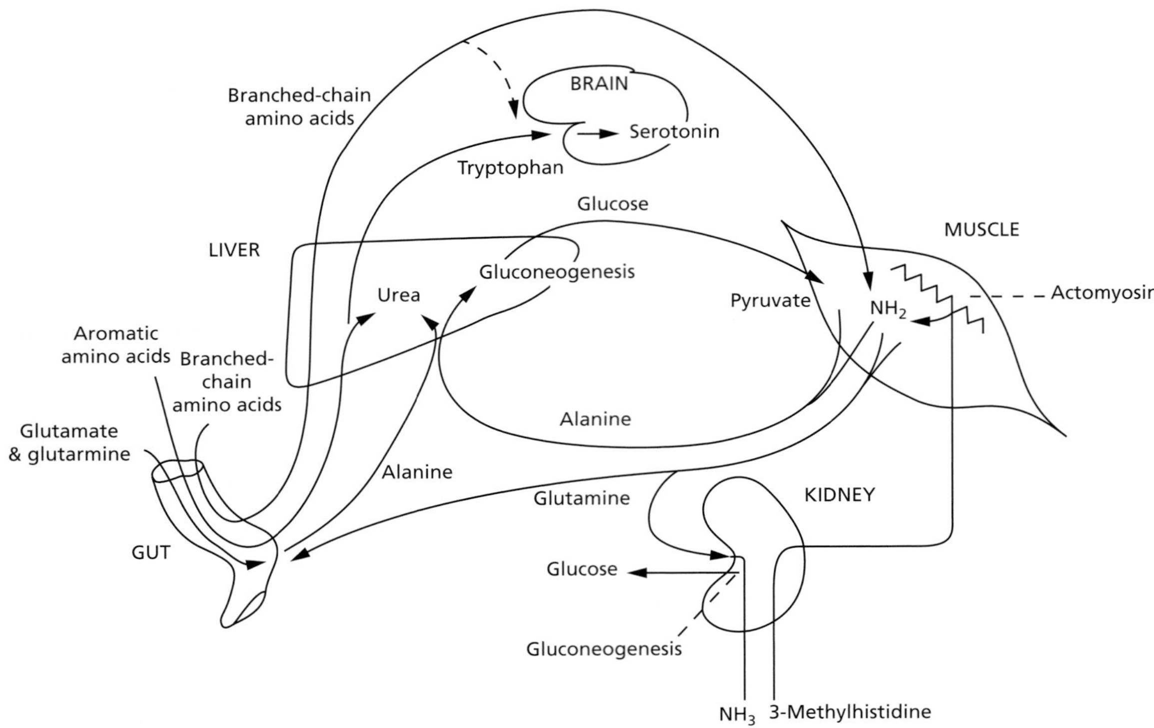

Figure 20.3 Interactions of organs in the metabolism of some major amino acids. Source: Adapted from Munro 1982 [112]. Copyright © 1982, Elsevier.

triglycerides and releases free fatty acids for local tissue uptake. Fatty acids are transported across the cell membrane by passive diffusion, facilitated diffusion, and active transport. Membrane and cytosolic fatty acid-binding proteins are important in transporting fatty acids across the cell membrane and in directing fatty acids from the cell membrane to different metabolic sites. This intracellular fatty acid transport system enhances fatty acid uptake by maintaining a fatty acid concentration gradient and prevents potentially toxic interactions between fatty acids and intracellular organelles. Long-chain fatty acids are delivered across the outer and inner mitochondrial membranes by a carnitine-dependent transport system. Inside the mitochondria, fatty acids are degraded by β-oxidation to acetyl-CoA, which enters the tricarboxylic acid cycle (see Figure 20.3).

Ketone bodies are produced solely by the liver and are generated by the partial oxidation of fatty acids. Ketone body production increases when the rate of fatty acid production is much greater than the rate of fatty acid oxidation, such as during starvation or uncontrolled diabetes mellitus. In these conditions, ketone bodies become an important fuel and are released into the bloodstream for delivery to extrahepatic tissues. Ketone bodies represent a water-soluble fuel derived from water-insoluble fatty acids. Ketone bodies can cross the blood–brain barrier to replace glucose as the major fuel for the brain, sparing plasma glucose for consumption by other tissues [113].

The biosynthesis of fatty acids is mediated by fatty acid synthase, a multienzyme complex embodied in a single polypeptide chain. It elongates the molecule by sequential addition of two-carbon units and stops with the formation of palmitic acid, a 16-carbon fatty acid. The formation of malonyl-CoA from acetyl-CoA is the committed step in fatty acid biosynthesis and the most important step of regulation. The enzyme that catalyzes this step, acetyl-CoA carboxylase, is stimulated by citrate. Citrate is abundant when ATP and acetyl-CoA are abundant, a condition appropriate for fat synthesis. Palmitoyl-CoA, the end-product of fatty acid synthesis, antagonizes the activation of acetyl-CoA carboxylase by citrate.

Nutrients

Carbohydrates

Carbohydrates, one of the three main dietary macronutrients, are important sources of metabolic fuel. Over the past 20 years, there has been a small decline of the estimated percentage of energy intake from total carbohydrates in the US adult population, from 52.5% to 50.5% [114], but it remains a major source of energy intake. The National Academy of Sciences recommends a minimum of 130 g (520 calories) of carbohydrates intake daily for adequate glucose supply to the brain. The dietary guidelines for Americans recommends that 45–65% of total daily calories should be derived from carbohydrates. Carbohydrates are found in a variety of natural and processed foods, including whole grains, starchy vegetables, fruits, sugars, juices, and refined grains such as bread, white rice, and pasta. Carbohydrates were classically classified as simple starches (monosaccharides, disaccharides) and complex starches (polysaccharides) based on the number of sugar molecules in the chemistry structure. Fiber, a type of complex starch, is a component of plant cell walls that is indigestible by the human gastrointestinal tract.

Carbohydrates undergo hydrolysis to yield glucose and other simple sugars, and glucose plays critical roles in various cell and organ functions. Some cells, including mature erythrocytes and leukocytes, do not contain mitochondria for citric acid cycle activity so rely solely on glucose as fuel for anaerobic glycolysis, while some tissues, including the inner medulla of the kidneys, cornea and lens of the eye, are poorly vascularized and rely heavily on glucose as a direct energy source despite the presence of mitochondria. The brain is the largest consumer of glucose. While the brain only accounts for ~2% of the bodyweight, it consumes ~20% of glucose. Absorbed glucose that is not oxidized can be converted to glycogen or fat and deposited in organs for storage. The physiological effects of dietary carbohydrates on human health have been research foci in nutrition since the mid-20th century. Both the quantity and quality of carbohydrates ingested have shown significant impacts on human health.

In the 1940s, it was first hypothesized that high saturated fat and cholesterol intake was associated with coronary heart disease in high-risk individuals. Low-fat diets became standard dietary recommendation for high-risk populations as well as for the general adult population as a preventive measure [115]. USDA guidelines adopted this dietary approach, famously as part of the USDA food pyramid [116], and a concordant reduction in the dietary intake of fat and an increase in carbohydrate intake resulted. However, despite these changes, the prevalence of obesity and its comorbidities, including type 2 diabetes, continued to rise [117,118].

In recent decades, serious concerns have been raised about these high-carbohydrate and low-fat diets. High carbohydrate consumption reduces high-density lipoprotein (HDL) cholesterol and raises blood concentration of sugar and triglycerides, thus causing insulin resistance, metabolic syndrome, and type 2 diabetes. These metabolic alterations contribute to the pathogenesis of coronary heart disease [119]. According to the carbohydrate-insulin model, carbohydrate restriction could impose a positive impact on insulin-adipocyte physiology [120]. As a result, during recent years, low-carbohydrate, high-fat diets have gained popularity. Although still controversial, some studies have shown that these diets could lead to a number of positive short-term effects, including improved insulin sensitivity, weight loss and corresponding decrease in various disease risk factors [121–123]. However, there has not been sufficient data supporting long-term efficacy, safety, and health benefits.

High-quality carbohydrates, such as whole grains and whole fruits, provide a wider spectrum of nutrients, including phytonutrients and antioxidants and rich source of fibers. Low-quality carbohydrates, such as refined grains, starchy vegetables and added sugars, lack the natural nutrients and fibers and may contain added sugars, preservatives, and other ingredients which make them even less healthy. The typical American diet is largely dependent on low-quality carbohydrates. These often contain refined grains with modified grain composition and natural dietary fiber stripped away. Increased intake of refined carbohydrate along with decreased intake of fiber were observed to parallel the upward trend in type 2 diabetes prevalence [117].

The public has now started to pay more attention to the quality of dietary carbohydrates. Researchers were able to demonstrate increases in estimated carbohydrate intake from high-quality carbohydrates during recent years, along with decreases in estimated carbohydrate intake from low-quality carbohydrates. However, low-quality carbohydrates still make up nearly 42% of the average American's calorie intake [114].

Fiber

Dietary fiber is generally defined as complex carbohydrates that are not hydrolyzed or absorbed by the small intestine enzymes in humans. The polysaccharide compounds originated from the plant cell walls, and primarily consist of a complex polymer of phenylpropanoid subunits. The adequate intake for fiber, suggested by the Food and Nutrition Board of the Institute of Medicine, is 14 g total fiber per 1000 kcal consumed, or, on average, 25 g/day for adult women and 38 g/day for adult men. For adults over 50 years old, the recommendation is 21 g/day for women and 30 g/day for men [124]. However, a national survey analysis concluded that the mean dietary fiber intake among Americans averaged 15.7–17.0 g, significantly lower than the recommended amount [125]. Hispanics was found to consume more fiber (18.8 g) compared with non-Hispanic white (16.3 g) and non-Hispanic black (13.1 g) subjects [125].

To date, most studies on the benefits of dietary fiber are observational while interventional data remain limited with short follow-up and weak evidence. Thus, it is challenging to define the causality between dietary fiber intake and various outcomes. Moreover, a significant number of studies examined the association between outcomes and high-fiber diet instead of fiber itself, which could introduce confounding factors including other bioactive components in fiber-rich foods.

Water-soluble fiber (e.g., pectin, gums, mucilage, fructans, β-glucan, some resistant starches) is present in barley, oats, mushrooms, some fruits (e.g., bananas, apples, berries) and vegetables (e.g., broccoli, onion, carrots). Soluble fiber is generally more subject to fermentation in the colon, where it is readily metabolized by the gut microbiota. Fermentation of the fiber by colonic bacteria generates gases and active by-products including short-chain fatty acids, acetate, propionate, and butyrate. These fats serve as an energy source and growth stimulant for the colonic microbiota [126–128]. Because of the role as fuel for bacteria, these fibers are called prebiotic fibers.

Recently, evidence has suggested that these active by-products have a regulatory effect on intestinal immune response and an antiinflammatory effect. This may be particularly important in the inflammatory bowel disease model [129,130]. Studies have also shown that not only does fiber increase gut microbial biomass, it also influences microbial diversity and predominance in a positive way by stimulating proliferation of beneficial bacteria and inhibiting growth of potentially pathogenic bacteria [131]. Some of the soluble fibers (e.g., β-glucan, raw guar gum) are viscous and absorb water, leading to gel formation. This delays gastric emptying and increases food transit time, resulting in a slowing of carbohydrate absorption and a lower glycemic index. Gels have also been touted as creating a greater sense of fullness which is theorized as beneficial for weight loss. However, while weight loss studies using fiber supplementation have shown some benefit, the effect is small (~3 kg) [132].

Insoluble fiber (e.g., cellulose, some hemicellulose, lignin) is present in whole grains, bran, nuts, and seeds and is poorly fermented in the colon. Insoluble fiber has rapid gastric emptying and thus decreased transit time. Some larger coarse fiber has a mechanical stimulating effect on the colonic mucosa, triggering mucus secretion, resulting in increased stool bulk, while small fiber does not have the irritating effect and may actually have a constipating effect by adding dry stool mass. Psyllium belongs to a special category of fiber that is soluble, viscous, and resistant to fermentation. It forms gel-like particles by absorbing water in the gut and retains water while moving along the digestive tract, resulting in soft stools and easy defecation.

While primary and secondary prevention randomized trials for prevention of coronary disease are lacking, soluble, viscous fiber has been shown to lower blood cholesterol and improve glycemic control by several mechanisms [133]. Studies showed that cholesterol (low-density lipoprotein [LDL]) lowering was highly correlated with the viscosity of soluble fiber [134,135]. It was proposed that by forming a gel, soluble fiber traps and prevents bile reabsorption close to the end of the ileum where it is normally recycled, thus eliminating bile via the stool. Hepatocytes compensate to synthesize more bile by increasing LDL cholesterol clearance from the blood and thus lower LDL and total cholesterol levels [133,136,137]. Psyllium, for instance, has been found to have time- and dose-dependent effects on lowering total and LDL cholesterol levels, and combining psyllium and statin resulted in enhanced efficacy in lowering LDL cholesterol concentrations [138,139].

Studies also showed decreased HbA1c values as well as fasting plasma glucose reduction in patients with type 2 diabetes who consumed high-fiber diets or supplements containing soluble viscous fiber compared with controls [140–143]. The mechanism is probably that viscous fiber forms gels and sequesters monoglycerides while moving along the gut lumen, thus decreasing glucose absorption in the proximal small intestine [127]. Nutrients delivered to the distal ileum can stimulate mucosal L-cells to release glucagon-like peptide-1 (GLP-1) which can stimulate pancreatic β cell growth, improve insulin production and sensitivity, slow gastric emptying via the ileal brake, and inhibit hunger and food intake [133,134]. Moreover, a metaanalysis pooled 17 prospective cohorts and found that the risk of developing type 2 diabetes was inversely associated with dietary intake of total fiber (≥25 g/day), cereal fiber, fruit fiber, as well as insoluble fiber, which indicates mechanisms other than the viscosity-associated benefits are likely involved in this protective effect [145].

Since type 2 diabetes and hyperlipidemia are both important risk factors of atherosclerosis and its complications, it is understandable that observational studies have shown the association between dietary fiber and decreased risk of coronary heart disease (CHD) and cardiovascular disease (CVD) [146]. Several earlier prospective cohort studies have shown the benefit of dietary fiber in CHD prevention among people of different sexes from different regions [147–149]. More recent metaanalyses showed that the amount of dietary fiber intake is inversely associated with both CHD and CVD risk, while soluble and insoluble fibers both appear effective in lowering the risk [150,151]. The mechanism of such effect is also likely multifactorial given that insoluble fibers do not have the viscosity that some soluble fibers have; however, they are still found to be associated with decreased risk of CHD and CVD.

Fiber has long been thought to protect against cancer, particularly of the gastrointestinal tract, based on correlations in observational trials and findings in mechanistic studies. However, randomized primary and secondary prevention trials are as yet insufficient to confirm a causal relationship. A large cohort study on the European Prospective Investigation into Cancer and Nutrition found protective associations between dietary fiber intake (fruit, vegetable, or total) and the risk of cancers in the upper gastrointestinal tract, CRC, liver cancer, lung cancer, and breast cancer [152]. Studies have shown convincing and linear dose–response negative correlation between fiber intake and CRC risk [153,154]. Similar correlation appears to exist between fiber intake and colorectal adenoma [155,156]. Several mechanisms have been proposed for this correlation. Fiber fermentation involves butyrogenic activity of the gut microbiota. This generates high amounts of butyrate, which has been shown to have antineoplastic effects [154]. Fiber decreases colonic transit time and increases stool volume, thus minimizing colonic mucosa exposure to carcinogens. Fiber also influences gut microbiota by improving gut dysbiosis associated with CRC [157]. Recently, a study showed that higher fiber intake after diagnosis of nonmetastatic CRC is associated with lower CRC-specific and overall mortality [158].

The evidence for recommending fiber in the treatment of gastrointestinal disorders is limited, but in certain gastrointestinal diseases the efficacy of fiber has been recognized [159]. Psyllium and other bulk-forming fibers are recommended in patients with constipation, especially those with diabetes mellitus, given the benefit of glycemic control associated with soluble fiber viscosity. The American College of Gastroenterology recommends a gradual increase in fiber intake in patients with chronic idiopathic constipation to limit adverse effects caused by insoluble fiber including bloating, flatulence, and cramping [160]. Soluble fiber has also shown beneficial effect in symptomatic management of irritable bowel syndrome (IBS) so is also recommended by the American College of Gastroenterology [160,161].

Lipids

Lipids are a group of biological substances that are soluble in organic solvents, including methanol and chloroform, but insoluble in water. Lipids include a heterogeneous group of compounds such as triglycerides, sterols, phospholipids, fatty acids, and fat-soluble vitamins. These compounds can serve as a major dietary source of energy, provide critical structural components of cell membranes, contribute to synthesis of steroid hormones and cell signals including inflammatory response, regulate gene expression, metabolism, and apoptosis. Triglycerides consist of a glycerol backbone with three fatty acids attached in ester linkage to the carbon positions. Fatty acids consist of a hydrocarbon chain that ends with a carboxylic acid group so the molecules have a polar hydrophilic end and a nonpolar hydrophobic end. Fatty acids can be categorized into saturated fatty acids (SFAs), monounsaturated fatty acids (MUFAs), and polyunsaturated fatty acids (PUFAs). The hydrocarbon chain in fatty acids usually contains 16, 18, or 20 carbon atoms, can be saturated or unsaturated, and may attach to biologically functional molecules.

The typical western diet contains 35% of calories from fat, and 90% of dietary fat are triglycerides [162]. The triglycerides in animal fat contain more saturated fatty acids while the triglycerides from certain plants (e.g., olive, avocados, nuts, seeds) and fish contain more unsaturated fatty acids. Dietary intake of total fat among the US adult population increased from 32.0% to 33.2% during recent years, along with increases in both saturated fat (11.5% to 11.9%) and unsaturated fat (monounsaturated and polyunsaturated fat, 20.5% to 21.3%) [114]. The 2002 Institute of Medicine Dietary Reference Intakes recommended 20–35% of total calorie intake from fat. However, current evidence found no significant difference in all-cause or coronary heart disease (CHD) mortality with dietary fat interventions [163]. In a large international cohort, higher intake of total fat and individual types of fat was related to lower total mortality [164].

The impact of total dietary fat intake on human health is unclear as most studies have confounding factors, making results difficult to interpret. The Women's Health Initiative Dietary Modification Trial, a randomized controlled trial conducted in postmenopausal women in the US back in the 1990s, implemented a low-fat diet modification, but showed no significant effect on overall risk of CHD, diabetes, CRC, or breast cancer over a mean follow-up of 8 years [165–167]. Different types of fat appeared to have different impacts on human health, so recent studies have focused more on the quality than the quantity of dietary fat. The 2015 Dietary Guideline Advisory Committee recommended no upper limit for dietary fat while retaining a 10% upper limit for saturated fat intake [168,169].

Saturated fatty acids

It remains controversial whether total intake of SFAs is associated with the risk of coronary and cardiovascular disease. While a prospective cohort among the US population showed an association between increased risk of CHD and higher dietary intake of saturated fatty acids [170], a larger cohort study did not prove an association between cardiovascular health and total fat intake or different types of fat intake [164]. Metaanalyses of prospective cohorts showed no significant evidence of such association as well [171,172]. Current evidence does support that replacing saturated fat with polyunsaturated fat may decrease the risk of CHD [173]. Interestingly, higher SFA intake has been associated with a lower risk of stroke [164]. Many guidelines recommend lowering total saturated fat intake below 10% and substituting PUFAs for SFAs to maintain optimal cardiovascular health.

It appears that SFAs from various food sources have different impacts on cholesterol levels. Lauric acid (12-carbon chain), a major component of tropical oils (coconut, palm kernel), was found to have the largest cholesterol-raising effect, but much of it was due to increase in HDL cholesterol, thus decreasing the total cholesterol to HDL cholesterol ratio. Stearic acid (18-carbon chain), from beef and cocoa butter, had a similar but smaller effect. Myristic (14-carbon chain) and palmitic acids (16-carbon chain), primarily found in dairy products and red meats, appeared to increase both LDL and HDL cholesterol, with little and less desirable effect on the ratio [174].

Monounsaturated fatty acids

Compared with SFAs, MUFAs have one double bond in the long chain. Oleic acid (18-carbon chain) makes up the majority of dietary MUFAs and comes from both animal (red meat, dairy) and plant (olive, nuts, avocados) sources. Studies have suggested that MUFAs may increase HDL cholesterol and decrease triglycerides, while the effect on LDL is inconsistent [175]. High MUFA diets, compared with carbohydrate substitute low MUFA diets, appeared to improve HbA1c in diabetics [176]. Current data do not provide sufficient evidence of a direct association between MUFAs and risk of CHD. However, some studies showed that replacing energy intake from saturated fats with equivalent from MUFAs was associated with a lower risk of CHD [177].

No dietary recommendations for MUFAs are given by most major guidelines, including that from the Institute of Medicine, while the Academy of Nutrition and Dietetics and the American Heart Association set a limit of 25% and 20%, respectively, of daily total energy intake [175].

Polyunsaturated fatty acids

Polyunsaturated fatty acids are categorized into two classes: n-3 (or omega-3) fatty acids and n-6 (omega-6) fatty acids, based on the location of the double bond in the fatty acid chain. The n-3 double bond is between carbons 3 and 4, and the n-6 double bond is between carbons 6 and 7. Unlike most other fatty acids, the 18-carbon n-6 (linoleic) and n-3 (α-linolenic) fatty acids cannot be synthesized by the liver due to lack of the specific type of desaturase enzyme. Thus, they are essential fatty acids (EFAs) and the parent fatty acids the liver needs to synthesize longer chain PUFAs such as arachidonic acid and eicosapentaenoic acid. Thus, low blood and tissue levels of EFAs usually indicate lack of consumption of these essential nutrients.

Essential fatty acid deficiency causes increased production of eicosatrienoic acid (a n-9 fatty acid synthesized by the same desaturase enzymes that synthesize n-3 and n-6 fatty acids), a fatty acid containing three double bonds (i.e., triene) derived from oleic acid (an 18-carbon n-9 fatty acid), and decreased arachidonic acid production, a tetraene derived from linoleic acid elongation. An elevated triene to tetraene ratio >0.2 (some suggest >0.4) is considered diagnostic for deficiency of essential fatty acids [178]. Essential fatty acid deficiency is rare in healthy adults because EFAs can be stored in adipose tissues and released slowly when intake is low. However, in patients receiving fat-free parenteral nutrition (PN), increased insulin in peripheral blood can inhibit lipolysis and release of EFAs, causing EFA deficiency even within 7–10 days [179,180].

Patients with gastrointestinal disorders were found to be at higher risk for EFA deficiency and the extent of deficiency appears to correlate with the degree of malabsorption [178,181]. Diseased small bowel in inflammatory bowel disease, massive bowel resection (distal jejunum, ileum), enterocutaneous fistulas involving the small bowel, and bariatric surgery (especially malabsorptive procedures) can all prevent normal absorption of fat, thus increasing the risk of EFA deficiency. Pancreatic insufficiency and cystic fibrosis are also risk factors due to impaired pancreatic enzyme secretion leading to poor fat absorption. Patients on fat-restricted diets, either voluntarily or in the setting of chyle leaks, and patients with carnitine deficiency are also more likely to develop EFA deficiency [182]. Clinical signs of EFA deficiency are generally nonspecific and can include dry, scaly rash, hair loss or depigmentation, poor wound healing, etc. [182].

Foods such as seafood, eggs, soybean, nuts, seeds, and canola oil are good sources of EFAs. Fatty fish, in particular, is rich in long-chain n-3 fatty acids including eicosapentaenoic acid (EPA) and docosahexaenoic acid (DHA). The American Heart Association recommends people without preexisting CHD eat fatty fish at least twice weekly. The National Institute of Medicine recommends adequate intake of 1.6 g/day n-3 fatty acids in adult males and 1.1 g/day in adult females, 17 g/day n-6 fatty acids in adult males and 12 g/day in adult females. In adults above age 50 years, the recommended n-6 daily intake is 14 g in males and 11 g in females.

N-6 and n-3 fatty acids have been extensively studied in the prevention and treatment of diseases. Prospective observational studies have shown that dietary linoleic acid intake was inversely associated with CHD risk in a dose–response manner. When comparing the highest category with the lowest category, linoleic acid was associated with a 15% lower risk of CHD events and 21% lower risk of CHD deaths [183]. However, metaanalysis of adequately controlled randomized trials failed to prove reduction of CHD events or mortality by replacing SFA with mostly n-6 PUFA [184]. Similarly, α-linolenic acid intake was inversely associated with risk of composite CHD outcomes and fatal CHD [185], while metaanalysis of moderate and high-quality randomized controlled trials did not show significant impact on CHD or CVD events or mortality with increasing dietary n-3 PUFA [186].

Hypertriglyceridemia is an independent risk factor for CVD and the hypotriglyceridemic effects of n-3 fatty acids from fish oils are well established. In 2002, the American Heart Association recommended n-3 fatty acids EPA and DHA (at a dose of 2–4 g/day) for reducing triglycerides in patients with hypertriglyceridemia. Since then, prescription agents containing EPA + DHA or EPA alone have been approved by the US FDA for treatment of hypertriglyceridemia [187]. In the recently published results of the Reduction of Cardiovascular Events with EPA Intervention Trial, EPA resulted in a 20% decrease of triglycerides compared with placebo among patients with elevated triglyceride levels despite the use of statins [188]. The risk of major adverse cardiovascular events was decreased by 25% in patients who received 2 g of icosapent ethyl (a purified EPA ethyl ester) twice daily compared with those who received placebo [188]. In a large trial studying the efficacy of icosapent ethyl, total atherogenic lipoproteins (non-HDL cholesterol and apolipoprotein B) were significantly decreased with 4 g/day prescription, suggesting a possible underlying mechanism of the protective effect of high-dose n-3 fatty acids in adverse cardiovascular, especially ischemic, events [189].

Nonalcoholic fatty liver disease (NAFLD) is a condition commonly associated with metabolic syndrome; it is caused by the toxic and inflammatory effect of excessive lipid deposits in the liver. The condition can progress to more severe inflammation in the setting of nonalcoholic steatohepatitis (NASH) and predispose patients to liver cirrhosis and hepatocellular carcinoma. In patients with NASH, hepatic PUFAs (EPA, DHA, arachidonic acid) in hepatic total lipids were lower than in simple steatosis; this change in hepatic lipid composition is associated with hepatic lipotoxicity, inflammation, and fibrosis [190]. Marine n-3 PUFAs have been suggested as an important tool for NAFLD treatment although high-quality evidence is lacking. A recent review examined 17 human studies investigating the effects of n-3 PUFAs on markers of NAFLD and 12 of them reported a decrease in liver fat and other markers of NAFLD. However, most studies are limited by small sample size, poor compliance, and short follow-ups [191].

Given the antiinflammatory effects of n-3 PUFAs on a biochemical level, studies have tried to explore the efficacy of n-3 supplementation in patients with Crohn's disease and ulcerative colitis. However, major trials showed no significant placebo-adjusted effect of n-3 supplementation on disease course [192,193]. Even though n-3 supplementation is generally benign, it has been shown to cause a higher rate of diarrhea and upper gastrointestinal tract symptoms [193].

Trans fatty acids

Trans fat is a type of unsaturated fat with trans configuration as opposed to the cis configuration found in the vast majority of dietary unsaturated fats. It occurs naturally in some foods such as dairy and meats but it exists in much higher levels in processed foods (i.e., margarine, deep-fried food, baked goods). The cis double bonds in the long hydrocarbon chain of an unsaturated fatty acid can be converted to trans double bonds during partial hydrogenation, producing a trans fatty acid. Industrially produced trans fat should generally be avoided given the negative health impacts. Studies have shown associations between higher intakes of trans fat and increased CHD risk as well as increased total cholesterol to HDL cholesterol ratio [194,195]. In 2003, the World Health Organization recommended that the total trans fat intake be limited to less than 1% of total energy intake; foods containing more than 2% total fat as trans fat were banned in Denmark in 2004; Dietary Guidelines for Americans 2015–2020 recommended limiting trans fat to as low as possible [196].

Proteins

Proteins are polymer chains composed of amino acids linked together by peptide bonds. Proteins have diverse three-dimensional configurations and unique functions based on their amino acid components and their sequence. They are the major component of all cells and are crucial in almost all functions and regulations of the tissues and organs in the human body. They can also serve as an energy source, providing 4 kcal per gram, the same as carbohydrates.

Twenty different amino acids are commonly found in human proteins. There are nine essential amino acids (histidine, isoleucine, leucine, lysine, methionine, phenylalanine, threonine, tryptophan, and valine) which humans must consume from dietary sources to prevent deficiency since their carbon skeletons cannot be synthesized by the body. The other 11 amino acids (alanine, aspartic acid, asparagine, glutamic acid, serine, arginine, cysteine, glycine, glutamine, proline, tyrosine) are considered nonessential because their carbon skeletons can be synthesized endogenously. Free amino acids exist in the human body in a dynamic state during anabolic and catabolic processes and can be utilized to synthesize nitrogen-containing compounds. Dietary sources of proteins are various, including meats, seafoods, eggs, dairy products, whole grains, nuts, seeds, legumes, high-protein vegetables (i.e., broccoli, brussels sprouts), etc.

Protein quality

Protein quality refers to the amino acid composition and bioavailability of the protein. These characteristics determine the value of a protein in human metabolic homeostasis and growth. The greater the ratio of essential to nonessential amino acids, the better the quality of the protein. The digestibility of the protein also affects protein quality. Animal proteins generally have higher absorption rate and essential to nonessential amino acid ratio compared with plant proteins, so are higher in quality [197]. The Digestible Indispensable Amino Acid Score (DIAAS) is a method of analyzing dietary protein availability and was proposed in 2013 by the Food and Agriculture Organization to replace the old standard, the Protein Digestibility Corrected Amino Acid Score (PDCAAS). The absolute protein content and levels of indispensable amino acids for a given food are required to calculate the score [198]. The DIASS reflects the true ileal digestibility of individual indispensable amino acids present within the food mixture, instead of the total tract digestibility of crude protein which was used to calculate the PDCAAS, and has been shown to be more accurate in estimating protein quality [199]. Vegetarian athletes were found to require an additional 10 g protein compared with nonvegetarian athletes to reach the recommended protein intake (1.2 g/kg/day) based on the DIAAS [200].

Gastric acid is important for the digestion of proteins. Protein is denatured by gastric acid, making it more susceptible to proteolysis, the breakage of peptide bonds. Proteolysis is initiated by the proteolytic enzyme pepsin. Pepsin activation requires that pepsinogen is converted to pepsin by the action of hydrochloric acid. The process continues in the intestine where the pancreatic proteases, including trypsin and chymotrypsin, further break down the peptide bonds. Essentially, all protein is absorbed as short peptides (dipeptides or tripeptides) or amino acids. Most peptides containing more than four amino acids are not absorbed in the small intestine and can be excreted in feces. The speed of protein digestion also influences postprandial amino acid gain and the anabolic response of skeletal muscle. Dietary proteins can be classified as "fast" or "slow" proteins based on their matrix food structure and biochemical reaction, which determine their absorption rate and metabolic profile [201,202]. "Fast" proteins have been shown to stimulate anabolism and improve muscle function in older patients, thus improving aging-related sarcopenia [201].

Nitrogen balance

Nitrogen is the fundamental component of amino acids and the vast majority of nitrogen in the human body is contained in amino acids. Nitrogen balance is the calculated difference between nitrogen intake and output and thus is an indicator of protein metabolism. Nitrogen can be excreted in different nitrogen-containing compounds such as urea (the primary source of urine nitrogen), creatinine, ammonia, porphyrins, and uric acid. Small amounts of exogenous dietary protein that is not absorbed by the gut and endogenous protein from sloughed intestinal epithelial cells and secretions can be passed as fecal nitrogen. Minor amounts of nitrogen can be lost through skin, hair, body fluids, and secretions. A positive nitrogen balance indicates a net increase in body protein and is usually associated with an anabolic state such as growth or pregnancy, while a negative nitrogen balance indicates a net loss in body protein and is usually associated with catabolism. Common conditions predisposing the human body to catabolism include starvation, surgery, trauma, burns, cancers, infections, inflammatory diseases, hyperthyroidism, etc. One gram of nitrogen represents 6.25 g of protein, which is equivalent to 30 g of hydrated lean body mass. Thus, negative nitrogen balance can manifest as muscle mass loss, which is a diagnostic criterion for malnutrition [4].

The western diet is rich in proteins. The majority of the US population exceeds minimum recommendations for protein intake while remaining below the upper end of the Acceptable Macronutrient Distribution Range. The average protein intake for adults aged 20 years and older is 98.3 g/day in men and 69.8 g/day in women [203]. The total protein intake in the US population has increased from 15.5% to 16.4% of total calorie intake [114]. The Dietary Reference Intake (DRI) for proteins, in order to meet the needs of healthy adults, is 0.8 g per kilogram bodyweight. For average-sized women (57 kg) and men (70 kg), the recommended intake is 46 g and 56 g, respectively [204]. This recommendation is based on baseline body needs without consideration of utilizing protein as energy source, physical activity, anabolic states such as pregnancy and growth during childhood, or recovery from surgery or trauma or other catabolic states. Therefore, athletes and people who are highly physically active require higher protein intake (1.2–2.0 g/kg), with intake spaced throughout the day. For pregnant women, the DRI is 1.1 g protein per kilogram bodyweight or an additional 25 g/day to meet anabolic needs. For lactating women with an average milk output, an additional 25 g/day protein is recommended [204]. Protein requirement also increases with illness severity. Current guidelines suggest 0.8–1.2 g/kg/day protein for patients with mild to moderate illness and 1.2–1.5 g/kg/day for patients with severe illness; even higher protein requirements can be seen in some ICU patients and burn victims [205,206].

Patients on chronic hemodialysis have increased proteolysis due to inflammation, chronic metabolic acidosis, and the dialysis procedure itself [207,208]. As a result, they require higher dietary protein intake to achieve a net balance between muscle protein synthesis and breakdown. The guidelines recommended 1.2 g/kg/day protein intake in chronic hemodialysis patients although studies have shown that most of the dialysis population do not have such high protein intake requirements [208,209]. On the other hand, a low-protein diet is often recommended in patients with chronic kidney disease since high protein may lead to increased intraglomerular pressure and hyperfiltration, thus, at least theoretically, causing glomerular damage and worsening kidney function [210]. Studies have shown that moderate protein restriction (0.6 g/kg) is generally safe and may be beneficial in the progression of kidney disease, while a very low-protein diet did not show benefit but increased mortality risk [211–213].

Patients with liver cirrhosis are often malnourished because the alterations in substrate utilization for energy production cause a catabolic state and predispose to protein-calorie malnutrition. Evidence suggests that a high-calorie (35–40 kcal/kg) and high-protein (1.2–1.5 g/kg) diet is effective in improving nutritional status and was associated with decreased hospitalization and mortality rates in this population [214]. There is also a growing consensus that patients with hepatic encephalopathy should not be on protein-restricted diets since there is no difference in clinical outcomes with protein restriction. Earlier recommendations for low protein intake were based on uncontrolled observations neglecting the lactulose-like impact of high fermentable fiber intake [215,216].

High-protein diets have been shown to increase satiety, enhance weight loss, and improve body composition [217]. It is generally accepted that the oxidation of excessive amino acids has a satiety effect. Increased satiety caused by high protein intake can result in reduced carbohydrate intake, and low-carbohydrate diets have been shown to result in clinically meaningful weight loss regardless of which macronutrients they emphasize [218]. High-protein diets alone, without change in carbohydrate intake, could cause decreased ad libitum caloric intake, likely mediated by increased central nervous system leptin sensitivity, resulting in weight loss [219]. High-protein diets, compared with isocaloric standard-protein diets, appeared to provide benefits through reductions in triglycerides and fat mass, and may improve insulin resistance, although the effects of reduced carbohydrate intake can be mixed in the results [220,221].

Protein restriction has been advocated for reducing the incidence of calcium-oxalate renal calculi based on observational and metabolic studies. The few randomized secondary prevention trials, however, are relatively small, and differ in both design and outcome. In one (n = 99), which included animal protein restriction, fiber supplementation, and an increase in fruit and vegetable intake, recurrent stones were significantly increased (odds ratio [OR] 5.6), the opposite of what was anticipated [222]. In another comparative trial (n = 120), one group was randomized to eat a diet with normal amounts of calcium (30 mmol per day), but reduced amounts of animal protein (52 g per day) and salt (50 mmol sodium chloride per day), while the other group was assigned to a low-calcium diet, without attention to protein intake. In this trial, the low-protein, normal-calcium group had fewer stones [223]. Other studies have suggested that calcium supplementation may significantly decrease oxalate absorption and stone risk [224].

Branched-chain amino acids

Branched-chain amino acids (BCAAs) are amino acids with a branched aliphatic side-chain, and are the most hydrophobic of the amino acids. Leucine, isoleucine, and valine are the three essential BCAAs and are abundant in meats and dairy products. BCAAs have a stimulatory effect on protein synthesis and an inhibitory effect on proteolysis, play an important role in promoting glucose metabolism, and have been shown to influence immunomodulation and brain function [225]. There is also some evidence showing the beneficial effects of BCAAs on cirrhosis-related complications. A randomized controlled trial among advanced cirrhosis patients showed decreased hospitalization rate, decreased combined rates of mortality and hepatic complications, improved liver function and nutritional markers and quality of life measures with a 1-year intervention of BCAA supplementation [226]. However, this trial and other similar studies had large withdrawal rates due to poor compliance and adverse reactions such as diarrhea and abdominal distension, adding potential bias to the results. There is no consensus regarding the therapeutic effectiveness of BCAAs. The optimal BCAA intake remains unknown, thus making it difficult to recommend appropriate doses for supplementation [214].

Micronutrients: minerals and vitamins

Micronutrients include minerals and vitamins that are essential elements required by the human body in small amounts (generally less than 1 gram) to maintain proper function. DRIs are reference values that are quantitative estimates of nutrient intakes introduced by the Institute of Medicine of the National Academies in the United States for diet planning and assessment. The Adequate Intake (AI) and Recommended Dietary Allowance (RDA) are based on the amount of a nutrient needed for an individual to avoid deficiency. The RDA is set as two standard deviations above the mean requirement for the population. Stated differently, it is the dietary intake level that is sufficient to meet the nutritional requirement of almost all (>97%) healthy individuals in the population, thus exceeding the needs of most individuals. The AI is a recommended value of nutritional intake based on observations and experiments in a group of healthy individuals assuming that their intakes are adequate, and is often used when an RDA cannot be determined.

The Estimated Average Requirement (EAR) is the estimated intake of a nutrient that covers the needs of half the healthy individuals in a population. The Tolerable Upper Intake Level (UL) reflects the highest level of nutrient intake that is likely to pose no adverse effects to the population [227]. Food labels usually contain percent daily values (DVs), reflecting the percentage of nutrient amount in one serving of the food based on the average levels of nutrients for a 2000 kcal diet, with 5% or less considered low in a nutrient and 20% or more considered high.

Minerals

Sodium

Sodium, the most prominent cation in extracelluar fluids, plays a crucial role in the maintenance of membrane potentials, intravascular fluid volume, and nutrient absorption and transport. Na/K-ATPase pumps are ion pumps that utilize energy to maintain the Na/K gradient across cell membranes, keeping sodium concentration 10 times higher and potassium concentration 30 times lower in extracelluar fluid compared with intracellular fluid. The Na/K-ATPase activity is crucial in neuron function, cardiac function, and muscle contraction, and is estimated to cost 50% of brain energy consumption and 20-40% of resting energy consumption in adults [228,229].

Most sodium absorption in the small intestine occurs via solute-dependent cotransport along with glucose and amino acids, making sodium a key element in nutrient absorption. Various hormones target sodium to regulate blood volume and blood pressure since sodium is the principal cation that maintains intravascular volume. The kidney maintains intravascular volume by regulating sodium excretion via the renin-angiotensin-aldosterone system. When intravascular volume is low, the kidneys release renin into circulation, which generates angiotensin I from angiotensin, then converts it into angiotensin II by angiotensin converting enzyme, while angiotensin II stimulates aldosterone production from adrenal glands which targets kidneys to increase reabsorption of sodium and water retention at the expense of potassium excretion, thus increasing intravascular volume in the absence of capillary leak. Antidiuretic hormone (ADH) can be released from the pituitary gland when there is a decrease in intravascular volume. ADH also targets kidneys and increases sodium and water reabsorption by stimulating epithelial sodium channels in distal tubules.

Atrial natriuretic peptide (ANP) and brain natriuretic peptide (BNP) are secreted by cardiac muscle cells in the atria and ventricles of the heart, respectively, when volume receptors of the cells sense increased stretching of atrial and ventricular walls due to increased blood volume. ANP and BNP cause increased sodium and water excretion via the kidneys, decreased aldosterone secretion via the adrenal glands, and relaxed vascular smooth muscle, thus decreasing blood volume and blood pressure.

Sodium is abundant in the diet in developed countries. Most dietary sodium comes from salt and processed foods while natural foods usually contain very little. The minimum daily sodium requirement to replace daily loss is about 0.18 g which is far below the dietary intake of the general population. Sodium deficiency is rarely caused by inadequate intake, and is usually caused by increased losses from the gut, kidneys, or skin.

The recommended daily intake for sodium included on most packaged foods labels is less than 2.4 g/day. Processed meat and seafood, frozen breaded meals, canned beans, pickled foods, and salted nuts are high in sodium content. Natural foods such as fresh meat and seafood, vegetables and vegetable oils, fruits, and whole grains are lower in sodium content. The Food and Nutrition Board of the National Academy of Medicine established an AI for sodium due to insufficient evidence to determine an RDA or EAR. The AI for sodium in male and female adults is 1.5 g/day which is equivalent to 3.8 g of salt per day. The NHANES 2007–2010 data suggested that sodium intake exceeded recommendations across all age and gender groups in the United States, with adults (age 19–50 years) consuming sodium at 3.8 g/day and older adults at 3.3 g/day. The American Heart Association continues to recommended that sodium intake should be no more than 2.4 g/day and ideally no more than 1.5 g/day for adults with high blood pressure [230].

The health risks of excessive sodium intake have been research foci for many years. The DASH-sodium (Dietary Approaches to Stop Hypertension) trial compared the DASH diet (diet rich in vegetables, fruits, and low-fat dairy products) to a typical US diet at high, intermediate, and low levels of sodium intake, and found that reduction of sodium intake significantly reduced blood pressure in hypertensive consumers of either diet [231]. Other studies indicate that sodium intake reduction decreased systolic and diastolic blood pressure in subjects with and without hypertension [232]. A randomized control trial showed that sodium restriction could also improve brachial artery flow-mediated dilation (FMD), which indicates endothelium-dependent response to shear stress and is utilized as a marker for endothelial function [233]. Even though observational data found greater risks of cardiovascular disease with higher sodium consumption, current evidence fails to prove the efficacy of dietary sodium reduction on lowering cardiovascular disease risks [234,235].

Overall, most studies on the effect of sodium intake reduction on various health risks face the common challenges of poor compliance [236] and inconsistent goal of reduction, thus making it difficult to interpret mixed study results.

Potassium

Potassium is the most prominent cation in intracelluar fluids. Along with sodium, it plays an important role in maintenance of membrane potential via ion pumps, especially Na/K-ATPase. Potassium ions are also present in a number of proteins and enzymes to facilitate their physiological functions. The 2% of total body potassium present in extracellular fluid influences resting membrance function and significantly impacts cardiac muscle function. Abnormal serum potassium concentrations outside the narrow normal range may cause muscle paralysis or abnormal heart rhythm, which can be fatal. The kidneys regulate potassium excretion using mechanisms closely related to sodium regulation. Potassium excretion is heavily influenced by aldosterone as well as pH in the distal tubule.

Normal people absorb about 90% of potassium intake. Roughly the same amount of potassium taken in is excreted by the kidneys, while the other 10% is excreted by the gut. The vast majority of potassium absorption occurs in the small intestine. Colonic absorption and secretion of potassium occur mainly by passive mechanisms, while enhanced active secretion, although still at a low level, may occur in the setting of hyperaldosteronism. Patients with hypokalemia can present with fatigue, weakness, muscle cramps, constipation, arrhythmias, etc. Potassium deficiency is usually due to increased losses from the gastrointestinal tract (vomiting or diarrhea), certain types of kidney diseases, and medications including potassium-wasting diuretics. Diarrheal diseases cause increased fecal potassium losses due to increased unabsorbed anions, electrochemical gradients secondary to active chloride secrection, and increased renal losses possibly resulting from secondary hyperaldosteronism due to sodium and fluid losses [237].

Fresh fruits and vegetables are rich in potassium. Meats, fish, nuts, and dairy products are also good sources of potassium. The anions in unprocessed foods are usually organic (e.g., citrate), whereas the anions in processed foods with added potassium are usually chloride. The minimum potassium intake to compensate for obligatory losses is 400–800 mg/day. The AI for potassium based on median intakes in a healthy population is 3.4 g/day in male adults and 2.6 g/day in female adults, with increased requirements during pregnancy (2.9 g/day) and breastfeeding (2.8 g/day) [238]. The NHANES 2009–2010 data suggested that the average dietary potassium intake was 3.2 g/day for male adults and 2.4 g/day for female adults, which are below the recommended AI. Potassium was identified by the 2015–2020 Dietary Guidelines Advisory Committee as a nutrient of public health concern due to the potential for negative health outcomes associated with potassium underconsumption. High dietary intake of potassium, especially increased intake of natural potassium-rich foods such as fruits and vegetables, has been associated with decreased risk of stroke and kidney stones, as well as increased bone mineral density [239]. Clinical trials such as the DASH trial provided evidence supporting the efficacy of a high-potassium diet rich in fruits and vegetables on lowering systolic and diastolic blood pressures in populations with and without hypertension [240].

Calcium

Calcium is the most abundant cation in the human body. About 99% of calcium is stored in the skeleton and teeth, the other 1% circulates in the body and plays a crucial part in cell signaling and regulation of protein functions. The homeostasis of circulating calcium is tightly controlled by vitamin D and parathyroid hormone (PTH) to maintain normal physiological functions involving calcium. Calcium circulates in blood as dissolved ions, complexed with anions, or bound to proteins. Only ionized serum calcium is regulated tightly by hormones. PTH is released by parathyroid glands when there is a drop in serum calcium level. It acts on bones to release calcium into circulation and stimulates the activation of vitamin D into its active form, calcitriol (1,25-dihydroxyvitamin D). Increased circulating 1,25-dihydroxyvitamin D levels can increase bone resorption by activating osteoclasts, increasing intestinal absorption of calcium and phosphorus, and decreasing calcium excretion and increasing phosphorus excretion in kidneys. The combination results in increased calcium levels, which decreases the secretion of PTH. On the other hand, calcitonin is secreted by the parafollicular cells in the thyroid gland when serum calcium level increases. Calcitonin inhibits PTH secretion, decreases bone resorption and intestinal calcium absorption, and increases calcium excretion in the kidneys, all of which result in decreased calcium levels.

Calcium absorption is relatively inefficient (usually approximately 30%) and occurs via both active and passive process, while an obligatory loss of calcium occurs in the intestine and kidneys. Active absorption is dependent on 1,25-dihydroxyvitamin D, which is converted from 25-hydroxyvitamin D and upregulates calcium transporters in the intestine when calcium intakes are low. Passive absorption occurs largely in the distal part of the small intestine and can be affected by various factors including luminal solubility, transit time, and passive diffusion rate. High sodium and low potassium intake seems to result in increased urinary calcium excretion and bone loss [241,242]. Caffeine intake at low doses (≤400 mg/day) may cause increased urinary calcium content but does not seem to impact calcium homeostasis or bone health [243,244]. High calcium and oxalate levels in the urine can predispose to stone formation but high calcium intake is associated with lower risk of kidney stone, likely due to reduced intestinal oxalate absorption with high calcium consumption [224].

When there is a net negative calcium balance, the skeleton serves as a reserve for maintaining circulating calcium levels. Given the large amount of calcium reserve in the skeleton, low calcium levels are usually not due to the lack of calcium but calcium dysregulation. Hypoparathyroidism along with impaired PTH regulation, vitamin D deficiency, chronic kidney disease, and hypercatabolic states including tumor lysis syndrome or massive trauma could all be potential causes of hypocalcemia. Hypomagnesemia is also a common cause of hypocalcemia, both by diminishing PTH secretion and downregulating osteoclast sensitivity to PTH, so correcting hypomagnesemia is the key to reversing hypocalcemia.

Dairy products are the richest and most absorbable source of calcium, and have been estimated to provide 75% of dietary calcium in Americans. Some vegetables (e.g., collard greens, kale, broccoli, bok choy) and seafood (sardines, salmon, shrimp) are also high in calcium with good calcium bioavailabilty. The RDA for calcium is 1000 mg/day for male adults aged 19–70 years and female adults aged 19–50 years, 1200 mg/day for male adults aged above 70 years and female adults aged above 50 years, 1300 mg/day during pregnancy and breastfeeding. The NHANES 2009–2012 data suggested that 37.7% of nonsupplemented adults and 19.6% of supplemented adults had inadequate calcium intake (below the EAR) [245].

The Dietary Guidelines for Americans identified calcium as one of the nutrients of public concern. Calcium supplements can be helpful for people who have difficulty consuming adequate calcium from diet alone. Calcium supplements come in different formulations such as calcium carbonate, calcium citrate, calcium gluconate, etc. Calcium citrate is preferred when there is concurrent use of H_2 blockers or proton pump inhibitors as acid improves absorption.

The maximum single dose of elemental calcium is 500 mg, while total calcium intake from diet and supplements should not exceed 1500 mg/day, given the potential increase in the risk of prostate cancer and cardiovascular disease mortality [246,247]. Data from randomized controlled trials showed increased bone mineral density with increased dietary calcium intake with or without vitamin D supplementation, while combined vitamin D and calcium supplementation appeared to reduce fracture risk among older adults [241,242]. Calcium supplementation is recommended by the World Health Organization for pregnant women in areas with low calcium intake, starting at the 20th week of pregnancy, since it has been shown to lower the risk of gestational hypertension and preeclampsia [248]. Prospective cohort studies identified a negative correlation between dietary calcium intake and risk of colorectal cancer, although evidence from randomized controlled trials is lacking. Data from one clinical trial failed to demonstrate any efficacy of calcium or vitamin D supplementation on lowering the risk of recurrent colorectal adenomas [249].

Magnesium

Magnesium is the second most abundant intracellular cation after potassium and is crucial in maintaining normal physiological function. Magnesium is a cofactor in more than 300 enzyme systems and is required for energy production, DNA and protein synthesis, ion transport, and cell signaling [250]. An adult body contains approximately 25 g magnesium, with 50–60% in the skeleton and the rest in soft tissues, primarily muscles [250]. Less than 1% of total manesium is in blood where 20–30% is protein bound with the rest in active ionized form. Magnesium absorption is usually 30–40% of dietary intake, and occurs primarily in the small intestion via a paracellular pathway, mostly in the ileum due to a relatively longer transit time compared with that in the duodenum and jejunum. Smaller amounts of magnesium can be absorbed in the colon mainly via a transcellular pathway [251].

Magnesium deficiency is relatively rare in people on a balanced diet since the kidneys regulate magnesium excretion based on intake and absorption, and obligatory intestinal loss is minimal. However, certain conditions of the gastrointestinal tract, kidneys, endocrine and metabolic conditions can predispose patients to magnesium deficiency. Crohn's disease, celiac disease, radiation enteritis, and short bowel syndrome commonly lead to malabsorption and deficiency. Prolonged use of certain diuretics, diabetes mellitus, parathyroid dysfunction, primary aldosteronism, and excessive lactation could all potentially cause magnesium depletion [252].

Food sources such as green leafy vegetables (e.g., spinach, Swiss chard, kale), legumes, nuts, seeds, whole grains, and seafoods are rich in magnesium. Some fortified foods and cereals may contain added magnesium. For young adults aged 19–30 years, the RDA for magnesium is 400 mg/day and 310 mg/day for male and female, respectively. The RDA for adults aged above 30 years is higher, at 420 mg/day and 320 mg/day for male and female, respectively. Analysis of data from NHANES 2003–2006 showed that the average natural magnesium intake among adults was 278 mg/day, while the combined intake considering fortified foods and supplements was 332 mg/day, indicating a significant proportion of the general population had inadequate intake [253].

Magnesium supplements come in various formulations such as magnesium oxide, magnesium hydroxide, magnesium citrate, etc. The upper supplemental magnesium intake recommended by the US Food and Nutrition Board is 350 mg/day, since a higher dose may increase the risk of diarrhea and other gastrointestinal disturbances. Inadequate magnesium intake has been associated with increased risk of multiple chronic diseases including cardiovascular diseases, hypertension, insulin resistance and type 2 diabetes, Alzheimer's disease, etc. [254]. The efficacy of magnesium supplementation has been explored in the management of a number of chronic conditions but the current data do not provide sufficient evidence to recommend supplementation of magnesium for disease prevention.

Phosphorus

Phosphorus is the major intracellular anion, an essential component of all cell membranes and nucleic acids, and plays an important role in cell signaling, energy production, and regulation of enzyme systems. Phospholipids are the major component of cell membranes, and require phosphorus in their structure. Nucleic acids (DNA and RNA) are long-chain molecules requiring phosphorus as part of their backbones. Phosphorylated compounds such as adenosine triphosphate (ATP) and creatine phosphate are crucial energy units for the production and storage of energy. The phosphorus-containing molecule 2,3-diphosphoglycerate regulates oxygen delivery to tissues by binding to hemoglobin in red blood cells. Approximately 85% of adult body phosphorus resides in bone in the form of hydroxyapatite, a calcium phosphate salt, while the remaining 15% is distributed in the soft tissue [255].

Phosphorus is predominantly absorbed as inorganic phosphate by passive diffusion in the upper small intestine, although active transport via sodium-dependent phosphate cotransporters is also important [256]. The expressions of these cotransporters are enhanced to some extent by 1,25-dihydroxyvitamin D. As in regulation of calcium homeostasis, PTH and vitamin D also play an important role in phosphorus regulation. Also, fibroblast growth factor (FGF)-23 secreted by osteoblasts and osteocytes plays an important role in phosphorus homeostasis by decreasing the active form of vitamin D and increasing urinary phosphorus excretion when phosphorus is high. Since the kidneys can be very efficient in phosphorus reabsorption (up to 99.8%) and phosphorus is abundant in various food sources, phosphorus deficiency is rare in the general population. However, alcoholism, diabetic ketoacidosis, severe starvation and anorexia, and refeeding syndrome could be risk factors for phosphorus deficiency [257].

Phosphorus can be found in most food sources since it is a crucial component of living organisms. Foods that are rich in proteins are generally rich in phosphorus: meats, fish, dairy, legumes, nuts, and whole grains are natural foods high in phosphorus. Carbonated drinks, particularly cola, are rich in added phosphorus. Vegetarian dietary phosphorus has lower bioavailability compared with phosphorus from animal protein sources so is recommended in chronic kidney disease given concern for hyperphosphatemia [258].

The RDA for phosphorus in the adult population is 700 mg/day, while the EAR is 580 mg/day and UL is 4000 mg/day for adults aged 70 years or below and 3000 mg/day for adults over 70 years old. Analysis of NHANES 2003–2006 data showed that the average phosphorus intake for adults far exceeds the EAR and RDA, while remaining far below the UL at 1308 mg/day with natural source only, and 1360 mg/day including fortified foods and supplements [253].

Observational data have shown an association between high serum phosphorus levels and increased risk of cardiovascular disease and mortality in patients with chronic kidney disease [259]. Higher phosphorus levels, even within normal range, appear to be correlated with an increased cardiovascular disease risk in patients without chronic kidney disease [260,261]. The underlying mechanism remains unclear but it is hypothesized that excessive phosphate may contribute to vascular calcification and endothelial dysfunction, thus increasing cardiovascular disease risk [262,263]. Observational data have also described a negative relationship between the amount of cola consumed and bone density in women [264].

Iron

Iron is an essential mineral and component of hundreds of proteins and enzymes involved in oxygen delivery, energy metabolism, and DNA synthesis, among others. Approximately three-quarters of iron is present as part of heme in hemoglobin and acts as an oxygen-carrying cofactor. Other heme proteins exist in organs and function to store oxygen (e.g., myoglobin) or in enzymes acting as cofactor to transfer electrons (e.g., cytochrome P450). Nonheme iron-containing proteins and enzymes also play an important part in catalytic reactions, energy metabolism, DNA replication, iron transport and storage, etc.

The human body can recycle iron in hemoglobin, thus maintaining iron storage despite low iron intake. Iron can be absorbed either in the form of heme or as inorganic iron. Absorption of dietary iron varies depending on whether the iron is in the form of heme or not. Foods rich in iron include red meat, poultry, seafood, green leafy vegetables, raisins, beans, and lentils [265]. Heme iron mainly comes from animal protein and is better absorbed and less affected by other dietary factors. Nonheme iron mainly comes from plants, dairy products, iron fortified foods, and dietary supplements. This nonheme iron in the diet is predominantly in ferric (Fe^{3+}) form.

The absorption of inorganic (nonheme) iron occurs primarily in the duodenum and upper jejunum and is relatively inefficient relative to heme iron, but is improved by an acidic environment. Concurrrent intake of vitamin C improves nonheme iron absorption by reducing ferric iron to ferrous (Fe^{2+}) iron and forming an iron–ascorbic acid complex which is highly absorbable. Other acids including gastric acid and other organic acids, including some amino acids, can also enhance the absorption of nonheme iron. Absorption is decreased when iron forms insoluble complexes in the lumen with phytates, polyphenolic compounds, and antiacids. Phytates are prevalent in seeds (grains, nuts, and legumes). Polyphenols are ubiquitous in plant-based foods, particularly fruits and some beans. Both may contribute to a higher incidence of iron deficiency in populations consuming plant-based diets.

In the duodenum, ferric iron is reduced to the ferrous form and transported into enterocytes along with a proton via the divalent metal transporter 1 (DMT1). In an iron-depleted state, iron in the enterocytes is transported out of the cells via ferroportin and then binds to transferrin in the circulation. In an iron-excessive state, iron binds to ferritin and is trapped in the enterocytes, which eventually slough with iron loss.

The human body lacks regulation of iron excretion, so regulation of absorption is the key for iron homeostasis. Hepcidin, a peptide primarily synthesized by the liver, is the primary modulator for iron absorption. When iron levels are high, hepcidin acts by inducing internalization and degradation of ferroportin, which is a transporter found in enterocytes, hepatocytes, and macrophages that recycle iron. When iron levels are low, hepcidin production is limited by the liver, resulting in increased iron absorption and release from cell storage. Hepcidin expression can be upregulated by inflammatory conditions and downregulated by anemia and hypoxia [266]. In type 2B hereditary hemochromatosis, hepcidin levels are inappropirately low due to mutations of the hepcidin gene, causing abnormal iron overload.

Loss of iron can occur from skin, urine, and gastrointestinal tract with enterocyte sloughing and fecal loss along with unabsorbed dietary iron. Uterine loss during menstrual periods in premenopausal women is another major source of iron loss.

Iron deficiency is the most common nutrient deficiency in the world. Iron deficiency can cause anemia and associated symptoms (e.g., fatigue, dizziness, dyspnea, pale skin), impaired immune response while more severe deficiency can cause brittle nails, tongue inflammation and soreness, pica, and esophageal webs in Plummer–Vinson syndrome. Patients with iron deficiency anemia (IDA) are frequently referred to gastroenterologists for evaluation.

Any condition that predisposes to bleeding or iron malabsorption in the gastrointestinal tract increases the risk of iron deficiency. IDA is one of the manifestations of *Helicobacter pylori* infection and *H. pylori* eradication has been shown to reverse IDA in interventional trials [267]. The underlying mechanisms include chronic occult bleeding due to mucosal microerosions, competition for dietary iron by bacteria, decreased iron absorption due to reduced ascorbic acid concentration in the stomach, and increased levels of hepcidin in the setting of chronic inflammation [268].

Autoimmune atrophic gastritis, caused by antibodies against parietal cells in the stomach, can impair vitamin B_{12} absorption, as well as iron absorption due to reduced or absent acid production. Autoimmune atrophic gastritis often presents as IDA before the depletion of vitamin B_{12} storage, particularly in patients with other risk factors for iron deficiency [269]. In some series, 20–30% of IDA is due to autoimmune atrophic gastritis and is refractory to oral iron supplementation [268]. Celiac disease and inflammatory bowel disease cause chronic inflammation of the intestinal mucosa and are commonly associated with iron deficiency due to impaired iron absorption, blood loss from inflamed intestinal mucosa, and systemic inflammation affecting hepcidin regulation. Early initiation of intravenous iron supplementation is important in patients with celiac disease who have IDA [268,270]. Some types of bariatric surgery, such as Roux-en-Y gastric bypass, increase the risk of malabsorption of multiple micronutrients, including iron, and also respond well to intravenous iron [265].

The RDA for iron in the adult population is 8 mg/day for males and postmenopausal females. The current recommendation for premenopausal females is 18 mg/day. Breastfeeding is associated with lower dietary requirements (RDA 9 mg/day) while pregnancy is associated with higher dietary requirements (RDA 27 mg/day). A national survey showed that the average intake of dietary iron in the US is 16–18 mg/day in males, 12 mg/day in pre- and postmenopausal females, and 15 mg/day in pregnant women [271].

Given the inadequate dietary iron intake among most premenopausal and pregnant women, iron supplementation is indicated to prevent iron deficiency. Oral iron supplements come in various forms such as ferrous sulfate, ferrous gluconate, ferrous succinate, ferrous fumarate, etc. There is no evidence that any one oral preparation is more effective or safer than the others. Intravenous iron also comes in various formulations including ferric gluconate, ferric carboxymaltose, iron sucrose, low molecular weight iron dextran, etc. Low molecular weight iron dextran has the advantage of low cost and can be administered in a single dose, so is preferred by clinicians [272]. Iron overload is rarely caused by prolonged supplementation even in healthy individuals without iron deficiency, unless there are underlying genetic or aquired conditions that predispose them to iron overload [273].

Zinc

Zinc is an essential trace element for the human body and is the second most abundant trace mineral after iron. The adult human body contains approximately 2.6 g of zinc, with the majority residing in bone and skeletal muscle (>85%), followed by skin and liver. Zinc plays a crucial role in the growth and function of cells. It is a cofactor for over 300 enzymes and 1000 transcription factors and is essential for cell proliferation and apoptosis, reproductive organ growth and function, energy metabolism, regulation of ion homeostasis, signal transduction, cellular defense against oxidative stress and detoxification. [274]

Zinc is absorbed inefficiently throughout the entire small intestine (16–50% inversely related to oral intake). A number of zinc transporters are involved in zinc absorption. A carrier named Zrt-, Irt-like protein (ZIP)4 imports ionic zinc from the intestinal lumen into enterocytes, while ZnT1, a basolateral membrane protein, exports zinc from enterocytes into the portal blood. Other important transporters include ZIP5 and ZIP14, which import zinc from the blood into entercytes, and

ZnT5 variant B on the apical membrance which can transport zinc bidirectionally between the enterocytes and the gut lumen [275].

The amount of zinc absorption is not only dependent on dietary zinc intake, but also heavily affected by its bioavailability. Zinc from plant sources generally has lower bioavailability compared with zinc from animal sources due to the effect of phytate, a common plant component. The phosphates of phytate can bind to zinc, forming an insoluble complex which is excreted with feces. The higher the ratio of phytate to zinc, the lower the zinc bioavailability. Dietary protein, however, has been shown to positively correlate with zinc absorption, likely due to enhanced compound solubility in the presence of amino acids [276]. Both heme iron and nonheme iron have been shown to negatively impact zinc absorption [277]. Copper does not seem to impact zinc absorption, but prolonged high-dose zinc supplementation can severely impact copper absorption, resulting in copper deficiency [278].

Shellfish, especially oysters, red meat, and poultry are rich in zinc; nuts, dairy products, and legumes also have fair amounts of zinc. The RDA for zinc is 11 mg/day for male adults and 8 mg/day for female adults. It is higher during pregnancy (11 mg/day) and breastfeeding (12 mg/day) [279].

Nearly 2 billion people worldwide are deficient in zinc. The NHANES 2003–2006 data showed that average zinc intake from both natural and fortified food in the US adult population was 12.3 mg/day and 11.9% had inadequate intake [253]. Symptoms of zinc deficiency are diverse and sometimes nonspecific: growth and development delay, delayed sexual maturation and sexual dysfunction, chronic diarrhea, cornea and skin lesions, alopecia, impaired wound healing, suppressed immune function, poor appetite, impaired taste and smell, night blindness, and altered cognition are all potential clinical manifestations. Severely malnourished patients and patients on chronic parenteral nutrition are at high risk of zinc deficiency. Other risk factors include older age, vegetarian diet, alcoholism, inflammatory bowel disease, chronic diarrhea and malabsorptive diseases including celiac disease and short bowel syndrome, etc. [280].

Zinc supplementation is available in various formulations and has been shown to be potentially beneficial in the management of chronic conditions such as age-related macular degeneration, Wilson disease, diabetes mellitus, etc. [281–283]. High-dose zinc supplementation has been consistently shown to reduce the duration of common cold symptoms; however, prolonged use of high-dose zinc supplementation of 50 mg/day or more should raise concern for development of copper deficiency [284].

Copper

Copper is an essential trace element that acts as a cofactor for multiple enzymes involved in energy metabolism, oxidation reduction, iron absorption, tissue formation, and nervous system development and function. The body contains about 100 mg of copper, 30 mg of which is bound to proteins and enzymes. The liver contains various copper-containing enzymes and about one-third of total copper is in the liver.

Copper can be absorbed relatively effciently (35–70%) in the stomach and along the small intestine. Animal protein, soluble carbohydrates, and organic acids other than ascorbic acid appear to have a positive effect on copper absorption [285]. High dietary zinc intake can increase synthesis of metallothionein, an enterocyte protein that binds to certains metals including copper and zinc. Metallothionein has higher affinity for copper than zinc, thus trapping copper in the cells and preventing absorption. Most absorbed copper is excreted in bile, while some biliary copper can be reabsorbed in the enterohepatic circulation.

Foods such as organ meats, shellfish, nuts, and seeds are rich in copper. Whole grains, lentils, and mushrooms are also good sources of copper. The RDA for copper is 900 μg/day for both male and female adults. The requirement is higher during pregnancy (1000 μg/day) and breastfeeding (1300 μg/day). The average dietary copper intake in the US is reported to be approximately 1.2–1.6 mg/day for male adults and 1.0–1.1 mg/day for female adults based on national surveys [271].

Clinically significant copper deficiency is relatively rare. The most common clinical presentation in such cases is microcytic anemia that does not resolve with iron supplementation but can be corrected by copper supplementation. Neutropenia can also occur with copper deficiency, resulting in impaired immune function. Other clinical manifestations such as osteoporosis and other bone abnormalities, neurological symptoms, and loss of pigmentation are relatively rare [286]. Severe myelopathy due to copper deficiency has been described in patients after Roux-en-Y gastric bypass with long Roux limbs and severe malabsorption [287]. Copper toxicity is rare, but patients with genetic conditions predisposing to copper overload, such as Wilson disease, are at high risk of copper toxicity even with low copper intake.

Other trace minerals

Selenium is an essential mineral required as a component of more than 25 selenoproteins, and is crucial for the normal function of the antioxidant system. Keshan cardiomyopathy is a congestive cardiomyopathy that occurs in selenium-deficient areas in Asia, and has been linked to coxsackievirus infection and selenium deficiency. Low ejection fraction cardiomyopathy with low selenium levels, responding to supplementation, has been reported [288].

Chromium is an ubiquitous trace element and has been shown to play a role in normal insulin function by being a cofactor for chromodulin which potentiates the action of insulin at the cell receptor level, improving tissue sensitivity to insulin [289]. Potential chromium deficiency cases have been linked to clinical manifestations resembling type 2 diabetes mellitus [289,290].

Manganese plays an important role in antioxidant function and macronutrient metabolism, but a deficiency state in humans has not been identified. Manganese toxicity may result from long-term parenteral nutrition and manifests as gait disturbances and tremors.

Iodine is an essential component of thyroid hormones and thus is crucial for metabolism, growth, and development. Iodine deficiency can cause a wide range of clinical manifestations from goiter to cretinism, but iodine-enriched table salt has made deficiency rare.

Fluoride is a structural component in bones and teeth. It is not generally considered essential for life but it improves structural stability and plays an important role in bone homeostasis and prevention of dental caries.

The minerals mentioned above are very rarely deficient in the general population in developed countries. With the exception of fluoride, supplementation is usually only recommended in the setting of long-term parenteral nutrition (PN).

Minerals including vanadium, nickel, cobalt, tin, and silicone are potentially essential in humans, but no deficiency state has been reported. Other minerals including cadmium, lead, boron, aluminum, arsenic, mercury, strontium, and lithium have not been proven essential. Supplementation of these minerals is not indicated. Contaminants in PN solutions contain some of these minerals and aluminum toxicity is a concern. Parenteral solutions stored in glass containers will leech aluminum from the glass. Most are sold in plastic but a few, such as potassium phosphate, are still only available in glass containers.

Vitamins

Thiamin (vitamin B_1)

Thiamin, also known as vitamin B_1, is a water-soluble B vitamin. Thiamin in its active form, thiamin pyrophosphate, functions as a coenzyme in the metabolism of carbohydrates, fatty acids, and branched-chain amino acids. For instance, enzymes critical for energy metabolism such as pyruvate dehydrogenase, α-ketoacid dehydrogenase, and transketolase all require thiamin pyrophosphate. Generally, the requirement for thiamin is related to energy intake, especially carbohydrate intake.

The human body acquires thiamin mostly from dietary sources with a small amount from microbiota in the colon. Whole-grain cereals, lean pork, legumes, and nuts are food sources that are rich in thiamin. Thiamin can also be added during fortification of foods and is available in various vitamin supplements. Although more than half the adult population in the US has inadequate thiamin intake (below the EAR) from natural foods, only 7% has inadequate intake if fortified foods are included, and the number is lower at 5% if including dietary supplements [253].

The RDA for thiamin in adults is 1.2 mg/day for males and 1.1 mg/day for females. The RDA is higher during pregnancy and breastfeeding at 1.4 mg/day [291]. An RDA of 0.5 mg thiamin for every 1000 kcal of dietary calorie intake is also appropriate.

Severe thiamin deficiency can affect multiple organs and result in beriberi, which can present as congestive heart failure, gastrointestinal distress, neuropathy, and neurological damage causing Wernicke encephalopathy and Korsakoff psychosis. Thiamin deficiency can result from poor dietary intake, increased requirement, decreased absorption, or increased loss. Chronic alcoholism is the most common cause of thiamin deficiency in developed countries. In refeeding syndrome, thiamin deficiency due to increased demand for glycolysis can be observed in starved individuals loaded with carbohydrates. Diuretics can decrease thiamin reabsorption in the kidneys by increasing urinary flow and may potentially worsen congestive heart failure among patients with existing diagnosis [292].

Riboflavin (vitamin B_2)

Riboflavin, also known as vitamin B_2, is an integral component of two flavocoenzymes: flavin adenine dinucleotide (FAD) and flavin mononucleotide (FMN). These enzymes are involved in oxidation-reduction reactions and are crucial for metabolism of macronutrients and energy production [293]. Flavoproteins are enzymes that utilize a flavocoenzyme to function, and are involved in the metabolism of iron and other vitamins such as niacin, vitamin B_6, and folate. Even though riboflavin is required for metabolic function, unlike thiamin, its requirement is not related to energy intake.

Most plant- or animal-derived foods have small amounts of riboflavin. Meats, fish, milk, eggs, almonds, and some green vegetables (e.g., spinach, asparagus) are relatively rich in riboflavin. Fortified food products including cereals, wheat flour, bread, and rice in the US are enriched with riboflavin. However, certain food processing and ultraviolet light can break down riboflavin and cause loss of this vitamin. The RDA for riboflavin is 1.1 mg/day and 1.3 mg/day for adult women and men, respectively. The RDA is higher at 1.4 mg/day and 1.6 mg/day during pregnancy and breastfeeding, respectively [294]. An average US adult consumes 1.7 mg/day of riboflavin from natural foods, 2.3 mg/day from all foods including enriched and fortified foods, 5.6 mg/day if adding dietary supplements [253].

Riboflavin deficiency is rare in developed countries and usually occurs with deficiencies of other water-soluble vitamins. Clinical symptoms of riboflavin deficiency can include angular stomatitis, cheilosis, glossitis, cornea vascularization and vision disturbances, etc. Alcoholics and anorexic patients are at high risk for riboflavin deficiency.

Niacin (vitamin B_3)

Niacin, also known as vitamin B_3, includes nicotinic acid and its amide form, nicotinamide. It is an essential component of nicotinamide adenine dinucleotide (NAD), which can be phosphorylated into nicotinamide adenine dinucleotide phosphate (NADP). NAD and NADP participate in various oxidation-reduction or other metabolic reactions. With the presence of riboflavin, vitamin B_6, and iron-containing enzymes, niacin can be synthesized from the essential amino acid tryptophan. In the human body, the conversion is quite inefficient, as roughly 60 mg of tryptophan is required to synthesize 1 mg of niacin [295].

Niacin is present in most foods, especially meat, fish, grains, and fortified foods such as cereals. Niacin equivalent (NE) is used to describe dietary intake of all elements that contribute to niacin available in the human body (1 NE = 1 mg of niacin = 60 mg of tryptophan). The RDA for niacin is based on the prevention of deficiency: 16 mg and 14 mg NE daily for adult men and women, respectively. The requirement is higher at 18 mg and 17 mg NE daily during pregnancy and breastfeeding, respectively [296]. The average US adult consumes 18.5 mg/day of niacin from natural food sources, 25.1 mg/day from all foods including enriched and fortified foods, and 37.3 mg/day if supplement use is accounted for.

Pellagra is the result of severe niacin deficiency. The clinical manifestations include photosensitive dermatitis, diarrhea, dementia, and potentially death. Niacin deficiency and pellagra can result from inadequate intake and defective absorption of NE, including tryptophan. Prolonged use of the antituberculosis drug isoniazid, immunosuppressive drugs, and chemotherapy can all increase risk of niacin deficiency. Alcoholism can cause decreased dietary niacin intake and tryptophan conversion to NAD, thus resulting in niacin deficiency [297]. Nicotinamide is recommended for the treatment of niacin deficiency to avoid flushing which is a common adverse effect of nicotinic acid.

Pyridoxine (vitamin B_6)

Vitamin B_6 refers to three pyridines (pyridoxine, pyridoxal, and pyridoxamine) and their phosphorylated forms. It is essential for the function of many enzymes involved in amino acid metabolism, hormonal regulation, and neurotransmitter synthesis. Requirement of vitamin B_6 is correlated to protein intake. Vitamin B_6 is rapidly absorbed primarily in the jejunum by passive diffusion, and excreted mostly in the urine in the form of metabolic products such as 4-pyridoxic acid. A small amount of vitamin B_6 is excreted in the feces.

Meat, fish, legumes, potatoes, bananas, and fortified foods are rich in vitamin B_6. Many plant-based foods contain vitamin B_6 in the form of pyridoxine glucoside, which has about half of the bioavailability of other forms of vitamin B_6, thus increasing the risk of inadequate intake among people who are strictly vegeterian [298]. The RDA for vitamin B_6 is 1.3 mg/day for adults up to 50 years old, 1.7 mg/day for males over 50 years old, and 1.5 mg for females over 50 years old. The requirement for vitamin B_6 is higher in older adults due to decreased absorption, increased catabolism, and impaired phosphorylation [299]. The requirement is also higher during peregnancy (1.9 mg/day) and breastfeeding (2.0 mg/day) [294]. Analysis of the NHANES 2003–2006 data showed that the average adult vitamin B_6 intake from natural foods was only 1.6 mg/day, with more than a quarter of the population having inadequate intake, or 2.0 mg/day if including enriched and fortified foods, and still 15% of the population had inadequate intake.

Vitamin B_6 deficiency can manifest as cheilosis and glossitis with ulceration, seborrheic dermatitis-like rash, peripheral neuropathy, confusion, irritability, and depression. Similar to other vitamins of the B complex, vitamin B_6 deficiency is common among alcoholics. Patients with chronic diseases and underlying systemic inflammation also seem to be at high risk for deficiency due to increased catabolism of vitamin B_6 [300]. Certain drugs such as antituberculosis drugs (isoniazid, cycloserine), penicillamine, and L-dopa are pyridoxine antagonists. Oral contraceptives have also been shown to negatively impact vitamin B_6 status, likely due to estrogen's effect on vitamin B_6 metabolism [301].

Folate (folacin, folic acid)

Folate, also known as folacin or vitamin B_9, refers to compounds sharing a similar structure and function with folic acid, a major synthetic form used for fortification and supplementation. Folic acid and other synthetic forms (folinic acid, levomefolic acid) need to be converted to folate which is biologically active. The many forms differ in the degree of reduction of the double bonds in the ring structure and the number of glutamyl residues in the peptide chain. Folic acid is a synthetic monoglutamate while dietary folates mostly come in the polyglutamyl form. Folate functions as a carrier of one-carbon units and folate coenzymes act as acceptors and donors of one-carbon units during various reactions involved in the synthesis and metabolism of nucleic acids, amino acids, acetylcholine, and methionine. Folate plays an important role in homocysteine metabolism. Folate and vitamin B_{12} are required as cofactors in the methionine synthase pathway of homocysteine metabolism, while the other pathway of homocysteine metabolism requires vitamin B_6 as cofactor. Folate polyglutamates need to be hydrolyzed into monoglutamates before being transported into enterocytes where they are further converted into 5-methyltetrahydrofolate and released into circulation, and eventually stored in the form of polyglutamates.

Total body stores of folate are relatively small and can be depleted in months if dietary intake is poor. Folate excreted in bile can be reabsorbed via enterohepatic circulation, which could be affected by the presence of malabsorption. Since the bioavailability of natural folates varies, folate requirements can be measured in dietary folate equivalents (DFEs). 1 µg of dietary folate provides a standard 1 µg of DFEs, while 1 µg of folic acid supplement can provide as much as 2 µg of DFEs, depending on absorption.

Folate is abundant in citrus fruits, legumes, green leafy vegetables, and fortified foods. However, significant dietary folate loss happens during food preparation and cooking. Since 1998, the US FDA has required that all refined grain products be fortified with 1.4 mg of folic acid per kg of grains to help prevent neural tube defects. The RDA for folate in DFEs is 400 µg/day for male and female adults. The RDA during pregnancy is 600 µg/day and during breastfeeding is 500 µg/day [294]. Analysis of the NHANES 1988–2010 data showed that the postfortification prevalence of low serum folate concentration in the US population was less than 1%, compared with 24% during the prefortification period [302]. Analysis of the

NHANES 2003–2006 data showed that 91% of the US adult population had inadequate folate intakes (<EAR) when only natural foods are considered. However, with fortified foods, only 13% had inadequate intake, and the number was further reduced to 9% if dietary supplements were added [253]. More recently, the FDA has approved folate supplementation in oral contraceptives to help improve folate status among women of childbearing age [303].

The clinical manifestation of folate deficiency is megaloblastic anemia, a form of macrocytic anemia due to impaired nucleic acid metabolism and inhibited cell division. Hypersegmented neutrophils can be seen due to similar reasons. Folate deficiency due to dietary insufficiency has become less common in countries where foods are routinely fortified with folate. Some malabsorptive conditions, such as inflammatory bowel diseases and celiac disease, can cause folate deficiency. Decreased dietary intake and intestinal absorption of folate is seen in alcoholism along with other vitamin B complex deficiencies. Smoking has also been shown to negatively impact folate status [304]. Cancers and systemic inflammation due to chronic diseases are associated with increased cell division and altered metabolism causing increased demand for folate, thus increasing the risk for folate deficiency [305]. Other rare causes of folate deficiency include hereditary folate malabsorption, which is caused by mutations in the SLC46A1 gene which encodes the proton-coupled folate transporter.

Cobalamin (vitamin B_{12})

Cobalamin, known as vitamin B_{12}, is the largest and most structurally complex vitamin. It contains a cobalt atom in the center of a corrin ring bound to chemically active components of the vitamin. Vitamin B_{12} is an essential cofactor for two enzymes: methionine synthase and methylmalonic coenzyme A mutase. Methionine synthase converts homocysteine to methionine, which can be utilized to synthesize S-adenosyl-methionine, an important methyl donor during methylation of nucleic acids and proteins. Methylmalonic coenzyme A mutase converts L-methylmalonyl-coenzyme A to succinyl-coenzyme A which enters energy production from lipids and proteins via the citric acid cycle.

Vitamin B_{12} is bound to proteins in natural foods. After ingestion, it is released by gastric proteases. It is then bound to haptocorrin, also known as the R-protein, a B_{12} binding protein that protects the vitamin from degradation in acidic environments. In the duodenum, haptocorrin is digested by pancreatic proteases, releasing the vitamin, which is then bound to intrinsic factor produced by the parietal cells of the stomach and forming a complex. This complex can then be efficiently absorbed in the ileum via a receptor-mediated pathway. The other pathway of vitamin B_{12} absorption is via passive diffusion, which is ineffecient but could potentially become the prominent pathway for absorption in the setting of conditions such as Roux-en-Y bypass, atrophic gastritis, or resection of the distal ileum. Very high oral doses of vitamin B_{12} may be adequate to replace normal absorption in these conditions, but parenteral B_{12} may be required.

Total body store of vitamin B_{12} in a healthy adult is 2–2.5 mg, most of which is in the liver. Daily losses average around 1.3 µg/day. Vitamin B_{12} deficiency usually does not occur in the absence of a prolonged period of poor intake or malabsorption. Since 5–10 µg of vitamin B_{12} undergoes enterohepatic circulation daily, malabsorption causes more rapid loss of vitamin B_{12} reserves.

Vitamin B_{12} is synthesized only by bacteria and is acquired by animals via ingestion of bacteria or production by microbiota [306]. Thus, animal products, including meat, poultry, and fish, especially shellfish, are rich in vitamin B_{12}. Eggs and dairy products are also good sources. Vitamin B_{12} is relatively stable during food processing and cooking. The RDA for vitamin B_{12} is 2.4 µg/day for male and female adults. The requirement is higher at 2.6 µg/day and 2.8 µg/day during pregnancy and breastfeeding, respectively. Due to increased risk of protein-bound vitamin B_{12} malabsorption in older adults, the Food and Nutrition Board recommended supplements as the primary source of vitamin B_{12} intake among adults aged 50 years or older [294]. The average American adult consumes 4.3 µg/day from natural foods only, 5.2 µg/day including fortified foods, and 30.1 µg/day when supplements are accounted for, all far above the RDA [253].

Vitamin B_{12} deficiency can cause megaloblastic anemia due to reduced activity of methionine synthase which converts folate from an inactive form into an active form, tetrahydrofolate. Other clinical manifestations include glossitis, gastrointestinal dysmotility (constipation), and neurological symptoms consistent with peripheral neuropathy (numbness, tingling, imbalance) and degenerative neuropathy (dementia). Most cases of vitamin B_{12} deficiency are associated with intestinal malabsorption. Dysfunction of stomach, pancreas, and small intestine can all affect vitamin B_{12} absorption. Pernicious anemia is an autoimmune condition due to autoantibodies against intrinsic factor or gastric parietal cells. Pernicious anemia or *H. pylori* infection can induce chronic inflammation of the gastric lining, resulting in atrophic gastritis with loss of gastric glands and decreased production of gastric enzymes, causing food-bound vitamin B_{12} malabsorption. Other conditions such as pancreatic deficiency, celiac disease, inflammatory bowel diseases, alcoholism, and vegan diet are also risk factors for vitamin B_{12} deficiency.

Ascorbic acid (vitamin C)

Vitamin C, also known as ascorbic acid, is a water-soluble vitamin that is an essential cofactor for multiple hydroxylation reactions and biosynthesis of collagen, carnitine, and neurotransmitters such as norepinephrine. It also acts as an essential antioxidant that protects molecules against oxidative damage and stabilizes vitamin E and folic acid. Humans cannot synthesize vitamin C endogenously so dietary intake is crucial. The body tightly controls vitamin C levels in tissue and plasma. Vitamin C is generally well absorbed in the small intestine by two sodium-dependent transporters (SVCT1 and SVCT2) at intakes up to 200 mg. Intake of larger amounts of vitamin C results in decreased absorption and increased proportion excreted in urine once plasma concentration saturates [307]. Thus, the vitamin C level in plasma is a better indicator of recent dietary intake, while the levels in tissues and cells (leukocytes) may be better indicators of body storage [308].

Citrus fruits (e.g., kiwi, orange, grapefruit) and vegetables (e.g., pepper, broccoli, brussel sprouts) are rich in vitamin C. The RDA for vitamin C in adults is 75 mg/day for females and 90 mg/day for males. Recommended intake is 35 mg/day higher for both female and male smokers due to increased oxidative stress [309]. The RDA is 85 mg/day during pregnancy and 120 mg/day during breastfeeding [310]. Analysis of the NHANES 2003–2006 data showed inadequate vitamin C intake from only natural foods in 52% of the adult population, decreasing to 43% considering fortified foods contribution, and 28% including supplements [253].

Severe vitamin C deficiency is rare but well known to cause scurvy, which is characterized by subcutaneous bleeding, impaired wound healing, gingivitis, arthralgias, etc. Alcoholics, the elderly, the chronically ill, and those who are severely malnourished or on extremely poor diet are at high risk for vitamin C deficiency. Vitamin C supplementation has long been touted for prevention and treatment of the common cold. However, metaanalysis of randomized controlled studies shows no benefit in reducing the incidence in otherwise well subjects. In the aggregate, vitamin C decreased the incidence by half in those with high levels of physical stress (marathon runners, skiers, and soldiers in Arctic training) [311]. Vitamin C supplementation prior to onset had small effects on shortening the duration of cold symptoms in adults (8%), with a larger decrease in children (14%). No benefit was seen with vitamin C supplementation after onset of symptoms [311].

Biotin

Biotin is a water-soluble vitamin and a cofactor required for various carboxylases. It plays an important role in the metabolism of carbohydrate, protein, and fat. Biotin is essential for all living organisms. Humans cannot synthesize biotin and rely on exogenous sources. In addition to dietary sources, colonic microflora synthesize biotin and release a substantial amount of free biotin for absorption [312]. Dietary protein-bound biotin is converted to free biotin prior to being absorbed. Uptake is via a sodium-dependent multivitamin transporter (SMVT) in the small and large intestine.

The dietary requirement of biotin is not known and an RDA has not been determined. The AI for adults is estimated at 30 μg/day. Healthy adults have an estimated biotin intake of 40–60 μg/day [294]. Egg yolk, liver, and yeast are food sources rich in biotin. Biotin deficiency is rare and can present with scaly red rash around orifices, hair loss, and neurological symptoms (lethargy, depression, paresthesias, seizures). Prolonged parenteral nutrition without adequate biotin supplementation can cause deficiency. Ingestion of large amounts of raw egg white over time is also a risk factor because avidin, an antimicrobial protein in raw egg white, can bind biotin and prevent its absorption.

Pantothenic acid

Pantothenic acid, also known as vitamin B_5, is a water-soluble vitamin and a precursor of coenzyme A, which is an essential coenzyme for the metabolism and synthesis of carbohydrate, protein, and fat. Pantothenic acid is well absorbed in the intestine via SMVT and can be excreted in the same form in the urine. Pantothenic acid is essential for all living organisms and is widely available in various food sources. Meat, liver, fish, eggs, dairy products, legumes, and some vegetables (sweet potato, avocado, mushroom) are rich sources of pantothenic acid. No RDA for pantothenic acid has been established. The AI for adults is estimated at 5 mg/day [294]. Pantothenic acid deficiency is extremely rare in humans and has only been observed in cases of severe malnutrition or starvation. Typical clinical manifestations include fatigue, muscle cramps, numbness and tingling in hands and feet.

Vitamin A

Vitamin A refers to a group of related fat-soluble compounds, the basic molecule of which is retinol, known as vitamin A alcohol. Vitamin A is present in foods of animal origin in its ester form combined with long-chain fatty acids. Retinol and retinyl esters are known as preformed vitamin A. Retinol can be converted to its aldehyde form, retinal, which is the active element of visual pigment, and then oxidized to retinoic acid, which is an intracellular messenger that modulates gene transcription. Retinol, retinal, retinoic acid, and other related compounds are referred to as retinoids. Plants also have various carotenoids, some of which, such as β-carotene, can be converted to retinol in the human body by an oxygenase. These plant-based carotenoids are referred to as provitamin A. Carotenoids, including the ones that cannot be converted to vitamin A, may possess antioxidant properties which are theorized to have benefit [313].

Vitamin A, ingested in the form of long-chain retinyl esters, is hydrolyzed to retinol by lipases and esterases before it gets absorbed, mostly in the upper half of the small intestine. Free retinol uptake likely occurs by a saturable carrier-mediated process at physiological doses, and by passive diffusion at pharmacological doses. Carotenoid uptake has been assumed to occur via passive diffusion but data have suggested that certain transporters might be involved [314]. Absorption is generally more efficient with retinol than carotenoids. The absorption efficiency is estimated at 75–100% for retinol and 3–90% for β-carotene [314]. Once absorbed by the enterocytes, retinol is esterified into retinyl esters. Carotenoids are converted to retinol and then retinyl esters, for the most part, but may stay intact. Retinols and carotenoids can be packed into chylomicrons and transported in the lymphatic circulation before being stored in the liver. Vitamin A released from the liver is transported in the circulation bound to retinol-binding protein and transthyretin (also known as prealbumin). Excessive vitamin A is excreted in urine and bile. A small amount of retinol is converted to retinoic acid and undergoes enterohepatic circulation.

Vitamin A is only synthesized by plants and microorganisms. Historically, its activity in dietary sources was expressed in international units (IUs). The value in IUs, however, does not reflect its bioavailability. The current international standard for measuring vitamin A is retinol activity equivalents (RAE), which is standardized to retinol activity. Reflective of lower absorption effeciency for dietary β-carotene and other provitamin A caroteniods, the conversions are 1 RAE = 1 μg of retinol = 2 μg of supplemental β-carotene = 12 μg of dietary β-carotene =24 μg of other carotenes (α-carotene, β-cryptoxanthin). 1 IU of retinol is equivalent to 0.3 μg RAE.

Animal products including organ meat, dairy products, and eggs are rich in vitamin A. Carotenoids, especially β-carotene, are found in yellow and green vegetables (i.e., sweet potato, pumpkin, carrot, spinach, kale, etc.). The RDA for vitamin A is estimated at 700 μg RAE/day for female adults and 900 μg RAE/day for male adults. It is higher, at 770 μg RAE/day, during pregnancy and 1300 μg RAE/day during breastfeeding [315]. Analysis of NHANES 2003–2006 data showed that 80% of the adult population had intakes of vitamin A from natural foods below the EAR. This was decreased to 51% by accounting for fortified food contribution, and further down to 37% when supplement use was included [253].

Vitamin A deficiency is the leading cause of preventable blindness in underdeveloped areas of the world. The typical symptoms include impaired vision adaptation to darkness, Bitot spots (conjunctiva changes with keratin build-up), and xerophthalmia (dry eyes). Vitamin A deficiency is also associated with increased susceptibility to infections, increased risk of iodine deficiency-induced goiter, and hyperkeratosis-related skin conditions [316,317]. Vitamin A deficiency is usually caused by inadequate dietary intake over time. Since it is a fat-soluble vitamin, patients with impaired lipid digestion and intestinal malabsorption are at high risk for deficiency. Conditions including bariatric surgery, pancreatic insufficiency, celiac disease, and Crohn's disease can all predispose patients to vitamin A deficiency.

Vitamin D

While vitamin D intake is essential to prevent deficiency, its metabolism and functions have led to some debate as to whether dietary vitamin D should be considered a prohormone.

Vitamin D is a group of fat-soluble sterols and their metabolites which play an important role in calcium homeostasis and bone metabolism. Active vitamin D increases intestinal absorption of calcium and phosphorus, increases renal reabsorption of calcium and excretion of phosphorus, as well as mobilizing calcium reserve in the bone. Vitamin D_3 (cholecalciferol) can be synthesized in the epidermis of skin from 7-dehydrocholesterol by the action of ultraviolet-B radiation from sunlight; about 100 IU/day can be synthesized endogenously in people living in the temperate zone [318]. Vitamin D_2 (ergocalciferol) is a vitamin D analog synthesized in a number of plants and fungi. Both vitamin D_2 and D_3 are absorbed with similar efficiency, likely through passive diffusion and membrane transporters in the small intestine, before being released and transported to the liver by vitamin D-binding protein. They undergo hydroxylation in hepatocytes to form 25-hydroxyvitamin D (25(OH)D; calcidiol), which is the major form of vitamin D in circulation and an indicator of vitamin D status [319,320]. In the kidney, 25(OH)D is further hydroxylated to 1,25-dihydroxyvitamin D (calcitriol) by 25-hydroxyvitamin D-1α-hydroxylase.

The hydroxylation of 25(OH)D is tightly regulated by various factors including serum calcium, phosphorus, PTH, and FGF-23. PTH secreted in the setting of low calcium levels can promote hydroxylation of 25(OD)D. FGF-23 secreted by osteoblasts can inhibit hydroxylation of 25(OH)D, thus decreasing bone breakdown. Calcitriol, the active form of vitamin D, also plays a positive role in the regulation of blood pressure, insulin secretion, immune response, and cell differentiation via its action through the vitamin D receptor [321].

Even though vitamin D_3 can be synthesized in the skin with exposure to ultraviolet light, the length of daily exposure to sunlight required for synthesizing a certain amount of vitamin D_3 varies with latitude, season, time of the day, skin type, and age. Higher latitude, winter season, darker skin type, and older age are associated with decreased sythesis of vitamin D_3.

Food sources rich in vitamin D include oily fish, certain organ meats, eggs, and fortified foods (cereal and dairy products). The current RDA for vitamin D recommended by the Institute of Medicine is 600 IU/day (15 μg/day) for all adults (including during pregnancy and breastfeeding) aged 70 years or below, and 800 IU/day (20 μg/day) for older adults aged above 70 years due to decreased capacity to synthesize vitamin D and decreased exposure to sunlight [322]. Analysis of NHANES 2003–2006 data showed that 100% of the US adult population had dietary intake of vitamin D from natural foods less than EAR. This changed to 95% when fortified foods were accounted for, and even with supplements, 68% had inadequate vitamin D intake [253]. This suggests that the current level of fortification in the US is likely ineffective in helping the population reach the recommended amount of vitamin D intake [323].

In the setting of vitamin D deficiency, calcium absorption in the intestine and calcium reabsorption in the kidney are impaired, causing increased calcium release from bone breakdown by the effect of PTH. Severe vitamin D deficiency in children can cause rickets, which is a consequence of bone mineralization failure. This had become quite rare, with supplementation of milk and public health efforts to increase milk intake. But there is concern over a possible resurgence of rickets, reported in at least one study [324], as supplemented milk intake has fallen from favor and has been substituted by sugary drinks and juices. In adults, excessive loss of bone minerals can cause softening of the bones, known as osteomalacia, and increases the risk of osteoporosis. Chronic musculoskeletal pain is also common in vitamin D deficiency.

Measurement of total serum 25(OH)D level is the best diagnostic test to assess vitamin D status. However, the cut-off levels for diagnosis of deficiency are still not quite clear, and the designation "insufficient" by commercial laboratories is of questionable clinical significance. Based on clinical trials of vitamin D supplementation to maintain bone health, the Institute of Medicine defined deficiency as serum 25(OH)D levels ≤12 ng/mL (≤30 nmol/L), and insufficiency as serum 25(OH)D levels of 12–20 ng/mL (30–50 nmol/L) [322]. Other societies such as the US Endocrine Society suggested a definition of deficiency as serum 25(OH)D levels ≤20 ng/mL (≤50 nmol/L), and insufficiency as 20–30 ng/mL (50–75 nmol/L) based on data from observational studies on low vitamin D-associated chronic diseases [325].

Apart from environmental factors and low dietary intake, patients with chronic kidney disease, fat malabsorption syndromes, Crohn's disease, and obesity (BMI ≥30 kg/m^2) are at increased risk for vitamin D deficiency [321]. Studies have shown that percentage of body fat content is inversely related to serum 25(OH)D levels [326]. This is likely due to vitamin D being squestered in body fat stores, making it less available for people with higher body fat mass to utilize. Observational data have shown that higher vitamin D intakes and predicted vitamin D levels were associated with significantly reduced risk of Crohn's disease in a cohort of 72 719 women [327]. A double-blinded trial randomized 108 patients with Crohn's disease to receiving either 1200 IU vitamin D_3 or placebo daily over 12 months and found significantly increased vitamin D levels and insignificantly reduced relapse risk in the study group (29% to 13%) [328]. Observational data also suggested an inverse association between vitamin D status and disease severity in Crohn's patients [329]. The underlying mechanism is likely related to the immunomodulatory effect of vitamin D.

As reviewed in the introduction of this chapter, vitamin D levels decrease in the presence of systemic inflammation, due to a decrease in carrier protein concentrations, and are thus unsurprisingly predictive of outcomes in such conditions as critical illness. However, randomized control trials of vitamin D supplementation have not shown an impact on clinical outcomes in critical illness or in the prevention or treatment of respiratory illness such as COVID-19.

Vitamin E

Vitamin E refers to a group of fat-soluble compounds that include four tocopherols (α-, β-, γ-, and δ-tocopherol) and four tocotrienols (α-, β-, γ-, and δ-tocotrienol). Humans cannot synthesize vitamin E so must obtain it from dietary sources. α-Tocopherol is the most predominant and biologically active form of vitamin E in the human body, and is the only form that meets the human vitamin E requirement [330]. α-Tocopherol and the other forms of vitamin E are important antioxidants and free radical scavengers. The fat solubility promotes incorporation of α-tocopherol into cell membranes where it acts to protect cells against lipid oxidation by free radicals. This protective effect stabilizes cell membrane structure and improves membrane function and also enhances T-cell immunity [331]. The antioxidant capacity of α-tocopherol can be regenerated by other antioxidants such as vitamin C.

The mechanism of intestinal absorption of vitamin E is unclear, but it likely involves passive diffusion and certain cholesterol transporters [332]. Absorption requires gastric lipase and pancreatic enzymes including esterases, as well as bile salt micelle formation, and requires a normal intestinal mucosa. Within the enterocytes, vitamin E is packed into chylomicrons along with dietary fat and apolipoproteins before it is released and transported to the liver. The efficiency of vitamin E absorption is dependent on dietary fat content. Within hepatocytes, chylomicrons are broken down and α-tocopherol is preferentially released into circulation bound to α-tocopherol transfer protein (α-TTP) and various lipoproteins. α-Tocopherol can then be transported to adipose tissue and stored. Excessive α-tocopherol can be excreted in bile or metabolized by cytochrome P450-dependent hydroxylases [333]. Vitamin E can protect the fats in low-density lipoprotein (LDL) against oxidation, thus potentially preventing ischemic cardiovascular damage [333].

All eight forms of vitamin E exist in natural plant-based foods at different levels. Food sources rich in α-tocopherol include vegetable oils, nuts, seeds, and green leafy vegetables. The RDA for α-tocopherol is 15 mg/day (22.5 IU/day) for male and female adults. The requirement is the same during pregnancy and higher at 19 mg/day (28.5 IU/day) during breastfeeding [334]. Analysis of the NHANES 2003–2006 data showed that the average US adult consumes 7.2 mg/day of α-tocopherol from the diet, including fortified foods, while 94% of the population had dietary intakes less than EAR. This number is improved to 58% when supplements were accounted for, indicating the importance of supplementation in vitamin E status among the general population [253].

Vitamin E deficiency is rare in humans and is usually a result of abnormal dietary fat absorption or metabolism rather than of poor intakes. Fat malabsorption syndromes can cause deficiency of vitamin E and other fat-soluble vitamins. Severe vitamin E deficiency has been associated with genetic defects affecting α-tocopherol transport by α-TTP and lipoproteins [334]. Severe vitamin E deficiency can present as peripheral neuropathy, myopathy, spinocerebellar ataxia, and pigmented retinopathy [335]. Low dietary intakes can cause marginal vitamin E deficiency, which is generally asymptomatic.

Vitamin K

Vitamin K refers to a group of fat-soluble naphthoquinone compounds with antihemorrhagic activity. They share similar structure with warfarin and other coumadin-like anticoagulants that function as vitamin K antagonists. Naturally occurring vitamin K comes in two forms: vitamin K_1 (phylloquinones), the predominant form of dietary vitamin K which is synthesized in green plants, and vitamin K_2 (menaquinones) which consists of several variants that are synthesized in bacteria and in humans by gut microbiota.

Vitamin K activates vitamin K-dependent proteins (VKDPs) by functioning as the essential cofactor for carboxylation of glutamic acid residues in the proteins. Vitamin K is crucial for the activation of factors II (prothrombin), VII, IX, and X which make up the coagulation cascade. It also plays an important role in bone formation and prevention of vascular calcification, among many others [336,337]. Intestinal absorption of vitamin K likely occurs via passive diffusion as well as membrane transporters. Similar to other fat-soluble vitamins, the absorption process requires pancreatic enzymes and bile salt micelles. Vitamin K is then incorporated into chylomicrons and transported to the liver via lymphatics before it is released into circulation bound to lipoproteins, while excessive vitamin K can be oxidized in hepatocytes or secreted in bile, stool, and urine. Unlike other fat-soluble vitamins, vitamin K is not stored in large amounts in adipose tissue, and the body recycles vitamin K via a oxidation-reduction cycle to maximize the use of the vitamin [338].

Dietary sources rich in vitamin K_1 include green leafy vegetables and some plant oils (e.g., soybean, canola, olive). Fermented foods and animal livers are rich in vitamin K_2. Due to the lack of data on which to estimate an average requirement, the RDA is not available; instead, the AI was set at 90 µg/day and 120 µg/day for adult women (including during pregnancy and breastfeeding) and men, respectively [339]. The average US diet contains about 80 µg/day of vitamin K and only about one-third of the population have intakes above the AI [253]. The human body hosts certain bacteria that synthesize vitamin K_2 in the gut. Most of these bacteria are located in the colon where bile salts are lacking to facilitate absorption, although absorption in terminal ileum can occur with backwash. The production and absorption of vitamin K_2 by the human body is highly variable [340,341].

Vitamin K deficiency is rare in the healthy population because the human body conserves vitamin K by recycling it, and a variable amount of K_2 is synthesized by gut bacteria. High-risk factors for vitamin K deficiency include fat malabsorption syndromes, cystic fibrosis, celiac disease, inflammatory bowel disease, biliary disease, and liver failure. Vitamin K antagonists, antibiotics, and high doses of vitamin E may also negatively impact vitamin K status. Similar to vitamin D, vitamin K is low in breast milk, and since vitamin K storage is also low due to limited transport through the placenta, newborns are at increased risk for vitamin K deficiency. Symptoms associated with vitamin K deficieny are caused by impaired coagulation and include easy bruisability, mucosal bleeding, melena, hematuria, and heavy menstrual bleeding. In newborns, intracranial hemorrhage is the most feared consequence which may be prevented by routine administration of vitamin K prophylaxis at birth [342].

Other nutrients

Choline

Choline can be synthesized endogenously in small amounts in the human body, but it is still generally considered an essential nutrient. Choline is a precursor for the neurotransmitter acetylcholine, the methyl donor betaine, and phospholipids [343]. Choline and its metabolites are involved in many crucial physiological functions. The majority of choline in the human body is in the form of phospholipids, the most common of which is phosphatidylcholine, an essential structural component of cell membranes. Choline is absorbed from the intestines via transporter proteins; the water-soluble compounds (choline, phosphocholine, glycerophosphocholine) are transported via the portal circulation whereas the lipid-soluble compounds (phosphatidylcholine, sphingomyelin) are absorbed into the lymphatic circulation in the form of chylomicrons [344].

Food sources including liver, eggs, meat, fish, and dairy products are rich in choline. Vegan diet is a high-risk factor for inadequate choline intake since animal products are the best sources of choline. Due to lack of evidence supporting a recommendation on RDA, the AI was set instead at 550 mg/day for adult men and 425 mg/day for adult women. The AI during pregnancy is 450 mg/day and during breastfeeding is 550 mg/day [344]. Analysis of the US NHANES 2013–2014 data showed that the mean dietary intakes of choline among adults aged 20 or above were approximately 278 mg/day for women and 402 mg/day for men [345].

The endogenous synthesis of choline in the human body is not sufficient to meet daily requirements and prolonged poor dietary intakes can cause choline deficiency. Symptomatic choline deficiency is rare in humans. Since phosphatidylcholines are required for the synthesis of very low-density lipoprotein (VLDL), choline deficiency causes decreased VLDL secretion, resulting in steatosis. A study showed that when deprived of dietary choline, 77% of men, 80% of postmenopausal women, and 44% of premenopausal women developed fatty liver, liver damage, or muscle damage, and these organ dysfunctions resolved with the addition of choline back into the diet [346]. Premenopausal women are less susceptible to organ damage in the setting of choline deficiency, likely due to the fact that estrogen stimulates endogenous synthesis of phosphatidylcholine. Postmenopausal women have a higher dietary requirement for choline [347].

Carnitine

Carnitine is a crucial compound involved in fatty acid metabolism and energy production. It is required to transport long-chain fatty acids into mitochondria to be oxidized for energy production and for transport of metabolic products out of mitochondria to prevent toxic effects from accumulation. Studies have shown that deficiency may cause insulin resistance, heart dysfunction, and peripheral neuropathy [348–350]. L-carnitine and D-carnitine are the two isoforms of carnitine, but only L-carnitine is biologically active in animals. The human body can synthesize sufficient L-carnitine in the liver and kidney, but when there is increased demand it becomes an essential nutrient. Meat, fish, and dairy products are food sources rich in L-carnitine. Carnitine deficiency is generally due to impaired mitochondrial energy metabolism or impaired kidney reabsorption and does not occur in healthy people without metabolic disorders.

The kidney is crucial in maintaining carnitine status via L-carnitine synthesis and tubular reabsorption. Impaired reabsorption in Fanconi syndrome and chronic renal failure results in increased urinary loss of carnitine. Patients on hemodialysis are also at risk for carnitine deficiency due to carnitine removal by dialysis, so L-carnitine is recommended for the treatment of carnitine deficiency in hemodialysis patients. Patients with liver cirrhosis normally are not carnitine deficient, whereas those with alcohol-induced cirrhosis have increased plasma carnitine levels, likely due to increased carnitine synthesis from high skeletal muscle protein turnover [351]. Rarely, patients on chronic parenteral nutrition have developed carnitine deficiency, initially manifesting as elevated liver enzymes [352].

Arginine

Arginine is a conditionally essential amino acid, depending on the developmental state and health status of the individual. Certain conditions such as metabolic or traumatic stress may produce a conditional deficiency due to increased demands. Arginine plays an important role in cell division, microcirculation regulation, T-cell function, and wound healing [353]. It is an intermediate metabolite in the urea cycle and is used for the treatment of hyperammonemia since it increases ammonia elimination in the urea cycle [354]. Arginine is a precursor for nitric oxide (NO) and part of its physiological function is dependent on the action of NO. Arginine is also required for the production of urea, creatine, and polyamines, among others. Common sources of arginine include meat, fish, eggs, dairy products, and nuts. Arginine supplementation is generally considered safe without significant adverse reactions. Recent studies have shown potential benefit in individuals with obesity, insulin resistance, and diabetes, as well as the surgical or critically ill population [355,356]. However, more data are needed to fully evaluate the safety and efficacy of arginine supplementation.

Glutamine

Glutamine is the most abundant extracellular amino acid in the human body and considered nonessential in healthy individuals. Glutamine is a precursor of glutathione, an important intracellular antioxidant and modulator of cell signaling. Glutamine availability and release into circulation is mainly determined by key organs such as the liver, intestine, and skeletal muscles. Glutamine plays an important role in synthesis of protein and lipids, as well as regulation of acid–base balance. It is essential for the immune system and is required for lymphocyte proliferation and cytokine production, macrophage activities, and neutrophil functions [357]. During catabolic states including exhaustion in athletes and critical illness, glutamine availability may be compromised.

While glutamine is considered a conditionally essential nutrient, a deficiency state has not been well described in these populations, and a decrease in production may be adaptive or a disease epiphenomenon. There has been little evidence supporting the efficacy of glutamine supplementation in stimulating immune function, reducing infectious complications, or improving catabolic states in athletes or critically ill patients. Glutamine is an important energy source for the small intestine and is approved for use in short bowel syndrome in combination with growth hormone and nutritional support. It is also approved by the FDA for use in sickle cell disease to prevent vasoocclusive pain in patients with frequent episodes, along with hydroxyurea, or as an alternative in patients who are intolerant to hydroxyurea [358,359].

Dietary supplements for general use

Fifty-four percent of US adults responding to the National Health and Nutrition Examination Survey (1999–2014) reported using a dietary supplement in the past 30 days [360]. This underscores the necessity for all practitioners to include questions related to supplement use for all patients. Supplement users in the US tend to be older, female, non-Hispanic whites, with higher than average educational attainment and income. They also tend to be physically active, maintain healthy weights, eat healthy diets, and are less likely to be current smokers or heavy drinkers [361]. Reported reasons for initiation and continuation of supplement use vary, with 33% of users taking supplements to maintain overall health, and 45% aiming to improve general health [362]. Only 23% of supplements taken are based on recommendations from a healthcare provider [362]. Despite their widespread use, a prospective cohort study utilizing NHANES data matched with National Death Index Mortality data found no association between dietary supplement use and mortality benefits, after controlling for differences in lifestyle factors [361].

Supplement use is not without risk. For example, the Selenium and Vitamin E Cancer Prevention Trial (SELECT) found that supplementation of 400 IU vitamin E daily significantly increased the risk of prostate cancer among healthy adult men [363]. Similarly, the Beta-Carotene and Retinol Efficacy Trial (CARET) found that supplementation of vitamin A (with 30 mg/day β-carotene and 25 000 IU retinyl palmitate) increased the risk of lung cancer mortality among smokers [364,365]. Herbal supplements, such as green tea extract, are known to cause liver injury [366].

Regulation of dietary supplements in the United States

Under the US Dietary Supplement Health and Education Act of 1994, dietary supplements are considered food, not drugs. Because of this distinction, manufacturers generally do not need to seek premarket approval from the FDA. The FDA must prove a supplement to be unsafe in order to remove it from the market. The FDA regulates product safety for supplements, but not efficacy, and safety need not be proven prior to bringing a supplement to market.

The Federal Trade Commission oversees dietary supplement advertising and product labeling. Manufacturers may make structure function claims (e.g., "supports immune function"), but may not claim to prevent or treat disease (e.g., "prevents the common cold").

The Office of Dietary Supplements (ODS; https://ods.od.nih.gov/) at the NIH promotes, conducts, coordinates, and compiles research about dietary supplements. The ODS has many resources available to consumers and health professionals, including dietary supplement fact sheets and databases of product labels and supplement ingredients.

Multivitamins

The term *multivitamin* does not have a standard definition; multivitamins contain different formulas, and often do not contain all vitamins and minerals. In 2014, 32% of adults reported taking multivitamins (defined as ≥10 vitamins and/or minerals) in the last 30 days [360]. Primary reasons reported for multivitamin use are to improve or maintain general health and supplement the diet [362]. Evidence does not show significant health improvements from multivitamin intake. The Cancer Prevention Study II found no significant association between multivitamin use and cardiovascular or cancer mortality [367]. Likewise, the Multiethnic Cohort Study found no association between multivitamin use and all-cause mortality [368], and NHANES data indicate no significant associations between multivitamin with mineral use and cardiovascular disease mortality [369]. The NHANES did report a significant association between multivitamin-mineral use for more than 3 years with a decreased risk of CVD mortality among women [10], but randomized data are lacking.

Vitamin B_{12}

As vitamin B_{12} is solely found in animal sources, vegans and, to a lesser extent, vegetarians are at risk of vitamin B_{12} deficiency. In a study of British men, 52% of vegans and 7% of vegetarians were B_{12} deficient (defined as serum vitamin B_{12} <118 pmol/L) [370]. Fortified foods, such as plant milk and nutritional yeast, or supplements are necessary to meet vitamin B_{12} needs in this population [371]. These may be marketed as "vegan" but the B_{12} added to these is from animal sources. The lack of non-animal B_{12} sources is often cited as a physiological argument against strict veganism.

Older adults are at risk of B_{12} deficiency, in part due to decreased production and/or suppression of hydrochloric acid and intrinsic factor [372]. Medications may also play a role in the development of B_{12} deficiency. A retrospective cohort study of older adults in long-term care facilities found that prevalence of B_{12} deficiency among residents with diabetes taking metformin was 53.2%, compared to 31% and 33% among residents with diabetes not on metformin and residents without a diagnosis of diabetes, respectively [373].

Vitamin D

As mentioned, vitamin D has received special attention as a preventive agent for cancer, cardiovascular disease, respiratory illness, and more. As of December 1, 2020, a search for "vitamin D and prevention" retrieved more than 17 000 publications on Pubmed.gov, "Vitamin D AND critical care" found 673, and "vitamin D AND COVID" already resulted in more than 300 publications, only one of which is a randomized trial.

Importantly, the data refute the theories of benefit for D supplementation. For example, a large cohort study using NHANES data found that vitamin D supplement use was associated with an increased risk of all-cause mortality [361]. A placebo-controlled study found no association between supplementation with 2000 IU cholecalciferol (vitamin D_3) and cancer or cardiovascular events [374]. A randomized controlled trial of older adults in New Zealand found that high-dose supplementation (200 000 IU, followed by 100 000 IU monthly) of vitamin D did not prevent acute respiratory infections [375].

As discussed in the section on deficiency in the introduction to this chapter, a deficiency does not result simply because there is a low serum concentration of a substance. The vast literature on vitamin D, however, largely misinterprets low vitamin D levels as deficiency in a multitude of disease states. We will discuss critical illness for illustration.

Most studies of vitamin D in the ICU are retrospective, observational, and highly flawed, often including only patients in whom D levels happened to be drawn [376]. That said, there is no question that low vitamin D levels are associated with an increase in length of stay and mortality in the critically ill [377]. However, it is highly likely that this relationship results simply because of a decrement in the levels of the main carrier for transporting vitamin D in the bloodstream.

Vitamin D-binding protein (VDBP) drops in the face of systemic inflammation just as albumin does. However, when VDBP and total, bioavailable, free vitamin D were measured prospectively, it was only VDBP that was associated with survival [378]. No effect of vitamin D level was seen when levels were tested at ICU admission [379].

Large randomized controlled studies have failed to demonstrate a morbidity or mortality benefit from vitamin D supplementation in critically ill patients, despite causing an increase in D levels [380] and biochemical changes suggestive of potential benefit [381]. Fortunately, since vitamin D is not without toxicity, they have also failed to demonstrate harm [382,383].

All these findings indicate that the low D levels seen in the critically ill and associated with morbidity and mortality do not constitute a deficiency state. Moreover, if vitamin D were truly deficient in these patients, it would be expected that ionized calcium and phosphate levels would be significantly decreased and PTH levels elevated. These expected changes are either not reported or occur equally in critically ill patients with and without low D levels [381].

There are clear and unsurprising relationships between COVID outcomes and vitamin D levels, but low D levels are not associated with an increased risk of COVID infection [384]. The broader literature does not support a role for vitamin D to prevent pneumonia [385,386] or upper respiratory infection [387].

Similar results have been seen in IBD [388] and other inflammatory diseases [389] in which vitamin D has been characterized as a negative acute phase reactant. In the absence of demonstrable benefit or other findings of deficiency (hypocalcemia, elevated PTH), a decrement in levels should be considered reflective of the level of systemic inflammation and capillary leak.

References are available at www.yamadagastro.com/textbook7e

CHAPTER 21

Nutrient digestion, absorption, and sensing

Shrinivas Bishu[1] **and Eamonn M. M. Quigley**[2]

[1] Division of Gastroenterology and Hepatology, Crohn's and Colitis Center University of Michigan, Ann Arbor, MI, USA

[2] Lynda K and David M Underwood Center for Digestive Disorders, Houston Methodist Hospital and Weill Cornell Medical College, Houston, TX, USA

Chapter menu

Nutrient digestion, absorption, and sensing are fundamental processes that are critical to the survival of biological organisms. In general, these topics are broad, overlapping, interconnected, nonredundant, and impact biological processes extending from metabolism at the cellular level to disease states at the macroscopic level. We have organized this chapter into two larger sections: (1) nutrient digestion and absorption, and (2) nutrient sensing. These sections are further split along natural divisions. We hope this organization eases the burden of reading and organizes the material in a systematic way. Given the depth of the topic, our goal here is to provide an overview with depth sufficient for the clinical gastroenterologist. For those interested in the granular details, we refer the reader to the cited references and any number of outstanding in-depth reviews covering each of the topics.

Nutrient digestion and absorption

Digestion of carbohydrates, proteins, and lipids

Digestion of carbohydrates

Structure of carbohydrates

Carbohydrates are composed of carbon, hydrogen, and oxygen with the formula $C_m(H_2O)_n$, where m refers to the number of carbon molecules and n the number of attached H_2O units. Carbohydrates are the major source of calories in the diet of the average adult human. Spatially, carbohydrates can be linear or arranged in pentose or hexose rings. Carbohydrates composed of a single moiety are termed monosaccharides. Disaccharides are composed of two monosaccharides, and larger units are oligosaccharides (3–9 units) or polysaccharides (>9 units). Linkages between monosaccharides to form these large units are either via α(1,4), α(1,6), or β(1,4) bonds, where α and β refer to bonds above or below the plane of the sugar ring, respectively. Human enzymes can readily hydrolyze α(1,4) bonds but have greater difficulty with β linkages.

The most important dietary disaccharides are sucrose, maltose, and lactose (Figure 21.1). Sucrose (table sugar) is the natural sugar of fruits and vegetables and accounts for ~30% of all dietary carbohydrate intake. Similarly, maltose is composed to two α(1,4) linked glucose molecules, while lactose is composed of β(1,4) bond linked glucose and galactose. Polysaccharides may be either linear or branched, and can be either absorbable or nonabsorbable. Starches, composed of amylose and amylopectin (~20:80 ratio), are the most important dietary polysaccharides. Amylose is a linear polymer of glucose bound by α(1,4) bonds. Amylopectin is a branched chain polymer composed of linearly bound glucose molecules attached by α(1,4) bonds with branching provided by α(1,6) bonds every 25–30 glucose molecules.

Luminal digestion of carbohydrates

Large polysaccharides such as starches cannot be transported across the enterocyte brush border membrane. Thus, the

Yamada's Textbook of Gastroenterology, Seventh Edition. Edited by Timothy C. Wang, Michael Camilleri, Benjamin Lebwohl, Anna S. Lok, William J. Sandborn, Kenneth K. Wang, and Gary D. Wu.

Companion website: www.yamadagastro.com/textbook7e

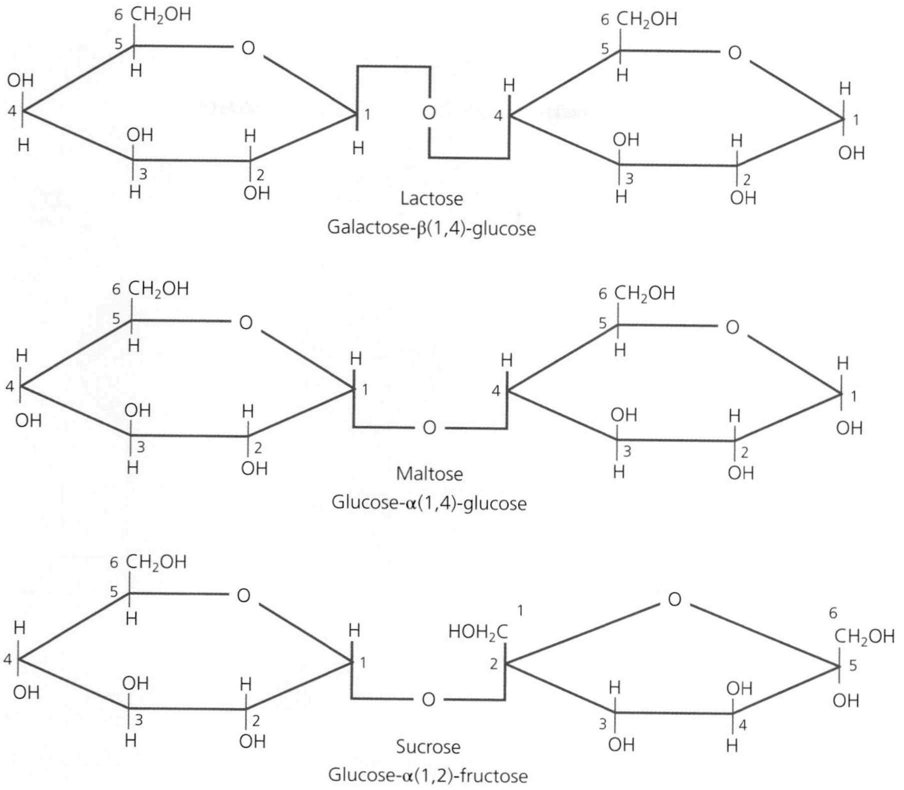

Lactose
Galactose-β(1,4)-glucose

Maltose
Glucose-α(1,4)-glucose

Sucrose
Glucose-α(1,2)-fructose

Figure 21.1 Structure of the three major nutritional disaccharides: lactose, maltose, and sucrose.

fragmentation of larger branched starches is a primary outcome of the luminal phase of carbohydrate digestion. Carbohydrate digestion begins with the action of α-amylase (hereafter referred to as amylase), which hydrolyzes α(1,4) glycosidic bonds [1]. Amylase is calcium dependent and acts on amylose and amylopectin in starches to generate constituent molecules. Amylase degrades amylose into maltose and maltotriose, which is a trisaccharide linked by α(1,4) glycosidic bonds [2]. Amylase degrades amylopectin into glucose, maltose, amylose, and α limit dextrins, which are glucose oligosaccharides with α(1,6) linkages [2]. Amylase exists in salivary and pancreatic isoforms produced by the parotid glands and pancreatic acinar cells, respectively. Pancreatic amylase is secreted with pancreatic juices at an alkaline pH and is the primary enzyme mediating the initial digestion of carbohydrates.

Mucosal digestion of carbohydrates

Luminal digestion of starches results in disaccharides, trisaccharides, and oligosaccharides, such as α limit dextrins. The mucosal phase of digestion further degrades the products of luminal digestion into constituent monosaccharides that are capable of being transported across the enterocyte brush border membrane. The mucosal phase is primarily executed by saccharidases, which are a group of hydrolytic enzymes expressed on the mucosal brush border of intestinal enterocytes. Saccharidases, which are important for human digestion, include sucrase-isomaltase, lactase-phlorizin hydrolase, maltase-glucoamylase, and trehalase (Figure 21.2).

Sucrase-isomaltase

Sucrase-isomaltase contains active sites for sucrase and isomaltase. It also has the capacity to hydrolyze α limit dextrins via the isomaltase site (and is, therefore, also known as α limit dextrinase) [3,4]. The sucrase site hydrolyzes α(1,4) bonds of disaccharides and short oligosaccharides, such as sucrose, maltose, and maltotriose, and is the only enzyme capable of hydrolyzing sucrose. The isomaltase site is unique in that it can hydrolyze α(1,6) in addition to α(1,4) bonds, which gives it the capacity to degrade the branching points in α-limit dextrans [4–6].

Although sucrase-isomaltase contains two active sites, it is synthesized as a single glycoprotein [7,8]. Sucrase-isomaltase is glycosylated postsynthesis and then transported to the apical brush border membrane of the enterocyte. This membrane-expressed complex is then cleaved by trypsin in the intestinal lumen, thus exposing the two active sites as a heterodimer on the enterocyte membrane [7,8]. Sucrase-isomaltase is primarily expressed in the jejunum with maximal activity in the lower to mid-villus cells, and almost no expression at the villus tip or in the crypt [9].

Sucrase-isomaltase is expressed at birth and facilitates digestion of sugars before weaning. Sucrase-isomaltase deficiency is

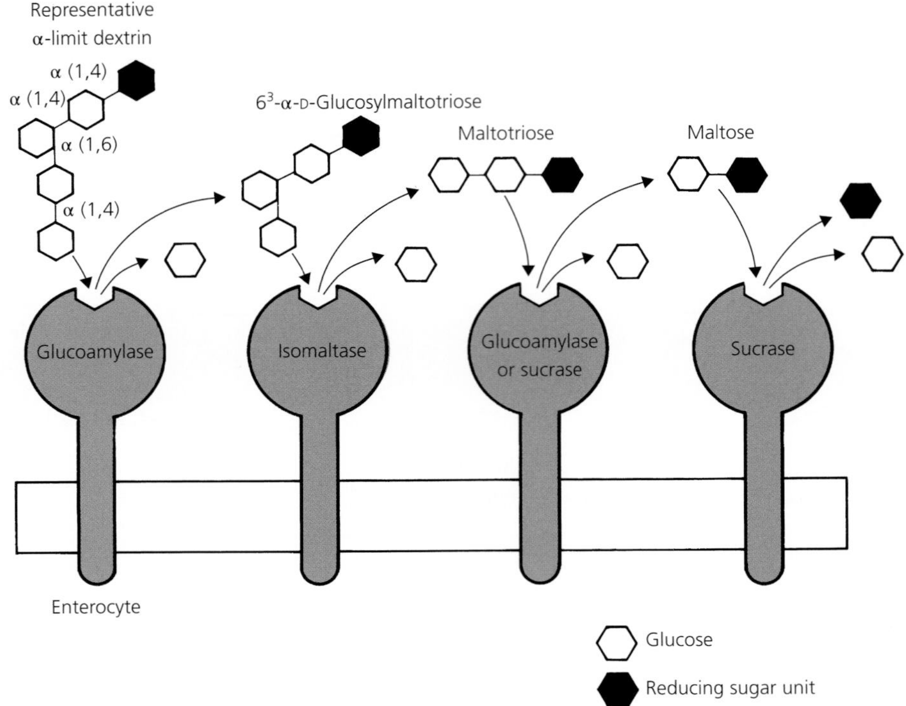

Figure 21.2 Overall process of digestion to monosaccharides. The hydrolysis of α limit dextrins is a collaborative effort among multiple brush border enzymes.

an autosomal recessive condition with variable incidence across populations (approximately 3–10% in Inuits in Alaska and Greenland to 0.2–0.5% in North American and European populations [10,11]). Consistent with its expression early in life, genetic deficiency presents in infancy as a malabsorptive condition that becomes symptomatic on introduction of sucrose-containing foods [5,10,12]. Avoidance of sucrose is the primary treatment modality. However, dietary supplementation with the enzyme sacrosidase, a β-D-fructofuranoside fructohydrolase produced by the yeast *Saccharomyces cerevisiae*, may be safe and effective [12]. More broadly, recent data suggest that a small minority of patients with irritable bowel syndrome have genetic mutations in the sucrase isomaltase gene that may be functionally significant [13].

Lactase-phlorizin hydrolase

Lactose, composed of glucose and galactose linked by a β(1,4) bond, is the primary carbohydrate in milk. Lactase-phlorizin hydrolase, or lactase, is the only brush border enzyme with activity for the β(1,4) bond of lactose, making it necessary for digestion of milk in humans. In addition, lactase-phlorizin also exhibits phlorizin hydrolase, glycosyl-ceramidase, and β-galactosidase activities [3,14,15].

Lactase-phlorizin is synthesized as a precursor peptide followed by posttranslational modifications (glycosylation and cleavage) before enterocyte membrane expression as a mature peptide [16]. Lactase is primarily expressed at the villus tips of the distal duodenum and proximal small intestine with lower expression in the remaining intestine [17]. Lactase is not expressed in crypts [15,17]. Humans express the highest levels of lactase before weaning, with declining expression thereafter. The age of onset of the decline varies considerably among human populations worldwide, ranging from the toddler years to young adulthood, and may be related to local population evolutionary pressures or epigenetic modifications of *LCT*, which is the gene for lactase. On average, most adult human populations worldwide demonstrate 5–10% of maximal activity [14].

Lactase deficiency can be either primary or secondary and should be regarded as a distinct entity from the aforementioned age-related decline in intestinal activity. Primary deficiency, termed primary congenital alactasia, is a rare autosomal recessive condition that has been described in specific populations (e.g., it affects up to 60% of the Saami population of Finland and Russia). Missense mutations in *LCT*, which encodes lactase, are the most common cause of congenital alactasia. However, other mutations, including frameshift, have been identified in affected patients. The net result of these mutations appears to be either the total absence or significantly reduced expression of lactase, with concomitant profound defects in enzymatic function [18,19]. Secondary lactase deficiency is the most common clinical condition associated with lactose malabsorption and occurs as a result of processes that damage the enterocyte brush border and reduce membrane enzyme expression, thereby reflecting the vulnerability of the enzyme conferred by its anatomical positioning on the villus tip. Secondary lactase deficiency is commonly associated with inflammatory, infectious, ischemic, toxic (e.g., cancer chemotherapy), and radiation-induced intestinal insults. For example, transient lactose intolerance is common among children in the aftermath of an enteric infection and may lead to an apparent failure to respond to a gluten-free diet in newly diagnosed individuals with celiac disease.

In contrast with primary and secondary lactase deficiency, age-related decline in lactase activity, termed lactase persistence (or nonpersistence), is variably present in most human populations. Lactase persistence is transcriptionally controlled, potentially via epigenetic mechanisms, ultimately resulting in reduced expression of lactase messenger RNA (mRNA) in enterocytes [20]. Thus, lactase persistence is not considered a deficiency, such as primary or secondary lactase deficiency. Some populations, such as those of northern European descent, do not exhibit the age-related decline in a lactase expression [18,21]. Several single-nucleotide polymorphisms in an enhancer of the *LCT* gene are associated with lactase persistence.

Primary and secondary lactase deficiency present with lactose intolerance. Undigested lactose in the gastrointestinal tract is fermented by bacteria in the distal ileum and colon to produce short-chain fatty acid (FAs), hydrogen, carbon dioxide, and methane. Thus, bloating, flatulence, and diarrhea with resulting abdominal discomfort are typical features of lactase deficiency. Those with age-related maturational decline in lactase expression typically present with symptoms of lactose intolerance on ingestion of a volume of lactose-containing foods that overwhelms their enzymatic capacity. Given the inherent variability in expression, what constitutes excess will vary from person to person and between populations. The prevalence of lactose malabsorption in the United States is highly variable and is generally lower in those of northern European ancestry (~25%) compared with other genetic backgrounds (~80–95% in those of African and Asian ancestry) [14,21]. Lactose intolerance is generally diagnosed clinically and is often assessed in practice by the response to empiric dietary lactose withdrawal. Objective confirmation can be provided by a lactose hydrogen breath test or direct assays of lactase activity on duodenal biopsy specimens. Treatment consists of avoidance of lactose-containing foods or supplementation with exogenous lactase.

Maltase-glucoamylase

Maltase-glucoamylase hydrolyzes short glucose chains at α(1,4) bonds to release glucose from polysaccharide chains (starches) [22]. Maltase-glucoamylase also has low activity for the hydrolysis of α(1,6) bonds. Maltase-glucoamylase is synthesized as a single precursor polypeptide that undergoes post-translational modification by glycosylation [23]. It is then expressed on the enterocyte brush border membrane as a mature protein. The strong homology between the genes for maltase-glucoamylase and sucrose-isomaltase suggests shared ontology with a common precursor. Maltase-glucoamylase is expressed prenatally with stable expression throughout life thereafter. Maltase-glucoamylase deficiency has been described in children with chronic diarrhea with a reported prevalence rate of 1.8% [24].

Trehalase

Trehalase hydrolyzes the disaccharide trehalose into its constituent glucose molecules. Trehalose is found in mushrooms, yeast, algae, and insect hemolymph and is composed of two glucose molecules linked by a unique α(1,1) bond that makes it resistant to hydrolysis. In mice, trehalase is maximally expressed in the proximal small intestine with lower levels of expression in other parts of the intestine. Levels of trehalase expression appear to be similar in fetal and adult intestine [25,26]. Trehalase deficiency is largely limited to Greenland, where it is reported to occur in 8% of the population [4,27]. Trehalase deficiency can result in severe diarrhea after ingestion of mushrooms.

Digestion of proteins

Carbohydrates must be hydrolyzed to constituent monosaccharides before they can be transported across the brush border. In contrast, enterocytes can transport amino acids or protein polypeptides; thus, these are the end products of protein digestion (Figure 21.3). Another important difference between carbohydrate and protein digestion is the site of expression of digestive enzymes. The hydrolytic enzymes that mediate carbohydrate digestion are expressed by enterocytes. In contrast, the proteolytic exopeptidases and endoproteases that mediate protein degradation are released from the pancreas. Thus, bile salts and lipids indirectly impact protein digestion by modulating secretion of pancreatic juices.

Luminal digestion of proteins

Protein digestion starts in the stomach with the action of pepsins, which are a family of aspartic proteases that are largely produced by gastric chief cells. Pepsins are produced as proenzymes but undergo autocleavage at low pH, thus exposing the active site. Pepsins are, therefore, optimally active at the acidic pH of the stomach. Pepsins are endopeptidases and hydrolyze internal peptide bonds with preferential activity for bonds between aromatic amino acids [28]. The activity of pepsin results in a mixture of large polypeptide fragments and small oligopeptides.

Pepsinogens possess positively charged cationic residues in the amino-terminal region and negatively charged acidic residues at the catalytic site. The negatively charged amino-terminal residues are folded into the catalytic site and are stabilized there by electrostatic interactions with the cationic acidic residues at neutral or alkaline pH [29,30]. The folded structure masks the catalytic site of pepsins and prevents their autoactivation. However, in the acidic pH of the stomach, the acidic residues are protonated, thus destabilizing the electrostatic interactions and exposing the active site. The catalytic site then autocleaves a 40-amino acid residue in the amino terminal, thus generating the active form of pepsin [29,30]. Pepsins also contain the anionic

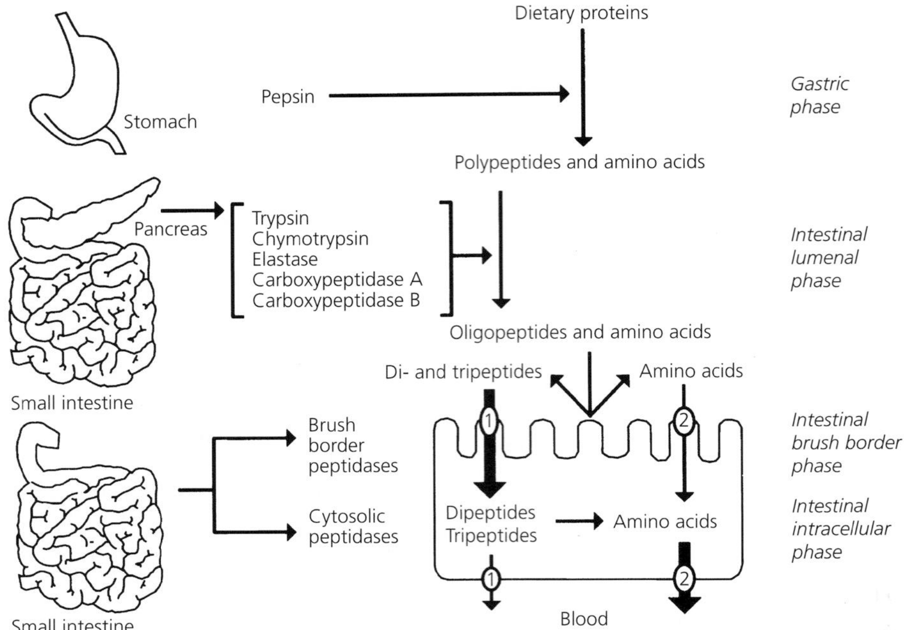

Figure 21.3 Digestion of dietary proteins and absorption of digestion products in the gastrointestinal tract. 1, Transport system for dipeptides and tripeptides; 2, transport systems for free amino acids.

amino acid aspartate at the catalytic site that is necessary for enzymatic activity. Pepsin is inactive at pH > 4 and is, therefore, neutralized rapidly in the small intestine by pancreatic and duodenal secretions [29,30].

In addition to generating pepsin, the acidic gastric environment denatures proteins, thus promoting susceptibility to enzymatic digestion. Pepsins and low gastric pH both contribute to protein digestion but are not absolutely necessary because patients who have undergone partial or total gastrectomy do not generally exhibit protein malnutrition. This is because the pancreatic proteases trypsin and chymotrypsin are the major enzymes of protein digestion [31,32]. The exocrine pancreas produces three endoproteases and two exopeptidases, all of which are released as inactive proenzymes (zymogens). They require cleavage for activation, which prevents autodigestion of pancreatic tissue [31,32]. The three endoproteases are trypsinogen, chymotrypsinogen, and proelastase. The exopeptidases are procarboxypeptidase A and B. In general, endoproteases and exopeptidases are so named because they cleave internal and terminal amino acid bonds in proteins, respectively [31,32].

The process of converting pancreatic zymogens to active enzymes begins with the conversion of trypsinogen to trypsin by enterokinase (also called enteropeptidase). Trypsin then activates the remaining pancreatic zymogens. Enterokinase is expressed on the duodenal brush border as a heterodimer of a disulfide-linked light and heavy chain [33]. The light chain contains the catalytic site, while the heavy chain anchors the protein to the cell membrane. Enterokinase cleaves a hexapeptide from the amino terminus of trypsinogen-generating trypsin. Trypsin

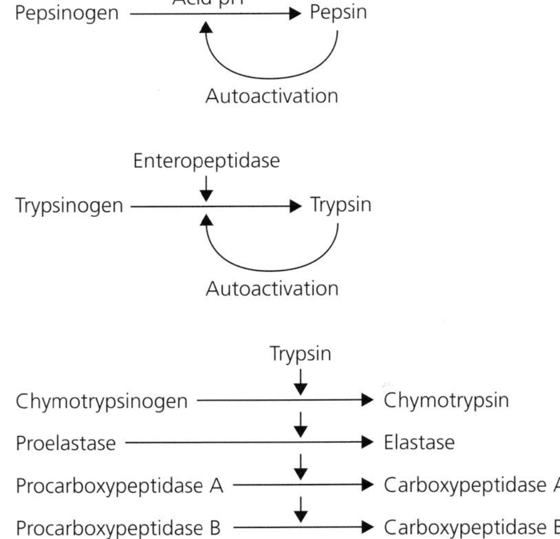

Figure 21.4 Activation of gastric and pancreatic zymogens.

can then autocatalytically activate trypsinogen itself, as well as the remaining pancreatic zymogens, to generate active pancreatic proteases (Figure 21.4).

Trypsin, chymotrypsin, and elastase all hydrolyze internal peptide bonds and are thus endoproteases. Trypsin hydrolyzes bonds flanked by the cationic (basic) residues lysine and arginine, chymotrypsin targets bonds formed by the carboxyl groups of aromatic amino acids (phenylalanine, tyrosine, and tryptophan), and elastase hydrolyzes bonds formed by the carboxyl group of aliphatic residues (glycine, alanine, valine, leucine, and isoleucine) [34]. Carboxypeptidase A and B are exopeptidases that hydrolyze terminal bonds on the carboxyl terminus of polypeptides [35]. Carboxypeptidase A cleaves bonds adjacent to neutral amino acids (aromatic or aliphatic residues), and carboxypeptidase B cleaves bonds adjacent to cationic amino acids (lysine or arginine). These endoproteases and exopeptidases function in unison in protein digestion. The endoproteases chymotrypsin and elastase liberate oligopeptides containing neutral amino acids at the carboxyl terminal, while trypsin generates oligopeptides with cationic residues [35]. The exopeptidases then act on oligopeptides generated by the action of chymotrypsin and elastase (carboxypeptidase A) and trypsin (carboxypeptidase B) to liberate amino acid residues.

Defects in the expression or activity of pancreatic proteases and peptidases result in impaired protein digestion. In particular, notable defects center on trypsin activation given that trypsin converts all other pancreatic zymogens, including trypsin itself. Congenital trypsinogen deficiency presents in infancy with failure to thrive, hypoproteinemia, and edema as a consequence of reduced intravascular oncotic pressure [36]. Treatment with protein hydrolysate-containing diets (rather than intact protein) results in dramatic clinical improvement. Enterokinase is required for the activation of trypsin. Thus, enterokinase deficiency results in severe malabsorption with a clinical picture similar to trypsinogen deficiency because of the similarly impaired activation of pancreatic proteases [37]. Treatment with activated pancreatic enzymes will improve protein digestion. Deficiencies of trypsinogen and enterokinase also affect fat and vitamin B_{12} absorption. Trypsin is necessary for the conversion of procolipase to colipase, which is necessary for the activity of pancreatic lipase and thus fat absorption. Trypsin is also necessary for cleaving vitamin B_{12} from R-binders.

Mucosal digestion of proteins

Brush border peptidases

Luminal digestion generates a mix of oligopeptides (~70%), dipeptides, tripeptides, protein-bound amino acids, and free amino acids. Oligopeptides cannot be transported into enterocytes; thus, they must be hydrolyzed into amino acids and tripeptides and dipeptides by brush border peptidases.

The intestinal brush border contains high levels of exopeptidases, endopeptidases, and dipeptidases. The major exopeptidases are aminopeptidase N, aminopeptidase A, dipeptidylcarboxypeptidase, and dipeptidylaminopeptidase IV [38–42]. Dipeptidylcarboxypeptidase is also known as angiotensin-converting enzyme because of its ability to convert angiotensin I to angiotensin II. In general, aminopeptidases hydrolyze terminal peptide bonds at the amino terminus of short peptides. As their names suggest, aminopeptidase N and A hydrolyze bonds adjacent to neutral and anionic amino acids, respectively, whereas the exopeptidases dipeptidylcarboxypeptidase and dipeptidylaminopeptidase IV hydrolyze bonds adjacent to carboxyl- and amino-terminal peptide bonds, respectively. Thus, aminopeptidases liberate free amino acids, while dipeptidylcarboxypeptidase and dipeptidylaminopeptidase IV generate dipeptides, typically of the X-proline type, from oligopeptides.

Intracellular peptidases

Tripeptides and dipeptides undergo further intracellular digestion within enterocytes by intracellular peptidases. Intracellular peptidase activity is closely linked with dipeptide and tripeptide transport systems. Aminotripeptidase is an intracellular peptidase that liberates amino acid residues from the amino terminus of tripeptides. Iminodipeptidase is also called prolidase because of its specificity for moieties of the X-proline or X-hydroxyproline type. These moieties are typically resistant to hydrolysis by brush border and luminal proteases in the intestinal lumen. Given that other types of peptide bonds are efficiently cleaved by these enzymes, it follows that the majority of peptide fragments and amino acids that are transported across the enterocyte membrane are of the X-proline or X-hydroxyproline type. Thus, iminodipeptidase within enterocytes is required to efficiently hydrolyze these bonds.

In general, intracellular peptidases comprise a heterogeneous group of enzymes that serve wide-ranging functions depending on the cell and tissue in which they are expressed. Deficiencies of intracellular peptidases in humans have been reported, but they are rare. Clinically, they result in a wide variety of impairments because of the fact that intracellular peptidases are expressed in wide-ranging tissues and cells [43].

Digestion of lipids

In contrast with carbohydrates and proteins, lipids are hydrophobic, which poses a major challenge to their digestion and absorption. The overwhelming majority of the internal contents and borders of the human body are aqueous and thus hydrophilic. The major hurdle for lipid digestion and absorption is that hydrophobic lipids must be "dissolved" into a hydrophilic environment. This is accomplished by bile salts and formation of micelles, which allow lipids to interact with hydrophilic interfaces.

Luminal digestion of lipids

Triglycerides (TGs), which are also called triacylglycerols, are the major form of dietary lipids. TGs are esters composed of glycerol and three FAs. Other forms of dietary lipids include phospholipids, free FAs, cholesterol, and fat-soluble vitamins. TGs are hydrolyzed to diacylglycerols (DGs), monoacylglycerols (MGs), and FAs. The length of TGs is determined by the length(s) of their constituent FA chains. TGs are considered "short chain" if their FA tails contain less than 6 carbon atoms, medium chain if they contain 6–12 carbons, long chain if they contain greater than 13 carbons, and very long chain if they contain greater than 21 carbons. Similarly, TGs saturation is determined by the status of their constituent FAs and how many double (unsaturated) bonds they contain.

Lipid digestion begins in the stomach with the action of lingual and gastric lipase, produced by the lingual serous glands and gastric chief cells, respectively [44,45]. These lipases are collectively termed "acid lipases" because they are optimally active at low pH (3–6), which is in contrast with pancreatic lipase [45,46]. Lingual and gastric lipase are thought to retain activity in the duodenum and to significantly contribute to lipid digestion in healthy humans and patients with pancreatic insufficiency states, such as cystic fibrosis [45–49]. Gastric lipase has higher enzymatic activity for hydrolyzing medium-chain TGs compared with long-chain TGs. Gastric lipase hydrolyzes TGs to liberate DGs and nonionized long-chain FAs, but it is inactive against phospholipids and cholesterol esters [44]. Gastric lipase is particularly important in neonates, whose primary nutritional source is milk fat, which is composed of medium-chain TGs. Because pancreatic lipase is not fully developed in neonates, gastric lipases are critical for neonatal digestion and absorption of milk fat. Gastric lipase also has an important role in patients with cystic fibrosis who have impaired pancreatic lipase activity because it preserves (to some degree) their ability to digest and absorb dietary lipids [47].

In addition to enzymatic degradation, the mechanical forces generated by gastric motor activity are also important in lipid digestion and absorption. Gastric peristaltic waves liquefy and emulsify dietary TGs, thus creating a lipid emulsion consisting of particles that are approximately 0.5 μm in diameter [50].

Pancreatic lipase is the major enzyme responsible for the digestion of dietary TGs in the proximal small intestine. Pancreatic lipase, accounting for 2–3% of the total protein content of pancreatic juice, is catalytically efficient and permits the absorption of >90% of dietary fat. Optimal enzymatic efficiency, however, requires colipase, which acts as a cofactor for pancreatic lipase [51]. TG emulsions covered with bile salts are not accessible to pancreatic lipase, making hydrolysis by pancreatic lipase inefficient. Colipase circumvents this problem by binding to the TG–aqueous interface, thus allowing pancreatic lipase to access the lipid–aqueous interface [51]. Pancreatic lipase acts on TGs to release 2-MGs and free FAs [52,53]. In general, MGs can exist as 2- or as 1-MG, the latter formed from 2-MGs by isomerization. In addition to acting on TGs, pancreatic lipase can act on both 1-MG and 2-MG to liberate glycerol and FAs. As is well known in general clinical practice, pancreatic insufficiency (of any etiology) can result in severe fat and fat-soluble vitamin malabsorption.

Phospholipid digestion is primarily accomplished by pancreatic phospholipase A_2 (PLA_2). Pancreatic PLA_2 is secreted as a zymogen and is activated by trypsin cleavage. Optimal enzymatic activity requires a basic pH (8–9) and the presence of bile salts, collectively consistent with activity in the proximal small intestine [54,55]. In the small intestine, phospholipids in the form of phosphatidylcholine (PC) are mixed in micelles with cholesterol and bile salts. Pancreatic phospholipase functions to release lysophosphatidylcholine (LPC) and FAs from intestinal PC [54]. Pancreatic PLA_2 acts on PC to release FA and LPC.

Most dietary cholesterol is in the form of free sterol, with a minority in ester form. Cholesterol is absorbed in the free form, and cholesterol esters must be hydrolyzed before absorption. Cholesterol esterase, also known as carboxylic ester hydrolase or sterol ester hydrolase, is the primary enzyme responsible for the hydrolysis of cholesterol esters. Cholesterol esterase is a 100-kD protein produced by the pancreas. The catalytic activity of cholesterol esterase depends on a serine at position 194, aspartic acid at position 320, and a histidine at position 452 [56–58]. In addition to acting on cholesterol esters, cholesterol esterase has broad activity and is capable of hydrolyzing TGs and phosphoglycerides. Cholesterol esterase function is dependent on the presence of bile salts containing 3a, 7a-hydrosy groups, such as cholate and chenodeoxycholate, which stabilize the active site of the enzyme [59,60]. Cholesterol esterase is also unique in its ability to polymerize in the presence of trihydroxy bile salts, which protects cholesterol esterase from proteolytic inactivation. The action of cholesterol esterase on cholesterol esters produces a free sterol and free FA [54,55].

Absorption of carbohydrates, proteins, and lipids

Absorption of carbohydrates

There are two components of carbohydrate absorption. First, they must be transported from the intestinal lumen into enterocytes. Second, they are transported from the enterocyte into the portal circulation. Glucose, galactose, and fructose are the primary products of carbohydrate digestion, and all of these monosaccharides must be actively transported into enterocytes before transfer into the portal circulation and systemic distribution. Glucose and galactose are transported across the apical membrane by the Na^+-dependent cotransporter sodium-glucose-linked transporter 1 (SGLT1) (Figure 21.5). Movement across the basolateral enterocyte membrane into the portal circulation is by facilitative diffusion mediated by glucose transporter type 2 (GLUT2). SGLT1 is expressed on the apical surface of enterocytes as a tetramer with 14 transmembrane domains. There is an electrochemical gradient across the enterocyte that is maintained by the Na^+,K^+-ATPase pump [61]. The SGLT1 uses this gradient to cotransport monosaccharides (glucose, galactose) and sodium in a 1:2 ratio [62]. SGLT1 also has a major role in the absorption of luminal water. Each monosaccharide molecule is transported with ~264 molecules of water, resulting in the net absorption of 5–6 L of water per day, and thus the rationale for adding glucose to oral rehydration solutions [63]. The physiological importance of SGLT1 in vivo has been demonstrated in families with disorders of glucose transport. These autosomal recessive disorders are due to mutations in *SGLT1* resulting in a nonfunctional protein and severe glucose-galactose malabsorption. Affected individuals present as neonates with life-threatening acidic diarrhea with dehydration on ingestion of breast milk or standard infant formula. Congenital SGLT1 deficiency can be treated with avoidance and substitution of glucose and galactose with fructose [64,65]. The new medication mizagliflozin is an inhibitor of SGLT1, and it is being developed for the treatment of chronic constipation [66].

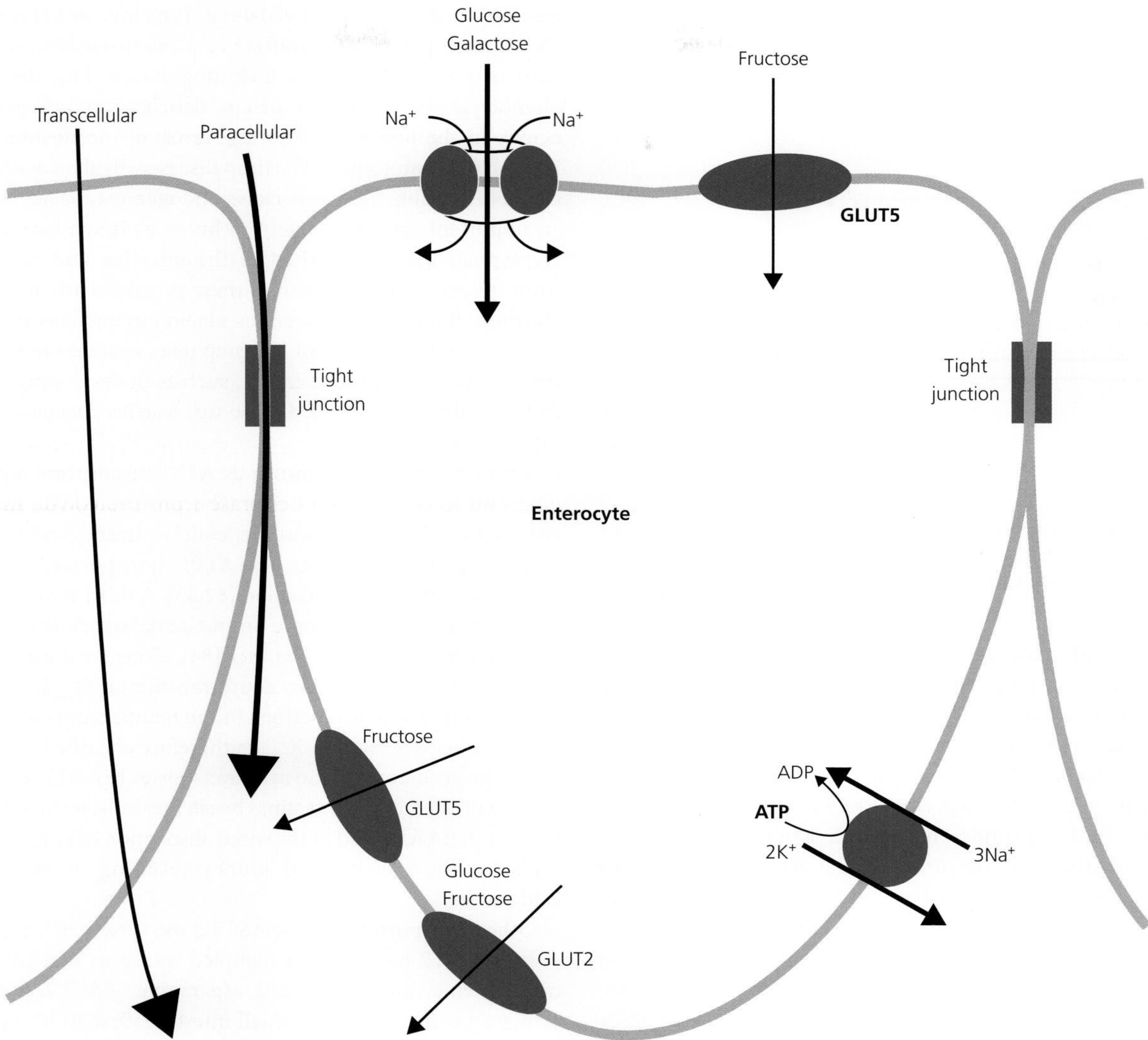

Figure 21.5 Transport processes in the enterocyte responsible for the movement of monosaccharides across the intestinal epithelium. Studies in some animals suggest that glucose transporter type 2 (GLUT2) may also exist in the apical membrane when luminal glucose levels are high.

Once inside the enterocyte, glucose and galactose must be transported into the portal circulation, which is accomplished by GLUT2. GLUT2 is expressed as a transmembrane protein with 12 membrane spanning domains on the basolateral membrane of the enterocyte and mediates Na^+-independent transport of monosaccharides via facilitative diffusion [67]. GLUT2 has an especially high affinity for glucose, and it can be recruited to the apical enterocyte membrane under conditions of high luminal glucose and fructose to aid in glucose absorption [67]. GLUT2 deficiency is due to mutations in *SLC2A2*, which is the gene encoding GLUT2. Patients present as neonates with hepatomegaly as a result of glycogen accumulation and characteristic tubular nephropathy, glucosuria, phosphaturia, bicarbonate wasting, and generalized amino aciduria resulting in rickets with impaired postprandial glucose regulation [68]. There is considerable phenotypic overlap with glycogen storage disease and unfortunately, there is no specific directed therapy.

Fructose is primarily transported across the apical membrane of the enterocyte by the GLUT5 transporter, which preferentially transports fructose (see Figure 21.5). GLUT5 is primarily expressed in the small intestine, kidney, testis, adipose tissue, and skeletal muscle [69]. Luminal fructose both induces expression of GLUT5, owing to the presence of a sugar response element in the *GLUT5* promoter, and stabilizes GLUT5 mRNA [70]. Although GLUT5 is the predominant fructose transporter, GLUT2 can transport excess fructose. In addition to mediating apical membrane transport, GLUT5 is expressed on the basolateral membrane, suggesting it also mediates fructose transport from the enterocyte into the portal circulation [71]. Fructose is slightly less well absorbed than glucose – absorption is 80% that of glucose in adults. In children, where fructose transport capacity may not be fully developed, excess fructose ingestion, in the form of juices, can result in carbohydrate intolerance, resulting in diarrhea, intestinal gas, and abdominal pain [72–74].

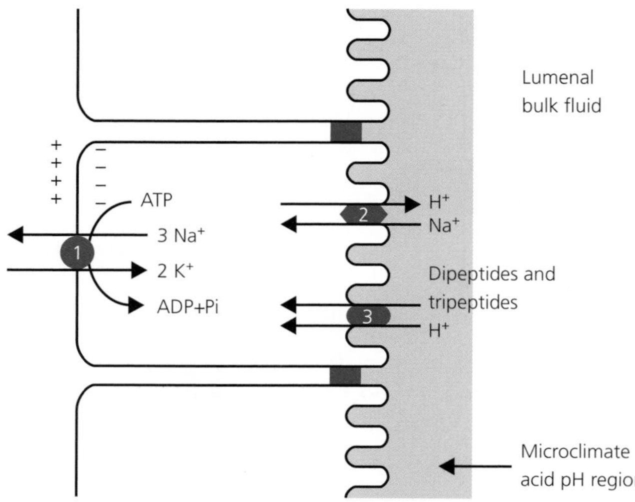

Figure 21.6 Generation of an electrochemical proton gradient across the intestinal brush border membrane. 1, Na^+,K^+-ATPase; 2, Na^+/H^+ exchanger; 3, H^+/peptide cotransporter.

Absorption of proteins

Carbohydrates must be degraded into constituent monosaccharides before transport. In contrast, proteins may be transported as dipeptides and tripeptides and free amino acids. Moreover, amino acid transporters can transport entire classes of amino acids. The peptide transporter PEPT1 (PepT1) transports dipeptides and tripeptides of neutral, anionic, and cationic amino acids (but not free amino acids) across the enterocyte brush border [75,76]. PepT1 is a 79-kD protein with 12 transmembrane domains that is primarily expressed in the duodenum, jejunum, and ileum with lower expression in the colon [77]. The intestinal brush border has an acidic microenvironment that is maintained by a Na^+/H^+ exchanger on the apical surface and a Na^+,K^+-ATPase in the basolateral membrane [78] (Figure 21.6). PepT1 couples peptide transport with the H^+ gradient across the apical membrane of enterocytes [75,76]. Interestingly, there is a net transfer of one positive charge into the enterocyte from the hydrogen ion regardless of the net charge on the transported peptide.

Free amino acids are transported by amino acid transport systems. Broadly speaking, amino acid transport systems exhibit variable substrate specificity and typically use a Na^+ gradient. Neutral amino acids are transported primarily via the Na^+-dependent system B^0, which is primarily expressed in intestinal and renal epithelial cells [79,80]. The transport protein for system B^0 is termed B^0AT1 and is expressed on the apical membrane of enterocytes [80]. Mutations in the gene *SLC6A19*, which encodes B^0AT1, result in Hartnup disease. These mutations are generally loss of function and produce defective B^0AT1 with concomitant impaired renal reabsorption and urinary hyperexcretion of neutral amino acids [79]. The neutral amino acids affected in Hartnup disease include alanine, serine, cysteine, threonine, glutamine, asparagine, valine, isoleucine, leucine, methionine, phenylalanine, tyrosine, and tryptophan. The disease primarily manifests as a photosensitive skin rash with neurological features, including ataxia. This disorder is phenotypically similar to niacin deficiency ("pellagra") but occurs in the presence of normal levels of niacin intake [81]. Indeed, the symptoms of Hartnup disease will abate with niacin supplementation. This is because endogenous niacin, which is an important source of niacin in humans, is synthesized from tryptophan that is absorbed in the intestine and reabsorbed from the renal tubules. Both of these processes are impaired in Hartnup disease, and exogenous niacin circumvents this problem. The manifestations of Hartnup disease are more profound with poor dietary protein intake, such as in developing nations. In this setting, untreated disease can lead to permanent intellectual disability.

Another transporter, known as $ATB^{0,+}$, transports both cationic and neutral amino acids. The protein $ATB^{0,+}$, which is encoded on the X chromosome, couples amino acid transport with Na^+ and Cl^- transport. The $ATB^{0,+}$ transporter is primarily expressed in the ileum and colon [82,83]. A third system, termed $X-_{AG}$, transports the anionic amino acids aspartate and glutamate in a Na^+-dependent manner [84]. Consistent with the role of glutamate as an excitatory neurotransmitter, X^-_{AG} is expressed in the brain, where it functions in the neural reuptake of glutamate at synapses. System X^-_{AG} is therefore classified as a member of the excitatory amino acid transporter (EAAT) family. The form expressed in the intestinal brush border is termed EAAT3. Defects in EAAT3 lead to impaired absorption of anionic amino acids in the intestine and kidney resulting in dicarboxylic aciduria [85].

Other transporters include ASCT2 and system $b^{0,+}$. The transporter ASCT2 mediates Na^+-coupled transport of alanine, serine, cysteine, glutamine, and asparagine. ASCT2 protein is primarily expressed in the small intestine. System $b^{0,+}$ is a Na^+-independent, high-affinity transporter of neutral and cationic amino acids, as well as the disulfide-linked amino acid, cysteine [83]. This transporter is a heterodimer composed of a light chain ($b^{0,+}$AT) and a heavy chain (rBAT). The light chain contains a transmembrane domain typical of transport proteins, while the heavy chain recruits the light chain to the apical border of the enterocyte. Defects in this transporter result in impaired transport of cationic amino acids and the disorder cystinuria.

Cystinuria is characterized by increased excretion of the cationic amino acids lysine, arginine, and cysteine [86]. Patients with cystinuria have impaired intestinal and renal tubular absorption of cationic amino acids [87]. Cysteine is poorly water soluble and must be reabsorbed by the renal epithelial cells to prevent precipitation in the renal tubules. Patients with cystinuria have impaired renal tubular reabsorption of cysteine and form cysteine stones when urinary concentrations of cysteine are high (>300 mg/L) [87]. System $b^{0,+}$ is composed of a light ($b^{0,+}$AT) and a heavy chain (rBAT), and cystinuria may result from mutations in either chain. The light and heavy chains are encoded on chromosomes 19 and 2, respectively. Cystinuria is transmitted in an autosomal recessive manner and can result from mutations in two genes (light or heavy chain) [88]. Treatment is directed at enhancing cysteine excretion by increasing urine volume or enhancing cysteine solubility by either alkalinizing the urine or using penicillamine.

Lysinuric protein intolerance is an autosomal recessive disorder due to impaired absorption of the cationic amino acids lysine, arginine, and ornithine in the intestine and kidney [89]. Patients with lysinuric protein intolerance exhibit increased urinary excretion with reduced serum levels of these amino acids. Arginine and lysine are essential amino acids that are necessary for protein synthesis. Arginine and ornithine are involved in the urea cycle and ammonia elimination. Thus, the major clinical manifestations are growth retardation, neurological complications, and hyperammonemia caused by impaired protein synthesis and ammonia excretion [89]. Dietary protein induces diarrhea and vomiting and can result in coma. Dietary protein restriction and ornithine supplementation are the treatments of choice. This disease is distinct from cystinuria, which also involves a defect in the absorption of cationic amino acids. The transport defect in lysinuric protein intolerance is restricted to the basolateral membrane in intestinal and renal epithelial cells, whereas transport across the brush border is not affected [89]. Lysinuric protein intolerance is caused by defects in isoforms of the amino acid transport system $y^{+}L$, which is composed of a heavy and light chain. Loss-of-function mutations in the light chain $y^{+}LAT1$ are thought to be causative, because mutations have been identified in affected patients [90,91].

Regulation of peptide absorption

Protein transport and absorption can be affected by targeted mechanisms impacting the expression and activity of transporters. Furthermore, as discussed in the next section, intestinal disorders can secondarily lead to nonspecific impairments in protein absorption.

Targeted regulatory mechanisms include alterations in the number and activity of the transporters themselves. Hormones can also regulate the activity of peptide transporters. Somatostatin and vasoactive intestinal polypeptide are negative regulators of transporter activity, whereas epidermal growth factor, neurotensin, cholecystokinin, and secretin all enhance transporter activity. Furthermore, in vitro data demonstrate that peptide transporters are stimulated by insulin, leptin, and growth hormone and are inhibited by thyroid hormones, protein kinase C, and cyclic adenosine monophosphate (cAMP) [92–94].

Peptide transporter expression can also be altered, thus serving as another mode of regulation. Animal studies have demonstrated that changes in dietary protein content, as well as in the intraluminal concentration of the products of protein digestion, impact peptide transporter expression [95]. Although peptide transporters are constitutively expressed along the length of the small intestine, there may be regional changes in the expression pattern that are subject to regulation. A high-protein diet not only increases transporter transcripts (mRNA) but also enhances the activity of small-intestinal peptidases (dipeptidylcarboxypeptidase and dipeptidylaminopeptidase IV) [95].

Peptide transporter expression may be altered in a number of clinical scenarios. Although, in health, the expression of peptide transporters is low in the colon, this can be upregulated in disorders that alter the absorptive surface area of the small intestine. Thus, enhanced colonic peptide transporter expression has been documented in the short gut syndrome and Crohn's disease [96]. In these circumstances, the upregulation of peptide transporters in the colon can be seen as adaptive responses that aim to preserve protein absorption. Enhanced colonic expression of peptide transporters has also been described in ulcerative colitis.

Secondary defects in protein absorption

A variety of diseases, including celiac disease, dermatitis herpetiformis, tropical sprue, and cystic fibrosis, can all result in secondary impairments of protein digestion and absorption. Cystic fibrosis is caused by defects in the cystic fibrosis transmembrane conductance regulator (CFTR) protein, which is a cAMP-regulated Cl^- channel. Defects in the Cl^- channel result in impaired secretion of salt and water into the pancreatic ducts, leading to retention of digestive enzymes in the pancreas. This ultimately results in destruction of pancreatic tissue and exocrine pancreatic insufficiency with impaired digestion of protein and fate.

In celiac disease, immune-mediated inflammation leads to the characteristic histological findings, which include villous blunting, increased intraepithelial lymphocytes, and villous flattening. Collectively, these structural defects result in a reduction in the absorptive surface of the intestine, which ultimately affects protein absorption. Dermatitis herpetiformis is related to celiac disease in being induced by gluten and is distinguished by the presence of pruritic bullous rashes. Intestinal involvement is generally milder compared with celiac disease but can result in protein malabsorption. Treatment for both celiac disease and dermatitis herpetiformis consists of dietary gluten avoidance.

Tropical sprue (also known as environmental enteropathy) is a gastrointestinal disease characterized by broad impairments of digestive and absorptive intestinal function. The disease has an unknown etiology but is thought to be infectious. It primarily occurs among residents of tropical regions.

Absorption of lipids

Lipids are generally hydrophobic, and long-chain FAs and MG, which have long hydrophobic tails, are particularly insoluble in water, which poses a major problem because they will need to traverse an aqueous medium. This problem must be overcome for FAs and MG to be absorbed across the apical membrane of the brush border. Micellar solubilization enhances the concentration of FAs and MG in an aqueous medium, thereby greatly increasing the number of molecules available for enterocyte

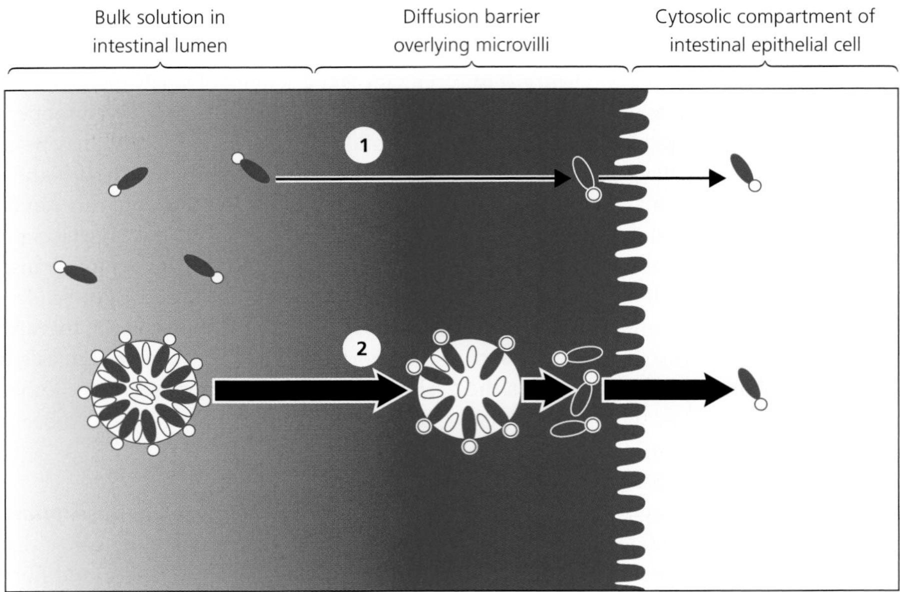

Figure 21.7 The effect of bile salt micelles (or vesicles) in overcoming the diffusion barrier resistance presented by the unstirred water layer. In the absence of bile acids, individual lipid molecules must diffuse across the barriers overlying the microvillus border of the intestinal epithelial cells (arrow 1). Hence uptake of these molecules is largely diffusion limited. In the presence of bile acids (arrow 2), large amounts of these lipid molecules are delivered directly to the aqueous–membrane interface so that the rate of uptake is greatly enhanced. Source: Westergaard and Dietschy 1976. [175]. Reproduced with permission of the American Society of Clinical Investigation.

uptake [97] (Figure 21.7). Solubilized FAs and MG can then be transported across the brush border as monomers by simple diffusion [52]. However, recent data also suggest roles for carrier-mediated transport systems [98].

A number of lipid binding proteins have been identified, including GP330, CD36, and caveolin [52,99]. However, whether they facilitate gastrointestinal uptake of fats, lipids, and cholesterols in vivo in humans has not been definitively proved. GP330, also called megalin, is a member of the low-density lipoprotein receptor gene family. It is an endocytic receptor that is primarily expressed in epithelial cells, including the proximal tubules of the kidneys, type II pneumocytes, mammary epithelium, and thyroid follicular cells [100]. Whether GP330 is expressed in the intestine or is involved in small-intestinal cholesterol uptake remains unknown. GP330-deficient animal models exhibit impaired forebrain development, which is thought to be due to impaired cholesterol supply [101].

Other well-characterized FA transporters include CD36, plasma membrane-associated FA-binding protein (FABPpm), and the FA-binding transport protein family (FATP1–6). CD36 is an 88-kD transmembrane protein that binds to multiple ligands, including FAs and lipoproteins [102]. CD36 expression is upregulated by dietary fat, as well as being upregulated in obesity and diabetes mellitus. It is widely expressed in muscle, the vascular endothelium, and adipose tissue in addition to the intestine [103]. The highest levels of expression of CD36 are found in duodenal and jejunal villi with very low expression in the ileum and colon [104]. Polymorphisms in CD36 in humans have been associated with obesity, metabolic syndrome, and elevated low-density lipoprotein cholesterol levels. These patients have impaired peripheral uptake of FAs that is thought to partially contribute to the abnormal lipid levels [105]. They also have impaired intestinal FA uptake.

FATP4 may also be an intestinal FA transporter. FATP4 is highly expressed in jejunal enterocytes and possesses endogenous acyl coenzyme A (CoA) synthetase (ACS) activity [106]. ACS activity allows it to convert trapped long-chain FAs to fatty acyl CoA, which is converted into other intracellular lipids [107]. ACS activity also enhances the diffusion gradient for luminal FAs from the intestinal lumen into enterocytes. FATP4 may be partially inducible because animals fed a high-fat diet have increased expression compared with those on a low-fat diet.

In contrast with FAs, carrier-mediated transport is important for cholesterol absorption. Mutations in the transporters ABCG5 and ABCG8 cause sitosterolemia, characterized by cholesterol deposition in peripheral tissues as a result of increased intestinal absorption and decreased biliary clearance of plant sterols [108]. These heterodimeric apical membrane transporters function as efflux pumps for cholesterol and plant sterols. Interestingly, there is an inverse relationship between the expression of ABCG5 and ABCG8 and cholesterol transport in the jejunum and ileum, but not in the duodenum. Niemann–Pick C1-like 1 (NPC1L1) protein, encoded by the gene *Npc1l1*, is another recently discovered cholesterol transporter [109,110]. In mice, *Npc1l1* is primarily expressed in the small intestine with maximal expression in the jejunum. The NPC1L1 transporter mediates cholesterol transport via vesicular endocytosis [109,110].

Bile acids are critical to the digestion and absorption of lipids because they form micelles, which facilitate the solubilization of lipids [97]. Conjugated bile salts form small-diameter (3-nm) simple micelles. FAs, MGs, and phospholipids are readily soluble in simple micelles to form mixed micelles. Mixed micelles are larger than simple micelles and have a variable size depending on the mix of bile acids and phospholipids. In contrast with simple micelles, mixed micelles can solubilize cholesterol. Mixed micelles also form when bile acids combine with fat-soluble vitamins, DGs, and triacylglycerols. Mixed micelles enhance lipid digestion by facilitating the interaction of pancreatic lipase with FAs [97]. Mixed micelles are critical in lipid absorption because they transport lipids, which are relatively insoluble in water, across the unstirred water layer of the brush border into the apical surface of the enterocyte.

Nutrient sensing

Control of metabolism at a molecular level is fundamental to cellular homeostasis. This process, termed *nutrient sensing*, regulates cellular energy expenditure in a nutrient-dependent manner to balance anabolic and catabolic processes with nutrient availability. Sensing of nutrients can be direct or indirect via surrogate molecules. Regardless of the mode of detection, proteins are considered "sensors" if they detect nutrients or their surrogates in situ within physiological concentration ranges.

In general, nutrient sensing encompasses sensing of lipids and sterols, glucose, cellular energy, and amino acids (among others). Nutrient sensing converges on key transcription factors that are fundamental to cellular survival. These transcription factors effectively act as nodes integrating multiple upstream stress responses and executing multiple downstream responses. It is critical to understand that these nodal transcription factors are not acting in vacuo, but rather are interacting to achieve a balance.

Nutrient sensing and downstream signaling encompass broad processes that are overlapping but nonredundant. These responses are likely to be tissue and cell specific to meet local needs. In this section, we focus on three key and well-described processes: (1) sensing of cellular energy by 5′ adenosine monophosphate-activated protein kinase (AMPK), (2) sensing of amino acids by general amino acid control nonderepressible 2 (GCN2), and (3) regulating cellular energy and metabolic state by the transcription factor mammalian target of rapamycin (mTOR).

AMPK

AMPK is a highly conserved serine/threonine kinase that functions as an intracellular energy sensor. AMPK is activated when energy levels are low, and it functions to conserve energy by initiating adenosine triphosphate (ATP)-generating catabolic processes and inhibiting anabolic ATP-requiring processes [111,112]. High cellular energy is characterized by an abundance of ATP with a low AMP/ATP ratio (~1:10). In contrast, AMP and adenosine diphosphate (ADP) are relatively more abundant when intracellular energy stores are depleted. AMPK is a heterotrimer composed of a catalytic α subunit and regulatory β and γ subunits, constructed in a manner that facilitates its activation in low-energy states (high AMP/ATP ratio) and inhibition in high-energy states (high ATP) [113]. The α subunit contains the kinase domain in the N terminus and is responsible for the phosphorylation of target proteins. The β subunit contains a carbohydrate-binding module that mediates association with glycogen. The γ subunit contains four cystathionine β-synthase motifs that play key roles in the activation of AMPK [114]. Although all four cystathionine β-synthase motifs can theoretically bind adenosine nucleotides, site 2 lacks a key aspartate residue, rendering it nonfunctional (site 2). Site 4 can bind either AMP or ATP but has higher affinity for AMP and constitutively binds it. The remaining sites (sites 1 and 3) provide the energy-sensing component by competitively binding AMP, ADP, or ATP (Figure 21.8).

In high-energy states, ATP binds to sites 1 and 3. In contrast, the concentration of AMP (or ADP) rises with increasing cellular energy stress. This results in sequential binding of AMP or ADP to sites 1 and 3 [113]. Binding of AMP to these sites on AMPK promotes the phosphorylation of a conserved threonine residue (Thr172) that is required for AMPK activation. AMP binding also prevents the dephosphorylation of this Thr172 residue and causes an additional allosteric activation. Thus, AMP results in a trifold activation of AMPK: (1) through

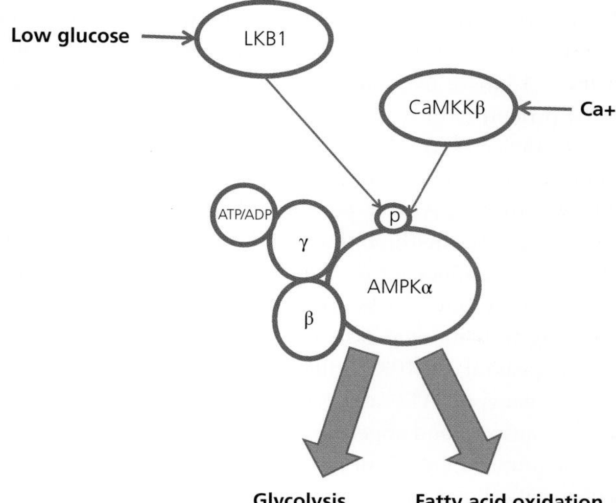

Figure 21.8 The 5′ adenosine monophosphate-activated protein kinase (AMPK) pathway. The heterotrimeric kinase AMPK senses low-energy states and the proteins liver kinase B1 (LKB1) and CAMKK2 to activate adaptive processes resulting in regeneration of intracellular adenosine triphosphate (ATP). Source: Mihaylova and Shaw 2011 [176]. Reproduced with permission of Macmillan Publishers Ltd.

facilitating phosphorylation of Thr172, (2) through preventing dephosphorylation of Thr172, and (3) in causing allosteric activation of AMPK [115]. Collectively, this results in a greater than 100-fold increase in AMPK activity (at least in vitro) [111,116–118]. Moreover, there are multiple isoforms of AMPK because humans express genes encoding two isoforms of the α (α1, α2), two of the β (β1, β2), and three of the γ subunit (γ1, γ2, γ3) [111]. This leads to 12 potential combinations of the AMPK protein, each with differing degrees of activation.

The liver kinase B1 (LKB1) and Ca^{2+}/calmodulin-activated protein kinases (CaMKKβ) are the major kinases that phosphorylate Thr172, the key event in activating AMPK. LKB1 is a heterotrimer composed of LKB1 with the proteins STRAD (STE-20 related kinase binding protein) and MO25 (calcium binding protein 39) [119–121]. Murine experiments indicate that LKB1 is the major kinase that regulates activation of AMKP in response to energy stress in most tissues [119]. Similarly, CaMKKβ phosphorylates Thr172 as a result of increases in intracellular Ca^{2+} independent of LKB1 or nucleotide levels. Thus, CaMKKβ is thought to mediate activation of AMPK downstream of hormones and cellular stressors that increase intracellular calcium [120]. Interestingly, *LKB1*, also called *STK11*, is a tumor suppressor gene that is mutated in many lung and cervical cancers and in Peutz–Jeghers syndrome.

Canonical AMPK activation occurs in response to energy stress with subsequent alterations in nucleotides or in intracellular Ca^{2+}. In addition, AMPK may also be activated by drugs and xenobiotics, including metformin, resveratrol, epigallocatechin gallate (found in green tea), capsaicin, curcumin, and garlic [111,112]. AMPK can also be activated in vitro by reactive oxygen species and hydrogen peroxide via poorly understood mechanisms [122]. DNA damage by chemotherapeutic agents, including etoposide, doxorubicin, and ionizing radiation, also appear to activate AMPK via the cytoplasmic form of phosphoinositide 3-kinase-like kinase ataxia telangiectasia mutated (ATM) protein (which is the product of the gene mutated in ataxia telangiectasia). This DNA damage-dependent activation of AMPK is ATM dependent but LBK1 independent [123].

Once activated, AMPK phosphorylates target substrates at characteristic serine/threonine residues that are flanked by hydrophobic residues at the −5 and +4 positions and basic residues at the −4 and −3 positions, with the best substrates also possessing an additional basic residue at the −6 position [124]. Broadly speaking, AMPK regulates catabolic and anabolic processes to generate ATP and regulates whole-body energy via glucose transport and appetite. In addition, AMPK also signals to the mammalian target of rapamycin complex, itself a master regulator of cellular energy utilization and state.

Regulation of catabolic and anabolic processes by AMPK

Two important and model ATP-generating catabolic pathways regulated by AMPK are glycolysis and FA oxidation. AMPK activates glycolysis by sequentially enhancing glucose uptake followed by activating glycolytic pathways. AMPK promotes intracellular glucose uptake by increasing plasma membrane localization of GLUT1 and GLUT4 (discussed in detail in the following sections). AMPK then activates glycolytic pathways by phosphorylating the enzyme 6-phosphofructo-2-kinase/fructose-2,6-bisphosphatase (PFKFB), leading to the generation of fructose-2,6-bisphosphate. AMPK phosphorylates the PFKFB2 and PFKFB3 isoforms of PFKFB and, therefore, activates these pathways only in tissues that express these isoforms [125]. PFKFB is an important allosteric activator of 6-phosphofructo-1-kinase (PFK1), which is the rate-limiting enzyme in glycolysis.

Analogous to promoting glycolytic pathways, AMPK promotes FA oxidation by first enhancing cellular uptake and then oxidative pathways. AMPK promotes FA uptake, particularly in cardiac myocytes, by enhancing translocation of the FA transporter CD36 from the cytoplasm into the cell membrane [126]. AMPK then promotes FA β-oxidation by enhancing mitochondrial FA transport, which is the rate-limiting step of β-oxidation. This is due to AMPK-mediated inactivation of acetyl-CoA carboxylase (ACC) β via phosphorylation, leading to decreases in malonyl-CoA [112,117]. This has the collective effect of enhancing FA transport because malonyl-CoA is an inhibitor of FA transport into mitochondria.

AMPK conserves ATP by inhibiting anabolic processes, including synthesis of lipids, carbohydrates, proteins, and ribosomal RNA (rRNA). Similar to the role of the regulatory motif of AMPK in controlling catabolic processes, regulation of the anabolic process occurs via AMPK-dependent phosphorylation of key enzymes. AMPK acts to phosphorylate or regulate enzymes involved in FA synthesis (ACC1), TG and phospholipid synthesis (glycerol phosphate acyl-transferase), cholesterol synthesis (3-hydroxy-3-methylglutaryl CoA reductase), glycogen synthesis (glycogen synthase), and rRNA synthesis (transcription initiation factor IA). In addition, AMPK also signals to the mTOR complex (mTORC) via the intermediary molecules tuberous sclerosis 2 (TSC2) and regulatory-associated protein of mTOR (RAPTOR) [111,112,116,117,127].

Regulation of glucose uptake and appetite by AMPK

Muscle tissues take up glucose during contraction via GLUT4. Intracellular glucose is then converted into ATP; thus, muscle uptake of glucose is considered a catabolic process. AMPK promotes this conversion of glucose to ATP in active muscle cells by enhancing the translocation of GLUT4 from cytoplasmic vesicles into the plasma membrane, which facilitates glucose uptake. AMPK mediates this translocation by phosphorylating and thus inactivating the protein TBC1 domain family member 1 (TBC1D1) [128]. TBC1D functions to inhibit the fusion of GLUT4-containing vesicles with the cell membrane, thus effectively acting as a negative regulator of GLUT4. Phosphorylation of TBC1D1 by AMPK identifies TBC1D1 as a target of the 14-3-3 family of regulatory proteins, ultimately leading to degradation of TBC1D1 [128]. Thus, AMPK positively regulates glucose uptake by muscle by promoting the degradation of a negative regulator of glucose transport (TBC1D1).

In addition to these effects, AMPK may enhance total body glucose uptake. The ventromedial hypothalamus reportedly senses low blood glucose levels with resultant AMPK-dependent release of adrenaline and glucagon [129]. These hormones then stimulate gluconeogenesis in the liver, which increases serum glucose. Data from in vitro experiments indicate that hormones that promote feeding, such as ghrelin and adiponectin, as well as cannabinoids, activate AMPK, whereas those that inhibit feeding, such as leptin, inhibit AMPK (α2 i3soform). There is also evidence that these effects are mediated in presynaptic neurons through release of intracellular calcium with subsequent AMPK activation via CaMKKβ [111,112,116,117].

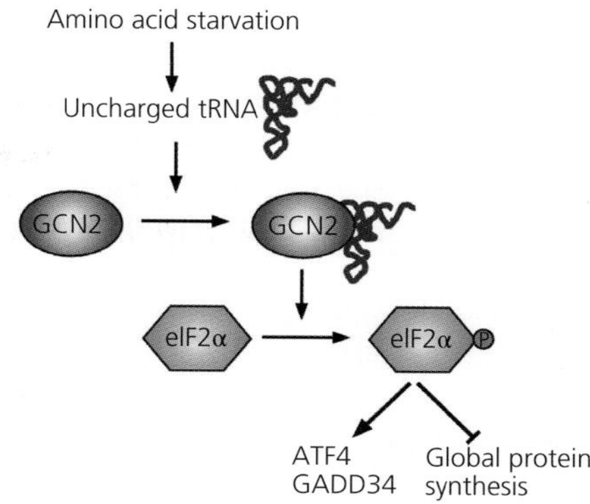

Figure 21.9 General amino acid control nonderepressible 2 (GCN2) and the amino acid response. GCN2 is an α subunit of eukaryotic initiation factor 2 (eIF2α) kinase that is activated on binding to uncharged transfer RNA, which accrues in states of amino acid starvation. Phosphorylation of eIF2α by activated GCN2 inhibits global protein translation while selectively increasing translation of activating transcription factor 4 (ATF4) and growth arrest and DNA damage-inducible 34 (GADD34) to mediate adaptive responses to amino acid starvation. Source: Towle 2007 [177]. Reproduced with permission of Elsevier.

Sensing of amino acids and the GCN2/ATF4 pathway

Amino acids are biologically critical molecules with pleiotropic roles in vivo, including acting as the building blocks of proteins and functioning as neurotransmitters and hormones and as sources of cellular energy. In general, amino acid deficiencies are contextual. This is because the absence of one amino acid, even with an abundance of all others, still represents a deficiency state that impedes biological processes. The detection and regulation of amino acids and proteins at both cellular and organismal levels is thus essential for life. Nine amino acids are considered essential in humans, meaning that our cellular synthetic machinery cannot endogenously generate them. All organisms have developed signal transduction cascades that recognize protein and amino acid deprivation and function as global transcriptional and translational regulators. Molecular sensors of nitrogen in bacteria and plants are the most basic forms of amino acid sensing. In mammals and humans, sensing of amino acid and protein deprivation is housed under several pathways alternatively termed the amino acid response (AAR), the unfolded protein response (UPR), and the integrated stress response (ISR). These pathways have similar but nonredundant functions and, broadly speaking, are active in different tissues, cells, and cellular organs. The AAR, UPR, and ISR also include a vast array of signal transduction pathways. Given the broad nature of this topic, we will focus here on two well-characterized pathways: the GCN2 and the activating transcription factor 4 (ATF4) cascades [130,131] (Figure 21.9).

Protein synthesis is initiated when mRNA transcripts are translated into proteins in ribosomes, a process that requires conjugation of mRNA with amino acid-bound transfer RNA (tRNA). tRNA thus provides the physical link between the genetic message and individual amino acids. Protein and amino acid deprivation manifests as tRNA that is not bound to amino acids, which is termed *uncharged tRNA*. The first step in translation involves binding of the small ribosomal subunit (40S) with the methionine tRNA (met-tRNA) that serves as the initiator tRNA. Importantly, all eukaryotic translation is initiated by the met-tRNA [132]. The complex composed of the 40S ribosomal subunit, met-tRNA, and associated binding proteins is termed the 43S ribosomal preinitiation complex (PIC). The PIC then scans mRNA transcripts beginning from the 5′ cap to the 3′ tail screening for the initiation codon (AUG), which begins protein synthesis [132]. The eukaryotic initiation factor (eIF) family of proteins performs critical functions along the various stages of protein translation, as well as rRNA, tRNA, and mRNA interactions [132–134]. Of these, the eIF2 protein functions to bring the initiator met-tRNA to the peptidyl binding (p site) on the 40S ribosomal subunit (see Figure 21.9). An important regulatory component of this complex is the protein eIF2B, which is a guanine nucleotide exchange factor that is necessary for continued activity of eIF2 (discussed in detail later) [132–134].

GCN2 is a kinase that senses amino acid deprivation by detecting uncharged tRNA, and subsequently activates proteins that suppress transcription and translation [135]. The kinase activity of GCN2 is initiated on binding of the GCN2 protein with uncharged tRNA and functions to phosphorylate the α subunit of eIF2 (eIF2α) [136]. As noted earlier, eIF2 brings the initiator met-tRNA into the 40S complex and is necessary for assembly of the PIC. The protein eIF2 is a guanine triphosphate (GTP) binding protein that hydrolyzes GTP to guanine diphosphate (GDP) on deposition of the initiator met-tRNA at the P-site of the 40S ribosomal subunit. The hydrolysis of GTP to GDP also activates additional eIFs and provides the signal to begin the elongation phase of translation. Although GTP-GDP hydrolysis by eIF2 is necessary, eIF2-GDP does not bind met-tRNA, and translation is repressed unless eIF2-GTP is (re)generated by the guanine exchange factor eIF2B [137]. eIF2 is a heterotrimeric protein composed of α, β, and γ subunits [132]. When the α subunit is phosphorylated by GCN2, eIF2α functions as an inhibitor of eIF2B, and translation is repressed.

Activated GCN2 functions as a negative regulator of translation by phosphorylating eIF2α, thus conserving amino acids and proteins in times of deprivation. However, although GCN2 globally suppresses translation, it, paradoxically, increases translation of selected mRNAs. In particular, translation of mRNAs for the ATF4 and ATF5 transcription factors is increased. In addition, the protein growth arrest and DNA damage-inducible 34 (GADD34) is also induced (*PP1R15A*, the gene encoding GADD34, is a target of ATF4) [138]. ATF4 mRNA contains two upstream open reading frames (uORFs; uORF1 and 2). In the basal state, both uORFs are translated, which suppresses synthesis of the ATF4 protein because the uORF2 is frameshifted. In the stressed state, however, GCN2-mediated suppression of translation results in the bypassing of uORF2 by the ribosome, resulting in synthesis of ATF4 [139]. ATF4 is a basic leucine zipper transcription factor that globally functions to increase transcription and responds to the stressed state; a response that includes reactivation of translation (via GADD34) [140]. ATF4 enhances transcription by binding to the CCAAT/enhancer binding protein-ATF4 (C/EBP-ATF4) response elements (CARE) [140–143]. The gene products of the CARE elements mediate a wide variety of cellular processes and stress responses, including upregulating select amino acid transporters. Thus, amino acid-induced GCN2-mediated activation of ATF4 results in activation of processes that should counteract the deprived state (upregulation of amino acid transporters, reinitiation of translation via GADD34). Should these responses fail, cellular apoptosis will occur.

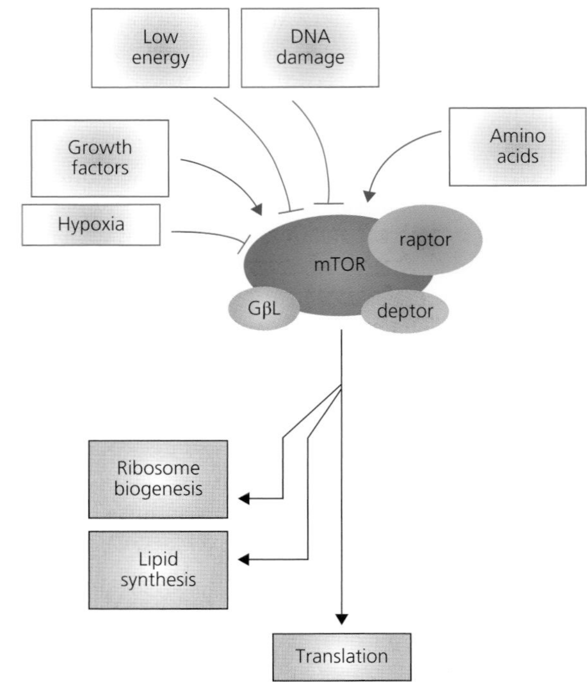

Figure 21.10 Activators of mechanistic target of rapamycin complex 1 (mTORC1). The mTORC1, composed of the serine/threonine kinase mTOR and the proteins raptor, deptor, and GβL (also known as mLST8), is activated by varied inputs, including DNA damage, low energy via 5′ adenosine monophosphate-activated protein kinase (AMPK), amino acids, and growth factors. mTORC1 activation results in enhanced lipid synthesis, translation, and ribosomal biogenesis. Source: Efeyan et al. 2012 [178]. Reproduced with permission of Elsevier.

Global regulation of cellular state and mTOR

The protein mTOR is a serine/threonine kinase that responds to a variety of environmental inputs, including nutrient deprivation and cellular stress, to regulate a broad array of activities that control anabolic and catabolic processes and the cell cycle (Figure 21.10). The importance of the mTOR pathways arises from the central position that mTOR occupies in regulating these processes; indeed, the AMPK and GCN2 pathways that respond to energy and amino acid deprivation both signal to mTOR. The mTOR protein was so named because it was identified as mediating the biologic effects of the macrolide antibiotic rapamycin. Interestingly, rapamycin was originally isolated from the soil of Rapa Nui (Easter Island) as a molecule with potent antifungal and immunosuppressive properties.

In humans, the mTOR kinase, encoded by the gene *MTOR*, exists in two distinct complexes: mTOR complex 1 (mTORC1) and complex 2 (mTORC2) [144–147]. mTORC1 controls many nutrient sensing properties, including the regulation of anabolic and catabolic processes, as well as the synthesis of proteins, lipids, nucleotides, and ribosomes [144–147]. mTORC2 primarily regulates cell survival and cytoskeleton activation; the regulation and function of mTORC2 is relatively poorly understood compared with mTORC1 [145–147]. This section focuses on mTORC1 because it is the primary mTOR complex involved in nutrient sensing. Complex 1 is composed of the mTOR protein, along with the proteins: raptor, target of rapamycin complex subunit LST8 (mLST8), proline-rich AKT1 substrate of 40 kD (PRAS40), and DEP domain-containing mTOR-interaction protein (deptor) [148,149]. The mTORC2 complex shares the proteins mLST8 and deptor but has the specific proteins rapamycin-insensitive companion of mTOR (rictor), mammalian stress-activated map kinase-interaction protein 2 (mSin1), and protein observed with rictor 1 and 2 (protor1/2) [144,150].

The complexity of the mechanisms that control mTORC1 activation is commensurate with the biological importance of this complex in controlling cellular states. Broadly, mTORC1 activation is a two-step process involving: (1) cellular localization of mTORC1, and (2) activation of its kinase function. In the nutrient and growth factor starved state, mTORC1 is inactive in the cytoplasm. However, in the nutrient and growth factor replete state, mTORC1 translocates to the lysozyme membrane where its kinase activity is activated.

Sensing of amino acids by mTORC1

Sensing of lysosomal amino acids by mTORC1

Activation of mTORC1 is complex, and as described in detail later, involves translocation of mTORC1 to the lysosomal membrane. Mammalian lysosomes are involved in autophagy and protein degradation and can store amino acids, suggesting that mTORC1 may sense intralysosomal amino acids [151]. Consistent with this concept, in vitro experiments found that mTORC1 can be recruited to the lysosomal membrane by intralysosomal amino acids. Furthermore, it was also discovered that the lysosomal transmembrane protein SLC38A9, which has homology with amino acid transporters, is a positive regulator of the mTORC1 pathway. SLC38A9 has a unique 119-amino acid extension at its N terminus that binds another lysosomal membrane-bound protein called Ragulator [152–154]. As detailed in later sections, Ragulator is a guanine exchange factor that is involved in sensing of amino acids to mTORC1. Gain-of-function mutations in SLC38A9 confer cells with resistance of mTORC1 to amino acid withdrawal. In contrast, SLC38A9 deficiency causes impaired mTORC1 activation in response to amino acids, especially arginine [152–154]. Consistent with this, SLC38A9 has (low) affinity for arginine and possibly higher affinity for other amino acids in vitro [152–154]. Collectively, this suggests that SLC38A9 is a putative sensor for arginine (and other amino acids) and links mTORC1 to sensing of intralysosomal amino acids [151] (Figure 21.11, right panel).

Sensing of cytosolic amino acids by mTORC1

In addition to sensing lysosomal amino acids, it appears that mTORC1 can sense cytosolic amino acids via the intermediary Sestrin proteins [151] (see Figure 21.11, right panel). As detailed in the next section, the protein Sestrin2 negatively regulates mTORC1 by inhibiting the protein complex GATOR2, which itself is a positive regulator of mTORC1. Under leucine-deficient conditions, Sestrin2 binds GATOR2, thus inhibiting mTORC1 activation [155–157]. However, when leucine is abundant, leucine stimulation causes the disassociation of Sestrin2 from GATOR2, thereby relieving the inhibition of mTORC1. This process appears to be specific because arginine deficiency does not induce the Sestrin2-dependent mTORC1 inhibition [155–157]. Importantly, sensing of cytosolic and lysosomal pathways appears to be entirely distinct [151] (see Figure 21.11).

Activation of mTORC1 by amino acids

Amino acid deprivation is a potent inhibitor of mTORC1 activation and results in the induction of autophagy whose aim is to replete diminished intracellular amino acid stores in the starved state. Amino acids activate mTORC1 by inducing mTORC1 translocation to the lysozyme membrane, a process mediated by the Rag family of guanine triphosphatases (Rag GTPases). The Rag GTPases consist of the molecules Rag A–D, which, on sensing amino acids, bind to cytoplasmic mTORC1 and recruit it to the lysozyme membrane.

The Rag GTPases exist as heterodimers (Rag A or B bound to Rag C or D) that bind GTP or GDP [158]. Of the combinations, the Rag A/B^{GTP}-$RagC/D^{GDP}$ states provide the greatest degree of activation for mTORC1, whereas $RagA/B^{GDP}$-$RagC/D^{GTP}$ are the most suppressive. Amino acids and, in particular, leucine promote formation of the active Rag A/B^{GTP} state. The RagA/B--RagC/D-mTORC1 complex is bound to the lysozyme membrane by the action of the proteins, Ragulator, and vacuolar ATPase (v-ATPase) [159,160]. Ragulator is a guanine exchange factor for Rag A and B, meaning that it promotes the release of GDP to allow GTP binding [160,161]. Rag GTPase function is also

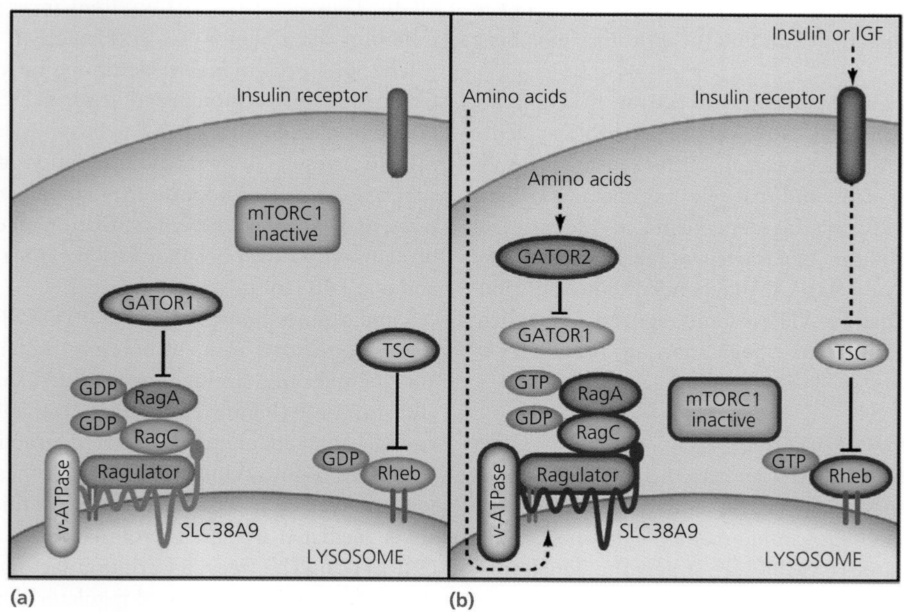

Figure 21.11 Activation and regulation of mechanistic target of rapamycin complex 1 (mTORC1). Inactive mTORC1 is recruited from the membrane to the lysosome by the Rag guanosine triphosphatase (GTPase) proteins when activated by growth factors and amino acids. The mTORC1–Rag complex associates with proteins Rheb, regulator, vacuolar adenosine triphosphatase (v-ATPase), and the amino acid transporter, SLC38A9, on the lysosome membrane. Guanosine triphosphate (GTP)-bound Rheb potentiates the kinase function of mTORC1, while SLC38A9 is thought to mediate amino acid sensing to mTORC1. Source: Chantranupong et al. 2015 [145]. Reproduced with permission of Elsevier.

regulated by two GTPase-activating protein (GAP) complexes, GATOR1 (acts on Rag A/B) and Folliculin-FNIP2 (Rag C/D), which hydrolyze Rag GTPase bound GTP to GDP. Additional layers of complexity are added by the protein complexes GATOR2, which is a negative regulator of GATOR1, and the Sestrins, which function as guanine nucleotide dissociation inhibitors that inhibit amino acid-induced Rag guanine nucleotide exchange [145,147]. Collectively, GATOR1 and Sestrins negatively regulate mTORC1 activation by maintaining the RagA/B complex in GDP-bound states (GATOR1 and Sestrins) and preventing Rag-mTORC1 docking to the lysozyme membrane (Sestrins). Similarly, RAG-ulator (a guanine nucleotide exchange factor inhibitor) and GATOR2 (a GATOR1 inhibitor) positively regulate mTORC1 activation by effectively promoting the formation of RagA/B GTP-bound states.

The second step in the induction of mTORC1 is the activation of the kinase function. The ras homolog enriched in brain (Rheb) GTP binding protein is a lipid membrane-bound GTPase that is active in the GTP-bound and inactive in the GDP-bound state [144,146,147]. Rheb is anchored to the lysozyme membrane, and the GTP-bound form of Rheb ($Rheb^{GTP}$) potently activates the kinase function of mTORC1 [162]. Rheb is regulated by the TSC composed of the proteins TSC1 (hamartin), TSC2 (tuberin), and TBC1D7 (TSC–TBC complex). The TSC–TBC complex collectively functions as a GAP for Rheb, thus maintaining Rheb in the inactive GDP-bound state ($Rheb^{GDP}$) [163]. Growth factors and amino acids inhibit the TSC–TBC complex, allowing Rheb to bind GTP and thereby activate the kinase function of mTORC1 [164]. Importantly, Rheb is required for all forms of mTORC1 activation, and to date, no Rheb-independent mTORC1 activator has been identified.

The mechanisms by which amino acids activate mTORC1 are not completely characterized. However, the available evidence suggests that there are distinct mechanisms for sensing cytosolic and lysosomal amino acids, and that select amino acids differentially activate mTORC1 via Rag-dependent and -independent pathways [151]. In addition, glutamate was recently discovered to activate mTORC1 in a RagA/B-independent but ADP ribosylation factor-1 GTPase-, v-ATPase-, and regulator-dependent manner, suggesting differential regulation of mTORC1 by amino acids [165].

Activators/Regulators of mTORC1

The mTORC1 complex integrates an extremely diverse array of inputs. Growth factors (e.g., insulin and other hormones), hypoxia, inflammation (e.g., inflammatory cytokines), DNA damage, and energy stores (AMPK) are among the signals integrated by the mTORC1 pathway. An important mediator of mTORC1 activation downstream of many of these signals is the TSC (TSC1–TSC2–TBC) (see Figure 21.11). Growth factor tyrosine kinase receptor signaling and energy sensing (via AMPK) can activate or inactivate the TSC–TBC with resultant mTORC1 inhibition or activation, respectively [163]. As described earlier, amino acid interactions with mTORC1 are TSC–TBC independent. Thus, the TSC–TBC complex may be a potentially powerful target for therapeutic manipulation of the mTORC1 pathway.

As previously discussed, AMPK is an important energy sensor that functions by sensing low-energy states (via ATP/ADP/AMP) to increase energy stores. The proteins TSC2 and raptor (a component of the mTORC1 complex) are phosphorylated by activated AMPK [127]. Phosphorylation likely augments the GAP activity of TSC2, resulting in inactivation of Rheb (i.e., maintaining the $Rheb^{GDP}$ state) and thereby inhibiting mTORC1 activation. Similarly, phosphorylation of raptor results in its association with the 14-3-3 proteins with resulting allosteric inhibition of mTORC1 [166].

Downstream effects of mTORC1

Regulation of protein and lipid synthesis by mTORC1

The control of protein synthesis is a critical and well-characterized process downstream of mTORC1 [167]. The proteins eukaryotic translation initiation factor 4E (eIF4E)-binding protein (4E-BP1) and S6 kinase 1 (S6K1) both function to stimulate protein synthesis when activated by mTORC1. The eIF proteins are deeply involved in the initiation phase of protein synthesis, and eIF4E specifically functions to direct the ribosome to the 5′ cap of mRNA in the initiation complex [132]. The 4E-BP1 protein binds to eIF4E, thereby inhibiting eIF4E and, in this manner, negatively regulating protein synthesis. Activated mTORC1 phosphorylates 4E-BP1, which prevents its binding to eIF4E. Thus, activated mTORC1 enhances protein synthesis by inhibiting the inhibitor (4E-BP-1) of eIF4E [144].

The S6K1 protein is a serine/threonine kinase that has pleiotropic functions in protein synthesis, including interacting with ribosomes and eIFs. S6K1 phosphorylation by activated mTORC1 results in increased translation of the 5′ TOP mRNA subclass (so named because they contain a 5′ oligopyrimidine tract) and enhanced protein translation mediated by a variety of proteins, including phosphorylation of the ribosomal protein S6 and of eIF4B [168].

Lipid synthesis downstream of mTORC1 is primarily via the sterol regulatory element-binding protein 1/2 (SREBP1/2) and peroxisome proliferator-activated receptor γ (PPARγ) [145,147,169] (Figure 21.12). Inactive SREBP resides on the endoplasmic reticulum. However, when activated (via insulin or low levels of intracellular cholesterol), these transcription factors are freed by proteolytic cleavage. In this instance, proteolysis is mediated by site 1 protease (S1P) and site 2 protease (S2P) [170]. The free transcription factors then translocate to the nucleus and bind to sterol regulator elements on DNA, and thereby direct the synthesis of cholesterol and lipid-generating enzymes [170]. Inhibition of mTORC1, via unknown mechanisms, results in reduced SREBP1/2 expression and processing, resulting in inhibition of induction of lipogenic genes [171].

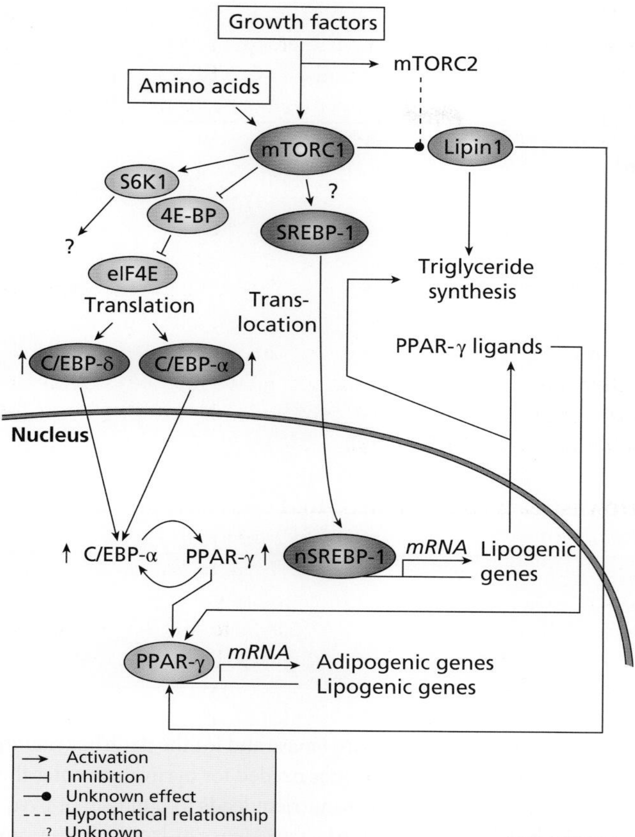

Figure 21.12 Mechanistic target of rapamycin complex 1 (mTORC1) regulation of peroxisome proliferator-activated receptor γ (PPARγ), sterol regulatory element-binding protein (SREBP), and adipogenesis. Inhibition of mTORC1 results in inhibited translation of PPARγ via 4EBP-mediated inhibition of the CCAAT/enhancer binding protein (C/EBP) transcription factors. mTORC1 positively regulates cleavage and activation of the SREBP proteins via an unknown mechanism. Source: Laplante and Sabatini 2009 [179]. Reproduced with permission of Elsevier.

Although the complete mechanism behind mTORC1 regulation of SERBPs is unknown, S6K1 is thought to play a role.

PPARγ belongs to a family of nuclear receptors that also function as transcription factors. PPARγ is induced during the process of adipogenesis (differentiation of cells toward mature adipocytes), by the C/EBP family of transcription factors (C/EBP/β, C/EBP/δ, and C/EBP/α) [172,173]. PPARγ activates adipogenic and lipogenic genes and promotes uptake and synthesis of FAs. Inhibition of mTORC1 results in reduced PPARγ translation and expression with subsequent impairments of adipogenesis [174]. These mTORC1-dependent effects on PPARγ are thought to be mediated by the protein 4E-BP1. Although our understanding of the mechanisms that underlie mTORC1 regulation of SREBP1/2 and PPARγ remain incomplete, the physiological importance of mTORC1 in lipid metabolism is evidenced by the marked abnormalities in serum TGs that can occur in patients treated with rapamycin (sirolimus) or its analogs (tacrolimus).

Conclusions

The gastrointestinal tract plays its most fundamental role in the homeostasis of the complete organism through its many contributions to the digestion and absorption of nutrients derived from our dietary intake. Complex adaptations of the anatomy and physiology of the gastrointestinal tract have evolved to facilitate and promote absorption of molecules that are in a form that can be used by the organism for energy, growth, and development. Although many of the elegant processes that lead to the digestion and ultimate absorption of the end products of the carbohydrates, proteins, and lipids that we ingest were described in detail decades ago and the clinical consequences of their disruption recognized, more recent research has revealed the cellular and molecular mechanisms that regulate the utilization of these molecules and appropriately adapt to nutrient deprivation and excess. These new findings related to what has come to be referred to as nutrient sensing complete the circle and place the processes of nutrient digestion and absorption in the much broader context of nutrient supply and demand.

References are available at www.yamadagastro.com/textbook7e

Further reading

Chantranupong L., Wolfson R.L., Sabatini D.M. Nutrient-sensing mechanisms across evolution. Cell 2015;161(1):67.

Drozdowski L.A., Thomson A.B.R. Intestinal sugar transport. World J Gastroenterol. 2006;12(11):1657.

Gudmand-Hoyer E., Skovbjerg H. Disaccharide digestion and maldigestion. Scand J Gastroenterol Suppl 1996;216:111.

Hardie D.G., Ross F.A., Hawley S.A. AMPK: a nutrient and energy sensor that maintains energy homeostasis. Nat Rev Mol Cell Biol 2012;13(4):251.

Kilberg M.S., Balasubramanian M., Fu L., Shan J. The transcription factor network associated with the amino acid response in mammalian cells. Adv Nutr 2012;3(3):295.

Ko C.W., Qu J., Black D.D., Tso P. Regulation of intestinal lipid metabolism: current concepts and relevance to disease. Nat Rev Gastroenterol Hepatol 2020;17(3):169.

Laplante M., Sabatini D.M: mTOR signaling in growth control and disease. Cell 2012;149(2):274.

Mueckler M, Thorens B. The SLC2 (GLUT) family of membrane transporters. Mol Aspects Med 2013;34:121.

Rubio-Aliaga I., Daniel H. Peptide transporters and their roles in physiological processes and drug disposition. Xenobiotica 2008;38(7-8):1022.

Wang T.Y., Liu M., Portincasa P., Wang D.Q. New insights into the molecular mechanism of intestinal fatty acid absorption. Eur J Clin Invest 2013;43(11):1203.

CHAPTER 22

Vitamins and minerals

Berkeley N. Limketkai[1], Laura E. Matarese[2], and Gerard E. Mullin[3]
[1] UCLA School of Medicine, Los Angeles, CA, USA
[2] East Carolina University, Greenville, NC, USA
[3] Johns Hopkins University School of Medicine, Baltimore, MD, USA

Chapter menu

Introduction

Vitamins and minerals are essential micronutrients needed in small amounts to maintain the body's metabolic functions. Vitamin and mineral deficiencies most commonly arise from malnutrition, malabsorption, and medication effects. As physiological disruptions among patients with gastrointestinal and liver diseases often place them at increased risk for vitamin and mineral deficiency, the clinician caring for these patients should remain vigilant about the clinical manifestations, potential complications, diagnostic methods, and treatment of vitamin and mineral deficiency (or deficiencies). On the other hand, many individuals with digestive disorders consume dietary supplements that may place them at risk for vitamin and mineral toxicity. In this chapter, we review the function, structure, dietary sources, manifestations of deficiency and toxicity, and treatment of important vitamins and minerals.

Water-soluble vitamins

Thiamin (B_1)

Function, structure, sources, and requirements

Thiamin (vitamin B_1) plays a key role in carbohydrate and branched-chain amino acid metabolism [1]. Thiamin is phosphorylated to its active form thiamin pyrophosphate, which acts as a coenzyme for pyruvate dehydrogenase and for the decarboxylation of α-ketoacids. Because thiamin is needed for pyruvate to enter the Krebs cycle, a lack of the micronutrient leads to build-up of pyruvate, which is then converted to lactate. Hence, D-lactic acidosis can be seen with severe thiamin deficiency. Thiamin is present in significant amounts in pork, legumes, and fortified cereals. The Recommended Dietary Allowances (RDA) for thiamin, based on the amount needed to maintain normal erythrocyte transketolase activity, are 1.2 mg/day for men, 1.1 mg/day for women, and 1.4 mg/day during pregnancy and lactation (Table 22.1) [1]. Thiamin is absorbed by a dual process in the jejunum. At low concentrations (0.2–2.0 mM), thiamin is absorbed by an active Na^+-dependent transport that involves phosphorylation, and at higher concentrations, it is absorbed by passive diffusion [2].

Deficiency

Thiamin deficiency is common among chronic alcoholics because of a combination of poor intake and reduced absorption – alcohol interferes with active transport absorption across the basal enterocyte membrane [3]. Other causes of thiamin deficiency include extensive diuretic use and extreme malnutrition from causes such as chronic recurrent vomiting, anorexia, malabsorption syndromes, and gastric bypass surgery [4]. Mild inadequate intake of thiamin may result in nonspecific symptoms, while thiamin deficiency is associated with

Yamada's Textbook of Gastroenterology, Seventh Edition. Edited by Timothy C. Wang, Michael Camilleri, Benjamin Lebwohl, Anna S. Lok, William J. Sandborn, Kenneth K. Wang, and Gary D. Wu.

Companion website: www.yamadagastro.com/textbook7e

Table 22.1 Water-soluble vitamins.

	Thiamin (B1)	Riboflavin (B2)	Niacin (B3)	Pantothenic acid (B5)	Pyridoxine (B6)	Biotin (B7)
Dietary source	Whole-grain, fortified cereals, pork, organ meats	Milk, eggs, fortified cereals	Tryptophan, fish, liver, meat, legumes, fortified cereals	Wide variety of foods: meat, vegetables, unprocessed grains	Meat, fish, poultry, noncitrus fruit, fortified cereals	Peanuts, almonds, soy, eggs, yogurt
Daily requirement	Men 1.2 mg; women 1.1 mg; pregnancy and lactation 1.4 mg	Men 1.3 mg; women 1.1 mg; pregnancy 1.4 mg, lactation 1.6 mg	Niacin equivalents (NE is 60 mg tryptophan): men 16 NE; women 14 NE; pregnancy 18 NE, lactation 17 NE	Men and women 5 mg; pregnancy 6 mg; lactation 7 mg	Men and women 1.3–1.7 mg; pregnancy 1.9 mg, lactation 2.0 mg	Men and women 30 μg; pregnancy 30 μg; lactation 35 μg
Absorption	Active Na^+-dependent transport, passive diffusion higher dose	Active Na^+-dependent transport	Active tryptophan; passive niacin	Passive diffusion; and active transport in jejunum	Hydrolysis and passive transport	Carrier-mediated diffusion
Function	Carbohydrate and energy metabolism	Redox, especially glutathione reductase; cofactor for MTHFR	NAD and NADP redox reactions, DNA repair	Carbohydrate and energy metabolism, manufacture of red blood cells and adrenal hormones	Heme synthesis, cofactor for alanine transaminase, cystathione β-synthase	Carboxyl carrier for enzymatic reactions related to gluconeogenesis and fatty acid formation
Clinical signs of deficiency	High-output heart failure, peripheral neuropathy, Wernicke–Korsakoff syndrome	Glossitis, peripheral neuropathy, elevated homocysteine in TT homozygous MTHFR 677C→T	Pellagra in malnutrition, AIDS, Hartnup disease, carcinoid syndrome	Fatigue, insomnia, depression, irritability	Elevated homocysteine, altered cognition, glossitis, peripheral neuropathy	Rare, but can be induced by avidin (raw egg whites). Also in setting of incomplete parenteral nutrition: dermatitis, glossitis
Toxicity	None known	None known	Flushing, exacerbation of peptic ulcer	Diarrhea at intakes of 10–20 g	Sensory neuropathy in gram amounts	None known
Method of assessment	Erythrocyte transketolase	Erythrocyte glutathione reductase	Urine metabolites	Urinary excretion, and blood levels	HPLC	HPLC

HPLC, high-pressure liquid chromatography; MTHFR, methylenetetrahydrofolate reductase; NAD, nicotinamide adenine dinucleotide; NADP, nicotinamide adenine dinucleotide phosphate.

clinical manifestations of anorexia, weight loss, weakness, cardiovascular compromise, and neurological dysfunction. Deficiency can also result in one of two forms of beriberi. Classical wet beriberi, which often accompanies starvation, is characterized by cardiomyopathy with high-output cardiac failure. In contrast, dry beriberi is characterized by progressive stocking–glove polyneuropathy of the lower extremities. The extensive use of diuretics promotes thiamine deficiency in patients with congestive heart failure, whereas the left ventricular ejection fraction improves with thiamine replacement [5]. Additional neurological features of thiamin deficiency occur in chronic alcoholics and are classified as the Wernicke–Korsakoff syndrome, where manifestations range in relation to the severity and duration of the deficiency from nystagmus and ocular paresis to cerebellar dysfunction with a wide-based gait, global confusion, and, ultimately, permanently impaired mentation [6].

Because body stores of thiamin are regulated by carbohydrate metabolism, the administration of intravenous dextrose to a malnourished patient may precipitate an acute demand for residual endogenous thiamin with resultant overt thiamin deficiency manifested by cardiac failure and confusion. When presented with an alcoholic patient or one who has experienced prolonged starvation, it is critical to empirically supplement with thiamin prior to administration of intravenous carbohydrates.

Toxicity

There are no known adverse effects of excessive thiamin consumption.

Assessment of status

Thiamin status is most accurately assessed by a functional assay of erythrocyte transketolase before and after the addition of thiamin pyrophosphate [7].

Riboflavin (B_2)

Function, structure, sources, and requirements

Riboflavin (vitamin B_2) supports the metabolism of all macronutrients and antioxidant protective mechanisms. Riboflavin exists in coenzyme forms as flavin mononucleotide (FMN) and flavin adenine dinucleotide (FAD), each of which is involved in redox reactions. Rich food sources of riboflavin include milk, eggs, and fortified cereals. The RDA for riboflavin are 1.3 mg/day for men, 1.1 mg/day for women, 1.4 mg/day during pregnancy, and 1.6 mg/day during lactation (see Table 22.1) [8]. Riboflavin requirements in the elderly appear to decline with a lower fat and higher carbohydrate diet content, although these changes have not yet been studied at other ages [1].

Absorption and homeostasis

During the process of assimilation, dietary FAD and FMN are released from food protein by gastric acid and then hydrolyzed by intestinal phosphatases. Most absorption of riboflavin occurs in the proximal small intestine by a Na^+-independent, carrier-mediated system [9]. Riboflavin circulates in the plasma bound to albumin and enters cells by carrier-mediated transport; it is excreted in the urine [10]. Riboflavin metabolism appears to be unaffected by liver disease [11]. A major function of flavin coenzymes is the regulation of redox reactions. For example, FAD is essential as a cofactor for glutathione reductase, which regenerates glutathione, the principal antioxidant substrate for the protection of cellular functions [12,13]. In addition, FMN is required for the generation and activation of pyridoxal phosphate from nonphosphorylated forms of pyridoxine [14]. FAD plays a role as a cofactor for methylenetetrahydrofolate reductase (MTHFR) in reducing homocysteine (Figure 22.1), particularly in individuals who are homozygous for the 677C→T polymorphism [15].

Deficiency

Riboflavin deficiency often stems from similar causes of other water-soluble vitamin deficiencies, such as malnutrition associated with chronic alcoholism, celiac disease, and anorexia. The clinical manifestations include sore throat, hyperemia and edema of the oropharyngeal mucosa,

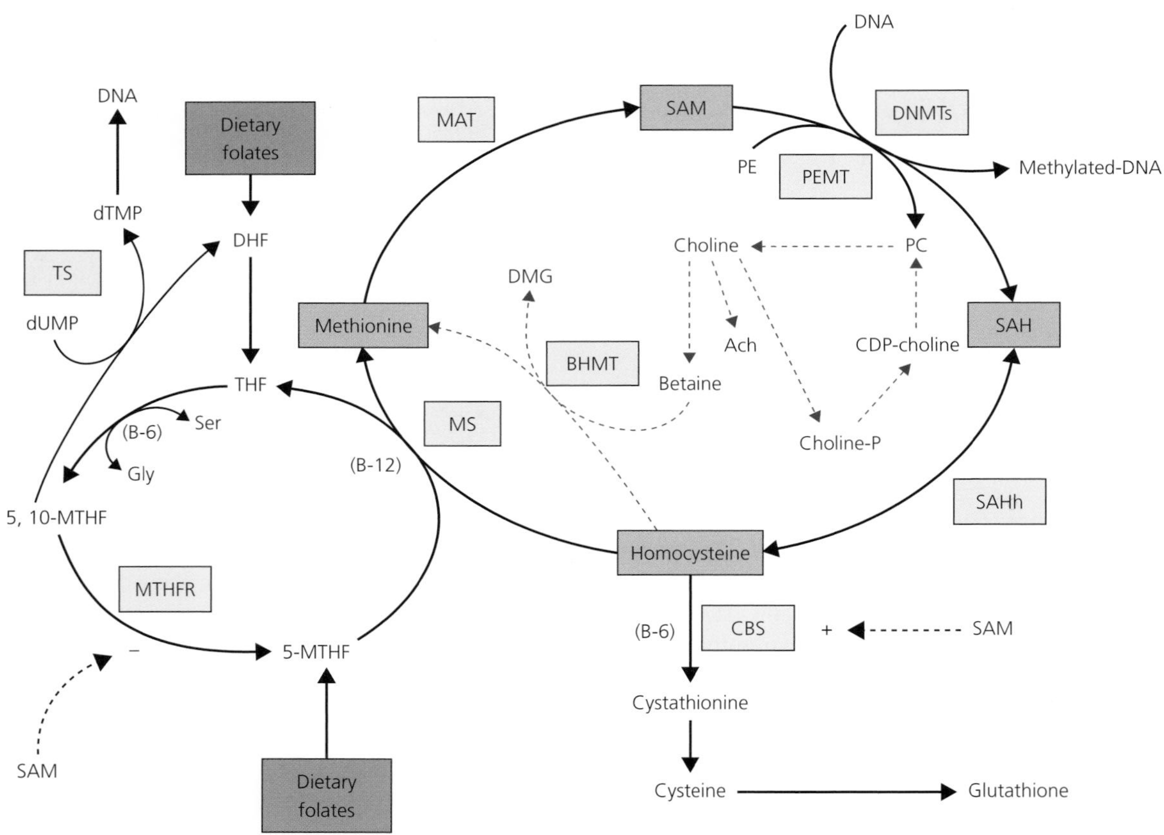

Figure 22.1 Interactions of folate and methionine metabolism. BHMT, betaine homocysteine methyltransferase; CBS, cystathionine β-synthase; CDP-choline, cytidine diphosphorylcholine; choline-P, phosphoryl choline; DHF, dihydrofolate; DNMTs, DNA methyltransferases; dTMP, deoxythymidine monophosphate; dUMP, deoxyuridine monophosphate; GSH, glutathione; MAT, methionine adenosyltransferase; MS, methionine synthase; 5-MTHF, 5-methyltetrahydrofolate; 5,10-MTHF, 5,10-methylenetetrahydrofolate; MTHFR, methylenetetrahydrofolate reductase; PC, phosphatidylcholine; PE, phosphatidylethanolamine; PEMT, phosphatidylethanolamine methyltransferase; SAH, *S*-adenosylhomocysteine; SAM, *S*-adenosylmethionine; SAHh, SAH hydrolase; THF, tetrahydrofolate; TS, thymidylate synthase.

glossitis, cheilosis, angular stomatitis, seborrheic dermatitis, and peripheral neuropathy [1].

Toxicity

There are no known toxicities, but elevated levels have not shown benefit. Some hypothesize riboflavin's poor solubility and absorption to explain the lack of toxicity at higher doses.

Assessment

Riboflavin status is assessed by determining the level in the urine using high-pressure liquid chromatography (HPLC) or by colorimetric measurement of erythrocyte glutathione reductase before and after the addition of FAD [7].

Niacin (B_3)

Function, structure, sources, and requirements

Niacin (vitamin B_3) – essential in all cells for metabolism – is expressed biologically by its two coenzymes, nicotinamide adenine dinucleotide (NAD) and nicotinamide adenine dinucleotide phosphate (NADP). Both forms are involved in a vast number of redox reactions in the generation of energy from carbohydrates, fats, proteins, and ethanol. NADP is also involved in fatty acid and cholesterol biosynthesis, and NAD is the substrate for poly (ADP-ribose) polymerase, which is involved in DNA replication and repair [16]. Dietary niacin is derived from animal protein as tryptophan, and as nicotinic acid and nicotinamide from enriched or whole-grain cereals, leafy vegetables, and legumes. The Dietary Reference Intake (DRI) for niacin is measured in units called niacin equivalents. Because niacin is derived from tryptophan, 1 mg niacin equivalent is equal to 60 mg tryptophan. The RDA of niacin is 16 mg/day of niacin equivalents for men, 14 mg/day for women, 18 mg/day during pregnancy, and 17 mg/day during lactation (see Table 22.1) [17].

Absorption and homeostasis

The two coenzyme forms of niacin – NAD and NADP – need to be digested to release nicotinic acid and nicotinamide, which are absorbed in the stomach and the small intestine via carrier-mediated and passive diffusion.

Deficiency

Pellagra is the classical disease of niacin deficiency and occurs in populations whose diets contain insufficient animal protein as a source of tryptophan, particularly if corn is used as a grain staple. Once prevalent as a cause of mental illness among the very poor in the southern United States, pellagra was eliminated after Goldberger's classic finding that the missing vitamin was present in grains other than corn [18]. It still occurs in persons living in areas of Africa and other less developed countries where there is a scarcity of animal protein, in malnourished chronic alcoholics [19], and sometimes in patients with acquired immunodeficiency syndrome [20]. Pellagra is clinically manifest by the "three Ds" of diarrhea, dementia, and dermatitis – and in the most severe cases, the "fourth D," death. The dermatological manifestation is a scaly red rash of sun-exposed areas. Characteristic signs of pellagra may also occur in Hartnup disease of congenital impaired tryptophan absorption and in the carcinoid syndrome, in which endogenous tryptophan is diverted into serotonin synthesis [21].

Toxicity

There are no known adverse effects from consumption of niacin in unfortified foods, although toxicity can occur through excessive dietary or pharmacological supplementation. Common toxic effects include flushing (which is related to the absorption rate) and exacerbation of peptic ulcer disease. Some suggested interventions to help ameliorate these adverse effects include: (i) the use of lower doses of niacin together with a statin medication [22]; (ii) use of concomitantly administered low-dose nonsteroidal antiinflammatory agents (NSAIDs) [23–25]; (iii) use of an extended-release formulation, which has the efficacy of its immediate-release counterpart but without the adverse effects [26].

Assessment

Niacin status is assessed by measurement of the urinary ratio of its metabolites, *N*-methyl-2-pyridone-5-carboxamide and *N*-methylnicotinamide [7].

Pyridoxine (B_6)

Function, structure, sources, and requirements

Vitamin B_6 includes six compounds: pyridoxine, pyridoxal, pyridoxamine, and their phosphorylated analogs. Vitamin B_6 has a variety of functions in enzymatic reactions involving metabolism of glycogen, lipid metabolism, erythrocyte metabolism and function, metabolism of tyrosine- and tryptophan-derived neurotransmitters (dopamine, serotonin, epinephrine, norepinephrine), and hormone modulation. Vitamin B_6 is widely distributed in foods, occurring in greatest concentrations in meats, whole-grain products (especially wheat), vegetables, and nuts. The RDA of pyridoxine is 1.3 mg/day for men aged 19–50 years, 1.7 mg/day for men above 50 years old, 1.3 mg/day for women aged 19–50 years, 1.5 mg/day for women above 50 years old, 1.9 mg/day during pregnancy, and 2.0 mg/day during lactation (see Table 22.1) [1].

Absorption and homeostasis

Vitamin B_6 in its dephosphorylated forms is readily absorbed by passive diffusion in the jejunum [27, 28]. A related compound, pyridoxine-5′-β-D glucoside, was found to be taken up by Caco-2 cells in a pattern consistent with passive diffusion across a wide range of pyridoxine-5′-β-D glucoside extracellular concentrations [29]. The exchange of sodium for other monovalent cations did not change pyridoxine-5′-β-D glucoside uptake by Caco-2 cells. The results suggest that pyridoxine-5′-β-D glucoside is taken by a Na^+-independent process by passive diffusion. Some evidence also demonstrates the existence of a specialized, carrier-mediated system for pyridoxine uptake [30]. This system is Na$^+$ independent but highly dependent on acid-buffered pH and is amiloride sensitive [31].

Deficiency

Clinical manifestations of deficiency may include seborrheic dermatitis, microcytic anemia, epileptiform convulsions, depression, and confusion. Isolated deficiency of vitamin B_6 is uncommon. However, the tuberculosis drug isoniazid and penicillamine bind it and may induce iatrogenic deficiency. Alcoholism and preeclampsia have been associated with decreased pyridoxal 5′-phosphate concentrations, although their clinical relevance is currently unclear.

Toxicity

There are no known adverse effects from consumption of pyridoxine from foods, although toxicity from excessive supplementation may lead to peripheral neuropathy.

Cobalamin (B_{12})

Function, structure, sources, and requirements

Vitamin B_{12} refers to a family of cobalamin compounds. In its active coenzyme forms, the cobalt atom is bound to specific moieties, resulting in methylcobalamin and adenosylcobalamin, whereas cyanocobalamin is the pharmaceutical and interchangeable form of the vitamin.

Cobalamin serves a role in two major enzymatic reactions: methylcobalamin participates in the transfer of the methyl group from 5-MTHF to total homocysteine (tHcy), producing methionine and tetrahydrofolate (THF) (see Figure 22.1), and adenosylcobalamin is a cofactor for methylmalonyl-coenzyme A (CoA) mutase in the conversion of methylmalonyl-CoA to succinyl-CoA. In this section, the term *cobalamin* is used to describe dietary sources, metabolic pathways, and clinical manifestations of deficiency. The term *vitamin B_{12}* is used to describe the pharmacological and supplemental forms of the vitamin.

The most abundant source of cobalamin is from food: animal products, including meat, fish, shellfish, poultry, eggs, milk, and other dairy products. The adult RDA for cobalamin is 2.4 μg/day (2.6 μg/day during pregnancy and 2.8 μg/day during lactation), which accounts for an average 50% absorption from all dietary sources.

Absorption and homeostasis

Cobalamin enters the stomach bound to food and is released in the presence of gastric acid and pepsin. Free cobalamin then binds R protein (also called haptocorrin), a protein secreted by salivary and parietal cells and useful to protect cobalamin from denaturation by strong acids in the stomach [32] (Figure 22.2). Cobalamin is again released in the duodenum when R protein undergoes degradation by pancreatic proteases and free cobalamin then binds intrinsic factor (IF). IF is secreted by parietal cells, but is ineffective at binding cobalamin at the acidic pH of the healthy stomach; IF binds cobalamin more effectively at the neutral pH of the duodenum [32,33].

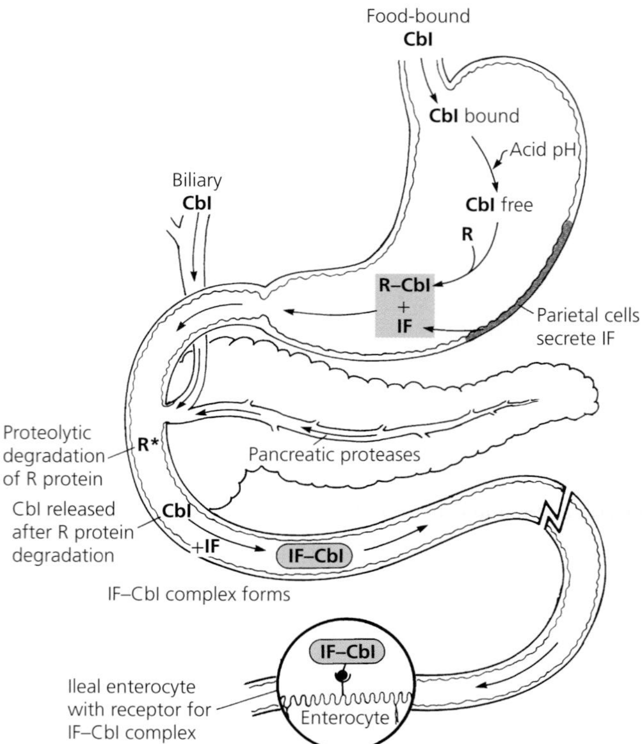

Figure 22.2 Sequential steps in the gastrointestinal absorption of dietary protein-bound cobalamin (Cbl). Gastric acid is required to liberate both methylcobalamin and adenosylcobalamin from dietary protein. In the acidic gastric environment, cobalamin is then bound to salivary R proteins, and gastric parietal cells secrete intrinsic factor (IF). After neutralization of the gastric contents in the upper duodenum and pancreatic protease digestion of the R protein–cobalamin complex, free cobalamin then binds to IF. After transit to the terminal 50 cm of ileum, the IF–cobalamin complex interacts at the microvillus surface with the specific ileal receptors cubulin and amnionless, and is then internalized and binds to megalin and transcobalamin II. Source: Sitrin 1996 [405]. Reproduced with permission of Dr Eugene B. Chang.

The absorption of cobalamin by ileal enterocytes requires several binding proteins. First, the cobalamin–IF complex is bound to a specific membrane receptor on the ileal enterocyte called cubulin, which arranges itself next to another enterocyte receptor called amnionless (AML). Subsequent transfer across the ileal enterocyte involves the intracellular cleavage of the cobalamin–IF/cubulin/amnionless complex [34]. Cobalamin then binds to transcobalamin II, which carries cobalamin out of the ileal mucosa to the portal circulation [35,36]. The transcobalamin II–cobalamin complex, known as holotranscobalamin, accounts for 10–20% of all circulating cobalamin and is essential for its transport to all cells of the body. Holotranscobalamin is taken into cells by endocytosis, which is followed by liberation of the two coenzyme forms methylcobalamin and adenosylcobalamin [32]. In an enterohepatic cycle, about 1.4 μg/day of endogenous cobalamin is secreted into the bile as a complex with R protein [37]. Circulating cobalamin is then released from biliary R protein by pancreatic trypsin and then rapidly bound to IF for subsequent passage to the ileal receptor site, where about half (0.7 μg/day) is reabsorbed and the other half is excreted in the stool [38].

Deficiency

The daily cobalamin requirement of 2.4 μg is very small compared to its body pool size (1–2 mg); therefore, it takes several years to become deficient from dietary inadequacy alone and only true vegans are at risk for dietary inadequacy. The worldwide incidence of vitamin B_{12} deficiency is substantial due to dietary insufficiency. However, in the United States, vitamin B_{12} deficiency is more common in older adults who have a higher prevalence of achlorhydria and in those with digestive diseases associated with malabsorption [39].

The clinical expression of cobalamin deficiency as megaloblastic anemia and hyperhomocysteinemia is indistinguishable from that of severe folate deficiency (Box 22.1). However, because cobalamin also participates in the methylmalonyl-CoA mutase reaction, its deficiency may also be expressed in the nervous system as subacute combined degeneration of the posterior columns of the spinal cord, which is characterized by the loss of position and vibratory sensation and other features of peripheral neuropathy of the lower extremities. Cobalamin deficiency also has more subtle and frequent effects on the central nervous system that include neuropsychiatric disorders such as ataxia, paresthesias, memory loss, cognitive dysfunction, and more severe dementia, even in the absence of anemia [40].

Gastric acid is required for the release of food-bound cobalamin from dietary protein, so achlorhydric individuals are at risk for cobalamin deficiency. Achlorhydria of aging is the most common cause of cobalamin deficiency in the United States. According to the criteria of elevated levels of methylmalonic acid and tHcy and a serum cobalamin level of less than 222 pmol/L (300 pg/mL), at least 15% of ambulatory individuals older than 65 years are vitamin B_{12} deficient in the United States, with greater prevalence in Hispanic Americans and less in African Americans [39,42]. A similar incidence of age-related cobalamin deficiency has been reported in European countries [32]. The increasing prevalence of age-related cobalamin deficiency, which is 40% in persons older than 80 years [32], could be related to a greater prevalence in that age cohort of *Helicobacter pylori*, which predisposes to more severe gastric atrophy and malabsorption of food-bound cobalamin [43].

Box 22.1 Relationship between vitamin B_{12}, folate, and homocysteine.

Because folate and vitamin B_{12} work in conjunction, a deficiency in either vitamin can result in high serum homocysteine levels. However, vitamin B_{12} deficiency can result in a secondary folate deficiency due to trapping the folate as 5-methyl-FH4 (so called the methyl-folate trap) [41]. Giving folate to a person with vitamin B_{12} deficiency can therefore actually precipitate the vitamin B_{12} deficiency, which can result in neurological damage.

Pernicious anemia was first described by Thomas Addison in the early 19th century and is recognized as an autoimmune disorder characterized by the absence of IF in the gastric juice in association with achlorhydria. Almost all patients have gastric and serum antibodies to either parietal cells or IF, and most have elevated serum gastrin levels [32]. Pernicious anemia may be associated with other autoimmune diseases, including Hashimoto thyroiditis, adrenal atrophy, and Sjögren syndrome, and carries increased potential for the development of gastric adenocarcinoma, lymphoma, and carcinoid tumors. While the overall incidence of pernicious anemia in the United States is about two cases per 1000 per year [39], it increases with age [44]. Because IF is also required for the absorption of endogenous cobalamin in the enterohepatic circulation, cobalamin deficiency develops more rapidly in patients with untreated pernicious anemia than in strict vegans or elderly persons with achlorhydria. There is an associated increased risk of gastric neoplasms so persons with proven pernicious anemia should have endoscopic surveillance every 3 years [32].

Many other clinical conditions involving the stomach or small intestine cause cobalamin malabsorption. Chronic use of proton pump inhibitors is associated with a greater risk of cobalamin deficiency [45]. Surgical causes of cobalamin deficiency include total gastrectomy and gastric bypass surgery for obesity, each associated with malabsorption of food-bound cobalamin secondary to achlorhydria. A survey performed early in the era of gastric bypass surgery found that two-thirds of patients developed cobalamin deficiency within 12 months of surgery, though this is thought to be a result of blind loop syndrome and resulting bacterial overgrowth [46]. However, a more recent survey found a 12% incidence of postoperative cobalamin deficiency among routinely screened patients [47]. Persistent duodenal hyperacidity may inactivate pancreatic trypsin and prevent the transfer of cobalamin from gastric R protein to IF; thus, cobalamin deficiency is a recognized component of Zollinger–Ellison syndrome [48].

Abnormal pancreatic and upper intestinal events

The dissociation of vitamin B_{12} from R protein relies on pancreatic proteases and bicarbonate to increase the pH of the acidic gastric effluent entering the duodenum. Pancreatic insufficiency can therefore lead to reduced dissociation of vitamin B_{12} from R protein. Although cobalamin malabsorption was described in 50% of patients with pancreatic insufficiency, including those with cystic fibrosis, actual deficiency is uncommon in these patients [49]. During passage through the jejunum, the cobalamin–IF complex is susceptible to bacterial cleavage or uptake; cobalamin deficiency with megaloblastic anemia is an increasingly recognized clinical expression of bacterial overgrowth syndromes in the elderly [50,51]. Intestinal infestation with the fish tapeworm *Diphyllobothrium latum* also causes cobalamin deficiency through competition for the cobalamin–IF complex [52].

Abnormal ileal events

According to retrospective studies of patients with ileal resections of various lengths, at least 50–80 cm of the terminal ileum participates in the ileal uptake and transfer of cobalamin, so that patients with inflammatory disease affecting longer lengths of intestine or those who have had surgical resection of the terminal ileum are at increased risk for cobalamin deficiency [53]. Diseases that interrupt enterohepatic cycling, such as Crohn's disease affecting the terminal ileum, radiation enteritis [54], and ileal bypass surgery or resection [55], promote increased loss of endogenous cobalamin in the feces. Surgical resection of the ileocecal valve increases the risk for cobalamin deficiency by permitting the migration of colonic bacteria and subsequent small intestinal bacterial overgrowth (SIBO). Because the terminal ileum is the site for both dietary cobalamin absorption and the reabsorption of endogenous cobalamin from its enterohepatic circulation, cobalamin deficiency may become evident within several months of surgical resection of more than 50 cm of terminal ileum [55].

Small intestine bacterial overgrowth

Vitamin B_{12} deficiency from SIBO occurs through competitive consumption of the micronutrient by bacteria instead of allowing ileal absorption.

Diagnosis of cobalamin deficiency

Cobalamin is conventionally measured in the serum by a radioassay with high specificity and sensitivity, with values less than 250 pmol/L considered subnormal [42,56]. The measurement of holotranscobalamin is potentially a more accurate assessment of the amount of cobalamin that is available for cellular uptake, but its utility relative to the cobalamin assay is still uncertain [57]. Measurements of the metabolites tHcy and methylmalonic acid (MMA) are both useful to confirm cobalamin deficiency. An elevated tHcy is nonspecific and does not distinguish between cobalamin deficiency and folate deficiency, whereas the measurement of MMA is costly and often not easily available. MMA measurement has been recommended to confirm cobalamin deficiency when the serum cobalamin level is in the intermediate range between 125 and 250 pmol/L. However, there is also a gray area of uncertain MMA normality; a value greater than 0.75 μmol/L is confirmatory of cobalamin deficiency [56].

The Schilling test of cobalamin deficiency, which was widely available until recently, involved measuring the 24-h urine excretion of radiolabeled cobalamin with and without the inclusion of exogenous IF. This test was used to differentiate among dietary causes (normal absorption), pernicious anemia (low absorption corrected with exogenous IF), ileal malabsorption (low in either case), and intestinal bacterial overgrowth (low then corrected with oral antibiotics). However, this "gold standard" test is seldom available because of limited availability of exogenous IF, the need for the use of radioactive dosages, and cumbersome urine collections. The clinician must now rely on a careful history to distinguish potential causes before determining the best approach to the treatment of cobalamin deficiency.

Treatment of cobalamin deficiency

The treatment of cobalamin deficiency is based on both its detection and the identification of its cause. Because cobalamin deficiency secondary to the achlorhydria of aging or gastric surgery is caused by malabsorption of food-bound dietary cobalamin but not of unbound crystalline pharmaceutical vitamin B_{12}, it can usually be treated by supplemental oral vitamin B_{12} at over-the-counter doses of 350 μg/day crystalline vitamin B_{12} supplement [58]. Because patients with pernicious anemia lack both IF and gastric acid, they can absorb neither crystalline cobalamin nor dietary food-bound cobalamin and must be treated with intramuscular injections of vitamin B_{12}, starting at 1000 μg/day for a week, then weekly for a month, and then in monthly 1000 μg doses, ideally after training on self-injection. A study of 33 patients with cobalamin deficiency caused by atrophic gastritis with or without pernicious anemia reported that an oral dose of 2000 μg/day was as effective in correcting the deficiency as an intramuscular dose of 1000 μg/month [59]. Patients who develop cobalamin deficiency in the presence of bacterial overgrowth, ileal disease, or surgical resection, each of which limits the absorption of the cobalamin–IF complex, should be similarly treated with regular parenteral cobalamin injections.

Folate

Function, structure, sources, and requirements

Folate is a coenzyme necessary for the synthesis of nucleic acids and amino acids. The metabolism of folate is intrinsically tied to methionine metabolism and to the synthesis, nucleotide balance, and methylation of DNA. Figure 22.1 depicts these interactions in the liver. There are two key functions of folate: one is the conversion of homocysteine to methionine in the synthesis of *S*-adenosylmethionine (SAM), the other is the methylation of deoxyuridylate to thymidylate in the formation of DNA.

Folate is found naturally in a wide variety of foods. Dark green leafy vegetables (spinach, Brussels sprouts) liver, yeast, and asparagus are among the foods with the highest folate content, though folate is also a component of fruits and fruit juices, nuts, beans, peas, dairy products, poultry and meat, eggs, seafood, and grains. The DRI for folate from all sources is expressed in dietary folate equivalents (DFEs). This term accounts for the fact that folic acid (the form in supplements and additives) is 1.7 times more bioavailable than the folates that naturally occur in foods [60]. The RDA for folate is set at 400 μg of DFE per day for adults, 600 μg/day during pregnancy, and 500 μg/day during lactation.[1] Since 1998, all grain products in the United States have been fortified with folic acid at 140 μg/g to ensure a daily intake equal to or more than the RDA for folate.

Absorption and homeostasis

Folates are absorbed in the duodenum and upper jejunum. During the process of intestinal absorption, dietary folylpolyglutamates are hydrolyzed at the epithelial cell (enterocyte) brush border membrane, followed by active transport of the folylmonoglutamate derivative into the absorbing enterocyte. In adult human volunteers, the absorption of monoglutamyl folic acid was about 85%, compared to about 50% absorption of complex dietary polyglutamyl folates [61].

Two intestinal brush border proteins – glutamate carboxypeptidase II (GCP2, or folate hydrolase) and the reduced folate carrier – are required, respectively, for the sequential hydrolysis of dietary folylpolyglutamates and the transport of folylmonoglutamate derivatives across the enterocyte brush border and basolateral membranes [62,63]. Folate in its reduced and methylated forms is more easily absorbed [64–66].

The uptake of 5-MTHF by hepatocytes involves binding to the liver plasma membrane and carrier-mediated transport into the cell. The binding step is regulated in part by the high-affinity folate receptor, folate-binding protein. Within hepatocytes, uptake of 5-MTHF is followed by conversion to folylpolyglutamates for storage and metabolism. After reconversion to monoglutamyl forms for membrane transport, about 10% of the liver folate pool undergoes biliary secretion as 5-MTHF to an enterohepatic folate circulation, while the remaining nonhepatic folate pool circulates in the blood to other tissues [67]. About 1% of the total body folate pool is excreted daily in the urine and 0.1% in the feces of nonhuman primates [68].

Causes of folate deficiency and aberrant folate metabolism

Assessment of folate deficiency

Folate deficiency should be confirmed by measurement of a low concentration of red blood cell folate. The serum folate level is more labile and dependent on recent dietary intake, whereas the red blood cell folate level is a more accurate measure of tissue stores. Depending on the laboratory, folate deficiency is defined by a serum folate concentration less than 7 nmol/L (3 ng/mL), while a concentration of red blood cell folate level less than 305 nmol/L (140 ng/mL) is predictive of tissue folate deficiency [60]. Measurement of the plasma tHcy concentration is a more sensitive functional assay for folate deficiency. A low folate concentration is represented by an increased tHcy concentration. However, cobalamin deficiency is also reflected by an elevated tHcy concentration, as well as by the same tissue expressions found in folate deficiency. Therefore, folate deficiency can be defined metabolically by high tHcy and normal cobalamin status, as described in the vitamin B_{12} section.

Causes of folate deficiency

Isolated folate deficiency is uncommon; it usually coexists with other nutrient deficiencies because of its strong association with poor diet, alcoholism, intestinal malabsorptive disorders, and altered metabolism as a result of genetic aberrations and toxins such as alcohol. Folate deficiency can also arise from medication effects, such as methotrexate, sulfasalazine, high-dose NSAIDs, anticonvulsants, pyrimethamine, trimethoprim, and triamterene [1]. Since mandatory fortification of the US diet in 1998, the incidence of folate deficiency in the United States has decreased from 22% to 1.7% of the population [69]. However, folate deficiency as the result of inadequate diet is common in impoverished populations, in developed countries where the diet does not contain fortified grains, and in susceptible populations including infants, elderly people, and chronic alcoholics whose diets are inadequate [70]. The body stores of folate are sufficient for about 4 months.

Malabsorption

Intestinal folate malabsorption and deficiency are associated with diseases and surgical procedures that affect absorption by enterocytes in the duodenum and jejunum, such as celiac disease, severe Crohn's disease, extensive gastric bypass surgery for severe obesity, and extensive small bowel surgery. A Finnish study found that about one-third of adolescents with celiac disease had low serum folate concentrations, which was double the incidence in control subjects [71], but concentrations have been shown to normalize after treatment with a gluten-free diet [61]. Multivitamin supplementation after gastric bypass surgery has lowered the potential for folate deficiency [47]. Whereas folate deficiency is not considered a risk for patients with inflammatory bowel disease who use mesalamine drugs, sulfasalazine inhibits the absorption of both monoglutamyl and polyglutamyl dietary folates [72]. Studies in the prefortification era identified a high incidence of folate deficiency in chronic alcoholics, mainly ascribed to poor diet [73] and intestinal folate malabsorption [74].

Genetic abnormalities of methionine metabolism

Clinically significant MTHFR polymorphisms can affect folate metabolism. A thermolabile form of MTHFR occurs in TT homozygotes of the 677C→T variant, who represent 10–15% of the general population and express moderate hyperhomocysteinemia, especially when the polymorphism is combined with low folate concentrations [75]. A second MTHFR polymorphism at 1298A→C was thought to cause neural tube defects [76], but does not appear to interact with 677C→T nor to cause elevated homocysteine concentrations [77]. While functional polymorphisms have been described in the folate metabolizing genes, *GCP2* and *RFC1* (reduced folate carrier 1), their single or combined effects on folate absorption and status appear to be insignificant [77].

Clinical effects of folate deficiency and aberrant methionine metabolism

Because folate ultimately is required to maintain nucleotide balance during DNA synthesis, its deficiency is expressed by increased apoptosis with compensatory increased proliferation of cells, including rapid turnover in the blood-forming bone marrow and the intestinal mucosa. As indicated in Figure 22.1, folate deficiency also affects the methionine metabolic cycle, resulting in elevated circulating tHcy. Several common clinical conditions have been linked to folate deficiency with abnormal DNA metabolism and aberrant methionine metabolism.

Anemia and diarrhea

The main clinical expression of overt folate deficiency is megaloblastic anemia, with findings of macrocytic red blood cells with increased mean corpuscular volume and hypersegmented neutrophils in the peripheral blood, which are expressions of reduced levels of DNA and delayed erythropoiesis. Macrocytic enterocytes are evident in small intestinal biopsy specimens from alcoholic patients with folate-deficient megaloblastic anemia [78], and are associated with the diarrhea of chronic alcoholism caused in part by abnormal fluid and electrolyte transport in the intestine [79].

Folate deficiency and neural tube defects

Neural tube defects (NTD) are errors of fetal spinal cord development that occur within the first 2 weeks of pregnancy and result in anencephaly and spina bifida. The association of neural tube defects with folate deficiency is based on findings that red blood cell folate levels in early pregnancy correlate with the risk for delivery of a child with a neural tube defect [80], and on the results of trials in which neural tube defects were prevented by periconceptional supplementation with folic acid [81]. Public health policy of folic acid fortification of the US food supply has reduced the incidence of neural tube defects by only about 50% [82].

Cardiovascular disease

Hyperhomocysteinemia increases the risk for stroke and coronary heart disease [83]. The prevention of cardiovascular disease by lowering homocysteine concentrations with folic acid supplements has been the focus of many clinical trials. A metaanalysis of 12 randomized clinical trials involving 17 000 patients with preexisting vascular disease concluded that folic acid supplementation had no effect on the risk of recurrent stroke or coronary heart disease or on mortality. The authors do not exclude the possibility that lowering homocysteine concentrations by folic acid supplementation may reduce the incidence of primary cardiovascular events in susceptible populations [84].

Colon cancer

Data from epidemiological studies show that higher folate status correlated with decreased risk of colorectal cancers. Though the mechanism is not fully elucidated, it is thought that folate influences the development of cancer through its role in one-carbon metabolism and subsequent effects on DNA replication and cell division [85]. Additional research is needed to understand the role of dietary folate and supplemental folic acid in the prevention of various cancers. Although adequate folate status has been shown to be protective, there are subsets in which supplementation is not recommended. In individuals with colorectal adenomas, folic acid supplementation is not advised because there is some evidence that it does not prevent, and may even increase, the risk of recurrence.

Alcoholic liver disease

The contributory role for folate deficiency with consequent elevated liver homocysteine and *S*-adenosylhomocysteine (SAH) in the pathogenesis of alcoholic liver disease has been well established and is summarized in a 2007 symposium report [86]. In addition to poor diet and intestinal malabsorption, folate deficiency in alcoholism is caused by decreased uptake of folate by the liver and enhanced excretion in the urine [70]. Because liver folate stores are reduced in alcoholic liver disease [87], the combination of these factors accelerates the risk for folate deficiency in these patients.

Neural function

Recently, there has been renewed interest in the ability of vitamin B_{12} and folate supplementation to improve neurological function. The results of an analysis of a randomized, controlled trial found that supplementation with folic acid at 400 µg daily plus 100 µg of vitamin B_{12} over a 2-year period improved immediate and delayed memory in older men and women [88]. While orientation, attention, verbal memory, and processing speed remained unchanged, greater improvements from baseline in immediate and delayed recall scores were observed among those who received folic acid and vitamin B_{12} compared with the placebo group. Having a high homocysteine level at the beginning of the study was associated with reduced cognitive performance and higher depression scores at 24 months.

Toxicity

Evidence suggests that a considerable portion of supplemental folic acid is absorbed unchanged and that high circulating concentrations of folate may alter immune function, increase cancer risk, and promote worsening of cognitive function in elderly subjects [89]. At least 40% of aging Americans take supplemental folic acid at 400 µg/day and consequently their serum folate concentrations often exceed 40 nmol/L, which is at least double the highest serum folate concentrations in those who do not use supplements [90], and their concentration of unmetabolized folic acid constitutes more than 15% of serum folate that exceeds 50 nmol/L [91]. A study of postmenopausal women showed that immune function as measured by natural killer cell toxicity was improved by folic acid supplementation at 400 mg/day, but worsened in linear fashion with the increasing concentrations of unmetabolized serum folic acid in those who took larger doses of supplemental folic acid [92]. Furthermore, the risks for prostate cancer in men and breast cancer in postmenopausal women increased significantly in relationship to increasing plasma folate concentrations [93,94], especially when associated with the use of folic acid supplements [94]. A study of 1300 elderly people reported an increased risk for megaloblastic anemia and reduced cognitive function in those persons with low vitamin B_{12} status who took supplemental folic acid [95]. Supplemental folic acid can correct megaloblastic anemia, but not the neurological damage, that can result from vitamin B_{12} deficiency.

Vitamin C

Function, structure, sources, and requirements

Vitamin C plays an important role in a host of biochemical reactions, where it functions as either a cofactor for reactions requiring a reduced iron or copper metalloenzyme or a protective antioxidant. It has been identified as an electron donor for eight human enzymes – three of which participate in collagen hydroxylation, three in hormone and amino acid biosynthesis, and two in carnitine biosynthesis [96]. Vitamin C plays a role in expression of the collagen gene, cellular procollagen secretion, and the biosynthesis of other connective tissue components besides collagen (e.g., elastin, fibronectin, among others) [97]. It is involved in the biosynthesis of some of the hormonal components of the nervous system, including the formation of norepinephrine, and α-amidating monooxygenase enzymes, while also modulating neurotransmitter receptors, functions of dopaminergic and glutaminergic neurons, and synthesis of glial cells and myelin [98]. Vitamin C functions as an antioxidant because of its inherent ability to donate electrons. It scavenges reactive oxygen and nitrogen species [99] and also functions as a reducing agent for some mixed function oxidases found in the microsomal drug metabolizing system that inactivates a variety of substrates [100]. Biosynthesis of corticosteroids, aldosterone, and carnitine requires vitamin C [101]. The vitamin has been shown to modulate prostaglandin synthesis and, as such, is purported to exert bronchodilatory, vasodilatory, and anticlotting effects [102]. Ascorbic acid is involved in the absorption of dietary nonheme iron, via two mechanisms, preventing formation of insoluble and unabsorbable iron compounds, and reduction of ferric to ferrous iron a necessary requirement for uptake of iron into the mucosal cells [103].

Vitamin C exists in two forms: ascorbic acid (the reduced form) and dehydroascorbic acid (the oxidized form). It is an essential micronutrient in humans due to our inability to convert glucose to ascorbic acid in the absence of L-gulono-1,4-γ-lactone oxidase, unlike most other animals. Exogenous sources of vitamin C include the diet and supplementation. Vitamin C is present in some amount in all fruits and vegetables, although it is more abundant in citrus fruits and juices (orange, tangerine, grapefruit), kiwi, mango, cantaloupe, papaya, pineapple, berries (strawberries, raspberries, blueberries, cranberries), and watermelon. Vegetables with high concentrations of vitamin C include broccoli, Brussels sprouts, cauliflower, green/red peppers, leafy greens (spinach, cabbage, turnip greens, others), potatoes (sweet and white), tomatoes, and winter squash. Vitamin C-fortified foods and beverages are also available. Cooking vitamin C-rich foods can reduce the amount of the vitamin available and the best sources of the vitamin are raw fruits. The RDA for vitamin C is 90 mg/day for men, 75 mg/day for women, 85 mg/day during pregnancy, and 120 mg/day during lactation to maintain near-maximal neutrophil concentration with minimal urinary excretion [101].

Homeostasis and regulation

Vitamin C uptake and distribution in the body is under close homeostatic control by tissue-specific sodium-dependent vitamin C cotransporters (SVCT) 1 and 2 [104–106]. The close homeostatic regulation of vitamin C is controlled by four regulatory systems: intestinal uptake; tissue accumulation and distribution; rate of utilization and recycling; and renal-mediated excretion and reabsorption [105]. Vitamin C has been shown to display nonlinear pharmacokinetics as well as differential tissue distribution [105] (the brain, which depends on the SVCT2 receptor, can retain the vitamin at the expense of other tissues in states of chronic deficiency) [107].

Absorption and transport

Absorption of the vitamin occurs mainly in the ileum, with some absorption in the jejunum via passive diffusion, facilitated diffusion, and the SVCT 1 and 2 active cotransport systems [105]. The active transport system has been shown to be both saturable and dose dependent, meaning that as intake increases, the absorption decreases. Serum levels rise with dietary intake, with saturation levels of about 70 μmol/L suggested in humans [108]. Transport of vitamin C occurs mainly via facilitated diffusion through four of the glucose transporters (GLUT1–4) and is competitively inhibited by glucose [109].

Excretion

Once the serum saturation levels are reached and exceeded, renal excretion increases proportionately. Products of oxidation of vitamin C beyond dehydroascorbic acid include oxalic acid, threonic acid, L-xylose, and ascorbate 2-sulfate, and excretion of these products has been shown to rise with increased intakes of vitamin C [110].

Deficiency

An adequate intake of vitamin C is necessary for normal development, with symptoms of deficiency developing with too little intake. Scurvy is the pathognomonic disease associated with vitamin C deficiency, characterized by follicular hyperkeratosis, petechial hemorrhages, ecchymosis, coiled hairs, inflamed and bleeding gums, perifollicular hemorrhages, joint effusions, arthralgia, and impaired wound healing [111,112]. Scurvy had historically led to high mortality rates particularly among sailors on long-term sea voyages, until James Lind, a Royal Navy surgeon, discovered in the 18th century that citrus fruits could treat scurvy. Other signs and symptoms associated with vitamin C deficiency include anemia, impaired ability to fight infections, epistaxis, possible weight gain due to slowed metabolism, rough, dry scaly skin, and weakened tooth enamel.

Toxicity

Toxicity of vitamin C is rare. Symptoms that have been noted in individuals taking high doses include nausea and vomiting but more noteworthy is a dose-dependent osmotic diarrhea. Certain populations should exercise caution when considering supplemental vitamin C. Most notable are those with a history of renal failure, nephrolithiasis (increased oxalate formation), iron overload disease (increases the absorption of iron), and those on anticoagulation therapy; all should avoid ingestion of high doses of supplemental vitamin C [113].

Vitamin C and chemoprevention

Two-time Nobel Laureate Linus Pauling first proposed that vitamin C had chemopreventive properties in the 1970s. Subsequently, a number of investigations have been conducted regarding a possible chemoprotective effect of vitamin C on gastrointestinal cancers, but the findings to date have been discordant.

Colorectal cancer

A case–control study looking at vitamin C intake from both food and supplements found that increased intake from these sources was associated with a decreased risk of rectal cancer [114]. On the other hand, the Iowa Women's Cohort Study found no association between vitamin C intake and risk of colorectal cancer, although when they compared women taking supplements (more than 60 mg/day) versus no supplements, they found a 30% risk reduction [115].

Gastric cancer

Increased vitamin C status has been associated epidemiologically and experimentally with decreased reactive oxygen species/reactive nitrogen species activity and oxidant damage in the gastric mucosa, suggesting a possible protective effect against development of gastric cancer [116–118]. However, some studies found that vitamin C supplementation did not decrease the incidence of gastric cancers in the populations studied [116,119].

Pancreatic cancer

Some studies have shown that an increased intake of vitamin C was associated with a decreased risk of pancreatic cancer [120–122]. A multinational case–control study with 802 cases and 1669 controls corroborated prior studies when they found an inverse relationship between vitamin C and pancreatic cancer [123].

Fat-soluble vitamins (Table 22.2)

Vitamins A, D, E, and K are unlike the water-soluble vitamins due to their solubility in lipid solvents, their predominant roles as cell-signaling molecules, and their sequestration or storage in cellular organelles. Because of their nonpolar properties, the fat-soluble vitamins are usually found in the lipophilic core or domain of proteins, cellular membranes, or micellar structures. As a consequence, the essential features of digestion and assimilation of the fat-soluble vitamins involve the interaction of receptors and transporters for fat-soluble vitamins with intestinal mixed micelles and lipoprotein particles [124]. Symptoms of mild deficiencies of the fat-soluble vitamins may develop as a consequence of decreased absorption of dietary lipid or abnormal systemic metabolism of lipids [125].

Vitamin A

Function, structure, sources, and requirements

Vitamin A includes dietary retinol in its esterified form and the provitamin carotenoid precursors of retinal. The most important of the vitamin A precursors are β-carotene and the essential retinoids that include retinal, retinol (vitamin A), and retinoic acid. Vitamin A is essential for normal vision, for dark adaptation, and for epithelial cell differentiation [126,127]. Retinal is a necessary structural component of rhodopsin, the light-sensitive pigment within the rod and cone cells of the retina.

Carotenoids comprise a group of more than 700 compounds that most often contain red, yellow, and orange pigments in their isolated states and are found in many fruits and vegetables [128]. In plants and many single-cell organisms, carotenoids serve as mediators of photoenergy-related processes. β-Carotene is abundant and therefore is an excellent biomarker of the intake of fruits and vegetables. Lycopene is another carotenoid found in fruits and vegetables, especially tomatoes. Lutein and zeaxanthin are carotenoids found in green leafy vegetables that are associated with a decrease in the risk of cataracts. Other sources of vitamin A in animal products include retinol in its retinyl ester form, which is found in liver, eggs, and milk products [124,128]. The RDA for vitamin A as retinol equivalents (RE) is 900 μg/day for men, 700 μg/day for women, 750 μg/day during pregnancy, and 1200 μg/day during lactation [126].

Absorption and homeostasis

Carotenoids and retinoids that are released from food during digestion are first partitioned into micelles within the intestinal lumen. The retinoids in the micelles are hydrolyzed by specific pancreatic esterases to retinol, whereas the carotenoids are cleaved to form retinal. The movement of retinyl esters and carotenoids into the enterocytes involves both active and facilitated transport mechanisms. Within the enterocyte, retinol is transported to the smooth endoplasmic reticulum for reesterification and eventual incorporation into chylomicrons in preparation for subsequent transport as retinyl esters via the lymphatic vessels to the liver. In contrast, retinoic acid, which constitutes less than 5% of the total vitamin-related products, can be transported through the portal circulation by mechanisms similar to those for free fatty acids [124].

Retinyl esters are stored in the liver as fat droplets in the hepatic stellate cells. Carotenoids that reach the liver intact are transported together to the circulation in association with very-low-density lipoprotein and are eventually converted to retinoids by tissue oxygenases. In the liver, active exchange of retinyl esters and other retinoids occurs between hepatic stellate cells and parenchymal hepatocytes [124]. Excess vitamin A is rapidly converted to retinyl ester and is sequestered in lipid vacuoles within the hepatic stellate cells. As vitamin A is needed, retinyl ester is hydrolyzed and released as retinol bound to retinol-binding protein (RBP). When released into the circulation, RBP exists as a complex not only with vitamin A, but also with another protein, transthyretin, which binds thyroxine. The primary targets for the RBP–transthyretin complex are the epithelial cells of the fetus, gastrointestinal mucosa, reproductive tract, pulmonary secretory cells, and

Table 22.2 Fat-soluble vitamins.

	Vitamin A	Vitamin D	Vitamin E	Vitamin K
Dietary source	Carotenoids: green, yellow vegetables Vitamin A: liver, kidney, milk, butter, egg yolk	Fish oils, liver, fortified milk and cereals, egg yolk	Soy, corn, sunflower, safflower oils, almonds, avocado	Dark green leafy vegetables, liver, intestinal bacteria
Daily requirement	900 μg RE men, 700 μg RE women, 750 μg pregnancy, 1200 μg lactation	600 IU, age 70 or younger 800 IU, older than age 70	15 mg adults 19 mg lactation	120 μg men, 90 μg women, 90 μg pregnancy and lactation
Absorption	Pancreatic esterase, micelle incorporation, facilitated transport, carotenoids cleaved by intestinal monooxygenase	Micelle incorporation, facilitated diffusion	Micelle incorporation, passive and facilitated diffusion	Phylloquinone: micelle incorporation, passive and facilitated diffusion Menaquinone: uncertain
Function	Vision, cell differentiation, immune (particularly T and B cell) function	Calcium absorption and homeostasis	Antioxidant	Blood clotting: γ-carboxylation of clotting factors II, VII, IX, X; bone mineralization through osteocalcin
Clinical signs of deficiency	Night blindness, xerophthalmia, corneal ulceration, hyperkeratosis, infection risk	Rickets (children), osteoporosis, potential for immune compromise	Abnormal peripheral vision, peripheral neuropathy, hemolysis (newborns)	Decreased blood clotting, osteoporosis
Risks for deficiency	Protein malnourishment in infants, chronic alcoholism, intestinal malabsorption (e.g., short bowel syndrome, celiac disease)	Lack of sunshine, intestinal malabsorption (e.g., short bowel syndrome, celiac disease)	Intestinal malabsorption, especially short bowel syndrome, cholestasis	Intestinal malabsorption, prolonged use of antibiotics
Overconsumption	Nausea and irritability, blurred vision, growth retardation, enlargement of liver and spleen, hair loss, bone pain, increased spinal fluid pressure, skin changes	Nausea and weight loss, irritability, soft tissue calcification, kidney damage	Possible increase in coagulation/ prothrombin time	Few signs
Diagnosis	HPLC	Competitive protein binding of 25(OH)D	HPLC	Prothrombin response to vitamin K

HPLC, high-performance liquid chromatography; RE, retinol equivalent: 1 μg retinol or 24 μg mixed carotenes.

salivary gland. Within targeted cells, vitamin A interacts with cellular-binding proteins that control its subsequent cellular translocation and metabolism; for example, oxidation to retinal or to retinoic acid [124].

Deficiency

If inadequate quantities of vitamin A are present, vision is impaired. The identification of two families of nuclear receptors, retinoic acid receptors (RAR) and retinoid receptors (RAX), has helped to delineate the role of vitamin A in cell differentiation. RAX and RAR are essential for the regulation of several hundred genes, particularly those involved in epithelial and immune cell differentiation. Skin lesions and increased susceptibility to infection are common signs of vitamin A deficiency [124,129]. Further, the epithelial layers of cells become hyperkeratotic and may undergo metaplasia. Defects in the corneal epithelium can result in xerophthalmia, which may progress to the appearance of conjunctival white deposits known as Bitot spots, and eventually corneal ulceration, scarring, and permanent blindness. Vitamin A deficiency also results in decreased fluid secretion and phagocytic activity of natural killer cells. International vitamin A supplementation programs yield improvements in innate immune function and have significantly reduced life-threatening infections, especially pathogen-induced diarrhea, in children worldwide [124]. Nevertheless, much of the world's preventable blindness continues to be the result of vitamin A deficiency [130].

Individuals with gastrointestinal diseases that result in poor absorption of lipids, including impaired pancreatic or biliary secretions, Crohn's disease, celiac disease, radiation enteritis, and short bowel syndrome, are at risk of vitamin A deficiency. Vitamin A status may also be influenced and augmented by other dietary factors. Protein deficiency contributes to decreased RBP production [124]. Vitamin A deficiency is also common in patients with alcoholic liver disease [125]. Conversely, the signs of supplemental vitamin A hepatotoxicity are enhanced by chronic alcoholism [131].

Excessive alcohol consumption can also interfere with the metabolism of supplemental carotenoids and result in the production of carcinogens, particularly in alcoholics who smoke [124]. In the setting of chronic alcoholism, vitamin A deficiency may also induce the development of esophageal squamous cell cancer [132]. In spite of evidence that retinoids may prevent carcinogenesis in vitro, the use of vitamin A and carotenoids in cancer prevention is unproven. The incidence of lung cancer was increased by 28% among smokers participating in the Carotene and Retinol Efficacy Trial (CARET) [133]. While the incidence of breast cancer was found to be inversely proportional to total daily vitamin A intake in one study of premenstrual women [134], another study showed no relationship between serum retinol concentrations and breast cancer risk [135]. The increased consumption of dietary lycopene from tomatoes may be associated with a reduced risk of prostate cancer [136].

Toxicity

Vitamin A toxicity can occur with long-term daily ingestion of 25 000–50 000 IU, amounts that are easily obtained from over-the-counter supplements. Because vitamin A can be teratogenic in high doses, women who are pregnant should not exceed the RDA.

Symptoms of acute toxicity include nausea, headache, abdominal pain, fatigue, loss of appetite, dizziness, loss of skin, and cerebral edema. Chronic toxicity (chronic hypervitaminosis A) typically occurs after long-term ingestion of vitamin A in excess of 50 000 IU/day for more than 3 months. Doses of vitamin A in this range can lead to bone and muscle pain because of increased periosteal resorption. Other less specific symptoms include dry, itchy and cracking skin, desquamation, dry lips, scaling, anorexia, headache, psychiatric changes, cerebral edema (excess fluid), bone and joint pain, osteoporosis (bone loss), and hip fracture [126] (Box 22.2). Carotenoids, in contrast, are generally nontoxic, and may be ingested in gram amounts on a daily basis with no deleterious effects [124].

Box 22.2 Vitamin A toxicity and pseudotumor cerebri.

Pseudotumor cerebri is a condition of increased intercranial pressure in the absence of a mass lesion. It can occur as a manifestation of acute hypervitaminosis A [137,138]. The condition is seen in only 1–2 per 100 000 but is more frequent in the obese and in females. Many diseases have been associated with pseudotumor cerebri, including sleep apnea syndrome, anemia, Behçet syndrome, Addison disease, polycystic ovarian syndrome, and systemic lupus erythematosus. Use of tetracycline and growth hormone has also been linked to increased risk of pseudotumor cerebri. Clinical suspicion should be raised in an individual with a history of excessive vitamin A intake presenting with severe headache, diplopia, dizziness, and brief episodes of blindness or flashing lights. Blurring of the optic disk can be seen on fundoscopic examination and, although not pathognomonic, supports the diagnosis [139,140].

Method of assessing status

Vitamin A is measured by HPLC of plasma or serum. Radial immunodiffusion assays are also available. A liver biopsy provides the most accurate assessment but this is not done on a routine clinical basis. Levels of plasma RBP are decreased in severe protein–calorie malnutrition, acute and chronic infection, and trauma.

Vitamin D

Function, structure, sources, and requirements

Vitamin D represents a group of secosteroid compounds that are necessary for the homeostasis of calcium. They include ergocalciferol (vitamin D_2, mainly derived from plant sources), and cholecalciferol (vitamin D_3, mainly endogenously produced and found in animal products) (Box 22.3). Vitamin D has multiple functions as listed in Box 22.4, but its principal function is to maintain serum calcium and phosphorus at normal physiological levels. According to the National Health and Nutrition Examination Survey (NHANES) of 2005–2006, approximately 41.6% of participants aged >20 years had 25-hydroxyvitamin D concentrations below 20 ng/mL [141].

There are currently three main sources of vitamin D: dietary intake, supplementation, and endogenous production from exposure to ultraviolet light (see Box 22.3). The body can

Box 22.3 Sources of vitamin D.

Endogenous production: occurs when the skin is exposed to solar or artificial ultraviolet light. 7-Dehydrocholesterol (usually found in epidermal keratinocytes and dermal fibroblasts) on exposure to ultraviolet light is converted to previtamin D, and subsequently isomerized to cholecalciferol (D3)

Dietary intake:

- Seafood: swordfish, salmon, tuna, sardines
- Dairy: milk (fortified), yogurt, margarine, cheese
- Orange juice (fortified)
- Beef liver
- Supplements

Box 22.4 Functions of vitamin D.

1. *Maintenance of calcium and phosphorus serum levels*

   Increases intestinal absorption of calcium and phosphorus [150]

   Direct suppression of parathyroid hormone (PTH)

   Regulation of osteoblast function [150]

   Permissively allowing PTH-induced osteoclast activation/maturation [150]

   Increasing bone resorption of calcium and phosphorus

2. *Cell differentiation*

   Promotes enterocyte differentiation

   Growth and maturation of hematopoietic and immune cells [168]

3. *Immune functions* [169]

   T lymphocytes

   Antigen or lecithin stimulated human and murine T-lymphocyte proliferation, cytokine secretion and cell cycle progression from G1a to G1b are inhibited by vitamin D_3 [170]

   Inhibition of IL-12, IFN-γ, and IL-2 release [171]

   Inhibition of antigen-specific T-cell activation [172,173]

   IL-4, IL-5, IL-10 production increased [174]

   B cells

   Vitamin D receptor (VDR) expression in B cells [175]

   Suppression of IgE secretion [175]

   Natural killer cells

   IFN-γ downregulation [176,177]

   Antigen-presenting cells (APCs): monocytes, macrophages, dendritic cells

   Downregulation of the surface expression of costimulatory receptors (CD40, CD80, and D86) and other maturation-induced proteins (CD1a, CD83) [178]

   Downregulation of MHC class II molecule expression on APCs [179–181]

   Inhibition of the dendritic cell maturation [179,182,183]

   Increase the chemotactic and phagocytic capacity of monocytes, and the tumor cell cytotoxicity and microbial activity of monocytes [178,184,185]

   Induction of tolerogenic dendritic cells that are able to induce T-regulatory cells [186]

4. *Antiinflammatory function*

   Increasing its possible utility in prevention and management of disease conditions including cancer, autoimmune diseases, and heart disease [187–190]

IFN, interferon; IL, interleukin.

synthesize adequate amounts of D_3 with reasonable exposure to sunlight, more commonly occurring in people living in the tropical and temperate regions of the world. There is nonetheless a relative concern that overexposure to ultraviolet radiation can lead to increased incidence of skin cancer.

The RDA for vitamin D, assuming the absence of sun exposure, is 15 μg/day (600 IU/day) for adults below the age of 70, 20 μg/day (800 IU/day) for adults above the age of 70, and 15 μg/day (600 IU/day) during pregnancy or lactation [142]. Dietary or supplementation needs may be higher during states of chronic inflammation or malabsorption, although there are no guidelines to quantitatively specify requirements in these disease states.

When adequate serum concentrations of 25(OH)D cannot be maintained by sun exposure and/or dietary sources alone, the use of vitamin D supplements is necessary [142]. Vitamin D is available as vitamin D_2 (ergocalciferol) and vitamin D_3 (cholecalciferol), although ergocalciferol has been shown to be only 30% as effective as cholecalciferol in its ability to maintain 25(OH)D levels [143]. Given the lower efficacy of ergocalciferol, a dose three times that of cholecalciferol can be considered. However, studies have provided recommendations [144–148]. One study recommended a dose of 50 000 IU of vitamin D_2 weekly for 8 weeks, followed by 50 000 IU of D_2 every 2–4 weeks [149]; another study suggested a dose of 50 000–100 000 IU of D_2 taken weekly [145]; and a third study proposed a dose of at least 600 000 IU of D_2 given over a period of 60 ± 40 days [144]. Pepper et al. retrospectively looked at three repletion regimens: 50 000 IU of D_2 once weekly for 4 weeks followed by 50 000 IU monthly for 5 months; 50 000 IU of D_2 once monthly for 6 months; and 50 000 IU of D_2 three times weekly for 6 weeks. They found that each of the three regimens significantly increased serum vitamin D levels, but this occurred in 38%, 42%, and 82%, respectively, of the populations reviewed [144]. More studies are needed to determine reliable repletion regimens and duration of treatment using vitamin D_2, as these are currently being guided by laboratory results, which can be both inconvenient and expensive.

Homeostasis and regulation

Vitamin D homeostasis is closely tied to that of calcium and phosphorus and is mediated via parathyroid hormone (PTH). Vitamin D undergoes two hydroxylation reactions – at the carbon 25 and the carbon 1 positions – before it becomes biologically active [150]. The first hydroxylation reaction occurs in the endoplasmic reticulum of the hepatocyte when vitamin D is delivered to the liver and converted by the enzyme 25-hydroxylase to 25-hydroxyvitamin D_3 (also known as calcidiol) [150]. This enzyme is regulated by overall vitamin D status and has been observed to be upregulated in states of vitamin D deprivation [151]. The second and final hydroxylation reaction occurs in the kidneys, catalyzed by 25-hydroxy-D3-1-α-hydroxylase, to form 1,25-dihydroxyvitamin D_3 (also known as calcitriol), the physiologically active form of the vitamin. This enzyme is tightly regulated and affected by factors that influence calcium homeostasis. Stimulating factors include a decrease in serum calcitriol, low serum calcium, and low PTH levels; inhibiting factors include an accumulation of calcitriol, high serum calcium, high dietary intake of phosphorus, and fibroblast growth factor 23 (FGF23) [152].

Absorption and transport

Most vitamin D absorption occurs in the distal small intestine, with a slightly more rapid uptake occurring in the duodenum [150]. About 80% of dietary vitamin D is absorbed after incorporation into micelles; it then undergoes passive (facilitated) diffusion into the enterocytes with fat and bile salts. Once in the enterocyte, vitamin D is incorporated into chylomicrons and moves to the lymphatic system from where it is transported to the blood and finally to the liver. Some of the vitamin D in chylomicrons is transferred to a vitamin D-binding protein (DBP) for transport to extrahepatic (muscle and adipose) tissue. DBP (also known as group-specific component [Gc] and vitamin D-binding α-globulin) is a member of the albumin, α-fetoprotein, and albumin/afamin gene family [153]. After binding to DBP, endogenously produced vitamin D is primarily transported to the liver, with some being transported to muscle and adipose tissue along the way.

Excretion

A major proportion of vitamin D excretion occurs via the biliary system and the GI tract, with minimal amounts lost via the renal system in urine.

Deficiency

Clinical signs of vitamin D deficiency include rickets in children, osteomalacia in adults, hypocalcemia (which can cause tetany and seizures), low bone mineral density, and osteoporosis. In the past, severe vitamin D deficiency was common and resulted in a high prevalence of rickets in children. However, with the introduction of formula and food fortification and vitamin supplementation, the prevalence of rickets has dramatically declined in industrialized nations. Certain populations and disease states have been firmly associated with vitamin D deficiency, while some have been postulated to be associated with vitamin D deficiency, although without definitive proof of a causal relationship. These are listed in Box 22.5.

Box 22.5 Conditions associated with vitamin D deficiency.

Populations/disease states associated with vitamin D deficiency

- Elderly
- Exclusively breastfed infants
- Gastric surgery, e.g., resection, bypass
- Hepatic disease
- High-altitude dwellers
- Malabsorptive states, e.g., celiac disease, primary biliary cirrhosis, short gut syndrome
- Malnourished children, children with chronic illnesses
- Medications: antiepileptic medications phenobarbital, phenytoin
- Nursing home residents
- Parenteral nutrition long term
- Renal disease
- Sunlight: populations with minimal exposure to sunlight, including total covering of skin, sedentary indoors, daily sunscreen use

Postulated conditions associated with vitamin D deficiency

- Multiple sclerosis [191]
- Type 1 diabetes mellitus [192]
- Rheumatoid arthritis [193]
- Inflammatory bowel disease [194]
- Mood disorders [195]
- Cancer: breast [196,197], colon [198,199], prostate [200]
- Hypertension [201]
- Hyperglycemia [201]
- Metabolic syndrome [201]
- Upper respiratory tract infections [202]
- Asthma [203,204]

Toxicity

Vitamin D toxicity tends to occur from inappropriate intake of supplements. The DRI was updated in 2010 by the Food and Nutrition Board (FNB), Institute of Medicine of the National Academies, and the recommended "tolerable upper intake levels" for vitamin D are 100 μg/day (4000 IU/day) for any person >9 years old [142]. For ethical reasons, there have been no studies performed on humans evaluating the effects of vitamin D toxicity, but there have been published reports of vitamin D toxicity, usually from accidental ingestion [154–165]. Most of the reports had measured 25(OH)D, which were reported as elevated, ranging from 710 to 1587 nmol/L. Two reviews of the reports on vitamin D toxicity concluded that hypercalcemia will only result when the 25(OH)D_3 concentrations have been consistently above 375–500 nmol/L [166,167]. Clinical symptoms of acute intoxication of vitamin D, summarized in Table 22.2, are for the most part related to hypercalcemia and include polyuria, polydipsia, anorexia, nausea, emesis, muscle weakness, confusion, nephrocalcinosis, bone demineralization, and pain.

Assessment of status

The FNB of the Institute of Medicine recommends that the most reliable biochemical marker of vitamin D status is serum 25(OH)D [142]. The half-life of serum 25(OH)D is 15 days and encompasses endogenously produced vitamin D as well as dietary and supplemental vitamin D. It does not indicate the amounts of vitamin D stored in body tissues. Serum 1,25$(OH)_2$D is not recommended as an indicator of vitamin D status, because amounts present in serum are tightly regulated by osteometabolic pathways and may not adequately reflect overall vitamin D status [142]. According to the FNB, levels of 25(OH)D in excess of 50 nmol/L (>20 ng/mL) are sufficient to promote bone and overall health in most people. Concentrations of 25(OH)D below 30 nmol/L (<20 ng/mL) are associated with rickets in children and osteomalacia in adults, whereas evidence suggests an increased risk of adverse effects when serum 25(OH)D concentrations exceed 125 nmol/L [142].

Chemoprevention

Vitamin D may theoretically have chemopreventive effects on cancers through regulation of its involvement in cell differentiation, proliferation, and apoptosis. Laboratory investigations suggest that vitamin D may aid in chemoprevention of colon cancer by promoting apoptosis, especially in upper regions of mucosal crypts [205]. In view of these and other regulatory effects, several studies suggest that vitamin D supplementation may be beneficial in the prevention of certain malignancies and may also influence the course of autoimmunity [187,188,206]. A small study showed preventive benefits in recurrence of prostate cancer [207] and a case–control study found an inverse association of plasma levels of 25(OH)D_3 with the risk of precancerous colonic adenomas [208]. However, a Women's Health Initiative (WHI) trial involving 36 282 postmenopausal women – the largest randomized, placebo-controlled trial to date – did not find that 1000 mg of calcium and 400 IU of vitamin D_3 per day, when compared with placebo, reduced the incidence of primary colorectal cancer (168 vs 154 cases; hazard ratio 1.08; 95% confidence interval [CI] 0.86–1.34; $p = 0.51$) over a 7-year study period [209]. Another large multinational randomized placebo-controlled trial involving 427 patients with one or more sporadic adenomas did not find 3-year adenoma recurrence rates to differ between patients receiving the combination of 0.5 µg/day calcitriol, 75 mg/day acetylsalicylic acid, and 1250 mg/day calcium carbonate, or placebo [210].

Nonetheless, a subsequent metaanalysis found that higher doses of vitamin D (1000–2000 IU/day) might reduce the incidence of colorectal cancer with minimal risk [211]. A metaanalysis by Lee et al. reported that serum 25(OH)D levels are inversely associated with colon and rectal cancer, with a stronger association for rectal cancer [212]. Gandini et al. demonstrated an inverse association between serum levels of 25(OH)D and risk of colorectal cancer [213]. In a metaanalysis of dietary vitamin D status and colorectal cancer incidence, Ma et al. concluded that a 10 ng/mL increment in serum 25(OH)D reduced the risk of colorectal cancer by approximately 25% (relative risk 0.74; 95% CI 0.63–0.89) [214]. The currently available data on the association of vitamin D and the risk of colorectal cancer are inconsistent, but the evidence seems to suggest that vitamin D and the vitamin D receptor (VDR) genotype affect colorectal cancer risk differently in various gender, racial, and ethnic groups.

Crohn's disease

Vitamin D has been suggested to play a role in the pathogenesis, prevention, and treatment of inflammatory bowel disease (IBD) (see Chapter 64). Local activation of vitamin D coordinates the activity of the innate and adaptive arms of immunity and of the intestinal epithelium in a manner that promotes barrier integrity, facilitates the clearance of translocated flora, and diverts CD4 T-cell development away from inflammatory phenotypes. Vitamin D deficiency aggravates IBD in mouse models, while administration of vitamin D has a therapeutic benefit [194,215,216]. Several polymorphisms have also been identified in the *VDR* gene [217].

Clinical data on the role of vitamin D in IBD are nonetheless inconsistent. Results of the Nurses' Health Study revealed that higher estimated concentrations of 25(OH)D are associated with a lower risk of developing Crohn's disease, but not for ulcerative colitis [218]. However, the only three studies thus far that directly measured 25(OH)D concentrations prior to diagnosis of Crohn's disease did not find an association between vitamin D and incident Crohn's disease [219,220,221]. Vitamin D levels were nonetheless found to be low after diagnosis of Crohn's disease. This is not surprising, as patients with IBD are generally at risk for vitamin D deficiency from alteration of diet (e.g., avoidance of vitamin D-fortified milk), malabsorption, and limitations on outdoor activity while ill. Inflammation can also lead to increased utilization/consumption of vitamin D [222].

Clinical trials have evaluated the effects of vitamin D in patients with Crohn's disease. In the largest double-blind placebo-controlled trial involving 94 patients with quiescent Crohn's disease, participants were randomized to either receive 1200 IU/day vitamin D or placebo in addition to 1200 mg calcium daily. The study found that vitamin D insignificantly reduced the risk of clinical relapse from 29% to 13% ($p = 0.06$) [223]. In an open-label pilot study, vitamin D_3 oral therapy was initiated at 1000 IU/day and after 2 weeks, the dose was escalated incrementally until patients' serum concentrations reached 40 ng/mL 25(OH)D_3 or they were taking 5000 IU/day [224]. Vitamin D oral supplementation significantly increased serum 25(OH)D_3 levels from 16 ± 10 ng/mL to 45 ± 19 ng/mL ($p < 0.0001$) and reduced the unadjusted mean Crohn's disease activity index (CDAI) scores from 230 ± 74 to 118 ± 66 ($p < 0.0001$). Quality-of-life scores also improved following vitamin D supplementation ($p = 0.0004$). Twenty-four weeks' supplementation with up to 5000 IU/day vitamin D_3 effectively raised serum 25(OH)D_3 and reduced CDAI scores in Crohn's disease patients, suggesting that restoration of normal vitamin D serum levels may be useful in the management of patients with mild-to-moderate Crohn's disease. At the moment, the role of vitamin D as a treatment for IBD is still unclear.

Patients with IBD are at risk for metabolic bone disease due to restrictive dietary habits, malabsorption, and/or the use of glucocorticoids. Vitamin D and calcium supplementation should be considered in this patient population when deficiency has been identified based on routine assessments for bone health.

Vitamin E

Function, structure, sources, and requirements

Vitamin E comprises eight tocopherols, two of which, α-tocopherol and γ-tocopherol, are the most important in human nutrition. The predominant natural form of vitamin E is the *RRR*-α-tocopherol isomer [225]. The major food sources of vitamin E include polyunsaturated vegetable and seed oils, whole grains, nuts, and green leafy vegetables. The RDA of vitamin E is 15 mg/day for adults of all ages, 15 mg/day during pregnancy, and 19 mg/day during lactation [226].

Absorption and homeostasis

The intestinal absorption of dietary vitamin E includes deesterification by pancreatic esterases, followed by bile-dependent incorporation into intralumenal micelles, diffusion, or facilitative transport into enterocytes, and incorporation into chylomicrons for transfer in lymphatics. After peripheral hydrolysis of chylomicrons, vitamin E as *RRR*-α-tocopherol returns to the liver with chylomicron remnants and is then transferred by hepatic α-tocopherol transfer protein to high-density or low-density lipoprotein. The subsequent transfer to tissues occurs by receptor-mediated endocytosis of low-density lipoprotein. As a consequence, plasma levels of α-tocopherol vary according to the total plasma lipid concentration and often correlate with values for total cholesterol. Once within cells, vitamin E is incorporated into lipid membranes, about 40% into nuclear membranes, and the remaining 60% into lysosomal, mitochondrial, and outer cell wall membranes. The efflux of vitamin E from cells is less well understood, but it appears to be dependent on the ATP-requiring transporters associated with the cholesterol transporter family [227].

Tocopherols are unique because they act as chemical antioxidants, although possible roles in cell signaling have also been described [227,228]. Vitamin E protects unsaturated fatty acids found in the phospholipids of cell membranes. Cell membranes contain vitamin E at a concentration of about 1 mg per 5–10 g of membrane lipid, a concentration sufficient to retard membrane lipid oxidation. Membrane lipids are constantly engaged in the process of turnover and repair, and vitamin E in membranes is consumed while inhibiting the formation of lipid-derived oxidation products. By prolonging the initiation time before a free-radical chain reaction occurs, vitamin E gives cells time to replace damaged membrane lipids through the process of normal cell turnover [228].

Deficiency

Vitamin E deficiency is rare, although it occurs mainly in patients with malabsorptive disorders involving the biliary circulation, pancreas, and intestinal mucosa. Some infants can also be at risk because their body stores of vitamin E are lower. Children with biliary atresia or other causes of cholestasis become depleted more rapidly than older children and adults with malabsorption diseases [229]. Vitamin E deficiency is manifested by neurological damage involving the posterior columns, cranial nerves, brainstem, and peripheral nerves, with loss of balance and peripheral neuropathy, and by retinal damage with visual field defects [227]. A water-soluble form of vitamin E, *RRR*-α-tocopherol glycol (Aquasol E), is better absorbed than the dietary, fat-soluble natural vitamin and hence is more effective in the treatment or prevention of vitamin E deficiency in malabsorption diseases such as short bowel syndrome [229].

Toxicity

Vitamin E toxicity has not been demonstrated to occur through consumption of natural food sources, although elevated levels of vitamin E can occur through consumption of fortified foods and supplements. Few adverse effects have been documented in short-term doses below 2100 mg/day of *RRR*-α-tocopherol, although the threshold for toxicity is believed to be lower when taken chronically. Vitamin E toxicity has been associated with an increased risk of mortality and hemorrhagic stroke.

Method of assessing status

Vitamin E status is assessed by HPLC measurement of plasma concentrations. Normal concentrations of α-tocopherol are greater than 12 μmol/L (5 μg/mL). However, because the plasma level of vitamin E is regulated in part by plasma lipid concentrations, more correct values include α-tocopherol at greater than 8 mg per the sum of triglycerides and total cholesterol concentrations, or 2.8 mg per g total cholesterol [227].

Supplementation studies

Vitamin E supplementation in the form of *RRR*-α-tocopherol at daily doses up to 800 IU has been used in several trials for the prevention of cardiovascular disease, with conflicting and nonconclusive results; furthermore, vitamin E carries the risk of increasing bleeding when combined with aspirin [227]. Other diseases associated with an inconclusive preventive effect of vitamin E supplementation include Alzheimer disease, several cancers, and cataracts [227]. One study suggested a positive effect of vitamin E over placebo in improvement of nonalcoholic steatohepatitis [230]. Although many food sources of vitamin E contain both α and γ forms of tocopherol, the functional potency of supplemental γ-tocopherol is only about 10% that of α-tocopherol [227].

Vitamin K

Function, structure, sources, and requirements

The major function of vitamin K is to activate blood clotting by serving as a cofactor for microsomal synthesis of γ-carboxyglutamic acid (Gla) residues, which permit the formation of specific calcium-binding sites in prothrombin (factor II) and factors VII, IX, and X. Gla residues are also found in proteins C and S, which are anticoagulants by virtue of their ability to inhibit factor V [231]. Vitamin K is also essential for the γ-carboxylation of osteocalcin, an osteoblast protein that is upregulated by $1\alpha,25(OH)_2D_3$. Vitamin K activity is associated with phylloquinone (K1) and menaquinone (K2–5) derivatives of

1,4-naphthoquinone [231]. The main dietary sources of phylloquinone are dark green leafy vegetables and some vegetable oils. There is no precise RDA for vitamin K. The recommended adequate intake for dietary phylloquinone is 120 μg/day in men, 90 μg/day in women, 90 μg/day during pregnancy, and 90 μg/day during lactation. Uncertain amounts are derived from intestinal bacterial synthesis of menaquinone (see Table 22.2) [232].

Absorption and homeostasis

As a fat-soluble vitamin, phylloquinone requires micellar solubilization before diffusion into enterocytes and uptake with chylomicrons. Phylloquinone circulates with chylomicrons with a high triglyceride level and very-low-density lipoproteins, and blood concentrations are dependent on plasma lipid concentrations. In contrast, menaquinones are synthesized by anaerobic intestinal bacteria and their route of absorption remains unclear [231].

Deficiency

Vitamin K deficiency may occur in neonates as a result of immature metabolic pathways, insufficient intestinal bacterial synthesis, and low levels in breast milk. Hemorrhagic disease of the newborn is prevented by a single injection of phylloquinone to all neonates, as recommended by the American Academy of Pediatrics [233]. Phylloquinone deficiency in adults occurs in biliary diseases, malabsorption disorders such as the short bowel syndrome, and celiac disease. Ineffective use of vitamin K occurs in individuals adhering to long-term regimens of the antagonist warfarin and in patients with severe liver disease that leads to impaired synthesis of coagulation factors irrespective of vitamin K adequacy. Also, long-term oral regimens of antibiotics may suppress menoquinone-synthesizing anaerobic bacteria and lead to vitamin K deficiency [231]. A large study of elderly people found that those in the highest quartile of dietary vitamin K intake had a reduced risk of hip fracture compared with those in the lowest quartile of vitamin K intake, although there was no relationship of these findings to bone mineral density measurements [234]. There is some evidence to suggest that high intake of menoquinone can inhibit coronary calcification, though optimal levels are not known, and intake has not been correlated with stroke risk [235]. Given vitamin K's role in the carboxylation of osteocalcin, a deficiency of vitamin K may contribute to osteoporosis, while vitamin K supplementation has been shown to prevent bone fractures [236].

Method of assessing status

Vitamin K deficiency can be assessed by a prolonged prothrombin time that responds to parenteral vitamin K administration [231] and by direct measurement of plasma concentrations of phylloquinone by HPLC.

Minerals

Minerals constitute about 5% of our diet and some are essential for normal health and bodily functions. Classification of minerals is somewhat controversial but one scheme that has been utilized by nutritionists is prioritization based upon the DRI for the mineral required with macrominerals (>100 mg/day required), microminerals (1–100 mg/day required), and trace minerals (<1 mg/day required) (Box 22.6).

A comprehensive discussion of each of these minerals could in itself constitute a textbook; this section will focus on a select group especially relevant to gastrointestinal tract disease. The healthcare provider caring for the patient with digestive disease should be familiar with calcium, magnesium, iron, zinc, copper, chromium, and selenium. The source, homeostasis/regulation, absorption/transport mechanism, excretion, functions, deficiency, and toxicity are discussed for each of these minerals. It is important to note that the minerals can influence the absorption and biological activities of each other and this should be taken into account when evaluating patients with potential mineral deficiencies.

Table 22.3 shows some dietary sources, recommended daily requirement, mechanism of absorption, primary functions, deficiency signs, and etiology of key minerals discussed in this section. Table 22.4 lists clinical signs and symptoms of deficiency and toxicity of the minerals discussed.

Box 22.6 Classification of minerals.

Macrominerals
- Calcium
- Chloride
- Magnesium
- Potassium
- Phosphate
- Sodium

Microminerals
- Copper
- Fluoride
- Iron
- Manganese
- Zinc

Trace minerals
- Arsenic
- Boron
- Chromium
- Iodine
- Nickel
- Selenium
- Silicon
- Vanadium

Table 22.3 Dietary sources, recommended daily requirement, mechanism of absorption, primary functions, deficiency signs, and etiology of selected minerals.

	Calcium	Magnesium	Iron	Zinc	Copper
Dietary source	Milk, dairy products, fortified juices, green vegetables, beans	Vegetables, fruits, dairy, animal products	Meat, fish, poultry, fortified cereals	Animal protein, seafood, especially oysters	Meat, grain, nuts
Daily requirement	1000 mg men and women 19–50 years 1200 mg females 51+ years and all adults >51 years	400–420 mg men 310–320 mg women	8 mg men 18 mg women 8 mg postmenopause	11 mg men 8 mg women	0.9 mg men and women
Absorption	Active transport by way of vitamin D; passive diffusion	Active transport, passive diffusion	Active transport, passive diffusion	Active transport, passive diffusion	Active transport, passive diffusion
Function	Bone formation; muscle and nerve function	Bone metabolism; nerve, muscle, cardiac functions	Oxygen transport as heme, energy metabolism, neurotransmitter synthesis	Cofactor for many enzymes involved in nucleic acid, protein, lipid, carbohydrate metabolism	Connective tissue synthesis, bone growth, ferroxidase activity
Causes of deficiency	Malabsorption, dietary inadequacy	Malabsorption, alcoholism, surgery, renal disease	Blood loss, malabsorption, achlorhydria, hookworm	Diarrhea, surgery, malabsorption, alcoholism	
Diagnosis	Bone density scan	Serum magnesium	Hemoglobin, iron-binding capacity, ferritin, transferrin receptor	Serum zinc	Serum copper, red cell superoxide dysmutase

Calcium

Calcium is considered a macromineral; it has been characterized as one of the most abundant ions in the body and is thought to constitute 1–2% of the total adult human body weight [237]. A large proportion (99%) of the calcium in the body is stored in teeth and bones, with the remaining 1% in the serum and distributed throughout the rest of the body. Only the calcium in bone is available for resorption when needed.

Dietary sources and requirements

The dietary sources of calcium are vast, with the main sources listed in Box 22.7. The RDA is 1000 mg/day for men below 70 years, 1200 mg/day for men above 70 years, 1000 mg/day for women up to 50 years, 1200 mg/day for women above 50 years, 1000 mg/day during pregnancy, and 1000 mg/day during lactation.

The dietary reference intake for calcium is shown in Table 22.3.

Homeostasis and regulation

The homeostasis and regulation of calcium for the most part involves the 1% of calcium in the serum and body tissues. Serum calcium exists in three forms: complexed calcium (calcium that is bound to nonprotein anions, including phosphate, citrate, and carbonate); protein-bound calcium (a high percentage of serum calcium is bound to some protein, with albumin being the major protein); and ionized calcium (the most physiologically important part of the calcium in serum, and considered the metabolically active form of calcium).

Serum calcium is influenced by a variety of metabolic conditions, most notably hypoalbuminemia. Serum calcium parallels serum albumin concentrations as calcium is extensively bound to albumin. Hypoalbuminemia is associated with a decrease in serum calcium due to a decrease in the available protein-bound calcium. It is important to note that although hypoalbuminemia will affect the total serum calcium, it does not cause changes to the ionized calcium levels. Factors that affect concentrations of the ionized calcium include changes in body pH (metabolic alkalosis will lead to a decrease in the ionized calcium as calcium binds more easily to proteins and vice versa in states of metabolic acidosis), and phosphorus (hyperphosphatemia leads to a decrease in the percentage of ionized calcium and hypophosphatemia increases ionized calcium).

Calcium is regulated via a complex mechanism involving PTH, vitamin D, calcitonin, and phosphorus [238]. PTH acts by increasing bone resorption of calcium, augmenting renal conservation of calcium, and activating vitamin D, which enhances the intestinal absorption of calcium. Conversely, calcitonin released by the thyroid gland acts by inhibiting bone resorption of calcium and augments renal excretion of calcium. PTH is released in response to low serum calcium levels and calcitonin is released in response to high serum calcium levels.

Table 22.4 Clinical signs and symptoms of mineral deficiencies and toxicity.

	Deficiency	Toxicity
Calcium (Ca^{2+})	Cardiovascular: hypotension, decreased myocardial contractility, prolonged QT interval Neuromuscular: tetany, distal extremity paresthesias, Chvostek sign, Trousseau sign, muscle cramps, seizures	Gastrointestinal: anorexia, nausea, emesis, bowel dysmotility, constipation, pancreatitis, peptic ulcer disease Cardiovascular: hypertension, bradycardia, shortening of the QT interval Musculoskeletal: generalized weakness, bone pain, osteopenia, osteoporosis Renal: polyuria, polydipsia, nephrolithiasis, nephrocalcinosis, distal renal tubular acidosis, nephrogenic diabetes insipidus, renal insufficiency Neurological: confusion, poor concentration, fatigue, stupor, coma
Magnesium (Mg^{2+})	Neuromuscular: hyperexcitablity (e.g., tetany: Trousseau and Chvostek signs, spontaneous carpal–pedal spasms, tremors, convulsions), weakness, fatigue, delirium, apathy, involuntary movements (athetoid/choreiform movements), coma Cardiovascular: QRS widening, peaked T waves, PR interval widening, diminution of T waves, atrial and ventricular arrhythmias, hypomagnesemia also potentiates the development of digoxin toxicity Electrolyte abnormalities: hypocalcemia, hypokalemia Gastrointestinal: loss of appetite, nausea, emesis	Gastrointestinal: nausea, emesis, Cardiovascular: bradycardia, hypotension Neuromuscular: drowsiness, muscle weakness, alteration in mental status Miscellaneous: diaphoresis, flushing, heat intolerance
Iron (Fe)	Hematological: anemia, poor capillary refill, pallor, Neuromuscular: weakness, fatigue, lightheadedness, headache, irritability, impaired intellectual and behavioral performance, restless leg syndrome Cardiovascular: exercise intolerance, shortness of breath, dyspnea on exertion, tachycardia, reduced work performance Immunological: decreased resistance to infections Miscellaneous: increased lead absorption, pica, pagophagia, beeturia	Gastrointestinal: nausea, emesis, hemorrhagic gastroenteritis Endocrine: hyperglycemia with metabolic acidosis
Zinc (Zn)	Dermatological: skin lesions (mostly located at the eyes, nose, mouth, gluteal region, and perianal skin) Ophthalmic: night vision dysfunction Endocrine: hypogonadism, dysguesia, anosmia, alopecia, Gastrointestinal: anorexia, diarrhea Immunological: immune dysfunction (especially T-cell dysfunction), impaired wound healing Neuropsychiatric: personality changes	Gastrointestinal: gastric distress, nausea, emesis Neurological: dizziness Immunological: decreased immune function Miscellaneous: copper deficiency
Copper (Cu)	Dermatological: skin depigmentation Neuromuscular: muscle weakness (myeloneuropathy), ataxia, neuropathy, and cognitive deficits Hematological: hepatosplenomegaly, anemia (usually microcytic and hypochromic), leukopenia, neutropenia, thrombocytopenia Endocrine: hypercholesterolemia Miscellaneous: fragile, brittle hair, peripheral edema	Gastrointestinal: abdominal pain, diarrhea, nausea, emesis, hepatic necrosis, cirrhosis Neurological: encephalopathy, Cardiovascular: cardiac failure Renal: renal failure Miscellaneous: death
Chromium (Cr)	Endocrine: impaired glucose tolerance, unfavorable lipid profiles	Dermatological: contact dermatitis, skin ulcers Pulmonary: bronchogenic cancers
Selenium (S)	Endocrine: thyroid hormone dysfunction Metabolism: metabolic effects of oxidative injury, alteration in biotransformation enzymes Musculoskeletal: skeletal muscle dysfunction Cardiovascular: cardiomyopathy Neuropsychiatric: mood dysfunction Hematological: macrocytosis Miscellaneous: whitening of the nail beds	Gastrointestinal: nausea, emesis, diarrhea Neurological: alteration in mental status, irritability, fatigue, peripheral neuropathy Miscellaneous: tooth decay, hair loss, nail deformity and loss

Absorption, transport, and excretion

Serum calcium accumulates for the most part via bone resorption and dietary intake. Active absorption dominates in times of low calcium intake, while passive absorption dominates in high-intake states. Absorption of calcium is possible once it is in the ionized form, which occurs in the stomach, followed by active absorption in the duodenum [239]; passive diffusion takes place in the ileum [239], and both active and passive processes in the

Box 22.7 Dietary sources of calcium.

Dairy products: milk, yogurt, ice cream, pudding, cheese (cream cheese, mozzarella, cheddar, cottage)

Seafood: sardines, pink salmon

Leafy vegetables: spinach, rhubarb, turnip greens, kale, Chinese cabbage

Nuts: almonds

Orange juice (fortified)

Corn tortilla, bread (white, whole wheat fortified)

colon [240]. Active transepithelial transport of calcium in the upper part of the duodenum is highly vitamin D dependent and is thought to involve three mechanisms: a group of nonvoltage-gated calcium channels [239]; a carrier-mediated facilitated diffusion via calcium-binding proteins (calbindin 3 [CALB3 or D9K] [241,242] and calbindin 1 [CALB1 or D28K], which is induced by vitamin D) [243]; and finally, calcium ATPase and the Na/Ca exchanger [243]. Passive calcium absorption is thought to occur via paracellular diffusion down a chemical gradient in all areas of the small intestine [239]. Several factors affect calcium absorption, including presence of oxalates, insufficient amounts of vitamin D, renal disease, alkalinity of the blood, and some medications (glucocorticoids and phenytoin have been implicated in decreasing the absorption of calcium, while thiazide diuretics increase the renal absorption of calcium).

The body maintains a delicate balance between excretion and absorption. The excretion of calcium usually occurs via renal mechanisms. Other vehicles of calcium excretion include sweat and feces. A few mechanisms are responsible for increased calcium excretion. Phytic acid combines with calcium to form unabsorbed calcium phytate excreted through the feces. Excess dietary protein [244], high caffeine intake [245], high sodium intake [245], and chronic alcohol intake [246] have also been implicated in increased calcium excretion.

Functions, deficiency, and toxicity

Calcium has been found to be essential for many physiological functions, including preservation of cell membrane integrity, neuromuscular activity, regulation of endocrine secretory activities, blood coagulation cascade, activation of the complement system, and invariably bone metabolism [247]. Normal serum calcium ranges from 8.5 to 10.5 mg/dL (2.12–2.62 mmol/L) with hypocalcemia defined as serum calcium concentrations below 8.5 mg/dL. Serum calcium is strictly maintained within a narrow range optimal for the many extra- and intracellular functions regulated by calcium.

Because of the ubiquitous binding of calcium to proteins (especially albumin), fluctuations in protein concentrations usually cause a decrease in the total calcium concentration, but usually not the ionized calcium level. The calculation for adjusting total calcium in states of hypoalbuminemia is given below. The corrected total calcium is usually higher than the measured level as the formula adjusts for the missing calcium–albumin binding complex and tries to estimate what the calcium concentration would be if the albumin concentration were normal.

$$\begin{aligned}&\text{Corrected total calcium}\left(\text{mg / dL}\right)\\&\quad=\text{measured total calcium}\left(\text{mg / dL}\right)+0.8\left[4-\text{albumin}\left(\text{g / dL}\right)\right]\end{aligned}$$

When the body pH fluctuates, it also affects the calcium concentrations by primarily affecting the calcium–albumin binding complex. Acidosis reduces the binding of calcium to albumin and alkalosis has the opposite effect. Hypocalcemia can occur when PTH is low (primary hypoparathyroidism), high (secondary hyperparathyroidism), or ineffective (either low or high). The possible etiologies of hypocalcemia are listed in Box 22.8.

The clinical manifestations of hypocalcemia are usually limited to the cardiovascular [248] (hypotension, decreased myocardial contractility, prolonged QT interval), and neuromuscular systems [248] (tetany, distal extremity paresthesias, Chovstek sign, Trousseau sign, muscle cramps, seizures), and symptoms related to the disease-specific condition.

Box 22.8 Etiology of hypocalcemia.

Hypocalcemia with low PTH

- Parathyroid gland destruction: postsurgical, autoimmune, irradiation, infiltration of gland (granulomatous, hemochromatosis, metastases)
- Hungry bone syndrome (postparathyroidectomy)
- HIV

Hypocalcemia with elevated PTH

- Renal disease (acute)
- Hyperphosphatemia
- Tumor lysis syndrome
- Acute pancreatitis
- Osteoblastic metastases
- Sepsis
- Respiratory alkalosis

Hypocalcemia with ineffective PTH

- Vitamin D deficiency
- PTH resistance: pseudohypoparathyroidism, hypomagnesemia
- Chronic renal disease
- Intestinal malabsorptive states (celiac, Crohn's disease, short bowel, etc.)
- Drugs: Bisphosphonates, Calcitonin, Cinacalcet, Citrate, Denosumab, EDTA, Foscarnet, Furosemide, Phenytoin, Phenobarbital

EDTA, ethylenediaminetetraacetate; PTH, parathyroid hormone.

The management of hypocalcemia initially takes into account whether the patient is symptomatic or not. In cases where the patient is asymptomatic, daily oral calcium repletion can be suggested. If the patient is symptomatic, treatment is usually required and the magnitude of the deficiency will determine the appropriate modality of repletion of calcium. Severe hypocalcemia (defined as serum calcium below 7.5 mg/dL) or acute symptomatic hypocalcemia usually requires quick correction with intravenous (IV) calcium gluconate or calcium chloride [249]. Continuous IV infusion of calcium may be required if intermittent boluses are not effective in correcting the hypocalcemia, as bolus doses have been shown to be effective for only 2 h or less [249]. Hypomagnesemia can also lead to calcium loss as it is necessary for PTH secretion and function. Indeed, in some patients with hypocalcemia due to low magnesium, magnesium repletion alone may lead to correction of low calcium concentrations [250,251]. When the etiology of the hypocalcemia is due to hyperphosphatemia, use of phosphate binders before calcium supplementation has been advocated to prevent formation of soft tissue calcification. Oral supplementation with calcium and vitamin D can be used to manage patients with chronic and asymptomatic hypocalcemia [252].

Hypercalcemia is defined as a total serum calcium concentration of >10.2 mg/dL. The two most common causes are hyperparathyroidism and malignancy. The clinical manifestations of hypercalcemia in the early stages are mostly nonspecific. If not recognized and treated, persistent or worsening hypercalcemia can lead to more serious consequences. The addition of serum calcium concentrations to the standard basic metabolic panel in most emergency rooms has generally resulted in quicker diagnosis and treatment. Clinical manifestations associated with hypercalcemia are myriad and include gastrointestinal (anorexia, nausea, emesis, bowel dysmotility, constipation, pancreatitis, peptic ulcer disease), cardiovascular (hypertension, bradycardia, shortening of the QT interval), musculoskeletal (generalized weakness, bone pain, osteopenia, osteoporosis), renal (polyuria, polydipsia, nephrolithiasis, nephrocalcinosis, distal renal tubular acidosis, nephrogenic diabetes insipidus, renal insufficiency), and neurological (confusion, poor concentration, fatigue, stupor, coma).

Hypercalcemia can be mediated by PTH or non-PTH mechanisms. The etiologies under each mechanism are listed in Box 22.9.

Box 22.9 Etiology of hypercalcemia.

Parathyroid hormone (PTH) mediated

- Primary hyperparathyroidism
- Multiple endocrine neoplasia I and IIa
- Familial hypocalciuric hypercalcemia
- Familial isolated hyperparathyroidism
- Tertiary hyperparathyroidism – renal failure

PTH independent

- Malignancy related: PTH-related protein (PTHrp), osteolytic bone metastases
- Multiple myeloma
- Vitamin D intoxication
- Chronic granulomatous disorders: activation of extrarenal 1α-hydroxylase (leads to increased calcitriol)
- Medications: thiazides, lithium, teriparatide, excess vitamin A, theophylline toxicity
- Hyperthyroidism
- Acromegaly
- Pheochromocytoma
- Adrenal insufficiency
- Immobilization for prolonged periods
- Parenteral nutrition
- Milk alkali syndrome

Calcium and disease outcomes

Calcium concentrations have been associated with a variety of disorders including colorectal cancer (CRC), cardiovascular disease (CVD), and obesity.

Colorectal cancer

The relationship between calcium intake and CRC risk remains unclear. Several studies have suggested a 20–30% reduction in adenoma and CRC risk when comparing high- and low-intake categories of calcium and vitamin D [253–263]. It appears that most of the protective effect noted in some of the studies was related to supplemental intake and not dietary intake only [253,254,258–260]. A metaanalysis of five randomized trials also found calcium supplementation to possibly reduce the risk of recurrent colorectal adenomas [264]. In contrast, a trial conducted as part of the Women's Health Initiative study did not reveal any protective effect of calcium supplementation for CRC risk [209].

Cardiovascular disease

The relationship between calcium intake and CVD risk is also controversial. A systematic review and metaanalysis of observational studies and randomized trials that included data on the effect of dietary or supplementary calcium intake on CVD risk found inconsistent results [265]. Dietary intake of calcium did not appear to be associated with CVD risk. However, a metaanalysis of pooled RCTs found calcium supplementation to be associated with a marginal increase in the risk of CHD and MI. These data are concerning given the recommendation of the Institute of Medicine to supplement all postmenopausal women with oral calcium to prevent osteoporosis [266]. In contrast, a study from

China suggested that higher intake of dietary calcium was associated with reduced risk of all-cause mortality and possibly CVD mortality in older people with low habitual calcium intake (defined as daily dietary calcium intake of <700 mg/day) [267].

Obesity

An association between obesity and calcium intake has been postulated and studied, but there is still no concrete evidence to suggest calcium supplementation has a long-term effect on obesity. A systematic review of eight studies [268–276] evaluated the relationship between calcium and weight [277]. The authors recommended that primary care providers target postmenopausal women and overweight/obese adults and children for extra counseling about calcium intake (strength of recommendation level C: expert opinion) [278]. Most of the more recent studies have focused on dietary calcium intake from dairy sources, as this has shown the most promising results to date [279–282]. A 2009 metaanalysis of randomized controlled studies, looking at the effect of calcium from dairy and dietary supplements on fecal fat excretion, concluded that dietary calcium has the potential to increase fecal fat excretion, which could be relevant in the prevention of weight gain [280].

Magnesium

Magnesium is considered one of the macrominerals and is distributed mostly in the intracellular fluid (ICF). Magnesium has been estimated to be needed in close to 300 biochemical reactions in the body across all major organ systems [283]. The body magnesium content has been estimated at approximately 25 g (2000 mEq) with 50–60% found in the bones [283,284]; the remaining 40–50% is distributed between cardiac muscle, skeletal muscle, liver, and the extracellular fluid (ECF). Only about 2% of the latter half of the magnesium is found in the ECF.

Dietary sources and requirements

The dietary sources for magnesium are listed in Box 22.10. The magnesium content of food varies considerably. The RDA is 400 mg/day for men aged 19–30 years, 420 mg/day for men above 30 years, 310 mg/day for women aged 19–30 years, 320 mg/day for women above age 30. Based on the mother's age, the RDA is 350–360 mg/day during pregnancy and 310–320 mg/day during lactation.

Box 22.10 Dietary sources of magnesium.

Legumes: navy beans, tempeh (fermented soybeans), pinto beans, lima beans, kidney beans

Nuts: cashews, almonds

Seeds: sunflower seeds, sesame seeds, pumpkin seeds

Grains: barley, buckwheat, brown rice, quinoa, millet

Drinking water

Green leafy vegetables: spinach, turnip greens, green peas, kale, green beans, mustard greens, leeks, parsley

Fruits: papaya, watermelon, cantaloupe, strawberries

Sea food: scallops

Homeostasis and regulation

Serum-based magnesium exists in three forms, similar to calcium: protein-bound magnesium (33%; mostly to albumin), complexed magnesium (5%; bound to other compounds including phosphate and citrate), and free magnesium (>60%; ionized or physiologically active forms).

The dietary reference intake for magnesium is shown in Table 22.3. In certain situations, the dietary reference intake for magnesium can vary, including pregnancy (400 mg/day) and lactation (360 mg/day).

Unlike most other ions, magnesium does not have a specific hormone that regulates its serum levels. Intracellular fluid and extracellular fluid magnesium levels are closely maintained by the combination of the gastrointestinal tract, kidney, and bone. Magnesium in bone is rarely available for use, but the importance of bone in magnesium homeostasis becomes more apparent in cases of progressive magnesium depletion. Following progressive decline in the serum concentrations of magnesium, the exchangeable magnesium in bone becomes available for use (only after several weeks) [285] and helps restore the ECF levels; overall, both bone and ECF magnesium are usually sacrificed to maintain ICF magnesium levels [286].

Absorption, transport, and excretion

Approximately 21–27% of dietary magnesium (which has been estimated at 240–360 mg/day) is usually absorbed [151,287]. This occurs primarily in the distal jejunum and ileum and varies inversely with intake. The colon has also been shown to absorb some of the ingested magnesium with only a small portion being absorbed in the duodenum [288]. Both active transport and passive diffusion have been proposed to play a role in magnesium absorption [287].

Approximately one-third of absorbed magnesium is normally excreted via the kidney, which is also the main route of excretion of excessive dietary magnesium [237]. Magnesium is also lost from the feces, but only 1–2% is thought to be lost via this means. Due to this renal-dependent excretion of magnesium, with loss of renal function, there is no protection against elevated magnesium concentrations, and continued intake of magnesium in patients with end-stage renal disease leads to hypermagnesemia.

Functions, deficiency, and toxicity

Magnesium is necessary for many biochemical reactions in the body and has been shown to be important for proper functioning of some physiological processes and biochemical reactions [289]. Physiological functions of magnesium include glucose metabolism, fatty acid synthesis and breakdown, DNA and protein metabolism, immunomodulation (suppresses interleukin [IL]-1), CNS function (plays a key role in *N*-methyl-D-aspartate receptor transmission), energy production (magnesium is a cofactor in a host of enzymatic reactions in the body leading to production of energy), and bone metabolism [289].

Hypomagnesemia is defined as serum magnesium concentrations less than 1.8 mg/dL (0.75 mmol/L); it has been reported in 7–47% of hospitalized patients [290–294] and in as many as 65% of intensive care unit patients [295]. Symptoms associated with low magnesium include neuromuscular hyperexcitablity (e.g., Trousseau and Chovstek signs, spontaneous carpal–pedal spasms, tremors, convulsions, weakness, fatigue, delirium, apathy, involuntary movements athetoid/choreiform movements, coma), electrocardiac derangements (QRS widening, peaked T waves, PR interval widening, diminution of T waves, atrial and ventricular arrhythmias; hypomagnesemia also potentiates the development of digoxin toxicity) [296], electrolyte abnormalities (concomitant electrolyte abnormalities can be seen with low magnesium and include hypocalcemia [22–28%] and hypokalemia [38–61%]), and gastrointestinal symptoms (loss of appetite, nausea, emesis).

Possible causes of hypomagnesemia are listed in Box 22.11. Hypomagnesemia predominantly arises from gastrointestinal or renal losses. Other possible mechanisms include decreased oral intake or redistribution into the ICF. Hypomagnesemia due to decreased or ineffective PTH hormone has been reported; it is usually associated with hypocalcemia as PTH is one of the hormonal regulators of calcium. One study that prospectively followed patients undergoing total thyroidectomy found that hypomagnesemia and hypocalcemia were transient. Most patients were more likely to be symptomatic if both cations were low, and repletion of both cations usually resulted in better outcomes [297]. An entity associated with neurological damage and failure to thrive due to a loss of function mutation in the transient receptor potential channel melastatin 6 gene (*TRPM6*) leads to hypomagnesemia with secondary hypocalcemia [298].

With only 1–2% of total body magnesium present in the ECF, there is difficulty correlating the total body and intracellular magnesium concentrations; there is thus no real evidence-based treatment algorithm for magnesium deficiency. Magnesium supplementation in cases of deficiency can be done intravenously, intramuscularly, or orally, with the preferred route being intravenous due to the associated issues with the other routes, including gastrointestinal intolerance, compliance, absorption, and skin reactions. Some suggested repletion regimens based on the concentration of serum magnesium have been proposed: 8–32 mEq [1–4] magnesium sulfate, up to 1 mEq/kg, for mild to moderate deficiency (serum magnesium concentration 1–1.5 mg/dL); and 32–64 mEq [4–6] magnesium sulfate, up to 1.5 mEq/kg, for severe deficiency [299–301].

Hypermagnesemia is defined as a serum magnesium level >2.3 mg/dL (0.95 mmol/L) and has been associated with renal insufficiency or administration of a large magnesium load (e.g., preeclampsia/eclampsia, laxative abusers, Epsom salt overuse, enemas). Clinical symptoms associated with hypermagnesemia generally begin to appear when the serum magnesium concentration reaches 4.8 mg/dL (2 mmol/L) [291,292]. Reported symptoms include nausea, emesis, diaphoresis, flushing, heat intolerance, alteration in mental status, drowsiness, muscle weakness, bradycardia, and hypotension.

Box 22.11 Etiology of hypomagnesemia.

Gastrointestinal loss

- Diarrhea or emesis (the former is a greater risk than the latter due to higher magnesium concentrations of stool)
- Malabsorptive disorders
- Steatorrhea
- Small bowel bypass surgery
- Primary intestinal hypomagnesemia
- Acute pancreatitis
- Proton pump inhibitor use
- Protein–calorie malnutrition
- Parenteral feeding

Renal loss

- Volume expansion, prolonged administration of IV fluids (low in magnesium)
- Alcohol
- Uncontrolled diabetes mellitus
- Hypercalcemia
- Familial magnesium renal wasting
- Gitelman syndrome: an autosomal recessive renal tubular disorder characterized by hypokalemia, hypomagnesemia, hypocalciuria, metabolic alkalosis, and hyperreninemic hyperaldosteronism
- Medications: loop diuretics, thiazide diuretics, aminoglycosides, amphotericin B, cisplatin, pentamidine, cyclosporine, cetuximab, panitumumab

Iron

Iron is essential in the maintenance of health and has been identified as a component of all living cells. Iron content has been shown to vary based on the age, sex, weight, and nutritional status of the person, but the normal total body content of iron is approximately 3000–4000 mg. Iron is one of the better understood trace minerals due to its ubiquitous availability and has been studied extensively due to its relationship to one of the most common causes of anemia (iron deficiency anemia). Analysis of the data from the NHANES III (1988–1994) showed that iron deficiency anemia is present in at least 1–2% of all US adults [302]. When evaluated based on age and sex, iron deficiency and iron deficiency anemia were more prevalent in younger individuals of both sexes (1–11 years 2–9% of iron deficiency, <1–3% of anemia) and women of child-bearing age (16–49 years 9–11% of iron deficiency, 2–5% of anemia), when compared with men (>12 years old 1–4% of iron deficiency, and 1–2% of anemia) [302].

Dietary sources and requirements

Dietary sources of iron contain both heme and nonheme sources of iron. As discussed in further detail below, absorption and metabolism of these two forms vary. Heme iron is found in animal sources while nonheme iron is found in plant sources, and these are listed in Box 22.12. RDA for iron is 8 mg/day for men, 18 mg/day for women aged 19–50 years, 8 mg/day for women above 50 years old, 27 mg/day during pregnancy, and 9 mg/day during lactation.

Homeostasis and regulation

Iron in the human body exists in four forms: hemoglobin (found in circulating red blood cells and erythroblasts and accounting for 2.5 g of total body stores); bound to serum transferrin (accounting for 3–7 mg of body stores); bound to other iron-containing proteins (such as myoglobin, catalase, and cytochrome complexes, which account for 400 mg of stores); and the storage forms of iron (ferritin and hemosiderin).

Iron homeostasis is regulated through a complex interplay between alterations in absorption, recycling, and loss of iron, and also interactions between a host of specific proteins, listed in Box 22.13. When iron stores are high, absorption is decreased and vice versa.

Absorption, transport, and excretion

Absorption of most of the dietary iron occurs in the duodenum and jejunum. Dietary iron, as mentioned above, comes in two forms (heme and nonheme); the absorption mechanism and the amounts absorbed differ for each form depending on additional factors. Heme iron constitutes about 18.5% of iron in the typical diet, and about 30–40% of this is absorbed, while nonheme constitutes slightly more than 80% of iron in the typical diet with a wide range from <10% to 50% being absorbed depending on other associated factors. Heme iron is absorbed directly, probably via a heme iron transporter named heme carrier protein 1 [303]. Nonheme iron absorption occurs after it has been converted to the ferrous (Fe^{2+}) form by gastric acid, from the usually released ferric (Fe^{3+}) form, which is poorly soluble above a pH of 3. The mechanism of absorption of ferrous iron is thought to be via the divalent metal transporter 1 (DMT1, Nramp2, DCT1, solute carrier family 11), discussed briefly in Box 22.13.

Increased acidity (vitamin C, hydrochloric acid, lactic acid, acidic amino acids like aspartate and glutamate) and presence of heme iron enhance absorption of nonheme iron. Factors that inhibit the absorption of nonheme iron include presence of tannates (found in teas), phytate (found in grains), oxalate (found in spinach, chard, tea, and chocolate), polyphenols (found in coffee, tea, cocoa, cereals), reduced acidity (antacids, H_2 antagonists, proton pump inhibitors, achlorhydria), and malabsorptive states (celiac disease, Crohn's disease).

Following absorption, iron is transported to where it is needed, depending on the iron requirements at the time. Two paths are usually dictated physiologically depending on low iron need/full stores versus high iron need/depleted stores. In states of low iron need/full iron stores, the absorbed iron is not released immediately into the bloodstream, but is stored in the cell bound to apoferritin, leading to the formation of the aforementioned ferritin, a short-term storage form for iron. When the amount of iron in the body exceeds the storage capacity of ferritin, some ferritin is then switched to the iron–protein complex, hemosiderin, another storage form of iron. In states of high iron need/low iron stores, the opposite occurs; iron is absorbed into the bloodstream with the help of the protein ferroportin and then bound to transferrin. The number of transferrin receptors to which iron can bind depends on the state of iron need in the body. With high iron need, more receptor sites are expressed and more iron is bound; with low iron needs, fewer receptor sites are expressed. As such, iron storage levels will determine to a great extent how much iron is absorbed. The interplay between some of the proteins described above and the regulation of iron is shown in Figure 22.3.

There is no mechanism that has been identified as regulating the loss of iron. It has been shown to be lost via sweat, shed skin cells, gastrointestinal losses (defecation, urine), and bleeding.

Functions, deficiency, and toxicity

Iron is required for a host of highly complex processes that are indispensable to the normal physiological functioning of the body. Some of these functions include hematopoiesis, transport of oxygen and carbon dioxide, conversion of glucose to energy (as a component of cytochromes), enzyme production, immune system functioning, reducing free radical production and oxidative damage to DNA [324,325], and it is also a component of myoglobin.

Box 22.12 Dietary sources of iron.

Heme sources

- Beef: chuck, corned, liver, ground, etc.
- Chicken: liver, ground
- Turkey
- Pork
- Seafood: clams, cod, flounder, salmon, shrimp, oysters, tuna

Nonheme sources

- Vegetables: broccoli, lentils, spinach
- Grains: rice
- Legumes: soybeans, pinto beans, peas, navy beans, lima beans, kidney beans, black eyed peas
- Tofu
- Fruits: raisins, prunes, apricots, dates
- Nuts: almonds
- Oatmeal
- Bagels, bread

The dietary reference intake for iron is shown in Table 22.3.

Box 22.13 Proteins involved in iron metabolism, regulation, and homeostasis.

Transferrin: binds tightly to 1–2 ferric (Fe^{3+}) molecules and is the main transporter protein for serum iron. It is synthesized in the liver, and is upregulated in states of iron deficiency [304,305]. In the steady state about one-third of serum transferrin is usually saturated with iron – known as the transferrin saturation, expressed mathematically as iron/TIBC (total iron binding capacity) = 1/3. See text for conditions that affect the transferrin saturation.

Transferrin receptor: transmembrane protein that is capable of binding to two molecules of transferrin, hence can carry four Fe^{3+} molecules of iron. Following endocytosis of the receptor the iron is released into acidified vacuoles, and it is then recycled back onto the cell surface with repetition of the process [306].

Ferritin: an acute phase reactant and the storage protein for cellular-based iron. Each ferritin complex can store as much as 4500 atoms of iron [307]. As an acute phase reactant it works in conjunction with transferrin and transferrin receptors to institute the cellular defense against oxidative stress and inflammation [308,309].

Iron regulatory protein 1 and 2 (IRP1, IRP2): cellular iron-sensing proteins that work in conjunction with iron-responsive elements (IRE). Binding of the IRPs to IRE target sequences usually occurs in states of cellular iron deficiency [310].

Divalent metal transporter 1 (DMT1, Nramp2, DCT1, solute carrier family 11) duodenal iron transporter: located on the brush border membrane, and involved in the transport of ferrous iron across the brush border and glycocalyx of the enterocytes [311,312].

Ferroportin (Ireg1, SLC11A3, Mtp1): cellular iron exporter responsible for exporting absorbed iron from the basolateral membrane of the cell and also recycled iron from red blood cells located in the macrophages into the bloodstream. It has also been shown to help transport iron from mother to fetus during pregnancy [313–315].

Hephaestin: a ferroxidase thought to be necessary for the recycling of iron in the liver, reticuloendothelial system, and blood. After iron is transported by ferroportin across the basolateral membrane, it is oxidized from the ferrous form back into the ferric form for binding to transferrin. Hephaestin is thought to be involved in this oxidative process [316].

Ceruloplasmin: a known ferroxidase involved more importantly in copper metabolism, but also plays a role in iron metabolism as it helps in the oxidizing of ferrous iron (released from ferroportin) into the ferric form, which is subsequently loaded on transferrin.

HFE protein: role in iron regulation is not clearly understood, but it has been shown to be involved in a complex with the transferrin receptor (but its role in this complex is poorly understood). Mutations associated with this protein are responsible for most of the patients with hereditary hemochromatosis.

Transferrin receptor 2 (TFR2): similar to transferrin 1, but does not have an IRE element. Mutations in this protein are responsible for a rare hereditary form of hemochromatosis [317].

Hemojuvelin (HJV): regulates hepcidin production. Mutations in this protein have been implicated in development of the common form of juvenile hemochromatosis [59-utd] [318].

Hepcidin: liver-expressed antimicrobial peptide (LEAP-1) is another acute phase reactant the liver expresses. It is in two forms, hepcidin-25 and hepcidin-20, of which hepcidin-25 is involved in iron metabolism [319–322].

Bone morphogenic protein 6 (BMP6): this is a cytokine, which is produced in states of iron overload and has been shown to be involved in the main pathway for activation of hepcidin [323].

Iron deficiency usually manifests as a microcytic and hypochromic anemia, due to the intricate relationship between iron, hemoglobin, and hematopoiesis. This develops in stages, starting with iron deficiency and, following depletion of the body stores, anemia becomes evident. It is the most common nutrient deficiency worldwide, estimated to affect up to 1 billion people; iron deficiency anemia is estimated to affect close to 500–600 million people worldwide.

Clinical symptoms associated with iron deficiency anemia include weakness, fatigue, exercise intolerance, lightheadedness, shortness of breath, dyspnea on exertion, headache, irritability, tachycardia, poor capillary refill, pallor, reduced work performance, impaired intellectual and behavioral performance, decreased resistance to infections, increased lead absorption, pica, pagophagia (form of pica involving compulsive consumption of ice or iced drinks), beeturia (Box 22.14), and restless leg syndrome.

For diagnosis, blood tests including serum ferritin, iron, total iron binding capacity, and transferrin are usually ordered. A peripheral blood smear showing the classic microcytic red blood cells can help make the diagnosis. Certain conditions predispose individuals to iron deficiency anemia including women of child-bearing age, menstrual disorders (menorrhagia, metromenorrhagia, etc.), hospitalized individuals with excess blood draws, and malabsorptive states (celiac, IBD, gastric or intestinal surgery).

Iron toxicity usually arises from short- or long-term exposure to iron levels that exceed the body's physiological protective mechanisms for handling iron (including antioxidants, iron binding proteins) and ranges from acute toxicity to chronic iron overload. Acute iron toxicity/poisoning is still a common problem in the pediatric population with almost 16 000 events reported yearly in children less than 6 years old in the USA [329]. It is also the most common cause of poisoning-related deaths in this age group.

Iron toxicity can initially present as vomiting and gastrointestinal distress, followed by dysfunction in one or more organs with clinical manifestations of neurological, cardiovascular, hematological, hepatic, and renal dysfunction. The most common chronic iron overload state is hereditary hemochromatosis, and in the homozygous hereditary variant of the disease it is thought that the absorption of iron is not regulated by iron stores as occurs physiologically (see Chapter 93). Other situations in which iron overload occurs include transfusion-dependent conditions such as β-thalassemia major, sickle cell anemia, and myelodysplastic syndromes.

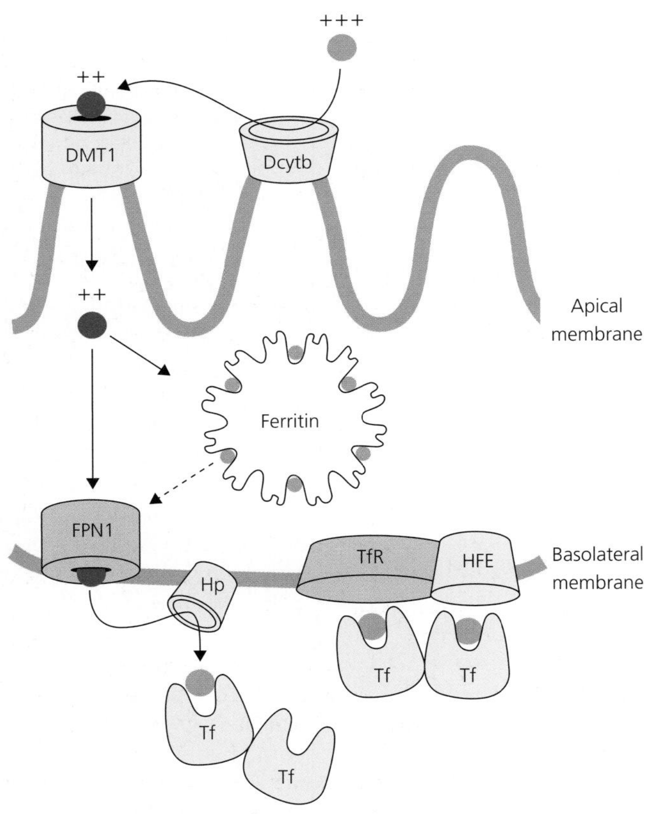

Figure 22.3 Interaction of potential mechanisms for the regulation of iron absorption by the mucosal cell. Dcytb, duodenal cytochrome b; DMT1, divalent metal transporter 1; FPN1, ferroportin 1; HFE, hemochromatosis gene product; Hp, hephaestin; Tf, transferrin; TfR, transferrin receptor.

Box 22.14 Beeturia.

Beeturia is defined as pink or red urine (or sometimes feces) after the ingestion of beets and is due to excretion of betalain (betacyanin) pigments, estimated to affect about 10–14% of the population [326,327]. It has also been found to be more common in people with enhanced iron absorption, and has been reported at a rate of 66–80% in patients with untreated iron deficiency anemia, and close to 45% in patients undergoing treatment for pernicious anemia [326,328].

Zinc

Zinc has been implicated as a catalyst for close to 100 enzymatic reactions and is bound to cellular proteins in virtually all cells in the body [330,331]. In 1961, a link was found between zinc deficiency and endemic hypogonadism and dwarfism in rural areas of Iran [332,333]. It was, however, not until the 1990s that zinc was identified an essential mineral.

Dietary sources and requirements

The dietary sources for zinc are listed in Box 22.15. The RDA is 11 mg/day for men, 8 mg/day for women, 11 mg/day during pregnancy, and 12 mg/day during lactation.

Box 22.15 Dietary sources for zinc.

Seafood: oysters (tops the list), crab, lobster, flounder

Meat: beef, poultry, pork

Legumes: beans (baked, plain), kidney beans, peas, lentils

Nuts: almonds,

Fortified cereals, oatmeal

Dairy: milk, cheese

The dietary reference intake for zinc is given in Table 22.3.

Homeostasis and regulation

Total body zinc content has been estimated at about 1.5–2.5 g in adults [334]. About 60% of this amount is found in the bones and muscles. Approximately 95% of total body zinc content is intracellular. Zinc homeostasis is closely regulated by the protein metallothionein, a metalloprotein that binds both copper and other divalent cations, but has been shown to be more avid for copper than zinc. Plasma zinc levels have been shown to vary in certain conditions, including variations with dietary zinc intake, during states of acute infections, in fasting states, and following injuries to the body (concentrations have been shown to drop by as much as 10– 69% depending on the extent and form of injury) [335].

Absorption, transport, and excretion

About 15–35% of ingested zinc is absorbed by the body [336] via a carrier-mediated process and also a noncarrier-mediated diffusion process utilizing metallothionein [337]. Most zinc is absorbed in the small intestine, mainly at the duodenum and jejunum, and to a lesser extent the ileum. The absorptive process of zinc involves transport from the enterocyte to the liver, which involves binding of zinc to albumin; the liver then releases the zinc into the bloodstream as needed. Zinc absorption can be affected by other factors, including the presence of other minerals (calcium, iron, copper), vitamins, proteins (certain milk proteins), phytic acid, physiological factors, disease processes (inflammatory conditions), and alcohol.

The ZIP (Zrt-like, Irt-like protein) family has been implicated in the transport of zinc from the ECF space or organelles into the cytoplasm [338]. ZIP4 transporter was discovered when it was shown that mutations in its gene were linked to the recessive genetic disorder acrodermatitis enteropathica. Zinc is transported in the blood bound to both albumin (at least 70% of plasma zinc) and α-macroglobulins (20–40%) [337].

Zinc excretion occurs via the following organ systems: the gastrointestinal tract (feces), the kidney (urine), and the skin (integument and sweat).

Functions, deficiency, and toxicity

Zinc functions in many biochemical reactions, as noted above, and these functions are shown in Box 22.16.

Box 22.16 Key functions of zinc [337].

Catalytic functions

Zinc has been shown to be an important catalyst for enzymes including:

Alkaline phosphatase

Carbonic anhydrase

Alcohol dehydrogenase

RNA polymerases I, II, III

Structural functions

Metalloenzymes

Zinc finger motif in proteins – the zinc finger proteins

Regulatory functions

It has also been shown to have a regulatory function in expression of some genes, including metallothionein expression

Other functions

Peroxidation of lipids

Cellular apoptosis

Cellular proliferation and differentiation

Immune function

Zinc deficiency occurs but is difficult to diagnose for a few reasons, including lack of validated biomarkers for zinc status in the body, effect of changes in albumin on zinc status (serum zinc depends on albumin for transport), and the diverse nonspecific clinical symptoms associated with zinc deficiency. Assessment of zinc status in the context of systemic inflammatory response syndrome (SIRS), which can occur in a wide variety of situations, is complicated because it is depressed by nearly half until the insult resolves. Clinical signs associated with zinc deficiency include growth delay, skin lesions (mostly located at the eyes, nose, mouth, gluteal region, and perianal skin), night vision dysfunction, hypogonadism, dysguesia, anosmia, anorexia, diarrhea, immune dysfunction (especially T-cell dysfunction), alopecia, personality changes, and impaired wound healing [337,339,340].

Zinc deficiency can contribute to vitamin A deficiency because zinc aids the absorption of vitamin A from the diet [341] (via its regulatory role in vitamin A transport, and in the oxidative conversion of retinol to retinal leading to decreased mobilization of retinol from the liver). A deficiency of zinc also decreases work capacity of the muscles, which can cause respiratory impairments [342]. Hepatic dysfunction has also been associated with zinc deficiency [343], as has glucose intolerance through an as yet unidentified mechanism [344]. Certain conditions and populations have been associated with zinc deficiency, such as the elderly, alcoholics, postoperative patients (especially intestinal bypass or resection), burn patients, other wound drainage (gastrointestinal fistulas, draining decubitus ulcers), pregnant and lactating women, pancreatic insufficiency, chronic corticosteroid use, and traumatic brain injury.

Acrodermatitis enteropathica is an autosomal recessive disorder of zinc metabolism. It usually presents in the first year of life, although can also present in adolescents and adults. It is thought to result from mutations in the *SLC39A4* gene located on chromosome 8q24.3, which encodes the ZIP14 protein involved in zinc transportation [345,346]. Clinical symptoms include eczema, dermatitis, anorexia, immunocompromised state, dysguesia, poor growth, delayed sexual maturation, delayed wound healing, photophobia, and night blindness [332]. Zinc repletion is usually the treatment, with higher levels required during periods of rapid growth (e.g., puberty).

Zinc toxicity has been linked to excessive use of denture adhesives and fixatives, as they earlier contained high amounts of zinc [347,348]. Currently, most acute cases of zinc toxicity result from supplemental intake, with instances of death reported after large intravenous doses of zinc [337]. Clinical manifestations of zinc toxicity include gastric distress, nausea, emesis, dizziness, decreased immune function, and copper deficiency.

Copper

Copper is a trace mineral and necessary for physiological functions of different body systems.

Dietary sources and requirements

Copper can be found in a wide variety of dietary sources shown in Box 22.17. The RDA is 900 μg/day for men and women, 1000 μg/day during pregnancy, and 1300 μg/day during lactation.

Homeostasis and regulation

The homeostasis and regulation of copper stores and levels are thought to occur mainly by excretion, not absorption, and via a biliary-mediated process. Homeostasis at the cellular level

Box 22.17 Dietary sources of copper.

Legumes: lentils, Lima beans, garbanzo beans, soybeans, tempeh, black beans, pinto beans, dried peas, green beans, navy beans, green peas, kidney beans

Nuts: cashews, sesame seeds, sunflower seeds, walnuts, peanuts, almonds

Mushrooms: shitake, crimini

Meats: liver

Seafood: shrimp, sardines

Greens: turnip greens, spinach, asparagus, kale, mustard greens, Brussels sprouts, broccoli, parsley, romaine lettuce, leeks, collard greens, bok choy, cucumber

Fruits: orange, apricot, grapefruit, watermelon, strawberries, cantaloupe, banana, papaya, grapes, raisins, pear, avocado, kiwi fruit, tomatoes, egg plant, raspberries, plum, pineapple

The dietary reference intake of copper is shown in Table 22.3.

involves a delicate balance of uptake and efflux mediated by membrane proteins [349], including the copper-transporting P-type ATPases [350]. The copper-transporting ATPase ATP7A has been implicated in exporting copper from the enterocyte [351], while ATPase7B transports copper into the secretory pathway for incorporation into apoceruloplasmin [352]. Most dietary copper is present in the ionic Cu^{2+} form bound to organic compounds, hence the need for gastric acid and pepsin to cleave the copper from these compounds before it can be absorbed.

Copper is mostly absorbed in the stomach, duodenum, and to a lesser extent the jejunum and ileum [353,354]. Copper absorption [353] occurs by both an active transport system (saturable), which operates during low copper intake, and a passive system (nonsaturable) that operates during high copper intake. Certain conditions have been shown to affect copper absorption, including phytates, dietary fiber, zinc, calcium gluconate in large doses, molybdenum, iron, and vitamin C in large doses (have all been shown to negatively impact copper absorption).

Copper interacts with two proteins in the liver. Ceruloplasmin transports copper from the liver to the peripheral tissues and 60–95% of postprandial circulating copper exists as a component of ceruloplasmin [355]. The other protein is metallothionein, which is thought to act as a storage protein for copper. Approximately 50% of copper excretion occurs through the biliary system and the other half is secreted through other gastrointestinal secretions [353,354].

Functions, deficiency, and toxicity

Copper has multiple biological functions [356,357], some of which are listed in Box 22.18.

Copper deficiency has been known to occur, although clinically evident deficiency is fairly uncommon [357,358]. Some of the mechanisms that can lead to this include poor intake, decreased absorption, and increased losses from the GI tract [359]. Clinical symptoms of copper deficiency include fragile, brittle hair, skin depigmentation, muscle weakness (myeloneuropathy), neurological abnormalities (ataxia, neuropathy, and cognitive deficits), peripheral edema, hepatosplenomegaly, anemia (usually microcytic and hypochromic), leukopenia, neutropenia, thrombocytopenia, and hypercholesterolemia (Box 22.19). Laboratory findings include low serum copper level, low ceruloplasmin, low erythrocyte copper–zinc superoxide level, and decreased 24-h urine copper excretion [355,360].

Certain conditions have been associated with an increased risk of development of copper deficiency, including abdominal surgery (e.g., gastrectomy, gastric bypass, small intestine resection), administration of formula without adequate copper supplementation to premature infants, undernutrition, chronic diarrhea, malabsorptive conditions (e.g., steatorrhea, celiac disease), dialysis (peritoneal or hemodialysis), excessive zinc ingestion, treatment of Wilson disease, treatment with copper chelator (clioquinol), and treatment with tetrathiomolybdate.

Menkes disease is a congenital X-linked genetic disorder caused by a mutation in the transport protein mediating copper uptake in the intestine (encoded by the *ATP7A* gene). Clinical features are similar to copper deficiency but occur in early childhood. If untreated, the condition leads to death during early childhood. Characteristic features include "kinky" hair, growth retardation, skin hypopigmentation, osteoporosis, and spur formation.

Copper toxicity is not very common because the mode of regulation of copper is via excretion from the bile. Mechanisms that lead to impaired biliary excretion or cholestasis can lead to accumulation of copper in the hepatocytes and toxicity [355,359]. While uncommon, clinical features of copper toxicity include abdominal pain, diarrhea, nausea, emesis, hepatic necrosis, cirrhosis, encephalopathy, and end-organ damage – cardiac failure, renal failure, and death. Sources of copper toxicity, apart from the mechanisms described above, can be accidental ingestion, contaminated food/beverage sources, suicide attempts, and use of topical burn creams that contain copper salts [355].

Wilson disease is an autosomal recessive disorder caused by a mutation in the copper ATPase enzyme closely related to the Menkes disease gene (*ATP7B* or the WD protein) [369,370]. Here, excessive amounts of copper accumulate in the body (especially the liver and brain). Clinical symptoms include cirrhosis, eye problems (with the pathognomonic Kayser–Fleischer

Box 22.18 Functions of copper.

Oxidation reduction and electron transfer reactions involving oxygen via cytochrome-c oxidase [355]

Antioxidant defense via zinc–copper superoxide dismutase

Neurotransmitter synthesis via dopamine monooxygenase

Collagen cross-linking and bone formation via lysyl oxidase

Manganese and iron oxidation via ceruloplasmin

Activation/deactivation of peptide hormones via peptidylglycine α-amidating monooxygenase

Clot formation/thrombosis via factor V

Melatonin production via tyrosinase

Important for cholesterol and glucose metabolism [355,361]

Box 22.19 Interplay between copper and zinc.

Copper deficiency and elevated zinc levels associated with degeneration of the neurological network of the central and peripheral nervous systems, resulting in myelopolyneuropathy with associated hematological dysfunction (pancytopenia), have been increasingly recognized and reported in the literature [362–368]. High zinc levels have been associated with copper deficiency thought to be due to expression of metallothionein that binds copper [329–333]. It appears that zinc-containing denture adhesive overuse is associated with zinc excess. The etiological role of excessive zinc supplementations as the cause of the zinc overload has now been confirmed [364].

rings), kidney dysfunction, and neurological manifestations [371] (see Chapter 94).

Chromium

Chromium is an essential trace mineral, which was initially identified in 1957 following extraction from pork kidney and was called "glucose tolerance factor" because it corrected hyperglycemia in rats [372]. It exists in several ionic states ranging from Cr^{2+} to Cr^{6+}, but trivalent Cr^{3+} is the biologically relevant state found in dietary sources, and Cr^{4+} to Cr^{6+} are strong oxidizing and toxic agents that are easily reducible to Cr^{3+} in an acidic environment.

Dietary sources and regulation

Dietary sources of chromium are varied and are listed in Box 22.20. Depending on the age, adequate intake of chromium is 30–35 μg/day for men, 20–25 μg/day for women, 30 μg/day during pregnancy, and 45 μg/day during lactation.

Homeostasis and regulation

The homeostasis and regulation of chromium are still unclear, but it is thought that the total body store of chromium is one of the main regulatory controls of further absorption by the GI tract.

Absorption, transport, and excretion

Chromium is absorbed throughout the intestine, but occurs predominantly in the small intestine (jejunum). The main underlying mechanism of chromium absorption is still unclear, but one postulated adjunct mechanism is a nonmediated passive diffusion process [151,373]. The absorption of chromium has a dose-dependent relationship: as intake increases, absorption decreases. Absorption of dietary chromium is in general quite poor with only an estimated 0.4–3% being absorbed into the bloodstream [374–376]. Some minerals have been shown to affect the absorption and uptake of chromium, including zinc and iron, where states of deficiency are associated with an increased absorption and uptake of chromium [373]. Other factors that affect chromium absorption include gastric acid [377] (which can form insoluble salts leading to decreased absorption), vitamin C [378] (appears to enhance uptake), drugs (indomethacin enhances uptake while prostaglandin E2 decreases uptake of chromium in murine models) [379]; antacids containing magnesium, calcium, or aluminum salt and NSAIDs decrease absorption of chromium.

Chromium is transported via the iron transport system, where trivalent chromium binds competitively to transferrin and is transported from the blood into cells and is then transferred from the transferrin to chromodulin, which can bind four molecules of trivalent chromium, and was formerly referred to as "glucose tolerance factor" [374–376]. It is thought that a majority of ingested chromium is excreted via feces [380], while urinary and biliary excretion are other routes. Conditions associated with increased secretion of chromium in the urine include diabetes mellitus type 2 and pregnancy [381].

Box 22.20 Dietary sources of chromium.

Grains: whole wheat (bread, English muffins)

Fruits: grape (juice), orange (juice), apple, banana

Vegetables: broccoli, green beans

Meats: processed meats, beef, turkey

Potatoes

Basil, garlic

Red wine

The dietary reference intake for chromium is 20–35 μg/day

Functions, deficiency, and toxicity

Chromium is thought to potentiate the action of insulin as its biologically active form, chromodulin, serves a role in insulin signaling, amplifying the tyrosine kinase activity of the insulin receptor [374–376]. With this it has a role in glucose, protein, and lipid metabolism, and is therefore also required for growth. There is very little evidence of chromium deficiency in humans, and the only documented cases have been seen in patients receiving parenteral nutrition without adequate supplementation [382]. Other patient populations at risk for chromium deficiency include hospitalized patients (with increased catabolism and metabolism), short bowel syndrome, burns, and traumatic injuries. Some authors have postulated an association between chromium deficiency and impaired glucose tolerance and unfavorable lipid profiles [383], and studies seem to suggest that chromium supplementation improved glycemia among patients with diabetes but not among those with normal glucose tolerance [384]. Clinical signs observed in patients with chromium deficiency include weight loss, peripheral neuropathy, hyperglycemia refractory to insulin, glucosuria, impaired amino acid utilization, and dyslipidemia (increased plasma LDL-cholesterol levels).

A large proportion of the evidence presently available does not support chromium supplementation in patients without a proven deficiency. It is also important to note that iron levels can be affected with chronic chromium supplementation because iron and chromium compete for transferrin. Serum ferritin levels decrease when chromium intake is more than or equal to 200 μg/day [385].

Chromium toxicity is not common, and there have not been any reports of toxicity of dietary or trivalent chromium. Although animal studies suggest that high doses of trivalent chromium are nontoxic because of the poor bioavailability [386], others think that poor absorption of chromium, especially if taken as a supplement, can lead to accumulation of chromium in body tissues leading to adverse effects [387]. Some of the possible side-effects include rhabdomyolysis, and liver and renal dysfunction [387–391]. The higher forms of chromium, including the pentavalent and hexavalent forms, are known toxic agents and industrial pollutants, and are not usually found in the diet. Exposure to these toxic agents can lead to lung (bronchogenic) cancer [375,392,393], contact and allergic dermatitis, and skin and nasal septal lesions/ulcers.

Selenium

Selenium is a trace mineral and exists in several ionic states (Se^{2+}, Se^{4+}, and Se^{6+}). It is a constituent of more than 30 selenoproteins, which play essential roles in various bodily functions [394]. Selenium found in foods is usually complexed with derivatives of two main amino acids, methionine and cysteine, with selenomethionine being predominantly from plant sources and selenocysteine from animal sources.

Dietary sources, requirements, homeostasis, and regulation

Dietary sources of selenium are shown in Box 22.21. The RDA is 55 mg/day for men and women, 60 mg/day during pregnancy, and 70 mg/day during lactation. Mechanisms underlying the regulation or homeostasis of selenium are still unclear, but it is thought to occur through a balance between fecal and urinary excretion.

Absorption, transport, and excretion

Once ingested, the bioavailability of dietary selenium is high and ranges from 50% to 100%, dependent on luminal factors [395]. Selenium absorption occurs mainly in the duodenum, and to a lesser extent the rest of the small intestine. Selenomethionine absorption occurs via an active methionine absorptive pathway, while the pathway of selenocysteine absorption is still unclear. Selenomethionine appears to serve as the storage pool for selenium, and in vivo both selenomethionine and selenocysteine are catabolized to release selenium. Following absorption, selenium is bound to the plasma protein, selenoprotein P, whose role in the transport of selenium in the body is still unclear [151]. The main route of excretion of selenium is via the urine but, as already noted, some excretion does occur via the gastrointestinal tract (via feces).

Box 22.21 Dietary sources of selenium.

Nuts: brazil nuts,[a] cashews

Seafood: halibut, sardines, shrimp, tuna

Meats: ham, beef steak/ground/liver, turkey, chicken

Dairy: milk, yogurt, cottage cheese

Fruits: peaches, bananas

Eggs

Bread, spaghetti, macaroni, corn flakes, potato, oatmeal

Baked beans, lentils, green peas

The dietary reference intake for selenium for adults (>14 years old) is 55 μg/day.

[a] Selenium from one Brazil nut/day is suggested to be close to the DRI. However, the selenium content has been found to vary considerably based on the region: the mean, standard deviation, and range of selenium concentrations in ppm, for Brazil nuts from Acre-Rondonia and Manaus-Belem regions were, respectively, 3.06 ± 4.01 (0.03–31.7) and 36.0 ± 50.0 (1.25–512.0).

Functions, deficiency, and toxicity

Selenium has been found to be a necessary cofactor for certain enzymatic reactions, including glutathione metabolism (glutathionine peroxidase which catalyzes reactions to remove hydrogen peroxide), iodine and thyroid metabolism (iodothyronine deiodinase which catalyzes the deiodination of iodine, triiodothyronine, and reverse triiodothyronine), oxidative defense (selenoprotein P), the other selenoproteins [395–397]. Selenium deficiency has been associated with metabolic effects of oxidative injury, thyroid hormone dysfunction, alteration in biotransformation enzymes [395], skeletal muscle dysfunction, cardiomyopathy [398,399], mood and immune dysfunction [400,401], macrocytosis, and whitening of the nail beds [402]. Keshan disease is an endemic cardiomyopathy that affects women of childbearing age and children in geographic areas of China with local diets nearly devoid of selenium [395,403].

Selenium toxicity, otherwise known as selenosis, usually occurs following excess dietary intake or high-dose supplementation. Clinical symptoms associated with selenosis include nausea, emesis, diarrhea, tooth decay, hair loss, nail deformity and loss, alteration in mental status, irritability, fatigue, and peripheral neuropathy [395]. In China, chronic increased consumption of selenium in Enshi County has been associated with most of the symptoms listed above [404].

References are available at www.yamadagastro.com/textbook7e

Further reading

Battistini C., Ballan R., Herkenhoff M.E., et al. Vitamin D Modulates Intestinal Microbiota in Inflammatory Bowel Diseases. Int J Mol Sci. 2020 Dec 31;22(1):362. doi: 10.3390/ijms22010362. PMID: 33396382; PMCID: PMC7795229.

Institute of Medicine of the National Academies. Dietary Reference Intakes: The Essential Reference for Dietary Planning and Assessment. www.nationalacademies.org/our-work/summary-report-of-the-dietary-referenceintakes

García-Montero C., Fraile-Martínez O., Gómez-Lahoz A.M., et al. Nutritional Components in Western Diet Versus Mediterranean Diet at the Gut Microbiota-Immune System Interplay. Implications for Health and Disease. Nutrients. 2021 Feb 22;13(2):699. doi: 10.3390/nu13020699. PMID: 33671569; PMCID: PMC7927055.

Green R., Allen L.H., Bjørke-Monsen A.L., et al. Vitamin B12 deficiency. Nat Rev Dis Primers. 2017 Jun 29;3:17040. doi: 10.1038/nrdp.2017.40. Erratum in: Nat Rev Dis Primers. 2017 Jul 20;3:17054. PMID: 28660890.

CHAPTER 23

Nutrition Support

Dong Wook Kim[1] **and David S. Seres**[2]
[1]Department of Medicine, Boston University School of Medicine, Boston, MA, USA
[2]Department of Medicine, Columbia University Irving Medical Center, New York, NY, USA

Chapter menu

Nutrition support is the provision of nutrients by medical means, usually enterally by tube or parenterally. Definitions for nutrition support vary, however, and sometimes include not only enteral nutrition (EN) or parenteral nutrition (PN) but also oral calorie and protein supplements, or even dietary alterations.

Irrespective of cause, or defining characteristics, malnutrition correlates with higher morbidity and mortality, decreased functional status and quality of life, and higher healthcare costs [1–7]. However, identifying patients for whom nutritional intervention will result in improved outcomes remains difficult. Only recently have data emerged showing outcomes benefits from nutrition support in select patients with malnutrition [8–11].

This chapter will review the classification and diagnosis of malnutrition, the assessment for and provision of nutrition support, as well as specific conditions that require special nutritional intervention.

Diagnosis of malnutrition and nutritional assessment

As stated earlier, malnutrition is associated with elevations in morbidity, mortality, and high healthcare costs [1–7]. The term has been variably defined but is generally considered to be present when there is imbalance (deficiency or excess) of macronutrients (e.g., calories and protein), micronutrients (e.g., vitamins, minerals, essential fatty acids, and trace elements), or both (Figure 23.1). Some definitions refer strictly to deficiency of calories or other nutrients. For example, the World Health Organization defines malnutrition as "Deficiencies, excesses or imbalances in a person's intake of energy and/or nutrients" [12]. However, others conflate malnourishment with disease processes and include changes in body components irrespective of cause, such as wasting as a result of cancer that occurs despite adequate nourishment [13,14]. These latter schemata have become widely adopted in the hospital setting but may cause confusion. One cannot assume that patients with malnutrition are malnourished. In other words, these diagnostic methods do not readily identify individuals in need of nutrition intervention [15,16].

Etiology-based malnutrition diagnosis

Recent efforts to standardize the definition of malnutrition have included criteria to distinguish between malnutrition caused by malnourishment and that as a result of disease process. In 2012, The Academy of Nutrition and Dietetics (AND) and the American Society for Parenteral Enteral Nutrition (A.S.P.E.N.) together published proposed etiology-based malnutrition criteria [13]. A multinational consortium (Global Leadership Initiative on Malnutrition [GLIM]) then approved in 2018 updated guidance for diagnosing malnutrition in the hospital [17]. Both have been specifically validated to predict adverse outcomes [3–6], but not the response to nourishment interventions.

Yamada's Textbook of Gastroenterology, Seventh Edition. Edited by Timothy C. Wang, Michael Camilleri, Benjamin Lebwohl, Anna S. Lok, William J. Sandborn, Kenneth K. Wang, and Gary D. Wu.

Companion website: www.yamadagastro.com/textbook7e

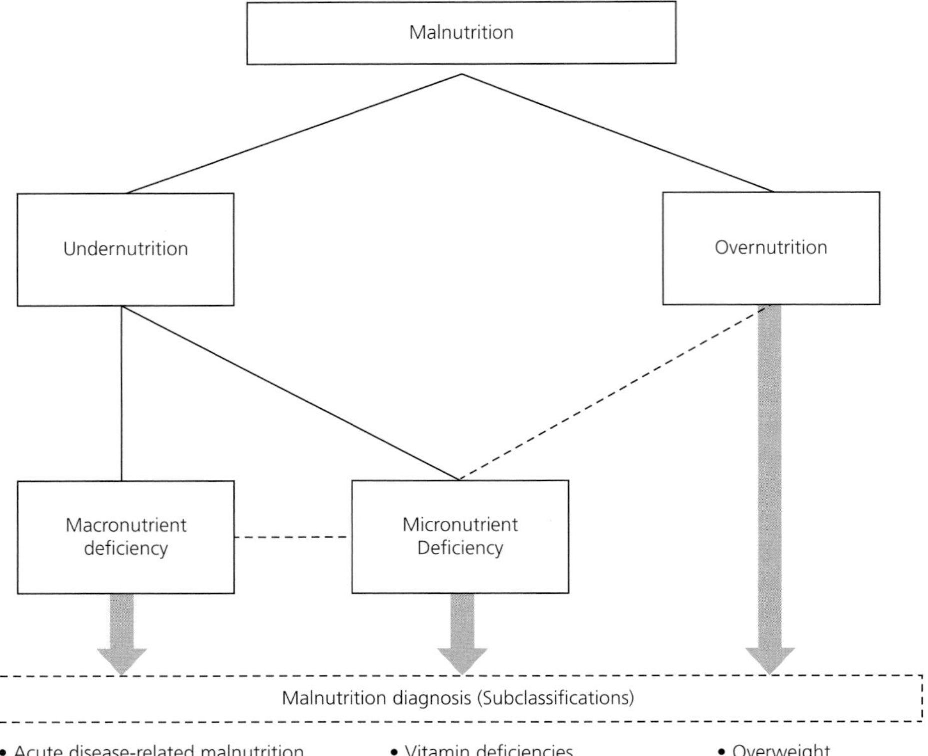

Figure 23.1 Malnutrition classification.

The AND/A.S.P.E.N. guidelines classify malnutrition into three categories based on the degree of systemic inflammatory response: (1) starvation-related malnutrition, (2) chronic disease-related malnutrition, and (3) acute disease-related malnutrition. Starvation-related malnutrition is a state of chronic insufficient nourishment without any systemic inflammation. Anorexia nervosa and simple starvation as a result of socioeconomic status are examples of this type of malnutrition. Chronic disease-related malnutrition is associated with mild-to-moderate disease-related inflammation. Wasting associated with malignancy and autoimmune disease, for example, define this condition. Acute disease-related malnutrition is an acute wasting caused by acute illness. Patients who are catabolic after trauma or major burns are examples of this category of malnutrition. Notably, disease-related malnutrition may or may not include poor intake and may therefore not have a nutritional cause or require nutritional intervention other than closer monitoring [13,14].

The diagnosis of malnutrition, based on AND/A.S.P.E.N. guidelines, includes the assessment of six parameters and the inflammatory state of the patient. These parameters include the presence of:

1. insufficient energy intake,
2. weight loss,
3. loss of muscle mass,
4. localized or generalized fluid accumulation,
5. loss of subcutaneous fat, and
6. diminished functional status as measured by handgrip strength

The patient is considered at nutritional risk if they have two or more of the six parameters. The patient's inflammatory status then determines which of the etiology-based malnutrition diagnoses apply [13] (Figure 23.2).

The AND/A.S.P.E.N. [13] guideline is limited in its applicability. It is designed for use by nutrition practitioners trained in physical examination for muscle and fat mass. Further, it was intended for use in hospitalized patients. Last, micronutrient deficiencies are not considered as criteria for diagnosing malnutrition in this definition. Therefore, vitamin and mineral deficiencies must be considered separately. The GLIM [17] criteria was created to be more universally applicable by untrained healthcare professionals. Like AND/A.S.P.E.N., GLIM conflates starvation and wasting, and includes direct markers for systemic inflammation, such as hypoalbuminemia.

Last, although overnutrition is also considered malnutrition and is associated with comorbid conditions, obesity is not included in these etiology-based malnutrition criteria. Moreover, muscle wasting, so-called sarcopenic obesity, may be present in obese patients with systemic inflammation and may be missed if

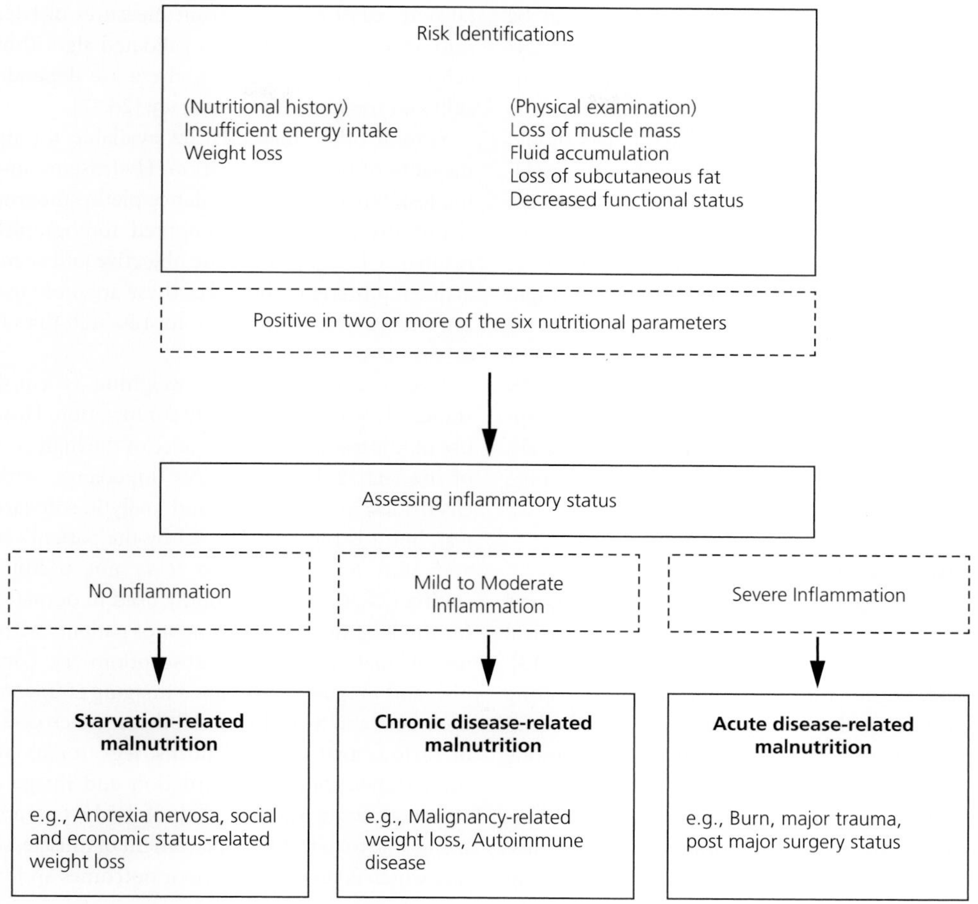

Figure 23.2 Etiology-based malnutrition diagnosis. Source: Modified from White et al. 2012 [13].

practitioners are not attentive to examining muscle mass. Sarcopenic obesity is poorly studied, and there is no consistent definition [18].

Nutritional and medical history

Clinically significant weight loss, and the rate of loss, are the most important clinical measures for diagnosing malnutrition and determining its severity. "Significant" weight loss has been variably and arbitrarily defined. Blackburn et al. [19] proposed a definition based on percentage weight loss. Although, to our knowledge, these parameters have never been directly validated, they have been widely adopted into guidelines that have been, as a whole, validated to predict morbidity and mortality [3–6]. Weight loss is usually defined as significant when more than 5% weight is lost unintentionally over 6–12 months [20]. Unintentional weight loss of either 5% in a 1-month period or more than 10% in a 6-month period is diagnostic criteria of severe malnutrition [13,17]. A history of hospitalizations, operations, major injury or burn, and acute and chronic illnesses are meaningful clinical factors in raising suspicion for systemic inflammation and nutritional risk.

Because signs and symptoms of micronutrient deficiencies are usually late to manifest, screening for risk for deficiency is important. Chronic diseases predisposing to deficiency include those with chronic nutrient loss, such as diarrheal illness, or poor intake, including highly restrictive diets. Other less obvious conditions may result in nutrient deficiencies. Notably, a poorly described syndrome of systemic inflammation and multiple nutrient deficiencies has been observed as a late complication in patients who have undergone Roux-en-Y surgery, and is thought to be due to bacterial overgrowth in the nonalimentary limb. Bile is deconjugated and rendered inactive by the bacteria, interfering with its ability to form micelles, which in turn hampers fat digestion and absorption, and chronic steatorrhea ensues. Although most reports focus on thiamine deficiency [21] as the predominant nutritional feature, we have observed multiple instances of fat-soluble vitamin deficiency, as well as deficiencies in other water-soluble vitamins.

Assessment of intake

Commonly used dietary assessment methods include such tools as dietary history and 24-hour diet recall [22]. Diet history is an unstructured and subjective assessment of intake and can be obtained from the patient, caregivers, and medical records. A 24-hour diet recall is a structured interview designed to more accurately assess food intake and to identify the general pattern of the patient's quantity and quality of daily intake. Practitioners should be facile, at a minimum, at performing cursory dietary assessments. There are readily available resources for obtaining these skills [22]. Referral to a nutrition practitioner (e.g., registered dietitian) should be made at the first sign of a decrease in intake or at the time of diagnosis of any gastrointestinal disease that might hamper intake or absorption, or cause systemic inflammation.

Assessment of intake extends beyond oral intake and must be performed on an ongoing basis in patients receiving EN or PN support. These patients are often underfed because of interruptions for diagnostic or therapeutic procedures, or, inappropriately, for minor gastrointestinal symptoms. Without careful ongoing assessment of intake, these patients are often underfed [23].

Physical examination

Muscle mass, localized or generalized fluid accumulation, and loss of subcutaneous fat can be identified with careful physical examination and are criteria for diagnosing malnutrition [13]. A systemic physical examination is required for detecting micronutrient deficiencies. These findings are described in Table 23.1. There is much overlap of clinical findings among micronutrient deficiencies. For example, glossitis is seen in vitamin B_1, vitamin B_{12}, iron, and zinc deficiencies. Therefore, physical findings, nutritional history, and laboratory findings must all be considered in confirming the presence of micronutrient deficiencies. Symptoms and signs are often late manifestations.

Anthropometry

Anthropometry refers to the measurement of the human body. These measures are used to describe body composition, which, in turn, is used to assess the state of health and risk for morbidity and mortality. Indices such as height, weight, triceps skinfold thickness, and mid-arm circumference are used commonly and are noninvasive.

Height is used to calculate ideal bodyweight and body mass index (BMI). Ideal bodyweight is used as a comparator for assessment of measured weight or BMI, and for estimating calorie needs. BMI is commonly used to subclassify the status of underweight ($<18\,kg/m^2$), overweight ($25–30\,kg/m^2$), and obesity ($>30\,kg/m^2$). However, a patient can have malnutrition in any BMI range. Therefore, BMI itself is not considered as a clinical parameter in the etiology-based malnutrition diagnostic methods. BMI is independently correlated with life span and mortality [24,25].

Subjective assessments of subcutaneous fat and muscle mass, based on physical examination, are important criteria in the new malnutrition guidelines [13,17]. However, subjective assessment of muscle size and quality is often challenging, especially in patients who are difficult to examine (e.g., those super obese or with severe anasarca). An estimated quantification of lean and fat mass can be derived from measures of triceps skinfold and mid-arm circumference via validated algorithms. Despite using calipers and tape measures, these are dependent on examiner skill and fraught with inaccuracy [26,27].

Several other methods are available for more quantitative measure of body composition. Hydrostatic underwater weighing test, bioelectrical impedance plethysmography, dual-energy X-ray absorptiometry, computed tomography, and magnetic resonance imaging are more objective and accurate than is mid-arm circumference, but all of these are more useful for monitoring change over time and/or for research than for point-in-time assessments.

Hydrostatic underwater weighing is considered the gold standard for measuring body composition. However, the clinical use of this test is limited because of the high cost and complexity of the test [28]. Bioelectrical impedance, which requires four electrodes, an ohmmeter, and analytic software, is the simplest test, but it is highly impacted by the patient's state of hydration and skin temperature, so it is not useful in the hospital setting [29,30]. It is commonly used in outpatient clinic settings for the longitudinal assessment of patients with obesity. Clinical use of dual-energy X-ray absorptiometry, computed tomography, and magnetic resonance imaging is uncommon because of their cost and availability. All three use cross-sectional imaging of various anatomy [31] (arms, legs, torso), with and without three-dimensional reconstruction and image analysis, to construct accurate models [32] of body components, including being able to detect fat replacement of muscle, so-called sarcopenia, which is predictive of poor outcomes and frailty [33].

Laboratory testing

Although a simple laboratory test for diagnosing malnutrition is desirable, no such parameter exists. The levels of many blood components, such as albumin, are highly predictive of morbidity and mortality, but none predicts which patient will respond to nourishment interventions. This, however, is true of many of the parameters used to diagnose disease-related malnutrition. Traditional protein makers, such as serum albumin, transthyretin (otherwise known as prealbumin), transferrin, and retinol-binding protein, were excluded from the AND/A.S.P.E.N. definition [13], but albumin has been included in the GLIM criteria [17]. Inflammation alters serum protein distribution, as well as increases the protein catabolic rate [34]. Protein shifts between intravascular and extravascular compartments in the presence of inflammation, which causes capillary leak [35] (Figure 23.3). Ironically, low serum albumin may be a common reason for referral of a patient to nutrition support teams. Low serum proteins should be considered acute phase responders. Because malnutrition is diagnosed based on disease processes, such as weakness and wasting, serum proteins may also be considered by some as being diagnostic of malnutrition. However, they do not indicate whether the patient is malnourished.

Nitrogen balance is often used to determine dietary protein requirements in a hospital setting by assessing the difference

Table 23.1 Physical findings and associated nutritional disorders.

System	Physical findings	Nutritional disorder
General	Loss of subcutaneous fat and weight loss	Macronutrient deficiency
	Loss of appetites (anorexia)	Zinc deficiency
Skin	Petechiae, purpura	Vitamin C deficiency, vitamin K deficiency
	Poor wound healing	Zinc deficiency, vitamin C deficiency
	Desquamation, erythema, scaling, and keratosis of sun exposure	Niacin or tryptophan deficiency, leucine excess
	Eczematous scaling	Essential fatty acid, zinc, or biotin deficiency
	Corkscrew hairs	Vitamin C deficiency
	Thin hair, hair loss	Zinc deficiency, essential fatty acid deficiency, macronutrient deficiency
	Koilonychia (spoon nails)	Iron-deficiency anemia
Head, eyes, and neck	Night blindness, Photophobia, blurring	Vitamin A deficiency, riboflavin deficiency
	Angular stomatitis	Riboflavin, pyridoxine, niacin deficiency
	Cheilosis	Riboflavin, niacin deficiency
	Gingival enlargement, gum bleeding	Vitamin C deficiency
	Loss of lingual papillae	Riboflavin, niacin, folate
	Glossitis	Vitamin B_{12} deficiency, iron deficiency, riboflavin deficiency
	Goiter	Iodine deficiency
Respiratory	Acute respiratory failure	Refeeding syndrome (most causes are nonnutritional)
Circulatory	Heart failure (cardiomyopathy)	Thiamine deficiency, refeeding syndrome, selenium deficiency, carnitine deficiency, pyridoxine deficiency
Gastrointestinal	Diarrhea	Niacin deficiency
	Hepatomegaly	Macronutrient deficiency (protein deficiency)
Musculoskeletal	Bone tenderness, joint pain	Vitamin D deficiency, vitamin C deficiency
	Muscle casting	Macronutrient deficiency (chronic disease- or starvation-related malnutrition)
Neurological	Confabulation, disorientation	Thiamine deficiency
	Dementia, degenerative neuropathy	Niacin deficiency, vitamin B_{12} deficiency, manganese excess
	Peripheral neuropathy	Thiamine deficiency, pyridoxine deficiency, vitamin B_{12} deficiency, copper deficiency, chromium deficiency
Hematological	Signs of anemia (fatigue, pale skin, dizziness)	Iron deficiency, vitamin B_{12} deficiency, folate deficiency, copper deficiency

between nitrogen intake and loss. Most nitrogen excretion in humans is in the urine, and 3–5 g of nitrogen is excreted by feces, skin, and sweat. A 24-hour urine collection is performed to calculate nitrogen loss. Note that 6.25 g of protein contains 1 g of nitrogen [36] (Box 23.1).

Micronutrient levels are not routinely measured during nutritional screening and assessment. However, patients who are at risk for development of micronutrient deficiency, or who have clinical and physical signs of micronutrient deficiency, should be investigated and routinely monitored for micronutrient levels. For example, serum levels of iron, ferritin, zinc, copper, vitamin A, vitamin B_1, vitamin B_{12}, and folic acid are routinely monitored for the patients who have undergone gastric bypass surgery for weight loss [37].

Overview of nutrition support

EN versus PN support

EN is defined as nutrition provided through the gastrointestinal tract, whereas PN is defined as nutrition provided through an intravenous route. EN is generally preferred, and the advantages of EN over PN are well established by multiple randomized clinical trials in diverse clinical conditions, including critical illness, trauma, burn, and acute pancreatitis [38–41]. EN, when compared with PN, is associated with less infectious morbidity and shorter length of hospital stay [39,42–44].

EN also has several theoretical benefits compared with PN. EN can support gut integrity by maintaining the tight junctions between the intestinal epithelial cells [45]. EN can also stimulate

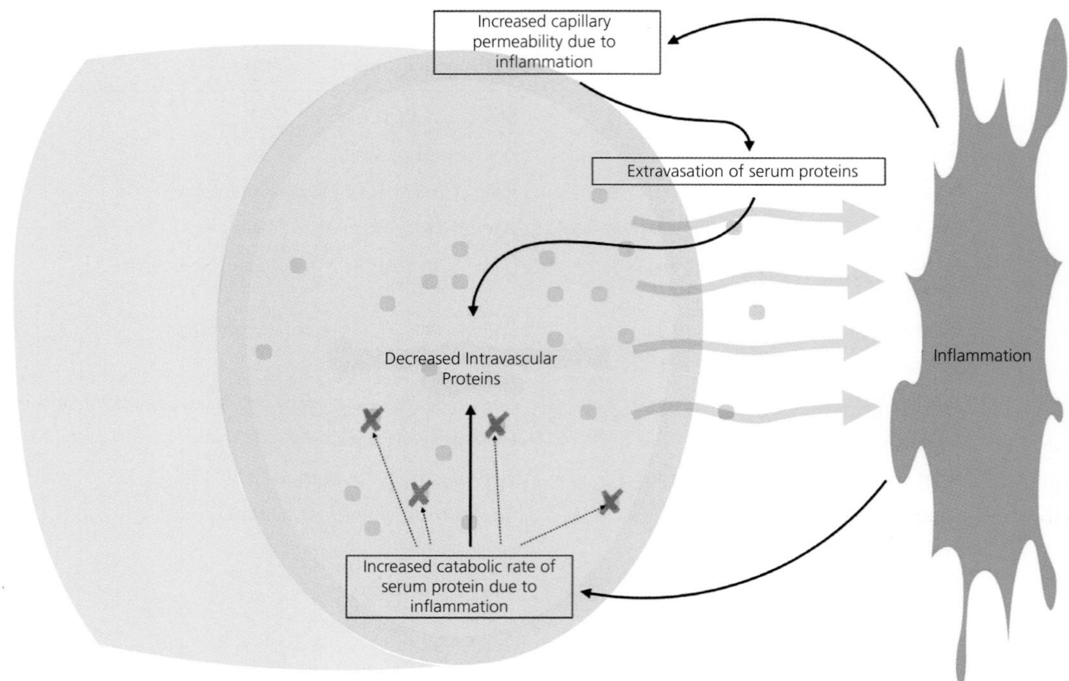

Figure 23.3 Pathogenesis of hypoproteinemia. Source: Based on Lee and Slutsky 2010 [35].

the release of secretory immunoglobulin A (IgA), which can prevent bacterial adherence to the intestinal epithelium [46]. Moreover, long-term PN can alter the gut microbiome [47], which may contribute to complications. The absence of enteral feeding can result in villous atrophy and bacterial overgrowth. In rat models, PN for up to 3 weeks resulted in a 73% reduction in small-intestinal weight compared with controls on a standard enteral diet. Although less dramatic, this has also been demonstrated in humans, with a 20% reduction in small-intestinal weight [48,49].

Box 23.1 The formula for calculating nitrogen balance.

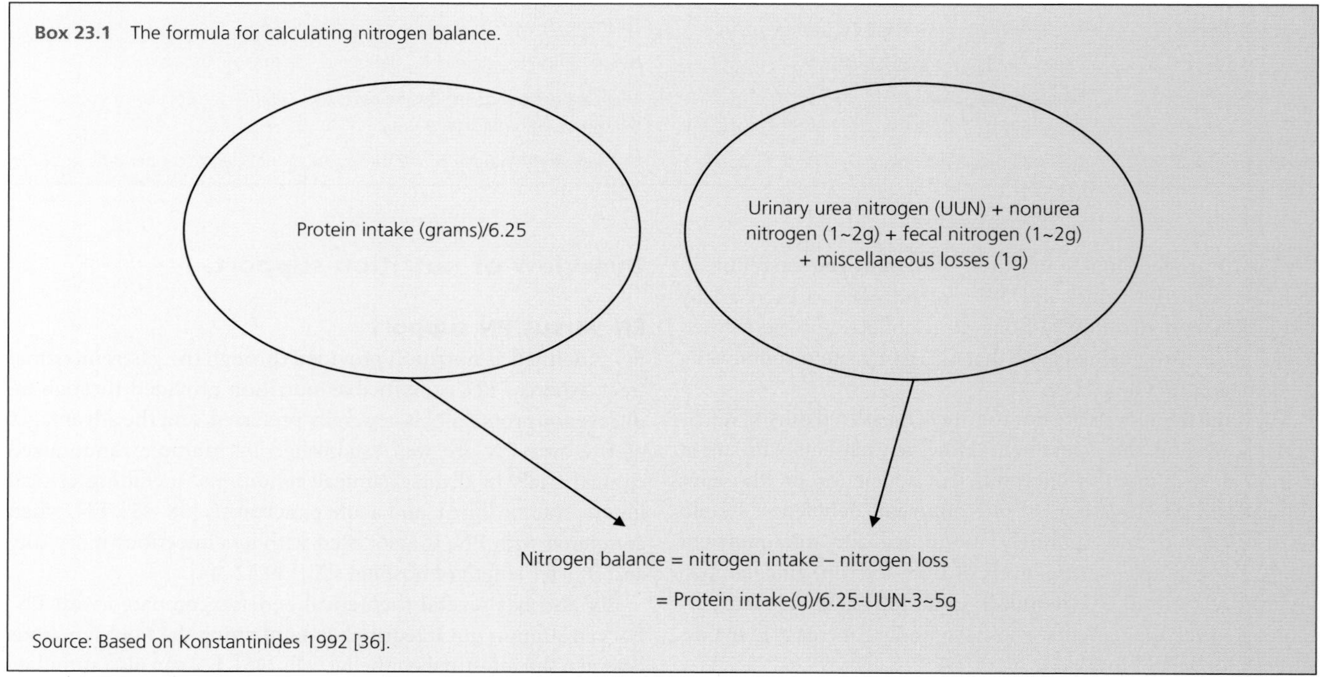

Source: Based on Konstantinides 1992 [36].

In its early use, PN was often extremely high in calories. This caused serious complications, such as hyperglycemia, liver steatosis and failure, and hypercapnia. This practice stemmed, in part, from the high-calorie burn rate seen in critically ill patients. With improvements in critical care, the calorie burn in critically ill patients is closer to basal metabolic rate. This reduction in calorie requirements is due to better practice in ventilation and sedation, and control of pain, temperature, and anxiety, all of which contributed to reducing calorie consumption. With reduction of calories in PN, overfeeding-induced complications have been reduced. Sterile central line placement techniques have significantly improved, and central catheter-related complications have been reduced [50]. In one series, excess central line infections occurred in hospital inpatients only once every 100 patient-days [51]. There are randomized control trials that have shown that hypocaloric PN is as safe as EN [52,53]. However, other studies show clear risk of adding PN [54]. Regardless, it is undisputed that EN provides a more physiological means to deliver nutrients and is less costly than PN; therefore, "If gut works, use it" determines the route of nutrition support.

Estimation of energy and protein requirements

Total energy expenditure consists of three major components: (1) resting energy expenditure, (2) the thermogenic effect of food, and (3) physical activity. Resting energy expenditure contributes the largest portion of total energy expenditure in healthy individuals. Digestion and absorption of the foods can increase the metabolic rate. This approximate 5–10% increase is referred to as the thermogenic effect of food [55]. However, the thermogenic effect becomes negligible in patients who receive EN or PN support [56]. In healthy individuals, physical activity is an unpredictable component in total energy expenditure. In hospitalized patients, physical activity is measured to be approximately 5–10% of total energy expenditure [57]. Therefore, calculation or measurement of resting energy expenditure is used to estimate calorie requirements in nutrition support for the hospitalized patient [58].

Indirect calorimetry is considered to be the gold standard for measuring resting energy expenditure [59]. Continuous measurement of oxygen consumption (VO_2) and carbon dioxide production (VCO_2) is required. The Weir equation,

$$\left[\text{Resting energy expenditure} = \left(3.94 \times VO_2\right) + \left(1.1 \times VCO_2\right)\right],$$

is used to calculate energy expenditure and respiratory quotient [60]. Respiratory quotient is the ratio of VCO_2 and VO_2 and is useful in determining nutrient utilization. Carbohydrate metabolism generates more CO_2 than of the metabolism of fat. Thus, the respiratory quotient is low in underfeeding, which can promote lipolysis of fat stores, or when excess fat is provided. It is high in overfeeding, which can induce lipogenesis. Indirect calorimetry is recommended for patients for whom it is difficult to use calorie estimation equations because of their clinical conditions. For example, patients who are underweight, are obese, have amputation, have fluid overload, or are critically ill are good candidates for indirect calorimetry (Figure 23.4).

Many predictive equations are available for calculating resting energy expenditure. These are usually validated against oximetry but are valid only in specific conditions. Moreover, they mostly cluster around a weight-based estimation of 25–30 kcal/kg/day.

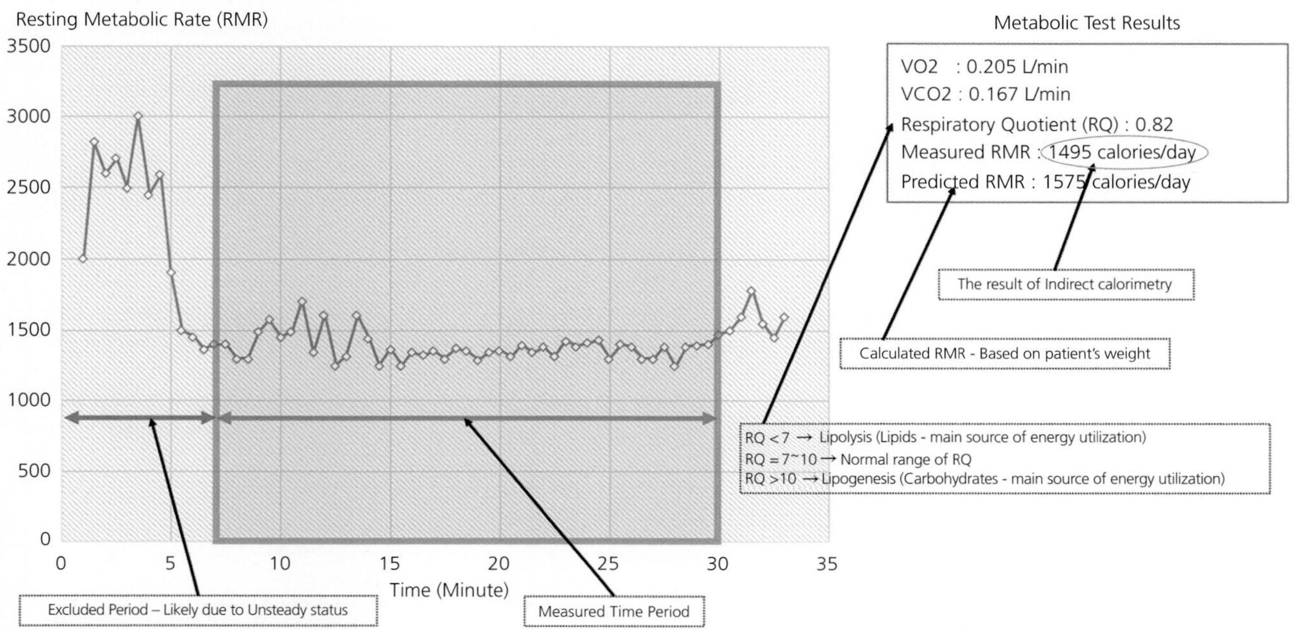

Figure 23.4 Result interpretation of indirect calorimetry.

This is often used for calculating daily energy requirements in view of its simplicity. This estimation of needs should be modified dependent on the patient's clinical condition. For example, hypocaloric feeding (20 kcal/kg/day) is recommended for critically ill patients who need PN. Needs for critically ill obese patients may be estimated using ~11–14 kcal/kg/day if indirect calorimetry is not available [59].

Protein requirements can be estimated based on weight. Prescriptions vary from 0.8 g/kg/day for the healthy to 2.0 g/kg/day for the severely catabolic patient, such as those suffering from significant burn injury or who are severely critically ill. A moderately supplemented prescription at around 1.2–1.3 g/kg/day should suffice for most hospitalized or chronically ill patients [59,61].

These simplified methods for estimating calorie consumption are useful as starting points. Nutrition professionals, such as registered dietitians, make use of far more sophisticated estimates, such as the Modified Penn State equation and others. These practitioners can help determine when direct measurement, such as indirect calorimetry, is needed, and they should be involved in verifying the appropriateness of all nutrition prescriptions.

Enteral nutrition support

Timing of EN

Generally, early initiation of EN is recommended. However, because of the poor quality and risk for bias in these studies, this strong consensus is still subject to verification [62]. Specifically, it is recommended that EN be initiated within 24–48 hours in critically ill patients. Multiple metaanalyses have shown a trend toward reduced mortality when EN was initiated within 48 hours of the onset of the critical illness [59]. The historical practices of delaying EN until bowel movement or bowel sounds appear after gastrointestinal surgery are associated with greater risk. Early initiation of EN is recommended for all postsurgical patients regardless of the presence of signs of gastrointestinal contractility because it is associated with enhanced recovery and reduced complications postoperatively, even in critically ill patients [63].

Enteral feeding formulas

Enteral formulas (Table 23.2) can be divided into two major categories: (1) standard formulas and (2) disease-specific formulas. Standard feeding formulas are most widely used for patients who require EN. The composition of macronutrients and micronutrients in the standard feeding formula is quite similar to what is recommended for healthy individuals. They are polymeric (i.e., not predigested), and the electrolyte levels are not restricted relative to other formulas. Patients with normal electrolyte needs can maintain their electrolytes without any supplementation with standard feeding formulas. Standard formulas can be divided into multiple subcategories based on the concentration and the presence of fiber. The concentrations vary from 1 to 2 kcal/mL. Concentrated standard formulas are recommended for patients who require volume restriction without electrolytes restriction, such as patients with congestive

Table 23.2 Specialized enteral feeding products.

Disease	Special formula content	Outcomes	Recommendation
Diabetes	High fiber, complex carbohydrates, lower total carbohydrates, higher fat	No improvement in glycemic control in continuous feeding	Consider for patients with diabetes being bolus fed; otherwise, use standard formula
Predigested	Protein and carbohydrate provided vary from individual amino acids and simple sugars to oligomers of each Fat either restricted or altered structure	Poor evidence of improved absorption Variable results on improved gastrointestinal tolerance	Avoid use in short gut due to theoretic decrease in adaptation
Renal	Electrolyte and volume restricted	Useful in patients with poor electrolyte clearance No impact on underlying renal disease	Use when electrolyte restriction is needed
Immune modulating	Supplemented with arginine, glutamine, ω-3 fats, and various micronutrients	Decreased postoperative complications	Consider for postoperative patients in the surgical intensive care unit or patients with severe trauma
Obesity	High protein with supplemental micronutrients	None	Consider use in obese patients for whom restriction of calories and supplementation of protein are desired
Acute respiratory distress syndrome	High fat and high in ω-3 fats	Improved outcomes compared with pulmonary formula May be harmful compared with standard formulas	Use standard formula
Hepatic encephalopathy	Supplemented with branched-chain amino acids Electrolyte restricted	No impact on encephalopathy or mortality	Use standard formula

heart failure, ascites, or edema. It should be noted that the sodium concentration is low for all of these products, approximately 40 mEq, or 700 mg, per 1000 kcal. Fiber-containing formulas provide fermentable and nonfermentable fiber. The former is converted to short-chain fat, the preferred fuel source for colonocytes [64]. The latter helps regulate stool quality. It is recommended that noncritically ill patients who do not have feeding intolerance receive fiber-containing tube feeds. The recommendations to avoid fiber in the critically ill have been eased [59]. Fiber-containing formulas may be beneficial for patients with persistent diarrhea or constipation [59,65].

Disease-specific formulas are specialized and targeted formulas designed for patients with specific organ dysfunction or metabolic conditions. Most have proved to have no benefit. These are summarized later and in Table 23.2.

Diabetes formulas

Diabetes formulas are lower in carbohydrate, higher in monounsaturated fat, and have more soluble and insoluble fiber than standard formulas. These formulas have a low glycemic index and are beneficial for glycemic control when administered orally. However, a large body of clinical evidence refutes the value of diabetic formulas in hospitalized patients with diabetes to improve glycemic control [66]. This is thought to be due to tube feeds being administered as a continuous infusion, rather than as a meal. Thus, glucose appearance is equal to glucose delivery (feeding plus gluconeogenesis), which reaches equilibrium in continuously fed patients. Glycemic index measures glucose increase after meals. Due to the high fiber content of these products, they should be used with caution in patients who have a high risk for bowel ischemia or severe dysmotility [59] (see later *Intestinal ischemia/intestinal bezoar* section).

Predigested formulas

Predigested formulas are designed for use in patients with malabsorption and persistent feeding intolerance. These can be elemental or semielemental formulas. The former is characterized by individual amino acids and simple sugars and is usually extremely low in fat. Semielemental formulas have oligopeptides and oligosaccharides. All have some amount of long-chain triglyceride. Some contain medium-chain triglyceride oil, which can be directly absorbed into the portal circulation, bypassing digestion and gut lymphatics. Predigested formulas can be considered for patients with chronic malabsorption who are not able to be managed with standard feeding formula and exogenous pancreatic enzyme supplements. These are not appropriate as substitutes for pancreatic enzyme supplementation in those with pancreatic insufficiency because all fat is provided as a triglyceride which requires lipase for absorption. The routine clinical use of these formulas is not recommended because of a lack of evidence of outcomes benefit. In particular, these formulas are not recommended for the early stage of short bowel syndrome because they may delay the adaptation process [67].

Renal formulas

Renal formulas are designed for the patient with chronic kidney disease who is receiving intermittent hemodialysis, when fluid and electrolyte restrictions are required. The protein content of these products is usually slightly higher than in standard feeds to compensate for the catabolic effect of dialysis, although there is no supporting evidence that there is an outcome benefit from providing this additional protein. Unless patients receiving dialysis require the electrolyte restrictions provided by these formulas, a standard product is preferred [59]. These formulas may also be useful for patients with hyperkalemia and/or hyperphosphatemia without renal failure. Highly protein-restricted formulas are also available. These are also concentrated and have lower concentrations of electrolytes, including potassium, phosphate, and calcium. In fact, there are no proven outcomes benefits from protein restriction for patients with acute or chronic renal failure. Protein restriction may have the effect of decreasing blood urea nitrogen levels, but this is a matter of reduced substrate. Neither progression of acute renal disease nor the need for dialysis is impacted by protein restriction. Moreover, the impact of protein restriction on long-term progression of renal disease is small at best, is associated with poor patient compliance, and does not impact mortality [68].

Immune-modulating formulas

Arginine, glutamine, nucleic acids, and ω-3 fatty acids are all important in immunity and inflammation and are added to immune-modulating formulas in supplementary amounts. These nutrients are thought to have the potential to enhance the immune response and modulate the metabolic response to severe inflammation. Multiple clinical studies and metaanalyses have demonstrated a small but significant improvement of clinical outcomes in surgical patients using these formulas [69–72]. Whether clinical outcomes in nonsurgical patients with severe inflammation are improved is still controversial [59,73]. Therefore, these formulas should not be used routinely in medical intensive care units. Currently, these formulas deserve consideration for postoperative patients in the surgical intensive care unit or patients with severe trauma [59].

Formulas for obese patients

Based on very little prospective data, hypocaloric and high-protein feeding has been recommended for obese patients, particularly those who are critically ill [74]. One such product is semielemental (predigested) and contains supplemental amounts of ω-3 fats, as well as other nutrients that are reported to be at lower levels in the obese based on observational studies. The proportion of protein is very high in these formulas (35–40% of calories). The rationale for these alterations is that obesity-related inflammation can be reduced with ω-3 oils, and that lean body mass can be preserved with high-protein feeding. However, clinical evidence is very weak or lacking, and these products require more and higher-quality clinical studies.

Formulas for acute respiratory distress syndrome

In the past, a formula that contained large amounts of ω-3 oils was recommended for patients with acute respiratory distress syndrome and severe acute lung injury based on multiple randomized clinical trials [63]. However, these studies have been strongly criticized. The controls used in these trials were very high in fat, entirely ω-6 oils. These ω-6 fats in turn may be proinflammatory and are theorized to be potentially harmful. Thus, the benefit seen from these formulas may have been the result of *not* using the control high ω-6 product, rather than a direct benefit from the high ω-3 intervention. Recent multicenter clinical trials, moreover, revealed no clinical benefit using high-dose antiinflammatory lipids for acute lung injury or patients with acute respiratory distress syndrome [75], and these formulas are no longer recommended [59].

Formulas for hepatic encephalopathy

Branched-chain amino acids leucine, isoleucine, and valine are essential amino acids that cannot be produced by the human body. Supplementation of these can reduce ammonia levels in the brain and skeletal muscles [76]. In animals, they can suppress hepatocyte apoptosis and promote hepatocyte proliferation [77,78]. Concentrations of BCAAs can be decreased in advanced liver cirrhosis, whereas levels of aromatic amino acid, such as phenylalanine and tyrosine, are increased. The ratio of branched-chain amino acids to aromatic amino acids, called Fisher's ratio, is considered to be an important parameter for assessing liver metabolism, hepatic functional reserve, and the severity of liver dysfunction [79]. Further, the metabolic by-products of the aromatic amino acids mimic neurotransmitters and were theorized to be part of the cause of hepatic encephalopathy.

Formulations and supplements high in branched-chain amino acids were promoted to use in hepatic encephalopathy. However, clinical outcomes were not significantly improved when compared with standard feeding formula [80] and supplementation of branched-chain amino acids for hepatic encephalopathy remains controversial. Supplementation may have some small beneficial effects on hepatic encephalopathy. However, the recurrence of hepatic encephalopathy or mortality were not reduced [81,82]. Therefore, standard feeding formulas are recommended for hepatic encephalopathy [59]. In the past, restriction of protein intake was recommended for patients with liver failure. However, there is concern that this restriction can exacerbate lean mass loss and may actually result in high ammonia levels. Therefore, this approach is no longer recommended [59,83].

Enteral access

Enteral access is discussed in Chapter 123.

Parenteral nutrition

PN is a complex, hypertonic solution, infused via central or, less commonly, peripheral vein, which requires appropriate administration and safety precautions to prevent complications [84,85]. The Institute for Safe Medication Practices considers PN a high-alert medication; similar to chemotherapy and neuromuscular blockade medications. These medications "bear a heightened risk of causing significant patient harm when they are used in error" [86]. Published guidelines exist with which any practitioner involved in the administration of PN, from assessment to ordering to monitoring to compounding, should be familiar [84,85]. Complications may include catheter-related infections, phlebitis, thrombosis or sclerosis of veins, electrolyte abnormalities, and hepatic dysfunction. Central venous access is used for PN in most clinical situations because of the frequency of pain and phlebitis and the relatively larger volume required to avoid exceeding the theoretical limit of 900 mOsm when using peripheral veins [84].

Nomenclature

PN has undergone numerous changes in nomenclature. Originally, it was referred to as hyperalimentation, reflecting the dextrose concentration [87]. This was misconstrued as reflecting a need to overfeed. Later, the terms "partial" and "total" PN were used. As mentioned earlier, PN administered via a peripheral vein must be relatively dilute. Because the amounts of calories and protein provided were relatively high, it was believed that full nourishment could not be provided via peripheral vein because of the required volume for dilution. Now, because we recognize that "total" PN can often be administered peripherally, the accepted nomenclature is "parenteral nutrition," with specification as to route contained in the orders [84,85]. The terms "central PN" and "peripheral PN" are also sometimes used. Because of the ease of obtaining and the safety of peripherally inserted central catheters (PICCs) and the frequent damage to peripheral veins, PN is much less often administered peripherally.

Indications and timing of PN

PN provides nourishment to those patients who are not able to tolerate or absorb enough macronutrients via the gastrointestinal tract to maintain adequate nourishment. Common indications for PN support include short bowel syndrome, bowel obstructions, high-output enterocutaneous fistula, prolonged ileus, severe acute pancreatitis, and chronic malabsorptive conditions (Box 23.2).

Box 23.2 Indications for parenteral nutrition in specific clinical conditions.

Common indications	Potential indications
Short bowel syndrome	Inflammatory bowel disease
High-output enterocutaneous fistula	Hyperemesis gravidarum
Complete bowel obstruction	Severe mucositis
Prolonged ileus	Preoperative severe malnutrition
Chronic malabsorption	Chyle leak
	Severe pancreatitis

Guidelines suggest that the timing for initiation of PN differs from that of EN and depends on the patient's nutritional status [59]. It is incontrovertible that patients will starve to death if those with prolonged gut failure are not fed parenterally. As stated earlier, critically ill patients with malnutrition are at higher risk for mortality and increased risk for morbidity and prolonged length of stay [3]. A recent systematic review suggests that stratification of patients to receive EN based on the presence of malnutrition improves outcomes [11]. However, analyses are inconsistent in demonstrating benefit from shorter-term PN in hospitalized patients, whether compared with EN [42] or compared with no intervention [88].

In general, if gut failure is anticipated for less than 1 week, PN is not indicated, unless the patient has severe malnutrition. In the presence of chronic starvation, PN should be initiated carefully because of risk for refeeding syndrome (reviewed later). In patients without severe malnutrition, PN support can be considered after 1 week of limited enteral intake.

If enteral feeding is chronically insufficient to meet the patient's calorie requirements goal (e.g. <60%), supplemental PN can be considered. The practice of "topping up" calories with PN has been much promoted, based on the association between calorie "deficit" and outcomes in observational studies. However, early PN and early supplemental PN should be avoided, even for malnourished patients, because this has been shown to increase medical costs and length of hospital stay [54,89]. A large, multicenter, randomized trial was conducted to attempt to better define the role and timing of PN [90]. Data indicate that early PN and early supplemental PN are associated with an increased risk for infections [91] in general and invasive fungal infections [92] specifically. In one small cohort, early PN did not slow muscle wasting and resulted in an increase in fat deposition in muscle in the critically ill [93]. Therefore, we believe that supplemental PN support should be considered only after ~7–10 days, regardless of the presence of malnutrition.

Routes of PN

Central venous access

Direct central access (internal jugular venous central line or subclavian central venous line) or PICCs are commonly used for hospitalized patients who are receiving PN. Trials comparing complications between catheter type in hospitalized patients receiving PN are scant. Subclavian venous access is related to increased risk for stenosis [94]. Therefore, it may be advisable to avoid subclavian access in patients who experience renal failure and may require hemodialysis.

PICC is increasingly used for home PN patients [95,96]. Tunneled central catheters (e.g., Hickman, Broviac, Groshong) and ports are reserved for longer-term use, because their insertion and removal are more complex than is that for PICCs. The notion that the risk for catheter-related bloodstream infection (CRBSI) is less with tunneled catheters has been seriously challenged. Observations [97] and a meta-analysis [98] indicate noninferiority for PICCs. Moreover, a recent analysis of a registry of a large number (n = 1046; 223,493 PN days) of home PN patients found a strong negative association between PICC and CRBSI when compared with tunneled central catheters or port. The overall CRBSI rate was 0.87 per 1000 PN days. For PICCs, which made up nearly half of the cohort, the CRBSI rate was 0.41 per 1000 PN days. For ports and tunneled catheters, the rates were 0.66 and 0.51 per 1000 PN days, respectively. In contrast, the frequency of thrombosis has been reported to be higher with PICC, thought to be due to the longer length of the indwelling catheter [99].

Certain patients tend to have recurrent CRBSI. Techniques such as ethanol or antibiotic lock, in which an antiinfective is instilled and left to remain in the catheter when it is not in use, can be considered to reduce subsequent infections [100–102].

Peripheral venous access

PN can be administered via peripheral vein. As mentioned earlier, the amount of macronutrients delivered in peripherally infused PN can be the same as that infused centrally. However, peripheral PN must have a maximum osmolality of <900 mOsm/L. Peripheral veins can develop phlebitis and be sclerosed by a hypertonic solution. The site for peripheral PN often needs to be changed daily, or more, even when kept <900 mOsm/L, and should be changed at least every 2–3 days, so it is useful only in patients with plentiful peripheral veins. Peripheral PN cannot provide full calories in patients who need volume restriction. The amount of electrolytes added to a peripheral PN solution is also limited. Because central access is rarely delayed more than a few days, peripheral PN is rarely necessary.

Prescribing PN

Macronutrients

Protein

As with EN, protein requirements can be estimated based on the patient's weight. Prescriptions vary from 0.8 g/kg/day for the healthy to 2.0 g/kg/day for the severely catabolic, such as after burn or severely critically ill. A moderately supplemented prescription around 1.2–1.3 g/kg/day should suffice for most hospitalized or chronically ill patients [59,61]. In PN, 1 g of protein provides 4 kcal. Amino acid solutions range in concentration from 5% to 15% (grams percent, or grams solute per 100 g solution). Specialized formulations are available, such as high branched-chain/low aromatic amino acids for hepatic encephalopathy; however, these have not proved to provide benefit over much less expensive standard amino acid mixtures.

Lipid

Daily recommended fat intake in normal adults is between 20% and 35% of total daily calorie requirements [103]. Triglyceride, however, need only make up 1–2% of calories to prevent essential fatty acid deficiency, which can develop in a matter of weeks when PN is given without lipids [104]. Lipid emulsions (properly termed lipid injectable emulsion and abbreviated ILE [84]) are relatively contraindicated for patients with severe hypertriglyceridemia. Therefore, serum triglyceride level must be checked before their use. They must be used with caution in patients with abnormal liver function, because lipid injectable emulsion has been associated with hepatic dysfunction [105,106]. Lipid injectable emulsion should be avoided in patients with severe sepsis because they have been associated with adverse outcomes in these patients.

Until recently, the only lipid emulsion available in the United States was a 100% soybean oil-based formula. This formula contains plant sterols, proposed to be involved in lipid injectable emulsion-related hepatic dysfunction [107]. These also contain a large amount of the fatty acid linoleic acid. This is one of two essential fatty acids and a polyunsaturated ω-6 fatty acid. Newer formulas, available in Europe for some time, have been recently approved for use in the United States. These have less plant sterol and may have less hepatic toxicity [108].

These new lipid injectable emulsions also contain more ω-3 fatty acids. ω-6 fats are considered proinflammatory, whereas ω-3 fats anti-inflammatory. Although this theoretical benefit has been touted by proponents of their use, there is some disagreement as to their benefit [108,109].

The two newly approved formulations include a four-oil source mixed lipid emulsion and one that is solely from fish oil. The first contains soybean oil (30%), medium-chain triglyceride (30%), olive oil (25%), and fish oil (15%). The concentration of linoleic acid in this mixed emulsion is much lower than the concentration in the soybean-based emulsion. Thus, patients may require more of the mixed emulsion than that of the traditional emulsion to prevent essential fatty acid deficiency. This mixed emulsion may have clinical benefits in PN-associated liver disease [108]. Fish oil-based lipid emulsion is also proposed to help decrease PN-associated liver disease. It is approved by the US Food and Drug Administration for pediatric patients with PN-associated cholestasis [110]. Fish oil-based emulsions, however, contain very little linoleic acid and thus may put patients at risk for essential fatty acid deficiency if these are the sole source of fat.

Egg phospholipid is used as an emulsifier to make the triglyceride water miscible. All of these lipid emulsions are used with caution in patients with egg, soy, and/or fish allergies (in the mixed or fish oil-based lipid injectable emulsion).

One gram of dietary fat provides 9 kcal. One gram of triglyceride, in lipid injectable emulsion, provides 10 kcal in 20% lipid injectable emulsion and 11 kcal in 10% lipid injectable emulsion. This is due to extra calories contained in the glycerol and other emulsifiers. The 20% lipid injectable emulsion is commonly used in PN.

Carbohydrate

The recommended macronutrient distribution range for carbohydrates is 45–65% of total daily calorie requirements. Dextrose is the most commonly used carbohydrate form for PN. One gram of dietary carbohydrate provides 4 calories, whereas 1 g of hydrated dextrose, used in making dextrose solutions used in PN, provides 3.4 calories. A minimum of calories must be provided to avoid ketosis, and the theoretical maximum for dextrose is approximately 5 g/kg/day [84].

Macronutrient prescription

After the estimation of daily calorie requirements, protein and lipid amounts should be calculated. The remaining calories, after subtracting protein and lipid calories from total daily calories, are provided by carbohydrates. The minimum total volume required to compound the PN is calculated based on the concentrations of the macronutrients, plus an allowance of 100–150 mL for electrolytes. The final volume should be calculated based on an assessment of the patient's daily needs. Detailed methods for the creating the PN order can be found in Tables 23.3 and 23.4.

Electrolytes are added to the PN formulation to maintain normal serum levels. Sodium is a major cation in serum and PN formulation. The amount of sodium in PN will be determined by estimating needs and monitoring serum sodium levels. Normal requirements are approximately 1–2 mEq/kg/day. It is recommended that sodium content in PN not exceed sodium concentration level (154 mEq/L) found in normal saline.

The daily dose of potassium in PN formulation is 1 mEq/kg in patients with normal renal function. This dose of potassium should be adjusted based on the patient's clinical condition. Normal calcium and magnesium requirements for adults are between 10 and 20 mEq/day.

The major anions in PN are acetate and chloride. They are adjusted dependent on the patient's acid–base balance. Nonanion gap metabolic acidosis can be seen in hospitalized patients because of administration of chloride-based maintenance fluid, such as normal saline and half normal saline [111]. Acetate is a buffer that is metabolized to bicarbonate. In patients with acidosis, larger amounts of acetate may be added to PN. Phosphorus, provided as a phosphate anion, is added to adult PN at approximately 10–30 mmol/day. Both sodium and potassium are available as chloride, acetate, or phosphate. It is recommended that only one anion of potassium be used, to avoid calculation errors [85].

Multivitamins and trace elements should be added to PN daily. Injectable multivitamin mixtures include retinol, ergocalciferol, alfa tocopheryl acetate, phytonadione, thiamin, riboflavin, pyridoxine, niacin, dexpanthenol, biotin, folic acid, cyanocobalamin, and ascorbic acid. Additional vitamins can be added, in the event that additional supplementation is required. For example, additional thiamin can be added to PN for the first few days for patients with refeeding syndrome or at high risk for thiamine deficiency. The combined multitrace elements may include zinc, copper, chromium, manganese,

Table 23.3 Writing a parenteral nutrition prescription—macronutrients.

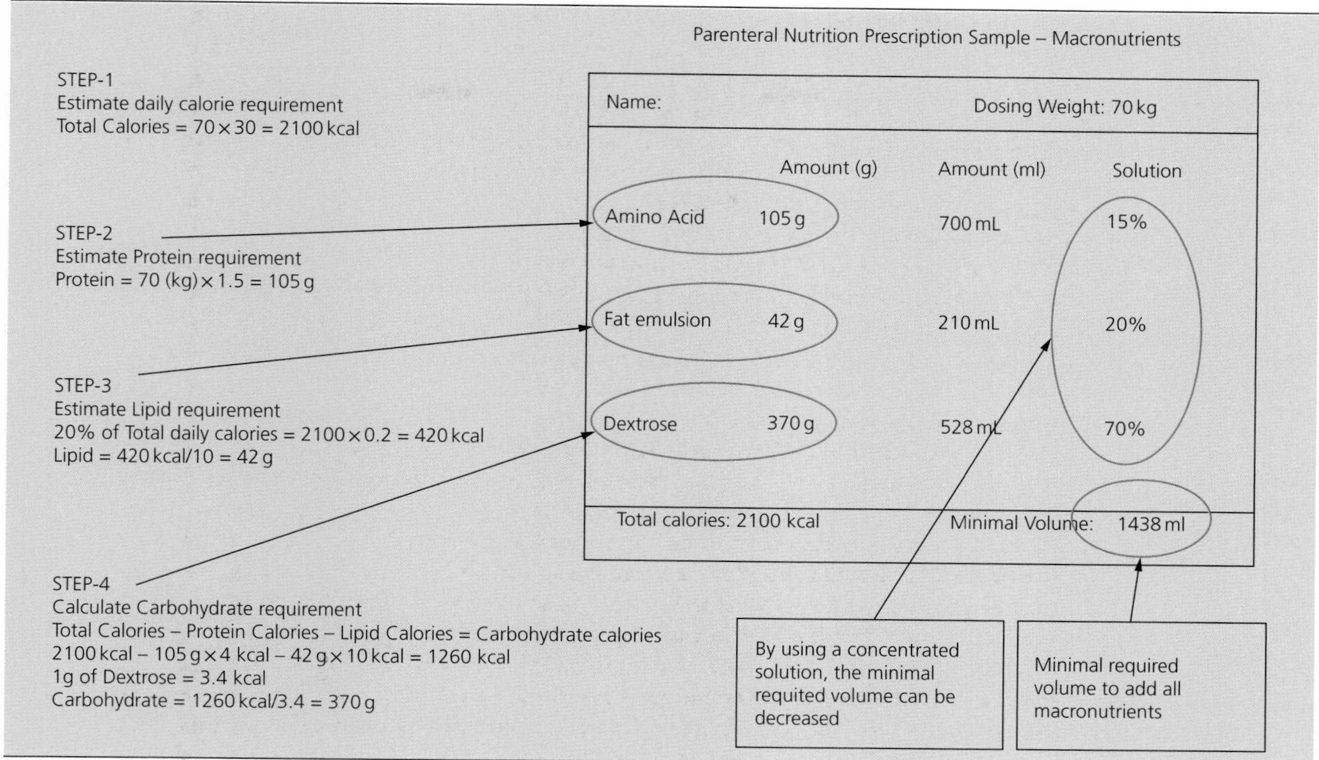

and selenium. Copper and manganese are excreted mainly in the bile, so these are withheld, and the other trace elements are ordered individually, when the patient has cholestasis. Moreover, a high manganese level itself can be a contributing factor for cholestasis [112].

Insulin

Hyperglycemia is common in patients receiving PN. The American Diabetes Association recommends conventional blood glucose control (target blood glucose goal, ~140–180 mg/dL) for critically ill patients [113]. In relatively stable patients, or those with previously established insulin need, regular insulin can be added to PN to obtain target blood glucose levels. We advise against attempting to tightly control glucose with insulin added into the PN in the critically ill, especially those who are not chronically receiving insulin. Insulin sensitivity can fluctuate widely and acutely in these patients, and measures such as continuous insulin infusions are more appropriate in this population.

The initial daily dose of insulin can be estimated by the dose of dextrose on PN. One unit of regular insulin per 11 g of dextrose can be added on the PN solution for patients with diabetes and 1 unit per 20 g of dextrose can be added for patients without diabetes. The insulin dose should be adjusted based on previous day's additional insulin dose or by calculation of insulin sensitivity factors. The calculation of insulin sensitivity factors is described in Box 23.3.

Medications

Addition of any medication to PN is discouraged, given the limited data on compatibility [85]. Histamine H_2-receptor antagonists, such as famotidine (~20–40 mg) or ranitidine (~200–300 mg), are commonly added to PN solutions. However, proton pump inhibitors are not compatible with PN. Proton pump inhibitors are weak

Box 23.3 Insulin sensitivity factor.

Definition: "How much does 1 unit of insulin lower the blood glucose level?"

Insulin sensitivity factor = 1500/total daily dose of insulin

Example

Daily insulin dose in total parenteral nutrition (PN): 35 units
Previous daily requirement of subcutaneous dose of insulin: 15 units

Insulin sensitivity factor = 1500/(35 + 15) = 30
1 unit of insulin will lower blood glucose by 30 mg/dL (estimation)

Current blood glucose level: 250 mg/mL
Target blood glucose: 130 mg/mL

Correction bolus dose = (250 – 130)/30 = 4 units

Table 23.4 Writing a parenteral nutrition prescription—micronutrients.

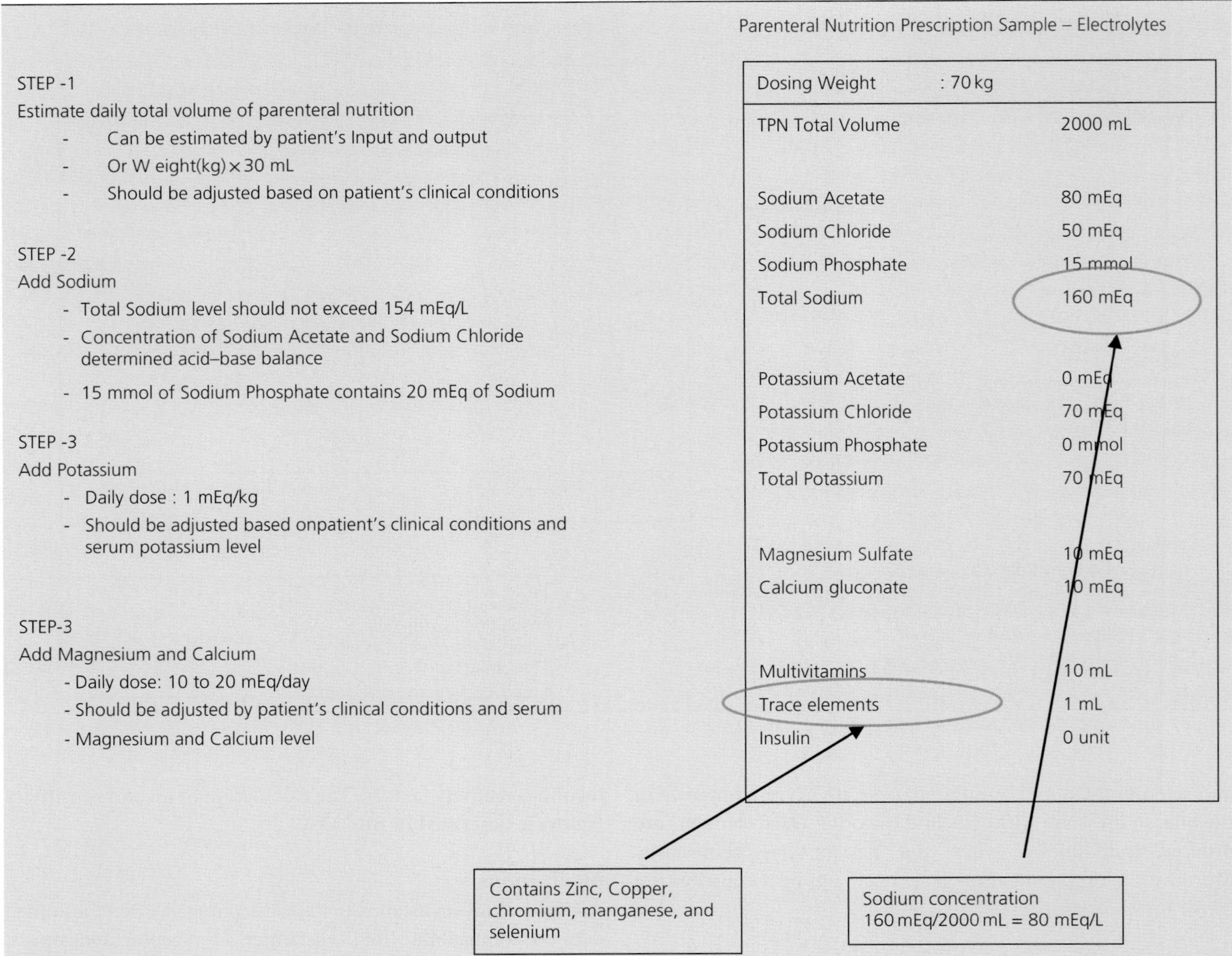

STEP -1
Estimate daily total volume of parenteral nutrition
- Can be estimated by patient's Input and output
- Or W eight(kg) × 30 mL
- Should be adjusted based on patient's clinical conditions

STEP -2
Add Sodium
- Total Sodium level should not exceed 154 mEq/L
- Concentration of Sodium Acetate and Sodium Chloride determined acid–base balance
- 15 mmol of Sodium Phosphate contains 20 mEq of Sodium

STEP -3
Add Potassium
- Daily dose : 1 mEq/kg
- Should be adjusted based onpatient's clinical conditions and serum potassium level

STEP-3
Add Magnesium and Calcium
- Daily dose: 10 to 20 mEq/day
- Should be adjusted by patient's clinical conditions and serum
- Magnesium and Calcium level

Parenteral Nutrition Prescription Sample – Electrolytes

Dosing Weight	: 70 kg
TPN Total Volume	2000 mL
Sodium Acetate	80 mEq
Sodium Chloride	50 mEq
Sodium Phosphate	15 mmol
Total Sodium	160 mEq
Potassium Acetate	0 mEq
Potassium Chloride	70 mEq
Potassium Phosphate	0 mmol
Total Potassium	70 mEq
Magnesium Sulfate	10 mEq
Calcium gluconate	10 mEq
Multivitamins	10 mL
Trace elements	1 mL
Insulin	0 unit

Contains Zinc, Copper, chromium, manganese, and selenium

Sodium concentration
160 mEq/2000 mL = 80 mEq/L

bases and can become destabilized in PN [114]. If patients are receiving oral or intravenous proton pump inhibitors, additional H_2-receptor antagonists are not required in PN solutions, nor are they required "on principle" when patients are receiving PN. Octreotide should not be added to PN.

Complications of nutrition support

Refeeding syndrome

Refeeding syndrome is a decrease in serum potassium, phosphorus, and/or magnesium, which occurs when calories, especially carbohydrate, are resumed or increased after a significant period of inadequate or absent nourishment. In severe cases, refeeding syndrome results in organ failure. Wernicke syndrome is often included as one of these. Others include respiratory failure, rhabdomyolysis, arrhythmia, and others. Refeeding syndrome was first reported after World War II, when severely malnourished Japanese prisoners were refed and then experienced electrolyte abnormalities and in some cases sudden death [115]. Refeeding syndrome can occur as a result of calories provided orally, enterally, or parenterally. Many, if not most, patients for whom EN or PN is indicated might be considered as being at risk for refeeding syndrome [116].

During starvation, fatty acids and amino acids become the main fuel sources. Intracellular minerals and electrolytes are depleted because of lack of intake. Despite depletion, serum electrolyte levels can remain normal. Refeeding syndrome is induced by the reintroduction of carbohydrates, which become a major fuel source again. In the refeeding period, insulin secretion is stimulated. This stimulates sodium–potassium ATPase to exchange intracellular sodium and extracellular potassium, reducing potassium levels. Phosphate is consumed in the process of glycolysis. The mechanism for hypomagnesemia is unknown and may exacerbate hypokalemia. Thiamine is a cofactor for pyruvate dehydrogenase, and pyruvate cannot enter the Krebs cycle without thiamine. Consequently, thiamine requirements are significantly increased during the refeeding period (Figure 23.5).

Nutrition support should be initiated slowly to prevent refeeding syndrome, for example, providing only 50% of the energy requirements the first day in patients at risk. For patients receiving PN, providing only 50% of the dextrose the first day is also an

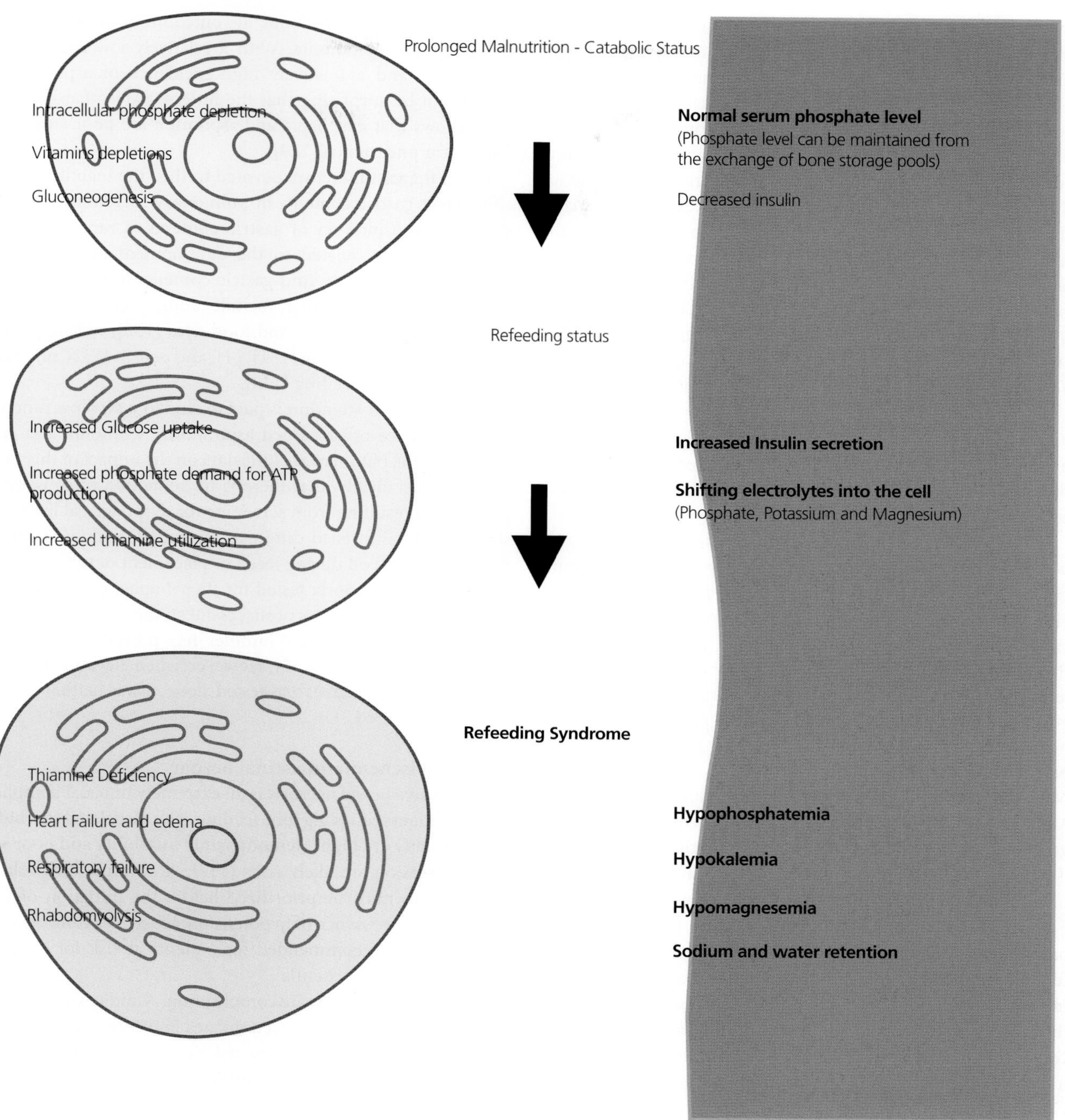

Figure 23.5 Pathogenesis of refeeding syndrome.

option for increased safety. Additional thiamine can be provided to patients deemed at risk. Serum electrolytes, including phosphorus, potassium, and magnesium, should be closely monitored and aggressively repleted during the initiation of nutrition support in patients at risk or who demonstrate shifts in electrolyte levels [117]. Patients at highest risk (e.g., those with prolonged starvation and chronic electrolyte losses as a result of diarrhea or fistulas) and those with rapid declines in levels may benefit from initial restriction of total calories to less than 10 kcal/kg/day.

Although there are no universally accepted and validated means for risk stratification, no commonly accepted diagnostic criteria, and no uniform guidelines for the management of refeeding syndrome, recent consensus guidelines have been published [118].

Complications of EN support

Diarrhea

Diarrhea is commonly reported as a gastrointestinal side-effect during EN support. Because definitions vary, so do the reports of incidence of diarrhea with EN. Medication side-effects are likely the most common cause. These include antibiotic- and other drug-related diarrhea, with or without bacterial overgrowth (e.g., *Clostridium difficile*). Enteral electrolyte supplementation introduces a large osmotic load into the gut. Liquid medications are often supplied in a suspension of sorbitol.

Underlying gastrointestinal disease, bacterial overgrowth, and overall state of illness are other conditions associated with diarrhea in tube-fed patients. The manner of tube feeding administration or types of feeding formula are often blamed for the presence of diarrhea; however, all other causes of diarrhea should be addressed before attributing it to the type of tube feeding [119,120]. Randomized trials have for the most part failed to demonstrate a difference in diarrhea incidence between isotonic and more concentrated feeds [121]. The osmolality of the most concentrated tube feed products is only in the range of 700–800 mOsm/L, whereas the osmolality of oral sodium/potassium phosphate is in the range of 8000 mOsm/L.

The practice of diluting concentrated feeds by mixing water into the formula bag is discouraged, to avoid bacterial contamination, which is itself associated with an increased risk for diarrhea [122]. Where additional water is needed, separate bolus or coinfusion of sterile water is acceptable.

Unless *Clostridium* infection is suspected, antidiarrheals may be used. Adding fiber or changing to fiber-containing formula can be considered if the patient has persistent diarrhea [59]. However, in patients with high risk for bowel ischemia or severe critical illness, fiber-containing formula should be avoided. Predigested formulas can be considered for patients with persistent diarrhea or clinical signs of malabsorption [59], but their effects are poorly documented or minimal [123].

Nausea and vomiting

Nausea and vomiting are not uncommon during tube feeding. Medication side-effect and underlying illness may cause delayed gastric emptying and decreased bowel motility. Adjusting or discontinuing motility-suppressing agents should be the first intervention for tube feeding-related nausea and vomiting [124]. Fiber-free, low-fat and isotonic tube feeding formulas are recommended for improving tolerance of tube feeding, because fiber and fat slow gastric emptying, and higher osmolality may increase gastric fluid production [59]. Temporary reduction of tube feed administration rate or trial of prokinetic agent can be considered for persistent nausea and vomiting, but run the risk for chronic underfeeding if symptoms are poorly controlled. Changing from gastric to small-bowel access is often effective in the presence of delayed gastric emptying [125]. In addition, antinauseant medications may be beneficial in persistent nausea with low gastric residual volume.

Aspiration

Aspiration ranges in severity from a normal daily occurrence [126] to life-threatening pneumonitis. EN support has long been recognized as an independent risk factor for aspiration pneumonia [127,128]; however, whether the presence of the tube or the feeding is causal is still a matter of speculation. Moreover, aspiration, unless large enough to cause hypoxia and/or pneumonitis, is itself not an outcome. Rather, the focus should be on pneumonia. With a relatively low incidence of pneumonia and a relatively high incidence of aspiration, it should not be surprising that the little research that has been done shows that dysphagia and aspiration are poor surrogates for risk for pneumonia [129].

Given the vast literature devoted to this, the inability to reliably detect gastric contents in pulmonary secretions may also suggest that aspiration of gastric contents is rare and/or not strongly causally related to the development of pneumonia. Methods attempted to find gastric contents in the pulmonary tree during tube feeding include adding colored markers, including methylene blue and food dyes [130], testing pulmonary aspirates for glucose [131], pH, and pepsin [132], and radiolabeling the tube feeding [133].

A great deal of attention is paid to studying swallow function in the presence of presumed aspiration pneumonia and after critical illness, but there are little data on the impact of this practice, and specifically, that there is no reduction of subsequent pneumonia resulting from screening for dysphagia, at least after stroke [134]. Efforts to diminish aspiration, including raising the head of the bed during feeds or placement of tubes into the small bowel, are poorly tested for their impact on pneumonia. There are many examples of successful studies in which instituting guideline-based order bundles has prevented ventilator-associated pneumonia [135]. However, when elevating the head of the bed to 45° degrees was tested alone, it was neither feasible nor effective [136].

Intestinal ischemia/intestinal bezoar

Nonocclusive bowel necrosis is an extremely unusual complication in patients receiving tube feeding. The associated morbidity and mortality are high. Hemodynamic instability and poor systemic perfusion are likely risks [137]. At a minimum, volume resuscitation must be prioritized before the initiation of tube feeding in the presence of hypotension. Fiber-free isotonic feeding formula is recommended for patients at risk for development of intestinal ischemia.

Intestinal bezoar is a rare complication. Nondigestible fiber in fiber-containing formula accumulates and forms accretions in the gut of patients with intestinal hypomotility as a result of medications that suppress motility, such as vasopressors or opioids [138,139].

Because of the rarity of either of these complications, guidelines have become far less proscriptive regarding feeding hemodynamically compromised patients [59].

Complications of PN

Catheter-related infection

Catheter-related infection is one of the more serious PN-related complications. Catheter-related infections are subcategorized by the Centers for Disease Control and Prevention (CDC) based on the site and type of infection: exit site, tunnel, or bloodstream infection [140].

Exit site infection is defined as erythema within 2 cm of the catheter exit site without bloodstream infection. Blood and drainage cultures should be obtained before the administration of empiric antibiotics. Exit site infections are treated with antibiotics for 7–14 days, depending on the microorganism isolated.

Tunnel infection is erythema or site induration in the subcutaneous track of a tunneled catheter without a bloodstream infection. Blood and drainage cultures should be obtained, and the catheter should be removed. A new catheter should be placed at a different site. Exchanging the catheter over a wire is not recommended. Tunnel infections are usually treated with a 14-day course of antibiotics depending on the microorganism isolated. The duration of the treatment can be changed if the bloodstream infection is concurrent with tunnel infection [140,141].

CRBSI is defined by the CDC as a laboratory-confirmed growth of bacteria from the bloodstream in which a central line was in place for more than 2 consecutive calendar days. The diagnosis of laboratory-confirmed bloodstream infection is described in Box 23.4 [140,142]. Fever and chills are the common clinical manifestations in CRBSI but may be masked if the patient is immunocompromised.

The catheter exit site, and tunnel track when appropriate, must be examined regularly for signs of infection and inflammation. This is usually done weekly at the time of dressing changes in patients receiving home PN. Empiric therapy should be initiated based on the clinical picture when CRBSI is suspected. At least two sets of blood cultures should be obtained from the separate sites before the initiation of empiric antibiotics [143]. In most cases of CRBSI, catheter removal is recommended, especially if the patient has signs of sepsis, endocarditis, thrombophlebitis, persistent bacteremia after antimicrobial treatment, or infected tunnel. Catheter removal should be immediate when the patient is in septic shock [144–146]. Salvage of the catheter can be considered for the patients who do not have the complications mentioned earlier and the source of infection is coagulase-negative staphylococci or drug-susceptible Enterobacteriaceae [144].

Prevention of CRBSI in PN support

The best choice of central venous access device to prevent CRBSI in long-term use is a single-lumen PICC [95,97–99]. In addition, the CDC recommends the following strategies for

Box 23.4 Laboratory-confirmed bloodstream infection.

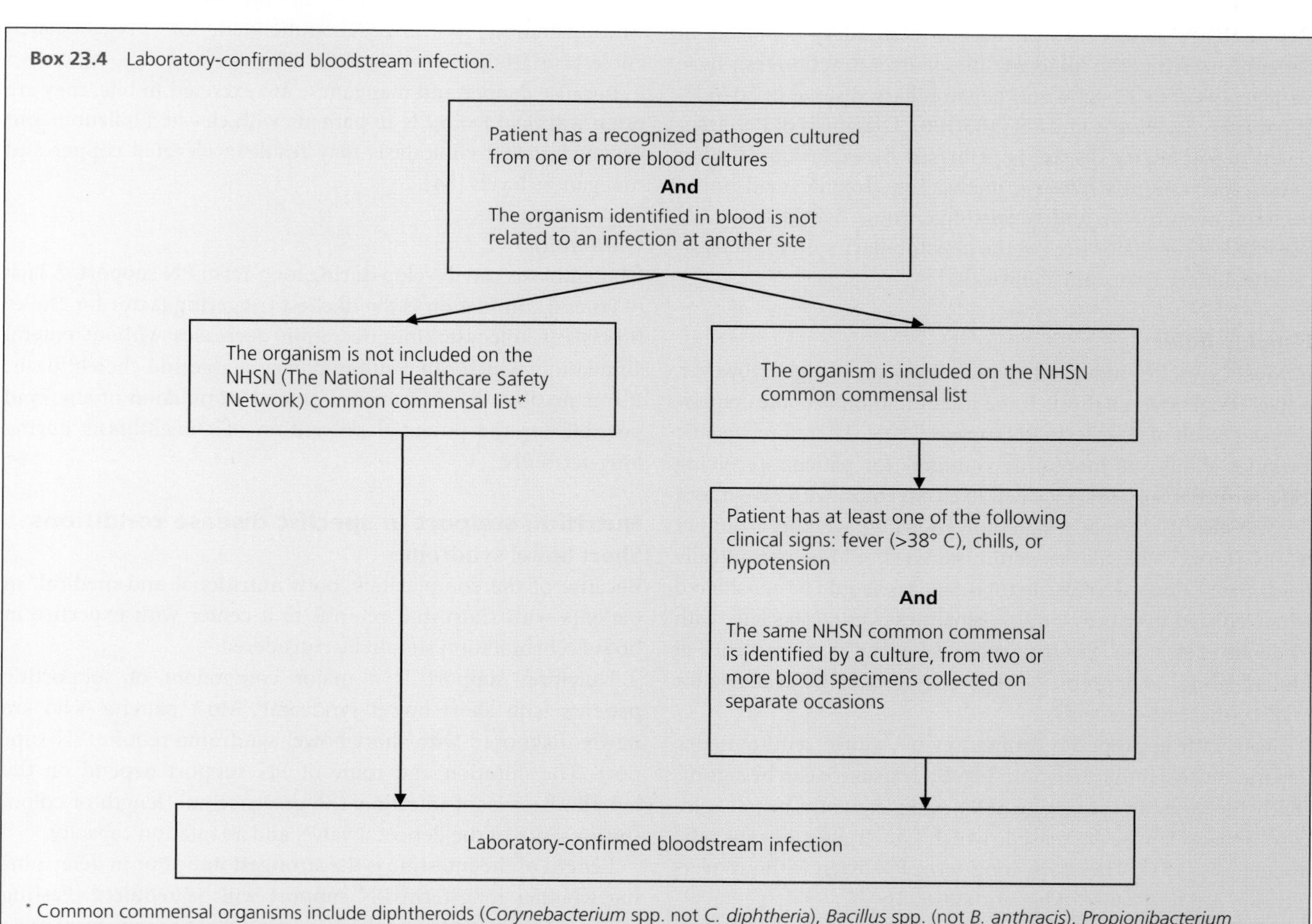

* Common commensal organisms include diphtheroids (*Corynebacterium* spp. not *C. diphtheria*), *Bacillus* spp. (not *B. anthracis*), *Propionibacterium* spp., coagulase-negative staphylococci (including *S. epidermidis*), viridans group streptococci, *Aerococcus* spp., *Micrococcus* spp., and *Rhodococcus* spp.
Sources: O'Grady et al. 2011 [140] and Marschall et al. 2014 [142].

central line placement to prevent CRBSI infection: (1) hand hygiene, (2) skin antiseptic, (3) completely dried skin prep agent before inserting the central line, and (4) maximal sterile barrier precautions [140,142]. Addition of ethanol and/or antibiotic lock can be considered in patients with a history of or at elevated risk for CRBSI [101,147].

Insertion site is also an important risk factor in the development of CRBSI. Femoral catheterization doubles the incidence of infections in patients receiving PN compared with subclavian or internal jugular catheterization [148]. The risk can be increased by any manipulation of the line. Using the central venous catheter lumen (e.g., for blood drawing or for coinfusion, or Y-siting/piggybacking of medications) through which the PN is administered is not advised, because of both infection risk and incompatibility. The exception to this is lipid injectable emulsion. When given separately from the rest of the PN, it should be Y-sited/piggybacked into the same line as the remainder of the PN. However, total nutrient admixture (three-in-one, in which lipid injectable emulsion is mixed in with the rest of the PN) is favored [85,149].

PN-associated hepatobiliary disease

Hepatobiliary biliary dysfunction is commonly reported in patients receiving PN. Abnormalities in liver function tests have been reported in 15–85% and hepatobiliary disease in 50–65% of patients receiving home PN [105,106]. Diagnosis of PN-associated hepatobiliary disease is primarily by exclusion of other causes, such as sepsis, hypoxia, medications, toxins, small-bowel bacterial overgrowth, and coexisting chronic liver disease. PN can affect three major sites of the hepatobiliary system: hepatocellular, biliary tract, and gallbladder.

Hepatocellular

In most cases, PN-induced hepatic steatosis is benign. However, it may progress to cirrhosis if the inflammation becomes persistent as a result of long-term PN support [106]. Therefore, hepatic enzymes should be monitored routinely for patients receiving long-term PN support. Elevated liver enzymes, with or without hepatic steatosis, can be a sign of overfeeding, whether from EN or PN [150]. Total calories administered should be periodically reestimated, and a decrease in total calories should be considered when isolated liver enzyme abnormalities occur, especially with evidence of steatosis. Steatosis may also occur in the presence of underfeeding, so appropriate expertise needs to be available for making these assessments.

Even with appropriate estimation of calorie requirements, hepatic steatosis still can occur. Insulin resistance can be significantly increased in the setting of PN. Consequently, hepatic glucose uptake can be increased, which can trigger intrahepatic lipogenesis [151]. Therefore, long-term PN, even without overfeeding, can be a cause of hepatic steatosis.

Carnitine is not routinely added to PN solutions. Chronic carnitine deficiency can develop in long-term PN support, and it may be associated with hepatic steatosis [152]. Cyclic PN infusion, that is, infused over 12 hours, is a standard of care for long-term PN. It has long been theorized that the continuous "postprandial" state, with elevated insulin, accompanying 24-hour PN infusion may be causal of hepatic steatosis [153]. However, demonstration of benefit for this practice in randomized controlled studies is lacking.

Biliary tract

Long-term use of soybean-based lipid has been strongly associated with PN-associated cholestasis. The soybean-based emulsion contains phytosterols, which are metabolized and excreted through the bile duct. These can lead to impaired bile drainage. However, serum phytosterol level is not associated with cholestasis, and it does not need to be checked [154,155]. The high content of ω-6 fatty acids in soybean-based lipid is another proposed contributing factor in developing cholestasis. Chronic PN-associated cholestasis can also progress to hepatic cirrhosis and failure. Although in most cases this is not feasible, discontinuation of PN can be a definitive treatment. Both decreasing the total amount of lipid and/or switching from soybean-based lipid emulsion to the mixed oil-based emulsion can be considered part of management and prevention of PN-associated cholestasis. For pediatric patients, fish oil-based lipid emulsion, which was approved recently by the US Food and Drug Administration, is now recommended for PN-associated cholestasis [156].

Because copper and manganese are excreted in bile, they are often withheld from PN in patients with elevated bilirubin, out of concern that cholestasis may result in elevated copper and manganese levels [84].

Gallbladder

Cholelithiasis can develop during long-term PN support. A lack of enteral stimulation is the likeliest triggering factor for cholelithiasis. Cholecystokinin secretion decreases without enteral simulation, which can result in biliary sludge and cholelithiasis. If it is feasible, we recommend enteral stimulation of any kind possible for the potential prevention of cholelithiasis during long-term PN.

Nutrition support in specific disease conditions

Short bowel syndrome

Because of the complexities, both nutritional and medical, in patients with short gut, referral to a center with expertise in bowel rehabilitation should be considered.

Nutrition support is a major component of supporting patients with short bowel syndrome. Most patients who are newly diagnosed with short bowel syndrome require PN support. The duration and route of PN support depend on the length of remnant intestine, the presence and length of colon, the presence of the ileocecal valve, and adaptation capacity.

Length of the intestine is the strongest indicator in determining whether long-term PN support will be required. Fasting serum citrulline levels are highly reflective of the mucosal mass of the intestine, and a serum level greater than 20 μmol/L is strongly predictive of eventual independence from PN [157]. Citrulline is a nonessential amino acid that is produced by enterocytes of the small intestine.

Glucagon-like peptide-2 analog (teduglutide) has been used with success for patients with short bowel syndrome to improve intestinal absorption and decrease the dependency on PN [158].

Oral diet or EN support should be attempted for patients who are diagnosed with short bowel syndrome. Stimulation of the remnant of the intestine with intact macronutrients is an essential nutritional treatment during the adaptation period. A standard polymeric isotonic formula is an appropriate choice of enteral feeding formula in short bowel syndrome. Predigested (elemental or semielemental) formulas are not recommended for routine use in short bowel syndrome [159].

Short bowel syndrome is covered in more depth in Chapter 59.

Severe acute pancreatitis

Severe acute pancreatitis is a highly catabolic state, and most patients with severe acute pancreatitis have a negative nitrogen balance. EN is recommended over PN for patients with severe acute pancreatitis. Early EN can improve clinical outcomes in severe acute pancreatitis [160]. Multiple randomized clinical trials and metaanalysis comparing EN with PN demonstrate a reduction in infectious complications, length of hospital stay, needs for surgical intervention, and mortality in those receiving EN [161–163]. EN support should be initiated within 24–48 hours of admission for the critically ill patients [59].

A.S.P.E.N. recommends a standard isotonic polymeric formula in this case. Immune-enhancing or predigested formulas may have theoretical benefits in decreasing inflammation and decreasing pancreatic stimulation. However, clinical evidence is equivocal and does not support their routine use in patients with severe acute pancreatitis [59]. Previously, jejunal tube feeding was recommended for routine use because it was thought to allow for pancreatic rest. However, three randomized clinical trials and a meta-analysis showed that there is no difference in clinical outcomes between jejunal and gastric tube feeding [164–167]. Therefore, either jejunal or gastric tube placement can be used. In the presence of an inflammatory phlegmon causing compressive duodenal obstruction, gastroparesis, or pseudocysts, nasojejunal intubation via endoscopic placement may be considered. If enteral or oral feeding is not possible, PN can be considered after 1 week from onset of the severe acute pancreatitis.

More details about acute severe pancreatitis are described in Chapter 74.

Chylous ascites

Chylous ascites refers to the presence of lymphatic fluid in the peritoneal cavity that derives from gut lymphatics. It is caused by traumatic injury or obstruction of lymphatic outflow. Common causes of chylous ascites are postoperative complications, traumatic injury, infection, malignancy, and cirrhosis. Chyle has a high content of fat, but only if the patient is eating. Long-chain dietary triglycerides are packaged into chylomicrons that travel via lacteals into the intestinal lymphatic system. In contrast, medium-chain triglycerides are directly absorbed into the portal venous circulation.

The main purpose of nutritional intervention in chylous ascites is to minimize the chyle output from the leaking site. Two approaches, a very low-fat diet or nothing by mouth with PN support, have been proposed [168,169], but neither has been tested in randomized trials. Because chyle appears serous when the patient is not eating and turns dramatically milky once fat is consumed, a very low-fat diet is theorized to reduce chyle flow. These diets are supplemented with medium-chain fat as a calorie source, because these diets are hard to consume and very low in calorie content and because medium-chain fat does not enter the lacteals. It should be noted that medium-chain fats do not have any known therapeutic effect in this setting and are solely given as a concentrated calorie source. Furthermore, these diets are not viable long term because of the difficulties mentioned and because these patients risk essential fatty acid deficiency.

PN, which has been in and out of favor in this setting, may well be the better choice if a reduction in chyle flow is desired. Whether containing measurable fat or not, chyle is gut lymph, and the goal of lymph flow reduction may require that no nourishment be put into the gut. Lymphatic flow is mostly dependent on blood flow, and the presence of food is the most important stimulant to mucosal blood flow. Thus, nothing by mouth, with PN, aligns with the physiology of lymphatic flow reduction. Certainly, PN should be considered when enteral dietary interventions fail to decrease the chyle output. It is worth noting that intravenous lipid emulsions can be used in patients with chylous ascites because these do not enter the gut lymphatic circulation.

Status after bariatric surgery

Macronutrient deficiency can be considered as the purpose or consequence of bariatric surgery. Proper protein intake is believed to be the most important factor to minimize the complications from macronutrient deficiency in postbariatric status. The minimum intake of protein should be more than 60 g/day. The intake can go up to 1.5 g/kg (ideal bodyweight) in uncomplicated patients [170] and 2.0 g/kg in the critically ill [59].

In contrast, micronutrient deficiency is a common complication of bariatric surgery. Micronutrients should be routinely monitored, and daily micronutrient supplementation is required after bariatric surgery. The detailed recommendations are described in Table 23.5 [37].

Less commonly, particularly in patients who have had bypass surgery, bacterial overgrowth of the nonalimentary limb can lead to deconjugation of bile and increase steatorrhea. In our experience, patients present with multiple nutrient deficiencies, particularly fat-soluble vitamins, copper and zinc, low albumin, vague gastrointestinal symptoms, and sometimes severe and irreversible nutritional neuropathy or myelopathy (e.g., with copper deficiency). These often require nutrition support (to rapidly reverse existing deficiencies) and systemic antibiotics, because nonabsorbed antibiotics do not reach the nonalimentary limb [21,171].

Enterocutaneous fistula

Enterocutaneous fistula is most commonly a complication of surgery (75–80%) [172]. One of the most important risk factors for development of enterocutaneous fistula is the presence of

Table 23.5 Recommended micronutrient screening and supplementation after bariatric surgery.

Micronutrients	Postoperative screening	Postoperative supplementations
Thiamine	• Routine postoperative screening • Should be assessed at least within first 6 months, then every 3–6 months	• Preferable daily dose: 50 mg • Minimum daily dose: 12 mg
Vitamin B_{12}	• Routine postoperative screening • Frequent screening in the first postoperative year (every 3 months) • Annual screening after 1 year	• Oral dose: 350–500 µg daily • Parenteral dose: 1000 µg monthly • Nasal spray: 500 µg weekly
Folate	• Routine postoperative screening	• Preferable daily dose: 400–800 µg • Women of childbearing age: 800–1000 µg daily
Iron, ferritin, and TIBC	• Routine postoperative screening within 3 months after the surgery, then every 3–6 months until 12 months • Annual screening after 1 year	• Minimum daily dose: 18 mg of elemental iron • Menstruating females: 45–60 mg of elemental iron
Vitamin D and calcium	• Routine postoperative screening	• Preferable daily dose: 1200–1500 mg • BPD/DS: 1800–2400 mg daily
Vitamin A	• Routine postoperative screening within the first postoperative year	• Preferable daily dose: 5000–10 000 IU • BPD/DS: 10 000 IU daily
Vitamins E and K	• Screening only for symptomatic patients	• Vitamin K: 90–120 µg daily (300 µg daily for BPD/DS) • Vitamin E: 15 µg daily
Zinc	• Routine screening for the patient who received gastric bypass or BPD/DS	• Preferable daily dose: 8–22 mg • BPD/DS: 16–22 mg daily
Copper	• Routine postoperative screening	• Preferable daily dose: 1–2 mg

BPD/DS, biliopancreatic diversion with duodenal switch.
Source: Modified from Parrott et al. 2017 [37].

presurgical or postsurgical malnutrition. Moreover, enterocutaneous fistula, especially with high output, is itself a contributing factor for developing malnutrition, and nutrition plays a major role in its management [173]. The location of the fistula and volume of fistula output are two clinical components for determining the route of feeding. PN support should be considered when patients have high-output enterocutaneous fistula (>500 mL/day). Proximally located enterocutaneous fistulas should be evaluated for intubation and used as feeding ostomies (so-called fistuloclysis) [174,175]. The total volume of PN should be adjusted based on fistula output to ensure adequate hydration. If the enterocutaneous fistula output is controlled, and it is located distally, EN support or diet can be considered. Quantitation of fat content of fistula output can help determine the degree of absorption when the position of the fistula is unclear.

Home and long-term EN support for nonhospitalized patients

EN support is provided at home or in out-of-hospital facilities to nonhospitalized patients who cannot meet their macronutrients and micronutrients requirements via a regular oral diet. They must be stable enough to receive EN support and have an adequate gastrointestinal tract that can absorb the nutrients. Appropriate home EN support can improve clinical outcomes and quality of life [176,177]. Severe gastrointestinal dysfunctions, such as obstruction, active bleeding, and malabsorption, are contraindications to home EN support. In patients at the end of life with advanced terminal illness, home EN support is not recommended [178].

The choice of route and device for nonhospitalized patients receiving EN is somewhat controversial. In certain regions of the United States, and contrary to the availability of supporting data [179], skilled nursing facilities and home nursing agencies refuse to accept patients with nasally placed feeding tubes [180]. In a survey comparing skilled nursing facilities in New York City with a large random sample throughout the United States, 82% of facilities refused nasal tubes in New York versus 38% nationwide. A systematic review suggests the possibility that gastrostomy might be favorable to nasal tube for long-term EN, based mostly on a higher incidence of "treatment failure" (e.g., clogging) with nasal tubes. However, overall complication rates are similar between nasal tube and gastrostomy, and the severity of complications was worse with gastrostomy. There are cosmetic concerns with nasal tubes, but quality-of-life scores did not differ between nasal and percutaneous tubes [179]. Because of the prevalence of these policies, preemptive gastrostomy placement (e.g., placing gastrostomy at the time tracheostomy is placed) has become increasingly common, resulting in placement earlier during hospitalization and in sicker patients [181]. In our experience, the percentage of patients who require tube feeding at discharge was only approximately 30% of those who required tracheostomy [182], strongly suggesting that routine preemptive placement of gastrostomy should be reconsidered.

Bolus feeding, in which feeds are given in three to six rapid infusions per day, is thought to be a more physiological way to provide nutrients than is continuous feeding. Bolus feeding is often recommended for use only with gastric tubes, as opposed to jejunal tubes, because of volume reserve capacity [183]. However, patients with enteric (duodenal or jejunal) tubes can often build up tolerance for bolus infusion [184]. In hospitalized patients, continuous tube feeding is commonly used. For longer-term EN, overnight continuous feeding (i.e., infusing for 12 hours) is often favored. Overnight feeding is believed to allow for more freedom of activities. Overnight feeding can be combined with daytime bolus feeding if the patient is not able to reach the calorie requirements with a single method [185].

Commercial tube feed products are traditionally favored over homemade blenderized formulas, but this is debatable. Despite concerns about blenderized feeding not meeting nutrient requirements if not properly supervised, being contaminated with bacteria if not properly cooked, or at increased risk for clogging the feeding tube if not properly liquefied, there is evidence that a large segment of patients receiving home EN are using self-prepared feeds for at least some of their nourishment [186]. Insurance coverage is notoriously poor for home tube feeding in the United States, and access to commercial products is lacking in less affluent regions of the world. Blenderized feeds may be far more viable economically, and acceptable formulas have been tested and published [187]. Importantly, practitioners caring for patients receiving home EN should be aware of their patient's practices and provide nutritional expertise to help oversee the balance of the homemade tube feed.

Clogging of the enteral tube is a frequent complication that occurs in the outpatient setting. Inadequate flushing of the tube, using a blenderized formula, flushing with acidic fluids (e.g. juice, soda) and the injection of crushed medications down the tube increase risk for clogging. Simple water flushing will be the first step in managing the clogged tube. If the obstruction is persistent, carbonated drinks or pancreatic enzyme infusion can be tried [188].

Home EN support should be decreased and/or discontinued when oral intake resumes and normalizes, and/or patients reach their weight goal. Feed calories should be adjusted in response to an assessment of oral intake and weight trajectory.

Home PN support

Home PN support is recommended for outpatients who cannot meet their requirements of macronutrients and micronutrients by EN. Patients who require home PN should be referred to centers expert in their care or, at a minimum, infusion companies with experience with caring for patients on home PN and with in-house clinicians who can help monitor and advise ordering practitioners in the absence of those with expertise.

Common clinical conditions that cause chronic intestinal failure that requires home PN include obstruction or protracted ileus, complications of inflammatory bowel disease, postsurgical complications, bowel ischemia, radiation enteritis, short gut, fistula, and motility disorders. Prognosis of home PN depends on the patient's primary diagnosis. For example, 1-year survival rate for patients receiving PN support as a result of malignancy-induced intestinal failure rate is close to 20%. In contrast, the 5-year survival rate for patients receiving PN support because of Crohn's disease is close to 90% [189]. Like EN support, PN is not recommended for patients at the end of life with advanced terminal illness. However, PN can be used for patients with incurable cancer, if expected survival is longer term (i.e., several months) [190].

Safe practices for home PN require a close collaborative relationship among the prescriber, the patient, the infusion pharmacy, and the nursing agency. Patients and/or their caregiver must be trained, preferably before discharge, and demonstrate competence in safe self-administration and catheter care. The home environment should be assessed for appropriate social and physical support of the patient, the availability of proper equipment, such as refrigeration, and space that can be designated as clean. The ordering process should include clear and ongoing handoff between providers.

Cyclic infusion (i.e., overnight for 12 hours) is commonly used in home PN support. However, it can decrease patients' quality of sleep because of frequent nocturnal urination or noise from the infusion pump. As discussed earlier, the evidence for a metabolic benefit from cycled PN is theoretical. PN may be infused 8–24 h/day, dependent on patient's preference and tolerance. Cycled infusions may be given at night or during the day, and they are portable. The pump operates on battery power, and most infusion companies can provide patients with specially designed backpacks to carry the pump and PN.

Routine monitoring of electrolytes, liver functions, and complete blood counts is required. The frequency of monitoring varies dependent on the patient's condition. Most patients start with weekly electrolytes, magnesium, calcium, and phosphorus and liver enzymes every 2–4 weeks. In our experience, stable patients receiving PN for long periods may require only laboratory testing every 3–12 months. The levels of trace elements (zinc, copper, selenium, iron, manganese, and chromium) and vitamins (A, D, E, K, B_1, B_2, B_6, niacin, folic acid, B_{12}, and C) should be checked initially, then every 3–6 months, and then less frequently when stable.

References are available at www.yamadagastro.com/textbook7e

Further reading

Burgermaster M., Slattery E., Islam N., Ippolito P.R., Seres D.S. Regional comparison of enteral nutrition-related admission policies in skilled nursing facilities. Nutr Clin Pract 2016;31(3):342.

Casaer M.P., Van den Berghe G. Nutrition in the acute phase of critical illness. N Engl J Med 2014;370(13):1227.

Hiura G., Lebwohl B., Seres D.S. Malnutrition diagnosis in critically ill patients using 2012 Academy of Nutrition and Dietetics/American Society for Parenteral and Enteral Nutrition standardized diagnostic characteristics is associated with longer hospital and intensive care unit length of stay and increased in-hospital mortality. JPEN J Parenter Enteral Nutr 2020;44:256.

Ippolito P., Larson E.L., Furuya E.Y., Liu J., Seres D.S. Utility of electronic medical records to assess the relationship between parenteral nutrition and central line-associated bloodstream infections in adult hospitalized patients. JPEN J Parenter Enteral Nutr 2015;39(8):929.

Koretz R.L. Death, morbidity and economics are the only end points for trials. Proc Nutr Soc 2005;64(3):277.

CHAPTER 24
Control of food intake

Andres Acosta
Mayo Clinic, Rochester, MN, USA

Chapter menu

Introduction

The control of food intake is a tightly regulated homeostatic process. The key stages of food intake regulation are hunger, satiation, and satiety. These different stages are regulated by the brain–gut–fat axis. Many etiologies that disrupt this homeostatic process result in either decrease or increase of food intake, and these pathophysiological changes can lead to diseases such as anorexia or obesity. This chapter discusses the key aspects, phases, and mechanisms illustrating how the control of food intake is a homeostatic process by which the central nervous system, in tight interaction with the gastrointestinal system, responds to multiple hormonal and metabolic cues to regulate food intake, body weight, and glucose homeostasis. Thus, the key aspects of food intake regulation are usually targeted to treat food intake-related diseases. Additionally, hedonic eating behavior may override the physiological homeostatic regulation of food intake.

Maintaining energy homeostasis and storing calories when food is available is fundamental for survival. All species have faced the challenge of adapting to scarcity of food, and thus strategies to deal with major discrepancies in food availability have evolved to allow propagation of the species. Thus, the human, throughout evolution, has developed a very complex mechanism of autoregulation of energy balance, mainly driven by energy intake and energy expenditure. These complex, redundant, survival-essential mechanisms quickly adapt to preserve energy and change to a food-seeking behavior in the context of any reduction of energy intake or with the minimal increase in energy expenditure.

In the modern world, a disruption in energy balance from an increase in calories consumed compared to energy expended is more common than food scarcity. Unfortunately, overnutrition can lead to obesity, diabetes, nonalcoholic fatty liver disease, colon cancer, and many other significant chronic diseases. Clearly, obesity is an increasing public health problem, since more than two-thirds of the US population is now overweight or obese and parallel increases in prevalence are being recorded virtually worldwide [1].

Stages of food intake regulation

Food intake regulation is a tightly controlled homeostatic process. The key stages of food intake regulation are hunger, satiation, and satiety (Figure 24.1). Hunger is the stimulus that promotes the initiation of food consumption in an individual. Satiation is the sensation of fullness during a meal that aids in inducing the termination of a meal [2]. Satiety is the time the subject has with the sensation of fullness [3]. These different stages are regulated by the brain–gut–fat axis [4,5]. Homeostatic (physiological) and hedonic (psychological) components coalesce to regulate eating behavior.

Yamada's Textbook of Gastroenterology, Seventh Edition. Edited by Timothy C. Wang, Michael Camilleri, Benjamin Lebwohl, Anna S. Lok, William J. Sandborn, Kenneth K. Wang, and Gary D. Wu.

Companion website: www.yamadagastro.com/textbook7e

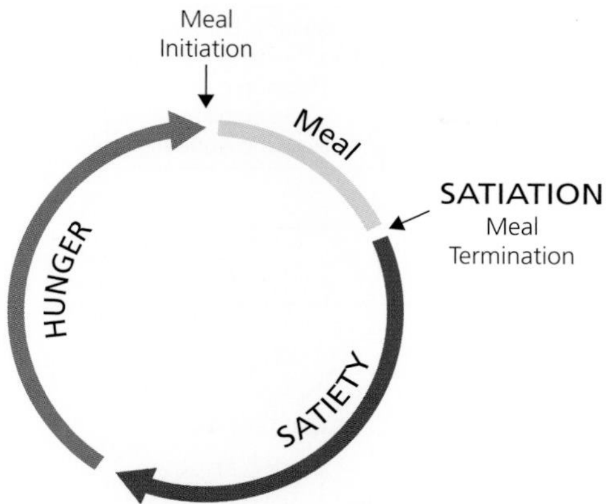

Figure 24.1 Key stages of food intake regulation are hunger, satiation, and satiety in relationship with a meal.

Homeostatic control of food intake

The homeostatic control of food intake has three stages which are tightly regulated by the brain–gut–fat axis (Figure 24.2). The nervous system and the closely coordinated mechanisms in the periphery, mainly the gut and adipose tissue, are in constant communication with the current nutritional status of the body. This communication is mediated by the peripheral nervous system and key hormones that send signals to the central nervous systems. The central nervous system's role in regulating energy balance in a coordinated fashion with the constantly adjusting energy intake, expenditure, and storage was first demonstrated by studies in which selective surgical lesions of certain hypothalamic areas were found to result in extreme obesity in rats [6].

Numerous recent discoveries have substantially extended our understanding of the importance of central control of energy balance and metabolism. Delineation of the underlying central and hormonal mechanisms that coordinate food intake, bodyweight, and glucose homeostasis has accelerated in recent decades. The discovery of leptin by Friedman and colleagues in 1994 was a key breakthrough that linked peripheral hormones from the adipose tissue and the central nervous system (CNS) [7]. In addition, the cloning of the melanocortin receptors and subsequent elucidation of this system in regulating energy balance by Cone and colleagues was a key discovery [8]. Definition of the effects of additional critical metabolic hormones such as ghrelin and insulin, as well as the role of neurotransmitters such as serotonin, on coordinated control of energy balance responses has underscored the importance of the CNS in maintaining homeostasis.

The hypothalamus is the key region of the brain that is required to maintain homeostasis. The hypothalamus is made up of clusters of neurons (referred to as nuclei) that act in conjunction to regulate nearly all the basic functions of the body. These include coordinated control of energy balance and blood glucose levels (Figure 24.3). As outlined later in this chapter, several hypothalamic nuclei have been demonstrated to play essential roles in regulating food intake and bodyweight. In addition, key groups of neurons in the brainstem are important in regulating energy balance. These neurons include vagal sensory neurons, the neurons that are primary targets of the sensory neurons, as well as the parasympathetic motor neurons of the vagus nerve. As will be discussed, the vagal innervation of key metabolic visceral organs, including the liver, portal vein, and small intestine, is important in regulating energy balance. Moreover, it is now appreciated that the vagus nerve serves as a critical link between changing energy availability and coordinated control of glucose homeostasis [9]. Put simplistically, the nervous system senses peripheral metabolic cues, resulting in coordinated energy homeostasis. Recent studies primarily done in animal models, especially mice, have provided an avenue to genetically dissect and define the neuronal circuits and important hormonal cues that regulate energy homeostasis. As discussed below, the importance of these genes has been confirmed in human subjects.

The vast majority of the peripheral signals originate in the gastrointestinal system (see Figure 24.2), which communicates with the central nervous system through two different processes: neuronal and hormonal [4]. Gastric function influences all three stages in the control of food intake (hunger, satiation, and satiety) and merges the signals from gastrointestinal hormones, autonomic and enteric nervous system, and mechanical receptors of the stomach. Gastrointestinal functions are, therefore, essential in obesity, as the stomach is the reservoir that determines entry of calories into the body and contributes to satiation or postprandial fullness that signal the need to cease consumption of calories. Changes in gastric function could lead to the ingestion of more calories, contributing to weight gain and obesity. Gastrointestinal hormones have an essential role in regulating appetite and satiety in coordination with the brain–gut axis. Thus, alterations in gastric function or in any of these mechanisms can alter the response to food intake and may lead to caloric overconsumption.

The communication between the brain–gut–fat axis is represented in three stages of food intake control to maintain energy homeostasis. Each stage has an additional importance for nutrient digestion, gastrointestinal function, food-seeking (or not) behavior and overall well-being. The key stages of food intake regulation are hunger, satiation, and satiety.

Hunger

Hunger, defined as the stimulus that promotes the initiation of food consumption in an individual, and also called appetite or desire to eat, is mainly controlled by the hypothalamus. The ultimate, absolute goal of hunger sensations, mechanisms, and drivers is to trigger a food-seeking behavior that will culminate in the consumption of nutrients. The hunger sensation gradually increases with time in the setting of food deprivation.

The "hunger centers" in the hypothalamus are always "on." These centers are driven by the agouti-related protein and neuropeptide Y neurons (AgRP and NPY neurons), known as the "hunger neurons," located in the arcuate nucleus of the

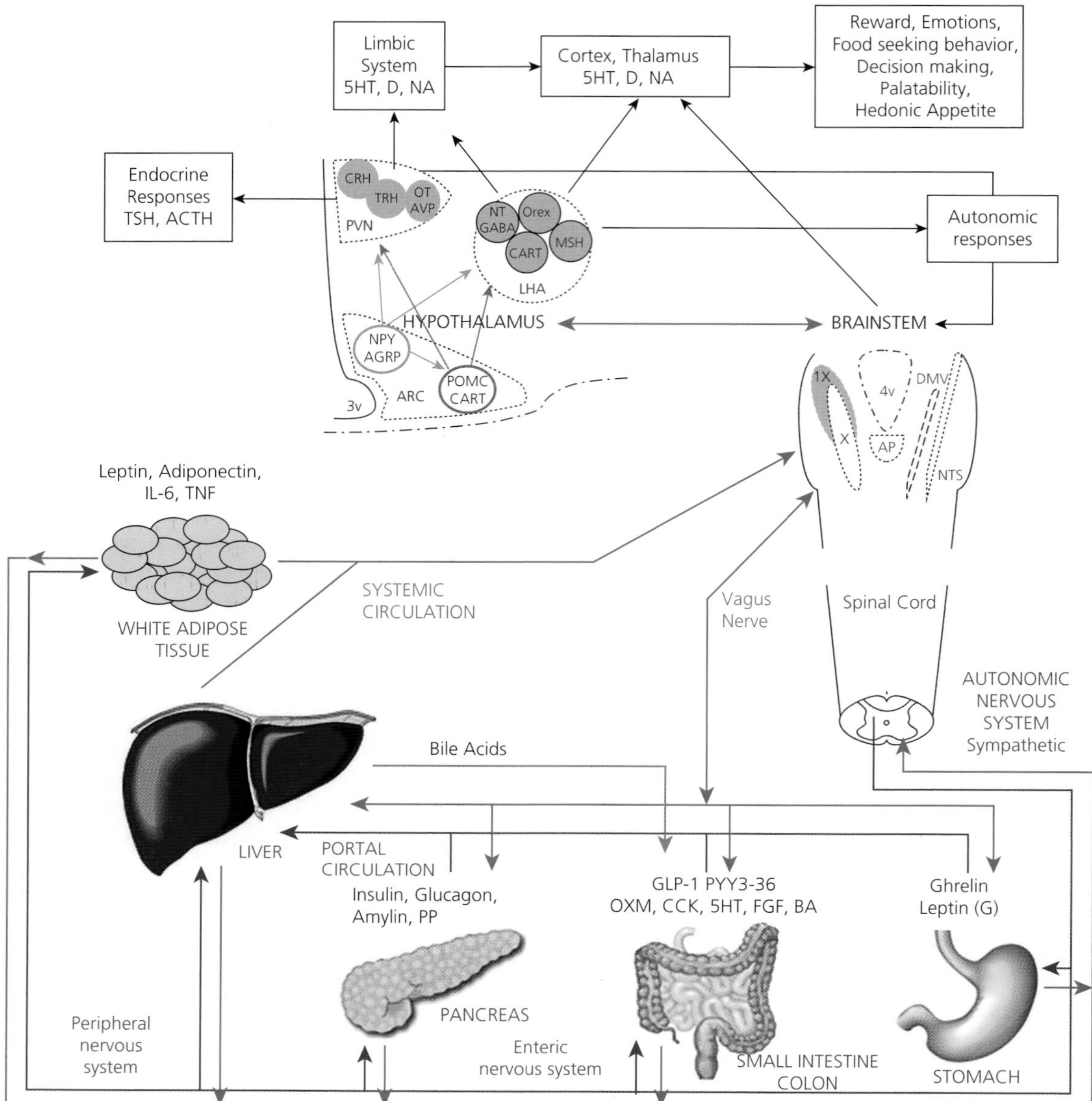

Figure 24.2 Complex mechanism of food intake regulation. The food intake process initiates when nutrients enter the GI tract. Digestion starts when the nutrients enter the stomach and produce mechanic-dilation, decreasing acyl-ghrelin and increasing desacyl-ghrelin and gastric leptin. Stomach dilation sends signals through the vagus nerve and peripheral nervous system to the brainstem and hypothalamus. The digested nutrient passes to the small intestine and colon, producing further mechanic-dilation, GI hormones release, bile acid and pancreatic juices secretion. These GI hormones have a local (paracrine) and peripheral effect, when secreted into circulation and passed through the liver, and affect the muscle, adipose tissue, GI motility and function, and nucleus of the hypothalamus and brainstem. The paracrine and endocrine effect induces satiation and satiety. The muscle and adipose tissue release hormones which affect similar nuclei in the brain. The effect on the hypothalamus and brainstem trigger higher brain area responses, modulating behavior and enhancing nutrient-related reward. In the hypothalamus, first-order neurons in the arcuate nucleus (ARC) modulate appetite by the NPY/AGRP pathway and satiation by the POMC/CART pathway. The neurons interact with second-order neurons in the paraventricular nucleus (PVN) and lateral hypothalamic area (LHA) to send signals to higher brain areas and the brainstem. In the brainstem, the nucleus of the tractus solitarius (NST) and dorsal vagal complex (DMNV) interact with the periphery and GI system and bring signals to the higher brain areas and hypothalamus. 5-HT, serotonin; ACTH, adrenocorticotropic hormone; AGRP, agouti-related peptide; ARC, arcuate nucleus; AVP, arginine vasopressin; BA, bile acids; CART, cocaine- and amphetamine-regulated transcript; CCK, cholecystokinin; CRH, corticotropin-releasing hormone; D, dopamine; DMNV, dorsal vagal complex; FGF, fibroblast growth factor-19; GABA, γ-aminobutyric acid; GLP-1, glucagon-like peptide-1; IL-6, interleukin-6; LHA, lateral hypothalamic area; MSH, melanocortin-stimulating hormone; NA, noradrenaline; NPY, neuropeptide Y; NST, nucleus of the tractus solitarius; NT, neurotensin; OT, oxytocin; Orex, orexin; OXM, oxyntomodulin; PP, pancreatic polypeptide; PVN, paraventricular nucleus; peptide tyrosine-tyrosine (PYY3)-36, peptide tyrosine-tyrosine 3-36; POMC, proopiomelanocortin; TNF, tumor necrosis factor; TRH, thyroid-releasing hormone; TSH, thyroid-stimulating hormone. Source: Reproduced with permission from Acosta et al. 2014 [4] with permission from *Gut*.

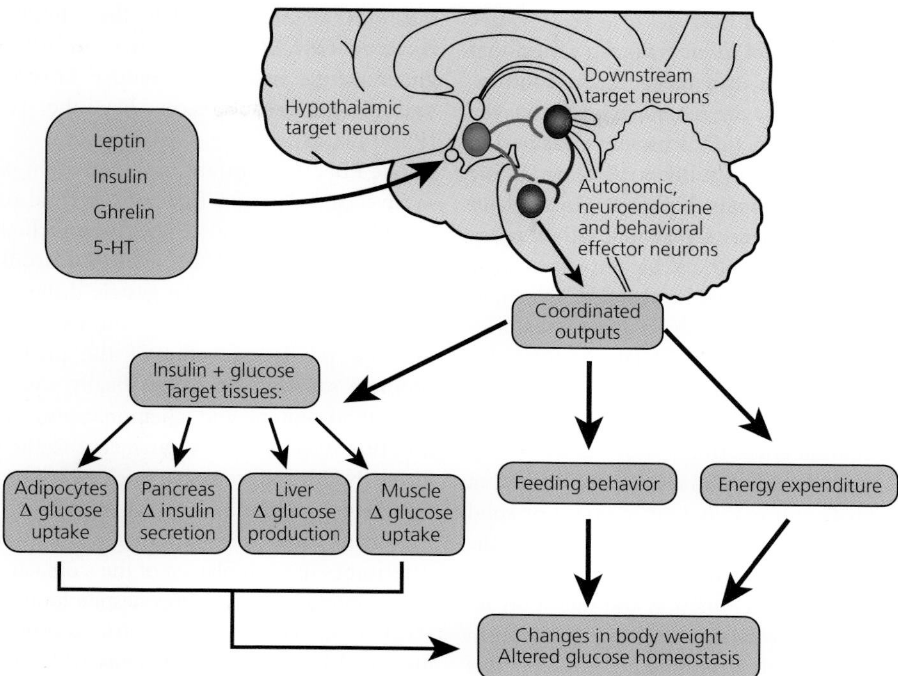

Figure 24.3 Neurons in the hypothalamus, including those in the arcuate nucleus, are targets of a number of key hormones and metabolic cues. These neurons target several downstream sites to influence complex circuits in the central nervous system (CNS). The downstream effector circuits mediate the coordinated autonomic, behavioral, and endocrine responses to changing levels of metabolic signals. Diminished responses of first-order neurons such as those in the arcuate nucleus may contribute to the pathogenesis of obesity and type 2 diabetes. This includes increased bodyweight, uncontrolled glycemia, and altered insulin secretion and insulin sensitivity in target tissues such as liver, adipose tissue, pancreas, and skeletal muscle. Thus, the CNS not only regulates food intake and bodyweight, but also plays a key role in regulating glucose homeostasis in peripheral tissues. Source: Adapted from Elmquist and Marcus 2003 [10]. Reproduced by permission of Springer Nature.

hypothalamus (ARH), and send signals to the lateral nuclei of the hypothalamus (LH), the "hunger center." The NPY/AgRP neurons stimulate hunger by secreting neuropeptide Y (NPY), and antagonizing the melanocortin-4 receptors (MC4Rs), respectively. These neurons are constantly sensing the nutrient load in plasma and are also influenced by different peripheral signals or signaling molecules.

One of the key signals is ghrelin, a hormone mainly secreted by the P/D1 cells in the gastric fundus, that acts in AgRP neurons to promote hunger [11,12]. Ghrelin is unique in that the hormone requires the addition of an octanoate group (an eight carbon fatty acid) for it to have agonist activity at the ghrelin receptor. The enzyme that catalyzes the addition of the octanoyl group is ghrelin O-acyltransferase (GOAT), which is also expressed in the ghrelin-producing cells of the stomach [13].

The identification of the hormone ghrelin was accomplished using a "reverse" pharmacology approach as the receptor was identified using synthetic ligands long before the endogenous hormone was discovered. Ghrelin was ultimately identified as the endogenous ligand for the growth hormone secretagog receptor (GHSR; ghrelin receptor) [14]. Over the intervening years, ghrelin has emerged as a potential regulator of energy balance and glucose homeostasis. Plasma ghrelin levels vary throughout the day, with a characteristic premeal spike and a subsequent postprandial decline in plasma levels. These patterns have led to predictions that ghrelin plays a physiological role in hunger and meal initiation in humans. Consistent with a role of ghrelin in regulating energy balance, levels of ghrelin rise following fasting and after chronic deprivation of food. Notably, ghrelin levels rise during periods of negative energy balance. Ghrelin levels are elevated following weight loss, chronic and intense exercise, cancer cachexia, and in eating disorders such as anorexia nervosa [15].

The rise in ghrelin levels that occurs following diet-induced weight loss has been proposed to serve as a response to chronic periods of negative energy balance. It has also been hypothesized that this weight loss-induced rise in ghrelin provides a potential mechanism for the rebound weight gain that is often observed in subjects following dieting and exercise-induced weight loss. Moreover, following bariatric surgery, plasma ghrelin levels are lowered, which may contribute to the ability of this procedure to maintain long-term weight loss, although other studies have not found this reduction. An elevation of ghrelin has also been found in patients with Prader–Willi syndrome. This condition results from defects of imprinting of several genes located on chromosome 15 and is associated with several disorders including a voracious appetite and morbid obesity. Thus, high ghrelin levels may contribute to the pathophysiology of this disorder [15].

Satiation

Satiation is defined as a sensation of fullness during a meal that aids in inducing the termination of a meal [2]; in contrast, satiety is the feeling of fullness or satiation prior to the consumption of the next meal. Satiation is usually measured in calories consumed prior to reaching fullness. A Mayo Clinic study reported that in 509 individuals, higher BMI correlates with higher calories consumed prior to reaching satiation, i.e. for every 5 kg/m^2 of BMI, there was 50 kcal higher caloric consumption prior to reaching comfortable satiation. Normal-weight participants consumed an average of about 650 calories prior to reaching satiation (Figure 24.4). Additionally, participants with abnormal waist circumference consumed 140 more calories prior to reaching maximal fullness compared to those with normal circumference [16].

Reaching satiation is mediated by many mechanisms that occur simultaneously. First, nutrient content in liquid or solid form produces a distension of the stomach, which stimulates the vagal afferents to conduct the signal to the satiation brain centers. The initial studies of gastric function and sensation are more than a century old and involved distending a balloon in the stomach and noting the feeling of fullness [18–20]; this sensation of satiation was calorie independent. However, nutrients do play a major role as well. When the enteroendocrine cells in the stomach and duodenum sense the content of nutrients, they release satiation hormones such as cholecystokinin as the first stop signals [21]. The signals from the gastric distension, nutrients and hormones convolute in the brainstem and hypothalamus. Here, the inhibitory neurons are the proopiomelanocortin and the cocaine and amphetamine-related transcript (POMC/CART) neurons. These sets of neurons are located in the ARH too, and send their downstream signaling to the "satiety center," the ventromedial nucleus of the hypothalamus (VMH) and the paraventricular hypothalamus (PVH). POMC/CART neurons secrete α-melanocyte-stimulating hormone (α-MSH), which then binds to melanocortin-4 receptors (MC4Rs) in the VMH and PVH and stimulates the glutamatergic neurons to induce satiation, and send downstream signals to places like the parabrachial neurons (PBN) [22,23].

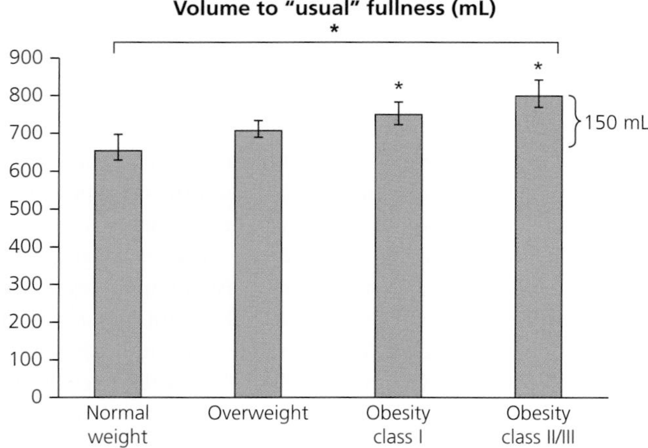

Figure 24.4 Obesity is associated with higher volume to experience fullness during a nutrient drink test (*$p < 0.05$). Source: Reproduced with permission from *Gastroenterology* [16,17].

The PBN is important in the satiation process, as it not only receives signals from first- and second-order neurons in the hypothalamus; but also, the parabrachial nucleus calcitonin gene-related peptide (PBN CGRP) neurons are related to direct satiation mechanisms like gastric distension [24,25] and hormones like CCK [21]. These neurons are responsible for receiving and mediating some of the physiological signals that promote satiation [26]. Specifically, the afferent signals from mechanoreceptors and chemoreceptors in the stomach and intestine travel via the vagus nerve to the nucleus tractus solitarius (NTS), and from that nucleus, anorectic signals are transmitted to the PBN [27] and the hypothalamus [28,29].

Normal gastric accommodation is important in satiation as it determines the compliance of the stomach and the maintenance of low intragastric pressures despite food intake. There is a correlation between reduced gastric accommodation and weight loss, as demonstrated in patients with functional dyspepsia or cancer [30,31] and enlarged fasting gastric volume in patients with obesity [16]. Stomach distension and increased intragastric pressure enhance satiation by stimulating the mechanosensitive receptors of the stomach [32,33]. These effects might be mediated mainly by the antral area and antral distension, as both are positively correlated with the sensation of fullness – satiation [34,35].

This constellation of signals is able to turn "off" the hunger neurons and turn "on" the satiation signals and induce the sensation of fullness, and therefore meal termination. Patients with genetic disorders that affect the satiation pathway may suffer from hyperphagia and subsequent severe obesity; this includes the Prader–Willi syndrome, as discussed below. Satiation can be overcome by hedonic mechanisms as well as conditioned or trained reflexes or behaviors such as in bulimia nervosa eating disorder [36]. Additionally, the sensation of hunger, gastric emptying rate, and gastric accommodation predict the quantity of calories ingested in a satiation test [37].

Satiety

Once the individual has reached satiation and completed the meal, satiety starts. Satiety is defined as the duration of the sensation of fullness [3] or the time before the return of hunger. However, there is also a period, not defined as a clear stage in the food intake process, in which the individual may feel neither significant fullness nor hunger.

In the stage of satiety, our brain is in the "off" mode for hunger, and slowly over time, the satiation signal experienced during the meal which led to cessation of food intake is wearing off. However, peripheral signals, mainly from the distal gut and adipose tissue, communicate with the brainstem and hypothalamus, to retain the sensation of fullness. These signals from the distal gut are key to nutrient ingestion and digestion as these satiety hormones signal to the brain centers to evoke satiation and also slow down the upper gut motor function to enhance digestion, nutrient and calorie absorption, and maximize the energy availability through calories recently consumed. This slowing of upper digestive function that slows gastric emptying and upper small bowel motility is known as the ileal brake [38–40].

When nutrients reach the small bowel, they interact with enteroendocrine cells (EEC), which are gut-specific cells that are constantly sensing the intraluminal and circulatory nutrient status. In response to a meal, there is mechanical stimulation as well as nutrient stimulation that result in the release of satiety hormones (summarized in Table 24.1). The L-type EECs coexpress and cosecrete glucagon-like peptide (GLP-1) and peptide YY (PYY), which are key to the induction of satiety and inducing the ileal brake [41] These gut hormones enhance satiety via a paracrine effect in the vagus nerve and an endocrine effect in the NTS and hypothalamus. The paracrine and endocrine effects of satiety gut hormones, such as CCK, obestatin, GLP-1 or PYY, also delay gastric emptying and inhibit antral contractility, pancreatic secretions and gastrointestinal motility [42–47], contributing to the sensation of fullness and satiety.

The EECs are constantly sensing and interacting with the luminal content, including the microbiome. There is emerging evidence suggesting interaction of the human gut microbiome, the gastrointestinal system, and the control of food intake [48–50]. Gut bacteria are essential in deconjugation, dehydrogenation, and dehydroxylation of primary bile acids in the colon [51]. The microbiota contributes to breaking down otherwise indigestible carbohydrates or the 5–10% of complex carbohydrate that reaches the colon even in health each day [52], and this results in the increase in short-chain fatty acid absorption in the colon, providing additional energy and increasing fat storage in adipose tissue [48,49]. The metabolites of the gut microbiome induce the secretion of gut hormones by intermediate metabolites such as bile acid and short-chain fatty acids. Additionally, the microbiome may produce inflammatory changes and increase the production of lipopolysaccharide (LPS) which will stimulate the synthesis of CCK and PYY in enteroendocrine cells [53]. Further studies are needed to understand the role of the gut microbiome in human regulation of food intake.

Delay of gastric emptying is linked to increased feelings of satiety, which then increases over time until the next meal, and decreases caloric intake during that meal [37,54]. Decreasing gastric emptying could conceivably result in a larger intragastric volume over time, resulting in sensation of gastric distension and feelings of satiety and a delayed return of hunger.

Satiety gut hormones result in inhibition of food intake signals from the hypothalamus, akin to switching food intake "off" by first counteracting the orexigenic gastrointestinal hormones such as ghrelin, which activate the NPY/AGRP appetite pathway in the arcuate nucleus of the hypothalamus. Concurrently or sequentially, the anorexigenic gastrointestinal satiety hormones, such as GLP-1 or PYY3-36, inhibit the NPY/AGRP and stimulate the POMC/CART pathway in the arcuate nucleus of the hypothalamus to induce satiation and satiety and stop food intake. The arcuate nucleus sends signals to the paraventricular nucleus and the lateral hypothalamic area. In the brainstem, orexigenic and anorexigenic gastrointestinal hormones modulate the nucleus of the NST and dorsal vagal complex (DMNV) and signal to the higher brain areas and the hypothalamus. The effect on the hypothalamus and the brainstem triggering of higher brain areas result in modulation of behavior and enhancement of nutrient-related reward [4]. Leptin (predominantly from adipose tissue) stimulates POMC and CART neurons via leptin receptors (LepRs) to promote satiation [55,56] and stimulates GLP-1 neurons in the brainstem [57].

Table 24.1 Enteroendocrine cell types, peptide(s)/hormone(s) secreted, predominant location, and proposed physiological role of peptide(s)/hormone(s).

Cell type	Hormone(s)	Predominant location	Function
X/A[a] **P/D1[b]**	Ghrelin, nesfatin-1	Gastric oxyntic mucosa and proximal small intestine	Appetite control, food intake, glucose homeostasis, growth hormone release, sleep, and mood
Chief cells P cells	Gastric leptin	Gastric mucosa	Short-term regulation of food intake
D	Somatostatin	Stomach, small intestine	Gastrointestinal hormone inhibition
I	CCK	Duodenum, proximal jejunal mucosa, enteric nervous system	Stimulates gallbladder contraction, inhibits stomach emptying, and food intake
K	GIP	Proximal small intestine	Insulin release, gastric acid secretion
L	GLP-1, GLP-2, PYY, OXM, NT	Along the entire small intestine with ileal and colonic predominance	Nutrient sensing, GI motility, stimulation of insulin release, inhibition of glucagon release, appetite suppression, and promotion of energy expenditure

[a] Rodents.
[b] Humans.
CCK, cholecystokinin; GI, gastrointestinal; GIP, glucose-dependent insulinotropic polypeptide; GLP, glucagon-like peptide; NT, neurotensin; OXM, oxyntomodulin; PYY, peptide tyrosine tyrosine.
Source: Reproduced from Monteiro and Batterham 2017 [80] with permission from *Gastroenterology*.

Hedonic control of food intake

The signals emanating from the hunger–satiety circuitry that are activated by food intake can be overridden by the hedonic components of food intake, or by environmental factors [58,59]. Studies in mice demonstrate that the circuitry is extremely interconnected, with an excess of compensatory circuits that are tightly connected with the reward brain centers. These higher brain centers which regulate emotions, mood, desire, and many other positive and negative sensations can override the homeostatic control of food intake (see Figure 24.2). This phenomenon, known as emotional eating, could bypass the brain–gut signals to control food intake and lead to either anorexia or hyperphagia.

Key organs contributing to the regulation of food intake

Hypothalamus

Arcuate nucleus of the hypothalamus and the central melanocortin system

The arcuate nucleus of the hypothalamus plays a fundamental role in regulating feeding and glucose homeostasis. This is due in large part to the role of melanocortin neurons whose cell bodies reside in the arcuate nucleus. The central melanocortin system is composed of POMC neurons and AgRP neurons. POMC neurons produce α-MSH, an endogenous agonist of MC4Rs [6,60]. The word "melanocortin" is a collective term for a series of peptides that are cleaved from POMC. One of the products cleaved from POMC is the anterior pituitary gland hormone, adrenocorticotropic hormone (ACTH), which is a key regulator of the stress axis. In the CNS, POMC neurons are located only in the ARH, and the nucleus of the solitary tract in rodents and humans. Considerable attention has focused on α-MSH and other MC4R agonists and their regulation of food intake, bodyweight, and glucose homeostasis [60]. Conversely, AgRP neurons secrete AgRP, the endogenous MC4R antagonist (see Figure 24.2). These neurons also express and secrete the orexigenic neuropeptide Y (NPY). Notably, complete ablation of AgRP neurons results in anorexia. In addition, acute activation of AgRP neurons increases food intake and bodyweight [6,61]. Serotonin is an important neurotransmitter in the arcuate nucleus.

Serotonin regulates food intake and bodyweight

In addition to circulating metabolic signals, classic neurotransmitters in the brain are critical regulators of energy balance and food intake [61]. One excellent example is the central serotonin system, which is an important regulator of feeding, energy balance, and glucose homeostasis [62]. Pharmacological compounds that target central serotonin [5-hydroxytryptamine (5-HT)] signaling potently regulate energy homeostasis and have been used effectively as antiobesity drugs in humans. Dexfenfluramine (d-Fen) increases serotonin content by stimulating synaptic release of serotonin and blocking its reuptake into presynaptic terminals. This class of drugs showed a potent anorexigenic activity in rodents and humans. Conversely, treatments that suppress central serotonergic signaling, such as paroxetine, a selective serotonin reuptake inhibitor, produce hyperphagia and weight gain in humans and rodents [63].

Dexfenfluramine was widely used in combination with phenteramine (Fen-Phen) to successfully induce weight-loss. Unfortunately, d-Fen and other nonspecific serotonergic agonists were associated with cardiac valve lesions as well as adverse cardiovascular events and were withdrawn from clinical use [64]. Subsequent work has focused on dissecting how serotonin and d-Fen modulate a complex central 5-HT system, composed of 14 different 5-HT receptor (5-HTR) isoforms in multiple cell types, to stimulate weight loss. These efforts have pinpointed that serotonin and d-Fen act predominantly via central 5-HT_{2C} receptors [65,66] and downstream melanocortin pathways to suppress feeding, thus reducing bodyweight. The selective 5-HT_{2C} receptor agonist locarserin (Belviq®) was shown to reduce bodyweight and improved glycemia in patients with obesity and type 2 diabetes, respectively [67]. This drug, approved in 2012 by the FDA, was recently withdrawn from clinical use due to increased overall cancer risk.

Ventromedial hypothalamic neurons (VMH)

Recently, physiologically important targets of leptin in regions outside the ARH have been identified. These include neurons in the VMH [61,68]. The VMH has historically been linked to the regulation of bodyweight based on lesion studies that led to the view that the VMH was a satiety center. Several recent studies have established that the VMH is a physiologically important site regulating bodyweight homeostasis. Steroidogenic factor 1 (SF-1) is an orphan nuclear receptor transcription factor expressed exclusively in the VMH [69]. Mice lacking SF-1 develop late-onset obesity. Notably, leptin receptors are abundantly expressed in the VMH and selective deletion of leptin receptors from SF-1 neurons produces obesity. Thus, the VMH is a critical site in the brain regulating bodyweight.

Ventromedial hypothalamic neurons can also regulate insulin sensitivity in peripheral tissues, including skeletal muscle, white adipose tissue, and brown adipose tissue. Leptin action in the VMH significantly increases glucose uptake in the skeletal muscle and brown adipose tissue without affecting blood insulin levels, which suggests that leptin acts on VMH neurons to enhance peripheral insulin sensitivity [70]. This and other findings suggest that nonmelanocortinergic neurons outside the arcuate nucleus are important in the antidiabetic actions of leptin. In addition, mice lacking leptin receptors in SF-1 neurons in the VMH show insulin resistance that precedes the development of obesity [68]. In contrast, selective deletion of suppressor of cytokine signaling 3 (Socs3, a negative regulator of leptin signaling) in SF-1 neurons prevents insulin resistance induced by high fat feeding.

Vagus nerve

A key concept is that the control of energy balance results from the coordinated actions of long-term and short-term metabolic cues. Simplistically, one can consider the actions of hormones such as leptin as long-term regulators of food intake and bodyweight with relatively little in the way of meal-to-meal changes in leptin levels. In contrast, short-term (meal-to-meal) regulation of food intake is thought to be importantly regulated by peripheral sensing mechanisms, prominent among them being sensory neurons of the vagus nerve. The vagus nerve, the 10th cranial nerve, has both sensory and motor fibers and innervates the viscera. It is thought to be important in regulating energy balance, appetite, and liver gluconeogenesis that are altered in obese patients [5].

The vagus nerve innervates organs in the thoracic and abdominal cavities. It is a mixed nerve and, importantly, more than half of the fibers are sensory and thus serve a key role in conveying information from the viscera to the brain. The vagus nerve also provides the cholinergic (parasympathetic) motor innervation to the thoracic and abdominal viscera. The cell bodies of the sensory neurons reside in the nodose ganglion located in the jugular foramen at the base of the skull. The sensory neurons terminate in the NTS in the medulla oblongata.

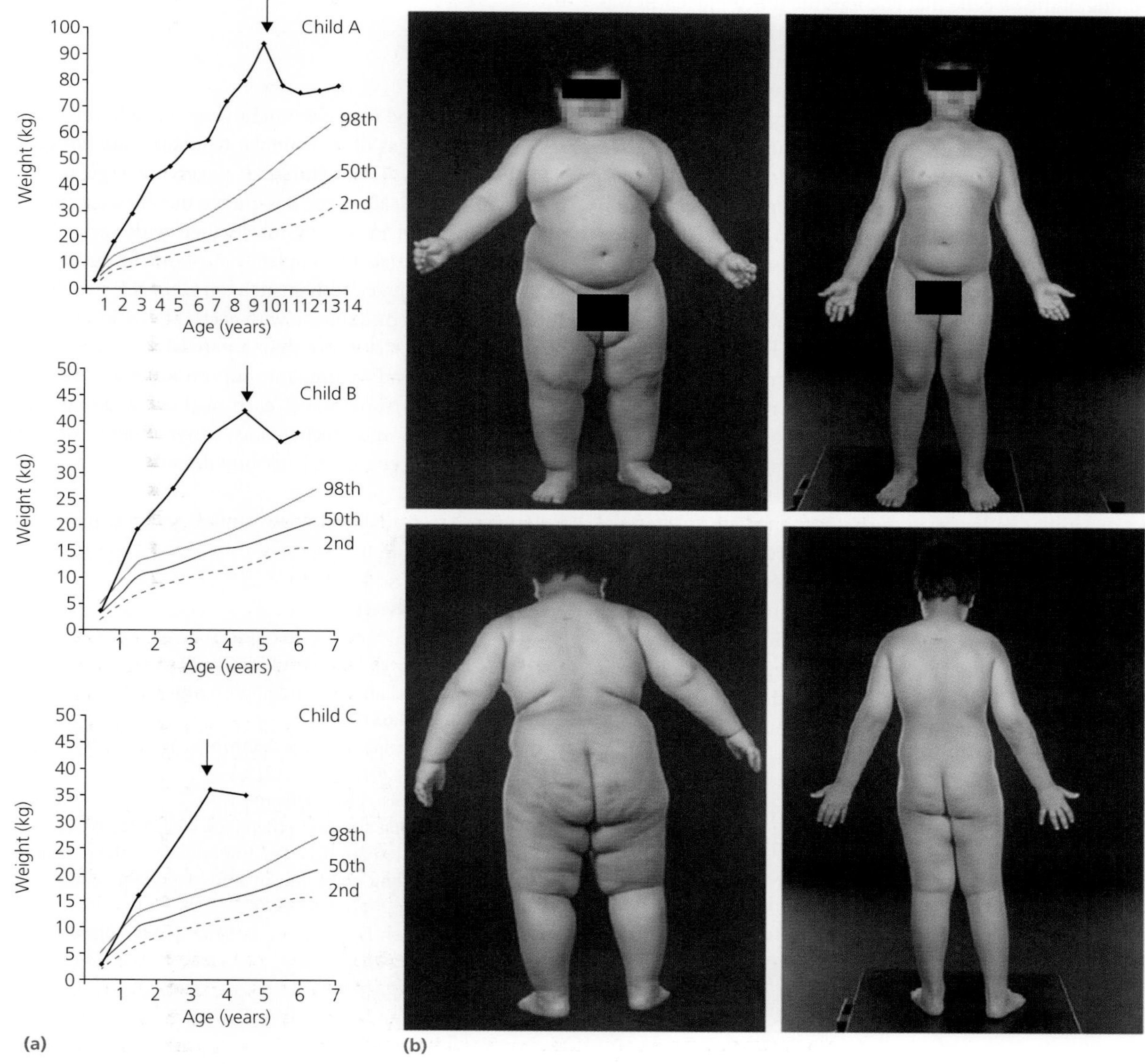

Figure 24.5 Congenital leptin deficiency [75]. Three children are illustrated. **(a)** Weights of child A compared with normal centiles for girls, and of child B and child C, compared with normal centiles for boys. Arrows indicate the start of leptin therapy. **(b)** Clinical photographs of child B before (height = 107 cm) and 24 months after leptin therapy (height = 124 cm). Source: Farooqi et al. 2002 [81]. Reproduced with permission from the American Society for Clinical Investigation.

The vagal sensory neurons innervate the length of the gastrointestinal tract up to the right colon and thus are ideally positioned to convey information from the GI tract back to the brain [4,5]. For example, vagal afferents regulate multiple postprandial functions. One excellent example is the role of vagal afferents in regulating food intake following a meal. Cholecystokinin, an endogenous peptide released by duodenal enteroendocrine cells during meals, is the prototypical gut-derived satiety peptide [71]. CCK acts (at least in part) via vagal afferents in the gut through the CCK-A receptor. This reduces meal size and initiates meal termination or satiation [72].

Adipocyte influence in energy balance: leptin

The cloning of the *ob* gene that encodes the hormone leptin was the catalyst that led to our current understanding of the molecular and neural mechanisms controlling energy balance [7]. Leptin deficiency in mice (*ob/ob*) causes myriad disturbances including a ravenous appetite, morbid obesity, diabetes, reduced energy expenditure, cold intolerance, immune defects, delayed onset of puberty, and various neuroendocrine abnormalities [61]. Leptin is produced and secreted primarily by white adipose tissue. The circulating levels of leptin plasma levels are positively correlated with total body fat mass [73,74]. Notably, several cohorts of leptin-deficient patients have also been identified [75]. The phenotypic abnormalities found in the *ob/ob* mice are also present in humans who lack leptin (Figure 24.5). While these mutations are extremely rare, they are nonetheless very important as they demonstrate that leptin is required for appropriate control of energy balance and glucose homeostasis in humans. Moreover, the similarities of the physiological responses of human subjects to leptin administration suggest that leptin may act on similar pathways in the brain to mediate its effects.

A key to understanding the biological importance of any hormone is to assess the response of hormone replacement in individuals who are deficient or lacking the hormone. Importantly, replacement of leptin in *ob/ob* mice, and in humans with leptin deficiency, essentially normalized all the reported phenotypic abnormalities (see Figure 24.5). This included decreased food intake, which resulted in greatly reduced bodyweight in both mice and leptin-deficient patients. In the *ob/ob* mice, leptin administration also increased baseline energy expenditure and greatly improved cold intolerance [75,76]. The dramatic results of replacing leptin in leptin-deficient patients and mice led to the hope that the administration of leptin to obese individuals would result in weight loss by reducing food intake and increasing energy expenditure. Unfortunately, obese individuals actually have higher levels of circulating leptin compared to normal-weight individuals, so it appears that "leptin resistance" develops in obesity in a manner similar to insulin resistance [77]. Consistent with this model, administration of leptin to obese subjects showed varied effects and did not result in significant weight loss [78].

Actions of leptin in peripheral tissues have been identified that may play important roles in regulating diverse processes such as immune function [76]. However, as it relates to energy balance and glucose homeostasis, the brain is thought to be the primary and most important site of leptin action. For example, injection of leptin into the brains of leptin-deficient mice is sufficient to normalize bodyweight, feeding, energy expenditure, and glucose metabolism [79].

Summary

The control of food intake is a tightly regulated homeostatic process. The key stages of food intake regulation are hunger, satiation, and satiety. These different stages are regulated by the brain–gut–fat axis. However, it is known that these circuits are not unidirectional but intricately intertwined with each other, such that it is inappropriate to completely attribute the entire control of food intake to a single mechanism as an ON/OFF switch. The two sets of neurons communicate with each other within the arcuate nucleus, showing that more than a parallel process, most of it is interconnected and redundant (an evolutionary necessity to ensure survival). Nonetheless, each of these stages and the key regulatory organs and mechanisms, when altered, contribute to disequilibrium in energy balance and disease.

References are available at www.yamadagastro.com/textbook7e

Further reading

Acosta A., Abu Dayyeh B.K., Port J.D., Camilleri M. Recent advances in clinical practice challenges and opportunities in the management of obesity. Gut 2014;63:687.

Camilleri M. Peripheral mechanisms in appetite regulation. Gastroenterology 2015;148(6):1219.

Gautron L., Elmquist J.K., Williams K.W. Neural control of energy balance: translating circuits to therapies. Cell 2015;161(1):133.

Monteiro M.P., Batterham R.L. The importance of the gastrointestinal tract in controlling food intake and regulating energy balance. Gastroenterology 2017;152(7):1707.

Myers M.G. Jr, Olson D.P. Central nervous system control of metabolism. Nature 2012;491:357.

CHAPTER 25

Eating disorders

Leslie Sim[1], Jocelyn Lebow[1], and Janna R. Gewirtz O'Brien[2]

[1] Department of Psychiatry and Psychology, Mayo Clinic, Rochester, MN, USA
[2] Department of Pediatrics, University of Minnesota, Minneapolis, MN, USA

Chapter menu

Eating disorders are associated with a host of adverse medical morbidities that affect every organ system [1,2]. Because eating disorders involve behaviors associated with altered consumption or absorption of food, gastrointestinal (GI) symptoms are common. Consequently, many patients with eating disorders seek gastroenterological healthcare during some point in their illness. In fact, many individuals with eating disorders seek gastroenterological care even before they seek treatment for their eating disorder. As such, the gastroenterologist is often in a unique position to diagnose an eating disorder early in its illness course. Without adequate diagnoses, eating disorders can progress in severity and become increasingly difficult to treat [3]. Moreover, it is unlikely that medical management of GI symptoms will be effective without first addressing eating disorder symptoms.

The Fifth Edition of the *Diagnostic and Statistical Manual of Mental Disorders* (DSM-5) provides diagnostic criteria for anorexia nervosa (AN), bulimia nervosa (BN), binge eating disorder (BED), avoidant/restrictive food intake disorder (ARFID), pica, and rumination syndrome [4]. Because patients with eating disorders were historically perceived to "refuse" to gain weight, their restrictive eating was thought to be considered evidence of an underlying psychological disorder. The associated traits and symptoms of obsessiveness, perfectionism, altered body image, anxiety, and depression further support this viewpoint. Accordingly, patients with eating disorders are commonly referred to a mental health provider for treatment. There is now, however, a growing body of evidence showing that many of the features of eating disorders may be maladaptive physiological responses to caloric restriction. In this chapter, we will review in depth AN, BN, BED, and ARFID, emphasizing this biological perspective. Because rumination syndrome is frequently seen in gastroenterology settings, this eating disorder will be briefly discussed.

Epidemiology of eating disorders

About 0.5–1% of adolescent and adult women in the United States have a diagnosis of AN, with a lifetime incidence rate as high as 3.7% [4]. Boys and young men represent approximately 10% of individuals with AN. The prevalence of BN is reported to be at least 1% of the population [5], and BED affects at least 3.5% of women and 2.0% of men [6]. Given that it is a recently

Yamada's Textbook of Gastroenterology, Seventh Edition. Edited by Timothy C. Wang, Michael Camilleri, Benjamin Lebwohl, Anna S. Lok, William J. Sandborn, Kenneth K. Wang, and Gary D. Wu.

Companion website: www.yamadagastro.com/textbook7e

added diagnosis with less research, the prevalence of ARFID is less clear.

Although eating disorders are more common in women [7], it is possible that some of this discrepancy is due a relatively poor understanding of eating disorder presentations in male individuals, and that the majority of screening tools and clinical interviews have been developed with predominantly female samples [8]. Nearly 75% of individuals manifest features of their eating disorder while in adolescence [9], with the average age of onset for AN being 15 years [7]. In addition, although the prevalence rates for full syndrome eating disorders are relatively low, robust data suggest subclinical eating disorder behaviors are relatively common in adolescents. A large community-based study conducted by Croll and colleagues [10] found that 57% of female adolescents and 33% of male adolescents report using unhealthy weight control behaviors, including concerning behaviors such as fasting and smoking for weight control. In the same sample, 12% of female adolescents and 5% of male adolescent report using extreme weight-control behaviors such as intermittent self-induced vomiting, laxative use, or diet pill abuse [10]. These subsyndromal behaviors are not less serious than full syndrome eating disorders, and the conditions of patients who do not meet the full criteria for AN or BN are no less severe. In particular, studies suggest a comparable rate of mortality and morbidity for idiosyncratic and subclinical eating disorders as compared with full-spectrum AN and BN [11,12].

Although there is a common misconception that eating disorders largely affect young Caucasian females from families of middle to upper socioeconomic status [8], there is increasing evidence that they affect groups more broadly than initially assumed [13]. Eating disorders in ethnic and racial minority groups have become increasingly researched, as well as those across the socioeconomic spectrum. In addition, it has become recognized that eating disorders affect patients of all ages, including younger children and members of the geriatric population [14]. Finally, it is also coming to the field's attention that eating disorders affect individuals of every body habitus and weight [15]. Although early diagnostic criteria associated AN with a low absolute body mass index (BMI), recent modifications to the DSM reflect the growing understanding that serious restrictive eating disorders can be present in individuals at every BMI. Similarly, although it is a common misperception that individuals with binge eating present at higher BMIs, these individuals also can present at every size.

Although the etiology of eating disorders is complex, specific factors have been identified that increase one's risk for development of an eating disorder. Individuals with type 1 diabetes, or with another medical disorder characterized by dietary restriction, or those with symptoms that affect appetite and eating, such as abdominal pain or nausea, have a higher rate of eating disorders than the general public [16,17]. Psychological characteristics, such as perfectionism, deficits in emotion regulation, anxiety, or body image dissatisfaction, are also associated with increased risk for an eating disorder [18–22]. There also appears to be a strong genetic predisposition [23]. Social factors, such as a history of experienced weight stigma or weight-related teasing [23–25] and a history of dieting behavior, is strongly linked to all types of eating disorders [26]. Finally, there is increasing research on neurobiological characteristics of eating disorders, including disruption of hypothalamic–pituitary–adrenal (HPA) axis functioning, catecholamine disturbances, and central nervous system anomalies, particularly in the insular cortex and reward pathways.

Recognizing eating disorders

Anorexia nervosa

Cases of AN have been described in medical writings dating back 300 years [27]. Increasing attention was given to AN in the 1900s, with various etiologies for the condition proposed during that time [28]. Hilde Bruch [29], a pioneer in the field of eating disorders, proposed that the hallmarks of the disease included a distorted body image, alterations in the perception of signals of hunger and satiety, and an overwhelming feeling of ineffectiveness. In other writings, she describes a preoccupation with eating and food in individuals with AN [27]. In the absence of an underlying organic disease, she proposed that AN is a mental disorder [29]. However, modern research supports the neurobiological underpinnings of the disease, as well as the physiological contribution of malnutrition and starvation [30,31].

Under DSM-5, the overarching psychopathology that characterizes AN is persistent energy intake restriction leading to weight loss or failure to make expected gains in weight. A second criterion involves an intense fear of gaining weight or becoming fat, or persistent behavior that interferes with weight gain. The third criterion is a body image disturbance, disproportionate influence of weight or shape on one's self-image, and/or a persistent lack of recognition of the seriousness of the disorder (Box 25.1).

In a shift from previous versions of the DSM, the DSM-5 no longer requires that patients meet a specific "low weight" threshold; instead, weight loss and underweight status is determined based on physical health consequences of low weight and an individual's own historic weight and growth history, in the context of their developmental trajectory. This change in the definition of low weight has implications for higher weight status individuals who have lost a large percentage of their bodyweight, in that they still may meet criteria for AN. In addition, although previous versions of the DSM required postmenarcheal females to be amenorrheic to qualify for a diagnosis of AN, the DSM-5 has eliminated that criterion.

AN has different subtypes, including AN-restrictive subtype and AN-binge/purge subtype. Whereas the former is characterized by dietary restriction, the latter can include symptoms of binge eating (or perceived binge eating wherein the patient eats an objectively small amount of food, or any food at all, and feels a distinct loss of control) and purging.

Box 25.1 *Diagnostic and Statistical Manual of Mental Disorders, Fifth Edition* (DSM-5) diagnostic criteria for anorexia nervosa, bulimia nervosa, binge eating disorder, avoidant/restrictive food intake disorder, and other specified eating disorder.

DSM-5 criteria for anorexia nervosa [4]

Criterion A. Restriction of energy intake relative to requirements leading to a significantly low bodyweight in the context of age, sex, developmental trajectory, and physical health. Significantly low weight is defined as a weight that is less than minimally normal or, for children and adolescents, less than that minimally expected.

Criterion B. Intense fear of gaining weight or of becoming fat, or persistent behavior that interferes with weight gain, even though at a significantly low weight.

Criterion C. Disturbance in the way in which one's bodyweight or shape is experienced, undue influence of bodyweight or shape on self-evaluation, or persistent lack of recognition of the seriousness of the current low bodyweight.

DSM-5 criteria for bulimia nervosa [4]

Criterion A. Recurrent episodes of binge eating. An episode of binge eating is characterized by both of the following:

1. Eating, in a discrete period (e.g., within any 2-hour period), an amount of food that is definitely larger than what most individuals would eat in a similar period under similar circumstances.
2. A sense of lack of control over eating during the episode (e.g., a feeling that one cannot stop eating or control what or how much one is eating).

Criterion B. Recurrent inappropriate compensatory behavior to prevent weight gain, such as self-induced vomiting; misuse of laxatives, diuretics, or other medications; fasting; or excessive exercise.

Criterion C. The binge eating and inappropriate compensatory behaviors both occur, on average, at least once a week for 3 months.

Criterion D. Self-evaluation is unduly influenced by body shape and weight.

Criterion E. The disturbance does not occur exclusively during episodes of anorexia nervosa.

DSM-5 criteria for binge eating disorder [4]

Criterion 1. Recurrent episodes of binge eating. An episode of binge eating is characterized by both of the following:

a. Eating, in a discrete period (e.g., within any 2-hour period), an amount of food that is definitely larger than most people would eat in a similar period under similar circumstances.
b. The sense of lack of control over eating during the episode (e.g., a feeling that one cannot stop eating or control what or how much one is eating).

Criterion 2. Binge eating episodes are associated with three (or more) of the following:

a. Eating much more rapidly than normal
b. Eating until feeling uncomfortably full
c. Eating large amounts of food when not feeling physically hungry
d. Eating alone because of being embarrassed by how much one is eating
e. Feeling disgusted with oneself, depressed, or very guilty after overeating

Criterion 3. Marked distress regarding binge eating is present.

Criterion 4. The binge eating occurs, on average, at least 1 day a week for 3 months (DSM-5 frequency and duration criteria).

Criterion 5. The binge eating is not associated with the regular use of inappropriate compensatory behavior (e.g., purging, fasting, excessive exercise) and does not occur exclusively during the course of anorexia nervosa or bulimia nervosa.

DSM-5 criteria for avoidant restrictive food intake disorder [4]

Criterion A. An eating or feeding disturbance (e.g., apparent lack of interest in eating or food; avoidance based on the sensory characteristics of food; concern about aversive consequences of eating) as manifested by persistent failure to meet appropriate nutritional and/or energy needs associated with one (or more) of the following:

1. Significant weight loss (or failure to achieve expected weight gain or faltering growth in children)
2. Significant nutritional deficiency
3. Dependence on enteral feeding or oral nutritional supplements
4. Marked interference with psychosocial functioning

Criterion B. The disturbance is not better explained by lack of available food or by an associated culturally sanctioned practice.

Criterion C. The eating disturbance does not occur exclusively during the course of anorexia nervosa or bulimia nervosa, and there is no evidence of a disturbance in the way in which one's bodyweight or shape is experienced.

Criterion D. The eating disturbance is not attributable to a concurrent medical condition or not better explained by another mental disorder. When the eating disturbance occurs in the context of another mental disorder, the severity of the eating disturbance exceeds that routinely associated with the condition or disorder and warrants additional clinical attention.

DSM-5 criteria for rumination syndrome [4]

1. Repeated regurgitation of food over a period of at least 1 month. Regurgitated food may be rechewed, reswallowed, or spit out.
2. The repeated regurgitation is not attributable to an associated gastrointestinal or other medical condition.
3. The eating disturbance does not occur exclusively during the course of anorexia nervosa, bulimia nervosa, binge eating disorder, or avoidant/restrictive food intake disorder.
4. If the symptoms occur in the context of another mental disorder (e.g., intellectual disability or another neurodevelopmental disorder), they are sufficiently severe enough to warrant additional clinical attention.

DSM-5 criteria for other specified feeding and eating disorder [4]

This category applies to presentations in which symptoms characteristic of a feeding and eating disorder that cause clinically significant distress or impairment in social, occupational, or other important areas of functioning predominate but do not meet the full criteria for any of the disorders in the feeding and eating disorders diagnostic class. The other specified feeding or eating disorder category is used in situations in which the clinician chooses to communicate the specific reason that the presentation does not meet the criteria for any specific feeding and eating disorder. This is done by recording "other specific eating disorder" followed by the specific reason (e.g., bulimia nervosa of low frequency).

Examples of presentations that can be specified using the "other specified" designation include the following:

1. Atypical anorexia nervosa: All of the criteria for anorexia nervosa are met, expect that despite significant weight loss, the individual's weight is within or above the normal range.
2. Bulimia nervosa (of low frequency and/or limited duration): All of the criteria for bulimia nervosa are met, except that the binge eating and inappropriate compensatory behaviors occur, on average, less than once a week and/or for less than 3 months.
3. Binge eating disorder (of low frequency and/or limited duration): All of the criteria for binge eating disorder are met, except that the binge eating occurs, on average, less than once a week and/or for less than 3 months.
4. Purging disorder: Recurrent purging behavior to influence weight or shape (e.g., self-induced vomiting; misuse of laxatives, diuretics, or other medications) in the absence of binge eating).
5. Night eating syndrome: Recurrent episodes of night eating, as manifested by eating after awakening from sleep or by excessive food consumption after the evening meal. There is awareness and recall of the eating. The night eating is not better explained by external influences, such as changes in the individual's sleep/wake cycle or by local social norms. The night eating causes significant distress and/or impairment in functioning. The disordered pattern of eating is not better explained by binge eating disorder or another mental disorder, including substance use, and is not attributable to another medical disorder or to an effect of medication.

Avoidant/restrictive eating disorder

ARFID is a new classification under DSM-5 describing patients who restrict their dietary intake due to concerns regarding the aversive consequences of eating, and this restriction interferes with nutrition or sufficient energy intake. For diagnostic criteria to be met, one or more of the following features must be present: "significant weight loss, significant nutritional deficiency, dependence on enteral feeding or oral nutritional supplements or marked interference with psychosocial functioning" [4]. In addition, the disturbed eating is not due to an explainable external factor, such as food being unavailable or in short supply, or another physical or mental illness. Finally, the restriction and weight loss must occur in the absence of any weight or shape concerns or distorted body image.

Both AN and ARFID involve prominent symptoms of restrictive eating. The primary distinction between the two disorders is an individual's motivation for restrictive eating. Although those with AN typically endorse weight and shape concerns and fear of weight gain as a primary driver of symptoms, those with ARFID restrict their eating because of concerns that eating will be unpleasant or painful and/or feelings of aversion or disgust around food. Patients with ARFID may endorse an intolerance of textures, taste, or somatic experiences anticipated with eating, such as feelings of fullness, nausea, vomiting, abdominal pain, and the like. Although it is a diagnosis encompassing heterogeneous symptom presentations ranging from extreme picky eating to those with low appetitive drive to others who show concern about potential aversive somatic experiences of eating (e.g., stomach pain, nausea, risk of vomiting), the defining feature is restrictive eating that interferes with physical health and/or functioning. Individuals resembling those with AN are commonly diagnosed with ARFID when they do not endorse fear of weight gain. There is some controversy over whether these patients actually fit better under AN and suggest that ARFID may be a variant or an atypical form of AN and share similar pathophysiology.

Bulimia nervosa

BN was first described as a clinical entity in 1979 [32]. In addition to excessive concern about weight or body shape, which is similar to AN, patients diagnosed with BN also have recurrent episodes of binge eating followed by inappropriate compensatory activities, such as vomiting. There are five criteria for the diagnosis of BN under DSM-5 [4]. The first criterion requires "recurrent episodes of binge eating." It is important to note that binge eating is defined as both eating a quantity of food in a discrete period that would be considered objectively large in the circumstances, as well as experiencing a marked feeling of loss of control during the eating episode. The second criterion, "recurrent compensatory behaviors to prevent weight gain" includes behaviors such as self-induced vomiting, laxative/diuretic/medication abuse, or fasting. The third criterion requires the binge eating and compensatory behaviors to occur, on average at least once per week for 3 months. Finally, the fourth criterion requires "self-evaluation that is unduly influenced by body shape or weight" (see Box 25.1), and the fifth criterion indicates that the disturbance cannot occur exclusively during episodes of anorexia nervosa. In general, binge eating and BN symptoms are characterized by a substantial amount of shame and as such, patients may be prone to underreport or hide the size or frequency of their symptoms. Because fasting behavior is common in BN, and binge/purge behavior can be seen in the AN-binge/purge subtype, there is considerable overlap between these conditions, although patients cannot have both disorders simultaneously. The differentiating feature between AN and BN is the presence of significantly low bodyweight in AN, assessed in the context of age, sex, and developmental trajectory.

Binge eating disorder

BED is defined by DSM-5 as "recurring episodes of eating significantly more food in a short period of time than most people would eat under similar circumstances, with episodes marked by feelings of lack of control." Someone with BED may eat rapidly, even when they are not hungry. "The person may have feelings of guilt, embarrassment, or disgust and may binge eat alone to hide the behavior. This disorder is associated with marked distress and occurs, on average, at least once a week over 3 months" [4]. Although patients with BED may be underweight, normal weight, or overweight [33], many have a distorted body image similar to patients with other eating disorders [34]. BED is associated with shame and significant depression and, as such, is often underreported or minimized by patients.

Although both BN and BED are characterized by the presence of binge eating, it should be noted that both typically have restrictive eating or attempts at restrictive eating as maintenance factors in their cycle of binge eating [35].

Rumination syndrome

Because the primary feature of rumination syndrome involves "the repeated regurgitation of food occurring after feeding or eating over a period of at least 1 month, the condition is frequently seen in gastroenterology settings. Previously swallowed food that may be partially digested is brought up into the mouth without apparent nausea involuntary retching or disgust. The food may be rechewed and then ejected from the mouth or reswallowed" [4]. It may also resemble intractable vomiting. Weight loss is present in a portion of patients, but most patients show normal weight. Using manometry and a gastric barostat, Thumshirn et al. [36] reported a number of abnormalities in 12 patients with rumination disorder, including exaggerated relaxation of lower esophageal sphincter in response to distension of the stomach and greater than normal discomfort with gastric distension. Impaired relaxation of the stomach in response to meals was also found in half of the subjects. Gastroduodenal manometric features of rumination include "an abrupt rise in intragastric pressure (strain) followed by an increase in intraesophageal pressure in all channels (common cavity) and primary or secondary peristalsis" [37]. Such a finding is not universal. When gastroduodenal manometry was performed on 65 children and adolescents diagnosed with rumination syndrome, only 40% had "simultaneous pressure spikes across all sensors" [38]. In another study involving 12 adolescents, simultaneous pressure increased across all sensors suggesting rumination was found in eight patients [39]. However, manometry may be useful in distinguishing rumination disorder from belching and regurgitation. When 16 patients (aged 15–71 years) who were referred for rumination were tested with combined esophageal impedance and manometry, only 50% of the patients had objective findings supporting the clinical diagnosis of rumination. Other patients were diagnosed to have postprandial belching and regurgitation. Habit reversal treatment emphasizing diaphragmatic breathing, an incompatible physiological process with regurgitation, is the standard of care [40].

Could anorexia nervosa, avoidant/restrictive food intake disorder, bulimia nervosa, and binge eating disorder share an underlying pathophysiology?

Although cycles of binge eating and subsequent compensation, such as purging and vomiting, are necessary for the diagnosis of BN, a large subset of patients with AN show regular binge eating and/or purging behavior. In addition, as noted, all eating disorders typically include some sort of attempted dietary restriction or a history of these behaviors [35]. Could there be a common etiology? There is research to suggest that AN and BN represent a continuum of the same underlying process [41]. Notably, 33% of patients will shift from AN to BN in their lifetime [42].

Furthermore, eating disorder diagnostic systems have always included a category/categories for presentations that are more idiosyncratic or meet criteria in between several other diagnoses [4]. In the DSM-4, this was "eating disorder not otherwise specified (EDNOS)," and in DSM-5, two categories were created: "other specified feeding and eating disorder (OSFED)" and "unspecified feeding and eating disorder." The necessity to devise such categories highlights the difficulty that is encountered in drawing a clear distinction between the diagnostic criteria for eating disorders as they pertain to some individuals.

It should be noted that EDNOS and OSFED are actually the most common of any eating disorder with prevalence rates of 11.5% overall and are the diagnoses most often seen in clinical settings [43]. Although the changes reflected in DSM-5 were intended to reduce the prevalence of an "other specified diagnosis," research suggests that the prevalence of OSFED still remains high [44]. Further, these broader categories should not be seen as less serious or severe as AN or BN. In fact, research suggests that OSFED has a higher all-cause mortality rate than AN and BN [45].

Cardinal features of eating disorders associated with dietary restriction

The classifications of eating disorders put forth in the DSM-5 highlight the significant overlap in eating disorders, particularly because all diagnoses may include some degree of restrictive eating behavior. In this chapter, we will discuss both antecedents and consequences of unhealthy dietary restriction, as seen in AN, BN, and BED. Interestingly, although ARFID also is characterized by dietary restriction and weight loss, the fact that this loss is not characterized by weight or shape concerns suggests that these features are likely less relevant for this population.

Distorted body image

Since Bruch described a distorted body image as a core feature in AN [29], debate exists as to the specific nature of this disturbance [46]. Generally, two components have been described as making up this body image dysfunction, namely, a perceptual body size distortion and a cognitive evaluation dissatisfaction [46]. A perceptual distortion is manifested as an abnormality in accurately gauging one's body size. A negative cognitive evaluation encompasses a negative attitude toward one's size and shape. Because many patients with AN deny body image dissatisfaction or distortion, DSM-5 has revised criteria for AN to include a denial of the seriousness of the low weight. That is, on clinical interview, many patients with AN will admit that they are too thin. Yet, they are often indifferent to why their low weight is a problem. Other researchers describe body dissatisfaction as a normative discontent among girls and young women [47] and therefore not a unique feature of an eating disorder. There are also some data to suggest that the experience of body dissatisfaction is magnified by dieting and caloric restriction [48–52], and therefore may be a feature of starvation rather than specific to a psychological condition. Patients with BN and BED often report substantial body image distress as well, and in fact studies suggest body image dissatisfaction is highly correlated with urges to binge eat, particularly in female individuals [53].

Alterations in processing of signals of hunger and satiety

Patients with eating disorders, including ARFID, have reported low levels of hunger and heightened levels of fullness [32]. Although these findings suggest an alteration in how the brain processes signals of hunger and satiety as a contributing cause of their eating disorder, experiments in obese participants suggest the possibility of another explanation [54]. Specifically, after a 3-week, near-fasting diet of only 200 Kcal/day, hunger scores in these obese patients decreased to nearly zero, which argues that prolonged food deprivation leads to physiological loss of the desire to eat [55]. In states of malnutrition, delayed gastric emptying may account for early satiety [56], raising the possibility that loss of hunger and greater satiation may not be unique to patients with an eating disorder.

Observations from prisoners of war after World War II have provided some insight into feelings of satiety during the resumption of eating after prolonged starvation. When these prisoners were refed, they demonstrated lower levels of satiety and dramatically increased rates of food intake, with this increased drive to eat lasting for several weeks [57]. Similarly, in the seminal Minnesota Starvation Experiment, young men put on a severe calorically restricted diet with the goal of having them lose 25% of their bodyweight in 24 weeks developed profound mental health symptoms, including symptoms of an eating disorder [30,58]. In addition, resumption of caloric intake after long-term food deprivation was associated with diminished satiation and binge eating in some instances until the men achieved weight restoration [57,59].

Psychological features and comorbidities of eating disorders

Bruch [60] described a paralyzing feeling of "ineffectiveness" in her patients with AN, creating a sense of helplessness, passivity, and fear of losing control. Many other psychological disturbances have been associated with AN, BN, and BED, including irritability, depression, phobias, inertia, magical thinking, difficulty with concentration, and insomnia [61,62]. The coexistence of depression or dysthymia has been reported in 50–75% of patients [63]. In one series, about two-thirds of patients with an eating disorder had one or more lifetime anxiety disorders, with obsessive–compulsive disorder (OCD) being the most common, affecting 40% of those with AN [64] and 32% of those with BN [65]. An increased risk for substance abuse and personality disorders have also been described [61,66].

It should be noted that although patients with eating disorders almost uniformly present with significant psychiatric comorbidities, such as mood and anxiety symptoms, including, but not limited to, urges to self-harm and suicidality, the majority of these comorbidities are likely to partially or fully resolve after weight restoration and normalization of eating, without any separate psychotherapeutic or medication intervention [67].

Natural history of eating disorders

There are no formal definitions regarding what constitutes recovery from an eating disorder [68]. This adds some ambiguity when comparing data on long-term outcomes. The goals of treatment are generally said to be twofold: weight gain and normalization of eating patterns. It is reported that about half of individuals with AN will recover from their illness, whereas about 30% will demonstrate residual symptoms, which may fluctuate over time, and 10% will demonstrate more severe, persistent, and unrelenting symptoms. The final 10% will eventually die of the complications of their disease [69], with an overall mortality rate of 0.56% per year [70]. Others report rates of sustained remission of only 33% [71]. A longer-term follow-up study of 21 years reported a 16% mortality rate related to disease complications [72]. In younger adolescents with a short history of the disease who are offered evidence-based treatment, the outcomes are considerably more favorable, with full recovery from AN at 60% at long-term follow-up.

For BN specifically, studies suggest that patterns of aberrant eating usually wax and wane over the course of many months to years. Similar to AN, 50% of individuals with bulimia will eventually recover from their illness. Twenty to thirty percent suffer continued, persistent symptoms. An additional 30% who had achieved remission will experience a relapse [73]. Mortality in eating disorders is most commonly associated with complications of severe malnutrition. Accordingly, an important part of treating eating disorders is reversing malnutrition. Data regarding the long-term rates of recovery and relapse for BED and ARFID are relatively scarce and as such, it is still unclear how frequently patients are able to fully recover from these illnesses.

The biology of caloric restriction and disordered eating

Energy expenditure

A fluctuating food supply challenges the homeostasis of all animals. As such, semistarvation is a key stressor (see Chapter 106). What is the expected response to this stress? How does this response compare with the changes seen in AN? Similarities between the biology of malnutrition of the underfed, normal individuals and those with eating disorders have been described [74]. The body's two main physiological adaptations necessary for survival during starvation are providing a continual supply of energy to the brain, in the form of glucose, and conserving the body's protein stores [58,75,76]. The physiological changes described from the starvation associated with AN are analogous to those seen in other noninflammation-induced states of malnutrition and starvation.

The resting energy expenditure (REE) of the body is decreased as lean body mass is reduced during the starvation of AN. This may, at least partly, be influenced by diminished secretion of thyroid hormone. The muscle unit in a patient with AN also expends less energy than normal muscle; there is a decreased efficiency in work performed as a result [77]. After refeeding, undernourished muscle demonstrates a "super efficiency." One study reported that total energy expenditure was similar in those with AN and control subjects, but as REE is reduced in AN, an increased activity-related energy expenditure accounted for the difference [78]. The decreased REE and improved economy of muscle function allows individuals with AN to maintain an increased level of activity with relative conservation of energy.

Role of low blood glucose

The stress of restricted-feeding regimens on rats and the resulting hyperactivity has received significant attention since it was first reported in 1954 [79]. In this original description, the rats demonstrated abnormal behaviors similar to obsessive–compulsive behaviors witnessed in semistarved humans with AN. In these experiments, gastric ulcers were seen as another sign of stress. More recently, Takeda et al. [80] subjected rats to 7 days of a food-restricted diet while allowing for continued access to either water or a glucose solution of varying concentration. Prevention of hypoglycemia with glucose consumption inhibited many of the stress-induced outcomes in the rats. The authors interpreted their results to suggest that hypoglycemia is one of the driving forces for the abnormal behavioral and physical responses in this rat model.

Obsessive behavior and OCD have long been recognized in individuals with AN [63,69]. Diminished food intake, weight loss, and hyperactivity are often elements of OCD, as they are in AN. Elevated cerebrospinal fluid levels of corticotropin-releasing hormone (CRH) and vasopressin are found in patients with AN and patients with OCD, suggesting a common disturbance [81,82]. Based on positron emission tomography scans showing alterations in glucose metabolism in the brains of individuals with OCD [83], abnormally low serum glucose levels may play a role in the pathogenesis of OCD.

Role of hypoleptinemia

As the neuroendocrinology of the body's adaptation to starvation has become better understood, there is increased appreciation of the important role of leptin in this process. When first discovered in 1994 as a secretory product of adipose tissue, leptin was assumed to mediate a negative feedback mechanism to prevent overeating. It suppresses feeding behavior by stimulating expression of anorexigenic proopiomelanocortin in the nucleus of the hypothalamus, while inhibiting the expression of orexigenic neuropeptide Y (NPY) and agouti-related peptide in hypothalamic neurons. The original studies showed that leptin-deficient mice were subject to overeating and obesity [82]. Subsequent studies in humans failed to confirm an association between leptin concentrations in serum and human obesity [84]. Our understanding of leptin has since evolved, and it is now appreciated to be an important mediator of biological changes that occur during starvation [84–86].

Leptin is the protein product of the *OB* gene and is produced primarily by white adipose tissue and to some degree in the stomach, placenta, and mammary glands [86,87]. Plasma concentrations generally correlate with the amount of adipose tissue in the body and, thus, are generally higher in obese individuals [84]. In contrast with obesity, which is recognized as a high-leptin state, periods of starvation are associated with low levels of leptin. Leptin levels decrease dramatically after only 2–3 days of restricted nutritional intake [87,88]. In low-body-weight patients with AN, plasma and cerebrospinal fluid leptin concentration are low and well correlated with the body fat mass [89,90]. Hypoleptinemia below a cutoff value of 2 μg/L has been proposed as a laboratory diagnostic test for AN [91]. As leptin acts through OB receptors in the brain and elsewhere, hypoleptinemia is accompanied by upregulated expression of these receptors, as demonstrated by elevated circulating concentrations of OB receptors [92,93]. Increased severity of depression is correlated with decreased plasma concentration of leptin in women with AN [94]. A low leptin level signals a state of low-energy availability to the hypothalamus and the hormonal pathways it controls [85,88]. The body attempts to shift from a state of energy use to one of energy conservation. As part of this shift, levels of thyroid and reproductive hormones decline, accounting for the amenorrhea commonly seen in women with AN. Studies of healthy men who fasted for as little as 2–5 days reported reduced serum luteinizing hormone and testosterone concentrations [95,96]. The role of leptin in hormonal feedback control was demonstrated when exogenously administered recombinant leptin (r-metHuLeptin) prevented the decline in luteinizing hormone and testosterone levels seen with fasting [88]. In contrast with the decrease in sex hormone concentrations, stress hormone levels increase as part of an attempt to mobilize energy stores. Growth hormone (GH) levels also increase, but without an accompanying increase in insulin-like growth factor-1 (IGF-1). During starvation, GH can induce lipolysis, which allows the body to use some of its alternative energy reserves. Because IGF-1 levels remain low, the body's energy-consuming, growth-related pathways are not stimulated [88]. As a whole, the body is diverting energy to pathways most critical for survival.

Intense exercise is associated with amenorrhea in female athletes [97]. These athletes create a relative energy deficit by a combination of their high physical activity level and inadequate nutritional intake. This energy imbalance results in a hypothalamic amenorrhea similar to AN. Leptin has been implicated as a regulatory agent in this pathway. These athletes have a low-leptin state, as is the case in the semistarved state of an eating disorder, which results in lower levels of sex hormones, thyroid hormones, and IGF-1, but increased secretion of cortisol and GH [98–100]. Correspondingly, hyperactivity in women with AN is correlated with a low plasma concentration of leptin [89]. A relationship between hypoleptinemia in hyperactivity and impulsivity has been shown in other studies in rats and humans [101,102]. A mechanistic role for low leptin in AN was suggested when intracerebroventricular administration of leptin suppressed the hyperactivity associated with a semistarvation state in rats [103]. This inhibitory effect on hyperactivity was shown in rats to be dependent on leptin acting on the ventral tegmental area of the brain via stimulation to the mesolimbic award system [104].

Leptin secretion increases with the resumption of eating after a prolonged fast [88]. This enhanced secretion plays a role in limiting food intake and arresting weight gain to avert obesity as the undesirable outcome of overcorrection after a period of caloric deprivation. Because of this action, it was suggested that leptin might also be responsible, in some, for a relapse of AN [105].

Role of adiponectin

In addition to leptin, adipose tissue secretes a number of other biologically active proteins. Because of structural similarities to cytokines, these are sometimes referred to as adipocytokines, or just adipokine. Adiponectin is one such protein and is involved in regulating energy hemostasis and glucose and lipid metabolism [106]. Plasma concentration of adiponectin is lower in obese individuals [107], and weight reduction increases the plasma concentration of adiponectin in obese rats and humans [108,109]. Several studies have reported elevated plasma adiponectin in AN [106,110,111]; however, there are conflicting data regarding plasma adiponectin concentrations in AN. Lower adiponectin has also been reported in AN and BN compared with normal-weight control subjects, regardless of BMI [106]. Because adiponectin levels were restored with weight gain in the anorexic group, variable feeding behavior may account for the discrepancy in adiponectin levels in eating disorders. In addition, measuring isoforms of adiponectin rather than just total adiponectin may affect the result, because the percentage of high-molecular-weight to total adiponectin was low in patients with AN, but the percentage of low-molecular-weight to total adiponectin was high in this group when compared with control subjects [112]. Interestingly, patients who have AN with binge or purging behavior had higher serum adiponectin concentration than other patients with AN, suggesting a role of this peptide in determining specific disordered eating behavior [113]. A complex interplay of low leptin and high adiponectin exists in AN, mediating insulin sensitivity, neuroendocrine abnormalities, and osteopenia [114]. Adiponectin remains under investigation as a possible marker of weight restoration [115].

Role of elevated neuropeptide Y

The body strives for homeostasis with regard to its weight by either stimulating or suppressing the drive to eat via changes in the signals from the gut and energy stores [116]. These mechanisms do not function in this manner in AN. AN is a condition of starvation, yet these individuals are not intrinsically stimulated to eat. Some have suggested that actions of the various orexigenic and anorexigenic peptides are more complex than initially appreciated and may be partially dependent on the physiological context [117].

NPY is one of the peptides that has been best established to have orexigenic (stimulating food intake) effects. High leptin levels reduce the production of NPY by the hypothalamus, which would be the expected result from the hyperleptinemia of obesity [118]. Yet, this does not lead to less eating for many of these individuals. The classic theory of bodyweight regulation asserts that external signals are processed by hypothalamic centers, which then adjusts food intake, whereas reduced leptin levels induce an upregulation of orexigenic peptides, including NPY, resulting in increased nutritional intake [119–121]. In AN, however, these changes do not stimulate eating [118,122]. Additional biological actions of NPY, yet to be defined, may explain why higher levels of an orexigenic peptide may not be associated with stimulatory food intake.

This insight is derived primarily from animal data. Food deprivation increases the level of NPY mRNA in the hypothalamic arcuate nucleus of female rats. The most striking characteristic of these rats was that they engaged in progressively more running as food deprivation continued. Rats on a calorie-restricted diet that are provided an exercise wheel lost more weight than animals without access to an exercise wheel [123]. Administration of an NPY Y1 receptor antagonist to rats blunted the effect that food deprivation had on stimulating wheel running, demonstrating the role of NPY in the hyperactivity response [124]. Correspondingly, increased physical activity was reproduced with intracerebroventricular administration of NPY to these rats without stimulating increased food intake. Interestingly, in food-deprived rats that did not have access to an exercise wheel but did have continual access to food, exogenous NPY stimulated food intake [123]. These results are consistent with Morley's suggestion, in 1987, that NPY may have a stimulatory effect on behavior [125]. These findings in experimental animals, whereby NPY, an orexigenic peptide, paradoxically decreases food intake in the setting of stimulating physical activity, fit into a model of a complex interplay of behavioral, physiological, and biochemical adaptations to starvation in humans [126].

NPY has been implicated in food-anticipatory activities, including hoarding behavior [127,128]. Evolutionarily, such anticipatory behavior has been explained as a logical precursor to the impending search for food. Patients with AN have been reported as engaging in similar anticipatory behavior [129].

Role of reduced sensitivity to ghrelin

Ghrelin, a potent orexigenic peptide, is normally secreted by the stomach before meals. Ghrelin is also an endogenous ligand for the GH receptor. This peptide drives food intake by stimulating the orexigenic hypothalamic nuclei to release NPY and agouti-related peptide while inhibiting the anorexigenic hypothalamic proopiomelanocortin nucleus to suppress the release of α-melanocyte stimulating hormone. Because the plasma concentration of ghrelin is inversely proportional to the bodyweight, abnormally thin patients with an eating disorder have elevated plasma ghrelin [130]. Plasma concentration of ghrelin is higher in patients with AN when compared with constitutionally thin women who have normal eating behavior. An abnormal response to ghrelin in AN was demonstrated when intravenous administration of this orexigenic to patients with AN associated with very low bodyweight failed to stimulate appetite [131]. Depending on dietary composition, insulin is released after ingestion of food. In an experiment using a euglycemic hyperinsulinemic clamp in women with AN, elevating the insulin concentration led to an exaggerated inhibition of serum ghrelin [132]. This finding points to a mechanism for excessive suppression of appetite or greater signaling of satiety in AN.

The body's response to starvation: neuropsychiatric and physical manifestations of eating disorders

Eating disorders manifest with a range of serious neuropsychiatric and medical symptoms, which typically result directly from the malnutrition associated with food deprivation and indirectly from metabolic derangements following purging behaviors common to these patients [133]. The medical complications of eating disorders are generally identical to those reported in healthy individuals placed on a semistarvation diet, with changes affecting nearly every organ system [1,2] (Boxes 25.2 and 25.3). In the following section, we will highlight typical neuropsychiatric manifestations of eating disorders, as well as changes seen across nearly every body system, specifically highlighting GI, cardiac, and endocrine manifestations. This section also includes more detailed lists of common medical manifestations (see Box 25.3) and laboratory abnormalities (see Box 25.2).

Neuropsychiatric manifestations

Irritability, impulsivity, obsession, and mood changes

In the face of caloric restriction, independent of the inciting cause, individuals experience many of the cognitions and preoccupations characteristic of eating disorders, including a preoccupation with food, irritability, and impulsivity. This heightened sensitivity to risk is thought to be an evolutionary adaptation to resource scarcity. As a self-protective mechanism, impulsive behavior may convey an advantage, as the appropriate adaption to scarcity of food [134].

Box 25.2 Laboratory abnormalities seen in eating disorders.

Disorders characterized by dietary restriction and weight loss (e.g., AN and ARFID)

Hypokalemia, hyponatremia, metabolic alkalosis
Metabolic acidosis
Hypoglycemia
Mildly increased creatinine
Anemia, thrombocytopenia
Mild leukopenia
Low erythrocyte sedimentation rate
Mildly increased hepatic aminotransferases
Mildly increased serum proteins
Hypercholesterolemia
Low alkaline phosphatase
Decreased TSH, T_3, and T_4
Decreased FSH, LH, and prolactin
Elevated cortisol
Low magnesium, phosphorus, and zinc levels
Carotenemia

Disorders characterized by binge eating and purging (e.g., BN and BED)

Hypokalemia, hyponatremia, hypochloremic alkalosis
Metabolic acidosis
Hypoglycemia
Azotemia
Elevated cortisol
Increased prolactin
Low magnesium

AN, anorexia nervosa; ARFID, avoidant/restrictive food intake disorder; BED, binge eating disorder; BN, bulimia nervosa; FSH, follicle-stimulating hormone; LH, luteinizing hormone; T_3, triiodothyronine; T_4, thyroxine; TSH, thyroid-stimulating hormone.

Box 25.3 Medical complications of eating disorders.

Disorders characterized by dietary restriction and weight loss (e.g., AN, ARFID)

Neurological

- Depression
- Sleep disorders
- Decreased attention and concentration
- Diminished learning and problem-solving
- Decreased short-term memory
- Labile moods

Cardiovascular

- Cardiac arrhythmias
- Sudden death
- Bradycardia
- Hypotension
- Mitral valve prolapse
- Left ventricular dysfunction

Pulmonary

- Aspiration pneumonia
- Ventilatory failure

(*Continued*)

Gastrointestinal
- Impaired gastric emptying/early satiety
- Postprandial bloating
- Constipation
- Decreased motility
- Hypogeusia
- Abdominal pain
- Pancreatitis
- Peptic ulcer disease
- Superior mesenteric artery syndrome

Renal
- Prerenal azotemia
- Mesangial sclerosis
- Nephrolithiasis

Endocrine
- Amenorrhea
- Decreased libido
- Osteopenia and pathological fractures
- Impaired functioning of the hypothalamic–pituitary–adrenal axis
- Diabetes insipidus
- Hypothermia
- Increased growth hormone accompanying low levels of IGF-1
- Decreased insulin production

Metabolic
- Decreased metabolic rate
- Increased β-hydroxybutyrate

Immunological
- Decreased cell-mediated immunity
- Granulocyte dysfunction
- Decreased serum complement
- Altered cytokine levels

Musculoskeletal
- Decreased muscle mass and weakness
- Proximal myopathy

Dermatological
- Lanugo hair
- Brittle nails
- Pruritus
- Acrocyanosis

Disorders characterized by binge eating and purging (e.g., BN, BED)

Neurological
- Seizures (diet pill toxicity)
- Neuromyopathy (ipecac toxicity)
- Depression

Cardiovascular
- Arrhythmias
- Hypotension
- Mitral valve prolapse
- Palpitations

Pulmonary
- Aspiration pneumonia
- Pneumomediastinum

Gastrointestinal
- Constipation
- Cathartic colon
- Dysphagia
- Esophagitis
- Esophageal ulcer, stricture
- Mallory–Weiss tear
- Abdominal pain/dyspepsia
- Gastroparesis
- Pancreatitis
- Gastric rupture

Renal
- Pseudo–Bartter syndrome
- Hematuria
- Proteinuria
- Azotemia

Endocrine
- Amenorrhea or irregular menses
- Absence of follicular development
- Luteal phase dysfunction
- Increased rates of birth complications and miscarriages

Oral/dental
- Caries
- Perimolysis – lingual and occlusal surfaces
- Cheilosis
- Pharyngeal soreness
- Sialadenosis
- Salivary hyperamylasemia

Dermatological
- Russell sign (i.e., calluses over fingers)

AN, anorexia nervosa; ARFID, avoidant/restrictive food intake disorder; BED, binge eating disorder; BN, bulimia nervosa; IGF-1, insulin-like growth factor-1.

Keys et al. [30] published one of the sentinel works examining the effects of starvation in humans. The study enrolled 36 male conscientious objectors to significant caloric deprivation (40% of normal intake) for an average of 168 days. These individuals were normal weight at baseline and young (range 20–33 years), with the subjects losing 24% of their baseline bodyweight down to an average BMI of 17.5 kg/m^2. The effects of prolonged semistarvation were recorded in detail. This landmark study demonstrated this pattern of markedly altered behavior in previously healthy young adult participants, who experienced hyperirritability, impulsive behavior, and violent ideations with progressing weight loss on a semistarvation diet [30,41].

Keys et al. [30] also reported depression in his semistarved subjects, and during their refeeding there was a linear relationship between resolving malnutrition and improved feelings of depression. Södersten et al. [41] explain that an "obsession" with food would make sense during a period of significant food deprivation. With ongoing starvation, a preoccupation with food would prompt the individual to devote more time to searching for food. Södersten et al. [41] have posed the question, might obsessive thinking in an eating disorder represent an understandable adaptation to food deprivation rather than indicate a true psychiatric illness?

Anxiety

The presence of anxiety in those with eating disorders is also well described. A fear of becoming fat is listed as a key diagnostic criterion in DSM-5 [4]. Can the anxiety in AN be explained as a correlate of a fear of becoming fat? Södersten et al. [41] propose that the cognitive recognition of an obsession with food, which arises with extreme fasting, may transform into a fear of acting on this obsession, in which case obesity becomes the undesirable outcome to avoid. The desire to avoid an aversive outcome, like becoming fat, can become reinforced with the continual preoccupation with food seen in eating disorders, and this ever-present desire becomes very anxiety provoking. Although anxious individuals may be more likely to experience development of an eating disorder, numerous studies have shown that malnutrition alone may trigger symptoms of anxiety, even among those without a prior history. Although anxious individuals may be more likely to develop an eating disorder, numerous studies have shown that malnutrition alone may trigger symptoms of anxiety, even among those without a prior history.

Hyperactivity

Remarkably, despite weight loss and food deprivation, patients with eating disorders often exhibit exaggerated levels of activity [58,135]. During their caloric restriction, Keys et al.'s [30] participants were reported to have increased levels of hyperactivity, among the other symptoms described previously. An increase in physical activity has been observed in several different animal models as a response to food deprivation [136]. For instance, the imposition of food restriction on rats leads to a similar pattern of increased activity. When an exercise wheel is available, rats deprived of food will use the wheel to the point of markedly accelerating weight loss. From an evolutionary perspective, this would be an advantageous response in the face of a food shortage, but in the setting of eating disorders, this is quite maladaptive and may explain the hyperactivity and urge to exercise common to individuals with eating disorders.

Gastrointestinal symptoms

Abnormal gastric functions, dyspepsia, constipation, hepatitis, and hypogeusia are among the common digestive tract manifestations of eating disorders [137–139].

Abnormal gastric functions

Numerous studies have documented a delay in gastric emptying in association with eating disorders [138,140–142], which seems to worsen with increasing malnutrition. A lack of food in the stomach [142], gastric smooth muscle atrophy caused by protein malnutrition [136], the presence of gastric dysrhythmias [140], and the rectal distention seen with constipation reflexively inhibiting gastric emptying [143] have all been implicated as potential underlying mechanisms causing the delayed gastric emptying in AN. Although delayed gastric emptying is associated with symptoms of bloating, early satiety, and abdominal distention, the severity of symptoms do not correlate with the degree of physiological abnormality [144]. These symptoms may prove to be an impediment to refeeding and weight gain, because eating may increase physical discomfort and exacerbate bloating and distention, reinforcing a perception of feeling "fat" [145]. Several studies support an association of delayed gastric emptying with BN [146,147], whereas others do not [6,142,148]. Geliebter et al. [146] reported that patients with BN require a larger volume of gastric balloon distention to produce a feeling of fullness. Proposed explanations for this include abnormalities in gastric relaxation and diminished release of the anorexigenic signal cholecystokinin [149–151]. It is also unclear how to best manage gastroparesis in the setting of eating disorders. The data are somewhat conflicting as to whether weight gain improves the delay in gastric emptying. Some studies demonstrated improvement after weight gain [152–154] and others did not [140,142]. There are even fewer studies examining the role of medications, such as metoclopramide or motility agents, in the treatment of gastroparesis in the setting of eating disorders [149].

Dyspepsia

Patients with eating disorders commonly report upper abdominal discomfort. Although it is sometimes attributed to gastroesophageal reflux, endoscopic findings suggest similar rates of gastroesophageal reflux between those with eating disorders and the general population. It is also unclear whether medications, such as proton pump inhibitors, are beneficial in the setting of eating disorders [155,156]. Pancreatitis occasionally occurs in the setting of eating disorders and can manifest with upper abdominal pain.

Constipation

Constipation is a common problem encountered in anorexia, which is at least partially due to diminished oral intake. Patients often report associated bloating and abdominal distention [143,145]. Constipation may also be related to chronic stimulant laxative use in some patients. Whole-gut transit times were found to be delayed in patients with AN and BN compared with control subjects when using a radiopaque-marker technique [143]. An association with abnormalities in anal canal resting pressure and rectal sensation suggestive of pelvic floor dysfunction has been suggested by some studies [157], but not by others [158]. The delayed colonic transit times did improve with refeeding.

Hepatitis

Liver dysfunction, manifested by transaminitis and abnormal liver function tests, is common in AN. Although the mechanism for starvation-related liver cell injury and death is unclear, some have proposed that it is related to autophagy among those with severe AN. Among hospitalized patients with severe AN, elevation in alanine aminotransferase was the most common abnormal liver test, followed by aspartate transaminase [159]. Elevations in bilirubin and international normalized ratio were less common. Importantly, in this study, patients with elevated liver enzymes were at significantly higher risk for hypoglycemia. In addition, hepatitis can occur in the setting of refeeding, but by a different proposed physiological mechanism. Refeeding hepatitis is characterized by hepatic fat deposition, resulting in steatosis on sonographic imaging [155,159].

Hypogeusia

Hypogeusia, or decreased taste acuity, has been described for both those with AN and those with BN. A reduced sensitivity to sweet, salty, sour, and bitter flavors was demonstrated in individuals with AN [156]. Another study of individuals who specifically used vomiting as their primary means of purging also demonstrated a similar loss of sensation on the tongue [160]. In conjunction with hypogeusia, most of these individuals demonstrated low serum levels of zinc, copper, and triiodothyronine (T_3 hormone), which all have been implicated as influencing taste [156]. In those patients who repeatedly purge by vomiting, the surfaces in the mouth endure frequent exposure to the acidity of the gastric contents. Often, there is also a loss of dental enamel [161,162], with an increased rate of caries formation and increased sensitivity to hot, cold, and acidic foods [163,164].

Electrolyte abnormalities and refeeding syndrome

Electrolyte abnormalities, including hypokalemia, hypophosphatemia, hypomagnesemia, and acid/base disturbances, are commonly associated with eating disorders, particularly in the setting of severe malnutrition and in cases involving bingeing and purging. Refeeding syndrome, a well-documented and feared complication of nutritional rehabilitation and weight restoration, is associated with rapid shifts in fluids and electrolytes, associated with significant mortality. In brief, when a malnourished person is refed, there are intracellular shifts in potassium and phosphorus, resulting in decreased serum concentrations of these electrolytes, which places the patient at high risk for cardiac arrhythmias and other complications related to electrolyte depletion [155]. Although additional research is needed regarding risk factors for refeeding syndrome among patients with eating disorders, hypokalemia and low serum prealbumin are associated with increased risk [165].

Hyponatremia is also commonly seen in patients with eating disorders. The causes are likely to be multifactorial, and the type of hyponatremia (e.g., hypotonic vs hypertonic) may depend on the specific implicated eating disorder behaviors. The optimal management in the setting of eating disorders remains unclear. Rapidly correcting hyponatremia can lead to potential serious neurological complications, warranting slow correction and close monitoring of those with severe hyponatremia [165].

Cardiovascular complications and the risk for sudden death

Patients with eating disorders are known to be at high risk for sudden death [155]. Although the etiology for sudden death is not entirely clear, it is suspected that it is at least in part related to cardiac changes in the setting of malnutrition. These include documented changes in cardiac structure, autonomic dysregulation, and arrhythmias. In particular, prolongation of the QT interval, likely related in part to common electrolyte abnormalities, is a known marker for certain arrhythmias and sudden cardiac death [166]. Several studies have linked AN, a prolonged QT interval [167–170], and an increased risk for ventricular arrhythmias [169]. Cardiac imaging studies have also revealed pathological ventricular remodeling suggesting that myocardial fibrosis, documented in autopsies of people with AN, could be a source of ventricular arrhythmias [155]. It is important to note that the literature has also suggested that hypoglycemia may contribute to the increased risk for sudden death among young people with eating disorders as well and, as such, glucose should be monitored closely during treatment [155].

Bradycardia and hypotension are common in young people with eating disorders. One series showed that 100% of patients with AN had a sinus bradycardia with heart rate less than 60 beats/min compared with control subjects [155]. Several mechanisms for this have been proposed, including vagal hyperactivity of starvation [155,167,171–173] and reduced secretion of T_3 hormone [167]. Other influencing factors may include electrolyte abnormalities, decrease in myocardial glycogen stores, and myocardial cell atrophy [170].

Endocrine complications

Strong evidence exists of an association of AN with reduced bone mineral density in female adolescents and adults [174–177]. Although the degree of estrogen deficiency may be similar in AN and other causes of hypothalamic amenorrhea, individuals with AN have a much greater reduction in bone density, arguing for other contributory factors [178], such as malnutrition, low levels of IGF-1, acquired resistance to GH, excessive exercise, and hypercortisolemia [176]. In healthy subjects, GH is secreted by the pituitary and is nutritionally regulated. GH then stimulates the liver to secrete IGF-1, which is an identified bone trophic factor. IGF-1 levels are normally low during starvation. They decline to half during a 5-day fast [179]. In AN, resistance to GH exists, so IGF-1 levels remain low despite elevated levels of GH.

The hormonal changes that are observed in AN are best understood as an adaption to malnutrition and starvation rather than a manifestation of a primary endocrinopathy. Although amenorrhea is no longer included in the diagnostic criteria for

AN, it is a common manifestation of malnutrition during eating disorders due to an alteration in the normal hypothalamic–pituitary–ovarian axis. In the setting of a significant energy deficit, normal secretion of gonadotropin-releasing hormone from the hypothalamus is impaired, resulting in altered secretion of luteinizing hormone and follicle-stimulating hormone from the pituitary and low estradiol secretion from the gonads [180]. This amenorrhea without evidence of ovarian malfunction is termed hypothalamic amenorrhea. Both males and females may also manifest a diminished libido [181,182]. The body is attempting to divert energy from the reproduction pathway, which is not critical for survival in the face of starvation.

The hypothalamic dysfunction of AN also disrupts the hypothalamic–pituitary–thyroid axis through a similar mechanism to hypothalamic amenorrhea. In the setting of malnutrition, TSH levels may be low, with correspondingly low T_4 and T_3. This malnutrition-related hypothyroidism may contribute to lower body temperature, lethargy, dry skin, constipation, and bradycardia. This illness does not require thyroid hormone replacement, which can potentially be harmful because of the risk for additional weight loss and the abuse potential of thyroid hormone in patients with eating disorders. These thyroid abnormalities typically improve with weight restoration [183,184].

Feeding is one of the chief regulators of the daily rhythms of the HPA axis, mediating secretion of plasma corticosteroids [49]. Persistently elevated serum cortisol levels are commonly seen in patients with AN with an abolition of the normal, daily circadian rhythm observed in healthy individuals. Hypercortisolemia may be related to chronic malnutrition and could also be required for the maintenance of euglycemia [175,184]. There is blunting of the response of adrenocorticotropic hormone (ACTH) and cortisol to CRH [185,186]. In highlighting many of the clinical similarities between AN and depression, CRH hypersecretion is proposed as a common pathogenic mechanism in both AN and depression [186]. Notably, CRH is anorexigenic and could exacerbate weight loss [184,187]. Most of the disturbances may be secondary to malnutrition [184,187].

Abnormalities in the HPA axis and cortisol secretion have also been reported in BN, including an elevated 24-hour cortisol level, diminished CRH effect on ACTH and cortisol secretion [188], and a blunting of normal dexamethasone suppression of cortisol [189]. Because patients with BN are normal in weight, the changes appear to be independent of BMI. However, these changes do largely reverse with increased nutritional intake.

Psychological treatment of eating disorders

When evaluating treatment strategies for AN, the primary outcome goal is weight gain. Thus, treatment of eating disorders begins with appropriate nutritional assessment and treatment of identified malnutrition with the goal of nutritional repletion and weight restoration. Weight, eating, and nutritional improvement have been shown to have benefit on psychological features (e.g., body dissatisfaction), decreased pathological activity (e.g., overexercising), and resumption of menses. In addition, as noted earlier, weight restoration and normalization of eating have also been shown to have substantial benefits on comorbid mood and anxiety symptoms [67]. In the subgroup that engages in binging and purging, normalization of eating is an initial goal of treatment to reduce binge eating and purging.

Many forms of behavioral interventions have been tried for AN in adults, including cognitive, dynamic, family, individual, and group therapy. Although one study suggested that cognitive behavioral therapy (CBT) reduced the rate of relapse and led to improved outcomes in those who had already achieved inpatient weight gain [190], its efficacy in the more acute setting of the still-underweight patient with AN is less clear [191]. In general, individual therapy in the absence of weight restoration has not been shown to be effective for underweight patients.

For adolescents with AN, the first-line treatment is an outpatient psychological intervention, family-based treatment (FBT) [192–198]. FBT, sometimes known as the Maudsley approach, has been evaluated in eight randomized controlled trials (RCTs) for adolescent AN and has been found to be associated with approximately 40–50% of patients reaching full remission [192,193,195–198]. The treatment is a three-stage intervention in which the first phase focuses entirely on empowering parents or caregivers to prepare and monitor all meals, comparable with nursing staff on an inpatient unit. The primary goal is weight restoration, after which point phase II includes transitioning developmentally appropriate control over eating back to the patient. Phase III focuses on normative adolescent development and relapse prevention. In contrast with previous adolescent-focused individual therapies for eating disorders that required longer hospital stays and frequently blamed families, FBT takes a blame-free, agnostic approach that emphasizes the neurobiological basis of eating disorders and empowers families to support their children and adolescents to heal. FBT uses language that externalizes the eating disorder from the patient and intentionally medicalizes the disorder, highlighting the seriousness of malnutrition. Pediatric patients who do not respond to FBT often require a more intensive level of care, such as inpatient or day hospital treatment. The focus of these treatments is nutritional restoration and establishing preliminary weight gain. Although data from these programs is inconsistent, there are promising findings from both intensive outpatient and residential programs that incorporate elements of FBT programming [199].

For BN, adults have several evidence-based treatment options, including outpatient therapies such as individual, group, and self-help forms of CBT [200,201], enhanced CBT [202], and integrative cognitive affective therapy [203]. Individual, group, and self-help CBT have also been shown to be effective for adults with BED [53,204]. All are associated with significant improvement in binge eating and purging behavior, as well as psychological functioning. For adolescents with BN, both CBT and FBT for BN have been shown to reduce binge eating and purging behaviors [195]. Dialectical behavior therapy has also been shown to have preliminary effectiveness in treating adolescents with BN or BED [205].

Given that ARFID is a newer diagnosis, evidence-based treatments are largely in development [206], although there are some promising programs that combine elements of psychology, occupational therapy, and physical therapy to address the complex issues patients sometimes have with aspects of the disorder, such as disgust around food texture, issues swallowing, and complex family dynamics that inadvertently maintain avoidant eating behaviors. Modifications of CBT that include elements of exposure therapy for food phobias, vomit phobias, and other eating aversions driven by anxiety are also promising [206,207]. Given that ARFID tends to present earlier, in younger children, the majority of these interventions are pediatric focused and include family components as well.

Psychiatric and hormonal treatments of AN

In contrast with other psychiatric disorders, combining CBT with pharmacotherapy does not improve treatment effectiveness for AN [208]. Although selective serotonin reuptake inhibitors (SSRIs) are commonly used in the treatment of AN, RCT data do not support their efficacy for improving core symptoms of AN. In an RCT of hospitalized women with AN, there was no difference in weight gain, depression, or anxiety measures with fluoxetine treatment [209]. Another RCT did not show a noticeable difference in eating, psychological, or other biological markers at follow-up in a cohort that was randomized to fluoxetine or placebo treatment just before discharge, following hospitalization [210]. There was a notable overall dropout rate at 52 weeks of follow-up, indicating a failure to sustain a remission on placebo and on fluoxetine. An additional case–control study also suggested no difference in readmission rates after initiation of an SSRI [69]. A 2006 Cochrane Systematic Review of four placebo-controlled trials showed no benefit of antidepressants for the treatment of AN, which was later corroborated by a 2014 metaanalysis [211,212]. As such, the American Psychiatric Association does not endorse the use of SSRIs in the treatment of underweight patients with AN [213].

Based on its significant weight gain side-effect profile, together with perceived benefit to address the distorted thinking characteristic of AN, antipsychotic medications such as olanzapine and risperidone have been trialed for use in AN. In spite of this, a metaanalysis of existing RCTs suggested no benefit for improving BMI or core symptoms of AN [214].

In terms of hormonal management in the prevention of bone loss in AN, several treatments have been considered. A metaanalysis of estrogen preparations, such as oral contraceptives, in AN suggest that they had a mild-to-moderate effect on bone density. However, because studies were considered of small sample size and low quality, recommendations for their use in preventing bone loss could not be made. An RCT of physiological estrogen in adolescent girls suggests that bone mineral density scores in the spine and hip increased in the estrogen group compared with the placebo group even after controlling for baseline age and weight, suggesting that physiological estradiol replacement may be beneficial in preventing bone loss. However, because a regular menstrual cycle is an important sign of adequate weight restoration, full nutritional and weight restoration to mitigate bone loss is recommended before consideration of hormonal management, particularly for those with an early onset and good chance of full recovery [215].

Psychiatric treatment of BN and BED

There have been several randomized placebo-controlled studies demonstrating the efficacy of fluoxetine to treat BN [216,217]. One large study of women with BN randomized patients to either 60 mg fluoxetine, 20 mg fluoxetine, or a placebo [217]. The higher dose of fluoxetine reduced binge eating episodes by 67%, whereas the placebo and the lower dose did not result in a reduction in binge eating. Similar findings were demonstrated by a longer-term study comparing 60 mg with a placebo, suggesting that fluoxetine was significantly more effective for treating BN than placebo. These results suggest that high-dose fluoxetine may be an effective adjunct treatment for BN [216]. A 2003 Cochrane Systematic Review of 19 placebo-controlled trials of antidepressants further support the effectiveness of antidepressants in the treatment of BN [218]. There have also been several controlled trials of SSRIs for the treatment of BED, revealing reductions in binge eating episodes, decreased BMI, and clinical improvements associated with treatment, which was enhanced in combination with CBT [219].

In 2015, the US Food and Drug Administration approved lisdexamfetamine dimesylate as the only medication available for the treatment of moderate-to-severe BED. Efficacy for this medication was based on two studies [220,221]. In the first trial, patients randomized to 50 and 70 mg/day lisdexamfetamine dimesylate achieved a significant reduction compared with placebo. Those receiving a lower dose (30 mg/day) were not significantly different from a placebo. The second trial randomized patients to receive placebo or lisdexamfetamine (50 or 70 mg/day based on their tolerability during 3-week dose optimization period). At 12 weeks, lisdexamfetamine resulted in a significant mean reduction in binge eating from baseline and compared with placebo. Another study found the relapse rate was significantly lower for lisdexamfetamine (3.7%) than for placebo.

In spite of these findings supporting the effectiveness of lisdexamfetamine in reducing binge eating episodes, the outcomes must be weighed against the side-effect profile. In trials to obtain US Food and Drug Administration approval, serious adverse events leading to discontinuation ranged from 3% to 9% of patients [220–222]. Dry mouth, decreased appetite, insomnia, headache, and anxiety were the most common adverse effects of the medication. Notably, one study found there were electrocardiogram changes from baseline to 52 weeks in 98.1% of participants. As such, before considering this medication, an adequate trial of CBT should be considered [222].

Considerations for the gastroenterologist

Given that gastroenterology patients frequently struggle with symptoms such as abdominal pain, bloating, nausea, vomiting, constipation, loss of appetite, and early satiety, eating can become aversive and challenging. Side-effects from medications can also affect eating and weight. In some cases, medications suppress appetite and weight, and in others, weight gain side-effects can often be a precipitant of intentional dietary restriction and weight loss. Not surprisingly, in a gastroenterology population, restrictive eating and weight loss is common [223–225]. Unfortunately, acute and chronic effects of semistarvation may exacerbate GI distress and worsen preexisting GI disorders [226]. In addition, starvation-related changes to the brain can set the stage for depression and other psychiatric concerns, as well as difficulties with fatigue, concentration, and cognition.

In addition to the exacerbation of physical and psychological symptoms, as noted earlier, restrictive eating and weight loss can lead to the development of an eating disorder. In this vicious cycle, some GI patients have been observed to "back into" an eating disorder such as AN or BN through the effects of starvation caused by pain-related restrictive eating and weight loss [225]. For many patients, restrictive eating was not initially motivated by weight or shape concerns. Instead, these concerns developed through the effects of starvation on the central nervous system.

Besides the risk for the development of AN or BN, many of the eating-related challenges that these patients display meet criteria for ARFID, particularly if a medical cause for the restrictive eating and weight loss has not been identified. Even if a medical cause explains why eating might be difficult, if the disordered eating is greater than what would be expected based on what most individuals with the condition would demonstrate, then it may be classified as ARFID. For example, a patient with irritable bowel syndrome may be diagnosed with the condition if they do not eat all day because of fears of having to go to the bathroom and this restriction is causing impairments in functioning and/or nutritional status.

Not surprisingly, studies suggest that the prevalence rate of disordered eating and eating disorders in gastroenterology patients is high, ranging from 5.3% to 44.4% [224]. In addition, studies that use food diary assessment found that compared with healthy control individuals, patients with GI disease have significantly lower caloric intake and evidence of malnutrition [227,228]. In spite of the high prevalence of eating-related concerns, there has been a lack of research attention on the screening and treatment of this population.

Identifying eating disorders in patients with gastrointestinal symptoms

Although identifying eating disorders is already difficult, screening for eating disorders within the gastroenterology population represents an even greater challenge. In many cases, abdominal pain and GI symptoms can mask an eating disorder. That is, abdominal pain and symptoms may be seen by patients, family members, and providers as an acceptable excuse for dietary restriction and weight loss. In fact, a study of adolescents with eating disorders and comorbid chronic pain and symptoms found that more than a third of patients had developed their eating disorder before their pain. Although the pain and symptoms were the focus of the original diagnostic workup, it is possible that these symptoms were the consequence of an eating disorder that had developed earlier [225].

In this same study, another third of patients with chronic pain and eating disorders had developed the eating disorder subsequent to their pain and symptoms, and had essentially "backed into" the eating disorder through the pathway of restrictive eating and weight loss [225]. Unfortunately, patients with chronic pain and physical symptoms take much longer for their eating disorder to come to the attention of a medical professional [225]. In addition to pain and symptoms potentially disguising an eating disorder, it is likely that family members and providers become distracted by the physical complaints and assume that identifying and treating the origin of these complaints will resolve the restrictive eating. Unfortunately, as the workup to identify a medical cause for pain and restrictive eating continues, the eating disorder can progress in severity. Once disordered eating and weight loss begin, they become maintained by factors other than GI symptoms and warrant their own specific treatment. In particular, even if they developed from abdominal pain, once an eating disorder develops, treating the pain is unlikely to help the patient resume eating without additional eating disorders treatment [225].

In a gastroenterology setting, general screening measures that focus on intentional restrictive eating, drive for thinness and weight, and shape concerns may underestimate the number of patients struggling with eating disorders. In particular, these patients often deny or minimize weight and shape concerns and tend to be overly focused on the physical consequences that drive restrictive eating. As a result, measures that are focused on classic eating disorder symptoms may not resonate with these patients. In fact, prevalence studies that rely on the Eating Attitudes Test, a widely used screening measure for classic eating disorders, tend to find a lower prevalence of eating disorders than in the general population [229].

To address this clinical dilemma among gastroenterology patients with eating concerns, clinical assessment of eating disorders involves assessing a patient's eating habits, extent of weight loss, concerns about weight gain, as well as physical and psychological symptoms. In addition, examining a person's level of concern about their restrictive eating and weight loss may also help to identify an eating disorder. In particular, those with eating disorders may express some indifference to the seriousness of their low weight. To identify ARFID, it is helpful to examine a patient's overestimation of negative consequences of eating, as well as their level of preoccupation and rigid adherence to dietary management strategies for reduction of symptoms.

With regard to clinical interview, it is important to note that for patients with AN, symptoms of restrictive eating and maintaining a low weight tend to be ego syntonic, or are reinforcing to the patient. In addition, as described in the diagnostic criteria for AN, patients often demonstrate a lack of insight into the severity of the low weight. This means patients may underreport or minimize their restrictive behaviors or eating disordered cognitions. In addition, although patients can initially have little or no weight or shape concerns, these can develop in the context of weight loss, and thus an individual who initially lost weight secondary to a medication change or an illness may now be resistant to weight regain. Finally, it is important for the physician to remain aware that many patients deny concerns about weight or shape and instead express a preoccupation with healthy eating. This preoccupation is common in AN and warrants screening for an eating disorder.

Because patients with eating disorders often deny restrictive eating and/or claim uncertainty regarding the cause of weight loss, it is recommended that together with the clinical interview, clinicians use a behavioral assessment. The first step of a behavioral assessment involves providing psychoeducation about the effects of restrictive eating and low weight and the need for a high-calorie diet to gain weight. In this manner, clinicians can emphasize how weight loss and malnutrition can pose a greater harm to the patient's physical health and well-being than the GI symptoms themselves. To remedy this risk, patients are advised to eat in spite of pain or lack of hunger to increase or maintain their weight within a healthy range.

In this way, clinicians may liken eating and weight gain to a medical intervention. It can be helpful to describe how similar to refeeding, medical interventions commonly have adverse side-effects and/or are difficult to tolerate. Gastroenterologists should recommend that patients gain a specified amount of weight per week. To assess their progress, follow-up on eating and weight is essential. On follow-up, if patients struggle to make these improvements, the risk for the development of an eating disorder is high, and potential referral for an eating disorder assessment by a specialized provider is warranted.

Body mass index in eating disorder identification and treatment

As noted previously, a common misconception that hinders eating disorders identification is the notion that eating disorders are associated with low absolute BMI. There is strong evidence to dispel this myth, with studies finding that individuals with eating disorders present at all shapes and sizes [15]. In fact, data suggest that approximately one-fourth to well more than half of adolescent and adult patients presenting with restrictive eating disorders have a history of overweight or obesity [15]. Due to the tendency of higher-weight-status individuals to diet, it is possible that being overweight is a risk factor for the development of an eating disorder [26].

To reflect the finding that patients with AN can present at any BMI, in the revised DSM-5, the criteria for low weight no longer involves falling below a specific weight threshold. Yet, DSM-5 also distinguishes between "atypical" and full syndrome AN, with the atypical presentation representing symptomatic individuals presenting with a higher absolute BMI. In light of research finding that no differences exist in severity or consequences of low weight versus atypical anorexia, this distinction tends to be misleading [15].

It is important to note that many patients with a history of obesity and overweight are likely to present with eating disorder symptoms at a higher weight and may not appear cachectic and in need of refeeding and weight restoration. Unfortunately, research suggests that higher-weight-status individuals with AN take longer to be identified [15]. In addition, compared with lower-weight-status patients with AN, these patients tend to experience a larger decrease in BMI before presenting to treatment [15]. Because early detection is associated with a better prognosis in eating disorder treatment [230], this substantial discrepancy has important clinical implications and suggests that serious eating disorders in patients with a history of overweight may be overlooked until symptoms have progressed and become potentially more intractable.

In addition, there is a common misperception that the rate, method, or intent of weight loss makes a difference in diagnosing AN. In fact, as is supported by studies such as Keys and colleagues' 1950 starvation study [30], AN behaviors and cognitions can be present regardless of whether weight loss was slow or rapid, purposeful or accidental. It also suggests that weight restoration to higher-than-average levels may be needed for some patients.

It is recommended that eating disorders are assessed in any patient with restrictive eating and/or weight loss regardless of their BMI presentation. There is a growing understanding in the field that weight suppression, which is defined as the difference between an individual's highest historical weight and current or lowest weight [231,232], may be a better way to capture eating disorder severity than absolute low BMI. In particular, weight suppression is associated with increased eating disorder pathology, higher levels of distress, increased physiological abnormalities, longer time to remission, and poorer treatment outcomes [231,232].

Because child and adolescent patients are expected to make increases in BMI over their development, absolute weight or BMI is not an appropriate measure of severity or an estimate of weight restoration. Instead, it is recommended that the clinician review the patient's pediatric growth chart to examine the BMI percentile where the patient historically tracked and to also remain aware of stunted height secondary to malnutrition, which may artificially inflate BMI. Again, due to variability in each patient's genetic heritage, it is not appropriate for each child to restore to the 50th percentile for BMI. Instead, the child's former BMI percentile where their BMI trended is a more accurate measure of weight restoration, and deviations from that trend are a better estimate of severity than absolute BMI or amount of weight lost. In cases where a child's BMI trended higher, to achieve a full recovery, clinicians must be comfortable helping the patient restore weight to above the average range.

Weight restoration in a gastroenterology setting

Given that restrictive eating and/or weight loss may exacerbate preexisting GI conditions and produce thoughts and behavior patterns of an eating disorder, normalizing eating and/or weight gain is essential. In fact, normalizing eating is generally the first step of all evidence-based eating disorder treatments. The gastroenterologist is in a unique role to be able to support patients with this intervention. In particular, they have the ability to rule out and treat conditions that may make it difficult to eat and to help patients understand the effect of their restrictive eating on their physical health and well-being.

Patients who are unable to make necessary changes in eating may require alimentation to increase calories and weight. Unfortunately, in clinical practice, it is common to underestimate the calories required for weight gain that can keep patients from making progress even when they are on alimentation or compliant with oral caloric expectations. Although patients with AN are hypometabolic when in a starved state, they quickly become hypermetabolic with refeeding [233]. Even after refeeding and weight restoration, studies suggest that women with AN require nearly twice as many kilocalories immediately after treatment and one-third more calories at long-term follow-up to maintain a minimally healthy weight [224].

Common concerns about refeeding syndrome have informed recommendations for conservative feeding protocols, advising providers to start the patient on low calories and to advance calories slowly. However, recent research has examined more aggressive feeding regimens in hospitalized adolescents with AN and found no incidents of refeeding syndrome. In addition, patients on higher calorie diets experience faster weight gain, shorter hospitalizations, and fewer complications [234]. Additional studies of aggressive refeeding of patients with AN found similar results [235,236]. As such, aggressive refeeding regimens with electrolyte monitoring and prophylactic electrolyte repletion is recommended.

Addressing eating disorder risk in the setting of dietary management

Patients with GI disorders often require dietary management of symptoms and their disease process. Although some patients with certain conditions, such as celiac disease or lactose intolerance, require lifelong dietary modifications to manage disease, other conditions, such as irritable bowel syndrome and inflammatory bowel disease, may involve a system of trial and error to identify foods that trigger symptoms with recommendations to eliminate those foods from their diet. Although in some cases dietary modifications may be vital for optimizing health outcomes and disease management, they also may place individuals at risk for disordered eating and the development of a full-blown eating disorder [17,224,237].

A review of the literature on chronic illnesses that involve adherence to strict dietary regimens (i.e., celiac disease, diabetes mellitus, cystic fibrosis, inflammatory bowel disease) suggests that these individuals have a greater risk for disordered eating and eating disorders than the general population [17]. A recent comprehensive systematic review on the relationship between diet-treated pediatric chronic illness and eating disorders also found that diet-treated chronic illness was associated with the development of disordered eating and eating disorders. The study also found that in most cases, the onset of the chronic illness predated the onset of the eating disorders, suggesting that dietary management may have placed these individuals at risk for unhealthy dietary management practices. Finally, the study found that unhealthy dietary management practices placed children at risk for poor medical outcomes [237].

Satherley et al. [224] in 2015 conducted a systematic review examining disordered eating practices in dietary-controlled GI conditions in children, adolescents, and adults. Among studies that assessed the prevalence of eating disorders using a validated structured interview, prevalence rates averaged 23%, which vastly exceed that of the general population. They also found a relationship between the level of dietary adherence and the presence of disordered eating patterns such that those with both high and low adherence to dietary management recommendations were at risk for the development of an eating disorders. Not surprisingly, across studies, disordered eating was associated with psychological distress, poor quality of life, anxiety, and depression [224].

Because the symptom severity of the GI condition was strongly linked to disordered eating across studies, these authors highlight two potential pathways for the development of disordered eating and eating disorders among patients with dietary-controlled GI conditions [224]. In one pathway, individuals with severe symptoms who have a favorable response to dietary management practices become anxious about reexperiencing these symptoms and consequently become highly rigid and vigilant in their dietary practices [224]. Another pathway represents individuals who do not adapt well to their diagnoses and react with anxiety when prescribed regimens restore weight [224]. These individuals may believe that dietary management is associated with weight gain and consequently become nonadherent to dietary regimens, which is involved with ongoing distress and increased symptom severity [224]. Those patients in the first pathway seem to be at risk for ARFID and those in the second may be at risk for AN, BN, or BED.

Based on the research on the overlap between dietary-controlled GI disease and eating disorders, it is important for the gastroenterologist to consider the risk of disordered eating associated with restriction and recommend dietary management and elimination diets only when necessary. For those whose disease management depends on dietary restriction of food groups (i.e., celiac disease), providers should follow patients closely and help them to adhere to the regimen, while working with them to maintain a healthy relationship with food and decrease stress around eating. In some cases, working with a dietician to help patients find ways to broaden their food repertoire in the context of food restrictions and also find ways to ensure that this does not limit their social functioning may be helpful. Among patients with nonalcoholic fatty liver disease or other weight-related GI illnesses, for whom dietary changes are a critical element of management, gastroenterologists should work closely with dieticians to support necessary lifestyle changes while discouraging disordered eating behaviors, such as fad diets, and monitoring for eating disorder symptoms. When patients describe food sensitivities (i.e., gluten intolerance) rather than true malabsorption problems or food allergies, elimination diets should be recommended with caution. If foods do not diminish symptoms or help with functioning, they should be discontinued. As gastroenterologists navigate discussions regarding dietary management with patients, they are well positioned to promote positive body image, encourage healthy relationships with food, discourage unhealthy weight-control or disordered eating behaviors, and avoid unnecessary restrictions or dietary changes.

Summary

The significant overlap among various eating disorders suggests they may represent a continuum of the same underlying physiological changes that represent a biological adaptation to caloric restriction. Both dieting for weight loss and unintentional weight loss related to GI symptoms may begin the cascade of physiological and psychological changes related to malnutrition, characteristic of an eating disorder. Treatments that focus on normalizing eating, as well as nutritional and weight restoration, show the most benefit. It is recommended that gastroenterologist assess weight loss and malnutrition, manage complications, and attempt to normalize eating and weight. Moreover, in the absence of underlying disease that explains weight loss, providers should refer patients for evidence-based eating disorder assessment and treatment. Dietary therapy should be recommended when necessary and monitored closely, recognizing the potential risk of disordered eating associated with restrictive eating patterns.

References are available at www.yamadagastro.com/textbook7e

Further reading

American Psychiatric Association. Diagnostic and Statistical Manual of Mental Disorders, 5th edn. Arlington, VA: American Psychiatric Association; 2013.

Crow S.J., Peterson C.B., Swanson S.A., et al. Increased mortality in bulimia nervosa and other eating disorders. Am J Psychiatry 2009;166(12):1342.

Lebow J., Sim L.A., Kransdorf L.N. Prevalence of a history of overweight and obesity in adolescents with restrictive eating disorders. J Adolesc Health 2015;56(1):19.

Lock J., Le Grange D., Agras W.S., et al. Randomized clinical trial comparing family-based treatment with adolescent-focused individual therapy for adolescents with anorexia nervosa. Arch Gen Psychiatry 2010;67(10):1025.

Mitchell J., Crow S. Medical complications of anorexia nervosa and bulimia nervosa. Curr Opin Psychiatry 2006;19:438.

Neumark-Sztainer D., Wall M., Story M., Sherwood N.E. Five-year longitudinal predictive factors for disordered eating in a population-based sample of overweight adolescents: implications for prevention and treatment. Int J Eat Disord 2009;42(7):664.

Quick V.M., Byrd-Bredbenner C., Neumark-Sztainer D. Chronic illness and disordered eating: a discussion of the literature. Adv Nutr 2013;4(3):277.

Satherley R., Howard R., Higgs S. Disordered eating practices in gastrointestinal disorders. Appetite 2015;84:240.

Södersten P., Bergh C., Zandian M. Understanding eating disorders. Horm Behav 2006;50(4):572.

CHAPTER 26

The aging gastrointestinal tract: digestive and motility problems

Michael Camilleri
Mayo Clinic, Rochester, MN, USA

Chapter menu

Introduction

Changes in structure and function of the gastrointestinal tract result in specific changes leading to diseases specific to aging or to an increased propensity to develop diseases also observed in younger adults.

Pathobiological mechanisms associated with aging which impact the digestive tract

Aging has been defined as a series of changes that occur with time during postmaturational life, that underlie an increasing vulnerability to challenge, thereby decreasing the ability of the organism to survive. At the organ level, aging is associated with metabolic, genetic, neuroendocrine, and immunological changes that may contribute to the processes of cell death from apoptosis or phagocytosis. These mechanisms may lead to neural injury or morphological or functional changes in the digestive tract. Examples include gastric mucosal atrophy leading to atrophic gastritis and vitamin B_{12} deficiency due to lack of intrinsic factor or atrophic pancreatitis leading to pancreatic exocrine insufficiency.

Specific examples related to the loss of neural control that may contribute to a well-known consequence of constipation in the elderly are the reductions in the colon (of elderly humans as well as animal models) in the number of Hu-positive (marker of all neurons) and ChAT-positive neurons with age with no reduction in nNOS-positive neurons. As a result, the proportion of nNOS (inhibitory) to all neurons Hu increases. Moreover, older colonic muscle cells respond less to a variety of stimuli (e.g., acetylcholine and electrical field stimulation) than do cells from younger adult animals. These differences appear to reflect changes in L-type calcium currents in smooth muscle with aging. Such changes with aging may affect the entire digestive tract, including motor, sensory, and absorptive functions, and are illustrated by the examples discussed here.

Effects of aging on gastrointestinal physiology

Motor and sensory

Esophagus

Aging has effects on motor and sensory physiology throughout the gut, starting with dysfunction of the pharynx and esophagus which result in dysphagia and aspiration in the elderly. As people age, swallow is slower, which is attributed to delay in the oral phase of swallowing, reduced tongue propelling force, diminished

Yamada's Textbook of Gastroenterology, Seventh Edition. Edited by Timothy C. Wang, Michael Camilleri, Benjamin Lebwohl, Anna S. Lok, William J. Sandborn, Kenneth K. Wang, and Gary D. Wu.

Companion website: www.yamadagastro.com/textbook7e

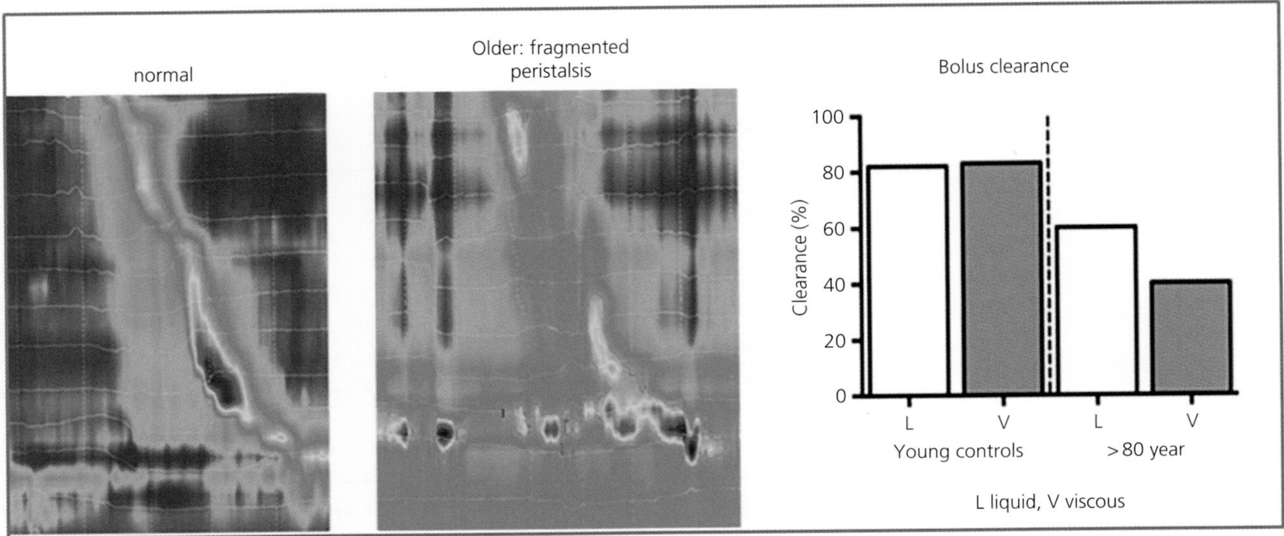

Figure 26.1 Presbyesophagus: fragmented peristalsis in an older subject without clearance. Source: Cock C., Besanko L., Kritas S., et al. Impaired bolus clearance in asymptomatic older adults during high-resolution impedance manometry. Neurogastroenterol Motil 2016;28:1890. Reproduced with permission of John Wiley & Sons.

pharyngeal lubrication, and delayed upper esophageal sphincter relaxation and opening. The term "presbyesophagus" describes disorganized and inefficient peristalsis, typically in nonagerani-ans. It is characterized by nonpropagated contractions occurring as frequently as well-propagated, normal-amplitude contractions (Figure 26.1).

Stomach and small bowel

In the elderly, solid foods empty from the stomach at a normal rate, while liquid emptying may be delayed or accelerated. Even in healthy elderly people, there is decreased perception of gastric distension without any change in fasting gastric compliance; there is also reduced gastric tone late in the postprandial period and this may contribute to discomfort or satiety and to the anorexia frequently observed in the elderly.

Small bowel motility patterns in the seventh and eighth decades show modest reduction in contraction frequency after feeding and propagation velocity of the fasting migrating motor complex. The significance of these changes is unclear but they may conceivably contribute to development of abdominal discomfort.

Colonic and rectoanal motor functions

The effects of aging on colonic transit and biomechanical properties of the colon in asymptomatic elderly are incompletely documented; most reports document normal overall colonic transit but delayed rectosigmoid transit, which may result from specific regional impairment of motor function or the frequently encountered pelvic floor dysfunction. Thus, elderly patients experience incomplete stool evacuation, with longer time to expel content from the rectum, partly due to excessive perineal descent which is more likely in multiparous elderly women.

Given the decline in skeletal muscle mass, strength, and fatigability that accompanies aging, squeeze anal sphincter pressures decline with aging in subjects without rectoanal symptoms. In asymptomatic females, aging has been reported to be associated with reduced anal resting and squeeze pressures, reduced rectal compliance, reduced rectal sensation, and perineal laxity. All of these factors may predispose to fecal incontinence in elderly females.

In addition to gender, parity and obstetric trauma, the effect of aging on rectoanal function is also modified by concomitant disease, medications, hormonal changes during menopause, and pudendal neuropathy secondary to excessive straining during defecation.

Aging has been associated with changes in smooth muscle function, loss of excitatory (cholinergic) neurons leading to constipation and possibly inhibitory neurons leading to uncoordinated contractions and discomfort.

Pelvic floor and anal sphincter dysfunction are detailed further below.

Small intestinal absorptive functions

Aging does not alter small intestinal anatomy, enterocyte height, or intraepithelial lymphocyte counts or permeability of lactose and mannitol. Changes in the absorptive function for carbohydrates, fats, and vitamin B_{12} result from disease rather than age-related processes. Calcium absorption declines over 60 years of

Table 26.1 Changes in absorptive functions of carbohydrates, fats, and vitamin B_{12}.

Reduced absorption	No change	Increased absorption
Carbohydrate	Thiamine	Cholesterol
Protein	Riboflavin	Vitamin A
Triglycerides	Niacin	Vitamin C
Folate, vitamin B_{12}	Vitamin K	
Vitamin D, calcium	Zinc, magnesium, iron	

Source: Morley J.E. The aging gut: physiology. Clin Geriatr Med 2007;23:757. Reproduced with permission of Elsevier.

age, with decreased intestinal responsiveness to vitamin D, and contributes to increased bone loss with aging. Multiple small, probably clinically insignificant, changes in nutrient absorption have been described, as summarized in Table 26.1.

Epidemiological studies of gastrointestinal symptoms in older people

Functional gastrointestinal disorders

These are addressed extensively in Chapters 31 (Approach to the patient with dyspepsia and related functional gastrointestinal complaints) and 67 (Irritable bowel syndrome).

Older people have a high prevalence of symptoms consistent with functional gastrointestinal disorders. The age- and sex-adjusted prevalence (and 95% confidence interval) per 100 persons were as follows: frequent abdominal pain 24.3 (19.3–29.2], irritable bowel syndrome 10.9 (7.2–14.6), chronic constipation 24.1 (19.1–29.0), chronic diarrhea 14.2 (10.1–18.2), and fecal incontinence >1 per week 3.7 (1.6–5.9). Constipation and, to a lesser extent, fecal incontinence were significantly more prevalent in 65–93 year-old residents of Olmsted County, Minnesota, compared to adults aged 30–64 years. In contrast, frequent abdominal pain, irritable bowel syndrome, and chronic diarrhea were not more prevalent in the elderly.

Similarly, in a Danish cohort, overall prevalence data were only slightly higher in older compared to younger adults (e.g., diarrhea 17.9% and constipation 24.1%) or not different at all (e.g., irritable bowel syndrome). In a medical outcomes survey of the physical function status and quality of life in 704 Olmsted County residents over 65 years old, functional bowel disorders interfered with daily living and quality of life. Similarly, in Copenhagen, Denmark, functional dyspepsia and IBS reduced functional ability at baseline and 5 years later.

Several factors predispose to constipation in the elderly: inactivity, inappropriate diet, depression, medications, neuromuscular disorders, and poor rectal sensation and evacuation dynamics.

Diverticulosis

This is discussed extensively in Chapter 69 (Diverticular disease of the colon). Diverticulosis is more prevalent with increasing age; about 56% of people >70 years of age have diverticulosis on postmortem examination, as well as a greater density of diverticula on colonoscopic examination. The increase in diverticula with age suggests that this is a progressive disease, although the mechanisms are unclear. Predominant location of diverticula differs by country: predominantly in the sigmoid and left colon in western countries, whereas in Japan 70–80% of people with diverticulosis have predominance of right-sided diverticula. A study in US black subjects showed a greater percentage of the diverticula in the proximal colon and fewer in the distal colon compared with white subjects.

Foregut diseases of motility in elderly

Gastroesophageal reflux disease

Gastroesophageal reflux disease (GERD) is highly prevalent (daily symptoms in 8% of men and 15% of women) and poses special diagnostic and therapeutic challenges in the elderly. GERD symptoms at least once a month are reported by 54% of men and 66% of women. Patients with GERD are more likely to consult their healthcare providers with increasing age and coexisting upper abdominal symptoms. Elderly patients may not report classic symptoms such as dysphagia, chest pain, and heartburn, and may therefore present with severe GERD or complications such as esophageal ulceration and bleeding.

The most common primary presenting symptoms of GERD in the elderly are regurgitation, dysphagia, dyspepsia, vomiting, and noncardiac chest pain, rather than heartburn. Typical reflux symptoms are often associated with atypical symptoms, such as abdominal symptoms, chest pain, or respiratory symptoms (e.g., hoarseness, chronic cough, wheezing). When elderly patients have sufficiently severe heartburn to require upper GI endoscopy, they are more likely to have more significant mucosal disease in the esophagus (e.g., erosive esophagitis, Barrett esophagus) compared to patients younger than age 60.

"Pill esophagitis"

Pill-induced esophagitis results from ingestion of certain drugs and is the cause of many cases of erosive esophagitis in the elderly. Among more than 70 drugs that induce esophageal disorders, antibacterial agents (such as doxycycline, tetracycline, and clindamycin) account for >50% of cases of pill esophagitis. Other medications resulting in pill esophagitis are aspirin, potassium chloride, ferrous sulfate, bisphosphonates, quinidine, alprenolol, steroids, and NSAIDs. Capsules or tablets are commonly delayed in their passage through the esophagus and may cause damage from the caustic contents of the drug in contact with the esophagus for a sufficiently long time. Taking medications at bedtime or without fluids is a common cause of esophagitis. Drug-related damage presents with esophagitis, chest pain, and dysphagia in the elderly.

Midgut and hindgut diseases

Weight loss, protein-energy malnutrition, and anorexia

Weight loss occurs commonly in the elderly, and is associated with functional decline, loss of skeletal muscle mass (sarcopenia), and mortality, the latter being more likely when there is a 10% or greater reduction in bodyweight over 10 years. A 4% or greater loss in bodyweight over 1 year warrants investigation for underlying causes including depression, cancer, benign GI conditions, and medication toxicity.

Protein-energy malnutrition is relatively common in the elderly; it is important to note that even in grossly undernourished patients, the results of hematological and biochemical tests (e.g., serum transferrin, transthyretin [prealbumin], and retinol-binding protein) can be normal.

A decline in food intake or "physiological anorexia" occurs with aging; there are many potential causes: alterations in satiation after food ingestion, elevated leptin levels (especially in men), depression, changes in central nervous system neurotransmitters, loss of adipose tissue and sarcopenia associated with age >70 years or dieting, and increase of cytokines (which are associated with anorexia and protein wasting).

The cause for early satiation in the elderly is unclear; the most attractive hypothesis is based on reduced gastric accommodation following ingestion of food despite normal fasting gastric compliance. Gastric emptying and satiation in the elderly have not been extensively studied.

Malabsorption

Among nonmalignant GI causes, celiac disease, chronic pancreatic exocrine insufficiency, and small intestinal bacterial overgrowth (SIBO) are the most common causes of malabsorption in the elderly. Age >65 years and female gender are associated with a positive lactulose-hydrogen breath test (LHBT) (1.02, 95% CI 1.01–1.03, $p<0.001$) based on a study of 791 subjects, 54% of whom had a positive LHBT. However, it is important to note (see Chapter 58, Bacterial overgrowth) that it is not clear whether a positive LHBT represents true SIBO or accelerated delivery of the substrate to the colon. Patients with a methane-positive lactulose breath test generally have slower small bowel and colonic transit, suggesting there is a subset of patients with SIBO who do have an underlying motility disorder.

The clinical effects of bacterial overgrowth can be equally severe in the elderly with or without an anatomical defect of the small bowel such as segmental dilation or diverticulosis. Tests of absorptive capacity may be normal, but empiric antibiotic treatment may positively impact nutritional state. However, unless there is positive evidence in support of bacterial overgrowth such as dilation, diverticulosis or a positive LHBT test with a peak in breath hydrogen within 1 hour of lactulose ingestion, such a therapeutic approach should be short and carefully monitored for positive response (e.g., weight gain) rather than being pursued over the long term because of the potential adverse responses to the antibiotics such as antibiotic-associated colitis, *C. difficile* infection, or peripheral neuropathy with long-term metronidazole.

It is estimated that 5% of people >70 years old and 10% >80 years old have pancreatic exocrine insufficiency (PEI) that may lead to maldigestion, malnutrition, steatorrhea, diarrhea, abdominal pain, weight loss, and fat-soluble vitamin deficiency.

Constipation, irritable bowel syndrome, and diverticulosis

Constipation, IBS, and diverticulosis are, at least in part, manifestations of impaired colonic motor functions. Extracolonic pelvic floor muscles also contribute to these syndromes. The mechanisms involved in IBS and constipation are detailed in other chapters (Chapters 55 and 69). There are several factors that are considered to predispose to *constipation* in the elderly and these include inactivity, inappropriate diet, depression, medications, neuromuscular disorders (including Parkinson disease), poor rectal sensation and evacuation dynamics, especially in multiparous women, and fecal impaction.

Diverticulosis and its complications are the more relevant colonic pathology in the elderly.

Pathology of diverticulosis

The effects of diverticulosis on colonic motility and transit in the absence of a stricture are unclear although dense diverticulosis can be associated with spasm and thickening of colonic circular muscle which may conceivably retard colonic transit. Uncoordinated colonic motility and colonic segmentation may lead to IBS and diverticulosis, respectively. It is possible that these pathophysiological findings result from disorders of inhibitory control of neuromuscular function or changes in the collagen structure in the wall of the colon as a manifestation of aging in patients with diverticulosis.

The total number of neurons in the myenteric plexus is decreased, and collagen deposited in the distal colon is increased with aging in humans; however, the one formal study performed in colon harboring diverticular disease reported upregulated nitrergic neuromuscular transmission. In vitro studies conducted with sigmoid colon muscle strips showed an altered motor pattern with reduced spontaneous motility and enhanced neurally mediated colonic responses involving both excitatory and inhibitory motor pathways. Conversely, smooth muscle (circular and longitudinal layers)and myenteric neurons densities were unaltered in one study. Different studies provide contradictory information about interstitial cells of Cajal and glial cells.

Table 26.2 Subtypes of fecal incontinence.

Type	Clinical description	Potential mechanism(s)
Passive incontinence	The involuntary discharge of stool or gas without awareness	Weak IAS and EAS Neuropathy Rectal hyposensitivity
Urge incontinence	The discharge of fecal matter despite active attempts to retain bowel contents	Weak IAS and EAS Rectal hypersensitivity Impaired rectal compliance
Fecal seepage	The leakage of stool following otherwise normal evacuation	Dyssynergia Rectal hyposensitivity Neuropathy

EAS, external anal sphincter; IAS, internal anal sphincter.

High intraluminal pressure in diverticulosis

The prevailing hypothesis to explain diverticulosis is that isometric contraction of individual haustra results in high intraluminal pressure and segmentation. This facilitates development of pulsion diverticula at points of weakness in the colonic wall corresponding to the site of perforating arteries. Greater collagen and elastin deposition with aging may contribute to reduction of compliance of the aging colon. It is conceivable that, given the fact that the compliance of the colon is lowest in the sigmoid region, the latter generates the highest intraluminal pressures and may be most prone to the development of diverticulosis. The high pressures may also lead to compensatory hypertrophy of the circular muscle layers, further increasing the pressure, reducing compliance, and possibly narrowing the lumen and increasing the likelihood of diverticulum formation.

Pelvic floor and sphincter dysfunctions: effects on colonic symptoms

The pelvic floor and anal sphincters are essential for continence and facilitation of defecation. The resting pressure (internal anal sphincter tone) and the voluntary contractile anal pressure (external anal sphincter tone) tend to decrease nonsignificantly with age, and both are lower in women than in men. Anorectal function in older compared to younger persons showed decreased anal pressures, lower rectal volume required to cause desire to defecate, inability to expel a solid 18 mm sphere or 50 mL balloon, and lower maximum tolerated volume. The degree of perineal descent is also greater in older women due to laxity in support structures and multiparity.

It is important to assess the evacuatory functions rather than assume constipation is an inevitable consequence of aging. Retraining of the pelvic floor muscles with biofeedback may be safe and effective in these patients, though not as effective as in younger patients with spastic (dyssynergic) rectal evacuation disorders.

Fecal incontinence

Age- and gender-related changes in anal sphincter function provide confirmation that the smooth and skeletal muscle components of the internal and external sphincters respectively are subject to degeneration. Anal resting and, to a lesser extent, squeeze pressures both decline with age in asymptomatic women. Rectal compliance is also lower with aging and may predispose to urge incontinence as the “reservoir capacity” related to relaxation of the rectum is reduced. Subtypes of fecal incontinence are described in Table 26.2.

Examples of sphincter weakness are shown in Figure 26.2 based on standard and high-definition manometry and pressure topography during rest and voluntary squeeze.

High-resolution manometry alone and together with anorectal descent during evacuation (as in barium or MR defecography [Figure 26.3]) may identify rectal prolapse and large rectoceles, which may sometimes occur in patients with fecal incontinence, especially in elderly and multiparous women.

Conclusions

Aging per se affects functions throughout the gut, particularly after the seventh decade, but these changes are relatively modest and often asymptomatic, perhaps due to the vast reserve of neuromuscular functional elements in the gut. The regions with reduced functional reserve are the proximal esophagus, anus, and pelvic floor and that is probably why the main motility disturbances in the elderly are high dysphagia, constipation, and

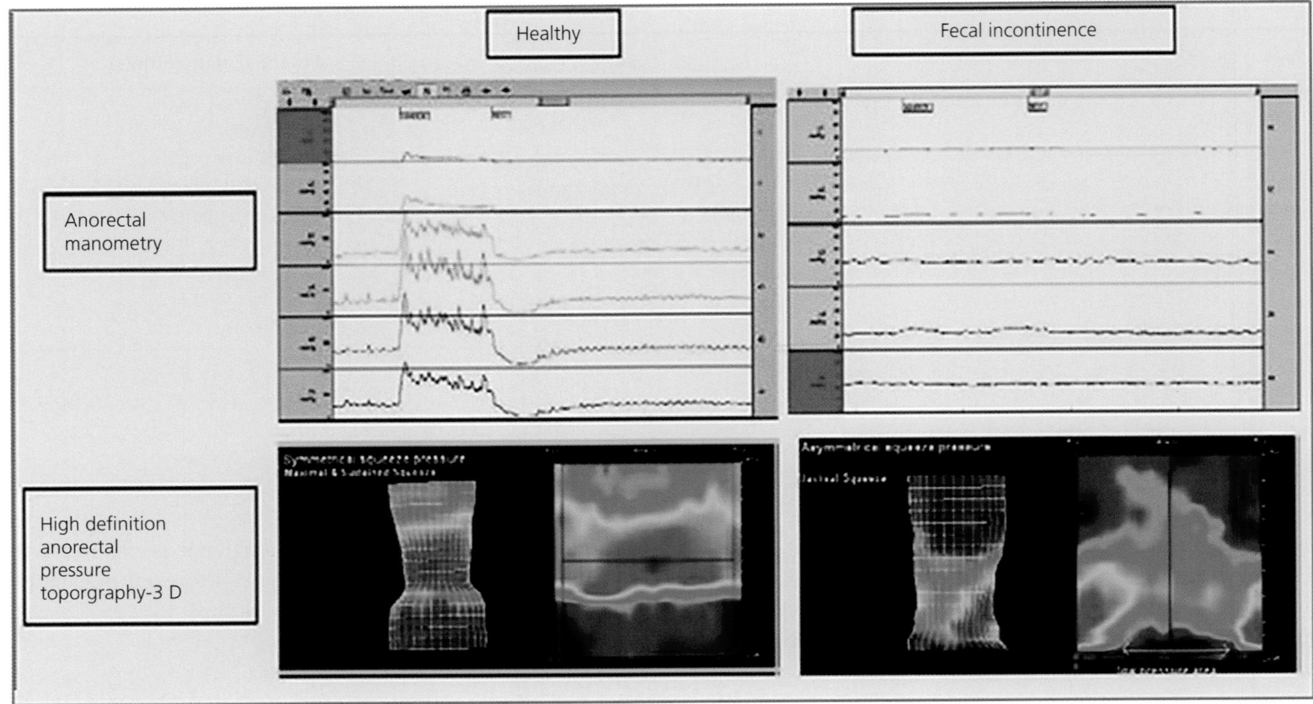

Figure 26.2 Standard and high-definition manometry and pressure topography during rest and voluntary squeeze. In the healthy subject (left), normal resting and normal increase in sphincter pressure are seen whereas in the incontinent subject, the sphincter is weak during squeeze. Source: Rao S.S. Advances in diagnostic assessment of fecal incontinence and dyssynergic defecation. Clin Gastroenterol Hepatol 2010;8:910. Reproduced with permission of Elsevier.

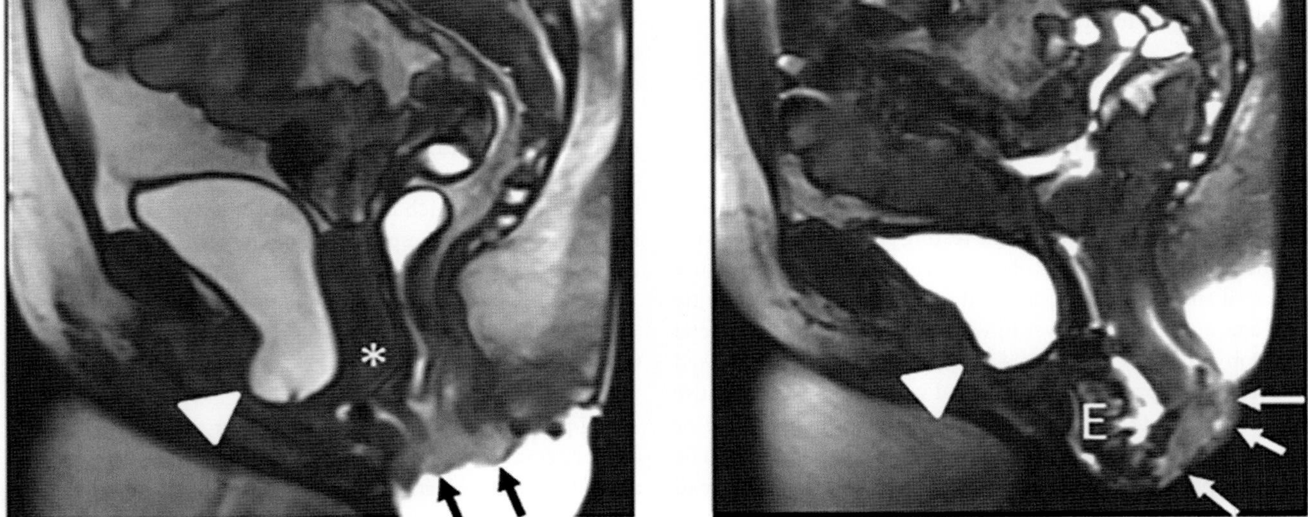

Figure 26.3 MRI shows small and large rectal prolapse (arrows), a cystocele (arrowhead), enterocele (E), and uterine prolapse (asterisk). Source: Reproduced from Prichard D.O., Lee T., Parthasarathy G., Fletcher J.G., Zinsmeister A.R., Bharucha A.E. High-resolution anorectal manometry for identifying defecatory disorders and rectal structural abnormalities in women. Clin Gastroenterol Hepatol 2017;15:412–420.

Table 26.3 Cross-references to other chapters.

Topic	Chapter #	Chapter title
Gastroesophageal reflux disease (GERD)	43	Gastroesophageal reflux disease
Barrett esophagus	46	Barrett esophagus and esophageal adenocarcinoma
Chronic atrophic gastritis	51	Gastritis and gastropathy
Peptic ulcer disease	49	Peptic ulcer disease
Celiac disease	56	Celiac disease
Mesenteric ischemia	114	Intestinal ischemia and vasculitides
Angiodysplasias	113	Gastrointestinal vascular malformations and neoplasms
Small intestinal bacterial overgrowth	58	Bacterial overgrowth
Pancreatic insufficiency	76	Chronic pancreatitis
Constipation	36	Approach to the patient with constipation
Diverticular disease	69	Diverticular disease of the colon
Irritable bowel syndrome	67	Irritable bowel syndrome
Clostridium difficile colitis	144	Bacterial, viral, and toxic causes of diarrhea
Inflammatory bowel disease	62–64	Inflammatory bowel diseases, Ulcerative colitis, Crohn's disease

fecal incontinence. The combination of aging, ischemia, and other factors, including obstetric damage, contributes to these manifestations. Elderly patients may have reversible, nonmalignant disease and can be restored to health through proper management. Table 26.3 shows cross-references where other gastrointestinal diseases identified in older age people are discussed in this textbook.

References are available at www.yamadagastro.com/textbook7e

Further reading

Bernard C.E., Gibbons S.J., Gomez-Pinilla P.J., et al. Effect of age on the enteric nervous system of the human colon. Neurogastroenterol Motil 2009;21:746.

Camilleri M., Lee J.S., Viramontes B., Bharucha A.E., Tangalos E.G. Insights into the pathophysiology and mechanisms of constipation, irritable bowel syndrome, and diverticulosis in older people. J Am Geriatr Soc 2000;48:1142.

Cock C., Besanko L., Kritas S., et al. Impaired bolus clearance in asymptomatic older adults during high-resolution impedance manometry. Neurogastroenterol Motil 2016;28:1890.

Dumic I., Nordin T., Jecmenica M., Stojkovic Lalosevic M., Milosavljevic T., Milovanovic T. Gastrointestinal tract disorders in older age. Can J Gastroenterol Hepatol 2019;2019:6757524.

Fox J.C., Fletcher J.G., Zinsmeister A.R., Seide B., Riederer S.J., Bharucha A.E. Effect of aging on anorectal and pelvic floor functions in females. Dis Colon Rectum 2006;49:1726.

Löhr J.M., Panic N., Vujasinovic M., Verbeke C.S. The ageing pancreas: a systematic review of the evidence and analysis of the consequences. J Intern Med 2018;283:446.

Peery A.F., Keku T.O., Martin C.F., et al. Distribution and characteristics of colonic diverticula in a United States screening population. Clin Gastroenterol Hepatol 2016;14:980.

Prichard D.O., Lee T., Parthasarathy G., Fletcher J.G., Zinsmeister A.R., Bharucha A.E. High-resolution anorectal manometry for identifying defecatory disorders and rectal structural abnormalities in women. Clin Gastroenterol Hepatol 2017;15:412.

Rao S.S. Advances in diagnostic assessment of fecal incontinence and dyssynergic defecation. Clin Gastroenterol Hepatol 2010;8:910.

CHAPTER 27

Neoplasia of the gastrointestinal tract

E. Ramsay Camp[1], Denise I. Garcia[2,3,4], and Raymond N. DuBois[5]

[1] Division of Surgical Oncology, Baylor College of Medicine, Houston, TX, USA
[2] Department of Surgery, Medical University of South Carolina, Charleston, SC, USA
[3] Hollings Cancer Center, Medical University of South Carolina, Charleston, SC, USA
[4] Ralph H. Johnson VA Medical Center, Charleston, SC, USA
[5] College of Medicine, Medical University of South Carolina, Charleston, SC, USA

Chapter menu

Introduction

Cancer is caused by uncontrolled growth of cells in a part of the body, often spreading to other vital organs, disrupting their function and ultimately leading to death. It is widely accepted that cancer is a result of genetic alterations either acquired over time or inherited. These genetic alterations include point mutations, small deletions and insertions, inversions, copy number alterations (CNAs), and chromosomal rearrangements [1–3]. Hereditary malignancies have been identified in every GI organ that are associated with several well-characterized inherited gene mutations such as familial adenomatous polyposis (FAP) in colorectal cancer (CRC) and CDH1 in gastric cancer [4]. With the advent of genomic sequencing, researchers have dissected cancers such as CRC and pancreatic adenocarcinoma (PDAC) at the molecular level to new depths. There is now a greater understanding of the cancer molecular subtypes and oncogenic signaling pathways that drive cancer. In addition, landmark studies have highlighted the critical relationship between the tumor, the surrounding microenvironment and immune system that is closely linked with the underlying cancer genetic alterations. Our expanded understanding of the cellular and molecular drivers of GI cancers has led to a dramatic increase in therapeutic strategies that have impacted clinical practice.

Mechanisms of genomic instability

Cancer is initiated by and progresses due to a series of genomic alterations. These alterations confer a selective survival advantage leading to the proliferation of dominant clones to establish a tumor. Using CRC as an example, three principal mechanisms leading to genomic instability have been identified – chromosomal instability (CIN), microsatellite instability (MSI), and CpG island methylator phenotypes (CIMP) – that we will discuss in more detail [5].

Chromosomal instability

Chromosomal instability has been associated with a variety of GI cancers. In particular, about 65–75% of sporadic CRC and about 49% of gastric cancers have CIN. CIN is defined by chromosomal defects leading to abnormal telomere stability, chromosomal segregation, DNA damage response, and loss of heterozygosity [5,6]. CIN is manifested by an imbalance in chromosome number, i.e., aneuploidy, and/or chromosome structure, e.g., subchromosomal genomic amplifications and loss of heterozygosity (LOH) [7]. These defects result in a variety of mutations in common protooncogenes and/or tumor suppressor genes (TSG). One well-described pathway of CIN is the multiple steps from adenoma to carcinoma sequence described

Yamada's Textbook of Gastroenterology, Seventh Edition. Edited by Timothy C. Wang, Michael Camilleri, Benjamin Lebwohl, Anna S. Lok, William J. Sandborn, Kenneth K. Wang, and Gary D. Wu.

Companion website: www.yamadagastro.com/textbook7e

by Vogelstein [8]. As a common example, isolated KRAS oncogene mutations can result in formation of precancerous polyps and are found in 30–60% of adenomas >1 cm. If a mutation to the tumor suppressor gene *APC* precedes the KRAS mutation, it is much more likely to result in neoplasia.

Microsatellite instability

The second type of genetic instability, MSI, is due to alterations in DNA mismatch repair (MMR) genes (*MLH1, MSH2, MSH6* or *PMS2*) that lead to accumulation of errors in DNA within short, repetitive sequences, termed microsatellites. MSI was discovered in Lynch syndrome (LS) patients. LS, also known as hereditary nonpolyposis colon cancer (HNPCC), is the most common form of hereditary colon cancer, accounting for 2–4% of all CRC cases [9]. LS is caused by a germline mutation in one of the MMR genes.

The MSI phenotype is also observed in around 10–15% of sporadic CRCs [10–12]. The mechanism responsible for MSI-H in sporadic CRCs is different from that in LS. The most common abnormality associated with MSI in sporadic CRC is epigenetic silencing of MMR genes due to hypermethylation of CpG islands in the promoter region [12]. Notably, MSI status in sporadic CRCs is of clinical importance, as it serves as a marker for a favorable prognosis and a decreased benefit, possibly even a detrimental effect, from adjuvant therapy in patients with stage II CRC [13,14]. Therefore, MSI/MMR testing is important in stage II patients as part of the decision making regarding the consideration of adjuvant therapy. The reason for the unexpected improved survival of MSI-H CRC patients, who harbor dramatically more mutations than MSS CRC patients [15], is an intriguing subject for future studies.

Early studies investigating MSI tumors established a strong relationship between MSI-high status and increased immune infiltration [16,17]. These studies also suggested that patients with MSI-high tumors have improved prognosis, highlighting the association between an immune phenotype and favorable biology. Patients with MSI-high tumors demonstrate increased expression of neo-antigens and increased infiltration of cytotoxic T cells [18]. Furthermore, MSI-H tumors are exceptionally sensitive to immune checkpoint therapy which is discussed in more detail later in the chapter [19]. A recent clinical trial of PD-1 blockade in patients with advanced MMR-deficient tumors, including CRC, demonstrated an objective response rate of 53%, with a complete response in 21% of patients [18].

CpG island methylation phenotype

The most common form of epigenetic instability in CRC is the CpG island methylation phenotype (CIMP), characterized by gene silencing due to hypermethylation of CpG islands found in promoter regions of genes throughout the genome [20]. Several groups have used different sets of promoters in order to define CIMP-positive tumors, some of which identified CIMP-high and CIMP-low subcategories [20–24]. In sporadic CRCs, biallelic hypermethylation of *MLH1* was first linked to the MSI-H phenotype [25–28], and later shown as part of the CIMP phenotype [22,23]. The CIMP phenotype is also present in gastric cancer (GC), where it is similarly associated with *MLH1* and *CDKN2A* hypermethylation [29] and MSI-H [30]. As in CRC, the link between hypermethylation of *MLH1* and MSI-H GC was also established [31]. However, in contrast to CRC, the clinical relevance of MSI-H in gastric cancer is unclear [32]. In addition, CIMP was noted in duodenal carcinoma, where it is associated with *MLH1* hypermethylation and MSI-H [33].

Oncogenic signaling pathways

The most basic hallmark of malignancies is their ability to maintain constant proliferation. To acquire this trait, cancer cells usually dysregulate pathways originating from cell surface growth factor receptors (GFRs). This chronic proliferation is achieved mainly by one or more of these four mechanisms: (1) overexpression of GFRs, (2) acquiring gain-of-function mutations in one of the intracellular components downstream of the GFRs, leading to constitutive activation of the pathway, (3) overproduction of growth factors which bind to and activate their corresponding receptors, and (4) induction of neighboring normal cells to produce growth factors which will bind to GFRs present on the cancer cells. Of these, the most studied alterations in GI malignancies are the first two, overexpression of GFRs and gain-of-function mutations in one of their downstream targets. Overexpression of GFRs can be due to increased transcription of the gene, decreased turnover of the protein following ligand binding to the receptor or increased copy number of the gene. The main pathway by which GI malignancies sustain proliferative signaling is the EGFR pathway and its two downstream pathways, namely, the KRAS-BRAF-MEK-ERK and the PI3K-AKT-mTOR pathways (Figure 27.1). Activation of this pathway results in sustained proliferation, as well as increased cell survival, cell cycle progression, angiogenesis, and invasion. In addition, the Wnt-β-catenin pathway plays a major role in promoting GI malignancies, particularly CRC and HCC. We will now describe in detail these pathways and their involvement in promoting GI malignancies.

EGFR pathway

Epidermal growth factor receptor (EGFR), also known as HER1 or ErbB1, is a member of the ErbB family of transmembrane receptor tyrosine kinases (RTKs), which includes three other members: HER2-ErbB2, HER3-ErbB3, and HER4-ErbB4. Overexpression of EGFR has been detected by immunohistochemistry (IHC) in 49–82% of CRCs [34–37], 32–71% of esophageal cancers (ECs) [38–40], 13–34% of GCs [41–44], and 53–66% of HCCs [45–47]. Several EGFR ligands like TGF-α are overexpressed in esophageal cancer (EC) [48] and GC [49].

Being the first and most studied component of these pathways, EGFR has long been a target for drug development. There are two classes of drugs targeting EGFR: monoclonal antibodies (mAbs) and tyrosine kinase inhibitors (TKI). mAbs bind to the extracellular domain of EGFR, thereby preventing other ligands from binding to the receptor. TKIs bind to the intracellular ATP-binding domain of EGFR, thereby competing with ATP and inhibiting EGFR autophosphorylation. Two anti-EGFR

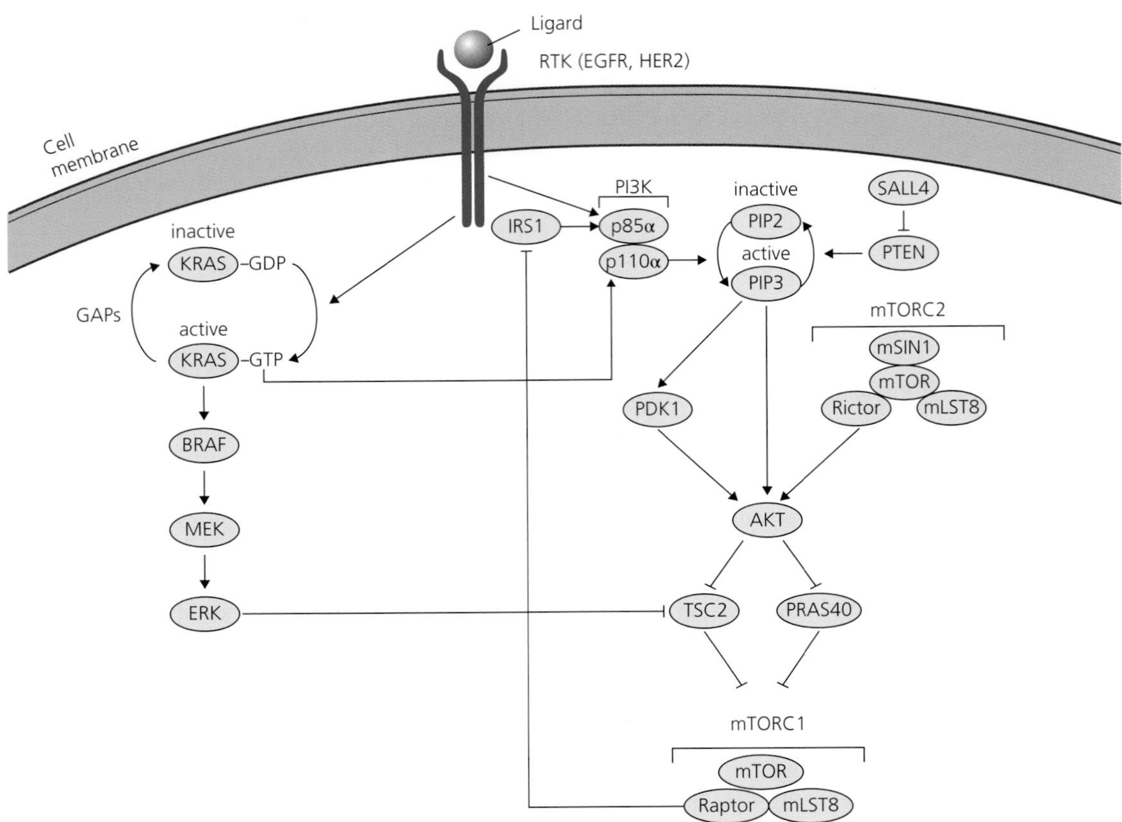

Figure 27.1 EGFR-mediated signaling pathways, KRAS-BRAF-MEK-ERK and PI3K-AKT-mTOR. Binding of a receptor-specific ligand activates epidermal growth factor receptor (EGFR), which in turn activates KRAS, and its following downstream targets BRAF, MEK and ERK, resulting in increased proliferation, cell survival, angiogenesis, and invasion. EGFR also activates phosphatidylinositol 3-kinase (PI3K) by binding to the p85α regulatory unit and removing its inhibitory effect on the p110α catalytic unit. This binding of PI3K to p85α can either be directly or through the adaptor molecule insulin receptor substrate 1 (IRS1). p110α then generates phosphatidylinositol-3,4,5-triphosphate (PIP3) from phosphatidylinositol-4,5-biphosphate (PIP2), while the reverse process is regulated by the phosphatase and tensin homologue [196] TSG. The oncofetal protein SALL4 inhibits PTEN. PIP3, along with its downstream target 3-phosphoinositide dependent protein kinase 1 (PDK1) and mammalian target of rapamycin (mTOR) complex 2 (mTORC2), activates AKT. Following AKT activation, the mTOR complex 1 (mTORC1) is activated through inhibition of two of its inhibitors, tuberous sclerosis complex 2 (TSC2) and PRAS40. mTORC1 activation eventually results in increased proliferation, cell growth, and angiogenesis. mTORC1 also activates a negative feedback loop through inhibition of IRS1. Components of the KRAS pathway also activate the PI3K pathway, i.e., KRAS activates the p110α catalytic unit of PI3K and ERK activates mTORC1 through inhibition of TSC2.

mAbs, cetuximab and panitumumab, are FDA approved for treating metastatic CRC patients [50,51]. In addition, the EGFR TKI erlotinib is FDA approved for use in combination with gemcitabine as first-line treatment for locally advanced and metastatic PDAC [52].

KRAS-BRAF-MEK-ERK pathway

When KRAS is mutated, it remains constitutively activated, leading to aberrant signaling of downstream pathways involved in invasion, apoptosis, and proliferation [53]. Mutations in the *KRAS* gene are found in approximately 40% of CRCs [54,55] and >95% of PDACs [56,57]. Most commonly, KRAS mutations are primarily at codons 12, 13, or 61. The specific mutation has implications for a biological effect and aggressiveness of the RAS mutation. The clinical relevance of the KRAS status of GI tumors is highlighted by the convincing evidence that mutations in RAS are good predictors for resistance to EGFR mAB in patients with CRC [50,58].

Immediately downstream of KRAS is BRAF, a member of the Raf serine/threonine kinases family. The most prevalent *BRAF* mutation, V600E, is found in around 8% of CRCs [59] and is less prevalent in HCCs and PDACs (4% and 2%, respectively) [60]. Interestingly, V600E *BRAF* mutation and *KRAS* mutations are mutually exclusive in CRC [59,61], suggesting that these events are genetically redundant, and that alterations in both genes do not confer a further advantage in CRC.

Downstream of BRAF is MEK, also known as mitogen-activated protein kinase (MAPK), a dual-specificity tyrosine and serine/threonine kinase, and ERK, also known as mitogen-activated protein kinase (MAPK). ERK is a serine/threonine kinase, which upon activation dissociates from MEK and translocates into the nucleus. ERK then phosphorylates and activates numerous targets, including transcription factors (TFs), leading to increased proliferation, as well as promoting cell survival, angiogenesis, and invasion.

Due to the high frequency of KRAS mutations across multiple cancers, it has been researched as a potential target although it has proven to be difficult due to the number of protein–protein interactions [53]. One approach to target KRAS-mutated cancers is to employ the concept of synthetic lethality [62]. Inhibiting a protein that is synthetic lethal to KRAS-mutated cancer cells should selectively kill them, while sparing normal cells. This approach led to the identification of the noncanonical IκB kinase TBK1 as a possible synthetic lethal protein to KRAS [63]. Other synthetic lethal targets being explored as a therapy strategy include BCL2 and CDK4 [62,64].

Encouragingly, recent novel strategies targeting mutant KRAS either directly or against essential mediators of KRAS-mediated signaling have demonstrated positive therapeutic effects. The breakthrough development of synthetic RAS protein–protein inhibitors that can effectively block mutant KRAS signaling has gained enthusiasm [53]. Although early in development, a recent $KRAS^{G12C}$ specific inhibitor, ARS-1620, demonstrated in vivo; antitumoral activity in PDAC [65]. Perhaps more immediately clinically relevant, novel combination therapeutic strategies incorporating inhibitors of downstream signaling mediators such as ERK have demonstrated promise in targeting KRAS-driven PDAC [66]. Evidence suggests that autophagy is upregulated in KRAS-driven PDAC and is critical for cancer progression [67]. In parallel, one group determined that ERK inhibition could block alternative essential KRAS-dependent metabolic processes. Taking advantage of this observation, a recent investigation convincingly demonstrated that combination of ERK inhibition with an autophagy inhibitor, chloroquine, targeted multiple metabolic processes to synergistically blocked in vivo; PDAC growth [66]. This concept holds great promise for future clinical trials in PDAC as well as other KRAS-driven cancers.

PI3K-AKT-mTOR pathway

The PI3K-AKT-mTOR pathway is the second most commonly abrogated pathway in cancer, after the p53 tumor suppressor pathway, and as such is the target of many investigational drugs, most of which are small inhibitors targeting kinases in this pathway. Phosphatidylinositol 3-kinase (PI3K) phosphorylates phosphatidylinositol-4,5-biphosphate (PIP2), thereby catalyzing the production of phosphatidylinositol-3,4,5-triphosphate (PIP3) (see Figure 27.1). PIP3, along with 3-phosphoinositide-dependent protein kinase 1 (PDK1) and mammalian target of rapamycin (mTOR) complex 2 (mTORC2), a complex composed of mTOR and other factors, participates in activation of AKT through its phosphorylation (see Figure 27.1). Mutations in the *PIK3CA* gene, encoding for the p110α catalytic subunit, were found in 14–32% of CRCs [68–71], 4–11% of GCs [71–73], and 36% of HCC [72]. In addition, *PIK3CA* amplifications were found in 36% of GCs [74]. Interestingly, in PDAC, 80% of mutations of the TSG PTEN, either through deletion of at least one copy (15%) or low to absent expression (70%), were associated with overactivation of AKT [75].

Wnt-β-catenin pathway

The Wnt-β-catenin pathway is one of the most often dysregulated pathways in CRC, with one report documenting mutations in one or more members of this pathway in over 94% of cases, predominantly in the adenomatous polyposis coli (*APC*) TSG [76] (Figure 27.2). The signaling cascade begins with Wnt ligands binding to a receptor complex composed of LRP5/6 and Frizzled (Fzd), with the latter being overexpressed in 18% of CRC cases [76]. Activation of the receptor complex leads to inhibition of the kinase activity of a "destruction complex" which then targets β-catenin for phosphorylation, leading to its proteasomal degradation [77]. Wnt signaling results in β-catenin accumulation and translocation to the nucleus, where it converts the T-cell factor/lymphoid enhancer factor (TCF/LEF) family into transcriptional activators (see Figure 27.2) [77,78].

The Wnt-β-catenin pathway is also known to be involved in HCC pathogenesis [79,80]. Studies revealed that this pathway is the most frequently altered pathway in HCC, with activating mutations in *CTNNB1* and inactivating mutations in *AXIN1* and *APC* found in 16–33%, 5–15% and around 2% of HCCs, respectively, in a mutually exclusive pattern [81,82]. In addition, a combined analysis of mutations and CNAs showed that this pathway was dysregulated in around 60% of HCCs [82]. Similar results were reported analyzing CNAs only, showing that the Wnt-β-catenin pathway is altered in 38% of HCCs [83]. Accumulation of β-catenin, reported in 10–50% of HCC tumors, has been linked to poor prognosis and disease progression [84]. The development of sorafenib, a multikinase inhibitor that targets several pathways, resulted in decreased β-catenin protein levels as well as reduction of mRNA levels of other genes targeted by Wnt [85,86]. Sorafenib has since become the approved standard of care monotherapy but studies have demonstrated prolonged overall survival by only 2.8 months [87].

APC role in CRC

Hyperactivation of the Wnt-β-catenin pathway in CRC is usually the result of inactivation of the *APC* TSG, which is found in 77% of CRCs [76]. The *APC* mutation was originally discovered by virtue of its association with the inheritance of FAP autosomal dominant syndrome [88,89]. FAP patients inherit one defective *APC* allele, usually harboring a truncating mutation, and then acquire a similar inactivating mutation in the other allele or lose the other allele (LOH) [90]. In accordance with the "two-hit" hypothesis introduced by Knudson [91], cancers develop once a TSG is hit in both alleles. As a result of complete loss of APC, classic FAP patients develop multiple colorectal adenomatous polyps (typically >100) by their early 20s. This burden of adenomas inevitably progresses to colon cancer by the age of 50, through accumulation of mutations in other TSGs or oncogenes, such as *TP53*, *SMAD4*, and *KRAS*. Therefore, prophylactic removal of the colon is the mainstay of clinical management of classic FAP patients. Similar to FAP, the *APC* gene is most commonly inhibited by a truncating mutation which is found in the majority of sporadic colorectal adenomas and cancers [92]. Hypermethylation of the *APC* promoter was also reported as a mechanism of *APC* inactivation, noted in 18% of sporadic CRCs [93]. These data emphasize the major role of the Wnt-β-catenin pathway in CRC pathogenesis.

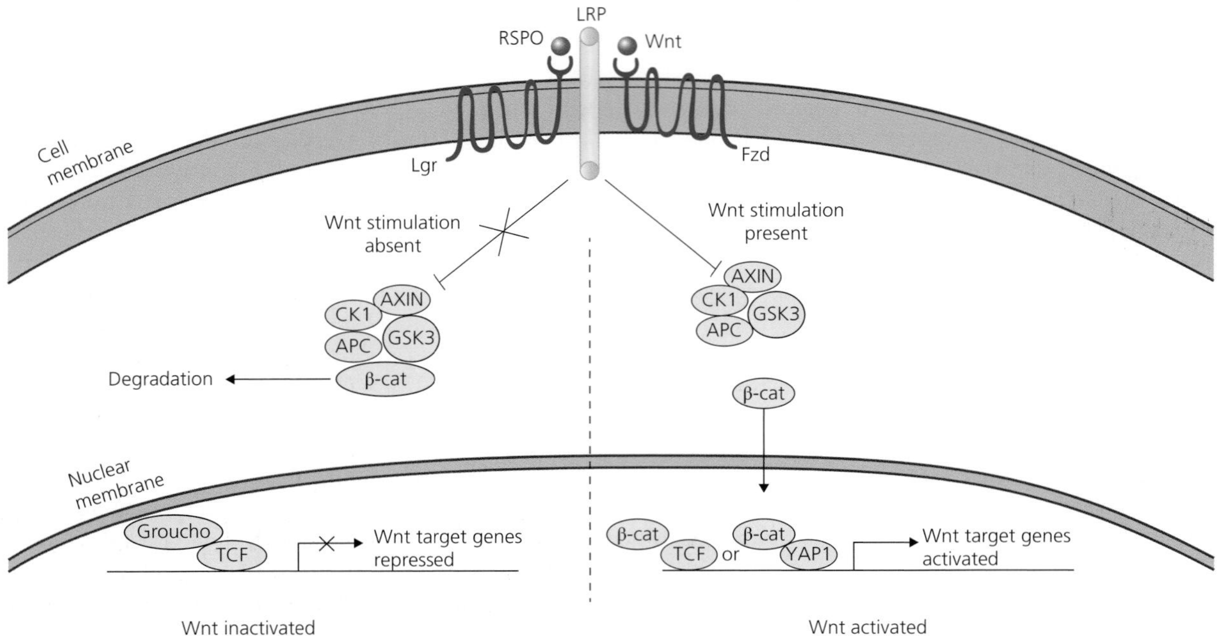

Figure 27.2 Wnt-β-catenin signaling. Wnt signaling is activated mainly by Wnt ligands binding to the Frizzled (Fzd) receptor, but also by R-spondins (RSPOs) binding to the Lgr receptor. In the absence of Wnt signaling, a "destruction complex" composed of AXIN, casein kinase (CK1), glycogen synthase kinase 3 (GSK3), and adenomatous polyposis coli (APC) targets β-catenin for proteasomal degradation. This is achieved through β-catenin phosphorylation by CK1 and GSK3, leading to its recognition and ubiquitination by an E3 ubiquitin-ligase. In this scenario, the T-cell factor (TCF) transcription factor is bound by the corepressor Groucho, leading to transcriptional repression of Wnt target genes. In the presence of Wnt signaling, the destruction complex is inhibited, allowing β-catenin to translocate to the nucleus. Following entry into the nucleus, β-catenin displaces Groucho and, together with TCF or possibly with Yes-associated protein 1 (YAP1), activates transcription of Wnt target genes, such as MYC and Cyclin D1.

Molecular classifications of gastrointestinal cancers

Large multiomic databases such as the Cancer Genome Atlas have redefined classification of cancers such as CRC and PDAC by identifying distinct molecular subtypes related to anatomy [76,94–99] (Figure 27.3). These large database studies stratified CRC as well as PDAC into various subtypes based on genetic signature and histology that have demonstrated significance to clinical practice. These studies demonstrated that most GI cancers are nonhypermutated with low number of methylated genes. The International CRC subtyping consortium has characterized four molecular subtypes (CMS): CMS1 which is MSI immune and consists of about 15% of CRC; CMS2 known as the canonical subtype which makes up 37%; CMS3 which is metabolic occurring in 13%; and CMS4 which is mesenchymal in 23%. CMS1 includes most of the MSI tumors and is highly hypermethylated and hypermutated but associated with lower rates of mutation in somatic copy number (SCNAs). CMS2 is found more frequently originating from the left colon but has higher survival rates following relapse than CMS1 tumors. CMS3 cancers often contain high numbers of KRAS-activating mutations and are more metabolically stable. CMS4 is associated with worse survival and is found in more advanced stages of CRC. In addition, CMS4 cancers tend to have a mesenchymal phenotype with overexpression of genes related to stromal infiltration.

Similarly, multiple studies have stratified PDAC into various subtypes based on genetic signature and histology. Early on, classical and quasi-mesenchymal subtypes were categorized based on their improved responses to EGFR inhibitor or gemcitabine respectively [97]. Another group of researchers further subtyped PDAC by characterizing the aberrantly differentiated endocrine exocrine subtype (ADEX), the squamous subtype which was found to have p53, KDM6A, and TP63DN mutations, and finally the immunogenic subtype which is more likely to respond to immunotherapy [98].

The potential value of molecular subtypes was recently highlighted by the PDAC COMPASS prospective clinical trial. This trial demonstrated the feasibility and predictive value of pretherapy genetic analysis by genome sequencing of PDAC biopsies to categorize tumors before starting FOLFIRINOX therapy. This study revealed that classic tumors were more responsive to FOLFIRINOX than basal-like tumors [99]. The continued expansion of the molecular/cellular classification of GI cancers holds great promise for more successful precision medicine application to improve clinical outcomes.

Tumor microenvironment

There is a growing appreciation of the relationship between tumor genomics and the tumor microenvironment. Whole-genome and multiplex analyses provide a high-resolution view of this phenomenon, showing that different areas within a

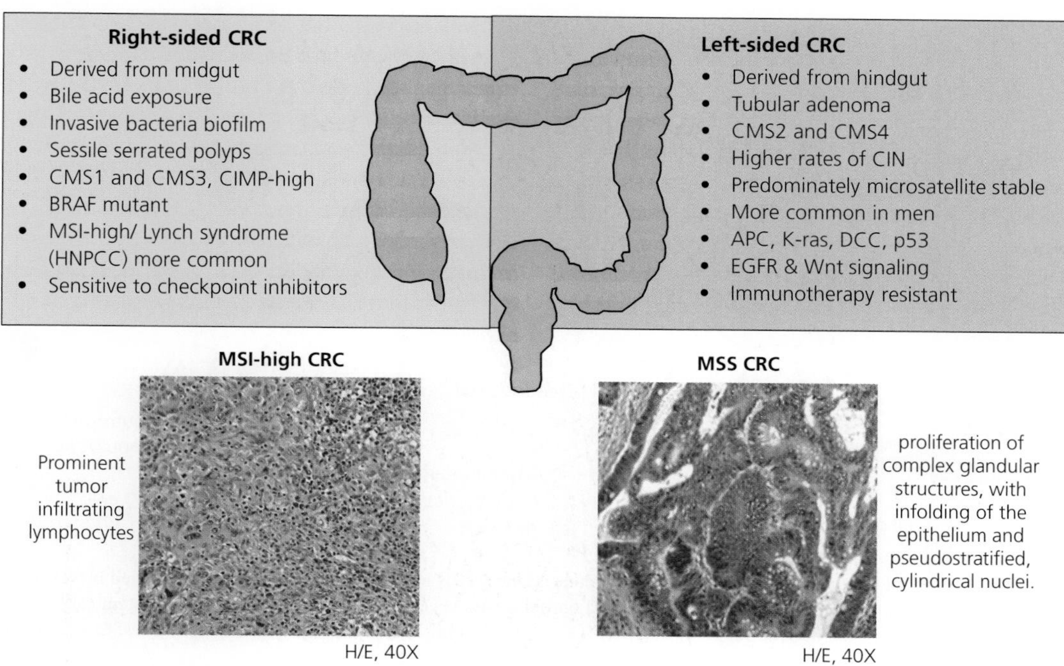

Figure 27.3 Characteristic molecular subtypes of CRC by anatomical location. The upper panel demonstrates the variation in CMS subtypes and tumor characteristics based on colorectal cancer location. The lower panel displays the central pathological differences between MSI-high and MSS colorectal cancers.

specific tumor display varying landscapes and interactions between malignant and nontransformed cells in what is referred to as the tumor microenvironment (TME) [100]. The impact of the TME on cancer progression and response to treatment has been well established in various GI malignancies including CRC [101], HCC [102], and PDAC [103, 104]. Specific components of the TME that this section will focus on are the immune landscape, the stroma, and tumor vasculature.

Tumor immune microenvironment

The fact the endogenous immune system has a built-in antitumor function has been well studied and documented. In fact, the principles around immunotherapy, which will be discussed further at the end of this chapter, focus on amplifying or turning on this cancer-targeting immune function [105]. The contribution of various immune cells such as macrophages, T cells, natural killer (NK) cells, and cytokines like IFN-γ and IL-12 to tumor immunogenicity has been shown in many studies over the past few decades (Figure 27.4). Pioneering studies in CRC have strengthened the association between the tumor immune landscape and clinical prognosis [106–109]. Investigations in CRC demonstrated the clinical significance of the tumor infiltrating lymphocyte (TIL) [110] highlighted by the development of the Immunoscore, which is a scoring system that focuses on density of CD3 and CD8 cell populations in the TME [111]. This histology-based analysis has been validated internationally as the strongest prognostic feature for CRC [112]. Unfortunately, the vast majority of GI cancers are "cold" tumors with a small population of TILs and low antigenicity. This feature has limited the clinical impact of current immunotherapy strategies that seek to harness the antitumor immune cell populations.

Cancers also recruit immunosuppressive cells to establish a favorable supportive microenvironment that works against the adaptive immune response [113–116]. Cell populations such as T regulatory (TReg) cells, tumor-associated macrophages (TAMs), marrow-derived suppressor cells (MDSCs), cancer-associated fibroblasts (CAFs), and tumor-associated neutrophils (TANs) are involved in immunosuppressive effects that result in inhibition of antitumor activity [102]. As demonstrated in multiple GI malignancies, high levels of these immunosuppressive cells in tumors are often associated with poor prognosis or poor immunotherapeutic response. The mechanistic effects of these tumor-associated inflammatory cells and mediators include promoting survival, angiogenesis, migration and invasion of cancer cells and mediating immunosuppression [113,115–117]. The close relationship between the immunosuppressive TME and chronic inflammation to promote cancer is discussed later in the chapter.

The growing interest in the tumor immune microenvironment has led to discoveries revealing the immune escape tactics of various cancers. In particular, PDAC is known to utilize multiple mechanisms that aid in immune evasion, such as downregulating MHC I molecules, thereby preventing CD8+ T-cell recognition [118]. This method of avoiding immune detection has also been observed in CRC [119]. Pancreatic exosomes are another immune escape mechanism that results in transfer of miRNA to dendritic cells, ultimately decreasing MHC II expression [120]. PDAC also has very low antigen expression for immune detection which is further compounded by inhibited MHC molecule expression. Our expanding knowledge of immune escape strategies used by cancers will hopefully shed light on next-generation immunotherapy strategies.

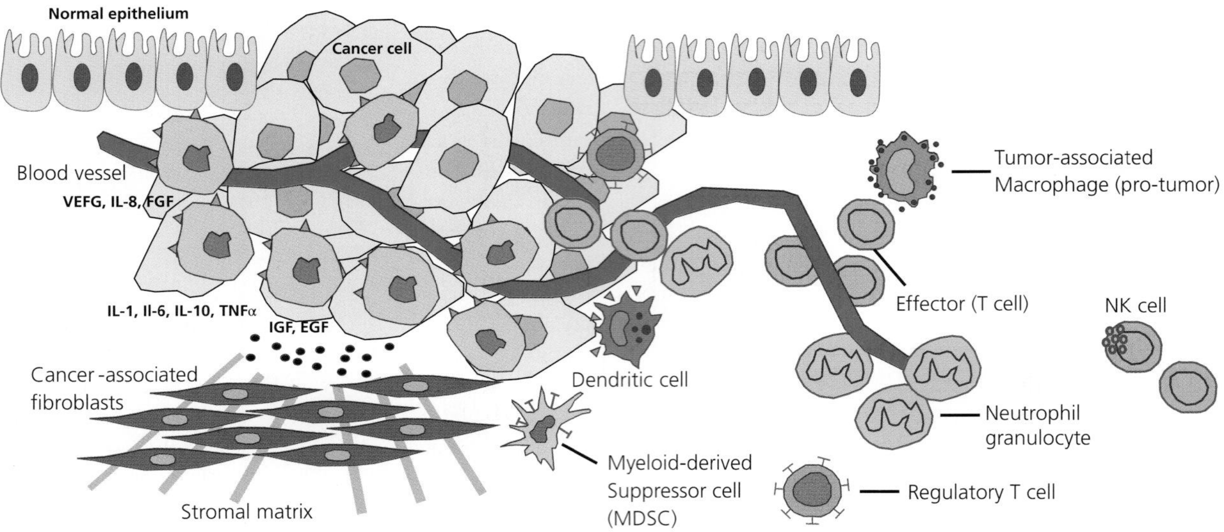

Figure 27.4 Schematic diagram of the primary tumor microenvironment. Cancer cells in the primary tumor are surrounded by various cells comprising the tumor microenvironment, including cancer-associated fibroblasts (CAFs), endothelial cells, mesenchymal stem cells (MSCs), tumor-associated macrophages (TAMs), myeloid-derived suppressor cells (MDSCs), neutrophils, and various B and T lymphocytes. Extensive cross-talk between tumor cells and the microenvironment regulates growth and progression.

Stroma

Stroma, primarily composed of connective tissue, is the functional support for all organs as well as cancer. Found within stroma are fibroblasts, osteoblasts, chondrocytes, mesenchymal stromal cells, and extracellular matrix (ECM). The ECM consists of proteoglycans, glycoproteins, and other fibrous molecules and is generated by fibroblasts.

In recent years, tumor stroma has been identified as a crucial component of the tumor microenvironment and alterations within the stroma can aid in cancer development, progression, and metastasis [121] (see Figure 27.4). In PDAC, the microenvironment consists of reactive desmoplastic stroma that can constitute up to 80% of the volume of the tumor [122]. Conceptually, the desmoplastic tumor stroma is thought to contribute to cancer aggressiveness and immunosuppression [123]. The density of the stroma results in an impenetrable obstacle to immune infiltration, preventing penetration of T cells into the TME to support tumor progression [124]. Furthermore, hyaluronic acid (HA), the major component of normal ECM, is significantly increased in several GI malignancies such as PDAC and has been implicated in tumor progression, treatment resistance, and poor prognosis. The pegylated recombinant human hyaluronidase (PEGPH20) was first investigated in PDAC patients to target the stroma with early promising results as reported in the phase II HALO 202 trial [125]. Subsequently, PEGPH20 efficacy was investigated in the SWOG S1313 trial, a phase Ib/II study of modified FOLFIRINOX plus PEGPH20 in PDAC patients. Unfortunately, the addition of PEGPH20 to FOLFIRINOX was detrimental [126]. These conflicting results have slowed the concept of targeting the stromal compartment, but it remains an active investigational strategy.

Cancer-associated fibroblasts (CAFs) further promote tumorigenesis by producing many growth factors and proinflammatory cytokines to support angiogenesis and modulate the immune microenvironment [127]. CAFs have the ability to both recruit immunosuppressive cells and inhibit cytotoxic T cells to promote cancer [128,129]. In addition, they can modify the ECM to serve as a physical barrier to immune infiltration. As a result of their promotion of tumorigenesis in the TME, CAFs have become an appealing target for immunotherapy in cancer [130].

Tumor vasculature

The tumor vasculature represents another critical component of the TME that cancers have harnessed to support growth and progression [131]. Blood vessels within the TME are generally functionally abnormal and have been found to promote the hypoxic, acidic and high-pressure environment to promote tumorigenesis and progression [132]. The development of the highly abnormal vasculature is driven by tumor-secreted proangiogenic factors. Angiogenesis cytokines such as vascular endothelial growth factor (VEGF), interleukin (IL)-8, and fibroblastic growth factor (FGF) are secreted within the TME and overpower the antiangiogenesis factors [131]. The resulting network of vasculature created is disorganized and porous with relatively poor perfusion and high interstitial fluid pressure within the tumor. Another major impact of this aberrant vasculature is prevention of secretion of signaling molecules to recruit immune cells and allow infiltration, therefore aiding in immune evasion [100]. With respect to therapeutic strategy, aberrant vasculature also acts as a barrier to delivery of any chemo or immunotherapeutic regimen to the tumor [100].

Considering the divers roles that the tumor vasculature plays to promote cancer, it remains a popular therapeutic target with several agents at various stages of clinical development. The most widespread and first-used clinical therapy to target the VEGF pathway is the humanized mAB bevacizumab [133]. Currently, it is approved for first-line therapy for metastatic CRC in combination with chemotherapy. Other agents such as aflibercept, a decoy VEGF receptor, and ramucirumab, a mAB targeting VEGF-2, have growing indications for GI cancers [134,135].

Inflammation, cancer, and the microbiome

Chronic inflammatory conditions of various etiologies predispose to cancer types throughout the GI tract. Approximately 20% of all cancers are preceded by infection, or chronic inflammation at the same organ site [115]. Barrett esophagus, caused by chronic gastroesophageal reflux disease (GERD), confers an 11-fold increased risk of esophageal cancer [136]. Similarly, microbial infection with H. pylori confers a sixfold increased risk of GC [137], and HCV infection increases risk of HCC by 20–70-fold [138–140]. Patients with ulcerative colitis (UC), an autoimmune disease, have an increased risk of CRC, depending on the extent, duration, and activity of disease. Specifically, pancolitis confers a 15–19-fold increase in risk, while disease limited to the left side of the colon is associated with about a threefold relative risk [141,142]. Primary sclerosing cholangitis (PSC), an idiopathic disease, confers a >100-fold risk of CC [143]. Collectively, these observations suggest a significant role for inflammation in initiation of carcinogenesis.

Evidence at the cellular and molecular level has strengthened the convincing link between chronic inflammation and cancer initiation and progression. For instance, mouse models of colitis-associated CRC have convincingly demonstrated that nuclear factor κB signaling as a central mediator of inflammation is closely linked to cancer development [144]. In addition, inflammatory macrophages and neutrophils release reactive oxygen species (ROS) and reactive nitrogen species (RNS) which can induce DNA breaks and mutations, potentially accelerating the genetic instability of cancer cells [115,145–147]. Evidence implicates chronic intestinal inflammation as a driver of p53 and additional mutations in epithelial cells [148]. Proinflammatory cytokines can also stimulate tumor progression and drive DNA methylation, leading to suppression of TSGs and DNA repair genes [149]. In CRC, the expression of inflammatory cytokines and myeloid cell subsets is associated with poor prognosis [150].

Inflammatory cells such as macrophages, neutrophils, and MDSCs are now considered an essential component of the tumor microenvironment that can be protumorigenic [113,115,116,147]. Recently, MDSCs have been characterized as immature myeloid cells that can impair antigen-presenting capabilities and generate an immunosuppressive environment by promoting expansion of TRegs via oxidative stress and amino acid deprivation [151]. Studies using colitis-induced CRC models supported a central role for the MDSC by demonstrating that depletion of MDSCs significantly reduced tumorigenesis. In addition, the ability of PDAC to recruit myeloid cells confers resistance to gemcitabine. The mechanistic effects of these tumor-associated inflammatory cells and mediators include promoting survival, angiogenesis, migration and invasion of cancer cells, and mediating immunosuppression [113,115–117].

NSAIDs can reduce colorectal initiation and progression

The above molecular and observational studies were the basis for the hypothesis that antiinflammatory drugs could possibly be used for CRC prevention and treatment. As inflammation plays a critical role in cancer development, antiinflammatory therapy has been investigated as a means of prevention. In fact, RCTs with long-term follow-up have shown that daily aspirin taken for at least 5 years reduced the risk of proximal colon cancer and rectal cancer by around 65% and 40%, respectively [152]. In addition, metaanalysis of observational studies of CRC, esophageal and gastric cancer showed that daily aspirin reduced the incidence of each of these cancers by around 40% [153]. Furthermore, metaanalysis of eight RCTs showed that daily aspirin also reduced mortality from CRC and esophageal cancer after 20 years of follow-up by around 40% and 60%, respectively [154]. The use of aspirin is limited, however, by the significant incidence of GI hemorrhage.

Aspirin exerts its antiinflammatory effect through inhibition of cyclooxygenase (COX)-1 and COX-2, with most of the aspirin-associated side-effects related to inhibition of COX-1 (Figure 27.5). Therefore, COX-2 selective inhibitors (COXIBs) have also been assessed for CRC prevention and treatment. Indeed, three large RCTs using COXIBs showed a reduction of risk of colorectal adenoma recurrence [155–157]. Unfortunately, COXIBs also confer unacceptable cardiovascular and thrombotic adverse side-effects [158,159], particularly in patients with preexisting atherosclerotic heart disease [160].

There are several ongoing and planned phase III RCTs addressing the possible use of NSAIDs in cancer prevention and treatment. The ongoing AspECT trial is studying the use of a combination of aspirin with a proton pump inhibitor (PPI) in preventing esophageal cancer in patients with Barrett esophagus (NCT00357682). The ongoing ASCOLT trial is studying aspirin use in improving survival of CRC patients with local or regional spread (NCT00565708). Following a successful phase IIb/III trial [161], combination of the NSAID sulindac with DFMO, an inhibitor of ornithine decarboxylase, in preventing colorectal adenoma recurrence is being evaluated in the ongoing phase III PACES trial (NCT01349881). Similarly, an active RCT in FAP patients is testing this combination for prevention of FAP-related events, including cancer (NCT01483144). In LS patients, the active CAPP3 trial seeks to establish the optimum dose and duration of aspirin treatment needed to prevent CRC [162]. Results from these trials, to be completed several years from now, will hopefully lead to the approved use of these regimens for the corresponding indications.

Tumor microbiome

Long associated with chronic inflammation, the human microbiota has recently been implicated as an important mediator of GI cancer progression. The human microbiota, consisting of multiple bacteria, viruses, fungi and other microorganisms and the corresponding collective genomes of which it is made, the microbiome, has recently come into focus in cancer biology [163]. Interestingly, microbiota are present in about 20% human tumors including colorectal and pancreatic

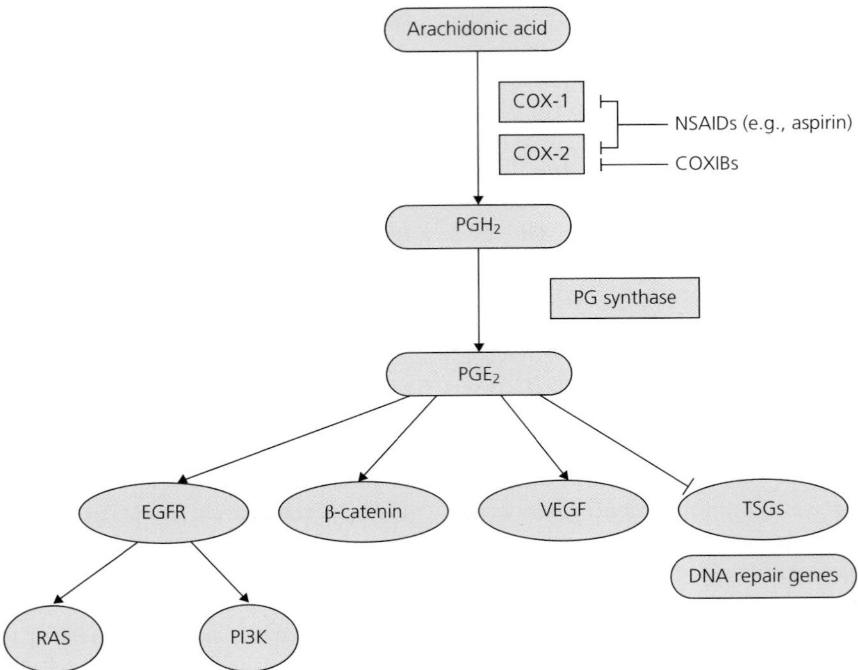

Figure 27.5 Overview of the mechanisms underlying the tumor-inhibitory effects of nonsteroidal antiinflammatory drugs (NSAIDs) and cyclooxygenase-2 (COX-2) selective inhibitors (COXIBs). Cyclooxygenase-1 (COX-1) and COX-2 are responsible for the enzymatic conversion of arachidonic acid to prostaglandin H_2 (PGH_2), which is later metabolized to prostaglandin E_2 (PGE_2). Both COX-1 and COX-2 are inhibited by NSAIDs, whereas COXIBs inhibit only COX-2. In the absence of COX inhibition, PGE_2 promotes proliferation, survival, invasion, and angiogenesis through activating epidermal growth factor receptor (EGFR) and its downstream pathways, β-catenin signaling and VEGF, and also by promoting epigenetic silencing of certain tumor suppressor genes (TSGs) and DNA repair genes.

cancers [163]. In fact, multiple bacterial species have been linked to the process of carcinogenesis [164]. For example, Fusobacterium nucleatum has been found in colorectal cancer tumors and has been shown to promote proliferation and tumor growth. One mechanism that F. nucleatum could contribute to tumorigenesis is through activation of the Wnt-β-catenin pathway via the binding of F. nucleatum adhesis (FadA) to E-cadherin on the surface of the CRC tumor cells [165]. Inflammation resulting from gram-negative bacteria causes an imbalance of oxidative stress which has been linked to development of cancer, resulting in altered metabolism and DNA damage that can promote tumorigenesis [163,166]. F. nucleatum has also been found to bind T-cell immunoreceptor with an Ig and ITIM domain (TIGIT) which is an immune inhibitory receptor, leading to dysfunction of TILs and NK cells [164].

Already the significance of microbiota in development of cancer is becoming relevant in clinical applications. Intriguingly, microbiota within tumors may confer resistance to specific chemotherapeutic agents. One investigation demonstrated that the presence of intratumoral Gammaproteobacteria was responsible for gemcitabine resistance and that specific antibiotics could reverse this effect [167]. Additionally, recent studies have associated the composition of the microbiome to the immune response against PDAC [168,169]. For example, loss of bacteria from the gut results in upregulated PD-1 expression. Conversely, gut microbiota ablation with antibiotics can reprogram the immune microenvironment to favor T-cell activation and improve immunotherapy response [170]. Intriguingly, the transplantation of fecal microbiota administered in pill form is being studied as a possible means of remodeling a PDAC nonresponder's GI microbiome to that of a responder [163].

Advances in therapy for gastrointestinal cancers

Our improved understanding of both the molecular drivers and the cellular components of GI cancers has led to notable advances in therapeutic strategies. As we have noted throughout this chapter, recent investigations have led to therapeutic approaches targeting the TME components such as the stroma, vasculature, and microbiota as well as specific novel strategies for KRAS mutant cancers. The significant clinical impact of the immune landscape not only in tumor progression but also with respect to predicting prognosis and survival has refueled interest in immunotherapy strategies. In addition, the recent landmark discovery of immune checkpoint molecules like programmed death-1 (PD-l), programmed death ligand-1 (PD-L1), and cytotoxic T-lymphocyte antigen 4 (CTLA-4) has dramatically changed the field of tumor immunology, resulting in therapeutic approaches that have revolutionized clinical oncology.

The concept of immune surveillance has been evolving since the early 1990s when it was noted by several scientists that components of the immune system engaged in antitumor activity [171–173]. As far back as 1996, studies reported increased antitumor activity against transplanted colon carcinoma in mice in response to blockade of CTLA-4 as well as slowed growth of established tumors [174]. Investigations have demonstrated that cancers harness immune checkpoint mediators such as PD-1 and CTLA-4 to escape an antitumor immune response [175]. In the cancer microenvironment, immune checkpoints can be overexpressed on either immune cells or the tumor itself to diminish tumoral immunity [176].

The FDA has approved use of PD-1 and PD-L1 checkpoint inhibitors in advanced liver, colorectal, and gastric cancers. Checkpoint inhibitors enable cytotoxic T cells (CD8+ effector) as well as CD4+ T cells to maintain an effective immune response and kill antigen-expressing cancer cells [175]. Unfortunately, most CRC and PDAC tumors are microsatellite stable and nonhypermutated with low TILs, rendering this strategy less effective [177]. In contrast, PD-1 blockade is very effective in MSI-high GI cancers and tumors with high tumor mutational burden. In CRC, for example, one study investigating PD-1 blockade in patients with advanced CRC with MMR-deficient tumors reported 53% objective response rate and 21% complete response rate [178]. Additionally, a phase II trial looking at refractory metastatic CRC reported a 40% objective response rate in MSI-high tumors compared with a 0% response rate in MSS tumors [179].

Despite some response in particular subsets of patients, results of monotherapy with checkpoint inhibitors in GI malignancies have been largely disappointing. As a result, investigations into combination therapies have begun and appear more promising, especially for GI cancers [180]. Combination therapies with conventional therapies such as chemotherapy or radiation have potential to promote tumor immunogenicity, increase tumor antigen recognition, and reduce immunosuppressive components. Combination of immunotherapy with chemotherapy improved response in an in vivo; CRC model where mice treated with CTLA-4 inhibitor in combination with ixabepilone or paclitaxel demonstrated a tumor rejection rate of 50–70% [181].

Clinical trials involving immunotherapy combinations for GI cancer are rapidly expanding. In PDAC, for example, there are currently more than 20 clinical trials combining immunotherapy with radiation therapy [104]. One combination immunotherapy of note that has just recently been approved by the FDA for metastatic CRC is the combination of 0pilumumab (anti-CTLA-4) and nivolumab (anti-PD-1). The CHECKMATE-142 study results showed that progression-free survival was 76% at 9 months and 71% at 12 months with overall survival rates of 87% and 85% respectively [182,183]. Another combination therapy breakthrough in HCC was recently reported from the phase III IMbrave150 study which showed that the PD-L1 inhibitor atezolizumab and the VEGF inhibitor bevacizumab resulted in improved overall survival and response compared to sorafenib. This is particularly noteworthy as it is the first new treatment to improve survival in HCC compared to the standard of care, sorafenib [184].

Novel immunotherapy approaches

The success of immune checkpoint inhibitors in oncology has fueled research into additional immunotherapy strategies, especially for tumors with low TILs. One strategy that has been explored in PDAC is the use of tumor vaccines such as GVAX vaccine (irradiated allogeneic PDAC cells that express the immunostimulatory cytokine GM-CSF) [185]. In preclinical and clinical trials, the GVAX vaccine has induced cytotoxic T-cell infiltration, increased PD-L1 expression in the tumor, and demonstrated promising in vivo; tumor responses [186–188]. Several ongoing trials have incorporated GVAX in combination strategies (NCT02243371, NCT03161379, NCT03190265, NCT02451982, NCT03767582). Additional vaccine strategies delivering specific cancer antigen-carrying dendritic cells are in various stages of clinical trials.

Utilization of autologous immune cells and genetically engineered antigen receptors for oncologic therapy is well under way. Adoptive cell therapy (ACT) with endogenous TILS and chimeric antigen receptor (CAR) T cell therapy are two methods that have had very promising results with high response rates in multiple malignancies [189,190]. ACT relies on TILS identification of nonself antigen through MHC molecules which is problematic in cancers like PDAC that actively downregulate MHC expression. In contrast, CAR T cells are composed of an antibody linked to the CD3ζ TCR signaling domain. Thus, this approach does not depend on antigen presentation by MHC molecules, but rather recognizes the unprocessed protein on the cell surface [191]. A phase I clinical trial using mesothelin-targeted CAR T cells resulted in tumor responses in three of six PDAC patients (NCT01897415) [192]. Additional phase I clinical trials targeting mesothelin (lentiviral transduced; NCT03323944) and PSCA (NCT02744287) are also currently under way. Based on promising preclinical trial results, multiple clinical trials involving ACT and CAR T cell therapy are ongoing in CRC, HCC, and PDAC [193–195].

Conclusions

Gastrointestinal malignancies are a very diverse group of cancers, each with a very unique genome, classification structure, and set of therapeutic challenges. However, constant themes still prevail such as the role of the TME and the impact of tumor mutational profile on TILs that can be translated across tumor types. This complex network in the TME of malignant and nontransformed cells and signaling pathways that promote cancer is becoming more appreciated. As a result, cancer biology and therapeutic interventions have shifted focus from the tumor epithelial cancer cell to the multicellular network that promotes cancer. Our greater understanding of this complex interaction and the relationship with cancer genomics has directly led to the development of new therapeutic strategies for GI cancers. In parallel, the shift in focus on tumor immunology as highlighted by the advent of checkpoint inhibitors has brought new-found optimism and hope even for devastating diseases such as PDAC.

References are available at www.yamadagastro.com/textbook7e

CHAPTER 28

Drug metabolism, transport, and pharmacogenomics

Ann M. Moyer and Joel M. Reid
Mayo Clinic College of Medicine and Science, Rochester, MN, USA

Chapter menu

General principles

Numerous physicochemical and biochemical processes influence the absorption, distribution, metabolism, and excretion of drugs and other xenobiotics. Following oral administration, small lipophilic molecules cross the intestinal mucosa by passive diffusion. Without subsequent chemical modifications, these compounds tend to sequester in adipose tissue or bind to plasma proteins, potentially accumulating to toxic concentrations. As such, elimination frequently includes metabolic events that convert hydrophobic compounds into hydrophilic, inactive metabolites to facilitate excretion into bile or urine. The typical sequence of events divides xenobiotic metabolism into two categories: phase I (oxidation or reduction) and phase II (conjugation). The liver is the main organ involved in xenobiotic metabolism and the intestinal tract is the main extrahepatic organ. A major breakthrough promoting the study of drug metabolism was the development of techniques to isolate endoplasmic reticulum, the organelle containing multiple drug-metabolizing enzymes, from whole tissue. During this process, the endoplasmic reticulum fractures into small spheres termed microsomes, which can reproduce most of the metabolites generated from drugs by metabolic organs in vivo.

Historically, researchers assumed that drug molecules cross cellular membranes via passive diffusion and that this process was dictated by the physicochemical properties of the compound [1]. The identification of P-glycoprotein (P-gp) in the 1970s challenged this notion. Subsequently, specialized proteins referred to as transport proteins (i.e., transporters), including P-gp, were recognized to transfer some xenobiotics and endogenous compounds into and out of cells [2]. Hundreds of transporters have since been identified in the human genome [3,4]. Substantial progress has been made in cloning, characterizing, and determining the tissue and cellular membrane domain localization of many transporters.

The location and structure of the genes that encode drug-metabolizing enzymes and transporters have been elucidated. Early studies revealed individual variation leading to differences in enzyme or transporter activity. As the genes encoding many enzymes and transporters were identified and studied, it became apparent that these genes were highly polymorphic and a portion of the individual differences in metabolism and transport could be attributed to genetic variation. This led to the field of pharmacogenomics, which is the study of the impact of genetic variation on drug metabolism. Genetic variation can impact drug metabolism through several mechanisms. Nucleotide sequence changes could lead to disruption of the translation initiation codon, a premature stop codon, or alteration of a splice site, while substitution of an amino acid within the protein may lead to a change in the active site or substrate channel or alteration in protein stability that could result in changes in protein quantity [5]. Variants in the promoter of the gene or other

Yamada's Textbook of Gastroenterology, Seventh Edition. Edited by Timothy C. Wang, Michael Camilleri, Benjamin Lebwohl, Anna S. Lok, William J. Sandborn, Kenneth K. Wang, and Gary D. Wu.

Companion website: www.yamadagastro.com/textbook7e

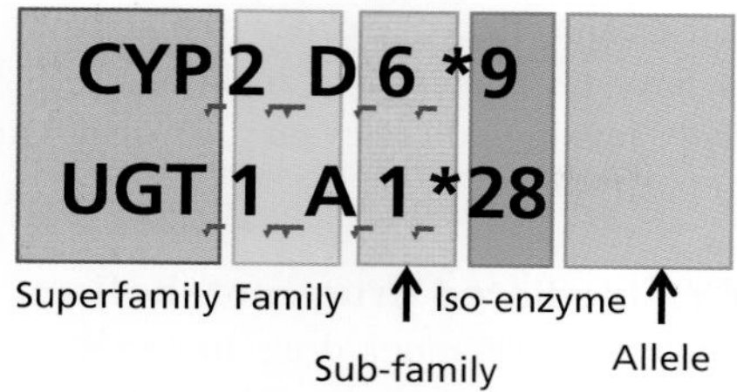

Figure 28.1 Pharmacogene nomenclature.

regulatory regions could lead to altered transcription, which may in turn lead to a higher or lower quantity of protein. In addition, several pharmacogenes are known to be duplicated or deleted, resulting in individuals having more or fewer copies of the gene, which may also lead to higher or lower protein quantity [6,7].

Many pharmacogenes and their corresponding enzymes are part of larger superfamilies, such as the cytochrome P450s (CYPs) or the UDP-glucuronosyltransferases (UGTs). These enzymes are named by the superfamily, then the family, subfamily, isoenzyme, and finally star allele (Figure 28.1).

At present, some pharmacogenomic associations are well established and genetic testing for those genes has been incorporated into routine clinical care to guide therapy of relevant medications. These tests typically detect presence or absence of relatively common single nucleotide variants, small insertions and deletions, or copy number alterations (whole-gene deletion/duplication). Thus, the test can establish the patient's genotype that is then used to predict the enzyme or transporter activity, which is referred to as the phenotype. Depending on the specific gene, phenotypes may be reported as poor, intermediate, normal, rapid, or ultrarapid metabolizer. Of note, the normal metabolizer phenotype was historically referred to as an "extensive" metabolizer.

The phenotype of an individual can be predicted by genetic testing but many other variables may also influence individual enzyme activity. Individuals with rapid or ultrarapid metabolizer phenotypes typically have one or two alleles, respectively, with a promoter variant resulting in increased activity; ultrarapid metabolizers may also be due to duplication or multiplication of a normal function allele. Individuals with poor metabolizer phenotypes typically have two alleles with variants or a deletion that result in a lack of or severely decreased enzyme activity. Intermediate metabolizers have enzyme activity that is between that of normal metabolizers and poor metabolizers, and this is typically due to either a heterozygous variant that abolishes or severely reduces enzyme activity or biallelic variants that moderately decrease enzyme activity.

In many cases, multiple variants may be detected that are inherited together as a haplotype, which is described in pharmacogenomics as a star allele (e.g., *2). In the star allele system, *1 is designated as the reference sequence. Typically, *1 was the first sequence described but may not be the most common allele in all populations. For example, the *CYP3A5*3* nonfunctional allele is the most common *CYP3A5* allele among Caucasian populations, while the *CYP3A5*1* allele that is functional is the most common among African populations. Thus, the poor metabolizer phenotype is the most common CYP3A5 phenotype among Caucasian individuals. As additional haplotypes containing one or more variant are identified, a new number is assigned. When additional variants that do not change the function of the encoded enzyme are identified, these sequences are designated as suballeles, which were historically denoted by a letter (e.g., *3B) and are now denoted by a decimal and additional number(s). Several databases, such as PharmVar (www.pharmvar.org), maintain the allelic designations to ensure consistent use of the star allele nomenclature [8–10].

When using a pharmacogenomic report, healthcare providers should still consider nongenetic factors that impact drug response, such as drug–drug interactions, renal function, etc. A general approach to use of a pharmacogenomic test report may involve the provider first identifying which gene(s) have a clinically significant association with the medication of interest. Then, if the medication is an active drug (e.g., does not require metabolism to the active metabolite), the provider may consider a decreased dose for individuals with reduced enzyme activity, an increased dose for individuals with increased enzyme activity, or potentially an alternate medication in either scenario. In contrast, if the medication is a prodrug that the enzyme will metabolize into the active form, the provider may consider an increased dose for individuals with decreased enzyme activity, a decreased dose for individuals with increased enzyme activity, or an alternate medication. The report may include specific recommendations for the medication, or the provider may refer to the FDA label or published practice guidelines.

It is important to be aware that most pharmacogenomic tests currently used are based on targeted genotyping and can only detect variants included in the test design. The *1 allele is assigned when no variants are detected. Therefore, if the patient has a rare variant that was not included in the design of the test, the result will likely be *1/*1, corresponding to a normal metabolizer phenotype, which may represent a false negative. Pharmacogenomic tests should be considered a predictive tool, and providers should continue to monitor for adverse effects and lack of efficacy as they would have done prior to the availability of pharmacogenomic tests.

While pharmacogenomic testing can be a useful clinical tool for a subset of medications, other pharmacogenomic relationships remain less established and more research is necessary to determine whether the genetic variation observed has a clinically significant impact on pharmacotherapy. Throughout the chapter, established pharmacogenomic associations that are relevant in the practice of gastroenterology will be highlighted.

Phase I drug metabolism

Phase I metabolism introduces functional groups to a molecule through oxidation or reduction. The majority of reactions are mediated by the cytochrome P450 enzyme (CYP) superfamily, with some contribution by other enzymes including flavin monooxygenases (FMOs). CYPs are membrane-bound hemoproteins, with a peak absorbance at 450 nm. Originally named for the reactions catalyzed, CYP substrate specificities became recognized as broad and overlapping. As such, current classification is based on protein sequence homology. Within each Arabic-numbered CYP family (>40% homology), a subfamily (>55% homology) is designated by a capital letter. Each subfamily generally contains multiple members, designated by Arabic numbers that often reflect the order of discovery. While 57 CYP genes have been identified in humans [11], only 10 enzymes are considered relevant to drug metabolism (Table 28.1) [12,13].

Sites of CYP-mediated drug metabolism

Following oral administration, drug molecules are exposed initially to CYP enzymes in the gastrointestinal (GI) tract, including those in the esophagus, stomach, small intestine, and colon (Figure 28.2a) [14]. CYP expression generally is highest in the duodenum and jejunum, declining progressively in the ileum and colon. CYPs usually are not expressed in intestinal crypt (nondifferentiated) cells, but as these immature epithelial cells migrate towards the villus tip, the cells mature and begin to express CYPs, most likely as a result of transcriptional activation. This location is particularly conducive to drug metabolism, as absorption is believed to occur primarily in the upper part of the villus.

Drug molecules escaping metabolism in the intestine enter the portal vein and either passively diffuse or are transported

Table 28.1 Select substrates, inhibitors, and inducers of major human hepatic and intestinal drug-metabolizing cytochrome P450 enzymes (CYPs).

CYP	Gene	Substrates	Inhibitors	Inducers
CYP1A2	*CYP1A2*	Caffeine, dihydralazine, phenacetin, tacrine, theophylline, tolcapone	Cimetidine, ciprofloxacin, fluvoxamine	Chargrilled meat, cigarette smoke, omeprazole
CYP2A6	*CYP2A6*	Acetaminophen, halothane, nicotine	Ketoconazole, 8-methoxypsoralen	Phenobarbital, rifampicin
CYP2B6	*CYP2B6*	Bupropion, carbamazepine, efavirenz, methadone	Orphenadrine, thioTEPA, ticlopidine	Carbamazepine, phenobarbital, phenytoin, rifampicin, St John's wort
CYP2C8	*CYP2C8*	Paclitaxel, repaglinide, rosiglitazone	Gemfibrozil, montelukast, trimethoprim	Carbamazepine, phenobarbital, phenytoin, rifampicin, St John's wort
CYP2C9	*CYP2C9*	Celecoxib, diclofenac, flurbiprofen, phenytoin, siponimod, tafenoquine, tolbutamide, (*S*)-warfarin	Fluconazole, sulfamethoxazole, sulfaphenazole, tienilic acid	Carbamazepine, phenobarbital, phenytoin, rifampicin, St John's wort
CYP2C19	*CYP2C19*	Amitryptyline, citalopram, clopidogrel, dexlansoprazole, doxepin, escitalopram, diazepam, imipramine, fluoxetine, (*S*)-mephenytoin, omeprazole, pantoprazole, rabeprazole, sertraline, trimipramine, voriconazole	Fluvoxamine, pantoprazole, sulfinpyrazone, ticlopidine	Carbamazepine, prednisone, rifampicin
CYP2D6	*CYP2D6*	Amitriptyline, aripiprazole, atomoxetine, codeine, debrisoquine, dextromethorphan, eliglustat, fluvoxamine, mirtazapine, metoprolol, ondansetron, paroxetine, pimozide, tamoxifen, tramadol, tropisetron	Fluoxetine, quinidine	None identified
CYP2E1	*CYP2E1*	Acetaminophen, ethanol, halothane, isoniazid, tolcapone	Disulfiram, ethanol	Ethanol, isoniazid
CYP3A4/5	*CYP3A4/5*	Carbamazepine, cyclosporine, docetaxel, erythromycin, lovastatin, midazolam, saquinavir, tacrolimus, troglitazone	Grapefruit juice,[a] ketoconazole, ritonavir, clarithromycin	Carbamazepine, phenobarbital, phenytoin, rifampicin, St John's wort

[a] Effect localized primarily in intestine.
thioTEPA, N,N′N′-triethylenethiophosphoramide.

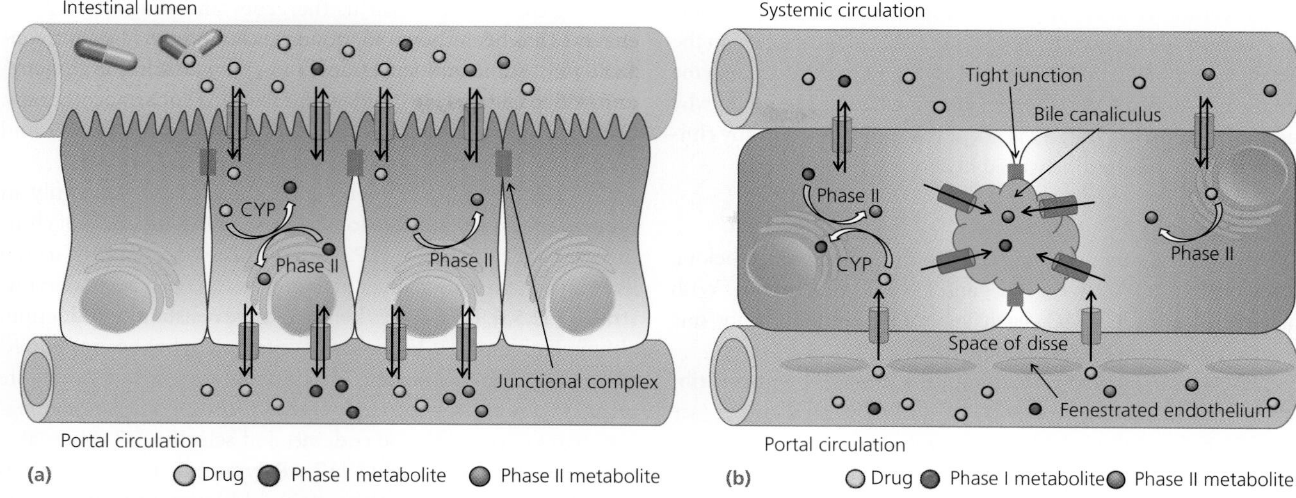

Figure 28.2 Drug metabolism in human enterocytes and hepatocytes. (a) Following oral administration, drug molecules traverse the apical (luminal) membranes of enterocytes via passive diffusion or active uptake. Within the enterocyte, drug molecules can undergo phase I metabolism, primarily by cytochrome P450 enzymes (CYPs), and phase II conjugation. Once formed, metabolites diffuse or are transported through either the apical or basolateral membranes, entering the intestinal lumen or portal circulation, respectively. (b) Drugs and metabolites can diffuse out of the portal circulation through the endothelial cell fenestrations into the space of Disse and enter hepatocytes via passive diffusion or active uptake. Within the hepatocyte, drugs and metabolites can undergo both phase I and phase II metabolism. Once formed, metabolites diffuse or are transported through the apical (canalicular) or basolateral (sinusoidal) membranes, entering the bile or systemic circulation, respectively.

actively into hepatocytes in the liver. Due to the particularly high expression of CYP enzymes in the perivenous (zone III) region, the liver is the prime organ for drug metabolism. Elimination occurs both upon "first pass" and during subsequent passes through the liver (Figure 28.2b).

Cytochrome P450 reductase (POR)

Cytochrome P450 reductase (POR) is a flavoprotein that serves as an electron donor for many CYP enzymes. The POR protein includes a membrane-bound domain, a flavin mononucleotide (FMN)-binding domain, a flavin adenine dinucleotide domain (FAD), an NADPH-binding domain, and a CYP-binding domain.

When a substrate binds in the active site of a CYP, near the heme group, a conformational change often occurs, which facilitates transfer of an electron. First, the electron is transferred from NADPH to the FAD associated with POR. This elicits a conformational change bringing the FMN and FAD domains closer to allow the electron to transfer to FMN. Along with another conformational change, the electron is then transferred to the P450 heme iron, which is reduced, allowing for oxygen binding. Next, a second electron can be transferred from either POR through a similar mechanism or through cytochrome b_5 to form an intermediate compound. After reaction with protons, the oxygen can then be transferred to the substrate, leading to hydroxylated substrate.

Rare genetic variants have been described in POR that lead to POR deficiency, which is an autosomal recessive disorder characterized by altered sex steroid synthesis and accompanying disorders of sex development, cortisol deficiency, and Antley–Bixler syndrome (ABS) skeletal malformations [15]. In addition, some variants have been reported to impact CYP-mediated metabolism. POR variants that impact binding of cofactors result in decreased or absent activity for all CYP enzymes that interact with POR, while other variants that cause more subtle structural changes may have variable interactions that differ among CYP partners, leading to different effects [16].

CYP enzymes

CYP1 family

The CYP1 family members most relevant to xenobiotic metabolism are CYP1A1 and CYP1A2. While substrate specificity of these enzymes generally overlaps, CYP1A1 favors planar aromatic hydrocarbons whereas CYP1A2 favors aromatic amines [17]. CYP1A1 has been detected in the intestinal mucosa [18,19], although basal expression is low. Compared to CYP1A1, CYP1A2 is more relevant to drug metabolism, contributing to the metabolism of ~10% of clinically used drugs [17]. In addition to metabolizing drugs, CYP1As bioactivate some xenobiotics to reactive intermediates [20,21]. CYP1 transcription occurs via activation of the aryl hydrocarbon receptor (AhR) via polycyclic aromatic hydrocarbons found in chargrilled meat and cigarette smoking (see Table 28.1) [22,23]. Clinically relevant CYP1A2 substrates include acetaminophen, lidocaine, clozapine, duloxetine, and propranolol (see Table 28.1) [24–26]. CYP1A2 inhibitors include the antidepressant fluvoxamine (see Table 28.1).

While both CYP1A1 and CYP1A2 are polymorphic, with 13 and 21 alleles reported respectively [27], the pharmacogenomics of CYP1A2 has been studied more extensively. Many promoter variants have been reported in CYP1A2, which may interaction with medications and environmental substances to lead to differences in enzyme induction [28]. While CYP1A2 is involved in the metabolism of many medications, it is often not the only enzyme nor the rate-limiting step in metabolism, which may explain why genetic variation in CYP1A2 is not currently included in any clinical guidelines nor routinely used in clinical practice.

CYP2 family

CYP2 family members associated with drug metabolism belong to the CYP2A, CYP2B, CYP2C, and CYP2D subfamilies. With the exception of CYP2C, each subfamily contains only one enzyme relevant to drug metabolism.

CYP2A6 is expressed primarily in the liver [29] and contributes to the metabolism of ~3% of clinically used drugs (see Table 28.1) [17,30]. CYP2A6 transcription is mediated via the pregnane X receptor (PXR) and CAR [31]. Increased transcription also has been observed with dexamethasone-mediated glucocorticoid receptor (GR) activation [32] and oral contraceptive-mediated estrogen receptor (ER) activation [33,34]. In addition to transcriptional regulation, genetic variation may contribute to interindividual differences in CYP2A6-mediated clearance. Currently, 45 allelic variants [35] have been identified that result in altered protein expression or function [17] and have been shown to influence cigarette smoking behavior [36].

Hepatic CYP2B6 expression is relatively low and contributes to ~5% of the total hepatic CYP pool [17]. In addition to drugs (see Table 28.1), CYP2B6 metabolizes a large number of environmental chemicals [17]. The gene encoding CYP2B6 is polymorphic, with at least 38 allelic variants [27]. Low-activity alleles have demonstrated clinical importance with substrates such as efavirenz [37,38], nevirapine [39], and cyclophosphamide [40].

The CYP2C subfamily contains four enzymes which, in aggregate, contribute to the metabolism of ~25% of clinically used drugs [41]. Hepatic messenger RNA (mRNA) expression of CYP2C18 is relatively high, but inefficient translation yields low protein expression and, consequently, CYP2C18 is a minor contributor to drug metabolism [17]. Protein expression of CYP2C9 is roughly twofold and 10-fold greater, respectively, than that of CYP2C8 and CYP2C19. CYP2C8, CYP2C9, and CYP2C19 are inducible via PXR, CAR, GR, and vitamin D receptor activation. CYP2C9 induction also is influenced by hepatocyte nuclear factor (HNF)-α [17].

Despite highly conserved protein sequences, substrate specificities of the CYP2C subfamily members vary widely. CYP2C8 metabolizes rosiglitazone, paclitaxel, and amodiaquine (see Table 28.1) [17]. CYP2C9 prefers weak acids such as losartan, nonsteroidal antiinflammatory drugs (NSAIDs), and phenytoin (see Table 28.1) [42]. Some substrate specificity overlap exists between CYP2C8 and CYP2C9 with drugs such as ibuprofen [43]. CYP2C19 metabolizes (*S*)-mephenytoin, omeprazole and other proton pump inhibitors, and clopidogrel (see Table 28.1). All three of these CYP2C enzymes have clinically relevant decreased function polymorphisms. The CYP2C8 gene has 14 known allelic variants, while CYP2C9 has 61 and CYP2C19 has 37 [27]. Genetic variation in the genes encoding the CYP2C enzymes has been shown to influence clopidogrel [44], voriconazole [45], some antidepressants [46,47], warfarin [48], phenytoin [49], paclitaxel [50], and omeprazole [51] pharmacotherapy. Clinically, genetic tests are widely available for CYP2C9 and CYP2C19, with fewer available for CYP2C8.

CYP2D6 is the only member of the CYP2D subfamily in humans and is responsible for the metabolism of ~20% of clinically used drugs [17]. CYP2D6 is expressed primarily in the liver, although some intestinal expression has been demonstrated [52,53]. CYP2D6 is believed to be resistant to induction, although phenotypic induction by rifampicin has been reported [54]. CYP2D6 metabolizes drugs from multiple therapeutic areas, including the antiarrhythmic propafenone, antidepressant paroxetine, analgesic codeine, and selective ER modulator tamoxifen (see Table 28.1) [17]. Polymorphisms of CYP2D6 contribute to the more than 1000-fold variability in enzyme activity, ranging from null activity splice variants to enhanced enzyme activity due to copy number variants [29]. Currently, there are over 130 known CYP2D6 alleles [27].

The incidence of CYP2D6 genetic diversity varies substantially among populations [55]. For example, ~5% of Caucasians lack CYP2D6 activity due to either full gene deletions or null alleles and are deemed CYP2D6 "poor metabolizers," whereas the poor metabolizer phenotype is present in less than 1% of Japanese [56]. Approximately 5% of Caucasians have gene duplication of CYP2D6, resulting in an "ultrarapid" metabolizer phenotype [56]. These individuals exhibit unusually rapid clearance of some CYP2D6 substrates, which can account for the therapeutic failure of those medications.

While clinical CYP2D6 genetic tests are widely available, laboratory interpretation of results has varied widely, and, there has been a drive toward increased standardization [57]. When reviewing the literature and clinical CYP2D6 genetic test results, it is essential to recognize that different methodologies have been utilized for phenotype prediction from genotype and to understand which strategy was used in that specific instance.

CYP3 family

The human CYP3 family consists of a single subfamily, CYP3A, which comprises CYP3A4, -3A5, -3A7, and -3A43 [12]. CYP3A7 is expressed predominantly in fetal liver, with enzyme expression decreasing markedly after birth [58,59]. A subset of individuals carry the CYP3A7*1C allele, which contains the proximal PXR/CAR element of CYP3A4, and express CYP3A7 beyond fetal life [60]. This may result in greater CYP3A activity and impact levels of some medications. CYP3A4 is the most abundant single human CYP in both the liver and intestine [29,52,53] and has been estimated to be involved in the metabolism of ~30% of drugs used clinically [17]. Aggregate CYP3A4 protein content in the intestine has been estimated to be less than 10% of that in the liver [61]. Intestinal CYP3A4 does not correlate with hepatic CYP3A4, indicating that the enzyme is regulated differently in the two organs [62,63]. As the presystemic clearance of CYP3A4 substrates may be mediated by both intestinal and hepatic extraction, the site of first-pass metabolism can be difficult to delineate. This conundrum is especially true for substrates that undergo extensive intestinal extraction, such as verapamil [64], cyclosporine [65], and midazolam [66,67].

The importance of intestinal CYP3A4 also has been highlighted by drug interactions perpetrated by grapefruit juice [68–70]. The grapefruit constituents (i.e., furanocoumarins) [71–73] responsible for this interaction efficiently "knock out" intestinal CYP3A4 [71,74–76], but do not reach sufficient concentrations in the liver to inhibit hepatic CYP3A4 [69,74]. Drugs that undergo significant metabolism in the intestine are metabolized rapidly by CYP3A4, administered in relatively small amounts, and/or have a prolonged absorption phase (i.e., prolonged contact with the enzyme).

While CYP3A4 has been extensively studied, few genetic variants have been identified that result in significant changes in expression and/or activity. The CYP3A4*22 haplotype is present at a frequency of approximately 5–7% among Caucasians and results in low hepatic CYP3A4 expression and activity due to formation of a nonfunctional splice variant with partial retention of intron 6 [77,78]. In addition, the CYP3A4*1B allele has been reported to impact activity although this may be due to linkage disequilibrium with the CYP3A5*1 allele [79]. Additionally, ~20% of Caucasians and ~50% of African Americans exhibit CYP3A5 expression in the liver and intestine; this enzyme metabolizes several of the same substrates as CYP3A4 [80]. CYP3A5 expressors carry at least one CYP3A5*1 allele and generally have increased dosing requirements for tacrolimus and other drugs, in part because dosing recommendations are often based on a Caucasian population, which includes many individuals who do not express CYP3A5 [81].

Several genetic variants have been described that result in no CYP3A5 expression, such as the *3 and *6 alleles that cause splicing defects [82]. Consistent with in vitro observations, CYP3A5 carriers have demonstrated a lower extent of CYP3A inhibition compared to CYP3A5 noncarriers [83].

While several CYP3A43 variant alleles have been described, this gene has not been thoroughly studied and limited information is available about its potential clinical significance . Clinical pharmacogenetic tests are widely available for both CYP3A4 and CYP3A5, but not CYP3A7 or CYP3A43.

Flavin monooxygenases

Five members of the flavin monooxygenase (FMO) family (FMO1–5) are expressed in humans, although the contributions of FMO2, FMO4, and FMO5 to drug metabolism are not completely defined. As with CYPs, the FMOs have broad and overlapping substrate specificity [84]. Despite expression in the fetal liver [85], FMO1 is expressed primarily in the adult kidney and intestinal tract and is not expressed in human adult liver [86,87]. FMO1 metabolizes drugs including the antidepressant imipramine [88] and the antihistaminics promethazine and brompheniramine [89,90]. FMO3 is expressed primarily in the liver at a level comparable to that of CYPs, and is also expressed in skin, pancreas, adrenal cortex and medulla [87,91,92]. Substrates of FMO3 include the H_2 receptor antagonists cimetidine [93] and ranitidine [94], sulindac sulfide, itopride, olopatadine, albendazole, and ethionamide.

The ability of FMOs to oxidize a broad range of substrates may in part be due to their unusual mechanism of action, where the enzyme can activate oxygen as part of a stable FAD derivative C4a hydroperoxide. This is accomplished by NADPH binding and reducing FAD to $FADH_{2;}$ the $NADP^+$ that is generated can then stabilize the C4a hydroperoxyflavin that is created when molecular oxygen binds. The enzyme is then able to oxygenate any nucleophile that can access the active site. This mechanism differs from that used by the CYPs, in that FMOs accept electrons from NADPH directly rather than using an accessory protein (such as POR), and CYPs are not able to activate oxygen until an appropriate substrate has bound [87].

A number of single nucleotide polymorphisms (SNPs) in the FMO1 gene have been identified, but the clinical significance of these polymorphisms remains to be determined [84]. Interindividual variation in the expression of FMO3 in adult human liver ranging from 10- to 20-fold has been reported [87]. Because FMO3 is not thought to be readily inducible or subject to irreversible inhibition by other chemicals or mediations, genetic variation or other factors may lead to the high degree of variation in expression. Over 40 FMO3 variants resulting in severely decreased or absent function have been identified [95,96] and cause trimethylaminuria, which is inherited in an autosomal recessive manner, and may impact ranitidine clearance [94].

Genetic testing for variation in FMO genes in the setting of pharmacogenomics is not routinely performed.

Dihydropyrimidine dehydrogenase (DPD)

Dihydropyrimidine dehydrogenase (DPD) catalyzes the first step in metabolism of endogenous pyrimidines. DPD forms a homodimer with each subunit including a FAD domain, FMN domain, and four iron-sulfur (Fe-S) clusters to accomplish electron transfer. There are binding sites for NADPH and the substrate. Upon binding, NADPH first reduces FAD, then the electrons are transferred via the Fe-S clusters to FMN for reduction of the substrate.

Capecitabine and 5-fluoruracil, chemotherapeutic agents used in the treatment of colorectal carcinoma and other malignancies, are also metabolized by DPD. In phase III studies, 30–40% of patients treated with monotherapy with these agents developed severe toxicity that was fatal in 0.5–1% of patients [97–99]. DPD is expressed in many cell types, including the liver and peripheral blood. While there is a strong correlation between DPD protein level and enzyme activity when measured in the liver, there is limited correlation between peripheral blood mononuclear cell (PBMC) DPD activity and hepatocyte activity [100]. Therefore, clinical assays to measure enzyme activity using a peripheral blood sample to guide fluoropyrimidine dosing have not been developed.

Genetic variants in DPYD, which encodes DPD, have been demonstrated to reduce DPD activity, and patients with these variants are at increased risk of toxicity when treated with fluoropyrimidines [101]. DPYD genetic testing to predict fluoropyrimidine toxicity risk is clinically available through many laboratories and guidelines for the use of the results have been published [102]. While most patients with DPD deficiency are asymptomatic until treated with fluoropyrimidines, severe DPD deficiency can present in rare individuals as an autosomal recessive condition characterized by neurological problems. Factors in addition to genetics may contribute to risk for this presentation.

Phase II drug metabolism

Compared to the CYPs, phase II enzymes are less well characterized, partly reflecting the fact that these enzymes are generally colorless (making purification more difficult) and tend to lose catalytic activity during purification. The most extensively studied phase II enzymes are the uridine 5′-diphosphate (UDP)-glucuronosyltransferases (UGTs), glutathione-*S*-transferases (GSTs), and sulfotransferases (SULTs), which catalyze conjugation to glucuronic acid, glutathione, and sulfate, respectively [103]. Other phase II enzymes include the *N*-acetyltransferases (NATs) and thiopurine methyltransferase (TPMT). Reactive functional groups produced by oxidative metabolism are common loci for phase II metabolism; however, many drugs can be conjugated directly. Except for glucuronidation, all phase II reactions are mediated by cytosolic enzymes.

UDP-glucuronosyltransferases

Conjugation with glucuronic acid generally results in enhanced water solubility, promoting excretion of the conjugated metabolites. Glucuronide conjugates commonly are excreted into the bile and eliminated via the stool. Glucuronidation usually, but not always, reduces pharmacological activity. A notable exception is morphine-6-glucuronide, which has up to 650-fold greater opiate activity than morphine [104].

As with CYPs, UDP-glucuronosyltransferases (UGTs) constitute a multigene family of microsomal enzymes, some of which are inducible [105,106]. Human UGTs are part of four families (UGT1, UGT2, UGT3, and UGT8) that correspond to 22 enzymes. Nearly all drug glucuronidation reactions are catalyzed by nine enzymes in the UGT1A subfamilies and seven enzymes in the UGT2B subfamily. The catalytic specificity of UGTs toward drugs and endogenous substrates is considerable (Table 28.2), and characterization of these pathways is an active area of research [105–108].

Unlike CYPs, which are located on the cytosolic side of the endoplasmic reticulum, UGTs are located on the luminal side. Accordingly, in vitro assessment of UGT activity with microsomes requires addition of agents to permeabilize microsomal membranes, which can confound data interpretation. Recent advances have improved methods to accurately extrapolate in vitro glucuronidation data to predict in vivo behavior [109].

UGTs are expressed throughout the human body but appear to be most abundant in the liver and GI tract. The complement of UGTs expressed in liver and intestine are not identical [106– 109]; some UGTs expressed in the liver are not expressed in the GI tract (e.g., UGT2B4), whereas others expressed in the intestine are not expressed in the liver (e.g., UGT1A8 and UGT1A10). UGTs present in the colon have been proposed to provide protection by conjugating reactive compounds that are deconjugated by colonic bacteria [110]. UGTs expressed along the GI tract also may limit the bioavailability of phenolic xenobiotics, including some drugs [111].

The human UGT1 locus includes many unique first exons accompanied by promoter elements upstream from four common exons, such that each UGT1A gene has a unique 5' portion and a shared 3' end. Multiple variants in the UGT1 family have been identified [109]. Pathogenic variants in the common exons can result in decreased or no activity of the entire family of isozymes, while a variant in one of the unique exons would only be expected to impact that specific isozyme.

Genetic variants in UGT1A1, which encodes the enzyme chiefly responsible for bilirubin conjugation, are some of the most well studied. Variations in UGT1A1 can lead to Gilbert and Crigler–Najjar (types 1 and 2) hyperbilirubinemia and have been associated with irinotecan toxicity [112]. UGT1A1 variation is also associated with risk of jaundice among individuals prescribed atazanavir [113] and reduced clearance of nilotinib, pazopanib, and belinostat [114].

Drug–drug interactions due to alterations in UGT activity have been described. For example, anticonvulsants have been shown to induce some UGTs and may account for some drug–drug interactions, particularly in patients treated for HIV [115]. Induction of UGTs can involve several receptors, including PXR, CAR, and AhR [116]. Inhibition of UGTs has been proposed to account in part for the pharmacokinetic interaction between gemfibrozil and cerivastatin [117]. Regardless, drug–drug interactions due to induction or inhibition of UGTs are generally low in magnitude and are rarely clinically significant [118,119]. This observation is underscored by the relatively high capacity of UGTs, coupled with overlapping substrate specificities that provide compensatory pathways for drug elimination.

Some glucuronides, particularly acylglucuronides, have been shown to be reactive molecules and may be involved in drug-induced liver injury [120]. For example, a glucuronide metabolite of diclofenac has been shown to bind covalently to multiple proteins in the hepatocyte, potentially causing a rare hepatotoxicity [121].

Glutathione-*S*-transferases

Glutathione-*S*-transferases (GSTs) are cytosolic enzymes involved in hepatic and intestinal drug metabolism and belong to seven separate gene families designated α, μ, θ, π, ζ, σ, and ω

Table 28.2 Select substrates, inhibitors, and tissue expression of major human phase II drug-metabolizing enzymes.

Enzyme	Gene	Substrates	Inhibitors
Microsomal			
UGT1A1	UGT1A1	Acetaminophen, atazanavir, bilirubin, irinotecan (SN-38), buprenorphine	Diclofenac, tangeretin, ketoconazole
UGT1A3	UGT1A3	Ezetimibe, naproxen, quercetin	Diclofenac
UGT1A4	UGT1A4	Amitriptyline, endoxifen, imipramine	Bilirubin, hecogenin
UGT1A6	UGT1A6	Acetaminophen, 1-napthol, valproic acid	Diclofenac, indomethacin, troglitazone
UGT1A7[a]	UGT1A7	Acetaminophen, mycophenolic acid	Phenylbutazone, probenecid, magnolol, quinidine
UGT1A8[a]	UGT1A8	Mycophenolic acid, propofol, raloxifene	Diclofenac, probenecid, phenylbutazone
UGT1A9	UGT1A9	Acetaminophen, fenofibrate, quercetin	Diclofenac, phenylbutazone, magnolol
UGT1A10[a]	UGT1A10	Entacapone, mycophenolic acid, raloxifene	Diclofenac, phenylbutazone, probenecid
UGT2B7	UGT2B7	Morphine, oxazepam, zidovudine	Fluconazole, phenylbutazone, quinidine, valproic acid
UGT2B15	UGT2B15	Acetaminophen, (S)-oxazepam, tolcapone	Amytriptyline, quinidine, valproic acid
Cytosolic			
GSTs	Multiple	Busulfan, ethacrynic acid, NAPQI	Artemisinin, quinidine
SULT1A1	SULT1A1	Acetaminophen, minoxidil	Curcumin, grapefruit juice, piroxicam, quercetin
SULT1A3[a]	SULT1A3	Dopamine, norepinephrine	Grapefruit juice
SULT1E1	SULT1E1	Estrogen, naringenin, 4-hydroxytamoxifen	Ibuprofen, sulindac
SULT2A1	SULT2A1	Dehydroepiandrosterone, androgens	Genestein, quercetin
NAT1	NAT1	Isoniazid, sulfamethoxazole	Genestein, quercetin
NAT2	NAT2	Dapsone, isoniazid, sulfasalazine	Coumarin
TPMT	TPMT	6-Mercaptopurine, azathioprine, thioguanine	Naproxen, sulfasalazine

[a] Expressed in GI tract but not liver.
NAPQI, *N*-acetyl-*p*-benzoquinone imine.

[122]. Each family has several members designated by Arabic numbers. For example, GSTM1 is the first of five members of the μ gene family. GSTs are expressed in many organs in addition to the liver and intestine. While the GSTs have overlapping substrate specificity, the complement of GSTs present in each organ is not identical [123]. GSTs typically function to detoxify electrophilic metabolites of drugs (see Table 28.2), such as *N*-acetyl-*p*-benzoquinone imine (NAPQI) produced from acetaminophen. In general, the reactions catalyzed are not rate limiting in drug elimination. An exception may be busulfan, which requires glutathione (GSH) conjugation catalyzed by GSTA1 for elimination. Studies have suggested that busulfan oral availability is limited by GSTA1 activity in the intestine [124]. GSH depletion also has been implicated as a potential mechanism underlying acetaminophen hepatotoxicity [125]. During acute acetaminophen overdose, the glucuronidation pathway is overwhelmed, resulting in excess formation of NAPQI. GSH can be depleted as the liver attempts to eliminate NAPQI via GSH conjugation, perpetuating toxic effects of NAPQI.

Polymorphisms in GSTs are common [126], with GSTM1 and GSTT1 being absent in 40% and 15% of Caucasians, respectively. Polymorphisms in these and other GSTs have been linked to susceptibility to a variety of illnesses, including asthma, cancer, diabetes, heart disease, and drug-induced liver injury. An example of the latter is the anti-Alzheimer agent, tacrine. Patients who lack both GSTM1 and GSTT1 appear to have increased incidence of treatment-associated ALT elevations [127]. Some studies have also suggested that genetic variation in several GSTs (GSTP1, GSTM1, and GSTT1) may be associated with differential response to antineoplastic therapy with platinum-containing compounds [128]; however, these variants are currently not typically included in clinical testing.

Sulfotransferases

The human liver and intestine conjugate sulfate to a variety of xenobiotics via sulfotransferases (SULTs) (see Table 28.2). These reactions, which catalyze the transfer of the sulfonyl group from 3'-phospho-adenosine-5'-phosphosulfate (PAPS) to acceptor molecules, usually enhance solubility and result in decreased biological activity, but exceptions exist. For example, morphine-6-sulfate is 30 times more potent an analgesic than morphine [129]. Sulfation also may produce chemically reactive metabolites [130,131]. SULTs are involved in the metabolism of potential carcinogens, some medications, and endogenous hormones.

Three SULT gene families in humans, SULT1, SULT2, and SULT4, encode at least 13 members [130]. SULT1A1 is the most abundant SULT in the liver, whereas SULT1B1 predominates in the intestine [132]. SULT catalytic activity varies considerably among individuals, and polymorphisms in specific SULTS have been identified [131]. SULT1A1 genetic variation has been most widely studied, particularly with respect to risk of a variety of malignancies [133]. Several SULT family members, including SULT1A1, are known to be duplicated or deleted, so copy number variation has also been studied with respect to drug metabolism as well as disease risk [7]. Some SULTs are inducible, at least in liver, by the same nuclear receptors as those for CYP and UGT induction [134]. For example, one study suggested that the loss of efficacy of birth control pills during treatment with antiseizure medications or rifampin reflected induction of SULTs, in addition to CYP3A4 (see Table 28.1) [135].

N-acetyltransferases

Two *N*-acetyltransferases (NATs), NAT1 and NAT2, have been implicated in human drug metabolism. Both enzymes are polymorphic, although the prevalence and functional relevance of NAT2 polymorphisms surpass those identified for NAT1 [136,137]. Up to 50% of Caucasians lack NAT2 activity and are termed slow acetylators. Slow acetylators have reduced clearance of multiple xenobiotics (see Table 28.2) and may have increased risk of dose-dependent toxicities. For example, slow acetylators may be more susceptible to idiosyncratic hepatotoxicity from isoniazid, especially when risk is adjusted for a CYP2E1 polymorphism [138]. NAT2 polymorphisms also have been linked to cancer. Slow acetylators appear to be at higher risk for bladder cancer but at lower risk for colon cancer [139]. Overexpression of NAT1 in several cancer types has prompted research targeting the enzyme as a means to overcome chemotherapeutic resistance [140].

While rarely used today, NAT2 genetic testing is available through a small number of clinical laboratories to predict risk of isoniazid toxicity.

Thiopurine methyltransferase

Thiopurine methyltransferase (TPMT) catalyzes the *S*-methylation of the thiopurine drugs 6-mercaptopurine, azathioprine, and thioguanine to pharmacologically inactive metabolites. Approximately 0.3% of Caucasians harbor genetic polymorphisms of TPMT that result in null enzyme activity, with an additional 10% having reduced activity. Children with certain leukemias and deficient in TPMT have a higher incidence of myelosuppression when receiving standard doses of thiopurine drugs [141]. Screening for TPMT deficiency prior to initiating thiopurine drugs, either by use of a biochemical or a genetic test, is becoming standard clinical practice [142,143]. While leukopenia impacts up to 35% of Asians taking thiopurine medications, only 1–3% of Asians have TPMT variants that would lead to reduced activity [144]. Genetic variants in NUDT15, which encodes nudix hydrolase 15 (NUDT15), have recently been found to be common among individuals of Asian descent and may in part explain the high incidence of thiopurine toxicity in these populations [145]. NUDT15 is responsible for dephosphorylation of the active triphosphate metabolites of thiopurines. Genetic testing for NUDT15 is available for clinical use, often coupled with TPMT testing.

Transport proteins

In addition to phase I and II drug metabolizing enzymes, transporters have become well-recognized determinants of drug disposition, contributing not only to absorption and elimination, but also tissue distribution [146–149]. Localization of these proteins within cellular membranes, particularly of enterocytes (Figure 28.3a) and hepatocytes (Figure 28.3b), facilitates the uptake and efflux of drugs and associated metabolites, as well as other xenobiotics and endogenous substrates.

The transporters responsible for these functions belong to two major superfamilies: ATP binding cassette (ABC) and solute carrier (SLC) [2–4,150,151]. ABC family members are primary active transporters, relying on ATP hydrolysis to pump substrates against a concentration gradient. In contrast, SLC family members typically are secondary or tertiary active transporters (i.e., substrate movement is dependent upon energy created from the transport of a cosubstrate(s), typically an ion, with its own concentration gradient). Substrate and ion movement can be coupled either in the same direction, as for symporters, or in the opposite direction, as for antiporters/exchangers. Other SLC family members transport substrates via facilitated diffusion.

Transporters are classified further according to localization within cellular membrane domains and function. Intestinal transporters reside within the apical, or brush border, membrane facing the intestinal lumen and the basolateral membrane, whereas hepatic transporters reside in the apical membrane facing the bile canaliculus and the basolateral/sinusoidal membrane [1,146,152,153]. Based upon function, transporters are grouped into two categories: uptake and efflux. Uptake transporters facilitate drug absorption into enterocytes from the intestinal lumen (with subsequent entry into the portal circulation) and into hepatocytes from the portal circulation. Efflux transporters transfer drugs/metabolites from enterocytes into the intestinal lumen or portal circulation and from hepatocytes into the bile or systemic circulation.

Similar to drug-metabolizing enzymes, characterization of intestinal transporters lags behind hepatic transporters [152]. The current general knowledge of intestinal and hepatic transporters that are clinically relevant to drug disposition, some of which has been highlighted by the International Transporter

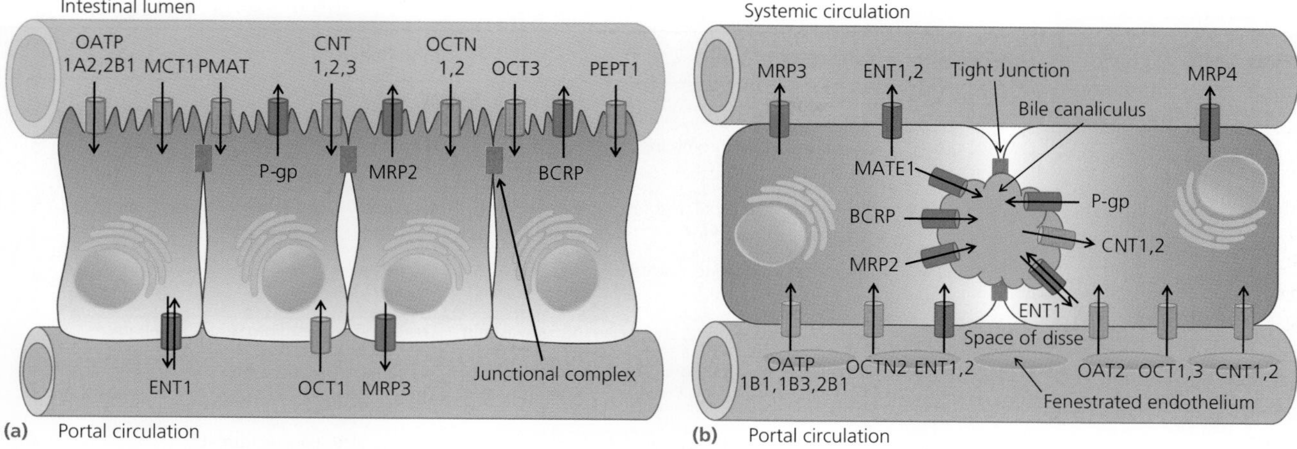

Figure 28.3 Transport proteins in human enterocytes and hepatocytes considered important in drug disposition. Schematic representations of adjacent enterocytes **(a)** and hepatocytes **(b)** show transporter membrane domain localization: apical (luminal or canalicular, respectively) and basolateral (blood; sinusoidal for hepatocytes). Transporters marked in gray are considered primarily uptake transporters, green are efflux transporters, and purple are bidirectional. Arrows denote the direction of substrate transport. BCRP, breast cancer resistance protein; CNT, concentrative nucleoside transporter; ENT, equilibrative nucleoside transporter; MATE, multidrug and toxin extrusion protein; MCT, monocarboxylate transporter; MRP, multidrug resistance-associated protein; OAT, organic anion transporter; OATP, organic anion transporting polypeptide; OCT, organic cation transporter; OCTN, organic cation/carnitine transporter; PEPT, peptide transporter; P-gp, P-glycoprotein; PMAT, plasma membrane monoamine transporter.

Consortium, is summarized in Table 28.3 and Figure 28.3 [147,154,155].

Similar to enzymes, interindividual differences in transporter expression and function due to naturally occurring genetic polymorphisms are important areas of study. Some transporters have been studied extensively (e.g., P-gp and OATP1B1), whereas investigation of others has been limited to date (e.g., OCTs). Research encompasses determining the effect (i.e., decreased expression or activity) of the identified polymorphisms on transporter function in vitro and then conducting association studies in humans to assess the clinical impacts on pharmacokinetics and pharmacodynamics, as well as on the etiology and prognosis of disorders/diseases [156]. A large number of genetic variants have been linked to decreased expression and/or activity; however, similar to the influence of genetic variation on enzymes, the impact of genetic variation on transporter function may differ for different substrates. Depending on the function of the transporter, decreased drug absorption, and ultimately decreased exposure and efficacy, could result; alternatively, increased drug absorption and an increase in the risk of toxicity could result. Genetic variation impacting transporters differs among racial groups for most transporters [156–164]. Genetic variants that are known to impact transporter function will be highlighted throughout the remainder of this chapter.

Uptake transporters

Organic anion transporting polypeptides

Organic anion transporting polypeptides (OATPs) constitute the SLCO (formerly SLC21A) superfamily. Eleven OATPs have been identified in humans, four of which are important in drug disposition [146–148,152]. OATP1A2 is expressed in the apical membrane of enterocytes, among numerous other tissues, but at a much lower level than OATP2B1 [165,166]. OATP2B1, also widely expressed, localizes to the apical membrane of enterocytes and basolateral membrane of hepatocytes [167,168]. Unlike other OATPs, OATP1B1 and OATP1B3 are expressed predominantly in the liver, localized to the basolateral membrane of hepatocytes [169–172].

Organic anion transporting polypeptides are considered primarily as uptake transporters, although evidence suggests bidirectional function [173]. The mechanism of substrate transport remains under investigation and appears to vary between isoforms. Research indicates that transport occurs by electroneutral exchange, but the driving force(s) has yet to be elucidated completely [151,174–178]. OATP1B1 and OATP1B3 have been shown to function via facilitated diffusion [173]. Most OATPs have broad substrate specificity [148,151,157]. Overlaps exist between isoforms but none are identical. OATPs are considered multispecific due to multiple binding sites on the protein [179–181]. Substrates include amphipathic compounds with a relatively high molecular weight (>350 Da) [151,152]. Most are anionic in nature, but some are neutral or cationic. Substrates may contain a steroidal or peptide structural backbone [2]. Therapeutic substrates include statins (HMG-CoA reductase inhibitors), anticancer agents, antihypertensives, and HIV protease inhibitors (see Table 28.3).

SLCO1B1 encodes the OATP1B1 transporter. Through a genome-wide association study, heterozygous and homozygous carriers of the C allele at rs4149056 in SLCO1B1 (which is present in the *5, *15, and *17 alleles) were found to be at increased risk of myopathy when taking high-dose

Table 28.3 Select substrates, inhibitors, and inducers of major human hepatic and intestinal drug transporters.

Transporter	Gene	Other names	Substrates	Inhibitors
Uptake transporters				
OATP1A2	SLCO1A2	OATP-A, OATP	Ciprofloxacin, erythromycin, fexofenadine, pravastatin	Grapefruit juice,[a] orange juice,[a] verapamil
OATP1B1	SLCO1B1	OATP-C, OATP2, LST-1	Atorvastatin, enalapril, fexofenadine, repaglinide, saquinavir, simvastatin	Atazanavir, cyclosporine, rifampicin, ritonavir
OATP1B3	SLCO1B3	OATP-8, LST-2	Digoxin, fexofenadine, paclitaxel, rosuvastatin, valsartan	Cyclosporine, rifampicin, ritonavir
OATP2B1	SLCO2B1	OATP-B	Aliskiren, fexofenadine, glibenclamide, pravastatin	Cyclosporine, gemfibrozil, grapefruit juice[a]
PEPT1	SLC15A1		Cephalexin, enalapril, valaciclovir	Lisinopril
ENT1	SLC29A1		Adenosine, capecitabine, gemcitabine	Dilazep, dipyridamole, draflazine
ENT2	SLC29A2		3′-Azido 3′-deoxythymidine, didanosine	Dilazep, dipyridamole, draflazine
CNT1	SLC28A1		5-Fluorouridine, gemcitabine, zidovudine	Phloridzin
CNT2	SLC28A2		Cladribine, didanosine, ribavirin	Phloridzin
CNT3	SLC28A3		Anthracyclines, c ytarabine, 5-fluorouridine, 6-mercaptopurine	Phloridzin
PMAT	SLC29A4	ENT4	Dopamine, epinephrine, metformin	Desipramine, fluoxetine, quinidine
OAT2	SLC22A7		Aciclovir, erythromycin, 6-fluorouracil, zidovudine	Hydrochlorothiazide, phenacetin
OCT1	SLC22A1		Aciclovir, desipramine, metformin	Prazosin, quinidine, verapamil
OCT3	SLC22A3		Lidocaine, oxaliplatin	Desipramine, phenytoin, tenofovir
OCTN1	SLC22A4		Acetylcarnitine, acetylcholine, ergothioneine, carnitine, tetraethylamonium, pyrilamine, quinidine, verapamil	Cimetidine, lidocaine, procainamide
OCTN2	SLC22A5		Betaine, L-carnitine, cephaloridine, tetraethylamonium, quinidine	Grepafloxacin, levofloxacin
OCTN3	OCTN3		Acetylcarnitine	
MCT1	SLC16A1		Naproxen, propicillin, salicylic acid	AR-C15585,[b] stilbene disulfonates
Efflux transporters				
P-gp	ABCB1	MDR1	Digoxin, fexofenadine, loperamide, losartan, methotrexate, vinblastine	Amiodarone, cyclosporine, quinidine, verapamil
MRP2	ABCC2	cMOAT	Cisplatin, irinotecan, methotrexate, pravastatin	Cyclosporine, efavirenz, emtricitabine, probenecid
MRP3	ABCC3		Acetaminophen glucuronide, etoposide, methotrexate, morphine-3-glucuronide	Efavirenz, emtricitabine, indomethacin
MRP4	ABCC4		Furosemide, tenofovir, topotecan	Celecoxib, losartan, sulindac
BCRP	ABCG2	MXR, ABCP	Doxorubicin, gefitinib, glyburide, imatinib, irinotecan, methotrexate, mitoxantrone,nilotinib, prazosin, rosuvastatin, sulfasalazine	Cyclosporine, elacridar, gefitinib, imatinib, nelfinavir, nicardipene, nilotinib, ritonavir, saquinavir
MATE1	SLC47A1		Cimetadine, metformin, oxaliplatin, topotecan	Cimetidine, imatinib, pyrimethamine, quinidine

[a] Effect localized primarily in intestine.
[b] Developed by AstraZeneca.

simvastatin [182]. This variant is associated with decreased OATP1B1 activity and increased plasma simvastatin and rosuvastatin concentrations and may also be associated with toxicity and efficacy of atorvastatin [183]. Decreased hepatic uptake of these compounds may result in insufficient hepatic concentrations needed to inhibit HMG-CoA reductase and lower lipid concentrations. Other statins may also be impacted by variants in SLCO1B1, but have not been as well studied to date. In addition to the pharmacogenomic significance, autosomal recessive inheritance of deleterious variants simultaneously in both SLCO1B1 and SLCO1B3 results in Rotor syndrome, which is characterized by hyperbilirubinemia.

Having one functional copy of either gene is sufficient to prevent Rotor-type hyperbilirubinemia [184].

Additional uptake transporters

Peptide transporter 1

Peptide transporter 1 (PEPT1; SLC15A1), a low-affinity, high-capacity symporter, is localized to the apical membrane of enterocytes [185,186]. Transport activity is dependent upon pH and is optimal at pH 4.5–6.5 [187]. PEPT1 has broad substrate specificity for di- and tripeptides and peptidomimetic drugs [188]. Clinically relevant substrates include antibiotics, angiotensin converting enzyme inhibitors, and renin inhibitors (see Table 28.3).

Equilibrative nucleoside transporters

The SLC29A family comprises equilibrative nucleoside transporters (ENTs), which are low-affinity, bidirectional transporters that mediate substrate movement by facilitated diffusion [189]. ENT1 and ENT2 are localized to the basolateral membrane of enterocytes and hepatocytes; however, the extent of ENT2 expression in enterocytes is unclear [190,191]. ENT1 also is expressed at the canalicular membrane of hepatocytes. Both isoforms transport a diverse array of purine and pyrimidine nucleosides and nucleobases [189]. ENT1 has a higher affinity for substrates than ENT2 but ENT2 appears to predominate for the transport of antiviral nucleosides and nucleobases [154]. Substrates include the anticancer agents capecitabine and azacytidine and the antivirals zidovudine and 2′,3′-dideoxyinosine (see Table 28.3) [192]. A 3′-hydroxyl group on the sugar moiety of a substrate is important for ENT1 recognition [193,194].

Concentrative nucleoside transporters

Concentrative nucleoside transporters (CNT; SLC28A) 1, 2, and 3 are sodium-dependent, high-affinity symporters [195–197]. All three CNTs are localized to the apical membrane of enterocytes, whereas CNT1 and CNT2 are localized to both the apical and basolateral membranes of hepatocytes [190,191]. Substrates include anticancer agents and antivirals (see Table 28.3) [198]. CNT1 favors pyrimidine nucleosides, including gemcitabine and zidovudine; CNT2 favors purine nucleosides, including 5-fluorouridine and ribavirin. CNT3 substrate specificity overlaps with those of CNT1 and CNT2, as both pyrimidine and purine nucleosides are transported by CNT3. Similar to ENT1, a 3′-hydroxyl group on the sugar moiety of a substrate has been shown to be important for CNT recognition [198].

Several variants in SLC28A3, which encodes CNT3, have been associated with reduced risk of cardiotoxicity among pediatric patients treated with anthracyclines. While this gene is not commonly tested clinically, the Canadian Pharmacogenomics Network for Drug Safety recommends testing all childhood cancer patients with an indication for doxorubicin or daunorubicin therapy for SLC28A3 (rs7853758), along with RARG (rs2229774) and UGT1A6*4 (rs17863783) [199].

Plasma membrane monoamine transporter

Plasma membrane monoamine transporter (PMAT; SLC29A4), also known as ENT4, is a low-affinity symporter localized to the apical membrane of enterocytes [189,200]. Transport activity is stimulated at acidic pH due to the coupling of substrate transport with an inward proton gradient [201,202]. Substrates are predominantly organic cations (see Table 28.3), exhibiting specificity overlap with organic cation transporters (OCTs) [200,201,203]. Metformin is one clinically relevant PMAT substrate.

Organic anion transporters

The SLC22A family comprises organic anion transporters (OATs), OCTs (described in the section on Organic cation transporters), and organic cation/carnitine transporters (OCTNs; described in the section on Organic cation and carnitine transporters). OATs are expressed in

multiple tissues, including liver and kidney [204]. Two OATs are expressed in the liver: OAT2 and OAT7. OAT2, an antiporter, is believed to localize to the basolateral membrane of hepatocytes based on observations in the kidney [205,206]. Substrates include antineoplastics, H_2 receptor antagonists, and antivirals (see Table 28.3). OAT7 also is localized to the basolateral membrane of hepatocytes [207]; the contribution of this isoform to drug disposition is not known.

Organic cation transporters

Organic cation transporters 1 and 3 (OCT1 and OCT3) are localized predominantly to the basolateral membrane of hepatocytes and the apical membrane of enterocytes [208–210]. OCT1 mRNA in the small intestine and colon is much lower than that in the liver. OCTs, like OATPs, are considered primarily as uptake transporters but can be bidirectional [211,212]. Transport occurs by facilitated diffusion. Substrate specificity overlaps between isoforms with some distinct differences. In general, substrates consist of hydrophilic, low molecular weight (<500 Da), positively charged organic cations or weak bases that are positively charged at physiological pH [210]. Clinically relevant substrates include antidepressants, antiinflammatory agents, antineoplastics, and antihistaminics (see Table 28.3).

SLC22A1 encodes the OCT1 transporter. Several genetic variants are known to influence transporter function and may impact response and toxicity of metformin, tropisetron, ondansetron, morphine, and tramadol; however, more research is required as findings of many of the initial studies have not been replicated [213].

Organic cation and carnitine transporters

Organic cation and carnitine transporters 1, 2, and 3 (OCTN1, OCTN2, and OCTN3) represent a subfamily of the SLC22 family. The physiological role of OCTN1 is unclear but acetylcholine has been identified as a physiological substrate. OCTN2 is important in carnitine absorption and distribution throughout the organism [214]. OCTN3 catalyzes sodium-independent carnitine transport. OCTN1 and OCTN2 are widely expressed, including the apical membranes of intestine, kidney, placenta, and mammary gland as well as other tissues such as liver, heart, testis, skeletal muscle, and brain [214]. OCTN3 is present in the apical membrane of renal cells, the basolateral membrane of intestinal cells, and in breast myoepithelial cells. OCTN1 employs different mechanisms to transport substrates, and bidirectionality has been demonstrated [151,215]. OCTN2 can function as either a polyspecific transporter or a high-affinity transporter. Each isoform has a limited substrate list with some overlap; no specific drug classes are represented (see Table 28.3) [152,215].

Several genetic variants have been reported that alter function of OCTN family members. While no pharmacogenomic associations are known, these variants may lead to human pathology. For example, deleterious variants in SLC22A5, which encodes OCTN2, cause autosomal recessive primary carnitine deficiency. Other alterations in OCTN function that impair carnitine homeostasis have been proposed to be related to a variety of conditions including diabetes, Alzheimer's disease, male infertility, and cancer [214]. Finally, while inflammatory bowel disease is multifactorial, with contributions from both the environment and underlying genetic variation, alterations in SLC22A4 and SLC22A5 (OCTN1 and 2) have been implicated [214,216,217].

Monocarboxylate transporter 1

Monocarboxylate transporter 1 (MCT1; SLC16A1), located on the apical membrane of enterocytes, is a low-affinity, high-capacity symporter/exchanger [218–220]. MCT1 primarily mediates substrate uptake but has bidirectional function [221]. Substrates are weak organic acids with a relatively small lipophilic or hydrophilic *R*-group attached to a carboxyl and include some β-lactam antibiotics (see Table 28.3) [218,222].

Efflux transporters

P-glycoprotein

P-glycoprotein (P-gp; ABCB1), also known as multidrug resistance protein 1 (MDR1), is the most extensively studied and best characterized transporter. P-gp was identified initially in the 1970s in colchicine-resistant Chinese hamster ovary cells and later found to confer resistance to a variety of other amphiphilic drugs [223–225]. P-gp is expressed extensively throughout the body [2,226]. Within the intestine, P-gp is localized to the apical membrane of enterocytes, increasing from proximal to distal regions of the intestinal tract [227,228]; expression is sevenfold lower than that in the liver [63]. Within the liver, P-gp is localized to the apical/canalicular membrane of hepatocytes [228].

Based on location, predominantly in regions that serve as barriers, P-gp acts as a protective mechanism for the body by extruding drugs/metabolites into the intestinal lumen and bile in an ATP-dependent manner [229]. However, decreased drug efficacy can result due to limited oral absorption and systemic exposure. P-gp is nonspecific, with substrates of varying size, structure, and function [230]. Preference has been noted for amphipathic, hydrophobic, and cationic molecules ranging in size from 200 to 2000 Da and containing a planar ring system [231,232]. However, substrates can be neutral or anionic. Clinically relevant P-gp substrates include anticancer, antihypertensive, immunosuppressive, and antihistaminic agents (see Table 28.3). Multiple binding sites for substrates and inhibitors, which can switch between high- and low-affinity conformations, have been identified [230]. P-gp overexpression can lead to treatment failure in epilepsy, acute myeloid leukemia, childhood neuroblastoma, sarcoma, and other cancers [233].

Genetic variations in many members of the ABC superfamily have been described and associated with human diseases (e.g., CFTR, also known as ABCC7, variants lead to cystic fibrosis), but no clear associations between ABCB1 variants and human disease have been established. Several genetic variants have been associated with efficacy and/or toxicity of a variety of drugs, including simvastatin, methotrexate, atazanavir, ondansetron, and other medications; however, clinical testing is not in widespread use.

Multidrug resistance-associated proteins

Multidrug resistance-associated protein 1 (MRP1) was the second multidrug resistance-conferring transporter isolated and identified, observed in doxorubicin-resistant human lung cancer cell lines that had negligible to no P-gp expression [234–236]. MRPs belong to the ABCC gene family, and 12 additional family members have since been identified, of which four are important in drug disposition [152,154,237,238]. MRP1 normally is present at very low levels within the liver and intestine, localized to the basolateral membrane, but can be expressed at much higher levels in proliferating hepatocytes and Paneth cells of the colon [239–242]. MRP2 is expressed on the apical membranes of hepatocytes, enterocytes, and colonocytes [243–246]. Gene expression analysis indicates that MRP2 decreases from proximal to distal regions of the intestinal tract [247]. MRP3 is localized to the basolateral membrane of hepatocytes and enterocytes, and expression can vary as much as 80-fold between individuals [248–250]. MRP4 localizes to the basolateral membrane of hepatocytes but has yet to be detected in healthy tissues from the GI tract [251]. Expression can vary greatly among individuals [252].

Multidrug resistance-associated proteins exhibit substrate overlap [253]. MRP substrates generally are amphiphilic organic anions, ranging from 300 to 1000 Da [238], and can be glucuronide, sulfate, and GSH conjugates [152,237,238]. MRP1 and MRP2 substrates overlap extensively; differences may be detectable only in kinetic constants [254,255]. MRP3 favors glucuronide conjugates [253]. MRP4 exhibits broad substrate specificity, transporting nucleoside and nucleotide analogs, amongst numerous other compounds [253]. Clinically relevant MRP substrates include anticancer agents, antibiotics, antivirals, and diuretics (see Table 28.3). Transport is ATP dependent but the transport of some compounds by MRP1 and MRP2 requires the presence of, or is stimulated by, GSH [237,256]. MRP4-mediated transport also may require GSH. The underlying mechanism(s) is unknown, but it has been proposed that GSH binds to the transport protein and induces a conformational change, rendering the substrate binding site more accessible [257].

Genetic variants in ABCC2 (MRP2) that result in a transporter protein with reduced or absent activity are known to cause Dubin–Johnson syndrome [184]. This syndrome is inherited in an autosomal recessive manner and is characterized by impaired excretion of organic anions, including bilirubin glucuronides, resulting in conjugated hyperbilirubinemia and jaundice. Individuals may also have a black liver due to accumulation of other substances that cannot be transported out of the liver.

From a pharmacogenomic standpoint, ABCC2 has been extensively studied and genetic variants have been implicated as potentially associated with toxicity and/or efficacy of a wide variety of medications. However, many of these findings have not been replicated in independent cohorts and therefore clinical testing for ABCC2 variants is not routinely performed. The ABCC4 rs1751034 variant has been associated in several studies with tenofovir exposure [258].

Breast cancer resistance protein

Breast cancer resistance protein (BCRP; ABCG2) was identified through its ability to confer drug resistance to human cancer cell lines in the absence of P-gp and MRP overexpression [259,260]. BCRP was reported to be highly expressed in the placenta [261] and has since been detected in a number of nonmalignant tissues [262–265]. Within the intestine and liver, BCRP is localized to the apical membranes of enterocytes and hepatocytes. Protein expression is relatively uniform throughout the small intestine [266]. Both hepatic and intestinal BCRP expression vary greatly among individuals [266,267].

Breast cancer resistance protein is an ATP-dependent half-transporter, containing a single ATP-binding site and six transmembrane domains, rather than the two ATP-binding sites and 12 transmembrane domains associated with other ABC family members [268]. BCRP forms oligomers, predominantly homotetramers, to function [269–271]. Like P-gp and MRPs, BCRP limits the cellular accumulation of a wide variety of compounds. Substrates are diverse, both structurally and functionally, and include hydrophobic compounds and hydrophilic compounds that are charged or conjugated by phase II enzymes [2,152,156,272]. Some chemical moieties (e.g., hydroxy or amino group) have been identified as important for interaction with BCRP [273–275]. There is considerable overlap in substrate specificity among P-gp, MRP1, and MRP2 [152,276]. Therapeutic BCRP substrates include statins, antivirals, calcium channel blockers, and anticancer agents (see Table 28.3).

ABCG2, which encodes BCRP, is a highly polymorphic gene. Altered intracellular distribution, decreased transport efficiency, and reduced BCRP stability or expression are reported effects of ABCG2 variants that have been functionally characterized [277]. The ABCG2 rs2231142 A allele, which results in reduced expression, has been associated with increased serum uric acid levels and risk for gout. The same variant has also been implicated in lower rosuvastatin, atorvastatin, and simvastatin clearance as well as increased risk of developing dose-dependent atorvastatin adverse effects. Additionally, this variant has been associated with increased exposure to sulfasalazine, rosuvastatin, and topotecan, but no alterations in the pharmacokinetics of pravastatin and irinotecan [278–283]. In addition to genetic alterations, other variables contribute to variation in BCRP expression, such as microRNAs, epigenetic modifications, and other clinical parameters [277].

Additional efflux transporters

Multidrug and toxin extrusion protein 1

Multidrug and toxin extrusion protein 1 (MATE1; SLC47A1), an antiporter, localizes to the apical membrane of hepatocytes [284]. Substrates are either cationic or weak bases that are positively charged at physiological pH and belong to numerous therapeutic classes, including antibacterials and antivirals (see Table 28.3) [2,285]. Substrate specificity partially overlaps with OCTs; together, OCTs and MATE1 form an hepatic organic cation transport system. Substrate overlap with P-gp provides cells with an alternative elimination route for potentially harmful compounds. Several variants in SLC47A1 have been reported to influence metformin efficacy but findings have not been consistent across studies [286].

Transporter regulation

Transporter expression and function are regulated at multiple levels, including transcription and post translation. Transcriptional regulation appears to be dependent upon isoform, tissue localization, and activated transcription factor [2]. The transcription factors responsible for transporter regulation are similar to those for phase I and II enzyme regulation. These factors include xenobiotic-sensing (e.g., PXR and CAR) and sex hormone-dependent (e.g., ERα) nuclear receptors; stress-related transcription factors such as nuclear factor E2-related factor 2 (Nrf2) and Y-box protein 1 (YB-1); and a number of other transcription factors influenced by growth hormones and cytokines [2,151,287–294].

Several mechanisms contribute to the posttranslational regulation of transporters. Correct localization and expression at cellular membranes are critical for proper function. The localization of some transporters to cellular membranes occurs within membrane rafts (e.g., P-gp) [295–297]. The correct organization of lipids and proteins in these rafts is dependent upon cholesterol. When cholesterol is decreased, P-gp activity is decreased, possibly due to altered protein interactions or substrate binding, or disassembly of the membrane rafts [298,299]. Other transporters, such as OATPs and possibly MRP2, rely on interactions with PDZ (postsynaptic density 95/disc-large/zona occludens) proteins, which are scaffold proteins that help anchor other proteins to the cytoskeleton [237,300,301]. Additionally, posttranslational modifications can influence localization, stability, turnover, and function with diverse outcomes.

Glycosylation, the addition of a sugar moiety, may be required for proper transport activity, as is the case for P-gp, BCRP, and MRP2; the absence alters protein stability or localization [302–305]. Glycosylation may not alter localization but substrate recognition, which is the case for OAT1 [306]. Phosphorylation may result in internalization of the protein and reduced transport activity, as has been reported for OATP2B1 following protein kinase C (PKC) activation [307]. Conversely, phosphorylation can sometimes increase transport activity. ENT1 activity is increased following phosphorylation, which was hypothesized to be due to either activation of the transporter or changes in substrate affinity [308]. Finally, transporters such as P-gp and BCRP can undergo ubiquitination, a process of targeting proteins for proteosomal degradation. Increased ubiquitination results in increased protein turnover and decreased substrate transport [278,309,310].

Transporter expression, and ultimately function, are influenced by various disease states. For example, MRP1 in the intestine is elevated in patients with inflammatory bowel disease, whereas with cholestasis, hepatic MRP2 is downregulated and MRP3 and MRP4 are upregulated [237,239]. Disease effects can be widespread, not just localized to the affected tissue/organ. For example, uremic serum obtained from end-stage renal failure patients decreased MRP2 and OATP1B1 in human intestinal (Caco-2) and hepatic (Hep3B) cell lines, respectively [311].

Transporter-mediated drug interactions

Transporter-based drug interactions occur similarly to drug-metabolizing enzyme-based interactions, and the clinical relevance of transporter-mediated interactions has garnered increased attention in recent years [312]. Of concern is the ability of drugs and various dietary substances, including herbal supplements, to inhibit activity, resulting in an increased risk of drug interactions [148,152]. Similar to genetic variants, these interactions could lead to decreased drug efficacy or increased toxicity.

A well-studied interaction is the decreased hepatic uptake of statins (e.g., pravastatin and lovastatin) by OATPs in the presence of cyclosporine [313]. This interaction results in increased systemic concentrations of the statin and potentially an increased risk of rhabdomyolysis (muscle toxicity). A second example is offered by a clinical study involving endoxaban, an oral factor Xa inhibitor under development for thromboprophylaxis [314]. Administration of endoxaban with quinidine, a strong P-gp inhibitor, resulted in an increased endoxaban maximum concentration (C_{max}) and area under the plasma concentration–time curve (AUC), indicative of increased absorption. This information could be useful in determining dosing algorithms for patients already taking xenobiotics that inhibit P-gp, decreasing potential bleeding risks. A final example is the decreased intestinal absorption of fexofenadine by grapefruit juice [315]. This interaction results in a lower systemic exposure to fexofenadine, possibly decreasing efficacy. In vitro studies indicate that the underlying mechanism is inhibition of intestinal OATP1A2 and/or OATP2B1 by the grapefruit juice constituent naringin.

Both the US Food and Drug Administration and the International Transporter Consortium have suggested frameworks that can serve as starting points when evaluating possible interactions of new molecular entities with transporters [147,154,316]. Decision trees are provided for hepatic OATP1B1 and OATP1B3; renal OCT2, OAT1, OAT3, MATE1, and MATE2K; and broadly based P-gp and BCRP. As the field of transport proteins continues to evolve, so will these decision trees.

In addition to drug–drug and dietary component–drug interactions, drug–endogenous substrate interactions also are of emerging importance. Many of the transporters discussed transport various endogenous substrates (e.g., bilirubin and bile acids) in addition to drugs. As described in a number of reviews, another host of transporters not mentioned in this chapter almost solely transport endogenous substrates and can be inhibited by drugs and/or dietary components [1,148,154].

Pharmacogenomics in clinical gastrointestinal practice

Pharmacogenomics may be used to guide medical therapy of many disorders that are commonly encountered within gastroenterology practice. This section will highlight several classes of medication to demonstrate how pharmacogenomics can be used to guide therapy.

Thiopurines

Thiopurines, including azathioprine and 6-mercaptopurine, are inexpensive medications commonly prescribed to maintain corticosteroid-free remission of inflammatory bowel disease. Use of these medications has been limited due to adverse events, such as myelosuppression, hepatotoxicity, and pancreatitis. As discussed in the phase II drug metabolism section on thiopurine methyltransferase earlier in this chapter, myelosuppression is a common adverse reaction that disproportionately affects individuals of Asian descent (approximately 15%) compared to individuals of European descent (approximately 4%) despite the lower standard doses utilized in Asian countries.

Historically, TPMT testing – either through a biochemical activity assay or through genetic testing – was performed prior to administration of thiopurine medications to predict which individuals were at higher risk of toxicity, followed by dose adjustments as needed. The three most common variant TPMT alleles, *3A, *3C, and *2, have a minor allele frequency (MAF) among individuals of European descent of 3.43%, 0.47%, and 0.21%, respectively, for a collective frequency of 4.11%. These same three alleles, which are commonly included in clinical

TPMT tests, only have a MAF of 0.03%, 1.64%, and 0.01%, respectively, for a collective frequency of 1.68% among individuals of East Asian descent. Among African American populations, these variants have a MAF of 2.40% (*3C), 0.80% (*3A), and 0.53% (*2), while the *8 and *24 alleles, which are not typically included in clinical tests, have a MAF of 0.7% and 3.3%, respectively [317].

Genetic variation in the NUDT15 gene was identified as an additional contributor to thiopurine toxicity through a genome-wide association study [318]. The most common variant NUDT15 alleles among individuals of East Asian descent include *3, *2, *6, and *5 with 6.1%, 3.5%, 1.3%, and 1.1% MAF, respectively. The *2 allele is also relatively common among Latino populations, with a MAF of 3.7%. In contrast, these alleles are less frequently encountered among populations of European descent, with a MAF of <0.1% (*2, *5), 0.2% (*3), and 0.3% (*6). All of the alleles described thus far in both TPMT and NUDT15 lead to decreased enzyme activity. Interestingly, TPMT activity assays sometimes detect individuals with higher than expected activity but the underlying mechanism is not understood at this time.

Now that genetic variation in NUDT15 has also been recognized as contributing to thiopurine toxicity, particularly for Asian and other non-Caucasian populations, it is increasingly common to test both TPMT and NUDT15 prior to thiopurine use. Historically, a TPMT activity assay or genetic test could be used and were considered equivalent, though each test had unique benefits and limitations. The activity assays in clinical use today typically cannot detect variable NUDT15 activity; therefore, if a TPMT activity assay is used, an NUDT15 genetic test may be added.

While TPMT and NUDT15 are independent genes with differing frequencies among populations, individuals may have variants in one or both genes. Therefore, current dosing recommendations take into consideration both genes simultaneously [317]. Generally, for individuals who have one TPMT or NUDT15 decreased activity allele, a dose reduction is recommended. Individuals with two or more decreased activity alleles (impacting one or both genes) require a more significant dose reduction or an alternate therapy. Information on TMPT and NUDT15 genotype-guided dosing is also available in the FDA label. Of note, genetic testing does not replace the need for clinical monitoring with laboratory tests such as a complete blood count and liver function tests.

Proton pump inhibitors

Proton pump inhibitors (PPIs) are another class of medications often utilized in gastroenterology. While the medications comprising this class share a similar mechanism of action, their pharmacokinetics vary.

The first-generation PPIs, omeprazole, lansoprazole, and pantoprazole, are predominantly cleared by CYP2C19 along with a smaller contribution by CYP3A4. Dexlansoprazole, a second-generation PPI, also undergoes significant CYP2C19-mediated metabolism, while rabeprazole and esomeprazole are metabolized to a lesser degree by CYP2C19. As such, genetic variation in CYP2C19 has less influence on rabeprazole and esomeprazole. Rabeprazole is cleared predominantly through nonenzymatic reduction to a thioether metabolite, with a smaller contribution from CYP3A4 and CYP2C19 [319]. Esomeprazole and, to a lesser degree, omeprazole autoinhibit CYP2C19, which results in an increased area under the concentration-time curve with repeated administration [320].

While PPIs are considered to have an excellent safety profile, emerging evidence suggests that there may be more adverse events particularly with long-term use than previously appreciated, such as electrolyte imbalances, bone fractures, renal disease, and infections [319].

Genetic variation in CYP2C19 can lead to either increased or decreased activity, and the activity of variant alleles differs among populations [321]. The *17 allele includes a promoter variant that is thought to lead to increased transcription and increased activity. This allele is common among individuals of European, African American, Central/South Asian, and Latino descent (MAFs of 21.6%, 20.7%, 17.1%, and 16.7%, respectively), but rare among individuals of East Asian descent (MAF 2.05%). Individuals with increased CYP2C19 activity are expected to metabolize most PPIs, with the exceptions of rabeprazole and potentially esomeprazole, more quickly and may be at risk of lack of efficacy when used at standard doses. In contrast, the *2 and *3 alleles, which lead to decreased enzyme activity, are common across multiple populations but particularly those of East Asian descent. Specifically, the *2 and *3 alleles collectively have a MAF of 35.6% among East Asians, 28.6% among Central/South Asians, 18.4% among those of African American descent, 14.8% among individuals of European descent, and 10.5% among Latinos. Individuals with decreased CYP2C19 are expected to metabolize most PPIs (again, with the exceptions of rabeprazole and potentially esomeprazole) slower and may be at increased risk of adverse events, particularly with long-term use.

The Clinical Pharmacogenetics Implementation Consortium (CPIC) published a guideline for the use of CYP2C19 genetic information to guide PPI dosing [321]. In this guideline, recommendations are made for CYP2C19-based dosing of omeprazole, lansoprazole, pantoprazole, and dexlansoprazole. For ultrarapid metabolizers, consideration of an increased starting dose (100% greater than the standard dose) is recommended. Similarly, an increased starting dose (increased by 50–100% of the standard dose) is recommended for rapid metabolizers, particularly in the setting of treatment of *H. pylori* infection or erosive esophagitis. In both cases, monitoring for efficacy is recommended. For most indications, the guideline recommends starting normal metabolizers with a standard dose; however, similar to the recommendation for rapid metabolizers, for treatment of *H. pylori* or erosive esophagitis, consideration of an increased dose (50–100% increased) for normal metabolizers is recommended. For intermediate and poor metabolizers, initiating PPI therapy with a standard dose is recommended. For long-term treatment, consideration of a dose reduction by 50% is recommended once efficacy has been achieved. In addition, monitoring for continued efficacy is recommended.

Prokinetic agents

Metoclopramide is a dopamine type 2 receptor agonist that has been commonly used as a prokinetic agent since it was approved by the FDA in 1979. In addition to CYP2D6-mediated oxidation, metoclopramide is also metabolized by glucuronide and sulfate conjugation. In 2009, the FDA issued a boxed warning indicating that individuals taking metoclopramide are at increased risk from tardive dyskinesia, a severe movement disorder that is often irreversible. Older patients, those on a dose of 30 mg or more per day, and those on long-term (>2 years) metoclopramide therapy were found to be at higher risk [322,323]. Additionally, given that metoclopramide is a CYP2D6 substrate, genetic variation in CYP2D6 is also associated with risk of tardive dyskinesia.

While no practice guidelines for pharmacogenomic-based dosing of metoclopramide currently exist, the FDA label suggests a reduced metoclopramide dose for CYP2D6 poor metabolizers. A standard adult dose for the indication of gastroesophageal reflux is 10–15 mg four times daily, for a total of 60 mg. For CYP2D6 poor metabolizers, the label recommends 5 mg four times daily or 10 mg three times daily, with a maximum recommended daily dose of 30 mg. For the indication of acute and

Table 28.4 Examples of medications used in gastroenterology practice where genetic variation and/or pharmacokinetic interactions may necessitate an altered dosing strategy.

Medication	Enzyme	Allele frequency	Effect on medication
Thiopurines	TPMT	Reduced function alleles: European 4.1% African American 2.4% East Asian 1.7%	Increased risk of toxicity; dose reduction should be considered
	NUDT15	Reduced function alleles: East Asian 12.0% Latino 3.7% European 0.5%	
Proton pump inhibitors	CYP2C19	Reduced function alleles: East Asian 35.6% Central/South Asian 28.6% African American 18.4% European 14.8% Latino 10.5%	Increased risk of toxicity, particularly for those on long-term therapy; dose reduction once efficacy is achieved should be considered
		Increased function alleles: European 21.6% African American 20.7% Central/South Asian 17.1% Latino 16.7% East Asian 2.1%	Increased risk of lack of efficacy; dose increase should be considered
Metoclopramide	CYP2D6	Reduced function alleles: European 22.7% African American 15.4% African 13.8% South/Central Asian 9.2% East Asian 5.7%	Increased risk for toxicity; dose reduction should be considered
Cisapride	CYP3A4	Reduced function alleles: European 4.4% African 0.95%	Increased risk of toxicity, but most cases due to drug–drug interactions

recurrent diabetic gastroparesis, the FDA label recommends a dose of 10 mg four times daily and a maximum daily dosage of 40 mg for adult patients. For CYP2D6 poor metabolizers, the recommendation is only 5 mg four times daily and a maximum daily dosage of 20 mg. While genetic variations in KCNH2, HTR4, and ADRA1D have also been suggested to potentially influence risk of tardive dyskinesia or metoclopramide efficacy, these genes are not included in routine clinical testing [324].

Cisapride is also a prokinetic agent that stimulates 5-hydroxytryptamine (serotonin) receptors, resulting in an increase in lower esophageal sphincter tone, gastric emptying, and intestinal motility. Cisapride is metabolized in the liver predominantly by CYP3A4, with a smaller contribution of CYP2A6 [325]. In 1995, only two years after its 1993 approval, there were approximately 5 million prescriptions for cisapride filled in the US but in addition, the FDA had been informed of 23 cases of prolonged QT interval, 34 cases of torsade de pointes, and four deaths among cisapride users [326]. Many of the individuals who experienced adverse cardiac events had an underlying cardiac disorder, were taking medications that prolonged the QT interval (e.g., amitriptyline), or were also taking other medications or foods that inhibit CYP3A4 (e.g., erythromycin, clarithromycin, and grapefruit). As a result, in 1995, the FDA added a boxed warning to the cisapride label and the manufacturer sent a “Dear Health Care Professional” letter to inform ordering providers about the risk of adverse reactions with concurrent use of CYP3A4 inhibitors. Despite the growing concerns, widespread cisapride use continued and additional cases were reported. In 1998, the FDA expanded the boxed warning to include a contraindication in individuals taking medications that prolong the QT interval and patients with baseline cardiac disease and a follow-up “Dear Health Care Professional” letter was sent. Ultimately, in 2000, the manufacturer withdrew cisapride from the market, though it is still available for special uses in humans as well as in veterinary medicine.

The cisapride story highlights the potential impact on medication safety of altered drug metabolism through drug–drug interactions. While CYP3A4 genetic variation was not a feature of the cisapride story, the common CYP3A4*22 allele (MAF 4.4% among those of European descent, 0.95% among those of African descent, and rare among those of Asian descent) is defined by a deeply intronic variant that leads to aberrant splicing and decreased enzyme activity. Had genetic studies been performed, perhaps this variant may have also increased risk.

Summary

Taken together, these examples highlight the importance of considering pharmacokinetics when prescribing medications in clinical gastroenterology practice (Table 28.4). Pharmacokinetics can be altered through drug–drug (or drug–food) interactions or through genetic alterations. Pharmacogenetic testing is of increasing importance but the traditional variables considered when prescribing medications (e.g., renal function, hepatic function, age, body mass index, etc.) remain applicable and must be considered.

References are available at www.yamadagastro.com/textbook7e

Further reading

Bailey D.G., Dresser G., Arnold J.M. Grapefruit–medication interactions: forbidden fruit or avoidable consequences? *CMAJ* 2013;185:309.

Brantley S.J., Argikar A.A., Lin Y.S., et al. Herb–drug interactions: challenges and opportunities for improved predictions. *Drug Metab Dispos* 2014;42:301.

Gardiner S.J., Begg E.J. Pharmacogenetics, drug-metabolizing enzymes, and clinical practice. *Pharmacol Rev* 2006;58:521.

Giacomini K.M., Balimane P.V., Cho S.K., et al. International Transporter Consortium commentary on clinically important transporter polymorphisms. *Clin Pharmacol Ther* 2013;94:23.

Gurley B.J. Pharmacokinetic herb–drug interactions (part 1): origins, mechanisms, and the impact of botanical dietary supplements. *Planta Med* 2012;78:1478.

Gurley B.J., Fifer E.K., Gardner Z. Pharmacokinetic herb–drug interactions (part 2): drug interactions involving popular botanical dietary supplements and their clinical relevance. *Planta Med* 2012;78:1490.

Hillgren K.M., Keppler D., Zur A.A., et al. Emerging transporters of clinical importance: an update from the International Transporter Consortium. *Clin Pharmacol Ther* 2013;94:52.

Weinshilboum R.M., Wang L. Pharmacogenomics: precision medicine and drug response. *Mayo Clin Proc* 2017;92(11):1711.

Won C.S., Oberlies N.H., Paine M.F. Mechanisms underlying food–drug interactions: inhibition of intestinal metabolism and transport. *Pharmacol Ther* 2012;136:186.

Zanger U.M., Klein K., Thomas M., et al. Genetics, epigenetics, and regulation of drug-metabolizing cytochrome P450 enzymes. *Clin Pharmacol Ther* 2014;95:258.

CHAPTER 29

Medical decision making

John M. Inadomi
Department of Internal Medicine, University of Utah School of Medicine, Salt Lake City, UT, USA

Chapter menu

Medical decision making is a formal process that aims to optimize patient care using decision analytic techniques to weigh the benefits and harms of competing management strategies. Secondary goals include increasing patient participation in healthcare decisions to incorporate their healthcare preferences and minimizing unnecessary evaluation and treatment. This chapter will examine the tools available to synthesize published data and translate the information into clinical practice. The use of systematic reviews and metaanalyses to summarize evidence across multiple studies will be demonstrated. Incorporation of these data into medical decision models that synthesize benefits, harms, patient preferences, and costs will be illustrated. Development of clinical practice guidelines using methods that are valid and mitigate the risk for bias will be described. Finally, real-world examples of how clinical decision analysis has changed patient care will be presented.

Systematic reviews and metaanalysis

A systematic review examines a specific clinical management question using explicit methods to identify, select, and critically appraise relevant research, and to collect and analyze data from included studies [1]. Systematic reviews aim to present these findings in a transparent, unbiased manner. The first stage of a systematic review involves construction of a clinically relevant, focused question. The questions should be developed in the PICO format (Patient population, Intervention or exposure, Comparator, Outcome or endpoint). Study inclusion and exclusion criteria are declared, including the type of study design, participants, interventions, and outcome measures that will be included. A literature search is conducted using appropriate search terminology, such as Medical Subject Headings (MESH), in all appropriate electronic libraries (PubMed, Embase, Ovid, etc.) within a specified time frame in sufficient detail to allow others to replicate findings. Authors should also supplement the electronic search with manual searches of references lists of retrieved papers, trial registries, and regulatory agency websites. Titles and abstracts of search results may be screened for relevance, but full manuscript examination must be performed in all papers that meet entry criteria. Data extraction should be performed using standardized formats, and a minimum of two independent reviewers should abstract data using consensus to resolve discrepancies. Risk for bias of included studies should be assessed and reported. Finally, the primary and secondary summary measures and comparisons should be reported in the manner established before study initiation [2].

A systematic review may provide the data necessary to conduct a metaanalysis through which a summary estimate of the effect of an intervention or exposure is presented [1–3]. If the

Yamada's Textbook of Gastroenterology, Seventh Edition. Edited by Timothy C. Wang, Michael Camilleri, Benjamin Lebwohl, Anna S. Lok, William J. Sandborn, Kenneth K. Wang, and Gary D. Wu.

Companion website: www.yamadagastro.com/textbook7e

results are homogenous (i.e., answers to the clinical question across multiple studies are similar), a summary estimation of the size of the effect of the intervention or exposure is calculated using appropriate statistical tests; if, however, the data are heterogeneous, the reasons underlying the heterogeneity are sought.

Policy makers highlight the value of systematic reviews and metaanalyses as means to summarize evidence [4]. Despite this recognition, they are underutilized in clinical decision making [5]. A Cochrane review identified the following list of facilitators to increase the use of systematic reviews: (1) they clearly enhance knowledge, research, clinical protocols, and evidence-based medicine skills; (2) the content includes benefits, harms, and costs and is current, transparent, and timely; (3) the format includes staged access and an executive summary (different levels of detail are available); (4) there exists training in use of systematic reviews; and (5) peer-group support to understand and use systematic reviews is available [6]. The difficulty in translating knowledge into practice remains a persistent barrier to quality healthcare and is discussed later in this chapter.

Cost-effectiveness and medical decision making

Healthcare costs in the United States have increased from $1.4 trillion in 2000 to $2.6 trillion in 2010 and $3.5 trillion in 2017 [7]. The proportion of gross domestic product (GDP) spent on healthcare has increased in this time period from 13.4% to 18%. This rate of spending increase is unsustainable because these expenditures impact growth in other vital areas of the economy, such as education and research. Moreover, it is estimated that $700 billion each year are wasted in the United States, being used for interventions that do not improve health [8,9]. As the costs of providing healthcare increase in the face of limited available resources, it is increasingly essential to identify management strategies that are both effective and cost-effective. There are increasing requirements to validate practice patterns to patients, insurers, and regulatory agencies, including demonstration of cost-efficient management. Based on these realities, it is imperative that today's clinicians possess a solid understanding of healthcare economics.

Forms of economic analysis

Medical decision analysis uses a set of mathematical tools based on probability theory to quantitatively compare the expected outcomes of competing medical management strategies [3,10–12]. Economic analysis includes costs in the comparison of competing strategies to identify optimal management strategies in the context of limited economic resources [13]. Guidelines directing the conduct and interpretation of economic analysis in healthcare have been previously published [14–18]. The simplest form of economic analysis is a *cost-minimization analysis*, also known as a cost-identification analysis. The objective of a cost-minimization analysis is to calculate the least expensive manner in which to treat a specific disorder. For this type of analysis to be valid, the clinical benefits of competing strategies must be equivalent. The economic resources expended through each strategy are summed, considering the costs of the disease and its complications in addition to the costs of treatment. The results of a cost-minimization analysis are expressed in terms of the resources expended through implementation of each strategy.

If the clinical benefits between competing management strategies differ, a cost-minimization analysis is an inappropriate tool and more complex analytic methods should be used. A *cost-effectiveness analysis* aims to measure the cost incurred in relation to the benefit achieved and may be used to compare strategies that are expected to yield different outcomes. The result of a cost-effectiveness analysis is typically reported as the cost required to achieve each unit of benefit, such as the cost per life-year gained or the cost per symptom-free day achieved. When comparing competing strategies of management, the difference in net costs between strategies can be compared with the difference in net benefits to calculate the incremental cost-effectiveness ratio (ICER). Because this ratio represents the increase in resource expenditure per unit of benefit achieved with one strategy compared with another, lower ICERs are desirable, or more "cost-effective."

For some diseases, time spent in one state of health may not be viewed equal to time spent in other health states. Whereas a cost-effectiveness analysis assigns the same measure of outcome to all states in which the patient is alive, a *cost-utility analysis* varies the outcome to reflect patient preferences associated with each health state. To incorporate the differences in the quality of life between various states of health, a cost-utility analysis uses a conversion factor or weight that is assigned to each health state. These weights can range in value from 1, representing the state of perfect health in which full credit for time spent in this state is accrued, to 0, representing the state of death in which no credit is accrued. These factors, or *utilities*, represent the preferences that patients report for these various health states. The results of a cost-utility analysis include a unit of measurement that reflects the quality adjustment to the outcome, such as a quality-adjusted life-year (QALY). Comparison between strategies will yield an incremental cost-utility ratio that combines the quantity and quality of the outcome measure in one metric.

A fourth type of economic analysis is the *cost-benefit analysis*. This type of analysis differs from cost-effectiveness or cost-utility analysis in that all outcomes are expressed in monetary terms. Although this allows the results of the analysis to be expressed as a single value, it requires assumptions that all benefits can be assigned specific monetary units. The results of a cost-benefit analysis are calculated by subtracting the costs accrued from implementation of the strategy from the economic benefits gained; if the result is positive, a net gain is perceived to be achieved, whereas a negative result indicates that the strategy is not cost beneficial [19].

A final form of economic analysis is a *cost-consequence analysis*, in which the components of costs and benefits of competing programs are calculated and presented individually, without an attempt to aggregate the results.

Costs

An important distinction must be made between costs and charges. Costs are defined as the resources required to provide a particular service that represents the foregone opportunity to provide another service. Because resources expended for one service cannot be used for another purpose, this "opportunity cost" is defined by the value of that resource in its next best use to society [13]. Charges may deviate from cost estimates based on inclusion of profit margins, the relative bargaining power of payers and providers, and inaccuracies of accounting systems [20].

Different components of costs are included depending on the perspective of the economic analysis. Cost components include direct and indirect (productivity) costs. Direct costs are further subdivided into direct healthcare costs and direct nonhealthcare costs [13]. Direct healthcare costs are generally borne by *insurers and patients* and include the costs of procedures, tests, drugs, supplies, healthcare personnel, and medical facilities. Direct nonhealthcare costs are additional costs accrued by patients and include child care, elder care, and transportation costs required to attend healthcare encounters. Indirect or productivity costs represent resources lost by *society* resulting from the inability to work or engage in leisure activities because of morbidity or death from disease [13].

Evidence-based approach to economic studies

Criteria defining valid economic analyses have been previously published [13,18,21], including the Evidence-Based Medicine Working Group series "Users' Guide to the Medical Literature" [14,15]. Before accepting the conclusions of an economic analysis, three main issues should be considered: validity of the methods, presentation of the results, and implications for patient care.

Validity of the methods

Did the analysis provide a full economic comparison of healthcare strategies?

To answer this question, all clinically relevant strategies must be included in the analysis and an appropriate perspective of the analysis be chosen.

Was a broad enough viewpoint adopted?

When an economic model is constructed, the perspective, or vantage point from which costs and benefits are observed, must be established. A societal perspective is preferred whereby all costs borne by the healthcare system, the patient, and society are included; thus, direct healthcare costs, direct nonhealthcare costs, and indirect (productivity) costs are included [13,18,21]. Because direct nonhealthcare costs and indirect costs may be difficult to identify, perspectives less comprehensive than the societal perspective are commonly used. These perspectives include a third-party payer (insurer) perspective, the perspective of a hospital or clinic, or the patient perspective [13].

In addition to costs, outcomes include the effects examined, such as life-years gained or the number of cancer cases detected or prevented. If the analysis includes patient preferences for the various health states included in the model (a cost-utility analysis), the outcome will be described in units of QALYs. By examining more global benefits, such as life-years or QALYs, an economic analysis may compare resource expenditures among differing disease states; if outcomes are limited to those specific to a disease process, such as the numbers of cancers detected, such comparisons are not possible.

Were all the relevant strategies compared?

All clinically reasonable strategies available to manage a clinical problem should be considered. Moreover, each strategy should be scrutinized to ensure it conforms to a logical sequence of events. Generally, investigators will provide a figure summarizing their proposed model so readers can critique the model's structural and variable assumptions. Although it is beyond the scope of this chapter to discuss construction of decision models in detail, it should be noted that decision trees are designed to model the temporal flow of clinical events from one initial decision point to subsequent events, branching in a treelike fashion that aims to capture the probabilistic nature of a disease process. In contrast, Markov models allow for movement of hypothetical patients back and forth between various health states in a recursive fashion based on time. Discrete event simulation, conversely, assigns the probability of events occurring independently of time.

Were the costs and outcomes properly measured and valued?

Was clinical effectiveness established?

The clinical effectiveness of management strategies must be established before any comparison of the cost-effectiveness of these strategies. Results from a single trial, a range of values from multiple trials, or a summary estimate derived from a quantitative analysis of published studies (i.e., a metaanalysis) are generally accepted to approximate effectiveness. It should be noted that *efficacy*, which represents outcomes achieved in research settings using idealized subjects under optimal conditions, may differ from *effectiveness*, which reflects outcomes achieved in "real-life" settings using patients who may not have been represented in clinical trials, under varied management conditions. Thus, although published results from randomized clinical trials are considered the best evidence for establishing efficacy of therapy, economic studies may be more valid if based on effectiveness data that reflect clinical practice [14].

Were costs measured accurately?

Depending on the identified perspective of the analysis, different direct and indirect cost components should be included in the economic model. Specifically, a societal perspective that incorporates all direct (healthcare and nonhealthcare) and indirect (productivity) costs is optimally desired. However, because direct nonhealthcare and indirect costs are generally not available, many economic models are based on the third-party payer or insurer perspectives.

Were costs and outcomes data appropriately integrated?

The most common metric used to integrate results of a cost-effectiveness analysis is the ICER, which describes the additional cost incurred by providing an alternative strategy to achieve increased effectiveness [14]. Thus, in addition to reporting the costs of tested strategies and their associated outcomes, such as life-years or QALYs gained, an economic study should present the ICER between competing strategies. In this manner, the resources required to implement management strategies to improve outcome in one disease may be compared with interventions proposed to manage unrelated disease states.

Economic analyses commonly incorporate discounting or time preferences for outcomes. Discounting reflects people's preference for having money and material goods in the present rather than in the future, independent from the effect of inflation [18,21]. This concept accounts for the opportunity cost of spending money now to derive benefit at some later time and is generally based on the financial gain that could have been achieved had the resources required to implement an intervention instead been invested. In a similar manner, health benefits must also be adjusted to reflect time preferences of patients; if not, delaying implementation of an intervention would always appear more cost-effective [18].

Was appropriate allowance made for uncertainties in the analysis?

This is arguably the most important question to answer when assessing decision analysis studies, including those focusing on health economic questions. Uncertainty in the assumptions of the model may induce variability in the results that may cause the conclusions of the analysis to change. Uncertainty may be present in the parameter estimates (numerical values used for the model variables), as well as in the structural assumptions of the model, that is, how the model is constructed [13]. The conventional manner used to examine uncertainty is through sensitivity analysis. Values used as parameter estimates may be tested to observe whether variation within clinically relevant extremes alters the results. The structural assumptions may be tested by changing the relationship between various parts of the model and observing whether differences in conclusions arise. If variations of these factors are associated with substantial changes in conclusions, the model is reported to be sensitive to these factors. One of the major functions of decision analysis is to identify critical factors necessary to define a clinical problem. The variables to which a model is sensitive identify the priority areas in which further investigation should be pursued.

Uncertainties in parameter estimates may be examined through one-way sensitivity analysis in which a range of clinically plausible values are assigned to a single variable and the results are examined to determine whether the overall conclusions of the analysis change. In two- or three-way analyses, two or three variables are varied simultaneously to assess their joint influence on the outcome of the model. Multiple (n-way) sensitivity analysis can be accomplished through specialized modeling techniques, such as Monte Carlo simulation, in which the values assigned to multiple variables are varied simultaneously [22].

Are estimates of costs and outcomes related to the baseline risk in the treatment population?

It is important to understand the population simulated in an economic model. Specifically, the generalizability of the results of an analysis depend heavily on whether the hypothetical subjects are representative of the population as a whole, or represent only a subpopulation at high or low risk for the outcomes assessed by the model.

Presentation of the results

If serious methodological flaws are identified through the process outlined earlier, there is little need to examine the results of the study. However, it is hoped that published studies are of sufficient quality to achieve favorable responses to the criteria presented and warrant examination of the results of the analysis.

What were the incremental costs and outcomes of each strategy?

Results of an economic analysis are best understood by presenting the costs and health outcomes of each strategy, identifying dominated strategies (strategies costing more despite providing less benefit than other strategies), and calculating the incremental cost-effectiveness between successively more effective nondominated strategies [15].

Do incremental costs and outcomes differ between subgroups?

Much of outcomes research concerns identification of populations in which costs or health outcomes differ substantially from the average results. Subgroup analysis allows formation of models that can determine whether certain interventions are cost-effective only if limited to populations at high risk for development of poor outcomes or, conversely, may be cost-effective for the general population except for those identified at low risk for poor outcomes.

How much does allowance for uncertainty change the results?

As stated previously, one of the most important functions of a health economic analysis is to identify critical areas of research needed to establish whether proposed interventions are cost-effective. A sensitivity analysis illustrates whether variation in the baseline assumptions of a model substantially alter the conclusions of an analysis. Because uncertainty exists in the estimates used to populate the variables of all models, it is imperative that the range of clinical plausible values be examined in a systematic fashion. These values are generally obtained through systematic reviews and metaanalysis of existing literature. There may be insufficient data with which to conduct the analysis of some variables; in this case, the use of expert opinion may be the only method available to generate values.

If the conclusions of an analysis substantially change with variation in the assumptions of the model, the model is defined to be sensitive to these assumptions. If these assumptions are parameter estimates for variables, then clinical research is needed to more precisely define the value of these variables. If these assumptions are structural assumptions of the model, additional data are required to define the interactions between the variables of the model. The latter generally requires progress in understanding of the biology and etiology of a disease process, or the mechanism by which interventions may provide benefit.

Implications for patient care

An economic analysis will not be useful unless it addresses a clinical question that has the potential to improve patient management. It is essential to critically appraise the actual benefits, harms, and costs associated with implementation of tested strategies and to determine whether the results of an analysis based on data derived from a research environment can be extrapolated to real-world populations.

Are the treatment benefits worth the harms and costs?

When comparing competing strategies in terms of their costs and benefits, three outcomes are possible. First, a strategy may be less costly and provide greater benefit than an alternative strategy, in which case it is defined to be a *dominant* strategy. Conversely, the strategy itself may be *dominated* by being both costlier and less beneficial than the alternative. Lastly, a strategy may be costlier but more beneficial than the alternative; in this case the incremental cost-effectiveness or incremental cost utility may be calculated to determine whether the benefit is worth the expense. Implementation of the costlier strategy depends on the willingness or ability of the healthcare system (or appropriate perspective of the analysis) to commit the required resources to achieve the greater benefit.

Table 29.1 illustrates these possibilities. The difference in cost between strategies is aligned in rows, whereas the difference in effectiveness is listed in columns. When strategy A is less expensive than (or the same cost as) strategy B and possesses greater effectiveness, strategy A is defined to dominate strategy B. If the converse is true and strategy A is both more expensive and associated with less (or equal) effectiveness compared with strategy B, strategy A is defined to be dominated by strategy B. The remaining cells depict situations in which one strategy is associated with greater costs but also greater effectiveness. In these cases, the ICER may be calculated, representing the additional resources required to improve outcome by using one strategy instead of another.

Table 29.1 Interpretation of cost-effectiveness analyses.

		Effectiveness	
		A > B	**A ≤ B**
Costs	A > B	ICER A vs B	B dominant
	A ≤ B	A dominant	ICER B vs A*

* If costs and effectiveness are equal, strategies are equivalent.

Could my patients expect similar health outcomes?

This question addresses the generalizability of findings from research studies to clinical practice. One must consider the potential difference between the efficacy of an intervention in a clinical trial and the effectiveness of that intervention in a general practice setting. Because clinical trials are usually performed in highly selected patient populations at specialized research institutions, it must be questioned whether patients in one's own practice are similar enough to those in clinical trials to warrant extrapolation of the findings. In addition, the infrastructure to successfully implement the intervention must be shown to function as effectively as that available in the clinical trial [15].

Could I expect similar costs?

The perspective of the analysis dictates what types of cost are included in the model. However, even when limiting an economic analysis to direct healthcare costs, considerable differences may exist between costs used in a study and the costs inherent to one's own health system. The reasons are varied but include differences in the resources required to render services in different geographies or by the type of healthcare system (government, private insurer, HMO), or because variations in clinical practice may induce cost differences that prevent translation of study costs to one's own practice environment [18].

Clinical practice guidelines

In addition to data synthesis through systematic review, metaanalysis, and cost-effectiveness analysis, additional steps are needed to impact clinical management. Clinical practice guidelines are intended to create this link and are defined as "systemically developed statements to assist practitioner and patient decisions about appropriate healthcare for specific clinical circumstances" [23]. The goals of systematically developed clinical practice guideline are multiple: to improve patient care and health outcomes, to reduce inappropriate variations in practice, to promote efficient use of resources, and to help define and inform public policy. Although there has been a steady increase in the number of guidelines over the past decade, uptake and adoption of guidelines has been hindered by a number of factors, notably, lack of transparency in the development process, lack of a uniform system for rating the evidence that informs the guideline, lack of trust in the recommendations, and ineffective management of conflict of interest of guideline authors. Recognizing these deficiencies, an Institute of Medicine report defined standards for the development of high-quality guidelines [24].

Although several development frameworks have been used, the most widely accepted are the GRADE (Grading of Recommendations Assessment, Development and Evaluation) and the US Preventive Services Task Force. Because much of gastroenterology and hepatology care is not focused on prevention but rather diagnosis and treatment, GRADE is the preferred framework. GRADE's methodologically rigorous framework and binary classification of strong versus conditional (weak) recommendations provides a clear and actionable direction to patients, clinicians, and policy makers [25]. Strong recommendation means that most patients should receive the recommended course of action, whereas a conditional recommendation means that different choices may be appropriate for different patients (Table 29.2).

Developing a guideline using GRADE

The first step in the GRADE process is to define the clinical questions that will be addressed by a guideline. Each question should be framed using the PICO format. Since clinical outcomes often do not share equal importance, GRADE differentiates outcomes as those critical for decision making, others that are important but not critical for decision making, and those that are less or not important for decision making. Ranking of outcomes is important because the quality of evidence is determined separately for each outcome across studies.

The next step in GRADE is to conduct or identify a high-quality systematic review of the literature using Medline or the Cochrane Library for each PICO [25]. Each systematic review should examine data across individual studies used to generate a best estimate of the effect for each outcome. GRADE defines the quality of evidence as the confidence in the summary estimate, specified as high, moderate, low, and very low (Table 29.3). Unlike other quality assessments that are based exclusively on the study design, GRADE has explicit criteria allowing the assessor to rate up or down the quality of evidence (Table 29.4). Evidence from randomized controlled trials starts with a high confidence, and observational studies begin with an initial low confidence in the estimate. However, if a randomized controlled trial has major methodological limitations, such as inadequate allocation concealment, lack of blinding, high losses to follow-up, or absence of an intention-to-treat analysis, the quality of the evidence may be down-staged. If there is large variation in the effects observed across studies it is important to try to identify the cause for these inconsistent results, which may result from differences in the study populations, intervention, comparators, outcome measures, or study methodology. If no explanation for

Table 29.2 GRADE quality of evidence, strength of recommendations, and implications.

Strong recommendations

Patients: Most people in this situation would want the recommended course of action and only a small proportion would not. Formal decision aids are not likely to be needed to help individuals make decisions consistent with their values and preferences.

Clinicians: Most patients should receive the recommended course of action. Adherence to this recommendation according to guidelines could be used as a quality criterion or a performance indicator.

Policy makers: The recommendation can be adapted as a policy in most situations.

Conditional (weak) recommendations

Patients: The majority of people in this situation would want the suggested course of action, but many would not. Decision aids are useful in helping individuals make decisions consistent with their values and preferences.

Clinicians: Examined a summary of the evidence to help patients make a decision that is consistent with their own values and preferences (shared decision making).

Policy makers: There is a need for substantial debate and involvement of stakeholders.

GRADE, Grading of Recommendations Assessment, Development and Evaluation.

Table 29.3 Conceptualizing quality of evidence supporting a recommendation.

- High quality: We are very confident that the true effect lies close to that of the estimate of the effect supporting the recommendation.
- Moderate quality: We are moderately confident in the estimate of effect supporting the recommendation. The true effect is likely to be close to the estimate of effect, but the possibility exists to be substantially different.
- Low quality: Our confidence in the effect supporting the recommendations is limited. The true effect may be substantially different from the estimate of the effect
- Very low quality: We have very little confidence in the effect estimate supporting the recommendation. The true effect is likely to be substantially different from the estimate of effect.

Table 29.4 Rating the quality (confidence) of evidence.

Factors that can decrease our confidence (rating down)
1. Limitations in study design
2. Inconsistency of results
3. Indirectness of evidence
4. Imprecision of results
5. Publication bias

Factors that can increase our confidence (rating up)
1. Large magnitude of effect
2. Dose–response gradient
3. All plausible confounding would increase the effect of the intervention

the inconsistency can be identified, the evidence may be downgraded. In addition, it may not be possible to directly compare competing management strategies with other patient populations, or there may be low numbers of study participants or rare study outcomes that reduce certainty and may lead to downgrading evidence quality. Finally, the presence of wide confidence intervals that include benefit and no effect, or even potentially harms, may require further downgrading of quality.

Conversely, evidence derived from observational studies, such as retrospective cohort or case–control studies, may be upgraded if the effect size is large, if there is a dose-response gradient that supports a causal role of the intervention, or if all plausible confounding works to increase the observed effect.

The overall quality of evidence supporting a specific PICO is based on outcomes that are a priori deemed critical for decision making, and less so on outcomes that are deemed to be less critical. Importantly, however, there are additional factors that influence the strength of recommendations. The balance between desirable and undesirable effects of interventions, accounting for differences between individual patients' values and preferences, and consideration of the healthcare resources required to implement an intervention or strategy also influence the strength of a recommendation.

Real-world examples of medical decision making influencing clinical practice

The American Cancer Society's updated guidelines (2018) recommend initiating colorectal cancer screening in individuals at average risk for development of cancer at age 45 years [26]. There are no clinical studies reporting data for screening outcomes in this population; instead, this recommendation is based on computer simulation modeling that extrapolated the benefits and harms of studies of screening individuals aged 50 years and older and incorporated these assumptions into an existing framework of screening. Several independent computer models that had been calibrated to Surveillance, Epidemiology, and End Results cancer incidence and validated in prior studies to accurately represent the screening outcomes observed in clinical trials were used for this analysis [27,28]. The investigators belong to a National Institutes of Health-funded consortium of biostatisticians, epidemiologists, gastroenterologists, and computer scientists (Cancer Intervention and Surveillance Modeling Network) whose robust simulation methods have been replicated in many other cancer types (lung, breast, prostate, esophagus, cervix). The analysis supporting this recommendation calculated that colonoscopy screening every 10 years beginning at age 45 years provided an increase of 15–28 life-years per 1000 screened individuals compared with beginning screening at age 50 years [29]. Costs were not evaluated in this analysis, but the number of colonoscopies required to implement each strategy was used as a proxy for resource use. Starting colonoscopy screening at age 45 years compared with 50 years requires an additional 827–856 colonoscopies per 1000 individuals. Although this may be a reasonable use of resources, it is not possible to compare this with other cancer screening strategies.

A formal cost-effectiveness analysis of initiating screening at an early age has been published in which the costs of treatment and loss of life-years and quality of life resulting from colorectal cancer were balanced with the costs and harms associated with screening initiation at age 45 years instead of 50 years [30]. This analysis reported that initiating screening colonoscopy at age 45 years averted four cancers and two cancer deaths per 1000 persons, gaining 14.4 discounted QALYs compared with screening initiation at age 50 years. A total of 758 additional colonoscopies would be needed for screening and surveillance through age 75 years, with total costs of $33 900 per QALY gained. Similarly, initiating screening with annual fecal immunochemical testing (FIT) at age 45 years instead of age 50 years prevented four cancers and one cancer death, and gained 14.0 QALYs per 1000 persons; this required 267 more colonoscopies and 3242 additional FIT at a cost of $7700 per QALY gained.

One may evaluate the validity of this cost-utility analysis using the criteria presented earlier in *Evidence-based approach to economic studies*. The viewpoint of the analysis was the "health sector perspective" defined as costs of third-party payers and paid out of pocket by patients, related and unrelated to the condition under consideration. These included the costs of screening tests and procedures (FIT and colonoscopy) plus the costs of managing colonoscopy complications and the costs associated with cancer management; however, these did not include direct nonhealthcare costs (child-care or transportation costs to attend colonoscopy) or indirect costs (wages lost because of screening complications or cancer) that would be necessary to provide a "societal perspective." This may be considered a limitation of the analysis; however, including indirect costs requires monetizing the value of life through lost wages, which is controversial and requires assumptions that could reduce the validity of the results.

A wide variety of clinically feasibly strategies were considered, not only including standard strategies such as annual FIT or colonoscopy every 10 years but also "hybrid" strategies in which sigmoidoscopy or FIT was modeled between the ages of 45 and 49 years, followed by colonoscopy every 10 years after age 50 years. For this reason, it seems that all clinically relevant options were considered in this study. The clinical effectiveness for screening was based on published literature reporting the sensitivity and specificity of individual screening tests for detection of polyps and cancer. Costs and outcomes data were integrated in a standard cost-effectiveness analysis using the ICER to evaluate the added costs required to implement successively more expensive strategies in relation to the increase in benefit (QALYs gained) with each strategy. Both costs and benefits (QALYs) were discounted at the standard annual rate of 3% to account for the opportunity cost foregone to implement screening in a healthy population and patient preferences for benefits to be achieved sooner than later.

Most importantly, an extensive sensitivity analysis was presented in which variation in the model inputs was tested to observe the thresholds at which the conclusions of the analysis changed. In particular, this analysis found that the results were highly sensitive to the cancer risk in the population and the costs of colonoscopy and cancer management. If the cancer risk was reduced to half of the observed rate in 45- to 49-year-old individuals, initiating screening colonoscopy would not be a cost-effective alternative to waiting to initiate screening at age 50 years. This analysis also identified that the costs and outcomes of the analysis were directly related to the baseline risk in the treatment population.

Moving to the presentation of the results, this study presented the costs and health outcomes of each screening strategy and identified dominated strategies, including no screening that was both costlier and less effective than screening with annual FIT or colonoscopy every 10 years. The main point of the study was that the subgroup of younger adults (45–49 years of age) had sufficiently elevated risk for colorectal cancer to warrant screening irrespective of the screening strategy chosen. The authors chose to consider an alternative use of the additional screening tests in a sensitivity analysis: if the 758 additional colonoscopies per 1000 persons needed to initiate screening in 45-year-old individuals was instead used to screen currently unscreened 55-year-old persons, 13 cancers and 6 cancer deaths could be prevented. This highlighted the fact that although screening may be cost-effective in younger adults, the risk for cancer is still greater in older adults, rendering screening opportunities in older adults more effective and cost-effective. Finally, the implications for patient care are clear from this analysis: lowering the age at which colorectal cancer screening is initiated to 45 years is cost-effective compared with other healthcare interventions that society has adopted.

Despite the validity of the model structures, analysis, and reporting, a number of considerations should be made when evaluating the use of medical decision models in clinical practice and policy. In addition to the categories discussed previously (see earlier *Evidence-based approach to economic studies*), there are several issues that may be explored with this specific example. There is an assumption that the natural history of the transition from polyp to cancer is identical between younger and older adults, that screening tests behave similarly, and that the effectiveness of screening is equal between these age groups. There are reasons to question these assumptions. The increasing incidence of colorectal cancer in younger adults (<50 years old) has peculiar characteristics that have not been fully explained. For example, the increase is predominantly observed in distal colon and rectal cancers, especially among younger white individuals, compared with older adults in whom proximal cancers are more common [31]. The striking birth cohort effect seen in the early-onset colorectal cancer strongly suggests an environmental factor that influences cancer risk at a young age [32]. In contrast, a greater proportion of early-onset colorectal cancers have germline mutations and half are in genes associated with Lynch syndrome [33], although a germline mutation was not identified in 80% of patients with early-onset colorectal cancer [34].

For this reason, the public policy to change the age at which to initiate screening to age 45 years should be carefully scrutinized. It is possible that some colorectal cancer screening tests may not possess the same characteristics (sensitivity, specificity) in the younger versus older population if, for example, the genetic alterations are not identified similarly with a stool DNA test because the underlying genetic pathogenesis differs between younger and older adults. Likewise, colonoscopy may not be as effective in detecting and removing neoplasia if the polyp characteristics are flatter (sessile) and susceptible to misses or incomplete resection. Simulation models can be a powerful tool to extend the results of clinical trials to populations and positively influence clinical practice and policy; however, they should be thoughtfully implemented with regards to the limitations of the models to ensure they accurately calculate the outcomes of interventions.

Problems implementing guidelines into clinical practice

Practice guidelines have not yet achieved the goal of increasing quality while reducing unnecessary expenditures. A Cochrane review of 45 studies comparing the effectiveness of provider-focused educational material versus no intervention revealed that these had only a small beneficial effect on professional practice outcomes (median absolute risk difference in categorical practice outcomes = 0.02 [0–0.110]) [24]. A cluster-randomized trial testing whether dissemination of published guidelines, algorithms, stratification scoring systems, and written reminders with performance feedback improved adherence to guideline recommendations for management of ulcer bleeding failed to show a significant difference compared with control groups [35]. A qualitative study of Dutch general practitioners identified several barriers to adherence to clinical practice guidelines: lack of agreement with the recommendations due to lack of applicability or lack of evidence; environmental factors, such as organizational constraints; lack of knowledge regarding the guideline recommendations; and guideline factors, such as unclear or ambiguous guideline recommendations [36]. Additional research has shown that controversial recommendations are less often followed than noncontroversial recommendations, and recommending a change in practice is difficult but is made easier if recommendations are based on research evidence [37]. Conversely, the features of guidelines that have been shown to be associated with greater uptake included recommendations that required acquisition of new skills, absence of a complex decision tree, compatibility with existing norms and values and practice, and support from published evidence [38].

In addition to these empirically identified barriers, it seems apparent that there exists a lack of adequate incentives to implement recommendations and motivate change in behavior. The emerging focus on "value-based purchasing" of healthcare insurance attempts to provide financial incentives for providers to pursue management strategies that are based on best evidence and have been demonstrated to be cost-effective. The shift from reimbursement based on quantity to payment based on quality represents the next step in the evolution of healthcare payment reform. In the United States, the National Quality Forum establishes quality measures on which the Centers for Medicare & Medicaid Services may employ differential reimbursement to reward programs that achieve or exceed these metrics, and penalize programs that either do not meet these requirements or are unable to measure, document, and report their outcomes.

Conclusions

The ultimate goal of medical decision making is to provide a framework through which clinicians may translate best evidence into optimal management for patients under their care. This starts with rigorous systematic reviews and metaanalyses, which may be complemented by cost-effectiveness or similar economic analyses. Clinical practice guidelines are designed to synthesize information to assist clinicians improve healthcare decisions. However, it is imperative that guidelines are constructed in a transparent fashion that demonstrates the rationale for recommendations and mitigates potential bias and author conflict of interest. Guidelines must provide clear guidance to practicing physicians and form the basis for metrics upon which we agree to be judged. The GRADE framework is an internationally recognized method through which clinical practice guidelines may be developed, taking account of not only the quality of the evidence but also the relative benefits and harms associated with competing management strategies, potential ambiguity in patient preferences for treatments and outcomes, and the healthcare resources necessary to implement interventions or strategies.

References are available at www.yamadagastro.com/textbook7e

Further reading

Gold M.R. Cost-Effectiveness in Health and Medicine. New York: Oxford University Press; 1996.

Guyatt G.H., Oxman A.D., Vist G.E., et al. GRADE: an emerging consensus on rating quality of evidence and strength of recommendations. BMJ 2008;336(7650):924.

Heitkemper M.M., Jarrett M.E., Levy R.L., et al. Self-management for women with irritable bowel syndrome. Clin Gastroenterol Hepatol 2004;2(7):585.

Institute of Medicine. In: Field M, Lohr K, editors. Guidelines for Clinical Practice: From Development to Use. Washington, DC: The National Academies Press; 1992.

Institute of Medicine. The Healthcare Imperative: Lowering Costs and Improving Outcomes: Workshop Series Summary. Washington, DC: The National Academies Press; 2010.

Liberati A., Altman D.G., Tetzlaff J., et al. The PRISMA statement for reporting systematic reviews and meta-analyses of studies that evaluate health care interventions: explanation and elaboration. Ann Intern Med 2009;151(4):W65.

Palmblad M., Tiplady B. Electronic diaries and questionnaires: designing user interfaces that are easy for all patients to use. Qual Life Res 2004;13(7):1199.

Richardson W.S., Detsky A.S. Users' guides to the medical literature. VII. How to use a clinical decision analysis. A. Are the results of the study valid? Evidence-Based Medicine Working Group. JAMA 1995;273(16):1292.

Richardson W.S., Detsky A.S. Users' guides to the medical literature. VII. How to use a clinical decision analysis. B. What are the results and will they help me in caring for my patients? Evidence Based Medicine Working Group. JAMA 1995;273(20):1610.

Weinstein M.C., Siegel J.E., Gold M.R., Kamlet M.S., Russell L.B. Recommendations of the Panel on Cost-effectiveness in Health and Medicine. JAMA 1996;276(15):1253.

PART 2

Symptom management

CHAPTER 30

Approach to the patient with dysphagia, odynophagia, or noncardiac chest pain

Albert J. Bredenoord
Academic Medical Center, Amsterdam, The Netherlands

Chapter menu

Definition

Despite its relatively simple anatomy and function, the esophagus can generate a variety of symptoms. Probably the most commonly encountered esophageal symptoms are heartburn and regurgitation. These are most frequently associated with gastroesophageal reflux disease (GERD), but can occur in many other disorders as well. Reflux symptoms and GERD will be discussed elsewhere in this book (see Chapter 43). In this chapter, three other esophageal symptoms – dysphagia, odynophagia, and chest pain – will be discussed. As will be outlined, the pathophysiology of these symptoms is diverse and their recommended management is highly dependent on the underlying abnormality.

Dysphagia

The term *dysphagia* is derived from the ancient Greek words δυς (dys, bad, disordered) and φαγέίν (fagein, to eat). Dysphagia is often translated as "difficulty with swallowing" but this is frequently incorrect because in many patients with dysphagia, the swallowing act (deglutition) is normal. It is essential to distinguish between oropharyngeal dysphagia and esophageal dysphagia. In oropharyngeal dysphagia, the patient perceives difficulty in transporting the bolus from the mouth to the esophagus; in esophageal dysphagia, the patient experiences delayed transit of the bolus through the esophagus. Oropharyngeal dysphagia is also referred to as "high" or "cervical" dysphagia and can be associated with aspiration, cough during eating, and drooling. It should be noted that in some patients with an esophageal cause of dysphagia (e.g., achalasia), the history suggests a disturbance in proximal esophageal function because of the patient's perception of the area of hold-up. These patients point at the region of the upper esophageal sphincter as the site of bolus hold-up. This can be misleading; it can be the cause of referral to an ear-nose-throat (ENT) specialist rather than to a gastroenterologist and may lead to a delay in diagnosis.

Dysphagia (both oropharyngeal and esophageal) can be limited to solid or liquid boluses or can occur with both.

Odynophagia

The term *odynophagia* is mostly used to indicate that transit of swallowed material through the esophagus is associated with retrosternal pain. The word is derived from the Greek οδυνη (odyno, pain) and φαγέίν (fagein, to eat). Odynophagia can occur with all types of food and drink but often certain foods are more painful than others. The symptom is less common than dysphagia.

The term odynophagia can also be used to denote pain in the pharynx or throat that occurs during swallowing. Management

Yamada's Textbook of Gastroenterology, Seventh Edition. Edited by Timothy C. Wang, Michael Camilleri, Benjamin Lebwohl, Anna S. Lok, William J. Sandborn, Kenneth K. Wang, and Gary D. Wu.

Companion website: www.yamadagastro.com/textbook7e

of this type of odynophagia ("oropharyngeal odynophagia") is usually in the domain of the ENT specialist.

Chest pain

Angina-like chest pain is a retrosternal oppressing pain that is usually described as severe and can be frightening. The characteristics of this pain are similar to those of angina pectoris and acute myocardial infarction, including radiation to jaw and left arm. The adjective "noncardiac" should only be used when a cardiac origin of the pain has been excluded or made highly unlikely by evaluation by a cardiologist.

Organic versus functional disorders

Whereas the symptoms dysphagia, odynophagia, and noncardiac chest pain point to the esophagus as a cause, it is not always possible to prove the esophageal origin of symptoms. If an esophageal cause is identified, the correlation between the severity of the abnormal findings and the severity of these symptoms is often poor. If a clear origin of the symptoms cannot be found, the symptoms are categorized as "functional." The Rome IV classification of functional gastrointestinal disorders encompasses criteria for "functional dysphagia" and "functional chest pain" [1].

Pathophysiology

The symptoms of dysphagia, odynophagia, and chest pain can result from a multitude of diseases and disorders, not only of the esophagus but also of neighboring organs. Whereas there clearly is overlap between the pathophysiology of the three symptoms, specific pathophysiological mechanisms appear to be involved in the development of each symptom.

Dysphagia

In the pathophysiology of *oropharyngeal* dysphagia, factors that may play a role include poor dentition, neurological diseases that impair mastication and diminish saliva production because they affect the oral preparation phase of swallowing. Neurological disorders, such as stroke, malignancy or Parkinson disease, and cerebral trauma may also lead to disordered bolus transit from the mouth to the pharynx and disordered delivery of the bolus to the proximal esophagus. Even if the contractile forces are in the normal range, loss of coordination between the pharyngeal peristaltic contraction and relaxation of the upper esophageal sphincter resulting from a neurological disorder can cause severe oropharyngeal dysphagia.

Esophageal dysphagia is caused by either luminal obstruction or by abnormal motor function of the esophagus and/or the lower esophageal sphincter (LES). Not infrequently, a combination of obstructive and motility factors can be identified, as in eosinophilic esophagitis (EoE) [2].

Obstruction of the esophageal lumen can be caused by an intrinsic (esophageal) abnormality, such as a tumor or peptic stricture, or by an extrinsic (extraesophageal) process, such as a tumor in the mediastinum or an aneurysm of the thoracic aorta or rarely dysphagia lusoria caused by the aberrant subclavian artery crossing and compressing the esophagus.

Motor disorders of the esophageal body that can cause impaired esophageal transit and dysphagia are of two types: those with diminished or absent peristalsis and those associated with spastic esophageal contractions. In addition, dysphagia can be caused by insufficient relaxation of the LES ("esophagogastric junction dysfunction"), either as an isolated abnormality or in combination with disordered or absent peristalsis, as occurs in achalasia. In Figure 30.1 the Chicago classification of esophageal motor disorders is presented [3].

In the pathophysiology of achalasia, loss of neurons in the esophageal myenteric plexus is a key mechanism, the most plausible explanation for which being the development of autoantibodies against the neurons. Rarely, achalasia occurs as a paraneoplastic effect of a distant tumor. In some regions of South America, achalasia-like motor abnormalities are brought about by Chagas disease, resulting from an infection with Trypanosoma cruzi. There are increasing numbers of patients who acquired such infections while living in South America and who now reside in the United States. Indeed, increasing numbers of endogenous infections have been documented in Texas and elsewhere in the southern states. Esophagogastric junction outflow obstruction (EGJOO) is the condition where LES relaxation is insufficient but peristalsis is preserved such that the criteria for achalasia are not met. EGJOO can be a precursor state of achalasia but in most patients, it is not associated with impaired bolus transit and symptoms of dysphagia.

As in other parts of the gastrointestinal tract, there is usually a poor correlation between the severity of a motility disorder and the severity of the patient's symptoms. This is certainly true for the symptom of dysphagia. Even in patients with complete absence of peristalsis, as in scleroderma, dysphagia is frequently absent. At the other end of the spectrum, patients may experience severe dysphagia but have completely normal esophageal peristalsis, LES function, and bolus transit on barium studies.

The pathophysiological events underlying dysphagia in eosinophilic esophagitis are incompletely understood. In some cases, narrowing of the esophageal lumen, often at more than one site, plays a role. In others, eosinophilic esophagitis is associated with disordered esophageal motility. Studies also suggest that impaired distensibility of the esophagus is involved in the pathophysiology in a subset of patients with the disorder [4].

Odynophagia

Organic causes of odynophagia usually seem to have in common a lesion of the esophageal mucosa; in a minority of cases, the pain with swallowing is caused by esophageal spasms. The assumption is that the lesion leads to increased exposure of chemo- and thermonociceptors within the mucosa and submucosa. When activated, these nociceptors transmit their impulses through unmyelinated C-fibers or myelinated Aδ-fibers, the

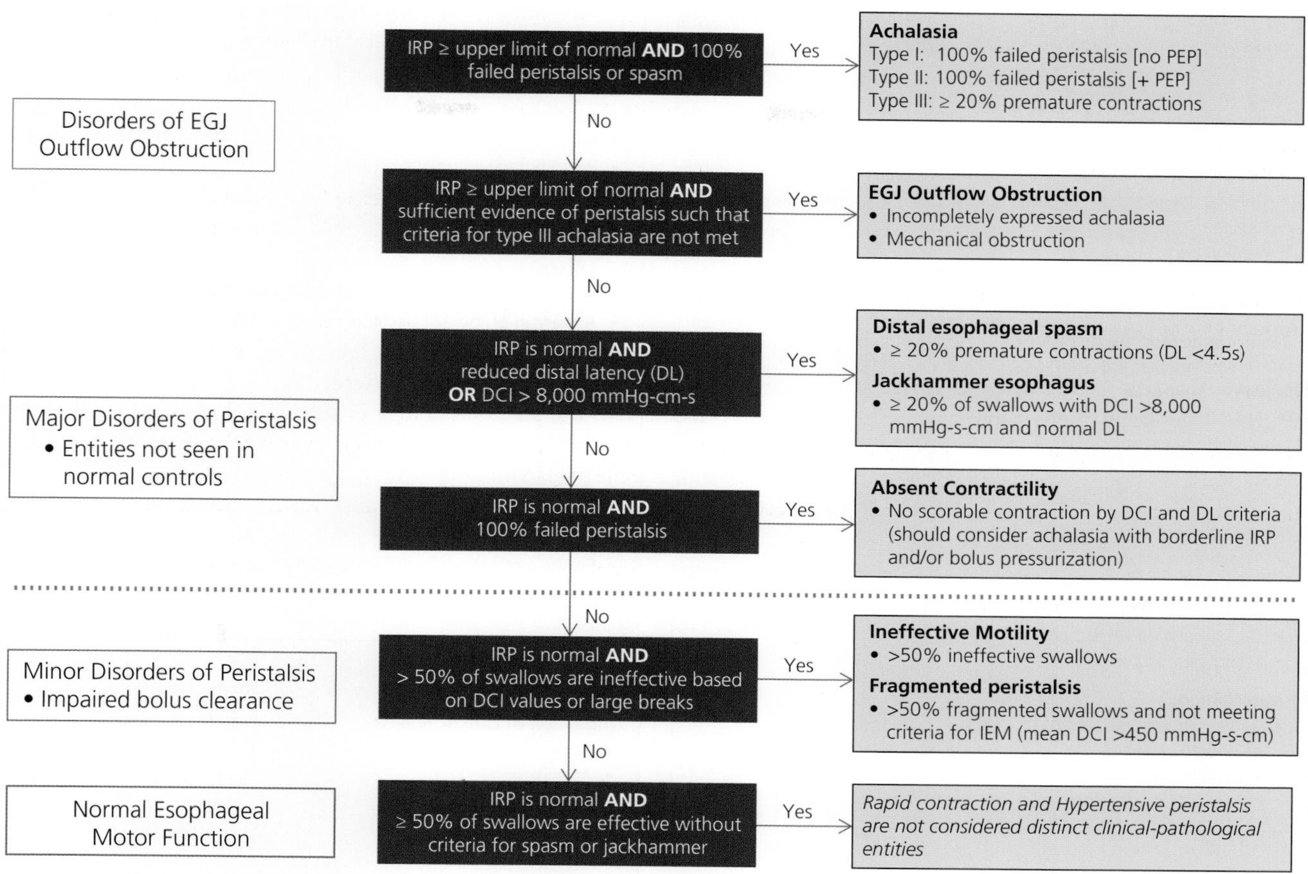

Figure 30.1 Chicago Classification of Primary Esophageal Motor Disorders v3.0. The conditions below the red dotted line are not considered to be clinically significant. IRP, integrated relaxation pressure; EGJ, esophagogastic junction; DL, distal latency; PEP, panesophageal pressurizations; DCI, distal contraction integral.

latter leading to sharper and better localized pain than the former [5]. Odynophagia can also be functional in nature.

Noncardiac chest pain

Most patients with episodic chest pain do not have an organic cause of their symptoms, so their symptoms are deemed to be functional. Episodic chest pain of esophageal origin can be elicited by gastroesophageal reflux and spastic motor disorders, with the former being more frequent. It is unclear why most patients experience reflux as heartburn and a minority as angina-like chest pain. The mechanisms through which presence of gastric contents in the esophagus elicits heartburn or chest pain have not been fully elucidated. It is intuitively plausible that a defective mucosal barrier makes it possible for hydrogen ions to penetrate deeper in the mucosa than is the case in health [6]. The discovery that the intercellular spaces between the surface epithelial cells are wider in patients with reflux disease than in healthy subjects lends support to this hypothesis [7].

The mechanisms through which esophageal spasm, jackhammer esophagus, and achalasia can lead to chest pain are far from clear. Three theories have been proposed as being responsible for the pain: stimulation of stretch-sensitive mechanoreceptors in the deeper layers of the esophageal wall [5]; ischemia of the esophagus takes place during prolonged and abnormally strong esophageal contractions; and sustained longitudinal muscle contractions [8]. None of these mechanisms explains the relatively poor correlation between chest pain episodes and episodes of abnormal contractility.

The pathogenesis of the chest pain in patients with "functional chest pain" (Rome IV) is still obscure. Whereas there are data showing that visceral hyperalgesia and central sensitization may be involved, recent findings do not support the notion that esophageal hypersensitivity plays a role [9,10].

Etiologies

Oropharyngeal dysphagia

The causes of *oropharyngeal* (cervical) dysphagia are listed in Box 30.1. As in esophageal dysphagia, obstruction of the lumen by an intrinsic or extrinsic lesion or structure is high on the list of possibilities. Since most of the causes of oropharyngeal

Box 30.1 Causes of oropharyngeal dysphagia.

Mechanical obstruction
- Cricopharyngeal bar
- Neoplasms
- Retropharyngeal abscess
- Cervical osteophyte
- Goiter
- Foreign body
- Zenker diverticulum
- Any esophageal stenosis or obstruction

Neurogenic motility disorder
- Cerebrovascular accident
- Parkinson disease
- Amyotrophic lateral sclerosis
- Multiple sclerosis
- Brainstem tumors
- Peripheral neuropathies

Myogenic motility disorder
- Myasthenia gravis
- Polymyositis
- Myotonic dystrophy
- Oculopharyngeal dystrophy
- Esophageal motor disorders

Miscellaneous
- Decreased saliva secretion
  - Sjögren syndrome
  - Radiotherapy
  - Medication with anticholinergic side-effects

dysphagia lie within the realm of the otolaryngologist and the neurologist, these will not be discussed in detail here. However, every gastroenterologist must have sufficient knowledge of these disorders to recognize them and to refer the patient to the most appropriate specialist.

Functional dysphagia

The causes of *esophageal* dysphagia, listed in Box 30.2, clearly differ from those of oropharyngeal dysphagia, but they share the subdivision into two broad groups: mechanical obstruction and motility disorders.

A few decades ago, fibrotic stenosis (stricture) of the distal esophagus caused by reflux esophagitis was one of the most common causes of dysphagia. Since the advent of drugs that inhibit acid secretion, in particular proton pump inhibitors, the prevalence of peptic esophageal stenosis has declined considerably. Likewise, the prevalence of Schatzki ring, an easily disruptable superficial circular stricture, has become less common, with the widespread use of acid inhibitors. In contrast, malignant strictures of the esophageal lumen are increasingly relevant as a cause of dysphagia, not only because acid-peptic causes have become less prevalent but also because the incidence of esophageal adenocarcinoma is increasing. There has also been a huge increase in prevalence of eosinophilic esophagitis, making it now the most common cause of dysphagia in young adults and adolescents [11].

Box 30.2 Causes of esophageal dysphagia.

Mechanical obstruction
- Eosinophilic esophagitis
- Peptic stricture
- Radiotherapy-induced stricture
- Esophageal adenocarcinoma
- Esophageal squamous cell carcinoma
- Benign esophageal tumor
- Schatzki ring
- Aberrant subclavian artery (dysphagia lusoria)
- Aneurysm of thoracic aorta
- Mediastinal abnormalities
- Foreign body

Motility disorders
- Achalasia
- Distal esophageal spasm
- Jackhammer esophagus
- Scleroderma
- Chagas disease
- Severe ineffective esophageal motility

Box 30.3 Causes of odynophagia.

Ingestion of caustic agents
- Acid
- Alkali[xbl]

Pill-induced esophagitis
- Doxycycline
- Nonsteroidal antiinflammatory drugs
- Bisphosphonates
- Slow-release potassium chloride

Foreign body

Radiation esophagitis

Infectious esophagitis
- Candida albicans
- Viral infections (herpes simplex virus, cytomegalovirus, HIV)
- Mycobacteria (tuberculosis, avium complex)

Erosive esophagitis in gastroesophageal reflux disease
Eosinophilic esophagitis
Esophageal carcinoma

Odynophagia

The causes of odynophagia are listed in Box 30.3. The clinical picture of pill-induced odynophagia is characteristic: a history of ingestion of a drug with corrosive properties, midesophageal odynophagia, and a localized mucosal lesion at endoscopy, usually at the level of the aortic impression [12]. The odynophagia associated with esophagitis caused by Candida albicans, herpes simplex virus or cytomegalovirus is most frequently found in patients who are immunocompromised [13]. Candida albicans infection can also occur in patients who use an inhalation corticosteroid for obstructive lung disease and in those with severe esophageal stasis, for example in achalasia. Rarely, odynophagia

Box 30.4 Causes of chest pain.

Cardiac abnormalities
- Angina pectoris
- Myocardial infarction
- Pericarditis
- Mitral valve prolapse
- Microvascular angina

Gastroesophageal reflux

Eosinophilic esophagitis

Musculoskeletal causes
- Costochondritis
- Fibromyalgia

Esophageal motor disorders
- Esophageal spasm
- Jackhammer esophagus
- Achalasia

Neuropsychiatric causes
- Panic disorder

is the first symptom of esophageal squamous cell carcinoma, which need not be advanced to cause the symptom.

Chest pain

The causes of noncardiac chest pain are listed in Box 30.4. In contrast to popular belief, GERD is a far more common cause of noncardiac chest pain than so-called spastic motor disorders such as diffuse spasm or jackhammer esophagus [14]. Musculoskeletal causes of chest pain can usually by identified by physical examination, revealing tenderness on palpation. Panic attacks in the context of panic disorder may be accompanied by a variety of somatic symptoms, chest pain being one of the most frequently encountered [15]. In most patients with noncardiac chest pain, a clear cause of their symptom will not be identified and their symptoms will be deemed functional.

Diagnosis

History and physical examination

In patients presenting with dysphagia, odynophagia, or chest pain, the diagnostic process must start with meticulous history taking. It is of the utmost importance to obtain information about the onset of the complaint. In general, a symptom with long duration is less reason for concern than a symptom with a recent onset. It is also important to inquire about potential factors that led to the development of the symptom, for example the ingestion of a sharp object or a caustic substance.

Functional chest pain of esophageal origin

In the case of dysphagia, it is of primary importance to find out whether there is a problem with the act of swallowing (oropharyngeal dysphagia) or with the transit of a successfully swallowed bolus through the esophagus (esophageal dysphagia).

In patients with episodic angina-like chest pain, it is pivotal to ascertain whether or not the pain is exercise related. If this is the case, gastroesophageal reflux can still be the cause of the pain, but it is essential to exclude a cardiac origin of the symptom before any gastroenterological work-up is begun.

Laboratory tests

In the diagnosis of disorders associated with dysphagia, odynophagia, or noncardiac chest pain, laboratory tests rarely contribute to the management and are therefore not recommended in the work-up. In patients with severe esophagitis or esophageal carcinoma, iron deficiency and anemia can sometimes be found.

Imaging tests

Endoscopy

Endoscopic examination of the esophagus plays a pivotal role in the management of patients with dysphagia, odynophagia, or noncardiac chest pain. In patients with dysphagia or a history of food impaction, eosinophilic esophagitis should be ruled out by taking an adequate number of biopsies along the length of the esophagus, even if the mucosa is macroscopically normal [16]. There is no evidence that taking biopsies from macroscopically normal mucosa is useful in patients with odynophagia or chest pain in the absence of dysphagia and food impaction.

Barium swallow

The barium esophagogram is still a useful technique in the work-up of patients with unexplained dysphagia [17]. Detection of subtle changes in esophageal diameter (dilation or stenosis) is better with radiography than with endoscopy. In addition, and most importantly, the barium esophagogram provides information about esophageal transit. It is controversial whether swallowing of a solid bolus, such as a marshmallow or a piece of bread impregnated with barium, should be part of the examination. It is normal for a solid bolus to remain in the esophagus for several peristaltic waves and use of a solid bolus therefore easily leads to overdiagnosis of a problem in esophageal emptying [18].

Function tests

It is of the utmost importance that structural lesions of the esophagus, in particular cancer, have been ruled out before considering function testing.

Esophageal manometry

Manometry is the gold standard for the detection and classification of esophageal motility disorders. With manometry, even subtle impairment of esophageal peristalsis can be detected. In recent years, high-resolution manometry has largely replaced conventional manometric techniques. With this technique, intraesophageal pressures are measured at 1–2 cm intervals, rather than at 3 cm or 5 cm intervals. This innovation has led to new algorithms for graphical display and interpretation of the recorded signals [3]. High-resolution manometry is felt to be easier, more intuitive, and better able to identify achalasia.

Esophageal manometry can be combined with intraluminal impedance measurement which allows assessment of the functional impact of esophageal contractions; it is uncertain if this helps in the clinical work-up of a patient and findings with impedance monitoring are not part of the classification system. The use of solid swallows, a test meal or a rapid drinking test in the manometric study have been advocated but it should be realized that it may also complicate interpretation and "abnormal findings" are often seen in healthy subjects [18,19].

Esophageal transit scintigraphy

Esophageal emptying scintigraphy involves ingestion of a liquid or solid bolus labeled with a radionuclide and recording of radionuclide transit by a gamma-camera [20]. Scintigraphy does not provide structural information and although the technique allows detailed quantification of esophageal transit, it has largely been abandoned as the same can be done with barium swallows and these also add structural information.

Differential diagnosis

In all patients presenting with dysphagia, odynophagia, or noncardiac chest, the underlying cause should be sought. As is apparent from Box 30.1 through Box 30.4, the differential diagnosis is different for each of these symptoms, and it is different for oropharyngeal and esophageal dysphagia.

Principles of management

The most important principle of the management of patients presenting with dysphagia, odynophagia, or chest pain of potential esophageal origin is that a definite diagnosis must always be made. An initial judgment should be made regarding the urgency with which the diagnostic process should be carried out. As described above, a detailed history should be taken because this will provide clues not only regarding the possible cause but also regarding the degree of urgency that is required in diagnostic testing. Only when the history is long and alarm symptoms such as weight loss are absent is delay in the performance of diagnostic tests justifiable.

A second important principle specifically applies to the management of patients with angina-like chest pain. In these patients, it is essential that cardiac causes of the symptoms be ruled out before proceeding with any investigation of the gastrointestinal tract. In most cases this includes the involvement of a cardiologist.

Endoscopy plays a pivotal role in the management of patients with dysphagia, odynophagia, and noncardiac chest pain and is the first test that should be performed. Endoscopy is more sensitive for the detection of mucosal abnormalities than barium esophagogram and has the advantage of offering the possibility to take biopsy specimens. In patients presenting with dysphagia, biopsies from the esophageal body should be taken even when no abnormalities are seen in order to rule out eosinophilic esophagitis [16]. As is apparent from the algorithms in Figures 30.2–30.4, the findings made during endoscopy largely determine the subsequent management strategy.

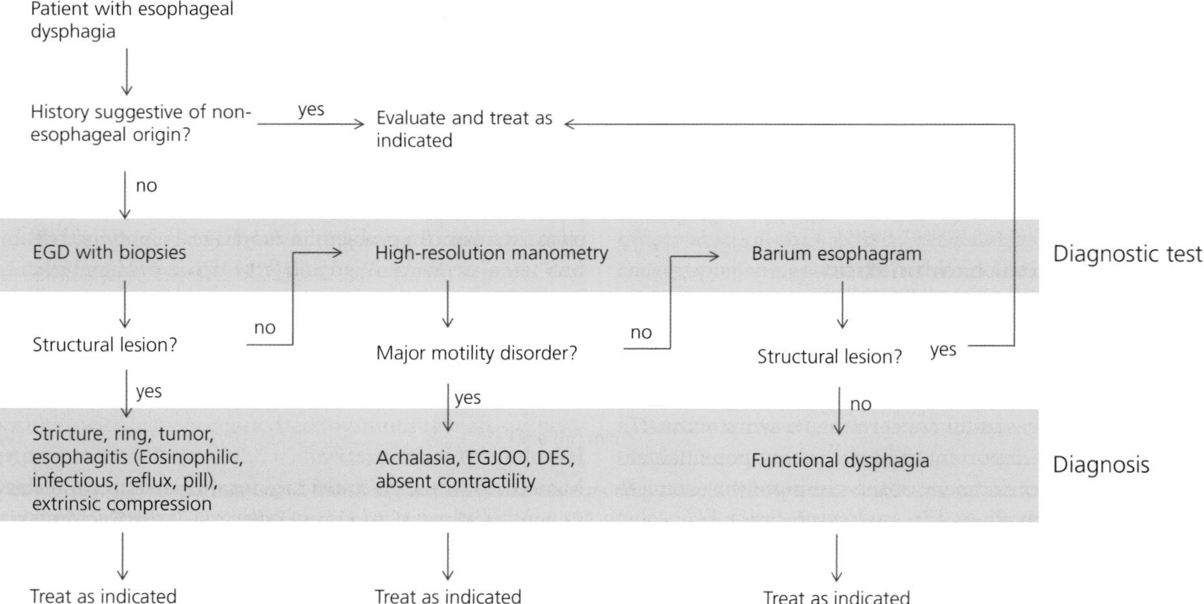

Figure 30.2 Algorithm for the management of esophageal dysphagia. DES, diffuse esophageal spasm; EGD, esophagogastroduodenoscopy; EGJOO, esophagogastric junction outflow obstruction.

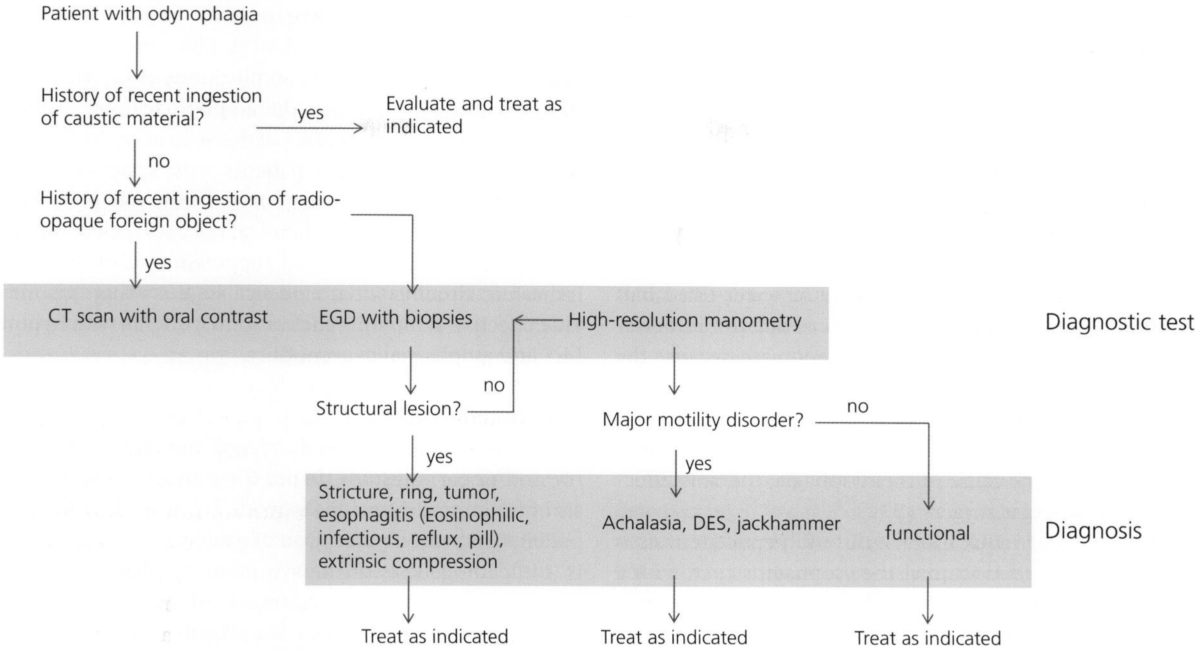

Figure 30.3 Algorithm for the management of odynophagia. DES, diffuse esophageal spasm.

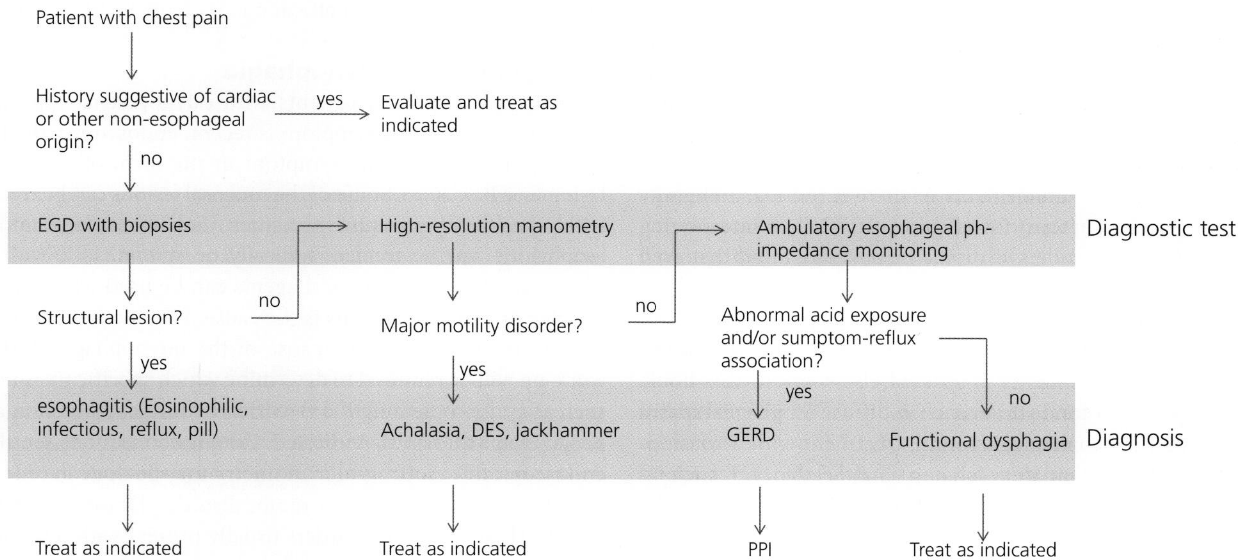

Figure 30.4 Algorithm for the management of (noncardiac) chest pain. DES, diffuse esophageal spasm; PPI, proton pump inhibitor; GERD, gastroesophageal reflux disease.

Management of dysphagia

As outlined above, the management of a patient with dysphagia must be based upon an established diagnosis and therapy must consist of treatment of the cause of the dysphagia.

In this chapter the management of *oropharyngeal* (cervical) dysphagia will not be discussed because treatment of the underlying disorders – listed in Box 30.1 – generally lies in the purview of otolaryngologists or neurologists. There are two exceptions. First, some gastroenterologists have specialized in the endoscopic treatment of Zenker diverticulum. They use a flexible endoscope and electrocautery to incise the tissue bridge between the diverticulum and the main esophageal lumen [21]. Second, stenosis in the proximal esophagus, leading to esophageal dysphagia, causes symptoms that are often indistinguishable from oropharyngeal dysphagia. In most centers, dilation of such a stenosis will be performed by a gastroenterologist rather than by an ENT specialist. A typical example is the stenosed anastomosis between the proximal esophagus and a gastric remnant in patients who underwent esophagectomy.

In the management of *esophageal* dysphagia, therapy will be guided by the cause of the symptom. If esophageal carcinoma is found, treatment will depend on localization and size of the tumor, presence or absence of metastases, and the condition or general health of the patient. This is discussed elsewhere in this book. When a benign stricture is the cause of the symptoms, endoscopy-guided dilation, with a bougie or water-filled balloon, is usually carried out. If the stricture is due to radiotherapy, dilation should be carried out with great care because the risk of perforation is higher than with other types of stricture. This will be described in other chapters of this book. In the rare cases in which the arteria lusoria syndrome or an aneurysm of the thoracic aorta is the cause of the dysphagia, the only effective treatment is vascular surgery [22].

If a combination of reflux esophagitis and peptic stenosis is found, it is recommended to treat the esophagitis first, with a proton pump inhibitor. When the dysphagia subsides upon healing of the esophagitis, dilation may not be necessary.

In patients with dysphagia in whom endoscopy does not reveal a cause, biopsies should be obtained to exclude eosinophilic esophagitis, and then esophageal manometry is often the most useful next investigation. It may demonstrate an unequivocal cause, such as achalasia, or an abnormality that may or may not be a causative factor, such as diffuse esophageal spasm or jackhammer esophagus. Some prefer to do a barium swallow first, prior to esophageal manometry. However, most experts advise pursuing the barium swallow when esophageal manometry has revealed no abnormality or there is residual ambiguity in the cause of symptoms (see Figure 30.2). When interpreting solid bolus transit studies, it should be borne in mind that even in asymptomatic healthy subjects, temporary hold-up of the bolus occurs quite frequently and may not be pathological [18].

If achalasia is diagnosed, several effective therapeutic options are available. These will be discussed elsewhere in this book. When a spastic motor disorder such as diffuse esophageal spasm or jackhammer esophagus is found, treatment with a spasmolytic drug, in particular a calcium channel blocker such as nifedipine or a nitric oxide donor such as nitroglycerin, is the first choice but side-effects often outweigh the beneficial effects. The reader is referred to Chapter 42 on esophageal motor disorders for a more detailed discussion.

If esophageal manometry indicates absent contractility, typically in the presence of systemic sclerosis, the therapeutic options are limited. Dietary and lifestyle advice combined with effective control of acid reflux, if present, are the mainstays of clinical management. Patients should favor liquid and semisolid nutrition over solids, consume meals in the upright position, chew all food well, and drink plenty of fluids, as these measures are likely to promote esophageal clearance. There is no prokinetic drug that improves smooth muscle contractility and esophageal function to a clinically relevant degree.

Patients with hypotensive motility of the smooth muscle portion of the esophagus and weak LES function often experience severe symptoms and complications of GERD in addition to dysphagia. This is largely due to poor clearance, which leads to prolonged acid exposure, particularly at night. These problems are most marked in patients with systemic sclerosis in whom the combination of poor motility and poor salivation impacts both volume and chemical (i.e., acid) clearance [23]. In these patients, high-dose acid suppression taken twice a day is indicated; circumstantial evidence suggests that this may provide effective symptom relief in some patients with hypotensive LES and esophageal hypomotility.

Functional dysphagia

When patients experience dysphagia and endoscopy, manometry, and/or barium study do not show an abnormality, a diagnosis of functional dysphagia is made [1]. It is likely that, in these patients, increased perception of esophageal stimuli is involved in the pathogenesis of the symptom dysphagia. There are no data on the effective treatment of functional dysphagia. Explanation and reassurance are probably the most useful contributions that the physician can make to the well-being of patients with this disorder. An antidepressant such as amitriptyline or citalopram may be used to reduce visceral perception, but there is no evidence of efficacy.

Management of odynophagia

As discussed above, in patients with odynophagia, especially when the onset of this symptom is recent, endoscopy will often identify the cause of the symptom in the form of a mucosal lesion (see Box 30.3). Some of the mucosal lesions can be treated with specific therapeutic measures. For instance, Candida esophagitis can be treated, topically or systemically, with an antifungal drug, and antiviral agents can be used when herpes simplex or cytomegalovirus is the cause. When esophageal carcinoma is found to be the cause of the odynophagia, further work-up will be required to determine which specific treatment, such as endoscopic mucosal resection or surgical resection and neoadjuvant therapy, is indicated. If no lesion can be identified endoscopically, esophageal manometry may be done in order to rule out achalasia or a spastic motor disorder. However, patients with the latter type of disorders usually present with dysphagia and spontaneous chest pain, rather than with odynophagia. It is doubtful whether nonerosive reflux disease can be the cause of odynophagia, but empiric treatment of odynophagia with a gastric acid secretion inhibitor can be considered if not already performed.

Management of noncardiac chest pain

In patients presenting with angina-like chest pain in whom a cardiac cause has been ruled out, and in whom another nonesophageal cause is felt to be unlikely, upper endoscopy is done to search for esophagitis (reflux, pill-induced, or infectious) as a cause of the symptoms. If no other symptoms such as dysphagia or food impactions are present, eosinophilic esophagitis is very unlikely. Because gastroesophageal reflux is a common esophageal cause of noncardiac chest pain, many clinicians would use empiric treatment with a gastric acid secretion inhibitor to rule out or establish this cause. Indeed, there are at least four systematic reviews suggesting that this empiric approach would be acceptable practice [24–27]. However, the placebo effect of such treatment is considerable, so that it is difficult to draw conclusions as to the definite cause of the noncardiac chest pain. Therefore, in centers where esophageal manometry and 24-h esophageal pH monitoring are available, there is often preference to carry out these tests first. If esophageal manometry identifies achalasia or a spastic motor disorder, specific treatment can be instituted. During esophageal pH measurement, an effort must be made to assess the temporal association between the pain episodes and reflux episodes. If available, impedance monitoring should be done in addition to pH monitoring because nonacid reflux can also be the cause of the symptoms [28] and can be identified by change of impedance reflecting the reflux of fluid content to the esophagus. Unfortunately, the yield of 24-h monitoring is likely to be limited if the chest pain occurs infrequently. Using catheter-free capsule pH-metry, reflux monitoring can easily be prolonged to 48 h or more, which increases the chance that a chest pain episode will occur during the observation period [29].

Some centers provide the service of 24-h esophageal manometry, in conjunction with 24-h pH monitoring. This technique makes it possible to determine whether chest pain episodes are associated with episodic spastic motor abnormalities, if chest pain episodes occur during the observation period. However, the yield of prolonged esophageal manometry for this indication is low; a new diagnosis is made in less than 5% of patients [30].

If none of the known causes of chest pain can be identified, a diagnosis of functional chest pain ("chest pain of presumed esophageal origin") is made. This is one of the functional disorders of the gastrointestinal tract defined by the Rome IV criteria [1]. In functional chest pain, as in functional dysphagia, increased visceral perception is thought to play a role. Limited evidence suggests that treatment with an antidepressant such as amitriptyline or citalopram may be effective [25].

References are available at www.yamadagastro.com/textbook7e

Further reading

Aziz Q., Fass R., Gyawali C.P., et al. Functional esophageal disorders. Gastroenterology 2016;150:1368.

Gyawali C.P., Bredenoord A.J., Conklin J.L., et al. Evaluation of esophageal motor function in clinical practice. Neurogastroenterol Motil 2013;25:99.

Kahrilas P.J., Smout A.J. Esophageal disorders. Am J Gastroenterol 2010;105:747.

Kahrilas P.J., Bredenoord A.J., Fox M., et al. International High Resolution Manometry Working Group. The Chicago Classification of esophageal motility disorders, v3.0. Neurogastroenterol Motil. 2015;27:160.

Kopelman Y., Triadafilopoulos G. Endoscopy in the diagnosis and management of motility disorders. Dig Dis Sci 2001;56:635.

CHAPTER 31

Approach to the patient with dyspepsia and related functional gastrointestinal complaints

Jan Tack
Department of Gastroenterology, University of Leuven, Belgium

Chapter menu

Definitions

Dyspepsia is one of the most common gastrointestinal conditions seen in both primary and specialist care. The term dyspepsia, which is derived from Greek and literally means "difficult digestion," has been used to refer to a heterogeneous group of symptoms, located in the upper abdomen. These symptoms may include postprandial fullness, early satiation, epigastric pain, upper abdominal bloating, nausea and even heartburn, regurgitation, anorexia, belching, or vomiting [1–6]. Up to 20% of the general population may experience regular dyspeptic symptoms in the broad sense, but only a minority will seek medical care [7–9]. Patients usually present with several of these symptoms, making it one of the most variable clinical syndromes. The severity and intensity of symptoms may range from very mild to interfering with daily activities and food intake. Hence, dyspepsia may be a challenging problem in clinical practice.

In patients with dyspepsia, additional investigations may identify an underlying organic disease that is likely to cause the symptoms. These patients are referred to as having an *organic cause of dyspepsia*. However, in the majority of patients with dyspeptic symptoms, routine clinical work-up reveals no organic abnormality, and these patients are said to have *functional dyspepsia* (FD). The term *uninvestigated dyspepsia* refers to patients with dyspeptic symptoms in whom diagnostic investigations have not (yet) been performed [4–6] (Figure 31.1).

The definitions of dyspepsia and of functional dyspepsia have undergone major changes over the last few decades. Factors underlying these variations include inclusion or exclusion of symptoms suggestive of gastroesophageal reflux disease (GERD), and the type and number of symptoms that were proposed to be indicative of dyspepsia, which has become more restrictive over time. The earliest definitions considered dyspepsia to comprise all upper abdominal and retrosternal sensations [2]. Later, Rome I and II consensus criteria defined dyspepsia as *pain or discomfort centered in the upper abdomen* [3,4]. In these definitions, discomfort refers to a wide range of symptoms which include postprandial fullness, upper abdominal bloating, early satiety, epigastric burning, belching, nausea, and vomiting. The Rome II consensus decided that esophageal disorders are not part of the dyspepsia symptom cluster, and that the presence of heartburn as a predominant symptom should label the patient as having GERD and not dyspepsia [4].

The Rome III consensus criteria, published in 2006, introduced two major and significant changes. First, the number of cardinal dyspeptic symptoms was reduced to only four that are considered to consistently originate from the gastroduodenal region. According to the same Rome III consensus, FD is defined as the presence of early satiation, postprandial fullness, epigastric pain or epigastric burning, in the absence of underlying organic or metabolic disease that is likely to explain the symptoms [5]. This definition gave a clear-cut identity and

Yamada's Textbook of Gastroenterology, Seventh Edition. Edited by Timothy C. Wang, Michael Camilleri, Benjamin Lebwohl, Anna S. Lok, William J. Sandborn, Kenneth K. Wang, and Gary D. Wu.

Companion website: www.yamadagastro.com/textbook7e

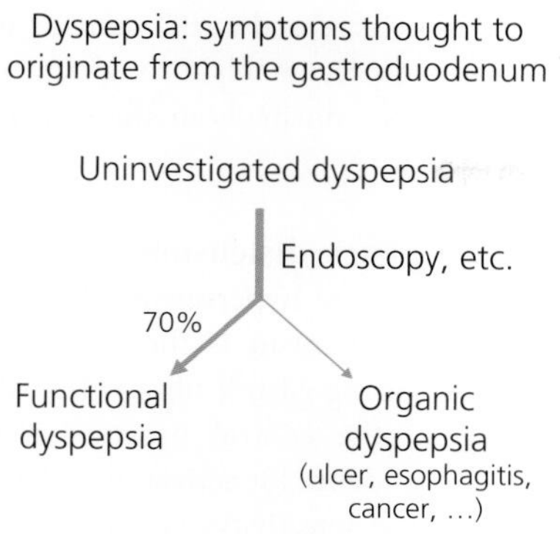

Dyspepsia: symptoms thought to originate from the gastroduodenum

Uninvestigated dyspepsia

Endoscopy, etc.

70%

Functional dyspepsia

Organic dyspepsia (ulcer, esophagitis, cancer, ...)

Figure 31.1 Uninvestigated, organic, and functional dyspepsia. Source: Based on Talley N.J., Stanghellini V., Heading R.C., et al. (1999). Functional gastroduodenal disorders. Gut 45(Supplement 2), ii37–ii42.

focus to FD, compared to previous consensus criteria which also included a multitude of symptoms within the dyspepsia spectrum. A second significant change was the introduction of a distinction between meal-related and meal-unrelated FD symptoms. Beginning with Rome III, these categories were respectively referred to as postprandial distress syndrome (PDS) and epigastric pain syndrome (EPS) [5].

The changes that were introduced by Rome III were largely based on expert opinion and on observations in tertiary care patients. Nevertheless, epidemiological studies conducted soon after the publication of Rome III confirmed the existence of PDS and EPS as two well-separated entities in the general population [10]. In clinical practice, however, the majority of FD patients fulfilled criteria for both groups as defined by Rome III, and given the dominance of a group with symptom overlap (that is, with components of both EPS and PDS), this subdivision has little use in patient management. It was soon established that using the "meal relationship" criterion more rigorously allowed a better separation of the subgroups [11].

The Rome IV consensus implemented this rigorous application of the meal relationship criterion for FD subgroups, and a good separation between meal-related and meal-unrelated groups is now identified both in epidemiological studies and in clinical practice [6,9]. Moreover, pathophysiological studies and symptom analysis studies reveal increasingly clear differences between PDS and EPS according to Rome IV, suggesting that a meaningful subgroup concept for FD has now been reached [12,13].

Etiologies and pathophysiology

Organic causes of dyspepsia

The most prevalent organic causes of dyspeptic symptoms, including epigastric burning, are peptic ulcer disease and GERD. Upper GI tract malignancies and celiac disease are less common but clinically relevant causes of dyspeptic symptoms [5,6,14–17]. These conditions are addressed in more detail in other chapters in this textbook (see Chs 51 and 55). The key investigation in patients with (chronic) dyspeptic symptoms is endoscopy, which may identify erosive esophagitis, peptic ulcer or gastric or esophageal cancer.

Peptic ulcer is a well-known cause of dyspeptic symptoms, but the prevalence of peptic ulcer in dyspeptic patients is estimated to be only 5–10%, with decreasing incidence [15–17]. The two main causes of peptic ulcer disease are H. pylori infection and intake of nonsteroidal antiinflammatory drugs (NSAIDs). Features indicative of peptic ulcer disease are a history of improvement of symptoms with meals, nocturnal pain and symptomatic relief by a course of H_2 receptor antagonists or proton pump inhibitors (PPIs). However, the symptom pattern does not adequately discriminate peptic ulcer disease from FD, and hence, differentiation requires endoscopy [15–17].

Gastroesophageal reflux disease is the most important condition overlapping with and requiring distinction from FD. Heartburn and regurgitation are the most typical symptoms associated with GERD, but often dyspeptic symptoms in the form of epigastric burning coexist with those typical symptoms [18]. A systematic review reported that erosive esophagitis was the most common abnormality encountered upon endoscopy in dyspeptic patients (pooled prevalence 13.4%), followed by peptic ulcer (pooled prevalence 8.0%) [19]. The prevalence of erosive esophagitis was lower when the presence of dyspepsia was based on the Rome criteria compared with a broad definition incorporating all upper gastrointestinal symptoms (6% vs 20%). It is likely that at least a similar number of patients with dyspeptic symptoms has nonerosive reflux disease, even in the absence of typical GERD symptoms, based on pH monitoring [19–21].

The risk of *gastric or esophageal* cancer in patients presenting with dyspeptic symptoms is probably below 1% (22), but is higher in patients who are infected with H. pylori, immigrants from areas with high prevalence of gastric cancer, such as eastern Asia, and those with a family history of gastric malignancy. Unfortunately, it seems that alarm symptoms and age are not adequate predictors of the risk of finding malignancy at endoscopy, and clinicians should remain alert to those with a family history or rapidly evolving symptoms with high impact to exclude malignancy by endoscopy [15,16,19,22,23].

Biliary tract disorders are rarely found in patients presenting with dyspepsia, and are not really thought to mimic the dyspepsia symptom pattern [5,6]. The clinical presentation of biliary colic is easily distinguishable from that of dyspepsia; therefore, patients with dyspepsia in the absence of biliary colic do not require routine biliary tract ultrasound. *Pancreatic disease* is less prevalent, but both chronic pancreatitis and pancreatic cancer may initially present as dyspepsia. The further evolution of pancreatic disorders with more severe pain and development of jaundice or weight loss usually distinguishes them from dyspepsia.

Lifestyle factors. Contrary to popular belief, studies have failed to establish ingestion of specific foods (spicy foods, coffee, alcohol) as a cause of dyspepsia [24]. On the other hand, ingestion of capsaicin triggers dyspeptic symptoms in FD patients [25].

Dyspepsia is also a common side-effect of several drugs, such as iron supplements, narcotics, antibiotics, digitalis, estrogens, theophylline, levodopa, and many others. NSAIDs may induce dyspepsia in up to 20% and peptic ulcers or erosions in up to 10% of patients [26]. Compared to NSAIDs, cyclooxygenase-2 inhibitors are associated with a lower frequency of dyspepsia and peptic ulceration [27].

Several other gastrointestinal disorders may also cause dyspeptic symptoms. These include infectious (Giardia lamblia and Strongyloides stercoralis), ischemic (arcuate ligament, atheromatosis of the celiac artery), inflammatory (celiac disease, Crohn's disease, sarcoidosis, lymphocytic gastritis, eosinophilic gastroenteritis) or infiltrative (amyloid, lymphoma, Ménétrier disease) upper gastrointestinal disorders. Most of these will be identified by upper gastrointestinal endoscopy with biopsies. Gastroparesis (idiopathic or secondary to drugs, metabolic, systemic or neurological disorders) is also associated with a dyspepsia-like symptom pattern [28], and the distinction between idiopathic gastroparesis and FD with delayed gastric emptying is a matter of controversy [29].

Functional dyspepsia

Several pathophysiological mechanisms have been implicated in symptom generation in functional dyspepsia, including impaired gastric accommodation to a meal, hypersensitivity to gastric distention, delayed gastric emptying, H. pylori infection, low-grade duodenal inflammation, altered duodenal sensitivity to lipids or acid, abnormal intestinal motility, and central nervous system dysfunction [1–6,30–34].

Impaired gastric accommodation to a meal

Accommodation of the stomach to a meal is a vagally mediated reflex relaxation of the proximal stomach, triggered by ingestion of a meal; accommodation serves to provide the meal with a reservoir. The accommodation reflex enables the stomach to handle large meal volumes without a rise of intragastric pressure [35]. Studies using intragastric high-resolution manometry have demonstrated that ingestion of a meal is associated with a drop in intragastric pressure, followed by a gradual recovery of pressure during ongoing nutrient ingestion which parallels the occurrence of meal-induced satiation [36].

Studies using a variety of methods indicate that approximately 40% of FD patients have impaired accommodation: These studies have been conducted using diverse methods (gastric barostat [a balloon device in which air insufflation is kept under constant pressure and a change in tone is reflected in the volume of air insufflated or aspirated to maintain constant balloon pressure], scintigraphy, ultrasonography, single photon emission computed tomography), or noninvasive surrogate markers (nutrient drinking test) [1,5,6,30,31,35]. In cases of impaired accommodation, meal ingestion is associated with increased intragastric pressure and activation of mechanoreceptors, leading to early satiation and potentially weight loss [35,36]. The causes of impaired accommodation are unknown, but its prevalence seems to be increased in FD patients with a postinfectious symptom onset, presumably through impaired nitrergic nerve function [37] which normally mediates vagally mediated gastric relaxation.

Hypersensitivity to gastric distension

As a group, FD patients are hypersensitive to gastric balloon distension, and this mechanism is thought to contribute to symptom generation during gastric filling [1,5,6,35]. Although altered processing by the central nervous system may be involved, there is also evidence for activation of tension-sensitive mechanoreceptors in hypersensitivity to gastric distention [34,35].

Disordered gastric emptying

Between 20% and 50% of FD patients have delayed rate of solid gastric emptying, with the largest studies showing delayed emptying in approximately 30% [,1,5,6,28,29,31]. Whether delayed gastric emptying underlies symptom generation or is an epiphenomenon is a matter of ongoing controversy [28,29]. In three large single-center studies from Europe, patients with delayed gastric emptying for solids were more likely to report postprandial fullness, nausea, and vomiting [38–40]. One study reported rapid gastric emptying in a relevant subset of FD patients [41] but this was a rare finding in the other studies [30,31,38–40].

Altered duodenal sensitivity and integrity

A number of studies have reported increased sensitivity to duodenal lipid or acid perfusion in FD [30,32]. Duodenal pH monitoring revealed increased duodenal acid exposure in FD compared to controls, which was attributable to impaired acid clearance [42]. More recently, altered mucosal integrity of the duodenum in FD was reported, attributable to changes in tight junction protein expression and correlated to low-grade inflammatory changes [43]. Several papers have now confirmed that FD patients as a group have significantly elevated eosinophil counts and, in some studies, mast cell counts in duodenal mucosal biopsies, compared to age-matched controls [33]. Elevated eosinophil counts are associated with early satiation and seem, at least in part, to be driven by duodenal acid exposure, as they decrease with acid-suppressive therapy [33]. To what extent and how the duodenal inflammatory changes correlate with altered gastric sensorimotor function remain to be explored. Besides duodenal acid exposure, acute stress has been identified as a potential cause of loss of intestinal mucosal integrity, and the duodenal bile acid pool is also altered in FD and correlated to duodenal mucosal resistance [44,45]. Finally, a preliminary report suggests a potential for altered duodenal microbiota composition to be associated with symptom impact in FD [46].

Diagnosis

In patients presenting with dyspeptic symptoms, clinical history should identify the major complaint, and determine whether symptoms are related to meal ingestion, and whether they are intermittent or continuous. The site, mode of onset, intensity, character, and precipitating/relieving factors should be determined. The duration and severity of symptoms may help to distinguish dyspepsia from symptoms related to organic disorders such as peptic ulcer, acute cholecystitis, and acute pancreatitis, as addressed below. In patients with long-standing symptoms, the reason for the current presentation should be elicited, to recognize specific fears and concerns. The use of medications should be reviewed, and drugs commonly associated with dyspepsia (especially NSAIDS) should be discontinued, if possible.

In most instances, physical examination of the dyspeptic patient will not reveal any abnormality except for mild tenderness upon deep epigastric palpation in some cases. The onset of symptoms (acute or more chronic), evidence of weight loss, dysphagia, vomiting, bleeding, a family history of gastric or esophageal cancer, anemia, lymphadenopathy, or an abdominal mass are all so-called alarm features or red flags. While these may indicate an increased likelihood of an organic disorder, and prompt further technical investigations, their predictive value is limited [5,6,15,16,22,23].

The clinician may choose to approach the symptoms as "uninvestigated dyspepsia" and to start empiric treatment without additional investigations, especially endoscopy (Figure 31.2). This approach is chosen when there are no alarm symptoms, a low likelihood of organic disease, and no easy access to diagnostic endoscopy. In all other cases, prompt upper gastrointestinal endoscopy is recommended as the additional examination of choice. In most cases, this will be sufficient to distinguish functional dyspepsia from organic causes of dyspepsia [5,6].

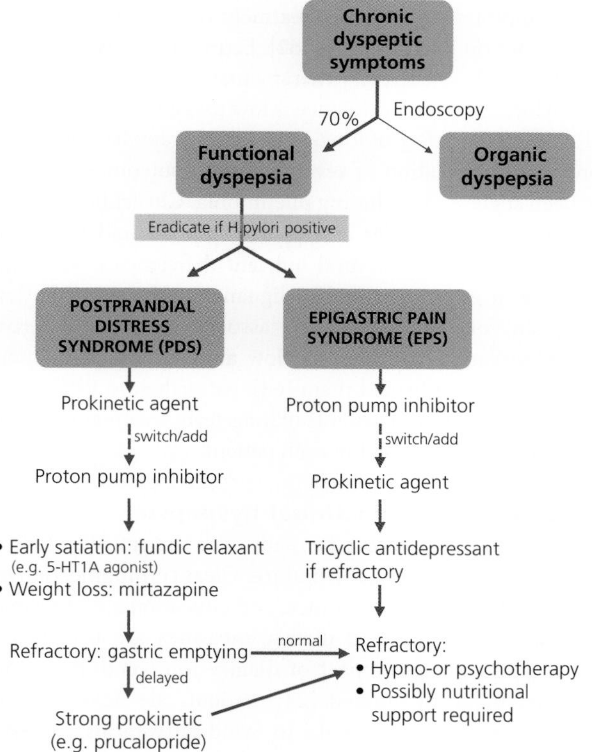

Figure 31.2 Proposed management algorithm for functional dyspepsia.

Differential diagnosis

The differential diagnosis of dyspepsia is extremely broad, including virtually all upper gastrointestinal tract diseases (Box 31.1). Even after detailed history taking and clinical examination, there is usually no diagnostic certainty. Dyspeptic symptoms may be attributed to a large variety of organic diseases ("organic" dyspepsia), where an identifiable cause for the symptoms exists, and where symptoms improve if the disorder is treated. The other large group includes patients with FD, where no definite structural or biochemical substrate underlying the symptoms is identified.

Heartburn, the typical symptom of GERD, is recognized by its occurrence after meals, the burning character of the pain, and its associated radiation to the retrosternal region. A word-picture questionnaire may be helpful to recognize the typical symptom pattern [18,20]. Peptic ulcer may be suggested by localized epigastric pain which is relieved by food or antacids and which may awaken the patient at night. A short history of new-onset dyspepsia in a patient over the age of 50, especially with weight loss, should raise the suspicion of gastric cancer, while nagging upper abdominal pain with irradiation to the back may indicate chronic pancreatitis or pancreatic cancer. The typical history of a biliary colic (sudden onset of severe epigastric pain with nausea and vomiting) should be recognized. The classic triad of upper abdominal pain induced by eating, fear of eating, and weight loss should raise suspicion of intestinal ischemia.

As indicated above, upper gastrointestinal endoscopy is the key investigation and will identify the most relevant organic disorders. In select cases, based on the clinical history and the clinician's evaluation, additional tests can be considered such as testing for celiac disease and Giardia lamblia infection

Box 31.1 Differential diagnosis of dyspepsia.

Gastroesophageal reflux disease
Chronic peptic ulcer
Drug-induced dyspepsia
Infectious disorders (Giardia, Helicobacter)
Symptomatic cholelithiasis
Chronic pancreatitis
Biliary dyskinesia
Malignant disease (gastric, pancreatic, colonic)
Mesenteric vascular insufficiency
Metabolic disorders (e.g., renal failure, hypercalcaemia, hyperthyroidism)
Abdominal wall pain
Ischemic heart disease (referred pain)
Others

(especially in association with acute onset), abdominal ultrasound or CT scan (in case of severe pain or weight loss), screening for stenosis of large abdominal arteries (history suggestive of ischemia), and psychological or psychiatric assessment in case of long-standing refractory or debilitating symptoms. Advanced motility testing may also be considered in refractory patients, by means of gastric emptying testing in cases of important nausea or vomiting (followed by small bowel x-ray or CT enterography in case of severe delay) or esophageal pH/impedance monitoring for refractory intermittent pain or epigastric burning.

Principles of management

Management of uninvestigated dyspepsia

The diagnostic approach to FD is relatively simple. Generally, medical history and physical examination are used to identify dyspeptic symptoms, to look for alarm features and to explore the presence of symptoms or signs that are more suggestive of esophageal, pancreatic or biliary disease [5,6].

Although the yield is hampered by the poor predictive value of alarm symptoms, the available guidelines advocate prompt endoscopy in cases of alarm features or risk factors like age above a threshold (usually 45 or 50 years) or NSAID intake [5,6,14–18,22,23]. The finding of organic disease generally leads to well-established diagnostic and treatment steps.

Furthermore, for those patients who do not fulfill risk or alarm criteria, different management strategies for "uninvestigated dyspepsia" are available. These include prompt diagnostic endoscopy, noninvasive testing for H. pylori infection followed by eradication therapy if positive ("test and treat") and initial empirical acid-suppressive therapy [47]. In theory, empirical prokinetic therapy could also be considered as an initial option, but this is not viable due to a lack of widely available prokinetic drugs with established efficacy and safety. A firm diagnosis of FD is only established after a negative upper gastrointestinal endoscopy, and this can be done before or after empirical symptomatic therapy [5,6].

No cost-effectiveness has been established for routine laboratory testing in patients with uncomplicated dyspepsia, but most clinicians will perform some limited routine tests (complete blood count, routine electrolyte measurement, serum calcium, liver biochemical tests, and thyroid function), especially in patients over the age of 40.

Prompt endoscopy has the advantage of immediate detection and rapid treatment of organic causes of dyspepsia such as peptic ulcer, erosive esophagitis or malignancy. Furthermore, biopsies allow diagnosis of H. pylori infection, if present. While this approach may provide a reassurance to both physician and patient, it is invasive, expensive and probably not cost-effective, and will often not dramatically alter therapeutic choices which will, in most cases, be based on acid suppression [47–50]. A network metaanalysis of 15 management trials of uninvestigated dyspepsia concluded that initial endoscopy was the patients' preference, but that none of the approaches (test and treat, empirical acid suppression, prompt endoscopy) was associated with a significant difference in outcome [47].

Test and treat for H. pylori allows identification of the cause of the majority of peptic ulcers and the most important risk factor for gastric cancer [51]. This is advocated for dyspeptic patients below the age of 45, and those with a positive test are prescribed standard eradication therapy (a proton pump inhibitor and two or more antibiotics for 10–14 days (see Chapter 49). Patients with a negative test result are treated empirically, usually with a proton pump inhibitor. The "test and treat" strategy leads to cure of peptic ulcer disease, prevention of future peptic ulcers, and also the cure of a small subset (approximately 7%) of patients with H. pylori-related dyspepsia in the absence of ulceration. Furthermore, eradication of H. pylori may reduce the risk of gastric cancer [51–54].

However, there are also some disadvantages to this approach, including a low yield when the community prevalence of H. pylori infection is low and concerns about allergy or development of resistance to antibiotics. Controlled studies show only a modest reduction in dyspeptic symptoms after a "test and treat" approach and no major difference in symptom resolution or costs compared to empirical PPI therapy [55–59].

Empirical antisecretory therapy with proton pump inhibitors as initial therapy is attractive because it controls symptoms and lesions in most patients with underlying GERD or peptic ulcer disease, and may be beneficial for a subgroup of FD patients [60,61]. Disadvantages of empirical proton pump inhibitor therapy include rebound hypersecretion which may cause symptom relapse upon treatment interruption and hence dependence on long-term use [62]. Economic analyses indicate that empirical antisecretory therapy may be more cost-effective if H. pylori infection prevalence is low [58,59].

Recently, the safety of long-term PPI therapy has been questioned and association of several adverse outcomes with PPIs has been suggested, including pneumonia, Clostridium difficile infection, cardiovascular events, osteoporosis and bone fractures, kidney disease, several nutrient deficiencies, Alzheimer disease, and gastrointestinal malignancies. However, the level and quality of evidence of these associations, mainly derived from observational studies, are low and the available clinical trials have not confirmed them [63]. Nevertheless, PPI overuse should be avoided and benefits of long-term treatment continuation should be evaluated in each patient.

Management of functional dyspepsia

A firm diagnosis of FD can be made after a negative endoscopy in patients with dyspeptic symptoms. Clear communication of a confident diagnosis, reassurance, and education are of primary importance. Lifestyle and dietary measures are usually prescribed although the impact of dietary interventions has not been systematically studied [24]. Patients are advised to eat more frequent, smaller meals, to avoid fatty meals and spicy foods. Limitation of coffee and alcohol and stopping smoking are proposed to be helpful, and NSAIDs should be avoided.

For many, but not all, patients pharmacotherapy will be considered. The therapies of choice are acid-suppressive therapy, prokinetics, H. pylori eradication and psychotropic agents.

Eradication of H. pylori in FD generates a small but statistically significant benefit, as evident from metaanalyses [64–67]. With an estimated number needed to treat of 12.5, a late occurring superiority of eradication over placebo (after 6–12 months), and a gradually declining subgroup of infected FD patients, the benefit is limited [64]. On the other hand, H. pylori eradication is the only therapy that may induce sustained remission, may protect against peptic ulcer and gastric cancer, and is relatively inexpensive [64,65]. Based on these considerations, an international consensus recommended H. pylori eradication in infected FD patients, and proposed to refer to those with a sustained symptomatic response as having "H. pylori-associated dyspepsia" [67]. Hence, treatment is recommended early on in the management cascade of FD patients if they are found to be H. pylori infected (see Figure 31.2).

Acid-suppressive therapy is a popular first-line treatment approach, and a metaanalysis of placebo-controlled, randomized trials with PPIs in FD showed a benefit, with a number needed to treat of 10 [63]. No significant difference in efficacy between different PPIs, and no dose-effect was found, arguing against dose escalation in cases of insufficient response [64,68]. The few available studies evaluating the response to PPI therapy in PDS or EPS according to Rome III or Rome IV definitions show no significant difference in response [64]. However, in older studies, the best response to PPIs was found in patients with concomitant heartburn, followed by FD patients with epigastric pain and patients with motility-like symptoms [68] (see Figure 31.2).

Prokinetics, drugs that stimulate gastric motility, are popular on a global scale for the treatment of FD. Metaanalyses showed significant benefit for prokinetics over placebo, with a number needed to treat of 12.5 [53]. As they are most beneficial to symptoms of postprandial fullness, early satiation and nausea, they seem best used in the management of PDS patients (see Figure 31.2). However, these results are mainly driven by studies using cisapride and domperidone, two drugs with limited availability due to cardiovascular safety concerns; in addition, the quality of studies is low and there are indications of publication bias in the literature [64]. Most importantly, with most of the drugs studied being available in selected countries only, a truly global treatment option with prokinetics is lacking.

Prokinetic agents are in fact a heterogeneous class of drugs, and although they are grouped for their ability to enhance gastric emptying, this aspect does not seem to predict the symptomatic benefit they may convey [69]. A relationship with enhancement of gastric emptying rate is only found when a high-quality emptying test is used and when the analysis is limited to selected prokinetic agent categories and agents [70]. Traditional prokinetic agents include dopamine$_2$ receptor (D_2) antagonists and 5-hydroxytryptamine $(5\text{-HT})_4$ receptor agonists. Metoclopramide and domperidone enhance gastric contractility through dopamine receptor antagonism, but metoclopramide has received a black box warning for neurological adverse events and domperidone has been associated with QT interval prolongation which may facilitate cardiac arrhythmias [71,72]. Cisapride, a 5-HT_4 receptor agonist, was withdrawn for QT prolongation and fatal arrhythmias [73]. Hence, the results of the metaanalysis should be interpreted cautiously. More recent studies indicate the potential to establish efficacy in FD for newer motility-modifying agents [74].

Acotiamide is a first-in-class antagonist of acetylcholinesterase and of presynaptic M1 and M2 muscarinic receptors, which are involved in the negative feedback inhibition of acetylcholine release. Overall, acotiamide induces an increased level of acetylcholine at synapses of the enteric nervous system and the vagus nerve [75]. Mechanistic studies showed that acotiamide enhances gastric accommodation and gastric emptying rate in animals and humans, and inhibits effects of stress on the gastrointestinal tract through the vagus nerve [75]. Acotiamide is well tolerated and safe in both short- and long-term studies. Although studies were also conducted in Europe and the USA, acotiamide has only been available since 2016 in Japan and since 2018 in India, where it is approved for the treatment of functional dyspepsia [76–78].

Tegaserod is a partial 5-HT_4 agonist indicated for women with constipation-predominant irritable bowel syndrome (IBS-C) [79]. A phase IIb program showed that 6 mg BID tegaserod was efficacious in females suffering from moderate and severe meal-related FD symptoms, a patient description reminiscent of what later would become PDS according to Rome III [80]. Both pivotal phase III trials failed to confirm these results, although one of the studies was statistically significant, but the patient selection criteria were changed for phase III, eliminating the meal-relationship connotation and including patients with only mild symptoms whose response to drug was not superior over placebo [81]. Tegaserod should probably be reevaluated in PDS patients according to the Rome IV criteria, using a validated instrument.

Prucalopride is a highly specific and potent 5-HT_4 agonist indicated for the treatment of refractory chronic constipation. Recently, in a controlled cross-over study, prucalopride enhanced gastric emptying rate, and improved symptoms mainly in idiopathic gastroparesis [82]. Prucalopride was generally well tolerated, indicating a rationale for evaluation of its use in PDS according to Rome IV criteria [78].

Psychotropic drugs, especially antidepressants, are often used as second-line drugs in functional gastrointestinal disorders. Systematic reviews suggest that psychotropic drug therapy in FD is associated with significant symptom improvement over placebo and a number needed to treat of 6, but most of the individual trials are small and of poor quality [83,84]. Moreover, psychotropics are a heterogeneous class of agents, with specific variable pharmacological profiles and actions, and differential therapeutic potential in FD. The available evidence from controlled trials indicates lack of efficacy of selective serotonin reuptake inhibitors and serotonine/noradrenaline reuptake inhibitors, while tricyclic antidepressants are effective mainly for the EPS group or FD patients with normal gastric emptying [83–87].

Mirtazapine is a tetracyclic antidepressant, with affinities for several serotonin and other receptors. A recent study showed that mirtazapine improved symptoms and promoted weight recovery in FD patients with weight loss and no major psychiatric comorbidity. Mirtazapine was well tolerated and also improved quality of life and visceral specific anxiety [88].

Buspirone and *tandospirone* (both azapirones) are 5-HT_{1A} receptor agonists with anxiolytic properties. Both were shown to provide symptomatic benefit in FD patients not explained by actions on anxiety or depression [89,90]. The main adverse event was drowsiness due to the central action of the products. Mechanistic evaluation in the study with buspirone suggests that enhanced gastric accommodation underlies the therapeutic benefit [89].

Several other therapeutic approaches have been evaluated in management of FD. In a controlled study in H. pylori-negative FD patients, the nonabsorbable broad-spectrum antibiotic rifaximin significantly improved FD symptoms such as postprandial bloating, fullness, and belching [91]. In two controlled trials, capsules of peppermint and caraway oil were superior to placebo in alleviating FD (both EPS and PDS) symptoms, with good tolerance [92,93]. A mechanistic study in healthy people showed the ability of peppermint oil to relax the proximal stomach [94]. Several herbal preparations have also been studied for their ability to improve FD symptoms. The main agents with evidence of efficacy over placebo are the Japanese Kampo preparation Rikkunshito and STW-5 (iberogast), although with the latter a case of potentially drug-induced liver failure was reported [95–99]. An algorithm that can guide the management of FD is shown in Figure 31.2.

References are available at www.yamadagastro.com/textbook7e

Further reading

Masuy I., Van Oudenhove L., Tack J. Review article: treatment options for functional dyspepsia. Aliment Pharmacol Ther 2019; 49(9):1134.

Moayyedi P., Lacy B.E., Andrews C.N., Enns R.A., Howden C.W., Vakil N. ACG and CAG clinical guideline: management of dyspepsia. Am J Gastroenterol 2017;112(7):988.

Stanghellini V., Talley N., Chan F., et al. Functional gastroduodenal disorders. Gastroenterology 2016;150(6):1380.

Vijayvargiya P., Camilleri M., Chedid V., Mandawat A., Erwin P.J., Murad M.H. Effects of promotility agents on gastric emptying and symptoms: a systematic review and meta-analysis. Gastroenterology 2019;156(6):1650.

Wauters L., Talley N.J., Walker M.M., Tack J., Vanuytsel T. Novel concepts in the pathophysiology and treatment of functional dyspepsia. Gut 2020;69:591.

CHAPTER 32

Approach to the patient with unintentional weight loss

Anupam Rej and David S. Sanders
Royal Hallamshire Hospital, The Sheffield Teaching Hospitals, Sheffield, UK

Chapter menu

Introduction

Unintentional weight loss remains a diagnostic challenge, as no guidelines exist for the approach to these patients, and it is frequently not recognized [1]. It is important that individuals with unintentional weight loss are appropriately assessed, as often they have malignancies, other organic disorders or psychiatric illness. The pathophysiology, as well as the approach to unintentional weight loss will be discussed. In patients presenting with isolated involuntary weight loss, there may be no clear lead from the history or examination and the choice of diagnostic approach may present a dilemma when there is no obvious organ focus. A logical approach to diagnosis needs to be based on probabilities; thus age, past medical history, and family history may all be highly relevant in determining the best approach. Management, particularly when no malignant underlying cause of weight loss is found, is also discussed.

Definition

There is no unanimous definition of unintentional weight loss. Clinically important unintentional weight loss is usually defined as loss of more than 5% of usual bodyweight over 6–12 months. If there is a family history of relevant illness, investigation may be appropriate with less than 5% weight loss. Loss above 10% of bodyweight is commonly associated with protein energy malnutrition and impaired physiological function [2], and loss of >20% weight with nutritional deficiencies and multiorgan dysfunction [3]. Percentage weight loss is used rather than absolute, as this is more clinically relevant [4]. It is important to note that these definitions do not distinguish between losses to lean body mass (sarcopenia) or body fat. Loss of muscle mass in elderly patients is likely to lead to frailty and functional decline [5] whereas loss of body fat with retention of muscle mass is usually associated with better clinical outcomes [6].

In a representative sample of over 9000 adults in the United States, 5% of adults aged 45–54 years reported involuntary weight loss of at least 5% of their usual bodyweight during the preceding year [7]. The strongest independent predictors of involuntary weight loss were age, smoking, and poor self-reported health. Involuntary weight loss is much more common amongst older people, with 15–20% incidence over 65 years of age [8] and 50–60% incidence among nursing home residents [9]. Unintentional weight loss is associated with 22–39% excess mortality rate, probably reflecting the underlying pathology [10]. Smoking status and body fat distribution may help identify those at risk of unintentional weight loss in early old age (60–64 years), with never smoking being associated with a lower

Yamada's Textbook of Gastroenterology, Seventh Edition. Edited by Timothy C. Wang, Michael Camilleri, Benjamin Lebwohl, Anna S. Lok, William J. Sandborn, Kenneth K. Wang, and Gary D. Wu.

Companion website: www.yamadagastro.com/textbook7e

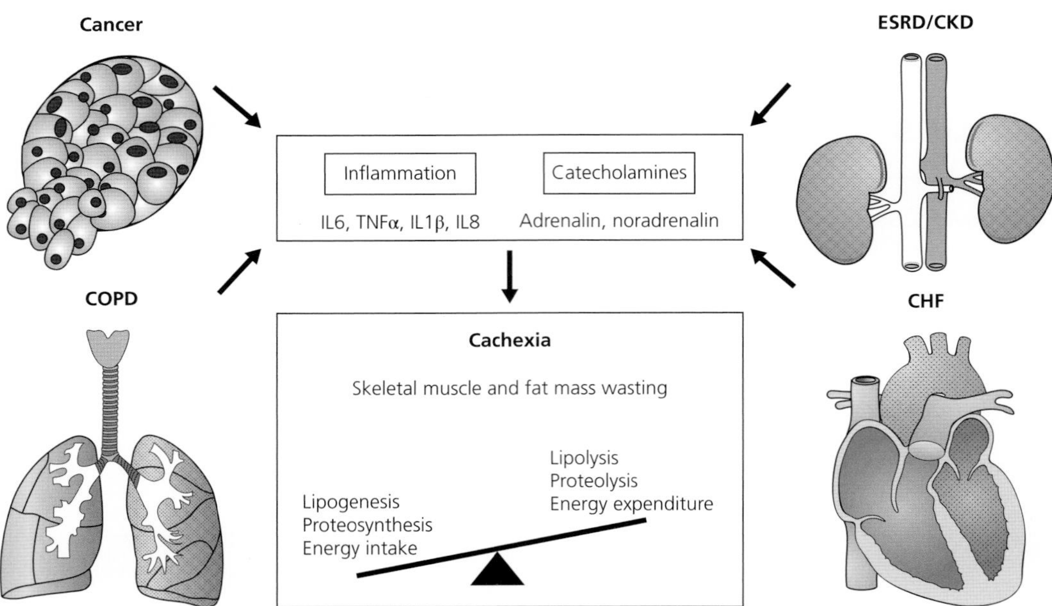

Figure 32.1 Molecular mechanisms of cachexia. Typical metabolic changes associated with the development of cachexia are an increased release of proinflammatory cytokines and an overactivity of the sympathetic nervous system, as indicated by increased plasma concentrations of catecholamines. Both proinflammatory cytokines and catecholamines promote catabolic processes, leading to skeletal muscle and fat mass wasting, such as stimulation of lipid utilization and skeletal muscle protein breakdown while decreasing energy intake and increasing energy expenditure. CHF, chronic heart failure; CKD, chronic kidney disease; COPD, chronic obstructive pulmonary disease; ESRD, end-stage renal disease; IL, interleukin; TNF-α, tumor necrosis factor α. Source: Müller et al. 2010 [12]. Reproduced with permission of Springer Science + Business Media.

risk of unintentional weight loss, as well as a greater waist:hip ratio and body fat-lean mass ratio, from a study in 2234 individuals in the United Kingdom [11].

Pathophysiology

Weight loss is induced by disease processes that affect appetite or nutrient absorption, or cause a catabolic state (Figure 32.1). Common molecular mechanisms often underlie these processes, irrespective of etiology, but have been best studied in cancer (Figures 32.2 and 32.3).

Cancer-related cachexia and altered lipid metabolism

Cachexia affects up to 80% of patients with gastrointestinal and pancreatic cancer and is reflected by anorexia, weight loss, loss of white adipose tissue, and loss of muscle mass, all of which can only partially be corrected by nutritional supplementation. Loss of white adipose tissue generally precedes loss of muscle and there may be important and specific underlying changes in lipid metabolism [13]. In white adipose tissue, triacylglycerol is the main storage fat and fat loss in cancer-related cachexia is due to loss of triacylgycerol rather than loss of lipocytes. Although there may be some reduction in lipid synthesis, the loss of triacylglycerol is predominantly due to increased lipolysis. It is probably related to increased activity of both hormone-sensitive lipase and adipose triglyceride lipase (see Figure 32.2). Cachexia is associated with a poor prognosis, regardless of tumor nature [14].

Cytokines and cachexia

Cytokines are implicated in both cancer-associated and other causes of weight loss. Excessive activity of proinflammatory cytokines, such as interleukin (IL)-1, IL-2, IL-6, interferon-γ, and tumor necrosis factor-α (TNF-α), is probably the most common underlying cause of cachexia in acutely ill patients (see Figure 32.1) [15]. Cytokines activate nuclear transcription factor-κB (NF-κB), which results in decreased muscle protein synthesis [16]. Cytokine activation is also responsible for the reduced expression of MyoD, a transcription factor that modulates signaling pathways involved in muscle development [17]. Cytokines also activate the ubiquitin-mediated proteolytic system, which is the principal mechanism for protein catabolism in disease-related catabolic states, including cancer [18], and induce lipolysis. Cumulatively, these processes result in negative energy balance and weight loss [13].

Etiology

There are many possible causes of unexplained weight loss (Box 32.1 and Table 32.1).

- Malignancy accounts for around 16–40% of cases and around 50% of malignancies presenting as weight loss are gastrointestinal [19–21].

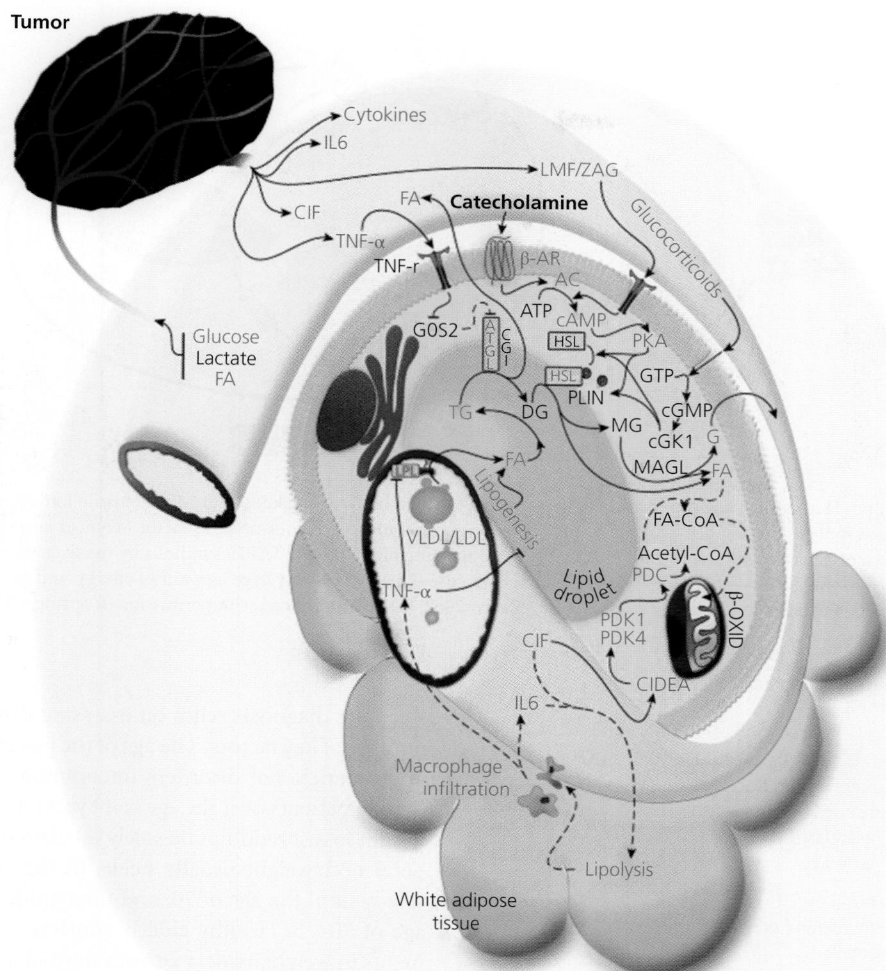

Figure 32.2 Altered lipid metabolism in cancer-associated cachexia (CAC). Malignant tumors release various cytokines including interleukin (IL)-6 and tumor necrosis factor-α (TNF-α), lipid-mobilizing factor (LMF)/Zinc-a2 glycoprotein (ZAG), and an unknown cachexia-inducing factor (CIF) in circulation. All these factors act on white adipose tissue (WAT) and deregulate lipid metabolism. TNF-α acts through the TNF receptor (TNF-r) and downregulates G0S2 (G0/G1 switch gene 2), which binds to and negatively regulates adipose triglyceride lipase (ATGL) activity. Therefore, TNF-α can increase ATGL activity. ATGL, along with its coactivator CGI-58 (comparative gene identification-58), catabolizes the first step of lipolysis by converting triacylglycerol (TAG) present in lipid droplets to diacylglycerol (DAG). DAG is further acted upon by activated (phosphorylated) hormone-sensitive lipase (HSL) and is converted into monoacylglycerol (MAG). As the final step of the lipolytic process, monoglyceride lipase (MAGL) converts MAG into glycerol (G) which can be released into circulation. One molecule of free fatty acid (FFA) is generated in each of the steps. HSL is phosphorylated by protein kinase A (PKA) or cGMP-dependent protein kinase 1 (cGK1). PKA can be activated by catecholamine or LMF/ZAG through various mechanisms. Similarly, glucocorticoids activate cGK1 by various processes. FA generated by increased lipolysis can be transported out of the adipocytes or β-oxidized in mitochondria. CIF induces cell death activator (CIDEA), which in turn increases the level of pyruvate dehydrogenase complex (PDC) and, hence, assists in β-oxidation. Along with TNF-α, IL-6 also induces lipolysis, although the mechanisms are unknown. In addition to inducing lipolysis, TNF-α downregulates lipogenesis and impairs FA uptake by inhibiting lipoprotein lipase (LPL) activity, leading to decreased TAG concentration in adipocytes and increased very-low-density lipoprotein/low-density lipoprotein (VLDL/LDL) levels in circulation. Increased lipolysis also attracts macrophages and results in macrophage infiltration in WAT often seen in cachexia. Factors in red are upregulated in cachexia, those in green are downregulated in cachexia, and factors in black have no change or have not yet been determined in cachexia. Solid lines indicate pathways confirmed in CAC and dotted lines expected but unconfirmed ones. Source: Das and Hoefler 2013 [13]. Reproduced with permission of Elsevier.

- 11–23% have a psychiatric disorder [21].
- At least 10% of people over 65 years of age have Alzheimer disease, rising to 25–45% over 85, and this is almost universally associated with weight loss in its later stages and may present with weight loss particularly if depression is present.
- Despite extensive evaluation, a cause cannot be found in 5–28%. In these patients, there is often spontaneous recovery of weight.

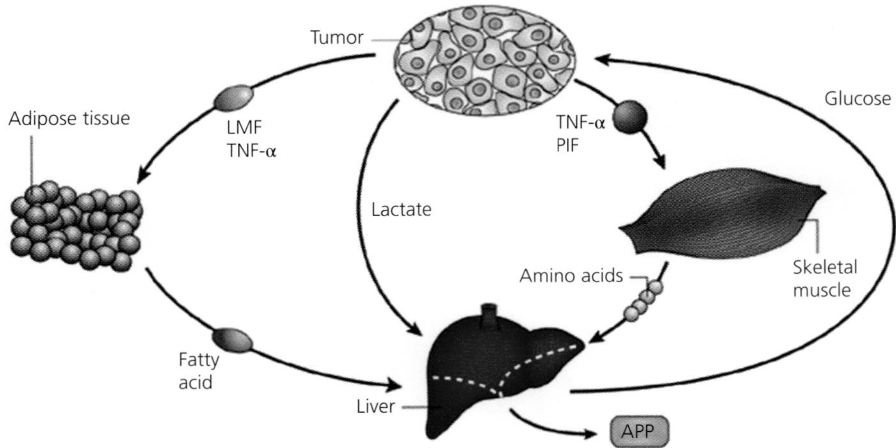

Figure 32.3 Tumors produce factors such as lipid-mobilizing factor (LMF), which induces breakdown of adipose tissue into fatty acids, and proteolysis-inducing factor (PIF), which induces protein degradation (amino acids) in skeletal muscle. Tumor necrosis factor (TNF)-α also contributes to these processes. These are important gluconeogenic substrates that can be used in acute phase protein (APP) synthesis by the liver. Tumors convert glucose to lactate, which is transferred to the liver, where it is converted back into glucose. This cycle uses a large amount of energy, and might contribute to cachexia. Source: Tisdale M.J. Cachexia in cancer patients. Nat Rev Cancer2002;2:862. Reproduced with permission of Springer Nature.

Box 32.1 Nonmalignant etiologies of involuntary weight loss.

Gastrointestinal
Malabsorptive syndromes (of gut or pancreatic origin), inflammatory bowel diseases, peptic ulcer disease, diabetic enteropathy, liver disease, partially or completely obstructing gastrointestinal lesion of any cause (all of which are usually associated with some gastrointestinal symptoms), mesenteric ischemia

Metabolic/endocrine/renal
Diabetes mellitus, hyperthyroidism, adrenal insufficiency, hypopituitarism, renal failure of any etiology

Cardiopulmonary
Chronic obstructive pulmonary disease, interstitial lung disease, cystic fibrosis, cardiac cachexia from heart failure, infective endocarditis

Neurological
Dementia, cerebrovascular disease, motor neuron disease, Parkinson disease

Psychiatric
Anxiety, depression, bipolar disorder, schizophrenia, psychosis of any cause

Inflammatory/infectious
Acute or chronic microbial infection (bacterial, viral, parasitic or fungal, e.g., human immunodeficiency virus, hepatitis, tuberculosis), chronic inflammatory disorders (rheumatoid arthritis, other autoimmune disorders such as systemic lupus erythematosus, giant cell arteritis, sarcoidosis, polyarteritis nodosa)

Pharmacological changes or misuse
- *Prescription medications* (e.g., metformin, antimitotic agents, liraglutide, exenatide, nonsteroidal antiinflammatory drugs, antiretroviral drugs) or cessation of drugs that increase weight, e.g., antidepressants
- *Over-the-counter remedies* (e.g., dandelion, aloe, cascara, chitosan, dandelion, ephedra, garcinia, guar gum, herbal diuretics, nicotine, pyruvate, St John's wort)
- *Substance misuse* (e.g., opiates, alcohol, psychotropic drugs such as cannabis, amphetamines, ecstasy)

Diagnosis

Accurate diagnosis relies on assessing probabilities based on a number of key factors. The age of the patient is especially important – functional disorders uncommonly present for the first time in patients over the age of 40 years. However, unintentional weight loss should not be solely attributed to the aging process. Total bodyweight usually peaks in the sixth decade, remains steady until the age of 70, and then gradually declines after the age of 70–75. Healthy elderly subjects only have small decrements in weight associated with normal aging [22].

Consideration of the likely prevalence of different diagnoses in a patient with unexplained weight loss (see Table 32.1) should influence the approach to diagnosis. A multivariate regression model based on age, white blood cell (WBC) count, serum albumin, alkaline phosphatase, and lactate dehydrogenase has been found to predict a malignant cause with sensitivity of 69% and specificity of 93% [19], and helps the clinician to understand how much emphasis can be put on these factors.

History and physical examination

A thorough history is essential and should first address the magnitude and time course of weight loss. Weight loss requires investigation if 5% of previous bodyweight has been lost. Weight loss over a very long period (>12 months) is less likely to be due to a malignant cause. There may be some instances where an accurate history of weight loss is challenging. In these circumstances, such as in individuals with cognitive impairment, a collateral history should be obtained.

The physician should ascertain whether there have been any significant changes in diet including:

- avoidance of specific foodstuffs due to perceived or actual food intolerance.
- significant changes in alcohol consumption.

Table 32.1 Representative studies evaluating the various etiologies of unintentional weight loss.

	Hernandez et al. 2003 [19], *n* = 276, %	Lankisch et al. 2001 [20], *n* = 158, %	Metalidis et al. 2007 [31], *n* = 101, %	Baicus et al. 2006 [32], *n* = 431, %
Malignancy	38	24	22	24
GI tract	20	13	10	–
Upper GI	7	–	–	5
Colorectal	3	–	–	3
HPB	11	–	–	–
Respiratory	0.3	4	2	3
Hematological	5	2.5	4	–
Unknown	7	1.3	1	–
Genitourinary	5			–
Prostate	–	1.3	1	–
Breast	–	0.6	–	–
Ovarian	–	0.6	–	–
Bladder	–	0.6	–	–
Renal	–	–	3	–
Uterine	–	–	1	–
Psychiatric disorder	23%	11%	16%	12%
GI disorders	10%	19%	15%	32%
Endocrine	8%	11%	2%	–
Cardiopulmonary	0%	10%	5%	–
Alcohol	0%	5%	0%	–
Rheumatic/inflammatory	7%	2.5%	4%	–
Infections	5%	–	8%	9%
Unknown	5%	16%	28%	–

GI, gastrointestinal; HPB, hepatopancreaticobiliary.

The history should assess whether there are any symptoms that might point to a specific organ/system. This includes soliciting possible difficulty in swallowing, nausea, vomiting, belching, satiety, pain with eating, or diarrhea, which might indicate a gastrointestinal problem, or shortness of breath that might indicate chronic obstructive airways disease (COPD). Weight loss occurs in about 50% of patients with severe COPD and chronic respiratory failure and about 10–15% of those with milder disease [23]. Cachexia has been demonstrated to confer an increased mortality in COPD, driven by the unintentional weight loss component [24]. "Cardiac cachexia" and relevant symptoms should be elicited.

The clinician should inquire about headaches, unsteadiness, and changes in gait, which may indicate an underlying neurological problem such as an intracranial tumor or parkinsonism. In the course of obtaining the history, the possibility of memory loss should be determined as dementia is commonly associated with weight loss and may warrant a mini mental score. The weight loss in dementia is multifactorial, and can include the cognitive impairment associated with loss of appetite and reduced food intake, as well as other features linked to Alzheimer dementia such as alterations of energy consumption due to olfactory changes, hypothalamic feeding dysregulation, and apraxia of swallowing [25]. Symptoms of depression are also essential to solicit. Cough or chest pain could suggest lung cancer which accounts for about 4% of cases of unexplained weight loss, while bony pain could indicate neoplastic infiltration due to metastases or myeloma. A history of excess thirst may suggest diabetes mellitus or hypercalcemia while muscle weakness may suggest a neurological or endocrine problem such as thyrotoxicosis.

Because weight loss can be a sign of chronic infection, inflammatory, or lymphoproliferative illness, it is pertinent to know if the patient has experienced night sweats or fever. Risk factors for infections, such as HIV and travel history should also be elicited.

Changes in medication may be highly relevant. Prescribed drugs can cause anorexia and weight loss (see Box 32.1) either as an idiosyncratic effect or related to their mode of action (e.g., biguanides such as metformin, or excessive thyroxine replacement). Occasionally, cessation of a drug associated with weight gain (e.g., tricyclic and some other antidepressants) can cause "unexplained" weight loss.

Inappropriate use of medicinal drugs–particularly laxatives –can be associated with marked weight loss and in severe cases with frank malabsorption and clubbing. This may be difficult to elicit from the history. Use of some "recreational" drugs, particularly amphetamines, also commonly causes weight loss.

Assessment of socioeconomic factors is important, as social isolation or poverty can contribute to unintentional weight loss, through a lack of access to adequate food intake and malnutrition [26].

Psychiatric illness and emotional stress are frequent reasons for unexplained weight loss, and it is important to obtain relevant history, including possible perceptible life stresses [27].

In a younger patient, it may be important to ascertain whether symptoms of an underlying eating disorder are present, including secondary amenorrhea in women. Soliciting a history of self-induced vomiting, laxative abuse, and anomalous eating habits can be challenging and requires sensitivity on the part of the physician.

Symptoms presenting for the first time in someone over 40 years of age are rarely functional, and age is the most important factor determining the probabilities of different causes of unexplained weight loss. Accordingly, this should influence any diagnostic plan. For example, in younger patients, psychiatric, gastrointestinal conditions (e.g., celiac disease), and cancers with a younger age of onset (e.g., leukemia) may be more prevalent. Likewise, cardiovascular conditions (e.g., heart failure), neurological conditions (e.g., Parkinson disease) or cancer may be more likely to present in older individuals.

Physical examination should include inspection for lymphadenopathy or thyroid enlargement and inspection of the oral cavity for evidence of glossitis/stomatitis and other features to suggest iron deficiency or immunodeficiency. Abdominal examination should include auscultation for bruits over the liver (present in around 30% of hepatocellular carcinoma) and splenic artery (pancreatic carcinoma). Percussion over the spine may detect local tenderness if metastases are present. A simple neurological examination should include inspection for nystagmus or ataxia, and assessment of peripheral sensation. Breasts and genitalia should be examined. If dyspnea is reported, a peak flow rate should be checked and if abnormal should be followed up with lung function testing.

Laboratory tests

Evaluation should encompass a complete blood count and ferritin (any suggestion of iron deficiency such as low mean corpuscular volume or ferritin should be followed by thorough gastrointestinal investigation), biochemical profile (raised serum alkaline phosphatase and raised γ-glutamyl transpeptidase should be followed by liver imaging, e.g., computed tomography [CT]), and thyroid function test.

C-reactive protein (CRP) and erythrocyte sedimentation rate (ESR) may also be helpful. CRP will be increased in most symptomatic chronic inflammatory disorders with a sensitivity of about 95% for patients with symptomatic Crohn's disease but a lower sensitivity for endoscopically active, asymptomatic Crohn's disease.

Erythrocyte sedimentation rate is also useful as there are conditions, such as systemic lupus erythematosis and multiple myeloma, where the ESR is often elevated despite a normal CRP.

Lactase dehydrogenase (LDH) may also be considered, with an elevated LDH possibly suggesting malignancy as an etiology for weight loss.

Other tests may be helpful depending on the specific circumstances. These include celiac-related antibody (tissue transglutaminase antibody) and tumor markers. Serological testing for the presence of immunoglobulin A antibodies against tissue transglutaminase has a sensitivity of approximately 95% for untreated celiac disease and should be performed. Testing for IgA deficiency, in conjunction with celiac serology, should be performed, as 2.6% of individuals with celiac disease have IgA deficiency [28].

The appropriateness of serological testing for tumor-associated antigens and other tumor markers depends on the patient population. None has sufficient sensitivity or specificity to be relied on as the sole test but they may be useful adjuncts to imaging in a symptomatic patient providing that the clinician is familiar with their reliability. These include, depending on circumstances, CA19.9, CA125, carcinoembryonic antigen (CEA), and prostate-specific antigen (PSA). Cancer screening should be performed if appropriate (e.g., colorectal).

Tests for pancreatic exocrine insufficiency, bacterial overgrowth, malabsorption, and protein-losing enteropathy will also be appropriate for some patients as dictated by the history and physical examination. Fecal fat estimation remains the gold standard for diagnosis of malabsorption but is unpopular with both patients and laboratory staff. In most patients, a diagnosis of a small intestinal cause of malabsorption can be made by endoscopic biopsy or alternatively a diagnosis of pancreatic enzyme insufficiency (PEI) made by fecal elastase determination, thus obviating the need for fecal fat estimation. Whilst a normal fecal elastase (below 200 μg/g) can rule out PEI in individuals with a low probability of the disorder, a normal level can miss approximately 10% of individuals with a high probability of PEI [29].

Small intestinal bacterial overgrowth (SIBO) can be difficult to diagnose because there is no "gold standard" test. Duodenal aspiration and culture (using a specially designed endoscopic cannula to avoid contamination) is probably the most reliable test but an empirical trial of antibiotics (such as tetracycline or metronidazole) may be warranted if there is a strong clinical suspicion, e.g., because of underlying achlorhydria or systemic sclerosis. Breath hydrogen (or methane) excretion after dextrose or lactulose can also be used but the results should be interpreted with caution – it is within normal limits to see a rise in breath hydrogen 30 min after ingestion of lactulose and only a very early rise, e.g., within 20 min, should be considered suggestive of proximal small intestinal overgrowth. The current tests used to assess SIBO lack sensitivity and specificity, highlighting the challenges of diagnosing this condition [30].

Protein-losing enteropathy should be suspected if there is marked hypoalbuminemia, usually associated with edema and, if more severe, with ascites and/or pleural effusion, in the absence of proteinuria, liver disease, or sepsis. Fecal α1-antitrypsin assay is the most appropriate test to confirm this suspicion [33].

Immunoglobulins and electrophoresis are useful when multiple myeloma, an autoimmune disease, or chronic infection such as tuberculosis is suggested.

Imaging tests

Chest x-ray

This should be performed as an initial screen in all patients with unexplained weight loss to identify possible carcinoma or lymphoma, tuberculosis, or chronic lung disorder such as bullous emphysema. If normal, the chest may need to be assessed more thoroughly, e.g., by CT scan, if other investigations fail to reveal a cause for weight loss.

Upper gastrointestinal endoscopy

Approximately 80% of gastric cancers present with advanced disease (stage II or more) [34], and even when weight loss is present other gastric symptoms may be absent or mild. Benign gastric ulceration is associated with weight loss of 4.5 kg (10 lb) or more in 80% of patients [35]. Upper gastrointestinal endoscopy should therefore be an early test in patients with unexplained weight loss. Duodenal biopsy to exclude rare cases of antitissue transglutaminase (TTG) antibody-negative celiac disease should be considered at the same time. Significant pathology, such as severe inflammation, ulceration, achalasia or neoplasia, has been demonstrated in up to 10% of individuals with both unintentional weight loss and foregut symptoms on upper gastrointestinal endoscopy. However, the yield is much lower in individuals with weight loss alone [36].

CT and MRI scanning

In most centers, a CT scan will be the imaging modality of first choice for investigation of possible intraabdominal malignancy following negative upper gastrointestinal endoscopy. Ovarian cancer is well known for its common lack of specific symptoms and it is important that scanning includes the pelvis in females undergoing investigation for weight loss. Whole-body CT imaging has been demonstrated to have a diagnostic yield of 33.5% for unexplained weight loss, with a good sensitivity and specificity for the detection of organic pathology [37]. MRI scanning probably has similar sensitivity. Positron emission tomography (PET)/CT may soon replace conventional CT and MRI for this indication.

F18-fluorodeoxyglucose and PET/CT

Although not available at all care delivery sites, PET/CT probably has the greatest sensitivity for detection of many disorders likely to be relevant to weight loss (e.g., neoplasia, infection, vasculitis). It has greater sensitivity than conventional CT or MRI for diagnosis of pancreatic and ovarian malignancy [38,39]. If available, it is an appropriate investigation if simpler investigations (chest x-ray and upper gastrointestinal endoscopy) have failed to provide an explanation. However, it has low specificity and cannot reliably differentiate between malignancy, infection, and inflammation. As a result, a positive result needs to be followed by additional imaging and possible biopsy. A delayed or dual time point scan may improve sensitivity for cancer detection substantially, for example from 77% to 94% [40].

Isotope bone scan

Isotope bone scan has been the standard technique for diagnosis of bony metastases but is being superseded by PET/CT due to its substantially better sensitivity [41].

Angiography/magnetic resonance angiography

Polyarteritis nodosa may present with weight loss and raised ESR/CRP but without localizing symptoms or signs. Diagnosis may be aided by identification of typical microaneurysms in hepatic and renal arteries. Again, fluorodeoxyglucose (FDG)/PET and PET/CT are superseding angiography as an initial imaging test for diagnosis with sensitivities reported of 77–92% and specificities of 89–100% for large vessel vasculitis.

Mesenteric ischemia, classically associated with abdominal pain after eating, is relatively uncommon and usually associated with at least 50% occlusion of at least two of the three relevant arteries – celiac, superior mesenteric, and inferior mesenteric.

Mammography

Breast cancer is unlikely to cause weight loss without metastases but mammography is appropriate in a woman over 50 years of age if initial investigations have not provided a diagnosis.

Testing for tuberculosis and human immunodeficiency virus

Positron emission tomography/CT may accurately distinguish between intraabdominal malignancy and tuberculosis. Biopsy, culture, and sensitivity are most reliable but may not always be feasible. Interferon-γ release tests are being used increasingly because of their greater convenience than tuberculin skin testing but still require further evaluation. Sensitivities for the diagnosis of active tuberculosis may only reach 70% [42] although higher sensitivities have also been reported [43]. Although interferon-γ release tests have a higher specificity than tuberculin skin testing, neither can accurately differentiate between latent tuberculosis infection and active tuberculosis [44].

Approximately one-quarter of patients with undiagnosed human immunodeficiency virus (HIV) present with weight loss, often with a high rate (e.g., 40% in India) for concomitant tuberculosis [45], so there should be a low threshold for requesting HIV and tuberculosis testing in any patient with unexplained weight loss.

Differential diagnosis

Malignancy

Anorexia and weight loss are present in over 50% of cancer patients at the time of diagnosis. Some intraabdominal cancers –particularly gastric, hepatic (primary), renal and ovarian–are particularly prone to present with unexplained weight loss and no localizing symptoms.

Early gastric cancer is sometimes completely asymptomatic. In Japan, where endoscopic screening of symptom-free individuals is undertaken, 30% of patients undergoing gastric resection for cancer were symptom free at diagnosis [46]. Making an endoscopic diagnosis of early gastric cancer can be challenging, as often there are very subtle changes [47].

Hepatocellular cancer in western countries usually affects patients known to have cirrhosis who should be in a screening program but in parts of the world such as Africa or Asia where hepatitis B is endemic, around 30% of hepatitis B-related hepatocellular cancer occurs in noncirrhotic livers and often presents late with associated weight loss.

Ovarian cancer is asymptomatic at 7% on diagnosis and symptoms are commonly vague such as bloating or loss of appetite. Weight gain (around 46%) is more common than weight loss (around 11–16%) [48].

Renal cancers are often clinically silent. In one study of 430 patients with renal cancer, 55% were asymptomatic at presentation and diagnosed as an incidental finding, typically after screening for microscopic hematuria. Only 29% had localizing abdominal or flank pain, and 19% had weight loss [49]. Patient-reported weight loss also predicts the recurrence rate in renal cell cancer cases after nephrectomy [50].

Small intestinal tumors, including adenocarcinoma, lymphoma, neuroendocrine tumors, and gastrointestinal stromal tumors (GIST), often present with nonspecific symptoms and may be easily missed or misdiagnosed on conventional barium studies. PET/CT scan should perform better but the tumors are rare. Prospective series looking at its utility in the diagnosis of small bowel tumors have not yet been reported, although it has been shown to be useful in assessing cases with an established diagnosis of small bowel neoplasm [51]. However, only 3% of neuroendocrine tumors present with weight loss [4].

Endocrine disorders

Diabetes mellitus (DM) and thyroid disorders are commonly associated with unintentional weight loss. Weight loss in type 1 DM is accompanied by polydipsia, polyphagia, and polyuria. There is a loss of lean body mass as well as loss of extracellular and cellular water due to the osmotic diuresis from glucosuria. Patients with type 2 diabetes may rarely develop *diabetic neuropathic cachexia* [52], characterized by a symmetrical peripheral neuropathy associated with profound weight loss and painful dysesthesias. Most patients recover spontaneously, although residual neurological deficits may persist.

Weight loss in hyperthyroidism is due primarily to increased catabolism, but compounded by increased intestinal motility and malabsorption. Weight gain occurs quickly with treatment. Greater vigilance and testing should be performed in elderly individuals, as they tend to present with a paucity of symptoms and signs [53].

Chronic primary adrenal insufficiency often presents with weight loss, but is usually associated with other features such as dehydration, anorexia, lassitude, fatigue, and weakness. Five percent of patients with pheochromocytomas report weight loss, which may present as part of multiple endocrine neoplasia type 2 [54].

Gastrointestinal diseases

Nonmalignant gastrointestinal conditions account for 10–20% of patients with involuntary weight loss [19,20,55] which can arise as a result of anorexia, early satiety, swallowing difficulties, dysmotility, diarrhea, malabsorption, chronic inflammation, chronic ischemia, obstruction from any cause, or fistulas. In most cases, these will present with symptoms suggestive of a specific gastrointestinal disorder.

Weight loss is common in peptic ulcer disease, affecting over 50% of patients in a study of 650 patients with gastric ulcers [35]. Chronic duodenal ulcer can cause gastric outlet obstruction although this has become more uncommon in recent decades.

Celiac disease in adults often presents with very nonspecific symptoms that often include weight loss, and is very common, with a prevalence of 1% [56]. Other causes of malabsorption such as giardiasis or Whipple disease usually present with weight loss and diarrhea although concomitant symptoms are usually present in patients with Whipple disease, including arthritis or encephalopathy.

Pancreatic exocrine insufficiency can present with weight loss, with diarrhea also being a presenting feature. Inflammatory bowel disease can also present with unintentional weight loss, and most commonly presents in younger individuals, although it can also occur in an elderly population.

Chronic mesenteric ischemia, although infrequent, is an important cause of weight loss, particularly in the elderly. Abdominal pain typically occurs half an hour after eating and lasts 1–3 h [57]. Patients limit their own food intake to avoid the pain of abdominal angina ("sitophobia"). By contrast, superior mesenteric artery syndrome is almost always a consequence of weight loss rather than its cause.

Human immunodeficiency virus and other chronic infections

These may account for about 5% of patients with involuntary weight loss [19]. Infection with HIV and hepatitis C virus (HCV) should be considered, especially in high-risk groups. Tuberculosis presents frequently with weight loss [58]. Bacterial endocarditis, fungal infections, parasitic infections, and intraabdominal abscesses may all present with weight loss.

Cardiopulmonary disease

Up to 50% of patients with New York Heart Association class III or IV heart failure lose lean body mass and meet the criteria for malnutrition [59]. In unselected patients with chronic heart failure, mortality rates were 50% in the cachectic subset compared to 17% in the noncachectic subset at 18 months of follow-up [60].

Chronic obstructive pulmonary disease

Malnutrition is a common and often underrecognized problem in patients with COPD. The prevalence of malnutrition is about 20–40% in outpatients and up to 70% in inpatients with acute respiratory failure or in patients awaiting lung transplantation [61]. Multiple factors contribute to malnutrition, including increased secretion of inflammatory mediators (TNF-α, IL-6, IL-8, CRP), increased metabolic rate due to ventilatory effort, and the therapeutic use of sympathicomimetic drugs, together with reduced appetite. Mortality rates are substantially higher in underweight patients than in overweight patients with COPD [61]. Individuals with COPD and unintentional weight loss must be evaluated for lung cancer, as both have the common etiological agent of smoking.

Renal disease

Uremia as a cause of weight loss is usually symptomatic (e.g., nausea), but nephrotic syndrome often leads to a negative caloric balance and may have a more subtle presentation. Hemodialysis is accompanied by swings in metabolic balance that may cause weight loss.

Neurological diseases

Weight loss is seen in patients with stroke, dementia, Parkinson disease, multiple sclerosis (MS), and amyotrophic lateral sclerosis. Weight loss may be due to one or more of anorexia, altered cognition, motor dysfunction, and dysphagia. It may be an early feature in Parkinson disease where, in addition to swallowing problems, rigidity, tremor, and levodopa-induced dyskinesia may increase energy expenditure. Levodopa may enhance glucose metabolism, resulting in enhanced energy expenditure. Depression also contributes to weight loss in Parkinson disease [62]. Depression and fatigue are common in MS and may be a contributing factor to weight loss.

Inflammatory disorders

Giant cell arteritis is a systemic immune-mediated disease that typically affects persons aged 50 years and over, with a 2–6-fold female preponderance. In addition to weight loss, giant cell arteritis patients present with fever, anorexia, and ischemic symptoms [63]. Patients with myocardial and pericardial disease may present with chest pain, palpitations, shortness of breath, and symptoms resembling myocardial ischemia or infarction. The manifestations of vasculitis include fever, weight loss, and fatigue, mimicking infectious or malignant processes.

Systemic sclerosis is commonly accompanied by weight loss and malabsorption. This is sometimes due to treatable small intestinal bacterial overgrowth but is also commonly due to severe dysmotility and mucosal ischemia, neither of which is readily treatable.

Psychiatric disorders

Involuntary weight loss due to psychiatric illness affects 11–44% of outpatients [19,55,64] and 58% of nursing home residents [65]. Depression is present in approximately 13% of individuals 55 years and older [66]. Depression can lead to weight loss due to loss of appetite or reduced motivation to prepare and consume food, and is commonly associated with weight loss in those 65 years or older in whom it contributes to increased mortality (OR 1.73, 95% CI 1.53–1.95) [67].

Patients with cognitive impairment and features of agitation and restlessness can expend substantial energy leading to weight loss. Others may forget that they need to eat or become suspicious and paranoid about food [8]. During the manic phases of bipolar disorder, hyperactivity and preoccupations may interfere with normal eating patterns. Patients with delusions or paranoia may develop peculiar ideations about food that lead to decreased food intake.

Anorexia nervosa and bulimia can present with weight loss, with careful probing required, as the history may not be forthcoming.

Drugs

Several prescription, over-the-counter, and illicit drugs can lead to weight loss. Some of these are listed in Table 32.1 [34,35]. Marked weight loss can also occur after reduction or withdrawal of antipsychotic drugs [68].

Substance abuse

Although moderate alcohol intake is common in overweight people, subjects who consume at least 100 g of alcohol a day have significantly lower body mass index than social drinkers [69]. Alcohol abuse causes weight loss through poor appetite, decreased oral intake, or malabsorption from pancreatic causes or rapid intestinal transit.

Stimulant use, such as cocaine and amphetamines, can result in both poor appetite and increased metabolic consumption, resulting in weight loss. Opiates directly inhibit the appetite center, decrease gastrointestinal motility, and can cause hyperalgesia with chronic abdominal pain. Discontinuation of chronic marijuana use can result in anorexia, weight loss, irritability, and strange dreams [70].

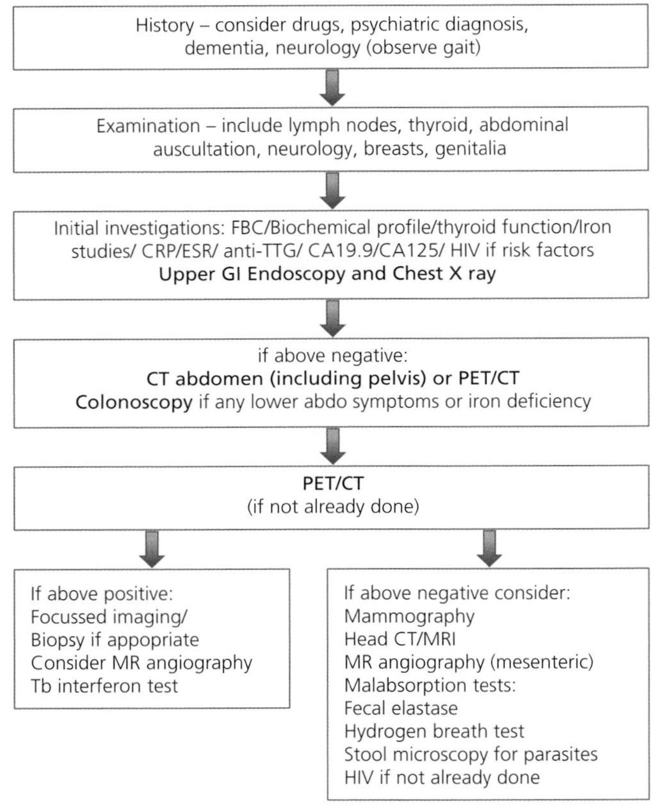

Figure 32.4 Flow chart. CRP, C-reactive protein; CT, computed tomography; ESR, erythrocyte sedimentation rate; FBC, full blood count; GI, gastrointestinal; HIV, human immunodeficiency virus; MRI, magnetic resonance imaging; PET, positron emission tomography; Tb, tuberculosis; TTG, tissue transglutaminase.

Unknown

Despite extensive evaluation, the cause of unintentional weight loss can be unknown. It is possible that these individuals have multiple medical conditions, psychological or social factors which may contribute to weight loss, but each factor may not be significant alone to cause clinically significant weight loss in its own right [26]. Therefore, a detailed history is essential to help elucidate these potential triggering factors (Figure 32.4).

Principles of management

Management will vary depending on the underlying cause but nutritional assessment should be performed and supplementation tailored accordingly. Nutritional support should be provided for all patients with a nonmalignant cause for weight loss. Nutritional supplementation can promote significant weight gain among patients with COPD, especially if malnourished [71]. Cancer-related malnutrition is almost universal, and occurs in 50–80% of patients with cancer [72]. Although cancer-related cachexia is largely irreversible, the degree of support should be assessed according to patient wishes. A metaanalysis concluded that there was no statistically significant difference in weight gain, energy intake, or mortality with oral nutritional supplementation [73].

Pharmacological interventions including progesterones and anabolic steroids have been tried in subjects with unintentional weight loss. Megesterol acetate is a synthetic derivative of a naturally occurring progestational agent and is currently the only pharmacological agent licensed for treatment of cachexia. However, it has been linked with a higher chance of developing deep vein thrombosis [74]. Placebo-controlled trials of megestrol (800 mg/day) have shown some improvement in quality of life but weight gain is modest and due to increased fat mass, without increase in lean body mass.

Ghrelin binds to the growth hormone secretagog-1a receptor in the arcuate nucleus of the hypothalamus to stimulate growth hormone release. Small studies of ghrelin mimetics have been performed in cancer-related cachexia with promising results but concerns that it may stimulate cancer growth persist [75]. A placebo-controlled trial of ghrelin in patients with COPD has shown mixed effects on respiratory function with no improvement in exercise tolerance or weight gain [76].

If investigations including baseline blood tests, chest x-ray, upper gastrointestinal endoscopy, and abdominal scan have not yielded an explanation for the weight loss then the patient can be reasonably reassured and followed up in clinic. In a series of 101 consecutive patients with unexplained weight loss, no cause was found on baseline investigations in 28% and at 6-month follow-up most (90%) had stable or increased weight [31].

Acknowledgments

The authors would like to acknowledge the previous authors of this chapter, Sreedhar Subramanian and Jonathan M. Rhodes, on which this chapter was based.

References are available at www.yamadagastro.com/textbook7e

Further reading

Alibhai S.M.H., Greenwood C., Payette H. An approach to the management of unintentional weight loss in elderly people. CMAJ 2005;172:773.

Das S.K., Hoefler G. The role of triglyceride lipases in cancer associated cachexia. Trends Mol Med 2013;19:292.

Maccio A., Madeddu C., Mantovani G. Current pharmacotherapy options for cancer anorexia and cachexia. Expert Opin Pharmacother 2012;13:2453.

McMinn J., Steel C., Bowman A. Investigation and management of unintentional weight loss in older adults. BMJ 2011;342:d1732.

Metalidis C., Knoickaert D.C., Bobbaers H., et al. Involuntary weight loss. Does a negative baseline evaluation provide adequate reassurance? Eur J Intern Med 2008;19:345.

CHAPTER 33

Approach to the patient with nausea and vomiting

Brian E. Lacy and David Cangemi
Mayo Clinic, Jacksonville, FL, USA

Chapter menu

Definitions

Nausea and vomiting are nonspecific symptoms that develop due to a wide variety of medical and surgical disorders.

- Nausea is a vague, unpleasant feeling of unease with the sensation that vomiting might occur.
- Vomiting (or emesis) is the forceful ejection of gastric contents from the mouth. Vomiting may occur with or without nausea.
- Retching involves a mechanism similar to vomiting; however, there is no oral discharge of gastric contents.
- Regurgitation is characterized by the effortless and involuntary movement of gastric contents into the mouth without abdominal wall contractions. It is a cardinal symptom of gastroesophageal reflux disease. Nausea is typically absent.
- Rumination is a process in which patients effortlessly bring up recently ingested food from the stomach into the mouth, where it is then rechewed and reswallowed. Nausea is typically absent.
- Anorexia is a loss of appetite.
- Early satiety is the sensation of being unable to complete a modest-sized meal. Often accompanied by epigastric pressure or fullness.

Introduction

Nausea and vomiting are two symptoms that frequently lead to medical consultation. Analysis of the National Ambulatory Medical (NAMCAS) data bank found that nausea and vomiting were the fourth and second most common reasons for an ambulatory care visit, respectively [1]. Nausea and vomiting can be classified as either acute or chronic in nature. Acute nausea and vomiting is generally defined by symptom duration of 7 days or less. Distinguishing acute nausea and vomiting from chronic is important, as the differential diagnosis is more limited, and includes a transient medical or surgical condition (e.g., an infectious gastroenteritis, medications, postoperative nausea), a self-limited somatic disorder (e.g., musculoskeletal trauma, myocardial infarction), or medications (Box 33.1).

The *epidemiology* of nausea and vomiting has not been extensively studied. A telephone survey of over 21 000 US adults reported that 7% suffered from nausea and vomiting in the prior 3 months [2]. Food poisoning, a common cause of nausea and vomiting, affects nearly one in six Americans each year [3]. There are better data for specific disease states. The Rochester (MN) epidemiology project estimated a prevalence rate of diagnosed gastroparesis – a disorder characterized by chronic nausea and vomiting – of 9.6 per 100 000 in men and

Yamada's Textbook of Gastroenterology, Seventh Edition. Edited by Timothy C. Wang, Michael Camilleri, Benjamin Lebwohl, Anna S. Lok, William J. Sandborn, Kenneth K. Wang, and Gary D. Wu.

Companion website: www.yamadagastro.com/textbook7e

Box 33.1 Etiologies of acute nausea and vomiting.

Infections
Viral gastroenteritis
Bacterial gastroenteritis
Opportunistic infections (immunosuppression)
Nongastrointestinal infections (e.g., pneumonia, peritonitis)

Somatic disorders
Musculoskeletal pain
Myocardial infarction

Medications
Nonsteroidal antiinflammatory agents/aspirin
Opiates
Antibiotics
- Macrolides
- Tetracycline
- Sulfonamides

Anticholinergic agents
Anti-Parkinsonian/restless legs drugs
Anticonvulsants
Cardiac antiarrhythmics/antihypertensive
Chemotherapy
Diuretics
Antidiabetes drugs
- Metformin
- Liraglutide, other GLP-1 analogs/agonists

Antidepressants (serotonin-norepinephrine reuptake inhibitors)
- Venlafaxine
- Duloxetine

Oral contraceptives
Estrogen
THC/marijuana
Smoking cessation drugs
- Nicotine
- Varenicline

Lubiprostone

37.8 per 100 000 in women [4]. Recurrent nausea and vomiting affects 50–75% of pregnant women [5,6], although only 0.5–1% of pregnant women suffer from the most extreme form of nausea and vomiting during pregnancy, hyperemesis gravidarum [7].

Nausea and vomiting can dramatically impair *quality of life*. Nausea during the first trimester of pregnancy reduces both physical and mental components of quality of life surveys. Women with hyperemesis gravidarum are 3–6-fold more likely to report low health-related quality of life than women with less severe symptoms [8]. Nausea and vomiting during pregnancy also are associated with fatigue, sleep disturbances, and irritability. Mental and physical function scores are reduced and psychological distress is increased by gastrointestinal consequences of cancer chemotherapy. Ninety percent of patients with uncontrolled chemotherapy-induced emesis have poor functioning [9]. In one study, nausea and vomiting reduced quality of life in ~40% of chemotherapy cycles [10]. Symptoms of nausea, which can occur frequently and be quite intense, may impact daily function more than vomiting, which is typically much less frequent. Nausea and vomiting after either chemotherapy or surgery reduce time spent on leisure and recreation, household tasks, and socializing and cause hardship to family members.

Nausea and vomiting also have a profound *socioeconomic impact*. Nausea of pregnancy can increase rates of job loss. It has been estimated that 8.5 million working days are lost in Britain yearly because of nausea of pregnancy and that severely affected women miss a mean of 62 work hours while pregnant [11]. In Sweden, 28% of sick leaves relates to nausea of pregnancy [12]. One percent of pregnant women are hospitalized because of nausea and vomiting with an average length of stay of 2.6 days. In a large US telephone study, nausea and vomiting led to an average of 6.6 work days, 9.0 leisure days, and 19.7 household days missed during the previous 3 months [2]. Nausea and vomiting after chemotherapy decrease employee productivity and increase healthcare costs due to prolonged hospitalization and home nursing needs. Analyses of a database of 11 495 patients found that total costs attributable to chemotherapy-induced emesis were $89 million, with an average cost of $1855 for daily treatment of the nausea and vomiting [13]. An investigation reported charges >$25 000 for treating 28 patients who returned to the hospital for persistent emesis after surgery [14]. Postoperative nausea and vomiting may potentially interfere with the ability of a surgery or endoscopy center to perform all scheduled surgeries or procedures due to prolonged recovery room stays and extra nursing requirements further exacerbating costs.

Etiology

The etiology of nausea and vomiting is diverse and not limited solely to the gastrointestinal tract. The first step in the evaluation of a patient with nausea and vomiting is to take a good history to understand the timeline of symptoms. This enables accurate categorization into either the acute category (symptom duration ≤7 days) or the chronic category (symptom duration >7 days). This is important because the vast majority of cases of acute nausea and vomiting are due to an infectious illness, recent medications, or somatic injury or inflammation. If symptoms are chronic in nature, then the next step is to exclude nongastrointestinal causes, such as long-standing medications, chronic renal insufficiency, cardiac disorders, vestibular disorders, neurologic disorders, and mechanical processes.

The etiology of chronic nausea and vomiting thought to be gastrointestinal in nature should be categorized as either gastroparesis or some other disorder (Box 32.2). This strategy is grounded in the fact that the vast majority of research in this field has focused on the diagnosis and treatment of gastroparesis [15]. Patients with functional dyspepsia (FD) frequently report nausea, especially in the postprandial period; vomiting as the predominant symptom is less common [16–18]. Cyclic vomiting syndrome (CVS) is characterized by recurrent, stereotypical, self-limited episodes of nausea and vomiting separated by symptom-free intervals [19]. A history of migraine

Box 33.2 Chronic nausea and vomiting.

Mechanical obstruction
Gastric/small bowel obstruction
Superior mesenteric artery syndrome
Volvulus
Antral web

Mucosal inflammation
Peptic ulcer disease
Crohn's disease
Pancreatitis
Cholecystitis
Appendicitis
Hepatitis

Motility disorders
Gastroparesis
Functional dyspepsia
Chronic intestinal pseudoobstruction (CIP)

Functional gastroduodenal disorders
Cyclic vomiting syndrome (CVS)
Chronic nausea and vomiting syndrome
Rumination syndrome

Cannabinoid hyperemesis syndrome

Nausea and vomiting of pregnancy (NVP)

Chemotherapy-induced nausea and vomiting (CINV): acute, delayed, anticipatory

Radiotherapy-induced nausea and vomiting

Postoperative nausea and vomiting (PONV)

CNS and peripheral neural conditions
Malignancy
Infarction
Hemorrhage
Infection
Migraine headaches
Motion sickness
Labyrinthine disease
Autonomic instability/neuropathy
Pseudotumor cerebri

Metabolic/endocrine causes
Diabetes (e.g., diabetic gastroparesis, DKA)
Uremia
Adrenal insufficiency
Thyroid disorders
Fatty liver of pregnancy

Miscellaneous
Myocardial infarction/heart failure
Ethanol intoxication
Graft versus host disease
Acute intermittent porphyria
Psychiatric disease
Eating disorders (anorexia, bulimia, conditioned vomiting)
Jamaican vomiting sickness

headaches is common and rapid gastric emptying is found in some patients [19,20]. The diagnosis of cannabinoid hyperemesis syndrome (CHS) can be made in some patients with

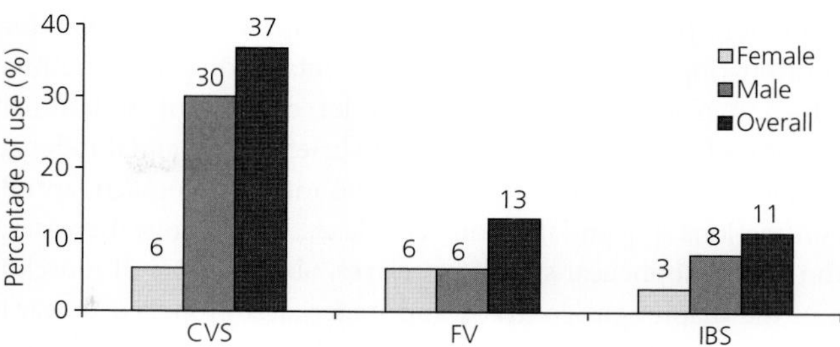

Figure 33.1 The proportions of cannabinoid users among patients with cyclic vomiting syndrome (CVS), functional vomiting (FV), and irritable bowel syndrome (IBS) are shown. Cannabinoid use was more prevalent with CVS, especially in men, compared to FV and IBS. Source: Choung et al. 2012 [79]. Reproduced with permission from John Wiley & Sons.

chronic cannabis use based on a history of compulsive bathing or showering during acute episodes [21]. Resolution of symptoms with cessation of cannabis use confirms the diagnosis (Figure 33.1).

Widespread use of proton pump inhibitors has led to a decrease in gastric outlet obstruction (GOO) secondary to peptic ulcer disease (PUD) as a cause of chronic nausea and vomiting; however, partial intermittent bowel obstruction needs to be excluded (see evaluation section below). A careful history and appropriate testing can identify chronic pancreatitis and hepatobiliary disorders as causes of chronic nausea and vomiting [22,23]. Chronic intestinal pseudoobstruction (primary or secondary) and connective tissue disorders should be considered as well [24,25]. Vascular disorders, such as median arcuate ligament syndrome (MALS) and superior mesenteric artery (SMA) syndrome, should be considered if other causes cannot be identified [26].

Pathophysiology

Symptoms of nausea and vomiting develop from complex neuroanatomical pathways that converge on the emetic center ("vomiting" center) located in the dorsolateral reticular formation of the medulla. The emetic center is a collection of closely linked nuclei that coordinate the complex series of events involved in vomiting [27]. Afferent pathways arise from the gastrointestinal tract, oropharynx, heart, musculoskeletal system, vestibular system, chemoreceptor trigger zone, and cerebral cortex, synapse on the solitary nucleus, and then travel to the emetic center [28]. One theory posits that mild stimulation of these pathways leads to nausea, while more intense stimulation leads to vomiting. However, it has also been proposed that each individual possesses an independent, dynamic threshold for nausea, which is subject to change and is dependent on interaction with certain modifiable factors, such as anxiety, anticipation, and adaptation [29]. This concept may explain the variability in symptom severity that can occur in response to a nausea-inducing stimulus.

Efferent pathways from the emetic center are responsible for coordinating the intricate series of events leading to vomiting, which involves the gastrointestinal tract, diaphragm, abdominal wall muscles, and oropharynx [30]. In brief, jejunal and duodenal retrograde contractions move material into the stomach, antral contractions stop and the stomach relaxes, pyloric tone increases, the lower esophageal sphincter relaxes, abdominal wall muscles and the diaphragm contract, and material is propelled upward into the mouth to be ejected. During the final step, respiration briefly ceases, the glottis and vocal cords close, and the soft palate rises, all to prevent aspiration. Key neurotransmitters and hormones involved in this process include histamine, dopamine, serotonin, norepinephrine, acetylcholine, substance P, NK1, cortisol, β-endorphin and vasopressin [31,32].

Medications

Medications are among the most common causes of nausea and vomiting, and symptoms typically present soon after initiating therapy. Emetogenic drugs exert their effects by acting in the periphery and within the CNS, including the vomiting center. Agents commonly producing nausea and vomiting include nonsteroidal antiinflammatory drugs (NSAIDs), opiates, antibiotics, anti-Parkinsonian agents and therapies for restless legs, cardiac antiarrhythmics, antihypertensives, diuretics, antidiabetics (metformin, exenatide, liraglutide), oral contraceptives, antidepressants (selective serotonin reuptake inhibitors, serotonin norepinephrine reuptake inhibitors, tricyclic agents), and treatments for smoking cessation (nicotine, varenicline) [33].

Chemotherapy (and radiation therapy)-induced nausea and vomiting (CINV)

Nausea and vomiting with cancer chemotherapy may be acute, delayed, or anticipatory. In data from a large registry, 26% of cases occurred after highly emetogenic chemotherapy, 46% after moderately emetogenic treatment, and 26% after milder therapies [13]. Acute nausea and vomiting are reported by 35% and 13% of patients, respectively; delayed emesis is noted by 50% and 28% receiving highly and moderately emetogenic agents respectively [34]. Risk factors for CINV include low social functioning, prechemotherapy nausea, young age, female sex, history of motion sickness, and use of highly emetogenic drugs (cisplatin, carmustine, high-dose cyclophosphamide, dacarbazine). Hematological malignancies are associated with more frequent CINV compared to solid tumors because of the young age of patients, the highly emetogenic nature of the chemotherapeutic agents, and the psychological impact of the diagnosis [35]. Risk scores predict CINV; those at high risk are 3–4-fold more likely to develop symptoms than those at low risk [36]. Anticipatory nausea and vomiting occur in 25–34% of patients by the fourth chemotherapy course, are more common in young patients, and impair quality of life. Patient expectations in concert with anxiety and coping mechanisms predict the onset of anticipatory nausea [37].

Mechanisms for CINV have been delineated from animal models and human studies. Highly emetogenic agents elicit acute vomiting with associated increases in plasma serotonin, urinary excretion of the serotonin metabolite 5-hydroxyindole acetic acid (5-HIAA), ileal tissue serotonin, and numbers of serotonin immunoreactive cells. One report proposed that an elevated 5-HIAA to creatinine ratio >70 is associated with CINV [38]. In contrast, less emetogenic agents evoke little rise in plasma serotonin or urinary 5-HIAA. Cisplatin-evoked emesis is reduced by vagotomy, suggesting peripheral afferent pathway involvement. However, the observation that intravenous administration of the CNS impermeant 5-HT_3 antagonist zatosetron (LY-277,359) does not block cisplatin-induced emesis while intracerebroventricular delivery has potent antiemetic action indicates an additional CNS site of action [39]. A polymorphism of one of the 5-HT_3 receptor genes (HTR3C) has been identified as a risk factor for developing CINV, further supporting a crucial role for serotonin pathways [40]. In contrast, delayed and anticipatory vomiting are mediated by serotonin-independent pathways. Delayed emesis after cisplatin is not associated with urinary 5-HIAA excretion and is poorly controlled by most 5-HT_3 antagonists. The ability of neurokinin NK_1 antagonists (e.g., aprepitant) to reduce delayed CINV indicates this phase is mediated by substance P pathways. Beneficial responses of delayed CINV to the long-acting 5-HT_3 antagonist palonosetron suggest interactions between 5-HT_3 and NK_1 pathways [41].

Radiation therapy for malignancy causes emesis due to its effects on gut structure and function. The incidence of nausea and vomiting increases to 80% when the upper abdomen is included in the radiation field. The ability of 5-HT_3 antagonists to reduce vomiting evoked by acute abdominal radiation indicates the participation of a serotonin pathway.

Infectious causes

Infectious illnesses commonly elicit acute nausea and vomiting. Acute enteric infection occurs most often in children <3 years old, but has a second peak incidence in the third decade. Norovirus from exposure to contaminated water is believed to be responsible for 68–90% of gastroenteritis attacks; its prevalence in winter is explainable by viral persistence at low temperatures [42]. Rotavirus is a common etiology of gastroenteritis leading to hospitalization of children from dehydration and lethargy. Viral gastroenteritis may also be caused by reoviruses, adenoviruses, and the Hawaii and Snow Mountain agents. An epidemic fever and vomiting syndrome has been related to an enterovirus (AU250G) that exhibits 95% homology to an echovirus that causes meningitis [43]. Nausea and vomiting also result from some bacterial infections (e.g., *Staphylococcus aureus*, *Bacillus cereus*, *Salmonella*, *Clostridium perfringens*). *S. aureus* produces a distinct enterotoxin. *B. cereus*, a bacterium found in starchy foods such as fried rice, contains an emesis-causing toxin, as well as three toxins that induce diarrhea. Nausea in immunocompromised patients may result from gut cytomegalovirus or herpes simplex infection. Nongastrointestinal infectious diseases that cause nausea include otitis media, meningitis, peritonitis, and hepatitis.

Mechanical obstruction and intraperitoneal inflammation

Gastric and small intestinal obstructions produce nausea that may be relieved by vomiting. Gastric obstruction often is intermittent, while small intestinal obstruction usually is acute and associated with abdominal pain. Superior mesenteric artery syndrome results from compression of the third portion of the duodenum by the overlying superior mesenteric artery as it originates from the aorta, causing anatomical obstruction. This condition is observed in patients who have had profound weight loss, undergone recent surgery, or been on prolonged bedrest. Other mechanical causes of chronic vomiting include subacute gastric volvulus, intussusception, celiac artery compression syndrome (also known as median arcuate ligament syndrome), and antral webs. Patients with inactive Crohn's disease can exhibit symptomatic delays in gastric emptying, presumably secondary to restricted gastric wall contractility [44].

Other intraperitoneal disorders produce nausea and vomiting. Biliary colic and inflammatory conditions (e.g., pancreatitis, appendicitis, cholecystitis, peritonitis) are associated with nausea a likely from activation of biliary or peritoneal afferent pathways. Nausea with fulminant hepatic failure is likely multifactorial in nature, including inability to eliminate toxins, stretching of the hepatic capsule, fluid shifts, accompanying kidney disease and increased intracranial pressure.

Gastroparesis and chronic intestinal pseudoobstruction

Gastroparesis is characterized by symptoms of nausea, vomiting and abdominal pain in the absence of mechanical obstruction with a documented delay in gastric emptying [15]. More than 90% of patients note nausea, 68–84% have vomiting, 60% report early satiety, up to 90% experience pain (predominant in 21%), and 80% note bloating (predominant in 7%) [45]. Other manifestations include heartburn, glycemic excursions (in diabetics, including significant hyper- and hypoglycemia), and pronounced fatigue. Bezoars – either phyto- or trichobezoars – may occur but are not common. Inadequate nutrient intake is common; significant weight loss is less common [46]. Systemic conditions causing gastroparesis include diabetes, connective tissue disorders (scleroderma, lupus), amyloidosis, neurological conditions (Parkinson disease, muscular dystrophy), and cancer (paraneoplastic gastroparesis).

Delayed gastric emptying has been found in 27–65% of those with long-standing type 1 *diabetes* (usually considered to be >10 years in duration) and in up to 30% of type 2 diabetics [47–50]. It is important to note that many of these studies examined referral populations which may not reflect true population prevalence. Among diabetics followed longitudinally, gastroparesis develops at a rate five times higher in type 1 versus type 2 patients [51]. Gastroparesis symptom differences between diabetic subtypes are minimal. Postsurgical gastroparesis develops as a consequence of intentional or inadvertent vagotomy; currently, the most common procedures with this complication include fundoplication for acid reflux and bariatric surgery. Rare causes of gastroparesis include gastric ischemia and median arcuate ligament syndrome, which results in compression of the celiac axis. Thirty percent to 60% of patients with gastroparesis exhibit no underlying systemic disease causing their symptoms.

Patients with *idiopathic gastroparesis* have a mean age of 41 years and are predominantly women; 46% are overweight and 50% had an acute onset of symptoms [52]. Nineteen percent of cases are preceded by prodromal symptoms (diarrhea, fever, headache, myalgias) suggesting a viral etiology; this form of disease may have a better prognosis than noninfectious gastroparesis. The responsible agent is rarely identified; rotavirus was implicated in a small study of 11 children [53]. Patients with idiopathic gastroparesis report lower vomiting severity and fewer daily vomiting episodes than diabetics with gastroparesis. The prevalence per 100 000 persons of definite gastroparesis (defined by typical symptoms with delayed emptying) is 9.6 for men and 37.8 for women [54]. Age-adjusted incidences per 100 000 person-years are 2.4 for men and 9.8 for women. Data suggest that inpatient admissions for gastroparesis more than quadrupled between 1997 and 2013, and the aggregate charges or "national bill" for gastroparesis increased by 1026% during this time [55]. Triggers of hospitalization include infection, poor glycemic control, and noncompliance with or intolerance of medications [56].

The *pathogenesis of gastroparesis* is multifactorial. Although needed for diagnosis, the relationship between extent of delay in gastric emptying and symptom correlation is controversial [57]. Electrical conduction defects (propagation blocks, abnormal initiation sites) are prominent on high-resolution serosal mapping of gastric pacemaker activity, providing a mechanism for contractile impairments [58]. Anxiety and depression scores relate to symptom severity in both diabetics and idiopathic patients, and women with idiopathic disease may report prior physical or sexual abuse, suggesting possible contributions from psychological dysfunction [59]. Symptoms may be increased during the luteal phase of the menstrual cycle, reflecting hormonal (such as progesterone) influences on disease severity [60]. On regression analyses, obesity is predictive of gastroparesis symptom severity [61]. Full-thickness gastric biopsies from patients with severe gastroparesis exhibit loss of interstitial cells of Cajal and inflammatory infiltrates in approximately half of patients, with a small number showing neuronal damage, neurotransmitter deficits, or smooth muscle fibrosis [62]. On electron microscopy, nerve endings are large and empty, the smooth muscle is damaged by lipofuscin and lamellar bodies, and fibrosis may be prominent around nerves [63].

Patients with *chronic intestinal pseudoobstruction* (CIP) report similar symptoms as those with gastroparesis but they often have more severe nutritional consequences and bowel habit disturbances. CIP etiologies are similar to gastroparesis and include connective tissue disorders, infiltrative disease, neurological conditions, paraneoplastic manifestations, and idiopathic disease. The majority of cases are neuropathic in origin. Some myopathic and neuropathic forms of CIP are hereditary. Full-thickness intestinal biopsies may show neuronal degeneration, inflammation, loss of interstitial cells of Cajal, and smooth muscle fibrosis.

Cyclic vomiting syndrome (CVS)

Cyclic vomiting syndrome (CVS) is characterized by discrete episodes of intractable emesis with stereotypic onset and duration and intervening well periods.

Diagnostic criteria for CVS have been defined by the Rome Foundation (Box 33.3) [20]. To be diagnosed with CVS, patients should report stereotypic episodes of vomiting with the following characteristics: at least three acute-onset episodes in the prior year and two episodes in the past 6 months, each occurring at least 1 week apart, and persisting for less than 1 week. Furthermore, there should be an absence of vomiting between episodes, but other milder symptoms can occur between cycles. A personal and/or family history of migraine headaches further supports a diagnosis of CVS. Four distinct phases characterize CVS: (1) a preemetic period with pallor, diaphoresis, and nausea; (2) a period with intense vomiting of up to 30 episodes daily; (3) a recovery period; and (4) an interepisodic period with few symptoms (although >50% report some intervening nausea) [20,64]. CVS attacks often are associated with abdominal pain and diarrhea. Adult CVS flares are longer in duration (5.9 days vs 3.4 days) and occur more often (14.4 vs 9.6 episodes/year) than in children [65]. Many patients show gradual symptom improvement over time (7 years in one study), but a subset (mostly adults) progresses to a coalescent pattern of daily nausea and vomiting. In some children, CVS can evolve into other functional bowel disorders, chronic headaches, or extraintestinal somatic symptoms.

Common CVS triggers include stress, sleep deprivation, infection, motion sickness, and food (allergies to milk, soy, and eggs and intolerances to chocolate, cheese, or monosodium glutamate) [20]. CVS may be exacerbated by menses (catemenial CVS) or pregnancy. Patients with diabetic gastroparesis report a cyclic vomiting pattern in 13–56% of cases [66]. Chronic cannabis exposure can cause recurrent vomiting, but the pattern is typically different from CVS, and vomiting resolves with cessation of marijuana use. The etiology of CVS is unclear, though recent evidence suggests there may be metabolic or genetic predispositions to development of CVS.

Cyclic vomiting syndrome is the cause of symptoms in 3–14% of adults with unexplained vomiting [67]. The condition shows

Box 33.3 Rome IV defined gastroduodenal disorders causing nausea and vomiting.

Chronic nausea and vomiting syndrome (CNVS)

Must include all of the following.

1. Bothersome (i.e., severe enough to impact on usual activities) nausea, occurring at least 1 day per week and/or 1 or more vomiting episodes per week
2. Self-induced vomiting, eating disorders, regurgitation, or rumination are excluded
3. No evidence of organic, systemic, or metabolic disease that is likely to explain the symptoms on routine investigations (including upper endoscopy)

Criteria fulfilled for the last 3 months with symptom onset at least 6 months before diagnosis

Cyclic vomiting syndrome (CVS)

Must include all of the following.

Stereotypical episodes of vomiting regarding onset (*acute*) and duration (*less than one week*)

1. At least three discrete episodes in the prior year and two episodes in the past 6 months, occurring at least 1 week apart
2. Absence of vomiting between episodes, but other milder symptoms can be present between cycles

Criteria fulfilled for the last 3 months with symptom onset at least 6 months before diagnosis

Supportive remarks

History or family history of migraine headaches

Cannabinoid hyperemesis syndrome (CHS)

Must include all of the following.

1. Stereotypical episodic vomiting resembling cyclic vomiting syndrome (CVS) in terms of onset, duration, and frequency
2. Presentation after prolonged excessive cannabis use
3. Relief of vomiting episodes by sustained cessation of cannabis use

Criteria fulfilled for the last 3 months with symptom onset at least 6 months before diagnosis

Supportive remarks

May be associated with pathological bathing behavior (prolonged hot baths or showers)

Rumination syndrome

Must include all of the following.

1. Persistent or recurrent regurgitation of recently ingested food into the mouth with subsequent spitting or remastication and swallowing
2. Regurgitation is not preceded by retching

Criteria fulfilled for the last 3 months with symptom onset at least 6 months prior to diagnosis.

Supportive remarks

- Effortless regurgitation events are usually not preceded by nausea
- Regurgitant contains recognizable food that might have a pleasant taste
- The process tends to cease when the regurgitated material becomes acidic

Source: Stanghellini 2016 [20]. Reproduced by permission of Elsevier.

a slight male predominance in adults, but pediatric patients are more often female [68]. The mean age of CVS onset in adults is 30–35 years (range 14–73 years); in children, it typically begins around age 5 [65]. Delays in diagnosis average 5–6 years in adults and are longer in pediatric patients [68]. Adults present to emergency departments a median of 15 times, including seven visits prior to diagnosis [69].

Since CVS represents a syndrome, rather than a single unique disease state, it should not be surprising that a number of different pathophysiological processes have been invoked as potential causes.

Pathophysiological process involved in CVS

When gastric emptying is measured in between attacks, it is rapid in 50–80% of patients with CVS, although it may be normal. If gastric emptying is delayed, other etiologies should be considered (e.g., gastroparesis, opioid use). Gastric emptying should not be measured during the acute phase of the attack. CVS is also associated with autonomic disorders, including complex regional pain syndrome and postural orthostatic tachycardia syndrome [70]. Autonomic function testing reveals orthostatic changes, impaired parasympathetic responses to deep breathing, absent sympathetic skin responses, altered responses on sweat testing, and impaired sudomotor function [71]. Fourteen percent of children have associated neurocognitive disorders, a subtype termed CVS plus [68]. Migraine headaches classically are reported by children with CVS, but 24–70% of adults also have a personal or family history of migraines [64]. In a systematic review, anxiety and depression were associated with CVS in 30% of cases [65].

In contrast to other chronic disorders associated with nausea and vomiting (e.g., gastroparesis), mitochrondrial dysfunction has been identified in some CVS patients. These abnormalities may include medium-chain acyl coenzyme A dehydrogenase deficiency, late-onset glutaric acidemia type II, mitochondrial encephalopathy, lactic acidosis, and stroke-like syndrome (MELAS) [20]. Maternal inheritance is observed in half of children with CVS, relating to mitochondrial DNA variants. Pediatric disease is associated with two mitochondrial DNA polymorphisms, 16519T and 3010A [72]. Mutations in the neuronal β-tubulin isotype 3 (TUBB3) gene produce hypogonadism, anosmia, midface hypoplasia, cognitive impairment, vocal cord paralysis, tracheomalacia, and CVS [73]. Another mitochondrial DNA deletion (nucleotides 10970–14118) is associated with CVS with neuromuscular disease and growth retardation [74].

Cannabinoid hyperemesis syndrome

Cannabinoid hyperemesis syndrome is a condition characterized by recurrent nausea and vomiting in chronic marijuana users. CHS typically presents after daily use of large quantities of marijuana (3–5 times daily) over a long duration (2–19 years) [75]. Young males comprise the majority of patients. The syndrome is divided into distinct phases: prodrome, hyperemesis during which patients may vomit up to five times hourly, and recovery. As with CVS, most patients with cannabinoid hyperemesis report associated abdominal pain. Patients also exhibit a learned behavior of frequent hot baths or showers during attacks (mean 5 ± 2 daily baths/showers; 5.0 ± 5.1 hours/day) that relieve the vomiting and pain during the hyperemetic phase [76]. Delays in diagnosis of up to 9 years are characteristic and emergency department visits prior to establishing the diagnosis are numerous (7.1 ± 4.3).

The pathophysiology of cannabinoid hyperemesis syndrome is poorly understood. Some cannabinoids in marijuana show potent antiemetic actions while others may contribute to recurrent vomiting. Δ^9-tetrahydrocannabinol (THC) exhibits antiemetic effects via action on CNS CB_1 receptors; cannabidiol shows a biphasic effect characterized by antivomiting actions at low doses and stimulation of emesis at high doses in animal models whereas cannabigerol acts as a CB_1 and 5-HT_{1A} antagonist to block antiemetic effects of cannabidiol [77]. CHS can be confused with CVS. Distinguishing characteristics of CHS are more persistent symptoms between acute episodes, reports of excessive bathing or showering, and marijuana use. Marijuana cessation leads to resolution of CHS, although effects may not be immediate in long-term users.

Chronic nausea and vomiting syndrome

Chronic nausea and vomiting syndrome is a relatively new diagnostic term, established by the latest Rome Foundation diagnostic criteria for functional gastrointestinal disorders (Rome IV) (see Box 33.3) [20]. CNVS replaces two prior diagnoses of chronic idiopathic nausea and functional vomiting, as these two symptoms are often associated and approached in the same manner. Though the prevalence of CNVS is not known, population data indicate that nausea occurring weekly is noted by 3% of individuals and vomiting monthly is reported by 2% of women and 3% of men [78]. There are no differences in age, body mass index, and smoking or alcohol use in those with functional vomiting compared to CVS [79]. The manifestations of CNVS are inferred from prior studies of functional vomiting.

The mechanisms underlying CNVS and cyclic vomiting are not well understood. Roles for gastric emptying delays have been proposed but are unproven. Reduced gastric accommodation and heightened perception during intragastric nutrient perfusion were observed in 19 patients with functional vomiting compared to 10 healthy controls [80]. However, these sensorimotor alterations have not been proved causative of symptoms in affected patients. Depression and conversion disorders have been related to unexplained vomiting, but similar psychiatric profiles have been noted in individuals with chronic vomiting and control patients with reflux disease or gastroparesis [20].

Because of the overlap of clinical manifestations of idiopathic gastroparesis and other functional gastroduodenal disorders, such as functional dyspepsia, it may be difficult to distinguish the different conditions associated with chronic nausea and vomiting symptoms. Furthermore, the relevance of making such diagnostic distinctions in directing subsequent clinical decision making requires additional confirmation. Percentages of patients satisfying the different Rome III gastroduodenal disorder definitions are similar among those with mild, moderate, and severe gastric emptying delays, confirming that diagnoses of these disorders do not relate to the degree of gastric retention. Furthermore, one modeling study concluded that only 10% of the variance in meal-induced functional dyspepsia relates to gastric emptying [81]. There is little evidence that testing to distinguish abnormal from normal gastric emptying facilitates managing unexplained dyspepsia. Thus, separating idiopathic gastroparesis from functional gastroduodenal disorders as independent entities may be an artificial distinction. This topic remains controversial, with some investigators reporting no benefits to gastric emptying testing in management of dyspepsia, and others observing important roles for such testing [82,83].

Rumination syndrome

Rumination syndrome is characterized by the repeated, effortless regurgitation of recently ingested food followed by its rechewing and reswallowing (see Box 33.3) [20]. The disorder is frequently misdiagnosed as GERD or gastroparesis. Regurgitation of gastric contents typically starts within minutes of starting a meal, often is preceded by a sensation of belching, and may occur within 1–2 hours after meal ingestion. The regurgitant contains recognizable food which may have a pleasant taste. Many individuals report nausea, heartburn, abdominal discomfort or pain, bloating, diarrhea, and/or constipation. Many patients show evidence of excess acid reflux on esophageal pH testing and may also have esophagitis on endoscopy [84]. Weight loss can be significant, especially in adolescents. The disorder was initially identified in infants and developmentally impaired individuals, but it is known to occur in adults of normal intellect. The prevalence of rumination syndrome in adults is not well defined, but 33% of patients with unexplained nausea and vomiting satisfied criteria for rumination syndrome with similar rates in both sexes in one report [52]. Others note a female predominance [85–87]. Rumination syndrome appears to be more prevalent in children, observed in 5.1% of one cohort, and causes increased school absenteeism [88].

Rumination occurs when gastric pressure increases due to volitional abdominal somatic muscle contractions that promote orad movement of gastric contents into the esophagus [89]. Lower esophageal sphincter (LES) relaxation is elicited at lower intragastric pressures in ruminators, some of whom also exhibit hypersensitivity to gastric distension [90]. Others hypothesize a role for voluntary diaphragmatic crural relaxation to facilitate retrograde flow during increased intraabdominal pressure [91]. Nontransmitted esophageal body contractions and low-amplitude contractions are found in 48% and 38% of cases, respectively [84]. Delayed gastric emptying is noted in 14% of patients. The pathogenic relevance of these factors is uncertain. Associations of rumination with psychological dysfunction, stressful life events, and eating disorders have been reported. Seventeen percent of female ruminators have a history of bulimia [85]. Patients may be diagnosed with upright reflux and differentiation from rumination syndrome may be challenging although subtle differences may be observed on esophageal impedance-pH monitoring [92]

Nausea and vomiting of pregnancy

Nausea and vomiting complicate 50–70% of pregnancies. Although nausea and vomiting of pregnancy (NVP) is referred to as "morning sickness," only 2% report symptoms restricted to the morning while 80% are symptomatic throughout the day [93]. NVP typically begins 39 days after the last menses, peaks in the 9th–11th gestational week, and persists for 35–45 days; symptoms continuing into late pregnancy are reported in 45% of cases [94]. NVP is more common in primigravida, younger, non-Asian, overweight, less educated, and more economically disadvantaged women and in those with pre-pregnancy nausea and vomiting. Dietary constituents associated with NVP include sugars, alcohol, and meats, whereas vegetables, fish, and vitamin supplements decrease the risk [95]. In most patients with NVP, there are no deleterious effects on the fetus or mother. Rather, it is associated with longer gestation and reduced incidences of miscarriage, preterm births, congenital heart defects, cleft lip and palate, and fetal demise. However, NVP leads to reduced protein and increased carbohydrate consumption as well as reduced intake of magnesium and zinc, raising the possibility of nutritional deficits during pregnancy [96].

Hyperemesis gravidarum, presenting with intractable vomiting, complicates 0.7–5% of pregnancies and causes dangerous fluid and electrolyte abnormalities. Although usually occurring in early pregnancy, up to one quarter of cases persist until delivery. Many with prior hyperemesis report severe vomiting in subsequent pregnancies; there is increased risk of hyperemesis in relatives of affected women [97]. Other risk factors include young age, first pregnancies, low socioeconomic status, assisted reproduction, hyperthyroidism, psychiatric disease, gastrointestinal disorders, asthma, and preexisting diabetes. Hyperemesis gravidarum is associated with an increased likelihood of premature delivery and having a low-birthweight baby (<2500 g) [98]. Other consequences of prolonged hyperemesis include maternal hematemesis, syncope, postpartum stress, motion sickness, muscle weakness, and infant irritability, colic, and growth restriction. Wernicke's encephalopathy (resulting from acute thiamine deficiency), osmotic demyelination syndrome, thromboembolism, gallbladder and liver dysfunction, renal insufficiency, and retinal hemorrhage are potentially severe complications. The condition leads to increased antiemetic use and frequent hospitalization; with recurrent hyperemesis, >75% require intravenous hydration and nearly one quarter need enteral or parenteral nutrition.

The cause of NVP is unknown. Symptoms parallel β-human chorionic gonadotropin (hCG) levels; one report showed correlation of elevated hCG levels and hyponatremia with length of hospitalization in hyperemesis gravidarum [99]. Others have shown associations of nausea severity in pregnancy with intolerance of oral contraceptives, correlation with levels of androstenedione, dehydroepiandrosterone sulfate, testosterone, leptin, prostaglandin E_2, vaspin (a novel serpin with insulin-sensitizing effects), and C-reactive protein, and inverse correlation with prolactin concentrations [100–105]. Reduced vitamin B_6 levels have been observed, providing a rationale for vitamin B_6 supplementation for NVP [106]. *Helicobacter pylori* exposure determined by serological testing has been associated with an increased risk of hyperemesis gravidarum. However, two studies employing fecal antigen testing observed no increase in the prevalence of active *H. pylori* infection and hyperemesis gravidarum [107]. Two single nucleotide polymorphisms of serotonin receptor [*HTR3C*] genes (rs6806362, rs6807670) are associated with NVP, providing a genetic correlate to the observed hereditary tendencies [108].

Postoperative nausea and vomiting

Postoperative nausea and vomiting (PONV) complicates 17–37% of operations, and is more common with general anesthesia compared to regional nerve blocks. PONV occurs more often after abdominal and orthopedic surgery than laparoscopic or other extraabdominal operations and is exacerbated by opiates. Other risk factors include female sex, increased age, obesity, nonsmoking status, prior PONV or motion sickness, prior *H. pylori* infection, history of migraines, preoperative anxiety, use of volatile anesthetics or nitrous oxide, and high-dose neostigmine [109]. A risk score comprising five factors (female sex, age <50 years, prior PONV, opioid administration after prior anesthesia, nausea in the postanesthesia care unit) is predictive of nausea and vomiting post discharge from the anesthesia care unit, with incidence increasing from 7% with one factor to 88% with all five factors [110]. Gene variants associated with PONV include one (rs2165870) upstream of the promoter for the muscarinic 3 receptor gene, two encoding 5-HT_3 receptors (HTR3A and HTR3B), and another with the Taq 1A polymorphism of the dopamine D_2 receptor gene [111,112].

Causes involving the central and peripheral nervous systems

Many emetic stimuli produce symptoms by action on the CNS. CNS causes (malignancy, infarction, hemorrhage, infection, congenital) produce maximal emesis at an intracranial pressure of 80 mmHg with or without nausea [113]. Diseases associated with vagal neuropathy such as diabetes may also result in emesis due to gastroparesis. Psychiatric conditions (anxiety, depression), eating disorders (anorexia nervosa, bulimia nervosa), and emotional responses to unpleasant smells or memories may be accompanied by nausea and vomiting.

Motion sickness evoked by repetitive movements activates the vestibular nuclei and is associated with autonomic activation that produces pallor, diaphoresis, and salivation. Motion sickness susceptibility in women increases during the menses [114]. Labyrinthine disorders (labyrinthitis, tumors, Ménière disease) produce nausea and vomiting with vertigo.

Syndromes of autonomic instability such as postural orthostatic tachycardia syndrome (POTS) often have associated nausea [115]. Other dysautonomias associated with nausea and vomiting include those after acute Epstein–Barr virus infection and Friedreich ataxia.

Miscellaneous conditions

Endocrinological and metabolic causes of nausea include uremia, diabetic ketoacidosis, hyper- and hypoparathyroidism, hyper- and hypothyroidism, and Addison disease. Acute fatty liver of pregnancy produces third-trimester vomiting and is complicated by liver failure, disseminated intravascular coagulation, and fetal or maternal death. Myocardial infarction produces nausea due to diaphragmatic irritation; inferior myocardial infarcts are more often associated with gastrointestinal complaints than anterior occlusions and are more common in women [116]. Nausea with congestive heart failure results from passive liver and gut congestion. Excess ethanol intake induces vomiting by action on the gut and brainstem. Acute graft-versus-host disease is a dominant cause of nausea and vomiting after bone marrow transplant. Excess vitamin intake as well as extended fasting or starvation also may cause nausea. Acute intermittent porphyria can manifest as intermittent vomiting and abdominal pain in association with neurological symptoms. Disorders of fatty acid oxidation produce cyclical emesis. Self-induced vomiting is reported by 36% of patients with eating disorders, especially in those with high body mass index or depression [117]. Jamaican vomiting sickness occurs after eating unripe ackee fruit containing the toxin hypoglycin A.

Diagnosis and differential diagnosis

Diagnosing the cause of nausea and vomiting requires conducting a careful history and physical complemented by directed laboratory, structural, and functional testing (Figure 33.2).

Historical features

A detailed history provides useful information that may help identify the cause of unexplained nausea and emesis. Before initiation and evaluation, it is helpful to first determine whether the symptoms are acute or chronic in nature, as the timing of symptoms may implicate certain diagnoses. As mentioned, acute vomiting (≤7 days) most often results from infection, a medication or toxin, endogenous toxins (uremia, diabetic ketoacidosis), or somatic injury. In contrast, chronic vomiting (>7 days) usually results from long-standing medical or psychiatric conditions.

Symptom profiles

The timing of symptoms provides clues to the underlying disease. Patients who vomit within minutes of ingesting a meal

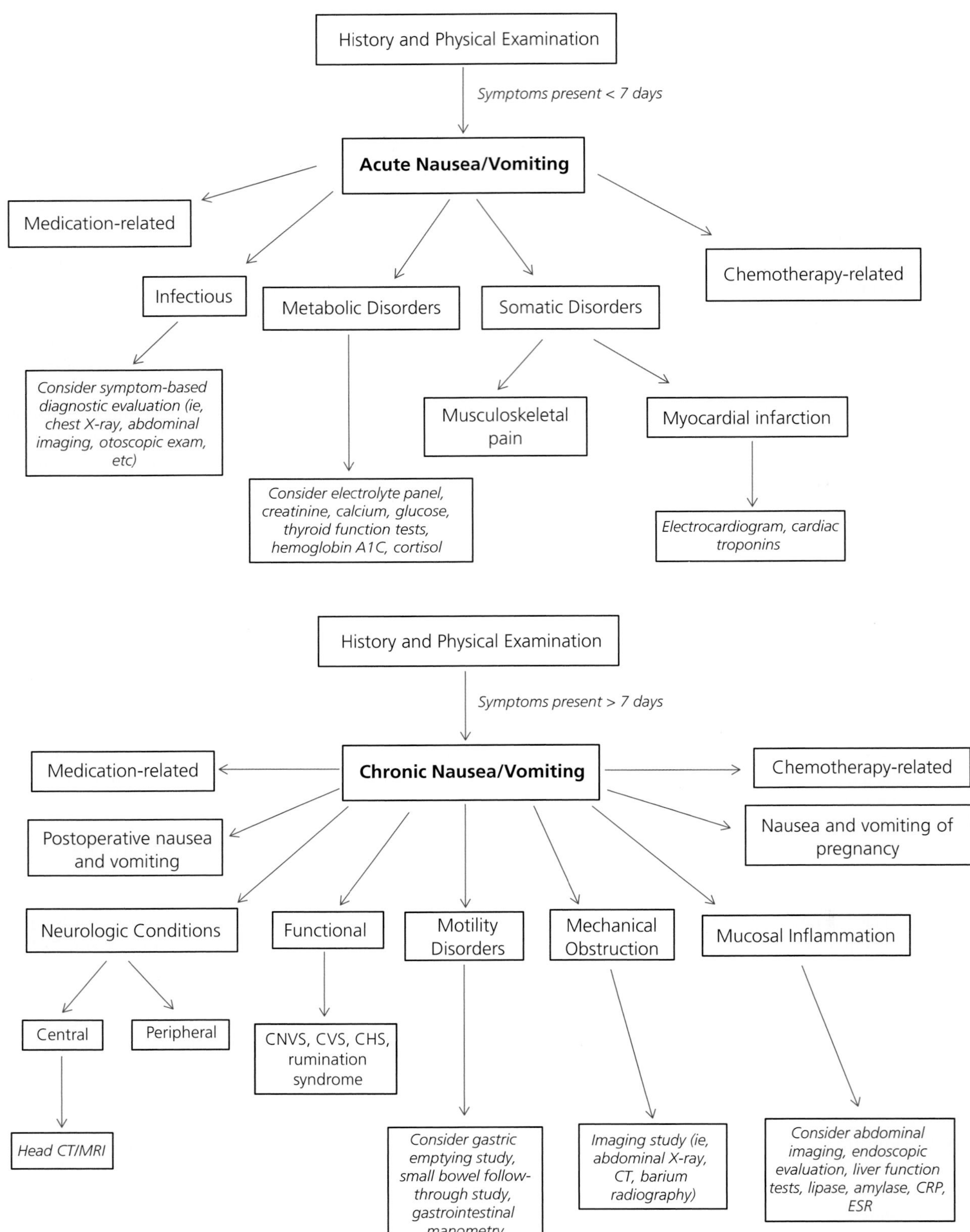

Figure 33.2 General approach to the evaluation of acute and chronic nausea and vomiting. Diagnostic testing is strongly dependent on the clinical suspicion derived from a careful history and physical examination.

generally have an esophageal disorder (e.g., achalasia, obstruction) or rumination syndrome. The latter group of patients can be quickly diagnosed by determining that they reswallow the regurgitated food, rather than spitting it out. Although patients with gastric obstruction or gastroparesis may report nausea within 5 minutes of eating, most vomiting occurs >1 hour after a meal. Nausea and vomiting from cholecystitis and pancreatitis may present in the first hour after eating. These are typically associated with abdominal pain in either the right upper quadrant or epigastric area. Conversely, nausea may abate with eating in some cases of esophagitis or ulcer disease. Morning emesis may be reported with pregnancy, uremia, or chronic alcoholism. Vomiting that occurs 3–5 hours after meal ingestion often reflects a small intestinal cause. Feculent vomiting generally indicates a distal small bowel process.

The characteristics of vomiting may assist in diagnosis. Undigested food return suggests achalasia, rumination, or a Zenker diverticulum; vomiting of partly digested or old food residue suggests gastric obstruction or gastroparesis. Emesis of bilious material only occurs in conditions in which there is no gastroduodenal obstruction proximal to the ampulla of Vater. Hematemesis usually reflects tissue injury. Gastrinoma patients may vomit voluminous clear acidic liquid; those with achlorhydria may expel odorless vomitus. Feculent emesis occurs with distal intestine or colon obstruction, bacterial overgrowth, and gastrocolic fistulas.

Related symptoms may clarify diagnostic considerations. In additional to functional and motor conditions, abdominal pain is noted with ulcer disease, obstruction, and inflammatory disorders (cholecystitis, pancreatitis). Vomiting may relieve nausea from ulcers or bowel obstruction, but has no effect in inflammatory conditions. Enteric infection may be associated with diarrhea, fever, or myalgias. Patients with cyclical vomiting should be queried about habitual marijuana use. CNS processes can produce effortless or projectile emesis without nausea and are suggested by headaches, visual changes, altered mentation, and neck stiffness. Labyrinthine diseases present with tinnitus or vertigo. Chest pain, dysphagia, or jaundice suggest cardiac, esophageal, or hepatobiliary disease, respectively.

Complications of nausea and vomiting

Chronic vomiting may lead to electrolyte disorders, malnutrition, weight loss, and loss of dental enamel. Violent retching or emesis may result in severe esophagitis or more rarely, cause a Mallory–Weiss tear or Boerhaave syndrome, with subsequent mediastinitis or peritonitis. In patients with impaired consciousness, emesis may be complicated by pulmonary aspiration of acidic material leading to chemical pneumonitis. Bezoars complicate cases of severe gastric retention, increasing gastroparesis symptoms or producing a palpable epigastric mass, gastric ulcers or perforation, or small bowel obstruction.

Validated symptom surveys

Quantification of symptom severity and characterization of disease subtypes in disorders with prominent nausea and vomiting, including gastroparesis, have been facilitated by validated symptom questionnaires. The Gastroparesis Cardinal Symptom Index-Daily Diary (GCSI-DD), comprising 11 questions in four domains (nausea/vomiting, fullness/early satiety, bloating/ distension, and pain/discomfort), shows good test-retest reliability, responsiveness to treatments, and relation to clinician-rated disease severity (Table 33.1) [118].

Table 33.1 The Gastroparesis Cardinal Symptom Index-Daily Diary to characterize and quantify symptoms.

Symptom	None	Very mild	Mild	Moderate	Severe	Very severe
Nausea (feeling sick to your stomach as if you were going to vomit or throw up)	0	1	2	3	4	5
Retching (heaving as if to vomit, but nothing comes up)	0	1	2	3	4	5
Vomiting	0	1	2	3	4	5
Stomach fullness	0	1	2	3	4	5
Not able to finish a normal-sized meal	0	1	2	3	4	5
Feeling excessively full after meals	0	1	2	3	4	5
Loss of appetite	0	1	2	3	4	5
Bloating (feeling like you need to loosen your clothes)	0	1	2	3	4	5
Stomach or belly visibly larger	0	1	2	3	4	5
Upper abdominal pain (above the navel)	0	1	2	3	4	5
Upper abdominal discomfort (above the navel)	0	1	2	3	4	5

Source: Data from Revicki et al. [118].

Physical examination findings

Physical examination provides diagnostic clues and facilitates management of nausea and vomiting. Fever suggests infection or inflammation. Tachycardia, orthostatic hypotension, poor skin turgor, absent sweating or dry mucous membranes indicate dehydration. The skin may show sclerodactyly in scleroderma or jaundice with hepatobiliary disease. Adenopathy (e.g., supraclavicular) or hepatomegaly raises concern for neoplasm. Absent bowel sounds signify an ileus. High-pitched hyperactive bowel sounds with a distended abdomen are consistent with a bowel obstruction. A succussion splash on side-to-side movement is found in gastric obstruction or gastroparesis. Ulcers, cholecystitis, pancreatitis, or peritonitis may produce abdominal tenderness or guarding. Gross or occult fecal blood prompts evaluation for a mucosal injury process. Focal neurological signs, papilledema, neck rigidity, or impaired mentation suggest a CNS process. Asterixis is present in metabolic disease (uremia, hepatic failure). Peripheral or autonomic neuropathy is found with many gut motor disorders.

Laboratory testing

Laboratory test findings complement the history and physical exam. Testing should be performed in patients with chronic symptoms for several reasons. First, measuring electrolytes may uncover hypokalemia, contraction alkalosis secondary to intravascular volume loss, or an elevated blood urea nitrogen level due to dehydration or persistent emesis. Second, a complete blood count may reveal anemia from inflammation or blood loss (which can be confirmed by low serum iron parameters), leukocytosis from an inflammatory source, or leukopenia from a viral infection. Hypoalbuminemia can occur with chronic diseases or with a protein-losing enteropathy; a low prealbumin suggests malnutrition. Pancreatic enzymes or liver chemistries can be used to identify pancreaticobiliary or hepatic disease. Endocrine and metabolic causes can be assessed by pregnancy testing, thyroid chemistries, serum calcium, and cortisol (fasting and post-ACTH) levels. Additional serological testing can be performed if there is clinical concern for a connective tissue disorder (lupus, scleroderma). Infiltrative disorders (amyloid, sarcoidosis) can be screened by checking serum protein electrophoresis, serum light chain testing, urine paraprotein levels, and angiotensin converting enzyme measurement. Paraneoplastic autoantibody panels (including type I antineuronal nuclear [also called anti-Hu] antibody, anti-Purkinje cell cytoplasmic antibody, ganglionic nicotinic acetylcholine receptor antibody) are positive with cancer-associated dysmotility and autoimmune ganglionitis [119].

Testing to exclude rare causes of cyclical emesis is indicated in some patients depending on other clinical factors. Urine δ-aminolevulinic acid and porphobilinogen can screen for acute intermittent porphyria. Urea cycle enzyme defects are considered for plasma ammonia levels >150 μM [120]. Fatty acid oxidation disorders are confirmed by plasma amino acid and urine organic acid quantification in cases with onset before age 2 years, neurological findings, or selected laboratory abnormalities (hypoglycemia, pronounced anion gap metabolic acidosis, hyperammonemia) [20].

Endoscopic and imaging evaluation

Radiographic and endoscopic studies may be required if initial testing is nondiagnostic. Plain abdominal radiography can screen for bowel obstruction (small intestinal air–fluid levels with absent colonic air), ileus or pseudoobstruction (diffuse luminal distension), or visceral perforation (pneumoperitoneum). Upper endoscopy or contrast upper gastrointestinal radiography may be performed for suspected ulcer disease or outlet narrowing. Endoscopy provides the capability to biopsy abnormal mucosa. Finding retained food on endoscopy without obstruction may be suggestive of gastroparesis. Suspected small intestinal obstruction may be further evaluated by computed tomography (CT), magnetic resonance imaging (MRI), or small intestinal contrast radiography.

Radiographic studies may employ either water-soluble contrast (which can screen for obstructions requiring surgery) or barium (which provides superior visualization of partial obstruction and can estimate small bowel transit time). If partial colonic obstruction is a consideration, contrast enema radiography should be performed before proceeding with small bowel imaging. CT and MRI enterography can characterize small intestinal inflammation with known or suspected Crohn's disease. Finding gastric or duodenal dilation on CT scanning with a diminished distance between the superior mesenteric artery and the aorta is consistent with SMA syndrome. Suspected pancreaticobiliary disease may be evaluated by a variety of modalities (CT, MRI, ultrasound, or scintigraphy) Generally, one should begin with an abdominal ultrasound as it is safe, inexpensive, and noninvasive without any radiation exposure. If visceral ischemia or median arcuate ligament syndrome are considerations, duplex ultrasonography, mesenteric angiography, CT or MRI angiography are useful. A CT or MRI of the brain is indicated for possible CNS disease.

Studies of gastrointestinal motor function

When obstruction has been excluded, motility and functional causes of nausea and vomiting should be considered. Clinicians can empirically treat with agents that stimulate gut motility or, alternatively, perform testing to better characterize gastrointestinal motility defects.

Quantification of gastric emptying

Gastric scintigraphy is the most widely performed test to diagnose gastroparesis. Most emptying scintiscans involve consumption of a ^{99m}Tc-sulfur colloid label bound to a solid food meal. A method using a consistent radiolabeled egg substitute meal has been promoted by major societies as a means of standardizing gastric emptying testing (Figure 33.3) [121,122]. With this technique, gastric retention >60% at 2 hours and/or >10% at 4 hours is consistent with gastroparesis. However, even

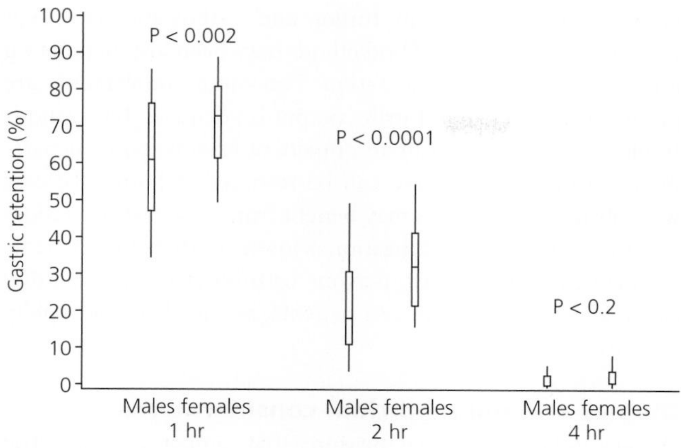

Figure 33.3 Rates of gastric emptying of a radiolabeled low-fat meal are shown for men and women using a standardized scintigraphic method. Using this technique, normal values for gastric retention are <60% at 2 hours after meal ingestion and <10% after 4 hours. Source: Tougas et al. 2000 [121]. Reproduced by permission of Wolters Kluwer Health, Inc.

standardized protocols do not eliminate the possibility of discordant results. In one investigation, 37% of patients with normal emptying at 2 hours exhibited delays at 4 hours, while 19% with delayed emptying at 2 hours showed normalization at 4 hours [123]. Moreover, another study demonstrated that gastric scintigraphy yielded a different interpretation (normal, delayed, or rapid) in 30% of patients when performed on two occasions, with an average interval of 15 days [124]. Quantifying emptying of a radiolabeled liquid may complement information provided by scintigraphy of emptying of the solid component of the meal. In a recent study, 26% with normal solid gastric retention showed prolonged liquid emptying [125].

The use of scintigraphy for diagnosing gastroparesis has not been rigorously subjected to outcomes analysis. One group reported that emptying scanning did not influence management decisions, but others have demonstrated that delayed gastric emptying can predict outcomes to treatments designed to have stimulatory effects on the stomach [126–128].

Controversy persists regarding the relationship between the extent of delay in gastric emptying and symptom generation. In analyses of a large standardized population of patients with symptoms of gastroparesis, severity of overall and individual symptoms, healthcare utilization, quality of life, and depression scores were similar with normal versus prolonged emptying at 2 and 4 hours [129]. However, in patients with idiopathic gastroparesis from the same database, those with severe emptying delays (>35% retention at 4 hours) had greater vomiting, anorexia, and overall symptoms [52]. Selected single-center studies do suggest correlations between symptoms and emptying profiles when symptom scores are quantified during performance of gastric emptying by scintigraphy (fullness, bloating, and pain are higher with delays) or when regional distributions of the meal are analyzed (symptoms relate to delayed proximal gastric emptying) [130,131]. Further, a recent study identified a significant association between gastric emptying and upper GI symptoms, when optimal gastric emptying test methods were utilized [57]. Finally, emptying delays may influence gastroparesis outcomes. Hospitalizations, clinic visits, and emergency department visits are greater for diabetics with upper gut symptoms and delayed emptying compared to similarly symptomatic individuals with normal emptying [132].

Gastric scintigraphy also detects rapid gastric emptying. This phenomenon is most often found in adults with CVS, but has also been described in some patients with functional dyspepsia, with diabetes, and with dietary "fat intolerance" [70,81,83]. Diabetics with unexplained symptoms exhibited delays in 36%, normal emptying in 42%, and rapid emptying in 22%, in one study [133]. Symptoms of patients with rapid and delayed gastric emptying are similar; distinguishing these two groups is important as therapies directed at accelerating gastric emptying in patients with gastroparesis will worsen symptoms in those with rapid emptying.

Other techniques to measure gastric emptying are available. A wireless motility capsule (WMC) continuously transmits data on luminal pH and pressure to a receiver worn by the patient. Gastric emptying, in addition to whole gut transit time (including the small intestine and colon), can be measured using the change in pH from the acidic stomach to the neutral or basic small intestine. Correlation coefficients between the WMC technique and gastric scintiscans for detecting delayed gastric emptying exceed 0.7 [134]. It should be recognized, however, that, as it is a large indigestible capsule, emptying of the WMC will occur independently of, and after completion of, emptying of the digestible solid meal consumed as part of the WMC test procedure. Some patients with gastroparesis show delayed colon transit on WMC testing, reflecting the common generalized transit defects in those with delayed gastric emptying [135].

Breath tests to measure $^{13}CO_2$ liberation in exhaled breath samples after consuming a nonradioactive ^{13}C-labeled nutrient substrate can assess gastric emptying of both solids (octanoate, *Spirulina platensis*) and liquids (acetate). These methods show good correlations with scintigraphy, but are reliable only with normal digestive, absorptive, and pulmonary function [136].

Ultrasound and MRI are not currently considered valid or reliable measures of gastric emptying due to variability related to meal composition and body position during testing.

Other tests of gastrointestinal function

The occasional patient with persistent nausea and vomiting may need further specialized testing to identify the cause. Testing may necessitate referral to an academic medical center or specialized motility center.

Combined esophageal impedance and high-resolution manometry can facilitate the diagnosis of rumination syndrome, characterizing nearly 90% of rumination events as elevations in intragastric pressure occurring before or concurrently with orad esophageal fluid propulsion [137].

Gastrointestinal manometry involves placing a catheter to monitor antroduodenojejunal pressures during fasting (4–6 hours, during which one or more fasting motor complexes are usually observed), and after eating a solid meal (2 hours, which should induce a fed pattern). In some institutions, manometry can assess the effects of motor stimulating drugs or record ambulatory motor activity for up to 24 hours. Manometry is considered for individuals who: (1) have unexplained symptoms; (2) have not responded to treatment; or (3) are being considered for surgery or enteral versus parenteral nutrition. Gastroparesis is characterized by loss of fasting migrating motor complexes, reduced antral contractions and, in some cases, pyloric spasm in the fed period. Manometry is useful to exclude small intestinal dysmotility including myopathic (duodenal contractile amplitude <20 mmHg with normal morphology), and neuropathic (intense, uncoordinated burst contractions with normal amplitude) patterns [138]. Small intestinal motor dysfunction is detected in 17–85% of patients with gastroparesis [139]. Manometric rumination (R) waves, characterized as simultaneous contractions in all recording sites in the early fed period after meal ingestion, are seen in 40% of patients with rumination [140].

Electrogastrography (EGG) employs electrodes placed on the skin overlying the stomach to measure activity of the gastric pacemaker. Under healthy conditions, EGG recordings exhibit uniform three cycles per minute waveforms that increase in amplitude after ingesting water or a meal. EGG abnormalities include tachygastria (frequency >4 cycles per minute), bradygastria (<2 cycles per minute), and lack of a signal amplitude increase with eating [141]. The utility of EGG is limited by lack of proven gastric antiarrhythmic therapies.

Satiety testing involves ingesting water or liquid nutrients until maximal fullness is reported. Volumes consumed in patients with functional dyspepsia and early satiety are reduced compared to healthy volunteers, reflecting either impaired proximal stomach relaxation or heightened sensitivity of gastric afferent pathways [142].

Single photon emission computed tomography (SPECT) employs intravenous ^{99m}Tc-pertechnetate that accumulates in the gastric wall rather than the lumen and provides a three-dimensional outline of the stomach. SPECT can measure gastric accommodation after eating [143]. Similar capabilities have been described for other methodologies (e.g., MRI).

Principles of management

Managing nausea and vomiting involves assessing disease etiology and severity, with prompt initiation of therapy to prevent complications.

Indications for hospitalization

Hospitalization should be considered for those with dehydration or electrolyte disturbances who cannot maintain oral replenishment. Poor skin turgor and orthostatic vital sign changes indicate >10% of body fluids have been lost, mandating intravenous fluid administration. Potassium supplements are given for hypokalemia if urine output is adequate. Intravenous fluids may be provided in an outpatient or emergency department setting if oral intake can be resumed at home. Patients with obstruction or ileus may benefit from nasogastric suction. The threshold for hospitalization is lower for diabetics, patients with concurrent diarrhea, persons with other debilitating diseases, and very young or old patients, as they become rapidly dehydrated.

Dietary and nonmedicinal considerations

Dietary and nonmedicinal measures that compensate for gastric motor impairment are recommended for most patients with nausea and vomiting. Nutritional deficiencies are prominent in some conditions. In a gastroparesis cohort, daily caloric intake averaged <60% of recommended levels and 64% of patients consumed calorie-deficient diets with associated deficiencies in vitamins A, B_6, C, and K, as well as iron, potassium, and zinc [46]. Ingesting 4–6 small daily meals enhances the efficiency of postprandial intragastric mixing. As liquids empty from the stomach rapidly, reducing solid food intake is desired. Some patients note that avoiding carbonated liquids improves symptoms as they cause gastric distension. Fats slow gastric emptying and should be avoided in patients with gastroparesis. Reducing indigestible fiber intake is advocated in those with gastroparesis as these products may promote bezoar formation [144]. A randomized controlled trial demonstrated improved symptoms in patients with gastroparesis who received a small particle diet compared to normal diet [145]. Medications which inhibit gut transit (e.g., opioids and GLP-1 agonists) should be discontinued if possible. In diabetic gastroparesis, maintaining euglycemia may avoid the inhibitory effects of hyperglycemia on gastric motor function. In a study of 28 diabetics with gastroparesis, provision of insulin pump therapy reduced hemoglobin A1c values by 1.8% with associated reductions in hospital stays [146].

Medications for nausea and vomiting

Medications used to treat nausea and vomiting include those that act in the CNS or periphery to suppress emesis, prokinetic agents that stimulate gut motor activity, and drugs that modulate gut sensory activity (Table 33.2).

Antiemetic medications

Antihistamines (meclizine, dimenhydrinate) are useful in conditions with labyrinthine activation (motion sickness, labyrinthitis), uremia, and PONV. Sedation and dryness of the mouth may limit their use. Less sedating antihistamines (astemizole, cetirizine, fexofenadine) have limited antiemetic activity [147].

Oral or transdermal muscarinic receptor antagonists (scopolamine) that act on vestibular pathways can be effective in treating motion sickness. However, these agents can retard

Table 33.2 Medications for treatment of nausea and vomiting.

Drug class	Examples (and typical initial doses in adults)	Clinical uses	Side-effects
Antiemetics			
Histamine antagonists	Dimenhydrinate (50 mg orally every 4–6 hours) Meclizine (25 mg orally every day) Promethazine (25 mg every 4–6 hours)	Motion sickness Labyrinthine disorders PONV Uremia	Sedation Dry mouth
Muscarinic antagonists	Scopolamine (1.5 mg transdermally every 72 hours)	Motion sickness Labyrinthine disorders PONV	Sedation Dry mouth and eyes Blurred vision Impaired concentration Urinary retention
Dopamine antagonists	Prochlorperazine (5 mg orally three times daily) Trimethobenzamide (300 mg orally three times daily)	Gastroenteritis Toxins PONV CINV Radiotherapy-induced	Sleep disturbances Constipation Blurred vision Anxiety Mood disturbances Dystonias Tardive dyskinesia Galactorrhea Sexual dysfunction
Serotonin antagonists	Ondansetron (4 mg orally three times daily) Granisetron (1 mg orally twice daily;or weekly transdermal patch) Dolasetron (50 mg orally once) Palonosetron (0.25 mg IV once)	CINV Radiotherapy-induced PONV Emesis in AIDS	Constipation Headache Fatigue Cardiac arrhythmias
Neurokinin antagonists	Aprepitant (40–80 mg prior to chemotherapy or surgery)	CINV PONV	Anorexia Diarrhea Constipation Fatigue
Cannabinoids	Dronabinol (2.5 mg orally twice daily)	CINV	Somnolence Weight gain Ataxia Hallucinations
Corticosteroids	Dexamethasone (4–5 mg IV prior to chemotherapy or surgery)	CINV PONV	Anxiety Depression Hyperglycemia Hypertension
Benzodiazepines	Lorazepam (1 mg IV prior to chemotherapy)	Anticipatory emesis	Sedation
Herbal remedies	Ginger (1 g orally daily) STW5 (20 drops in water orally three times daily before meals)	General indications	Heartburn
Prokinetics			
Dopamine antagonist/ serotonin agonist	Metoclopramide (5 mg orally three times daily before meals)	Gastroparesis	Sleep disturbances Anxiety Mood disturbances Dystonias Tardive dyskinesia Galactorrhea Sexual dysfunction
Peripheral dopamine antagonist	Domperidone (10 mg orally three times daily before meals)	Gastroparesis	Galactorrhea Sexual dysfunction Cardiac arrhythmias
Motilin agonist	Erythromycin (125 mg oral suspension three times daily before meals) Azithromycin (125 mg oral suspension three times daily before meals)	Gastroparesis CIP	Abdominal pain Nausea and vomiting Diarrhea Cardiac arrhythmias

Table 33.2 (Continued)

Drug class	Examples (and typical initial doses in adults)	Clinical uses	Side-effects
Acetylcholinesterase inhibitor	Pyridostigmine (60 mg orally three times daily)	Gastroparesis CIP	Abdominal pain Salivation Nausea Diaphoresis Cardiac arrhythmias
Somatostatin analog	Octreotide (50 μg subcutaneously at bedtime)	CIP with bacterial overgrowth	Diarrhea Altered glycemic control Gallstones Thyroid disease
Neuromodulators			
Tricyclic antidepressants	Amitriptyline (10 mg orally at bedtime) Nortriptyline (10 mg orally at bedtime) Desipramine (10 mg orally at bedtime)	CVS Functional causes	Sedation Constipation Lightheadedness Palpitations Cardiac arrhythmias
Tetracyclic antidepressant	Mirtazapine (15 mg orally at bedtime)	Functional causes	Sedation Constipation Weight gain
Atypical thienobenzodiazepine antipsychotic	Olanzapine (5 mg orally at bedtime)	Functional causes	Sedation Weight gain Tremor Peripheral edema Dizziness
GABA analog	Gabapentin (100–2700 mg orally daily in divided doses, typically 3 times daily)	CINV Functional causes	Sedation Dizziness Headache Weight gain

AIDS, acquired immune deficiency syndrome; CINV, chemotherapy-induced nausea and vomiting; CIP, chronic intestinal pseudoobstruction; CVS, cyclic vomiting syndrome; PONV, postoperative nausea and vomiting.

gastric emptying so their use in gastroparesis may be counterproductive. Side-effects include dryness of the mouth and eyes, sedation, impaired concentration, headaches, constipation, and urinary retention.

Dopamine D_2 receptor antagonists without stimulatory effects on gastric emptying in the phenothiazine (prochlorperazine, chlorpromazine) and butyrophenone (droperidol, haloperidol) classes are commonly prescribed to reduce emesis from gastroenteritis, medications, abdominal irradiation, surgery, toxins, and some chemotherapies. CNS side-effects include drowsiness, insomnia, anxiety, mood changes, confusion, dystonias, Parkinsonian symptoms, and irreversible tardive dyskinesia. These drugs also induce hyperprolactinemia by actions in the pituitary leading to breast engorgement, galactorrhea, and sexual dysfunction. Many antidopaminergic agents bind to other receptors and elicit antihistaminic and antimuscarinic side-effects as well.

Serotonin 5-HT_3 antagonists given orally (pills or sublingual tablets) or intravenously can prevent acute CINV, radiation-induced vomiting, and PONV but are less effective for delayed CINV. 5-HT_3 antagonists derive their antiemetic effects through central 5-HT_3 antagonism in the chemoreceptor zone and peripheral 5-HT_3 antagonism of vagal afferent nerves. A once-weekly granisetron patch may provide relief for those who cannot tolerate oral dosing. Other patients responsive to 5-HT_3 antagonists include adults with vomiting refractory to other antiemetics, hepatic or renal impairment, bulimia nervosa, gastroparesis, nausea from human immunodeficiency syndrome, and children with vomiting [148].

The 5-HT_3 antagonists ondansetron, granisetron, and dolasetron have similar efficacy. Palonosetron has a longer half-life, allosterically binds to the 5-HT_3 receptor, exhibits positive cooperativity, shows persistent inhibition of receptor function after drug withdrawal, and blunts substance P-mediated responses due to interactions with the 5-HT_3 receptor [41]. Consequently, palonosetron improves complete response rates in acute CINV and shows benefits with cases of delayed CINV as well. 5-HT_3 antagonist side-effects include constipation, headaches, and elevated liver chemistries. Cardiac rhythm disturbances can occur with 5-HT_3 antagonists given to patients with QTc prolongation on electrocardiography. Individuals with a single-nucleotide polymorphism (3435C>T) in the gene that codes for the drug efflux transporter adenosine triphosphate binding cassette subfamily B member 1 (ABCB1) show greater antiemetic responses to 5-HT_3 antagonists [149]. Patients with CPY2D6 allele duplications exhibit poorer responses to dolasetron than granisetron [150].

The neurokinin NK_1 antagonist aprepitant prevents acute and delayed CINV (especially coadministered with a 5-HT_3 antagonist), PONV, and motion sickness [151]. A prospective randomized, placebo-controlled trial of aprepitant in patients with chronic unexplained nausea and vomiting or gastroparesis identified some improvement in nausea using the validated Gastroparesis Cardinal Symptom Index [152]. Oral aprepitant is equivalent to an intravenous form, fosaprepitant. Side-effects include anorexia, constipation, diarrhea, and hiccups.

Cannabinoids (dronabinol) prevent CINV similar, or to slightly greater degrees, than antidopaminergics by acting on CNS CB_1 receptors [153]. Other proposed mechanisms of the cannabinoids include reduced prostaglandin synthesis and stimulation of endogenous endorphin production. Side-effects include somnolence, lethargy, euphoria, cognitive impairments, and in rare cases, syncope and hallucinations which may be prominent in the elderly. One study in healthy volunteers also demonstrated that dronabinol may slow gastric emptying, more so in women than men, thereby potentially worsening GI symptoms in patients with gastroparesis [154].

Other compounds have antiemetic actions. Corticosteroids and benzodiazepines often are included in antiemetic regimens for CINV or PONV prophylaxis, but their mechanisms of action are uncertain. Patients with nausea from narcotic withdrawal may respond to opiate antagonists such as naloxone. Ginger and ginger juice exhibit antivomiting actions in several clinical settings. The precise mechanism of action for ginger is unknown, but components of ginger (6-gingerol, 8-gingerol, 10-gingerol, 6-shogaol) have antagonist effects on 5-HT_3, dopamine, NK_1, muscarinic M_3, and histamine receptors [155]. The herbal extract STW5 (Iberogast® – which is composed of nine herbs) reduces symptoms in functional dyspepsia and gastroparesis [156].

Acupressure, with stimulation of the P6 pressure point (Nei Guan in traditional Chinese medicine), may improve nausea in some patients, although this has not been studied in large, sham-controlled trials.

Prokinetic agents

Metoclopramide stimulates gastric emptying by gastric 5-HT_4 receptor facilitation of cholinergic transmission and D_2 antagonism. CNS antiemetic actions of metoclopramide provide an additional means of symptom control. The prokinetic properties of metoclopramide do not extend into the distal gut, so the drug is not useful for small intestinal or colonic dysmotility. CNS side-effects (agitation, drowsiness, dystonia) and hyperprolactinemic manifestations (amenorrhea, galactorrhea, impotence) limit the drug's use in up to one-third of patients. A warning was issued for the risk of irreversible tardive dyskinesia with long-term metoclopramide use (average 1.5–2 years); women and patients >70 years old are at greatest risk [157]. Because this condition is disabling and can develop insidiously, metoclopramide complications should be explained (including description of the black box warning from the Food and Drug Administration [FDA]) and the discussions documented. Assessment of all the data available shows that the risk of tardive dyskinesia from metoclopramide is low, in the range of 0.1% per 1000 patient-years. This is far below a previously estimated 1–10% risk suggested in treatment guidelines by regulatory authorities [158].

Erythromycin and other macrolides (azithromycin, clarithromycin) elicit antroduodenal contractions and accelerate gastric emptying through action on receptors for motilin, the physiological regulator of fasting gastric contractility. Animal models of motion sickness suggest that low doses of erythromycin exhibit some additional antiemetic activity [159]. Macrolides have narrow dose ranges of efficacy, thereby limiting their utility; low doses are ineffective while high doses induce abdominal pain and nausea due to intense motor spasms. Erythromycin may be more useful for short-term use in gastroparesis due to development of tachyphylaxis and tolerance to its prokinetic action over time. Macrolides are associated with increased risks of sudden cardiac death. In a large Medicaid cohort, the sudden death rate of current erythromycin users was increased more than twofold overall and fivefold in those also on CYP3A inhibitors [160].

Domperidone promotes gastric evacuation by gastric peripheral D_2 antagonism and reduces vomiting by brainstem antiemetic actions. Prokinetic actions of domperidone are limited to the stomach, benefiting some patients with gastroparesis and functional gastroduodenal disorders. An intravenous form was responsible for sudden cardiac death in patients and was withdrawn. The oral form has been implicated as a potential cause of fatal cardiac arrhythmias in four case control studies in those with prolonged QTc EKG intervals [161]. Hyperprolactinemic side-effects also occur rarely as the drug can gain access to the anterior pituitary. Because the drug does not cross other regions of the blood–brain barrier, CNS side-effects are minimal. The drug is approved in most countries except the United States. Domperidone is obtainable from foreign pharmacies, US compounding pharmacies, and over the internet. The FDA discourages these practices, but does approve its use under the auspices of a program to clinicians who receive Investigational New Drug approval and obtain Institutional Review Board approval.

5-HT_4 agonists may improve symptoms of nausea and vomiting in some patients with gastroparesis. A small placebo-controlled, cross-over study demonstrated that prucalopride (which is approved for constipation) was efficacious and safe, while a larger prospective study showed some benefit for velusetrag [162,163], although it has not been approved by the FDA.

Other agents stimulate proximal gut transit and are used in selected cases of gastroparesis or small intestinal dysmotility. Cholinesterase inhibitors like pyridostigmine increase contractions in the stomach and small intestine and are employed in rare cases to treat gastroparesis and CIP. The somatostatin analog octreotide evokes propagative small intestinal motor patterns in some cases of CIP, and can reduce nausea, vomiting, and abdominal discomfort, and improve measures of intestinal bacterial overgrowth [164]. However, octreotide blunts antral contractions and can delay gastric emptying [165] as well as small bowel transit. Thus, it should be used judiciously in patients with associated gastroparesis.

Neuromodulating medications

Neuromodulatory agents that reduce luminal sensitivity benefit some conditions with nausea and vomiting.

Tricyclic antidepressants are proposed to reduce vomiting in this manner in functional vomiting and CVS [166]. Similarly, in a retrospective analysis of 24 diabetics with refractory nausea and vomiting, tricyclic use at a median 50 mg/day dose produced symptom reductions in 88% and near resolution in one-third [167]. Two-thirds of patients reported that the tricyclic therapy was the most effective treatment provided.

Mirtazapine (oral dose 15–30 mg) has shown efficacy in case reports of patients with gastroparesis, CINV, and PONV [168]. The antipsychotic olanzapine relieves nausea in some patients with drug refractory symptoms [169]. This agent has a complex mechanism of action including antagonism of dopamine, serotonin, α_1 adrenergic, histamine, and muscarinic receptors.

Gabapentin binds to the α-2/δ subunits of voltage-gated calcium channels and improves neuropathic pain. A metaanalysis of 12 studies found that gabapentin improved symptoms of nausea in patients with PONV and CINV; it was less useful in those with hyperemesis gravidarum [170].

Management approaches in selected clinical settings

Different approaches to nausea and vomiting are tailored to the etiology of symptoms.

Acute gastroenteritis

Because of its impact on resource utilization, controlling vomiting from gastroenteritis in pediatric populations has been the subject of clinical trials. In meta-analyses and systematic reviews of children and adolescents with gastroenteritis, reductions in vomiting, needs for intravenous hydration and hospitalizations, and improvements in overall well-being were greater with ondansetron (IV doses 0.15–0.3 mg/kg; oral doses 1.6–8 mg based on bodyweight) than placebo [171]. Likewise, dimenhydrinate reduced the time to cessation of vomiting by 0.34 days in children and adolescents.

Gastroparesis

A stratification of disease severity was proposed to facilitate gastroparesis treatment, in which disease severity is characterized by the percentage of gastric retention on a 4-hour gastric emptying scintigraphy study [172] (Figure 33.4). In general, medications that decrease gastrointestinal motility, such as opioids and GLP-1 analogs or agonists, should be discontinued in all patients with gastroparesis, and glycemic control should be optimized in diabetics. Additionally, patients with gastroparesis should be advised to consume small, frequent meals, which are low in fat and fiber. A blenderized (small particle) diet may be considered in patients with mild (10–15% gastric retention at 4 hours) or moderate (15–35% retention at 4 hours) gastroparesis on an as-needed basis, when symptomatic, but may be considered routinely in patients with severe gastroparesis (>35% retention at 4 hours) [145]. Nutritional support is rarely needed for patients with mild gastroparesis, but caloric liquids may be helpful in patients with moderate or severe gastroparesis; enteral nutrition via percutaneous jejunostomy tube or parenteral nutrition is typically only considered in patients with severe gastroparesis and malnutrition.

With regard to pharmacological treatment, treatment with a prokinetic, such as metoclopramide, and/or an antiemetic, such as ondansetron or promethazine, can be considered for patients with mild, moderate, or severe gastroparesis. Other prokinetic medications, such as domperidone and prucalopride, antiemetic medications, such as aprepitant, or neuromodulating medications, such as tricyclic antidepressants, may be considered in patients with severe gastroparesis, particularly those with symptoms refractory to traditional treatment measures. There have been 10 studies (seven randomized controlled trials of up 93 patients) of metoclopramide, and nine studies (three randomized controlled trials of up to 13 patients) of erythromycin in gastroparesis that report variable efficacy in the condition [47]. Two-thirds of 11 published articles and 16 abstracts reported benefits of domperidone in gastroparesis, but authors of a meta-analysis concluded there is insufficient evidence to recommend this agent because of study design flaws or small sample sizes [173]. A recent study found that prucalopride improved symptoms and enhanced gastric emptying in patients with idiopathic gastroparesis [162].

No controlled trials have been performed assessing antiemetic drug efficacy in gastroparesis. Based on retrospective data suggesting efficacy in diabetics with nausea and vomiting, tricyclic agents are often given for gastroparesis [167]. However, a controlled trial showed no overall benefits of nortriptyline in idiopathic gastroparesis, although secondary improvements in anorexia and body mass index were noted [174]. Factors predicting poor treatment response to medication therapy of gastroparesis include overall symptom severity and specific intensity of bloating or distension [175].

Botulinum toxin

Pyloric botulinum toxin injection can promote gastric emptying by reducing pylorospasm. In the largest series (which employed an uncontrolled, open label design), predictors of response included use of higher doses (200 units vs 100 units), idiopathic gastroparesis etiology, female sex, and age <50 years [176].

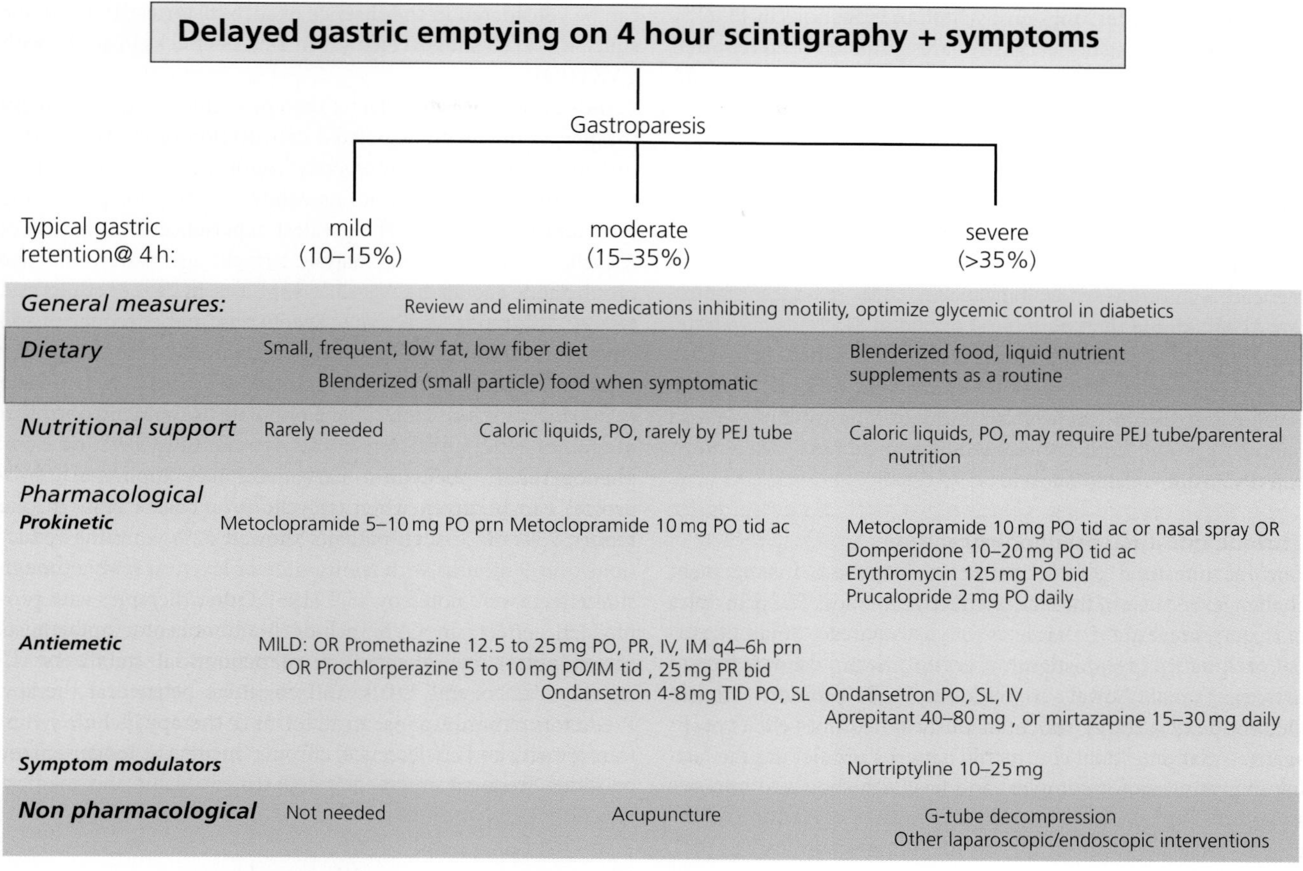

Figure 33.4 Summary of treatment strategy for patients with gastroparesis according to disease severity. Source: Lacy et al. [172]. Reproduced with permission of Wolters Kluwer Health, Inc.

However, two small, controlled trials showed no benefits of botulinum toxin compared to saline injection [177,178].

Gastric electrical stimulation

The FDA approved an implantable gastric electrical stimulator as a humanitarian use device to treat refractory diabetic or idiopathic gastroparesis in centers in which Institutional Review Board approval has been granted. In several, large uncontrolled series, gastric stimulation has shown efficacy in reducing nausea and vomiting, improving nutrition with less need for supplemental feedings, and improving glycemic control in diabetics [179]. Diabetics tend to respond better than those with idiopathic gastroparesis; pain and chronic opiate use are predictors of poor response [180].

Three small controlled trials of gastric stimulation have been published; the first showed nonsignificant trends to reduced vomiting in diabetics and no benefit in idiopathic patients, a second observed no benefit better than sham treatments in diabetic patients, and a third study with similar experimental design as the investigation in diabetics showed no difference in responses in patients with idiopathic gastroparesis when the device was ON or OFF as assessed in blinded fashion [181–183]. Two recent trials have also demonstrated relief of symptoms without improvement in gastric emptying. Thus, nausea was relieved in an open label experience that contrasted patients with those without a gastric electrical stimulator [184]. Vomiting was relieved in a cross-over study of 172 patients with refractory vomiting, with or without gastroparesis [185].

Gastric peroral endoscopic myotomy

Peroral endoscopic myotomy (POEM) was first performed in 2008 for the treatment of achalasia. During this procedure, an endoscope is used to create an incision in the distal esophagus with subsequent myotomy of the lower esophageal sphincter. Successful results in patients with achalasia stimulated researchers to evaluate this technique in patients with gastroparesis. Using similar techniques, endoscopic myotomy of the pylorus (pyloromyotomy) can be performed in the outpatient setting. A series of small case reports or small series of patients have demonstrated benefit in some patients with gastroparesis and refractory symptoms [186]. Large, randomized, sham-controlled studies are needed to confirm these preliminary results and determine which patients (e.g., idiopathic vs diabetic; moderate delay in emptying vs severe delay) are most likely to respond.

Gastric surgery

Retrospective series report benefit in up to 80% of gastroparetics undergoing surgical pyloroplasty [187]. Completion gastrectomy provides long-term symptom reductions in 43–67% of patients with postsurgical gastroparesis and has been reported to produce short-term improvements in up to 60% of those with other gastroparesis etiologies [188,189].

Nutritional supplementation

Enteral nutrition may be required on an intermittent basis for intermittent symptom flares or for permanent caloric and fluid support. Enteral feedings improve overall health with trends to reduced symptoms, hospitalizations, and enhanced nutrition [190]. Home total parenteral nutrition (TPN) is less desirable because of complication risks, but short-term TPN sometimes is offered to reverse rapid weight decline. Placing a venting gastrostomy affords the ability to intermittently release retained gas and liquid, thereby relieving fullness, discomfort, and distension-related nausea.

Chronic intestinal pseudoobstruction

Chronic intestinal pseudoobstruction can be a management challenge, because of the lack of effective therapy. The principles of management are the same as for gastroparesis. Small intestinal prokinetics (pyridostigmine, erythromycin) can be given to increase small bowel contractions and promote transit. Octreotide (25–200 μg subcutaneously at bedtime) elicits propagative small intestinal contractile patterns mimicking the fasting migrating motor complex, and has been shown to improve symptoms and decrease surrogate measures of bacterial overgrowth in selected causes of CIP, including scleroderma [164]. Control of small intestinal bacterial overgrowth with intermittent or rotating oral antibiotics can be crucial in limiting symptoms and maintaining nutrition. Rarely, decompressive stomas can reduce symptoms. Home TPN or small intestinal transplantation is considered for individuals who cannot sustain nutrition with oral or enteral supplements [191]. Outcomes often are poor with development of disabling complications on longitudinal follow-up.

Cyclic vomiting syndrome

Distinct approaches are offered to control acute attacks during the preemetic prodromal or hyperemetic phases and to prevent future emetic episodes.

Therapy of acute attacks includes supportive care and aggressive medication treatments. Intravenous hydration with 10% dextrose and potassium supplements as needed may be beneficial. Antiemetics tried for acute CVS episodes include prochlorperazine, metoclopramide, and haloperidol, but 5-HT_3 antagonists are prominently used for this indication. For attacks resulting in emergency department or inpatient care, intravenous benzodiazepines (e.g., lorazepam) provide substantial relief by induction of sedation [192]. Opiates can be used judiciously in the acute setting to help control abdominal pain; parenteral ketorolac also has benefits [65]. Antimigraine serotonin 5-$HT_{1B,1D}$ agonists (e.g., sumatriptan) are effective, especially in children with personal or family histories of migraines, but also can be considered in the absence of such histories [193]. In one study, this class showed efficacy in 54% of attacks in adults with CVS [194].

Indications for prophylactic therapy include frequent attacks (>1 per month) with associated dehydration or electrolyte disturbances, numerous emergency room visits or hospitalizations [20]. Several medications exhibit efficacy for preventing recurrent CVS attacks. The greatest experience is in the use of tricyclic agents. In a meta-analysis, tricyclic agents were effective prophylactic agents in CVS with responses in 76% of adults and 68% of children [65]. Tricyclic agents reduce the frequency and duration of CVS episodes for >2 years and decrease emergency room utilization [195]. Poor responses to tricyclic agents relate to psychiatric disease, marijuana or opiate use, and uncontrolled migraines [192]. Anticonvulsants (zonisamide, levetiracetam, phenobarbital, phenytoin, carbamazepine, topiramate, valproate) can be given when tricyclic prophylaxis fails. In one report, 75% of 20 such patients showed 62% vomiting reductions over 9 months with zonisamide or levetiracetam although side-effects were noted by 45% [196]. Other therapies with prophylactic effects in CVS include β-adrenoceptor antagonists (propranolol), cyproheptadine, mitochondrial stabilizers (L-carnitine, coenzyme Q10), and cognitive behavioral therapy. Predictors of nonresponse to all forms of therapy include symptom severity and coalescence, chronic opiate use, longer emetic episodes, frequent emergency department visits, and medication noncompliance [68].

Chronic nausea and vomiting syndrome

Limited research has been performed on therapies for CNVS. Older controlled trials of 5-HT_3 antagonists show modest reductions in nausea and vomiting in functional dyspepsia. Given their relatively greater reductions in vomiting versus nausea, it is conceivable these agents may be more effective for functional vomiting than nausea [197]. Tricyclic antidepressants show benefits in uncontrolled functional vomiting studies [166]. Furthermore, in a retrospective report of 94 patients fulfilling Rome III criteria for chronic idiopathic nausea or functional vomiting, 72% experienced at least moderate symptom decreases and 22% noted remission on neuromodulators (tricyclics 66 patients, norepinephrine dopamine reuptake inhibitors 10 patients, selective serotonin reuptake inhibitors five patients, serotonin norepinephrine reuptake inhibitors five patients, and others nine patients) [198].

Rumination syndrome

Lifestyle and behavioral therapies are offered for rumination syndrome with varying degrees of success. The most accepted treatment of rumination syndrome involves behavioral modification using diaphragmatic breathing techniques to compete with the urge to regurgitate [199]. This technique eliminated rumination in 30–66% of cases with reductions in many additional patients in older series, but a more recent study showed only incomplete symptom control in 43% [200]. However, diaphragmatic breathing has been shown to increase esophagogastric junction pressure and reverse the negative gastroesophageal pressure dynamic associated with rumination syndrome in a small study of patients with rumination who underwent esophageal manometry testing before, during, and after diaphragmatic breathing training [201]. Gum chewing has anecdotal benefits in children with rumination. Proton pump inhibitors protect the esophageal lining, but they may prolong rumination by limiting the meal acidification that often stops the postprandial regurgitations [202]. The γ-aminobutyric acid agonist baclofen reduces rumination events by half by increasing LES pressure and blunting transient LES relaxations [203]. Benefits of most prokinetics are unproved, but levosulpiride reduced rumination in one study when given in concert with education and psychotherapy [84].

Nissen fundoplication produced decreases in rumination events in one small series of patients unresponsive to behavioral approaches [204].The costs, risks, and potential complications of antireflux surgery (e.g., gas-bloat syndrome, rapid gastric emptying, delayed gastric emptying, chronic abdominal pain) should be thoroughly discussed with the patient.

Nausea and vomiting of pregnancy

Several agents are promoted to treat NVP, but pharmacological therapies provide benefits in only 31% of cases [205]. A Cochrane review of 27 trials of 4041 women reported no benefits of acupressure or acustimulation in NVP, and only limited evidence supporting utility of antiemetics including antihistamines, antidopaminergics, and antiserotonergics [206]. Others report benefits of mirtazapine in a subset of individuals with hyperemesis gravidarum [207]. Some studies observe benefits of corticosteroids in hyperemesis gravidarum, while others note no effect. Some older reviews suggest minor increases in adverse pregnancy outcomes with antiemetic treatments (odds ratio 1.03) [208]. One study reported an association of ondansetron given during pregnancy and cleft palate [209].

Because of concerns of potential antiemetic toxicity in NVP, dietary, complementary, and alternative strategies can be offered. Clinicians traditionally advocate ingesting dry crackers for relief, but some studies suggest greater benefits with proteins [210]. A systematic review reported superiority of ginger over placebo in four studies and equivalence of ginger and pyridoxine (vitamin B_6) in two others [211]. Pyridoxine may be given in concert with other drugs to optimize benefits. Acupressure and acustimulation also may have efficacy in NVP. Thiamine supplements are indicated to prevent Wernicke encephalopathy with hyperemesis gravidarum.

Aggressive measures are needed for some severe cases of hyperemesis gravidarum. Enteral feedings are indicated for persistent weight loss with this complication. In one series, jejunostomy placement for a mean of 19 weeks resulted in successful term pregnancies with mean birthweights of 2885g [212]. Intravenous hydration or parenteral nutrition may be needed, but these can be complicated by infection or thromboembolism in pregnancy.

Chemotherapy- and radiation therapy-induced nausea and vomiting

Extensive research has focused on antiemetic regimens to prevent or treat CINV. Most programs include multiple medications which act on distinct receptor sites. However, many regimens are more effective at controlling vomiting than nausea. Persistence of nausea may limit resolution of anorexia after chemotherapy [213]. Combining a 5-HT_3 antagonist, an NK_1 antagonist, and a corticosteroid provides significant control of both acute and delayed vomiting after chemotherapy [151]. The NK_1 antagonist aprepitant increases antiemetic responses by 20% with highly or moderately emetogenic chemotherapies compared to regimens without this agent [214]. In contrast to other drugs in the same class, the 5-HT_3 antagonist palonosetron exhibits efficacy at preventing delayed CINV, as does rolapitant (180 mg QD), an NK_1 antagonist; both are FDA approved for this indication [215]. Dexamethasone or a dopamine antagonist can be given before chemotherapy with low emetogenicity. Anticipatory emesis is poorly controlled by antiemetic medications and is best managed by relaxation therapy, systematic desensitization techniques, hypnosis, and intravenous anxiolytic medications such as benzodiazepines.

Predictors of failed response to antiemetic therapy of chemotherapy-induced emesis include female sex, nonhabitual alcohol intake, and nonsmoking status [216]. A variant of the 5-HT_3 receptor gene (rs6443930) is associated with nonresponse to antiemetic prophylaxis of CINV [217].

Miscellaneous therapies with reported benefit in CINV include olanzapine, gabapentin, electro-acustimulation, ginger, and therapeutic massage. One group has observed reductions in delayed nausea after chemotherapy in individuals on a high-protein diet [218].

As with CINV, guidelines for antiemetic therapy of radiation-induced emesis are based on emetogenicity of the radiation protocol [219]. Patients at high risk of radiation-induced emesis should receive prophylaxis with a 5-HT_3 antagonist plus dexamethasone. Those with moderate risk may receive either prophylaxis or rescue with a 5-HT_3 antagonist; those at minimal risk usually are given rescue antiemetics alone. 5-HT_3 antagonists may offer less benefit for radiation-induced nausea versus emesis.

Postoperative nausea and vomiting

Several regimens have been proposed to prevent or control PONV. A large systematic review of 737 studies in 103 237 subjects concluded that prophylactic antiemetic therapy provides benefit for 28% of patients [220]. In a factorial trial of six interventions for postoperative nausea and vomiting, antiemetic treatment with ondansetron, dexamethasone, and droperidol each produced similar benefits [221]. Selected genotypes for the adenosine triphosphate binding cassette subfamily B member 1 are reported to predict responses to ondansetron in PONV [222]. Other therapies with prophylactic efficacy in PONV include aprepitant, transdermal scopolamine, ginger, acustimulation, and electrical stimulation of the vestibular system.

Consensus guidelines suggest patients at low risk for PONV should not receive antiemetic prophylaxis while those at moderate risk should be given one or two agents [223]. Double and triple antiemetic drug regimens are considered for those at high risk. Other advocated measures to reduce risk include use of regional anesthesia, propofol for induction of anesthesia, intraoperative oxygen, intravenous fluids, avoidance of nitrous oxide and volatile anesthetics, and minimization of opioids and neostigmine. Use of nonsteroidal agents (e.g., ketorolac) to reduce postoperative opioid use can lead to a lower incidence of PONV [224].

Future treatments of nausea and vomiting

Several medication and nonmedication treatments are in testing and show promise as future treatments of nausea and vomiting. Novel investigational antiemetics include newer NK_1 receptor antagonists (rolapitant, netupitant) [151]. New agents acting as agonists on 5-HT_4, ghrelin, and motilin receptors are under consideration as prokinetics for gastroparesis. Drugs acting as ghrelin agonists exhibit abilities to accelerate gastric emptying in gastroparesis, and are in testing to determine their utility in this condition [225,226]. Next-generation gastric stimulators may exhibit pacing capabilities when delivered sequentially in antegrade direction across several electrode pairs [227]. Stimulation of the vagus nerve and transcranial electromagnetic stimulation are other modalities under investigation [228].

References are available at www.yamadagastro.com/textbook7e

Further reading

Abell T.L., Camilleri M., Donohoe K., et al. Consensus recommendations for gastric emptying scintigraphy: a joint report of the American Neurogastroenterology and Motility Society and the Society of Nuclear Medicine. Am J Gastroenterol 2008;103:753.

Camilleri M., Chedid V., Ford A.C., et al. Gastroparesis. Nat Rev Dis Primers 2018;4:41.

Carlisle J.B., Stevenson C.A. Drugs for preventing postoperative nausea and vomiting. Cochrane Database Syst Rev 2006;3:CD004125.

Das J.K., Kumar R., Salam R.A., et al. The effect of antiemetics in childhood gastroenteritis. BMC Public Health 2013;13 Suppl 3:S9.

Galli J.A., Sawaya R.A., Friedenberg F.K. Cannabinoid hyperemesis syndrome. Curr Drug Abuse Rev 2011;4:241.

Halland M., Pandolfino J., Barba E. Diagnosis and treatment of rumination syndrome. Clin Gastroenterol Hepatol 2018;16:1549.

Lee L.Y., Abbott L., Mahlangu B., et al. The management of cyclic vomiting syndrome: a systematic review. Eur J Gastroenterol Hepatol 2012;24:1001.

Navavi R.M. Management of chemotherapy-induced nausea and vomiting: focus on newer agents and new uses for older agents. Drugs 2013;73:249.

Revicki D.A., Camilleri M., Kuo B., et al. Evaluation symptom outcomes in gastroparesis clinical trials: validity and responsiveness of the Gastroparesis Cardinal Symptom Index–Daily Diary (GCSI-DD). Neurogastroenterol Motil 2012;24:456.

Stanghellini V., Chan F.K., Hasler W.L., et al. Gastroduodenal disorders. Gastroenterology 2016;150:1380.

Yokoe T., Hayashida T., Nagayama A., et al. Effectiveness of antiemetic regimens for highly emetogenic chemotherapy-induced nausea and vomiting: a systematic review and network meta-analysis. Oncologist 2019;24:e347.

CHAPTER 34

Approach to the patient with abdominal pain, gas, and bloating

Amrit K. Kamboj and Amy S. Oxentenko
Division of Gastroenterology and Hepatology, Mayo Clinic, Rochester, MN, USA

Chapter menu

Abdominal pain

Background and importance

As a sensation, pain is an integral component of the normal "defense" system, warning the organism about potentially noxious agents in the internal or external environment. Pain is also unique amongst sensations in that it can evoke, and to some extent be invoked by, complex alterations in the psychosocial state of humans. When pain becomes chronic, it can then dominate the clinical picture so that it is no longer regarded as a warning sensation, but instead, assumes the characteristics of a disease state by itself.

The gastroenterologist routinely has to address and manage abdominal pain, given it is one of the most common presenting gastrointestinal (GI) complaints. Prevalence rates of abdominal pain of greater than 20% have been reported, and women appear to be disproportionately affected [1,2]. In a population-based survey, the overall proportion (%) of any abdominal pain (mild, moderate, or severe) was 36%, with 5% of subjects reporting severe abdominal pain [3]. In the United States, abdominal pain accounts for 16.5 million visits annually [4], and of the nearly 122 million visits to the emergency room each year, about 15 million (12%) have a primary GI diagnosis, and of these, abdominal pain is the most common (4.7 million visits) [5]. Although abdominal pain is also a major reason for hospitalization, many patients may be discharged without a more specific diagnosis. In a consecutive group of 100 patients admitted with lower abdominal pain, 67% were diagnosed as having nonspecific abdominal pain; this represented about 13% of all general surgical admissions [6].

As can be expected, patients with abdominal pain consume significant resources. The annual healthcare expenditure for abdominal pain is approximately $10.2 billion [4] with mean annual direct healthcare costs per patient at $7646 [7]. Although only a small fraction of these individuals consult a physician, the symptom is severe enough to impair routine activities in many patients [8]. Further, chronic abdominal pain is an independent predictor of suicidal behavior after adjusting for comorbid psychiatric conditions, with a risk that is 3–11-fold greater than controls [9].

Neurobiology of pain

The perception of pain begins in the periphery with the stimulation of certain spinal sensory receptors of afferent neurons, also known as nociceptors. The nociceptor has to perform three key tasks (Figure 34.1): (1) transduction of noxious stimulus to an electrical signal; (2) conduction of that electrical signal from the peripheral to the central end of the nociceptor; and (3) encoding and relaying that signal to second-order neurons in the form of synaptic neurotransmitters. In general, nociceptors convert noxious stimuli to an electrical response via specialized receptors.

Thermal, mechanical, or chemical stimuli, acting via specific receptors, induce a change in the membrane potential of the nociceptor terminal, called a "receptor" or "generator"

Yamada's Textbook of Gastroenterology, Seventh Edition. Edited by Timothy C. Wang, Michael Camilleri, Benjamin Lebwohl, Anna S. Lok, William J. Sandborn, Kenneth K. Wang, and Gary D. Wu.

Companion website: www.yamadagastro.com/textbook7e

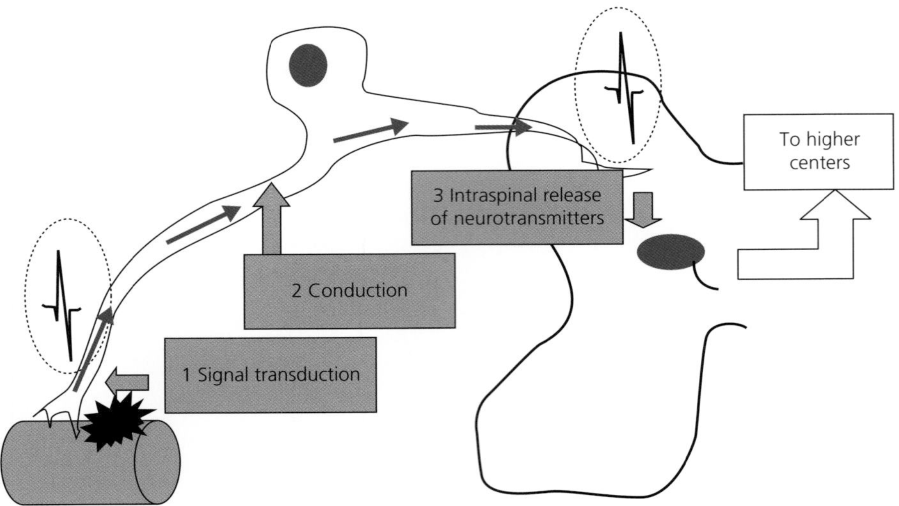

Figure 34.1 The primary nociceptor and its functions. Sensation from the peripheral organ is carried via fibers whose origin is in cell bodies within the dorsal root ganglia. The central projections of these neurons in turn relay information to second-order neurons in the spinal cord which transmit this information upwards to the brainstem and higher centers via distinct pathways. This diagram illustrates the three basic components of pain signaling at the level of the first-order neuron in the nociceptive pathway. A painful stimulus is translated into electrical activity, that is conducted centrally and eventually results in release of neurotransmitters at the central synapses, with stimulation of second-order neurons.

potential. Voltage-gated sodium and potassium channels play a fundamental role in controlling neuronal excitability in response to this relatively small change in membrane potential by setting thresholds for activation of an action potential. Finally, voltage-dependent calcium channels contribute to depolarization, but more importantly, mediate crucial nociceptor functions such as the release of neurotransmitters and long-term plasticity or adaptation [10]. Once generated, action potentials are conducted centripetally to the spinal terminals of the nociceptors, where they initiate neurotransmitter release and thereby relay nociceptive information to second-order neurons. Pain sensations are then transmitted through second-order neurons (e.g., in the spinothalamic tract) to the brainstem, from which a third-order neuron conveys the sensation to the higher centers for conscious sensation or to the limbic system (e.g., amygdala) which result in the emotional component of the pain experience.

Visceral and somatic pain

With the neurobiology of pain in mind, it is useful to briefly summarize the important differences in the clinically relevant features of pain originating in the viscera (internal organs) compared with that arising from somatic tissues (skin, soft tissue, muscle) [11]. First, visceral afferents are relatively few in number (compared with somatic structures) and diverge extensively in the central nervous system, with the result that the pain tends to be poorly localized and present at locations that do not intuitively correspond to structures conventionally associated with visceral sensation such as the insular cortex. Second, acute visceral pain is often accompanied by autonomic disturbances such as changes in blood pressure and heart rate, pallor, and sweating, and motor phenomena such as vomiting and diarrhea. Finally, humans rate visceral pain as more unpleasant and are more likely to react to it with anxiety and other emotions than cutaneous pain from the same spinal segment and of similar intensity [12]. In addition, there are several other clinically important features of visceral pain that need detailed description. These include the phenomena of referred pain, sensitization, and stress-induced exacerbation of pain.

Referred pain

Most clinically significant forms of visceral pain are referred to various somatic areas of the body. A patient with "pure" visceral pain is seldom seen in clinical practice, as this phase usually lasts only a few hours. When it begins, it is felt as a deep and dull discomfort in the midline, reflecting the embryogenic origin of the involved organ from the fore-, mid-, or hindgut, respectively (Figure 34.2). If the underlying insult persists, referred pain sets in. Referred pain is perceived as sharp and readily localized to the overlying or remote superficial somatic structures such as the skin or abdominal wall muscle. Referred pain can occur without hyperalgesia of the somatic structure (simple irritation) or can be accompanied by sensitization of these structures with resulting hyperalgesia (secondary somatic hyperalgesia) [13]. Examples of both are commonly seen in practice. For instance, gallstone-induced pain can felt in the right upper quadrant and epigastric regions, as well as in the shoulder and scapular area of the back, but hyperalgesia (painful to the touch or deeper palpation) is typically experienced at Murphy's point in the right subcostal area.

Pain and sensitization

Most clinically important painful conditions occur on a background of a nociceptive system that is no longer operating at a "normal" level, but rather, it occurs in a potentiated or

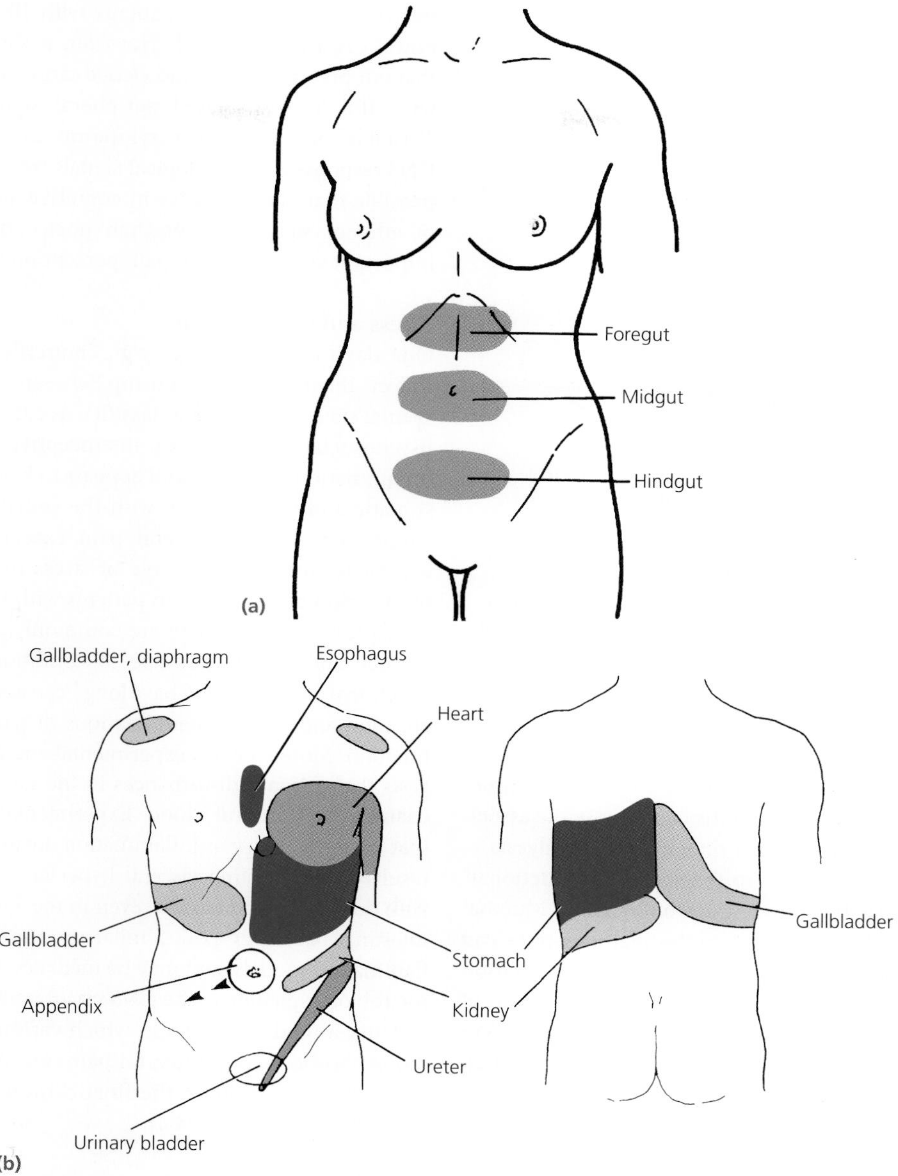

Figure 34.2 True visceral and referred pain patterns. **(a)** Approximate levels of the abdomen where "true" visceral pain is felt, according to its source. **(b)** Important skin areas for referral of visceral pain. Source: Snell 2000 [14]. Reproduced with permission of Wolters Kluwer Health.

"sensitized" state [10]. This concept can help explain many commonly encountered clinical situations.

Tissue injury or inflammation results in the local accumulation of several factors that can lead to a sustained and amplified (supranormal) activity of peripheral nociceptors, a phenomenon called *peripheral sensitization*. These factors may also result in a change in the responsiveness of previously dormant neurons ("silent nociceptors") such that they now start contributing to nociceptive activity. This increased "afferent barrage" over time leads to changes in second-order neurons within the spinal cord, causing an increase in their responsiveness with amplification and persistence of pain [15]; this is an example of central sensitization. The gain of the entire system is therefore reset upwards, with the result that noxious stimuli now elicit a pain response that is much greater when compared with the normal state, a phenomenon termed *hyperalgesia*. A further characteristic of the sensitized state is called *allodynia*, a phenomenon in which stimuli that are perceived as innocuous or physiological by healthy controls are perceived as painful by the patient. These manifestations of sensitization are graphically illustrated in Figure 34.3. As an example, patients with painful chronic pancreatitis may exhibit pancreatic neuronal sensitization and experience mechanical allodynia – pain in response to physiological changes in intraductal pressure (which would otherwise have not been

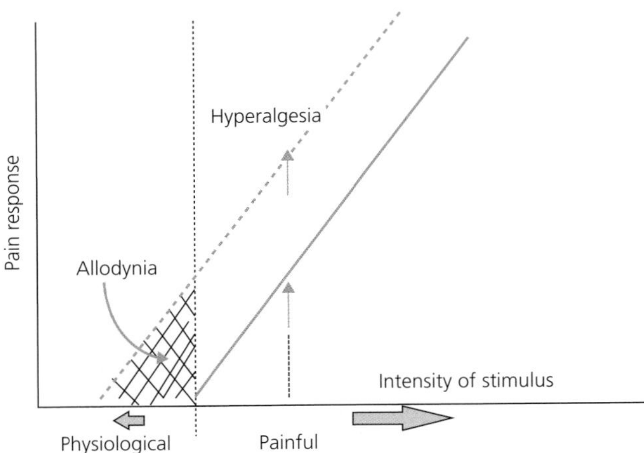

Figure 34.3 Basic concepts of pain sensitization, as illustrated in a theoretical stimulus–response curve. The right solid line represents a hypothetical control population while the left broken line represents the response in a sensitized population (e.g., patients with pancreatitis). The broken vertical line represents the threshold for painful stimulation in the control population. Note that the sensitized population experiences pain in response to stimulation that is in the nonpainful (physiological range) for the control population, a phenomenon known as allodynia (shaded area). Hyperalgesia refers to a response to painful stimulation that is greater than the control population (arrows).

perceived). Similarly, subsequent minor flare-ups of inflammation in patients with chronic pancreatitis could cause the associated pain to be noted as severe rather than mild (hyperalgesia).

This paradigm may also apply to the so-called "functional" disorders such as irritable bowel syndrome (IBS). Mucosal inflammation that accompanies gastrointestinal infections can produce visceral hyperalgesia by both peripheral sensitization and central hyperexcitability [16]. A significant number of patients develop IBS-like symptoms after a bout of acute infectious gastroenteritis [17,18]. According to this theory, the lack of overt inflammation or disruption of tissue architecture in patients with IBS is explained by the fact that the initiating event tends to be transient but leaves persistent changes in its wake that result in peripheral and central hyperalgesia. In such a sensitized state, even normal contractile events in the intestine or colon could be perceived as painful (i.e., allodynia).

It can be difficult to ascertain the relative importance of central and peripheral factors in patients with painful visceral conditions. In many patients, central sensitization is an expected and biologically predictable response to persistent noxious stimulation from the periphery. Thus, in patients with chronic pancreatitis, suppression of nociceptive signaling from the pancreas should turn down central sensitization. This is supported by studies on the effects of thoracic splanchnectomy/denervation on hyperalgesia in patients with chronic pancreatitis [19] as well as by the response to a peripherally acting κ-opioid agonist [20]. Central factors are often invoked as the "origin" of symptoms in patients with functional bowel disease, and imaging studies suggest morphological differences in the central nervous system between patients with IBS and inflammatory bowel disease (IBD) [21]. However, it should be emphasized that our present state of knowledge cannot determine if patients with IBS have increased peripheral signaling from a truly "irritable" bowel, or if their symptoms arise from changes in the CNS response to physiological signals from the bowel [22]. It is possible that abnormalities in cognitive–emotional processing of afferent signals, rather than nociception per se, may be important contributors to pain perception in these patients.

Stress and visceral pain

Our day-to-day language (e.g., "butterflies in the stomach") reflects the intimate relationship between gut sensation and our mental state. Stress can be classified as either exteroceptive (e.g., psychosocial in origin) or interoceptive (e.g., due to tissue inflammation or injury) and appears to have opposite effects on somatic and visceral pain, with the somatic component being suppressed and the visceral pain exacerbated [23]. Clinical experience attests to the role of stress in both the onset and modulation of symptoms in patients with IBS [24].

Depression and anxiety are commonly seen in patients with chronic abdominal pain due to conditions such as IBS and functional dyspepsia, and have long been assumed to lead to somatization and clinical manifestations of pain and disturbed gut function. More recently, experimental and clinical evidence suggests that primary disturbances in the gut can cause secondary changes in affect and mood. Experimental models have shown that transient injury or inflammation during the neonatal period results in long-lasting visceral hypersensitivity in adults, along with depression and anxiety, even in the absence of overt gastrointestinal pathology [25]. Similar processes accompany postinflammatory models, and may be mediated by changes in colonic microbiota signaling to the CNS via afferent vagal fibers [26,27].

Thus, a model emerges in which various components of the biopsychosocial continuum for pain can be seen to interact with each other and produce the final clinical picture in a bidirectional manner (Figure 34.4).

Classification of pain

Pain is a complex syndrome, and an attempt to classify it in a comprehensive manner poses a significant challenge. A commonly used approach classifies pain as either *nociceptive* or *neuropathic* based on the putative neurophysiological mechanism [29]. Nociceptive pain implies an ongoing stimulation of peripheral nociceptors by persistence of local painful conditions (e.g., injury and/or inflammation). Neuropathic pain, on the other hand, is pain that originates independent of nociceptor stimulation and implies structural or functional changes in the pain pathways (either peripheral or central) that result in persistent but aberrant signaling. The pain of some acute gastrointestinal conditions such as peptic ulcer, colonic ischemia, or acute cholecystitis can be considered to be predominantly nociceptive in nature. Neuropathic pain syndromes include post-stroke pain (central) or diabetic neuropathy (peripheral).

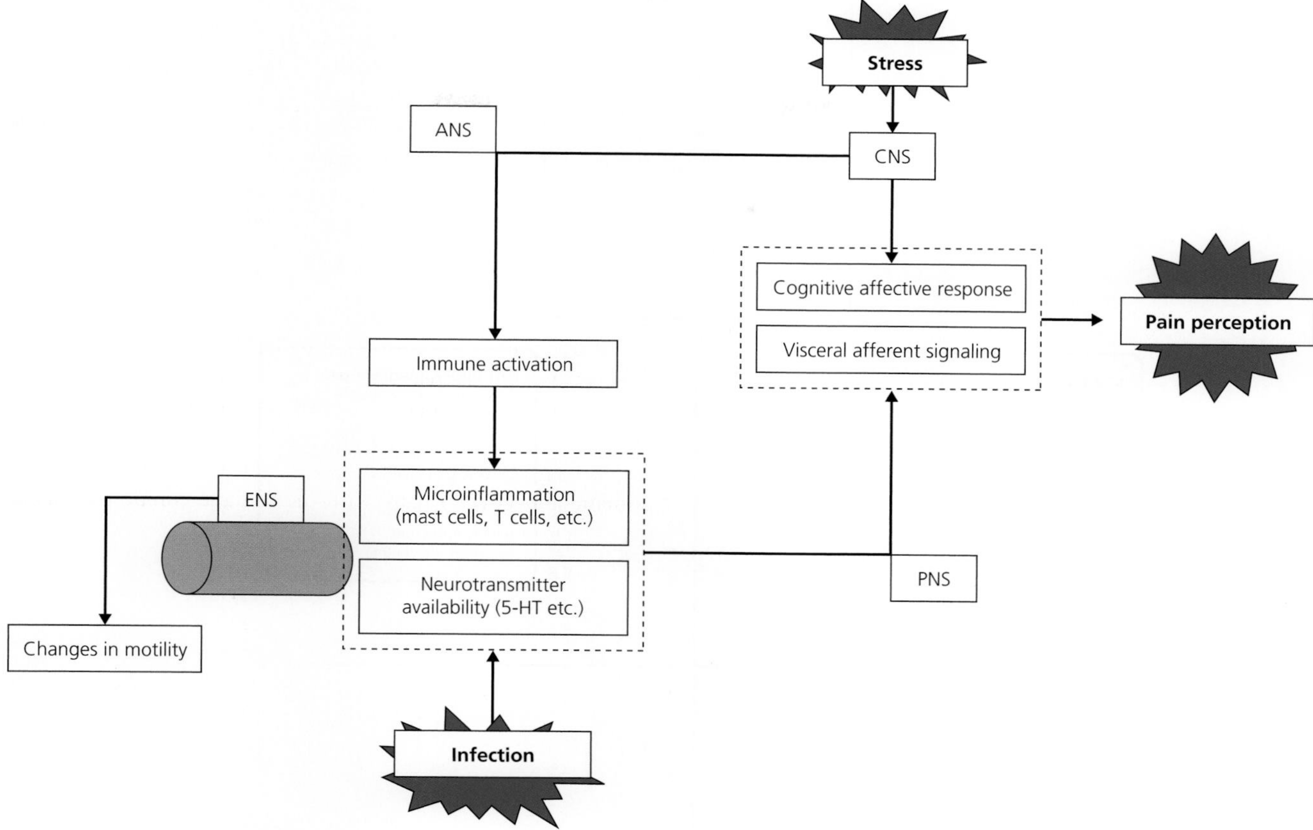

Figure 34.4 Current and emerging pathophysiological concepts on pain in irritable bowel syndrome (IBS). The figure assumes a vulnerable background (genetic, developmental phase) that is predisposed to developing a persistent state of activation in response to two major inciting factors, stress and infection, acting initially at central and peripheral sites, respectively. Subgroups of IBS patients may differ in the nature of the inciting factor, as well as activity of the various components that eventually lead to pain perception. Although changes in motility are shown separately, it is possible that in some instances they may also contribute to increased afferent signaling and discomfort. ANS, autonomic nervous system; CNS, central nervous system; ENS, enteric nervous system; PNS, peripheral nervous system (spinal afferents). Source: DuPont 2006 [28]. Reproduced with permission of Taylor & Francis.

Another way of classifying pain is by its temporal dimension. Acute pain serves a useful biological function, warning the organism of injury or impending injury. Chronic pain, arbitrarily defined as at least a month beyond the expected course of an injury to heal, can result in significant secondary morbidity in the form of physical, emotional, or socioeconomic stresses on the patient, family, and society [29]. The challenge for clinicians, therefore, is to recognize the various psychosocial attributes of chronic pain without overlooking the underlying problem.

Clinical assessment of the patient with abdominal pain

Acute abdominal pain

History

Acute abdominal pain may result from various etiologies, as outlined in Chapter 37. Taking a comprehensive history can help guide patient work-up and management. The patient history should be thorough and include details on the site of pain, onset, chronicity, temporal characteristics, character and intensity, and relieving and aggravating factors. An extensive review of systems should also be performed that includes gastrointestinal and nongastrointestinal signs and symptoms.

Site

Patients presenting with abdominal pain should be asked to point to the area of maximal tenderness using one finger. Most clinicians find it useful to divide the abdomen into four quadrants (Figure 34.5, Box 34.1) [30]. These general, if crude, inferences are supported by studies using balloon insufflation in various organs in conscious patients [31,32]. However, there is often considerable overlap between pain from various sites, such as the stomach, bile duct, pancreas, and proximal small intestine. When the abdominal pain does not easily lend itself to a quadrant-based approach, assessing whether it is focal or diffuse in nature can help narrow the differential diagnoses (see Figure 34.5). In acute abdominal pain, pain is often periumbilical at onset; the parietal peritoneum is later involved and identifies

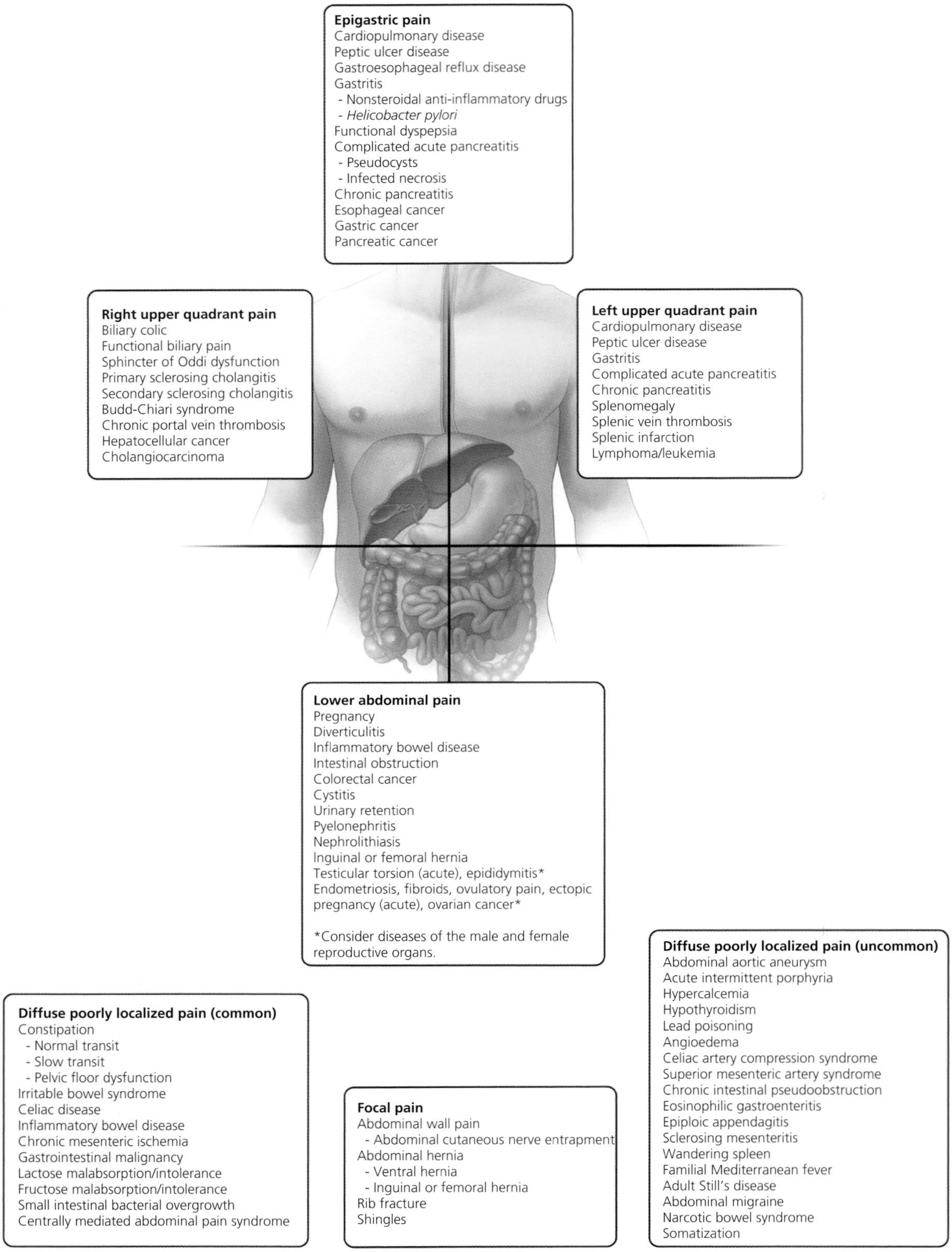

Epigastric pain
Cardiopulmonary disease
Peptic ulcer disease
Gastroesophageal reflux disease
Gastritis
- Nonsteroidal anti-inflammatory drugs
- *Helicobacter pylori*

Functional dyspepsia
Complicated acute pancreatitis
- Pseudocysts
- Infected necrosis

Chronic pancreatitis
Esophageal cancer
Gastric cancer
Pancreatic cancer

Right upper quadrant pain
Biliary colic
Functional biliary pain
Sphincter of Oddi dysfunction
Primary sclerosing cholangitis
Secondary sclerosing cholangitis
Budd-Chiari syndrome
Chronic portal vein thrombosis
Hepatocellular cancer
Cholangiocarcinoma

Left upper quadrant pain
Cardiopulmonary disease
Peptic ulcer disease
Gastritis
Complicated acute pancreatitis
Chronic pancreatitis
Splenomegaly
Splenic vein thrombosis
Splenic infarction
Lymphoma/leukemia

Lower abdominal pain
Pregnancy
Diverticulitis
Inflammatory bowel disease
Intestinal obstruction
Colorectal cancer
Cystitis
Urinary retention
Pyelonephritis
Nephrolithiasis
Inguinal or femoral hernia
Testicular torsion (acute), epididymitis*
Endometriosis, fibroids, ovulatory pain, ectopic pregnancy (acute), ovarian cancer*

*Consider diseases of the male and female reproductive organs.

Diffuse poorly localized pain (common)
Constipation
- Normal transit
- Slow transit
- Pelvic floor dysfunction

Irritable bowel syndrome
Celiac disease
Inflammatory bowel disease
Chronic mesenteric ischemia
Gastrointestinal malignancy
Lactose malabsorption/intolerance
Fructose malabsorption/intolerance
Small intestinal bacterial overgrowth
Centrally mediated abdominal pain syndrome

Focal pain
Abdominal wall pain
- Abdominal cutaneous nerve entrapment

Abdominal hernia
- Ventral hernia
- Inguinal or femoral hernia

Rib fracture
Shingles

Diffuse poorly localized pain (uncommon)
Abdominal aortic aneurysm
Acute intermittent porphyria
Hypercalcemia
Hypothyroidism
Lead poisoning
Angioedema
Celiac artery compression syndrome
Superior mesenteric artery syndrome
Chronic intestinal pseudoobstruction
Eosinophilic gastroenteritis
Epiploic appendagitis
Sclerosing mesenteritis
Wandering spleen
Familial Mediterranean fever
Adult Still's disease
Abdominal migraine
Narcotic bowel syndrome
Somatization

Figure 34.5 A location- and character-based approach to etiologies of chronic abdominal pain. Source: Kamboj A.K., Oxentenko A.S. A Diagnostic approach to chronic abdominal pain. In: Essential Medical Disorders of the Stomach and Small Intestine. Springer International Publishing; 2019: 209. Reproduced with permission of Springer Nature.

Box 34.1 Localization of common causes of acute abdominal pain.

Epigastric abdominal pain
- Esophagitis
- Gastritis
- Peptic ulcer disease
- Acute pancreatitis
- Cardiac ischemia

Right upper quadrant
- Acute cholecystitis
- Biliary colic
- Acute hepatic inflammation

Left upper quadrant
- Splenic infarct
- Splenic flexure ischemia

Right lower quadrant
- Appendicitis
- Infective terminal ileitis
- Crohn's disease
- Nephrolithiasis
- Pyelonephritis
- Tuboovarian disorders (in women)
- Ectopic pregnancy (in women)
- Ruptured ovarian cyst (in women)
- Salpingitis (in women)

Left lower quadrant
- Diverticulitis
- Infectious or inflammatory colitis
- Nephrolithiasis
- Pyelonephritis
- Tuboovarian disorders (in women)
- Ectopic pregnancy (in women)
- Ruptured ovarian cyst (in women)
- Salpingitis (in women)

Diffuse abdominal pain
- Acute peritonitis
- Spontaneous peritonitis in cirrhosis
- Inflammatory bowel disease
- Toxic megacolon
- Perforated ulcer (gastric or duodenal)
- Irritable bowel syndrome
- Complicated pancreatitis (with ileus, fluid collections, necrosis)
- Acute mesenteric ischemia
- Bowel obstruction
- Other (familial Mediterranean fever, porphyria, etc.)

the likely source of pain (e.g., right lower quadrant pain in appendicitis, left lower quadrant in diverticulitis, and Murphy's sign in acute cholecystitis).

Onset, chronicity, temporal characteristics

Duration and the pattern of variation with time are important features to elicit in taking the patient's history. Patients should be asked about when their pain first began as this can help distinguish acute from chronic abdominal pain. In general, acute abdominal pain tends to have a sudden onset and short duration. Immediate-onset, severe pain is suggestive of an acute obstruction of a hollow viscus (e.g., bile duct obstruction by a stone), perforation (e.g., free perforation of a duodenal ulcer), or a catastrophic ischemic condition. More commonly, onset of pain is gradual; the transition from a "glowing ember" to a "raging flame" may take hours or days depending upon the underlying condition and is typical of inflammatory conditions such as appendicitis, diverticulitis, pancreatitis, and cholecystitis.

Abrupt cessation of pain can occasionally occur and could suggest the relief of an obstructed organ; examples include passage of a biliary stone or resolution of a volvulus. However, in many cases, the pain is intermittent in that it wanes for varying intervals of time, only to wax to its original intensity subsequently. Such pain is typical of colic, usually intestinal in origin. Biliary pain, though traditionally labeled as colic, shows less variability than commonly thought (see Differential diagnosis).

In addition to intermittency, another pattern of temporal variation is periodicity, implying a long duration (weeks to months) of pain-free intervals. Such periodicity is seldom patterned or regular (unless pain is pelvic and related to the menstrual cycle) and, among others, used to be characteristic of peptic ulcer disease (PUD) before effective therapy was available. Other examples include patients with recurrent urinary stones and IBS. For the latter, the pain often varies with periods of psychosocial stress and associated disturbances in bowel function. Other conditions that can present with intermittent abdominal pain are highlighted in Box 34.2.

Finally, the duration of the pain should be mentioned as an important factor in that it has a direct bearing on the degree of difficulty in reaching a diagnosis. The clinical picture may be further clouded by the presence of confounding factors including referred hyperalgesia (see Neurobiology of pain above), secondary psychosocial morbidity, and aberrant illness behaviors.

Box 34.2 Some causes of intermittent abdominal pain.

Physical/obstructive
- Biliary colic
- Intermittent intestinal obstruction
  - Adhesions
  - Intussusception
  - Internal hernia
  - Abdominal wall hernia

Metabolic and/or genetic
- Acute intermittent porphyria
- Familial Mediterranean fever

Neurological
- Abdominal epilepsy
- Abdominal migraine
- Diabetic and other forms of radiculopathy
- Nerve entrapment syndromes

Miscellaneous
- Endometriosis
- Heavy metal (lead) poisoning
- Chronic mesenteric ischemia
- Recurrent pancreatitis

Intensity and character of pain

These attributes are sometimes less useful diagnostically because, by their very nature, they are subjective and may be influenced by the social and educational background of the patient as well as past personal experiences. Patients can be asked to rate their pain using a straightforward scale ranging from 1 to 10, typically using a previously encountered pain as a reference point. The clinician can clarify that a "10" on this scale refers to the worst pain in the patient's life. The pain scale, however, is seldom useful in distinguishing the cause of the pain or even whether the pain is organic or not.

Similar considerations apply to the description of the characteristics of the pain. For example, the pain associated with peptic ulcer disease has been described by such apparently contradictory terms as aching, gnawing, sharp, burning, tearing, and squeezing. Furthermore, patients often ascribe different meanings to common descriptors. While many patients often associate colic with any diarrheal illness, from a medical perspective, the pain of colic refers to a characteristic wave-like build-up in intensity culminating in severe pain, often associated with other symptoms such as sweating, nausea, and dizziness [33]. Colicky pain can also be described as having a crescendo-decrescendo pattern where the pain escalates in intensity over a period of time only to decrease thereafter. The pain of colic is the result of visceral obstruction and peristaltic contractions associated with increased intraluminal pressure and generally is similar in character regardless of the organ involved (Box 34.3). As previously noted, biliary disorders, although described as causing "colic," rarely cause the characteristic pain of colic, as the pain from biliary disease is often constant.

Relieving and aggravating factors

It is important to elicit the relationship, if any, between fluctuations in pain and physiological gastrointestinal activity. Such a relationship may allow the physician to more confidently link the pain to a hollow viscus (rather than musculoskeletal causes) as well as point towards a specific diagnosis. Thus, pain with swallowing (odynophagia) almost invariably points to an esophageal lesion. The pain of duodenal ulcer tends to improve with food or antacid use while gastric ulcer pain may be worsened by food intake. Relief after vomiting suggests a pyloric abnormality or proximal small bowel lesion. Colonic pain or distress may be relieved by a bowel movement, particularly in patients with IBS. In contrast, anorectal conditions such as proctitis or fissures may be aggravated by bowel movements.

Most inflammatory conditions of the bowel or solid organs (such as IBD or pancreatitis) are associated with varying degrees of systemic reaction including anorexia, malaise, and perhaps fever. The exception is duodenal ulcer, which may prompt the patient to increase food intake because of the perceived association with lessening of the pain. The specific nature of the food that either relieves or aggravates pain is seldom of diagnostic value, contrary to popular belief. Thus, the relationship between fatty foods and biliary pain or between spicy foods and peptic ulcer pain is dubious, at best [34].

Visceral pain by itself often induces restlessness in the patient, but when parietal or somatic structures become involved, aggravation by motion, coughing, or straining is characteristically noted. Retroperitoneal processes, including pancreatitis, tend to be somewhat relieved by maneuvers that increase the volume of this space (sitting up and bending forward).

Review of systems

An extensive review of systems, including GI and non-GI features, should be reviewed as these can provide important clues. Constitutional symptoms include fevers, chills, night sweats, weight loss, and fatigue. Important GI symptoms that should be discussed include dysphagia or odynophagia, nausea or vomiting, bloating or distension, jaundice, constipation, diarrhea, or change in bowel habits, as well as melena, hematemesis, or hematochezia. Cardiovascular etiologies can sometimes present with epigastric pain and it is important to elicit whether the patient has concomitant chest pain, shortness of breath, orthopnea, paroxysmal nocturnal dyspnea, lower extremity edema, or syncope; the relationship of symptoms to exertion and activity should also be sought.

Box 34.3 Common causes of colicky abdominal pain.

- Biliary colic
- Renal colic
- Gastrointestinal colic
- Acute gastroenteritis
- Small bowel obstruction
  - Crohn's disease
  - Postsurgical adhesions
  - Pseudoobstruction
  - Intussusception
- Colonic obstruction
  - Carcinoma
  - Diverticulitis
  - Postsurgical adhesions
  - Internal hernia

Physical examination

Acute, severe abdominal pain is best dealt with as an emergency and in many instances may warrant urgent surgical intervention (see Chapter 37). As with any acute medical condition, the physical examination should be directed first at the patient's vital signs in order to determine whether the patient is hemodynamically stable or is in need of emergency evaluation or resuscitation. These pseudoaffective responses are objective and reproducible signs of the severity of the patient's condition and should constitute the first part of clinical assessment of any patient with acute abdominal pain.

The remainder of the abdominal physical exam should be performed systematically as follows.

- *Inspection* noting any surgical scars, visible peristalsis, or the presence of abdominal distension.

- *Auscultation* of the abdomen is generally limited in utility but does provide broad clues as to the state of the bowels; in this regard, it is not necessary or helpful to auscultate all four quadrants. Hypoactive or absent bowel sounds are characteristic in the presence of peritonitis whereas hyperactive sounds throughout the abdomen may be heard with infectious gastroenteritis. Infrequent, prolonged rushes of high-pitched or "tinkling" peristalsis are often heard over the distended loops of bowel seen with intestinal obstruction.
- *Palpation and percussion* can identify localized masses, free peritoneal fluid such as ascites, or areas of tenderness. It can also determine whether localized or diffuse peritoneal inflammation is present. Eliciting rebound tenderness, a sign of peritonitis, may be useful when positive but may not be always reliable [35]. The success of palpation and percussion depends on the examiner's technique as well on the patient's cooperation. It can be difficult to differentiate guarding and tenderness caused by peritoneal inflammation from voluntary guarding caused by the brusque contact of an examiner's cold hands. Palpation should be performed with warm hands and begin away from the area of maximal tenderness.
- *A rectal and/or pelvic examination* should strongly be considered in patients with abdominal pain depending on the patient and features of the pain, as conditions such as constipation or disorders of the female reproductive organs may be contributing.

There are several specialized physical examination signs associated with various conditions that present with acute abdominal pain. *Murphy's sign* can be elicited by palpating the subcostal region in the right upper quadrant during inspiration; Murphy's sign is considered positive if pain is elicited with an abrupt halt in inspiration and is suggestive of acute cholecystitis [36]. Characteristic findings associated with acute appendicitis include the *psoas sign* (pain on passive extension of the right thigh), *obturator sign* (pain on passive internal rotation of the flexed right thigh), and *Rovsing sign* (palpation of the left lower quadrant elicits increased right lower quadrant pain) [37].

Diagnostic work-up

The diagnostic work-up for acute abdominal pain is addressed in Chapter 37. The clinical differential generated by a careful history and physical examination should lead to appropriate laboratory and imaging tests to either confirm or refute the diagnosis. The main approaches are based on blood tests to assess infections, inflammation, and impact on general health (e.g., renal impairment, acidosis) and noninvasive imaging typically with ultrasound or computed tomography. However, despite the fact that acute abdominal pain is traditionally equated with a surgical diagnosis, less than 5% of adults presenting with acute abdominal pain will require hospital admission, and even less will need surgery [38]. Indeed, in a substantial proportion of patients with acute abdominal pain, particularly those seen in a primary care setting or emergency room, no definite abdominal pathology will be found to account for the symptoms [39].

Chronic abdominal pain

History and physical examination

Chronic abdominal pain can result from various organic and functional [40] conditions, as discussed in greater detail in other chapters. Many of the same principles related to the history and physical examination of acute abdominal pain outlined earlier apply to patients in less emergent settings. The patient history should be comprehensive and elicit various features of pain, related to the site, onset, chronicity, temporal characteristics, character and intensity, relieving and aggravating factors, and review of systems. Chronic abdominal pain typically occurs over several weeks to months. While a quadrant-based approach can be used, patients with chronic painful conditions (including IBS) often have distorted patterns of pain compared to healthy volunteers (possibly due to spinal sensitization of convergent pathways, see section on Neurobiology of pain), rendering inference about the site of pain less reliable [41]. If other episodes of pain have occurred previously, it can help a clinician understand which treatment options may or may not work for the patient based on their prior experience.

In patients with chronic abdominal pain, the physical examination should be guided by patient history and may include inspection, auscultation, palpation, and percussion of the abdomen and a rectal and/or pelvic examination. Given the long-standing nature of the pain, vital signs are less likely to be affected compared to acute abdominal pain. Similarly, abdominal palpation is less likely to elicit peritoneal signs such as rebound tenderness or guarding compared to acute pain. Attention should be paid to skin lesions or rashes, pallor, jaundice, edema, and other obvious signs of a more generalized disorder (Table 34.1).

Carnett's sign

Acute recurrent abdominal pain, characterized by repeated attacks of pain, the patient being entirely well between these episodic bouts, can prove very difficult to diagnose. It is important to try and see the patient during an attack, as it is frequently the only time when it is possible to identify the correct diagnosis. When no obvious clinical or laboratory clues to a specific disease process are seen, the Carnett's test (Figure 34.6) may help to determine whether chronic intermittent abdominal pain arises from the abdominal wall or has an intraabdominal origin [42–44]. In this test, the clinician first palpates the area of a maximal tenderness. Once the tender spot is identified, the patient is asked to raise their legs or lift their head, thus tensing the abdominal musculature. If there is greater tenderness on repeat palpation with tensing, the Carnett's test is positive and suggests a cause in the abdominal wall (see Chronic abdominal wall pain). Diminished tenderness, on the other hand, may suggest an intraabdominal process.

Differential diagnosis

The differential diagnosis of "abdominal pain" is immense. Familiarity with broad pathophysiological principles of visceral pain and knowledge of common gastrointestinal diseases and

Table 34.1 Clues to the etiology of abdominal pain on clinical examination.

Physical finding	Related conditions
Jaundice	Choledocholithiasis Gallstone pancreatitis Liver failure Acute hepatitis
Rash/skin lesions	Celiac disease (dermatitis herpetiformis) Inflammatory bowel disease (erythema nodosum, pyoderma gangrenosum) Henoch–Schönlein purpura (petechiae)
Distended abdomen	Bowel obstruction Ascites
Palpable fullness	Hernia Neoplasm
Focal neurological finding	Nerve root compression Vertebral body fracture
Anal fissure (lateral)	Crohn's disease
Dark red "port-wine" urine	Acute intermittent porphyria
Occult blood in stool	Bowel inflammation Peptic ulcer disease Gastrointestinal cancer
Positive Carnett's test[a]	Cutaneous nerve entrapment Myofascial pain syndromes Rectus sheath hematoma Rib tip syndrome

[a] Worsening abdominal pain on contraction of the abdominal wall muscle.Source: Adapted from Zackowski S.W. Chronic recurrent abdominal pain. Emerg Med Clin North Am1998;16:877.

their natural history serves as a foundation for an appropriate approach to the patient. Informed clinical suspicion then should lead to further laboratory and radiological testing. Individual diseases are dealt with in their entirety in other chapters throughout this textbook. There are specific clues to suspect some conditions (Table 34.2).

When a careful history and examination and routine laboratory tests fail to reveal a cause of abdominal pain, consideration should be given to rarer syndromes [45] (Table 34.3).

Diagnostic work-up

The clinical differential generated by a careful history and physical examination should lead to appropriate laboratory and imaging tests to either confirm or refute the diagnosis. A definitive diagnosis is often uncommon among those referred for evaluation of chronic abdominal pain, as many of these patients have already been seen and evaluated by other physicians, and the most straightforward diagnoses having already been excluded. Indeed, in the absence of obvious clinical or laboratory clues, it is relatively unusual to uncover a new pathophysiological basis for symptoms in these patients [46]. Tests to exclude other diagnoses must be carefully considered and be based on the individual presentation and the degree of suspicion for underlying pathology and the presence or absence of "red flags" (Box 34.4).

In general, tests such as capsule endoscopy [50–53], ERCP or MRCP [54,55], and measurements of gastrointestinal transit have low yield for chronic abdominal pain lasting >6 months. Laparoscopy with or without lysis of adhesions also has low utility and the validity of the diagnosis of adhesions as a cause of

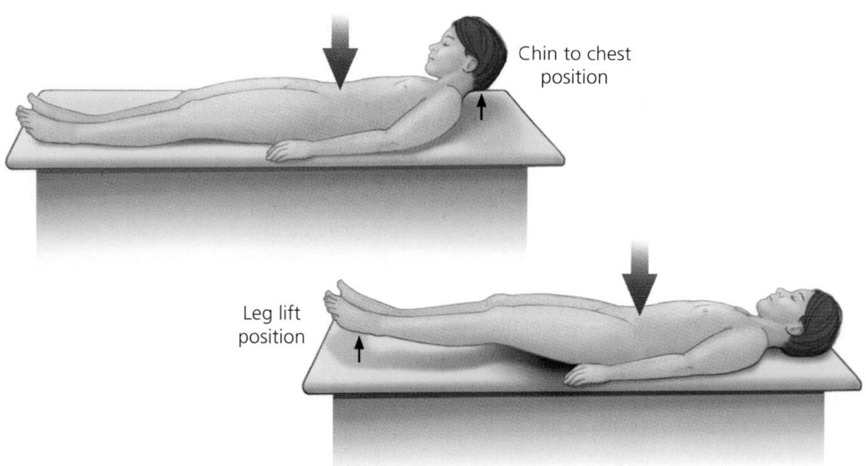

Figure 34.6 Presence of Carnett's sign can be used to diagnose chronic abdominal wall pain. Source: from Kamboj et al. [44]. Reproduced with permission of Elsevier.

Table 34.2 Characteristics of disease processes based on the origin of pain.

Origin of pain	Example of disease process	Location and radiation	Character	Aggravating or relieving factors
Gastroduodenal	Peptic ulcer (NSAIDs, *H. pylori* infection)	Midepigastric, left upper quadrant	Dull, "empty feeling," nocturnal	Food may aggravate (gastric ulcers) or relieve (duodenal ulcers); antacids relieve
Biliary	Biliary colic, acute cholecystitis	Midline (early), right upper quadrant (late), may radiate to the right infrascapsular region	Dull, colicky	May occur after a large, fatty meal
Pancreatic	Acute or chronic pancreatitis, pancreatic cancer	Midline, may radiate to the back	Sharp (acute), dull (chronic)	Alcohol may aggravate (acute pancreatitis)
Liver	Hepatitis, hepatic abscess, hepatocellular cancer	Right upper quadrant, diffuse	Dull	Alcohol, infection, and certain medications may aggravate (hepatitis)
Spleen	Splenomegaly (infectious mononucleosis, hematological disorders, malignancy, portal hypertension)	Left upper quadrant	Dull	
Small bowel	Duodenal ulcer, small bowel obstruction, ischemia	Midline, periumbilical, back, flank	Dull, colicky	Food may aggravate (obstruction/ischemia) or alleviate (duodenal ulcer)
Colonic	Constipation, IBD, colon cancer	Midline, lower abdomen	Dull	May vary with bowel movements
Rectal	Proctitis, hemorrhoids, rectal cancer, proctalgia fugax	Rectum	Tenesmus (urgency to defecate), sharp or dull	May vary with bowel movements

IBD, inflammatory bowel disease; NSAIDs, nonsteroidal antiinflammatory drugs.

unexplained abdominal pain is questionable [47]. Diagnostic laparoscopy often does not lead to a change in management [48]. Adhesions are very common in women, even in the absence of prior surgery [49] and are found in equal proportion in patients complaining of pelvic pain and those with other complaints [50]. In fact, randomized trials of laparoscopic adhesiolysis versus diagnostic laparoscopy alone have not shown any benefit from the former and the complication rate is high [51,52]. However, in cases where abdominal imaging suggests a partial or intermittent bowel obstruction from adhesions, this is a reasonable approach.

There is a risk of identifying incidental findings on these tests that are of questionable relevance to the patient's complaints (e.g., minimal changes in the secondary branches of the pancreatic duct). Before acting on these abnormalities, the prudent physician must carefully reevaluate the patient, going through an extensive checklist, such as that in Box 34.4, looking for "red flags."

Recognition and management of special abdominal pain syndromes

Chronic abdominal wall pain

Pain arising primarily in the abdominal wall can result from a heterogeneous and poorly defined group of conditions whose description remains largely anecdotal (Table 34.4) [53]. However, this condition is common and associated with significant healthcare costs, largely because it is so often overlooked [54]. In one report, chronic abdominal wall pain (CAWP) and IBS comprised 7.8% and 16.3% of symptomatic referrals, respectively [55]. As with other chronic abdominal pain syndromes, CAWP predominantly affects women; depression and obesity were comorbid conditions that were commonly present. The prevalence of CAWP has been reported to range from 10% to nearly 40% in referral clinics and up to 1% of all general surgical diagnoses [43,54,56]. An accurate diagnosis can result in marked decrease in physician visits and procedures with overall annual costs decreasing from around $1100 to $500 [55].

After Spigelian hernias or obvious traumatic tears are excluded, CAWP is often thought to result from some form of nerve entrapment, which has led to one of its many names in the literature – anterior cutaneous nerve entrapment syndrome (ACNES). This syndrome is also called myofascial pain syndrome and rectus syndrome, with little to suggest any phenotypic differences. The diagnosis is suggested when the pain is superficial, localized to a small area that is usually significantly tender, associated with dysesthesia in the involved region, and when Carnett's sign (see above) (see Figure 34.6) is positive. If there is an obvious scar from previous surgery or injury, a diagnosis of entrapment neuropathy (with or without a

Table 34.3 Rare or obscure causes of abdominal pain.

Condition	Characteristic features and diagnostic clues	Additional tests
Shingles (varicella-zoster)	Pain may precede rash by 5–7 days Dermatomal distribution	Appearance of rash Positive VZV testing
Compressive radiculopathy	Dermatomal distribution Tenderness/pain of spinal and paraspinal structures	CT or MRI
Lead poisoning	Crampy intermittent pain Bowel disturbance and nausea Dark blue pigment along gum line, anemia, and basophilic stippling	Elevated serum lead levels or urinary heavy metal screen
Narcotic withdrawal	12–36 h after abrupt cessation Nausea, diarrhea, and cramps Excessive secretion of tears, sweat, rhinorrhea, etc. Hyperdynamic bowel sounds	History of drug intake
Familial Mediterranean fever	Childhood onset Mediterranean ancestry Peritoneal signs and fever Meningitis, pericarditis, pleuritis, and arthritis may occur	Family history Genetic testing Exclusion of other causes
Acute intermittent porphyria	Diffuse "colicky" abdominal pain Associated changes in mental status, muscle weakness, and photosensitivity Port-wine urine False-positive urobilonogen (i.e., normal serum indirect bilirubin) reading on urine dipstick (due to porphobilinogen)	Urinary porphobilinogen
"Abdominal epilepsy" (temporal lobe seizures)	Pediatric patients Sharp abdominal pain, often periumblical in nature Accompanied by motor, psychic, or other sensory features	Electroencephalography
"Abdominal migraine"	Pediatric patients Associated migraine Nausea and occasional vomiting	Diagnosis of exclusion
Hereditary angioneurotic edema	Submucosal edema with intestinal obstruction Cutaneous manifestations	Measurement of plasma C1 esterase activity
Abdominal vasculitides	Poorly localized pain or tenderness GI bleeding Associated systemic disease (Henoch–Schönlein purpura, lupus, etc.)	Angiography (MR or direct) Diagnosis of systemic disease Rheumatological titers

CT, computed tomography; GI, gastrointestinal; MRI, magnetic resonance imaging; VZV, varicella-zoster virus.

Box 34.4 Questions to assess a patient with pain: red flags for referral to specialists in functional bowel disease.

Clinical issues

Does the patient:

Have pain that has persisted for 3 months or longer?

- despite appropriate interventions?
- in the absence of progressive diseases?

Have unrealistic expectations of:

- healthcare provider?
- treatment offered?

Complain about previous healthcare providers?

Have a history of substance abuse?

Display pain behaviors?

- grimacing
- rigid or guarded movement

Legal and occupational issues

Is litigation pending?

Is the patient receiving disability compensation?

Was the patient employed before the onset of the pain?

Is there a job to which the patient can return?

Does the patient have a history of frequent changes in occupation?

Psychosocial issues

Do other family members also suffer from chronic pain?

Excessive depression or inappropriate moods present?

Major stressful event before onset of pain exacerbation?

- high levels of marital or family conflict?

History of childhood abuse or other sexual trauma?

Activities given up because of pain?

- plans for renewed or increased activities if pain is reduced?

Source: Adapted from Turk and Okifuji 1999 [271].

Table 34.4 Etiology of abdominal wall pain.

Etiology	Comments	Diagnosis
Hernia	Protuberance in abdominal wall that usually decreases in size when patient is supine	Abdominal CT scanning, abdominal ultrasonography, herniography
Rectus nerve entrapment	Occurs along lateral edge of rectus sheath; worsening of pain with tensing of muscles	Injection of local anesthetic
Thoracic lateral cutaneous nerve entrapment	Occurs spontaneously, after surgery or during pregnancy	History and physical examination
Ilioinguinal and iliohypogastric nerve entrapment	Lower abdominal pain that occurs after inguinal hernia repair	History and physical examination
Endometriosis	Cyclic abdominal pain	Laparoscopy
Diabetic radiculopathy	Acute, severe truncal pain involving T6–T12 nerve roots	Paraspinal EMG
Abdominal wall tear	Occurs mainly in athletes	History and physical examination
Abdominal wall hematoma	Complication of abdominal procedures	Abdominal CT scanning, abdominal ultrasonography
Spontaneous rectus sheath hematoma	Presents as tender, usually unilateral mass that does not extend beyond midline	Abdominal CT scanning, abdominal ultrasonography
Desmoid tumor	Dysplastic tumor of connective tissue; occurs in young patients (females more often than males)	Surgical excision
Herpes zoster	Pain and hyperesthesia followed by vesicles along a dermatome	History and physical examination
Spinal nerve irritation	Caused by disorders of thoracic spine	CT scanning or MRI studies of thoracic spine
Slipping rib syndrome	Sharp, stabbing pain in upper abdomen caused by luxation of 8th–10th ribs	Hooking maneuver to pull lower ribs anteriorly, which reproduces the pain and sometimes a click
Idiopathic	Myofascial pain	History and physical examination

CT, computed tomography; EMG, electromyography; MRI, magnetic resonance imaging.Source: Adapted from Suleiman and Johnston 2001 [53].

"neuroma") is often entertained. In the absence of a scar, the pain is postulated to arise from so-called "myofascial trigger points" or abdominal cutaneous nerve entrapment due to a fibrous ring in the rectus muscle, through which the rectus neurovascular bundle travels [57] (Figure 34.7).

"Trigger" point injection (TPI) with local anesthetics is popularly regarded as a useful method to distinguish abdominal wall pain from that of visceral origin [58]. However, this approach may be subject to flawed interpretation. A characteristic of visceral pain is referral to somatic structures including the skin and abdominal wall. In some cases, these sites can in turn become sensitized and contribute to the overall pain sensation to varying degrees. It is conceivable that, in some patients, this contribution becomes dominant and its interruption by local anesthetics is sufficient to eliminate the pain nearly completely, giving rise to a false assumption about the source of pain. This may account for some of the observed inaccuracy in the predictive value of the abdominal wall tenderness test [59]. Nevertheless, clinical experience suggests that the diagnosis of CAWP by a combination of clinical findings and response to trigger point injection is surprisingly robust and does not change in 90–97% of patients over the long term [55,60].

Local neural blockade has been reported to be more successful in patients with chronic pain secondary to abdominal wall causes [53,61]. Once a trigger point has been identified by examination, a needle is inserted and a small amount of local anesthetic along with a corticosteroid (typically bupivacaine and triamcinolone) is injected at the site of greatest tenderness elicited by the tip of the needle. A placebo-controlled trial demonstrated that this is not simply a placebo response to an injection [62]. The response can be long-lasting and up to one-third of patients do not require another injection [63]. In those who have relief that is temporary, repeated injections may be necessary. However, patients may also benefit from surgical neurectomy, as shown in a randomized sham-controlled trial [64]. Other controlled studies suggest that these patients may respond to local lidocaine patches or even botulinum toxin [65,66]. Exacerbating activities such as abdominal crunches or plank exercises should be avoided. Thus, this is a relatively common and treatable condition.

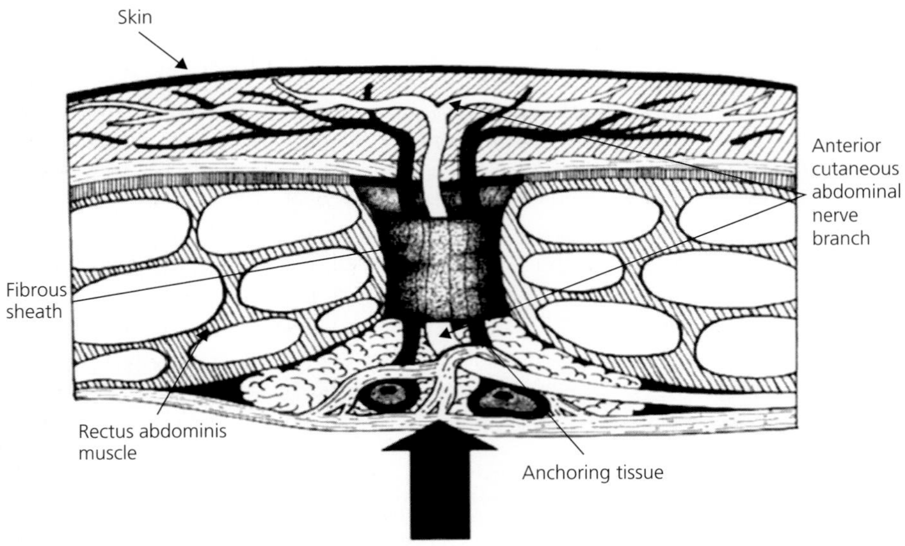

Figure 34.7 Schematized course of the anterior cutaneous nerve in the abdominal wall. Note the theoretical vulnerability to pressure-induced injury and hence generation of neuropathic pain. Source: Greenbaum 2006 [54]. Reproduced with permission of Taylor & Francis.

Centrally mediated abdominal pain syndrome

Patients who have chronic abdominal pain that remains unexplained despite a careful and detailed evaluation represent a significant clinical challenge to gastroenterologists who often become the de facto caretakers of these patients. In recent years, it has become evident that these patients as a group share enough common features to warrant consideration of a distinct descriptor, the centrally mediated abdominal pain syndrome (CAPS) [67,71] (Box 34.5). This was previously referred to as the functional abdominal pain syndrome or FAPS (Rome III); the name was changed to reflect the strong central component of this disease. It is not synonymous with other functional bowel disorders such as IBS or functional dyspepsia, which also feature pain. The distinction is based upon the lack of association with physiological gastrointestinal events such as eating or defecation in CAPS.

Box 34.5 Rome IV diagnostic criteria for centrally mediated abdominal pain syndrome. The criteria must be fulfilled for the last 3 months with symptom onset at least 6 months before diagnosis.

- Continuous or nearly continuous abdominal pain
- No or only occasional relationship of pain with physiological events (e.g., eating, defecation, or menses)
- Pain limits some aspect of daily functioning
- The pain is not feigned
- Pain is not explained by another structural or functional gastrointestinal disorder or other medical condition

Source: Keefer L., Drossman D.A., Guthrie E., et al. Centrally mediated disorders of gastrointestinal pain. Gastroenterology 2016;150:1408. Reproduced with permission of Elsevier.

In general, the features that are discussed below and attributed to CAPS are derived from prior studies of FAPS. Chronic abdominal pain in the absence of association with physiological GI events (which would now be categorized as CAPS) is relatively uncommon compared to typical IBS; in a US householder survey, it was found in only about 2% of respondents and appeared to increase with age, with women accounting for more than two-thirds of patients [72]. In other countries, the incidence has been even lower, ranging from 0.1% to 0.5% [73,74]. Nevertheless, patients with CAPS are heavy users of medical resources with a high morbidity [69].

Centrally mediated abdominal pain syndrome is a poorly understood disorder and is attributed to altered brain sensory processing with cognitive, emotional, or other sensory information, and genetic and environmental factors [71]. The responsiveness to tricyclic antidepressants has been said to indicate an underlying neuropathic process [68]. Patients with CAPS may have psychological disturbances or personality disorders and are often functionally impaired at many levels including work, family, and social settings [75]. They frequently suffer from depression, anxiety, sleep disturbances, withdrawal, decreased activity, fatigue, loss of libido, and morbid preoccupation with the chronic pain [76–78]. Many patients experienced abdominal pain in childhood, and often have relatives with abdominal pain [75]. A history of previous physical or sexual abuse is very frequent, up to 50% in some series [79]. The onset of pain may also be associated with the demise of a relative, spouse, or other figure important to the patient [80].

There is considerable overlap between CAPS and other somatoform pain disorders (physical complaints for which no adequate medical explanation exists) with heightened nociception, poor coping or response strategies that lead to aberrant illness behavior. This may be associated with specific neurophysiological abnormalities in the brain on experimental imaging; visceral sensitization does not appear to be as prominent as in patients with IBS [67]. Pain may serve many functions in these patients including a means of atonement, explanation for lack of success, and a morbid replacement for loss of relationships. Finally, it is possible that because of positive reinforcement, other behaviors (e.g., appearing uncomfortable and helpless, not reporting for work) may be reinforced by the gains the patient may feel, including increased or renewed attention and empathy from within the family structure, avoidance of the stresses associated with work and family responsibilities, and monetary compensation. Thus, in susceptible individuals, a set of behaviors becomes established that contributes to the maintenance of chronic pain.

Centrally mediated abdominal pain syndrome is associated with characteristic features: pain may be constant or nearly constant, occurs most days in bouts lasting from several hours to days or weeks, with residual pain, albeit not as severe or incapacitating between severe exacerbations. The abdominal pain is usually described in vague terms, sometimes through unusual, idiosyncratic, or even bizarre language, relatively unchanging in character, intensity, and location [80]. In contrast to other chronic pain related to a specific pathological diagnosis, which usually occurs with particular physiological activities (e.g., eating or defecation), this relationship is absent with CAPS. Lack of weight loss in the absence of significant depression and lack of fever also supports a diagnosis of CAPS. Although nocturnal pain is often assumed to be "organic," functional pain may also sometimes awaken patients from their sleep [81]. CAPS is also associated with various somatic complaints [82,83]. Other clues at the time of the interview may provide insight into social impairments contributing to the clinical presentation. These include the constant presence of a spouse or parent who assumes responsibility as a "go-between" with the physician and the patient, suggesting family "enmeshment" that may be contributing to illness behavior.

Physical examination findings that are suggestive but not diagnostic are absence of signs of autonomic activation (e.g., tachycardia, diaphoresis), inconsistent tenderness, discrepancy between tenderness elicited with pressure from the stethoscope and that from the examining hand, clutching of the physician's arm during the examination and the "closed eyes sign" (characterized by the patient keeping his or her eyes closed, often with a fixed, beatific smile, during abdominal palpation [84]).

If not established through the initial series of investigations, a gastrointestinal cause for the symptoms is rarely found through subsequent investigations (including surgical exploration) or follow-up visits [83,85]. Nevertheless, demands by patients and their families may lead to more invasive and costly tests in the hope of uncovering the elusive explanation for the patient's symptoms. Such activity ("furor medicus" [86]) in fact may be counterproductive as it reinforces the patient's conviction that there is something wrong to account for the pain that, if only found, could be successfully corrected. Often, when a "cause" is discovered, it is not clear whether it is truly the source of the pain, an incidental finding/epiphenomenon, or a consequence of the treatment, often surgical, used in an attempt to treat the original complaint [87]. In most of these cases, despite such "diagnosis" and treatment of the presumed cause of pain, the pain remains, or a new type of pain is manifest elsewhere.

Patients with chronic intractable abdominal pain are rarely substantially pain free after one or more years of follow-up [80], emphasizing the importance of focusing on adaptation to the pain rather than cure. Palliation is therefore an appropriate goal and it is achievable in most patients using a multidimensional approach used for other forms of chronic pain, with greater emphasis on the psychosocial dimensions [67,69]. These patients can be taxing in terms of time and resources and forming an effective patient–physician relationship can be challenging. Nevertheless, without such a relationship, little therapeutic gain can be expected. Familiarity with different neuromodulators is very important as many of these patients often complain of "intolerance" to one or more medications, which may be a component of their illness behavior rather than representing a true adverse effect [67]. One approach is illustrated in Figure 34.8. Regardless of what the caring physician believes is the origin of the pain (peripheral versus central, functional versus organic), the *suffering* is real, affecting the patient and everybody in the circle of people that care for him or her.

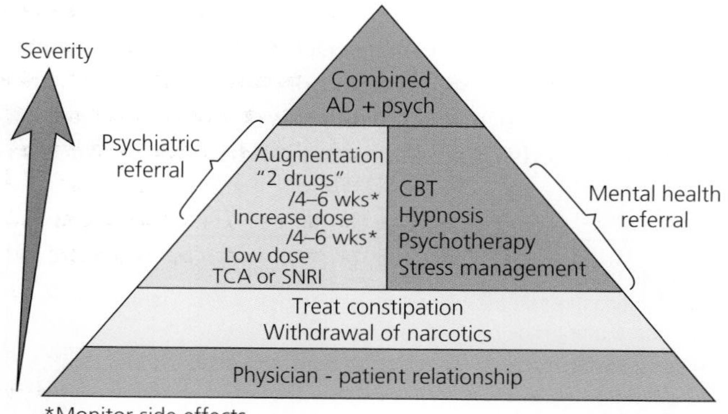

Figure 34.8 Treatment algorithm for functional abdominal pain syndrome. Beginning with an effective patient–physician relationship, treatments are added on the basis of the severity of the symptoms. Constipation if present is treated, and narcotics if present are withdrawn. Next, prescribe a low-dose tricyclic antidepressant (TCA) or serotonin/norepinephrine reuptake inhibitor (SNRI), and after 4–6 weeks this dosage can be increased while monitoring for clinical benefit and side-effects. If this is unsuccessful, psychiatric referral should be considered for augmentation treatment with another antidepressant (e.g., selective serotonin reuptake inhibitor [SSRI], bupropion), buspirone, or an atypical antipsychotic. On occasion, the patient might first be referred to a mental health counselor for psychological treatment. With more severe symptoms, combined pharmacological and behavioral intervention is needed. Source: Drossman 2008 [88]. Reproduced with permission of Elsevier.

Narcotic bowel syndrome

Narcotic bowel syndrome (NBS), also known as opiate-induced gastrointestinal hyperalgesia, refers to abdominal pain that occurs with continuous or increasing opioid use [89]. The diagnostic criteria for this syndrome are highlighted in Box 34.6 [71].

Opioids are a commonly prescribed medication class in the US and over the past two decades, their use has soared [90]. Patients may have been prescribed opioids for GI disorders (e.g., chronic pancreatitis and CAPS), non-GI disorders (e.g., fibromyalgia), malignancy, or after surgery. With time, the patient may require increasing doses of opioids for pain control due to development of tolerance or tachyphylaxis.

There are several mechanisms that have been postulated to describe the hyperalgesia associated with opioid use. Glial cell activation in the spinal cord may result in enhanced pain via release of neuroexcitatory substances in response to opioids [91]. Patients may present with poorly localizable abdominal pain. Other symptoms such as dysphagia, nausea, vomiting, constipation, and overflow diarrhea may be present and relate to opioid side-effects. Similar to CAPS, the cornerstone of management involves an effective patient–physician relationship. Treatment involves complete detoxification which requires patient trust and engagement given that opioids had originally been prescribed for "pain relief" [92]. Treatment is unlikely to be effective with continuation of opioids.

Approach to treatment of chronic abdominal pain

Whenever possible, healing of the underlying tissue insult or injury provides the most satisfactory approach to the control of pain. This is discussed in the respective chapters of this book dealing with specific painful conditions. However, in a significant number of patients with pain of suspected gastrointestinal origin, the underlying condition may not be reversible or even identifiable. Pain management then often becomes the primary therapeutic issue and in such patients, it is critical for the practicing gastroenterologist to become familiar with the general principles of pain management: exclusion of need for immediate surgical exploration (see Chapter 37 for management of pain in the context of the acute abdomen); make a confident working diagnosis; and provide effective pain relief, ideally without use of opioids.

For patients with chronic abdominal pain, a successful outcome requires consideration of several factors including psychological dimension, consisting of cognitive, emotional, and behavioral processes, and functional disability that affects the quality of life in most patients. A multidisciplinary approach is needed, including involvement of pain management physicians (internists, anesthesiologists, or neurologists), clinical psychologists/psychiatrists, nurses and, often, vocational rehabilitation specialists and nutritionists. The therapeutic interventions available are correspondingly diverse, including exercise programs, cognitive and behavioral therapies, traditional pharmacological agents, alternative therapies, and nerve blocking/ablation techniques. These should be applied either sequentially or in parallel, as part of a pain management continuum, beginning with the most innocuous and progressing to more invasive strategies. It is important for the gastroenterologist to broadly understand the entire spectrum of chronic pain management as this will facilitate appropriate referral to other specialists, promote a more meaningful interaction with them, and maintain a strong and supportive patient–physician relationship instead of leading to feelings of abandonment and other negative attitudes.

Pharmacological management of chronic abdominal pain

Although effective analgesia remains the foremost goal in the pharmacological approach to patients with chronic pain, it must be remembered that there is also a valuable role for medications that treat concomitant anxiety, depression, and insomnia.

"Neuromodulator" drugs

Although the term *neuromodulation* was originally used to describe a physiological process by which neurons influence each other, it is now increasingly applied to therapies that modulate activity of the nervous system at several different levels and can be used for treatment of a variety of conditions including neuropathic pain, seizures, and psychiatric disorders [93]. The term *neuromodulator* is preferred in the context of treating pain because it is less stigmatizing for the patient and analgesic effects may be independent of the psychotropic ones.

Neuromodulator drugs (chiefly antidepressants or anticonvulsants) are typically used for neuropathic pain, including functional abdominal pain, as they affect the excitatory or inhibitory pathways (or both) involved in nociception at any level,including neuronal hyperexcitability, neurotransmitter plasticity, and aberrant "rewiring."

Box 34.6 Rome IV diagnostic criteria for narcotic bowel syndrome. The criteria must be fulfilled for the last 3 months with symptom onset at least 6 months before diagnosis.

Must include all of the following.

- Chronic or frequently recurring abdominal pain that is treated with acute high-dose or chronic narcotics
- The nature and intensity of the pain is not explained by a current or previous GI diagnosis
- Two or more of the following.
  - The pain worsens or incompletely resolves with continued or escalating dosages of narcotics
  - There is marked worsening of pain when the narcotic dose wanes and improvement when narcotics are reinstituted (soar and crash)
  - There is a progression of the frequency, duration, and intensity of pain episodes

Source: Keefer L., Drossman D.A., Guthrie E., et al. Centrally mediated disorders of gastrointestinal pain. Gastroenterology 2016;150:1408. Reproduced with permission of Elsevier.

Antidepressants are perhaps the most useful drugs for the management of both somatic and gastrointestinal chronic pain syndromes: the pharmacology and therapeutic use of these agents are summarized in Tables 34.5 and 34.6 [94]. Although their usefulness in pain management was first suggested nearly half a century ago, these drugs have not been fully embraced by either gastroenterologists or their patients who are often fearful of being stigmatized as having "mental" problems. When patients also suffer from depression, anxiety, and disturbances of sleep, neuropsychiatric effects of the drug are beneficial. However, effective analgesic doses of these drugs are significantly lower than those required to treat depression [95]. From a mechanistic perspective, these drugs share ability to increase CNS monoamine (principally serotonin and norepinephrine) neurotransmitter levels (by inhibiting their reuptake), thereby dampening nociceptive signaling at the level of the second-order neurons; however, peripheral mechanisms may also contribute [96].

Tricyclic antidepressants (TCA) have the most proven track record in the management of chronic pain, both of somatic and visceral origin. *Selective serotonin reuptake inhibitors* (SSRIs), such as paroxetine, sertraline, and fluoxetine, have fewer side-effects and have been advocated particularly for patients with functional constipation as they can increase bowel movements and even cause diarrhea. However, at the present time, studies suggest that the efficacy of these agents for chronic pain is equivocal at best [97]. A metaanalysis of antidepressant treatment for IBS concluded that these agents were quite effective for pain, with a number needed to treat of 5 (i.e., five patients needing treatment for one patient to experience symptom improvement) [98]. TCAs were more effective in the treatment of pain than SSRIs, although the latter were able to significantly improve global well-being. TCAs have been found to be helpful in the patient with the epigastric pain syndrome type of functional dyspepsia [99].

Newer antidepressants offer greater promise for relief of pain [97], as they also inhibit the uptake of norepinephrine, which appears to be important for the analgesic effect. These include the *serotonin/norepinephrine reuptake inhibitors* (SNRIs) such as venlafaxine and duloxetine. Venlafaxine decreases pain in response to colonic distension in humans, but was not found to be effective for functional dyspepsia [100,101]. Duloxetine is approved for treatment of depression and anxiety as well as painful syndromes, including fibromyalgia, and may have benefit in patients with IBS as well [102,103]. There are also possible analgesic roles for *tetracyclic compounds* such as mirtazapine with a greater effect on the uptake of norepinephrine than serotonin (mirtazapine also has several postsynaptic effects including 5-HT$_2$, 5-HT$_3$, α_2, and H$_1$) [104]; other actions include a possible gastric prokinetic effect [105]. An older agent in the same class, trazodone, has been used with good effect in patients with noncardiac chest pain [106].

Finally, dyspeptic symptoms with predominant epigastric pain may respond to best to TCAs, while those with postprandial distress (fullness, satiety) may benefit more from anxiolytics such as buspirone, which have prominent 5-HT$_{1A}$ receptor agonist activity (in addition to several other potentially beneficial mechanisms) [107].

More recently, atypical antipsychotics such as quetiapine and olanzapine are being evaluated as possible agents for the treatment of pain in functional bowel syndromes [108]. However, their use should be considered only in refractory cases and preferably in consultation with a psychiatrist as they are not approved for these indications.

Other neuromodulator drugs

A variety of antiepileptic drugs with neuronal stabilizing (phenytoin, carbamazepine, gabapentin, pregabalin, topiramate, carbamazepine, lamotrigine, lacosamide) or GABA-enhancing properties (clonazepam, valproic acid) have some utility in somatic pain syndromes, particularly of the neuropathic variety [109,110]. In this regard, the N-type calcium channel blockers, gabapentin and pregabalin (see Table 34.6) show

Table 34.5 Receptor activity and dosages for selective serotonin reuptake inhibitor (SSRI) and serotonin/norepinephrine reuptake inhibitor (SNRI) antidepressants.

Drug	Receptor activity			Dosage (mg)	
	NE	5-HT	ACh	Initial	Range
Fluoxetine	–	+4	–	10–20	20–80
Fluvoxamine	–	+4	–	25–50	50–300
Paroxetine	–	+4	+1	10–20	20–60
Sertraline	–	+4	–	25–50	50–200
Venlafaxine	+4	+3	–	25–50	25–150
Duloxetine	+4	+4	–	20–40	20–80

5-HT, 5-hydroxytryptamine; Ach, acetylcholine; NE, norepinephrine.Source: Sperber and Drossman 2011 [67]. Reproduced with permission of John Wiley & Sons.

Table 34.6 Prescribing recommendations for first-line medications for neuropathic pain.

Medication class	Starting dosage	Titration	Maximum dosage	Duration of adequate trial	Major side-effects	Precautions	Other benefits
Antidepressant medications							
Secondary amine TCAs							
Nortriptyline Desipramine	25 mg at bedtime	Increase by 25 mg daily every 3–7 days, as tolerated, until pain relief	150 mg daily; if blood level of active drug and its metabolite is <100 ng/mL (mg/mL), continue titration with caution	6–8 wk with ≥2 wk at maximum tolerated dosage	Sedation, dry mouth, blurred vision, weight gain, urinary retention	Cardiac disease, glaucoma, suicide risk, seizure disorder, concomitant use of tramadol	Improvement of depression, improvement of insomnia, low cost
SSNRIs							
Duloxetine	30 mg once daily	Increase to 60 mg once daily after 1 wk	60 mg twice daily	4 wk	Nausea	Hepatic dysfunction, renal insufficiency, alcohol abuse, concomitant use of tramadol	Improvement of depression
Venlafaxine	37.5 mg once or twice daily	Increase by 75 mg each week, as tolerated until pain relief	225 mg daily	4–6 wk	Nausea	Concomitant use of tramadol, cardiac disease, withdrawal syndrome with abrupt discontinuation	Improvement of depression
Calcium channel α_2-δ ligands							
Gabapentin	100–300 mg at bedtime or 100–300 mg 3 times daily	Increase by 100–300 mg 3 times daily every 1–7 days, as tolerated, until pain relief	3600 mg daily (1200 mg 3 times daily); reduce if impaired renal function	3–8 wk for titration + 2 weeks at maximum dose	Sedation, dizziness, peripheral edema	Renal insufficiency	Improvement of sleep disturbance, no clinically significant drug interactions
Pregabalin	50 mg 3 times daily or 75 mg twice daily	Increase to 300 mg daily after 3–7 days, then by 150 mg/day every 3–7 days, as tolerated, until pain relief	600 mg daily (200 mg 3 times daily or 300 mg twice daily); reduce if impaired renal function	4 wk	Sedation, dizziness, peripheral edema	Renal insufficiency	Improvement of sleep disturbance, improvement of anxiety, no clinically significant drug interactions

Source: O'Connor and Dworkin 2009 [272]. Reproduced with permission of Elsevier.

promise and reduce hypersensitivity in both animal studies and patients with IBS as well as chronic pancreatitis [111–120]. These drugs inhibit the A2-δ subunit of the calcium channel on the presynaptic central terminals of spinal afferents, suppress the release of neurotransmitters in the synaptic cleft, and reduce neuropathic pain [121]. One clinical trial has demonstrated benefit for pain in IBS [122]. Benzodiazepines, which are frequently used by patients with chronic pain, including insomnia, anxiety, and muscle spasm, are associated with a significant risk for dependence and there is little evidence that they have any real analgesic effect.

Opioids

Gastroenterologists often see patients with functional bowel pain or IBD treated with opioids [123]. Opioids are thought to be more effective in nociceptive pain than in neuropathic pain, which may require considerably higher doses.

In general, opioid analgesics share a common adverse effect profile: constipation, nausea, sedation, and respiratory depression. An increasingly recognized problem with chronic opioid use is narcotic bowel syndrome or opioid-induced hyperalgesia, which is a paradoxical increase in pain and analgesic requirements induced by opioids themselves [124,125]. Moreover, in some gastrointestinal disorders such as IBD, opioids may even increase mortality [126]. Perhaps the problem most physicians fear with the use of narcotic analgesics is the potential for addiction. Opioids should not be used for functional abdominal pain syndromes. However, in some patients, such as those with chronic painful pancreatitis, these drugs may be used judiciously using rigid guidelines or protocols for narcotic use (Box 34.7), with sufficient evidence for an ongoing nociceptive component and reasonable psychological stability.

Box 34.7 Guidelines for narcotic use in patients with chronic noncancer pain.

1. Clear understanding that opioids are being used for a limited term in the first instance.
2. Only one practitioner takes responsibility for opioid prescription.
3. Opioid prescription is contingent upon certain agreed obligations or goals being met by the patient, e.g., return to work or alteration of inappropriate behaviors, etc. This could take the form of a written contractual arrangement.
4. Unauthorized demands for emergency injectable opioids will not be tolerated although some provision can be made for "rescue analgesia" for brief exacerbations of pain.
5. The patient understands that opioid dosage compliance will be checked at various random intervals, which may include drug screens and blood samples.
6. Physicians must be prepared to terminate the arrangement if the goals are not met or if there is evidence of misuse, even though this may lead to a confrontational meeting with the patient.

Source: Gourlay 1999 [273]. Reproduced with permission of Wolters Kluwer Health.

Other drugs

Smooth muscle relaxants, antispasmodics, fiber, and peppermint oil may be utilized for treatment of abdominal pain in IBS [127]; these agents tend to have a favorable adverse effect profile.

Neural blockade and neurolytic therapy

Theoretically, interruption of the pain pathways should provide relief of pain that is peripheral in origin. This has led to the development of various techniques such as trigger point injections (TPIs) and neural blockade, both for diagnostic and therapeutic purposes. TPIs are commonly used for treatment of CAWP, as discussed earlier. Celiac neurolysis may be effective for up to 85% of patients with pancreatic cancer pain and about 70% of patients with pain from nonpancreatic cancers [128]. By contrast, pain relief in nonneoplastic pain such as chronic pancreatitis is not routinely recommended because of low efficacy (50% or less) and the short duration of relief (around 2 months) even in those patients who initially respond [129].

Nonconventional treatment methods

Indwelling epidural and intrathecal access systems have been effectively used for some patients with intractable chronic pain to deliver opiates and other drugs such as clonidine and baclofen [130]. A variety of electrical stimulation techniques, including peripheral (transcutaneous electrical nerve stimulation or TENS), spinal, and cerebral stimulations, have been used for various somatic pain conditions as well as for angina pectoris with encouraging results [131]. This has also been shown to decrease esophageal pain sensitivity [132]. Spinal cord electrical stimulation via implantable electrodes is a recent technique with some promise in refractory visceral pain syndromes, particularly chronic pancreatitis [133–141]. Much more clinical experience is required before these techniques can be generally endorsed.

Acupressure and acupuncture (electrical or conventional) are alternative medicine techniques that have been widely used for somatic pain, with mixed results; there is limited clinical information on this technique in patients with IBS and other functional gastrointestinal disorders [142–144]. Hypnotherapy and other psychological measures have also been tested in functional pain syndromes, particularly IBS, and there is reasonable evidence to suggest overall improvement in symptoms, with fewer proven effects on pain itself [145–149].

Conclusions

The diagnosis and management of abdominal pain, particularly when chronic, is one of the most challenging clinical problems faced by gastroenterologists. Significant progress has been made in our understanding of the pathogenesis of somatic sensitization and it is hoped that this will lead to similar advances in visceral pain. While there is a clear role for pharmacotherapy, the successful management of pain requires an intensely engaged and compassionate physician who can interpret this symptom along with the psychosocial context of the patient.

Gas and bloating

Introduction

"Doctor, I am bloated" and "I have terrible gas" or "Please look at this photo" – a still image on a cell phone showing a protuberant abdomen – are complaints frequently encountered in the GI clinic. Although estimated at 20% [2], the actual prevalence of "gas" and "bloating" is unclear because patients use many other terms to describe such symptoms, like "belching," "cramps," "loud bowel sounds," and "flatus." Sometimes these symptoms can herald the onset of organic syndromes such as malabsorption, gastrointestinal obstruction, bacterial overgrowth, or alterations in sensorimotor function of the gut. For others, they can represent anxiety-related bowel dysfunction. The clinical challenge for the clinician is to identify an underlying cause so as to provide relief of symptoms to patients.

There has been significant interest in gas and bloating over the past decade because of new knowledge on the pathophysiology, including the role of the intestinal microbiome, diagnostic (breath) tests, and treatments including probiotics, antibiotics, and nutritional therapies.

Definitions

Bloating refers to the perception or sensation of fullness in the abdomen, with or without physical distension. *Distension* refers to the physical increase in abdominal girth with or without a sensation of bloating. Functional bloating is defined as: (1) recurrent bloating and/or distension occurring, on average, at least one day per week; abdominal bloating and/or distension predominates over other symptoms; and (2) there are insufficient criteria for a diagnosis of IBS, functional constipation, functional diarrhea, or postprandial distress syndrome [150]. *Flatulence* refers to the passage of excessive amounts of gas from the anus, particularly gas with an unpleasant odor. It is a frequent source of embarrassment to many patients. The clinical dilemma is often to determine whether the patient is producing or passing excessive amounts of gas or is unusually sensitive to normal amounts of flatus.

Sources and composition of gastrointestinal gas

There are four important sources of gas: (1) air that has been swallowed during ingestion of food or drink or at other times unrelated to meals; (2) carbon dioxide (CO_2) produced by digestion and enzymatic interactions; (3) CO_2, hydrogen (H_2), and methane (CH_4) produced by bacterial fermentation of food residues; and (4) diffusion of gas from the blood into the GI tract [151,152] (Figure 34.9). The normal GI tract contains approximately 200 mL of gas [153–155], although the volume released is influenced by the aforementioned processes, particularly the diet, and is estimated as 600–800 mL [153]. Below is a brief description of the important gases found in the gut.

Nitrogen (N_2) and oxygen (O_2)

Approximately 10–20 mL of air is swallowed with each bolus of food or drink [156]. Because there is little to no diffusion of N_2 between the GI lumen and the blood, the predominant source of N_2 found in the gut or in flatus is that which is swallowed with air. In contrast, O_2 diffuses freely between the blood and the GI lumen and consequently its concentration may vary depending on the amount of air swallowed and the metabolic processes occurring within the gut.

Hydrogen (H_2)

Germ-free rats [157], newborn infants, and mammalian cells [158] do not produce H_2. However, H_2 is produced within hours after bacterial colonization of the human gut. It has been estimated that between 30 and 150 g of carbohydrate normally escapes digestion in the small bowel and reaches the colon every day [159]. This unabsorbed carbohydrate serves as a substrate for fermentation by colonic anaerobic bacteria and H_2 is produced by this process. Endogenous substances such as glycoproteins (e.g., in mucins) may also serve as substrates for H_2 production [160]. The net volume of H_2 excreted from the body (breath and flatus) depends on the amount of H_2 produced in the colon and the volume consumed by bacteria within the gut [151,161]. Carbohydrate malabsorption, such as lactase deficiency, may also increase the volume and rate of H_2 production. Only 14–21% is absorbed into the bloodstream and eliminated through the lungs [162] (see Figure 34.9). While H_2 is generally considered to be inert, it can sometimes serve as metabolic fuel for intestinal archaea (single-celled prokaryotes genetically, biochemically, and structurally distinct from bacteria) and methanogens to produce methane (CH_4), and for acetogens and sulfate-reducing organisms to produce hydrogen sulfide (H_2S) [163,164].

Methane (CH_4)

Methane is also a product of the intracolonic metabolism of unabsorbed carbohydrate residues. It is primarily produced by single-celled organisms, the methanogens, that belong to the domain Archaea. The following reaction summarizes methanogenesis and also explains how H_2 is consumed during this process [165]:

$$4H_2 + CO_2 \rightarrow CH_2 + 2H_2O$$

As can be seen, 5 moles of gas (4 H_2 + 1 CO_2) are used to produce 1 mole of CH_4. Thus, methanogenesis serves as a mechanism for reducing the volume of gas produced in the colon.

It is estimated that one-third of the world's population has high concentrations of methanogenic flora in the colon. This appears to be a familial trait influenced by environmental rather than by genetic factors [166]. The prevalence of methanogenic flora is higher among Mexicans and Caucasians than Asians for reasons that are unclear [167]. Similarly, it is unclear why children under the age of 3 years do not have detectable levels of CH_4 in alveolar air [167]. Subjects who produce large amounts of CH_4 may have stools that consistently float in water because of gas entrapment in stool [168].

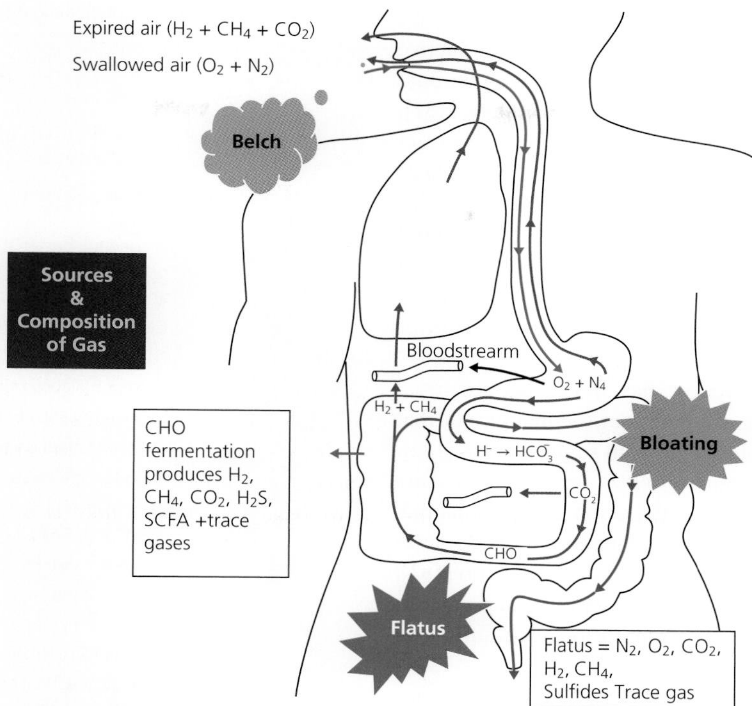

Figure 34.9 The sources for gas production in humans. (1) Air is swallowed; (2) a substantial portion is regurgitated (eructation); (3) O_2 and N_2 diffuse into the blood; (4) CO_2 is produced by the interaction of H^+ and HCO_3^-; (5) CO_2 diffuses into blood; (6) N_2 diffuses into the lumen; (7) unabsorbed carbohydrate (CHO) residues arrive in the colon and are fermented by anaerobic bacteria to produce short-chain fatty acids (SCFA), and H_2 + CO_2 + CH_2 + trace gases; (8) a proportion of these gases diffuses into the blood; (9) H_2 and CH_4 are excreted through the lungs; (10) O_2 + N_2 are consumed by colonic bacteria; (11) H_2 and O_2 are also consumed by colonic bacteria to produce CH_4, SO_2 and other gases, some of which are absorbed; (12) the remaining gases are expelled with stools or as flatus.

Carbon dioxide (CO_2)

Most CO_2 is formed during neutralization of acid by bicarbonate or other alkaline secretions [169,170]. Up to 2 L of CO_2 may be produced within 24 hours [169]. Other sources of CO_2 production include intestinal digestion of fat and protein. Hence, a large meal that is rich in fat and protein can produce significant amounts of CO_2 but most of this is absorbed in the small bowel. The bulk of CO_2 in flatus is derived from bacterial fermentation in the colon [171].

Hydrogen sulfide (H_2S)

Hydrogen sulfide is a toxic, pungent gas produced by both gut microbiota and mammalian tissues. H_2S has been recognized as an endogenous mediator for inflammation, motility, epithelial secretion, nociception, and neurotransmission [172–174]. Sulfate-reducing bacteria in the colonic lumen are also anaerobic H_2 consumers, like methanogens, and are part of the normal gut microbiota in healthy individuals [175]. Sulfate-reducing bacteria are the most efficient hydrogenotrophs, able to synthesize H_2S more efficiently at low H_2 concentrations. These H_2-consuming microbes are key for maintaining redox balance in the distal gut so that maximal energy extraction from efficient oxidation of food by the luminal microbes can occur.

Pathophysiology of bloating and gas

Bloating occurs in many organic and functional GI disorders. Some examples include lactose intolerance and small intestinal bacterial overgrowth (SIBO), where there may be excess gas production; IBS, where there may be altered or heightened perception; and constipation, where there may be excess retention of gas.

Bloating may arise from excessive production of intestinal gas during fermentation of meal residues or failure of evacuation of gas from the colon. Patients with bloating and IBS are more likely to report abdominal pain and distension coinciding with the arrival of meal residues in the colon compared to healthy controls [176]. However, in such cases, radiographic examinations have often failed to document a greater amount of gas than normal [177,178]. A systematic analysis of the intestinal gas contents using argon gas washout technique showed that the mean volume of gas in patients with bloating and in normal subjects was 176 mL versus 199 mL, respectively, and the mean composition of gases was similar [179]. However, the patients differed from controls in that more of the infused gas refluxed back into the stomach and they complained of abdominal pain more frequently [179].

Girth measurements have also been controversial [178,180] but electronic measurements of abdominal girth using inductive plethysmography show clear evidence of increased abdominal girth after each meal, and reduction of girth during sleep [181], presumably related to passage of gas out of the digestive tract during sleep. Other studies using more elegant techniques have confirmed that disturbed motility, including to and fro movements of gas with poor clearance within gut, was more frequent in bloaters (77%) and IBS (84%) but rare (<15%) in healthy controls [182]. This is most likely due to gas entrapment in the jejunum and proximal bowel rather than the ileum or colon.

Another intriguing observation has been the abnormal movement and configurational changes of the diaphragm that lead to accumulation and holding of gas in some bloaters [182]. This phenomenon of abdominophrenic dyssynergia occurs when normal upward movement of the diaphragm is impaired, leading to abdominal distension. Some patients may expel gas as soon as it is generated and thereby evade clinical detection [183]. This hypothesis is supported by the observation that gas can pass rapidly through the gut with a mouth to anus transit time of 15–20 min [184].

Flatus usually comprises N_2, O_2, CO_2, H_2, CH_4, and trace amounts of a few other gases (see Figure 34.9). Interestingly, those gases that are the major components of flatus do not have an odor. The unpleasant odor is believed to be related to sulfur-containing compounds such as methanethiol and dimethyl sulfide, which are present only in trace quantities in feces [185]. It is generally believed that <25 episodes/day of flatus emissions is normal [170]. A more frequent passage of flatus may suggest excess gas production, although frequency is only a rough guide to the volume generated.

A number of syndromes have been described in association with bloating. *Gas–bloat syndrome* may occur in 25–50% of patients following gastric fundoplication for a hiatal hernia [186,187], although it is less frequent after laparoscopic surgery [188]. This syndrome stems from the inability to belch and expel gas from the stomach after a meal. Usually, the problem resolves with time; rarely, surgical revision is required [189]. *Magenblase syndrome* arises from progressive and excessive accumulation of air swallowed during the course of a day, resulting in marked postprandial epigastric fullness and bloating, particularly after the evening meal. Symptoms can be chronic and sometimes severe and are often relieved by belching [155].

Diagnosis

The differential for a patient with bloating and gas is broad and includes both organic and functional etiologies (Table 34.7). The primary goal of investigating a patient should be to either confirm or refute specific diagnoses recognized through the history, physical examination, and review of systems and not to embark on a crusade of excluding every possible GI ailment.

Table 34.7 Common causes of bloating/distension.

Idiopathic	
Gastric disorders	Gastroparesis
	Gastric bezoar
	Gastric outlet obstruction/gastric cancer
Small bowel disorders	Lactose malabsorption/intolerance: Primary Secondary: bacterial overgrowth, celiac disease, giardiasis, tropical sprue, Whipple disease, *Taenia*, and other parasitic infestation
	Celiac disease
	Fructose malabsorption/intolerance
	Fructan malabsorption/intolerance
	Sucrose malabsorption/intolerance
	Small intestinal bacterial overgrowth
	Parasites: giardiasis, hookworm, tapeworm
	Fat malabsorption (chronic pancreatitis vs small bowel process)
	Crohn's disease
	Chronic intestinal pseudoobstruction
	Visceral neuropathy/myopathy
	Systemic sclerosis/muscular dystrophy
	Small intestinal obstruction (from adhesions, stricture, lymphoma, carcinoma)
	Jejunal diverticulosis with secondary small intestinal bacterial overgrowth
	Diabetic gastroenteropathy
Colonic disorders	Constipation (slow transit vs dyssynergic defecation)
	Colonic stricture (cancer, IBD, complication of prior diverticulitis)
	Amebiasis and other parasitic infestations
	Hirschsprung disease
	Chronic intestinal pseudoobstruction
	Bacterial/viral and parasitic infections
	Pneumatosis cystoides intestinalis
	Diverticular disease
	Colon cancer with obstruction
Miscellaneous	Drugs: narcotics, anticholinergics, antidiarrheals – kaolin compounds, atropine/dephenoxylate, loperamide, calcium channel blockers, psyllium supplements
	Metabolic: hypothyroidism, hypokalemia, hypercalcemia
	Diabetes mellitus with altered gastric emptying based on glucose control
	Ingestion of carbonated beverages
	Chewing gum, particularly those containing sorbitol
	Food intolerance
	Aerophagia

IBD, inflammatory bowel disease.

History and physical examination

The most important step in the evaluation of a patient with bloating and gas is to obtain a detailed history and perform a systematic physical examination (Table 34.8). The history should

Table 34.8 Clinical approach to bloating/distension.

History	Timing and duration of symptoms Presence of other associated gastrointestinal disturbances Dietary assessment Relationship of symptoms to meals and defecation Smoking, alcohol, and other habits, including carbonated drinks and chewing gum History of psychiatric disturbances Past medical history, including diabetes and hypothyroidism Medication history Family history of celiac disease, inflammatory bowel disease, malignancy Weight loss or other constitutional symptoms
Physical examination	Features of hyperventilation or aerophagia Abdominal and rectal examination • Confirm and exclude abdominal distension • Exclude organomegaly, intestinal obstruction, ascites • Evaluate for dyssynergic defecation in those with constipation

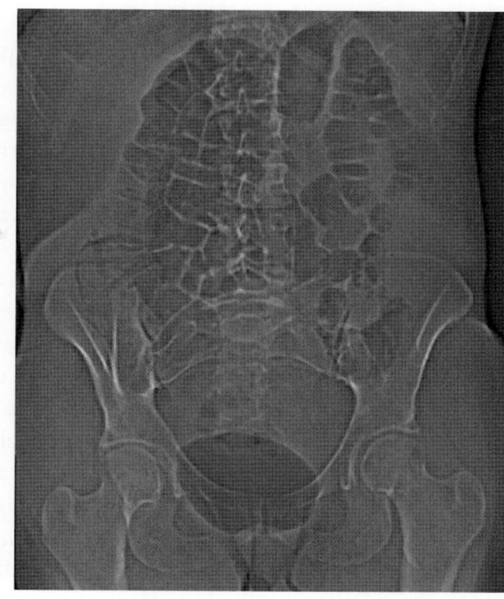

Figure 34.10 Plain abdominal radiograph demonstrating a "gas bubble" in the rectum. Source: Courtesy of Dr Amanda Johnson, Mayo Clinic, Rochester, MN.

seek to elicit the onset, chronicity, and temporal characteristics, character and intensity, and relieving and aggravating factors. The relationship of bloating and gas to intake of meals and bowel habits should be sought. The presence of other GI signs or symptoms, such as dysphagia, abdominal pain, constipation, diarrhea, melena, hematemesis, or hematochezia, should be noted. Additionally, patients should be asked about constitutional symptoms such as fevers, chills, night sweats, and weight loss.

An extensive dietary assessment should pay attention to recent changes in dietary habits and seek to identify potential food triggers, which may include dairy products, fructose, sucrose or sorbitol, beans, or fatty foods. The relationship of symptoms to defecation and changes in stool form and consistency is also important. Although smoking and alcohol consumption are usually reviewed, other habits such as the ingestion of carbonated drinks, artificially sweetened beverages, and chewing gum are often overlooked. A history of psychiatric comorbidities such as anxiety or depression and the presence of endocrine disorders such as diabetes and hypothyroidism may be important contributing factors. Consequently, the patient's past medical history should be carefully reviewed. A thorough medication assessment should be performed as drugs can have various GI side-effects and alter gut transit and motility. A family history of celiac disease, IBD, lactose intolerance, or malignancy may also provide important clues. A commonly overlooked problem is the association of bloating with inability to pass gas in association with constipation, especially in patients with pelvic floor dyssynergia; this can be identified on a plain abdominal radiograph showing a "gas bubble" in the rectum (Figure 34.10).

During physical examination, the following should be noted: the presence or absence of abdominal distension, and exaggerated lumbar lordosis with consequent protuberance of the belly. Flexion of the hips of the supine patient abolishes both the lordosis and the distension, quickly confirming the diagnosis of pseudocyesis. These patients should also be examined in the supine position. The abdomen must be carefully palpated and percussed to exclude organomegaly, signs of intestinal obstruction, and ascites. Patients who appear anxious with hyperventilation and cold skin and those who avoid eye contact and wince easily on gentle palpation may have anxiety, which can exacerbate functional symptoms including bloating [190]. Defecatory dysfunction, notably dyssynergic defecation with inability to expel gas and/or stool, may also cause significant bloating [191,192]. Therefore, a rectal examination needs to be performed in all patients presenting with bloating and constipation to exclude a rectal evacuation disorder (see Chapter 36) [190].

Diagnostic tests

Since recall of foods consumed and/or symptoms is often poor or unreliable, a prospectively recorded one-week food and symptom diary can be invaluable in the assessment of patients. Conventional blood tests such as complete blood count (CBC), thyroid function testing, calcium, and glucose measurements may be useful to exclude underlying metabolic disorders or serious organic diseases in select patients (see Table 34.6). Fresh stool samples (at least three) may be examined for ova/parasites and culture, but would only be indicated in the patient with at-risk travel. Checking for stool *Giardia* antigen is very reasonable, especially in the patient who may consume water that could be affected. The tissue transglutaminase (tTG) IgA antibody test is a useful screening measure for patients with suspected celiac disease. Plain x-rays of the abdomen may reveal excessive fecal loading in patients with constipation. A breath H_2 or CH_4 analysis can be helpful in diagnosing carbohydrate malabsorption or bacterial overgrowth and is discussed below.

A plain abdominal radiograph is a good first screening test to exclude intestinal obstruction and observe the gas pattern in the colon or rectum above the pelvic floor. Upper endoscopy with duodenal biopsy for celiac disease and/or small bowel aspirate of fluid for SIBO may be useful in recognizing these specific problems. Similarly, an upper GI series with small bowel follow-through versus cross-sectional imaging can be used to evaluate for intestinal strictures, malignant obstruction, or jejunal diverticulosis. While colonoscopy with biopsies can help to exclude inflammatory, infective, or ischemic conditions of the colon, these conditions are rarely associated with gas and bloating. Specific tests for evaluating GI motor dysfunction may include gastric emptying study, small bowel transit study, and a colonic transit study. Radionuclide studies that provide an overall assessment of GI transit may also be useful in refractory patients [193]. The wireless motility capsule has been shown to be quite useful in identifying a generalized GI motility disorder in patients with unexplained constipation, discomfort, bloating, and gas [194]. Importantly, these procedures should be obtained using patient history and physical exam as a guide and not performed on a routine or continuing basis.

Hydrogen breath tests

Breath sample analysis for H_2 and CH_4 has become an important tool to investigate carbohydrate malabsorption (lactose, fructose, sucrose) and bacterial overgrowth [195–199].

Rationale for the breath test

The breath test consists of administering an oral dose of a potentially offending carbohydrate, which serves as a substrate for bacterial fermentation, and measuring the breath H_2 and CH_4 responses. These two gases are used as they are principally produced by microbial fermentation in the gut [200]. Physiologically, the unabsorbed carbohydrate is fermented by colonic anaerobic bacteria to produce these gases, which are then rapidly absorbed together with salt and water into the abdominal venous circulation, transported to the lungs, and detected in the exhaled air [184,200–202]. As little as 2 g of carbohydrate that reaches the colon may produce an appreciable increase in breath H_2 values [162].

Principles of the breath test

After ingestion of the carbohydrate, H_2 and CH_4 are measured in expired air every 30 minutes for 3–5 hours [203]. Fructose and lactose malabsorption is defined by a ≥20 parts per million (ppm) increase in H_2 and ≥10 ppm increase in CH_4 compared to baseline [203]. Protocols used for breath tests are summarized in Table 34.9. A significant rise in breath values together with reproduction of the patient's typical symptoms is highly suggestive of carbohydrate malabsorption and intolerance whereas a rise without symptoms indicates malabsorption only. It is important to document the patient's symptoms during the study because the breath H_2 analysis technique has certain limitations and pitfalls (Table 34.10). In general, prior to breath testing, antibiotics should be avoided for at least 4 weeks, fermentable foods and smoking avoided the day before, and patients should be fasting for 8–12 hours prior to the test.

Rationale for methane analysis

Approximately 15–30% of people have methanogenic flora [175]. Following ingestion of unabsorbable carbohydrate, the breath H_2 values may not rise in these subjects and instead the CH_4 values may increase (Figure 34.11). In a study of 166 subjects with a negative lactose-H_2 breath test, 34% were found to be CH_4 excretors and 15% showed a significant rise in CH_4 levels after lactose ingestion [204]. Because colonic fermentation may produce one or both gases, simultaneous measurements of H_2 and CH_4 can improve the sensitivity and specificity of the breath tests.

Lactose hydrogen breath test

The purpose of the lactose H_2 breath test is to detect if symptoms of bloating, flatus, abdominal pain, or diarrhea are related to lactose malabsorption. Some clinicians overdiagnose this condition while others may underdiagnose it [205,206]. Many patients do not relate bowel symptoms to their oral consumption of lactose and, without an objective test, it is often difficult to convince a doubting patient that their symptoms are related to diet [207]. A 25 g dose of lactose is preferred for this test [200].

Table 34.9 Breath test protocols.

Indication	Test solution	Breath sampling interval	Duration of test	Interpretation (positive test)
Lactose malabsorption	25 g Lactose in 1 cup H_2O	Every 30 min	At least 3 h	H_2 >20 ppm or CH_4 >10 ppm compared to baseline
Fructose malabsorption	25 g Fructose in 1 cup H_2O	Every 30 min	As above	As above
Bacterial overgrowth	75 g Glucose in 1 cup H_2O; 10 g Lactulose in 1 cup H_2O	Every 15 min	At least 2 h	H_2 >20 ppm compared to baseline at 90 minutes; CH_4 >10 ppm compared to baseline

Normal range: fasting H_2 = 0–10 ppm; fasting CH_4 = 0–5 ppm.

Table 34.10 Precautions and limitations of interpreting breath tests.

Problem	Mechanism	Result
Active diarrheal disease	Lack of bacterial flora	False negative
Recent use of antibiotics	Lack of bacterial flora	False negative
Recent use of laxatives/enemas/colon cleansing	Lack of bacterial flora	False negative
Elevated fasting breath H_2 or CH_4 values	Poor preparation or SIBO	False positive or negative
Gastroparesis/gastric outlet obstruction	Delayed gastric emptying	False negative
Cigarette smoking	CO_2 effect	False positive
Sleeping	Hypoventilation	False negative
Contamination of stored samples or improper collection techniques.	Technical	False positive or negative
Administration of test solution after fiber-containing meal	Fiber fermentation	False positive
Use of opioids/anticholinergics	Slows gut transit/previous meal effects	False positive or negative

SIBO, small intestinal bacterial overgrowth.

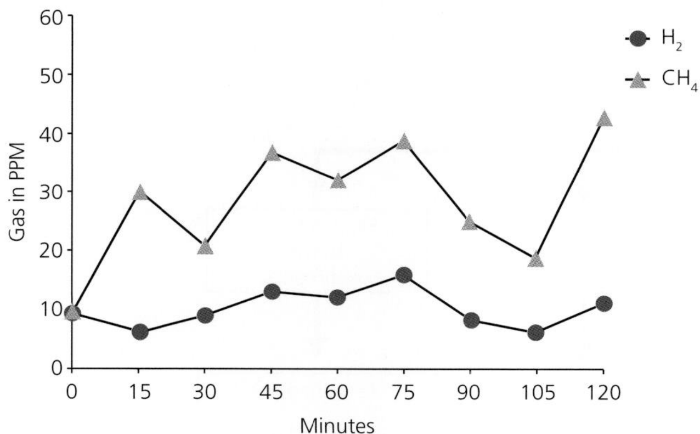

Figure 34.11 An example of the glucose breath test with significant elevation of CH_4 values, indicating SIBO, but a flat H_2 response. This graph also illustrates the need to sample both H_2 and CH_4, failing which the test may be misinterpreted as negative.

Fructose hydrogen breath test

The fructose H_2 breath test is useful for diagnosis of dietary fructose intolerance (DFI) [208,209]. A 25 g dose of fructose is administered and a diagnosis of DFI is made based on provocation of symptoms and positive H_2 breath test [203]. In a study of fructose absorptive capacity, healthy subjects completely absorbed a 15 g dose of fructose and nearly all absorbed a 25 g dose, whereas many exhibited malabsorption and intolerance with 50 g of fructose [210]. Hence, 25 g appears to be the optimal dose for assessment of DFI. However, the utility of a test that involves only fructose in solution has been questioned since fructose is most often ingested with food that delays emptying from the stomach, and with glucose that facilitates fructose absorption by facilitated carrier-mediated uptake [211].

Tests for small intestinal bowel overgrowth

Duodenal aspiration/culture

Small bowel sampling techniques available at this time are not considered satisfactory for assessment of SIBO and need to be further refined [200]. Using sterile precautions, a catheter is passed through the biopsy channel of an upper endoscope into the third or fourth portions of the duodenum. Approximately 3–5 mL of duodenal fluid is aspirated using gentle suction for aerobic/anaerobic and fungal cultures [212]. A bacterial concentration in the duodenum of $>10^3$ colony forming units (cfu)/mL is considered diagnostic of SIBO [200]. While previously a $\geq 10^5$ cfu/mL cutoff was used, this is usually indicative of stagnant loop conditions; most healthy controls have $\leq 10^3$ cfu/mL [200,213]. The most common pathogens include *Bacteroides*, *Enterococcus*, *Lactobacillus*, *Streptococcus*, *Klebsiella*, and *Escherichia coli* but mixed flora is reported rather than isolation of a single organism.

Glucose and lactulose breath test

The preferred substrates for the glucose and lactulose breath tests are 75 g and 10 g, respectively [200]. A rise of ≥20 ppm in H_2 compared to baseline by 90 minutes is considered positive for SIBO [200]. Glucose is readily absorbed in the proximal small bowel while lactulose is nondigestible and reaches the colon [200]. The sensitivity and specificity of the glucose breath test vary drastically between studies and range from 20–93% and 30–86%, respectively [213]. Similarly, the sensitivity and specificity of the lactulose breath test range from 31–68% and 44–100%, respectively [213]. However, the specificity of the breath hydrogen response to glucose or lactulose ingested in a solution in the fasting state is questionable since the substrate may easily reach the colon within 60 minutes or less. Therefore, some authors recommend concomitant radiolabeling of the solution with a radioisotope and obtaining gamma-camera images at the times of breath collection to determine whether the rise in hydrogen or methane in the breath was associated with isotope in the colon [214].

Differential diagnosis and principles of management

Because gas and bloating are nonspecific symptoms caused by a heterogeneous group of GI disorders or a consequence of dietary factors, there is no single therapy that will benefit all patients with these complaints. Hence, the best approach is to prioritize a differential diagnosis based on the clinical presentation and assessment, and then proceed to establish a diagnosis.

There are several different ways to approach a patient with bloating and gas. One such approach is outlined in Figure 34.12 [215]. Using this approach, conditions that present with nonintestinal distension or causes of "pseudobloat" such as ascites, adiposity, and pregnancy are first ruled out. Subsequently, the differential is narrowed based on whether bloating occurs with diarrhea, constipation, mechanical disturbance, or without bowel disturbance. A list of the various diagnoses for each of these categories and possible management strategies is given in Figure 34.11.

A different approach first focuses on identifying whether the patient has bloating or belching as the predominant symptom

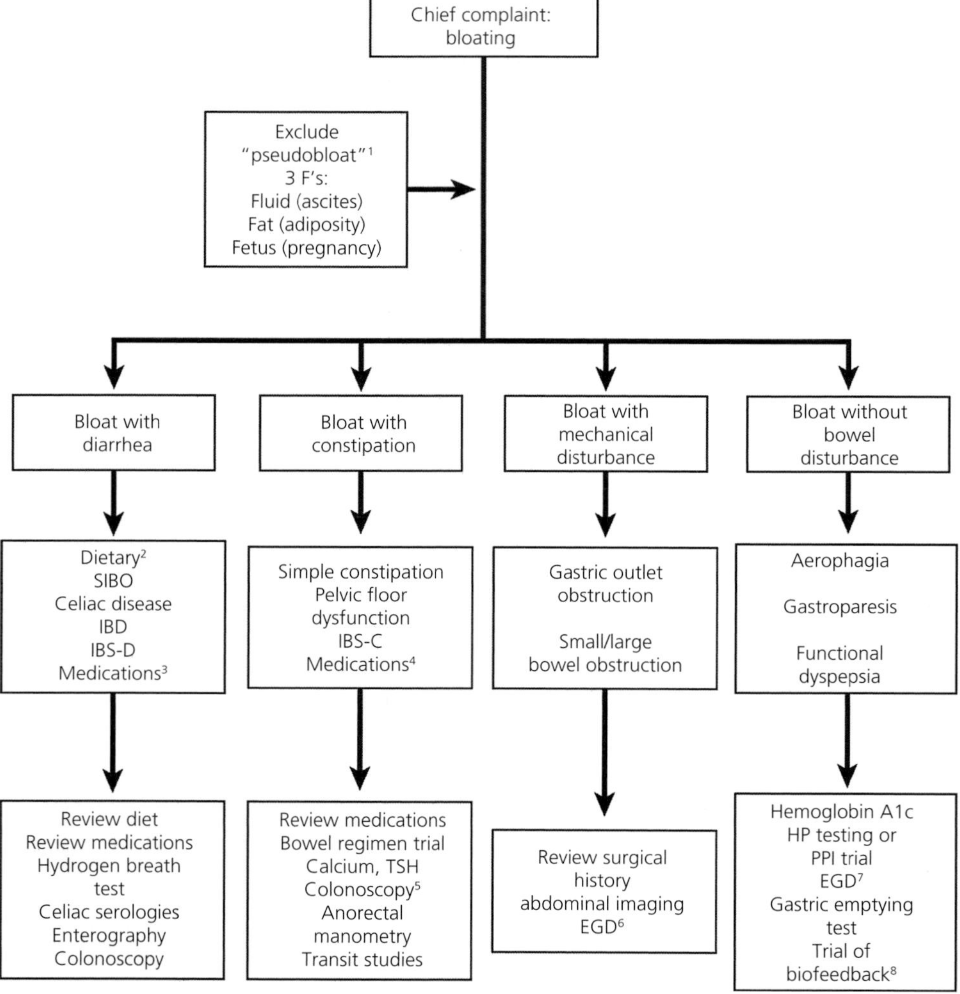

Figure 34.12 A systematic approach in the work-up and management of patients with bloating. 1.Pseudobloat refers to nonintestinal distention. 2.Carbohydrate malabsorption, osmotically rich sugars/sugar alcohols, enteral formulas, high-fiber foods. 3.Osmotic laxatives or agents (lactulose, magnesium, sorbitol, polyethylene glycol) or fiber products. 4. Narcotics. 5. If indicated based on presence of any alarm features, or if due for age-appropriate colorectal cancer screening/surveillance. 6. If features of gastric outlet obstruction, to help identify cause or for relief of obstruction. 7. Required before 4-hour solid food gastric emptying study if gastroparesis is considered to rule out gastric outlet obstruction; also consider if age ≥60 years. 8. If aerophagia felt to be from air swallowing not due to other etiologies such has dietary habits (fast eating, drinking carbonation), poorly fitting dentures, continuous positive airway pressure mask. EGD, esophagogastroduodenoscopy; HP, *Helicobacter pylori*; IBD, inflammatory bowel disease; IBS-C, irritable bowel syndrome with constipation; IBS-D, irritable bowel syndrome with diarrhea; PPI, proton pump inhibitor; SIBO, small intestinal bacterial overgrowth; TSH, thyroid stimulating hormone. Source: Kamboj and Oxentenko [215]. Reproduced with permission of Elsevier.

(Figure 34.13) [216]. If bloating is present, the clinical phenotype of the patient is further defined as "gastric bloater," "small bowel bloater," or "constipated bloater." The latter term refers to a patient with bloating secondary to constipation. The onset of symptoms soon after eating suggests a gastric origin while delayed symptoms may be more suggestive of a small bowel cause.

Management of common conditions with gas and bloating

The majority of the disorders outlined in the two algorithms above will be discussed in other book chapters. Below are a few common clinical problems and an approach to their management.

Lactose intolerance and malabsorption

Lactose, found in dairy products, is a disaccharide that is normally split in the small bowel into glucose and galactose by the enzymatic action of intestinal lactase. Deficiency of this enzyme leads to malabsorption of lactose, its fermentation to H_2 and CH_4, and resultant symptoms. It is the most common carbohydrate malabsorption problem, and worldwide, 75% of adults show some decrease in lactase activity during adulthood [217].

The breath H_2 test has been widely used for the detection of lactose malabsorption, and has superseded [218,219] other methods such as the measurement of blood glucose [220] or galactose levels [221]. The lactose-H_2 breath test is positive in about 90% of patients with lactose malabsorption. However, between 5–15% of patients with lactose malabsorption may have a false-negative breath test possibly due to an acidic pH in the colon, methanogenic flora, or deficiency of H_2-producing bacteria in the colon [161]. Patients with lactose malabsorption will benefit from complete elimination or restriction of dairy products. Educating the patient with the help of a dietitian is most useful because lactose is present in many popular food

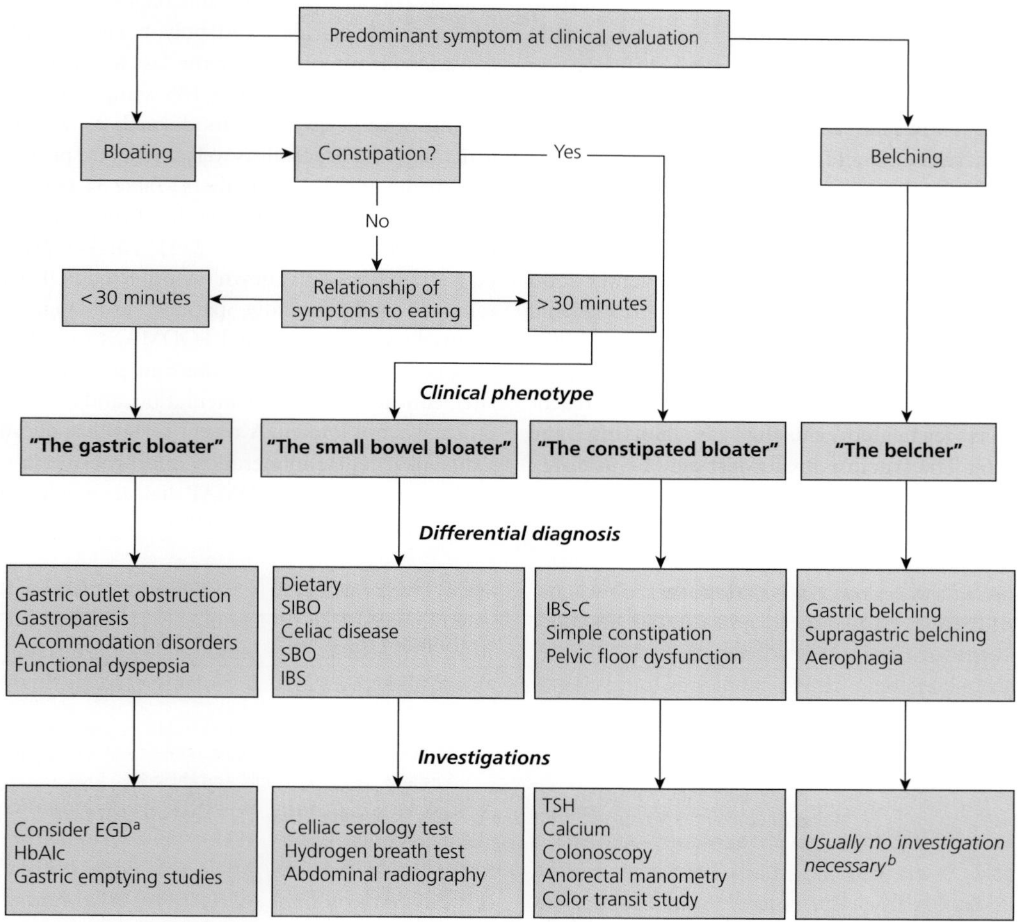

Figure 34.13 A simplified approach to the evaluation of the patient with gas-related symptoms. [a]Indicated in the presence of alarm features: age >50 years, upper GI malignancy in a first-degree relative, weight loss, GI bleeding, or iron deficiency anemia, dysphagia, odynophagia, persistent vomiting, abnormal imaging suggesting organic disease (American Society for Gastrointestinal Endoscopy). [b]Consider EGD (+/− gastric biopsies) and/or gastric emptying test to rule out an organic etiology, in certain patients. EGD, esophagogastroduodenoscopy; HbA1c, glycosylated hemoglobin; IBS, irritable bowel syndrome; IBS-C, irritable bowel syndrome – constipation; SBO, small bowel obstruction; SIBO, small intestine bacterial overgrowth; TSH, thyroid-stimulating hormone. Source: Cotter et al. [216]. Reproduced with permission of Elsevier.

items and its ingestion is often not recognized by the patient. Patients may benefit from lactase enzyme supplements (Lactaid®, McNeil Pharmaceuticals; Dairy-ease®, Sterling Health). Lactase enzyme tablets may help to better digest a lactose-containing meal but is not a panacea for all patients and at all times. Patients with secondary lactose intolerance require investigations to identify the primary problem.

The effective treatment of the underlying condition, such as a gluten-free diet for celiac disease, metronidazole or tinidazole for giardiasis, or oxytetracycline for tropical sprue, may not only serve to ameliorate symptoms but also improve tolerance to lactose-containing products.

Fructose intolerance and malabsorption

Fructose is a six-carbon sugar that occurs naturally in fruits and food additives. It is also present in high-fructose corn syrup, which is commonly used in many food sweeteners and soft drinks [222]. Unlike glucose, which is completely absorbed through an active transport mechanism in the small intestine via the GLUT2 and GLUT5 transporters, fructose is mostly absorbed through carrier-mediated facilitative diffusion via the GLUT5 transporter. This is an energy-independent process and consequently its absorptive capacity is limited [219,223]. Therefore, fructose malabsorption can occur with excess dietary intake of fructose, usually greater than 30–50 g/h, given the limited absorptive capacity [224]. Additionally, the passive diffusion of fructose is stimulated by glucose and inhibited by sorbitol [225]. Consequently, food products containing large amounts of both fructose and glucose can result in incomplete fructose absorption while sorbitol can worsen fructose malabsorption [224]. The unabsorbed fructose can serve as an osmotic load and, upon reaching the colon, is fermented, causing gas, bloating, and diarrhea [208,226]. The fructose breath test may be useful in the diagnosis of DFI [208,209].

A fructose-restricted diet, consisting of less than 10 g/day of fructose, can improve symptoms in patients with DFI [203,208,226,227]. This diet may require challenging dietary changes but, when adhered to, can confer significant relief [208,227]. Xylose isomerase, an enzyme that facilitates conversion of fructose to glucose, may help improve symptoms in patients with DFI [228].

Fructan intolerance and FODMAPs

Fructans are oligo- or polysaccharides consisting of short chains of fructose units with a single d-glucosyl unit. Because fructans are present in many common foods including wheat-based products like breakfast cereal, bread, and pasta, many people ingest high levels of fructans. Fructans may not be well tolerated by some subjects and its malabsorption may result in GI symptoms [229]. The mechanism for malabsorption is related to the inability to hydrolyze glycosidic linkages in the complex polysaccharide, resulting in the delivery of malabsorbed fructans to the large bowel.

Diets containing fermentable oligosaccharides, disaccharides and monosaccharides, and polyols (FODMAPs) have gained considerable attention over the last few years as an important cause of gas, bloating, and IBS symptoms [230–232]. These include several common foods such as wheat, onion, garlic, artichoke, and broccoli, as well as fructose products, dairy products, fruits, sorbitol, and others (Table 34.11).

A FODMAP-restricted diet has been tested and found to be useful in IBS patients [232–234]. The key principle is dietary education; firstly, all known or suspected FODMAPs are strictly removed and, secondly, patients are taught to rechallenge themselves with individual FODMAPs to test their own tolerance [231]. While effective, there are practical hurdles regarding such education and implementation, and its long-term safety or efficacy is not known. A recent review has questioned the relevance of fructose intolerance, and proposed a more personalized approach to the FODMAP diet, acknowledging the inability

Table 34.11 Constituents and common sources of FODMAPs.

FODMAP	Constituent	Sources
F = Fermentable		By colonic bacteria
O = Oligosaccharides	Fructans, galactooligosaccharides	Wheat, barley, rye, onion, leek, white part of spring onion, garlic, shallots, artichokes, beetroot, fennel, peas, chicory, pistachio, cashews, legumes, lentils, and chickpeas
D = Disaccharides	Lactose	Milk, custard, ice cream, and yoghurt
M = Monosaccharides	"Free fructose" (fructose in excess of glucose)	Apples, pears, mangoes, cherries, watermelon, asparagus, sugar snap peas, honey, and high-fructose corn syrup
A = And		
P = Polyols	Sorbitol, mannitol, maltitol, and xylitol	Apples, pears, apricots, cherries, nectarines, peaches, plums, watermelon, mushrooms, cauliflower, artificially sweetened chewing gum and confectionery

Source: Shepherd and Gibson 2006 [226]. Reproduced with permission of Elsevier.

to digest fructans in the human gut, the high world-wide prevalence of hypolactasia, and the facilitation of dietary fructose absorption (through GLUT2) by dietary glucose [211].

Sorbitol intolerance and sucrase-isomaltase deficiency

Sorbitol is a natural sugar found in fruits and artificial sweeteners. There is minimal absorption of sorbitol in the small intestine and patients may experience malabsorption with as little as 5–10 g of sorbitol [203,235–237]. Sucrase-isomaltase deficiency is an autosomal recessive disorder, due to mutations in the sucrose isomaltase gene [238,239]. It is a rare problem in adults and more commonly recognized in children. A sucrose breath test can help identify this problem [240]. Recognition and withdrawal of offending foods containing sorbitol and/or sucrose or maltose products with the help of a dietitian is the mainstay of therapy and appears to be successful [241–243].

Small intestinal bacterial overgrowth

Although a well-known cause of gas and bloating, there has been significant interest in SIBO over the past decade, largely spurred by the availability of breath testing and its linkage with IBS. SIBO results when there is excess bacteria in small bowel that may be causally linked with unexplained GI symptoms. Risk factors for SIBO include structural causes such as small bowel diverticular or strictures, surgical causes like gastric bypass, dysmotility from scleroderma, diabetes mellitus, and medications, and reduced gastric acid from acid-suppressive therapy and gastric resection.

The treatment for SIBO is multifactorial and involves addressing the underlying problem, eradicating bacterial overgrowth, and correcting vitamin deficiencies, if present. There are various antibiotic regimens available for treatment of SIBO; these cover both aerobic and anaerobic bacteria and include ciprofloxacin, metronidazole, trimethoprim/sulfamethoxazole, doxycycline, amoxicillin-clavulanic acid, and rifaximin. Antibiotics are typically given for 7–10 days. Rifaximin is sometimes used as first-line therapy as it may be superior to other antibiotics, although its high cost may be a prohibitive factor [244,245]. More than 40% of patients with SIBO treated with antibiotics have recurrent symptoms [246]. Patients with risk factors for SIBO and/or prior episodes may be empirically treated without undergoing additional testing, especially if they had a response previously.

Small intestinal fungal overgrowth

There is little information regarding gut fungi in humans. Small intestinal fungal overgrowth (SIFO) refers to excess fungal organisms in the small bowel [247]. SIFO predominantly involves *Candida* and most commonly presents in immunocompromised hosts. SIFO may play a role in the pathogenesis of unexplained symptoms including gas and bloating, but this is controversial and requires confirmatory studies [212]. Antifungal therapy may be helpful in improving symptoms in carefully selected patients [247].

Intestinal microbiome, probiotics, and prebiotics

The human colon has a multitude of bacteria but perturbations in type and balance of colonic flora may lead to GI symptoms [248]. Probiotics and prebiotics have been used to restore the intestinal microbiome, although research supporting their efficacy remains limited. Probiotics are generally considered safe although most studies to date have been small and used variable preparations. Multiple mechanisms have been postulated regarding benefits of probiotics and these include inhibiting pathogen growth, promoting intestinal barrier function, and immunomodulation [249–251]. Another approach has been to promote the growth of beneficial bacteria by administering prebiotic nutrients (poorly absorbed carbohydrates) such as inulin, lactulose, oligofructose, and fructans [252], which serve as substrates for rejuvenating growth of healthy intestinal microbiota. This merits further study.

Constipation, dysmotility, and dyssynergic defecation

Patients with concomitant constipation and bloating often find relief of their symptoms after they are placed on a bowel regimen and have regular bowel movements. Patients with delayed gastric emptying or those with disordered or sluggish small bowel transit may benefit from treatment with prokinetic drugs such as metoclopramide or erythromycin. In blinded controlled trials, metoclopramide [253] and prucalopride [254] improved symptoms of bloating compared to placebo. Likewise, patients with dyssynergic defecation and bloating improve with biofeedback therapy [255].

Other management strategies for gas and flatulence

Diet plays an important role in gas production. Hence, the elimination of offending foods such as beans, cabbage, lentils, Brussels sprouts, nuts, and legumes and high-fiber diets containing bran and fiber supplements may reduce bloating and gas. Some patients with refractory symptoms may benefit from elimination diets [256]. The essence of this therapy is to maintain a strict log of symptoms and foods consumed over a period of 1 month. If one or two food items are recognized, the patient is advised to try a diet without these food items. If several food items are recognized, an elimination diet may be required with the help of a dietitian.

There has been no systematic assessment of drugs that might reduce flatus production or alter the odor of flatus, although several compounds have been suggested. Following the ingestion of beans, patients who suffer from excessive bloating may obtain relief by taking an α-galactosidase preparation (Beano®, A.K. Pharma) [257,258]. Activated charcoal, administered prior to a meal, has been advocated [259,260], but remains controversial and its mechanism of action is not known [261,262]. Bismuth subsalicylate has also been suggested to help by decreasing H_2S [263,264]. Simethicone may act by altering the surface tension and elasticity of mucus-coated gas bubbles which causes the smaller bubbles to break down and coalesce [265,266]. Its usefulness and efficacy remain to be established. A chlorophyllin copper complex (Derifil®, Rystan Co Inc.), an agent that reduces fecal odor in patients with ileostomy, has been suggested as a useful adjunct to antiflatus therapy, particularly in patients with incontinence to flatus [267]. Controlled trials are, however, lacking. Patients with incontinence to flatus may benefit from biofeedback therapy [268] to help regain better control of their flatus expulsion.

Patients without definitive etiology

In those patients where an underlying cause is not demonstrable, reassurance together with drugs that bring about symptomatic relief may prove beneficial. Some patients may benefit from smooth muscle relaxants such as mebeverine, pinaverium, otilonium, cimetropium (all medications not currently approved in the US), dicyclomine, hyoscine, or peppermint oil [269], although controlled trials are lacking. Hypnotherapy with self-hypnosis has been shown to benefit some patients [270].

Conclusions

Bloating and gas are clinically challenging problems. Carbohydrate intolerance, SIBO, disturbed motility or visceral hyperalgesia are key etiological factors. Meticulous history and thoughtful work-up, including specific tests such as the breath hydrogen test, can identify malabsorption/intolerance of lactose, fructan, and SIBO and provide a basis for rational therapy, including dietary advice, antibiotics, and others.

References are available at www.yamadagastro.com/textbook7e

Further reading

Bharucha A.E., Chakraborty S., Sletten C.D. Common functional gastroenterological disorders associated with abdominal pain. Mayo Clin Proc 2016;91(8):1118.

Cotter T.G., Gurney M., Loftus C.G. Gas and bloating-controlling emissions: a case-based review for the primary care provider. Mayo Clin Proc 2016;91(8):1105.

Enck P., Aziz Q., Barbara G., et al. Irritable bowel syndrome. Nat Rev Dis Primers 2016;24;2:16014.

Ford A.C., Lacy B.E., Harris L.A., Quigley E.M.M., Moayyedi P. Effect of antidepressants and psychological therapies in irritable bowel syndrome: an updated systematic review and meta-analysis. Am J Gastroenterol 2019;114(1):21.

Kamboj A.K., Oxentenko A.S. Workup and management of bloating. Clin Gastroenterol Hepatol 2018;16:1030.

Kamboj A.K., Hoversten P., Oxentenko A.S. Chronic abdominal wall pain: a common yet overlooked etiology of chronic abdominal pain. Mayo Clin Proc 2019;94(1):139.

Keefer L., Drossman D.A., Guthrie E., et al. Centrally mediated disorders of gastrointestinal pain. Gastroenterology 2016;150:1408.

Malagelada J.R., Accarino A., Azpiroz F. Bloating and abdominal distension: old misconceptions and current knowledge. Am J Gastroenterol 2017;112(8):1221.

Mayer E.A., Tillisch K. The brain-gut axis in abdominal pain syndromes. Annu Rev Med 2011;62:381.

Peery A.F., Crockett S.D., Murphy C.C., et al. Burden and cost of gastrointestinal, liver, and pancreatic diseases in the United States: update 2018. Gastroenterology 2019;156(1):254.

Pimentel M., Mathur R., Chang C. Gas and the microbiome. Curr Gastroenterol Rep 2013;15:356.

Quigley E.M.M. The spectrum of small intestinal bacterial overgrowth (SIBO). Curr Gastroenterol Rep 2019;21(1):3.

CHAPTER 35
Approach to the patient with diarrhea

Gail A. Hecht and Judy A. Trieu
Loyola University Medical Center, Maywood, IL, USA

Chapter menu

Introduction

Diarrhea is derived from the Greek words meaning "flowing through." The illness is often self-limited in developed countries, but remains a significant cause of morbidity and mortality [1]. Diarrhea is defined as stool weight greater than 200 g per day but this definition has limited value in clinical practice. A more useful definition, which is employed by the World Health Organization, is three or more loose or watery stools per day or more frequently than an individual's baseline. Defining the duration of diarrhea is an important aspect of the initial evaluation as this provides invaluable information on the etiology. For the purposes of this chapter, the following definitions are used [2].

- Acute: less than or equal to 14 days in duration.
- Persistent: more than 14 days in duration.
- Chronic: more than 30 days in duration.

The majority of cases of acute diarrhea are self-limited infections caused by viruses and bacteria. As diarrhea persists, noninfectious etiologies become more prevalent. Evaluation for noninfectious etiologies should be considered in patients if the initial evaluation does not identify a pathogen and if the diarrhea worsens or becomes chronic. Approaches for assessing such patients are discussed in this chapter.

Acute diarrhea

Epidemiology

Diarrhea affects those in developed and developing nations differently. Diarrhea is the eighth leading cause of death worldwide, accounting for 1.6 million deaths annually [1,3]. The majority of deaths are among children and infants [4]. In the United States, it is often not much more than a "nuisance" disease. Despite this, it remains a significant cause of morbidity and mortality [2]. Diarrhea was the third most common outpatient visit complaint and the fourth most common reason for an emergency department visit in the US in 2016 [5,6]. Food poisoning accounts for 4000–5000 deaths annually [7]. In 2000, outpatient visits for diarrhea consisted of gastroenteritis (3.4 million), irritable bowel syndrome (1.6 million), Crohn's disease (725 000), and ulcerative colitis (488 000). The resultant burden on the US healthcare system is significant: diarrhea results in 300–400 child deaths per year, approximately 200 000 hospitalizations, and more than $1 billion in direct medical costs [8].

Various studies have aimed to estimate the incidence of acute diarrhea in the general population of developed countries [8–10]. Reported rates vary between 0.72 episodes/person-year and 1.3 episodes/person-year. However, the prevalence of acute diarrhea is likely highly underestimated as many, if not the majority, of those affected do not seek medical attention.

Yamada's Textbook of Gastroenterology, Seventh Edition. Edited by Timothy C. Wang, Michael Camilleri, Benjamin Lebwohl, Anna S. Lok, William J. Sandborn, Kenneth K. Wang, and Gary D. Wu.

Companion website: www.yamadagastro.com/textbook7e

Table 35.1 Epidemiological clues to infectious diarrhea. Source: Adapted from Parks and Giannella 1993 [335].

Vehicle	Classic pathogen
Water (including foods washed in such water)	*Vibrio cholerae*, Norwalk agent, *Giardia* organisms, and *Cryptosporidium* organisms
Food	
Poultry	*Salmonella*, *Campylobacter*, and *Shigella* species
Beef, unpasteurized fruit juice	*Enterohemorrhagic Escherichia coli*
Pork	Tapeworm
Seafood and shellfish[a] (including raw sushi and gefilte fish)	*Vibrio cholerae*, *Vibrio parahaemolyticus*, and *Vibrio vulnificus*; *Salmonella* species; hepatitis viruses A, B, and C; tapeworm and *Anisakis*
Cheese, milk	*Listeria* species
Eggs	*Salmonella* species
Mayonnaise-containing food and cream pie	Staphylococcal and clostridial food poisonings
Fried rice	*Bacillus cereus*
Fresh berries	*Cyclospora* species
Canned vegetables or fruits	*Clostridium* species
Sprouts, spinach	Enterohemorrhagic *E. coli* and *Salmonella* species
Animal-to-person (pets and livestock)	*Salmonella*, *Campylobacter*, *Cryptosporidium*, and *Giardia* species
Person-to-person (including sexual contact)	All enteric bacteria, viruses, and parasites
Day-care center	*Shigella, Campylobacter, Cryptosporidium, and Giardia species; viruses; Clostridium difficile*
Hospital, antibiotics, or chemotherapy	*C. difficile*
Swimming pool	*Giardia* and *Cryptosporidium* species
Foreign travel	*E. coli of various types; Salmonella, Shigella, Campylobacter, Giardia, and Cryptosporidium*

[a] Also includes fish poisonings such as scombroid, ciguatera, and paralytic, diarrheal, and neurotoxic shellfish poisonings.

Causes

While there are no specific data, experts believe that approximately 80% of acute diarrhea cases are infectious, with the remaining 20% attributable to drugs and/or chemicals. Causes of infectious diarrhea include various viruses, bacteria, and protozoa. Specific pathogens are discussed below. Noninfectious causes include medications, microbiota shifts, ischemic colitis, food allergy, fecal impaction, malignancy, and early manifestations of chronic diseases such as inflammatory bowel disease and thyrotoxicosis. Given the high incidence of infections as the cause of acute diarrhea, the work-up is initially tailored around evaluation/management of infectious conditions. If a patient's clinical history points towards a noninfectious cause, then the utility of certain diagnostic modalities becomes relevant (e.g., endoscopy or imaging).

Infectious diarrhea

Most causes of acute diarrhea in both developing and developed nations are secondary to infections, the majority of which are viral and less commonly bacterial and protozoan. Different studies have shown that bacterial stool cultures yield a bacterial pathogen in less than 10% of cases of patients with acute diarrhea. A more recent study that employed polymerase chain reaction (PCR) in addition to culture identified a bacterial pathogen in only 15% of over 1500 cases of acute diarrhea [11]. However, in cases of severe or bloody diarrhea or in food-borne outbreaks, the likelihood of a bacterial etiology increases, thus historical clues become instrumental in evaluating a patient with acute diarrhea (Table 35.1) [12,13].

Viruses

Viral gastroenteritis causes considerable mortality in developing countries, while in the US, viral gastroenteritis results in only a few hundred deaths per year, primarily due to norovirus and rotavirus [14,15]. Transmission of these common viral pathogens is via the fecal–oral route. Viral agents that are also important in causing acute diarrhea, besides norovirus and rotavirus (both discussed in further detail below in this section), are enteric adenoviruses and astrovirus. Enteric adenoviruses cause approximately 3–10% of pediatric gastroenteritis in endemic climates while astrovirus is responsible for 4–7% of diarrhea in day-care centers. Infections by astrovirus are typically less severe but can cause prolonged disease in immunocompromised patients.

Norovirus

Norovirus is a major cause of epidemic viral gastroenteritis and the most common cause of gastroenteritis in all adults. Over 90% of outbreaks are attributed to noroviruses [16]. Common outbreak settings include: (1) restaurants or events with catered meals, (2) long-term care facilities, (3) schools, day-care centers, and (4) vacation destinations including cruise ships [17]. Most patients develop both vomiting and nonbloody, nonmucous diarrhea. Systemic symptoms such as myalgias, headaches, and fevers are common [18]. Symptoms generally last 48–72 h and recovery is full.

Rotavirus

Infants and young children are by far most severely affected by rotavirus. Typical symptoms include vomiting, nonbloody diarrhea, and fever [19]. Adults present with similar but less severe symptoms. It has been estimated that the total economic impact of rotavirus diarrhea in the US is $1 billion yearly [20], undoubtedly one of the major reasons for the development of the rotavirus vaccine, which is now routinely given during infancy. In the prevaccine era, rotavirus was estimated to cause approximately 440 000 deaths, 2 million hospitalizations, and 25 million outpatient visits per year worldwide among children <5 years of age [21]. Since the advent of vaccination, there has been a significant decline in rotavirus infections, with one study reporting an 86% decline in positive tests [22].

Bacteria

Bacterial pathogens frequently cause acute infectious diarrhea but are not commonly isolated by stool culture. Enterotoxigenic *Escherichia coli* (ETEC) is a more common cause of diarrhea in developing countries. *Vibrio cholerae* is endemic along the Gulf Coast of the US but clinical cases are uncommon. Each of these organisms is discussed in further detail in Chapter 144.

The four most reported bacterial pathogens include *Campylobacter*, *Salmonella*, enterohemorrhagic *Escherichia coli* (EHEC) O157:H7, and *Shigella* [23]. Previously well known as "dysentery," these pathogens are also associated with bloody diarrhea, which likely prompts more patients to seek medical evaluation. Bloody diarrhea is an indication of inflammation. *Shigella* requires an inoculum of only 10 organisms to cause disease. This low inoculum allows *Shigella* to be transmitted person to person, as well as in food and water. EHEC is associated with undercooked ground beef and with systemic manifestations, such as thrombotic thrombocytopenic purpura (TTP) and hemolytic uremic syndrome (HUS). Other systemic symptoms and complications of enteric bacterial infections are shown in Table 35.2.

Food-borne

Food-borne illnesses account for over $7 billion in annual costs in the United States [24]. *Campylobacter* is generally contracted from undercooked poultry in developed countries and is the

Table 35.2 Systemic symptoms and complications of enteric infection.

Organism	Symptoms or complications	References
Vibrio cholerae and *Escherichia coli*	Dehydration, shock, and death	[5,347]
Bacillus cereus	Fulminant liver failure	[348]
Vibrio vulnificus	Shock and death in those with liver disease	[29,30,349]
Enteroadherent and enteroaggregative *E. coli*, *Cryptosporidium*, *Cyclospora*, and *Aeromonas* species	Prolonged (>6 weeks) diarrhea	[30,350–355]
Clostridium difficile	Relapse common, protein-losing enteropathy, colonectomy, death	[42–47,358–360]
Enterohemorrhagic *E. coli* (*E. coli* O157:H7)	Hemolytic uremic syndrome or thrombotic thrombocytopenic purpura	[357]
Salmonella species	Septicemia and invasive (extraintestinal) salmonellosis, e.g., peritonitis, cholecystitis, pancreatitis, intraabdominal abscess, mycotic aneurysm, osteomyelitis	[362,363]
Campylobacter species	Guillain–Barré syndrome	[365,366]
Shigella species	Seizures and encephalopathy	[363,364,367]
Salmonella, *Shigella*, *Campylobacter*, and *Yersinia* species	Postinfectious reactive arthritis and Reiter syndrome	[361,363,368]
Yersinia species	Thyroiditis, pericarditis, glomerulonephritis, myocarditis, extraintestinal infection, hemolytic uremic syndrome, Guillain–Barré syndrome	[355,356]

leading food-borne disease in the US, while nontyphoidal salmonellosis is a close second [25,26]. *Salmonella* is associated with the ingestion of poultry, eggs, and milk products. *Yersinia enterocolita* is common in the US and is associated with water-borne and food-borne outbreaks. Causes of food poisoning include heavy metals, monosodium glutamate, insecticides, and toxins found in seafood and mushrooms. Ciguatera, diarrheatic, paralytic, neurotoxic, amnestic, and pfiesteria fish poisonings are all caused by dinoflagellates ingested by fish or shellfish [27–32]. Puffer fish poisoning is caused by tetrodotoxin contained only in that fish. If certain fish are improperly stored, scombroid poisoning may occur, which is the release of toxic levels of histamine.

Clostridium difficile

While the primary risk factors for *C. difficile* remain antibiotic usage and hospitalization, the incidence of community-associated *C. difficile* infection is rising, having increased from less than one case per 100 000 in 1994 to 20–50 per 100 000 [33,34]. Given the increasing number of cases of *C. difficile* diarrhea in the community in the absence of traditional risk factors, clinicians should include this pathogen on the differential for any case of severe diarrhea. Compared to hospital-acquired *C. difficile* colitis, community-acquired infections are more commonly seen in younger females with few comorbidities and are typically less severe [35]. It is also important to note that *C. difficile* is a common cause of flares in patients with inflammatory bowel disease (IBD). Enteric infections account for about 10% of symptomatic relapses in IBD patients and nearly 50% of those are secondary to *C. difficile* [36]. It is therefore important to have a high index of suspicion for *C. difficile* in IBD patients presenting with a flare as failing to identify *C. difficile* infection may result in the inappropriate use of steroids and immunosuppressants that could exacerbate the infection and even result in death.

Although metaanalysis studies demonstrated that cure rates are lower in randomized trials compared to open-label trials (67.7% versus 82.7%), fecal microbiota transplantation (FMT) should still be considered for refractory and recurrent *C. difficile* colitis [37,38]. A single-center study showed that FMT after oral vancomycin was superior to oral vancomycin alone or to fidaxomicin alone in clinical and microbiological resolution [39]. There is no difference in clinical resolution of *C. difficile* between lower GI tract and upper GI tract delivery [37] but colonoscopy or oral modalities are more effective than enemas [38].

Protozoa

Protozoa can also cause acute diarrhea but less commonly than viral and bacterial pathogens. However, protozoan infections become more likely as an etiology when diarrhea progresses from persistent to chronic. The common parasites are *Cryptosporidium*, *Giardia*, *Cylospora*, and *Entamoeba histolytica*. In the US, *Cryptosporidium* is the most common parasitic cause of acute food-borne diarrhea [25]. Transmission occurs from an infected person or animal, or a fecal-contaminated food or water source. Numerous water-borne community outbreaks have occurred in the US. In immunocompetent hosts, infection with *Cryptosporidium* can cause severe dehydration but is generally self-limited. *Giardia lamblia* is the second most common gastrointestinal parasite in the US and an important cause of day-care center outbreaks. *Cyclospora* is a small bowel pathogen with symptoms often lasting longer than 3 weeks and is associated with intense fatigue. *Entamoeba histolytica* causes intestinal amebiasis and in developed countries is mainly seen in migrants from and travelers to endemic countries. Sexually active men who have sex with men are also at increased risk of this infection. Symptoms range from mild diarrhea to severe dysentery with abdominal pain and bloody diarrhea.

High-risk populations

Certain populations are at higher risk than others in acquiring diarrheal illnesses. Groups at high risk for infectious diarrhea are shown in Box 35.1. Special populations are further discussed below.

Recent travel

Traveler's diarrhea is the most common illness of people from developed countries traveling to developing countries [40]. Forty to 60% of people travelling to developing countries develop diarrhea. Episodes of traveler's diarrhea are almost always benign and self-limited. Greater than 90% of diarrheal illnesses are due to bacterial infections although viruses and parasites may also be the cause. Most infections are transmitted by food and water. ETEC is the most common cause [41] but other common bacterial pathogens include *Shigella*, *Campylobacter*, and *Salmonella*. The main preventive tool is education but useful medications include fluoroquinolones, rifaximin, and bismuth subsalicylate. Treatment is primarily

Box 35.1 High- risk groups for infectious diarrhea.

- Antibiotic use
  - Outpatient clinics
  - Hospital
- Recent travel
  - Developing nations
  - Peace Corps workers
  - Campers (ground water)
  - Cruise ships (norovirus)
- Homosexuals, sex workers, and intravenous drug users
  - Gay bowel syndrome
  - Acquired immunodeficiency syndrome
- Day-care facilities
  - Children
  - Secondary contacts (family members)
- Institutions
  - Mental institutions
  - Nursing homes
  - Hospitals

supportive with fluid and electrolyte repletion. In severe illness, the combination of antibiotics and an antimotility agent such as loperamide may be superior to either treatment alone [42].

Day-care centers

Diarrhea is extremely common in day-care settings. The most common organisms are those that colonize at a low inoculum dose (*Shigella*, *Giardia*, and *Cryptosporidium*) or that spread easily (rotavirus, astrovirus, adenovirus) [43,44]. The mode of transmission is person-to-person contact by fecal contamination of hands and fomites. In addition, up to 10–20% of parents and siblings of infected children become infected themselves [43,45].

Military personnel

As mentioned above, infectious diarrhea is a very common problem for all travelers. However, the risk and type of infection differ in those who travel for a short amount of time (i.e., less than 2 weeks) compared to those, such as military personnel, who live for extended periods of time remotely, often in locations where clean water and food are less available. Gastrointestinal illness is one of the top five reasons for clinic visits of military personnel deployed abroad [46]. In a systematic review of 49 articles on military personnel overseas, the median self-reported incidence of diarrheal illnesses ranged between 35% and 85%, of which approximately 25% sought medical treatment [47]. Increased incidence of diarrhea correlated with increased time off the military base and consumption of local food/water [48]. There were significant differences in the most common offending pathogen based on location. For instance, *Campylobacter* was the most common pathogen in Southeast Asia, while ETEC was the most common pathogen in Latin America and the Caribbean. Interestingly, specific pathogens were identified in the majority of cases with an overall estimate of 55%. Another study demonstrated that military personnel from the United Kingdom deployed to the Iraq war had a high prevalence of gastroenteritis and that this was highly associated with subsequent development of irritable bowel syndrome (IBS) [49]. Similarly, a study of US military personnel found that symptoms of gastroenteritis were significantly associated with the development of functional gastrointestinal disorders including IBS [50].

Hospitalized patients

Hospitalization is a risk factor for developing infectious diarrhea. *C. difficile* is the most common cause of hospital-acquired infectious diarrhea. Approximately 15% of hospitalized patients develop *C. difficile* colitis, increasing the average hospitalization by 3.6 days and costing an estimated $1.1 billion per year [51]. Acid suppression, particularly proton pump inhibitor use during hospitalization, is associated with developing *C. difficile* colitis [52]. Other causes of diarrhea in hospitalized patients include *Klebsiella oxytoca* and *Clostridium perfringens*, both of which are more commonly seen after antibiotic use [53]. Hospital outbreaks can also occur, primarily attributed to viruses as discussed above.

Immunocompromised patients

Patients with HIV/AIDS, on immunosuppressants, undergoing or post chemotherapy, and with primary immunodeficiencies are considered immunocompromised. Infectious diarrheas mentioned above that are typically short-lived and self-limited often are prolonged and severe in immunocompromised patients. Particularly in HIV/AIDS and post-solid transplanted patients on immunosuppressants, protozoa and viruses including cytomegalovirus must be considered [54]. Neutropenic patients who recently received chemotherapy can develop neutropenic enterocolitis, also known as typhlitis. Pathogenesis is unknown but suspected to be toxic injury to the mucosa allowing invasion of microorganisms; etiology is usually polymicrobial.

Protracted infectious diarrhea

Many of the organisms mentioned, as well as others, are difficult to diagnose and can cause a prolonged course of diarrhea. These include enteropathogenic *E. coli*, *Giardia*, *Amoeba*, *Cryptosporidium*, *Aeromonas*, *Yersinia enterocolitica*, and *Blastocystis hominis*. In addition, *C. difficile* is often difficult to clear, with multiple relapses being common.

Microbiota shifts

Changes in colonic microbiota have been shown to play a role in diseases such as antibiotic-associated colitis and inflammatory bowel disease [55]. Given this, it can be hypothesized that external factors that influence the colonic microbiota may cause symptoms such as diarrhea. In fact, changes in the colonic mucosa-associated microbiota occur following colonic lavage with polyethylene-glycol based regimens [56].

Noninfectious diarrhea

Nosocomial acute diarrhea

Antibiotic associated

Diarrhea occurs in up to 20% of patients receiving antibiotics, with only a portion of these being attributable to *C. difficile* (30–50%) [57]. *C. difficile* colitis on the other hand can cause severe diarrhea with significant morbidity and mortality, as discussed above [58–61]. Non-*C. difficile* but infectious diarrhea may occur with any antibiotic, but is more commonly associated with broad-spectrum antibiotics such as clindamycin, third-generation cephalosporins, and fluoroquinolones. These are mild and self-limiting, and generally clear spontaneously. Certain antibiotics have prokinetic effects on the bowel, such as erythromycin or amoxicillin-clauvulanate [57]. There is some evidence that the incidence of antibiotic-associated diarrhea may be decreased by the use of probiotics [62].

Drugs

Many medications can cause acute diarrhea and thus it is very important to obtain a full medication list from the patient, especially noting any new medications. Box 35.2 displays a list of medications to consider.

Box 35.2 Drugs associated with diarrhea.

Antibiotics: especially penicillins, cephalosporins, clindamycin
Selective serotonin reuptake inhibitors (SSRIs)
Angiotensin converting enzyme inhibitors (ACEIs)
Antacids that contain magnesium
Colchicine
Prednisone
Digoxin
Diuretics
Laxatives
Immunosuppressant medications (mycophenilic acid especially)
Chemotherapies
Metformin
Propranolol
Quinidine
Theophylline
Proton pump inhibitors (PPIs)
Lactulose
Acute alcohol ingestion
Benicar
Marijuana
Cocaine

Chemotherapy/radiation

The incidence of mild acute diarrhea with chemotherapy or radiation therapy is high, approaching 100% with some regimens [63]. Radiation therapy can also cause chronic diarrhea. Nausea, vomiting, and diarrhea are dose and age related. Chemotherapy-associated diarrhea is more common with the following agents: 5-fluorouracil, interferon, irinotecan, topotecan, and interleukin (IL)-2 [63–65]. Neutropenic enterocolitis is a serious diarrheal illness associated with chemotherapy for lymphoma and leukemia, as mentioned above. Radiation may induce diarrhea either through damage to segments of bowel during pelvic irradiation or through damage to the entire bowel if high-dose, total body radiation is received. Watery or bloody diarrhea occurs at dosages greater than 6 Gy. Treatment for both chemotherapy- and radiation-induced diarrhea is supportive with hydration and antimotility agents. Octreotide may be helpful in severe chemotherapy- or radiation-induced diarrhea.

Enteral feeding

More than one-third of patients receiving enteral feeding develop diarrhea [66–68]. Various causes of the diarrhea are hypothesized: bacterial contamination of the formula, hypertonic solutions that cause a "dumping syndrome," lactose-containing formulas in lactase-deficient patients, and sorbitol-containing mixtures. However, if it is needed and indicated for the hospitalized/critically ill patient, enteral feeding should not be stopped. Watery diarrhea occurring in those on enteral nutrition may be due to a multitude of other causes, which must be considered.

Ischemic colitis

Patients with ischemic colitis often present with bloody diarrhea within 24 h after the onset of abdominal pain (see Chapter 114). Three clinical stages have been described [69].

- Hyperactive phase
  - Occurs immediately after occlusion/hypoperfusion.
  - Severe pain predominates along with bloody diarrhea.
  - Blood loss is mild and generally does not require transfusion.
  - Symptoms resolve with conservative measures.
- Paralytic phase
  - Pain diminishes, becomes more continuous and diffuse.
  - Abdomen becomes more tender and distended.
- Shock phase
  - Massive fluid, electrolyte, and protein loss occur through a gangrenous mucosa.
  - Severe dehydration with shock requiring rapid surgical intervention.
  - Occurs in 10–20% of patients.

Fecal impaction

Chronic constipation may paradoxically present as acute and chronic diarrhea. Liquid stool passes around the obstruction, in this case impacted stool, causing an overflow diarrhea. This is often seen with fecal incontinence. Treatment is relief of the fecal impaction (i.e., manual disimpaction, enemas, laxatives). See section on Overflow diarrhea below.

Runner's diarrhea

A variety of gastrointestinal disturbances occur in those who exercise vigorously, especially marathon runners and triathletes [70]. Watery, self-limited diarrhea may occur in 10–25% and is especially common in women runners (40–70%). The mechanisms are unclear but possibly involve the release of gastrointestinal hormones such as gastrin, motilin, and VIP, or release of inflammatory mediators such as prostaglandins. There is also an increased incidence of ischemic colitis in marathon runners, and thus ischemia is postulated as a cause of runner's diarrhea [71,72]. No treatment regimens have been studied in the management of runner's diarrhea.

Food allergy

Gastrointestinal manifestations, particularly diarrhea, are common presentations of food allergies, both IgE- and non-IgE-mediated reactions. IgE-mediated reactions are typically acute, with diarrhea occurring within 2–6 h of ingestion, while nausea, vomiting, and abdominal pain can occur within minutes to hours. The term "GI anaphylaxis" is used when GI symptoms occur in the absence of other organ involvement, but this is very rare [73]. Non-IgE-mediated food allergies are more subacute/chronic in nature and are typically isolated to the GI tract and/or skin. These disorders include protein-induced enterocolitis syndrome, which manifests in infants, and celiac disease. Celiac disease is an immune disorder triggered by the gliadin component of gluten in genetically predisposed individuals. While celiac disease can present in a number of different ways, the classic signs are bulky, foul-smelling stools and flatulence due to steatorrhea related to malabsorption. Nonceliac gluten sensitivity is a clinical syndrome that is rising in prevalence. It manifests as irritable bowel-like symptoms that responds to gluten avoidance. There is currently no physiological explanation, histological changes, or serological markers that define nonceliac gluten sensitivity [74].

Early manifestations of chronic diseases

Early inflammatory bowel disease

While Crohn's disease and ulcerative colitis are chronic conditions with a relapsing and remitting course, they both can present initially as acute diarrhea. Consideration of either diagnosis should be given to patients who, while presenting with acute diarrhea, on further interrogation are noted to have chronic symptoms such as abdominal pain and weight loss. A family history of IBD may also provide a clue to this diagnosis.

Thyrotoxicosis

A common chronic manifestation of hyperthyroidism is diarrhea. However, in the acute case of thyroid storm, severe nausea, vomiting, and diarrhea can occur in addition to cardiovascular symptoms and hyperpyrexia.

Diagnostic approach

As has been described above, the majority of acute diarrhea is secondary to self-limited infections, most commonly viral. Therefore, it is not clinically necessary or economically feasible to perform extensive evaluation beyond the history and physical exam on every patient who presents with acute diarrhea. The most recent American College of Gastroenterology guideline regarding which patients should undergo additional medical evaluation is less restrictive than before. Those who are at high risk of spreading the disease or those involved in an outbreak warrant stool studies [75]. Diagnostic testing may also be warranted in incidences of dysentery, moderate to severe disease, and acute diarrhea occurring ≥7 days, with the goal of pathogen-directed therapy.

Historical clues

As for most presenting complaints, a thorough history can provide much insight into the etiology of diarrhea.

Symptoms

Presence of bloody diarrhea commonly indicates *Campylobacter*, *Salmonella*, EHEC O157:H7, and *Shigella*. Fever suggests invasive bacteria such as the aforementioned pathogens that cause dysentery, as well as other cytotoxic organisms such as *C. difficile* and *Entamoeba histolytica*. Table 35.3 provides a summary of important epidemiological clues [76].

Onset

The timing of symptoms also provides a clue to diagnosis. Symptoms that begin within 6 h of food ingestion suggest the presence of a preformed toxin of *Staphylococcus aureus* or *Bacillus cereus*. Symptoms that begin within 8–16 h are consistent with infection with *Clostridium perfringens*. Symptoms that begin after more than 16 h may be due to viral or bacterial infection.

Exposures

A thorough history of exposures can also lead to an accurate diagnosis, including recent travel history, food intake, identification of known contacts with similar symptoms, or new medications.

Laboratory testing

Stool studies

Fecal leukocytes/leukocytes The utility of fecal leukocytes in aiding in the detection of an inflammatory diarrhea is limited. A metaanalysis reported a sensitivity and specificity of only 70% and 50%, respectively [77]. However, if both fecal leukocytes and occult blood in the stool are positive, it is sufficient to support a bacterial cause of acute diarrhea [78]. Given the limitations of fecal leukocytes, a fecal lactoferrin latex agglutination assay was developed, which has a reported sensitivity and specificity greater than 90% in differentiating inflammatory diarrhea from noninflammatory causes [79].

Stool cultures As mentioned above, the rate of positive stool cultures in acute diarrhea is very low, except in patients with severe disease. Thus, it is only cost-effective to order stool cultures in the appropriate clinical scenarios, which include patients who are immunocompromised (especially HIV patients), patients with bloody diarrhea, patients at high risk of spreading the illness, patients involved in a suspected outbreak, and patients with underlying IBD.

Ova and parasites Similar to stool cultures, testing for stool ova and parasites is not indicated for all cases of acute diarrhea. In the following clinical scenarios, obtaining stool ova and parasites is justified: patients with persistent diarrhea, diarrhea in men who have sex with men, patients with AIDS, a community water outbreak (associated with *Giardia* and *Cryptosporidium*), and bloody diarrhea with few or no leukocytes (associated with intestinal amebiasis). Because parasitic excretion may be intermittent, obtaining three specimens on consecutive days is recommended.

C. difficile testing

If suspicion is high for *C. difficile* colitis, testing should be done, especially in high-risk patients (e.g., immunocompromised, hospitalized, recent antibiotic use) [80]. All toxigenic strains of *C. difficile* produce toxins A and B. Nucleic acid amplification tests (NAAT) targeting genes specific to toxigenic strains, commonly the gene for toxin B, are very sensitive but will not differentiate between active infections and asymptomatic carriers. Enzyme immunoassays (EIA) for toxins A and B and glutamate dehydrogenase (GDH) are used in conjunction to diagnose *C. difficile* infection. Current guidelines by the Infectious Diseases Society of America recommend a multistep algorithm that has increased positive and negative predictive values among high-risk groups and improves sensitivity to best detect the

Table 35.3 Correlation between pathophysiology and symptoms of infectious diarrhea.

Pathophysiology/microorganisms	Nausea and vomiting	Abdominal pain	Fever	Diarrhea
Toxin producers	2–4 + (within 4 h of ingestion)	1–2 +	0–1 +	3–4 +, watery
Preformed toxin				
Bacillus cereus, Staphylococcus aureus, Clostridium perfringens				
Enterotoxin	(Within 24–72 h of ingestion)			
Vibrio cholerae, enterotoxigenic Escherichia coli, Klebsiella pneumoniae, Aeromonas species				
Enteroadherent	0–1 +	1–3 +	1–2 +	1–2 +, watery
Enteropathogenic and enteroadherent *E. coli*, *Giardia* organisms, *Cryptosporidium* species, helminths				
Cytotoxin-producing	0–1 +	3–4 +	1–2 +	1–3 +, usually watery, occasionally or quickly bloody
Clostridium difficile, hemorrhagic *E. coli* O157:H7				
Invasive organisms	0–3 +	2–4 +	3–4 +	1–4 +, watery or bloody
Minimal inflammation				
Rotavirus and Norwalk agent, *Cryptosporidium* and *Cyclospora* species				
Variable inflammation				
Salmonella, *Campylobacter*, and *Aeromonas* species, *Vibrio parahaemolyticus*				
Severe inflammation				
Shigella species, enteroinvasive *E. coli*, *Entamoeba histolytica*, anthrax				
Systemic infection				
Hepatitis, measles, listeriosis, legionellosis, Rocky Mountain spotted fever, psittacosis, hantavirus, otitis media in infants, toxic shock syndrome, avian influenza (H5N1), severe acute respiratory syndrome (SARS)	Watery diarrhea may accompany these diseases but is often overshadowed by the other disease manifestations			

Numbers 0 to 4 + refer to the severity of symptoms.
Source: Adapted from Powell 1997 [334].

Box 35.3 Diagnostic modalities for detecting *C. difficile* infections.

Patient with increased risk (e.g., immunocompromised, immunosuppressed, hospitalized, recent antibiotic use) – use multistep algorithm:

- GDH *plus* toxin
  Or
- GDH *plus* toxin *followed by* NAAT
  Or
- NAAT *plus* toxin

Patients with clinical symptoms (3 or more watery stools per day):

- NAAT *alone*
  Or
- Multistep algorithm above

GDH, glutamate dehydrogenase; NAAT, nucleic acid amplification test.

infection among patients with clinical symptoms (Box 35.3). If clinical suspicion is high based on symptoms of three or more watery stools per day, NAAT alone may also be used.

Multiplex panels

The advent of multiplex PCR assays that can detect and identify multiple pathogens on one panel changed how we evaluate diarrhea in the inpatient and outpatient setting. Only a handful of multiplex assays have been approved by the Food and Drug Administration but several studies have demonstrated the cost-effectiveness of such assays, reducing the number of additional stool studies, diagnostic imaging, and days on antibiotics [81]. The sensitivities of these tests vary depending on the assay and the pathogen, typically ranging from 80% to 100%, but can be as low as 20% for adenovirus [82]. For enteropathogenic *E. coli* (EPEC), enteroaggregative *E. coli* (EAEC), and ETEC, the sensitivity and specificity are very high [83]. EPEC is one of the most common pathogens seen when utilizing the multiplex assays, both as single or coinfections [81,83]. However, these panels do not distinguish between typical (known diarrheal pathogen) and atypical (virulence profile not yet established) EPEC. Atypical EPEC comprise over 50% of EPEC-positive assays and its role in causing diarrhea is unknown, especially in adults [83,84]. This problem speaks to a larger issue with multiplex assays – as the rates of positive stool studies increase, providers are faced with how to interpret such results. Special care must be taken to apply positive results to disease severity and likelihood that the pathogen is the causative agent.

Endoscopic assessment

The role of endoscopy in acute diarrhea is overall quite limited. The settings in which endoscopy may be helpful are the following [85].

- Distinguishing IBD from infectious diarrhea (note that as mentioned above, early IBD can present as acute diarrhea) although the histopathology may not be able to differentiate these causes
- Determining the presence of pseudomembranes in toxic-appearing patients in order to diagnose *C. difficile* while awaiting the stool toxin assay; however, it should be noted that colonoscopy may be contraindicated in *C. difficile* patients due to the high risk of perforation in those with compromised integrity of intestine and pseudomembranes are not always present.
- Immunocompromised patients at risk for opportunistic infections such as CMV.

Treatment

The mainstay of treatment for acute diarrhea is hydration. Most deaths from diarrhea occur because of dehydration, therefore the most important part of the clinical assessment of such patients is their fluid status followed by treatment of hypovolemia and electrolyte disturbances. Severely dehydrated patients require intravenous fluid while those who are alert and only mildly dehydrated can be supported with oral rehydration, which is as effective as intravenous hydration in most instances [86]. An algorithm for a general approach to evaluating and treating patients with acute diarrhea is shown in Figure 35.1.

A few symptomatic treatment options also exist. Bismuth subsalicylate is safe and efficacious in bacterial diarrheas [85–87]. Loperamide can also be useful and safe in patients with traveler's diarrhea as long as it is not given to patients infected with an invasive pathogen (symptoms of high fever or blood in stool) [87–91]. Antiemetics are safe and make symptoms more tolerable. A systematic review found that probiotics can also be useful in treating traveler's diarrhea, but further research is needed to support this recommendation [92]. The use of antibiotics for acute infectious diarrhea is controversial [93]. Specific antibiotic recommendations are discussed in Chapter 144.

Complications of acute diarrheal diseases in adults

Guillain–Barré syndrome

Guillain–Barré syndrome (GBS) is an acute immune-mediated polyneuropathy resulting in ascending paralysis. A proposed mechanism for GBS is that an antecedent infection evokes an immune response whereby antibodies cross-react via molecular mimicry with peripheral nerve components [94]. The immune response may be directed towards the axon of the peripheral nerve. *Campylobacter jejuni* is the most commonly identified precipitant of GBS. One study reported that 26% of patients with GBS had a recent *C. jejuni* infection [95]. In addition, *Campylobacter*-associated GBS appears to have a worse prognosis with a slower recovery and more significant neurological dysfunction.

Thrombotic thrombocytopenic purpura–hemolytic uremic syndrome

Thrombotic thrombocytopenic purpura–hemolytic uremic syndrome (TTP-HUS) is an acute disorder that results in multiple organ dysfunction. While this syndrome is heterogeneous in terms of etiology, demographics, and response to treatment, the clinical features are similar and include thrombocytopenia and microangiopathic hemolytic anemia without another identifiable cause, and in many patients both renal and neurological abnormalities occur [96]. Most cases of HUS in children and occasional cases of TTP in adults are preceded by an episode of bloody diarrhea. Shiga toxin produced by *E. coli* O157:H7 or other bacteria is the etiology in these cases [97]. It is important to note that antibiotic treatment for *E. coli* O157:H7 is contraindicated given the increased incidence of HUS in patients receiving antibiotic therapy [93].

Postinfectious inflammatory bowel disease

Several observational studies have suggested an association between acute gastroenteritis and the development of IBD [98–101]. One of these studies showed a statistically significant increased risk of IBD in patients with a prior history of gastroenteritis [98]. A second study reported an increased risk of developing IBD in patients with documented *Salmonella* or *Campylobacter* infection versus a matched control group [99].

Reactive arthritis

Reactive arthritis is a spondyloarthritis that arises following an infection, although pathogens cannot be cultured from the affected joints. A variety of enteric infections are associated with reactive arthritis including *Salmonella*, *Shigella*, *Yersinia*, *Campylobacter*, and *C. difficile* [102].

Chronic diarrhea

Definition, classification, and epidemiology

Chronic diarrhea has classically been defined as loss of formed stool consistency occurring for greater than 4 weeks [103,104]. However, patients can present for evaluation of diarrheal syndromes without fitting this criterion. Two such examples are hyperthyroidism, in which case patients develop hyperdefecation of formed stool, and patients who report symptoms of fecal incontinence as diarrhea. Because of the heterogeneity that exists in diarrheal syndromes, in this chapter chronic diarrhea is

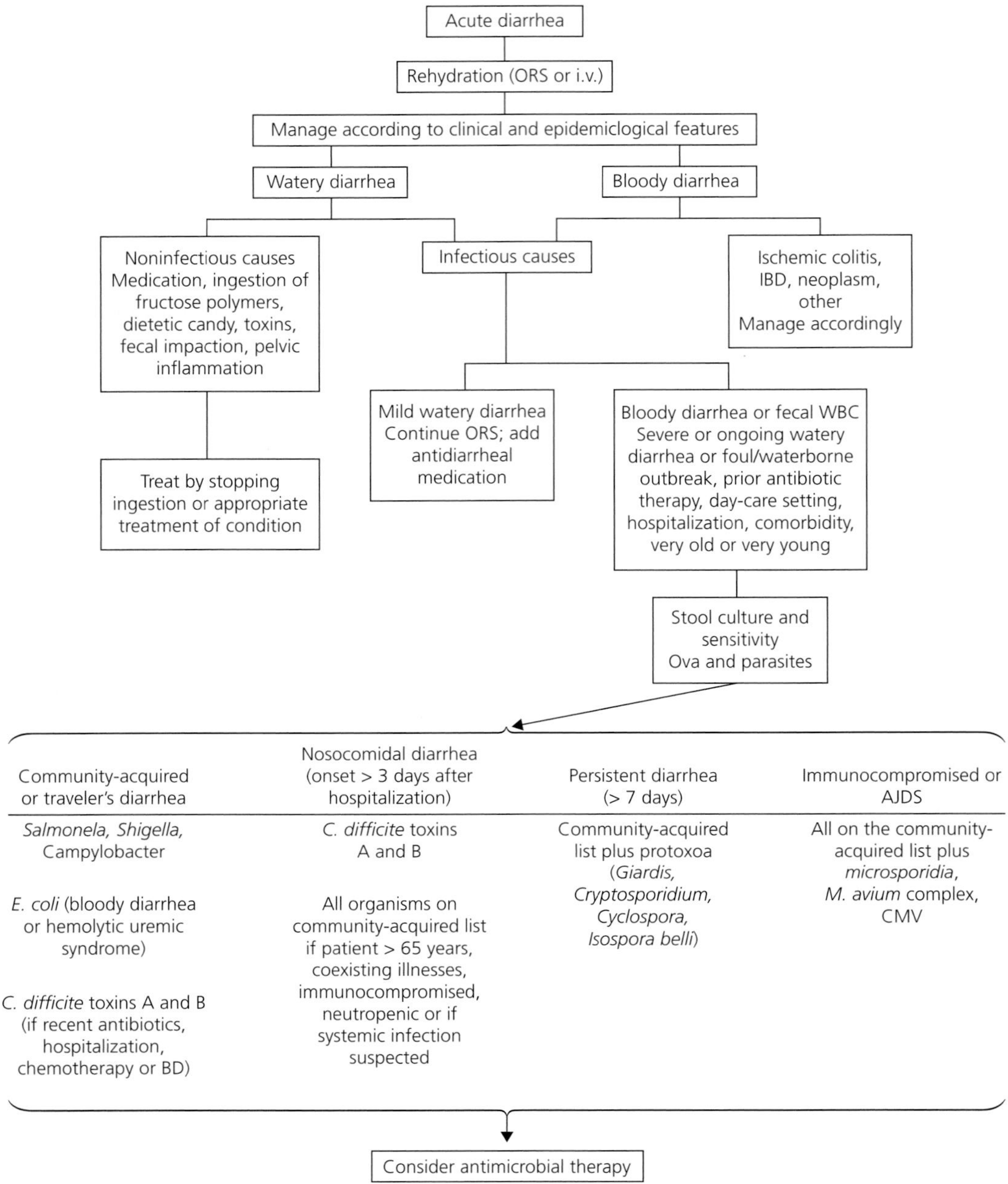

Figure 35.1 Algorithm for the diagnostic approach to acute diarrhea. CMV, cytomegalovirus; IBD, inflammatory bowel disease; i.v., intravenous; ORS, oral replacement solution; WBC, white blood cell count. Data from [89].

defined as the loss of formed stool, an increase in the frequency of bowel movements, or an increase in total daily stool volume that persists for greater than 4 weeks.

The majority of current literature supports the division of diarrheal syndromes into clinically defined subgroups, including watery, malabsorptive, and inflammatory diarrhea. Issues arise with this classification when a single disease presents in a variety of ways. For example, patients who suffer with chronic diarrhea from a gastrinoma may present with symptoms consistent with either secretory diarrhea or osmotic diarrhea. Thus, it is reasonable to develop a more expansive pathophysiology-based classification divided into the following categories: secretory, osmotic, malabsorptive, inflammatory, prolonged infectious, nosocomial, and functional (Table 35.4).

Evaluation of chronic diarrhea is a common reason for referral by primary care providers to subspecialists. Aside from the economic impact that occurs from loss of work hours, chronic diarrhea is a leading cause of impairment of mental health and a patient's overall quality of life [105,106]. Often times patients must interrupt social events secondary to frequent bowel

Table 35.4 Causes of chronic diarrhea.

Classification of diarrhea	Cause
Secretory	Carcinoid syndrome, VIPoma, gastrinoma, medullary carcinoma of the thyroid, bile acid diarrhea, villous adenoma, alcohol diarrhea, congenital diseases
Osmotic	Carbohydrate malabsorption, medications, consumption of alcohol, sugars (refer to Box 35.4)
Malabsorptive	Pancreatic insufficiency, celiac disease, small intestinal bacterial overgrowth
Inflammatory	Inflammatory bowel disease, celiac disease, microscopic colitis, eosinophilic enteropathies, systemic mastocytosis, protein-losing enteropathy
Prolonged Infectious	Whipple disease, tropical sprue (refer to Box 35.6)
Nosocomial	Medications, dumping syndrome, short bowel syndrome, overflow diarrhea, diabetic enteropathy, radiation enteritis/proctitis
Functional	Irritable bowel syndrome, postinfectious irritable bowel syndrome, factitious diarrhea

movements, refrain from taking long voyages, worry about the possibility of incontinence, and hesitate to use public restrooms.

Age, comorbidities, location, and socioeconomic status dictate the prevalence of chronic diarrhea syndromes [107]. Although difficult to accurately determine, the prevalence of chronic diarrhea in the US is estimated to be approximately 5% [103,108].

Clinical evaluation of chronic diarrhea

The first step in the evaluation of a patient presenting with chronic diarrhea is to obtain a thorough history and physical examination with the goal of acquiring significant clues that can inform the differential diagnosis and further testing (Figure 35.2). Questions related to symptomology should include onset of symptoms, abdominal pain, establishment of stool consistency, frequency, and volume, presence of nocturnal symptoms, and systemic symptoms such as fevers or weight loss. Rectal bleeding can be a sign of mucosal injury or may develop secondary to irritation of internal hemorrhoids. Important historical questions include any foreign or domestic travel, HIV risk factors, prior history of diarrheal syndromes, and family history of gastrointestinal disease. Special attention should be paid to current and past medications along with a review of prior hospitalizations, medical procedures, surgeries, and treatments.

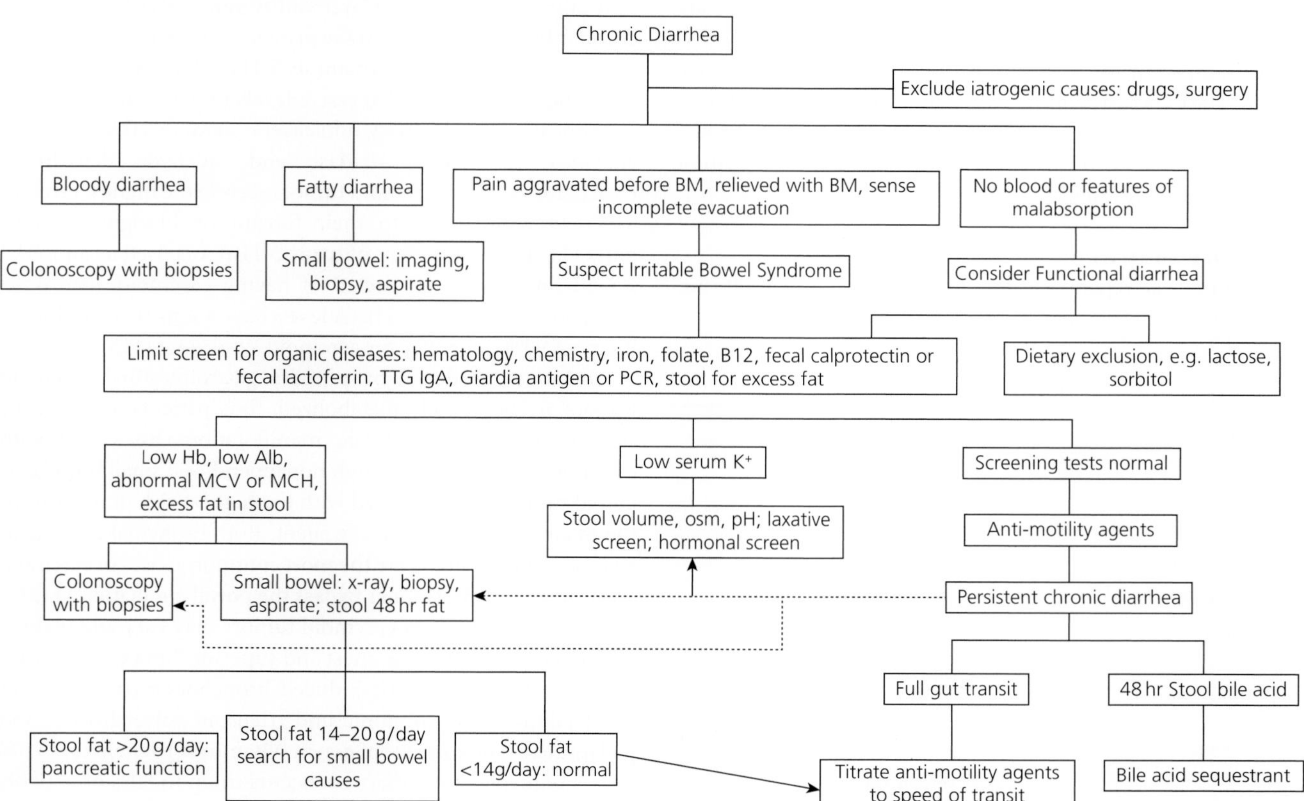

Figure 35.2 Approach to chronic diarrhea. BM, bowel movement; MCH, mean corpuscular hemoglobin; MCV, mean corpuscular volume; PCR, polymerase chain reaction; TTG, tissue transglutaminase. Source: Adapted from Camilleri et al. 2017 [371].

The physical exam should focus on searching for extraintestinal manifestations of chronic diarrheal syndromes and evidence of nutritional deficiencies. Because further testing will depend largely on the history and physical examination, there is no set protocol for laboratory, radiological, and endoscopic testing. Initial laboratory testing typically begins with a complete blood count with differential, electrolytes including renal function testing, liver function tests, and serum albumin with total protein levels. The American Gastroenterological Association's (AGA) Clinical Practice Guidelines for Chronic Diarrhea recommend using fecal calprotectin (>50 µg/g) or fecal lactoferrin (4.0–7.25 µg/g) to screen for inflammatory bowel disease and recommend against erythrocyte sedimentation rate and C-reactive protein levels [109]. The AGA further recommends screening for celiac disease with serum IgA tissue transglutaminase, as well as ruling out *Giardia* via the stool antigen test or polymerase chain reaction. Low serum albumin levels occur in patients with poor nutritional status as well as those with chronic inflammatory conditions through a decrease in protein synthesis [110]. Testing for vitamin and mineral deficiencies can provide clues to the localization of disease (Table 35.5).

Colonoscopy with terminal ileal and colonic biopsies is recommended in patients without an established diagnosis after initial testing, particularly those over the age of 50 [111]. Upper endoscopy is useful if a malabsorptive, inflammatory, or prolonged infectious process is suspected. Some situations may justify empiric treatment of patients if there is a high level of clinical suspicion for a specific cause. For example, one may elect to start cholestyramine in a patient who reports chronic diarrhea following ileal resection or gallbladder surgery. In such situations, response to treatment affirms the diagnosis without need for further testing.

Secretory diarrhea

Stool output is reliant on the maintenance of equilibrium between the secretion and absorption of water and electrolytes.

Table 35.5 Vitamin/mineral deficiencies in patients with chronic diarrhea.

Vitamin/mineral	Site of absorption
Vitamin A, D, E, K	Small intestine
Vitamin B-2 (Riboflavin)	Small intestine
Vitamin B-3 (Niacin)	Small intestine
Vitamin B-6 (Pyridoxine)	Small intestine
Vitamin B-12 (Cobalamin)	Ileum
Folate	Proximal small intestine
Calcium	Small intestine
Magnesium	Small intestine
Copper	Stomach; duodenum
Zinc	Proximal small intestine
Iron	Duodenum

Cyclic adenosine monophosphate (AMP) and cyclic guanosine monophosphate (GMP) pathways play a primary role in regulating electrolyte secretion. In the setting of acute infections, pathogenic enterotoxins bind to receptors that stimulate these pathways leading to chloridorrhea and subsequent luminal fluid shifts that clinically manifest as severe watery diarrhea [112]. Chronically, endogenous compounds such as neurotransmitters, hormones, and solutes can also stimulate intestinal electrolyte transporters to induce secretory diarrhea.

Although clinical presentations are variable, several historical clues can help clinicians distinguish between secretory and osmotic diarrheas. Classic findings associated with secretory diarrhea include frequent, watery, voluminous, bowel movements, night-time awakening, dehydration, altered serum electrolytes, and lack of response to fasting [113]. Laboratory findings in chronic diarrhea associated with increased electrolyte secretion include a stool sodium concentration greater than 90 mmol/L and an osmotic gap less than 50 mOsm/kg. Osmotic gap is calculated though the equation: 290 mOsm/kg $H_2O - 2 \times$ [stool Na^+ + stool K^+] mM (Figure 35.3).

Carcinoid syndrome

Although carcinoid tumors have been described since the late 19th century, identification of carcinoid syndrome as a manifestation of excess vasoactive substances did not occur until the mid-20th century [114]. Carcinoid tumors arise from enterochromaffin cells involved in the primary production and release of serotonin (5-hydroxytrypamine, 5-HT) along with other bioactive hormones [115]. Excessive levels of 5-HT are converted systemically to 5-hydroxyindoleacetic acid (5-HIAA) by the enzymes monoamine oxidase and aldehyde dehydrogenase [116]. Midgut carcinoid tumors secrete the highest levels of 5-HT in comparison to their foregut or hindgut counterparts [117]. Measurement of urine 5-HIAA is used as an initial screen for patients suspected of having carcinoid syndrome. Elevated 24-h urinary 5-HIAA levels have a sensitivity and specificity of 90% or greater for carcinoid syndrome [118].

Hormones produced by primary gastrointestinal carcinoid tumors are hepatically metabolized, thus patients are typically free of the classic systemic manifestations associated with carcinoid syndrome. Although nonappendiceal small bowel carcinoid tumors are associated with the highest risk of metastasis, the majority remain clinically silent. Both bronchial and metastatic carcinoid tumors are the most common causes of carcinoid syndrome as the hormones bypass the portal circulation [119].

Typical symptoms of carcinoid tumors may vary and include cutaneous flushing of the chest and superior thorax, respiratory wheezing from histamine-induced bronchoconstriction, right heart failure from pulmonic and tricuspid valve disease, and pellagra as a consequence of niacin (vitamin B_3) deficiency [120–122]. Frequent watery diarrhea occurs in up to 80% of patients with carcinoid syndrome. Hormonal and serotonergic activation of intestinal transporters along with local tissue effects lead to increased intestinal transit, thus overwhelming colonic

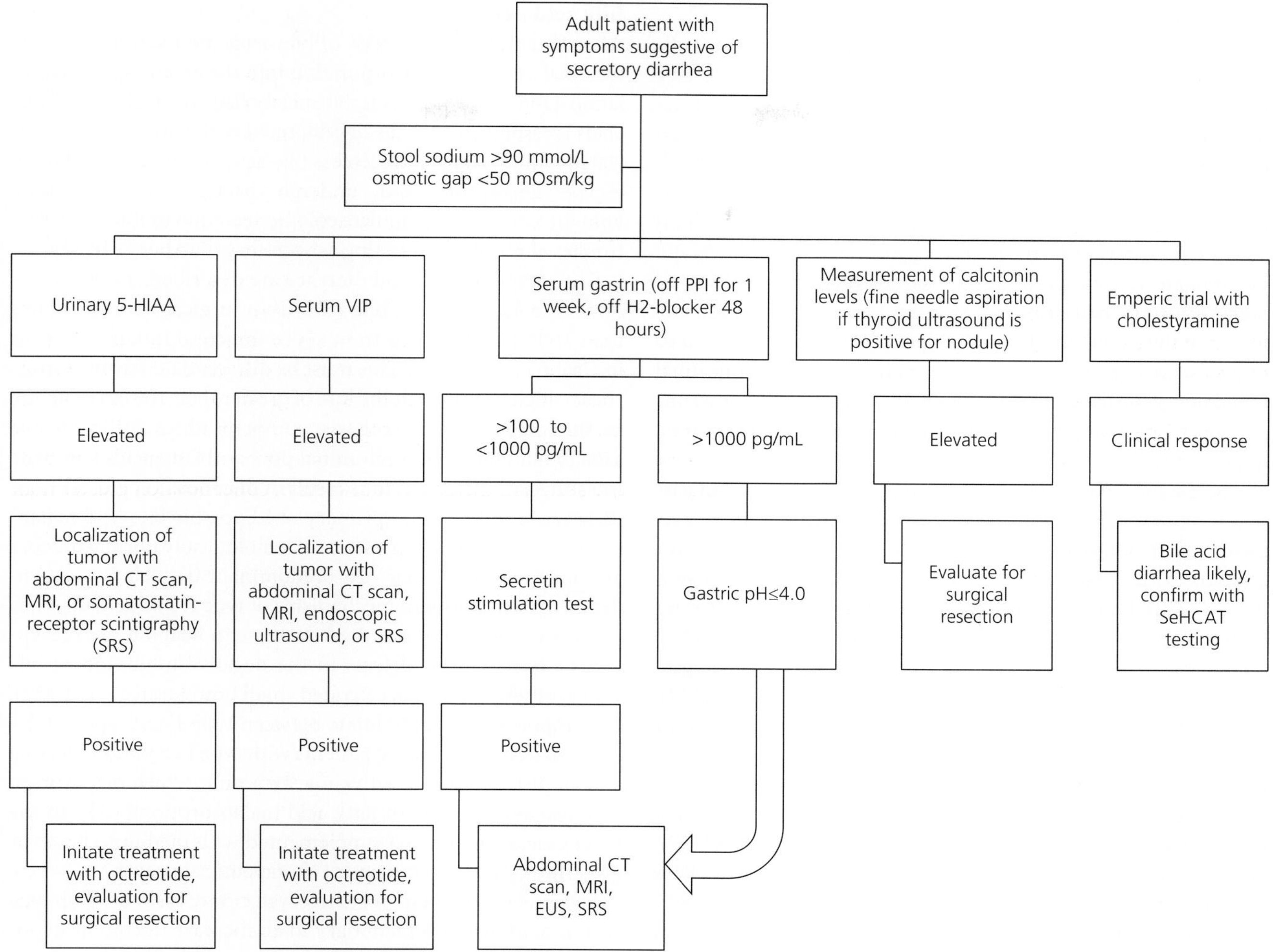

Figure 35.3 Algorithm for evaluation of secretory diarrhea. PPI, proton pump inhibitor.

absorptive capacity [123]. Diarrhea is typically managed with common antidiarrheal agents such as loperamide, diphenoxylate/atropine, and opiates [124]. Along with its effects on cutaneous and cardiorespiratory symptoms, ondansetron may be of use in patients with severe refractory diarrhea largely from its effects as a serotonin receptor antagonist [125,126].

VIPoma

Vasoactive inhibitory peptide (VIP) is an important gastrointestinal hormone, which plays a key role in smooth muscle relaxation. VIP binds to calcitonin-like G-protein coupled receptors, leading to activation of adenylyl cyclase and accumulation of cyclic AMP. This ultimately induces intestinal secretion of water and electrolytes including sodium, potassium, chloride, and bicarbonate [127]. VIPomas are pancreatic non-β islet cell tumors that express VIP in an unregulated fashion. They can occur sporadically or rarely in association with multiple endocrine neoplasia syndrome type I (MEN I) [128]. Overactivation of the aforementioned pathways leads to a constellation of symptoms associated with severe chronic watery diarrhea; hypokalemia was first described by Verner and Morrison in 1958 [129]. The terms watery diarrhea– hypokalemia–achlorhydria syndrome and pancreatic cholera describe the constellation of watery diarrhea and hypokalemia associated with elevated VIP levels presenting along with dehydration, achlorhydria, metabolic acidosis, flushing, hypercalcemia, and hyperglycemia [130].

The first step in the management of these patients is supportive care to correct fluid and electrolyte losses. Patients with VIPomas will have elevated VIP levels at least three times above the upper normal limit. Proper identification of the lesion requires imaging with computed tomography (CT) scan, magnetic resonance imaging (MRI), or endoscopic ultrasound [131]. The goal of imaging is to identify the potential for surgical resection. Octreotide has been shown to be effective in controlling diarrhea in patients with VIP-associated tumors [131–133].

Gastrinoma (Zollinger–Ellison syndrome)

As with VIP-secreting tumors, gastrinomas can occur sporadically or in association with MEN I syndrome [128,134] (see Chapter 50). Despite gastrinomas being a rare cause of refractory peptic and small bowel ulceration, 70% of patients with gastrinomas develop diarrhea as the initial symptom [135]. Diarrhea presents in one of two forms. Secretory diarrhea develops secondary to activation of channels responsible for sodium and water secretion in combination with increased pancreatic bicarbonate secretion [136,137]. Osmotic diarrhea results from the inability to neutralize excess acid being released into the lumen of the small bowel. Malabsorption of macronutrients also occurs secondary to the low intraluminal pH due to intestinal villi damage and inactivation of pancreatic enzymes. For example, inactivation of pancreatic lipase prevents the binding of fat to bile acids [138].

The diagnosis of gastrinoma requires an elevated serum gastrin level. It is important to note, however, that a gastrin level greater than 1000 pg/mL is diagnostic only when found in combination with clinical manifestations of Zollinger–Ellison syndrome. This holds true because serum gastrin levels greater than 1000 pg/mL may be present in patients with achlorhydria secondary to atrophic gastritis. Endoscopically, 94% of gastrinoma cases have evidence of thickened gastric folds [134]. Patients for whom there is a high level of clinical suspicion for Zollinger–Ellison syndrome but who have serum gastrin levels less than 1000 pg/mL should undergo secretin stimulation testing. Secretin is a hormone produced by the small intestine that binds primarily to pancreatic G-protein coupled receptors [139]. Under normal physiological conditions, secretin stimulates pancreatic fluid secretion and inhibition of gastrin release [140]. In an unexplained physiological phenomenon, administration of secretin in patients with a gastrinoma leads to an increase in serum gastrin levels.

Medullary carcinoma of the thyroid

Thyroid medullary carcinomas are rare malignancies associated with multiple endocrine neoplasia type II (MEN II) syndrome that account for only 4% of thyroid gland tumors [141,142]. They are classified as neuroendocrine tumors originating from parafollicular C cells involved in calcium level regulation by secretion of the hormone calcitonin [143,144]. Medullary carcinomas excrete excessive levels of calcitonin and calcitonin gene-related peptide. Activation of G-coupled calcitonin receptors in the small bowel causes a secretory diarrhea secondary to secretion of water and electrolytes [145,146]. This can be propagated by the release of other intestinal secretogogs such as prostaglandins, VIP, substance P, serotonin, and kallikrein [147]. Release of these hormones leads to the development of extraintestinal manifestations such as flushing. Measurement of serum calcitonin levels can be obtained but the gold standard is fine needle aspiration of a thyroid nodule with calcitonin immunohistochemical staining [145,147].

Bile acid diarrhea

After fat emulsification, 95% of bile acids are reabsorbed in the terminal ileum for reincorporation into the enterohepatic circulation [148]. Colonic bacterial metabolism of unabsorbed bile acids is responsible for the development of the brown color associated with normal stool. Excess bile acids in the colonic lumen escape absorption and undergo bacterial deconjugation. Dihydroxy bile salts stimulate colonic secretion of fluid and electrolytes clinically manifesting as secretory diarrhea [148,149].

Three types of bile acid diarrhea are described. Type I is secondary to ileal bypass of bile acids from surgical resection of less than 100 cm of ileum or from severe mucosal inflammation as in Crohn's ileitis [150]. This must be differentiated from steatorrhea, which occurs with the loss of greater than 100 cm of ileum. In this case, hepatic synthesis cannot produce sufficient bile salts to maintain the intraluminal pool and fatty acids stimulate intestinal secretion and thus result in diarrhea. Type II bile acid diarrhea, also known as primary or idiopathic bile acid malabsorption, occurs in the presence of histologically normal mucosa and may present as diarrhea-predominant irritable bowel syndrome [151]. Proposed mechanisms of type II bile acid diarrhea include congenital or acquired decrease in ileal bile acid receptors or transporters, defects in the negative inhibition of bile acid synthesis, and/or accelerated small bowel transit [151,152]. It is important to differentiate between type I and type II bile-induced diarrhea because patients with type I respond to fasting and empiric treatment with cholestyramine, which may worsen diarrhea associated with fatty acid malabsorption [153]. In the latter case, a low-fat diet supplemented with medium-chain triglycerides is the recommended therapeutic approach.

Seventeen percent of postcholecystectomy cases develop type III bile acid diarrhea secondary to an increase in colonic exposure to bile acids typically stored in the gallbladder [154]. Type IV bile acid diarrhea results from increased hepatic bile acid synthesis, which can be seen with metformin use [151]. Although testing for 23-seleno-25-homo-tauro-cholic acid (SeHCAT) and high-performance liquid chromatography of serum 7-α-OH-4-cholesten-3-one (C4) can be performed to assess for loss of bile acids, these tests may not be readily available, are time-consuming, and expensive. Instead, current recommendations include an empiric trial of cholestyramine in a patient who presents with an unexplained secretory diarrhea [151].

Congenital chloride diarrhea

Congenital chloride diarrhea is a rare autosomal recessive disorder caused by a mutation of the gene *SLC26A3* on chromosome 7. This mutation renders ileal and colonic Cl^-/ $HCO3^-$ transporters defective, thus leading to inadequate chloride absorption [155]. Congenital chloride diarrhea was first described by Gamble and Darrow in 1945 when evaluating infants whose severe diarrhea contained unusually high concentrations of chloride accompanied by systemic hypochloremia, metabolic alkalosis, and hypokalemia [156,157]. Diagnosis is typically suspected prenatally with findings of polyhydramnios on ultrasound and confirmed upon findings of excessive fecal chloride concentrations [158,159]. Treatment consists of high-dose chloride supplementation to allow for passive chloride absorption along with control of chloridorrhea by decreasing gastric chloride secretion with the use of proton pump inhibitors [160,161].

Villous adenoma

Villous adenomas account for 5–10% of all adenomatous polyps [162,163]. Although the majority of villous adenomas remain asymptomatic, a rare subset can cause severe secretory diarrhea leading to hypovolemia with acute renal failure, hyponatremia, hypokalemia, metabolic acidosis, and confusion [164]. Excess fluid and electrolyte secretion is thought to develop as a consequence of an elevation in prostaglandin E2 and adenylate cyclase activity [164–166]. Secretory villous adenomas are typically large and located in the rectosigmoid colon where they produce an excessive amount of mucus from hyperstimulated goblet cells [163,167]. Management of secretory villous adenomas includes fluid and electrolyte resuscitation with a plan for adenoma removal by endoscopic polypectomy, endoscopic mucosal resection, or surgery [168]. Medical management with indomethacin is aimed at decreasing fluid and electrolyte loss through inhibition of prostaglandin synthesis [169].

Alcohol diarrhea

Alcohol abuse is associated with multiple gastrointestinal diseases including alcohol-related gastritis, gastroesophageal reflux disease, pancreatic disease, and liver disease. Perhaps an underreported phenomenon is alcohol's effects on intestinal mucosa leading to diarrhea. Acutely, excess alcohol consumption can lead to an inflammatory response causing epithelial and microvascular damage [170,171]. One common cause of diarrhea relates to the effects of nonalcohol components including those containing high levels of wheat or rye products leading to symptom provocation in patients suffering from celiac disease. Chronic alcohol consumption can also cause cytotoxic endothelial cell damage within the small intestine, leading to villous blunting [172]. Other potential causes of diarrhea include bacterial overgrowth, decreased intestinal disaccharidase activity, and increased propulsive contractions leading to rapid intestinal transit [173–175]. Reversal of diarrhea related to alcohol consumption typically occurs with abstinence.

Osmotic diarrhea

The process of osmosis describes the flow of water across a semipermeable membrane from an area of hypotonicity towards an area of hypertonicity. The central mechanism of an osmotic diarrhea revolves around the osmotic reaction that occurs secondary to a nonabsorbable intraluminal substrate. An osmolar gap develops and subsequently the severity of the gap determines the degree of fluid shift as an effort to maintain an osmolarity equal to plasma (290 mOsm/kg). Stool osmotic gap is calculated through the formula: 290 mOsm/kg $H_2O - 2 \times$ [stool Na^+ + stool K^+] mM. Classic findings include the presence of a high stool osmotic gap (>100 mOsm/kg), representing the presence of nonelectrolyte solutes. Passive and ion channel-related sodium absorption occurs at the colonic lumen in an effort to promote water reabsorption [176]. This process is responsible for the characteristic laboratory finding of a low stool sodium level (<60 mmol/L). Measurement of stool osmotic gap and stool sodium concentration is necessary when attempting to distinguish between a secretory and osmotic cause of chronic diarrhea (Figure 35.4).

Common causes of osmotic diarrhea are described in Box 35.4. Ingestion of nonabsorbable ions such as magnesium, phosphorus, and sulfate accounts for a common cause of osmotic diarrhea. Purposeful induction of osmotic diarrhea for the treatment of chronic constipation occurs with ingestion of

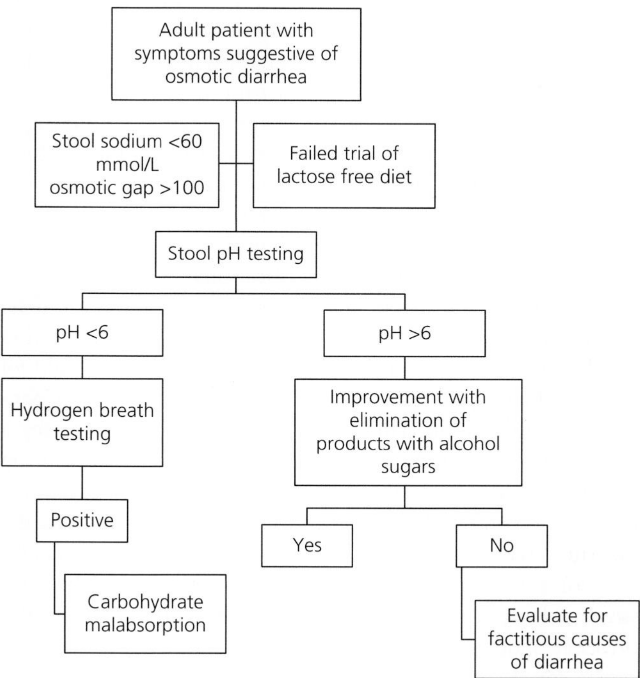

Figure 35.4 Algorithm for evaluation of osmotic diarrhea.

Box 35.4 Common causes of osmotic diarrhea.

Medications
- Lactulose, laxatives (magnesium citrate, magnesium phosphate, milk of magnesia, magnesium sulfate, sodium phosphate, polyethylene glycol), excessive magnesium supplementation, magnesium antacids, vitamin C

Carbohydrates (caused by enzyme deficiency)
- Lactose, fructose, maltase, sucrase, trehalase

Alcohol sugars
- Sorbitol, mannitol, xylitol

milk of magnesium and magnesium citrate. Patients suffering from dyspepsia, reflux, and peptic ulcer disease may develop diarrhea as an unexpected side-effect of overingestion of magnesium-containing antacids. Lactose intolerance is frequently encountered as a benign cause of chronic osmotic diarrhea [177]. Unlike monosaccharides, disaccharides require breakdown into fructose or lactose by small bowel brush border enzymes. In patients with lactase deficiency, undigested sugars are metabolized by colonic bacteria into short-chain fatty acids, carbon dioxide, and hydrogen [178]. Production of these intestinal gases causes bloating, flatulence, and abdominal pain. Colonic metabolism of undigested carbohydrates and production of short-chain fatty acids act as organic anions diagnosed clinically as a low stool pH (pH<6) [179].

Classically, patients suffering from osmotic diarrhea report having loose stools that improve or resolve with fasting. Because of this, nighttime symptoms are rare and patients may even report food avoidance prior to long trips in an effort to avoid diarrhea. An in-depth clinical history, including establishment of exacerbating factors, foods, and medications, is critical when evaluating a patient suffering from osmotic diarrhea. Among other factors, excess ingestion of sorbitol in patients adhering to diabetic diets and those consuming excessive amounts of low-calorie sodas and sugar-free gum should be considered.

Identification and elimination of causative agents are critical for the treatment of patients suffering from osmotic diarrhea. Education regarding dietary modifications can be helpful to avoid relapse or persistent symptoms. When elimination diets do not yield an adequate clinical response, laboratory testing provides objective evidence. Breath testing can be a useful tool when evaluating patients who are thought to suffer from disaccharide maldigestion. This procedure involves administering a dose of lactose or fructose after an 8–12-h fast, then measuring expired hydrogen or methane levels every 15–30 min for a minimum of 2–3 h. Hydrogen levels 10–20 ppm greater than the measured basal levels indicate positive testing and thus malabsorption [180]. Although hydrogen breath testing is highly sensitive and specific, false-positive results can occur in the presence of other diseases affecting carbohydrate digestion such as bacterial overgrowth, chronic pancreatitis, and celiac disease [181].

Malabsorptive diarrhea

Malabsorption is the lack of uptake of intraluminal nutrients across the intestinal epithelium and transport into the bloodstream. Maldigestion, on the other hand, refers to a dysfunction in the processing of nutrients into absorbable compounds. Although a variety of conditions cause malabsorption, this section concentrates on diseases that manifest as diarrhea. An algorithm outlining an approach to evaluating patients believed to suffer from intestinal malabsorption can be found in Figure 35.5.

Under normal physiological conditions, an adult absorbs 93–97% of ingested fats as long as the total intake does not surpass 200 g per 24 h [182]. Steatorrhea is defined physiologically

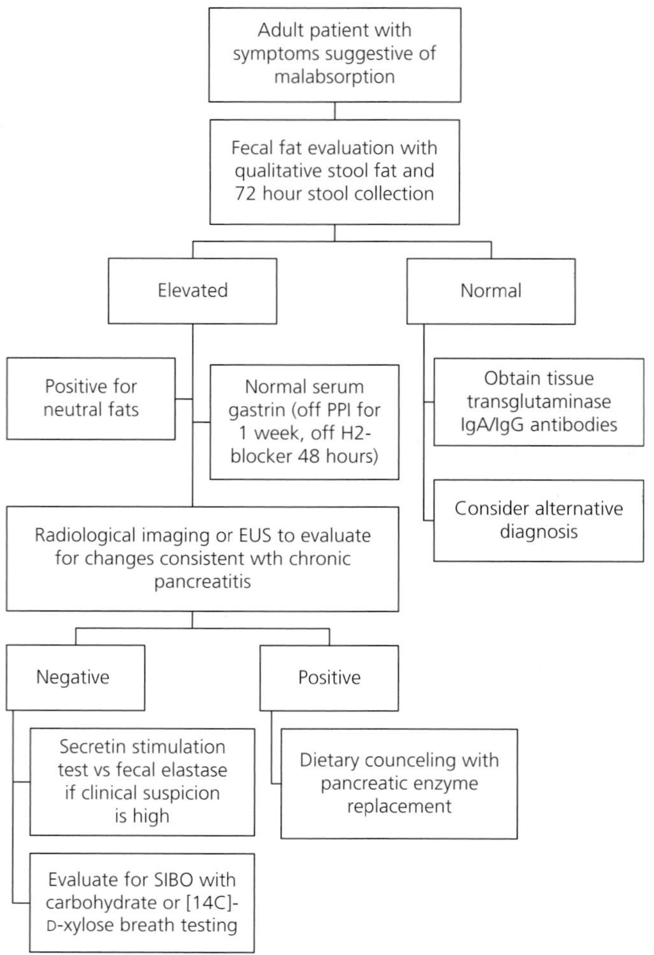

Figure 35.5 Evaluation of malabsorptive diarrhea. PPI, proton pump inhibitor; SIBO, small intestinal bacterial overgrowth.

as stool fat exceeding 7 g per 24 h and clinically by the presence of gross fat in stool [183]. The stool of patients with steatorrhea is typically described as greasy, floating, foul smelling, and with or without fat droplets. Screening of stool samples by Sudan III staining can indicate the presence of steatorrhea but this must be confirmed by quantitative fecal fat testing [183]. Fecal fat testing requires the ingestion of a diet containing 100 g of fat per day for 3 days followed by a 3-day collection of stool [184]. Determination of neutral versus split fats is helpful in determining the cause of steatorrhea. Neutral fats are detected in the presence of pancreatic disease while increased split fats (i.e., free fatty acids) are present if there is impairment of intestinal fat absorption [182].

Pancreatic insufficiency

Pancreatic exocrine production of lipase and protease is essential for the adequate digestion of fat and protein. In patients with cystic fibrosis, mutation of cystic fibrosis transmembrane conductance regulator leads to defective pancreatic ductal cell chloride and fluid secretion. This results in the development of thick and viscous pancreatic secretions that can cause obstruction of the pancreatic ducts [185]. Long-standing obstruction of the pancreatic duct induces an inflammatory response that may destroy pancreatic acinar cells and stimulate fibrosis, resulting in chronic pancreatitis.

Regardless of the etiology of chronic pancreatitis, pancreatic insufficiency occurs upon destruction of greater than 90% of acinar cells and pancreatic lipase production is less than 10% of normal [186]. In addition to steatorrhea, symptoms of pancreatic insufficiency become evident through the clinical findings associated with fat malabsorption including weight loss, fat-soluble vitamin deficiencies, and steatorrhea [187]. Further tests indicating the presence of pancreatic insufficiency include a fecal elastase of less than 100 μg/g [188]. Imaging, including plain abdominal films, CT, and MRI, may reveal the presence of classic features of chronic pancreatitis including pancreatic calcifications and ductal dilation. Pancreatography with magnetic resonance cholangiopancreatography or endoscopic retrograde cholangiopancreatography (ERCP) offers an opportunity to better evaluate for pancreatic duct changes when imaging is nondiagnostic and, in the case of ERCP, provides the opportunity for therapeutic intervention. Endoscopic ultrasound also provides a reliable tool for evaluating parenchymal and ductal changes in patients with chronic pancreatitis [189].

Management includes initiation of a diet meeting the daily recommended nutritional fat content in combination with pancreatic enzyme replacement [188,190].

Small intestinal bacterial overgrowth

The microbiota of the small and large intestine differ in both bacterial species present and the concentration of bacteria. While the colonic bacterial load can reach a concentration of 10^{12} colony-forming units (CFU)/mL, several protective mechanisms maintain a reduced bacterial load, approximately 10^3 CFU/mL, in the small intestine [191]. Aside from innate small intestinal immunological defenses, bactericidal salivary and gastric fluid decrease the bacterial content of food prior to duodenal arrival [192,193]. Also, the mean transit time through the small intestine, approximately 84 min, allows for frequent bacterial clearance while bile acids and intestinal mucosal secretions play a key role in limiting bacterial proliferation [194,195]. A condition that disrupts any of the aforementioned protective mechanisms places an individual at risk for the development of bacterial overgrowth (Box 35.5).

Common symptoms of small intestinal bacterial overgrowth (SIBO), such as bloating, flatulence, and abdominal pain, occur as a consequence of bacterial carbohydrate metabolism. The increased concentration of small intestinal bacteria can induce an inflammatory response resulting in enterocyte damage and villous blunting [191]. Because of the histological and pathological heterogeneity that exists in patients with SIBO, diarrhea may be secondary to fat malabsorption or maldigestion of carbohydrates [196]. Commonly associated findings include megaloblastic anemia secondary to bacterial consumption of vitamin B_{12} [197]. On the other hand, bacterial folate synthesis can result in elevated serum folate levels [198]. The American College of Gastroenterology recommends only testing patients with symptoms who have irritable bowel syndrome, suspected motility disorders, or previous luminal abdominal surgeries [199].

Diagnosis of bacterial overgrowth relies on indirect measures such as lactulose or glucose hydrogen breath testing, given the myriad of technical limitations with jejunal aspirate cultures [200]. Nonabsorbable rifaximin has been the most studied antibiotic in the treatment of SIBO, but evidence for its use is still lacking. Efficacy as defined by symptom improvement or normalization of breath testing ranged from 34% to 87.5%, with higher efficacy found in studies with smaller sample sizes (less than 100) [201]. Due to increasing resistance to antibiotics, empiric treatment of SIBO with antibiotics is not recommended.

Box 35.5 Conditions associated with small intestinal bacterial overgrowth.

Decreased motility/stasis
- Scleroderma
- Celiac disease
- Irritable bowel syndrome
- Diabetes
- Cirrhosis with portal hypertension
- Chronic renal disease
- Surgical blind loops
- Small bowel diverticulosis
- Acute pancreatitis
- Elderly patients

Anatomic obstruction
- Strictures (Crohn' s disease, radiation, nonsteroidal antiinflammatories, surgical)
- Malignant tumors (carcinoid tumors, adenocarcinoma, lymphomas, sarcoma)
- Benign tumors (adenomas, lipomas, leiomyoma)

Mechanisms that allow bacterial for alteration in bacterial load
- Fistulous connections
- Gastric surgery
- Surgery involving resection of the ileocecal valve
- Hypochlorhydria
- Chronic use of proton pump inhibitors
- Immune deficiency (IgA deficiency, acquired immune deficiency syndrome, common variable immunodeficiency)

Inflammatory diarrhea

Chronic inflammatory diarrhea results from the activation of intestinal inflammatory mediators leading to excessive cytokine production that disrupts epithelial function and integrity. Depending on the cause, location, and degree of mucosal inflammation, patients can present with a wide array of symptoms ranging from bloody diarrhea in colonic inflammatory bowel disease, to chronic malabsorption from celiac disease. Determining the diagnosis relies on historical clues in

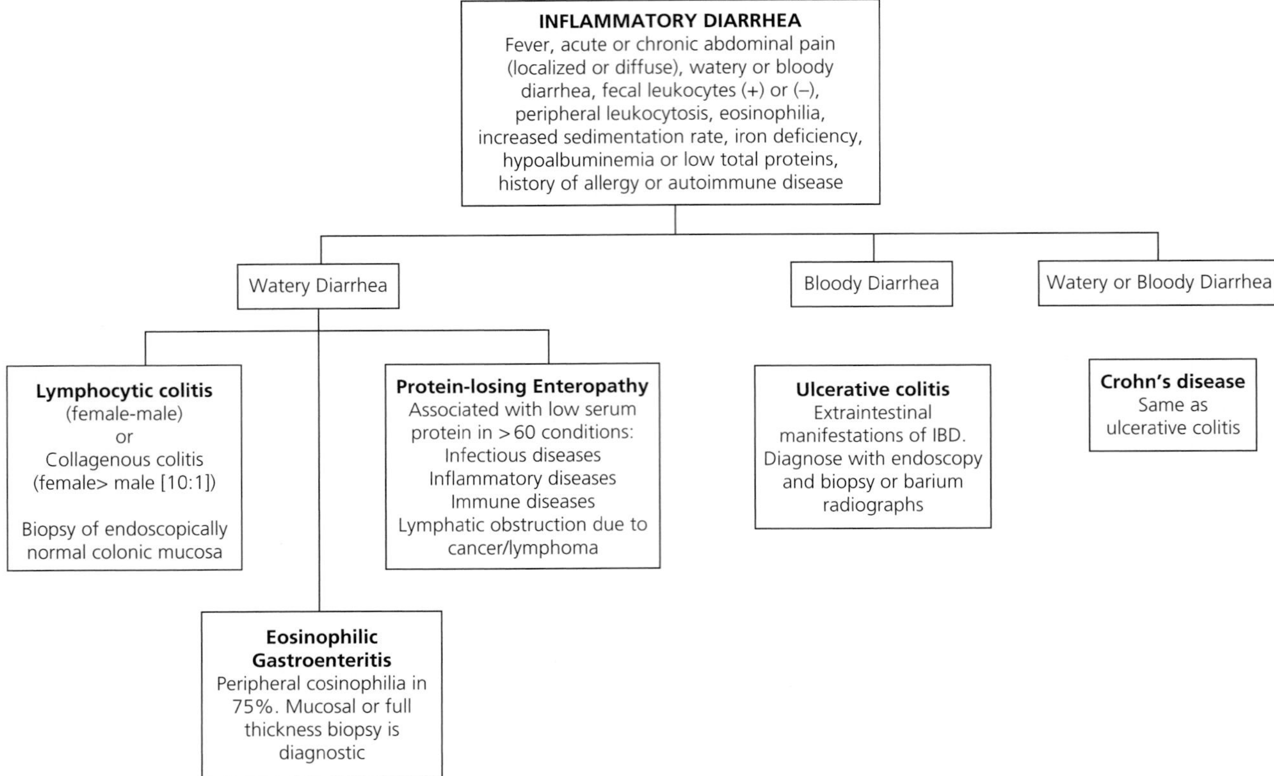

Figure 35.6 Approach to assessment of inflammatory diarrhea. IBD, inflammatory bowel disease.

combination with laboratory values and histology (Figure 35.6). Stool cultures, evaluation for ova and parasites, and *Clostridium difficile* testing should be obtained to rule out chronic infectious etiologies (Box 35.6). Endoscopy with biopsies is warranted in patients with persistent symptoms and negative initial testing, and when there is a high index of suspicion for mucosal disease or infection [202].

Box 35.6 Causes of chronic infectious diarrhea.

Bacterial
Campylobacter, Salmonella, Aeromonas, Plesiomonas, Clostridium difficile, Tropheryma whipplei, Enteropathogenic Escherichia coli, Yersinia enterocolitica
Mycobacterium: [a]*Mycobacterium tuberculosis, Mycobacterium avium intracellulare*
Protozoa
Giardia, amebiasis, *Cryptosporidium*[a], *Microsporidia*[a], *Isospora*, *Cyclospora*, blastocytosis
Viral
CMV [a], HSV [a], HIV [a]
Fungal
Candida, *Histoplasma*, coccidiomycosis
Parasitic
Schistosoma, Diphyllobothrium
Unknown etiology
Tropical sprue, Brainerd diarrhea

[a] HIV associated.

Inflammatory bowel disease

The human gut harbors a unique microbiota integral to the digestive process, nutrient production, host defense, etc. Host intolerance to the intestinal microbiota, driven by genetic susceptibility, results in an immune response that is believed to contribute to the development of inflammatory bowel disease. These theories are supported by the identification of specific mutations in genes (such as nucleotide oligomerization domain 2 [*NOD2*], the autophagy gene *ATG16L1* specifically in Crohn's disease, and the interleukin-23–type 17 helper T-cell pathway) that result in the dysfunctional response to intestinal microbiota by the intestinal epithelium and lamina propria [203]. Alterations in intestinal microvasculature and increased leukocyte recruitment prolong inflammation and delay mucosal healing [203]. Continuous inflammatory disease confined to the colon involving the mucosa and submucosa is pathognomonic for ulcerative colitis. Crohn's disease is characterized by transmural inflammation that can involve any site along the GI tract while sparing the rectum. Both diseases can include extraintestinal manifestations involving the joints (seronegative spondyloarthropathies, ankylosing spondylitis, sacroiliitis), skin (pyoderma gangrenosum, erythema nodosum), and eyes (episcleritis, uveitis), amongst others (see Chapters 63 and 64).

Table 35.6 Crohn's disease-related diarrhea.

Cause or site of disease	Dysfunction
Ileum	Steatorrhea, bile salt diarrhea
Small bowel strictures	Bacterial overgrowth
Small intestine	Lactose intolerance
Surgical resection	Short bowel syndrome

Diarrhea in ulcerative colitis is typically bloody and can occur with or in the absence of abdominal pain. Patients with rectal involvement may relate a sensation of incomplete stool voiding known as tenesmus. Gastrointestinal symptoms are variable in Crohn's disease and largely depend on the area affected (Table 35.6). There is also evidence of a disturbance in the normal absorption and secretion of electrolytes in patients with IBD [176]. The primary defect seems to be in the reduced capacity for sodium and chloride absorption, rather than increased secretion [204]. In addition, tumor necrosis factor (TNF) activates myosin light chain kinase, which phosphorylates myosin light chain, stimulating contraction of the perijunctional tight junction actomyosin ring, thus rendering tight junctions leakier. Dysfunctional tight junctions prevent the efficient absorption of fluid and electrolytes across a chemical gradient, leading to excess fluid in the intestinal lumen [205].

Celiac disease

Vincent Ketelaer, a 17th century Dutch physician, coined the word "sprouw" to describe oral inflammation thought to be secondary to stomatitis [206]. Celiac disease was first described in 1888 by English pediatrician Samuel Gee and further investigated by Dutch pediatrician Willem Dicke and colleagues when he noted an improvement in children with chronic diarrhea after elimination of breads, which had become sparse during the occupation in World War II [207]. In the following years, the etiology of celiac disease was identified with the discovery of gluten, a protein found in products containing wheat, barley, and rye. Gluten contains an undigestible gliadin component that is responsible for an inflammatory immune reaction after passage through intestinal epithelial cells (see Chapter 56). This inflammatory response is characterized by activated intraepithelial lymphocytes that in turn lead to epithelial cell destruction [208]. These changes may manifest endoscopically as scalloped mucosa, decreased epithelial folds, a mosaic mucosal pattern, and mucosal nodularity [209]. Histopathologically, celiac disease is graded based on the presence of intraepithelial lymphocytes with or without crypt hyperplasia and villous atrophy [210].

Clinical manifestations typically correlate with the severity of intraepithelial inflammation. Less than 50% of patients with celiac disease develop diarrhea and may present only with extraintestinal manifestations of the disease such as dermatitis herpetiformis, arthropathy, peripheral neuropathy, iron-deficient anemia, and elevated liver function tests [211]. In patients who present with diarrhea, symptoms are dependent on which portions of small bowel are affected. Malabsorption of nutrients can occur secondary to loss of surface area and intestinal enzymes from villous atrophy. Those who develop steatorrhea are thought to have coexisting defects in pancreatic enzyme production and bile salt secretion [212,213]. An osmotic form of diarrhea can develop in patients who develop lactose intolerance secondary to duodenal mucosal injury and, in one study, 24% of patients with lactose intolerance had coexisting celiac disease [214].

The initial work-up for celiac disease includes obtaining both IgA and IgG tissue transglutaminase antibodies as there is a higher prevalence of IgA deficiency amongst celiac disease patients compared to the general population (2.5% vs 0.2%) [215]. Except in patients with dermatitis herpetiformis shown to have granular IgA deposits in the dermis, all patients with positive serological testing should undergo endoscopy with the intent of obtaining a minimum of four biopsies from the first and second portion of the duodenum [216,217]. The mainstay of treatment continues to be maintenance of a gluten-free diet.

Microscopic colitis

Increased awareness of microscopic colitis as a cause of chronic watery diarrhea helps to explain the increase in prevalence since its description [218–220]. The term microscopic colitis is broad and used to define two conditions. Lymphocytic colitis denotes the presence of a lymphocyte-predominant mixed inflammatory condition with intraepithelial lymphocyte counts greater than 20 per high-power field. Collagenous colitis includes histological features of lymphocytic colitis accompanied by the formation of a subepithelial collagen band greater than 7 μm in size (normal 1–7 μm) [221]. Chronic inflammation leads to destruction of the surface epithelium and, in the case of collagenous colitis, the loss of epithelium above the collagenous zone [222,223]. The aforementioned colonic epithelial changes are associated with defects in electrolyte transporters as well as perturbation of intestinal epithelial tight junctions, manifesting as chronic watery diarrhea through the loss of electrolyte-rich fluid [223].

Although the exact etiology of this disease has not been established, there appears to be a relationship between the presence of microscopic colitis and the use of nonsteroidal antiinflammatory drugs, proton pump inhibitors, and selective serotonin inhibitors [219,224–227]. An association between coexisting celiac disease and microscopic colitis has also been established [228].

Initial treatment includes avoidance of possible causative medications and treatment with medications such as budesonide, mesalamine, bismuth subsalicylate, prednisolone/prednisone, and cholestyramine [227,229].

Eosinophilic enteropathies

Despite an increase in the clinical understanding, awareness, and management of eosinophilic gastrointestinal disorders in adults, the definitive causes of associated conditions are still debated. Two distinct eosinophilic enteropathies are eosinophilic gastroenteritis and eosinophilic colitis. In both, eosinophil-predominant inflammation of greater than 20 eosinophils per high-power field is associated with diarrheal symptoms when involving small bowel or colonic mucosal layers [230]. Patients may develop additional symptoms such as vomiting, nausea, weight loss, and intermittent bowel obstruction if there is involvement of the deeper muscular and serosal layers. Half of patients who develop eosinophilic gastroenteritis report a history of food allergies, with some patients exhibiting peripheral eosinophilia, elevated serum IgE levels, asthmatic symptoms, or eczema [230,231]. Diagnosis of either condition involves exclusion of parasitic infections and acquisition of multiple endoscopic biopsies.

For patients with eosinophilic gastroenteritis, initial treatment with the six-food elimination diet (milk, soy, eggs, wheat, peanuts/tree nuts, and seafood) for 6 weeks has been shown to provide symptomatic and histological remission [232]. Topical steroids (i.e., viscous formulations) such as fluticasone and budesonide are first-line therapies, followed by prednisone if topical steroids are ineffective [233]. Concerns over the short- and long-term effects of glucocorticoid therapy have led to further studies investigating the effects of alternative treatments. Steroid-sparing agents including mast cell stabilizers, leukotriene antagonists, antihistamines, immunomodulators, and biologics have shown positive outcomes, but further studies are needed to provide more evidence of efficacy [234,235].

A non-IgE-mediated process involving a CD4+ T helper (Th2) lymphocyte response is thought to be the pathogenic factor leading to eosinophilic colitis [236]. Endoscopic findings range from normal-appearing mucosa to colitis with erythema, ulcerations, and loss of mucosal vascular pattern [237]. Because eosinophilic colitis is less commonly IgE mediated, elimination diets are not as efficacious and management typically involves the use of steroid agents such as prednisone and budesonide [237–241].

Systemic mastocytosis

Gastrointestinal manifestations are common in patients with systemic mastocytosis and are due to organ damage resulting from mast cell infiltration [240]. Common symptoms include abdominal pain, nausea, and vomiting, with diarrhea occurring in 43% of patients [241]. Diarrhea in these patients occurs secondary to villous blunting leading to malabsorption and steatorrhea [242]. Other mechanisms that could contribute to villous damage and diarrhea include histamine-induced excess gastric acid production and increased intestinal transit [240,243]. Gastrointestinal symptoms occur in conjunction with other disease manifestations such as facial flushing, itching, and urticaria [241]. Symptomatic treatment includes the use of antihistamines, proton pump inhibitors, the mast cell mediator cromolyn sodium, and the antileukotriene drug montelukast [242,244]. Use of systemic or targeted steroids such as budesonide is recommended for treatment of diarrheal symptoms [245].

Prolonged infectious diarrhea

Whipple disease

An aura of mystery has surrounded Whipple disease from the time George Hoyt Whipple introduced "intestinal lypodystrophy" to the medical community in 1907 [246]. The causative organism, *Tropheryma whipplei*, is a unique gram-positive rod-like bacillus that affects tissues both intra- and extracellularly [247]. The development of chronic infection appears to occur in the setting of defects in the host immune response, particularly macrophage, monocyte, and T helper (Th1) cell function [248].

A systemic disease known for typically affecting Caucasian males over the age of 40, Whipple disease is characterized by migratory arthralgias with gastrointestinal manifestations of chronic diarrhea, abdominal pain, and weight loss [249,250]. Neurological manifestations occur alone or in combination with gastrointestinal disease and include the onset of dementia, oculomotor dysfunction, myoclonus, and cerebellar ataxia [251]. Cardiac involvement can lead to congestive heart failure, pericarditis, and endocarditis as a result of chronic valvular inflammation and fibrosis [252]. Endoscopic findings on upper endoscopy include mucosal congestion with erosions and whitish-yellow plaques. Multiple small bowel biopsies are necessary to establish the diagnosis and histological findings include villous atrophy with foamy macrophages that stain periodic acid–Schiff positive in the lamina propria [253,254]. Stool and salivary PCR testing is useful adjuncts to the initial diagnostic work-up while serum and cerebrospinal fluid monitoring is helpful in assessing the treatment response [255,256]. Immunofluorescence staining for the presence of IgM antibodies also offers a greater sensitivity for diagnosis of Whipple disease [257].

The current standard of treatment includes the use of antibiotics capable of crossing the blood–brain barrier. Initiation of therapy with parental penicillin G or ceftriaxone for 2 weeks followed by oral trimethoprim-sulfamethoxazole for 1–2 years is one recommended regimen, with higher doses required for CNS involvement [258]. Given the organism's ability to survive in phagosomes secondary to vacuole acidification, the recommended treatment of patients without neurological symptoms includes dual therapy with doxycycline and hydroxychloroquine [258,259].

Tropical sprue

Typically affecting long-standing travelers to tropical regions around the world, tropical sprue is a rare condition of unknown etiology described in the early 19th century when British soldiers stationed in India became afflicted with a severe form of diarrhea named diarrhea alba for its characteristic white color [260]. It is now understood that these findings occur secondary to steatorrhea accompanied by abdominal pain, bloating, weight loss, and megaloblastic anemia from vitamin B_{12} and folate deficiency [261]. Affected patients are inhabitants or travelers to endemic countries in the Caribbean, Central America, South America, and Southeast Asia [262]. The pathogenic organism is unknown and assumed to be bacterial [263]. Endoscopic and histological findings resemble those found in patients with celiac sprue but without the classic serological findings. Assessment for HLA-DQ2 and HLA-DQ8, found in 95% of patients with celiac disease, can be useful in excluding celiac disease, especially amongst travelers to endemic countries [264].

Antibiotic treatment with tetracycline and folate replacement for 3–6 months is recommended for patients with a history of travel to endemic regions and clinical findings after exclusion of celiac disease and infectious causes of diarrhea [263].

Nosocomial chronic diarrhea

Medication-induced diarrhea

With over 700 potentially causative medications (a list of common offenders can be found in Box 35.7), establishment of drug-induced diarrhea can be challenging if not clearly established in the initial patient history [265]. Factors that may come into play include lack of familiarity with certain medications and unawareness of diarrhea as a possible side-effect. Often times, investigation of a medication-induced condition occurs after an extensive negative work-up, especially in elderly patients and those with multiple comorbidities [266]. In an effort to avoid a potentially unnecessary, costly, extensive, and often invasive work-up, it is recommended that careful evaluation of the patient's medication list be performed on the initial consultation visit.

The causes of medication-related chronic diarrhea are diverse and can best be explained through a mechanistic subclassification system. Commonly encountered mechanisms include the development of osmotic and secretory diarrhea with the use of medications intended for treatment of constipation. Along with antibiotic use, patients on chronic proton pump inhibitors are at risk for development of *C. difficile* infection [267]. Less common drug-related pathophysiological phenomena are now being recognized. For example, olmesartan has been shown to cause villous atrophy much like that associated with celiac disease, accounting for up to 22% of idiopathic cases of sprue [268]. Understandably, treatment of the majority of these conditions involves discontinuation of the offending agent.

Box 35.7 Medications known to cause diarrhea.

Antiarrythmics
- Digitalis, procainamide, quinidine

Antihypertensives
- Furosemide, hydrochlorothiazide, acetazolamide, ethacrynic acid

Cholesterol
- Cholestyramine, clifibrate, gemfibrozil, statins

Central nervous system
- Alprazolam, meprobamate, levodopa, anticholinergic drugs, fluoxetine, lithium, tacrine

Endocrine
- Metformin, synthroid

Gastrointestinal
- Proton pump inhibitors, histamine-2 blockers, magnesium antacids, misoprostol, ursodeoxycholic acid, chenodeoxycholic acid, lactulose, cathartics, sorbitol, 5-aminosaliccylic acids, tetrahydrolipstatin, phenolpthalein, anthraquinone, bisacodyl, oxyphenisatin, senna, aloe, castor oil, dioctyl sodium, sulfosuccinate

Musculoskeletal
- Auranofin, ibuprofen, mefenamic acid, naproxen, phenylbutazone

Respiratory
- Theophylline

Ocular
- Timolol

Antibiotics
- Amoxicillin, cephalosporins, clindamycin, neomycin, tetracycline

Chemotherapy
- 5-fluorouracil, irinotecan, capecitabine

Vitamins/minerals
- Vitamin C, magnesium

Dumping syndrome

Dumping syndrome occurs in up to 10% of patients who undergo gastric surgery [269]. Denervation and gastric anatomical changes lead to an increase in small bowel delivery of hyperosmolar solutes, creating large fluid shifts. This in turn causes a release of gastrointestinal hormones, including VIP, peptide YY, and glucagon-like peptide, leading to a constellation of gastrointestinal and vasomotor symptoms including diarrhea, flushing, sweating, abdominal pain, bloating, and palpitations [269]. Diagnosis can typically be established in patients who report a history of a gastric surgery in conjunction with classic symptoms. Dietary changes are the first line of therapy and include avoidance of simple carbohydrates and liquids with meals while increasing intake of fiber, protein, and complex carbohydrates [269]. Refractory cases can be managed with subcutaneous somatostatin or surgical revision [269–271].

Short bowel syndrome

Small bowel dysfunction or extensive resection leaving less than 200 cm of viable tissue predisposes patients to the development of short bowel syndrome [272]. The consequences of this degree of small bowel loss by either surgical resection or mucosal damage include the malabsorption of fluids, bile salts, nutrients, and electrolytes, manifesting clinically as severe diarrhea with dehydration, weight loss, and electrolyte imbalances [273]. Diarrheal symptoms depend on the site and extent of affected tissue and can be augmented by the development of rapid intestinal transit, acid hypersecretion, and bacterial overgrowth [274]. Common acquired causes of short bowel syndrome include surgical resection from Crohn's disease, trauma, ischemia, and radiation injury. Associated congenital diseases include necrotizing enterocolitis, small bowel atresia, gastroschisis, and aganglionosis [272]. Dietary management also depends on the severity of the disease and ranges from dietary modifications to the need for total parenteral nutrition (TPN) in patients with less than 60 cm of small bowel [275] (see Chapter 59). Medical management of diarrhea includes the use of loperamide, opiates, opiate agonists, and octreotide subcutaneous injections [274].

Treatment of small intestinal bacterial overgrowth should be performed in susceptible patients while bile acid resins are beneficial only in patients with ileal resection of less than 100 cm [273]. Glucagon-like peptide-1 (GLP-1) delays gastric emptying and small bowel motility and glucagon-like peptide-2 (GLP-2) has trophic effects on villous heights and crypt depths, thereby increasing luminal absorption [276]. GLP-2 analog, teduglutide, can decrease TPN requirements and is FDA approved for short bowel syndrome. More recently, exenatide, a GLP-1 agonist, has shown promising results in reducing need for TPN and small bowel transplant [277]. Small bowel transplantation is an option for patients requiring lifelong TPN who either fail to meet adequate hydration or develop TPN-related complications, including catheter-related infections, cholestatic liver disease, or central vein thrombosis [278].

Post-bariatric surgery

Bariatric surgeries have become common in developed countries, as it is a treatment option for patients with morbid obesity and resultant comorbidities. Fecal consistency changes are common complaints of patients after bariatric surgery, with diarrhea being a significant symptom [279]. Short bowel syndrome and dumping syndromes, as discussed above, may occur in this patient population. Other causes of diarrhea include malabsorption of bile acids and exocrine pancreatic insufficiency, due to decreased contact time between bile acids and digestive enzymes with chyme, respectively [280]. There has also been an observed rise in SIBO after bariatric surgery, presumably due to the changes in gut microbiota [281].

Overflow diarrhea

Overflow diarrhea from severe constipation typically presents as incontinence when relaxation of the internal anal sphincter leads to passage of liquid stool contents [282]. The appearance of liquid stool often causes patients to report their symptoms as diarrheal in nature. Ascertainment of a prior long-standing history of constipation and incomplete evacuation unresponsive to aggressive laxative treatment is crucial to establishing the diagnosis. Risk factors associated with development of overflow diarrhea include elderly nursing home residents, individuals with severe neurological disorders, use of chronic narcotics, and patients with pelvic floor dysfunction [283]. "Bowel cleanses" with high-volume polyethylene glycol prior to starting a bowel regimen are often recommended, but there is no evidence to support this practice. Manual disimpaction of retained stool may be necessary if there is failure after treatment with hydration, fiber supplementation, osmotic laxatives, enemas, and suppositories. Distal colorectal cancers may also be accompanied by alternating episodes of constipation and diarrhea as stool leaks through a luminal obstruction. Associated symptoms can include rectal bleeding, weight loss, abdominal pain, and in severe cases may evolve to colonic obstruction [284].

Diabetic enteropathy

Long-standing diabetes can lead to gastrointestinal autonomic nerve damage and subsequent diarrhea. In animal studies, sympathetic trunk demyelination caused impaired absorption of fluids and electrolytes leading to unopposed cholinergic activity [285]. Watery diarrhea associated with nocturnal awakening is rare but occurs more commonly in patients with poorly controlled type 1 diabetes [286]. Neuropathic changes can also lead to impairment of anal sphincter tone, resulting in incontinence in a subset of patients [287]. Given the increased prevalence of celiac disease amongst type 1 diabetes, exclusion of gluten intolerance should be performed by screening for IgG and IgA antibodies to transglutaminase [288]. Initial therapy includes close glucose monitoring, appropriate changes in insulin requirements, and use of oral antidiarrheal agents. In refractory cases, somatostatin analogs are recommended [289]. However, in contrast to patients with type 1 diabetes, the majority of patients with type 2 diabetes who develop diarrheal symptoms do so from use of metformin [290].

Radiation enteritis/proctitis

Radiation therapy for abdominal or pelvic malignancies places patients at risk for both acute and chronic gastrointestinal disease. Acutely, radiation injury occurs secondary to a loss of mucosal surface area, inflammatory changes, and increased motility. This histological phenomenon manifests clinically as abdominal pain, nausea, tenesmus, and diarrhea [291,292]. These symptoms typically resolve spontaneously within 2–6 weeks after completion of therapy [293]. Chronic radiation injury is a process that depends on the total dose of radiation and can occur 1–30 years after radiation exposure [293,294]. Histological changes occur secondary to collagen deposition, progressive obliterative arteritis, and fibrosis [292]. These changes can endoscopically present as ischemic mucosal atrophy, stricture formation, and telangiectasias [295]. Bleeding as a consequence of rectal telangiectasias often requires endoscopic therapy with argon plasma coagulation or radiofrequency ablation for refractory cases [296]. Diarrhea related to chronic radiation injury can be multifactorial, occurring from factors such as bile salt malabsorption in the event of terminal ileal disease, bacterial overgrowth from small bowel stricture formation, inflammatory changes leading to water and nutrient malabsorption, or from an alteration in the gut microbiota [297,298]. Therapy for small bowel and proximal colonic injury can be challenging and aims at symptom control with antidiarrheal therapy and dietary modification including avoidance of lactose and high-fiber foods [299].

Functional diarrhea

Irritable bowel syndrome

In recent years, irritable bowel syndrome has ranked amongst the most prevalent gastrointestinal diseases in the US, with similar

Box 35.8 Rome criteria.

Recurrent abdominal pain or discomfort[a] at least 3 days/month in the last 3 months associated with two or more of the following:
1. Improvement with defecation
2. Onset associated with a change in frequency of stool
3. Onset associated with a change in form (appearance) of stool

[a] Criterion fulfi lled for the last 3 months with symptom onset at least 6 months prior to diagnosis.

rates in most European countries (see Chapter 67) [300,301]. Because of these epidemiological findings, IBS must be included in the differential diagnosis of any patient who presents for evaluation of chronic abdominal pain in conjunction with a change in bowel habits. Despite its prevalence and adverse impact on quality of life, little is known regarding its etiology [302]. It is presumed that the mechanisms which predispose an individual to develop IBS are multifactorial. Current findings include a predisposition to altered gastrointestinal motility, evidence of increased visceral hypersensitivity, and chronic low-grade mucosal inflammation [303–306].

Currently, the diagnosis of IBS is dependent on the clinical parameters outlined by the Rome IV criteria (Box 35.8). Four clinical subtypes have been determined, with diarrhea-predominant IBS constituting approximately one-third of cases [307]. Initial treatment of diarrhea-predominant IBS includes symptom control with either loperamide or bulk-forming fiber supplementation. Alosetron is a 5-HT_3 antagonist currently approved for treatment of diarrhea-predominant IBS [308]. The relationship between the aforementioned presumed pathophysiology in patients with IBS and dietary intake has expanded over the past decade, particularly with evidence showing that over half of patients with IBS report worsening symptoms after meal consumption [309]. One study has shown that coexisting lactose intolerance is present in 67% of patients with IBS [310]. Identification and elimination of such trigger foods can aid patients in improving their symptoms. Initiation of a diet low in fermentable oligosaccharides, disaccharides, monosaccharides, and polyols (FODMAPs) can also prove beneficial in reducing symptoms [311]. Probiotic therapy has been reported to ameliorate symptoms related to dysbiosis such as bloating and distension, but not diarrhea [312].

Randomized control studies have shown that cognitive behavioral therapies (CBT), whether in person, web-delivered, or via telephone, as well as hypnotherapy are superior to education alone [313–315]. Compared to drug therapy alone, CBT combined with exercise decreased IBS symptoms [316]. Few studies have examined biofeedback, but it has not been consistently effective in controlling IBS symptoms [317].

Postinfectious irritable bowel syndrome

Postinfectious IBS refers to a condition in which patients develop gastrointestinal symptoms fulfilling Rome criteria after resolution of an acute gastrointestinal infection. Preceding infections with viral, parasitic, and bacterial species including *Campylobacter*, *E. coli* 0157:H7, *Shigella*, and *Salmonella* have been associated with the development of postinfectious IBS [318–323]. A small study suggested that microscopic changes in duodenal mucosa persisted after *Giardia* infections in both patients with postinfectious functional gastrointestinal disorders and those without [324]. Although postinfectious histological changes may predispose patients to IBS, some studies are revealing that prior psychological disorders, such as anxiety and depression, increase the risk of having postinfectious IBS by 73% [325,326]. The pathophysiological etiology of postinfectious IBS may be related to increased intestinal permeability leading to an inflammatory response initiated by an alteration in the intestinal microbiota [327–329]. Given the lack of reliable laboratory, serum, or stool testing, diagnosis is dependent on disease exclusion and acquisition of functional gastrointestinal symptoms after a prior episode of infectious gastroenteritis.

A recent randomized placebo study of 106 patients demonstrated that glutamine therapy reduced IBS severity score by more than 50 points, reduced stool frequency, and decreased intestinal permeability as measured by urinary lactulose/mannitol ratio [330]. There is also a possible role for probiotics in treatment of postinfectious IBS, but prospective studies support spontaneous recovery of normal gastrointestinal function in some patients over ensuing years [331–333].

Factitious diarrhea

A factitious disorder occurs when a patient falsifies clinical information and strives to induce prolonged medical symptoms with the goal of portraying the role of a sick patient [334]. Laxative abuse represents a common cause of factitious diarrhea, occurring in 15% of tertiary care center referrals for diarrhea [335]. These cases commonly are reported as simulating secretory diarrheas with associated symptoms of abdominal pain, weight loss, nausea, vomiting, and electrolyte abnormalities [336]. Given objective clinical changes, an absence of historical clues can make diagnosis of factitious diarrhea very challenging. Stool studies can provide diagnostic clues helpful in establishing surreptitious laxative ingestion as a cause of diarrhea. As previously mentioned, an elevated osmolar gap (>100 mOsm/kg) is a characteristic finding of osmotic diarrhea whereas a low osmolar gap (<50mOsm/kg) is suggestive of secretory diarrhea. In cases of factitious diarrhea, ingested laxatives may cause a low or elevated gap, depending on the type of laxative. A diagnostic algorithm for factitious diarrhea is shown in Figure 35.7. Findings of a stool osmolality lower than plasma osmolality (<250 mOsm/kg) or extremely elevated (>400 mOsm/kg) may represent purposeful dilution with either hypotonic or concentrated urine, respectively. Confirmation can be done with testing for presence of creatinine in a stool sample [337].

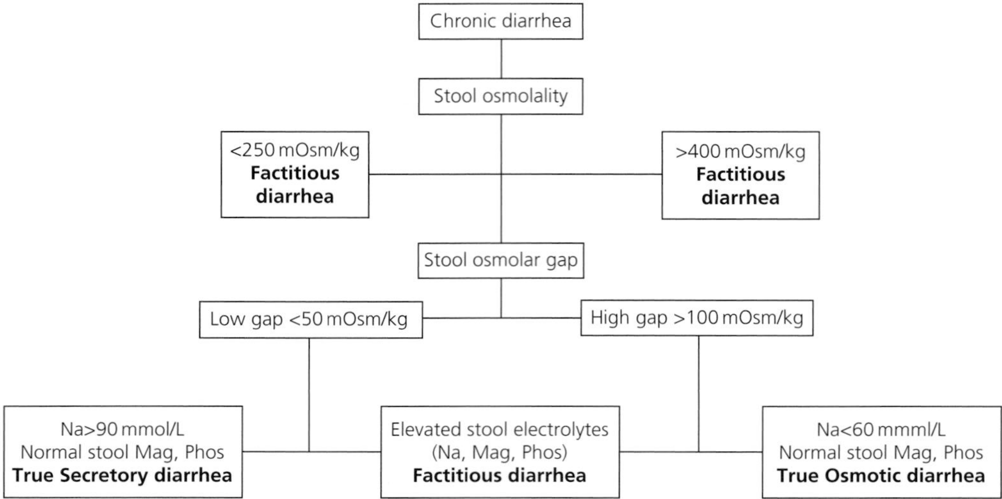

Figure 35.7 Diagnostic algorithm to differentiate types of factitious diarrhea via stool studies.

If clinical suspicion is high for factitious diarrhea, stool electrolytes can be tested; elevated stool magnesium and phosphate indicates magnesium- and phosphate-containing laxatives [338]. Stool laxative screening for bisacodyl, anthraquinones (senna), and castor oil may also be performed [339,340].

Congenital and neonatal diarrhea

This chapter has addressed a variety of adult causes of chronic diarrhea. As in the case of diabetic diarrhea and celiac disease, some of these etiologies begin to manifest during early childhood and adolescence. Others, such as congenital chloride diarrhea and congenital sodium diarrhea, present soon after birth. Patients with Hirschsprung disease can develop overflow diarrhea and soiling of stool after manual disimpaction [341]. Genetic mutations affecting microvilli and enterocytes include microvillus inclusion disease, tufting enteropathy, enteric anendocrinosis, and congenital bile acid diarrhea [151,342–344]. Osmotic diarrhea can develop from malabsorptive diseases as in the case of glucose–galactose malabsorption and congenital sucrase–isomaltase deficiency [345,346]. Steatorrhea may occur in patients with cystic fibrosis secondary to defects in pancreatic exocrine insufficiency [185].

References are available at www.yamadagastro.com/textbook7e

Further reading

Boland K., Nguyen G.C. Microscopic colitis: a review of collagenous and lymphocytic colitis. Gastroenterol Hepatol 2017;13:671.

Borbely Y., Osterwalder A., Kroll D., et al. Diarrhea after bariatric procedure: diagnosis and therapy. World J Gastroenterol 2017;23:4689.

Camilleri M., Sellin J.H., Barrett K.E., Pathophysiology, evaluation, and management of chronic watery diarrhea. Gastroenterology 2017;152(3):515.

Chang F. Irritable bowel syndrome: the evolution of multi-dimensional looking and multidisciplinary treatments. World J Gastroenterol 2014;20:2499.

Krones E., Hogenauer C. Diarrhea in the immunocompromised patient. Gastroenterol Clin North Am 2012;41:677.

Meehan A.M., Tariq R., Khanna S. Challenges in management of recurrent and refractory *Clostridium difficile* infection. World J Clin Infect Dis 2016;6:28.

Smalley W., Falck-Ytter C., Carrasco-Labra A., et al. AGA clinical practice guidelines on the laboratory evaluation of functional diarrhea and diarrhea-predominant irritable bowel syndrome in adults (IBS-D). Gastroenterology 2019;157(3):851.

Vijayvargiya P., Camilleri M. Current practice in the diagnosis of bile acid diarrhea. Gastroenterology 2019;156:1233.

Yalamanchili H., Dandachi D., Okhuysen P.C. Use and interpretation of enteropathogen multiplex nucleic acid amplification tests in patients with suspected infectious diarrhea. Gastroenterol Hepatol 2018;14:646.

CHAPTER 36

Approach to the patient with constipation

Satish S.C. Rao
Division of Neurogastroenterology & Motility, Department of Medicine, Augusta University, Augusta, GA, USA

Chapter menu

Constipation is a heterogeneous, multifactorial disorder that affects 15% of the global population and significantly affects healthcare burden and quality of life (QOL) [1–4]. Defined as two of six symptoms, notably straining, hard stools, incomplete evacuation, digital maneuvers, blockage sensation, or less than three bowel movements per week, pathophysiologically, it is subcategorized into evacuation disorders (dyssynergic defecation), slow-transit constipation (STC), irritable bowel syndrome (IBS) constipation, opioid-induced constipation, and other secondary causes. Rome diagnostic criteria are helpful. A detailed history, prospective stool diary phone app, digital rectal examination (DRE), together with colonic transit study, anorectal manometry, and balloon expulsion test are key for establishing diagnosis. Laxatives, secretagogues, prokinetics, and biofeedback therapy remain mainstays, although novel treatments are underway.

Constipation can be mild and transitory, or chronic and unresponsive to treatment, and is more prevalent and more severe in women [5]. It places a substantial burden on healthcare resources, including physician visits and over-the-counter and prescription medications, and affects QOL. Over the past few years, significant new knowledge has emerged on several aspects of constipation, including its epidemiology, pathophysiology, and treatment.

Definition

Chronic constipation is a heterogeneous disorder that encompasses many symptoms. It has several definitions [5,6], and up to 50% of patients define constipation differently from their physicians [7]. Patients often define constipation as excessive straining, a sense of incomplete bowel evacuation, failed or lengthy attempts to defecate, or hard stools, but rarely by stool frequency [7–10]. Also, patients' perception of constipation may be inaccurate. In one study, 51% of patients considered themselves constipated and reported three or fewer bowel movements per week for at least 6 months, but on prospective stool diaries, they averaged six bowel movements per week [11]. Recently, a mobile phone app has been shown to improve the accuracy of assessment and documentation of constipation symptoms [12]. Consequently, constipation stool app, stool diaries, and physiological measurements can provide a more reliable assessment of bowel function than history by recall. To improve the diagnosis of constipation and to facilitate clinical research, experts have proposed consensus criteria [13–17]. Rome IV criteria for functional constipation and diagnostic criteria for dyssynergic defecation are listed in Box 36.1 [13,17,18]. Observational studies find that many patients do not meet the Rome criteria, so the American College of Gastroenterology

Yamada's Textbook of Gastroenterology, Seventh Edition. Edited by Timothy C. Wang, Michael Camilleri, Benjamin Lebwohl, Anna S. Lok, William J. Sandborn, Kenneth K. Wang, and Gary D. Wu.

Companion website: www.yamadagastro.com/textbook7e

Box 36.1 Diagnostic criteria for functional constipation (Rome IV) and dyssynergic defecation.

Diagnostic criteria[a] for functional constipation (Rome IV)

1. Must include two or more of the following:
   a. straining during at least 25% of defecations
   b. lumpy or hard stools in at least 25% of defecations
   c. sensation of incomplete evacuation in at least 25% of defecations
   d. sensation of anorectal obstruction/blockage in at least 25% of defecations
   e. manual maneuvers to facilitate at least 25% of defecations (e.g., digital evacuation support of the pelvic floor)
   f. fewer than three defecations per week
2. Loose stools are rarely present without the use of laxatives
3. There are insufficient criteria for irritable bowel syndrome

Diagnostic criteria for dyssynergic defecation [13,17,18]

Patients must fulfill all three of the following criteria:

1. The diagnostic criteria for functional chronic constipation (Rome IV)
2. Demonstration of dyssynergia during repeated attempts to defecate and a dyssynergic or obstructive pattern of defecation (types 1–4), which is defined as a paradoxical increase in anal sphincter pressure (anal contraction) or less than 20% relaxation of the resting anal sphincter pressure or inadequate propulsive forces based on manometry, imaging, or electromyography
3. One or more of the following criteria during repeated attempts to defecate:
   a. Inability to expel an artificial stool (50-mL water-filled balloon) within 1 min
   b. A prolonged colonic transit time; i.e., more than five markers (≥20% marker retention) on a plain abdominal radiograph taken 120 hours after ingestion of one Sitzmarks capsule containing 24 radiopaque markers
   c. Inability to evacuate or ≥50% retention of barium during defecography

[a]Criteria fulfilled for the last 3 months with symptom onset at least 6 months before diagnosis.

Chronic Constipation Task Force recommended a broader definition: "unsatisfactory defecation characterized by infrequent stools, difficult stool passage, or both" [19].

Epidemiology

The prevalence rate of chronic constipation varies from 2% to 28% [1–4,20]. It is commonly encountered in primary care (Figure 36.1) [21]. Telephone interviews with 10018 individuals, aged at least 18 years, produced an estimated prevalence rate of 14.7% [2], and if this statistic is applied to the US population, constipation may affect more than 33 million adults. Most patients do not seek healthcare, so the prevalence of constipation has been underestimated [22]. Its natural history is not known, and it may not resolve quickly. In one study, 89% had similar symptoms 1 year apart [23]; in another, 45% of subjects interviewed reported having the condition for at least 5 years [2]. In a large metaanalysis of 45 cross-sectional surveys in 41 different adult populations, the global prevalence rate of chronic constipation using validated questionnaires was 14% [24].

Populations at greater risk for constipation

Constipation is more common in women, with an estimated female: male ratio of 2.2: 1 [8,25–27] and a pooled prevalence rate of 17.4% in women versus 9.2% in men [24]. Its occurrence increases with advancing age, particularly after age 65 years, with an odds ratio of 1.4 for those aged ≥60 years [24] and with elderly adults reporting more problems with straining and hard stools than with infrequency [8,26,27]. Its prevalence is twofold higher in African Americans [4,8], in those of lower socioeconomic status (annual income <$20000) [1,4,8], and in nursing home residents [8,9,28]. In a study based on a National Health and Nutrition Examination Survey database, the factors associated with constipation were low liquid consumption (among women and men), and among women, African American race/ethnicity, being obese, and (in contrast with earlier studies) having a higher education level were significantly associated with constipation [29]. Pregnancy is also associated with higher prevalence of constipation, but no differences were found between the first and the last trimester [30].

Familial tendency and other comorbid features

A survey has shown familial susceptibility, with a higher prevalence in sisters, daughters, and mothers of constipated women with an odds ratio of 3.8 [31]. Chronic constipation is also frequently associated with other functional gastrointestinal (GI) disorders, including chest pain [32], gastroesophageal reflux disease [33–35], IBS, and functional dyspepsia [33–35].

Economic and social impact

Chronic constipation has a significant impact on the use of healthcare resources, including the cost of inpatient and outpatient care, laboratory tests, and diagnostic procedures [36] (Box 36.2). In the United States, $1.43 billion was spent on over-the-counter laxatives alone in 2019 [6]. Constipation was a reason for seeking care in 5.7 million ambulatory physician visits per year [37], and almost 85% of physician visits resulted in a prescription for laxatives [36]. Laxatives are the most commonly prescribed medication in long-term care facilities [27]; about 58% of all patients in US nursing homes receive at least one laxative [27].

In a study of 76854 patients enrolled in the Medi-Cal program in California, the total healthcare expenditure for patients with constipation over a 15-month period was $18891008, with an average cost of $246 per patient [38]. Approximately 0.6% of patients were hospitalized, with an average cost of $2993 per admission [38]. In another study, expenditure for constipation was estimated at $235 million/year, with 55% incurred from

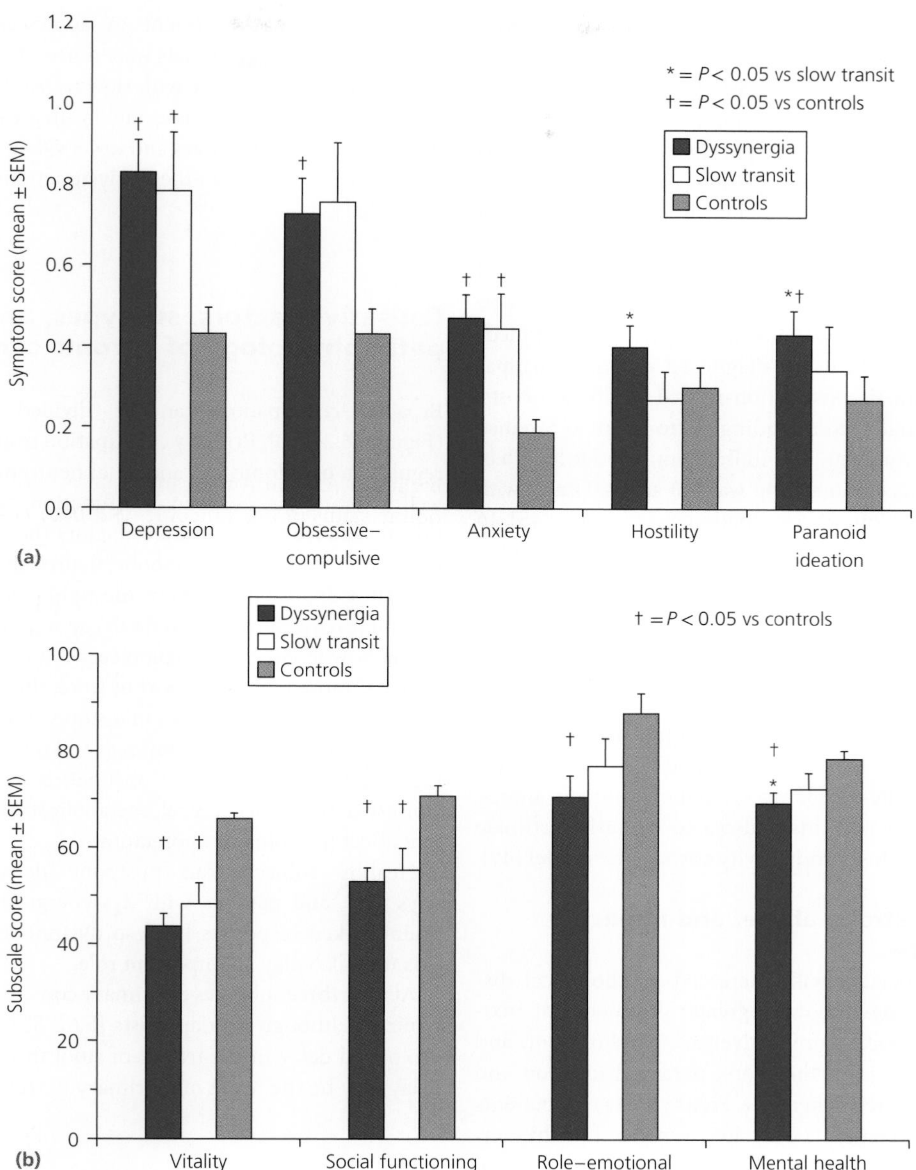

Figure 36.1 **(a)** Effect of chronic constipation on psychological symptoms and **(b)** impact of chronic constipation on quality of life. Source: Rao et al. 2007 [21]. Reproduced with permission of Elsevier.

Box 36.2 Socioeconomic and medical consequences of chronic constipation in the United States.

Mortality/year:	121 deaths (2002)
Hospitalizations/year:	398 000 (2002)
Ambulatory care visits/year:	1.8 million (2001)
Disability:	30 000 (1990–1992)
Physician cost:	$3 016 017
Healthcare cost:	$18 891 008
Over-the-counter laxatives cost:	$1.43 billion (2019)

inpatient, 23% from emergency department, and 22% from outpatient care [37]. In a tertiary-care center, average expenditure for diagnostic evaluation was $2752 [39]. A recent 5-year analysis showed that the frequency of constipation-related emergency department visits increased by 42%, and the mean cost per patient increased by 56%, from $1474 in 2006 to $2306 in 2011 [40]. The aggregate national cost for ED visits increased by 121% to $1.63 million in 2011, with infants and adults ≥85 years old contributing to most visits [40]. Constipation also resulted in 13.7 million days of restricted activity, missing work or school in 12% and impaired ability to work in 60% of patients [36].

In 2009, constipation was the third leading GI symptom prompting an outpatient clinic visit in the United States and the fourth leading physician diagnosis for GI disorders [41]. The number of inpatient discharges for constipation and associated costs ($17 518 mean in 2010 per discharged patient) has significantly increased between 1997 and 2010, with the most impressive change observed in children up to 17 years of age [42].

An international study showed that pharmacy and hospital care costs for chronic constipation-related comorbidities were the largest cost drivers for total constipation-related direct medical costs in patients with newly diagnosed chronic constipation [43]. Mean annual constipation-related healthcare costs, adjusted for potentially confounding factors, in a Swedish cohort were €951 per patient [44]. In Belgium, average length of stay in a full hospitalization setting was 7.0 and 4.0 days, with and without complications of constipation, respectively [45]. In almost 15 000 commercially insured patients in the United States, mean annual all-cause costs for patients with chronic constipation were $11 991 (2010 USD) [46].

There are graded increases in productivity losses and healthcare utilization with increasing severity of constipation [47]; suboptimal treatment responses may lead to substantial health resource utilization and healthcare costs [48]. Increasing dietary fiber consumption has been associated with considerable cost savings, potentially exceeding $12 billion annually among adults in the United States; this is also a conservative estimate given the exclusion of lost productivity costs in the model [49].

Psychological distress, abuse, and impact on quality of life

Constipation is associated with increased psychological distress. Several studies have shown a greater prevalence of anxiety, depression, obsessive–compulsiveness, psychoticism, and somatization [21,50,51]. Furthermore, paranoid ideation and hostility subscores were higher (see Figure 36.1a) in patients with dyssynergia than patients with slow transit or healthy control subjects, providing evidence for significant psychological distress, more so in subjects with dyssynergia than patients with STC.

Sexual abuse was reported by 22–48% of subjects, mostly women, and physical abuse was reported by 31–74% of patients with constipation who were evaluated at tertiary referral centers with special expertise in abuse [9,52]. Another study found greater incidence of sexual abuse in women with pelvic floor dyssynergia [53]. Also, patients with abuse were more likely to seek healthcare [22,54] and to report feelings of incomplete evacuation or urge to defecate, but did not demonstrate rectal hypersensitivity [55].

Patients with chronic constipation also showed significant impairment of health-related QOL (see Figure 36.1b) [21,28,56,57]. One study showed a greater impact of constipation on QOL in African Americans, especially the mental component summary scores [58]. Another recent study confirmed significant psychological maladjustment in adolescents with constipation [59]. Psychological traits were more affected in patients with dyssynergia than in those with slow transit [21], suggesting that dyssynergic defecation is associated with greater impact on QOL. Also, psychological distress and lower QOL were strongly correlated, suggesting that these dysfunctions have synergistic effects [21].

Causative factors, subtypes, and pathophysiology of chronic constipation

Broadly, constipation can be divided into two groups (Figure 36.2) [60]. Primary constipation results from disordered regulation of colonic and anorectal neuromuscular function, as well as brain–gut neuroenteric function. Secondary constipation results from a plethora of factors that include diet, drugs, behavioral, endocrine, metabolic, neurological, and other disorders (Box 36.3). Functionally, the right colon serves as a reservoir for mixing, fermentation, salvage, and transport of digestive residues, whereas the left colon serves as a conduit for desiccation and more rapid transport of stool; the rectosigmoid region acts as a sensorimotor organ that stores stool and facilitates defecation. Several neurotransmitters and intrinsic colonic reflexes regulate these functions. Constipation may therefore result from structural, mechanical, metabolic, or functional disorders that affect the colon or anorectum.

Healthy subjects can postpone defecation for several days [61], and patients with dyssynergia have impaired gut–brain-evoked responses [62], so dysfunction of the brain–gut axis may also play an important role.

At least three subtypes of primary constipation have been recognized, although overlap exists [5,6]. *STC* is characterized by prolonged delay in the transit of stool through the colon. This delay may be the result of a primary dysfunction of the colonic

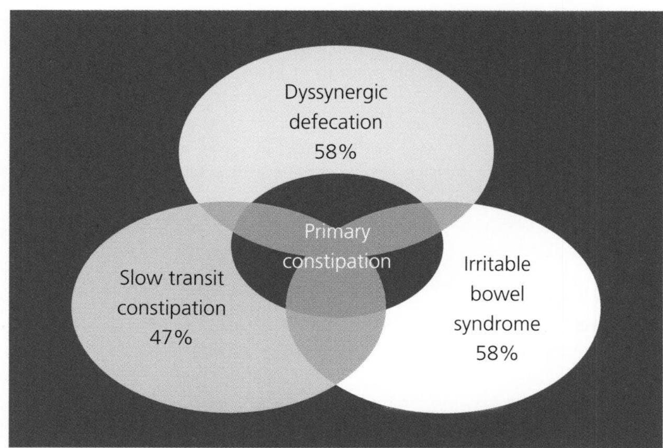

Figure 36.2 Pathophysiological subtypes of primary chronic constipation. Source: Adapted from Mertz et al. 1999 [60].

Box 36.3 Common causes of secondary constipation.

Anorectal and colonic disorders
- Anal fissure
- Hemorrhoids
- Colitis
- Ulcerative (proctitis)
- Diverticulitis
- Colorectal carcinoma
- Inflammatory, postoperative, and radiation strictures

Drugs
- Opioids and related agents
- Anticholinergic drugs and antispasmodics
- Antidepressants
- Antihypertensive drugs, particularly calcium channel antagonists, methyldopa
- Antiparkinsonian drugs
- Anticonvulsants
- Antihistamines
- Diuretics
- Metal ions, e.g., antacids (aluminum or calcium), iron supplements, and calcium
- Supplements
- Serotonin 5-HT_3 antagonists, e.g., with ondansetron or alosetron (for irritable bowel syndrome, diarrhea predominant)
- Progesterone drugs (e.g. Depo-Provera)

Endocrine and metabolic disorders
- Diabetes mellitus
- Hypothyroidism
- Hypokalemia
- Hypercalcemia
- Porphyria

Neuromuscular disorders
- Spinal cord lesions
- Parkinson disease
- Multiple sclerosis
- Stroke/cerebrovascular disease
- Chagas disease
- Hirschsprung disease
- Ehlers–Danlos syndrome
- Postural orthostatic tachycardia syndrome
- Systemic sclerosis

smooth muscle (myopathy) or its innervation (neuropathy), or both, and can be secondary to dyssynergic defecation. *Evacuation disorders* are characterized by either difficulty or inability with expulsion of stool from the anorectum. They include disorders of anorectal function, such as dyssynergic defecation [13,17], where the act of defecation is incoordinated or dyssynergic, as well as structural disorders, such as rectocele, rectal mucosal intussusception descending perineum syndrome, and rectal prolapse that cause a functional obstruction to defecation [13]. About 60% of patients with dyssynergic defecation have secondary STC [9,63]. In a series of 1411 patients evaluated by a single gastroenterologist at a tertiary-care center for chronic constipation over 15 years, 390 patients had evacuation disorders and 61 had STC without evacuation disorders; the remaining 960 had normal transit constipation [64].

Constipation-predominant IBS (IBS-C) is seen in patients in whom abdominal discomfort or pain is a prominent symptom together with symptoms of constipation [17]. These patients may or may not have coexisting STC or evacuation disorder. It accounts for 24–58% of chronic constipation cases [65]. Patients with IBS-C perceive a difficulty with evacuation or pass hard stools [5] despite normal stool frequency. Approximately 20% of patients with IBS have concurrent constipation [66], making it difficult to distinguish this from chronic constipation [56].

Pathophysiology of slow-transit constipation

In STC, the transport of stool across the colon is significantly slower than in healthy individuals. Consequently, there is prolonged retention of stool matter. This may occur because of either primary or secondary dysfunction of colonic smooth muscle or peristaltic activity, neurological innervation, colocolonic reflexes, pacemaker cell activity, or neurotransmitters that regulate colonic neuromuscular function. Altered absorption or secretion, as well as fluid and ion transport, including bile acid transport and alterations in the colonic flora, particularly the presence of methanogenic flora, may all play a role [67–71].

Colonic dysmotility

Colonic motor activity exhibits temporal and spatial variation [72] and can be influenced by sleep, waking, meals [73–75], physical [76] and emotional stressors [75,77,78], gender, aging, and regional variation [75,79]. Patients with STC exhibit significant reduction in overall colonic motor activity [73,75]. Furthermore, the increased motor activity after meals (gastrocolonic response) and after waking from sleep is significantly diminished or absent, but the diurnal variation of colonic motor activity is preserved (Figure 36.3) [79]. The colonic motor patterns, such as high-amplitude propagated contractions (HAPCs) and propagated and simultaneous contractions, are all decreased [79,80]. Furthermore, the velocity of propagation of HAPCs is slower, their amplitude is lower, and they abort prematurely in patients with STC [81]. Experimentally, the HAPCs can be induced by bisacodyl in adults [82] and by antegrade continence enemas in children [83]. The serotonin type 4 receptor (5-hydroxytryptamine [5-HT_4]) agonist, prucalopride, evokes HAPCs in dogs [84,85] and in patients with chronic constipation [86].

In contrast, the incidence of periodic rectal motor activity, a three cycles per minute activity of the rectosigmoid region [87–90] that is often seen at nighttime [88,91], is significantly increased and may serve as a nocturnal brake that retards colonic propulsion of stool [88]; these findings were further confirmed recently using high-resolution colonic manometry [92].

Colonic neuropathy

Studies of combined colonic manometry with barostat balloon maintained at constant pressure to record tone as changes in intraballoon volume have shown that meal-induced colonic

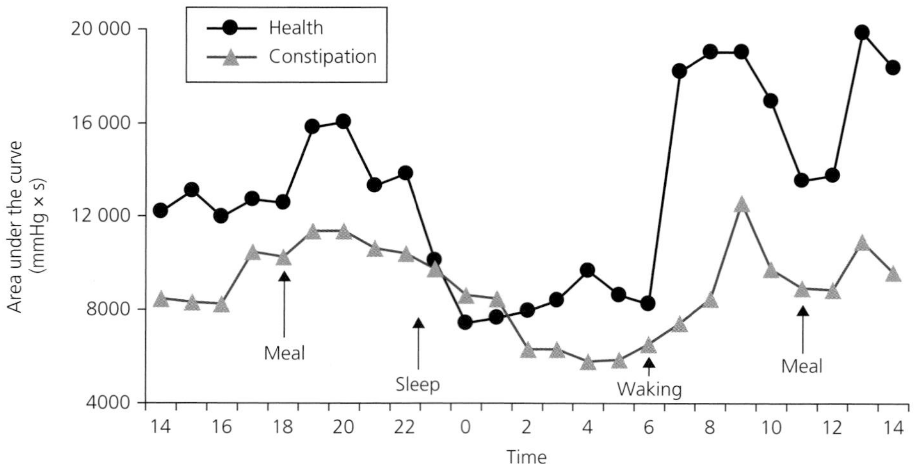

Figure 36.3 Ambulatory 24-hour colonic manometry profile in healthy subjects and in patients with chronic slow-transit constipation. Source: Rao et al. 2004 [79]. Reproduced with permission of Wolters Kluwer Health.

tonic and phasic responses are diminished [93–95] and colocolonic reflexes are impaired [94–98]. There was a greater tendency for retrograde propulsion of colonic contents [96]. Colonic responses to stimulation from a balloon [97] or bisacodyl were diminished [98]. STC may also be the result of dysregulation of the autonomic control of colonic neuromuscular activity [99–101].

Studies have consistently shown a paucity of interstitial cells of Cajal (ICCs), the intestinal pacemaker cells [102,103]. The ICC forms extensive networks of electrically coupled cells that are widely distributed in the submucosal, intramuscular, and intermuscular regions of the colonic wall and lie in close proximity to the enteric nerves [104,105]. Recent work reveals that ICCs, along with the platelet-derived growth factor receptor α-positive (PDGFRα^{+} symbol) cells, form a syncytial network with smooth muscle cells called the SIP syncytium [106,107]. The ICCs and SIP syncytium regulate the oscillatory electrical contractile activity of colonic smooth muscle cells [108]. Patients with STC not only exhibit a pancolonic decrease in the ICC volume across the circular and longitudinal muscle layers and submucosa but also in the number of myenteric ganglion cells [109]. These observations were made on colectomy specimens obtained from patients with chronic constipation, so it is unclear whether they represent a primary neuropathy or whether they are secondary to the use of drugs, cathartics, or behavioral changes over many years. Rarely, STC is associated with a more generalized dysmotility as a component of a pseudoobstruction syndrome [110,111].

Neurotransmitter and hormonal disturbances

Constipation is associated with hard stools, so one possible hypothesis is that excessive absorption of water from stool may desiccate the colonic contents. However, colonic absorptive function is relatively well preserved in patients with constipation [112]. In one study, abnormally impaired hormonal responses to ingested water load were reported, but its significance is unclear [113]. In younger adults, more women than men seek medical help for constipation, suggesting a possible role for endocrine or hormonal imbalance [113]. A decreased level of ovarian and adrenal steroid hormones has been suggested [114], but not confirmed. In fact, routine estrogen and progesterone levels are not altered. Also, the relationship between menstrual cycle and gut transit remains controversial [115]. Both slower transit and normal transit during the luteal phase [116] have been reported [117]. Studies of neurotransmitters have also provided conflicting data [118]. A decrease in vasoactive intestinal polypeptide levels [119], an increase in serotonin levels in the circular muscle [120], and alterations in enteroglucagon, pancreatic polypeptide [121,122], and other hormones have all been reported, but whether they are primary or secondary remains unknown [122]. An intriguing study examined G-protein-mediated smooth muscle contractility of colectomy specimens from women with STC. This study showed downregulation of progesterone-dependent contractile G proteins and upregulation of inhibitory G proteins, probably caused by an overexpression of progesterone receptors in patients with constipation when compared with control subjects without constipation [123,124]. This study offers some mechanistic insights as to why women are more prone to constipation.

The ICCs and the enteric nervous system largely govern inhibition of colonic smooth muscle activity and neuronal and neurotransmitter-mediated excitation. A number of studies suggest that alterations in 5-HT signaling may lead to constipation, but again inconsistencies exist [125]. Serotonin is synthesized and stored in the enterochromaffin cells that are located within the mucosal crypts and accounts for up to 95% of the total body serotonin [125]. When the mucosa is stimulated, either mechanically by stroking or chemically, the enterochromaffin cells release 5-HT and other peptides, including calcitonin gene-related peptide [126]. These paracrine neuromediators act on the intrinsic primary afferent neurons that synapse in the myenteric plexus with ascending excitatory and descending inhibitory interneurons. The activation of the ascending cholinergic interneurons releases acetylcholine and substance P, which produces smooth muscle contraction and initiates the peristaltic reflex [125,126]. Simultaneously, the activation of the descending cholinergic interneurons releases nitric oxide, vasoactive intestinal polypeptide, and adenosine triphosphate, which relax the circular muscle. Tegaserod, a 5-HT_4 receptor agonist, stimulates ascending contraction and descending relaxation [127] and accelerates small bowel and colonic transit [128]. In contrast, the gastrocolonic response and ascending contractions of the peristaltic reflex were impaired in patients with STC, and these effects were partially mediated by granisetron, a 5-HT_3 antagonist [129]. These observations support a role for serotonin and its receptors in the pathogenesis of constipation, but it is unclear whether there is decreased availability of serotonin, decreased receptor density, or altered function of the serotonin reuptake transporter [130].

Methanogenic flora and constipation

Methane is an inert gas produced by methanogens, which are present in the colon, especially *Methanobrevibacter smithii*, and belong to the family of Archaea [67–71]. Most recently, it has been observed that there is a higher prevalence of methanogenic flora in constipated patients [67–71], and that infusion of methane gas impairs muscle contractions, possibly causing constipation [131]. Also, the prevalence of methane was higher in women but was not influenced by age [69], the colonic pH was lower in methanogenic subjects, colonic motility was significantly diminished, but not small bowel motility, compared with patients without methanogenic flora, and methane patients had higher prevalence of rectal hypersensitivity [67,69]. Whether the presence of methanogenic flora predisposes an individual to development of constipation or whether excess methanogens is a consequence of altered colonic physiology merits further study.

Electrolyte and fluid transport

Each day, about 9 L of fluid enters the gut, of which 1–2 L reaches the colon, and most of this is absorbed, with the average stool containing 200 mL of fluid [132]. Recently, there has been a resurgence of interest in studying electrolyte transport because of drugs that can alter ion exchange, leading to secretion and improvement of constipation symptoms. Coupled NaCl absorption facilitated by Na^+/H^+ exchangers and anion exchangers [133] on the apical membrane of epithelial cells together with electrogenic Na^+ absorption [134] contribute to Na^+ absorption. Another important ion transport in intestinal, crypt epithelial cells is chloride secretion that is primarily regulated by eight types of chloride channels and the cystic fibrosis transmembrane conductance regulator (CFTR) [135].

Lubiprostone is a selective chloride channel-2 activator that leads to active secretion of chloride ions from intestinal epithelial cells and Na^+ and H_2O via a paracellular pathway [135]. Another mediator of intestinal secretion is through the guanylate cyclase C (GCC) receptor pathway. Activation of GCC receptors releases cyclic GMP that, in turn, activates CFTR, mediating chloride secretion [136]. Finally, the ileal bile acid transporter in the terminal ileum facilitates reabsorption of 95% of bile acids, but if excess bile spills over into the colon, the ensuing bile acid malabsorption can lead to colonic secretion and diarrhea [137,138]. Other ion transporters normally result in absorption of sodium ions, by intestinal epithelial cells; these include the sodium–hydrogen exchanger and the sodium–glucose transporter.

Clearly, further research is required to better understand the interplay between hormones, neurotransmitters, colonic flora, muscle function, and signaling from the enteric nervous system.

Pathophysiology of evacuation disorders

Evacuation disorders include a functional disorder of defecation, dyssynergic defecation, as well as structural disorders, such as Hirschsprung disease, rectocele, descending perineum syndrome, rectal mucosal intussusception, and rectal prolapse that can obstruct passage of stool.

Dyssynergic defecation

Dyssynergia or incoordination of the act of bowel movement is an acquired behavioral disorder of defecation. In two-thirds of adult patients, it stems from faulty toilet habit, or after prolonged painful defecation, obstetric or back injury, and brain–gut dysfunction [9,62]. In the rest, the process of defecation may not have been learnt since childhood (due to behavioral problems or parent–child conflicts) [9]. In a prospective study, most patients with dyssynergic defecation showed an inability to coordinate the abdominal, rectoanal, and pelvic floor muscles during attempted defecation [9,139]. This failure of rectoanal coordination consisted of either paradoxical anal contraction, inadequate anal relaxation, or impaired rectal/abdominal propulsive forces (Figure 36.4) [9,140]. A significant proportion of these patients exhibit rectal hyposensitivity [139,141] and others rectal hypersensitivity [142]. The hyposensitivity may result from rectal retention of stool, resulting in reduced sensation when tested with a latex balloon.

Earlier studies suggested that the paradoxical anal contraction resulted from an involuntary anal spasm (anismus) during defecation [143–145]. Of healthy subjects, 20–30% may also exhibit paradoxical anal contraction [146,147]. In a study of healthy subjects [148], in the lying position, one-third showed dyssynergia and half could not expel artificial stool, whereas in the sitting position and with a sensation of stooling, most subjects showed a normal pattern of defecation and an ability to expel stool [148]. This finding was further reaffirmed in a recent study of constipated patients where 85% showed dyssynergia in the lying position and 65% of the same group in sitting position using high-resolution manometry [149]. Also, a recent randomized controlled study of healthy subjects showed that a

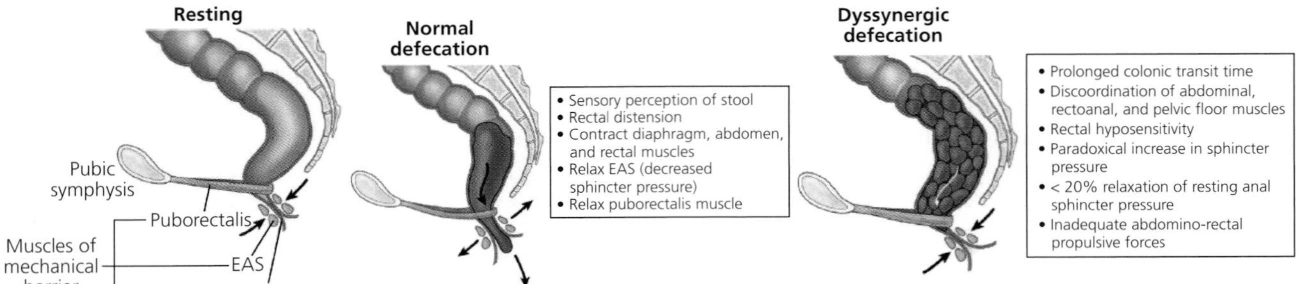

Figure 36.4 Continence is maintained by normal rectal sensation and tonic contraction of the internal anal sphincter (IAS) and the puborectalis muscle, which wraps around the anorectum, maintaining an anorectal angle between 80° and 110°. During defecation, the pelvic floor muscles (including the puborectalis) relax, allowing the anorectal angle to straighten by at least 15°, and the perineum descends by 1.0–3.5 cm. The external anal sphincter (EAS) also relaxes and reduces pressure on the anal canal. In dyssynergic defecation, the coordinated anorectal muscle function is dysfunctional. Source: Rao 2010 [140]. Reproduced with permission of Elsevier.

balloon filled with 50 mL water was expelled in a significantly shorter time and much easier than a Foley balloon; in fact, 43% could not expel the Foley balloon in the sitting and squatting position [150]. Thus, body position, sensation of stooling, and stool characteristics can each influence defecation. A recent systematic review addressed the probability of pretest and posttest utility of symptoms, DRE, and diagnostic tests for rectal evacuation disorders (REDs), including dyssynergia and STC in 3364 patients [151]. Objective tests identified REDs in 27%, normal transit constipation in 37%, STC in 19%, and REDs with STC in 17%. Also, the presence of urinary symptoms, findings of dyssynergia on DRE, a low rectoanal pressure gradient (−40 mmHg) during straining with high anal sphincter pressures had greater likelihood of detecting REDs, whereas lack of a call to stooling and absence of bloating and distension favored STC.

Anorectal myectomy involving puborectalis and external anal sphincter has been performed based on the notion that dyssynergia is a spasmodic dysfunction of the anal sphincter [144], but it helped only 10–30% of patients and some became incontinent [152]. Similarly, botulinum toxin injection has been ineffective [153,154]. Hence spasm or inability to relax the anal sphincter is unlikely to be the sole mechanism for dyssynergic defecation. Manometrically, at least four reproducible types of dyssynergia [13,18] have been recognized previously using wave form manometry, but recently with the advent of the more sensitive high-resolution anorectal manometry system, up to eight types of dyssynergia pattern have been described [149] (Figure 36.5) [155]. The recognition of these patterns allows the biofeedback therapist to offer patient-specific treatment programs, such as emphasis on pushing effort (type 2) or improved relaxation (type 3) or both (type 4), and may help to learn about predictors of response to therapy. In a prospective study of biofeedback therapy, there was no difference in the clinical outcome among the three groups of dyssynergia [156]. In addition, thresholds for first sensation or desire to defecate, or both, may be higher in 60% of dyssynergic patients, suggesting that rectal hyposensitivity [157] may play a role in the pathophysiology of constipation [139], or they may result from the enlarged rectum secondary to fecal retention. Likewise, constipated patients may also exhibit rectal hypersensitivity [158].

Hirschsprung disease

This classic neuroenteric disorder usually presents by 6 months of age and rarely in adults [159]. It is characterized by absence of intramural ganglion cells in the myenteric plexus of the rectum and stems from developmental arrest of the caudal migration of neural crest cells during embryonic development. Consequently, there is increased acetylcholinesterase activity and depletion of inhibitory neurotransmitter release, such as nitric oxide and vasoactive intestinal polypeptide [160]. Manometrically, it is characterized by an absent rectoanal inhibitory reflex (Figure 36.6) [161]. Studies have identified mutations in the *RET*, *GDNF*, *EDN3*, and *EDNRB* genes [162] (see Chapter 55).

Pathophysiology of constipation-predominant irritable bowel syndrome

Multiple pathophysiological mechanisms of IBS-C have been proposed and include genetic, environmental, social, biological, and psychological factors [163,164]. In addition, dietary factors such as fructose intolerance [146], small intestinal bacterial overgrowth [165,166], altered intestinal microbiome [167,168], or abnormal cortical perception and hypervigilance have all been proposed [169–171]. These and other factors [172] are discussed in Chapter 67.

Clinical evaluation of chronic constipation

Medical history

A detailed medical, surgical, and drug history can help to identify most organic and secondary causes of constipation [5,6]. Constipated patients present with a constellation of complaints, such as excessive straining, passage of hard, pellet-like stool, or decreased stool frequency, or they may misrepresent their symptoms or may feel embarrassed to describe the use of digital

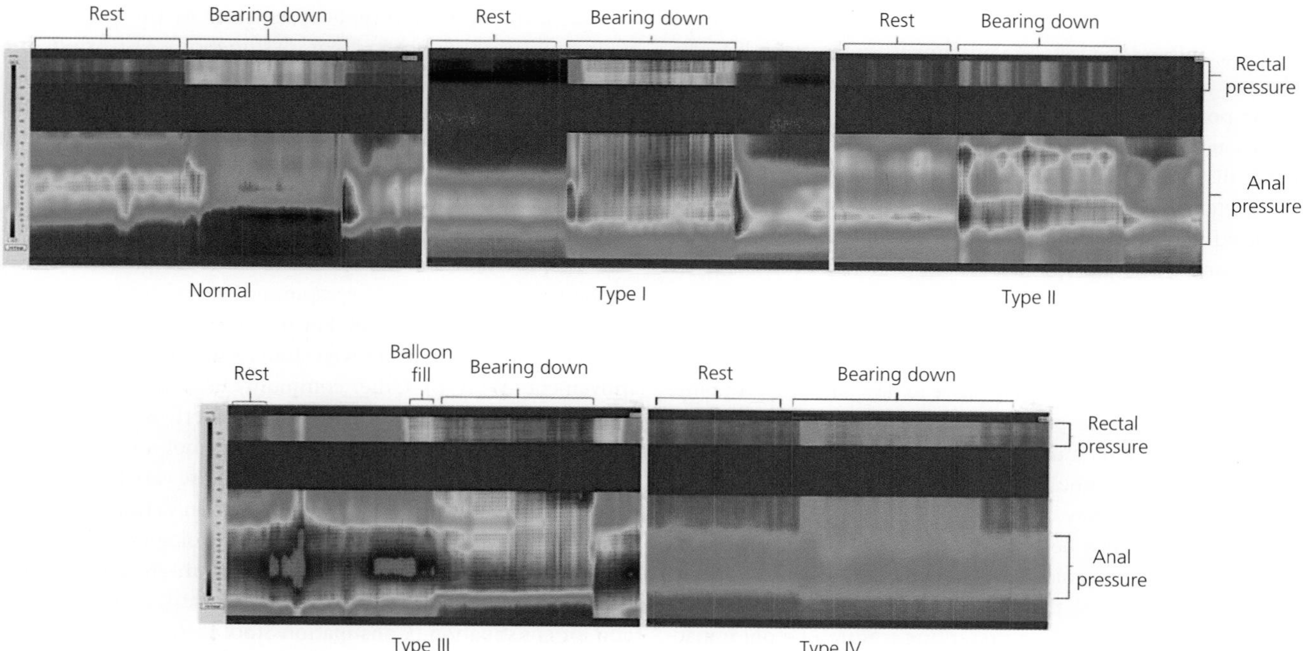

Figure 36.5 High-resolution anorectal manometry showing topographic images of anorectal pressure profiles during attempted defecation. The first image shows a normal defecation pattern comprising a good push effort (rise in intrarectal pressure) synchronized with anal relaxation (decrease in anal sphincter pressure). In contrast, the type 1 dyssynergia pattern shows an increased intrarectal pressure along with paradoxical anal contraction, type II dyssynergia pattern shows a poor push effort with paradoxical anal contraction, type III dyssynergia shows good push effort but impaired or incomplete anal relaxation, and type IV dyssynergia shows impaired push effort with impaired anal relaxation. Source: Rao 1998 [155].

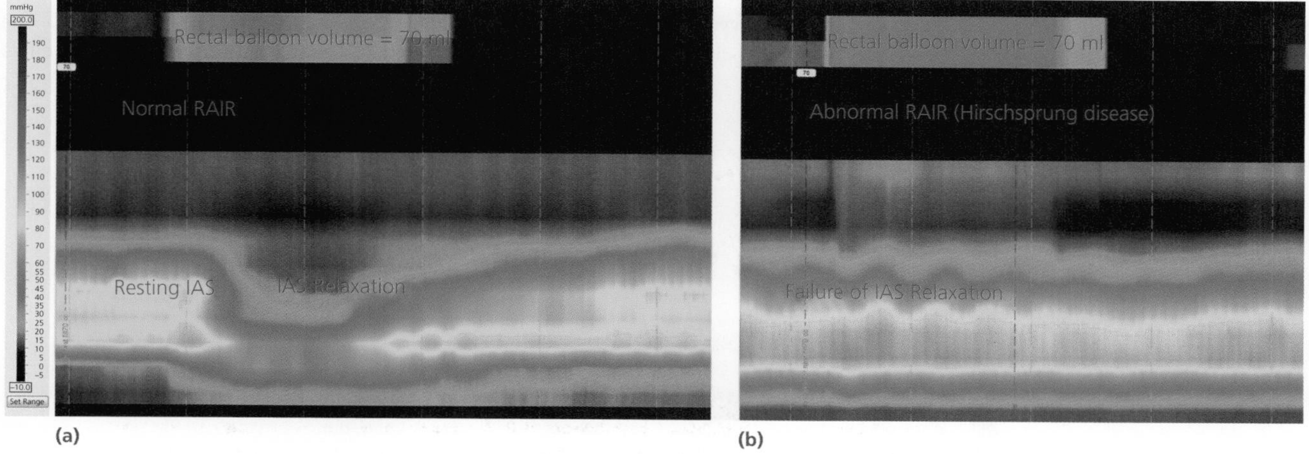

Figure 36.6 Example of normal rectoanal inhibitory reflex (RAIR) showing normal internal anal sphincter (IAS) relaxation **(a)** and a patient with Hirschsprung disease showing absent or failure of RAIR **(b)**. Source: Based on Tobon 1968 [161].

disimpaction or vaginal splinting [5,9,56]. However, by establishing a trusting relationship and through the use of symptom questionnaires or stool diaries [9,11], it is possible to define the nature of bowel dysfunction. A sensitive and compassionate approach is key for unraveling the mind–body interactions and the psychosocial issues of a constipated patient.

Patients should be encouraged to describe their bowel habit: How often they feel the urge to defecate and if they complete defecation in response to the urge; their definition of constipation – frequency, need for straining, stool consistency, and stool size; history of ignoring a call to stool; precipitating events; how their cultural beliefs and expectations affect their bowel patterns; what they believe is normal bowel habit [173]; and whether the problem began in childhood. The history should ascertain how the onset, severity, and duration of each symptom relate to the patient's normal bowel habit. A long history of recurring problems, which is refractory to dietary measures or laxatives, often suggests a functional colorectal disorder, whereas a history of recent onset (rectal bleeding, anemia, guaiac-positive stool, or mass in the abdomen) should alert the physician to seek and exclude an organic illness, including neoplastic disease.

A dietary history should include an assessment of the fiber and fluid intake, the number of meals and when they are consumed, and their caloric and nutrient content. A prospectively maintained food diary for a week and its appraisal by a dietician can be useful. Many patients tend to skip breakfast or do not allow time for defecation because of the "early morning rush" to get to work or school. This may prove to be a handicap. A failure to capitalize on these physiological stimulants, such as after waking [75] and after a meal [73,74], may predispose to constipation. The history should also include the number and type of laxatives and frequency of their use. A family history of bowel dysfunction may also be important [31]. Obstetrical, surgical, and back trauma, neurological problems, and drug history may provide clues regarding the cause of constipation. In the elderly, fecal incontinence may be a presenting feature of stool impaction. Symptoms alone do not appear to reliably differentiate among the three common pathophysiological subgroups of constipation [174]. In a prospective survey of 120 patients with dyssynergic defecation, the prevalence of constipation symptoms was similar between patients with or without dyssynergia [9]. In another study, two or fewer stools per week, laxative dependency, and constipation since childhood were associated with STC, whereas backache, heartburn, and anorectal surgery and lower prevalence of normal stool frequency were associated with pelvic floor dysfunction [56].

Thus, symptoms were good predictors of transit time but poor predictors of pelvic floor dysfunction. Also, stool frequency alone was of little value, whereas a sense of obstruction or digital assistance for evacuation was specific but not sensitive for difficult defecation [174]. Accordingly, symptom assessment should be combined with objective testing for optimal assessment of these patients.

Objective measures can facilitate the diagnosis of constipation by providing a common framework for physicians' and patients' understanding of symptoms. Several instruments are available. The Bristol Stool Form scale (Figure 36.7) allows patients to identify one of seven stool forms for any given bowel movement [175,176]. Other commonly used scales include the Constipation Assessment Scale and the Elderly Bowel Symptom Questionnaire [177]. The assessment of stool form can aid in the assessment of colonic transit time because very loose or hard stools correlate with rapid or slow colonic transit, respectively [178]. Likewise, assessments of psychological dysfunction or assessments of quality of life, Short Form-36, and a 1-week prospective stool diary can be useful. Recently, a mobile phone app for constipation (Constipation Stool Instrument; Neurogut Inc., Augusta, GA, USA) that records 10 key constipation symptoms has been evaluated in healthy control subjects and patients with constipation (Figure 36.8) [12]. The app was reproducible and valid when compared with a paper form stool diary, and a majority of subjects felt that it was user friendly and a preferred method of recording their bowel habit. Furthermore, it has two modules: a patient module that includes the app and a stool report, and a research module that provides detailed, day-to-day characterization of a subject's bowel habit over time, as well as calculation of complete spontaneous bowel movements per

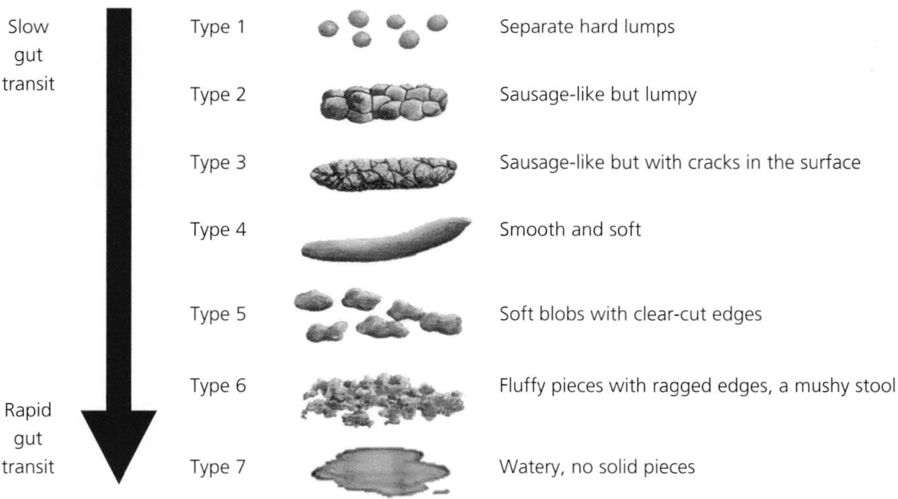

Figure 36.7 Bristol Stool Form Scale: a useful clinical scale for assessing and documenting stool consistency. Source: Heaton et al. 1994 [178]. Reproduced with permission of Wolters Kluwer Health.

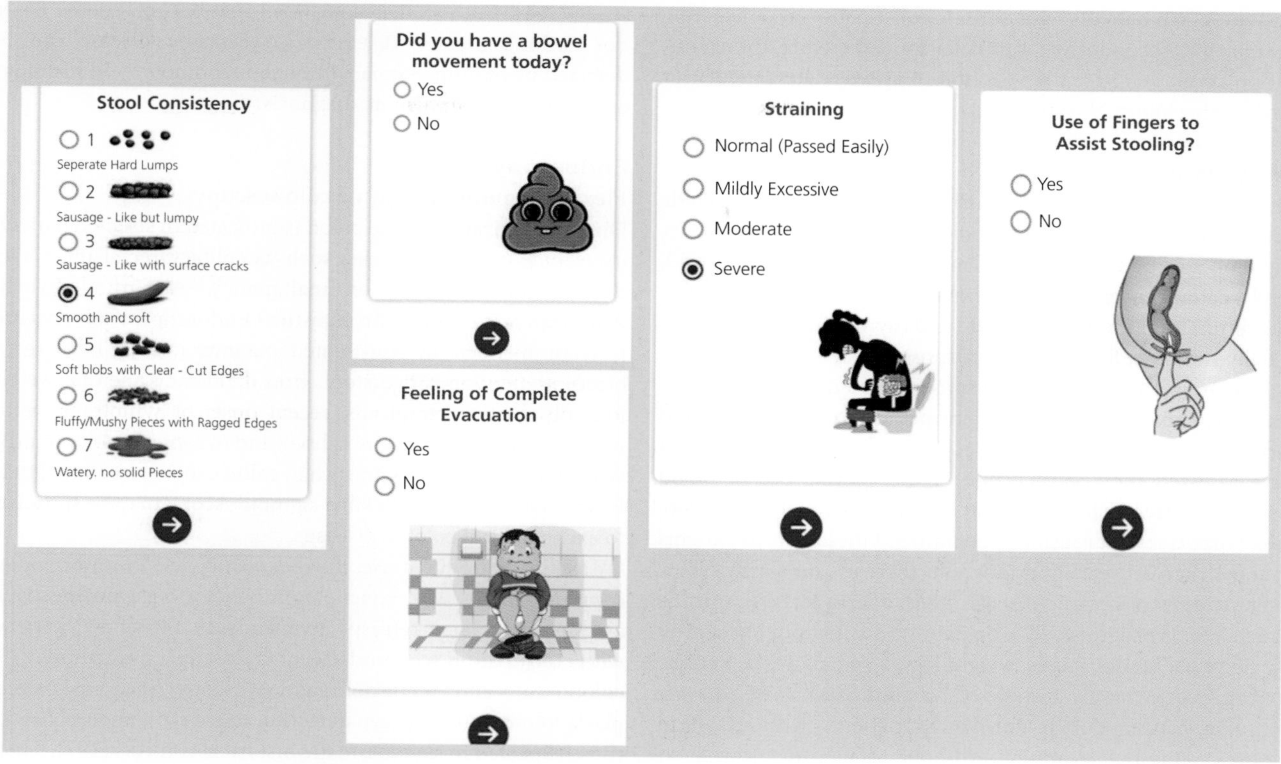

Figure 36.8 Examples of constipation stool app diary for prospectively recording constipation symptom. Source: Based on Rao et al. 2018 [324].

week and other stool parameters that can be useful to a researcher.

Physical examination

A thorough general physical examination that includes a detailed neurological examination should screen for most organic conditions that cause constipation. The abdomen must be carefully examined for the presence of stool, particularly in the left lower quadrant. A normal physical examination is common, but it is important to exclude a GI mass.

Digital rectal examination

A careful perianal and DRE is important and is often the most revealing part of clinical evaluation [5,13,179]. Anorectal inspection can detect skin excoriation, skin tags, anal fissures, or hemorrhoids. Assessment of perineal sensation and anocutaneous reflex by gently stroking the perianal skin with a cotton bud (Q-tip) or blunt needle in all four quadrants will elicit reflex contraction of the external anal sphincter. If this is absent, a neuropathy should be suspected. DRE may reveal a stricture, spasm, tenderness, mass, blood, or stool. If stool is present, its consistency should be noted and the patient should be asked if they were aware of its presence. A lack of awareness of stool in the rectum may suggest rectal hyposensitivity [179].

It is useful to assess the resting and squeeze tone of the anal sphincter and puborectalis muscle by asking the subject to squeeze. More importantly, the subject should be asked to push and bear down as if to defecate [179]. During this maneuver, the examiner should perceive relaxation of the external anal sphincter or the puborectalis muscle, together with perineal descent. A hand placed on the abdomen can gauge the abdominal push effort. An absence of these normal findings should raise the index of suspicion for an evacuation disorder such as dyssynergic defecation [12,179]. DRE has a high sensitivity of 75% and specificity of 87% for identifying dyssynergia [179,180].

Even though DRE is a useful clinical tool, many examiners lack knowledge on how to perform a comprehensive evaluation. A survey of 256 final-year medical students revealed that 17% had never performed a DRE and 48% were unsure of giving an opinion based on their findings [181]. Another US study confirmed that fewer medical students and internists perform DREs, and they lack confidence in using DRE to diagnose anorectal disorder [182]. Thus, improved training for DRE is needed. A recent article described in detail how to perform a DRE in a patient with suspected anorectal disorder and discussed its clinical utility [179]. A video demonstration of DRE is also available [183]. A recent study prospectively evaluated the ability of trainees to learn DRE under expert tutelage and showed that senior GI Fellows demonstrate significant improvement in accuracy and ability to identify normal DRE and dyssynergia in patients with constipation compared with junior trainees [184]. DRE appears to be a reliable tool for identifying dyssynergia in patients with chronic constipation and detecting normal, but not abnormal, sphincter tone; therefore, the examination could facilitate the selection of appropriate patients for further physiological testing and treatment [180].

Diagnostic tests

The first step in making a diagnosis of constipation is to exclude an underlying metabolic or pathological disorder, because constipation can be a symptom of many organic conditions and, rarely, colon cancer. A complete blood count, biochemical profile, serum calcium, glucose levels, and thyroid function tests are usually sufficient for screening purposes.

If there is a high index of suspicion, serum protein electrophoresis, urine porphyrins, serum parathyroid hormone, and serum cortisol levels may be requested. However, no studies have assessed the clinical value of the routine use of blood tests [185]. Hence the American College of Gastroenterology Task Force does not routinely recommend these tests in patients younger than 50 years and in whom there are no alarm symptoms or signs of organic disease [186]. Alarm features include new onset or progressively worsening constipation, onset after age 50 years, bloody stools, weight loss, fever, anorexia, nausea, vomiting, or a family history of inflammatory bowel disease or colon cancer [5,19]. For young patients without alarm features, empiric treatment without diagnostic testing is appropriate [19].

Once an organic disorder has been excluded, most patients have a functional neuromuscular disorder affecting the colon and/or the anorectum that merits appraisal through further investigation.

Radiographic studies

Plain abdominal radiograph

A plain radiograph of the abdomen is an inexpensive, frequently used test to complement clinical history and physical examination, both in children and adults with a suspicion of constipation [187]. However, systematic reviews have concluded that the evidence is conflicting in constipated children [188], and there is a lack of evidence in adults to support or reject its use [19,185]. A recent study showed that a computed tomography scan can provide useful diagnostic information regarding retention of excess rectal gas volume as a diagnostic marker for constipated patients, and a plain abdomen x-ray can also provide this information [189].

Barium enema

This test may be useful for the identification of redundant sigmoid colon, megacolon, megarectum, stenosis, extrinsic compression, and intraluminal masses. However, only two studies have evaluated its clinical utility [19,185]. In one retrospective study of 62 subjects, an organic lesion was not detected with barium enema [190]. In another retrospective study of 791 patients, constipation was reported in 22% and was equally present in those with an abnormal study as in those with a normal study [191]. Both studies concluded that barium enema could not exclude organic disease. Hirschsprung disease can be detected by barium enema, although manometry and histology are required to confirm its diagnosis.

Endoscopy

Flexible sigmoidoscopy or colonoscopy

Direct visualization of the colon is indicated in selected patients to exclude mucosal lesions, such as solitary rectal ulcer syndrome, inflammation, or malignancy. According to the American Society of Gastrointestinal Endoscopy, a colonoscopy is recommended in constipated patients if they have rectal bleeding, heme-positive stool, iron-deficiency anemia, weight loss, obstructive symptoms, recent onset of symptoms, rectal prolapse, or change in stool caliber, and in subjects older than 50 years who have not previously had colon cancer screening [192]. In younger patients, a flexible sigmoidoscopy may be sufficient to exclude distal colonic disease.

Despite its frequent use, the diagnostic yield of lower endoscopy in patients with constipation has not been prospectively assessed. In a large retrospective study, in 146 of 563 patients with constipation who underwent endoscopic evaluations (358 colonoscopy and 205 flexible sigmoidoscopy), the range of neoplasia found and the polyp detection rate were comparable with those expected in asymptomatic historical controls [193]. There is therefore little evidence to support the routine use of colonoscopy in patients without alarm features.

Specific diagnostic tests for functional constipation

Detailed physiological testing should be performed in patients whose constipation is refractory to laxatives and dietary changes, and in those with a suspected evacuation disorder. The following tests are routinely performed: colonic transit study, anorectal manometry, balloon expulsion test, and defecography. An evidence-based summary of the various diagnostic approaches for chronic constipation is provided (Table 36.1). Unfortunately, no single test is adequate to define the pathophysiology of constipation, given its multifactorial nature, and often more than one test is required [15,185].

Colonic transit study

An assessment of the rate of stool movement through the colon provides an objective measurement of infrequent defecation, because the patient's recall of stool habit is often inaccurate [11,15]. Colonic transit time can be measured using three general methods:

- Ingestion of radiopaque markers followed by abdominal radiographs [194]
- Radioisotopes and scintigraphy [195,196]
- Ingestion of pressure, pH capsule (SmartPill), and tracking its movement [197].

The radiopaque marker test is typically performed by administering a single capsule containing 24 plastic markers (Sitzmarks,

Table 36.1 Evidence-based summary of the utility of the diagnostic tests for chronic constipation.

Test	Clinical utility		Recommendation		
	Strength	Weakness	Evidence	Grade[a]	Comment
Blood tests (thyroid function tests, serum calcium, glucose, electrolytes)	Rule out systemic or metabolic disorder	Is not a cost-effective strategy	No evidence	C	Not recommended for routine evaluation, particularly in the absence of alarm features
Imaging tests					
Plain abdominal radiograph	Identifies excessive amount of stool in the colon, simple, inexpensive, widely available	Lack of standardization on how to review the image Lack of controlled studies	Poor	C	May be considered for routine evaluation, particularly in the absence of alarm features
Barium enema	Identifies megacolon, megarectum, stenosis, diverticulosis, extrinsic compression, and intralumenal masses	Lack of standardization, embarrassing for patients Radiation exposure Lack of controlled studies	Poor	C	Not recommended for routine evaluation, particularly in the absence of alarm features
CAT scan	Stool retention and rectal volume	Radiation exposure Cost	Fair	B3	May be useful given as adjunct test, CAT scan is commonly performed
Defecography	Identifies dyssynergia, rectocele, prolapse, excessive descent, megarectum, Hirschsprung disease	Radiation exposure, embarrassment, availability, interobserver bias, inconsistent methodology	Fair	B3	Used as an adjunct to anorectal manometry
Anorectal ultrasound	Visualization of the internal anal sphincter and puborectalis muscles	Interobserver bias, availability	Poor	C	Experimental
Magnetic resonance imaging	Simultaneously evaluates global pelvic floor anatomy, sphincter morphology, and dynamic motion	Expensive, lack of standardization, availability	Fair	B3	Used as an adjunct to anorectal manometry
Flexible sigmoidoscopy and colonoscopy	Direct visualization of the colon to exclude mucosal lesions, such as solitary rectal ulcer syndrome, inflammation, or malignancy	Invasive, risks related to the procedure (perforation, bleeding), and sedation	Poor	C	Indicated in patients younger than 50 years who have alarm symptoms Indicated in all subjects older than 50 years for colorectal cancer screening
Physiological testing					
Colonic transit study with radiopaque markers	Evaluate presences of slow, normal, or rapid colonic transit Inexpensive and widely available	Inconsistent methodology, validity has been questioned	Good	B2	Useful to classify patients according to the pathophysiological subtypes
Colonic transit study with scintigraphy	Evaluates presence of slow, normal, or rapid colonic transit Provides evaluation of whole gut transit	Expensive, time consuming, availability, lack of standardization	Good	B2	Useful to classify patients according to the pathophysiological subtypes
Colonic transit study with wireless motility capsule test	Evaluates slow colonic transit, as well as gastric emptying, small bowel, and whole gut transit Standardized test noninvasive No radiation Validated and Cost-effective	Limited availability Risk for capsule retention Contraindicated in dysphagia and multiple bowel surgeries	Excellent	A1	Increasing availability but limited outside United States Useful to identify regional and whole gut transit
Anorectal manometry high resolution and 3D high definition	Identifies dyssynergic defecation, rectal hyposensitivity, rectal hypersensitivity, impaired compliance, Hirschsprung disease	Lack of standardization Recent IAPWG protocol London protocol[b]	Good	B2	Useful to establish the diagnoses of Hirschsprung disease and dyssynergic defecation Identifies rectal hyposensitivity and hypersensitivity
BET	Simple, nonexpensive, bedside assessment of the ability to expel a simulated stool Identifies dyssynergic defecation	Lack of standardization	Good	B2	Normal BET does not exclude dyssynergia Should be interpreted alongside the results of the other anorectal tests
Colonic manometry	Identifies colonic myopathy, neuropathy, or normal function facilitating selection of patients for surgery	Invasive, not widely available, lack of standardization	Fair	B3	Adjunct to colorectal function tests

[a] Grade A1: excellent evidence in favor of the test based on high specificity, sensitivity, accuracy, and positive predictive values. Grade B2: good evidence in favor of the test with some evidence on specificity, sensitivity, accuracy, and predictive values. Grade B3: fair evidence in favor of the test with some evidence on specificity, sensitivity, accuracy, and predictive values. Grade C: poor evidence in favor of the test with some evidence on specificity, sensitivity, accuracy, and predictive values.

[b] Recent international experts consensus guidelines (London classification) have been proposed but have not been prospectively evaluated.

BET, balloon expulsion test; CAT, computed axial tomography; IAPWG, International Anorectal Physiology Working Group.

Konsyl Pharmaceuticals, Easton, MD, USA) on day 1 and by obtaining plain abdominal radiographs on day 6 (120 hours later) [15,198,199]. Retention of at least 20% of markers (more than six markers) on day 6 (120 hours) is considered abnormal [194,199] and is indicative of STC. Because 60% of patients with dyssynergic defecation demonstrate excessive retention of markers [139], a diagnosis of STC should be made only after excluding dyssynergia [13,185]. A multiple capsule technique has also been used, but its interpretation is variable, and its validity has been questioned [200]. Several studies have assessed the utility of colonic transit in the evaluation of constipation [185,198]. A systematic review of 10 studies found that the prevalence rate of STC varied from 38% to 80% [185], noting there were significant differences in study population, methodology, and interpretation, and a gold standard was lacking [185].

Colonic transit scintigraphy is a noninvasive and quantitative method of evaluation of total and regional colonic transit [195,196]. Here, an isotope (^{111}In or ^{99m}Tc) is administered either in a coated capsule that dissolves in the terminal ileum or colon, or it is included with a test meal. Subsequently, gamma-camera images are obtained at specified time points [195,196]. Assessment and interpretation of the colonic transit time varies among centers with summary measurements at 24, 48, or 72 hours. A high geometric center represents greater than normal retention of isotope and a low geometric center slower colonic transit time. In a study of 23 patients diagnosed with STC based on radiopaque marker studies and 13 healthy individuals, who underwent oral ^{111}In-diethylenetriaminepentaacetic acid scintigraphy [198], there was no difference in transit time in the right colon between patients and control subjects, whereas patients had significant delay in the left colon. The authors concluded that colonic scintigraphy may help to select patients with STC for hemicolectomy [198]. However, the results of segmental colectomy are less satisfactory [201]. Although scintigraphic studies have been validated and are reliable and reproducible, they are expensive, time consuming, and available in only a limited number of centers [185]. Studies at such a center show that patients with STC tend to have retention of isotope in the ascending and transverse colon at 24 and 48 hours [64], whereas patients with evacuation disorders have retention predominantly in the descending colon and rectum on 48-hour imaging (Figures 36.9 and 36.10) [202]. Sex differences in colonic transit by scintigraphy require comparison of data with sex-matched control subjects.

Assessment of colonic transit using an ambulatory wireless motility capsule (WMC) technique (SmartPill) provides a noninvasive method of measuring not only colonic transit but also gastric emptying and small bowel transit time (Figure 36.11) [197]. It also provides information regarding colonic contractile activity and the whole-gut pH profile. Studies in healthy control subjects show good correlation of the colonic transit time between the SmartPill and Sitz Marker techniques [203], and it appears to distinguish control subjects from patients with STC [203], as well as elderly healthy control subjects from elderly constipated patients [204].

WMC confirms a clinical suspicion for a motility disorder in approximately 60% of subjects with otherwise unexplained GI symptoms and provides a new diagnosis in approximately 50% of subjects that led to a change in management in many of these patients [205–210]. Patients who underwent a WMC test needed fewer additional diagnostic tests, and its use significantly impacted

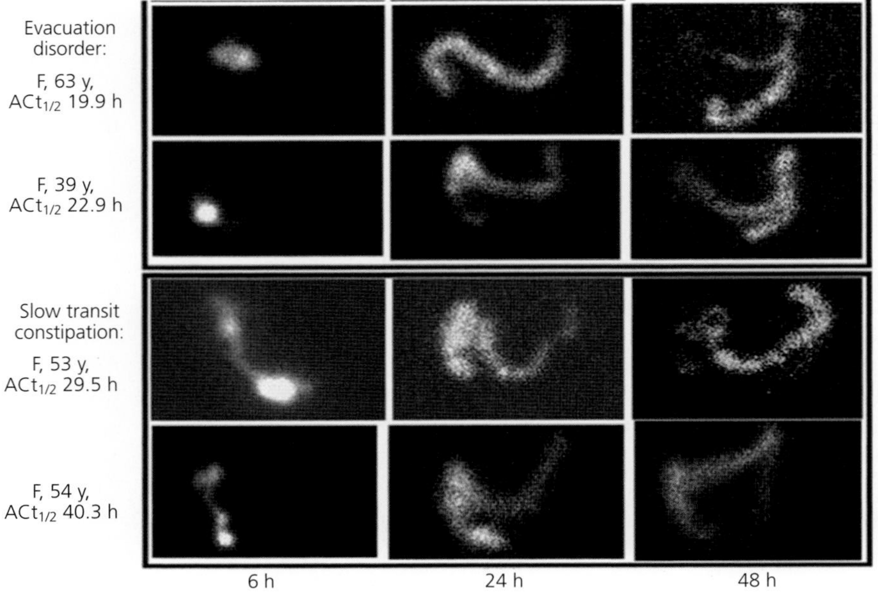

Figure 36.9 Examples of scintiscans at 6, 24, and 48 hours in patients with evacuation disorder and slow-transit constipation (STC). Note that delayed transit is also demonstrated at 48 hours in the patients with STC and the retention of isotope in the left colon in patients with evacuation disorder. Source: Nullens et al. 2012 [64]. Reproduced with permission of BMJ Publishing Group.

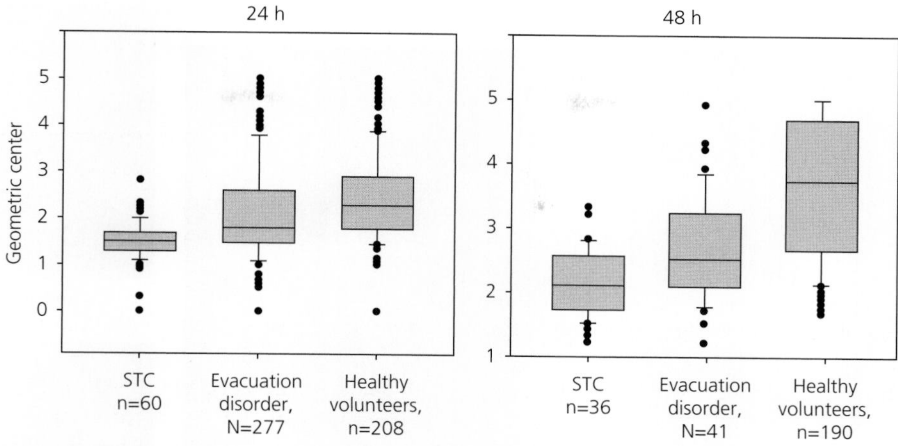

Figure 36.10 Distribution of geometric centers (median, interquartile range, 5th percentile, and 95th percentiles) at 24 and 48 hours in the different subgroups (*n* provided for each group). Note, however, that there is considerable overlap of overall transit in the evacuation disorder and slow-transit constipation (STC) groups. Source: Nullens et al. 2012 [64]. Reproduced with permission of BMJ Publishing Group.

clinical decision making, suggesting that this can be a very useful test in clinical practice and can be cost-effective [211,212].

Anorectal manometry

Anorectal manometry provides an integrated assessment of pressure activity in the anorectum together with an assessment of rectal sensation, rectoanal reflexes, and rectal compliance [15,147,207,208]. Manometry can detect dyssynergic defecation and Hirschsprung disease [161]. Normally, when a balloon is distended in the rectum, there is reflex relaxation of the internal anal sphincter. This rectoanal inhibitory reflex is mediated by the myenteric reflex [160] and release of nitric oxide and vasoactive intestinal peptide [213,214] and is absent in Hirschsprung disease [209]. A prospective study of 111 children showed that manometry had a sensitivity of 83% and specificity of 93% when compared with rectal suction biopsy (sensitivity 93% and specificity 100%) [210].

When healthy subjects attempt to defecate, they generate an adequate propulsive force that is reflected by a rise in intrarectal pressure. This movement is synchronized with relaxation of the puborectalis and the external anal sphincter, which is reflected by a decrease in anal sphincter pressure [13,139]. The inability to perform this coordinated maneuver represents the chief pathophysiological abnormality (see Figure 36.4) in patients with dyssynergic defecation [13,139]. However, some healthy subjects are also not able to produce a normal relaxation during attempted defecation [146,147]. The body position, whether sitting or lying down, the presence of stool-like sensation, and the consistency of stool may each influence the occurrence of dyssynergia and the ability to expel artificial stools [148,150]. Hence the finding of a dyssynergic pattern alone during manometry should not be considered as diagnostic of dyssynergic defecation. Additional features are usually recommended (see Box 36.1). By observing the manometric recordings during attempted defecation, it is possible to identify the sequence that most closely resembles a normal pattern of defecation (see Figure 36.5). Also, the manometry recording can be used to measure the intrarectal pressure, the anal residual pressure, and the percentage of anal relaxation [18,147,154]. From these measurements, one can calculate an index of the forces required to perform coordinated defecation – the defecation index, a simple and quantifiable measure of rectoanal coordination (normal index is at least 1.5) [13,147]. Furthermore, rectal sensory testing may reveal rectal hyposensitivity or rectal hypersensitivity [139,158,215–217]. Although several studies of anorectal manometry have been published, analysis of nine medium- to high-quality studies [185] has revealed differences in both methodology and interpretation, with the dyssynergia prevalence rate ranging from 20% to 95% [185]. This was further confirmed in a recent study [218]. Manometry detects only a dyssynergic pattern, and the diagnosis of dyssynergic defecation requires additional tests [13,16,18], so one should interpret manometric results with caution. Anorectal manometry provides confirmatory evidence for the diagnosis of dyssynergic defecation and helps to identify patients who may benefit from biofeedback therapy. The American and European Societies of Neurogastroenterology and Motility has proposed uniform standards for performing and interpreting anorectal manometry [219]. Newer manometric techniques, such as high-resolution anorectal manometry with multiple closely spaced circumferentially oriented solid-state sensors, provide a better delineation of the sphincter contours and pressure plots [220–223]. The 3D high-definition manometry system is useful for evaluating excessive perineal descent, rectal mucosal intussusception, or prolapse and anal sphincter defects, but has high false and positive rates and, therefore, is not suitable for detecting dyssynergia [224–226]. Recently, an international consensus panel has further modified the previous American and European Motility Societies recommendations [227], especially considering newer technology and emerging evidence, and has provided

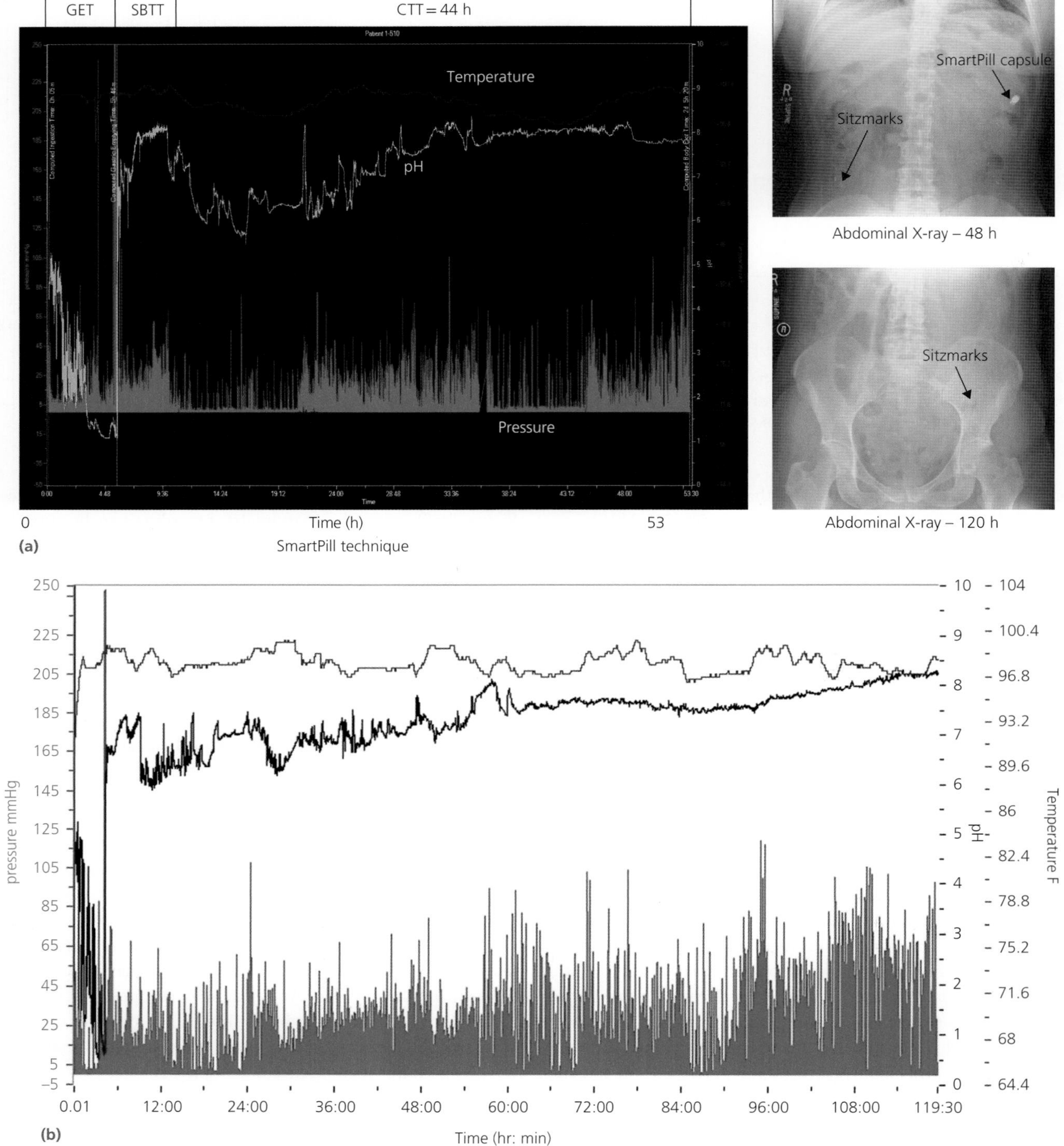

Figure 36.11 **(a)** Normal gastrointestinal transit as assessed by a wireless motility capsule. **(b)** Slow-transit constipation as assessed by wireless motility capsule showing delayed colonic transit of >144 hours in a patient with constipation. CTT, colonic transit time; GET, gastric emptying time; SBTT, small bowel transit time. **(a)** Source: Rao et al. 2009 [205]. Reproduced with permission of Elsevier.

new consensus guidelines for testing [227] and interpretation of findings [227]. However, these require further validation in prospective studies. In addition to diagnostic studies, anorectal manometry systems are also used routinely in many centers for performing biofeedback therapy. A new addition to anorectal physiology has been a 3D topographic representation of anorectal pressures, using either a solid-state 256 pressure sensor probe or software-configured 3D representation from a 10 sensor probe [228]. The normative data for the rigid 3D probe differs from conventional flexible probes, and hence results obtained from patient studies using this technique should be interpreted carefully, and the 3D rigid probe system has a high false-positive rate for detecting dyssynergia [228].

Balloon expulsion test

The balloon expulsion test provides a simple, bedside assessment of the subject's ability to expel an artificial stool. However, the methodology for this test has not been standardized. Several techniques have been used, including 25- or 50-mL balloons filled with warm water or air, 18-mm spheres, silicone-filled artificial stool, and weights attached to a pulley to assess the extra force required to expel a metal sphere in the lying position or a Foley catheter balloon [148,229]. The upper limit for normal balloon expulsion time has been variable. Some recommend 1 minute or longer, and others at least 5 minutes. In one author's laboratory, either a 4-cm-long balloon filled with 50 mL of warm water or a silicone-filled stool-like device (FECOM) is placed in the rectum; then the patient is asked to expel the device in the sitting position in privacy [147]. Most healthy subjects will expel the balloon filled with 50 mL water within 1 minute [147]. The prevalence rate of a positive test in favor of constipation varied between 23% and 67% [185]. A study suggested a specificity of 89%, negative predictive value of 97%, sensitivity of 88%, and positive predictive value of 67% [230]. However, this observation is confounded by other studies that have reported that many patients with dyssynergia can expel the balloon and that the test is insufficient to make a diagnosis [13]. Thus, although the failure to expel a balloon strongly suggests dyssynergia, a normal test does not exclude this possibility.

Nine studies of balloon expulsion showed impaired expulsion in 23–67% [185]. Hence this test should be interpreted in conjunction with other physiological tests. The most recent study in constipated patients confirmed that the balloon expulsion test using a Foley balloon catheter is reliable for analysis of pelvic floor dyssynergia; the optimal upper limit of normal is 2 minutes. Findings from the test have a high degree of agreement with those from anorectal manometry and electromyography [231]. Another recent study showed that 43% of healthy subjects could not expel the Foley balloon, whereas almost all expelled the 50-mL balloon, suggesting that the Foley balloon may not be an appropriate surrogate stool [150]. Another recent study suggested that a lower time limit of 22 seconds for balloon expulsion time had sensitivity and specificity of 78% and 70% and 1 minute had 39% and 93%, respectively [232]. Thus, the upper limit for a normal balloon expulsion test may vary up to 1 minute depending on the methodology and type of balloon.

Rectal barostat test

An assessment of rectal sensation, tone, and compliance using a highly compliant balloon that is placed in the rectum and connected to a computerized pressure-distending device (barostat) can be useful. Several studies have revealed rectal hyposensitivity in patients with constipation [215–217]. The test also can be useful for identifying patients with a normal, impaired, or hypercompliant rectum and can facilitate the detection of megarectum. The barostat system also can be used as a biofeedback device for treating patients with rectal hyposensitivity [157] and for treating patients with rectal hypersensitivity using a novel technique of sensory adaptation training [158].

Defecography

Defecography provides information regarding the anatomical and functional changes of the anorectum. It is performed by infusing 150 mL barium paste into the patient's rectum and having the subject squeeze, cough, and expel the barium. The most common findings are poor activation of levator muscles, prolonged retention of or inability to expel the barium, absence of a stripping wave in the rectum, mucosal intussusception, and rectocele [6].

According to the literature, the prevalence rate of normal defecography varies between 10% and 75% [185]. Although defecography revealed abnormalities in 77% of subjects, there was no relationship between symptoms and abnormalities [233]. Another prospective study found that the yield of defecography in the diagnosis of constipation was minimal [13]. Among 10 defecography studies, abnormalities were reported in 25–90% and dyssynergia in 13–37% [185]. Disadvantages of defecography include radiation exposure, embarrassment, limited availability, interobserver bias, and inconsistent methodology among centers [185]. As a result of these inherent limitations, it has been recommended that the test should be considered as an adjunct to clinical and manometric assessment of constipated patients whose symptoms have not responded to conventional therapy or in those with a history of excessive straining, prolapse, or use of digital maneuvers to facilitate defecation.

Colonic manometry

Colonic manometry provides a comprehensive assessment of overall motor activity at rest, during sleep, after waking, after meals, and after provocative stimulation, such as drugs, meal, or balloon distentions [75,79,85,234]. It is performed by using solid-state probes and portable recorders or water-perfused stationary systems [73,75,79]. It provides reproducible and reliable information regarding the pathophysiology of constipation [75,79,80] and can be used to explore the mechanisms and motor effects of pharmacological agents on the colon. The probes are often placed under endoscopic or fluoroscopic guidance, although other techniques have been described [85,86,234]. Prolonged recordings over 24 hours are preferred to optimally understand the overall colonic motor profile. Studies have confirmed that patients with STC exhibit a significant reduction of phasic colonic motor activity, the gastrocolonic and morning waking responses, and the number of HAPCs (see Figure 36.3) [79,80]. The application of multiple (up to 90) closely spaced sensors using fiberoptic catheters has further advanced our understanding of colonic motor function and revealed the importance of this spacing to detect colonic propagated contractions; tripling the distance between sensors reduced the number of contractions detected by 30% [85,234,235].

Thus, colonic manometry may reveal an underlying myopathy or neuropathy [79]. In some patients, despite slower colonic transit time, the colonic neuromuscular function is normal [79]. Similar to its utility in children [236], a study of 24-hour ambulatory colonic manometry in adults has shown that the test can facilitate the selection of patients for surgery [79]. In a case–control study, most patients with manometric features of colonic neuropathy (i.e., absence of any two of the three normal colonic motor responses: HAPCs, gastrocolonic response, and morning waking response) failed to respond to aggressive medical treatment and had a better clinical outcome after colectomy [79]. A prospective study of 80 patients with refractory STC showed that 59% had abnormal colonic manometry, with 26% showing features of colonic neuropathy, 33% features of colonic myopathy, and 41% normal colonic motility. Furthermore, 64% of patients with normal motility or colonic myopathy responded to aggressive medical or biofeedback therapy compared with 15% with colonic neuropathy; a majority of the latter group responded to surgery [237]. Colonic manometry is a useful technique to investigate colonic sensorimotor function in refractory constipation, helping to guide clinical management, and a recently published consensus paper provides improved metrics for nomenclature and for defining abnormalities that could help future research [85,234]. Newer high-resolution colonic manometry systems with more closely spaced sensors or noninvasive magnetic imaging technology may help to better define colonic abnormalities [85,234] in patients with constipation.

Magnetic resonance imaging

In the last few years, several uncontrolled studies have shown that endoanal magnetic resonance imaging (MRI) and dynamic pelvic MRI – "MR defecography" – can be useful [238–240]. This is the only imaging modality that can simultaneously evaluate global pelvic floor anatomy and dynamic motion. Endoanal MRI may reveal changes in the external anal sphincter that are not identifiable by endoanal ultrasound, whereas MRI fluoroscopy directly shows the pelvic floor and viscera during rectal evacuation and squeeze maneuvers [241]. The free selection of imaging planes, absence of radiation exposure, good temporal resolution, and the excellent soft tissue contrast are all advantages. Dynamic pelvic MRI in the sitting position provides a more physiological approach than in the supine position [242].

Dynamic MRI is useful for the diagnosis of rectal mucosal intussusception because it can differentiate between mucosal and full-thickness rectal prolapse [238]. In patients with dyssynergic, dynamic MRI reveals that the anorectal angle becomes more acute, confirming paradoxical contraction of the puborectalis [239]. In a controlled study, the degree of perineal descent was decreased in 35%, normal in 44%, and increased in 21% of constipated patients during rectal evacuation [243]. Increased perineal descent was associated with a hypertensive anal sphincter, a normal rectal balloon expulsion test, and a rectocele. Limitations of MRI defecography include its high cost, lack of standardization, wide range of normal values [244], possible lack of sensitivity [245], and general lack of availability.

Conclusions on diagnostic testing

Although several tests are performed to rule out structural and biochemical disorders that cause constipation, there is little evidence to support the use of hematological and biochemical tests, radiographs, or endoscopy in the routine management of constipated patients without alarm features [185]. The American College of Gastroenterology Task Force concluded that the routine use of a battery of diagnostic tests should be avoided in patients with chronic constipation, and that empiric treatment should be the initial approach [186]. Diagnostic tests are indicated to identify structural or functional causes of constipation in a subgroup of patients with alarm symptoms or signs, or in those who do not respond to empirical therapy, or where there is a suspicion of dyssynergia.

There is good evidence to support the use of physiological tests, such as anorectal manometry or colonic transit, in particular to define the pathophysiological subtypes and to guide the selection of treatment options. However, no single test will provide a pathophysiological basis for constipation because it is a heterogeneous condition that requires several tests to identify the underlying mechanism(s).

Treatment of chronic constipation

The treatment of chronic constipation should be customized for each individual, taking into consideration the cause of constipation, age, comorbid conditions, underlying pathophysiology, and the patient's concerns and expectations and previous use of over-the-counter products and prescription. A survey of 331 primary care physicians reported that 60% felt that there were inadequate treatments for constipation [246]. In another survey of 4680 patients with self-reported constipation and taking medication, 47% reported dissatisfaction with their current treatment [247]. Hence there is a large unmet need for the treatment of constipation, and the real challenge is to relieve the multiple symptoms and meet the patients' expectations. An algorithmic approach for the diagnosis and management of constipation is shown in Figure 36.12. Guidelines from the American Gastroenterology Association [248] and other reviews [71] provide additional approaches to constipation management.

Lifestyle changes, fluid intake, and exercise

Lifestyle changes, such as adequate fluid intake, regular non-strenuous exercise, and dedicated time for passing bowel movements, can be useful, but there is limited evidence to support these measures [122]. Patients should be encouraged to avoid postponing defecation [6], as the urge subsides after a few minutes and may not return for hours. Most patients who have a normal bowel pattern usually empty stool at approximately the same time every day [178]. This observation suggests that the act of defecation is, in part, a conditioned reflex. Hence ritualizing the bowel habit is worthwhile and could help establish a regular pattern of bowel movement. Physiologically, the colon is more active after waking and after a meal [75,79]. Accordingly, the optimal time for stool evacuation is within the first 2 hours

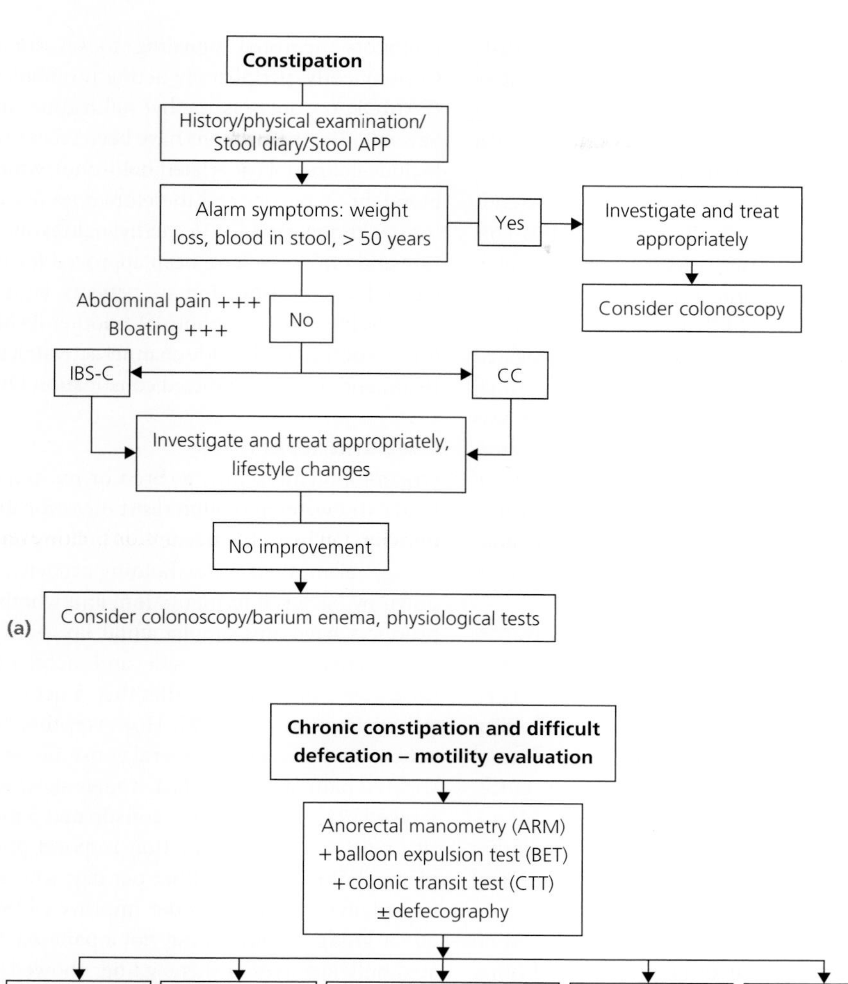

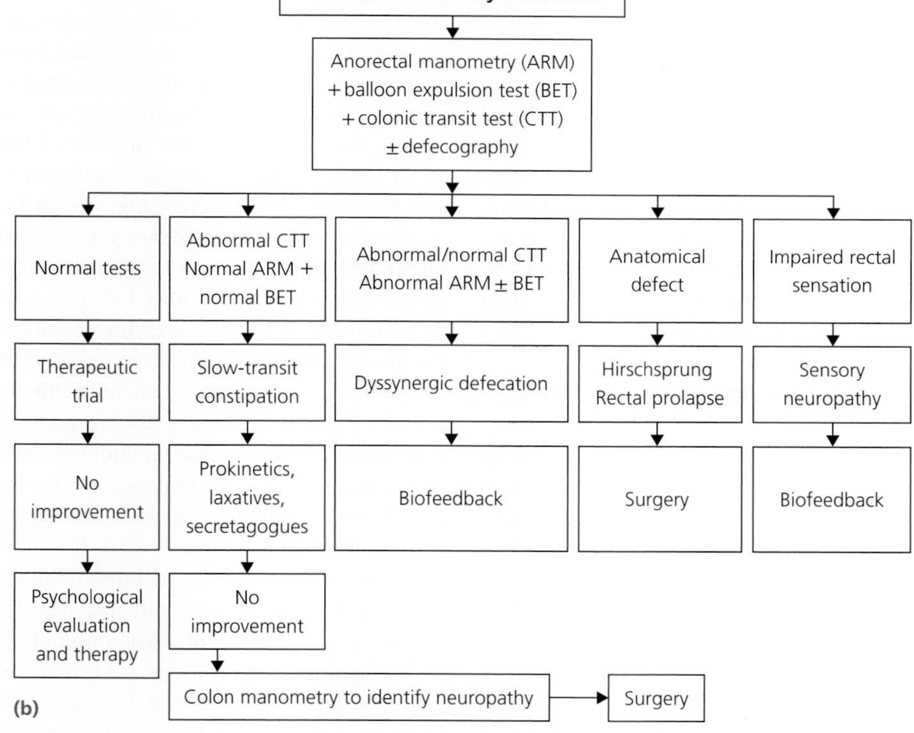

Figure 36.12 **(a)** Algorithmic approach to the management of chronic constipation and **(b)** algorithmic approach to the gastrointestinal motility evaluation and treatment of chronic constipation. CC, chronic constipation; IBS-C, irritable bowel syndrome with concurrent constipation. Source: Adapted from Rao 2003 [366].

after waking and after breakfast. Timed toilet training consists of educating the patient to attempt defecation for approximately 5 minutes, at least twice a day, usually 30–60 minutes after a meal, irrespective of whether they have an urge, and to push at a level of 5–7, assuming a maximum straining effort of 10.

Some research suggests that modest exercise can relieve constipation, especially if patients are generally inactive [249]. This recommendation is based on observations that bedridden patients are more prone to constipation and on the premise that exercise shortens GI transit time [249]. Exercise changes the colonic motor pattern by increasing the number of propagated contractions in the postexercise period [76]. In a longitudinal study of Australian women, the odds ratio for constipation was lower (0.76) in women who performed low-to-moderate exercise than in sedentary women [250]. In another study, of geriatric patients, the relative risks of constipation for those who walked 0.5 km/day, those who walked with help, or those who were chair or bed bound were 1.7, 3.4, 6.9, and 15.9, respectively [251].

Thus, bowel function may correlate with exercise activity, particularly in elderly adults, but other factors, such as diet, cognition, medications, and personality, may each play a role [122]. Acute graded exercise transiently diminishes colonic motility, and immediately thereafter, the return of propagating contractions can propel colonic contents, unimpeded, over long distances possibly resulting in exercise-induced bowel movements [76].

Constipation can be relieved in some patients by increasing daily fluid intake. In a study of 117 adults, intake of 2 L mineral water daily increased stool frequency when compared with control subjects [252], although baseline stool habit was based on recall, and the mineral water contained magnesium and other ions, compromising the validity of this study [122]. A study has further confirmed the equivalence of natural mineral water and magnesium sulfate-enriched mineral water, although hard stools decreased significantly in the latter group [253].

Treatment of drug-induced and opioid-induced constipation

Many patients with constipation are unaware that they are taking drugs that cause constipation. In a study of 329 individuals with self-reported constipation, 195 (59.3%) were using constipating medications [254]. A common list of drugs is shown in Box 36.3. The physician should seek out medications that cause constipation and, wherever possible, substitute agents that do not. In a study of 46 patients with cancer, the percentage of patients taking daily laxatives decreased significantly after patients were switched to a less-constipating analgesic [255]. Opioid-induced bowel dysfunction, in particular opioid-induced constipation, was reported in 47% of noncancer patients [256], and constipation itself has been reported in more than 80% of patients with cancer who are receiving opioids [257,258]. Both weak and strong opioids are equally bothersome [259]. Opioid-induced constipation primarily results from the effect of opioids on μ-opioid receptors in the enteric nervous system, resulting in suppression of excitatory and inhibitory neuronal signaling to GI smooth muscles [260]. Consequently, peripherally acting μ-opioid receptor antagonists (PAMORAs), such as methyl naltrexone, may be useful [261]. Several other medications have been recently approved [262] and include naloxegol (pegylated naloxone), which does not cross the blood–brain barrier and therefore does not reverse the effects of the opiate analgesia [263]. Methyl naltrexone subcutaneous injection and oral form have been approved for the treatment of opioid-induced constipation in patients with chronic noncancer pain. Naldemedine (Symproic), another PAMORA, and lubiprostone (Amitiza), a chloride channel activator, are also approved for treatment of opioid-induced constipation [264].

Diet and fiber

Organic polymers such as bran or psyllium have the ability to hold extra water and often resist digestion and absorption in the upper gut. Their effectiveness as bulking agents depends on the dosage taken, their water-holding capacity, the extent of breakdown by bacterial fermentation, and whether the fermentation products have any supplemental laxation [265]. A high-fiber diet increases stool weight and accelerates colonic transit time [266]. In contrast, a diet that is deficient in fiber may lead to constipation [266,267]. However, there is no evidence that constipated patients in general consume less fiber than nonconstipated patients, and in fact studies show similar levels of fiber intake [122]. Furthermore, constipated patients with slow transit or pelvic floor dysfunction respond poorly to dietary supplementation with 30 g fiber per day, whereas those without an underlying motility disorder improved [268]. A fiber intake of 20–30 g/day is optimal, but not a panacea. Six trials that evaluated bulk laxatives or dietary fiber showed an average weighted increase of 1.4 (95% confidence interval: 0.6–2.2) bowel movements per week, whereas seven trials that evaluated laxative agents other than bulk showed an increase of 1.5 (95% confidence interval: 1.1–1.8) bowel movements per week [269]. Both the American College of Gastroenterology Task Force [186] and a systematic review [269] concluded that psyllium, a natural fiber supplement, increases stool frequency, and they gave this compound a Grade B recommendation, but there were insufficient data to make a recommendation for the synthetic polysaccharide methylcellulose, or for calcium polycarbophil or bran in patients with constipation. A study has shown that dried plums (prunes) were superior to psyllium in the management of mild-to-moderate constipation, and that this effect may be in part because of the presence of other compounds in addition to fiber in dried plums [270]. Another study compared a mixed soluble, fruit-based fiber supplement (SupraFiber) with soluble fiber psyllium and showed that mixed fiber was better tolerated with less bloating, although both supplements were equally effective in improving complete spontaneous bowel movements [271].

The benefits of added fiber are not evident for days to weeks, and its fermentation can produce excessive gas, bloating, and flatulence [265]. It is important to recommend generous fluid intake along with fiber supplementation, failing which, stools could become hard and bulky and difficult to expel. Patients with an obstruction, gastroparesis, or fecal impaction, or those confined to bed or requiring fluid restriction should not be given fiber supplements. Inadequate calorie intake can cause constipation [272], and it is a common problem in patients with anorexia nervosa. Refeeding and restoration of normal weight normalize colonic transit [273].

Pharmacological treatments

Pharmacological treatments include laxatives, prokinetic agents, serotonergic compounds, chloride channel activators, and others. According to a recent report, $1.4 billion was spent yearly on over-the-counter laxatives in the United States [6]. A summary of these compounds, their mode of action, and evidence-based recommendations is presented in Table 36.2 [274].

Table 36.2 Summary of the pharmacological properties of conventional laxatives and newer therapies used in the treatment of constipation and related evidence-based medicine recommendations.

Laxative class	Medications	Mechanism of action	Side-effects	Level of evidence	Grade of recommendation
Bulk (fiber) laxatives	Psyllium, calcium polycarbophil, methylcellulose, bran	Retaining water in stool, increasing stool bulk, and improving consistency	Flatulence, bloating, abdominal distension, rarely causing mechanical obstruction of esophagus and colon	Psyllium II; Others III	B/C
Stool softeners or wetting agents	Docusate sodium, docusate calcium	Promoting luminal water binding by detergent-like action, increasing stool bulk	Intestinal cramping, irritation of throat (liquid formulation)	III	C
Stimulant laxatives	Senna, aloe, bisacodyl, sodium picosulfate	Increasing intestinal peristalsis by acting on myenteric nerve plexus; decreasing large intestinal water absorption	Abdominal discomfort, rarely electrolytes disturbance, melanosis coli	Sodium picosulfate II; Others III	A/C
Osmotic laxatives	PEG, lactulose, sorbitol, milk of magnesia, magnesium citrate	Osmotic water binding	Bloating, flatulence, abdominal cramping, in rare instances, electrolytes disturbances	PEG I	A
				Lactulose I	A
				Sorbitol/milk of magnesia III	B/C
Mixed laxatives	Dried plums	Stool bulking and osmotic action	Flatulence, bloating	II	B
Chloride channel activators	Lubiprostone (Amitiza)	Selective activation of intestinal epithelial chloride channel 2, increasing chloride secretion	Nausea, diarrhea, headache	I	A
GCC activators	Linaclotide (Linzess) Plecanatide (Trulance)	Activation of GCC receptor on enterocytes, increasing cyclic GMP, activating CFTR, increasing luminal chloride/bicarbonate secretion; ameliorating visceral hypersensitivity	Diarrhea	I	A
Opioid receptor antagonists	Methylnaltrexone (Relistor) Naloxegol (Movantik) Naldemedine (Symproic)	Enteric opioid receptor antagonism, with minimal absorption and not crossing blood–brain barrier	Abdominal cramping, flatulence, nausea	I	A
	Alvimopan (Entereg)		Nausea, vomiting	I	A
Serotonergic agonists	Prucalopride (Motegrity), Tegaserod, TD-5108, ATI-7505	Selective 5-HT_4 receptor activation with enhancement of gut motility by contraction of proximal smooth muscles and relaxation of distal smooth muscles; cAMP-mediated colonic chloride secretion	Headache, nausea, diarrhea, abdominal pain, tegaserod with unfounded concerns for ischemic colitis	I	A
Bile acid modulator	Elobixibat	Ileal bile acid transporter Antagonist	Diarrhea	II	A

cAMP, cyclic adenosine monophosphate; CFTR, cystic fibrosis transmembrane conductance regulator; GCC, guanylate cyclase C; 5-HT_4, 5-hydroxytryptamine; PEG, polyethylene glycol.

Source: Singh and Rao 2010 [274]. Reproduced by permission of Elsevier.

Stool softeners

Sodium and calcium docusate compounds (Colace, SURFAK) are anionic surfactants that lower the surface tension of stool and facilitate the mixing of aqueous and fatty substances and also stimulate intestinal fluid secretion [275]. There are four randomized controlled trials (RCTs) that have compared stool softeners with either placebo or other laxatives. The sample sizes were small and the data conflicting [269]. Consequently, these compounds were afforded a Grade B recommendation, and they were felt to be inferior to psyllium with regard to improvement of stool frequency [19]. Mineral oil is a lubricant used for the treatment of constipation [19]. It provides lubrication by emulsifying the stool mass [276]. There is no published study of the use of mineral oil in adults with constipation, although in children it appears to be more effective than senna-based compounds and less effective than osmotic laxatives [19]. Side-effects include lipid pneumonia from aspiration, a risk particularly in elderly subjects, malabsorption of fat-soluble vitamins, foreign-body reactions, and fecal incontinence [276].

Stimulant laxatives

This group consists of anthraquinones (senna, cascara sagrada, danthron, and casanthranol), diphenylmethane derivatives (bisacodyl, sodium picosulfate), and ricinoleic acid (castor oil). Stimulant laxatives affect electrolyte transport across the intestinal mucosa and enhance colonic transport and motility; they usually work within several hours of administration.

The anthraquinones increase fluid and electrolyte secretion in the small intestine [275] and are absorbed and metabolized by the liver. They cause melanosis coli, a brownish black pigmentation of the colonic mucosa as a result of cell debris inside submucosal macrophages. This is formed during apoptosis of colonic epithelial cells stained by the anthraquinones. Bisacodyl (Dulcolax; Correctol; Carter's Little Pills) is structurally similar to phenolphthalein, increases small intestinal fluid secretion and colonic motor activity, and is approved for the treatment of occasional constipation. It is a gastric irritant, so the tablets are enteric coated. It is also available as a suppository. A network metaanalysis together with systemic review found that the relative risk of having >3 complete spontaneous bowel movements per week was 2.46 (1.83,3.35) for bisacodyl and 2.83 (1.923, 4.16) for sodium picosulfate [277], although these results were based on single studies, and efficacy was assessed over 4-week trials [278].

Common side-effects include abdominal discomfort, cramps, and fecal incontinence [279]. Stimulant laxatives are best reserved for occasional or short-term use [177] and have been used as rescue agents in many clinical trials. Their long-term safety has not been established. Four RCTs were identified, but none of them were placebo controlled, leading to a Grade B recommendation [269]. A large RCT of 368 patients with constipation showed that 4 weeks of bisacodyl, 10 mg/day, was more effective than placebo in improving constipation and number of complete spontaneous bowel movements per week [280].

Osmotic laxatives

Osmotic laxatives include saline laxatives (salts of magnesium, phosphate, and sulfate), poorly absorbed synthetic disaccharides such as lactulose, sugar alcohols such as sorbitol or mannitol, and an inert polymer, polyethylene glycol (PEG-3350). This group includes ions or molecules that are not well absorbed by the intestine, driving retention of water by the intestinal lumen to maintain osmotic balance with plasma. Overuse of osmotic laxatives may induce abdominal cramps, diarrhea, and dehydration [19,269]. Magnesium compounds are commonly used. The typical adult dose of 1–2 tablespoons magnesium hydroxide contains 20–40 mmol magnesium ions and can produce an evacuation within 6–12 hours. A single, low-quality, 8-week crossover trial compared magnesium hydroxide with laxomucil and reported 2.8 more bowel movements with magnesium [19,269,281]. Citrate of magnesia is available as a carbonated drink in 300-mL (10-fluid ounce) bottles and contains 116 mmol magnesium ion, but there are no trials with this compound. Hypermagnesemia can occur in patients with renal failure. Likewise, sulfate compounds and phosphate salts (Fleet Phospho-Soda; C.B. Fleet Company, Lynchburg, VA, USA) serve as hyperosmolar agents causing laxation. The colon is less permeable to phosphate than is the small intestine, so phosphate salts can be used in an enema form to clean the lower colon. A standard phosphate enema (Fleet) contains 120 mL fluid and 1780 mmol/L phosphate ion.

Lactulose is a synthetic disaccharide that cannot be hydrolyzed in the small intestine and thereby serves as an osmotic agent. It is fermented in the colon by anaerobic flora. Significant diarrhea does not occur until more than 100 g/24 hours is consumed [282]; standard doses produce mild laxation [265]. Likewise, sorbitol and mannitol are sugar alcohols that are poorly absorbed. In one study of elderly constipated subjects, 70% sorbitol syrup was as effective as lactulose but was approximately one-tenth the cost [283]. Glycerin is another small molecule that can exert osmotic activity in the colon. It is not absorbed by the colon and is often used as a suppository to draw water into the rectum.

PEG 3350 (MiraLAX; Braintree Labs, Braintree, MA, USA; GlycoLax) is a large polymer that is poorly absorbed, metabolically inert, and not degraded by bacteria. It has been widely used as a lavage solution in preparation for colonoscopy. There are at least eight placebo-controlled randomized trials of PEG compounds and two randomized trials comparing PEG with lactulose [269]. PEG was superior to placebo in increasing stool frequency and stool consistency [284] and noninferior to prucalopride [285]. Its efficacy is often greatest in the second week of treatment, and a dose–response study showed that a 68-g dose produced reliable laxation within 24 hours [286]. Although generally safe, it can cause bloating or nausea. However, no electrolyte changes have been reported. In a 6-month multicenter study, stool frequency increased to 7.7 per week with PEG and 5.4 per week with placebo [287]. A study reported relief of constipation in 52% of patients receiving PEG-3350 versus 11% of patients receiving placebo [288].

Serotonergic agents

Serotonin is a neurotransmitter that is widely distributed in the body, although more than 90% is found in the GI tract [125]. Fourteen serotonin receptor subtypes have been identified, including type 4 receptors (5-HT_4), which when stimulated promote peristalsis, induce chloride secretion, and possibly reduce visceral hypersensitivity [289]. In many countries, including the United States, the 5-HT_4 receptor agonist, prucalopride (Motegrity), has been approved for the treatment of chronic constipation at a dose of 2 mg/day for adults and 1 mg/day for those older than 65 years. Metaanalysis demonstrates efficacy and safety of this selective 5-HT_4 receptor agonist [290]. Recently, 5-HT_4 partial agonist tegaserod (Alfasigma, Covington, LA, USA) that was previously shown to be effective and safe for both constipation and IBS-C has been reapproved for use in the United States for IBS-C in adult women younger than 65 years [291]. Unlike tegaserod, prucalopride is well tolerated with no significant cardiovascular effects or drug interactions [71].

Chloride channel activators

Chloride channels are located in the apical and serosal membranes of the enterocyte, and they facilitate chloride transport [135]. There are four subtypes [292]. Lubiprostone is a gastrointestinal-targeted bicyclic fatty acid that selectively activates type 2 chloride channels, resulting in increased secretion of chloride by the intestinal cells lining the small bowel. As the negatively charged chloride ion leaves the cell, sodium and water are also simultaneously excreted into the lumen paracellularly, to maintain enterocyte electrical gradient [135]. Thus, lubiprostone increases fluid secretion, secondarily increases intestinal motility, and enhances stool transport, alleviating symptoms of chronic constipation [235,293–295]. In a RCT involving 242 patients, 24 μg lubiprostone twice daily for 28 days was more effective than placebo in increasing the number of spontaneous bowel movements, decreasing straining, improving stool consistency, and relieving symptoms of chronic constipation [294]. Long-term studies show that the compound is efficacious and safe [296]. The most common adverse effects are nausea (31.1%), diarrhea (13.2%), and headache (13.2%) [296]. In guinea pigs, lubiprostone can cause fetal loss, so adequate contraceptive measures are recommended for young women taking lubiprostone, and it has been designated a pregnancy category C drug [297]. A recent study showed that lubiprostone does not cause any electrolyte imbalance when taken long term [298]. Most recently, lubiprostone has been approved for treatment of opioid-induced constipation and was shown to be effective in a large RCT [299].

Guanylate cyclase C agonist

Linaclotide (Linzess) is a novel drug with a novel mechanism of action (activation of chloride secretion through CFTR after binding to GCC receptor), low bioavailability, and local action in the intestinal epithelial cells. It accelerates colonic transit [300], relieves chronic constipation [301,302], and reduces pain sensation [303], thereby also relieving pain in IBS-constipation [304]. Plecanatide (Trulance) also activates GCC receptors, stimulating chloride and bicarbonate secretion, and inhibiting sodium absorption in intestinal enterocytes. In a 14-day treatment trial in 80 patients with chronic idiopathic constipation, plecanatide improved stool frequency and consistency, straining, and abdominal discomfort [305]. A preliminary report documented the efficacy of plecanatide (0.3, 1, and 3 mg) in 951 patients with chronic idiopathic constipation treated for 12 weeks [306]. Two large RCTs have demonstrated that plecanatide, 3 mg daily, was effective and safe in the treatment of chronic constipation [305,307].

Miscellaneous and emerging therapies

Colchicine, a plant alkaloid used to treat gout [265,276], and misoprostol, a prostaglandin analog used to treat peptic disorders, induce diarrhea as a side-effect [265,276]. Consequently, they have been tried in patients with chronic constipation [308,309]. A limited number of studies involving a small number of patients found that colchicine increased stool frequency and accelerated colonic transit, lessening the need for rescue laxatives [269]. Similarly, misoprostol increased intestinal motility, particularly of the left colon, and the rate of intestinal transit [269,309]. Misoprostol can trigger uterine contractions, so it should be avoided by women who are or who could become pregnant [265]. Severe abdominal cramping has also been reported [265].

Bile acid modulation

Delivery of bile acids into the colon results in diarrhea. Selective inhibition of the ileal bile acid transporter with elobixibat provides a novel approach to bile acid delivery to the colon. This drug accelerated colonic transit [310] to significantly increased stool frequency and improved constipation-related symptoms over 8 weeks of treatment in patients with chronic idiopathic constipation [311]. A recent RCT evaluated the short-term efficacy of elobixibat and separately its long-term safety in an open-label study and showed that the drug improved constipation in the short term and was well tolerated in the long term [312].

Treatment of evacuation disorders

Behavioral approaches using neuromuscular conditioning can be effective in the management of dyssynergic defecation [13].

Treatment of dyssynergic defecation

Treatment of dyssynergic defecation consists of diet, laxatives, timed-toilet training, and other measures outlined earlier, together with neuromuscular conditioning using biofeedback therapy techniques [13,139]. Biofeedback therapy has been shown to be efficacious [313–315]. Other approaches that have limited efficacy include botulinum toxin injection [153,154], anal myectomy, and surgery [144,316].

Biofeedback therapy is an instrument-based behavioral program that is based on "operant conditioning" techniques. The governing principle is that when any behavior is reinforced, its likelihood of being repeated and perfected increases several fold. In patients with dyssynergic defecation, the goal of neuromuscular conditioning is twofold:

1. To correct the incoordination or dyssynergic behavior during defecation, and restore normal coordination of the abdominal, rectal, puborectalis, and anal sphincter
2. To improve rectal sensory perception.

Rectoanal coordination training

Three techniques have been used:

1. Diaphragmatic muscle training with simulated defecation
2. Manometry-guided pelvic floor retraining
3. Simulated defecation training.

The biofeedback system consists of placing a manometry or electromyography probe into the anorectum [13]. These sensors pick up pressure or electromyographic signals from the anal sphincter, which are then displayed on a monitor. This provides visual feedback [155]. The simulated defecation technique consists of placing either a water-filled balloon or a silicone-filled balloon, called a FECOM [317], into the rectum, and the subject is trained to expel the device by coordinating the abdominal and pelvic floor muscles.

Typically, patients are instructed on diaphragmatic breathing techniques to improve their abdominal pushing effort. Thereafter, visual or auditory feedback techniques are used to provide input to the patient regarding their attempted defecation maneuvers. The patient's posture and breathing techniques are corrected. The number of training sessions is customized to the patient's need, but an average of six sessions is often required. Training is complete if a patient can demonstrate consistently, that is during two consecutive training sessions, a normal pattern of defecation with at least 50% of attempts, together with an improvement in symptoms of difficult defecation [13,315]. However, many patients tend to revert back to their previous pattern of defecation, so periodic reinforcement may be required. In a long-term assessment of biofeedback therapy, it was found that compliance with reinforcement sessions decreases with time [318]. Using any one or a combination of these methods, symptomatic improvement has been reported in about 80% of patients [13,313,319].

Sensory training

Sixty percent of patients with dyssynergic defecation have impaired rectal sensation [139,320,321], so rectal sensory conditioning may provide additional therapeutic benefit [318,320]. The goal is to enhance rectal sensory perception by training the patient to perceive a lower volume of rectal balloon distention, but with the same intensity as previously experienced with a larger balloon volume [320,321].

A recent study showed that barostat-assisted sensory training was more efficacious than syringe-assisted balloon training (78% vs 53%) and significantly easier to administer [157]. Also, another study compared escitalopram with sensory adaptation training, a novel method of progressive rectal balloon distension using a rectal barostat in patients with IBS-C and rectal hypersensitivity, and showed that sensory adaptation training was significantly more effective and better tolerated than escitalopram [158]. Simulated defecation is a maneuver performed by placing an artificial stool or water-filled balloon into the rectum [13,320]. The patient is asked to sit on a commode and to expel the device. Their posture and breathing techniques are continuously monitored and corrected, and a therapist assists the patient's efforts, if required, by applying gentle traction to the stool-like device while reinforcing their technique of defecation.

Four RCTs of biofeedback therapy have been reported. Rao and colleagues [315] showed that biofeedback therapy was superior to sham biofeedback and to the standard medical treatment of diet, exercise, and laxatives. Global bowel satisfaction was significantly higher with biofeedback compared with sham treatment (78% vs 48%; $p<0.05$). Also, the number of complete spontaneous bowel movements per week was significantly higher in the biofeedback group (Figure 36.13). In another study, Heymen and colleagues [322] showed that biofeedback was more effective than either 5 mg diazepam or a placebo. Response rates, defined by patients' self-report of "adequate relief" after 3 months of training, were 71% for biofeedback, 33% for placebo, and 20% for diazepam.

Chiarioni and colleagues [314] showed that five biofeedback sessions were more effective than continuous PEG (14 g/day) for treating dyssynergia, and benefits lasted for at least 2 years. Two RCTs have also reported sustained (1-year) improvement of symptoms [314,318] and colorectal function [318], confirming the long-term efficacy of biofeedback therapy. These studies indicate that biofeedback should be the preferred treatment for dyssynergic defecation. Unfortunately, biofeedback is a labor-intensive program that is not widely available. To treat the vast number of constipated patients, a home-based, self-training program may be required. Limited studies have demonstrated the feasibility of home training [319,323]. A recent RCT showed that 3 months of home biofeedback therapy using a novel device was as efficacious as office biofeedback therapy, with 68% and 70% responders in each arm [324]. Also, biofeedback therapy significantly improved QOL in patients with dyssynergic defecation, and home biofeedback was more cost-effective than office biofeedback [325], with an incremental cost effectiveness ratio of $20,753 favoring home biofeedback. These findings demonstrate that home biofeedback therapy is a preferred treatment option for patients with dyssynergia and if unavailable or patients do not respond successfully to this approach, then office biofeedback can be considered.

Treatment of stool impaction

Patients with stool impaction or those with hard stools that are difficult to expel require digital disimpaction. This can be painful and may require sedation or anesthesia. Once the colon has been cleaned, these patients require rigorous bowel conditioning

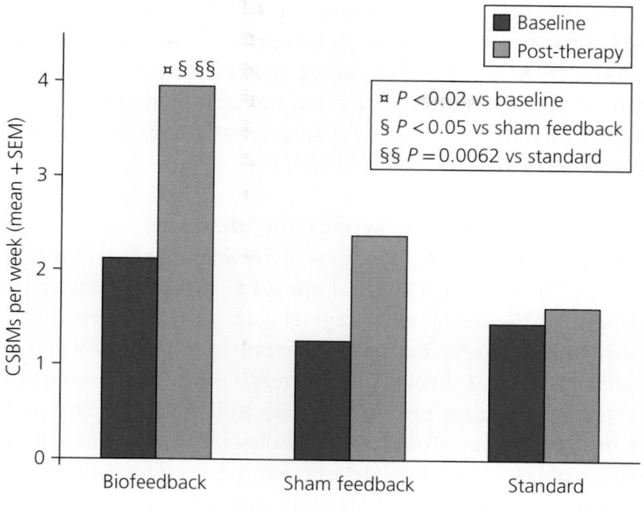

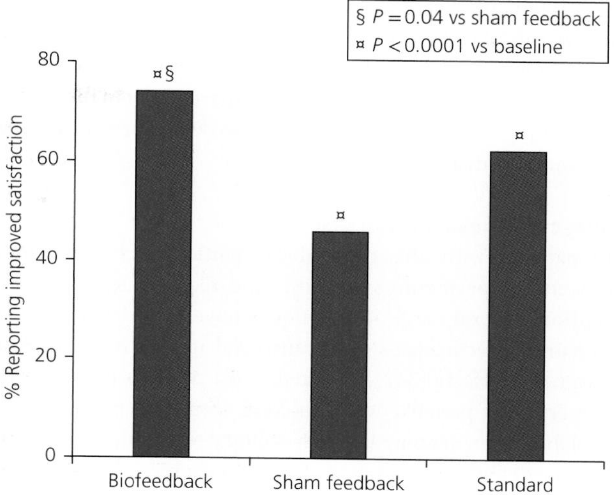

Figure 36.13 Effects of biofeedback therapy on the number of complete spontaneous bowel movements (CSBMs) and the proportion of subjects who reported improved bowel satisfaction in a randomized controlled trial that compared biofeedback therapy with sham feedback (relaxation) and standard treatment of diet and laxatives. Source: Rao et al. 2007 [315]. Reproduced with permission of Elsevier.

and a regimen of laxatives and suppositories or enemas to prevent stool impaction [326]. Glycerin or bisacodyl suppositories together with enemas (tap water or Fleet) are usually successful, but their efficacy has not been prospectively assessed. Additional measures include saline or osmotic laxatives or PEG solutions. After establishing a bowel regimen, it is important to assess these patients for secondary causes or an underlying colonic or generalized motility disorder, and they should be treated aggressively with either laxatives, secretagogues, prokinetics, or biofeedback therapies to prevent recurrence [326].

Surgical treatment

Surgery should be reserved for patients with unsuccessful aggressive medical and behavioral treatments under expert supervision, with demonstrable colonic neuropathy [79], and with motility dysfunction that is confined to the colon [327]. The latter two are best assessed by performing a gastric-emptying test, antroduodenojejunal manometry, and colonic manometry. Patients with a generalized motility disorder are more likely to have an unsatisfactory outcome [328,329]. Broadly, the surgical procedures may be considered under three categories: cecostomy, colectomy with anastomosis or construction of a stoma, and surgery for evacuation disorders. Recently, the American Society of Colon and Rectal Surgeons Clinical Practice Guidelines has summarized the evidence and indications for various surgical procedures except total colectomy with ileorectal anastomosis; overall, the evidence for most surgical procedures for constipation is weak [330].

Cecostomy

This procedure is analogous to a gastrostomy. Both surgical [331] and endoscopic [332] techniques have been described, and the results appear favorable. The procedure is generally preferred in children, institutionalized patients, and those with neurological lesions. The Malone or antegrade continent enema procedure consists of fashioning a cecostomy button or appendicostomy [331–333]. The principle is to perform periodic antegrade irrigation of the colon (once every 3 days) so that the colon is adequately cleansed and in a predictable manner. Solutions commonly used include a glycerin : saline solution in a ratio of 1 : 3; a volume of 500–1500 mL as tolerated is infused into the cecostomy. Alternatively, PEG solutions may be used. Satisfactory results range from 40% to 78% [332]. An ileal stoma is felt to cause fewer complications over time [332], but there are no controlled trials.

Colectomy

Several techniques for colectomy have been advocated that include segmental colectomy, ileorectal anastomosis, ileosigmoid anastomosis, cecorectal anastomosis, ileoanal anastomosis with proctocolectomy, and pouch formation or ileostomy [334]. Subtotal colectomy with ileorectal anastomosis is the most commonly performed technique. These surgeries can be effectively performed laparoscopically and could minimize adhesions [335]. A long-term study that compared the outcome of colectomy in patients with constipation, ulcerative colitis, and colon cancer concluded that patients with constipation fared poorly, had more complications, and had poorer QOL compared with other groups [336]. A more recent series of carefully selected patients reported that bowel symptoms improved in more than 80% of patients, and QOL scores normalized [329]. Segmental colectomy was felt to be unsuccessful in several case–control studies [337,338], although one report is more favorable [201]. There is no clear rationale for resection of a particular colonic segment, particularly because segmental retention of markers on a colonic transit study may not accurately predict colonic dysfunction in that segment. An ileostomy may be considered in patients with unsuccessful ileorectal anastomosis, but in one series a favorable outcome was seen in only 50% [339]. Many of these patients may have an underlying psychological dysfunction [327] or a generalized gut motility disorder [327].

Surgery for evacuation disorders

In patients with structural abnormalities, such as rectocele, descending perineum syndrome, and rectal mucosal intussusception, several surgical techniques have been tried [340,341]. Repair of a rectocele using a transrectal approach seems to have fewer side-effects [342], although most patients do not require surgery. For patients with mucosal intussusception or rectal prolapse often accompanied by solitary rectal ulcer, abdominal rectopexy with sigmoid resection has been recommended [340]. Local excision is not recommended because this procedure does not address the underlying pathophysiology, and the lesions tend to recur. Keighley and Shouler [343] described 14 patients who underwent posterior Marlex rectopexy for solitary rectal ulcer syndrome. The ulcer healed in five of six patients (83%) with full-thickness rectal prolapse. A similar result was noted in only two of eight patients (25%) with rectoanal intussusception. The authors concluded that only symptomatic ulcers should be treated by surgery and only after medical treatment has failed. Many of these patients have coexistent dyssynergia for which biofeedback can be effective [344]. A stapling procedure, stapled transanal rectal resection, has been advocated [345]. After initial experience, enthusiasm remains high [346], although in one multicenter series, several complications, including bleeding, incontinence, anal stenosis, and pain, have been reported. Controlled trials are awaited.

Sacral nerve stimulation and transabdominal electrical stimulation

Sacral nerve stimulation (SNS) was initially used for the treatment of fecal and urinary incontinence, but several studies have reported that sacral nerve stimulation may benefit patients with constipation [347–350]. The mechanism by which SNS improves bowel function is unclear; a study of six patients reported that S3, but not S2, nerve stimulation produced more HAPCs, suggesting that sacral nerve stimulation alters colonic physiology through neuroenteric pathways [347]. A prospective study of 62 patients who did not respond successfully to laxatives and biofeedback found that stool frequency and bowel satisfaction improved, whereas straining, time spent on the toilet, and pain decreased [350], colonic transit normalized in 50%, and QOL improved. However, a more recent RCT of SNS in 44 patients with chronic constipation, albeit for a shorter duration (3 weeks), found limited efficacy, with 11% of subjects reporting sustained symptom relief [351]. A recent study of 62 children with STC evaluated transabdominal electrical stimulation using a portable stimulator and 4 cm × 4 cm electrodes placed near the umbilicus and on the back, for 1 hour daily for 6 months. The stool frequency increased together with reduction in soiling episodes and improvement in QOL [352]. Another controlled study in 28 women also showed improvement with transabdominal electrical stimulation but was not different from control [353]. This noninvasive treatment option appears promising but requires rigorous trials.

Management of Hirschsprung disease

Surgery remains the cornerstone of treatment for Hirschsprung disease. The optimal surgical approach is determined by the length of the aganglionic segment, in particular whether it involves the anorectum, rectum, or colon. In patients with significant hindgut involvement, removal of the entire segment, as in the Swenson procedure [354] and the endorectal pull-through techniques of Soave and Boley [355], or bypassing the segment, as in the Duhamel operation, have all produced satisfactory results [356]. In patients with a short or ultra-short segment, anal myotomy with or without incision of a variable length of rectal smooth muscle has been reported to be useful [357].

Management of fecal impaction

Fecal impaction can be seen in a variety of clinical settings, including children with prolonged difficulty with defecation, adults with dyssynergia or STC, institutionalized patients, post-operative patients receiving opioids, patients with psychological and psychiatric comorbidities, and most importantly, elderly adults, many of whom may present with fecal soiling [358]. The first step is to confirm the diagnosis by DRE. A plain radiograph of the abdomen can reveal stool impaction. Initially, glycerin and bisacodyl suppositories together with phosphosoda or milk and molasses enema should be tried together with gentle disimpaction with fingers. If unsuccessful, manual disimpaction and evacuation should be performed, under sedation sometimes requiring anesthesia (particularly children). Once disimpaction has been achieved, the patient should be placed on an aggressive regimen of oral laxative, prokinetics, and suppositories to ensure frequent soft stools daily. Bulk laxatives and fiber supplements should be avoided [359,360]. Stimulant or osmotic laxatives such as PEG or magnesium compounds are preferred, although newer agents such as linaclotide, prucalopride, and lubiprostone may also be effective. After 1 or 2 months, efforts should be made to identify an underlying problem such as dyssynergic defecation, encopresis, mobility, or drugs, and appropriate steps should be taken to prevent a recurrence [361].

Gut dysbiosis and constipation

Over the last decade there has been significant interest in learning whether altered colonic microbiome or dysbiosis leads to chronic constipation [362], but there is a paucity of evidence. There are five controlled studies of colonic microbiome in constipation, three of which were in adults and provided inconsistent data, in large part, because of methodological problems.

Overall it appears that Bifidobacteria and Bacteroides species are decreased, whereas Firmicutes species may be increased, in the colonic microbiome of constipated patients, although these findings were not reproduced by other investigators [362]. Interventions including probiotics and synbiotics in a poorly characterized group of constipated patients may improve constipation symptoms [363]. However, rigorous placebo-controlled studies are lacking, and whether fecal microbiota transplantation is an option merits further study.

Complications of constipation

Several common anorectal conditions, such as anal fissure, hemorrhoids, megarectum, megacolon, fecal impaction particularly in elderly adults, fecal seepage, stercoral ulcer, solitary rectal ulcer syndrome, and rectoceles, may be a consequence of long-standing constipation [364]. Although a causal relationship can sometimes be difficult to establish, based on expert consensus, historical association of these problems, and recent evidence of altered anorectal physiology in many of these conditions, it is likely that long-standing constipation or difficulty with defecation, or both predispose to these common problems. Patients may not always describe or be aware of symptoms of coexisting constipation. Consequently, prevention and aggressive treatment of underlying constipation with diet, laxatives, behavioral and other approaches, and sometimes surgery may lead to longer-lasting relief or cure. Colorectal cancer has also been claimed as a potential side-effect, either because of long-standing constipation or as the result of unforeseen effects of the medications used to treat constipation [265,365], but there is no concrete evidence. With the recent advances in the pathophysiology of chronic constipation, these complications should be preventable.

References are available at www.yamadagastro.com/textbook7e

Further reading

Camilleri M., Ford A.C., Mawe G.M., et al. Chronic constipation. Nat Rev Dis Primers 2017;3:17095.

Carrington E.V., Heinrich H., Knowles C.H., et al. The international anorectal physiology working group (IAPWG) recommendations: standardized testing protocol and the London classification for disorders of anorectal function. Neurogastroenterol Motil 2020;32:e13679.

Luthra P., Camilleri M., Burr N.E., et al. Efficacy of drugs in chronic idiopathic constipation: a systematic review and network meta-analysis. Lancet Gastroenterol Hepatol 2019;4:831.

Rao S.S.C. Rectal exam: yes, it can and should be done in a busy practice! Am J Gastroenterol 2018;113:635.

Rao S.S. and Brenner D.M. Efficacy and safety of over-the-counter therpies for chronic constipation: An updated systematic review. Am J Gastroenterol 2021;doi:10.14309/ajg.0000000000001222

Rao S.S., Benninga M.A., Bharucha A.E., et al. ANMS-ESNM position paper and consensus guidelines on biofeedback therapy for anorectal disorders. Neurogastroenterol Motil 2015;27:594.

Rao S.S., Bharucha A.E., Chiarioni G., et al. Anorectal disorders. Gastroenterology 2016;150:1430.

Rao S., Lembo A.J., Shiff S.J., et al. A 12-week, randomized, controlled trial with a 4-week randomized withdrawal period to evaluate the efficacy and safety of linaclotide in irritable bowel syndrome with constipation. Am J Gastroenterol 2012;107:1714.

Rao S.S., Mudipalli R.S., Stessman M., et al. Investigation of the utility of colorectal function tests and Rome II criteria in dyssynergic defecation (anismus). Neurogastroenterol Motil 2004;16:589.

Rao S.S.C., Valestin J.A., Xiang X., et al. Home-based versus office-based biofeedback therapy for constipation with dyssynergic defecation: a randomised controlled trial. Lancet Gastroenterol Hepatol 2018;3:768.

Singh S., Heady S., Coss-Adame E., et al. Clinical utility of colonic manometry in slow transit constipation. Neurogastroenterol Motil 2013;25:487.

Suares N.C., Ford A.C. Prevalence of, and risk factors for, chronic idiopathic constipation in the community: systematic review and meta-analysis. Am J Gastroenterol 2011;106:1582.

Wald A., Bharucha A.E., Cosman B.C., et al. ACG clinical guideline: management of benign anorectal disorders. Am J Gastroenterol 2014;109:1141.

CHAPTER 37

Approach to the patient with acute abdomen

Courtney B. Sherman and Kenneth McQuaid
Department of Medicine, Division of Gastroenterology, University of California, San Francisco, CA, USA

Chapter menu

Definitions

Abdominal pain is a common patient complaint, accounting for a significant number of emergency department (ED) [1] and primary care visits [2] each year. In 2010–2014, the most common reason for an ED visit in the United States was abdominal pain, accounting for 11.8% of visits [3]. The differential diagnosis of acute abdominal pain is broad and ranges from benign to life-threatening etiologies. Although definitions vary, the term *acute abdomen* generally refers to the sudden onset of abdominal pain that requires prompt diagnosis and early management. Arbitrary time intervals can be used to differentiate the "acute abdomen" from acute abdominal pain, with an onset of less than 24 h for the former and up to several days for the latter. Although most cases do not require operative management, it is critical to have a systematic approach to the patient with abdominal pain to efficiently identify those who require expedited evaluation or urgent intervention. This chapter will review the pathophysiological mechanisms that determine how abdominal pain is sensed, provide a framework for understanding *acute* abdominal pain, and highlight special populations in whom the presentation of acute abdominal processes may be atypical.

Pathophysiology

Neuroanatomy

Neuronal sensory (afferent) pathway organization and embryological organ development play major roles in determining how abdominal pain is perceived. Sensory receptors in the digestive tract include mechanoreceptors, chemoreceptors, and thermoreceptors. Visceral chemoreceptors perceive a variety of chemical stimuli as noxious, including substance P, serotonin, prostaglandins, bradykinin, histamine, and hydrogen ions [4,5], whereas the principal mechanical stimulus for nociceptors is stretch. In hollow abdominal organs, afferents that respond to chemical and mechanical stimuli are located within the gastrointestinal mucosa and muscularis mucosa, between the smooth muscle layers, in the serosa (visceral peritoneum), and within the mesentery [6,7]. Solid organ nociceptive receptors generally are limited to the organ capsule and respond mainly to mechanical stimuli (stretch). Therefore, lesions within solid organs may not cause pain until they are of sufficient size to cause capsule stretch or traction.

There are three main patterns of abdominal pain: visceral, somatoparietal, and referred. Visceral and somatoparietal

Yamada's Textbook of Gastroenterology, Seventh Edition. Edited by Timothy C. Wang, Michael Camilleri, Benjamin Lebwohl, Anna S. Lok, William J. Sandborn, Kenneth K. Wang, and Gary D. Wu.

Companion website: www.yamadagastro.com/textbook7e

sensory pathways use a three-neuron chain [8]. The cell body of the first-order neuron resides in the dorsal root ganglion with one axon that projects centrally to the spinal cord and one axon that projects distally to either the visceral organs or the somatoparietal structures (parietal peritoneum, abdominal wall musculature, and skin). Visceral afferents projecting distally pass along the spinal nerve, exit via the white rami communicans to the sympathetic chain ganglia, and finally travel in association with the splanchnic (sympathetic) nerves to reach the visceral organ nociceptive receptors. Somatoparietal afferents pass along the spinal nerve to peripheral nerves that conform with cutaneous dermatomes (Figures 37.1 and 37.2). Both visceral and somatoparietal afferents projecting centrally enter the dorsal horn of the spinal cord and synapse with second-order neurons. Somatoparietal structures are densely innervated, and their afferent neurons synapse at the same level as their port of entry into the spinal cord. In contrast, visceral sensory afferents are fewer and synapse with second-order neurons located at, above, or below the level of spinal cord entry. As a result of this wider distribution of innervation, visceral pain often is more vague, diffuse, and difficult to localize than somatoparietal pain. Vagal sensory afferents primarily serve to regulate autonomic functions and have little role in pain sensation. The second-order dorsal horn neuron ascends through the spinal cord via two distinct pathways. The classic route for both visceral and somatoparietal pain is to cross the spinal cord and ascend in the spinothalamic, spinoreticular, and spinomesencephalic tracts to synapse with third-order neurons in the thalamus, reticular formation, and midbrain. Another second-order neuron pathway, which is relatively specific for visceral pain, ascends ipsilaterally in the dorsal column [9]. Tertiary neurons then project from the thalamus or reticular formation to the postcentral gyrus and cortex for somatic sensation and to the anterior cingulate gyrus and sensory cortex for visceral sensation. Projections to subcortical centers are thought to contribute to the affective aspects of pain [8].

Visceral pain

Visceral pain is mainly transmitted via neurons composed of slowly conducting unmyelinated C fibers. These fibers are stimulated by noxious chemicals and by distension, strong muscular contractions, mesenteric traction, or torsion. Heightened mechanoreceptor sensitivity to stretch may have pathophysiological importance in some conditions, such as irritable bowel syndrome, in which minor contractions or stretch may be perceived as painful [10]. Visceral pain is generally perceived as dull, deep-seated, cramping, poorly localized, and more gradual in onset when compared with somatoparietal pain. Patients may also note concomitant autonomic symptoms, including nausea, emesis, diaphoresis, and restlessness.

The location of visceral pain perception is correlated with the embryological origin of the diseased organ. During normal

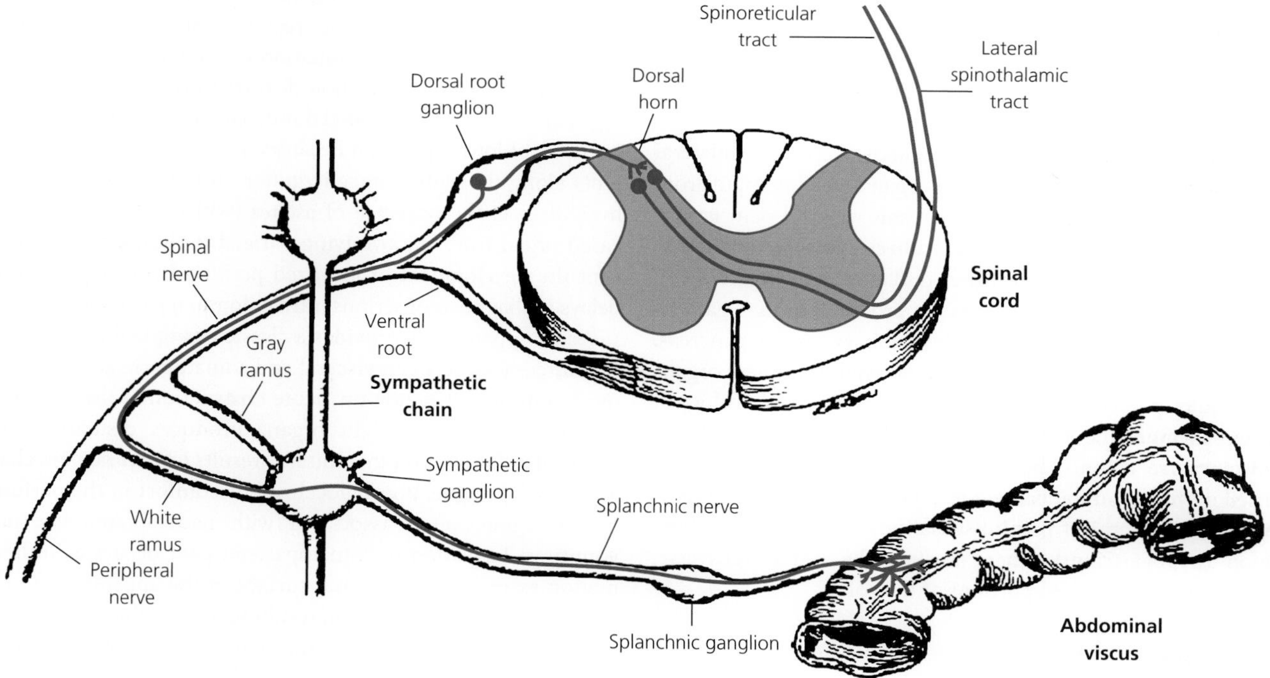

Figure 37.1 Classic neuronal pain pathways (blue), such as the spinothalamic and spinoreticular tracts, mediating abdominal visceral pain sensation leave the dorsal horn, cross the midline, and ascend to higher centers. Nociceptive information from visceral organs is relayed to cells near the central canal. These postsynaptic dorsal horn cells send their axons in the midline of the dorsal column to synapse in the nucleus gracilis. The pathway then crosses the midline in the lower brainstem to ascend to the ventral posterolateral nucleus of the thalamus. Source: Price 2000 [112].

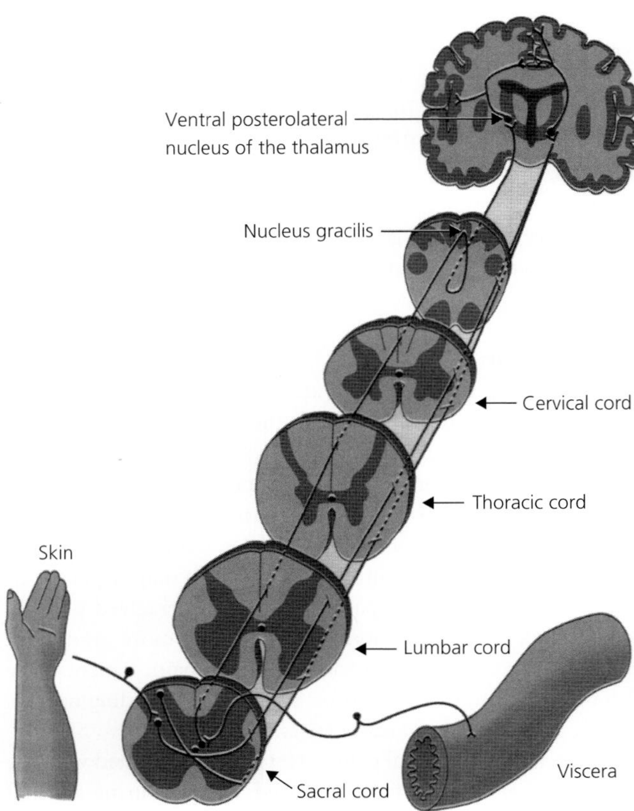

Figure 37.2 "Visceral-specific" pain pathways in the spinal cord. Artist's drawing showing how nociceptive input from the pelvic viscera arrives in the dorsal horn of the spinal cord, where it is relayed to higher centers by cells near the central canal. Source: Adapted from Willis and Westlund 1997 [113].

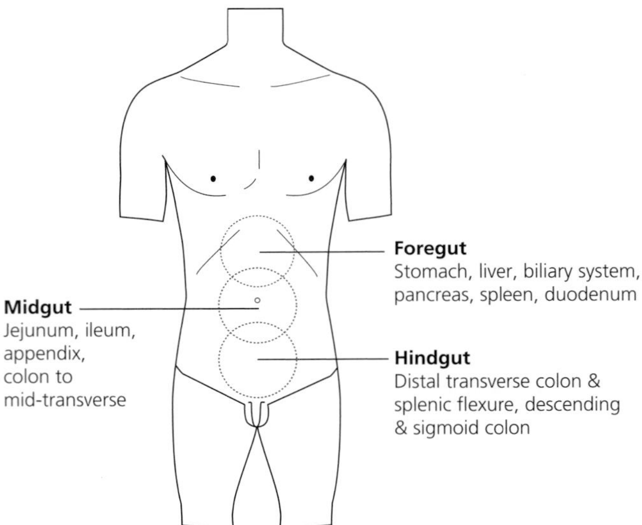

Figure 37.3 Areas of visceral pain perception based on embryological organ derivation.

embryological development, abdominal organs receive bilateral sympathetic innervation, with each organ receiving input from several adjacent spinal levels. As a result, visceral pain is perceived as a midline sensation that localizes poorly to the epigastrium, periumbilical area, or lower midabdomen (Figure 37.3). The embryonic foregut structures are proximal to the ligament of Treitz and include the stomach, liver, biliary system, pancreas, spleen, and duodenum. Visceral pain derived from these organs is generally perceived in the epigastrium. The embryological midgut includes the jejunum, ileum, appendix, and right and midtransverse colon. These structures transmit pain that is sensed in the periumbilical region. The embryological hindgut-derived organs project painful sensations to the lower midline region (hypogastrium). These include the distal transverse, descending, and sigmoid portions of the colon.

Somatoparietal pain

Somatoparietal pain is mediated by dense, rapidly conducting A-δ nerve fibers with small receptive fields. In contrast with visceral pain, somatoparietal pain is sharp and well localized (unless generalized peritonitis has developed). Furthermore, somatoparietal structures (including the parietal peritoneum) are innervated in a unilateral, dermatomal distribution by the sixth thoracic (T6) to the first lumbar (L1) nerves [11]. Parietal peritoneum afferent receptors may be stimulated by contact with an adjacent inflamed visceral organ or by direct chemical irritation (e.g., gastrointestinal secretions from perforated viscus, bile, urine, or pus). This results in localized peritoneal inflammation (localized peritonitis), which usually causes pain that is sharp, lateralized, and better localized than visceral pain. In some cases, chemical irritation or inflammation of the parietal peritoneum may result in pain at a location distinct from the site of pathology. For example, a perforated duodenal ulcer may produce pain in the right lower quadrant because of migration of gastric contents along the right paracolic gutter. In patients with chronic liver disease, the presence of ascites (which separates the diseased organ from the overlying parietal peritoneum) may prevent the development of localized peritonitis, often leading to delays in diagnosis of serious intraabdominal pathology.

Acute appendicitis provides a classic example that illustrates the differences between visceral and somatoparietal pain. In its most common presentation, acute obstruction of the appendix (an embryological midgut organ) produces distention and mucosal inflammation that initially results in visceral pain characterized by vague, poorly localized discomfort in the periumbilical region, often associated with nausea, anorexia, and vomiting. Transition to somatoparietal pain occurs as inflammation extends to the serosal surface of the appendix and the adjacent parietal peritoneum, resulting in pain that is sharp and well localized at McBurney point in the right lower quadrant.

Referred pain

Pain may be perceived in areas remote from the affected viscera [12], a phenomenon known as referred pain. This occurs when visceral afferents carrying noxious stimuli from a diseased

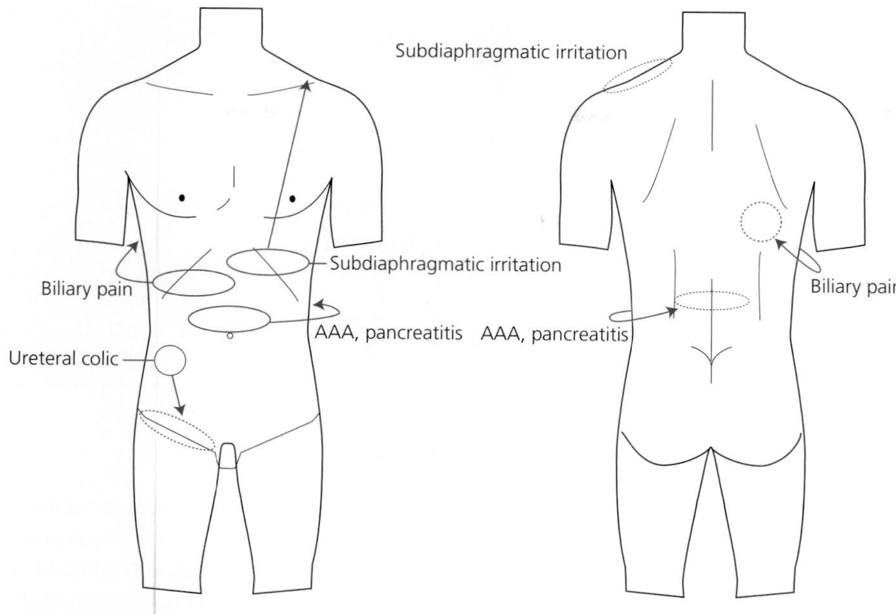

Figure 37.4 Patterns of referred pain. AAA, abdominal aortic aneurysm.

organ enter the spinal cord at the same level as somatic afferents from a distant anatomic site, resulting in pain that is perceived ("referred") in cutaneous dermatomes sharing the same spinal segments. Referred pain is often described as aching in quality and located near the body surface. Referred pain patterns are often stereotypical enough to provide useful diagnostic information (Figure 37.4). For example, pain from pancreatic disease often is referred to the posterior midline in the region of the first vertebra.

Acute cholecystitis provides an example of how a single affected organ can lead to all three patterns of abdominal pain [7]. Initial impaction of a stone in the cystic duct causes distention and mucosal inflammation in the gallbladder (an embryological foregut organ), resulting in an initial visceral pattern of vague, midline pain in the epigastrium. If inflammation progresses to involve the serosal surface, irritation and inflammation of the adjacent parietal peritoneum results in somatoparietal pain that is more intense, well localized, and lateralized to the right upper quadrant. In addition, pain from cholecystitis may be referred to the right scapula or shoulder.

Etiologies

The majority of patients with acute abdominal pain are evaluated in the ED or urgent care setting. Because most patients with typical presentations of common pathology are quickly recognized by ED or surgical providers, gastroenterologists are more likely to be consulted in cases in which the diagnosis is elusive or the presentation atypical. As such, it is important for gastroenterologists to understand the diverse causes and presentations of acute abdominal pain, including extraabdominal causes. For example, herpes zoster that involves thoracic dermatomes may cause neuropathic pain that precedes the development of the classic vesicular rash and can result in right upper quadrant pain mimicking acute cholecystitis. Boxes 37.1 and 37.2 provide examples of abdominal and extraabdominal etiologies of acute abdominal pain.

Box 37.1 Abdominal etiologies of acute abdominal pain.

Gastrointestinal
- Dyspepsia (food intolerance, gastroesophageal reflux, peptic ulcer, functional)
- Gastric outlet obstruction
- *Gastric volvulus*
- Gastritis (e.g., alcoholic, drug induced)
- Gastroenteritis
- *Perforated peptic ulcer*
- *Meckel diverticulitis*
- Gastroparesis
- Inflammatory bowel disease
- *Appendicitis*
- *Small bowel obstruction*
- *Large bowel obstruction*
- *Bowel perforation*
- *Bowel ischemia*
- *Strangulated hernia*
- *Colonic diverticulitis*
- Mesenteric adenitis

Hepatobiliary
- *Acute cholecystitis*
- Symptomatic cholelithiasis
- Acute hepatitis
- Acute cholangitis

(Continued)

Acute portal vein thrombosis
Hepatic abscess
Hepatic tumor rupture or hemorrhage

Pancreatic and splenic
Acute pancreatitis
Splenic rupture
Splenic infarct

Vascular
Ruptured aortic aneurysm
Acute mesenteric ischemia

Urological
Nephrolithiasis
Pyelonephritis
Renal infarct

Gynecological
Ruptured ectopic pregnancy
Ruptured ovarian cyst
Ovarian torsion
Acute salpingitis
Ruptured tuboovarian abscess
Pelvic inflammatory disease
Endometriosis

Peritoneal
Intraabdominal abscess
Infectious peritonitis (e.g., tuberculous, spontaneous bacterial)

Retroperitoneal
Retroperitoneal hemorrhage

Disease processes in italics often require urgent surgical or interventional radiology management.

Box 37.2 Extraabdominal causes of acute abdominal pain.

Cardiac
Myocardial infarction
Pericarditis
Myocarditis

Pulmonary
Lower lobe pneumonia
Empyema
Pulmonary embolism and infarction
Pneumothorax

Hematological
Sickle cell crisis
Acute leukemia

Neurological
Herpes zoster
Spinal nerve root compression
Tabes dorsalis (tertiary syphilis)
Abdominal epilepsy and abdominal migraine

Metabolic
Diabetic ketoacidosis
Acute adrenal insufficiency, Addisonian crisis
Acute porphyria
Uremia
Hyperparathyroidism, hypercalcemia

Toxin or medication related
Lead poisoning
Narcotic withdrawal

Rheumatological
Familial Mediterranean fever
Henoch–Schönlein purpura
Abdominal vessel vasculitis

Miscellaneous
Psychiatric disorders
Hereditary angioedema

Source: Data are from Purcell 1989 [114] and Mulholland and Debas 1997 [115].

Diagnosis

Acute abdominal pain presents a significant challenge to providers because its differential diagnosis is vast, ranging from benign to life-threatening, intraabdominal to extraabdominal, and organic to nonorganic. Understanding the anatomy and innervation of abdominal viscera assists in creating an initial differential diagnosis. To narrow the differential diagnosis and triage patients appropriately, it is critical to approach acute abdominal pain in a systematic fashion. This stepwise approach begins with a detailed history and physical examination that pays close attention to special populations who may present with common pathology in an atypical manner. These include the elderly, immunocompromised individuals, and pregnant women. In addition, the medical setting where patients present influences the differential diagnosis.

History

When investigating the etiology of acute abdominal pain, it is crucial to characterize the pain and its associated symptoms as precisely as possible. One must also consider the patient's age, sex, medical and surgical histories, medications, and social history to frame the differential diagnosis.

Characterization of pain

Acute abdominal pain typically is characterized by the following key information: location, onset, quality, and aggravating or alleviating factors.

Location

As previously described, the embryological origins of abdominal organs, as well as the visceral and somatoparietal sensory networks, help determine where patients perceive abdominal pain. While keeping the three pain patterns (visceral, somatoparietal, and referred) in mind, dividing the abdomen into anatomic regions can be useful when creating a differential diagnosis for acute abdominal pain (Figure 37.5). The use of abdominal regions to assist in identifying the likely diseased organ has shown highest specificity in patients with epigastric pain caused by gastroduodenal diseases, right subcostal pain

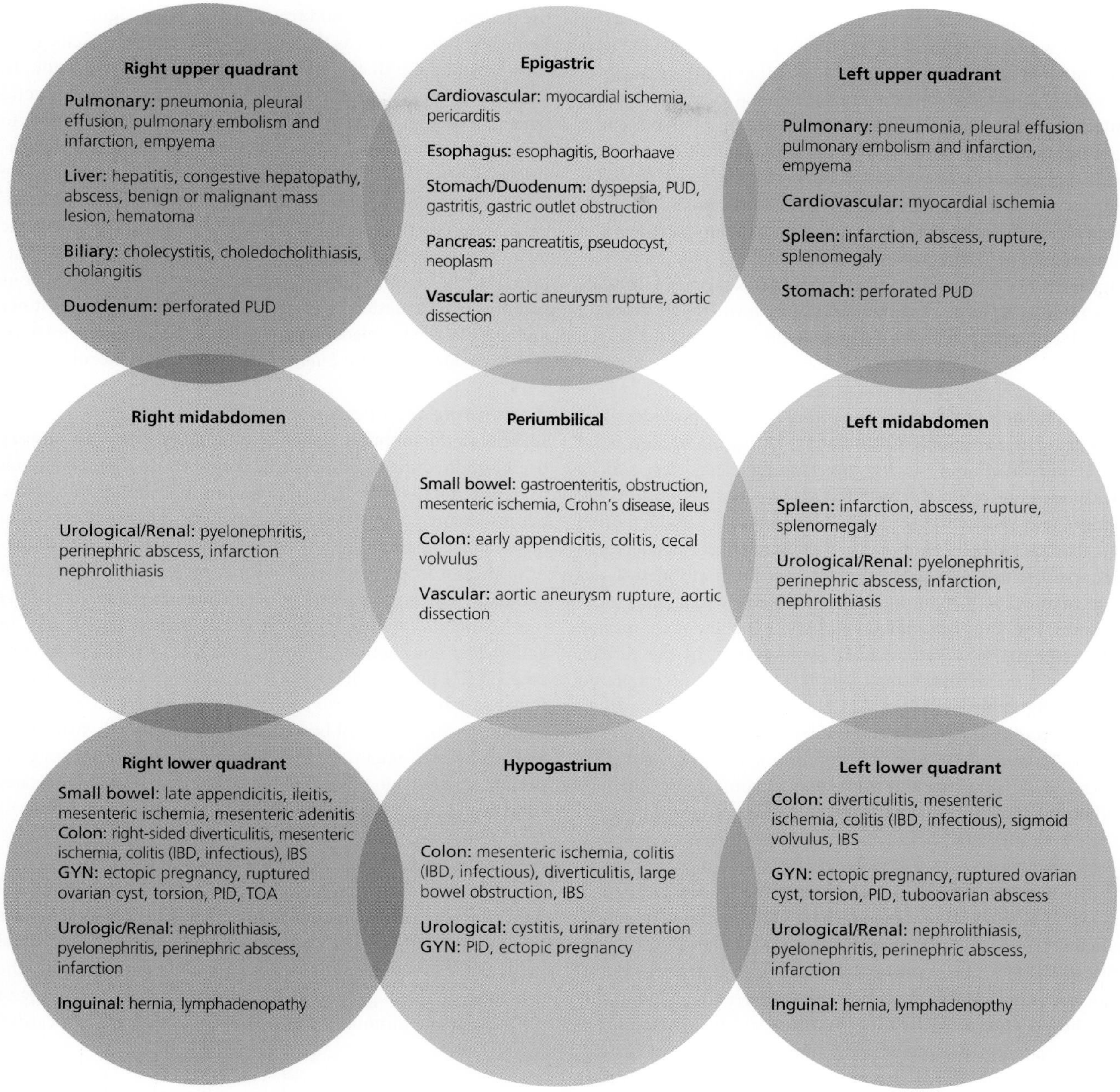

Figure 37.5 Differential diagnosis of acute abdominal pain by region of pain presentation. GYN, gynecological; IBD, inflammatory bowel disease; IBS, irritable bowel syndrome; PID, pelvic inflammatory disease; PUD, peptic ulcer disease; TOA, tuboovarian abscesses.

caused by hepatobiliary diseases, and midlower pain caused by gynecological diseases [13]. It is important to note that the location of abdominal pain within different anatomic regions, as shown in Figure 37.5, serves only as a rough guide to the etiology. Location alone should not be the sole consideration when creating a differential diagnosis. "Typical" patterns of abdominal pain have been shown to yield a correct diagnosis in only 60%–70% of patients, resulting in a 30%–40% misdiagnosis rate [14]. For example, appendicitis may be missed in patients with right upper quadrant pain if the clinician fails to consider the possibility of retrocecal appendicitis. In addition, dividing the abdomen into anatomic regions may miss conditions that can present with back pain, including pathology within retroperitoneal structures, such as the kidneys and aorta [15].

When evaluating pain location, it is important to consider patterns of radiation and referral. Pain location also can change over time as a result of progression of the underlying disease process. As such, it is important to distinguish the site of pain at onset from the site at presentation. For example, the onset of pain in acute appendicitis typically is periumbilical but later migrates to the right lower quadrant as inflammation extends to the adjacent parietal peritoneum. Additional examples include migration of pain in ongoing aortic dissection or passage of a ureteral stone [1]. In cases that progress to generalized peritonitis, the development of severe, diffuse pain can mask the location of the precipitating event [11]. The previously discussed interplay between visceral and somatoparietal innervations also can result in predictable patterns of referred pain (see Figure 37.4). One characteristic example is Kehr's sign, initially described in reference to splenic rupture, in which left shoulder pain develops after left-sided diaphragmatic irritation [16].

Onset

The timing of pain onset and symptom duration provides valuable clues to the underlying etiology. The timing of pain onset can be divided into several overlapping categories: *sudden* (within seconds to minutes), *rapidly progressive* (within 1–2 hours), and *gradual* (over several hours) [11,17]. Sudden onset of excruciating pain should alert the clinician to consider catastrophic events, such as esophageal rupture, perforated viscus (e.g., peptic ulcer), ruptured abdominal aortic aneurysm (AAA) or aortic dissection, ruptured ectopic pregnancy, acute mesenteric ischemia, or acute myocardial infarction. In these cases, systemic signs of shock may supplant abdominal complaints and highlight the need for rapid triage and urgent interventions. Several conditions begin with mild pain that rapidly progresses over 1–2 hours, becoming more intense and localized because of progression from visceral to parietal pain. Causes include inflammatory disorders (e.g., pancreatitis, cholecystitis, appendicitis), strangulated blood supply resulting in viscus ischemia (e.g., strangulated hernia, volvulus, torsion), or acute viscus obstruction (e.g., small bowel obstruction, renal or ureteral colic). Less severe pain that develops gradually over several hours more often is a result of medical rather than surgical conditions. This broad category includes upper gastrointestinal processes (e.g., dyspepsia), intestinal disorders (e.g., inflammatory bowel disease, gastroenteritis, diverticulitis), liver diseases (e.g., hepatitis), or gynecological and urinary disorders (e.g., cystitis, pyelonephritis, pelvic inflammatory disease [PID]). However, it is important to remember that some surgical disorders, such as acute cholecystitis or intraabdominal abscesses, also may progress over many hours.

Quality

When assessing pain quality, one must distinguish between the dull, poorly localized sensation associated with visceral innervation and the sharp, more localized somatoparietal pain caused by irritation of the parietal peritoneum or other somatically innervated organs. Patients with visceral pain may appear restless or try to have a bowel movement in an attempt to alleviate pain. This is in sharp contrast with patients with peritonitis, who tend to remain still to avoid activities that move or stretch the parietal peritoneum and trigger severe pain. Significant peritoneal irritation, such as that seen with a ruptured viscus, typically yields pain that is sharp, superficial, and constant. In contrast, acute bowel obstruction often begins with visceral pain that is vague and intermittent with later progression to parietal pain that is sharp, relentless, and more discrete in location. Obstruction of smaller hollow viscera (e.g., ureters, bile ducts) results in pain that is often perceived as rapid onset of paroxysms of agonizing pain followed by periods of relief. The term *colic* is appropriately used when describing this pain pattern, which reflects intermittent smooth muscle contractions (i.e., bowel obstruction or ureteral stones). Unlike the intestines and ureters, the gallbladder and bile ducts do not undergo peristalsis, making the term *biliary colic* technically inaccurate [11].

Aggravating and alleviating factors

Identifying factors that influence abdominal pain can be very useful in directing the differential diagnosis. It often is difficult to determine the role of meal ingestion in symptom causation, because many patients will have eaten within hours of symptom onset. Meals may precipitate acute pain in patients with cholelithiasis and in patients with chronic mesenteric ischemia. In cholelithiasis, acute pain may occur after ingestion of a fatty meal, which stimulates cholecystokinin release and results in gallbladder contraction. Dyspepsia caused by peptic ulcer disease (PUD) may be either exacerbated or alleviated by eating. Relief of pain with emesis and increased pain with eating are highly specific for small bowel obstruction [18,19]. Worsening of pain by movement, such as walking or coughing, suggests peritoneal irritation. Pleuritic upper abdominal pain implicates cardiopulmonary processes.

Associated symptoms

The presence of symptoms associated with acute abdominal pain can assist in narrowing the differential diagnosis. This is particularly true in patients with difficult-to-describe visceral pain, as well as extraabdominal complaints. For example, the presence of chest pain, cough, and/or dyspnea may suggest pneumonia, pulmonary embolism [20], or myocardial infarction.

Emesis

Nausea and vomiting are common nonspecific complaints; however, the timing, progression, and quality of emesis may provide useful clues to the diagnosis. Emesis that occurs after the onset of abdominal pain more likely stems from a surgical condition [21]. Vomiting associated with benign conditions, such as viral gastroenteritis or food-borne illness, usually is self-limited. In contrast, emesis is recurrent and progressive in mechanical small bowel obstruction, although frequently absent with large bowel obstruction. The character of emesis can be diagnostically useful. In small bowel obstruction, emesis may transition from gastric contents to bilious to feculent as a result of bacterial proliferation proximal to the site of obstruction as the disease progresses. Bilious emesis suggests an obstruction distal to the duodenum. Recurrent nonbilious emesis may signify gastric outlet obstruction. Mild-to-moderate epigastric pain or discomfort (dyspepsia) with coffee-ground emesis or hematemesis implicates upper gastrointestinal etiologies, including PUD or erosive gastritis (e.g., alcohol induced). In patients with prior AAA repair presenting with hematemesis, aortoenteric fistula should be considered [22,23].

Anorexia

This nonspecific symptom is present in a variety of medical and surgical abdominal syndromes but may be absent early in the course of the acute abdomen. For example, anorexia is seen at presentation in only 68% of patients with acute appendicitis [24].

Bowel symptoms

Although bowel symptoms are common and nonspecific in patients with abdominal pain, a complete absence of anorexia, vomiting, and constipation or obstipation weighs strongly against the diagnosis of an acute surgical condition involving the luminal gastrointestinal tract. Cessation of bowel movements and flatus, called *obstipation*, is common with acute, surgical gastrointestinal conditions. Obstipation is usually associated with functional ileus or mechanical obstruction of the small or large intestine. In contrast, diarrhea often is associated with benign, nonacute abdominal pathology, although its presence does not exclude surgical conditions. Copious watery diarrhea associated with acute abdominal pain suggests acute gastroenteritis or noninvasive infectious colitis. In early small bowel obstruction, diarrhea may occur as the hyperactive bowel distal to the obstruction reflexively empties [1]. Both acute appendicitis [25] and mesenteric ischemia [26,27] also may present initially with diarrhea. Abdominal pain with bloody diarrhea implicates inflammatory bowel disease, invasive infectious colitis, or colonic ischemia. However, in ischemic colitis caused by superior mesenteric artery occlusion, bloody diarrhea notably may be absent [11].

Medical and surgical history

A careful history of past and ongoing conditions can provide useful information regarding a patient's risk for disorders causing acute abdominal pain. Prior episodes of similar pain may suggest recurrent disorders, such as diverticulitis, cholelithiasis with biliary obstruction, pancreatitis, or sigmoid volvulus. In the presence of atrial fibrillation or heart failure, clinicians should consider mesenteric ischemia from an embolic source or low-output state, respectively. A preexisting history of cardiovascular and/or peripheral vascular disease increases the risk for mesenteric ischemia, acute myocardial infarction, and AAA. Previous history of intraabdominal or bowel surgery increases the risk for adhesions and resultant bowel obstruction. In women, it is crucial to obtain menstrual, genitourinary, and sexual histories to evaluate for possible gynecological etiologies of acute abdominal pain (e.g., ectopic pregnancy, PID).

Medications

Numerous medications are associated with adverse gastrointestinal events and conditions that can result in acute abdominal pain. Hence a careful review of all prescribed and nonprescribed medications, including herbal formulations, is warranted. Nonsteroidal antiinflammatory use predisposes to PUD [28] and intestinal ulcers. Corticosteroid use can mask the signs of intraabdominal disease, including peritonitis, and is associated with an increased risk for perforated diverticular disease [29]. Opiate analgesics can also increase the risk for colonic diverticular perforation [29] and may lead to narcotic bowel syndrome that results in acute or recurrent abdominal pain. Anticoagulants, including warfarin, may cause acute retroperitoneal [30] and intramural small bowel hematomas [31], resulting in abdominal pain or bowel obstruction. Patients with recent antibiotic use or healthcare exposure are at risk for *Clostridium difficile* colitis [32]. Numerous medications may cause acute pancreatitis or hepatitis.

Social history

Several features of the social history can be particularly useful. Excess alcohol use is associated with gastritis, pancreatitis, and hepatitis. Opiate withdrawal can present with significant abdominal cramping, nausea, and diarrhea. Mesenteric ischemia may be a complication of cocaine or methamphetamine use [33,34]. Obtaining a travel history or similar symptoms in friends or family may be useful evidence to suggest an infectious, nonsurgical process. It is also important to elicit information regarding atypical foods that may have been consumed. For example, the ingestion of raw or improperly cooked seafood can result in *Anisakis simplex* infection, which can cause sudden onset of severe abdominal pain mimicking an acute abdomen [35].

Physical examination

A systematic approach to the physical examination is required to appropriately triage patients with acute abdominal pain. Major goals of the examination are to assess for life-threatening illness, identify peritonitis, and detect localized areas of tenderness. The first step is direct observation of the patient, paying close attention to general appearance, preferred resting position, and the presence or absence of spontaneous movements. The patient who is anxious, pale, diaphoretic, and has rapid, shallow breathing should raise concerns for a serious intraabdominal process. The patient with peritonitis is more likely to remain still to avoid painful stretching of the peritoneum. In contrast, the patient with visceral pain may move restlessly about (e.g., early appendicitis) or writhe in agony (e.g., renal colic). Gentle shaking of the bed may elicit significant sharp pain in the patient with somatoparietal pain, but not visceral pain.

General examination

Abnormal vital signs should prompt the clinician to consider serious underlying pathology. Identification of hemodynamic instability should elicit immediate volume resuscitation and investigation for etiologies that may require urgent surgical consultation, such as perforated viscus or ruptured AAA. However, normal vital signs do not rule out significant diagnoses, particularly in the elderly or immunocompromised (see later *Special populations* section). For example, the sensitivity of fever for acute appendicitis is only 67% [24]. Hypotension can indicate significant dehydration, sepsis, or hemorrhage. Tachycardia may suggest pain, hemorrhage, hypovolemia, or sepsis but may be absent in patients taking β-blockers [19]. Tachypnea is a nonspecific finding that may be a clue to the presence of metabolic acidosis, as seen in diabetic ketoacidosis or mesenteric ischemia, or pulmonary disease [1]. A complete physical examination is required in all patients because numerous extraabdominal etiologies can present with acute abdominal pain.

Abdominal examination

One of the primary objectives of the abdominal examination is to determine the presence or absence of localized or generalized peritonitis. Signs of peritoneal inflammation (known colloquially as "peritoneal signs") include pain with movement, cough, percussion, and light touch, and the presence of involuntary guarding. The cough test can be used before physical examination as an indirect test for peritoneal irritation. This test is considered positive if sharp, localized pain is elicited by the act of coughing. This test has demonstrated sensitivities greater than 78% and specificities ranging from 79% to 95% in the diagnosis of peritonitis [36,37].

Inspection

Abdominal inspection allows for visualization of previous surgical scars, abdominal distension, liver disease (e.g., caput medusa), skin rashes (e.g., herpes zoster), and hemorrhage. Although rarely seen, Cullen sign describes periumbilical ecchymosis and Grey–Turner sign describes ecchymotic discoloration of the flanks, which are associated with conditions resulting in retroperitoneal hemorrhage, including acute hemorrhagic pancreatitis or ruptured AAA [38].

Auscultation

Auscultation should be performed before percussion or palpation on the undisturbed abdomen. Auscultatory findings have limited diagnostic utility (and may even be misleading) [39] in most patients with acute abdominal pain and are mainly helpful in two settings. The complete absence of bowel sounds suggests either peritonitis or adynamic ileus. Conversely, rushes of abnormally active, high-pitched bowel sounds that occur in synchrony with abdominal pain suggest a small bowel obstruction.

Percussion

Percussion of the abdomen provides several key pieces of information in the patient with acute abdominal pain. First, it is extremely valuable in the detection of localized or diffuse peritonitis. For this purpose, the elicitation of sharp pain with gentle percussion is preferred to both deep palpation and testing for rebound tenderness, which are unnecessarily painful [40]. Second, percussion provides accurate localization of pain before light (or deep) palpation. Third, percussion is useful in the presence of abdominal distension to help distinguish between distended bowel (tympanic) and ascites (dullness). Finally, percussion is helpful in determining the presence of liver, spleen, or bladder enlargement.

Palpation

Careful, slow, methodical gentle pressure with one or two fingers is the key to successful examination. In the patient with significant abdominal pathology, deep palpation may be incredibly painful, may induce patient apprehension that can limit the ability of subsequent examiners to obtain an accurate examination, and may be misleading to the physician. To gather useful information from palpation, several techniques can be used. Position the patient with both knees and hips flexed to allow for relaxation of abdominal musculature. Gentle, light palpation should begin in the area farthest from the point of maximum tenderness (as reported by the patient or determined by percussion) and gradually move toward the site of pain. In the patient who reports significant tenderness with palpation but who otherwise has a clinical presentation suggestive of a benign process, it is beneficial to use the stethoscope to replicate the pressure of palpation while seeming to auscultate bowel sounds. Notable discrepancies between tenderness elicited by manual palpation and the stethoscope can occur in patients who are anxious, seeking secondary gain, or have a functional disorder.

The presence of localized or diffuse pain with gentle percussion and/or light palpation is strongly suggestive of peritonitis. The traditional method of testing for peritoneal irritation by assessing rebound tenderness should be abandoned. This technique involves applying deep pressure to the abdominal wall over an area of tenderness before suddenly removing the palpating hand. The patient is then questioned to see whether the pain was greater with downward pressure or with its release. This test has limited accuracy in discriminating tenderness caused by peritonitis from other etiologies and causes unnecessary pain for the patient [41]. The term *guarding* describes an involuntary, reflexive increase in abdominal wall muscle tone, which often is present in the setting of peritoneal irritation and serves to "guard" the parietal peritoneum from pain caused by palpation, respiration, or movement. Even in the presence of severe peritoneal inflammation, guarding may be absent in certain cases (e.g., in the elderly because of laxity of abdominal wall musculature) [1,40]. To evaluate for guarding, the clinician assesses abdominal muscle tone during several respiratory cycles while gently resting the hand on the abdominal wall. When guarding is involuntary, there is continued abdominal muscle tension throughout the respiratory cycle. Voluntary guarding may be seen in normal patients who are anxious about the abdominal examination and is distractible. When guarding is voluntary, there is a notable decrease in abdominal muscle tone during inspiration or when the patient is distracted. "Rigidity" is considered a severe form of involuntary guarding.

On completion of light palpation, deeper palpation can be performed, if tolerated, to evaluate for more subtle tenderness, organomegaly, or abnormal masses. Although palpation of a tender, pulsatile epigastric mass suggests an AAA, the sensitivity of palpation is affected by the size of the aneurysm and the girth of the patient [42]. The inguinal and femoral canals, the umbilicus, and all surgical scars should be routinely evaluated for possible incarcerated hernias.

Additional maneuvers

Depending on the clinical presentation and suspected diagnosis, it can be useful to perform additional maneuvers, because a positive finding may suggest a specific diagnosis. For example, the psoas, obturator and Rovsing signs, which are associated with acute appendicitis, have demonstrated low sensitivity but high specificity, indicating utility if present; however, their absence does not exclude a diagnosis of appendicitis [19].

1. Murphy sign: Eliciting the Murphy sign is most useful when acute cholecystitis is suspected. For this test, the examiner deeply palpates the right upper quadrant (near the gallbladder) while the patient takes a deep inspiration. The sign is positive if the patient experiences pain and inspiration is arrested, presumably due to palpation of an inflamed gallbladder. Although this sign has a sensitivity of only 65% and specificity of 87% [43], it is considered one of the most reliable clinical indicators of acute cholecystitis.
2. Psoas sign: With the patient in the supine position, the patient is asked to lift the thigh against resistance imparted by the examiner's hand, which is placed just above the knee. Increased pain with this maneuver is a positive sign that suggests irritation of the ipsilateral psoas muscle by a contiguous inflammatory process. When elicited on the right side, the psoas sign is suggestive of acute appendicitis, although it may also be elicited in other retroperitoneal inflammatory processes, including psoas abscess or pyelonephritis [1,24].
3. Obturator sign: This sign is elicited by placing the patient in the supine position with the hip and knee both flexed to 90 degrees on the side being tested and performing passive internal and external hip rotation to stretch the obturator muscle. This sign is positive if pain is reproduced. A positive obturator sign on the right side suggests acute appendicitis or pelvic inflammatory processes, such as PID [1].
4. Rovsing sign: This maneuver is an indirect assessment for rebound in suspected acute appendicitis. The presence of pain in the right lower quadrant when the examiner applies or releases pressure in the left lower quadrant is considered a positive sign [24].

Genitourinary, rectal, and pelvic examination

Evaluating for costovertebral angle tenderness is useful when pyelonephritis is suspected. In men, it is important to inspect for testicular pathology, including torsion or infection, because pain radiation may cause abdominal discomfort. The female patient with acute lower abdominal pain must undergo a pelvic examination to investigate for gynecological etiologies, such as ectopic pregnancy, adnexal mass, or PID. The digital rectal examination is of limited value in most patients but nonetheless recommended to evaluate for obvious or occult gastrointestinal bleeding and to locate perirectal tenderness or fluctuance when a perirectal abscess is suspected. Additional useful findings may include fecal impaction or a rectal mass.

Special populations

Certain patient populations with acute abdominal pain require increased diligence during evaluation because they may present atypically or have limitations in their ability to describe symptoms. Such populations include the elderly, immunocompromised individuals, pregnant women, patients with psychiatric disease, and those with spinal cord injuries.

Advanced age

The evaluation of older adults (defined as 65 years and older) with acute abdominal pain can be challenging and replete with diagnostic obstacles that may confuse and delay the diagnosis. As a result, morbidity and mortality are increased [44,45]. Geriatric patients who present to the ED for abdominal pain have higher rates of admission and longer lengths of stay [46]. Factors that complicate the diagnosis include preexisting comorbidities, difficulty in obtaining an accurate history in some, use of medications that may disguise or confound the underlying disease process, and misleading physical examination findings [45,47,48]. Pain perception is less sensitive in this population [46,49]. Elderly patients are more likely to present for evaluation after experiencing abdominal pain for a prolonged duration [50], resulting in more advanced disease. Some elderly patients may not report abdominal symptoms and, instead, present with "altered mental status," "failure to thrive," or sepsis. Physical examination and laboratory findings may further confuse the clinical picture. Examination findings suggestive of peritoneal irritation, such as localized guarding or percussion tenderness, may be diminished [50]. Because aging is associated with a decreased response to pyrogens, older adults with acute surgical abdomens may present with minimal or no fever or leukocytosis [51].

Immunocompromised host

Immunocompromised patients encompass a heterogeneous group, including those who are mildly immune deficient (e.g., diabetic, elderly, uremic) and those who are severely immunocompromised (e.g., acquired immunodeficiency syndrome, posttransplant, current immunosuppressive therapy, malignancy undergoing chemotherapy) [52–54]. These patients are at risk for the same processes that affect immunocompetent patients but also are susceptible to complications of their underlying primary disease and immunosuppression. In the severely immunocompromised, the acute abdomen differential diagnosis must be expanded to include opportunistic infections (e.g., cytomegalovirus colitis, neutropenic enterocolitis), treatment-related conditions (e.g., intestinal graft-versus-host disease, corticosteroid-associated pancreatitis, or peptic ulceration), opportunistic neoplasms (e.g., posttransplant lymphoproliferative disease), or complications of primary pathology (e.g., bowel perforation or obstruction) [52,53]. Due to their blunted immune response, this population requires special attention because characteristic clinical findings of acute abdominal processes may be attenuated or absent. Vague signs and symptoms of altered mental status or tachycardia may replace the classic finding of abdominal pain. Fever is often absent, and signs of peritoneal inflammation may not be apparent on examination. As a result of diminished symptomatology, these patients often seek care late in the course of their disease [52]. Septic shock may be the initial manifestation of intraabdominal infection. It is critical to maintain a broad differential diagnosis when evaluating this patient population, and cross-sectional abdominal imaging is often required [55].

Pregnancy

Acute abdominal pain in pregnancy presents diagnostic challenges because of anatomic and physiological changes that result in atypical presentations of common pathology. Beginning around 12 weeks of gestation, the enlarged gravid uterus becomes an abdominal organ, compresses underlying abdominal viscera, and complicates the localization of pain. Enlargement of the gravid uterus and laxity of the anterior abdominal wall may mask or delay signs of peritoneal inflammation [56]. In addition to altered physical examination findings, laboratory studies may be challenging to interpret because of physiological elevations in white blood cell (WBC) count, amylase, and alkaline phosphatase. Given these diagnostic obstacles, prompt imaging can be helpful in distinguishing medical versus surgical disease. The preferred imaging modalities are ultrasound and magnetic resonance (MR), which do not use ionizing radiation. Computed tomography (CT), standard abdominal radiographs, and fluoroscopy should be avoided whenever possible to minimize potentially harmful radiation exposure to the fetus. Ultrasound should be used first; however, in cases of inconclusive ultrasound, MR is preferred and has been shown to perform equally well when compared with CT in the diagnosis of acute nontraumatic abdominal pain during pregnancy [57]. Utilization of gadolinium-based contrast with MR during pregnancy is controversial. According to the American College of Obstetricians and Gynecologists, use of gadolinium-based contrast with MR should be limited, with use only if it significantly improves diagnostic performance and is expected to improve maternal or fetal outcomes [58].

Appendicitis is the most common reason for nonobstetrical surgery, affecting 1 in 1500 pregnancies [56,59]. The incidence is similar in pregnant versus nonpregnant women, but the risk for perforation is increased during pregnancy. Appendiceal perforation is associated with increased fetal morbidity and mortality [60,61]. Right lower quadrant pain is the most common presenting symptom regardless of gestational age. However, patients may present with nausea and vomiting alone – common and nonspecific symptoms during pregnancy that may delay timely diagnosis. Although ultrasound generally is the first-line imaging study, MR is preferred by some clinicians and is the test of choice after nondiagnostic ultrasound [60].

Development of acute abdominal pain in the hospitalized patient

The differential diagnosis of acute abdominal pain that develops in the hospitalized patient usually is limited and differs from that of a patient who presents in the outpatient setting (Box 37.3). The evaluation of hospitalized patients may be challenging because of the inability to provide an adequate history or cooperate with the abdominal examination as a result of altered mental status, sedation, or the need for mechanical ventilation. Clinicians must be vigilant for intraabdominal conditions that were overlooked or misdiagnosed at admission, especially in the elderly, patients with psychiatric illness, patients with altered mental status, or patients taking corticosteroids or narcotics, who may neglect to report abdominal complaints. Admitting diagnoses such as "failure to thrive," "altered mental status," or "fever of unknown origin" may be attributable to undiagnosed cholecystitis, cholangitis, diverticulitis, appendicitis, perforated viscus, or intraabdominal abscesses. It is also important to consider medical and surgical etiologies that are more specific to (and common in) hospitalized patients. In the hospitalized patient who has undergone surgery or a minimally invasive procedure (e.g., endoscopy, cardiac catheterization, angiography), a procedure-related complication should be considered, including

Box 37.3 Acute abdominal pain etiologies in the hospitalized patient.

Conditions arising as a consequence of hospitalization
- *Clostridium difficile*-associated colitis
- Postprocedural complications (e.g., bleeding, hollow viscus perforation, infection)
- Medication or drug-associated abdominal pain (e.g., opiate withdrawal)
- Constipation
- Typhlitis
- Coronary ischemia
- Pneumonia

Conditions resulting from critical illness and physiological stress
- Acalculous cholecystitis
- Nonocclusive mesenteric ischemia (e.g., secondary to hypovolemic or cardiogenic shock)
- Ischemic colitis
- Stress-associated peptic ulcers
- Pancreatitis (e.g., medication induced)
- Ileus
- Acute colonic pseudoobstruction (Ogilvie syndrome)
- Acute adrenal insufficiency

infection, perforation, or bleeding (intraperitoneal, retroperitoneal, or within the bowel wall).

Certain forms of inflammatory colitis may occur as a consequence of hospitalization. Patients who experience abdominal pain and diarrhea or ileus, particularly in the setting of antibiotic use, should be evaluated for *Clostridium difficile* colitis. In patients with severe neutropenia (<500 neutrophils/mL), neutropenic enterocolitis (also known as typhlitis) should be considered. This entity occurs in the setting of chemotherapy-induced neutropenia, acute leukemia, aplastic anemia, bone marrow transplantation, and organ transplant-associated immunosuppression, resulting in necrotizing inflammation of the cecum and a mortality rate of 50% [52,62].

As a consequence of severe physiological stress and need for pressor support that leads to reduced splanchnic blood flow, critically ill medical and surgical patients are at increased risk for acalculous cholecystitis [63,64], stress-related gastrointestinal mucosal disease, and nonocclusive mesenteric ischemia. Adynamic ileus or acute colonic pseudoobstruction should be considered in patients with diffuse abdominal pain and distension who are critically ill, in the postoperative state, or using opiate analgesics [65].

Diagnostic evaluation

History and physical examination rarely provide a conclusive diagnosis for acute abdominal pain alone, hence laboratory testing and imaging studies are usually required. In the evaluation of patients who may present atypically (see earlier *Special populations* section), the clinician should have a low threshold to obtain more definitive testing. When determining the appropriate tests to order, it is important to consider the most likely diagnoses and focus the workup on ruling in or ruling out specific conditions. Although the accuracy of newer imaging modalities has improved, it must be recognized that none is perfectly sensitive or specific, especially early in the disease course. When the initial diagnosis is uncertain, serial examination over 8–12 hours is warranted. A period of observation and serial examination provides the opportunity to assess the evolution of signs and symptoms that may lead to a specific diagnosis. This strategy can also lead to decreased rates of inappropriate interventions [66]. Patients who are discharged should be given strict instructions to return if pain persists, recurs, or worsens, or new symptoms of fever or vomiting develop.

As previously discussed, dividing the abdomen into anatomic regions (see Figure 37.5) can assist in creating the differential diagnosis and, in turn, can also be useful in establishing a logical workup. Figure 37.6 provides a diagnostic algorithm for the evaluation of acute abdominal pain.

Overview of laboratory testing

Laboratory tests can be useful in narrowing the differential diagnosis and confirming a suspected diagnosis; however, they can also confound the clinical picture because of incidental findings. As such, it is important to obtain laboratory studies with a specific question in mind and understand how the laboratory result, positive or negative, will impact management. For

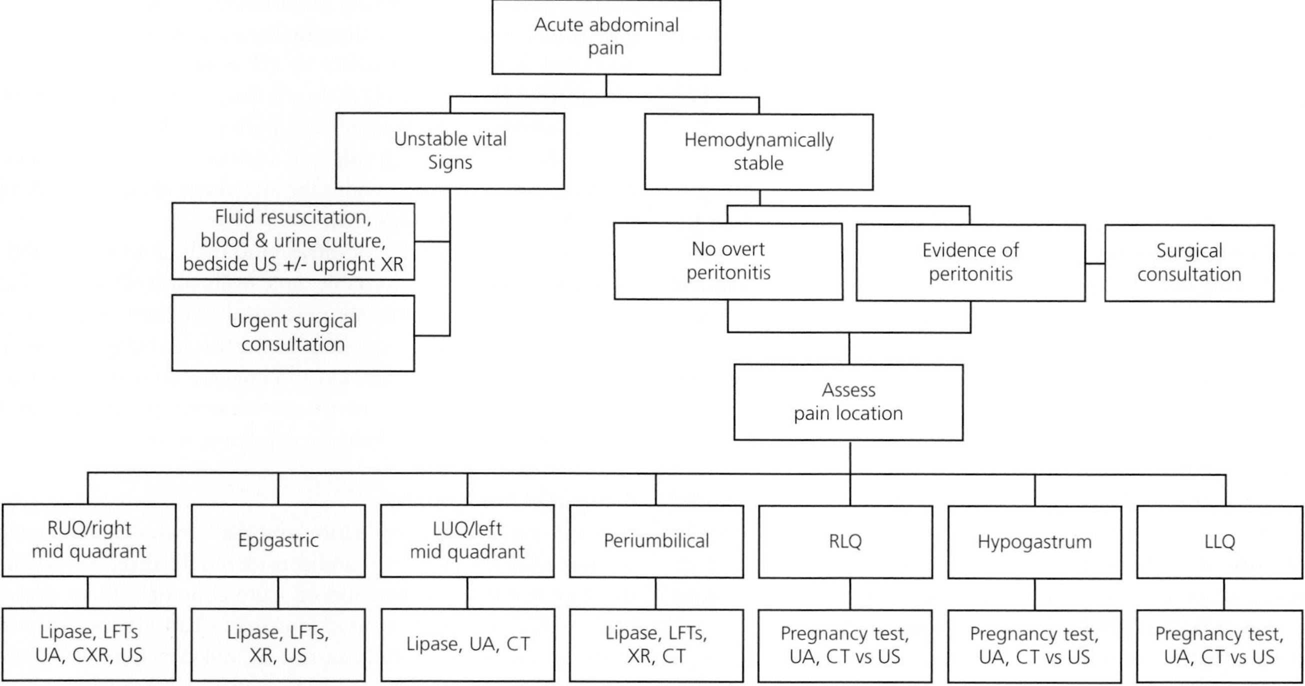

Figure 37.6 Diagnostic algorithm for acute abdominal pain. CT, computed tomography; CXR, chest x-ray; LFT, liver enzyme; LLQ, left lower quadrant; LUQ, left upper quadrant; RLQ, right lower quadrant; RUQ, right upper quadrant; UA, urinalysis; US, ultrasound; XR, x-ray.

the vast majority of patients with acute abdominal pain, a basic initial workup includes a complete blood count, serum electrolytes, blood urea nitrogen, creatinine, and glucose. Although these tests do not provide a specific diagnosis, they provide important insights to the patient's current health status and underlying physiology and can be useful in risk stratification. Patients with elevated lactate or metabolic acidosis, both associated with tissue hypoperfusion, are more likely to require a higher level of inpatient care or surgical intervention. C-reactive protein (CRP) and WBC count are inflammatory markers often tested in acute abdominal pain; however, elevated levels are nonspecific and have low diagnostic accuracy for a specific diagnosis. In addition, in a study evaluating the use of CRP and WBC count to discriminate between urgent and nonurgent conditions in patients with acute abdominal pain in the ED, these markers were deemed insufficient for use as a triage test in the selection for diagnostic imaging [67]. Procalcitonin, a precursor of calcitonin and marker of infection, has demonstrated high sensitivity (72–100%) and high negative predictive value (81–100%) for the diagnosis of intestinal ischemia [68]. Procalcitonin, however, can also be elevated in the setting of bacterial infection, sepsis, and other causes of systemic inflammation.

Laboratory studies that are more specific for direct organ damage are selectively ordered depending on diagnostic suspicion, including lipase, amylase, liver enzymes, and urinalysis. All women of childbearing age require pregnancy testing. Because geriatric and immunocompromised patients may have atypical presentations of common diagnoses, they often require broader laboratory testing. For example, it is useful to obtain liver chemistries in a geriatric patient with nonspecific abdominal pain to assess for an atypical presentation of biliary pathology. In addition, leukocytosis may be absent in geriatric or immunocompromised patients despite the presence of infection or intraabdominal surgical pathology.

Overview of diagnostic imaging

When ordering imaging, it is critical to remember that, in the setting of high pretest probability, a negative test does not absolutely rule out a diagnosis. In patients with acute abdominal pain (especially those presenting early), it may be necessary to repeat studies or order additional imaging after obtaining "negative" results if clinical suspicion is high or symptoms and signs persist or worsen.

Chest and abdominal radiography

Conventional radiography is often the initial imaging modality used for patients with acute abdominal pain who present to the ED. Although the major advantage is wide availability, its diagnostic accuracy is limited, and the majority of patients require further imaging [69], leading to increased cost, exposure to ionizing radiation, and diagnostic delay. Plain radiographs alone rarely (<5%) result in a change in patient management [70]. Furthermore, compared with conventional radiography, CT demonstrates significantly improved diagnostic accuracy [71]. For these reasons, the use of plain radiographs should be limited to specific clinical settings. The strongest indications are identification and localization of an ingested foreign body or confirmation of proper catheter placement. Additional indications may include suspected bowel obstruction or perforated viscus, particularly if CT availability is limited or delayed. When these diagnoses are suspected, plain radiographs should include an upright film to evaluate for dilated loops of small or large bowel in the case of intestinal obstruction and free (usually subdiaphragmatic) intraperitoneal air as a result of hollow viscus perforation. It is important to note that plain radiographs have relatively low sensitivity (71–77%) in detecting small bowel obstruction [19], and a nondiagnostic result can be misleading. In studies evaluating plain abdominal radiography for acute abdominal pain, the sensitivity ranged from 30% to 46% with specificity of 75% to 88% [72]. Given suboptimal test characteristics, patients often require further imaging with CT.

Ultrasound

Ultrasound is widely used to visualize the liver, gallbladder and biliary tree, aorta, urological tract, and gynecological viscera, and it is very useful in evaluating the pregnant patient with acute abdominal pain. However, it is of little value in diagnosing acute conditions involving the luminal gastrointestinal tract. In the diagnosis of acute appendicitis, ultrasound demonstrates lower sensitivity and specificity compared with CT or MRI and produces more nondiagnostic scans [73]. In the diagnosis of acute cholecystitis, abdominal ultrasound is the preferred initial imaging modality due to lower cost, better availability, lack of invasiveness, lack of ionizing radiation, and high accuracy for gallbladder stones [74–76]. Recent literature, however, has demonstrated improved sensitivity of CT over ultrasound in the diagnosis of cholecystitis [77]. In a retrospective review of adult ED encounters for right upper quadrant pain, CT was noninferior to ultrasound in both ruling in and ruling out the diagnosis of cholecystitis, and it provides the advantage of demonstrating nongallbladder pathology [78].

Overall, major benefits of ultrasound include wide availability and portability, which enable rapid evaluation of the unstable patient (e.g., to assess for intraperitoneal free fluid or an AAA) and lack of radiation exposure. Major disadvantages include operator-dependent acquisition and interpretation of images, as well as patient factors that may limit ultrasonic penetration and image quality (e.g., body habitus, overlying bowel gas).

Computed tomography

Given its rapid image acquisition and high degree of diagnostic accuracy, CT is widely used and considered the imaging modality of choice in the evaluation of acute abdomen. Main drawbacks to CT include the risks of ionizing radiation exposure and intravenous (i.v.) iodinated contrast, as well as its high cost compared with standard radiographs and ultrasound imaging.

The technique used with abdominal CT imaging generally involves scanning the entire abdomen with or without i.v.

contrast and with or without oral/rectal contrast. The use of i.v. contrast increases diagnostic accuracy for specific diagnoses but carries the risk for contrast-induced acute kidney injury. Although oral or rectal contrast may be useful in certain clinical scenarios (e.g., differentiating fluid-filled bowel loops from an intraabdominal abscess), the use of oral contrast is time consuming [79] and does not add considerably to the diagnostic accuracy in patients with nontraumatic acute abdominal pain [69,80].

Appropriate imaging plays an integral role in evaluating acute abdominal pain, narrowing the differential diagnosis, and guiding management. A prospective, multicenter ED study of patients with abdominal pain demonstrated that after CT imaging, physicians changed their leading diagnosis in 51% of cases, had increased diagnostic confidence (median increase of 25%), and changed the decision to admit in 25% of cases [81]. In another prospective study of patients presenting to the ED with nontraumatic abdominal complaints, the management plan was changed by CT in 42% [82].

Although CT imaging can increase physician diagnostic certainty in the evaluation of nontraumatic acute abdominal pain [83], the clinical utility, safety, and cost-effectiveness varies among patient populations. In the unstable patient or patient with overt peritonitis who may require immediate intervention, the risk of delayed treatment because of CT imaging may outweigh the diagnostic benefit. However, CT is highly accurate in localizing the site of a visceral perforation, which could impact surgical management [84]. CT imaging may not be warranted in the patient with a high index of suspicion for nonsurgical, medical illness. For most other patients who do not fit into these categories, CT can provide crucial information that directly affects management [85]. Clinicians should have a low threshold to obtain CT imaging in patients in whom the history, physical examination, and laboratory studies may be particularly unreliable (e.g., elderly patients, immunocompromised patients, or patients with altered mental status) [86].

Magnetic resonance

MR imaging is not widely used in the diagnostic evaluation of patients with acute abdominal pain; however, it has been shown to provide useful information for rapid diagnosis of acute bowel pathology and some gynecological emergencies [87]. The major advantages include lack of exposure to ionizing radiation and high intrinsic contrast resolution, which reduces the need for i.v. contrast [69]. Drawbacks to MR include specific contraindications (e.g., metal implants), reduced image quality in patients who are unable to lie still (e.g., due to restlessness), more limited availability, longer examination times, and increased cost compared with other imaging modalities. Because clinically valuable information can be obtained without contrast, MR is a useful imaging modality in the evaluation of pregnant women, particularly when ultrasound yields nondiagnostic findings.

Diagnostic evaluation by abdominal region

Generalized or diffuse

Important processes to consider in the evaluation of diffuse acute abdominal pain include generalized peritonitis, acute mesenteric ischemia, bowel obstruction, ruptured AAA, and medical conditions (narcotic withdrawal, sickle cell crisis, diabetic ketoacidosis, adrenal insufficiency, and infectious gastroenteritis) [88].

A host of disorders may progress to generalized peritonitis either quickly (e.g., ruptured viscus) or slowly, with the latter usually occurring when the underlying condition is not addressed in a timely manner (e.g., mesenteric ischemia, appendicitis). Spontaneous bacterial peritonitis may occur in the absence of an apparent source of infection in patients with ascites, usually in the setting of portal hypertension caused by chronic liver disease.

Any patient with severe generalized abdominal pain must be aggressively evaluated for a process requiring rapid surgical intervention ("surgical abdomen"), particularly when signs of peritonitis are present. Prior to the development of bowel infarction, mesenteric ischemia may present with severe, generalized pain without signs of peritonitis. In the geriatric population, nonspecific clinical presentation of mesenteric ischemia may lead to delayed diagnosis and higher mortality rate [89]. The clinician should maintain a high index of suspicion in patients with abdominal pain that appears out of proportion to the physical examination findings or with comorbid conditions that increase the risk for ischemia (e.g., atrial fibrillation, congestive heart failure). Early intervention with surgery or angiography may be lifesaving.

The workup is directed to rule in or out certain conditions based on the patient's clinical presentation, comorbidities, and most likely etiologies. In addition to the basic laboratory workup described earlier, liver enzymes and urinalysis should be obtained and the anion gap calculated. In the presence of unstable vital signs, blood and urine cultures should be obtained to evaluate possible sepsis. If viscus perforation or bowel obstruction is suspected, a flat and upright radiograph of the abdomen and chest is a rapid test that can be considered; however, CT imaging is more sensitive [90]. Bedside ultrasound to assess for intraperitoneal free fluid is useful in the unstable patient, in whom CT imaging may result in delays in definitive, potentially lifesaving treatment (e.g., acute AAA rupture). For suspected early mesenteric ischemia, no single serum test, including serum lactate, is sufficiently sensitive and specific [91]. When considering this diagnosis, signs, symptoms, and laboratory testing are insufficient [92], making imaging a necessity to confirm the diagnosis. CT angiography (CTA) with i.v. contrast of the abdomen and pelvis is the recommended initial imaging examination for patients with suspected acute mesenteric ischemia with reported sensitivity and specificity as high as 93–100%. As a rapid, accurate, and noninvasive test for acute mesenteric ischemia, CTA offers the potential to improve patient survival [93].

Right upper quadrant and right midabdomen

Right upper quadrant pain is most commonly attributable to processes involving the liver, gallbladder, and biliary tract, and less commonly the pancreas, right kidney and ureter, appendix, right colon, right lung, or the chest wall. Liver enzymes, lipase, and urinalysis should be obtained in addition to basic laboratory tests. Elevated liver enzymes may suggest hepatic disorders, cholecystitis, cholangitis, or extrahepatic biliary obstruction. It is important to remember that normal liver enzymes do not rule out acute cholecystitis [85]. As detailed earlier, abdominal ultrasound is the initial imaging modality of choice to evaluate right upper quadrant pain [94]. In the absence of findings of cholecystitis, the mere presence of gallstones does not prove that the symptoms are due to gallbladder disease. For suspected choledocholithiasis with cholangitis, abdominal ultrasound is sensitive for the detection of biliary dilatation but less sensitive (<75%) than CT, magnetic resonance cholangiopancreatography (MRCP), or endoscopic retrograde cholangiopancreatography (ERCP) for the detection of common duct stones. Thus, if there is a high clinical suspicion for common duct stones, ERCP is the preferred study because it is both diagnostic and therapeutic [95]. For patients in whom the suspicion for common ducts stones is low to intermediate, MRCP is an excellent option for further evaluation with a sensitivity of 95% and specificity of 100%. If MRCP is not immediately available, then CT is a suitable alternative with 80% sensitivity and 100% specificity [96]. Endoscopic ultrasound is an alternative strategy to confirm choledocholithiasis in patients at intermediate risk [97], although cost and procedure availability are important considerations. In addition, a chest radiograph can be useful to screen for pulmonary pathology if clinically appropriate.

Epigastric

Mild-to-moderate acute epigastric discomfort usually indicates visceral pain as a result of disorders of the foregut. In the absence of other worrisome symptoms, physical signs, or basic laboratory abnormalities, patients with symptoms characterized as dyspepsia may be tested for *Helicobacter pylori* infection, be given an empiric trial of an antisecretory agent (proton pump inhibitor), or undergo esophagogastroduodenoscopy. For symptoms suggestive of "biliary colic," abdominal ultrasound should be pursued, as described earlier.

In patients with the acute onset of severe epigastric pain, major considerations include pancreatitis, perforated viscus, and ruptured AAA. In diagnosing acute pancreatitis, lipase (sensitivity 90.3%, specificity 93%) has superior diagnostic accuracy to amylase (sensitivity 78.7%, specificity 92.6%) [98], although the degree of pancreatic enzyme elevation does not correlate with disease severity [99]. An elevation of alanine transaminase more than twice the upper limit of normal strongly suggests that pancreatitis is secondary to gallstone disease, with a sensitivity of 74% and specificity of 84% [100]. To make a clinical diagnosis of acute pancreatitis, two of the following three features are needed: (1) abdominal pain consistent with acute pancreatitis; (2) serum lipase or amylase levels at least three times the upper limit of normal; and (3) characteristic findings on contrast-enhanced CT, MRI, or ultrasound [101]. In a large majority of patients, a diagnosis of acute pancreatitis can be made via characteristic abdominal pain and elevated serum markers without the need for imaging to establish the diagnosis. In patients with abdominal pain that is atypical for acute pancreatitis or serum amylase or lipase less than three times the upper limit of normal, further evaluation with contrast-enhanced CT abdomen is the next step to confirm the diagnosis and exclude other causes of abdominal pain [102]. In addition to considering gastrointestinal etiologies, extraabdominal processes must be considered, particularly potentially life-threatening cardiovascular processes (e.g., myocardial infarction).

Left upper quadrant and left midabdomen

In the nontraumatic setting, the clinical history and physical findings guide the extent of laboratory testing and diagnostic imaging for left upper quadrant and left midabdominal pain. The differential diagnosis includes pathology of the spleen, stomach (e.g., PUD, gastritis), pancreas (e.g., malignancy, pseudocyst), left kidney, and left colon, in addition to extraabdominal processes (e.g., pneumonia, chest wall). Urinalysis and lipase should be ordered in addition to basic laboratory studies. CT may be helpful in evaluating for splenic abscess or infarction, pyelonephritis, or bowel inflammation.

Right lower quadrant

Right lower quadrant pain may be the result of various processes, including appendicitis, Crohn's disease with intestinal inflammation, stenosis, or abscess, gynecological processes (e.g., ovarian torsion), or ureteral colic. Basic initial laboratory workup must include a urine pregnancy test in women of childbearing age and urinalysis. Leukocytosis commonly is present with surgical disorders (e.g., appendicitis) but may be normal early in the course of presentation [103]. For the diagnosis of appendicitis, CT is the primary imaging modality given excellent diagnostic accuracy (sensitivities range from 85.7% to 100% and specificities range from 94.8% to 100%) [104] and is superior to ultrasonography [105,106]. Increasing use of CT imaging has coincided with a decrease in the negative appendectomy rate without increasing the rate of appendiceal perforation as a result of diagnostic delays in diagnosis [107]. CT has the added benefit of demonstrating alternative diagnoses when negative for appendicitis. US is preferred for diagnosis of gynecological pathology due to high sensitivity for tuboovarian abscesses, ovarian torsion, ovarian cysts, and ectopic pregnancy [85].

Left lower quadrant

The differential diagnosis for left lower quadrant pain includes diverticulitis, colitis (including inflammatory, ischemic, infectious), and gynecological processes. Laboratory testing is similar to that needed in patients with right lower quadrant pain.

Table 37.1 Typical presentations of abdominal etiologies of acute abdominal pain.

Condition	Location	Quality	Onset	Associated symptoms or signs	Diagnostic evaluation
Ruptured viscus and peritonitis (e.g., PUD)	Initially localized, then progresses to diffuse	Severe	Sudden[a] to rapidly progressive[b]	Anorexia, nausea, emesis, fever; minimal bowel sounds, focal or generalized peritoneal signs	Leukocytosis; early imaging with CT if stable; upright plain film if delay in obtaining CT
Acute bowel ischemia	Diffuse or localized Small bowel: periumbilical Proximal colon: periumbilical or RLQ Distal colon: LLQ	Severe pain out of proportion to physical examination findings	Sudden if embolic; may be more gradual[c] if thrombotic or nonocclusive	Nausea, blood in stool; peritoneal signs occur with progression of bowel infarction; associated factors (e.g., cardiac arrhythmias, hypotension)	Leukocytosis, lactic acidosis may be a late finding, CTA
Acute appendicitis	Initial periumbilical pain that later shifts to the RLQ	Initially vague, visceral pain; progresses to intense, localized parietal pain	Rapidly progressive to gradual	Anorexia, pain followed by nausea and/or emesis, fever is late finding	Leukocytosis, CT
Acute cholecystitis	Initially epigastric, then migrates to RUQ; may radiate to back	Steady and severe pain	Rapidly progressive to gradual	Anorexia, nausea, vomiting, fever	Leukocytosis, normal or minimally elevated liver enzymes with uncomplicated disease; US
Acute pancreatitis	Epigastric (sometimes RUQ, less often LUQ) with radiation to midback	Persistent, steady, severe pain	Rapidly progressive	Nausea, vomiting; fever, hypotension, tachypnea and/or hypoxia in severe disease; associated factors (gallstones, alcohol)	Elevated lipase
Diverticulitis	LLQ; may be suprapubic or RLQ	Steady or cramping; may be sharp or aching; moderate to severe	Gradual	Anorexia, nausea, may have constipation or diarrhea, abdominal distention, fever	Leukocytosis, CT
Bowel obstruction	Small bowel: periumbilical Proximal colon (right): periumbilical or RLQ Distal colon (left): left quadrants	Early: crampy, colicky, more diffuse Late: persistent, localized	Rapidly progressive to gradual	Abdominal distension, nausea, emesis, inability to pass flatus; nausea/emesis more severe in proximal small bowel obstruction (versus distal small bowel or large bowel)	Upright plain film or CT (to determine location of transition point, severity, etiology)
Ruptured ectopic pregnancy	RLQ or LLQ	Localized, severe	Sudden to rapidly progressive	Amenorrhea, abnormal vaginal bleeding; associated risk factors (e.g., previous ectopic, prior tubal surgery)	Serum β-human chorionic gonadotropin, US
Ovarian torsion	RLQ or LLQ; may radiate to back, flank, or groin	Moderate to severe; can be colicky, cramping, sharp, stabbing	Sudden to rapidly progressive	Nausea, emesis, unilateral tender adnexal mass	US
Ruptured AAA	May be diffuse or localized to the aneurysm site; may radiate to back, flank, or groin	Tearing, constant, severe	Sudden to rapidly progressive	Pulsatile mass; tachycardia, hypotension; associated factors (e.g., hypertension, peripheral vascular disease, known AAA)	Bedside US if hemodynamically unstable; CT preferred, if stable

AAA, abdominal aortic aneurysm; CT, computed tomography; CTA, CT angiography; LLQ, left lower quadrant; LUQ, left upper quadrant; PUD, peptic ulcer disease; RLQ, right lower quadrant; RUQ, right upper quadrant; US, ultrasound.
[a] Sudden = seconds to minutes.
[b] Rapidly progressive = 1–2 hours.
[c] Gradual = hours.

Acute sigmoid diverticulitis should be suspected in patients with the classic triad of left lower quadrant pain, fever, and leukocytosis; however, the absence of fever or leukocytosis does not rule out this diagnosis. Contrast-enhanced CT is the imaging modality of choice for suspected diverticulitis due to its excellent sensitivity [108] and ability to identify diverticulitis complications (e.g., abscess, perforation, fistula) and alternative diagnoses [85,108]. Imaging may be unnecessary if uncomplicated mild disease is suspected based on clinical presentation.

Hypogastrium/suprapubic

Because the differential diagnosis of hypogastrium pain includes urological conditions, colitis of various etiologies, and gynecological disorders, the laboratory workup is similar to that of left and right lower quadrant pain. Urinalysis plays a particularly important role to screen for urological disorders (e.g., cystitis). Ultrasonography often is performed initially to identify acute urinary retention and exclude gynecological pathology.

Differential diagnosis

When constructing a differential diagnosis for acute abdominal pain, the regions of the abdomen (see Figure 37.5) serve as a guide to assist in determining potential etiologies. Using this information, as well as that garnered from a focused history and physical examination, the differential diagnosis can be narrowed, tailoring the evaluation to rule in or rule out the most likely causes. Table 37.1 provides the typical presentations of common pathologies that result in acute abdomen or acute abdominal pain.

Principles of management

Empiric management and when to refer

Initiation of empiric therapy depends heavily on the diagnosis that is considered most likely. In the unstable patient with acute abdominal pain, the typical sequence of resuscitation (i.e., circulation, airway, breathing) is applied while simultaneously evaluating for life-threatening conditions (e.g., ruptured AAA, ruptured ectopic pregnancy). Intravenous fluids are routinely administered. Immediate surgical consultation is merited in any patient with findings of clinical instability thought to be secondary to a surgical condition or findings of peritonitis on physical examination. Prompt but less urgent surgical consultation is also warranted in stable patients with suspected surgical pathology, such as acute appendicitis or cholecystitis, in the absence of localized or generalized peritonitis.

Once the diagnosis is determined, treatment directed toward the underlying condition is begun. Historically, clinicians deferred administration of analgesic medications to patients with acute abdominal pain until the final diagnosis was determined. Hesitancy to administer these agents stemmed from fear of masking symptoms, altering physical examination findings, or obscuring the diagnosis of serious conditions that may require surgery. Studies have since concluded that clinicians should not be reluctant to provide appropriate pharmacological analgesia to patients with acute abdominal pain. Adequate analgesia improves patient comfort during the process of diagnosis and does not increase the risk for diagnostic errors or the risk for errors in treatment decision making [109].

For some patients, the diagnosis will remain indeterminate despite evaluation. Nonspecific acute abdominal pain (NSAP) is generally defined as pain lasting less than 7 days with uncertain diagnosis despite baseline examination and investigations. Studies have evaluated the performance of early laparoscopy compared with active observation for patients with NSAP. Although early laparoscopy has demonstrated enhanced performance in establishing a definitive diagnosis [110], no significant differences are noted with respect to complications, readmission rates, or length of hospital stay when compared with an active observation strategy [111]. Currently, data are insufficient to recommend early laparoscopy in the routine evaluation of patients with NSAP [110].

References are available at www.yamadagastro.com/textbook7e

Further reading

Doherty G. The acute abdomen. In: Doherty G. (ed). Current Diagnosis and Treatment Surgery, 13th edn. New York: McGraw-Hill; 2009: 451.

Gore R., Thakrar K.H, Wenzke R.I., et al. The acute abdomen. In: Gore R., Levine M. (eds). Textbook of Gastrointestinal Radiology, 4th edn. Philadelphia: Saunders; 2015: 2255.

O'Brien M. Acute abdominal pain. In: Tintinalli J., Stapczynski J., Cline D., et al. (eds). Tintinalli's Emergency Medicine: A Comprehensive Study Guide, 7th edn. New York: McGraw-Hill; 2011: 519.

Silen W. (ed). Cope's Early Diagnosis of the Acute Abdomen, 22nd edn. New York: Oxford University Press; 2010.

Squires R., Carter, S.N., Postier R. Acute abdomen. In: Townsend C.M., Beauchamp R.D., Evers B.M., et al. (eds). Sabiston Textbook of Surgery: The Biological Basis of Modern Surgical Practice, 20th edn. Philadelphia: Saunders; 2017: 1120.

CHAPTER 38

Approach to the patient with gastrointestinal bleeding

Kevin A. Ghassemi[1] and Dennis M. Jensen[1–3]

[1] David Geffen School of Medicine UCLA, Los Angeles, CA, USA
[2] CURE Digestive Diseases Research Center, Los Angeles, CA, USA
[3] VA Greater Los Angeles Healthcare System, Los Angeles, CA, USA

Chapter menu

Introduction

The annual hospitalization rate for any type of gastrointestinal (GI) hemorrhage in the USA is estimated to be 150/100 000 population, and the mortality rate is 2.5–3.5% [1]. Approximately 50% of admissions for GI bleeding are for upper GI (UGI) bleeding (from the esophagus, stomach, duodenum), 40% are for lower GI (LGI) bleeding (from the colon and anorectum), and 10% are for obscure (OGI) bleeding (source of bleeding has not been identified after esophagogastroduodenoscopy and colonoscopy have been performed).

This chapter focuses on overt GI bleeding that may be severe and prompts the patient to seek medical attention. The source of most GI bleeds can be suspected by the clinical symptoms and physical examination and confirmed by upper or lower endoscopy. Initial management focuses on medical resuscitation, followed by endoscopic diagnosis and interventions to halt acute bleeding and prevent recurrent bleeding. Pharmacological therapy has an increasingly important role in the management of UGI bleeding from peptic ulcers and varices. Optimizing outcomes depends on successful medical resuscitation, precise endoscopic diagnosis, and appropriate endoscopic therapy.

Severe GI bleeding is defined as documented GI bleeding (i.e., hematemesis, melena, hematochezia, or positive nasogastric lavage) accompanied by either shock or orthostatic hypotension, a decrease in the hemoglobin level of at least 2 g/dL, or the need to transfuse at least two units of packed red blood cells. Most patients with severe GI bleeding are admitted to hospital for resuscitation and treatment. Overt bleeding implies there is visible blood loss from the GI tract.

Hematemesis is defined as vomiting of blood, which indicates bleeding from the esophagus, stomach, or duodenum. Hematemesis includes vomiting of bright red blood, which suggests recent or ongoing bleeding, and dark material (coffee-ground emesis), which suggests recent bleeding. Melena is defined as black tarry stool and results from degradation of blood by digestive tract enzymes and intestinal bacteria. Melena usually indicates bleeding originating from an UGI or proximal small bowel source, but in rare instances it can originate from a proximal colonic source. Melena generally occurs when at least 50 mL of blood enters the GI tract (usually UGI tract), with passage of the characteristic stool several hours later. Hematochezia refers to bright red blood per rectum, and suggests either active UGI or small bowel bleeding or distal colonic or anorectal bleeding. Occult GI bleeding refers to subacute bleeding that is not clinically visible. Obscure GI bleeding is bleeding from a site that is not apparent after routine endoscopic evaluation with esophagogastroduodenoscopy (upper endoscopy), push enteroscopy, and colonoscopy.

Yamada's Textbook of Gastroenterology, Seventh Edition. Edited by Timothy C. Wang, Michael Camilleri, Benjamin Lebwohl, Anna S. Lok, William J. Sandborn, Kenneth K. Wang, and Gary D. Wu.

Companion website: www.yamadagastro.com/textbook7e

General assessment

History

Initial assessment of patients with acute GI bleeding includes taking the medical and surgical history, vital signs, performing a physical examination including a rectal examination, and possibly doing a nasogastric lavage. During history taking, patients should be questioned about factors that help identify diagnostic possibilities for the bleeding source. Peptic ulcer bleeding should be suspected in patients with history of an ulcer or those taking daily aspirin or other nonsteroidal antiinflammatory drugs (NSAIDs). Patients with chronic hepatitis or who are alcoholics may be bleeding due to a complication of portal hypertension. Patients with heavy alcohol intake, a feeding or chronic nasogastric tube, or a history of gastroesophageal reflux disease (GERD) are at risk for erosive esophagitis. Recent retching or vomiting may suggest a Mallory–Weiss tear. Prior surgical repair of an abdominal aortic aneurysm raises the possibility of an aortoenteric fistula. Patients with prior radiation to the abdomen/pelvis may have radiation enteritis or proctocolitis. Abdominal pain, weight loss, and stool caliber changes are nonspecific signs and symptoms, but could be due to inflammatory bowel disease, ischemic colitis, or a malignancy. Chest pain and syncope are potential cardiovascular complications of significant blood loss.

Physical examination

Initial evaluation should focus on vital signs, with attention to signs of hypovolemia such as hypotension, tachycardia, and orthostasis. The abdomen should be examined for surgical scars, tenderness, and masses. Signs of chronic liver disease include spider angiomas, palmar erythema, gynecomastia, ascites, splenomegaly, caput medusa, and Dupuytren's contracture. The skin, lips, and buccal mucosa should be examined for telangiectasias, which are suggestive of hereditary hemorrhagic telangiectasia (HHT). Purpuric skin lesions can be seen in a variety of vasculitides. Acanthosis nigricans may suggest underlying malignancy, especially gastric cancer. Stool should be examined, by digital rectal examination or bowel movement sample, to identify melena, maroon stool, and/or red stool. However, the subjective description of stool color varies greatly among both patients and physicians [2].

Nasogastric or orogastric tube placement allows for aspiration of gastric contents to visually determine whether red blood, coffee-ground material, or nonbloody fluid is present. Testing the nasogastric tube aspirate for occult blood is not useful because trauma from the tube placement may be sufficient to cause a false-positive result. Patients who have coffee-ground emesis or fresh bloody emesis that is witnessed do not require placement of a nasogastric tube for diagnostic purposes but may benefit from tube placement to help clear the gastric blood for better endoscopic visualization and to minimize the risk of aspiration.

Laboratory studies

Blood should be sent for standard hematology, chemistry, liver biochemical, and coagulation studies, as well as for a type and cross-match for packed red blood cells. The hemoglobin value immediately after the onset of bleeding may not reflect blood loss accurately because it can take at least 8 h for equilibration to occur between red blood cells in the vascular space and extravascular fluid, as well as from hemodilution resulting from intravenous fluid administration. The mean corpuscular volume (MCV) is an important indicator of the chronicity of blood loss; an MCV below 80 fL suggests chronic GI blood loss and iron deficiency, which can be confirmed by the finding of low ferritin and transferrin saturation levels. A high MCV (>100 fL) may be due to chronic liver disease or a folate or vitamin B_{12} deficiency. A low platelet count can contribute to the severity of bleeding and suggests chronic liver disease or a hematological disorder.

The blood urea nitrogen (BUN) and serum creatinine levels can help assess the patient for hemoconcentration (elevated levels) or chronic kidney disease, which may lead to chronic anemia because of decreased erythropoietin production. In patients with UGI bleeding, the BUN level typically increases to a greater extent than the serum creatinine level, because of increased intestinal absorption of urea after the breakdown of blood proteins by intestinal bacteria [3].

The prothrombin time (PT) and the international normalized ratio (INR) assess whether a patient has impairment of the extrinsic coagulation pathway. Values can be elevated in chronic liver disease or with the use of certain anticoagulants, most commonly warfarin. Liver biochemical test levels may indicate the presence of acute or chronic liver disease; a low serum albumin level suggests possible chronic liver disease, malnutrition, or protein loss via the intestine or kidney.

Clinical determination of the bleeding site

An UGI hemorrhage source is indicated by hematemesis, coffee-ground emesis, or nasogastric lavage with significant return of blood or coffee-ground material. A small amount of coffee-ground material or pink-tinged fluid that clears easily may represent mucosal trauma from the nasogastric tube rather than active bleeding from an UGI source. A clear (nonbloody) nasogastric aspirate does not necessarily indicate a more distal GI source bleeding, because 16% of patients with actively bleeding UGI lesions have a clear nasogastric aspirate [4]. The presence of bile in the aspirate makes UGI bleeding unlikely, but can be seen with an intermittently bleeding UGI source.

Melena usually indicates an UGI source but it can be seen with small intestinal or proximal colonic bleeding. Hematochezia typically implies a colonic or anorectal source of bleeding. However, if the patient is hypotensive, hematochezia could be the manifestation of a severe UGI bleed with rapid transit of blood through the GI tract [2]. Maroon-colored stool can be seen with active bleeding from the UGI tract, the small intestine, or proximal colon.

Hospitalization

Based on the patient's initial history, physical examination, and laboratory test results, the location of bleeding (upper or lower), suspected bleeding lesion, and severity of bleeding can be predicted. Patients with severe GI bleeding require hospitalization, whereas those with only mild acute bleeding (self-limited hematochezia or melena) and who are hemodynamically stable (not suspected to be volume depleted), have normal blood test results, and can be relied upon to return to the hospital if symptoms recur may be candidates for discharge and referred for a semi-urgent outpatient endoscopy rather than direct admission to the hospital [5]. Among patients requiring hospitalization, the intensive care unit is appropriate for those with large-volume hematemesis, nasogastric return or hematochezia, unstable vital signs, or severe acute blood loss that may exacerbate other underlying medical conditions. Patients who have had an acute GI bleed but are hemodynamically stable can be admitted to either a monitored bed or standard hospital bed, depending on their clinical condition.

Resuscitation

Resuscitation efforts should be initiated at the same time as the initial assessment and continue during the hospitalization. At least one large-bore (14 or 16 gauge) intravenous catheter should be placed. Normal saline is infused as fast as needed to keep the patient's systolic blood pressure greater than 100 mmHg and pulse lower than 100/min. The patient should be transfused with packed red blood cells, platelets, and fresh frozen plasma as necessary to keep the hemoglobin above 8 g/dL, platelet count greater than 50 000/mm^3, and INR at or below 1.5, respectively. The target hemoglobin may vary based on patient age and comorbidities, and the INR goal may vary based on whether the coagulopathy is intrinsic or drug induced. The hemoglobin threshold for transfusion of packed red blood cells generally should be 9–10 g/dL, depending on cardiovascular comorbidities.

A recent study evaluating blood transfusions for UGI bleeding found that a more restrictive transfusion threshold of 7 g/dL led to a significantly higher 6-week survival rate and lower rebleeding rate when compared to a threshold of 9 g/dL, However, poor risk patients with severe cardiovascular disease or very severe bleeding were excluded from the study, so caution is recommended to not undertransfuse those types of patients [6]. A physician with appropriate expertise should be consulted as soon as possible to expedite the patient's assessment and determine the optimal timing of endoscopy. In hospitals with a liver transplant program, it is usually appropriate to also notify the transplant hepatology service if the patient is known to have advanced liver disease and is a potential transplant candidate.

The patient's vital signs should be monitored frequently, as appropriate to the level of care in the hospital. The hemoglobin should be obtained every 4–8 h until it is stable. Endotracheal intubation should be considered in patients with active hematemesis or altered mental status to prevent aspiration pneumonia. Patients who are older than 60 years, have chest pain or a history of cardiac disease should be evaluated for myocardial infarction with electrocardiograms and serial troponin measurements. A chest x-ray should also be considered to assess for pneumoperitoneum prior to endoscopy.

Initial medical therapy

Administration of a proton pump inhibitor (PPI) is useful for reducing rebleeding rates in patients with peptic ulcer disease. Starting a PPI in the emergency department or intensive care unit before endoscopy is performed in patients with severe UGI bleeding has become common practice. Several clinical studies and metaanalyses have shown that infusion of a high-dose PPI (80 mg IV bolus and 8 mg infusion/h for 72 h) before endoscopy accelerates the resolution of endoscopic stigmata of bleeding in ulcers and reduces the need for endoscopic therapy but does not result in improved clinical outcomes, including the transfusion requirement, rebleeding rate, need for surgery, or death rate [7–10]. PPIs are also recommended if ulcer bleeding is suspected and a significant delay in endoscopy is anticipated [7]. Early PPI use may not be needed in patients who have mild self-limited bleeding, and is not indicated in patients who have suspected LGI bleeding. In patients with a strong suspicion for variceal bleeding, empiric intravenous octreotide should be started (50 μg IV bolus followed by 50 μg infusion/h). Octreotide can reduce the risk of rebleeding to a rate similar to that associated with endoscopic therapy [11].

Diagnostic and therapeutic modalities

Endoscopy

Gastrointestinal endoscopy can identify the bleeding site and permit therapeutic hemostasis in most patients with GI bleeding. Endoscopy should be done only when it is safe to do so and when the information obtained from the procedure will influence patient care. Ideally, the patient should be hemodynamically stable. Respiratory insufficiency, altered mental status, or ongoing hematemesis indicate the need for endotracheal intubation before emergency upper endoscopy to protect the airway. Proper medical resuscitation will not only allow safer endoscopy, but also ensure a better diagnostic examination for lesions, such as varices, that are volume dependent and will allow more effective hemostasis because of the correction of coagulopathy.

Patients with active hemorrhage (i.e., a high-volume bloody gastric lavage or ongoing hematemesis or hematochezia) should undergo emergency endoscopy soon after medical resuscitation. Appoximately 15–20% of noncirrhotic patients with severe, ongoing hematochezia without hematemesis have a foregut source of bleeding and this increases to over 50% in cirrhotic patients, so an early endoscopy or push enteroscopy is recommended in these subgroups of patients. Patients suspected of having cirrhosis or an aortoenteric fistula or who rebleed in the hospital should undergo emergent endoscopy, usually within 6 h of admission or rebleeding. Patients who are hemodynamically stable without evidence of ongoing bleeding can undergo endoscopy (within 12 h), often in the GI endoscopy unit rather than the intensive care unit or emergency department. Endoscopy should be avoided in the middle of the night, except for the most severely bleeding or high-risk patients, if well-trained endoscopy nurses, endoscopic equipment, and surgical back-up are not available at night. In the rare patient with massive bleeding and refractory hypotension, endoscopy can be performed in the operating room, with the immediate availability of surgical management, if necessary.

Intravenous administration of a prokinetic agent (erythromycin or metoclopramide) 30–90 min before upper endoscopy can push blood from the stomach into the small intestine and helps endoscopic visualization [12,13]. Therapeutic single- or double-channel endoscopes with large-diameter suction channels should be used to allow quick removal of fresh blood from the GI tract during endoscopy. Additionally, a water pump can be used to irrigate target lesions through the accessory channel and dilute blood for suctioning.

In patients with severe hematochezia and suspected active colonic bleeding, urgent colonoscopy can be undertaken after a rapid purge [14]. Patients should receive 6–8 L of a polyethylene glycol solution either orally or via a nasogastric tube over 4–6 h until the rectal effluent is clear of stool, blood, and clots. Additional polyethylene glycol may be required in some patients, particularly those with active bleeding, constipation, or the onset of hematochezia in the hospital. Metoclopramide, 5–10 mg, may be given intravenously before the purge and repeated every 4–6 h to facilitate gastric emptying and reduce nausea. In patients with severe or ongoing active hematochezia, urgent colonoscopy should be performed within 12 h, but only after thorough cleansing of the colon. Patients with self-limited hematochezia should undergo bowel purge and colonoscopy within 24 h of admission.

Patients with maroon stool in whom there is pretest uncertainty about the bleeding source should be considered for an urgent polyethylene bowel preparation as well. Colonoscopy immediately after push enteroscopy, while the patient is still sedated, will expedite a patient's care if push enteroscopy does not provide a diagnosis.

Wireless capsule enteroscopy (or capsule endoscopy) is recommended in patients with overt GI bleeding (and either melena or hematochezia) who have normal push enteroscopy and colonoscopy results and in whom a small bowel source of bleeding is suspected [15]. Capsule endoscopy has the advantage of directly visualizing the small intestine to identify potential sources or active bleeding. Disadvantages are that the procedure takes 8 h to complete, requires additional time to download and review the images, and does not have therapeutic capabilities. A follow-up endoscopic procedure, such as single- or double-balloon enteroscopy or retrograde ileoscopy, may be indicated for definitive diagnosis and treatment if a focal bleeding site is identified on capsule endoscopy.

Endoscopic hemostasis

Although details for the treatment of specific causes of hemorrhage are described below, there are general principles for use of the most common tools for endoscopic hemostasis.

Thermal contact probes have been the mainstay of endoscopic hemostasis since the 1970s. They come in diameters of 7 and 10 French and in lengths that can fit through various endoscopes. Contact probes effect hemostasis through two mechanisms: (1) tamponade of a blood vessel to stop bleeding and interrupt underlying blood flow; and (2) application of thermal energy to seal the underlying vessel (coaptive coagulation).

The most commonly used probe is a multipolar electrocoagulation (MPEC) probe, also referred to as bipolar electrocoagulation, in which heat is generated by current flowing between intertwined electrodes on the tip of the probe. Animal studies using MPEC probes to stop bleeding in mesenteric vessels have shown that optimal coagulation occurs with low-power settings (12–16 W), applied for 8–10 s, with moderate pressure on the bleeding site [16]. Thermal probes can provide a predetermined amount of joules of energy, which does not vary with tissue resistance. Animal studies have shown that heater and MPEC probes can effectively coagulate arteries up to 2 mm in diameter, a diameter that is considerably larger than most secondary or tertiary branches of arteries (usually ≤1 mm) found in resected bleeding human peptic ulcers [17]. The main risk of using a thermal probe is perforation with excessive application of coagulation or pressure, especially in acute or nonfibrotic lesions. Thermal probes can also cause coagulation injury that can make lesions larger and deeper, and may induce delayed bleeding in patients with a coagulopathy. Suggested MPEC technical parameters for treating various bleeding etiologies are described in Table 38.1.

Injection therapy is performed with a sclerotherapy needle to inject epinephrine, diluted to a concentration of 1:10 000 or 1:20 000, submucosally into or around the bleeding site or stigma of hemorrhage. Advantages of this technique are that it is widely available, relatively inexpensive, and safe for use in patients with a coagulopathy. Additionally, it is associated with a lower risk of perforation than thermal techniques. Its disadvantage is that it is not as effective for definitive hemostasis as thermal coagulation, endoscopic clips, or combination therapy [18]. Injection therapy can also be performed with a sclerosant, such as ethanolamine or alcohol, but these agents are associated with increased tissue damage and other risks.

Endoscopic clips (also known as hemoclips) apply mechanical pressure to a bleeding site, as is done with surgical clips or sutures. However, endoscopic hemoclips differ from surgical clips in that they do not have as much compressive strength, and the currently available clips do not close completely but leave a small space between the prongs. Hemoclips offer comparable efficacy to thermal probes in achieving definitive hemostasis [19]. By not causing thermal damage, they are especially useful in patients with malnutrition or coagulopathy [20]. Nevertheless, hemoclips can also be difficult to deploy depending on the

Table 38.1 UCLA CURE Center parameters for using multipolar electrocoagulation (MPEC) to treat bleeding lesions[a].

	Peptic ulcer						
	Arterial spurting	**Visible vessel**	**Adherent clot**	**Mallory–Weiss tear**	**Dieulafoy lesion***	**Colonic diverticulum with visible vessel**	**Vascular ectasia**
Epinephrine first?	Yes	No	Yes	+/–	Yes	No	+/–
Probe size (French)[b]	10	10	10	7/10	10	7/10	7/10
Power setting (W)	12–15	12–15	12–15	10–15	10–15	10–15	10–15
Pressure[c]	Firm	Firm	Firm	Moderate	Firm	Light	Light
Pulse duration (s)	8–10	8–10	8–10	4	8–10	2	2
Endpoint	Bleeding stops	Flat vessel	Flat stigmata	Bleeding stops	Flat vessel	Flat vessel	White

[a] Derived from experimental and randomized endoscopic studies. Power, pressure, and duration should be reduced for small or deep bleeding lesions.
[b] A 10 French probe fits through a 3.8 mm endoscope channel. A 7 French probe fits through a 2.8 mm channel.
[c] Tamponade pressure exerted by probe tangentially or en face on the lesion.
* A Dieulafoy lesion is a large artery protruding through the submucosa without a surrounding ulcer or other submucosal lesion. These can be found anywhere in the GI tract but are most common in the upper stomach.

bleeding location, the degree of fibrosis of the underlying lesion, and limitations to endoscopic access.

In most cases for which endoscopic hemostasis is appropriate, the combination of epinephrine injection and either thermal probe or hemoclips is more effective than epinephrine injection alone. This will be discussed in more detail in the section on treatment of peptic ulcer bleeding. Larger, over-the-scope, endoscopic clips (OTSC) will be discussed in this section as well.

Argon plasma coagulation (APC) uses ionized argon gas to transfer energy to target tissue. It uses a monopolar current, so a grounding pad is required. It has been used to ablate tissue (such as the edges of a postpolypectomy site), but also to treat superficial bleeding or sites for potential bleeding (such as isolated vascular ectasias, gastric antral vascular ectasia, and radiation proctitis) [21]. The depth of coagulation is superficial and it is a nontamponade device so coaptive coagulation is not possible, and this limits APC treatment of ulcers or Dieulafoy lesions with major stigmata of hemorrhage which have underlying arterial blood flow from arteries in the submucosa.

With band ligation, mucosal (with or without submucosal) tissue is suctioned into a cap placed on the end of the endoscope, and a rubber band is rolled off the cap and over the lesion to compress its base. This technique is widely used for the treatment of esophageal varices and can be used for other bleeding lesions. Band ligation's main advantage is that it is relatively easy to perform. Sufficient mucosa must be suctioned into the cap for successful ligation, so lesions involving or surrounded by fibrosis may be difficult to treat with this technique. Some band ligation devices can only fit on diagnostic endoscopes, so the endoscopist may need to switch from the therapeutic to the diagnostic endoscope after the bleeding lesion has been identified.

Radiological intervention and nuclear studies

Angiography may be useful to diagnose and treat severe bleeding, especially when the etiology cannot be determined by upper and lower endoscopy. Angiography can detect extravasation into the intestinal lumen when the arterial bleeding rate is at least 0.5 mL/min [22]. The sensitivity of mesenteric angiography is 30–50% (with higher sensitivity rates for active GI bleeding than for recurrent acute or chronic occult bleeding), and the specificity is 100% [23]. An advantage of angiography is that it permits therapeutic intraarterial infusion of vasopressin or transcatheter embolization for hemostasis if active bleeding is detected, without the need for bowel cleansing. Nevertheless, the rate of major complications, including hematoma formation, femoral artery thrombosis, contrast dye reactions, acute kidney injury, intestinal ischemia, and transient ischemic attacks, is 3% [24]. Another disadvantage of angiography is that it usually does not provide identification of the specific cause of bleeding, only its location.

Radionuclide imaging can help in cases of unexplained GI bleeding, although it is used less frequently now because of the widespread availability of endoscopy and lack of availability of nuclear medicine services for emergencies, particularly at night and on weekends. Radionuclide imaging can be performed relatively quickly and may help localize the general area of bleeding and thereby guide subsequent endoscopy, angiography, or surgery. The technique involves injecting a radiolabeled substance intravenously into the patient's bloodstream and then performing serial scintigraphy to detect focal collections of radiolabeled material. Radionuclide imaging has been reported to detect bleeding at a rate as low as 0.04 mL/min [25]. The overall rate of a positive diagnostic radionuclide scan is approximately 45%, with a 78% accuracy rate in the localization of the true bleeding site [26,27]. Up to 25% of bleeding scans suggest a site of bleeding that proves to be incorrect [27–29]. The rate of true-positive scans is higher for active bleeding with hemodynamic instability than for less severe bleeding [30]. The most common reason for a false-positive result is rapid transit of luminal blood, so that labeled blood is detected in the colon even though it originated from a more proximal site in the GI tract. Caution is recommended in utilizing the results of delayed scans to localize and target lesions for resective surgery [31].

Conventional radiographic imaging is usually not necessary for patients with GI bleeding, but occasionally it may provide some important information. In patients with a prior abdominal aortic aneurysm repair and graft, computed tomography (CT) with intravenous contrast may identify inflammation between the graft and duodenum that suggests fistula formation between the graft and duodenum [32]. CT scan may also identify a mass lesion or small bowel abnormalities that may suggest a cause of bleeding. Barium radiography is not indicated (and contraindicated if endoscopy or angiography is planned) in the emergency setting.

Surgery

Most patients admitted for acute GI bleeding have bleeding of mild-to-moderate severity and do not need surgical consultation or intervention. In selected patients with severe ongoing GI bleeding in whom a diagnosis is not made by urgent endoscopy or colonoscopy, surgical consultation is recommended. Patients with massive hemorrhage who cannot be stabilized hemodynamically should undergo either emergency angiography or urgent surgical exploration, either without prior endoscopy or with emergency endoscopy in the operating room.

Causes of upper gastrointestinal bleeding

Epidemiology

Despite advances in medical, endoscopic, and surgical care, the mortality rate of 2–10% for severe UGI bleeding has not changed over the past several decades [1,33]. The lack of improvement in the mortality rate may be explained by an increase in the proportion of elderly patients with GI bleeding, who may die as a result of exacerbation of other medical conditions rather than from exsanguination, as well as an increase in the number of patients with cirrhosis and variceal bleeding. Causes of UGI bleeding are listed in Table 38.2. Bleeding is self-limited in about 80% of patients with UGI hemorrhage, even without specific therapy. Of the remaining 20% who continue to bleed or rebleed, the mortality rate is 30–40% [34]. Patients at high risk for continuous bleeding or for rebleeding potentially can benefit the most from acute medical, endoscopic, and surgical therapy. Table 38.3 lists predictors of persistent or recurrent nonvariceal UGI bleeding.

Risk stratification

Scoring systems have been developed to identify patients with nonvariceal UGI bleeding potentially at greatest risk for

Table 38.2 Etiologies of severe upper gastrointestinal bleeding and their frequencies.

Diagnosis	Frequency (%)
Peptic ulcer	38
Gastric/esophageal varices	16
Esophagitis	13
No cause found	8
Neoplasm	7
Vascular ectasia	6
Erosions	4
Mallory–Weiss tear	4
Dieulafoy lesion	2
Other	2

Source: Adapted from UCLA CURE Center database.

Table 38.3 Statistically significant predictors of recurrent or persistent nonvariceal upper gastrointestinal bleeding. Source: Adapted from Barkun et al. 2003 [210].

Risk factor	Range of odds ratios for increased risk
Clinical factors	
Age >65 years	1.3
Age ≥70 years	2.23
Health status (ASA class 1 vs 2–5)	1.94–7.63
Shock (SBP <100 mmHg)	1.2–3.65
Comorbid illness	1.6–7.63
Erratic mental status	3.21
Coagulopathy	1.96
Presentation of bleeding	
Red blood on rectal examination	3.76
Melena	1.6
Hematemesis	1.2–5.7
Endoscopic factors	
Active bleeding	2.5–6.48
Diagnosis of gastric or duodenal ulcer	2.7
Ulcer size ≥2 cm	2.29–3.54
Ulcer high on gastric lesser curve	2.79
Ulcer on superior wall of duodenum	13.9
Ulcer on posterior wall of duodenum	9.2
High-risk stigmata	1.91–4.81
Clot over ulcer	1.72–1.9

ASA, American Society of Anesthesiologists; SBP, systolic blood pressure.

rebleeding and death. These tools could be used to triage patients to a higher level of hospital care or more urgent endoscopy. Scoring systems include those based on purely clinical parameters available on a patient's presentation to the hospital, and those that incorporate both clinical parameters and endoscopic findings.

Among many preendoscopy scoring systems for nonvariceal bleeding, the most commonly used are the Blatchford score and clinical Rockall score. The Blatchford score uses preendoscopy variables including pulse, systolic blood pressure, BUN, hemoglobin, syncope, melena, and major comorbidities to assess a patient's risk for requiring clinical interventions blood transfusions, endoscopic therapy, or surgery [35]. A modified Blatchford score only includes the vital signs and laboratory values from the Blatchford score, and appears to be as accurate for predicting clinical outcomes [36]. The clinical Rockall score uses the patient's age, the presence of shock, and coexisting illnesses [37].

The most commonly used postendoscopy scoring system is the Rockall complete score (Table 38.4) [37]. It includes the clinical Rockall score and endoscopic findings, including endoscopic stigmata of recent bleeding. The Rockall score after endoscopic therapy correlates well with mortality but does not correlate as well with the risk of rebleeding [38]. This risk stratification can be used not only to identify patients at highest risk for mortality, but also to identify those at low risk who should be considered for early discharge from the hospital [39].

Peptic ulcer (see Chapter 49)

Peptic ulcer, most commonly gastric or duodenal, is the leading cause of severe UGI hemorrhage in most countries and accounts for 38–50% of UGI bleeds and approximately 100 000 hospitalizations per year in the USA [40]. The hospitalization rate for peptic ulcer bleeding has not changed significantly over the past 20 years, likely due to the aging population and widespread use of NSAIDs [41]. The costs of hospitalization for peptic ulcer bleeding are estimated to be more than $2 billion per year in the USA [42]. For more details regarding peptic ulcers, see Chapter 49.

Pathogenesis

Peptic ulcers most commonly are caused by impairment of mucosal defense mechanisms due to NSAIDs or *Helicobacter pylori* infection (or both) [43]. *H. pylori* infection is common, with a prevalence of over 80% of the population in many developing countries and 20–50% in industrialized countries. Antral-predominant gastritis predisposes patients to duodenal ulcers, while body-predominant gastritis is associated with gastric ulcers. The lifetime risk of peptic ulcer disease from *H. pylori* infection ranges from 3% in the USA to 25% in Japan [44]. NSAIDs are the most widely used medication in the USA, with 11% of the adult population taking them on a daily basis [45]. NSAIDs, including aspirin, predominantly cause ulceration by inhibiting cyclooxygenase (COX)-mediated prostaglandin synthesis which impairs mucosal protection, rather than causing direct topical injury. Gastroduodenal ulcers are found at endoscopy in 1–45% of patients who take NSAIDs regularly [46].

Pathological examination of 27 surgically resected bleeding gastric ulcers with endoscopically visible vessels revealed an underlying artery in 96% of specimens. About half of the vessels protruded above the surface of the ulcer, whereas the other half had a clot in continuity with a breach in the vessel wall [47].

Endoscopic risk stratification

In addition to detecting a peptic ulcer, endoscopy can evaluate the ulcer for stigmata associated with an increased risk of rebleeding. The Forrest classification has been used in Europe and Asia to categorize findings during endoscopic evaluation of bleeding peptic ulcers. However, descriptive findings are used in the USA, and these are active spurting bleeding (Forrest IA); oozing blood (Forrest IB); pigmented protuberance or nonbleeding visible vessel (NBVV) (Forrest IIA); adherent clot (Forrest IIb); flat pigmented spot (Forrest IIC); and clean-based ulcer (Forrest III) [48,49].

Table 38.4 Rockall scoring system for risk stratification in nonvariceal upper gastrointestinal bleeding.

Score	0	1	2	3
Age (years)[a]	<60	60–79	≥80	
Shock[a]	None	Heart rate >100 beats/min	Systolic blood pressure <100 mmHg	
Comorbidity[a]	None		Congestive heart failure, ischemic heart disease, other major illness	Renal failure, liver failure, metastatic cancer
Endoscopic diagnosis	Mallory–Weiss tear, no major lesion	Peptic ulcer, esophagitis, erosive disease	UGI malignancy	
Stigmata of recent hemorrhage	Clean-based ulcer, flat pigmented spot		Blood in UGI tract, active bleeding, visible vessel, adherent clot	

The complete Rockall score consists of all variables.
[a] Variable needed to calculate the clinical Rockall score. A clinical Rockall score of 0 or a complete Rockall score of ≤2 indicates a low risk of rebleeding.
UGI, upper gastrointestinal.
Source: Rockall et al. 1996 [37]. Reproduced with permission of BMJ Publishing Group.

Endoscopic stigmata of recent hemorrhage from an ulcer are shown in Figure 38.1. Patients at high risk of rebleeding without treatment are those with active arterial bleeding (90%), a NBVV (50%), or an adherent clot (33%) [49]. These patients benefit from endoscopic hemostasis. An endoscopically identified NBVV, which has a translucent color, has a higher risk of rebleeding than a darkly colored pigmented protuberance (clot), because the translucent stigma likely represents the arterial wall [50,51]. Patients with high-risk stigmata of ulcer hemorrhage (spurting, NBVV, or adherent clot) benefit most from endoscopic hemostasis, whereas those with a flat spot or clean ulcer base do not. Patients with oozing bleeding and no other stigmata (such as a clot or NBVV) have an intermediate risk of rebleeding and may benefit from endoscopic hemostasis but not from high-dose PPI infusion [49].

For patients who start to hemorrhage as an outpatient, the risk of rebleeding from a peptic ulcer decreases significantly 72 h after the initial episode of bleeding. This is based on studies in which serial endoscopic examinations were performed and all nonactively bleeding stigmata observed [50,52,53]. Natural history studies of untreated such patients admitted with ulcer hemorrhage and NBVVs have found that these lesions resolve over 4 days, and adherent clots tend to resolve over 2 days [54]. In contrast, the time to rebleeding for patients with ulcer hemorrhage that starts as an inpatient may extend up to 30 days [55].

Doppler probe ultrasound

Portable Doppler ultrasound sound probes can be passed through the working channel of an endoscope and applied to an ulcer to determine if arterial blood flow is present beneath a stigma in the ulcer base [56]. The presence of an arterial flow signal correlates with the risk of rebleeding, both before and after endoscopic therapy. Although early data were conflicting regarding the utility of Doppler endoscopic probe (DEP), more recent studies have demonstrated efficacy of the DEP in identifying underlying blood flow and contributing to reduced rebleeding rates after endoscopic therapy.

In a prospective study of 163 patients with peptic ulcer bleeding and different stigmata of recent hemorrhage, DEP identified arterial blood flow in 87% of ulcers with high-risk stigmata (Forrest IA, IIA, and IIB) and 42% of ulcers with intermediate-risk stigmata (Forrest IB and IIC). After endoscopic hemostasis,

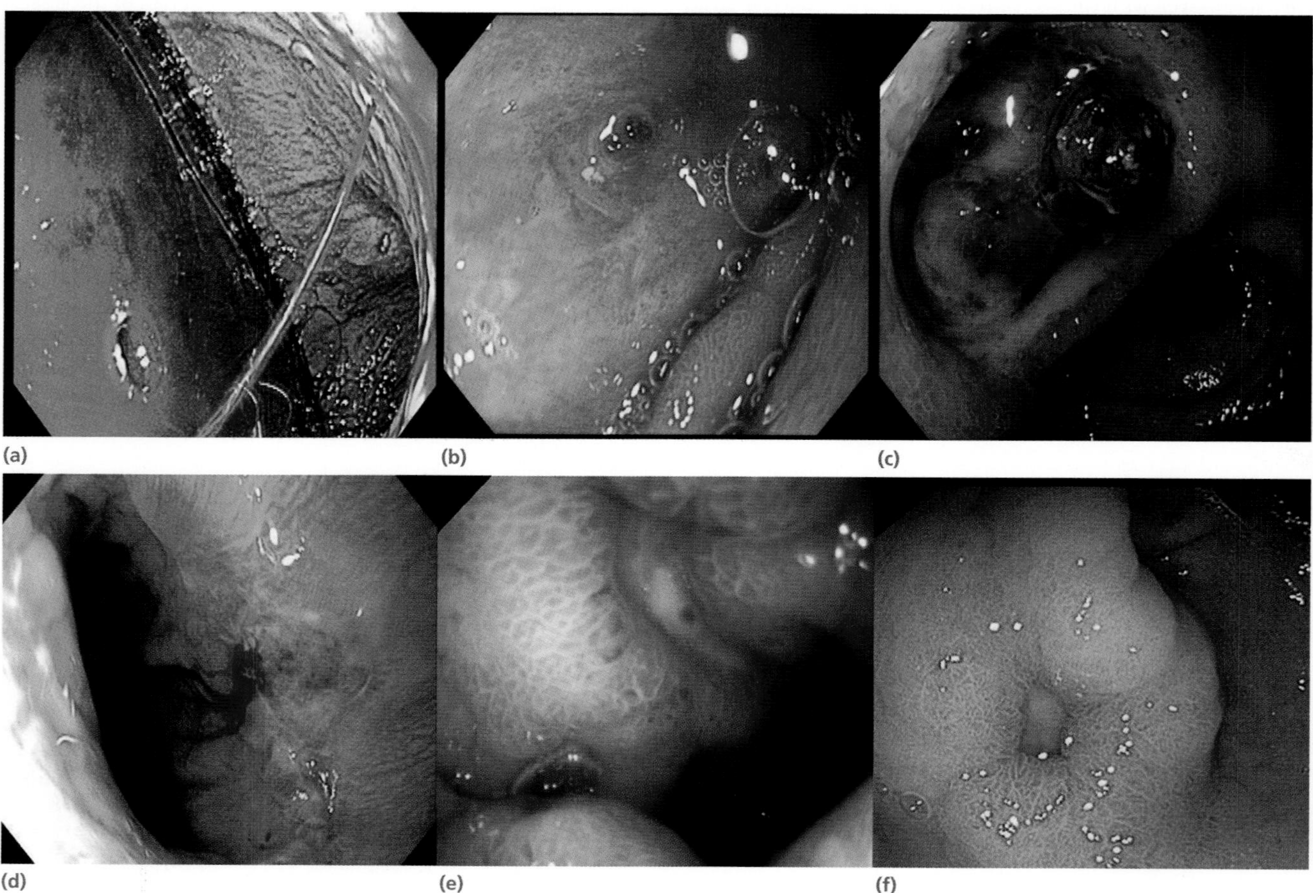

Figure 38.1 Endoscopic stigmata of recent hemorrhage in ulcers. **(a)** Arterial spurting; **(b)** nonbleeding visible vessel; **(c)** adherent clot; **(d)** oozing without other stigmata; **(e)** flat pigmented spot; **(f)** clean-based ulcer.

residual blood flow in the Forrest IA lesions was 36% and the 30-day rebleed rate was 30%. In the intermediate-risk stigmata lesions, posttreatment residual blood flow and 30-day rebleed rate were both 0% [57]. In a randomized controlled trial of patients with severe, nonvariceal upper GI bleeding, DEP-guided endoscopic hemostasis resulted in a significant reduction in the 30-day rebleed rate compared to standard, visually guided endoscopic therapy (11% vs 26%). There was also an arithmetic difference between the two groups in the rate of surgery and major complications (0% vs 5%) [58].

Based on these results, future guidelines should incorporate the use of DEP to improve outcomes for treating bleeding, nonvariceal, upper GI lesions.

Endoscopic hemostasis (see also Chapter 125)

Active bleeding and nonbleeding visible vessels (see Figure 38.1a,b)

Based on randomized controlled trials, metaanalyses, and consensus conferences, it has been concluded that endoscopic hemostasis with either epinephrine injection or coaptive thermal probe therapy significantly decreases the rates of ulcer rebleeding, urgent surgery, and mortality in patients with high-risk stigmata, such as active bleeding and NBVVs [59–61]. In general, for the lesions at highest risk, including those with active bleeding (90% risk of ongoing bleeding) or NBVVs (50% risk of ongoing bleeding), endoscopic hemostasis alone decreases the rebleeding rate to approximately 15–30% (Table 38.5). The adjunctive administration of a continuous infusion of high-dose PPI decreases this rate even further.

Worldwide, the most commonly used treatment for ulcer bleeding is epinephrine injection. Therapy with epinephrine alone may be more effective when used in high doses (13–20 mL) than in low doses (5–10 mL) [62]. Injection of epinephrine results in a fivefold increase in circulating plasma epinephrine levels but rarely is thought to cause clinically significant cardiovascular events [63]. Although epinephrine injection alone is effective compared with placebo, numerous studies and metaanalyses have shown that the addition of a thermal or mechanical hemostatic modality further decreases the rates of rebleeding, surgery, and mortality significantly [18,64,65]. Hemoclips have not been studied as well as injection and thermal probe techniques but seem to be more effective than epinephrine injection alone and overall are comparable to thermal probe therapy [19,66,67].

For actively spurting ulcer bleeding, injection of 0.5–1.0 mL aliquots of epinephrine (1:20 000 dilution) into four quadrants of the ulcer within 1–2 mm of the bleeding site is recommended. When combination therapy is performed, coagulation is performed with a large 10 French MPEC probe (7 French if a therapeutic channel endoscope is not available). After epinephrine injection, the probe is placed directly on the bleeding site in order to tamponade the site, and coagulation is applied with long (10 s) pulses and firm pressure at a low (12–15 W) power setting. The probe is then removed slowly from the ulcer with gentle irrigation to prevent pulling coagulated tissue, and thermal coagulation is repeated as needed to stop bleeding and flatten any underlying visible vessel. Epinephrine injection can be repeated if rebleeding persists. Alternatively, injection of epinephrine followed by hemoclip placement directly across the actively bleeding site is also effective. The same technique can also be used to treat ulcers with NBVVs.

Adherent clots (see Figure 38.1c)

An adherent clot is defined as a clot in the ulcer base that is resistant to being dislodged by vigorous target jet water irrigation. The rebleed rate for ulcers with an adherent clot with medical therapy alone is 8–35%, with most large studies reporting rebleeding rates of 30–35% [68–71]. Randomized controlled studies have shown that endoscopic treatment of adherent clots can decrease the rebleeding rate to less than 5% [70,71]. A metaanalysis found that endoscopic therapy is superior to medical therapy for preventing recurrent bleeding from peptic ulcers with an adherent clot, but there were no differences in other clinical outcomes [72].

The approach to treatment of an adherent clot on an ulcer is to inject epinephrine (1:20 000) in 1 mL increments in four quadrants around the pedicle of the clot followed by use of a cold snare to guillotine the clot piecemeal, without pulling it off

Table 38.5 Frequencies of stigmata of recent ulcer hemorrhage and the risk of rebleeding with and without endoscopic hemostasis.

Endoscopic appearance	Frequency (%)	Risk of rebleeding (%)	Risk of rebleeding after endoscopic hemostasis (%)
Active spurting	12	90	15–30
Visible vessel	22	50	15–30
Adherent clot	10	33	0–5
Oozing w/o stigmata	14	10	0–5
Flat spot	10	7	N/A
Clean base	32	3	N/A

N/A, not applicable.

the base, until an underlying stigma of hemorrhage is identified in the ulcer base or a clot pedicle ≤3 mm is left. MPEC coagulation or hemoclip placement can then be performed on the residual pedicle and/or if active bleeding or a visible vessel is seen.

Oozing of blood from an ulcer without other stigmata (see Figure 38.1d)

Minor bleeding from an ulcer base (without other stigmata) that continues despite water irrigation and observation warrants endoscopic treatment. Monotherapy with either probes or epinephrine injection reduces the rebleeding rate to <5%. In patients with oozing, the bleeding arteries may be small and the outcomes better than those in patients with active arterial bleeding. Patients with oozing and no other stigmata of hemorrhage (such as a clot or NBVV) can be treated effectively with epinephrine injection alone and have no added benefit from combination therapy, although those patients with active arterial bleeding do benefit presuming there are larger arteries underneath [73].

Clean-based ulcers (see Figure 38.1f)

Patients with clean-based ulcers at endoscopy after target irrigation have a rebleeding rate of less than 5% and do not require endoscopic therapy. There appears to be no difference in outcomes between patients who resume eating immediately after an UGI bleed and those who wait several days before eating [74]. Selected compliant and low-risk patients with clinically mild UGI bleeds and clean-based ulcers can be discharged safely to home with a significant saving in costs [5].

Over-the-scope clip

The over-the-scope clip (OTSC), introduced in 2007, has been used for closure of GI perforations and treatment of bleeding GI lesions. It has the ability to grasp the full thickness of the GI tract wall. The clip consists of a nitinol alloy, which provides significant elasticity. It fits onto a cylindrical cap in the open state, and the cap is mounted onto the tip of the endoscope. The clips are available in a variety of sizes to fit endoscopes with diameters ranging between 8 and 11.5 mm (cap sizes 11–14 mm). There are different teeth types, and the "atraumatic" type with its blunt teeth is used for treatment of GI bleeding. The clip is applied by stretching a cord with a hand wheel, installed on the suction channel of the endoscope, similar to rubber band ligation devices. The tip of the endoscope approaches the lesion, which is then suctioned into the applicator cap. Stretching the cord with the hand wheel then fires the clip (Figure 38.2).

There have been a few series evaluating the use of the OTSC in GI bleeding. A retrospective study assessed its effect after failure of conventional techniques (injection therapy along with through-the-scope hemoclips). Of 30 patients (23 UGI bleeding and seven LGI bleeding), primary hemostasis was achieved with the clip in 97% [75]. A prospective study evaluated the OTSC as first-line therapy for UGI bleeding in 40 patients. Hemostasis was achieved in all patients and there were no rebleeding events or complications at 30 days of follow-up [76]. In these studies, most patients had peptic ulcer bleeding, while Dieulafoy lesions were encountered in a small minority of patients.

A more recent, randomized controlled trial compared the OTSC to standard endoscopic therapy for initial endoscopic treatment of severe, nonvariceal upper GI bleeding (peptic ulcers and Dieulafoy lesions). In this study of 49 patients, the 30-day rebleed rate was significantly lower in the OTSC treatment group than in the standard therapy group (4% vs 28%). The results from this study appear to relate to the OTSC's superior ability to obliterate arterial blood flow underneath the stigmata of recent hemorrhage [77].

Pharmacological therapy

Acid suppression

In vitro; studies have shown that gastric acid inhibits platelet aggregation and promotes fibrinolysis. Platelet aggregation is impaired in a slightly acidic environment and is virtually absent when the pH is below 6. Gastric acid converts pepsinogen to pepsin, which digests blood clots [78]. Additionally, the acidic

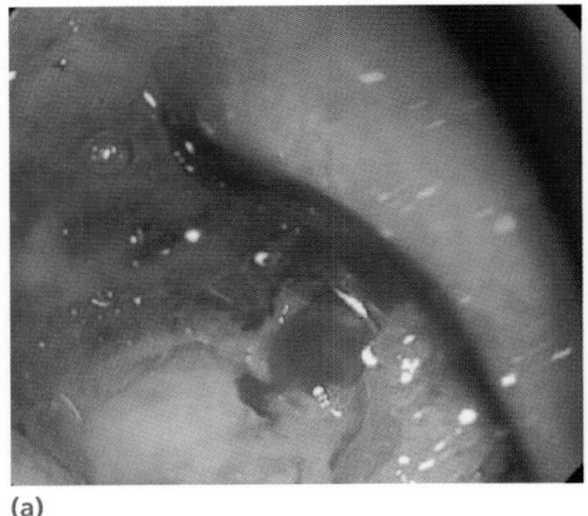
(a)

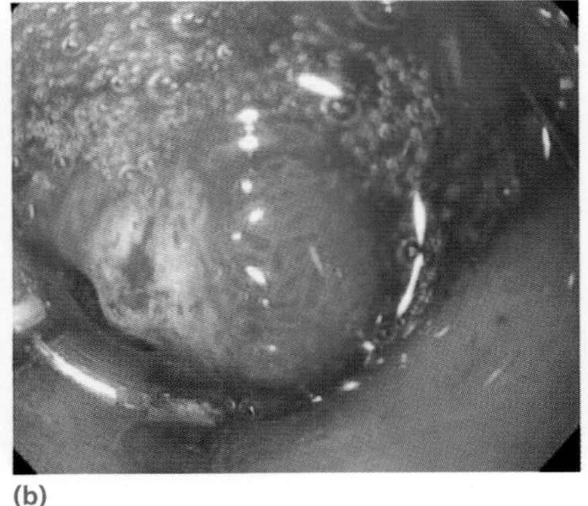
(b)

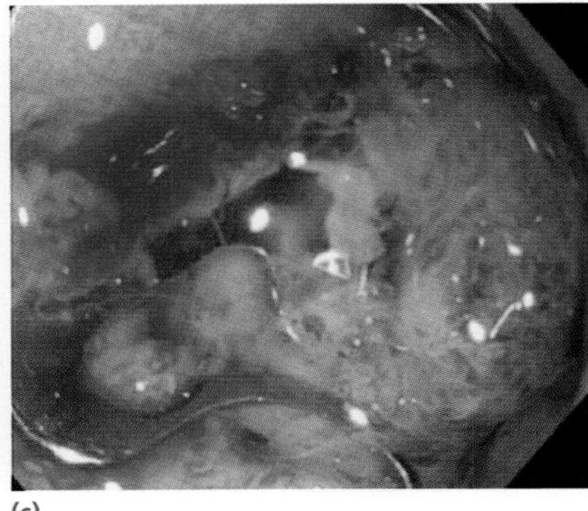
(c)

Figure 38.2 Endoscopic treatment of large duodenal bulb ulcer bleeding with over-the scope clip. (a) Active, arterial-type bleeding; (b) deployment of over-the-scope clip over bleeding focus; (c) post clip placement.

environment promotes plasmin-mediated fibrinolysis, and buffering the acidic medium reduces fibrinolytic activity [78,79]. These results suggest that raising the intragastric pH above 6 may improve hemostasis and reduce clot dissolution. Clinical studies have demonstrated that peptic ulcer rebleeding usually occurs within 72 h of the initial ulcer hemorrhage or after endoscopic hemostasis of ulcers with high-risk stigmata in patients with ulcer bleeding starting as an outpatient [43]. Collectively, these findings provide a rationale for maintaining pH above 6 for at least 72 h after successful endoscopic hemostasis. While intravenous H_2 receptor antagonists can raise the intragastric pH acutely, tolerance to these agents develops rapidly, and trials of intravenous H_2 receptor antagonists for the prevention of recurrent ulcer bleeding have shown no definite benefit [80].

Several studies of PPIs have shown that these agents are effective in reducing rebleeding rates from peptic ulcer. These studies have shown that administration of high-dose PPIs (orally twice a day or intravenous as a bolus followed by a continuous infusion) after endoscopy reduced the rebleeding rate with or without endoscopic hemostasis [81–84]. Another study found that intravenous omeprazole before upper endoscopy in patients with UGI bleeding resulted in a decrease in the number of high-risk stigmata found and the need for endoscopic therapy, but there was no difference in clinical outcomes such as red blood cell transfusions, recurrent bleeding, surgery, or mortality [7]. These findings have been confirmed in systematic and Cochrane reviews [85,86].

The results of PPI trials in Asian patients with peptic ulcer hemorrhage may not be generalizable to heterogeneous non-Asian populations. Asian patients are generally more responsive to PPIs than heterogeneous populations or Caucasians [87]. Asian patients have a smaller average parietal cell mass, are slower metabolizers of PPIs, and often have *H. pylori* infection, all of which increase the effectiveness of PPIs. These factors may explain why there are lower mortality rates in Asians compared with non-Asians in metaanalyses of PPI trials for peptic ulcer hemorrhage. However, one large international study in a predominantly Caucasian study population confirmed the benefit of high-dose intravenous PPI administration in high-risk patients with active arterial bleeding, a NBVV, or an adherent clot [88].

There are still several unresolved issues regarding PPIs and UGI bleeding. It is uncertain whether a PPI should be given before or after endoscopy. Although some randomized studies have not shown preendoscopy administration of a PPI to improve clinical outcomes, most modeling studies suggest that administration of a PPI prior to endoscopy is cost-effective [7,9,10,89,90]. Also, whether administration of an oral PPI is as effective as intravenous administration is unclear, although it has been shown that high-dose oral PPI administration (e.g., 160 mg or more in divided doses/day) reduces rebleeding to rates that would be expected from endoscopic hemostasis. Additionally, it has been shown that the increase in intragastric pH with high-dose oral PPI administration is similar to that with intravenous PPI administration [81,91]. Finally, intravenous administration of a PPI by high-dose continuous drip (e.g., 80 mg bolus and infusion of 8 mg/h for 72 h) or intermittent boluses (e.g., 40–80 mg every 6–12 h) is a matter of controversy, but most data favor continuous drip, with small comparative studies suggesting that continuous infusion decreases the rate of rebleeding and need for surgery compared with intermittent dosing [92].

Proton pump inhibitors post endoscopy based on stigmata

Patients who have undergone endoscopic hemostasis for active arterial bleeding, a NBVV, or an adherent clot should receive continuous intravenous PPI infusions. After successful endoscopic treatment and recovery from sedation, the patient can be started on a liquid diet, with subsequent advancement of the diet. The PPI infusion can be changed to a twice-daily oral regimen after 72 h, as long as the patient is tolerating oral or enteral nutrition. Patients with a clean-based ulcer in the ulcer base can generally resume a normal diet immediately, begin an oral PPI once daily, and be discharged from the emergency department or hospital when stable. Patients with intermediate-risk stigmata (oozing from an ulcer and with no other stigmata; or flat spot with underlying arterial blood flow detected by DEP) should receive oral PPI and observation in the hospital for 24–48 h after endoscopic hemostasis [76,77]. Such patients do not benefit from a high-dose intravenous PPI after successful endoscopic hemostasis. Oral PPI therapy may be continued for 8 weeks. Patients who need to take NSAIDs or antiplatelet agents chronically may need to continue taking a PPI indefinitely to protect against future peptic ulcer formation and bleeding.

Somatostatin and octreotide

Intravenous administration of somatostatin and its long-acting form octreotide has been shown to decrease the risk of rebleeding from peptic ulcers when compared with placebo or an H_2 receptor blocker. The proposed mechanisms of action include reductions in splanchnic and gastroduodenal mucosal blood flow, decreases in GI motility, inhibition of gastric acid secretion, inhibition of pepsin secretion, and gastric mucosal cytoprotective effects. However, these drugs have not been studied for this indication in the era of endoscopic therapy or PPIs and should not be considered for routine use [93].

Repeat endoscopy

Routine repeat, or "second-look," endoscopy 24 h after initial endoscopic hemostasis, with additional endoscopic hemostasis if persistent high-risk endoscopic stigmata are found, is not recommended for most patients with peptic ulcer bleeding [61]. However, this may be appropriate in patients who had an incomplete initial endoscopic examination because of excessive blood that obscured the view or technical problems with hemostasis. Patients with severe rebleeding should also undergo a repeat endoscopy. When endoscopic hemostasis is repeated in patients with hemodynamically significant rebleeding after initial endoscopic treatment, almost 75% of patients can achieve sustained hemostasis and not require surgery. Factors that predict failure of endoscopic retreatment include an ulcer size of at least 2 cm and hypotension on initial presentation [94]. Recently, a multicenter randomized controlled trial of peptic ulcer rebleeding reported significantly lower ulcer rebleeding rates for OTSC than with standard hemostasis retreatment [76].

Angiography and surgery

Patients with recurrent bleeding despite repeat endoscopic attempts to achieve hemostasis should be considered for angiographic or surgical therapy. Interventional angiography (IR) with embolization has become more widely available (Figure 38.3). Studies have reported no significant difference between angiographic embolization and surgery with regard to the rebleed rate and mortality, despite the older age of and greater medical comorbidities in patients treated by angiography [95,96]. These studies suggest that angiography can be considered for use before surgery. If embolization does not control the bleeding, surgery remains an option.

The ultimate choice between interventional angiography and surgery often depends on local expertise, as well as the patient's ability to undergo surgery safely or to tolerate the delay in surgery to permit a trial of angiography. In the future, deployment of the large OTSC as initial endoscopic treatment or for rebleeding of peptic ulcers or Dieulafoy lesions is expected to reduce the need for either surgery or IR because rates of further rebleeding, complications, and red blood cell transfusions are significantly lower than with standard endoscopic hemostasis [76,77]. Also, not all hospitals have the availability of emergency surgery or IR for treatment of severe GI bleeding [76,77].

Acute surgical intervention is indicated in patients who have exsanguination and/or cannot achieve hemodynamic instability despite medical resuscitation. Surgery should also be considered if the endoscopist does not feel a large or pulsating visible vessel (e.g., one in a deep, posterior duodenal ulcer that may represent the gastroduodenal artery) is amenable to endoscopic control. Another reason for surgery is a locally confined bleeding mass.

Ulcer hemorrhage in hospitalized patients

Hemorrhage from an ulcer or erosions (previously referred to as "stress ulcers") in hospitalized patients falls into two categories. The classic type is stress-related mucosal injury (SRMI or "stress ulcers"), which is characterized by diffuse bleeding from erosions and superficial ulcers. The second type is "inpatient ulcers," which are large focal chronic-appearing ulcers that are painless and present with severe inpatient UGI hemorrhage.

Stress-related mucosal injury in the UGI tract of severely ill patients in the intensive care unit is likely due to mucosal ischemia and decreased mucosal protection. SRMI usually occurs in the stomach but can also be seen in the duodenum and esophagus. Diffuse oozing is common, and patients have a high rebleed rate and poor prognosis, often related to impaired healing and multiorgan failure. The two main risk factors are severe coagulopathy and mechanical ventilation for more than 48 h. The incidence of clinically significant GI bleeding with either or both of these risk factors is 3.7% compared with 0.1% when neither risk factor is present [97]. Because SRMI is diffuse, endoscopic therapy is generally not feasible. If patients are supported hemodynamically, the lesions will heal as the overall medical status improves. By contrast, focal inpatient ulcer hemorrhage often requires endoscopic hemostasis for severe hemorrhage. Rebleeding rates are higher and healing rates are slower than those in patients in whom bleeding starts before hospitalization [55].

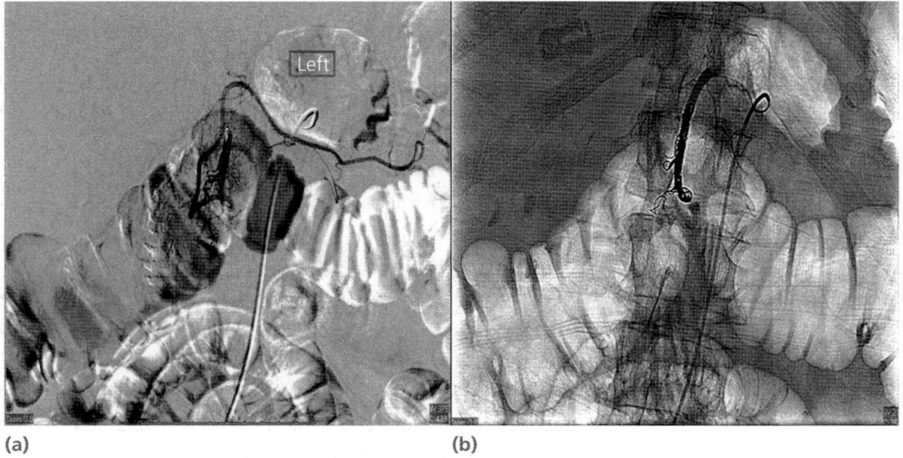

Figure 38.3 Angiography of a patient with a severe posterior duodenal bulb ulcer bleed that could not be stopped endoscopically. **(a)** Contrast is seen filling into the small intestine from a branch of the gastroduodenal artery. **(b)** After several coils were inserted transarterially, no further extravasation was observed.

Esophagitis (see Chapter 43)

Severe erosive esophagitis can present with hematemesis or melena and accounts for 8% of all UGI bleeding. Independent risk factors for bleeding include moderate to severe cirrhosis, a poor performance status, and anticoagulant therapy [98]. Endoscopy is critical to diagnosing severe erosive esophagitis, but endoscopic therapy generally does not have a role unless a focal ulcer with a stigma of recent hemorrhage is detected. These patients should be treated with a daily PPI for 8–12 weeks and undergo repeat endoscopy to rule out underlying Barrett esophagus.

Patients may present with mild UGI bleeding from esophagitis not related to GERD, such as infectious (*Candida*, herpes simplex virus, cytomegalovirus – see Chapter 43) or pill-induced esophagitis. A careful history, along with endoscopic biopsies and/or brushings, is critical for making the diagnoses and determining the appropriate pharmacological therapy.

Dieulafoy lesions

A Dieulafoy lesion is a large (1–3 mm) submucosal artery that protrudes through the mucosa, is not associated with a peptic ulcer, and can cause massive bleeding. Typically, it is located in the gastric fundus, although lesions in the duodenum, small intestine, and colon have been reported. The etiology is unknown.

A Dieulafoy lesion can be difficult to identify at endoscopy because of the intermittent nature of the bleeding, and the overlying mucosa may appear normal if the lesion is not bleeding. A NBVV or adherent clot without an ulcer may be seen on endoscopy. If a massive UGI bleed seems to be emanating from the stomach, then a careful inspection of the proximal stomach should be carried out to look for a protuberance that might be a Dieulafoy lesion. Because of the difficulty of identifying the bleeding site, if a Dieulafoy lesion is found and treated, the site may be marked with submucosal injection of ink to tattoo the area in case of rebleeding.

Endoscopic hemostasis of a Dieulafoy lesion can be performed with injection therapy, a thermal probe, a clip device or by band ligation. Studies have reported an initial hemostasis rate of approximately 90%, with the need for surgery in 4–16% of cases. Rebleeding after initially successful hemostasis is infrequent [99–102]. Randomized controlled trials of newer treatments such as DEP-assisted hemostasis or OTSC have reported lower rebleeding rates compared to standard endoscopic hemostasis [58,77].

Mallory–Weiss tears (see Chapter 48)

Mallory–Weiss tears are mucosal or submucosal lacerations that occur at the gastroesophageal junction and usually extend distally into a hiatal hernia. Patients generally present with hematemesis or coffee-ground emesis, and typically report preceding nonbloody emesis, although some patients do not recall any vomiting. It is likely due to the combination of increased intraabdominal pressure and shearing effect from the negative intrathoracic pressure above the diaphragm. Endoscopy usually reveals a single tear that begins at the gastroesophageal junction and extends several millimeters distally into a hiatal hernia sac. A retroflexed view in the stomach may provide better visualization than the forward-viewing position. The bleeding stigmata of Mallory–Weiss tears can include a clean base, oozing, or active spurting. Usually the bleeding is self-limited and mild, but occasionally it can be severe. Superficial (mucosal) Mallory–Weiss tears can start healing within hours and can heal completely within 48 h.

Although approximately 50% of patients hospitalized with UGI bleeding from a Mallory–Weiss tear receive blood transfusions, in a majority of patients, the tear manifests as mild, self-limited hematemesis for which medical care is not sought [103]. Patients with active bleeding from a Mallory–Weiss tear should undergo endoscopic therapy, which can be performed effectively with epinephrine injection, thermal probe, or hemoclip placement.

If they have persistent nausea or vomiting, patients with a Mallory–Weiss tear are often treated with antiemetics and a PPI to accelerate mucosal healing. The PPI may allow better natural hemostasis by raising the gastric pH to improve coagulation and possibly speed the healing of the tear, but most Mallory–Weiss tears heal within days even without PPI therapy.

Cameron lesions

Cameron lesions are linear erosions or ulcerations in the proximal stomach at the end of a large hiatal hernia near the diaphragmatic pinch [104]. Cameron lesions likely are caused by mechanical trauma and local ischemia, as the hernia moves against the diaphragm, and less likely due to acid and pepsin. More commonly, they present as slow GI bleeding and iron deficiency anemia. They are a common cause of obscure GI bleeding, and may be missed by an unsuspecting endoscopist. Although endoscopic management has been reported [105], the long-term medical management is usually with iron supplements and an oral PPI [106]. Surgery to correct a large hiatal hernia is indicated and can be curative in patients who fail medical therapy [107].

Upper gastrointestinal malignancy

Malignancy accounts for 1% of severe UGI bleeds. The tumors are usually large ulcerated masses. Endoscopic hemostasis with MPEC, APC, injection therapy, or hemoclips can temporarily control acute bleeding in most patients and allow time to determine the appropriate long-term management [108,109]. However, the rebleeding rate is high. Angiographic embolization should be considered for patients with severe UGI bleeding caused by malignancy that does not respond well to endoscopic therapy.

Angiodysplasia and gastric antral vascular ectasia (see Chapter 113)

Angiodysplasia, or vascular ectasia, is responsible for 5–7% of UGI bleeding cases. It is associated with chronic kidney disease, cirrhosis, prior radiation, hereditary hemorrhagic telangiectasia

(HHT), and possibly aortic valve disease. Endoscopically, these appear as superficial, red vascular lesions, ranging in quantity from single to innumerable [110–112]. Patients usually present with melena and a mildly decreased hemoglobin or iron deficiency anemia suggesting a slow UGI bleed.

Gastric antral vascular ectasia (GAVE), also described as "watermelon stomach," is characterized by rows or stripes of vascular ectasias that emanate from the pylorus and extend proximally into the antrum (see Chapter 113). The etiology is uncertain. GAVE has been associated with cirrhosis and systemic sclerosis. There are two endoscopic patterns of GAVE: linear arrays (classic GAVE) and diffuse type [113]. Because there are no effective medical therapies, the mainstay of palliative treatment is via endoscopy.

Endoscopic hemostasis with thermal heat modalities such as laser, MPEC, or APC has been used successfully. Endoscopic hemostasis and ablation with thermal modalities can result in good palliation with an increase in the hemoglobin and a reduced need for blood transfusions and hospitalization [113,114]. Usually several sessions, approximately 4–8 weeks apart, are needed to achieve eradication of the lesions and a reduction in bleeding from the ectasias. APC for GAVE is equally effective in cirrhotic and noncirrhotic patients [113,115]. Band ligation, radiofrequency ablation, and cryotherapy can also eradicate GAVE in selected patients [116–118].

Portal hypertensive gastropathy

Portal hypertensive gastropathy (PHG) is caused by increased portal venous pressure that leads to ectatic blood vessels in the gastric body and fundus with potential oozing of blood. Usually, patients with severe PHG present with chronic blood loss, but they occasionally manifest acute bleeding. Severe PHG with diffuse bleeding is treated by measures that decrease portal pressure, usually with β-blockers, transjugular intrahepatic portosystemic shunt (TIPS), or surgically created shunt. Endoscopic treatment has a limited role unless obvious focal bleeding sites are identified [113]. Liver transplantation provides definitive treatment.

Hemobilia and hemosuccus pancreaticus

Hemobilia may occur in patients who have undergone a liver biopsy, experienced liver trauma, manipulation of the hepatobiliary system (such as with endoscopic retrograde cholangiopancreatogram, percutaneous transhepatic cholangiogram, or TIPS) or have hepatocellular carcinoma, cholangiocarcinoma, or a biliary parasitic infection. The diagnosis is established by identification of blood emanating from the ampulla and demonstrable extravasation from a branch of the hepatic artery during angiography. Treatment is with angiographic embolization [119].

Hemosuccus pancreaticus is a rare form of UGI bleeding that occurs most commonly in patients with acute pancreatitis, chronic pancreatitis, pancreatic pseudocyst, pancreatic cancer, or after endoscopic retrograde cholangiopancreatogram with pancreatic duct manipulation. It can also result from rupture of a splenic artery aneurysm into the pancreatic duct [120]. CT may demonstrate the relevant pancreatic pathology. Blood may be seen from the ampulla at endoscopy, and angiography can demonstrate a splenic artery aneurysm with possible extravasation. Management of hemorrhage is usually best accomplished by angiographic embolization or surgery.

Aortoenteric fistula

Bleeding from an aortenteric fistula is usually acute and massive, and carries with it a high mortality rate [121]. A primary aortoenteric fistula is a communication between the native abdominal aorta (usually an atherosclerotic abdominal aortic aneurysm) and, most commonly, the third portion of the duodenum [122]. Secondary aortoenteric fistulas usually occur between the small intestine and an infected abdominal aortic surgical graft. The fistula usually forms between 3 and 5 years after graft placement. Patients often experience a "herald bleed" that is mild and self-limited, and occasionally intermittent, before massive bleeding occurs [123]. Occasionally, the diagnosis of an aortoenteric fistula is suspected by a history of abdominal aortic aneurysm or by palpation of a pulsatile abdominal mass. The diagnosis can be difficult to make on endoscopy in the absence of active bleeding, although a synthetic graft in the lumen of the third portion of the duodenum may be seen with an enteroscope in some patients. Changes in surgical technique and recognition of this complication, of aortic graft placement, have made this less common.

Patients with an acute UGI bleed and a history of an aortic aneurysm repair should undergo urgent CT or MRI with intravenous contrast, push enteroscopy to evaluate the third portion of the duodenum for compression or blood as well as to exclude other bleeding sources, and/or vascular surgery consultation. CT or MRI may show inflammation around the graft and may demonstrate the fistula. Surgical treatment is necessary to remove the usually infected graft. Therapeutic endoscopy does not play a role in the management of bleeding from an aortoenteric fistula.

Varices (see also Chapter 124)

Esophageal variceal bleeding caused by portal hypertension is the second most common cause of severe UGI bleeding. The acute mortality rate with each bleed is approximately 30%, and the survival rate in the past was less than 40% after 1 year with medical management alone [124]. Despite advances in medical therapy, endoscopic hemostasis, and IR procedures, overall long-term survival rates have not improved significantly for patients with variceal bleeding. While liver transplantation may improve survival in selected patients, survival in nontransplanted patients with variceal bleeding is heavily influenced by the severity of the underlying liver disease, with lower survival rates for patients with Child–Pugh class C cirrhosis. Treatment of gastric variceal bleeding remains a challenge. In contrast to esophageal varices, gastric varices tend to be larger and extend into the deeper layers of the gastric wall.

Management of acute variceal bleeding

Medical therapy

Somatostatin and octreotide cause selective splanchnic vasoconstriction and lower portal pressure, without causing the cardiac depressive complications seen with vasopressin (even in combination with nitroglycerin). Studies have yielded mixed results as to whether somatostatin is more effective than placebo in managing variceal bleeding, but it seems to be at least as effective as vasopressin and significantly safer. A metaanalysis showed that vasoactive drugs – octreotide, somatostatin, terlipressin (a long-acting vasopressin analog) – are as effective as sclerotherapy for controlling variceal bleeding and cause fewer severe adverse events [11]. No studies have shown a survival benefit from either vasopressin or somatostatin in patients with variceal bleeding. Given the potential ability to control acute variceal hemorrhage, and its low toxicity, octreotide (or possibly somatostatin where available outside the USA) appears to be the pharmacological drug of choice as an adjunct to endoscopic therapy for the treatment of variceal hemorrhage. It is frequently started before endoscopy when the physician suspects bleeding is due to a variceal source or other lesion related to portal hypertension, such as a postbanding ulcer. The dose of octreotide for acute variceal hemorrhage is a 50 μg bolus followed by a continuous infusion of 50 μg/h for up to 5 days.

Patients with an elevated INR that does not correct with fresh frozen plasma may benefit from infusion of human recombinant factor VIIa. However, a randomized controlled trial using recombinant factor VIIa in patients with advanced cirrhosis (Child–Pugh class B–C) and acute variceal bleeding failed to show better bleeding control rates (at 24 h and 5 days) compared to placebo [125].

Balloon tamponade

Although once essentially the only available modality, balloon tamponade of varices is seldom used now to control variceal bleeding. It may be used to stabilize a patient with massive bleeding prior to definitive therapy. Varices lie in the submucosa of the esophagus and cardia, and are amenable to physical tamponade.

Three types of tamponade balloons are available. The Sengstaken–Blakemore tube has gastric and esophageal balloons, with a single aspirating port in the stomach. The Minnesota tube also has gastric and esophageal balloons and has aspiration ports in the esophagus and stomach. The Linton–Nachlas tube has a single large gastric balloon and aspiration ports in the stomach and esophagus. The greatest effect comes from tamponade of varices at the gastroesophageal junction, which feed the esophageal varices. Most reports suggest that balloon tamponade provides initial control of bleeding in 85–98% of cases, but variceal rebleeding recurs soon after the balloon is deflated in 21–60% of patients [126].

The major problem with tamponade balloons is a 30% rate of serious complications, such as aspiration pneumonia, esophageal rupture, and airway obstruction. Patients should be intubated before placement of a tamponade balloon to minimize the risk of pulmonary complications.

Endoscopic sclerotherapy

Endoscopic variceal sclerotherapy involves injecting a sclerosant into or adjacent to esophageal varices. Ethanolamine oleate, sodium tetradecyl sulfate, sodium morrhuate, and ethanol have all been employed as sclerosants [127]. Cyanoacrylate is a glue that, when injected into esophageal or gastric varices, polymerizes and usually stops bleeding. However, it can be dangerous and difficult to use and has not been approved by the Food and Drug Administration. Although various techniques may be used, a combination of ethanolamine oleate and ethanol in a volume ratio of 2:1, injecting 2 cm^3 of sclerosant into the bleeding focus to achieve initial hemostasis has been effective in the authors' experience. Sclerotherapy is repeated every 1–4 weeks until all varices are obliterated [128]. Sclerotherapy can be used to treat acutely bleeding esophageal and gastric varices. Esophageal varices are more amenable than gastric varices to eradication with endoscopic therapy.

Studies suggest that sclerotherapy leads to improved immediate hemostasis and a reduction in acute rebleeding compared to medical therapy alone for bleeding esophageal varices. Although hemostasis can be achieved in 85–95% of cases, rebleeding occurs in 25–30% of patients [129]. Complications of endoscopic variceal sclerotherapy include esophageal ulcer bleeding, perforation, esophageal strictures, mediastinitis, pleural effusions, aspiration pneumonia, acute respiratory distress syndrome, chest pain, fever, and bacteremia. These potential complications have made band ligation the generally preferred endoscopic therapy for variceal bleeding

Endoscopic band ligation

Endoscopic band ligation is similar as a technique to that used to band ligate internal hemorrhoids. A rubber band is placed over a varix, which subsequently undergoes thrombosis, sloughing, and fibrosis. Ligation of varices has a significantly lower complication rate than sclerotherapy, and may further lower the rebleeding rate and improve survival [129–133]. Banding of varices is also faster and easier to teach trainees than sclerotherapy. Combination of band ligation and sclerotherapy may be more effective than either methodology alone [134–138]. However, band ligation may be more technically difficult to perform than sclerotherapy during active variceal bleeding. Generally, either sclerotherapy injection or banding is first used to control active bleeding and then additional bands are placed to ligate all the significant nonbleeding esophageal variceal columns.

Transjugular intrahepatic portosystemic shunts and surgical portosystemic shunts

Placement of a TIPS is an interventional radiological procedure in which an expandable metal stent is placed via percutaneous insertion between the hepatic and portal veins, thereby creating an intrahepatic portosystemic shunt. TIPS is effective in the short-term control of bleeding gastroesophageal varices. Initially considered as a bridge to liver transplantation, it is also used in nontransplant candidates who fail endoscopic hemostasis. Randomized trials that have compared TIPS with endoscopic sclerotherapy and band ligation suggest that TIPS is more effective for the long-term prevention of rebleeding [139]. Complications of TIPS include development of new or worsening hepatic encephalopathy and conversely shunt occlusion [140]. TIPS is usually not possible in patients with thrombosis of the portal vein and not feasible in patients with extensive neoplasia of the liver – either hepatocellular carcinoma or metastatic carcinoma. TIPS does not prolong survival of patients with variceal bleeding compared with endoscopic treatment. In patients with acute variceal bleeding, TIPS is usually reserved for those who fail endoscopic therapy.

A variety of portosystemic shunt operations can be performed to decompress the portal venous system, including mesocaval, portocaval, and splenorenal shunts. Compared to endoscopic therapy, surgical shunts significantly decrease the rebleeding rate but do not improve survival [141]. The distal splenorenal shunt can decrease the risk of hepatic encephalopathy [142]. Surgical shunts are considered in those few patients who have failed endoscopic therapy and who are not candidates for TIPS.

Lower gastrointestinal or colonic bleeding

Lower gastrointestinal bleeding, as defined here, originates in the colon or anorectum. The annual incidence of colonic bleeding is approximately 20/100 000 population, with an increased risk in the elderly [143]. The rate of hospitalization for colonic bleeding is lower than that for UGI bleeding. Patients usually present with painless hematochezia and a decrease in hematocrit but without orthostasis. The most common causes of colonic bleeding are shown in Table 38.6. Diverticulosis is generally the most common cause of acute colonic bleeding, accounting for approximately 30% of cases (see Chapter 69). Colonic polyps or cancer, colitis, and anorectal disorders each account for approximately 20% of cases. Delayed postpolypectomy induced ulcer bleeding is increasing in prevalence, related to screening colonoscopy and removal of larger polyps. The overall mortality rate from colonic bleeding is 3.9% [144]. Independent predictors of in-hospital mortality are age above 70 years, intestinal ischemia, two or more comorbid illnesses, inpatient bleeding after hospitalization for an unrelated condition, coagulopathy, hypovolemia, need for red blood cell transfusions, and male gender. Colorectal polyps and hemorrhoids were associated with a lower mortality risk.

Table 38.6 Causes of colonic bleeding and their frequencies.

Diagnosis	Frequency (%)
Diverticulosis	30
Hemorrhoids	14
Ischemic	12
Inflammatory bowel disease	9
Delayed postpolypectomy induced ulcer	8
Colon cancer/polyps	6
Rectal ulcer	6
Vascular ectasia	3
Radiation colitis/proctitis	3
Other	6

Source: Adapted from UCLA CURE Center database.

In most cases, acute colonic bleeding will stop spontaneously, thereby allowing nonurgent evaluation in most cases. For patients with ongoing or recurrent hematochezia, urgent diagnosis and treatment are required to control the bleeding. In a large patient series, 64% of patients with severe hematochezia required a therapeutic intervention to control continued bleeding or rebleeding [145]. Among these patients, 39% underwent endoscopic treatment, 1% underwent angiographic embolization, and 24% underwent surgery.

Several clinical factors are predictive of severe colonic bleeding (defined as continued bleeding during the first 24 h of hospitalization, with a drop in the hemoglobin of at least 2 g/dL and/or transfusion requirement of at least 2 units of packed red blood cells). These include antiplatelet drug or anticoagulant use, at least two comorbid illnesses, pulse greater than 100/minute, systolic blood pressure <115 mmHg, syncope, and bleeding within 4 h of evaluation [14,31,145,146].

Diagnostic approach

Patients with severe hematochezia should undergo the same careful history taking, physical examination, and laboratory testing described above for the general approach to the patient with UGI bleeding. The history should focus specifically on identifying sources of colon bleeding. Diverticular bleeding should be suspected in patients with painless severe acute hematochezia and a history of diverticulosis. Patients with a history of diverticulitis are not at increased risk of diverticular hemorrhage. However, profuse anal bleeding is often the first manifestation of diverticular disease. Ischemic colitis may be suspected in older patients with acute hematochezia. Although some may have associated abdominal cramping, most do not [147]. A recent polypectomy, particularly occurring 5–7 days prior, suggests a postpolypectomy bleed. A history of recent antibiotic use or inflammatory bowel disease and bloody diarrhea suggests colitis. The acute onset of bright red blood that drips from the anus suggests internal hemorrhoidal bleeding. Prior radiation suggests the possibility of radiation telangiectasia hemorrhage.

Patients should be medically resuscitated. Blood transfusion may not be needed because colon bleeding generally is less severe than UGI bleeding, and usually there is only a modest drop in the hemoglobin. Most patients should undergo initial evaluation with colonoscopy after bowel preparation, although in selected cases anoscopy or flexible sigmoidoscopy without any bowel cleansing or after an enema may be performed. Other diagnostic tests, including radionuclide bleeding scans or angiography, may be used in selected cases or when colonoscopy fails to detect a source of bleeding.

Colonoscopy

Urgent colonoscopy following a rapid bowel purge has been shown to be safe, and provides important diagnostic information, as well as therapeutic intervention in some patients [31,145].

Urgent colonoscopy for severe hematochezia is generally performed 6–18 h after the patient is admitted to hospital. Because most bleeding stops spontaneously, colonoscopy is often performed semi-electively within 24 h of initial hospitalization, to allow the patient to receive blood transfusions and bowel preparation.

The overall rate of identification of a presumed or definite cause of colonic bleeding by colonoscopy ranges from 48% to 90%, with an average of 68% [26]. The optimal time for performing urgent bowel preparation and colonoscopy is unknown. In concept, colonoscopy that is performed sooner should have a higher likelihood of finding a lesion with stigmata of hemorrhage that is amenable to endoscopic hemostasis. However, a retrospective study suggested that in patients with diverticular bleeding, the timing of colonoscopy (0–12 h, 12–24 h, or greater than 24 h after admission) was not significantly associated with finding active bleeding or other stigmata that would permit hemostasis [148]. Early colonoscopy (soon after admission) has been associated with a shorter length of hospitalization, principally because of improved diagnostic yield [149]. Consensus on the optimal approach to patients with severe hematochezia has not been achieved. With use of an urgent endoscopic approach, the diagnostic yield of definitive and presumptive bleeding sites is over 90%, and the estimated direct costs are significantly less than the costs associated with an elective evaluation [14].

Flexible sigmoidoscopy

Flexible sigmoidoscopy can evaluate the rectum and left side of the colon without a standard colonoscopy bowel preparation. Although inadequate for evaluation of the anal canal, flexible sigmoidoscopy alone will yield a diagnosis in approximately 9% of cases [150]. If the distal colon can be adequately cleansed with enemas, an urgent flexible sigmoidoscopy can be useful in patients suspected of having a solitary rectal ulcer, ulcerative colitis, radiation proctitis, distal colon ischemic colitis, postpolypectomy bleeding (in the rectosigmoid), or internal hemorrhoids. Therapeutic hemostasis can be provided with injection therapy, hemoclip placement, band ligation, OTSC, and MPEC. Monopolar electrocautery (i.e., APC, snare polypectomy, or hot biopsy forceps) should not be used in an unprepped or poorly prepped colon to avoid the risk of igniting flammable colonic gas.

Anoscopy

Anoscopy can be useful in patients in whom actively bleeding internal hemorrhoids or other anorectal disorders such as anal fissures are suspected. However, colonoscopy may still be necessary to exclude more proximal lesions.

Angiography

The diagnostic yield of angiography depends on patient selection, the timing of the procedure, and the skill of the angiographer, with positive results in 12–69% of cases. The major disadvantage of angiography is that only active bleeding can be detected. Nonbleeding stigmata (such as adherent clots, visible vessels, or flat spots) and specific lesion etiology cannot be identified [151]. An advantage of angiography is that embolization can be performed to control some bleeding lesions. Major complications occur in 3% of cases, including bowel ischemia, hematoma formation, femoral artery thrombosis, contrast dye reactions, acute kidney injury, and transient ischemic attacks [24].

Computed tomography

Multidetector CT can identify abnormalities in the colon that could be a source of bleeding, such as diverticulosis, colitis, masses, and varices. CT is often appropriate if the patient is having hematochezia with abdominal pain.

Surgery

Surgical management is infrequently needed in patients with colonic bleeding since most bleeding is either self-limited or easily managed with medical or endoscopic therapy. The most common indications for surgery are malignancy, diffuse bleeding that fails to cease with medical therapy (as in ischemic or ulcerative colitis), and recurrent bleeding from a diverticulum not controlled via colonoscopy or by angiographic embolization.

Diverticulosis (see Chapter 69)

Colonic diverticula are herniations of colonic mucosa and submucosa through the muscular layers of the colon. Histologically, they are actually pseudodiverticula, because they do not contain all layers of the colonic wall. Diverticula form when colonic tissue is pushed out by intraluminal pressure at points of entry of the small arteries (vasa recta), where they penetrate the circular muscle layer of the colonic wall. These are areas of relative weakness through which the mucosa and submucosa can herniate when intraluminal pressure is increased. Diverticula vary in diameter from a few millimeters to several centimeters and are located most commonly in the left colon. However, right-sided and pandiverticulosis are not uncommon. Most colonic diverticula are asymptomatic and remain uncomplicated. In Asia, it is reported that diverticula in the right colon are a common site of bleeding [152]. Two-thirds of definitive diverticular bleeds (with stigmata of hemorrhage) emanate from the region of the splenic flexure of the colon or proximally [151]. Bleeding may occur from vessels at the neck or base of a diverticulum, with the frequency of bleeding from each location being roughly equal [14,31,151,153].

Diverticular hemorrhage should be classified carefully based on findings at colonoscopy, particularly in the case of elderly patients with severe hematochezia who are likely to have colonic diverticulosis [14]. Definitive diverticular hemorrhage is diagnosed when stigmata of recent hemorrhage (active bleeding, visible vessel, adherent clot, or a flat spot with arterial blood flow detected underneath) are seen on colonoscopy. Presumptive diverticular hemorrhage is diagnosed when colonoscopy reveals diverticulosis without stigmata and no other significant lesions are seen in the colon and by anoscopy, terminal ileum examination, push enteroscopy, and capsule endoscopy. Incidental diverticulosis is the designation used when colonic diverticulosis is evident but another lesion is identified as the cause of hematochezia [14]. In a large prospective cohort study, colonic diverticulosis was incidental in 52%, presumptive diverticular hemorrhage occurred in 31%, and definitive diverticular hemorrhage was established in 17% of cases [151].

Stratifying the risk of recurrent diverticular bleeding, by applying the same endoscopic stigmata used in high-risk peptic ulcer bleeding (active bleeding, visible vessel, and clot), has been attempted, but the natural history associated with each of these stigmata is underreported. In at least 75% of patients with diverticular bleeding (presumptive or definitive), the bleeding stops spontaneously, and these patients require transfusion of less than 4 units of packed red blood cells [154]. When stigmata of recent hemorrhage in diverticula were found in patients in a CURE series of 125 patients, they were usually treated endoscopically and the rebleeding rate within 30 days was less than 5% and very few required surgery. However, among 37 patients with stigmata of recent diverticular hemorrhage (active bleeding in 18, visible vessel in five, and adherent clot in 14) who did not undergo endoscopic hemostasis, the rates of rebleeding with transfusion and emergency surgery within 30 days were 65% and 43%, respectively [155].

In long-term follow-up, the outlook for patients with diverticular bleeding is relatively good. In a large prospective cohort study of patients with documented colonic diverticular hemorrhage (definitive or presumptive), the overall rate of rebleeding was 18% in 4 years, but only 50% of these recurrent hemorrhages were due to a diverticular source [151].

Endoscopic hemostasis

The effectiveness of colonoscopic hemostasis for actively bleeding diverticula using MPEC, epinephrine injection, hemoclips, banding, or combination therapy similar to treatment of bleeding peptic ulcers has been reported [14,151,156–159]. If fresh red blood is seen in a defined segment of colon, then that segment should be irrigated vigorously with water in order to remove the blood and detect the underlying bleeding site. If bleeding is coming from the edge of a diverticulum or a pigmented protuberance is seen on the edge, then epinephrine (diluted 1:20 000 in saline) in 1 mL aliquots should be injected submucosally into four quadrants around the bleeding site. Subsequently, MPEC at a low-power setting (10–15 W) and light pressure can be carried out for a 1 s pulse duration to cauterize the diverticular edge and stop bleeding or flatten the visible vessel, or hemoclips can be applied. A nonbleeding adherent clot can be injected with 1:20 000 epinephrine in four quadrants, 1 mL per quadrant, after which the clot can be removed piecemeal with a cold polyp snare until a ≤3 mm pedicle is left above the diverticulum. The underlying stigma can be treated with MPEC or hemoclips, as described above. If the stigma of diverticular hemorrhage is in the base of the diverticulum, then hemoclipping is utilized (not MPEC) after preinjection of dilute epinephrine. This markedly reduces the risk of perforation from the base of the diverticulum after endoscopic hemostasis.

After endoscopic hemostasis of a bleeding diverticulum is completed, a submucosal tattoo should be placed around the lesion to allow identification of the site in case repeat colonoscopy or surgery is required for recurrent bleeding. Patients should be instructed to avoid aspirin and other NSAIDs and to take a daily fiber supplement indefinitely.

A landmark study evaluated urgent colonoscopic hemostasis of severe diverticular hemorrhage [14]. Colonoscopic treatment resulted in a rebleeding rate of 0% compared with 53% rebleeding and 35% requiring emergency hemicolectomy in historical controls with high-risk stigmata that did not receive colonoscopic treatment. No rebleeding had occurred after 3 years of follow-up in the patients who underwent hemostasis. Other studies have also suggested that endoscopic hemostasis is effective for immediate diverticular bleeding, although subsequent rebleeding and the need for surgery have been reported in some cases [160].

Angiography and surgery

Angiographic embolization can be performed in selected cases of diverticular bleeding, but with a risk of bowel infarction, contrast reactions, and acute kidney injury. One study found that routine angiography prior to surgical resection was not helpful in reducing the overall risk of complications [161].

Surgical resection for diverticular bleeding is rarely needed as primary intervention for initial acute bleeding and is reserved for recurrent bleeding [151]. The decision to operate is best guided by colonoscopic, angiographic, or nuclear medicine studies that identify the likely segment of colon from which the bleeding is emanating and the presence of medical comorbidities. Risks of surgical complications are increased in elderly patients. Although often performed in the past when a definite bleeding site could not be identified, blind subtotal colectomy should be avoided, if possible [14,31,151].

Colitis

The term colitis refers to any form of inflammation of the colon. Severe LGI bleeding may be caused by NSAID colitis, ischemic colitis, inflammatory bowel disease, or infectious colitis.

Ischemic colitis can manifest as painless or painful hematochezia. Painless hematochezia usually results from mucosal hypoxia due to hypoperfusion of the intramural vessels of the intestinal wall, whereas medium- to large-vessel occlusion is often painful, clinically more severe, and has worse outcomes [147]. The incidence of ischemic colitis ranges from 4.5 to 44 cases/100 000 person-years [162]. Risk factors associated with ischemic colitis have been reported to include older age, shock, cardiovascular surgery, congestive heart failure, chronic obstructive pulmonary disease, ileostomy, colon cancer, abdominal surgery, irritable bowel syndrome, constipation, laxative use, cocaine use, oral contraceptive use, and use of an H_2 receptor antagonist [162–164]. The colon has an abundant blood supply from the superior and inferior mesenteric arteries, but the watershed areas between the superior and inferior mesenteric arteries have the fewest collateral vessels and are at most risk for ischemia. The colon normally receives 10–35% of cardiac output, and ischemia can occur if blood flow decreases by more than 50%. Although ischemia is most likely to occur in the so-called watershed area of the splenic flexure, it can occur anywhere in the colon [165].

The diagnosis of ischemia is usually made by colonoscopy. However, it can be suspected by the demonstration of "thumb printing" on plain film radiographs or colonic wall thickening on CT. The colonoscopic appearance of the mucosa includes erythema, friability, and exudate. Mucosal biopsy specimens may suggest ischemic changes but are also used to exclude infectious colitis or Crohn's disease. If the underlying reason for hypoperfusion is corrected, the signs and symptoms of ischemic colitis generally resolve within days to weeks, and no further therapy is required. In contrast, patients in whom ischemic colitis develops in hospital or those with large-vessel mesenteric ischemia usually have worse outcomes, including higher rates of rebleeding, perforation, need for surgery, and death [143,147]. In the authors' experience, only about 10% of patients with ischemic colitis and severe hematochezia have a focal ulcer with a major stigma of hemorrhage on colonoscopy, and focal treatment of these lesions with epinephrine injection and hemoclip placement is recommended [147].

Inflammatory bowel disease that involves the colon rarely causes severe acute colonic bleeding. In a case series, the majority of patients with severe hematochezia had Crohn's disease, and most were successfully treated medically [166].

Infectious colitis should be excluded in any patient with LGI bleeding and imaging evidence that suggests colitis. Although significant bleeding is rare, it can be seen with infections caused by *Campylobacter jejuni*, *Salmonella*, *Shigella*, enterohemorrhagic *Escherichia coli* (O157:H7), *Clostridium difficile*, or cytomegalovirus. Diagnosis is made by stool cultures. Treatment is medical, with the use of antibiotics depending on the causative organism. Endoscopic management generally does not have a role in the management of infectious colitis.

Postpolypectomy bleeding

Bleeding occurs after approximately 1–2% of colonoscopic polypectomies; it is most common 5–7 days after polypectomy but can occur from 1 to 14 days after the procedure [167,168]. Although the bleeding is usually self-limited, 50–75% of patients require blood transfusions. Risk factors for delayed postpolypectomy bleeding include polyp size >2 cm, thick stalk, sessile type, location in the right colon, use of warfarin or heparin, and use of antiplatelet drugs (such as clopidogrel, aspirin or other NSAID) [168,169]. In most patients with delayed postpolypectomy bleeding, a chronic appearing ulcer at the site of the prior polypectomy is found on colonoscopy. In patients with severe bleeding, stigmata of recent hemorrhage may be found in the ulceration. Endoscopic management techniques for delayed postpolypectomy ulcer bleeding depend on the stigma found and are similar to those used for peptic ulcer hemorrhage, including epinephrine injection, thermal coagulation, hemoclip placement, and combination therapy.

Colon polyps and cancer

Patients with colon polyps and cancer can present with acute or chronic hematochezia. Often these patients have a microcytic iron deficiency anemia consistent with prolonged GI blood loss before more overt bleeding is manifest. At colonoscopy, epinephrine can be injected into the lesion to slow active bleeding, and hemoclips can be applied to treat ulcerated lesions that cannot be resected endoscopically. When possible, colon polyps should be removed to stop bleeding. Surgical resection is usually required to prevent rebleeding from a large ulcerated lesion.

Radiation telangiectasia

Radiation telangiectasia typically causes mild chronic hematochezia but occasionally can result in acute severe colonic bleeding. Ionizing radiation used to treat gynecological, prostatic, bladder, or rectal tumors causes acute and chronic damage to the normal colon and rectum. Chronic radiation effects occur 6–18 months after completion of treatment and manifest as bright red blood with bowel movements. Bowel injury resulting from chronic radiation is due to vascular damage, with subsequent mucosal ischemia, thickening, and ulceration. Much of this damage is thought to result from chronic hypoxic ischemia and oxidative stress. Flexible sigmoidoscopy or colonoscopy reveals numerous telangiectasia and often friability and/or ulceration in the rectum. Furthermore, active bleeding is observed, in conjunction with multiple non-bleeding telangiectasia in the field of prior radiation therapy.

Initial treatment includes avoidance of aspirin and other NSAIDs, consumption of a high-fiber diet, stool softeners, and iron supplementation if the patient is anemic. Medical therapy with topical or oral 5-aminosalicylic acid products, sucralfate, or glucocorticoids can be tried but generally is ineffective [170]. Focal thermal therapy of telangiectasia is usually successful, including repeated treatments with MPEC or APC [171].

Topical formalin applied directly to the rectal mucosa can reduce bleeding, as can the use of hyperbaric oxygen [172,173]. Radiofrequency ablation has been proposed as another endoscopic method for treatment [174]. Antioxidant, such as vitamins C and E, have also been reported to reduce bleeding from chronic radiation proctitis [175].

Vascular ectasia

A variety of vascular lesions may cause bleeding from the GI tract. Vascular ectasias (also referred to as angiodysplasia, telangiectasia, and angioectasia) are aberrant blood vessels found throughout the GI tract that develop with advancing age. They are distinct from arteriovenous malformations, which are congenital. Vascular ectasia results from dilation of the terminal aspect of a vessel. Any vascular lesions may cause overt or obscure GI bleeding in adults, particularly in the elderly and those who take antiplatelet and anticoagulant drugs. Acquired vascular lesions occur in association with various disorders, such as chronic renal disease, cirrhosis, rheumatoid disorders, and valvular heart disease [176]. Although vascular ectasias may present as overt bleeding, they more often manifest as occult bleeding or iron deficiency anemia. The most common locations are the colon and small intestine. Most angioectasias occur in patients older than age 60 years, and can involve any segment of the GI tract. These are usually multiple lesions in an affected segment of intestine. More than 20% of patients have vascular ectasias in at least two sections of the GI tract [177,178]. No bleeding occurred during a 3-year follow-up among asymptomatic persons found to have colonic angioectasias incidentally [179].

On endoscopy, vascular ectasias appear as 2–10 mm red lesions and may have an arborizing ectatic blood vessel that emanates from a central vessel. Application of pressure on an ectasia with an endoscopic probe may cause the lesion to blanch. Endoscopic treatment can be employed with a variety of modalities, including injection therapy with epinephrine, thermal probe coagulation, argon plasma coagulation, and band ligation. Assessing efficacy can be difficult given the intermittent nature of the blood loss. One older case series of patients with transfusion-requiring vascular ectasias found no difference in the frequency of continued bleeding whether surgery, endoscopic therapy, or blood transfusions alone were used for management [180].

Most patients with GI angioectasias that bleed intermittently require medical treatment in addition to endoscopic hemostasis. Aspirin and other NSAIDs, warfarin, and clopidogrel can exacerbate chronic low-level bleeding and should be avoided if possible. Many patients can be effectively managed with administration of iron (either orally or intravenously).

Internal hemorrhoids

Internal hemorrhoid bleeding is characterized by bright red blood per rectum that may coat the stool, drip into the toilet bowel, and be seen on tissue after wiping. Usually bleeding is mild, intermittent, and self-limited, but severe bleeding requiring transfusion may occur [181]. In a large study of patients with hematochezia discharged from hospital, 20% were thought to have had bleeding from hemorrhoids [144]. The diagnosis can be made by anoscopy, sigmoidoscopy, or colonoscopy.

Treating hemorrhoids (as described in detail in Chapter 68) typically begins with medical therapy, including fiber supplementation, stool softeners, and warm sitz baths. Anoscopic therapy, including injection sclerotherapy, rubber band ligation, cryosurgery, infrared photocoagulation, and MPEC, is used for larger hemorrhoids or those that do not respond to medical management. Surgical hemorrhoidectomy is reserved for treatment of large hemorrhoids not amenable to anoscopic treatment, complicated hemorrhoids in the setting of other anorectal disorders, and patient preference [182].

Anal fissures

Patients with anal fissures present with sharply painful bowel movements, with or without hematochezia. Generally, the bleeding is mild and noticed with wiping; rarely is it more severe. Treatment focuses on resolving the anal fissure, rather than using specific hemostasis techniques. Stool softeners and fiber supplementation are recommended for all patients. Topical therapies include diltiazem, nitroglycerin, and nifedipine. Botulinum toxin injections and lateral sphincterotomy are reserved for patients who do not respond to topical therapies [183].

Rectal varices

Varices may develop in the rectal mucosa between the superior hemorrhoidal veins (portal circulation) and the middle and inferior hemorrhoidal veins (systemic circulation) in patients with severe portal hypertension. In retroflexion, rectal varices are seen endoscopically as vascular structures located several centimeters above the dentate line and extending into the rectum, distinct from internal hemorrhoids. Rectal varices become more common as the severity of portal hypertension progresses. Approximately 60% of patients with a history of bleeding esophageal varices have rectal varices. However, hematochezia is rarely reported in patients with rectal varices. Similar to esophageal varices, bleeding rectal varices are treated with sclerotherapy, band ligation, or a portosystemic shunt [184–186].

Rectal ulcers

Solitary or multiple painless rectal ulcers occur in elderly patients with severe constipation, intensive care unit patients, and people who are bedridden, such as in nursing homes [187]. On colonoscopy, they appear as chronic, large, and single or multiple ulcers. They can be considered a type of stress ulcer of the rectum in extremely ill hospitalized patients. They often have stigmata of recent hemorrhage and can be treated endoscopically. Inpatients with hematochezia from a rectal ulcer have a higher rate of rebleeding than those who present from home. The pathology of the lesions revealed necrosis suggestive of mucosal ischemia, as seen with gastric stress ulcers [187].

Obscure gastrointestinal bleeding

Obscure GI (OGI) bleeding is defined as GI bleeding of uncertain etiology after upper endoscopy and colonoscopy. Obscure GI bleeding may have an overt or occult presentation. Overt OGI bleeding refers to patients who have visible acute GI bleeding (i.e., melena, maroon stool, hematochezia) and a nondiagnostic upper endoscopy and colonoscopy. Occult OGI bleeding refers to patients with a positive fecal occult blood test result, often in association with unexplained iron deficiency anemia. In most large series of GI bleeding, a diagnosis was not made by upper endoscopy and/or colonoscopy in 5% of hospitalized patients with overt GI bleeding, and in 75% of these patients a bleeding site was ultimately found in the small intestine [188]. While most cases of OGI bleeding have a bleeding source in the small intestine beyond the reach of standard endoscopes, other possibilities include: (1) the lesion was within reach of a standard endoscope and colonoscope but not recognized as the bleeding site; and (2) the lesion was within reach of the endoscope and colonoscope but was difficult to visualize (such as postbulbar duodenal lesions) or present intermittently (such as Cameron ulcers) [176]. Causes of OGI bleeding are shown in Box 38.1.

In a patient with recurrent severe unexplained hematochezia, without hypotension, a colonic source should be suspected, and a repeat colonoscopy is warranted. Colonic lesions that can bleed profusely and then stop, such as diverticulosis or hemorrhoids, should be considered. In patients with recurrent severe melena, push enteroscopy should be considered to reexamine the esophagus, stomach, and duodenum, as well as the proximal jejunum.

Box 38.1 Causes of overt obscure gastrointestinal bleeding[a].

Upper gastrointestinal tracta
Cameron lesions
Dieulafoy lesion
Gastric antral vascular ectasia (GAVE, "watermelon stomach")

Small intestine
Aortoenteric fistula
Dieulafoy lesion
Meckel diverticulum
Neoplasm
Pancreatic/biliary disease
Ulcer
Vascular ectasia

Colon
Diverticulosis
Hemorrhoids
Rectal varices
Vascular ectasia

[a] After excluding common causes of upper gastrointestinal bleeding.

Once it is certain that a bleeding lesion in either the UGI tract or LGI tract was not missed, the evaluation should focus on the small intestine. Because small bowel bleeding is often intermittent, nuclear medicine bleeding scans or angiography have limited value in the diagnostic evaluation. These procedures only visualize active bleeding and do not detect clean lesions or those with nonbleeding stigmata. Newer imaging techniques, including wireless capsule enteroscopy and deep enteroscopy, allow greater visualization and more therapeutic options than in the past.

Diagnostic tools

Push enteroscopy

Push enteroscopy can be performed with either a pediatric colonoscope (160 cm in length) or dedicated push enteroscope (220–250 cm). These endoscopes can be used to evaluate the esophagus, stomach, duodenum, and proximal jejunum approximately 50–150 cm beyond the ligament of Treitz [176]. Depth of insertion is often limited by looping of the endoscope in the stomach. Push enteroscopy identifies a potential bleeding site in approximately 50% of patients; 50% of lesions are actually within reach of a standard upper endoscope [176,189,190].

Capsule endoscopy

In patients with severe recurrent GI bleeding, capsule endoscopy can identify a transition point where fresh blood appears in the small bowel, defining a potential locus of bleeding. This can direct subsequent therapeutic procedures such as deep enteroscopy, angiography, or surgery. Although capsule endoscopy may occasionally detect gastric, duodenal, or colonic fresh blood of focal lesions, it is not a substitute for upper endoscopy, push enteroscopy, and colonoscopy.

Capsule endoscopy compares favorably to other small intestinal diagnostic methods. Compared to small bowel barium studies and CT enteroclysis, capsule endoscopy has a much better diagnostic yield [191,192]. Using intraoperative enteroscopy as the gold standard, capsule endoscopy has sensitivity, specificity, positive predictive value, and negative predictive values of 95%, 75%, 95%, and 85%, respectively [193]. The diagnostic yield of capsule endoscopy appears to increase in the setting of ongoing or recent (<2 weeks) overt GI bleeding or severe chronic GI bleeding (hemoglobin <10 g/dL, iron deficiency anemia, or >1 overt bleeding episode) [194,195].

Deep enteroscopy

Specially designed enteroscopes are used in conjunction with an overtube and/or balloons to advance the endoscope by pleating small intestine over it. Available systems include double-balloon enteroscopy (with a balloon on the tip of the endoscope and another balloon on the overtube), single-balloon enteroscopy (a balloon on the overtube only), and spiral enteroscopy. These enteroscopes can be inserted orally (antegrade) and advanced into the proximal/mid-ileum or inserted rectally (retrograde) and advanced to the distal/mid-ileum. On occasion, most often with double-balloon enteroscopy, complete enteroscopy can be performed unidirectionally. Deep enteroscopy allows both visualization and interventions such as biopsy, hemostasis, and tattooing of lesions. Endoscopes used for deep enteroscopy have standard working channels that allow passage of accessories, such as biopsy forceps, MPEC thermal probes, endoscopic hemoclips, and injection needles that fit through standard treatment channels. The risks of deep enteroscopy are similar to those for push enteroscopy or colonoscopy, with the additional small risk of pancreatitis.

Double-balloon enteroscopy has been shown to have a diagnostic yield in 56% in patients with obscure GI bleeding, and this yield increases to 75% if positive findings are first seen on capsule endoscopy [196]. Single-balloon enteroscopy has a diagnostic yield similar to that of double-balloon enteroscopy [197]. Spiral enteroscopy has been compared to single-balloon enteroscopy, and while depth of insertion is greater with spiral enteroscopy, the diagnostic yield is similar [198].

Intraoperative endoscopy and surgical exploration

Surgical exploration of the small intestine can be performed when other studies are nondiagnostic. At surgery, the small bowel should be palpated to detect mass lesions. In general, a standard exploratory laparotomy or laparoscopy is performed first to lyse any adhesions and to look for obvious tumors, a Meckel diverticulum, strictures, enteritis, or large vascular lesions. The small bowel is usually exposed through the abdominal incision to allow the surgeon to assist with advancement of an endoscope within the lumen of the GI tract, and facilitates mucosal visualization by the endoscopist as well as transillumination. The endoscope can be passed transorally for a natural orifice luminal examination or via an enterotomy with use of a sterile endoscope. The surgeon helps advance the endoscope by pleating the small bowel over the endoscope. Any lesion that is identified can then be assessed surgically or endoscopically, depending on the nature of the lesion.

Most series report complete intraoperative enteroscopy of the entire small bowel in 50–75% of cases [199]. The diagnostic yield of intraoperative enteroscopy is up to 88%, but rebleeding after intraoperative enteroscopy has also been reported in up to 60% of patients [188]. The risks of surgical exploration limit this procedure as a diagnostic tool, but in selected patients combined endoscopic and surgical evaluation can be useful and definitive, especially for focal lesions such as GIST tumors, focal ulcers, Crohn's ulcerations, or small bowel Dieulafoy lesions [200].

Approach to the patient with overt obscure gastrointestinal bleeding

A recommended approach to evaluating overt OGI bleeding is provided in Figure 38.4. For patients with unexplained overt GI bleeding and negative push enteroscopy and colonoscopy, capsule endoscopy should be undertaken if available. If a lesion is found in the mid- to small intestine, then deep enteroscopy or surgery may be considered, depending on the nature of the lesion. A lesion in the terminal ileum may prompt repeat colonoscopy or deep enteroscopy via the colonic route. If no

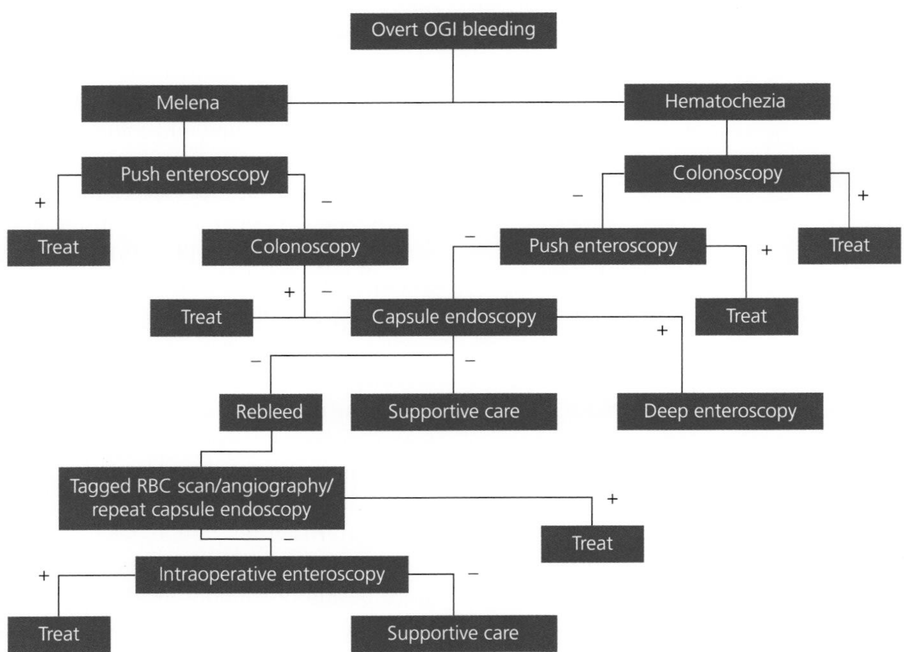

Figure 38.4 Algorithm for diagnostic approach to overt obscure GI (OGI) bleeding, including severe hematochezia. RBC, red blood cells.

lesion is detected on capsule endoscopy but a high suspicion for a lesion remains, repeat capsule endoscopy or enteroscopy should be considered. If deep enteroscopy is negative, intraoperative enteroscopy or supportive medical care (iron supplementation, blood transfusions, etc.) are reasonable alternatives [176, 200].

Causes

Patient age influences the differential diagnosis of obscure GI bleeding. Patients below the age of 40–50 years are more likely to bleed from a small intestinal neoplasm, as well as a Meckel diverticulum, Dieulafoy lesions, and Crohn's disease. Patients above 40–50 years are more likely to bleed from small bowel intestinal vascular ectasias or NSAID-induced ulcers.

Vascular ectasias

Vascular ectasias, including pathogenesis, risk factors, and treatment, are described in detail in the Lower gastrointestinal bleeding section above.

Meckel diverticulum

A Meckel diverticulum is a congenital blind intestinal pouch that results from incomplete obliteration of the vitelline duct during gestation. Meckel diverticula classically follow the "rule of twos": occurring in 2% of the population, found within 2 ft of the ileocecal valve, are 2 in long, result in a complication in 2% of cases, have two types of ectopic tissue (pancreatic and gastric) within the diverticulum, most commonly present at age 2 years (intestinal obstruction), and have a male-to-female ratio of more than 2:1. The most common complications of Meckel diverticula are bleeding, obstruction, and diverticulitis, which can occur in children or adults. Histopathological evaluation of bleeding diverticula reveals ectopic gastric mucosa in 75% of patients, leading to acid secretion and ulceration [201]. The diagnostic test for a Meckel diverticulum is a 99m technetium pertechnetate scan ("Meckel scan"). Meckel scans have a high specificity and positive predictive value, but they can be negative in the 25–50% of patients in whom the diverticulum does not contain gastric mucosa [202]. Meckel diverticula can also be diagnosed by capsule endoscopy and double-balloon enteroscopy.

Small intestinal neoplasms

Tumors of the small intestine make up 5–7% of all GI tract neoplasms, but are the most common cause of obscure GI bleeding in patients younger than age 50 years [203]. Such neoplasms include adenomas (usually duodenal), adenocarcinomas, carcinoid tumors, GI stromal tumors (GISTs), lymphomas, hamartomatous polyps (such as with Peutz–Jeghers syndrome), and juvenile polyps.

NSAID-induced small bowel ulcers and erosions

Mucosal ulcers or erosions develop in the small intestine in 25–55% of patients who take nonselective NSAIDs, and can be seen on capsule endoscopy. Patients who take selective COX-2 inhibitors have lower rates of mucosal ulcers on capsule endoscopy [204–207].

Blue rubber bleb nevus syndrome

Blue rubber bleb nevus syndrome is a rare condition characterized by venous malformations in the skin, soft tissues, and GI tract. Bleeding usually starts in childhood and continues into adulthood. It frequently results in iron deficiency requiring iron replacement and transfusions. Endoscopically, the lesions appear as large, protuberant, polypoid venous blebs. They can occur anywhere in the GI tract, but are more common in the small bowel and colon, and can be treated by endoscopic band ligation or surgical resection [208,209].

References are available at www.yamadagastro.com/textbook7e

Further reading

Barkun A.N., Bardou M., Kuipers E.J., et al. International consensus recommendations on the management of patients with nonvariceal upper gastrointestinal bleeding. Ann Intern Med 2010;152:101.

Jensen D.M., Ohning G.V., Kovacs T.O.G., et al. Natural history of definitive hemorrhage based upon stigmata of recent hemorrhage and Doppler blood flow monitoring for risk stratification and definitive hemostasis. Gastrointest Endosc 2016;83;416.

Kahi C.J., Jensen D.M., Sung J.J., et al. Endoscopic therapy versus medical therapy for bleeding peptic ulcer with adherent clot: a metaanalysis. Gastroenterology 2005;129:855.

Lau J.Y., Leung W.K., Wu J.C., et al. Omeprazole before endoscopy in patients with gastrointestinal bleeding. N Engl J Med 2007;356:1631.

Raju G.S., Gerson L., Das A., et al. American Gastroenterological Association (AGA) Institute technical review on obscure gastrointestinal bleeding. Gastroenterology 2007;133:1697.

Sung J.J., Barkun A., Kuipers E.J., et al. Intravenous esomeprazole for prevention of recurrent peptic ulcer bleeding: a randomized trial. Ann Intern Med 2009;150:455.

Teshima C.W., Kuipers E.J., van Zanten S.V., et al. Double balloon enteroscopy and capsule endoscopy for obscure gastrointestinal bleeding: an updated meta-analysis. J Gastroenterol Hepatol 2011; 26:796.

Villanueva C., Colomo A., Bosch A., et al. Transfusion strategies for acute upper gastrointestinal bleeding. N Engl J Med 2013;368:11.

CHAPTER 39

Approach to the patient with abnormal liver chemistries or jaundice

Yumi Ando and Joseph Ahn
Oregon Health and Science University, Portland, OR, USA

Chapter menu

Introduction

The liver is a complex organ with over 500 different functions. Some of the better-known functions of the liver include the formation and secretion of bile, maintenance of glucose homeostasis, metabolism of cholesterol and lipids, and breakdown of toxins. It has a large functional reserve capacity, with only 20–30% of liver volume needed to maintain hepatic function [1]. It is also a resilient organ as it can regenerate after injury or surgical resection. Nevertheless, despite these characteristics, the liver is highly susceptible to injury because drugs and toxins absorbed by the gastrointestinal tract are immediately presented to the liver through the portal vein. It is critically important to detect liver injury before significant or irreversible damage occurs. However, the challenge is that most liver diseases are asymptomatic until late stages and liver chemistries may remain normal even when there is substantial liver injury. Nonetheless, laboratory abnormalities are often the first clue to liver dysfunction and liver injury.

Alanine aminotransferase, aspartate aminotransferase, alkaline phosphatase, total bilirubin, direct bilirubin, protein, and albumin are often lumped together as a laboratory panel and are commonly referred to as the "liver function tests" (LFT). This is a misnomer as not all of these markers reflect hepatic function and thus, in this chapter they will be referred to as "liver chemistries" instead. The widespread availability of the liver chemistry panel has led to it often being obtained as part of routine physicals, health insurance screens, and during hospital stays for reasons unrelated to assessment for liver injury or disease. Prudent utilization of the liver chemistry panel as clinically indicated in Table 39.1 can help improve the value and yield of testing.

When evaluating a patient with abnormal liver chemistries, a thoughtful approach with the goal of providing high-value care should be emphasized. Not all patients with abnormalities in the liver chemistry panel have liver disease [2]. A population-based study in Scotland showed that when liver chemistries were obtained in asymptomatic patients without obvious signs of liver disease, over 20% had at least one abnormal liver chemistry, but only 1% developed liver disease after median follow-up of almost 4 years [3]. It is important to recognize that the liver chemistry values can be abnormal from nonhepatic causes, as will be elucidated in this chapter.

Of those who do have underlying liver disease, the majority will have common diseases. Though there is some variability depending on the country of practice, in general, nonalcoholic fatty liver disease (NAFLD) is the most common chronic liver disease. The global prevalence of NAFLD is estimated to be 25% based on currently available epidemiology data and is rapidly growing due to the obesity epidemic [4]. In the US, it will soon become the leading indication for liver transplantation [5]. Alcoholic liver disease also remains a common cause. In the US, it is currently the number one indication for liver transplant [6,7]. Globally, over 50% of mortality related to cirrhosis is attributable

Yamada's Textbook of Gastroenterology, Seventh Edition. Edited by Timothy C. Wang, Michael Camilleri, Benjamin Lebwohl, Anna S. Lok, William J. Sandborn, Kenneth K. Wang, and Gary D. Wu.

Companion website: www.yamadagastro.com/textbook7e

Table 39.1 When to order a liver chemistry panel.

1. Clinical suspicion for hepatobiliary disease or injury
2. Monitoring of known liver disease
3. Monitoring for hepatic adverse effects of certain drugs

to alcohol. Chronic hepatitis B and chronic hepatitis C are also common and account for most of the mortality related to viral hepatitis. Chronic hepatitis B is more prevalent than chronic hepatitis C globally while the inverse is true in the US [8].

In this chapter, each component of the liver chemistry panel will be reviewed. Guidance will be provided for how to approach different patterns of laboratory abnormalities that are commonly encountered in clinical practice. The goal is to obtain relevant patient-specific data in the most efficient and effective manner to reach a definitive diagnosis. There is currently no evidence-based "optimal" methodology or approach to the evaluation of abnormal liver chemistries or clinical jaundice. The algorithms provided in this chapter should never replace clinical judgment and should always be interpreted within the clinical context of the patient. Finally, the evaluation of specific liver diseases will be presented in subsequent chapters and will not be covered in depth in this chapter.

Biochemical basis of liver chemistries

A basic understanding of the biochemical processes that make up the liver chemistry panel is necessary before attempting to interpret their significance. The components of the liver chemistry panel can be divided into four broad categories–hepatocyte integrity, bile flow, bilirubin metabolism, and hepatic synthetic function.

Hepatocyte integrity

Loss of hepatocyte cellular integrity due to cell necrosis leads to leakage of hepatic enzymes into the systemic circulation. Aminotransferases are enzymes that catalyze the redistribution of nitrogen between an amino acid and a keto acid and are important in the synthesis and degradation of amino acids. In a healthy state, they are present in high concentrations within metabolically active cells such as hepatocytes and in low concentrations in the serum. Thus, elevated serum aminotransferase activity is a good indicator of a breach in cellular integrity. Alanine aminotransferase (ALT) and aspartate aminotransferase (AST) are the two aminotransferases of greatest clinical significance. ALT and AST catalyze the transfer of α-amino groups from alanine and aspartate to the α-keto group of ketoglutaric acid to form pyruvic and oxaloacetic acids, respectively. Both enzymes require pyridoxal-5'-phosphate (P5'P), the active form of vitamin B_6, as a coenzyme.

Alanine aminotransferase is predominantly found in the cytoplasm of hepatocytes and thus is a more specific marker of hepatocyte injury. Much smaller amounts are found in kidney, heart, and muscle. On the other hand, AST is ubiquitous and present in large quantities in the liver, heart, muscle, and kidney. It is also found in smaller quantities in the pancreas, spleen, lung, and red blood cells [9]. As a result, serum AST may be elevated in nonliver-related diseases such as myocardial infarction, rhabdomyolysis, and acute kidney injury. In fact, due to its rich activity in the cardiac muscle, AST was previously used as a biomarker for the diagnosis of myocardial infarction. An isolated AST elevation in the absence of other liver chemistry abnormalities should prompt work-up of nonhepatic organ injury. If rhabdomyolysis is suspected, creatine kinase (CK) is the serum enzyme of choice in estimating the degree of muscle injury because levels of CK in the muscle are much higher than the aminotransferases.

Table 39.2 Tissue activity of aspartate aminotransferase (AST) and alanine aminotransferase (ALT) and their ratios [57].

	AST activity	ALT activity	AST:ALT ratio
Liver	7100	2850	2.5
Kidney	4500	1200	3.8
Heart	7800	450	17
Muscle	5000	300	30
Serum	1	1	1

In a healthy state, the hepatic AST:ALT enzyme activity ratio is 2.5:1 (Table 39.2). However, the serum AST:ALT ratio is typically 1:1 because of the more rapid removal of AST by liver sinusoidal cells compared to ALT [10]. The half-lives of ALT and AST in the circulation are approximately 47 hours and 17 hours, respectively [11]. ALT is present in highest concentrations in periportal hepatocytes (zone 1) and lowest around the central vein (zone 3), whereas the concentration of AST is highest in zone 3 and lowest in zone 1 [12]. In ischemic hepatitis, hepatocytes around zone 3 are most prone to injury as it receives the lowest concentration of oxygen and is most sensitive to hepatic hypoperfusion. This results in centrilobular necrosis of the hepatic acinus and a high AST to ALT ratio. On the other hand, periportal hepatocytes are affected earlier in the course of viral and autoimmune hepatitis, resulting in a higher ALT to AST ratio.

It is worth noting that the reference range of AST and ALT varies greatly across different laboratories. One study that surveyed the interlaboratory variability of the upper limit of normal values of ALT found wide variability, ranging from 35 to 79 U/L in men and 31 to 55 U/L for women [13]. Due to technical reasons related to sample stability, universal validated standard values are not used to establish an upper limit of normal value. Instead, each laboratory uses a locally defined reference population to establish its own reference ranges [13]. The criteria defining a healthy control population are not standardized and can sometimes include patients with undiagnosed liver disease. The inclusion of such individuals may skew the "normal" range to inappropriately high levels. This is concerning as clinicians may be falsely reassured that a patient's lab value is within normal range and not pursue further evaluation despite the presence of risk factors for underlying liver disease. When more stringent criteria were used to define "normal" subjects by excluding subjects with known viral hepatitis, high-risk behaviors, alcohol use, and NAFLD risk factors, the true "normal" aminotransferase levels were found to be substantially lower [14–16].

Multiple population-based studies performed in several different countries have shown an association between elevated ALT levels and increased liver-related and all-cause mortality [17–20]. Because of this, using a more stringent ALT cut-off as a threshold to prompt further evaluation of liver disease is recommended as this can lead to earlier diagnosis of subclinical liver disease. Of note, the American Association for the Study of Liver Disease's Hepatitis B Virus (AASLD HBV) guidelines published in 2018 recommend using 35 U/L as the upper limit of normal for ALT in males and 25 U/L in females [21]. These numbers concur with the most recent American College of Gastroenterology practice guideline on the evaluation of abnormal liver chemistries [22]. Finally, it is also important to keep in mind that a normal ALT value does *not* exclude the existence of liver disease. Multiple studies have shown that ALT does not correlate with the degree of liver fibrosis [23,24]. Since the degree of hepatic fibrosis correlates with liver-related and all-cause mortality, ALT is a poor marker for assessing the severity of chronic liver disease [25].

Bile flow

Impairment of bile flow due to obstruction of the biliary tree leads to cholestatic liver injury, resulting in elevations in alkaline phosphatase (ALP) and, at a later stage, bilirubin. Bilirubin will be discussed in detail in the following section. ALP is a metalloenzyme that catalyzes the hydrolysis of organic phosphate esters in the extracellular space at alkaline pH environments [26]. Its physiological function is unknown except within the bone, where it participates in bone mineralization. Zinc and magnesium are important cofactors. Patients with Wilson disease may have unusually low serum ALP activity due to copper overload leading to displacement of zinc [27]. ALP is ubiquitous but particularly abundant in the placenta, small intestine, kidney, bone, and liver.[9] The majority of ALP in the serum is released from liver and bone, followed by intestine [28].

In the liver, ALP is found in the canalicular membrane of the hepatocyte. Bile duct obstruction stimulates increased canalicular synthesis of ALP and subsequent release into the circulation. ALP elevation is *not* due to reduced hepatobiliary excretion of the enzyme [26]. The degree of ALP elevation is not helpful in distinguishing between intrahepatic and extrahepatic etiologies of cholestasis. In acute biliary obstruction, there may be a delay in ALP elevation by 1–2 days since de novo synthesis of the enzyme is required. The liver ALP isoenzyme has a half-life of 3 days and clearance from the serum is independent of bile duct patency or hepatic function [9]. Thus, there can be a delay in ALP normalization after resolution of the biliary injury or obstruction.

Serum ALP level varies with age and, to a lesser extent, sex. Levels are highest in childhood when there is rapid bone growth. ALP is slightly higher in males in adulthood until later in life, when levels increase in postmenopausal females due to higher rates of bone turnover. Pregnancy increases serum ALP due to the rise in placental ALP and can be 3–4 times the upper limit of normal during the third trimester [29]. Subjects with blood type O and B demonstrate increased serum ALP for up to 12 hours after ingestion of a fatty meal due to an increase in the intestinal proportion of ALP [30]. Thus, for mild isolated elevation of ALP in an asymptomatic individual, repeat testing after fasting is recommended.

Isolated elevation of ALP necessitates further investigation to determine if it is of hepatic origin. γ-Glutamyl transferase (GGT) is a canalicular membrane enzyme that is present in the liver but *not* in bone and is useful in differentiating the origin of ALP elevation [9]. The serum GGT level is almost always elevated in the setting of cholestasis except in patients who have progressive familial intrahepatic cholestasis (PFIC) types 1 and 2. Patients with these rare hereditary disorders develop severe cholestatic liver disease due to defects in bile salt transport but have a normal serum GGT [31]. This is thought to be due to the reduced concentration of bile salts leading to preservation of GGT localization at the canalicular membrane [32]. Although GGT has an excellent negative predictive value for hepatobiliary disease, it lacks specificity. Elevated GGT can be seen in patients with myocardial infarction, renal failure, chronic obstructive pulmonary disease, diabetes, heavy alcohol intake even in the absence of alcohol-associated liver disease, and with ingestion of certain medications such as phenytoin and barbiturates [33].

Bilirubin metabolism

Bilirubin is a yellow pigment that is derived from the breakdown of heme-containing proteins including hemoglobin, myoglobin, and cytochromes. Heme is first broken down into biliverdin, which is then reduced to unconjugated bilirubin in the reticuloendothelial cells of the liver and spleen. Unconjugated bilirubin is lipid soluble and is bound to albumin for transport through the circulation. Once transported into hepatocytes, it is conjugated with glucuronic acid by uridine diphosphoglucuronosyltransferase (UGT) and made water soluble. Conjugated bilirubin within hepatocytes is transported across the hepatocyte canalicular membrane and secreted into bile. This is mediated by the multidrug resistance-associated protein 2 (MRP2) transporter expressed in the canalicular membrane. Bile then enters the small intestine. The majority of bile salts are reabsorbed into the bloodstream by the terminal ileum, but conjugated bilirubin is not absorbed by the small intestine. In the colon, bacteria deconjugate and metabolize bilirubin into urobilinogen. Most urobilinogen is excreted in feces, but a small amount is reabsorbed into the circulation and is excreted by the kidneys. For further details regarding bile formation and transport, please refer to Chapter 40 covering liver physiology.

The half-life of unconjugated bilirubin is only 5 minutes [34]. Conjugated bilirubin has a half-life of approximately 4 hours. In the serum, a proportion of conjugated bilirubin covalently bonds with albumin and is called δ-bilirubin. It has the same half-life as albumin, approximately 3 weeks, which explains why there is a delay in the improvement of jaundice and downtrend in the serum bilirubin level despite resolution of liver injury or biliary obstruction [35]. Although the terms direct bilirubin and conjugated bilirubin are often used interchangeably, they are not synonymous. The direct bilirubin assay measures δ-bilirubin and conjugated bilirubin, as well as a small percentage of unconjugated bilirubin [9].

Conjugated bilirubin is essentially absent from the blood in healthy people and thus, an increased level in the circulation is highly specific for hepatobiliary disease. Hepatocellular injury can cause a mixed unconjugated/conjugated hyperbilirubinemia due to impaired bilirubin conjugation, direct release of bilirubin from damaged hepatocytes, and impaired canalicular secretion. UGT activity is well preserved until the development of advanced liver disease [36]. Thus, jaundice is a hallmark of severe hepatocellular liver injury. Both extrahepatic and intrahepatic biliary obstruction also cause conjugated hyperbilirubinemia due to decreased bile flow resulting in an abnormal increase in conjugated bilirubin secretion into the bloodstream.

Isolated conjugated hyperbilirubinemia without abnormal AST, ALT, or ALP occurs in patients with rare inherited disorders of bilirubin transport. Rotor syndrome occurs due to a defect in sinusoidal reuptake of conjugated bilirubin. Dubin–Johnson syndrome is caused by a defect of canalicular organic anion transport [37]. Sepsis can also cause elevated conjugated bilirubin without other liver chemistry abnormalities. This is caused by inflammatory markers leading to a rapid but reversible decrease in the amount of MRP2 and other transport proteins on the canalicular membrane of hepatocytes, leading to decreased excretion of bilirubin into bile [38]. Typically, bilirubin levels are less than 5 mg/dL and will resolve with the treatment of the underlying infection and are not associated with liver injury.

Unconjugated hyperbilirubinemia is caused by several mechanisms. The most common is excess bilirubin production due to hemolysis. Note that AST may be elevated in the setting of severe hemolysis due to its release from damaged red blood cells (RBCs). Total bilirubin rarely exceeds 5 mg/dL even in profound hemolysis due to the efficiency of hepatic uptake and conjugation. Another common cause of mildly elevated unconjugated bilirubin is Gilbert syndrome. The prevalence of this condition is estimated to be 5–10% in the Caucasian population with worldwide prevalence ranging from 4% to 16% based on limited epidemiological data. This is a benign condition caused by mild decreased UGT activity causing mild jaundice and bilirubin elevation during times of physiological stress or fasting [37]. Some medications such as protease inhibitors and tyrosine kinase inhibitors can also cause temporary impairment of UGT [39]. Crigler–Najjar syndromes type I and II are rare autosomal recessive disorders due to mutations in the UGT1A1 gene encoding UGT [37]. Type I is most severe with complete loss of function of UGT. Liver transplantation is needed for definitive cure and avoidance of kernicterus. Type II is milder and has a much lower likelihood of developing neurological consequences.

Hepatic synthetic function

The liver is responsible for the synthesis of most plasma proteins. This includes albumin and other carrier proteins, globulins, coagulation factors, apolipoproteins, and hormones. Von Willebrand factor, made within endothelial cells, and immunoglobulins, made by plasma cells, are notable exceptions. Albumin and prothrombin time are the most common tests used to assess hepatic synthetic function.

Albumin

Albumin is synthesized solely by hepatocytes. On average, the adult liver synthesizes and secretes 10.5 g of albumin per day into the bloodstream [40]. It is the most abundant circulating protein found in plasma and represents approximately half of the total protein content in plasma. It functions as the main determinant of plasma oncotic pressure and transports many drugs, hormones, and waste products throughout the circulation. It also has antioxidant and immunomodulatory properties [40]. The rate of production of albumin by hepatocytes is influenced by the number of functioning hepatocytes, and thus can indirectly assess hepatic synthetic function.

A decrease in serum albumin does not always indicate hepatic synthetic dysfunction. Lower levels are caused by decreased synthesis, increased loss, increased catabolism, redistribution, and dilutional states (Table 39.3) [40]. The half-life of albumin is approximately 21 days. As such, it is not a sensitive marker for acute liver disease but can be helpful in assessing the severity of hepatic dysfunction in cirrhosis.

Table 39.3 Causes of low serum albumin.

Cause	Results
Decreased synthesis	Hepatic synthetic dysfunction Protein malnutrition
Increased loss	Malabsorption (i.e., protein-losing enteropathy) Nephrotic syndrome Burns
Increased catabolism	Chronic inflammation
Redistribution	Distributive shock
Hemodilution	Pregnancy

Prothrombin time

The prothrombin time (PT) measures the time it takes for plasma to clot after the addition of tissue factor and phospholipid. It is influenced by the activity of factors I, II, V, VII, and X, all of which are synthesized by hepatocytes [41]. Factors II, VII, and X require vitamin K as a cofactor in activation. Vitamin K deficiency can occur due to fat malabsorption. Vitamin K is a fat-soluble vitamin and its absorption is highly dependent on adequate bile flow into the small intestine. Therefore, vitamin K can be deficient in cholestatic liver disease, bile duct obstruction, and advanced liver disease. To assess whether PT elevation is due to true factor deficiency versus vitamin K insufficiency, supplemental vitamin K can be given subcutaneously [42]. Other factors that can prolong PT include medications (i.e., warfarin, antibiotics), disseminated intravascular coagulopathy, and hypothermia. PT does not become prolonged until less than 10% of the normal amount of any one factor is present [9], thus representing severe liver synthetic dysfunction. Because factor VII has a short half-life of 4–6 hours, PT can be much more sensitive in detecting liver synthetic dysfunction than albumin [43].

Platelet count

Although the platelet count is not classically considered a liver-related blood test, it should always be considered in the evaluation for chronic liver disease, particularly if there is suspicion for advanced fibrosis. The severity of thrombocytopenia correlates with the degree of liver fibrosis and portal hypertension. Moderate thrombocytopenia (platelet count of 50–75 000/microL) occurs in approximately 13% of patients with cirrhosis and severe thrombocytopenia (<50 000/microL) in about 1% [44].

The pathogenesis of thrombocytopenia in the setting of cirrhosis is multifactorial. The three main factors are decreased platelet production, splenic sequestration, and increased platelet destruction or consumption. Thrombopoietin (TPO) is a protein that affects platelet production by stimulating production and differentiation of megakaryocytes [45]. TPO is produced by the liver and kidneys. Patients with advanced liver disease may have decreased levels, leading to decreased platelet synthesis [46]. TPO levels rise immediately after liver transplantation, leading to improvement in the platelet counts, but typically without complete normalization [47]. Nutrient deficiencies and direct bone marrow toxicity from certain liver diseases such as alcohol and viral hepatitis also contribute to decreased production [48–50]. As liver fibrosis progresses, portal hypertension leads to congestive splenomegaly, causing further sequestration of the platelets from the circulation into the spleen. Normally, one-third of the platelets are sequestered within the spleen. In the setting of massive splenomegaly, this can increase to 90%. Thrombocytopenia may also occur due to immune-mediated destruction. Elevated levels of platelet-associated IgG are seen in patients with chronic liver disease and hepatitis C is associated with idiopathic thrombocytopenia purpura [48]. Cirrhosis results in imbalance between pro- and antifibrinolytic factors, which can lead to hyperfibrinolysis and increased platelet consumption. Cirrhosis promotes bacterial translocation from the intestinal lumen to the portal circulation, leading to increased levels of endotoxin [51]. Endotoxin triggers the release of proinflammatory cytokines and causes platelet aggregation and consumption due to disseminated intravascular coagulation [48].

Clinical approach and interpretation of abnormal liver chemistries

Three key questions should be explored when interpreting abnormal liver chemistries.

- What is the clinical context?
- What is the pattern, duration, and magnitude of liver injury?
- Is hepatic synthetic dysfunction present?

This diagnostic approach will help narrow the differential diagnosis considerably and minimize unnecessary testing. If hepatic synthetic function is disturbed, rapid and broad evaluation followed by close monitoring is needed. If hospital monitoring is deemed necessary, consideration should be given to transferring the patient to a liver transplant center as patients with severe liver injury can progress precipitately to liver failure and require urgent liver transplant evaluation. With the advent of telemedicine and electronic consultations, it may be expedient to interpret laboratory abnormalities based on chart history alone. However, this may limit the contextual data that can be gathered and thus delay appropriate diagnosis and management. Thus, it is preferable to evaluate a patient with abnormal liver chemistries in a face-to-face consultation. Potential etiologies can be narrowed considerably by identifying specific risk factors unique to each patient. Such risk factors are identified by taking the time to interview the patient thoroughly to elucidate detailed information regarding medical, drug/toxin exposure, psychosocial history, and family history. Developing rapport and a therapeutic relationship with a patient is often needed to obtain a candid drug and alcohol history. A physical exam focused specifically on identifying stigmata of chronic liver disease/portal hypertension and features indicative of extrahepatic manifestations should be performed.

What is the clinical context?

Demographics

Knowledge of specific epidemiological data based on geography, sex, age, and race/ethnicity of specific liver diseases will help inform the pretest probability prior to pursuing diagnostic testing. For example, women are nine times more likely to develop primary biliary cholangitis than men. HFE mutation-associated hereditary hemochromatosis is one of the most common genetic disorders in Caucasians and is extremely uncommon in Asians.

Table 39.4 Symptoms associated with specific liver diseases.

Disease	Symptoms
Primary biliary cholangitis	Sicca syndrome: dry eyes and dry mouth Pruritus
Primary sclerosing cholangitis	Bloody diarrhea, tenesmus, pruritus, fever, abdominal pain
α1-Antitrypsin deficiency	Wheezing, shortness of breath
Hemochromatosis	Impotence Joint pain
Wilson disease	Irritability Psychosis Difficulty speaking, swallowing, walking
Alcoholic liver disease	Decreased coordination Short-term memory loss Numbness and paresthesia

Table 39.5 Medical conditions associated with specific liver diseases.

Disease	Comorbid medical conditions
Nonalcoholic fatty liver disease	Diabetes Hypertension Dyslipidemia Obesity
Hemochromatosis	Diabetes Hypothyroidism Arthropathy Hypogonadism Dilated cardiomyopathy
Budd–Chiari syndrome	Occult malignancy Myeloproliferative disorder Primary hypercoagulable disorder
α1-Antitrypsin deficiency	Chronic obstructive pulmonary disease
Primary sclerosing cholangitis	Inflammatory bowel disease Ankylosing spondylitis
Primary biliary cholangitis/ autoimmune hepatitis	Autoimmune thyroiditis Type 1 diabetes Celiac disease Rheumatoid arthritis Inflammatory bowel disease

Prevalence of chronic hepatitis C is higher in people born between 1945 and 1965 in the US, though the recent opioid epidemic has led to an increase in hepatitis C infection in young adults [52]. The prevalence of chronic hepatitis B varies significantly by geographic area, and in western countries by country of birth. With the rise of globalization and increased immigration, familiarity with global epidemiological data is critical to develop a clinical context for evaluating abnormal liver chemistries.

Symptoms

In the outpatient setting, patients with abnormal liver chemistries are often asymptomatic. Symptoms, if present, are nonspecific and include malaise, fatigue, anorexia, and pruritus. Some hepatobiliary diseases have been associated with specific symptoms. Examples are listed in Table 39.4.

Medical history

Many chronic liver diseases are associated with comorbid conditions. Examples are listed in Table 39.5. Infectious disease risk factors are also important to elicit. These include travel to endemic regions, injection drug use, incarceration history, tattooing, history of blood transfusions, and history of hemodialysis. Finally, it is important to elicit any history suggestive of an immunocompromised state as this can greatly expand the possibilities of infectious causes of liver disease. Patients should be asked about history of organ or bone marrow transplantation, human immunodeficiency virus (HIV) infection, hematological disorders, and the use of immunosuppressive medications.

Ingestions

Medications

A detailed intake of all prescriptions, over-the-counter medications, dietary/herbal supplements, and illicit drug use should be obtained. The duration and timing of drug use in relation to the abnormal liver tests are critical in determining if drug-induced liver injury has occurred. Hepatotoxicity can occur in a dose-dependent or idiosyncratic way. It is important to be aware of common culprit medications and their characteristic pattern and timing of liver injury. It is also important to know what drugs are associated with autoimmune hepatitis as management includes steroids in addition to the discontinuation of the offending agent. Patients may not volunteer intake of herbal medications and dietary supplements unless specifically asked. In the United States, herbals and dietary supplements are not under the same rigorous Food and Drug Administration regulations that prescription and over-the-counter drugs must adhere to. As such, many potentially hepatotoxic supplements are readily available in natural food stores, naturopathic clinics, and online catalogs.

An excellent resource to help determine if a specific substance is the cause of liver injury is the LiverTox website: https://livertox.nih.gov. This is a comprehensive database maintained by the National Institute of Diabetes and Digestive and Kidney Diseases in collaboration with the National Library of Medicine and the Drug-Induced Liver Injury Network. The website is free to access and provides a wealth of information on the typical pattern and course of liver injury associated with various substances, with reference to case reports published in the medical literature. As of 2019, approximately 1200 drug records were available [53]. Drugs are categorized for the likelihood that they will cause clinically apparent drug-induced liver injury (DILI) based on published literature [54].

Alcohol

Obtaining an accurate alcohol use history can be challenging since patients may not want to disclose significant or surreptitious alcohol use. Establishing rapport and asking questions in a nonjudgmental manner are key to developing trust and an effective therapeutic provider–patient relationship to facilitate care. Patients should be asked about the pattern, quantity, and type of alcohol use. Alcohol quantity should be standardized in grams of alcohol rather than number of drinks. A standard drink is defined as 14 g of pure alcohol, and roughly equivalent to 12 fluid (fl) ounces of beer, 5 fl oz of wine, or 1.5 fl oz of hard liquor. Note that a typical serving size of an alcoholic beverage is more than one standard drink. "Risky use," defined as an amount of alcohol that puts an individual at risk for health consequences, is more than 14 standard drinks per week or two drinks per day for men, and more than seven drinks per week or one drink per day for women. There can be significant individual variability in the amount of alcohol that can cause chronic liver disease. Using validated screening tools such as the AUDIT-C for unhealthy alcohol use can be helpful in identifying patients who may benefit from further evaluation by a substance abuse psychologist/psychiatrist.

Family history

Patients should be asked whether any biological family members have heritable liver diseases. This includes hemochromatosis, α1-antitrypsin deficiency, Wilson disease, cystic fibrosis, and autosomal dominant polycystic kidney disease. Other information that is useful to obtain includes family history of chronic hepatitis B, chronic hepatitis C, hepatocellular carcinoma, alcoholism, and metabolic syndrome.

Focused physical exam

The physical exam is most useful in identifying the hallmark signs of end-stage liver disease but may be completely normal in patients with early-stage liver disease, including those with compensated cirrhosis. The development of ascites and splenomegaly supports the presence of portal hypertension. Palmar erythema, gynecomastia, spider angiomas, and reduced axillary/pubic hair can be manifestations of hyperestrogenism due to decreased metabolism of estrogen in patients with cirrhosis. Portosystemic shunting can be assessed by the presence of caput medusae, fetor hepaticus (due to thiols passing directly into the lungs), and hepatic encephalopathy. Asterixis, an involuntary flapping motion elicited in outstretched dorsiflexed hands, is sensitive in detecting overt hepatic encephalopathy. However, it is nonspecific as it can occur in other diseases such as renal failure and hypercapnia. Jaundice can be clinically detected in the sclera and sublingual area when the total bilirubin rises to >3 mg/dL [55].

Physical exam findings may also be helpful in pointing to specific liver disease. Obesity, particularly abdominal adiposity, is associated with nonalcoholic fatty liver disease. Dupuytren contracture can frequently be seen in alcoholics. Needle track marks from intravenous drug use should prompt work-up for hepatitis B and C. Bronzed skin due to hypermelanosis occurs in patients with untreated and late-stage hemochromatosis. Xanthomas and xanthelasmas can be seen in hypercholesterolemia, a common feature of primary biliary cholangitis (PBC). Purpuric rash on the lower extremities is seen in leukocytoclastic vasculitis from HCV-mediated mixed cryoglobulinemia. Kayser–Fleischer rings can be seen in Wilson disease due to copper deposition in the cornea, particularly in patients with neurological symptoms, though often slit lamp examination is necessary.

What is the pattern, duration, and magnitude of livery injury?

There are three main patterns of liver injury – hepatocellular, cholestatic, and mixed – and they can be defined by the R-value. The R-value is derived by dividing the ALT by the ALP using multiples of the upper limit of normal range for both values [56].

$$R = \left(\text{ALT value / ALT ULN}\right) \div \left(\text{ALP value / ALP ULN}\right)$$

Calculating the R-value is useful when the pattern of liver injury is not immediately evident. In most cases in clinical practice, it is sufficient to formulate a rough assessment of whether there is a predominance of aminotransferase elevation over alkaline phosphatase or vice versa.

Hepatocellular liver injury

Liver injury is characterized as predominantly hepatocellular if the R-value is >5. The magnitude of aminotransferase elevation is often classified as mild (<5× ULN), moderate (5–10× ULN), or marked (>10× ULN). These cut-offs are arbitrary and different guidelines use different cut-offs. However, the magnitude of aminotransferase elevation can narrow the differential diagnosis considerably (Figure 39.1). For example, aminotransferase levels >300 U/L are not typically seen in alcoholic liver disease despite extensive hepatocyte injury. This is thought to be due to vitamin B_6 deficiency, which leads to depressed AST and ALT activity [57]. The highest levels of aminotransferases (ALT >10 000) are seen only in toxin-mediated liver injury (i.e., amatoxin, acetaminophen) or ischemic hepatitis. Other diseases that can cause moderate to marked hepatocellular injury include acute viral hepatitis A–E, other viral hepatitis (i.e., herpes simplex virus, cytomegalovirus, adenovirus), acute hepatic venous outflow obstruction, acute biliary obstruction, autoimmune hepatitis flare, and Wilson disease.

For mild elevations in aminotransferases, a stepwise evaluation should be taken to avoid unnecessary testing (Figure 39.2). A detailed alcohol use history and medication review should always be performed. If excess alcohol use or ingestion of a potential hepatotoxic agent is identified, the

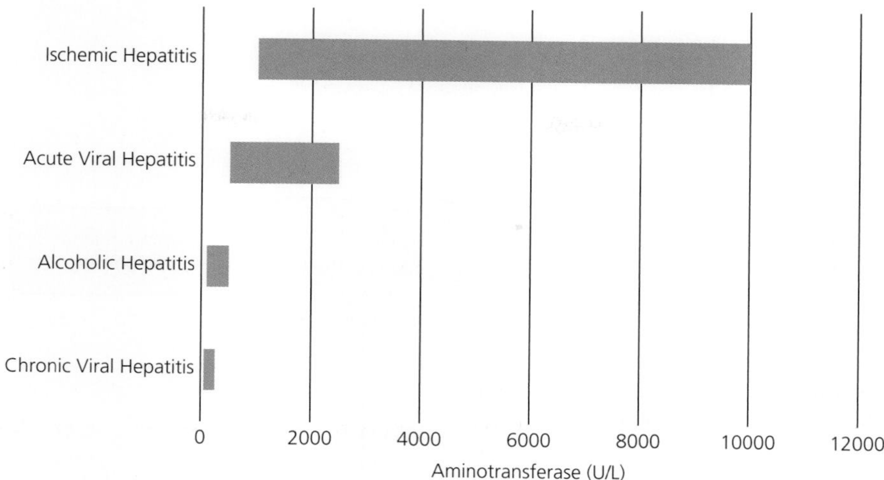

Figure 39.1 Typical serum aminotransferase levels in various liver diseases.

patient should be advised to discontinue their use. If elevations are <2× ULN in an asymptomatic patient, repeat blood work can be obtained in 3–6 months. In the National Health and Nutrition Examination Survey (NHANES) database, more than 30% of adults with elevated AST, ALT, or bilirubin were reclassified as having normal levels when retested, suggesting high intrapersonal variability with these tests in the absence of liver disease and when the values are only mildly elevated [58].

For elevations <5× ULN, evaluation should begin by considering the most common causes of chronic liver disease. These include alcoholic liver disease, NAFLD, chronic hepatitis C, and chronic hepatitis B. Hereditary hemochromatosis should also be considered early in Caucasian individuals due to the higher prevalence in this population. In addition, physical exam findings and laboratory data should be scrutinized for features suggestive of advanced liver disease. Patients with concern for cirrhosis should be referred to a hepatologist. Confirming the diagnosis of cirrhosis and staging the disease are critically important as they inform prognosis and hepatocellular carcinoma risk, and guide management strategies.

The gold standard for the diagnosis of cirrhosis is by histopathological examination of a liver biopsy specimen. However, liver biopsy is invasive and is susceptible to sampling error as the tissue specimen collected is only 1/50 000 of the entire liver parenchyma [59]. The advent of noninvasive assessment of hepatic fibrosis has greatly reduced the need for obtaining liver biopsies for the purposes of staging the degree of fibrosis. Advanced imaging techniques such as vibration-controlled transient elastography (VCTE) and magnetic resonance elastography (MRE) are validated in the staging of liver fibrosis in liver disease of varying etiologies and have predominantly replaced liver biopsy for this purpose. A detailed discussion regarding imaging modalities for the assessment of liver fibrosis is beyond the scope of this chapter, but will be covered in the chapter on assessment of liver fibrosis (Chapter 97).

If the initial serological work-up for liver disease is unrevealing, the next step is to look for less common causes. Celiac disease (CD) is associated with mild aminotransferase elevations. In one study, 9% of patients with chronic unexplained mild hepatocellular liver enzyme abnormalities were ultimately diagnosed with CD [60]. The mechanism of liver injury in CD is poorly understood, but since aminotransferases normalize with cessation of gluten exposure, there appears to be a causal relationship between gluten intake and liver damage. If no improvement in ALT is seen 1 year after strict gluten restriction, other etiologies of liver disease should be considered. This is especially important because CD is associated with autoimmune liver diseases such as autoimmune hepatitis (AIH) and PBC. Other causes to consider include Wilson disease and α1-antitrypsin deficiency. In certain clinical scenarios, other disease processes should be considered such as sinusoidal obstruction syndrome in bone marrow transplant recipients, or Budd–Chiari syndrome especially in pregnancy.

The diagnosis of most liver diseases can be made with a combination of clinical information and noninvasive testing. If the diagnosis remains in question, a liver biopsy is indicated, particularly if the diagnosis will require the use of chronic medication (i.e., immunosuppression for AIH, chelating agents for Wilson disease) or impact significant prognosis considerations (small duct primary sclerosing cholangitis). Histological analysis is also helpful in guiding treatment strategies for patients with AIH overlap syndromes and differentiating between NAFLD and nonalcoholic steatohepatitis (NASH). Figure 39.2 provides a diagnostic approach to elevated aminotransferases.

Severe elevations (>10× ULN) in aminotransferases require rapid evaluation and hospitalization if jaundice is present or liver synthetic function is impaired. In such scenarios, a nondirected work-up of liver injury may be preferred for rapid diagnosis to expedite treatment and prevent potential disease

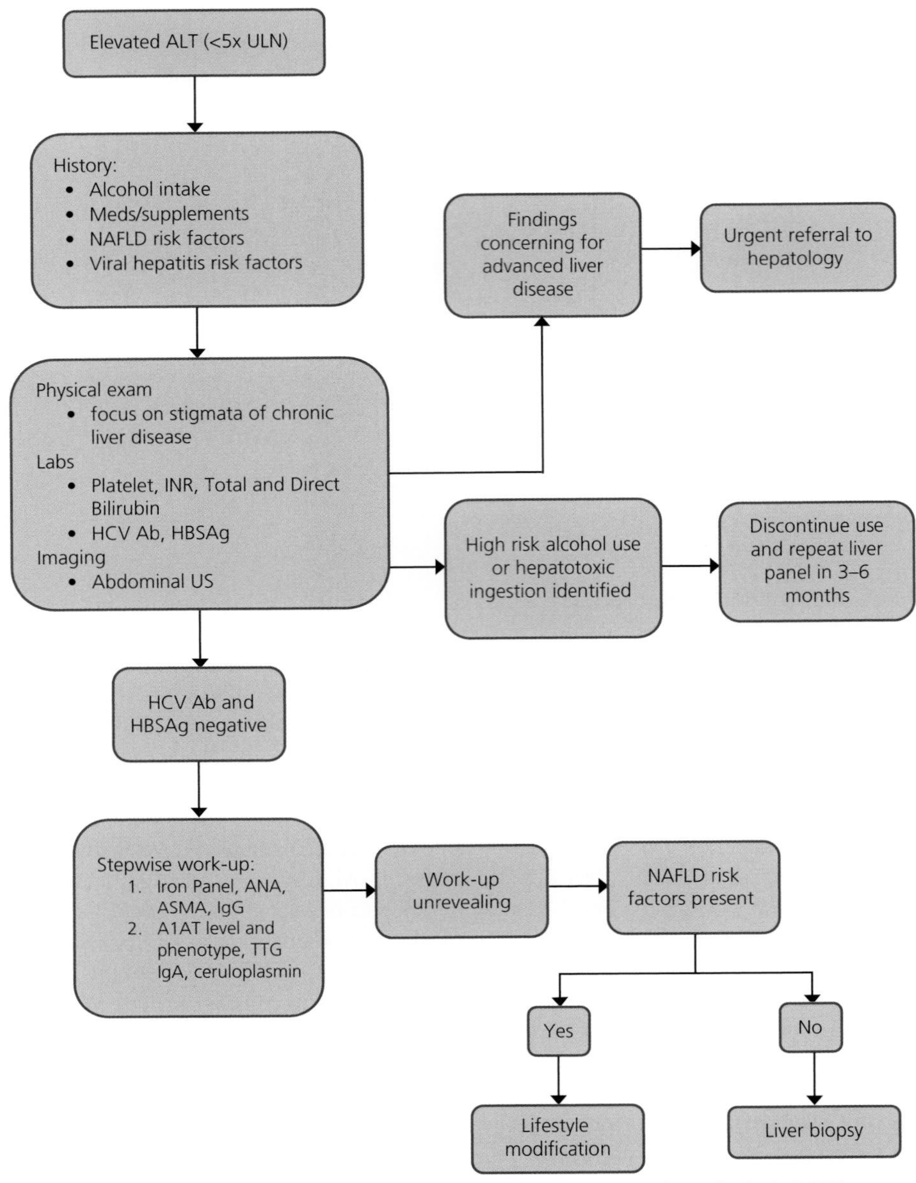

ALT alanine aminotransferase, NAFLD non-alcoholic fatty liver disease, INR international normalized ratio, HCV Ab hepatitis C antibody, HBSAg hepatitis B surface antigen, ANA antinuclear antibody, ASMA anti-smooth muscle antibody, IgG immunoglobulin G, A1AT alpha-1 antitrypsin, TTG IgA tissue transglutaminase antibody immunoglobulin A

Figure 39.2 Diagnostic approach to asymptomatic, mild elevations of aminotransferases.

progression. It is important to keep in mind that in acute liver injury, the degree of aminotransferase elevation will vary considerably depending on the time course in which the enzyme levels are tested (Figure 39.3). Some causes of liver injury such as ischemic hepatitis will have a characteristic acute rise and fall of aminotransferases that can be missed if only a single observation point of liver enzymes is obtained. Thus, aminotransferase levels should be checked immediately after liver injury is suspected and trended over time.

The clinical relevance of the AST to ALT ratio was first described by Fernando de Ritis in 1957 [57]. The de Ritis ratio is a useful tool in providing clues to the etiology of liver injury. A ratio ≥2 is suggestive of several liver diseases, of which the most well known is alcoholic liver disease. Patients with alcoholic liver disease often have malnutrition and vitamin B_6 deficiency. ALT activity is more dependent on vitamin B_6 than AST, which partly explains the high AST:ALT ratio. Another mechanism is that alcohol leads to direct mitochondrial injury which can

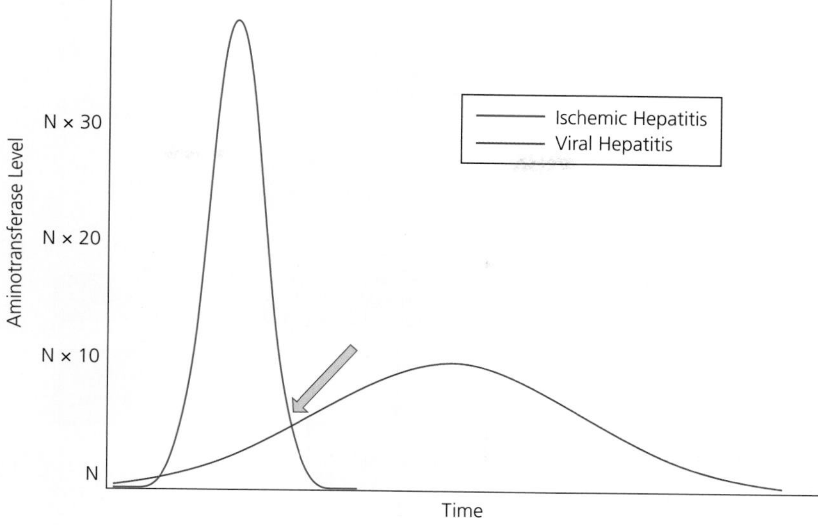

Figure 39.3 Schematic representation of the change in serum aminotransferase levels over time during ischemic and acute viral hepatitis. Aminotransferase levels can be similar at a single time point (arrow).

Table 39.6 Hepatobiliary and extrahepatic causes of elevated alkaline phosphatase (ALP).

Cause	

Hepatobiliary causes	**Intrahepatic cholestasis**
	• Medication/toxin
	• Primary biliary cholangitis
	• Alcoholic hepatitis
	• Infiltrative/space-occupying lesions
	  • Tuberculosis
	  • Granuloma/abscess
	  • Sarcoidosis
	  • Lymphoma
	  • Amyloidosis
	  • Liver metastases
	  • Hepatocellular carcinoma
	• Total parenteral nutrition
	• Chronic liver allograft rejection
	Intrahepatic and extrahepatic biliary obstruction
	• Choledocholithiasis
	• Biliary strictures
	  • Malignant: cholangiocarcinoma, pancreatic, ampullary, gallbladder cancer
	  • Primary sclerosing cholangitis
	  • IgG4-related sclerosing cholangitis
	  • Surgical: iatrogenic injury, biliary anastomosis
	  • Chronic pancreatitis
	  • Ischemic cholangiopathy
	• Infections
	  • Liver flukes (clonorchiasis, opisthorchiasis)
	  • Ascaris lumbricoides
	  • AIDS cholangiopathy

Extrahepatic causes	**Physiological** • Third trimester of pregnancy • Childhood **Bone turnover** • Osteomalacia • Paget disease • Bone metastases • Primary bone cancer • Hyperparathyroidism • Hyperthyroidism **Other** • The Regan isoenzyme of ALP is expressed in some types of malignant tumors without liver or bone involvement

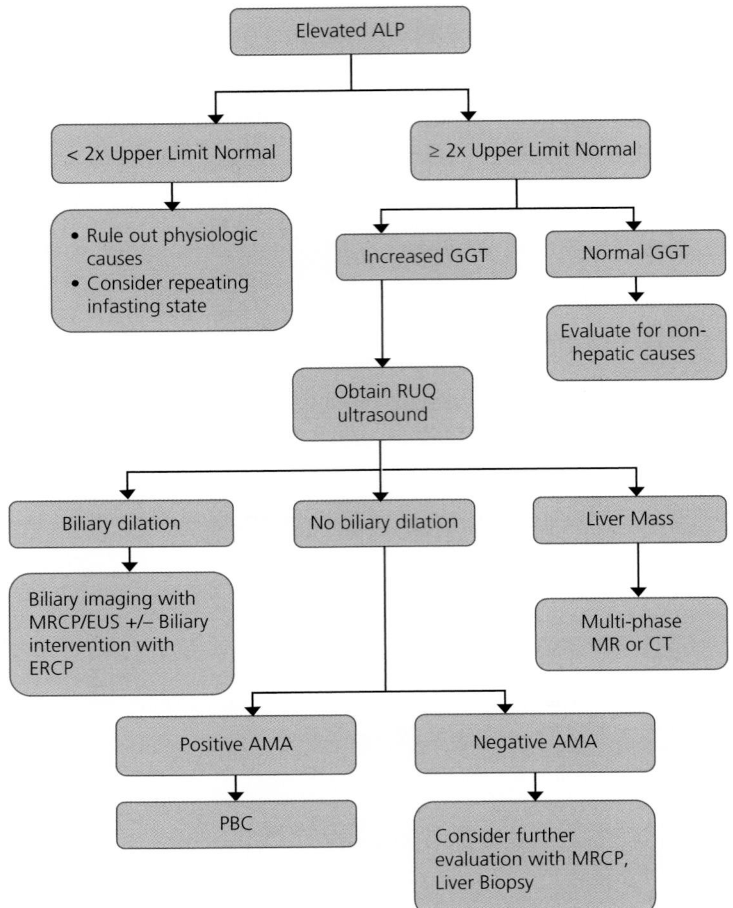

Figure 39.4 Diagnostic approach to elevated alkaline phosphatase. ALP, alkaline phosphatase; AMA, antimichondrial antibody; CT, computed tomography; ERCP, endoscopic retrograde cholangiopancreatography; EUS, endoscopic ultrasound; GGT, γ-glutamyl transferase; MR, magnetic resonance; MRCP, magnetic resonance cholangiopancreatography; PBC, primary biliary cholangitis; RUQ, right upper quadrant.

lead to higher levels of mAST leakage into the circulation [57]. Ischemic hepatitis also tends to result in serum AST > ALT, particularly in the first few days after the ischemic event. This is because of vulnerability of zone 3 hepatocytes to low flow states, leading to preferential necrosis of hepatocytes that have higher concentrations of AST compared to ALT. Progression of liver disease to cirrhosis will often lead to an AST:ALT ratio of >1 but no more than 2. This is theorized to be due to relatively reduced clearance of mAST or increased mitochondrial release. Patients with nonalcoholic steatohepatitis often have an AST:ALT ratio <1, particularly if they are morbidly obese. Serum aminotransferase levels increase with body weight, but the ALT rise is more prominent. In addition, insulin resistance is associated with elevated ALT independent of BMI and waist circumference [61].

Cholestatic liver injury

Liver injury is characterized as predominantly cholestatic if the R-value is <2. Cholestatic liver injury occurs due to impairment in the secretion of bile from the level of the hepatocyte to the ampulla of Vater in the duodenum. The first step is to assess if the ALP elevation is due to hepatobiliary pathology. If the etiology is unclear, GGT will clarify whether the ALP is of hepatic origin. Further investigation is then needed to determine whether the cholestasis is extrahepatic or intrahepatic. This requires abdominal imaging with visualization of the entire biliary tree. Table 39.6 outlines the common causes of elevated alkaline phosphatase and Figure 39.4 provides a suggested approach to elevated ALP.

Though jaundice often connotes hepatobiliary disease, hyperbilirubinemia in isolation cannot differentiate between

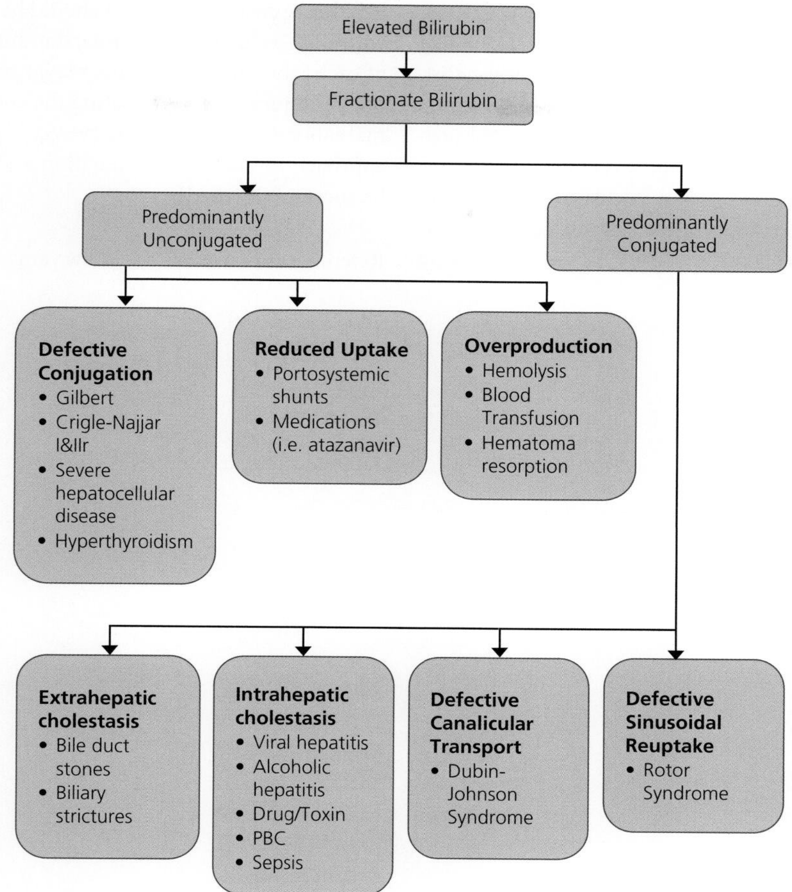

Figure 39.5 Diagnostic approach to elevated bilirubin. PBC, primary biliary cholangitis.

hepatocellular disease, impaired canalicular secretion, or biliary obstruction. The pattern of ALP and aminotransferase elevation as described in this section will help narrow the differential diagnosis. If hyperbilirubinemia occurs in isolation, hepatobiliary disease is unlikely. Rather, hemolysis or inherited/acquired disorders of bilirubin metabolism are likely culprits. Figure 39.5 presents a suggested diagnostic approach to elevated bilirubin in the blood.

Is hepatic synthetic dysfunction present?

When assessing abnormal liver chemistries, evaluating the degree of hepatic synthetic dysfunction is key in triaging the severity of illness. In patients with known chronic liver disease, severe synthetic dysfunction should prompt hepatology referral and consideration for possible liver transplantation. In a patient without history of liver disease, severe impaired synthetic function as evidenced by jaundice and coagulopathy should prompt hospitalization and referral to a liver transplant center in case of deterioration to acute liver failure (ALF). Frequent and careful neurological exams should be performed to detect the development of hepatic encephalopathy. A rapid and broad work-up should be initiated to provide timely treatments for reversible conditions, as clinical history is often difficult to elucidate in the setting of hepatic encephalopathy. Empiric therapy with N-acetylcysteine should be given if the cause of ALF is unknown as early administration improves transplant-free survival [62].

Conclusions

Abnormal liver chemistries are often the first indication of acute liver injury or underlying liver disease. They can provide clues to the cause, severity, and prognosis of liver disease. However, normal values do not preclude significant liver disease and abnormal values can occur in the absence of liver disease. Though it is one of the most common blood tests ordered by providers, interpretation of the results is challenging; hence it is the most common reason for referral to a liver specialist. However, it is impossible and often unnecessary for every patient with abnormal liver chemistries to see a liver specialist. Thus a basic understanding and a thoughtful algorithmic approach to these abnormalities will be useful to medical providers. No provider wants to miss a diagnosis but an indiscriminate approach to diagnostic evaluation is cost prohibitive and may generate harm due to complications associated with invasive diagnostic tests or false-positive results. In the era of rising healthcare costs, every effort should be made to provide patients with high-value care. By understanding the biochemical origin of each laboratory test value, recognizing the different patterns of liver injury, and appreciating the context in which the abnormal laboratory value is discovered, a pragmatic yet thoughtful approach to diagnostic evaluation and definitive diagnosis can be successfully made.

References are available at www.yamadagastro.com/textbook7e

CHAPTER 40

Approach to gastrointestinal and liver diseases in pregnancy

Stacy Menees[1] **and Grace L. Su**[1,2]
[1] Michigan Medicine, Ann Arbor, MI, USA
[2] Veterans Administration, Ann Arbor Healthcare System, Ann Arbor, MI, USA

Chapter menu

Introduction

The gastrointestinal (GI) system undergoes changes during pregnancy due to both hormonal and mechanical effects. Providing safe and effective care for women during pregnancy requires understanding of the physiological changes of pregnancy as this allows for differentiation between what is normal and what is pathological and may require treatment. It also requires awareness and understanding of the available safety data for medications and other therapies during pregnancy.

In June 2015, the Food and Drug Administration (FDA) updated the Pregnancy and Lactation Labeling Rule [1]. This update eliminated the prior A, B, C, D, X grading system for medication use in pregnancy and lactation. The prior FDA risk categories were often misinterpreted by clinicians to be a grading system for safety rather than a shorthand system for summarizing available data [2]. Furthermore, because they did not discuss the specific conditions for which the drug is used, an emphasis was placed on potential risk rather than potential benefit and/or potential harm from withholding the medication. They were also rarely updated to reflect new and reassuring data. The new pregnancy and lactation labeling rule ("the final rule") requires that the labeling include a summary of the risks of using a drug during pregnancy and lactation, a discussion of the data supporting that summary, and relevant information to help healthcare providers make prescribing decisions and counsel women about the use of drugs during pregnancy and lactation (Table 40.1) [3].

Upper gastrointestinal tract (esophageal and gastric diseases)

Esophageal and gastric function in pregnancy has been studied mainly in relation to nausea and vomiting of pregnancy and gastroesophageal reflux disease (GERD). Basal lower esophageal sphincter (LES) pressure decreases by as much as 50% in pregnancy, reaching a nadir at approximately 36 weeks gestation [4]. This decline is believed to be due to progesterone-mediated smooth muscle relaxation [5]. There is also early evidence that estradiol induces LES relaxation via potassium channels [6]. Loss of the intraabdominal segment of the LES and increased intraabdominal pressure from the physical effects of the expanding gravid uterus may also play a role. In addition, adaptive responses of the LES may be reversibly inhibited [7].

Esophageal motility is not known to be altered by normal pregnancy [8]; however, defective esophageal peristalsis resulting in delayed clearance of esophageal content may contribute to

Yamada's Textbook of Gastroenterology, Seventh Edition. Edited by Timothy C. Wang, Michael Camilleri, Benjamin Lebwohl, Anna S. Lok, William J. Sandborn, Kenneth K. Wang, and Gary D. Wu.

Companion website: www.yamadagastro.com/textbook7e

Table 40.1 Overview of new pregnancy and lactation labeling.

Section	Heading	Information
8.1 Pregnancy	Pregnancy exposure registry	Contact information if pregnancy registry available and general statement about background risk
	Risk summary	Provides "risk statements" that describe for the drug the risk of adverse developmental outcomes based on all relevant human data, animal data and the drug's pharmacology
	Clinical considerations	Provides information to inform prescribing and risk–benefit counseling using the following subheadings: • Disease-associated maternal and/or embryo/fetal risk • Dose adjustments during pregnancy and the postpartum period • Maternal adverse reactions • Fetal/neonatal adverse reactions • Labor or delivery (omit if not applicable)
	Data	Describes the data (human and animal) that provide the scientific basis for the information presented in the Risk Summary and Clinical Considerations
8.2 Lactation	Risk summary	Summarizes information on the presence of a drug and/or its active metabolite(s) in human milk, the effects of a drug and/or its active metabolite(s) on the breastfed child, and the effects of a drug and/or its active metabolite(s) on milk production
	Clinical considerations	Provides information to further inform prescribing and risk–benefit counseling using the following subheadings: • Minimizing exposure • Monitoring for adverse reactions
	Data	Describes the data that provide the scientific basis for the information presented in the Risk Summary and Clinical Considerations
8.3 Females and Males of Reproductive Potential	Pregnancy testing Contraception Infertility	Includes information for these populations when: • There are recommendations or requirements for pregnancy testing and/or contraception before, during, or after drug therapy; and/or • There are human and/or animal data suggesting drug-associated effects on fertility

Source: Data retrieved from [3].

the development of GERD in pregnancy [9]. The effects of pregnancy on gastric motility, on the other hand, are conflicting, possibly due to differences in the techniques used to assess motility, differences in the populations studied, and/or differences in the time point of pregnancy studied [10,11]. Studies by Koch and colleagues using elastogastrography have found altered gastric motility in women with nausea during pregnancy [12]. Nauseated women were more likely to have tachygastria (4–9 cycle-per-minute [cpm] waves) or bradygastria (1–2 cpm waves) compared to nonnauseated controls. Progesterone administration alone or in combination with estradiol demonstrates a slow-wave dysrhythmic effect. The exact mechanism is unclear. However, there is evidence that estrogen and progesterone cause relaxation of gastric smooth muscle [13–15]. Estrogen and progesterone via ERα and ERβ receptors and progesterone receptors, respectively, act on gastric smooth muscles leading to increased release of nitric oxide and higher production of cyclic guanosine monophosphate (cGMP).

Gastroesophageal reflux disease

Epidemiology

Gastroesophageal reflux disease with heartburn affects 30–80% of pregnant women [16,17]. Risk factors for heartburn in pregnancy include increasing gestational age, multigravidity, high pre-pregnancy body mass index, excessive pregnancy weight gain, and history of heartburn. Other associated factors include carbonated beverages, maternal age, smoking, race, and sleep-disordered breathing [9,17,18]. Most patients have a benign course, with only a few experiencing GERD-related complications. However, GERD in pregnancy can impact quality of life (see Chapter 43) [19].

Pathophysiology

The decrease in LES pressure, increased intraabdominal pressure, decreased esophageal peristalsis, and delayed gastric emptying described above are all likely to contribute to the pathophysiology of GERD in pregnancy.

Presentation

As with the general population, heartburn is the most common symptom of GERD in pregnancy. Patients may also report regurgitation, indigestion, epigastric pain, water brash, anorexia, and nausea and vomiting.

Diagnosis

Gastroesophageal reflux disease is a symptom-based diagnosis (see Chapter 43). Radiographic evaluation should be avoided due to the risks of radiation exposure to the fetus. Upper endoscopy is generally not necessary but can be considered in refractory cases.

Treatment

Treatment of GERD in pregnancy is recommended to follow a "step-up" approach, beginning with lifestyle and dietary modifications. Specific lifestyle interventions include tobacco and alcohol cessation, small, frequent meals, elimination of late night meals, and avoidance of recumbency within 3 hours after eating. Minimization of trigger foods or beverages including caffeinated or carbonated beverages, fatty or spicy foods, mints or chocolate, citrus or tomato products is recommended. In addition, medications known to provoke GERD, such as anticholinergics, sedatives, theophylline, prostaglandins and calcium channel blockers, should be discontinued, when possible. Twenty-five percent of patients with uncomplicated GERD experience symptom resolution after making these changes.

Patients who fail conservative measures can be treated with pharmacological treatment (Table 40.2). Antacids, alginic acid, and magnesium and sodium alginates can be considered first-line treatment. Aluminum, magnesium, and calcium-based antacids are generally considered safe in pregnancy. They do, however, have potential side-effects [20,21]. Use of magnesium-based antacids should be avoided in late pregnancy due to the additional potential side-effects of labor arrest and seizures. In addition, antacids can block absorption of iron so pregnant women should be advised not to take iron and antacids together. Sodium bicarbonate should be avoided due to the risk of metabolic alkalosis and fluid overload in the mother and fetus [22].

Alginic acid and the alginates (Gaviscon®) are not systemically absorbed. Two trials have demonstrated that these formulations are safe and efficacious in the treatment of heartburn and GERD symptoms in pregnancy [23,24].

Sucralfate has poor systemic absorption and provides local mucosal protection. Doses up to 50 times those used in humans were not teratogenic in rodent studies. In pregnancy, sucralfate at a dose of 1 g three times daily was found in a randomized controlled trial to provide greater relief from heartburn (90% vs 43%) and regurgitation (83% vs 27%) than lifestyle and dietary changes alone [25].

Metoclopramide can be used in the treatment of GERD [26]. However, a black box warning was issued by the FDA regarding metoclopramide use in 2009 due to the risk of tardive dyskinesia. Clinicians must exercise caution when prescribing this medication and avoid high-dose or long-term use (FDA approved for 4 weeks of use).

The H_2 receptor antagonists (H2-RAs) constitute the next tier of therapy. Ranitidine, cimetidine, famotidine, and nizatidine are considered safe in pregnancy. There is no apparent increase in risk for spontaneous abortions, preterm labor, or low birthweight after first-trimester exposure to an H2-RA [27]. A large metaanalysis found no increase in risk for congenital malformations, spontaneous abortion, preterm delivery, or small for gestational age births [28].

Among the H2-RAs, ranitidine is better studied, making it the preferred H2-RA in pregnancy [29]. At a dose of 150 mg twice a day, ranitidine reduced heartburn severity by an average of 55.6% (95% confidence interval [CI] 34.8–76.5%) compared with baseline and 44.2% (95% CI 15.4–72.9%) compared to placebo. Cimetidine and famotidine carry less safety data in pregnancy but in animal studies, there is no increase in risk of fetal toxicity or teratogenicity [26,30].

Proton pump inhibitors (PPIs) should be reserved for patients with severe symptoms refractory to lifestyle changes, antacids, and the H2-RAs. All the PPIs (lansoprazole, rabeprazole, esomeprazole, pantoprazole, and omeprazole) may be used when clinically indicated. The overall safety of PPIs in pregnancy was

Table 40.2 Pharmacological treatment of gastroesophageal reflux disease and peptic ulcer disease in pregnancy.

Drug class	Drug	Recommendations for pregnancy	Recommendations for lactation
Proton pump inhibitors	Omeprazole Lansoprazole Rabeprazole Esomeprazole Pantoprazole Dexlansoprazole	Data have not shown an increased risk of major birth defects following maternal use during pregnancy but there is conflicting human data. Caution advised	Omeprazole and pantoprazole are present in breast milk. Esomeprazole is the s-isomer of omeprazole, therefore likely present in breast milk. Unknown for lansoprazole, dexlansoprazole, and rabeprazole. Weigh risks/benefits for mother and infant
	Sucralfate	Only minimally absorbed. Use considered acceptable. No increase in the risk of adverse fetal events when used during the first trimester	Unknown if present in breast milk. No human data available. Use is considered acceptable
Dopamine receptor antagonist	Metoclopramide	May use during pregnancy. No increased risk of adverse pregnancy-related outcomes following maternal use. Extrapyramidal symptoms or methemoglobinemia may potentially occur in the neonate	Present in breast milk. Breastfeeding infants should be monitored for extrapyramidal symptoms or methemoglobinemia. Weigh risks/benefits for mother and infant
Histamine H_2 antagonists	Ranitidine Famotidine Nizatidine	All cross the placenta. May use during pregnancy. Renal clearance of famotidine may be increased. Adverse events have not been observed in animal studies	All excreted into breast milk. Weigh risks/benefits for mother and infant. Famotidine is the preferred agent due to its lower concentrations in breast milk

confirmed in a metaanalysis of seven studies by Gill et al. which found no increased risk for major malformations, spontaneous abortions, or preterm delivery with first-trimester use [31]. A Danish cohort study of 840 968 live births, of which 5082 were exposed to a PPI between 4 weeks before conception and the end of the first trimester, found a small increase in the risk of abnormalities in exposed newborns (odds ratio [OR] 1.23; 95% CI 1.05–1.44); however, in secondary analyses limited to the offspring of women who had filled PPI prescriptions and received enough doses to have a theoretical chance of first-trimester exposure, the risk of birth defects was not significantly increased [32].

Peptic ulcer disease

Epidemiology

Epidemiological studies suggest that the incidence of peptic ulcer disease (PUD) is decreased in pregnancy [33–37]. Cappell and Sidhom reported that of 29 317 pregnant women, less than 0.5% had severe upper gastrointestinal complaints and that only two of the 20 women who underwent endoscopy had PUD [38]. Whether the incidence of PUD is truly decreased in pregnancy or whether the available figures reflect underreporting of symptoms and/or the hesitancy by physicians to perform diagnostic tests during pregnancy is not clear.

Risk factors for the development of PUD in pregnancy are the same as for the nonpregnant population (see Chapter 49). These include smoking, nonsteroidal antiinflammatory drug (NSAID) use, alcoholism, genetic predisposition, gastritis, and *Helicobacter pylori* infection. Increased maternal age has also been associated with PUD.

Pathophysiology

The reasons for the decreased incidence of PUD in pregnancy are unknown. Several hypotheses have been proposed, including (1) mislabeling of PUD symptoms as GERD; (2) gastric hypochlorhydria due to lower maternal histamine and/or high estrogen levels; (3) an increased gastric mucous layer due to high progesterone; and (4) favorable behavioral changes in pregnancy such as avoidance of smoking, alcohol, NSAIDs, reduced stress, greater rest, and healthier diet [39].

Clinical presentation

Peptic ulcer disease presents similarly in the pregnant patient as in the general population; however, symptoms may be milder. Older studies suggest that while symptoms may improve during pregnancy, they frequently recur postpartum.

Diagnosis and evaluation

Esophagogastroduodenoscopy (EGD) is not necessary to diagnose PUD but can be performed safely in pregnancy, if necessary [38,40]. A recent population-based retrospective study utilizing the National Inpatient Sample databases from 1999 to 2015 demonstrated that pregnant women are less likely to undergo diagnostic or therapeutic EGDs without appearing to adversely affect their outcomes, thus justifying a conservative approach in this population [41]. Considerations regarding maternal and fetal monitoring, medication use, and hemostasis are discussed later in this chapter. Fluoroscopic and tomographic evaluation of the upper GI tract should be avoided except in medical emergencies.

Complications

Complications from PUD in pregnancy include GI bleeding, perforation, and strictures similar to that in the general population. PUD in pregnancy is associated with an increased risk for low birthweight, preterm birth, and small for gestational age deliveries [42]. In the aforementioned study by Rosen et al., pregnant women who underwent EGD were over eight times more likely to have a venous thromboembolism compared to nonpregnant women on multivariable analysis [41]. This novel finding is possibly explained by the hypercoagulable state of pregnancy and in this one paper, there was recommendation for thromboprophylaxis of pregnant women before EGD. However, further confirmatory studies are needed prior to implementation of this strategy.

Treatment

As with GERD in pregnancy, a sequential treatment regimen has been recommended for pregnant women with PUD, assuming no "red flag" symptoms such as dysphagia, weight loss, and gastrointestinal bleeding are present (see Table 40.2) [39]. Patients found to have active *H. pylori* infection during their PUD evaluation can defer treatment until after pregnancy [43]. Use of bismuth subsalicylate or tetracycline is not advised due to their possible harmful effects [43].

Nausea and vomiting of pregnancy and hyperemesis gravidarum

Epidemiology

Nausea and vomiting of pregnancy (NVP) is estimated to affect 70–80% of pregnant women [44]. Severe NVP is termed hyperemesis gravidarum (HG). In comparison to NVP, HG is rare, occurring in only 0.3–3% of all pregnancies [45]. HG typically is characterized by more than three episodes of vomiting per day with accompanying ketonuria and weight loss of more than 3 kg or 5% of bodyweight [46].

Risk factors for NVP include younger maternal age, nulliparity, low education achievement, nonsmoking status, obesity [47], and multiple gestation [48]. NVP is also associated with low income levels, part-time employment status [49], family history of NVP [50], and a personal history of motion sickness [51] and/or migraine headaches [52]. NVP in a prior pregnancy represents a risk factor for its development in subsequent pregnancies [50].

Risk factors for HG include type 1 diabetes mellitus, multiple gestations, trophoblastic disease, HG in prior pregnancy, fetal abnormalities such as triploidy, trisomy 21, and hydrops fetalis, and nulliparity [53,54]. Approximately 28–33% of women have a history of HG in their mothers and 19% have a history of HG in their sisters [55,56]. Cigarette smoking [53] and male gender of the fetus [54,57,58] may be protective.

Pathogenesis

The exact cause of NVP and HG is unknown. Human chorionic gonadatropin (hCG) levels peak around the time of maximal symptoms and may contribute to the development of NVP and HG by stimulating estrogen production from the ovary [59]. Symptoms are worse in pregnant women with conditions associated with elevated hCG levels such as molar pregnancies, multiple gestations, and Down syndrome [60], and concentrations of hCG correlate positively with symptom severity in women with HG in most but not all studies [46,61].

There is cross-reactivity between the α-subunit of hCG and the thyroid stimulating hormone (TSH) receptor [62]. "Biochemical thyrotoxicosis" characterized by a suppressed TSH and slightly elevated free T4 may be found in up to two-thirds of women with HG [46]. Despite these abnormalities, women with HG are generally euthyroid [63] and almost all women with HG normalize their TSH levels by 20 weeks gestation without intervention [64].

An increased incidence of infection with *H. pylori* has been observed in women with HG [65,66]. *H. pylori* may contribute to NVP and HG by worsening hormone-induced motility changes of the stomach [65]. The majority of infected pregnant women are asymptomatic [67–69]. However, there are case reports demonstrating *H. pylori* treatment alleviating severe HG symptoms [70,71]. Currently there are no guidelines for the evaluation or treatment of *H. pylori* during pregnancy and at this time delaying treatment is recommended [20].

Alterations in lower esophageal sphincter (LES) resting pressure, esophageal peristalsis, and gastric rhythmic activity may also contribute to NVP [72]. Estrogen and progesterone are the likely mediators of esophageal and gastric dysmotility in pregnancy [13–15,22]. Psychological disturbances including neurotic tendencies, hysteria, rejection of femininity, rejection of pregnancy as well as depression and psychological stress related to poverty and marital conflicts have been suggested to cause nausea and vomiting, but their importance has not been well defined [67,73–75].

History and physical examination

Although often termed "morning sickness," NVP typically persists throughout the day and is limited to the morning in less than 2% of women [49]. It begins within 4 weeks after the last menstrual period in most patients [59]. Symptoms usually peak between 10 and 16 weeks gestation and usually resolve by 20 weeks. Up to 10% of women, however, continue to be symptomatic beyond 22 weeks [49]. Patients with NVP may also complain of excess salivation [76] or GERD symptoms.

Most women with NVP have normal vital signs and a benign physical exam. Women with HG may demonstrate evidence of dehydration and orthostasis. A careful abdominal exam should be done to rule out peritonitis and other intraabdominal causes of nausea and vomiting. Women with suspected HG should be evaluated for muscle wasting and symptoms related to nutritional deficiencies.

Differential diagnosis

The onset of nausea and vomiting more than 8 weeks after the last menstrual period is atypical for NVP and should prompt investigation for other causes [59]. The differential diagnosis includes GERD, PUD, small bowel obstruction, and other causes of intraabdominal inflammation [77].

Diagnostic and laboratory tests

Once pregnancy has been established by a positive pregnancy test, no specific laboratory studies are needed for the clinical diagnosis of NVP. Laboratory studies may be helpful in excluding other causes of nausea and vomiting. A pelvic ultrasound can be helpful to document pregnancy and evaluate for conditions that increase the risk for NVP such as multiple gestation.

For women with suspected HG, serum electrolytes, blood urea nitrogen, creatinine, and hematocrit should be monitored. Urinalysis may reveal associated ketonuria and increased urine specific gravity. Hypochloremic metabolic alkalosis or metabolic acidosis with severe volume contraction is common [78]. Low prealbumin levels reflect poor protein nutritional status in the mother and may predict lower fetal birthweights [79]. Vitamin and mineral deficiencies are also possible [77].

Liver chemistries are abnormal in up to 40% of hospitalized patients with HG [80]. Mild hyperbilirubinemia (bilirubin <4 mg per deciliter) and/or a rise in alkaline phosphatase to twice the upper limit of normal (ULN) may be seen [81]. Alanine aminotransferase (ALT) levels are generally higher than aspartate aminotransferase (AST) levels. Aminotransferase levels are usually no more than 2–3 times ULN, although levels greater than 1000 U/mL have been reported [82]. The abnormal liver tests resolve promptly upon resolution of vomiting.

Serum amylase and lipase elevations are seen in 10–15% of women [78] and the increase in amylase is thought to be due to excessive salivary gland production [67].

Outcome

Nausea and vomiting of pregnancy is associated with a favorable outcome for the fetus, with no increase in risk for congenital abnormalities, miscarriage, or perinatal mortality [83–86]. Moreover, women without NVP deliver earlier compared to women with NVP [87]. NVP can cause substantial psychosocial morbidity in the mother [88,89]. It is also associated with depressed mood, consideration of pregnancy termination, and impaired relationships with partners.

Hyperemesis gravidarum, in comparison, is associated with adverse maternal and fetal outcomes, including low pregnancy weight gain (<7 kg), low birthweight (LBW) babies, small for gestational age babies, preterm birth, and poor 5-minute Apgar scores [90–93].

Common maternal complications include weight loss, dehydration, micronutrient deficiency, and muscle weakness. More severe, albeit rare, complications include Mallory–Weiss tears, Wernicke encephalopathy, retinal hemorrhage, spontaneous pneumomediastinum [94], and vasospasm of the cerebral arteries [95]. HG may also lead to psychological problems and termination of an otherwise wanted pregnancy [96].

Congenital malformations are more common [57], and fetal coagulopathy and chondrodysplasia have been reported from vitamin K deficiency [97] with third-trimester fetal intracranial hemorrhage [98].

Severity assessment

The Pregnancy Unique Quantification of Emesis (PUQE) score [99] and the Hyperemesis Impact of Symptoms Questionnaire (HIS) [100] can be used to assess the severity of symptoms.

Treatment

Early treatment of NVP is recommended to prevent progression to HG as it is thought to be on the continuum. Additionally, there is also emphasis on prevention with recommendations on the prophylactic use of prenatal vitamins prior to pregnancy. Studies have demonstrated a reduction in the incidence and severity of NVP in patients on prenatal vitamins one month before pregnancy [101,102].

Nonpharmacological therapy

Patients should avoid large meals and eat several small meals throughout the day [103]. Fatty foods may further delay gastric emptying and should be avoided. Protein-predominant or liquid meals may be beneficial [104]. Small volumes of salty liquids such as electrolyte replacement sport beverages are helpful [105]. Supportive psychotherapy, behavioral therapy, and hypnotherapy may be needed for women with severe symptoms and/or those in whom personality characteristics, marital, or family conflict play a role [106].

Ginger is the sole nonpharmacological intervention recommended by the American College of Obstetrics and Gynecology [45] as systematic reviews have demonstrated that ginger alleviates nausea for patients, although without any effect on actual vomiting [44,107,108]. Ginger may stimulate motility and one component of ginger has been shown to have similar activity to ondansetron [109].

Acupressure on the Neiguan or P6 point on the wrist may be helpful in treating HG [60]. Pressure may be placed manually or with elastic bands on the inside of the wrist. In a randomized, placebo-controlled trial, the ReliefBand®, a battery-operated electrical nerve stimulator, was associated with symptom relief and weight gain [110]. While studies regarding the benefits of acupressure have been limited, two systematic review found some benefit [44,108], thus some experts believe it should be offered given the absence of adverse side-effects [111].

Pharmacological treatment (Table 40.3)

Dicligis®, a combination of pyridoxine (vitamin B_6) and doxylamine, is the only medication specifically approved for the treatment of NVP by the FDA [112]. Previously sold under the brand name Bendectin®, the combination formulation was removed from the market in the US in 1983 due to concern over teratogencity with first-trimester use. There is now substantial follow-up data supporting its efficacy [59,113] and safety [114,115]. Combination doxylamine-pyridoxine is recommended by the American College of Obstetricians and Gynecologists (ACOG) as first-line therapy for NVP [45]. Patients intolerant to the antihistamine side-effects of doxylamine can also try pyridoxine alone [116,117].

The phenothiazines, chlorpromazine and prochlorperazine, are dopamine antagonists which have been shown to reduce symptoms in NVP and HG [118]. There are concerns regarding birth defects and other adverse effects [119–121], but the aggregate of studies demonstrates safety [122].

Metoclopramide is widely used for the treatment of NVP [123]. A recent study found 10 mg of metoclopramide given every 8 hours for 24 hours to be as effective in women with HG during their first hospitalization as 25 mg of promethazine given every 8 hours for 24 hours, and was better tolerated.

With regard to safety, in a study of 81 703 births involving exposure to metoclopramide, no increased risk of major congenital malformations, low birthweight, preterm delivery, or perinatal death was found [124]. Metoclopramide use is limited by its side-effect profile which includes dystonia, restlessness, and somnolence. In 2009, the FDA added a black box warning to metoclopramide due to the risk of tardive dyskinesia with chronic use.

Antihistamines, such as diphenhydramine and dimenhydrinate, indirectly affect the vestibular system, decreasing stimulation of the vomiting center [125]. Randomized controlled trials of antihistamine use in NVP are limited [118] but their use does not increase teratogenic risk [126].

Ondansetron is currently one of the most commonly prescribed antiemetics [125,127]. In women with HG, ondansetron is as effective as promethazine or metoclopramide [128,129] and less sedating [130]. When used in pregnancy, there is no significant increase in the number of miscarriages, major malformations, or birthweight between infants exposed to ondansetron and unexposed controls [131]. Oral and intravenous corticosteroids have been used for refractory cases of HG with variable results. In a randomized controlled trial of 40 women with HG treated with intravenous (IV) methylprednisolone, a lower rate of rehospitalization was found in the steroid-treated

Table 40.3 Pharmacological treatment of nausea and vomiting and hyperemesis gravidarum (HG) in pregnancy.

Drug class	Drug	Recommendations for pregnancy	Recommendations for lactation
Supplement	Vitamin B_6 (pyridoxine)	No known risk of fetal harm based on human data	Pyridoxine is present in breast milk. Effects on milk production inconclusive
	Vitamin B_6 with doxylamine	Adequate well-controlled studies in pregnant women have not shown an increased risk of fetal abnormalities	Pyridoxine is present in breast milk. Possible risk of infant CNS depression with doxylamine. According to the manufacturer, women using this combination should not breastfeed
Phenothiazines	Chlorpromazine Prochlorperazine	Use in third trimester of pregnancy has a risk for extrapyramidal symptoms and withdrawal symptoms in newborns following delivery. Low risk of teratogenicity based on human studies	Consider alternative. Concern for the potential for serious adverse reactions in the breastfeeding infant based on drug's mechanism of action
Dopamine receptor antagonist	Metoclopramide	See Table 40.2	
Antihistamines	Diphenhydramine Dimenhydrinate	Both cross the placenta. May use during pregnancy. Use prior to childbirth may cause respiratory depression in the newborn	Both are present in breast milk. Infant should be monitored for CNS depression
Serotonin 5-hydroxytryptamine type 3 receptor antagonists	Ondansetron	Consider avoidance in first trimester of pregnancy. Possible risk of teratogenicity, conflicting human studies	Caution advised. It is unknown if ondansetron is present in breast milk. Weigh risks/benefits for mother and infant
Corticosteroid	Methylprednisolone	The ACOG guidelines recommend its use with caution, as a last-resort treatment in HG, and it should be avoided before 10 weeks of gestation	
Antacids, histamine H_2 antagonists, proton pump inhibitors		See Table 40.2	

ACOG, American College of Gastroenterology; CNS, central nervous system.

group [132]. Other studies have not shown a statistically significant benefit of corticosteroids [133]. Three studies have demonstrated an association between oral clefts and methylprednisone use in the first trimester [134–136]. The ACOG guidelines recommend its use with caution, as a last-resort treatment in HG, and it should be avoided before 10 weeks of gestation [45].

Acid-reducing medications (i.e., antacids, H_2 blockers, and proton pump inhibitors) may be helpful in the treatment of NVP. One cohort study showed that women with NVP and heartburn had more severe nausea and vomiting than women without heartburn [137]. Follow-up studies have shown that treatment of GERD symptoms results in improved PUQE and quality of life scores [137].

Intravenous hydration and nutritional support

Women with symptoms unresponsive to dietary modification and pharmacological treatment who are unable to maintain weight require IV fluid therapy and/or nutritional support to prevent fetal intrauterine growth restriction, maternal dehydration and malnutrition. Women requiring multiple hospitalizations should be considered for in-home IV hydration [76,77]. Enteral feeding is preferred to total parenteral nutrition [138,139].

Disorders of the intestinal tract

Celiac disease

Celiac disease is an autoimmune disorder of the small intestine which is triggered by gluten ingestion (see Chapter 56). The only treatment available is lifelong adherence to a gluten-free diet (GFD). Obstetric and gynecological complications which have been associated with celiac disease include impaired fertility (both female and male) and an increased risk for adverse pregnancy outcomes [140].

Effect on fertility

Studies using serological screening have found significantly higher prevalence (4–8%) of celiac disease among women with unexplained infertility compared with the general population [141–143]. However, others have not confirmed this [144–146]. Whether a GFD improves fertility requires further investigation as studies to date have been inconclusive [147–149].

Effect on pregnancy

The effect of celiac disease on pregnancy outcomes is unclear [147,148,150–157]. However, withdrawal of gluten improves pregnancy outcomes, reducing risks for low birthweight, intrauterine growth retardation, and miscarriage in treated versus untreated women [152,153,158]. Consequently, some experts advocate screening for celiac disease in women with a history of recurrent spontaneous abortion, intrauterine growth retardation, and low birthweight [143].

Irritable bowel syndrome

Despite the prevalence of irritable bowel syndrome (IBS) (see Chapter 67) among reproductive-aged women, only a few studies of IBS in pregnancy have been conducted. One cohort study detected moderately increased risks for miscarriage (OR 1.21; 95% CI 1.13–1.30) and ectopic pregnancy (OR 1.28%; 95% CI 1.06–1.55) in women with IBS diagnosed before pregnancy, suggesting the need for high-quality prenatal care for this population [159].

Constipation

Epidemiology

After nausea, constipation is the next most common GI complaint and is experienced by up to 40% of pregnant women [160]. Risk factors include a prior history of treatment for constipation and iron supplementation. There is no clear association between dietary fiber intake and constipation during pregnancy [161,162].

Pathophysiology

The pathophysiology of constipation in pregnancy is multifactorial. Colonic motility is decreased [163,164]. Increased colonic transit time, in turn, leads to increased water absorption, causing stools to become small and hard. Decreased physical activity and supplementation with constipating agents such as iron and calcium may further worsen bowel function [165]. Later in pregnancy, pressure on the rectosigmoid colon from the gravid uterus may produce an additional mechanical barrier to evacuation [166].

Diagnosis

Low frequency of stools (<3 per week), hard stools, and/or difficulty evacuating feces have been suggested to be clinical criteria for constipation in pregnancy [166]. These symptoms along with the sensation of incomplete evacuation should trigger counseling and treatment for constipation. Patients should also be questioned about prolonged straining, perineal pressure or digital manipulation in order to defecate as these habits are suggestive of pelvic floor dysfunction [166].

The general approach to evaluation of constipation is similar to that for the nonpregnant patient (see Chapter 36), with specific consideration of imaging and other risks associated with pregnancy [167].

Treatment

Conservative treatment

The initial management includes patient education and reassurance about normal bowel function in pregnancy. Patients should be counseled to increase physical activity, practice Kegel exercises to gain better control of pelvic floor musculature, and take advantage of the gastrocolic reflex by scheduling defecation after meals [168]. Patients also should increase water intake [166]. Increasing dietary fiber to 20–35 g/d may prove helpful, but may also produce greater abdominal pain and distension [169].

Pharmacological treatment (Table 40.4)

Bulk-forming agents

Bulk-forming agents such as methylcellulose, psyllium, and unprocessed bran are considered safe during pregnancy and lactation. A Cochrane review of two studies found fiber supplements increased the frequency of defecation and lead to softer stools [160]. The daily dose of fiber should be titrated upwards gradually to avoid worsening abdominal bloating, gas, cramping and diarrhea, and adequate fluid intake should accompany use of these agents [169].

Osmotic laxatives

Polyethylene glycol (PEG) is the preferred treatment of the American Gastroenterological Association (AGA) for chronic constipation in pregnancy [43]. It is generally well tolerated, causing less abdominal bloating and gas than other osmotic laxatives. Lactulose can also be tried [170]. Osmotic laxatives such as magnesium citrate and magnesium hydroxide work rapidly, but only provide short-term, intermittent relief and should not be used daily [43]. In addition, the magnesium-containing salts can cause maternal sodium retention and should not be used by women with renal and cardiac disease [171].

Stimulant laxatives

Stimulant laxative use in pregnancy should be reserved for those not responding to other measures [169]. Stimulant laxatives are more effective than bulk-forming agents, but they also have more side-effects including abdominal pain, nausea, and bloating [160].

Senna was not found to be associated with a higher risk for congenital abnormalities or adverse birth outcomes [172]. Dantron and aloe are associated with congenital malformations [170,173] and should not be used in pregnancy. Castor oil is contraindicated in pregnancy as it may induce premature uterine contractions [168].

Emollient laxatives

Docusate sodium is frequently used to treat constipation in pregnancy but studies on efficacy are lacking. Safety has been demonstrated in several studies [174]. Mineral oil is contraindicated in pregnancy and may decrease maternal absorption of fat-soluble vitamins including vitamin K, increasing risk for neonatal hypoprothrombinemia and hemorrhage [175].

Secretagogs

For both tegaserod and prucalopride, studies confirming safety in pregnancy are limited [176], so routine use is not recommended in pregnancy [166]. Lubiprostone and linaclotide have also not been adequately studied in human pregnancy so their use in pregnancy is not recommended.

Table 40.4 Pharmacological treatment of constipation in pregnancy.

Drug class	Drug	Recommendations for pregnancy	Recommendations for lactation
Bulk-forming agents	Psyllium Methylcellulose Polycarbophil calcium Wheat dextrin	Administer with adequate fluids. Use is considered acceptable	NA
Osmotic laxative	Polyethylene glycol (PEG) PEG 3350	May use during pregnancy with minimal systemic absorption. Unlikely to cause fetal malformations	May use during pregnancy because only minimal amounts are absorbed. No human data available
	Lactulose	Adverse events have not been observed in animal reproduction studies. Lactulose is poorly absorbed following oral administration. Short-term use of lactulose is also considered to be safe/low risk when therapy is needed; however, side-effects may limit its use.	Unknown if excreted in breast milk; however, lactulose is poorly absorbed following oral administration. The manufacturer recommends that caution be exercised in nursing women
	Sorbitol	Animal reproduction studies have not been conducted	The manufacturer recommends that caution be exercised in nursing women
	Magnesium citrate Magnesium oxide	Crosses the placenta. Caution advised Although occasional use is OK, long-term use should be avoided	May use during breastfeeding. No known infant risk based on limited human studies
Stimulant laxative	Bisacodyl	May use during pregnancy. No known risk of fetal harm based on human studies	Unknown if present in breast milk, but may use based on minimal systemic absorption. No human studies
	Sennosides	May use during pregnancy. No known risk of fetal harm based on human studies	May use while breastfeeding. No known risk of fetal harm based on limited human studies
	Sodium picosulfate	Caution advised though no known fetal harm seen in animal data	May use while breastfeeding. No human studies available
	Castor oil Dantron Aloe	Contraindicated	Contraindicated
Emollient laxative	Docusate	Docusate sodium may be used if needed, but may not be as effective as other agents	May use while breastfeeding though unknown if present in breast milk. No human studies available
	Mineral oil	Contraindicated in pregnancy	Contraindicated in pregnancy
Guanylate cyclase-C agonists	Linaclotide Plecanitide	May use during pregnancy. No human studies available. Maternal use is not expected to result in fetal exposure	May use while breastfeeding, although unknown if either is excreted in breast milk. No human studies available
Chloride channel activator	Lubiprostone	May use during pregnancy. No human studies, though adverse events have been observed in animal studies	May use while breastfeeding, although unknown if present in breast milk. The manufacturer recommends that breastfed infants be monitored for diarrhea
Serotonin 5-HT_4 receptor agonist	Prucalopride	Caution in pregnancy as spontaneous abortions were observed in clinical trials. However, available data are insufficient to evaluate the risk of adverse maternal or fetal outcomes. Use of appropriate contraception in females of reproductive potential	Prucalopride is present in breast milk, therefore weigh risks/benefits for mother and infant
	Tegaserod	Caution in pregnancy as adverse events were observed in some animal reproduction studies	Unknown if present in breast milk. Use alternative due to potential serious adverse reactions in the breastfeeding infant

Diarrhea

Epidemiology

The prevalence of diarrhea in pregnancy is unknown, but 34% of pregnant women report more frequent bowel movements [168,177].

Pathophysiology

The causes of diarrhea in pregnancy are essentially the same as for the nonpregnant population (see Chapter 35). These include infection, medications, functional diarrheas, malabsorption, inflammatory bowel disease (IBD), and endocrine disorders such as hyperthyroidism and adrenal insufficiency.

Diagnosis

Patients presenting with diarrhea lasting more than a week with weight loss or with symptoms of hypovolemia, hematochezia, severe abdominal pain, a history of recent antibiotics use, or immuncompromise should undergo diagnostic evaluation (see Chapter 35) [168,178].

Treatment

Treatment of diarrhea in pregnancy should begin with conservative management, including oral rehydration, correction of electrolyte abnormalities, and dietary modification. Small, frequent meals which are low in fat and caffeine and do not contain artificial sweeteners are advised [179]. Bismuth subsalicylate as found in Kaopectate® and Pepto-Bismol® should not be used chronically as significant fetal adverse effects have resulted from chronic exposure to salicylates [180]. Alosetron should not be started in pregnancy but animal data suggest a low risk of teratogenicity. Therefore, if indicated, alosetron should not be withheld because of pregnancy [181].

Pharmacological treatment (Table 40.5)

Opioids

Loperamide is a peripherally acting opiate receptor agonist [182,183] and is the preferred antidiarrheal agent for use during pregnancy [168]. Loperamide is not known to be teratogenic but it has been associated with lower birthweights [183]. In comparison, diphenoxylate with atropine is teratogenic in animals and humans, and therefore is not recommended in pregnancy [179].

Bile acid sequestrants

Bile acid sequestrants can be used to treat some forms of diarrhea. As bile acid sequestrants interfere with the absorption of fat-soluble vitamins including vitamin K, they may lead to maternal coagulopathy. Women taking bile acid sequestrants for prolonged periods during pregnancy should be monitored for fat-soluble vitamin deficiency and disordered clotting function [184].

Irritable bowel syndrome/abdominal pain (Table 40.6)

Treatment

Tricyclic antidepressants

Amitriptyline, desipramine, nortriptyline, and imipramine are tricyclic antidepressants (TCAs) which in low dose are helpful

Table 40.5 Pharmacological treatment of diarrhea in pregnancy.

Drug class	Drug	Recommendations for pregnancy	Recommendations for lactation
Bismuth salts	Bismuth subsalicylate	Caution advised. Significant fetal adverse effects have resulted from chronic exposure to salicylates. Restricted use to <20 weeks gestation and then only in amounts that do not exceed recommended doses. Avoid use >20 weeks gestation	No human data. Potential toxicity. Use alternative
Selective 5-HT_3 receptor antagonist	Alosetron	No reports in human pregnancy have been located. Animal studies suggest low risk. The lack of human studies prevents assessment of risks. Therefore, if indicated, alosetron should not be withheld because of pregnancy	Unknown if present in breast milk. Use alternative while breastfeeding. Weigh risks/benefits for mother and infant. Monitor infants for severe constipation or blood in stools
Opioid	Loperamide diphenoxylate/ atropine	Caution advised as use in pregnancy is limited and data are conflicting. For acute diarrhea in pregnant women, loperamide in small amounts may be used only if symptoms are disabling	Loperamide may be present in breast milk. May use while breastfeeding, though no human studies available
	Diphenoxylate/ atropine	Caution in third trimester use with CNS depression risk at time of parturition. Limited human studies	Atropine is present in breast milk; diphenoxylic acid may be present in breast milk. Consider alternative during breastfeeding
Bile acid sequestrant	Cholestyramine Colestipol Colesevelam	Caution advised as they may interfere with maternal vitamin absorption; therefore, regular prenatal supplementation may not be adequate	Is not expected to be present in breast milk due to lack of systemic absorption. Caution advised as possible risk of infant fat-soluble vitamin deficiency with prolonged use

CNS, central nervous system.

Table 40.6 Pharmacological treatment of abdominal pain in pregnancy.

Drug class	Drug	Recommendations for pregnancy	Recommendations for lactation
Tricyclic antidepressant	Amitriptyline	Caution in third trimester. Teratogenicity has been noted in case reports (causal relationship not established). Possible risk of neonatal withdrawal symptoms	May use during breastfeeding. Low risk of infant harm based on drug properties and limited human studies
	Desipramine	Caution advised in third trimester. Animal studies are inconclusive. Possible risk of neonatal withdrawal symptoms	May use during breastfeeding. Low risk of infant harm based on drug properties and limited human studies
	Nortriptyline	Caution advised in pregnancy, particularly third trimester. Possible risk of neonatal withdrawal symptoms	May use during breastfeeding. Is present in breast milk. Infants should be monitored for signs of adverse events
	Imipramine	Caution advised in pregnancy, particularly third trimester. Congenital abnormalities have been reported in humans. Possible risk of neonatal withdrawal symptoms	May use during breastfeeding. Is present in breast milk. Infants should be monitored for signs of adverse events
Selective serotonin reuptake inhibitor	Fluoxetine	Caution advised in pregnancy, particularly third trimester. Possible risk of neonatal withdrawal symptoms	Is present in breast milk. Consider alternative during breastfeeding. Low risk of infant harm based on human studies
	Sertraline	Caution advised in pregnancy, particularly third trimester. Possible risk of neonatal withdrawal symptoms	SSRI of choice during breastfeeding. Low risk of infant harm based on human studies
	Escitalopram Citalopram	Caution advised in pregnancy, particularly third trimester. Possible risk of neonatal withdrawal symptoms	Consider alternative during breastfeeding. No studies to judge risk of infant harm
	Fluvoxamine	Caution advised in pregnancy, particularly third trimester. Possible risk of neonatal withdrawal symptoms	May use during breastfeeding. Low risk of infant harm based on human studies
	Vilazodone	Caution advised in pregnancy, particularly third trimester. Possible risk of neonatal withdrawal symptoms	Consider alternative during breastfeeding. No studies to judge risk of infant harm
	Vortioxetine	Caution advised in pregnancy, particularly third trimester. Possible risk of neonatal withdrawal symptoms	Consider alternative during breastfeeding. No studies to judge risk of infant harm
	Paroxetine	Paroxetine crosses the placenta. Discontinue paroxetine. Only indicated in menopausal females	Is present in breast milk. Only indicated in menopausal females
Antispasmodic	Dicyclomine	May be used in pregnancy. No known embryo-fetal risk based on human studies	Use is contraindicated in breastfeeding women due to possible infant apnea risk
	Hyoscyamine	Caution advised during pregnancy. Animal reproduction studies have not been conducted	Present in breast milk, so caution advised with breastfeeding women. No human studies to judge risk of infant harm
Calcium channel blocker	Nifedipine	May use during pregnancy. It crosses the placenta, but low risk of fetal harm based on limited human studies	Is present in breast milk though low risk of infant harm based on human studies
	Diltiazem	Adverse events have been observed in animal studies, so caution is advised. Other agents preferred	Is present in breast milk with caution advised during breastfeeding

SSRI, selective serotonin reuptake inhibitor.

for the treatment of IBS. Although neonatal withdrawal symptoms of cyanosis, respiratory distress, irritability, autonomic dysfunction, and hypoactivity have been reported after in utero exposure, a joint study of several European teratology information services found TCAs to be safe [185,186]. Nevertheless, TCAs are recommended for use in pregnancy only in women with severe gastrointestinal symptoms of IBS [184].

Selective serotonin reuptake inhibitors

The selective serotonin reuptake inhibitors (SSRIs) are generally considered safe in pregnancy [187]; however, use of paroxetine should be avoided due to the potential risk of fetal heart defects and other negative effects. Like TCAs, SSRIs have been associated with a neonatal withdrawal syndrome [188] and use for IBS in pregnancy should be limited to those with severe symptoms.

Antispasmodics

Antispasmodic medications should be avoided in pregnancy as their safety has not been established [184]. Drugs in this category include the anticholinergics, dicyclomine and hyocyamine, and calcium channel blockers such as nifedipine and diltiazem.

Inflammatory bowel disease

Inflammatory bowel diseases (IBD), Crohn's disease (CD), and ulcerative colitis (UC) are predominantly diseases of young adults, with peak incidence during the reproductive years [189]. Because fertility is, in most cases, preserved, many patients with IBD successfully conceive. This in turn may lead to challenges in the evaluation and management of IBD in pregnancy.

Fertility

Infertility rates for men and women with IBD of 5–14% are comparable to the general population [190–192]. Higher rates of infertility are observed in those who have undergone colectomy with ileal pouch construction and potentially other IBD surgeries [193]. A metaanalysis of eight studies confirmed that ileal pouch with anal anastomosis (IPAA) for UC increased the risk of infertility from 15% to 48% [194], likely due to impaired tubal function from adhesion formation after deep pelvic dissection. The effect appears to be permanent [193]. Ileorectal anastomosis and laparoscopic restorative proctocolectomy have been shown to improve pregnancy rates compared to standard open colectomy with IPAA [195,196].

Fertility in men with IBD is affected by sulfasalazine use which reversibly decreases sperm count, impairs motility, and alters morphology [197]. After two full cycles of spermatogenesis or 2 months after discontinuing the drug, sperm counts and quality should recover [198]. Methotrexate may also impact male fertility by causing oligospermia [199]. Impaired fertility has also been described in some men who have undergone IPAA due to retrograde ejaculation and erectile dysfunction [200]; however, overall pouch creation has been found to improve male sexual function [201].

Effect of pregnancy on IBD

Pregnancy has not been shown to increase the risk for flares in women with IBD. The risk of exacerbation during pregnancy (32–34%) is similar to that in nonpregnant women [202,203]. Notably, disease remission at the time of conception is very important for maintaining quiescent disease during pregnancy. Relapse rates in pregnancy and the puerperium were 34% and 27% for women with quiescent UC and CD at conception, respectively [204]. In contrast, up to two-thirds of women with active disease at conception will have persistent or worsening activity throughout pregnancy [205–207]. Thus, women with IBD should strive for disease remission prior to conception. They also should continue medications during pregnancy and not resume smoking after delivery to reduce the risk of flaring [197,208,209]

Alteration of ileoanal pouch function during pregnancy is common, especially in the third trimester [210]. Stool habits generally return to normal by 3 months postpartum [211].

Effect of IBD on pregnancy

Women with IBD are at increased risk for preterm birth, cesarean section, and having low-birthweight infants [212]. An increased risk for congenital anomalies among offspring of patients with UC has also been found, with an OR of 2.37 (95% CI 1.47–3.82); however, this may be more related to medication use than the disease itself [213] as other studies have not confirmed this finding [16,199].

Several studies indicate that the increased risk of adverse events is independent of disease activity [16,200]. In a population-based study from the US, women with IBD were found to be at increased risk for an adverse pregnancy outcome irrespective of disease activity (stillbirth, preterm birth, small for gestational age, spontaneous abortion, or complication of labor), compared to the general population [20].

Management

Treatment of active IBD in pregnancy follows the same guidelines as for nonpregnant patients given the potential adverse impact of disease activity on pregnancy outcomes (see Chapters 63 and 64). Mesalamine, corticosteriods, antibiotics, cyclosporine, and antitumor necrosis factor α (TNF-α) agents can all be initiated to control disease activity in pregnancy, if needed. Surgery should be performed for women with toxic megacolon, perforation, intestinal obstruction, or intractable bleeding. Only a few case studies and case reports have described the outcomes of women requiring surgery during pregnancy [214,215], In general, with the use of modern surgical and anesthetic techniques, the risks for maternal death and fetal loss appear to be low [216].

The mode of delivery in women with IBD, in general, is dictated by obstetric considerations. Women with active perianal disease, however, should undergo cesarean section as vaginal delivery may further disrupt the perineum and injure the anal sphincter [217].

Breastfeeding

Breastfeeding is not known to influence disease activity and may be protective for the future development of IBD [218]. Nevertheless, many women with IBD choose not to breastfeed [208]. Physician recommendations, the fear of medication transfer in breast milk, and personal preferences are the most common reasons why women with IBD do not breastfeed.

Treatment (Table 40.7)

Most patients with IBD require one or more medications to maintain disease remission. Since disease quiescence at conception is important for maintaining remission through pregnancy, women should not discontinue their medications while trying to conceive. With few exceptions, medications should be continued before and during pregnancy. It is important to carefully evaluate the risks and benefits of each medication with patients.

Table 40.7 Pharmacological treatment of inflammatory bowel disease in pregnancy.

Drug class	Drug	Recommendation for pregnancy	Recommendation for lactation
5-Aminosalicylic acid derivative	Mesalamine	Low risk	Limited human data; potential diarrhea in breastfed infants
	Sulfasalazine	Interferes with folate metabolism; give with 2 mg of folate	Limited human data; potential diarrhea in breastfed infants
Corticosteroid	Prednisone	Possible increased risk of oral clefts with first-trimester use; risk for fetal adrenal insufficiency, macrosomia, premature rupture of membranes	Compatible
Immunosuppressant agent	Azathioprine/6-mercaptopurine	Probably safe for continued use in pregnancy; avoid starting de novo in pregnancy	Not recommended
	Methotrexate	Contraindicated due to teratogenicity; stop 6 months prior to conception	Contraindicated
	Thalidomide	Contraindicated due to teratogenicity	Contraindicated
Anti-TNF agent	Infliximab	Low risk	Compatible
	Adalimumab	Low risk	Compatible
	Certolizumab pegol	Low risk	Compatible
	Golimumab	Limited evidence, likely low risk	Limited evidence, likely low risk
Integrin antagonist	Natalizumab	Discontinue 3 months prior to conception	Limited evidence, likely low risk
	Vedolizumab	Low risk	Limited evidence, likely low risk
Anti-IL-12/23 agent	Ustekinumab	Limited evidence	Limited evidence, likely low risk
Small molecules	Tofacitinib	Contraindicated due to possible teratogenicity	Contraindicated

Source: Lee et al. [301]. Reproduced by permission of Elsevier.

5-Aminosalicylates

The 5-aminosalicylates (5-ASAs) including sulfasalazine and mesalamine/mesalazine are considered low risk in pregnancy. A metaanalysis of seven studies of pregnancy outcomes in women with IBD exposed to 5-ASAs found no increased risk for congenital abnormalities, stillbirth, spontaneous abortion, preterm delivery or low birthweight [219]. Additionally, a large study of 1703 children born to women with IBD found no increased risk of congenital anomalies with 5-ASA exposure during pregnancy [220].

Women of childbearing age taking sulfasalazine should take 1 mg of supplemental folate twice daily if considering pregnancy [221]. Men on sulfasalazine should be informed about the reversible oligospermia and adverse changes in sperm motility and morphology associated with the drug [222,223]. It is advised that men taking sulfasalazine discontinue the drug for at least 3 months before attempting conception.

Both sulfasalazine and mesalamine are compatible with breastfeeding. Single case reports, however, suggest an association with watery diarrhea in the newborn with mesalamine use [224], and hematochezia with sulfasalazine use [225].

Corticosteroids

Corticosteroids are considered safe in pregnancy. There is inefficient transplacental transfer of prednisolone compared to other steroid preparations, so prednisolone is preferred for pregnant women [198].

Epidemiological studies have reported an increased risk for orofacial clefts in newborns exposed to steroids early in gestation [135,226,227]. A metaanalysis of 10 studies also found the risk for cleft palates to be increased [134].

Azathioprine/6-mercaptopurine

Previously, women were instructed to avoid pregnancy if they were taking the thiopurines, azathioprine and 6-mercaptopurine (6-MP). Studies in mice using 4–13 times the maximum human therapeutic dose demonstrate teratogenicity [228,229]. However, observational data from human pregnancies have not found a higher rate of major fetal malformations in women taking thiopurines compared to women on nonteratogenic medications ($p = 0.78$; OR 1.17; 95% CI 0.37–3.69) [230,231].

Overall, the thiopurine safety data from pregnant women with IBD is consistent with experience from the transplant literature where there is no evidence for higher rates or consistent patterns of malformations [232–234]. Thus, based on the best available data, continuation of thiopurines during pregnancy appears to be low risk.

The American Academy of Pediatrics (AAP) does not recommend breastfeeding while taking a thiopurine due to the hypothetical risk of immunosuppression in the neonate. However, thiopurine transfer via breast milk is exceedingly low [235], and no deleterious consequences of low-level transfer of thiopurine metabolites to the breastfed newborn have been found [236,237].

Methotrexate

Methotrexate is teratogenic and is contraindicated in pregnancy. Exposure to methotrexate during organogenesis (6–8 weeks after conception) is associated with multiple congenital anomalies collectively called methotrexate embryopathy or fetal aminopterin-methotrexate syndrome [238]. Thus, methotrexate should be used with extreme caution in reproductive-aged men and women and discontinued for 6 months before conception [192,198,221].

Methotrexate is excreted into breast milk at low levels [239]. The American Academy of Pediatrics advises against breastfeeding while on methotrexate [240].

Thalidomide

Thalidomide is teratogenic and contraindicated for use in pregnancy or during breastfeeding. Contraception should be employed while taking this medication if the patient is sexually active [192] and the drug should be discontinued for 6 months before conception.

Cyclosporine

Cyclosporine is known to cross the placenta [241]. Animal studies have not demonstrated teratogenic effects [242,243]. A metaanalysis did not find increased risk for major malformations, preterm birth, or low birthweight with cyclosporine use after solid-organ transplantation [242]. Similarly, in women treated with cyclosporine for steroid refractory UC in pregnancy, there was no increase in the rate of congenital malformations [244–246]. Cyclosporine is transferred at high levels into breast milk. The American Academy of Pediatrics advises against breastfeeding while on cyclosporine [247].

Tacrolimus

Most safety data regarding tacrolimus use in pregnancy are derived from posttransplant patients and have been largely favorable [238]. Tacrolimus use in pregnant women with IBD has not been adequately studied.

Tacrolimus is transferred in breast milk and its use by breastfeeding mothers is not advised [239].

Antibiotics

The antibiotics used most commonly in IBD, ciprofloxacin and metronidazole, should be used with caution in pregnancy. The quinolones are associated with an increased risk for cartilage defects in immature animals [240] but no adverse effects have been noted in women or infants [240,241]. Ciprofloxacin is compatible with breastfeeding.

Metronidazole has been previously associated with the risk for cleft lip and cleft palate when given during the first trimester [242]. However, a metaanalysis of 199 451 pregnant women with first-trimester exposure did not find an association between metronidazole and birth defects [248]. Additional studies have not found any association between metronidazole use and either adverse pregnancy or infant outcomes [249]. Short-term use of metronidazole can be safe in pregnancy. Breastfeeding while taking metronidazole is not advised.

Rifaximin has limited oral absorption. The exposure to the fetus is expected to be low. Currently, there are no data regarding safety in human pregnancy or lactation.

Biologics

Infliximab

Infliximab has been shown to cross the placenta and is detectable in cord blood and in the serum of exposed infants [246]. Nevertheless, use of infliximab has not been associated with adverse pregnancy or neonatal outcomes.[250,251]

Infliximab is detectable at low levels in breast milk [247–251]. However, it is felt to be compatible with breastfeeding as transferred drug should be inactivated by digestive enzymes in the neonate [252].

Adalimumab

Adalimumab use in pregnancy has not been associated with an increased risk of congenital malformations or miscarriage [252–254].

It is detectable in breast milk at levels lower than 1% of its level in serum [255]. Given that this small quantity is likely inactivated by intestinal enzymes, adalimumab is considered compatible with breastfeeding.

Certolizumab pegol

Certolizumab pegol enters the fetal compartment at low levels [246]. Absence of an Fc fragment may preclude active transport of certolizumab pegol across the placenta, thereby accounting for the lower levels found in exposed infants compared to the other anti-TNF-α agents. Review of the Union Chimique Belge UCB Pharma safety database for certolizumab found no increase in adverse pregnancy outcomes [253].

Certolizumab pegol is considered compatible with breastfeeding, although human data are lacking [256].

Golimumab

There are few reports describing the use of golimumab in pregnancy [254,255]. Animal data suggest that the embryo-fetal risk is low [256]. It is unknown if golimumab is excreted in breast milk. However, as it is similar to other immunoglobulins that are excreted into breast milk, exposure would be expected. Studies in monkeys demonstrated no impact on development and maturation with golimumab exposure [256].

Natalizumab

Natalizumab is one of the two anti-integrin medications and is approved for Crohn's disease. Studies of natalizumab safety in pregnancy are limited [255]. Some studies have shown adverse outcomes including anemia, thrombocytopenia [257], and lower birthweights in infants and higher rates of miscarriage in women exposed to natalizumab compared to disease-matched groups and healthy controls [258]. However, other prospective studies have not demonstrated adverse pregnancy or fetal outcomes [255,259]. Based on limited data, it is recommended that women treated with natalizumab use sufficient contraception or stop the drug 3 months prior to conception [256,257].

Natalizumab is excreted into human breast milk [260]. Breastfeeding while on natalizumab is not recommended due to lack of safety data.

Vedolizumab

Vedolizumab is the second anti-integrin medication. It is a monoclonal immunoglobulin G_1 (IgG_1) antibody to the $\alpha 4\beta 7$ integrin molecule that limits its actions to the gastrointestinal mucosa. Vedolizumab is anticipated to transfer across the placenta with increasing efficiency over the course of pregnancy, like other immunoglobulin G_1 therapeutic antibodies [258]. There are no controlled studies with vedolizumab in pregnant women. Mahadevan et al. provided data on 24 vedoluzimab-treated women from six studies and 81 pregnancies from a postmarketing program [261]. From the clinical trials (23 had IBD and one healthy volunteer), there were 11 live births, five elective terminations, four spontaneous abortions, and four undocumented outcomes. Postmarketing reports documented 81 pregnancies resulting in 11 spontaneous abortions, four live births, and 66 pregnancies that were ongoing or undocumented outcomes.

Data are limited for breastfeeding while on vedolizumab. Vedolizumab is present in breast milk at low concentrations [262,263].

Ustekinumab

Ustekinumab is a humanized IgG monoclonal antibody against interleukin (IL)-12 and IL-23 which crosses the placenta by an active transport process. In animal studies, no detrimental effects were noted in offspring [264]. There are limited pregnancy data regarding its safety. Of 176 patients, there were 122 live births while 31 gestations ended with miscarriage or fetal death [265]. The AGA Institute guideline on IBD in pregnancy clinical pathway recommends continuation of ustekinumab during pregnancy with the final pregnancy dose 6–10 weeks before estimated due date, with the caveat that limited pregnancy data are available [266].

Ustekinumab may be present in breast milk [267,268]. Exposure is thought to be low due to the large size of the molecule and degradation within the gastrointestinal tract, but this has not been verified.

Small molecules

Tofacitinib

Tofacitinib is an inhibitor of Janus kinases and it is unknown if it crosses the human placenta. However, in large doses, it was teratogenic in animal studies [269]. Guidelines recommend avoidance of this medication at least in the first trimester [266]. There is also a recommended 1-week washout period from the medication before attempting conception.

It is unknown if tofacinitib is excreted into breast milk. Guidelines recommend avoiding the use of tofacinitib in breastfeeding women until additional information is available.

Anorectal and perineal disorders

Hemorrhoids

Hemorrhoids occur in up to 85% of multiparous women [270]. Although they typically regress after delivery, they usually do not completely resolve [271].

Pregnancy is thought to increase the risk of hemorrhoid formation through both mechanical and hormonal factors. Mechanical factors include compression of the superior rectal vein and obstruction of the vena cava and portal vein by the gravid uterus causing venous stasis and congestion. In addition, pregnancy-induced increased intraabdominal pressure and mechanical pressure may cause venous blockage and arteriovenous shunting in the internal anal sphincter [271]. Hormonal factors include increased progesterone and decreased motilin levels [272].

Pregnant women with symptomatic hemorrhoids present with the same symptoms as nonpregnant patients: intermittent rectal bleeding, itching and pain (see Chapter 68), and the approach to diagnosis is analogous to nonpregnant patients [178,271].

Nonthrombosed external hemorrhoids do not require treatment. Patients with pain from thrombosed external hemorrhoids can generally be treated with conservative measures such as frequent sitz baths, stool softeners, and hemorrhoidal analgesics [179]. Patients not responding to conservative therapy can be treated with clot extraction or, more definitively, with surgical excision [273].

Internal hemorrhoids can also be treated conservatively in most patients with dietary changes, increased fluid intake, and fiber supplements. Patients with pain can be treated with topical local anesthetics containing benzocaine, dibucaine, or pramoxine [165]. Rubber band ligation can be performed in refractory cases. If the hemorrhoids are severely prolapsed or have associated ulceration, severe bleeding, fissure or fistula, hemorrhoidectomy should be considered [273].

Anal fissures

Up to 15% of women are affected by anal fissures postpartum [274]. In 313 primigravid women, only constipation was found to be associated with postpartum anal fissure development [275]. Notably, anal sphincter hypertonia was not observed [276–278]. None of the pharmacological therapies used to treat anal fissures have been studied for safety or efficacy in pregnancy. Thus, the primary goal in the management of anal fissures is prevention and treatment of constipation [279].

Anal sphincter injuries

Vaginal delivery is frequently associated with trauma to the anal sphincters. Obstetric anal sphincter injury (OASI), in turn, is the most common cause of fecal incontinence in women. The largest study using clinical examination at the time of delivery found that OASI occurred in 2.9% of primiparous women and 0.8% of multiparous ones [280]. In comparison, using anal endosonography, Sultan et al. found that 35% and 45% of primiparous and multiparous women, respectively, had a new sphincter defect after delivery [278]. Risk factors for sphincter damage include primiparity, birthweight greater than 4000 g, midline episiotomy, operative delivery, and prolonged second stage of labor [281,282].

Despite its prevalence, many women with OASI do not seek medical attention because of embarrassment [283]. Signs of OASI include fecal soiling, anal asymmetry, and poor sphincter tone on digital rectal examination. In addition, patients may report perineal pain, dyspareunia, incontinence of flatus, fecal urgency, and stool incontinence [284]. Symptoms generally resolve by 12 months postpartum [285]. Of those who remain symptomatic, most experience incontinence of flatus only [286].

It is recommended that all women who undergo an episiotomy or experience a perineal tear have a rectal examination to evaluate for a rectal or anal sphincter injury at the time of delivery [287]. Patients with suspected injuries which are not apparent on clinical examination should undergo additional testing with anorectal manometry, anal endosonography, or MRI with endoanal coil [178].

Primary repair of the external anal sphincter may be performed using an end-to-end (approximation) or overlap technique. Patients with persistent symptoms after primary repair may benefit from conservative therapy with diet modification, anal plugs, pelvic floor physical therapy, biofeedback, and/or sacral nerve stimulation [284]. Secondary repair may be needed in refractory cases. Women who have undergone secondary sphincter repair should deliver by cesarean section in future pregnancies [288].

Liver disease in pregnancy

Liver diseases occurring in pregnancy can be classified as those which occur uniquely in pregnancy or those which occur concurrent with pregnancy. In the latter category are liver diseases which occur more commonly because of pregnancy as well as preexisting liver diseases which require special consideration as a result of pregnancy (Figure 40.1). Because gestational age can have a significant impact on which liver diseases manifest, a convenient way to systematically approach abnormal liver enzymes or liver disease manifestations is to take into account the stage of pregnancy. In addition to diagnostic considerations, medications for liver disease which are used during pregnancy and breastfeeding may also have special considerations (Table 40.8).

Liver physiology during pregnancy

Pregnancy induces a progressive increase in serum estrogen and progesterone levels, peaking during the third trimester [289]. This increase leads to physiological changes that can be manifested by spider telangiectasias and palmar erythema [290]. Plasma volume increases by approximately 50% although hepatic blood flow is unchanged as systemic vascular resistance is lower and the liver receives a lower percentage of the cardiac output. Physical examination is compromised since the liver is forced into the chest as the gravid uterus expands. In late pregnancy a palpable liver is an abnormal finding.

Up to 3% of pregnancies are complicated by abnormal liver chemistries, which can be an early indicator of serious pathology. However, traditional liver chemistries can change significantly during normal pregnancy, making interpretation of these values difficult (Table 40.9). Separating normal physiological changes from significant disease is imperative [291,292].

With normal pregnancies, increased plasma volume leads to hemodilution and a subsequent decrease in serum protein concentrations. Serum alkaline phosphatase levels increase as a result of placental production as well as an increase in the bone isoenzyme, making this a poor diagnostic study especially in the third trimester [293,294]. Similarly, α-fetoprotein can be elevated due to production by the fetal liver [295]. γ-Glutamyl transpeptidase (GGT), on the other hand, may be lower, especially in late pregnancy. Bilirubin concentration is also lower in normal pregnancy, likely as a result of both hemodilution and lower concentration of albumin which transports bilirubin.

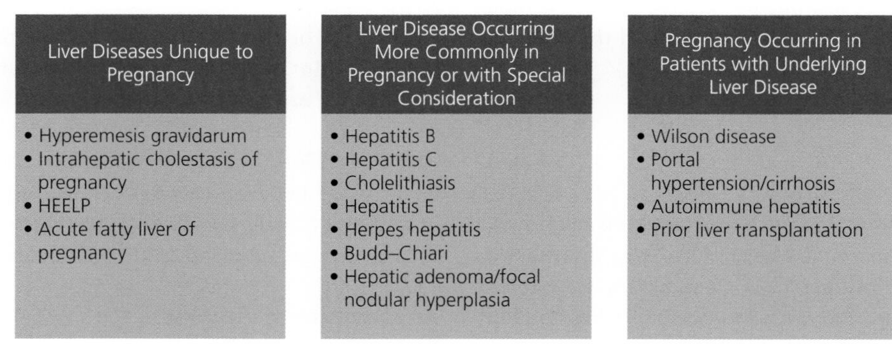

Figure 40.1 Liver disease occurring in pregnancy can be classified into three categories.

Table 40.9 Normal biochemical changes during pregnancy.

Test	Alteration
Albumin	L
Alkaline phosphatase	H
Alanine aminotransferase	U
Aspartate aminotransferase	U
γ-Glutamyl transferase	L
Total bilirubin	U/L
Conjugated bilirubin	L
5′-Nucleotidase	H
Total bile acids	U
Fibrinogen	H
Factors V, VII, VIII	H
α-Fetoprotein	H
Globulins:	
α and β globulin	H
γ globulin	L
Prothrombin time and activated partial thromboplastin time	U
Platelets	U
Ceruloplasmin	H
Hemoglobin	L
White cell count	H
Cholesterol and triglycerides	H

U, unchanged; H, higher; L, lower.

Serum ALT is the most commonly used measurement to assess liver disease [296]. ALT >19 U/L is considered abnormal in women [297]. ALT and AST activity are unchanged during pregnancy. Serum aminotransferase elevations and jaundice should initiate further evaluation.

Liver diseases unique to pregnancy

Several liver diseases are unique to pregnancy: hyperemesis gravidarum, intrahepatic cholestasis of pregnancy, acute fatty liver of pregnancy, and HELLP (hemolysis, elevated liver enzymes, and low platelets) syndrome. These diseases do not occur in the absence of pregnancy and generally improve with delivery of the fetus. They also occur in particular phases of pregnancy which can be used to guide the differential diagnosis of liver disease in pregnancy and thus patient evaluation and management (Table 40.10) [298,299]. HG can lead to increased liver enzyme elevations which need to be differentiated from other causes of increased liver injury. A thorough history and physical examination are essential, and in addition to the common risk factors for liver disease, the history should focus on prior pregnancies, high-risk behaviors, and medications.

Intrahepatic cholestasis of pregnancy (IHCP)

Intrahepatic cholestasis of pregnancy is one of the most common liver diseases unique to pregnancy and typically presents in the second or third trimester as persistent pruritus associated with elevated bile acid levels. Symptoms resolve after delivery.

Epidemiology

Prevalence in the US ranges from 0.3% to 5.6% but has been reported to be as high as 28% in Bolivia and Chile. Susceptibility may be higher in the colder months and varies between ethnic groups, with the highest occurrence in the US reported in a predominantly Latino Los Angeles population [300–304].

Risk factors include advanced maternal age, a history of cholestasis secondary to oral contraceptives, multiparity, and a personal or family history of IHCP. IHCP recurs in 60–70% of subsequent pregnancies. Although maternal outcomes are excellent, large retrospective studies from Finland found a higher incidence of preexisting hepatobiliary diseases such as hepatitis C, cholelithiasis, and nonalcoholic fatty liver in women with IHCP, suggesting that a thorough search for alternative explanations is essential [305,306].

Fetal complications

Intrahepatic cholestasis of pregnancy can lead to placental insufficiency, significantly increasing the risk of complications such as fetal distress, preterm labor, prematurity, and intrauterine death [307–310]. Neonatal respiratory distress syndrome is also twice as frequent. Although gestational age was the strongest risk factor in one study, a role for bile acids entering the fetal lungs and depleting surfactant is also hypothesized [311]. Intrauterine death is more common in the last month of pregnancy. The timing of parturition should always be matched to potential risks, but most obstetricians recommend early delivery at 37 weeks [312].

Etiology

The etiology of IHCP is multifactorial, with genetic, hormonal and environmental contributors. Bile acid levels are increased in both maternal and fetal serum and transplacental bile acid transfer is impaired in IHCP. IHCP is associated with morphological placental abnormalities that can be reproduced in vitro; with exposure to taurocholic and taurochenodoexycholic acid [313].

Several genomic variants in hepatobiliary transporters have been associated with IHCP [314–318]. The main transport protein that mediates movement of phospholipid across the canalicular membrane into bile is the multidrug resistance 3 P-glycoprotein (MDR3). Without phospholipids in bile, bile acids are poorly solubilized and can injure the canalicular membrane, causing cholestasis. Mutations in the ATP-binding cassette, subfamily B member 4 (ABCB4) gene, which encodes MDR3, are implicated in some cases of IHCP. In one study, 16% of Caucasian women with IHCP had ABCB4 gene mutations [319]. Defects in the ATP8B1 (ATPase, aminophospholipid transporter, class I, type 8B, member 1) gene

Table 40.8 Pharmacological treatment of liver disease during pregnancy.

Drug class	Drug	Recommendations for pregnancy	Recommendations for lactation
	Ursodeoxycholic acid	Adverse events have not been observed in animal studies. No observation of harm in human use known	Unknown if present in breast milk. Manufacturer recommends caution but limited data have not shown harm
Bile acid sequestrant	Cholestyramine	Is not absorbed systemically, but may interfere with maternal vitamin absorption; therefore, regular prenatal supplementation may not be adequate	Is not expected to be present in breast milk due to lack of systemic absorption
	Hydroxyzine	Caution is advised for use during pregnancy. The manufacturer recommends against use during pregnancy although risk of fetal harm may be low based on limited human data. Hydroxyzine crosses the placenta and possible withdrawal symptoms have been observed in neonates following chronic maternal use of hydroxyzine during pregnancy	Consider alternative medications while breastfeeding because of possible risk of infant CNS depression based on limited human data and concern that antihistamines may decrease maternal serum prolactin concentrations when administered prior to the establishment of lactation
	S-adenosyl-methionine	Few human studies have addressed safety of non-FDA approved herbal supplements in pregnancy so risk is unknown	Few human studies have addressed safety of non-FDA approved herbal supplements in breastfeeding so risk is unknown
Corticosteroids	Dexamethasone Prednisone Prednisolone	Dexamethasone crosses the placenta. Caution advised during pregnancy, especially with prolonged use. There are inadequate human data available to assess risk, although there is some controversial data that first-trimester use may be associated with cleft palate	Caution is advised while breastfeeding; no human data available, though risk of infant harm not expected based on no systemic absorption
	Eculizumab	Eculizumab crosses the placenta and thus risk/benefit needs to be assessed. Benefits may outweigh risks during pregnancy. The risk of fetal harm is low based on limited human data	Eculizumab may be present in breast milk. The manufacturer recommends weighing risk/benefit while breastfeeding
Antivirals	Interferon-α2b	Generally not advised given significant side-effects despite no known risk of teratogenicity based on limited human and animal data	Breast milk contains endogenous interferon that does not appear to be affected by exogenous interferon
	Ribavirin	Ribavarin is contraindicated during pregnancy due to risk of teratogenicity based on animal data. In addition, ribavirin is also contraindicated in male partners of women who are pregnant. Avoidance of pregnancy for 6 months after treatment	It is unknown if ribavirin is present in breast milk but caution should be used as the medication is known to cause hemolytic anemia
	Aciclovir	Aciclovir has been shown to cross the human placenta but limited human data show no adverse effects	Aciclovir has been found in breast milk but based on limited human data, there has been no infant harm known
	Lamivudine	There is no known risk for teratogenicity but risk/benefit need to be weighed when used during pregnancy	May use while breastfeeding
	Entecavir	Teratogenic effects have been observed in animal studies but limited data in humans have not shown teratogenicity. Risk vs benefit need to be weighed for use during pregnancy	It is not known if entecavir is present in breast milk. Manufacturer recommends weighing risk vs benefit
	Tenofovir disoproxil fumarate Tenofovir alafenamide	Tenofovir can cross the placenta but the benefits outweigh potential risks during pregnancy. Based on limited human data, there is no overall increase in birth defects for tenofovir disoproxil fumarate. There is possible risk of low birthweight based on limited human data and conflicting animal data	Tenofovir is minimally excreted in breast milk but limited human data do not suggest significant toxicity in the infant. However, the risk of long-term low-level exposure to the infant is unknown and thus risk vs benefit needs to be discussed
Immunosuppressives	Azathioprine	Azathioprine can cross the placenta. Risk/benefit should be weighed for use during pregnancy. Limited human data suggest that it may be reasonable to continue use during pregnancy if patient is already on treatment given risks for stopping to the mother. Caution is advised in 3rd trimester as there is possible low risk of neonatal myelosuppression	Azathioprine is rapidly metabolized to 6-mercaptopurine which is present in breast milk. Use during breastfeeding should weigh risk vs benefit although limited human data show low risk to infant

Table 40.8 (Continued)

Drug class	Drug	Recommendations for pregnancy	Recommendations for lactation
	Mycophenolate	Not recommended during pregnancy. There is a black box FDA warning due to teratogenic reports. Avoid use during pregnancy; risk of fetal harm, including teratogenicity and spontaneous abortion, based on human data	Risk/benefit should be weighed during breastfeeding. No human data available to assess risk of infant harm, though possible drug excretion into milk based on drug properties
Calcineruin inhibitors	Tacrolimus	Risk and benefit should be weighed for use during pregnancy although teratogenic potential appears low (4%), and rates of birth defects not different than in general population with present data	No known risk of infant harm based on limited human data
	Cyclosporine	Risk vs benefit should be weighed although limited human data suggest low fetal harm	Consider alternatives or otherwise monitor infant for signs and symptoms of cyclosporine toxicity while breastfeeding. There is a possible risk of infant toxicity, incl. hepatotoxicity, vomiting, and diarrhea based on conflicting human data
Copper chelators	Penicillamine	Risk vs benefit should be weighed, limited human data are conflicting, animal data suggest teratogenicity; however, in Wilson disease discontinuation can be detrimental so recommendation for continued use at minimum dose particularly in first trimester	Avoid breastfeeding; possible risk of infant harm based on conflicting human data and drug properties
	Trientene	Risk vs benefit suggest cautious use; limited human data do not show teratogenicity but animal data show teratogenicity. Risk of discontinuation in Wilson disease is high	Inadequate data in humans. Trientene is not known to be in breast milk; manufacturer recommends cautious use
	Zinc	Can be used in pregnancy based on limited human data	Zinc is excreted in breast milk; avoid breastfeeding due to possible infant risk of copper deficiency
Diuretics	Spironolactone	Spironolactone crosses the placenta and can cause feminization of male fetus and is not recommended during pregnancy	The active metabolite of spironolactone (canrenone) is present in breast milk. Risk/benefit should be assessed for use
	Furosemide	Furosemide can cross the placenta but limited human data have not shown significant harm although caution advised during pregnancy	Furosemide is present in breast milk and alternatives should be considered especially in high-risk infants
Hepatic encephalopathy medications	Lactulose	May use during pregnancy; no human data available, though risk of fetal harm not expected based on minimal systemic absorption	Not known if lactulose is excreted in breast milk but based on minimal maternal systemic absorption, can be used. However, caution should be exercised
	Rifaxamin	Consider avoiding use in first trimester, otherwise may use during pregnancy; no human data available, though risk of fetal harm not expected based on minimal systemic absorption; possible risk of teratogenicity in first trimester based on animal data at up to 33× recommended human doses	May use while breastfeeding; no human data available, though risk of infant harm and adverse effects on milk production not expected based on minimal maternal systemic absorption
β-Blockers	Propranolol Nadolol Carvedilol	Caution advised during pregnancy, especially in second and third trimesters; no known risk of teratogenicity, though risk of intrauterine growth restriction and neonatal adverse effects, including bradycardia and hypoglycemia, based on limited human data	May use while breastfeeding; no known risk of infant harm based on limited human data and drug properties
	Octreotide	Caution advised during pregnancy; inadequate human data available to assess risk; no known risk of teratogenicity based on animal data	Weigh risk/benefit while breastfeeding; no human data available, though risk of infant harm not expected based on drug properties

CNS, central nervous system; FDA, Food and Drug Administration.

Table 40.10 Liver diseases unique to pregnancy.

Disorder	Trimester	Diagnostic clues
Hyperemesis gravidarum (HG)	First through 20 weeks	Nausea, vomiting, mild AST, ALT elevations
Intrahepatic cholestasis of pregnancy (ICHP)	2nd/3rd	Pruritus, elevated bile acids, recurs in subsequent pregnancies
Eclampsia, preeclampsia	After 20 weeks	Abdominal pain, increased ALT, AST, ALP, and bilirubin
Hemolysis, elevated liver enzymes, low platelets (HELLP)	After 22 weeks	Platelets <100 000/mm^3 Increased AST, ALT, LDH. Risk of hepatic rupture
Acute fatty liver of pregnancy (AFLP)	3rd	Increased AST, ALT, and bilirubin. Low fibrinogen. Progresses to fulminant hepatic failure

ALP, alkaline phosphatase; ALT, alanine aminotransferase; AST, aspartate aminotransferase; LDH, lactate dehydrogenase.

associated with familial cholestasis, as well as in the ABCB11 (ATP-binding cassette, subfamily B member 11) gene which encodes the bile salt export pump (BSEP) have also been linked to IHCP [317]. Cases of IHCP in renal transplant patients on cyclosporine, which inhibits BSEP, have also been reported [320].

Female sex hormones may also contribute since estrogen inhibits the BSEP. There is a higher incidence during the third trimester when estrogen concentrations peak and in twin pregnancies which have higher circulating estrogen levels. Progesterone metabolites may saturate the hepatic transport system utilized for their biliary excretion. Progesterone administration to prevent premature delivery may trigger IHCP in predisposed women [307].

Presentation and diagnosis

Pregnant women with IHCP present with pruritus often involving the palms and soles before generalized itching. Jaundice occurs in 10–25% and fat-soluble vitamin deficiencies have been seen due to fat malabsorption [309,321]. The diagnosis can be confirmed by detection of fasting serum bile acid concentrations greater than 10 μmol/L. Cholic acid levels are increased while chenodeoxycholic acid level is decreased [81]. Bile acid levels also correlate with fetal distress – complications are rare until bile acid levels reach 40 μmol/L [309]. Aminotransferase levels can be elevated, reaching values greater than 1000 U/L, but alternative explanations should be excluded if elevations are significant. Elevation in alkaline phosphatase (ALP) is the most common lab abnormality in IHCP but results may be difficult to interpret due to physiological elevations in ALP secondary to pregnancy. GGT levels are usually normal and total bilirubin rarely exceeds 6 mg/dL [81]. Ultrasonography is normal without bile duct dilation and should be performed to exclude cholelithiasis. Liver biopsy is rarely needed but if performed, demonstrates bland cholestasis.

Treatment

The goals of therapy are twofold: one to alleviate symptoms and the other to improve fetal outcomes. Ursodeoxycholic acid (UDCA), given 10–15 mg/kg, may result in biochemical as well as symptomatic improvement [322]. Although the exact mechanism is unknown, UDCA increases expression of bile salt export pumps and increases placental bile transporters. While fetal toxicity is always a concern, treatment with UDCA has been shown to normalize serum bile acid patterns in babies with minimal accumulation in amniotic fluid and cord blood [322]. Some metaanalyses also found that women who received UDCA had better outcomes, with less pruritus, improved liver enzymes, and possibly improved fetal outcomes [323], while others have only shown some incremental benefit in symptomatic relief and no improvement in fetal outcomes [324]. A recent randomized controlled trial showed similar lack of effect on fetal outcome, calling into question the accepted use of UCDA as a first-line drug [325]. Other therapies have also been tried for symptomatic relief, including hydroxyzine, cholestyramine, and s-adenosyl-methionine [295]; however, the safety of these medications such as s-adenosyl-methionine and hydroxyzine is not well known. Cholestyramine can bind to other medications such as UCDA so administration should be well timed. Dexamethasone has been given with the idea of improving fetal lung maturity as timely delivery is warranted, usually by 37 weeks of gestation.

If cholestasis fails to resolve after delivery, evaluation for alternative explanations such as primary biliary cholangitis (PBC) and primary sclerosing cholangitis (PSC) may be warranted [326].

Preeclampsia and eclampsia

Preeclampsia is characterized by new-onset hypertension (systolic blood pressure [SBP] ≥140 mmHg or diastolic blood pressure [DBP] ≥90 mmHg), and proteinuria (≥300 mg/24 h) after 20 weeks of gestation [327–329]. Eclampsia is defined when grand mal seizures occur in the setting of preeclampsia. Clinical manifestations result from microangiopathy and can affect several organs. Severe preeclampsia/eclampsia is defined when there is evidence of organ dysfunction, including that of the liver. Up to 7.5% of all pregnancies are affected, but only 25% are severe [330]. Although generally mild, preeclampsia is one of four leading causes of maternal death in the United States [326].

Several factors increase the risk of preeclampsia, including a past history or family history of preeclampsia, nulliparity, twin pregnancies, advanced maternal age, pre-pregnancy diabetes, obesity, and antiphospholipid antibodies [330]. Recently, ethnicity has also been linked to the risk of preeclampsia, with African origin increasing the risk of onset before 28 weeks gestation. In contrast, symptoms related to hypertension including HELLP (hemolysis, elevated liver enzymes, low platelets) syndrome are more common in women of European origin [331].

Hepatic manifestations of preeclampsia can present with epigastric or right upper quadrant pain likely from stretching of Glisson's capsule from hepatomegaly. Hepatic involvement indicates severe preeclampsia and impacts management, as women are usually delivered promptly to limit maternal and fetal complications. Liver injury results as a consequence of vasoconstriction and fibrin precipitation in the liver [81]. AST and ALT elevations can be striking. ALP is elevated above normal pregnancy ranges and mild bilirubin elevations are also common. A liver biopsy is rarely necessary, but histological findings include periportal hemorrhage and fibrin deposition, ischemic lesions, and microvesicular fat deposits [81,332]. Hematoma below Glisson's capsule can develop and cases of hepatic rupture have been reported.

The magnitude of the liver chemistry derangements is associated with the risk of adverse maternal outcomes [333]. Analysis of a large cohort of births found that increased aminotransferase during the first 20 weeks of pregnancy was associated with a higher risk for severe preeclampsia in the second half of pregnancy. Unfortunately, no clinical cut-off value was identified [334].

HELLP syndrome

HELLP probably represents a severe form of preeclampsia but the relationship remains unclear. HELLP complicates up to 20% of cases of severe preeclampsia/eclampsia but a minority of total pregnancies (0.2–0.6%) [335]. Although felt to be an extreme manifestation of severe preeclampsia, 20% of patients lack antecedent hypertension and proteinuria [336]. The majority present between 28 and 36 weeks of gestation, but 30% develop the syndrome in the first week postpartum [335]. The most common symptom is abdominal pain especially in the epigastric area or right upper quadrant with associated nausea, vomiting, and malaise.

Risk factors include advanced maternal age, Caucasian ethnicity, and multiparity [328]. Although the exact cause is unknown, activation of the coagulation cascade is integral, resulting in fibrin deposition and microangiopathic hemolytic anemia and platelet consumption.

Diagnosis

The diagnosis of HELLP is made through recognition of the characteristic biochemical pattern. Similar to preeclampsia, hepatic injury is a manifestation of hypovolemia, intravascular fibrin deposition, and increased sinusoidal pressures. In addition to AST and ALT elevations, serum bilirubin and lactate dehydrogenase are increased. Signs of hemolytic anemia include schistocytes, elevated indirect bilirubin, and low serum haptoglobin. Thrombocytopenia is present with platelets less than 100 000 cells/microliter. Proteinuria and hypertension occur in about 85% [337]. Rarely is a biopsy necessary, as the results are unlikely to affect management. Efficient diagnosis is essential. The University of Tennessee or University of Mississippi criteria can aid in this process (Table 40.11) [338,339].

Progression can be rapid and maternal consequences severe, with mortality rates of 1–3% and high rates of disseminated intravascular coagulation (DIC) (21%), abruptio placentae

Table 40.11 Mississippi and Tennessee classification systems of HELLP syndromes.

HELLP class	Mississippi classification	Tennessee classification
Class 1 (Severe)	• AST and/or ALT >70 IU/L • LDH >600 IU/L • Platelets <50 × 10^9/L	• AST >70 IU/L • LDH >600 IU/L or bilirubin ≥1.2 mg/dL
Class 2 (Moderate)	• AST and/or ALT >70 IU/L • LDH >600 IU/L • Platelets 50–100 × 10^9/L	• Platelets <100 × 10^9/L • Evidence of hemolysis on peripheral blood smear
Class 3 (Mild)	• AST and/or ALT >40 IU/L • LDH >600 IU/L • Platelets 100–150 × 10^9/L	NA
Partial HELLP	NA	Severe preeclampsia and one of the following: • ELLP • HEL • EL • LP

Source: Martin et al. [340]. Reproduced by permission of Elsevier.
ALT, alanine aminotransferase; AST, aspartate aminotransferase; ELLP, absence of hemolysis; HEL, hemolysis and elevated liver enzymes absent thrombocytopenia; EL, elevated liver enzymes; LDH, lactate dehydrogenase; LP, low platelets.

(16%), acute renal failure (8%), and pulmonary edema (6%) [335,340]. Laboratory values typically begin to normalize within 48 hours postpartum [335]. Prematurity is common. Fetal prognosis is most strongly linked to gestational age at delivery and birthweight.

Hepatic consequences

Severe hepatic consequences are well recognized and include hepatic infarction, subcapsular hematomas, and intraparenchymal hemorrhage. Although increased liver enzymes are expected in HELLP, marked elevations are atypical. When ALT or AST is greater than 1000 IU/L, cross-sectional imaging can assist in excluding hepatic complications with more accuracy than ultrasound.

Right upper quadrant pain with fever increases concern for hepatic infarction. Although infarcts generally resolve after delivery, concomitant antiphospholipid syndrome should be considered [341,342].

Hepatic hematoma can also present as abdominal pain radiating into the right shoulder. Management of a contained hematoma is supportive with volume and transfusions as needed. Surgery is indicated for those with enlarging hematomas or evidence of rupture with hemodynamic instability. Successful percutaneous embolization of the hepatic arteries in stable women has been reported [343]. Liver transplantation has also been an effective salvage in patients with continued decompensation despite standard interventions [344,345].

Management

Prompt delivery is the management of choice, especially after 34 weeks gestation. Thrombocytopenia can be pronounced, and platelet transfusion to 40 000–50 000 cells/μL should be considered, especially if cesarean section is likely.

Corticosteroids are often used in the treatment of HELLP. The Mississippi protocol includes corticosteroids, magnesium sulfate, and control of systolic blood pressure. Early initiation of this protocol in 190 patients was associated with lower rates of progression and severity [346]. A recent Cochrane review found that although dexamethasone resulted in a greater improvement in platelet count, there was no difference in the risk of maternal morbidity and mortality or perinatal/infant death [347]. Glucocorticoids have a more established role in pregnancies less than 34 weeks where they accelerate pulmonary maturity during expectant management. Eculizumab, an inhibitor of complement protein C5 used for other diseases that affect hemolysis and increase thrombosis such as paroxysmal nocturnal hemoglobinuria, has also been used to prolong pregnancy [348].

Although HELLP in subsequent pregnancies is uncommon, there is a significant risk for preeclampsia, especially in those women with underlying hypertension [349].

Acute fatty liver disease of pregnancy

Acute fatty liver disease of pregnancy (AFLP) is a rare but life-threatening condition characterized by microvesicular fatty infiltration of the liver leading to hepatic failure. Originally felt to be universally fatal, maternal prognosis is excellent with early recognition, prompt delivery, and supportive care [350].

Epidemiology

Acute fatty liver disease of pregnancy does not discriminate by age, geographic location, or ethnicity. Although small retrospective cohorts reported high maternal (12–18%) and neonatal mortality (7–58%), a large national UK cohort involving 1 132 964 deliveries confirmed a much better prognosis. The incidence of AFLP was 5.0 cases per 100 000 pregnancies. Twin pregnancies and body mass index (BMI) <20 were found to be risk factors. The median gestation age at the time of identification was 36 weeks. Sixty percent were delivered within 24 hours after recognition and there was a high rate of cesarean section (74%). In this series involving 57 European women, only one woman died, and one received a liver transplant [350]. There were seven deaths among 67 infants (perinatal mortality rate 104 per 1000 births, 95% CI 43–203) [350]. Early recognition and improvements in supportive care improve mortality rates [351].

Presentation

Presentation is typically in the third trimester but may not be recognized until after delivery. Symptoms are nonspecific, with nausea, vomiting, and abdominal pain most commonly reported. Concomitant preeclampsia is present in roughly one half of affected women [352]. Criteria based on symptoms and laboratory derangements were proposed in 2002 by Ch'ng et al ("Swansea criteria") and validated in the UK population-based cohort [291] (Box 40.1).

Aminotransferases can be markedly increased and hyperbilirubinemia is common. As the disease progresses, hepatic failure ensues and can manifest with encephalopathy, coagulopathy, and hypoglycemia. The diagnosis is usually based on clinical presentation and laboratory studies. Liver biopsy can be diagnostic, but is rarely required as it infrequently impacts management.

Although considered a liver disease, extrahepatic manifestations are common. Infections, intraabdominal bleeding, and central diabetes insipidus have been described in association with AFLP [351,353]. Renal dysfunction is typical in advanced disease and severe pancreatitis can be a complication.

Pathogenesis

There is an association between AFLP and fetal deficiency of long-chain 3-hydroxyacyl- coenzyme A dehydrogenase (LCHAD). The LCHAD enzyme catalyzes the step in β-oxidation of mitochondrial fatty acid that forms 3-ketoacyl-CoA from 3-hydroxyacyl-CoA. Homozygous deficient offspring spill unmetabolized long-chain fatty acids into the maternal circulation. The accumulation of fetal or placental metabolites could then lead to hepatotoxicity. Case reports have suggested that women with AFLP are often heterozygous for LCHAD and carry heterozygous

Box 40.1 BoxSwansea criteria for diagnosis of acute fatty liver of pregnancy.

Six or more criteria required in the absence of another cause:

Vomiting

Abdominal pain

Polydipsia/polyuria

Encephalopathy

Elevated bilirubin >14 μmol/L

Hypoglycemia <4 mmol/L

Elevated urea >340 μmol/L

Leukocytosis >11 × 10^9/L

Ascites or bright liver on ultrasound scan

Elevated aminotransferases (AST or ALT) > 42 IU/L

Elevated ammonia >47 μmol/L

Renal impairment; creatinine >150 μmol/L

Coagulopathy; prothrombin time >14 seconds or APPT >34 seconds

Microvesicular steatosis on liver biopsy

Source: Ch'ng et al. [291]. Reproduced by permission of BMJ Publishing Group.ALT, alanine aminotransferase; APPT, activated partial thromboplastin time; AST, aspartate aminotransferase.

or homozygous infants [354]. However, not every series has confirmed this association. Several genetic defects can lead to LCHAD but not all may confer a risk for AFLP. LCHAD is one enzyme that resides in the mitochondrial trifunctional protein [355]. The offspring of mothers affected by AFLP should be monitored carefully as they may be at risk for manifestations of deficiency of LCHAD with hypoketotic hypoglycemia and fatty liver. All women with AFLP and their children should have molecular testing for LCHAD.

Oxidative stress in placental mitochondria and peroxisomes may contribute to hepatic injury. As the mother rapidly improves after delivery, Natarajan and colleagues hypothesized that the placenta may be responsible for the dysfunction. They found that placental mitochondria and peroxisomes showed oxidative stress in subjects with AFLP and that markers of oxidative and nitrosative stress were elevated in the serum [356].

Treatment relies on urgent delivery after stabilizing the mother. If hepatic function does not rapidly improve, efficient evaluation for liver transplantation offers the patient the best chance for survival [350]. There is risk for AFLP in subsequent pregnancies.

Liver diseases that can occur concurrent with pregnancy

Some liver diseases are exacerbated by the underlying physiological changes of pregnancy making them more common. Hormonal changes during pregnancy make cholelithiasis more common. Pregnancy is also a hypercoagulable state which may contribute to hepatic vein thrombosis or Budd Chiari syndrome. Liver diseases associated with a more fulminant course in pregnancy such as Hepatitis E and Herpes hepatitis may occur, in part, due to some level of immunosuppression during pregnancy. Other liver diseases such as hepatitis B and C may not occur more commonly because of pregnancy but the risk of perinatal transmission are important additional considerations. In patients with underlying liver disease such as cirrhosis, autoimmune hepatitis, and liver transplantation, special management approaches should be entertained.

Cholelithiasis and its complications in pregnancy

Gallbladder disease is the second most common nonobstetric surgical emergency after appendicitis. Pregnancy decreases gallbladder motility and increases the lithogenicity of bile, increasing the risk for gallstone formation. Increased levels of progesterone during pregnancy inhibit gallbladder motility, resulting in higher fasting and fed gallbladder volumes as well as a significantly reduced gallbladder ejection fraction in pregnant compared to nonpregnant women [357,358]. Bile also becomes supersaturated with cholesterol as a result of an estrogen-induced increase in cholesterol secretion, progesterone-induced reduction in bile acid secretion and a qualitative change in the bile acid pool as production of hydrophobic bile acids is increased [359,360].

Biliary sludge

Biliary sludge is present in up to 36% of pregnant women, but only 2–11% develop gallstones [361]. In a prospective study following women from the first trimester, biliary sludge generally remained asymptomatic but 28% of those who developed gallstones experienced biliary colic. The prevalence of sludge and stones initially increased during pregnancy, but resolved in 61% of women with sludge and 28% of those with stones after delivery [362]. Serious complications are less common, with an incidence of acute cholecystitis of 0.05–0.08% in pregnant women with gallstones [363,364].

Presentation is variable. Most symptomatic women will experience recurrent biliary colic with epigastric or right upper quadrant pain. Similar to nonpregnant subjects (see Chapter 81), it is often postprandial and resolves gradually after peaking in intensity approximately an hour after onset. When the pain is associated with fever, nausea, vomiting and Murphy's sign, acute cholecystitis must be suspected. Imaging and bloodwork are important in excluding alternative explanations such as fatty liver of pregnancy, HELLP, placental abruption, uterine rupture, appendicitis, and gastroesophageal reflux.

Ultrasound is the first-line diagnostic imaging test. Gallstones, sludge, and acute cholecystitis are easily confirmed with high sensitivity and specificity. Noncontrast magnetic resonance imaging (MRI) and magnetic resonance cholangiopancreatography (MRCP) can be considered if ultrasound is not diagnostic but suspicion is high. Laboratory studies are similar to nonpregnant patients with attention to the physiological increase in alkaline phosphatase in pregnancy.

Management of biliary colic is initially supportive with pain control and fasting to decrease the release of cholecystokinin. Recurrent episodes are common, with relapse rates as high as 69%. Subsequent episodes tend to be more severe and surgical intervention is appropriate when conservative therapy fails, preferably in the second trimester [365]. Nearly a third (27–30%) of women require cholecystectomy due to the failure of conservative treatment, although after the acceptance of laparoscopic cholecystectomy, there has been an increasing trend toward surgical management [366,367]. A retrospective evaluation of 36 929 pregnant women hospitalized with biliary tract disease found that 26% underwent cholecystectomy. Those who underwent cholecystectomy had lower rates of maternal (4.3% vs 16.5%), and fetal (5.8% vs 16.5%) complications when compared to those managed conservatively. However, length of stay and cost of hospitalization were higher. Laparoscopic procedures had better surgical, maternal, fetal, and economic outcomes compared to open cholecystectomy; however, as the study was retrospective, open procedures are likely biased toward a more complicated population [368]. A metaanalysis of 11 comparative studies of 10 632 women confirmed that laparoscopic cholecystectomy was associated with fewer maternal and fetal complications than open cholecystectomy during pregnancy [369].

Choledocholithiasis

Choledocholithiasis can result in obstructive jaundice, cholangitis or pancreatitis, increasing maternal and fetal risk. After stabilization including antibiotics, endoscopic retrograde cholangiopancreatography (ERCP) with sphincterotomy should be performed. Despite the use of fluoroscopy, ERCP has been performed without serious maternal or fetal complications [370]. If ERCP fails, then a percutaneous cholangiocatheter can be placed for decompression or cholecystectomy and stone removal performed.

Acute cholecystitis

Acute cholecystitis is treated surgically, with recommendations for cholecystectomy within 72 hours of presentation, after stabilizing the patient with antibiotics and hydration [371]. Even without surgery, symptoms can improve over 7–10 days. However, recurrence is common with a higher risk for severe complications including gangrene, perforation, and fistula formation. Given the technical difficulties in late pregnancy, management must be individualized [372].

Acute pancreatitis

Acute pancreatitis is rare in pregnancy, with an incidence of 1 in 1000 to 1 in 10 000 [373]. Historically, pancreatitis had significant impact on maternal and perinatal outcomes but with improved neonatal care, perinatal mortality has decreased to 3.6% [374]. Maternal mortality has also improved to <1%, likely linked to improvements in testing allowing earlier diagnosis. Incidence is highest in the third trimester and generally presents with epigastric pain, nausea, and vomiting. Radiation into the back is also common.

Mirroring nonpregnant adults, gallstones (66%), alcohol abuse (12%), idiopathic (17%), and hyperlipidemia (4%) are most common, with hyperparathyroidism, trauma, medications, and fatty liver of pregnancy as less common etiologies [374]. Diagnosis is confirmed by elevated serum amylase or lipase levels. Ultrasound has low diagnostic yield for acute pancreatitis but is an excellent study for gallstone detection or biliary dilation. MRCP can confirm suspicions when ultrasound is indeterminate. MRCP has been performed successfully during pregnancy and limits the use of ERCP to therapeutic procedures [375,376].

Pancreatic necrosis can progress to multiorgan failure and systemic inflammatory response syndrome (SIRS). If biliary pancreatitis is managed conservatively, up to 50–70% will experience recurrent episodes [377,378]. Small case series suggest that endoscopic sphincterotomy may be sufficient to prevent recurrence during pregnancy and allow cholecystectomy to be deferred [379]. In the nonpregnant population, sphincterotomy alone has been associated with 25–50% risk of gallstone-induced complications within 2 years [380].

Budd–Chiari syndrome (BCS)

Budd–Chiari syndrome (BCS) is a result of hepatic venous outflow obstruction generally related to prothombotic conditions leading to portal hypertension (see Chapter 103). High estrogen levels in pregnancy can be a risk factor for developing BCS in women with preexisting hypercoagulability, and high mortality rates (50%) have been reported in women diagnosed with BCS during pregnancy [381]. Patients can present with abdominal pain, hepatomegaly, and ascites. In women with established and treated BCS, successful pregnancy is possible. Retrospective data from 24 pregnancies involving 16 women with BCS found nine had decompressive procedures prior to pregnancy and the majority (17/24) received anticoagulant therapy during the pregnancy. Despite that, preterm birth and miscarriage (fetal loss before gestational week 20) were high, 76% and 29% respectively, and maternal complications included intrahepatic cholestasis, intrauterine hematoma, preeclampsia, and placenta previa. Limited data suggest that although maternal and fetal risk is higher, pregnancy is not contraindicated with portal vein thrombosis or BCS.

Hepatitis E virus (HEV)

Hepatitis E virus (HEV) is transmitted through fecal–oral exposure and typically is self-limited although fulminant hepatitis can occur (see Chapter 86). The highest incidence is in Asia, Africa, Middle East, and Central America [382]. Previously considered rare in industrialized countries, recent data suggest that HEV exposure in the US and Europe may be more common than previously suspected [383,384]. Using serum collected in the 2009–2010 National Health and Nutrition Examination Survey (NHANES), the seroprevalence of HEV exposure in the United States was found to be 6% [385].

Hepatitis E virus is typically a disease with minimal morbidity and mortality. However, when acquired during pregnancy, especially in the third trimester, HEV is associated with maternal fulminant hepatic failure with mortality rates of 20%. There is also a risk for vertical transmission resulting in significant infant morbidity and mortality [386,387]. Diagnosis is made by a positive serum or stool HEV RNA or by finding anti-IgM to HEV. The viral load of HEV is higher in pregnant women with acute liver failure, suggesting that viral titer may predict the severity of infection [388].

In the United States, commercial HEV RNA testing is not available and specimens should be sent to the CDC for testing (1-800-CDC-INFO, www.CDC.gov). Treatment is supportive. Ribavirin may be of benefit, mostly in those with chronic HEV which has been reported in immunosuppressed patients, but is contraindicated during pregnancy [389].

Herpes simplex virus (HSV) hepatitis

Acquisition of HSV during pregnancy is uncommon, with only 2% of susceptible pregnant women acquiring infection [390]. HSV is generally considered a benign disease except in immune-compromised individuals. However, there is a well-documented risk of disseminated disease and acute hepatic dysfunction when acquired in the third trimester of pregnancy [391]. Maternal mortality rates reach 24–39% [391]. Presentation is characterized by marked elevations in ALT and AST (may be >5000 U/L), fever, and abdominal pain. Jaundice is uncommon. Mucocutaneous lesions are only identified in half of cases. Concomitant HSV encephalitis can lead to lethargy and seizures [392]. Although generally presumed to be from primary infection, reactivation of latent virus is also possible.

Diagnosis

Either HSV serotype can cause hepatitis, although type 2 is responsible for most cases. PCR test for HSV DNA can distinguish acute HSV gestational hepatitis from alternative explanations [393]. Liver biopsy can be diagnostic but is rarely needed.

Therapy

Aciclovir has been shown to decrease the risk of death in both pregnant and nonpregnant adults with HSV hepatitis, with worse outcomes in those who had a delay in initiation of antiviral therapy [394]. In addition, some studies have shown that antiviral therapy delays delivery or rupture of membranes in pregnant women with HSV hepatitis [395]. Aciclovir is not FDA approved for use in pregnant women. A prospective epidemiological pregnancy registry accrued data involving 749 pregnancies exposed to aciclovir during the first trimester. Although the registry was insufficient to evaluate for less common defects, the overall birth defect rate was similar to that in the general populations [396].

No study has suggested that treating primary or reactivated HSV during pregnancy decreases the risk of severe maternal disease manifestations such as hepatitis.

Fetal outcomes

Fetal outcomes in women with HSV hepatitis are often poor, with mortality of 39%. Outcomes likely reflect both an increased risk for intrauterine fetal demise due to severe maternal illness and complications of prematurity [391].

Hepatitis B virus (HBV)

Epidemiology

Globally, mother-to-child transmission (MTCT) is the most common cause of chronic HBV infection because the risk of chronicity is 90% when infection is acquired perinatally.

Management of maternal HBV

Management of hepatitis B during pregnancy must be viewed from the perspective of the mother, the effect on the pregnancy, and the desire to reduce transmission to the infant (Figure 40.2). All pregnant women should be screened for HBV by testing for hepatitis B surface antigen (HBsAg) in the first trimester. Women who test negative should beconsidered for hepatits B vaccination especially if at high risk for infection. HBV vaccine is safe for use in pregnancy.

Those who test positive should be further evaluated for HBV replication by testing for HBV e antigen (HBeAg) and HBV DNA, and for liver injury by testing for liver chemistries (see Chapter 87). The criteria for treating a pregnant patient with chronic hepatitis B should be based on the general guidelines with the following considerations: risk of medication to the fetus, effect of hepatitis B on the pregnancy, and need for reduction of MTCT.

If antiviral therapy is needed, tenofovir disoproxil fumarate is preferred. No hepatitis B antiviral medication has been approved by the FDA for use during pregnancy but based on data from the antiretroviral registry which includes mostly patients with HIV/HBV coinfection and some patients with HBV monoinfection, tenofovir disoproxil fumarate appears to be safe (Table 40.12). A newer formulation, tenofovir alafenamide, was recently approved by FDA and while it has fewer side-effects that are important for fetal development such as bone density, there are at present limited safety data in pregnancy. Studies using lamuvidine and telbivudine have been performed in pregnant women and showed maternal and fetal safety as well as efficacy in decreasing MTCT, but the high risk of drug resistance makes these drugs a less attractive option [397,398]. There are limited data on the safety of entecavir during pregnancy, prompting experts to recommend switching women from entecavir to tenofovir disoproxil fumarate if they are planning to become pregnant or found to be pregnant [397,399]. Interferon-α is not recommended in view of significant side-effects in the mother and risks to the fetus [399].

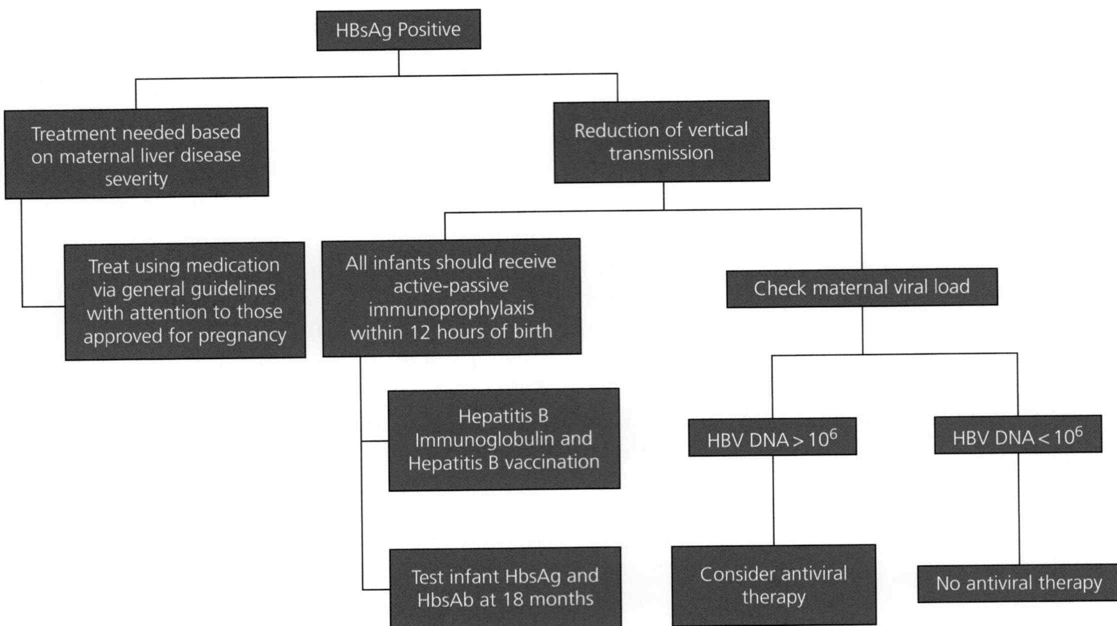

Figure 40.2 Management algorithm for assessment and treatment of chronic hepatitis B in pregnancy.

Although pregnancy invokes a relatively immunosuppressed state, HBV reactivation is rare [400,401]. During pregnancy, cortisol levels increase, peaking at term. After delivery, cortisol levels rapidly return to the pre-pregnancy range. It has been hypothesized that this is analogous to immune reconstitution after therapeutic withdrawal of oral steroids [402] and likely explains why nearly two-thirds of mothers experience an increase in ALT and 12.5–17% lose HBeAg or seroconvert in the postpartum period [401–403]. The ALT flares are typically well tolerated, although there have been case reports of fulminant hepatitis [404].

Fetal complications

Chronic hepatitis B does not increase the risk of fetal complications or overall maternal morbidity [405,406], though some studies observed higher rates of gestational diabetes, antepartum hemorrhage, and threatened preterm labor [407–409].

Even acute hepatitis B infection, acquired during pregnancy, is not associated with increased spontaneous abortion, stillbirth or congenital malformations [410,411]. Infection acquired during the last trimester has been linked with higher rates of low birthweight and prematurity [405,412]. The risk of MTCT transmission is also much higher if acute HBV infection occurs in the third trimester compared to the first (60–90% vs 10%) [405,412].

Prevention of mother-to-child transmission

One of the most important considerations for hepatitis B in pregnancy is the prevention of MTCT. Most MTCT occurs during delivery or postpartum. In utero transmission accounts for <2% cases and may explain some failures of standard immunoprophylaxis [413–415]. High maternal HBV DNA and positive HBeAg are the most important determinants of MTCT transmission, with transmission rates of 70–90% in HBeAg-positive mothers, compared to 5–20% in HBeAg-negative mothers [416]. Maternal HBV DNA (>200 000 IU/mL) is associated with increased risk of failure of passive-active immunoprophylaxis [398,417].

All infants born to HBsAg-positive mothers should receive hepatitis B immunoglobulins and the first dose of hepatitis B vaccination immediately after birth followed by completion of the three-dose series [416]. This passive-active immunoprophylaxis approach is 85–95% effective in preventing MTCT [416]. If the HBsAg status of the mother is not known, it is safest to offer prophylaxis against HBV.

Randomized controlled trials and metaanalysis have shown that antiviral therapy (lamivudine, telbivudine, and tenofovir disoproxil fumarate) administered to pregnant women with high viremia during the second or third trimester of pregnancy is safe for the mother and infant, and effective in further decreasing the risk of MTCT in infants who received passive-active immunoprophylaxis [417–420]. Because of the high risk of antiviral resistance to lamuvidine and telbivudine [421,422], tenofovir disoproxil fumarate is preferred. The American Association for the Study of Liver Diseases (AASLD) guidelines recommend the use of tenofovir disoproxil fumarate in early third trimester in mothers with HBV DNA >200 000 IU/mL [398,399]. Treatment can be stopped shortly after delivery but mothers should be monitored for 6 months after discontinuation given the risk of postpartum flare [398]. Although the AASLD recommends antiviral therapy for mothers with high HBV viral load, a recent multicenter double-blind placebo-controlled trial of tenofovir disoproxil fumarate did not show an incremental benefit of maternal antiviral therapy above the standard passive-active immunoprophylaxis [423], but all the infants received hepatitis B immunoglobulin and hepatitis B vaccination a median of 1.2 hours after delivery, suggesting that standard immunoprophylaxis alone can be very effective if early and strict adherence can be assured. These data need to be confirmed and the logistics of implementation in clinical practice determined.

The Antiretroviral Pregnancy Registry analyzed 13 711 cases of lamivudine or tenofovir disoproxil fumarate antiviral exposure during pregnancy. The overall birth defect prevalence was 2.8%, which is comparable to population-based data. Birth defect prevalence was similar between first and second/third trimester exposure [424] (see Table 40.12). Elective cesarean section (ECS) has been shown in some but not all studies to prevent MTCT of HBV. Until more definitive studies are available, routine elective cesarean delivery is not recommended [425].

There is no difference in perinatal infection rates between breastfed and formula-fed infants. The European Society of Pediatric Gastroenterology, Hepatology and Nutrition and the American Academy of Pediatrics do not consider HBV a contraindication to breastfeeding [426,427]. In addition, a metaanalysis did not find breastfeeding to be a risk for transmission in infants who received appropriate immunoprophyaxis [428]. Many mothers may be taking antiviral agents at the time of delivery. Exposure to lamivudine and tenofovir disoproxil is lower from breastfeeding than from in utero exposure, suggesting that their use during breastfeeding may be safe [429]. Benefits versus risks of continued antiviral therapy in breastfeeding mothers should be discussed. Antiviral therapy administered solely to reduce MTCT may be stopped immediately after delivery. Despite concerns about hepatitis flares after treatment withdrawal, clinical trials showed that they are rare and generally mild. Nonetheless, close monitoring of ALT and HBV DNA levels for 6 months is warranted.

A child born to an HBsAg-positive mother should be tested for hepatitis B surface antibody (anti-HBs) and HBsAg at 9–12 months or 1–2 months after the last dose of vaccination to confirm immunity. Testing should be performed after 9 months to avoid detection of anti-HBs from HBIG administered during infancy [430]. Hepatitis B core antibody (anti-HBc) testing is not recommended as passively acquired maternal anti-HBc can be detected even at 24 months.

Postpartum management

In mothers, the most common time to expect a flare of hepatitis is in the first months postpartum, especially if antiviral therapy is discontinued. Monitoring ALT and AST every 1–3 months during the first 6 months postpartum is recommended after antiviral therapy is discontinued. Virological rebound (increase in HBV DNA) is expected and does not necessitate resumption of antiviral therapy unless accompanied by severe or persistent increase in ALT and AST. All women found to be HBsAg positive during pregnancy should be referred for long-term management of chronic HBV infection.

Hepatitis C (HCV)

Epidemiology

Hepatitis C infection is reviewed in Chapter 88. Perinatal testing does not routinely include screening for hepatitis C, but cross-sectional studies estimate that 0.5–8% of pregnant women have anti-HCV [431–434]. With the recent increase in HCV prevalence, especially among younger individuals due to the opioid epidemic, there will likely to be a change in screening guidelines particularly among pregnant women [435].

Effects on pregnancy

Hepatitis C virus is generally well tolerated during pregnancy with minimal risk to the mother. ALT levels tend to decline during the second and third trimesters only to return to baseline postpartum. Conversely, HCV RNA peaks during the third

Table 40.12 Antiretroviral pregnancy registry data.

Agent	Earliest trimester of exposure	
	1st trimester birth defects/live births	**2nd/3rd trimester birth defects/live births**
Lamivudine	99/3481 (2.8%)	130/5194 (2.5%)
Adefovir	0/37	0/0
Telbivudine	0/5	0/3
Tenofovir disoproxil fumarate	19/879 (2.2%)	11/501 (2.2%)
Entecavir	0/12	0/2
Any HBV nucleoside/nucleotide	118/4414 (2.7%)	141/5700 (2.5%)

Source: Hepatitis B Therapy in Pregnancy, Curr Hepat Rep. 2010 Nov; 9(4): 197–204. Reproduced with permission of Springer Nature.
HBV, hepatitis B virus.

trimester but then returns to pre-pregnancy levels postpartum [436,437]. This pattern is consistent with relative immune suppression followed by immune reconstitution. Unlike HBV, postpartum flares of HCV have not been well described. HCV infection may be associated with a higher risk for premature rupture of membranes and gestational diabetes [408,438].

Perinatal transmission

Infants born to HCV-positive mothers have a small increase in rate of adverse neonatal outcomes including low birthweight, small for gestational age and neonatal intensive care admissions [438].

Transmission of hepatitis C is via parenteral exposure. MTCT rates are low, averaging 5–10%. Still, vertical transmission is the leading etiology for pediatric HCV in developed countries [439–441]. The risk of transmission is higher in those with higher viral loads and 4–5-fold higher in those coinfected with HIV [442,443].

Unlike HBV, there is no vaccine to prevent MTCT of HCV and none of the direct-acting antiviral drugs have been approved for use in pregnancy. Use of internal fetal monitoring devices and prolonged rupture of membranes (>6 hours) have been linked to increased transmission, and should be avoided [444]. A metaanalysis found that cesarean section did not reduce vertical transmission in HCV-RNA-positive HIV-negative mothers [445]. Children born with HCV have mild liver disease and approximately 20% will spontaneously clear the infection [446], especially those with the favorable IL28B CC polymorphism [443].

Hepatitis C virus is increasingly recognized in couples undergoing assisted reproduction techniques (ART). HCV viremia may have a negative impact on fertility, with reduced pregnancy rates in HCV PCR-positive subjects [447]. Because HCV is detectable in sperm, there is also concern that HCV-positive men may not be appropriate for ART procedures. However, studies show that with sperm washing, transmission is negligible [448].

With the advent of highly effective antiviral therapy for HCV, the approach for prevention is the testing and identification of infected persons. Antiviral therapy is recommended prior to pregnancy to prevent perinatal transmission [449]. If this is not feasible, antiviral therapy is recommended post-pregnancy as there is insufficient evidence to support the safety of use of the hepatitis C antiviral agents in pregnancy.

Nonalcoholic and alcoholic fatty liver disease

Nonalcoholic fatty liver disease (NAFLD) is common, with worldwide prevalence rates between 6.3% and 33% [450] (see Chapter 96). Risk factors for NAFLD include obesity, diabetes, and the metabolic syndrome. There is also an established link with polycystic ovarian syndrome [451]. NAFLD per se is not known to increase maternal or fetal risk during pregnancy. NAFLD should be considered in the differential diagnosis of abnormal liver chemistries [452]. In addition, animal and human studies have suggested that intrauterine environment in pregnant women with obesity or NAFLD impacts the risk for childhood and adolescent steatosis [453–455].

Independent of liver disease, alcohol use during pregnancy can lead to fetal alcohol syndrome, composed of a constellation of developmental and behavioral problems, heart defects, and learning disabilities. In mothers with established alcoholic liver disease, there is increased risk of preterm birth and small for gestational age children [456].

Autoimmune hepatitis (AIH)

Autoimmune hepatitis is a T cell-mediated immune hepatic injury that occurs in all races and all ages. Women are preferentially affected (3.6:1), especially in the childbearing age [457].

Historically it was felt that fertility was compromised in women with AIH. However, multiple case series of pregnancy in women with AIH have clearly shown that gestation is possible. High obstetric complications have also been reported, but more recent literature confirms that with well-controlled AIH, successful outcomes are possible [458]. Improvement in fertility and obstetric outcome in recent studies is likely related to earlier diagnosis and better control of liver disease. An update from King's College (81 pregnancies in 53 women) reported a live birth rate of 73%, 10% miscarriage, and 12 terminations. Mothers with cirrhosis had lower birth rates, higher risk for prematurity, and their children were more likely to require admission to the special care baby unit. The maternal complication rate was 38%, including one death during pregnancy and three in the 12 months after delivery, and was highest in women with cirrhosis. In addition, 33% had a flare in AIH disease activity, the majority (78%) of which occurred in the first 3 months postpartum, warranting closer monitoring during and shortly after pregnancy [459].

Immune suppression should be continued during pregnancy to prevent disease flares. Safety data are limited, with most information coming from case reports and registry records. Extrapolating data from transplantation, corticosteroids, azathioprine, cyclosporine, and tacrolimus have all been used successfully with low incidence of congenital malformations [232]. Mycophenolate mofetil should be avoided during pregnancy as it has been associated with malformations in both animal models and human case reports [460].

Benign hepatic lesions: hepatic adenoma and focal nodular hyperplasia

Hepatic adenoma is a benign hepatic tumor of epithelial origin. Often solitary, they occur in women four times more frequently than in men, presumably due to increased estrogen exposure, especially with long-term oral contraceptive use [461].

Tumors can be large, up to 30 cm, and involve the right hepatic lobe preferentially. They are heterogeneous in appearance on imaging due to areas of hemorrhage and necrosis. Most lesions are incidentally found during unrelated radiological evaluation of the abdomen. Abdominal pain, jaundice, hepatomegaly, increased alkaline phosphatase, rupture, and hemorrhage have been reported.

Diagnosis is usually made through histology after resection or contrast-enhanced CT or MRI, although differentiating adenoma from focal nodular hyperplasia can sometimes be difficult. Liver biopsy may not conclusively make the diagnosis and there is an increased risk of bleeding after the procedure (see Chapter 141).

Pregnancy is a state of high estrogen exposure, and poses a risk for hormone-induced growth. Cases of hepatic adenoma rupture have been documented with high maternal and fetal mortality [462]. Although the incidence of adenomas has increased with the use of oral contraceptives, hepatic adenomas remain a rare liver tumor. Most pregnant women with adenomas are unaware of the diagnosis. In women with known hepatic adenomas, management is controversial. Some women are counseled to avoid pregnancy, and others may be advised to have pre-pregnancy resection or ablation. This may also be recommended independent of pregnancy considerations as small series do support an 8–13% risk of malignant transformation [463,464]. A published series monitored 12 women with documented hepatocellular adenomas through 17 pregnancies. Growth of the tumor was documented in only four out of 17 cases. The authors concluded that only in women at high risk for bleeding complications should pregnancy impact the management of the adenoma [465]. Bleeding risk has been associated with prolonged oral contraceptive use, size (larger than 4 cm), and subcapsular location [466].

Focal nodular hyperplasia (FNH) is a common benign hepatic tumor, again preferentially affecting women. FNH is considered a regenerative response to hyperperfusion [467]. Some studies have reported that FNH may be responsive to estrogen but most have not. Routine management does not require discontinuation of hormone therapy and the incidence of this lesion did not increase in parallel with the increased use of oral contraceptives [468]. Case series suggest that pregnancy does not result in significant growth or complications in women with FNH [469].

Cirrhosis and portal hypertension

Fertility is reduced in patients with cirrhosis due to disturbed estrogen metabolism leading to anovulation and amenorrhea [470]. However, patients with compensated cirrhosis may become pregnant [471]. Unplanned pregnancies in patients with cirrhosis may lead to catastrophic consequences, particularly when portal hypertension is present, so it is important to discuss this possibility with women of childbearing age so that adequate planning can occur.

Overall, there are increased maternal and fetal risks but they have decreased in recent years, from maternal mortality as high as 10.5% in the early 1980s to 1.6% and decompensation of 10% [472]. Among the risks to the mother is the aggravation of existing diseases such as in autoimmune hepatitis and Wilson disease, particularly in the setting of inappropriate discontinuation of medications. Pregnancy is not known to alter the course of Wilson disease but discontinuation of medications has led to detrimental outcomes with maternal hepatic decompensation and copper deposition in placenta and fetal liver. Yet some of the medications such as penicillamine or trientine can have maternal and fetal consequences so it is important to have a planned approach with appropriate conversion of medications as indicated [473]. The most important risk in cirrhosis is that associated with portal hypertension.

Fetal risks are also increased in patients with cirrhosis. There is an increased rate of spontaneous pregnancy loss, preterm labor, and perinatal death [474]. In one study, the live birth rate was 58% (36/62). Miscarriage occurred in 19%, stillbirth 6%, and 15% elective termination. Prematurity occurred in 67%. There are limited data to suggest that preconception decompressive procedures may lower the risk of spontaneous abortion [475].

Variceal bleeding

Variceal bleeding has been reported in about half of pregnancies affected by portal hypertension and in 5–32% with cirrhosis. The risk is as high as 78% in those with preexisting varices [470,476–478], and carries substantial mortality [470]. Bleeding is most common in the second and third trimesters as a result of increased maternal blood volume and compression of the inferior vena cava from a large gravid uterus. Risk of bleeding is highest during labor due to repeated Valsalva maneuvers. For those with large varices, elective cesarean section can decrease this risk, but can also be complicated by bleeding from pelvic or abdominal wall collaterals ligated during surgery [479].

The prognostic models MELD (model for end-stage liver disease ≥10), UKELD (United Kingdom end-stage liver disease ≥47), and Child–Pugh can be used at the time of conception to predict clinical outcomes. In one center, maternal complications occurred in only 10% of 62 pregnancies involving 29 women with cirrhosis. There was one death related to variceal bleeding. The live birth rate was 58% with a median gestational age of 36 weeks. If the MELD score was ≤6 or the UKELD score was ≤42, no woman had any significant liver-related complication. MELD and Child–Pugh scores were also associated with preterm delivery [474].

Women with known portal hypertension and cirrhosis contemplating pregnancy should be informed of the increased risk of variceal bleeding and should have a screening endoscopy prior to conception. Screening should otherwise be done early in the second trimester. As in the nonpregnant population, prophylaxis with a nonselective β-blocker or band ligation can be considered; however, because of fetal risk with β-blockers, there may be a decision for band ligation more often than in nonpregnant populations. Active bleeding should be managed with band ligation with transjugular intrahepatic portosystemic shunt (TIPS) as a salvage therapy. Octreotide, which causes splanchnic vasoconstriction, has not been well studied in pregnancy and should be used with caution. There is controversy around its use given potential placental ischemia and abruption.

Ultimately, each patient should be considered individually as the risk benefit will vary.

Pregnancy and liver transplantation

Fulminant hepatic failure in pregnant women

Women with severe pregnancy-related liver disease such as HELLP and AFLP are at risk for liver failure and death. Liver transplantation (LT) has been performed in this population with good outcomes. Prompt delivery is the best treatment. In the rare patient whose liver failure does not reverse after delivery, prompt evaluation for transplant is imperative. All patients displaying signs of hepatic failure such as encephalopathy and coagulopathy should be assessed for transplant. A retrospective evaluation of 54 admissions with pregnancy-related liver disease found that the traditional King's College criteria were not effective in predicting outcome. An admission lactate greater than 2.8 mg/dL had 73% sensitivity and 75% specificity for predicting death or LT. The addition of encephalopathy increased sensitivity and specificity to 90% and 86%, respectively [480]. This classification should be validated in larger populations, but potentially helps to identify women at greatest risk.

Pregnancy in posttransplant women

Liver transplantation restores fertility for patients with end-stage liver disease, making pregnancy possible for recipients with childbearing potential [295]. A metaanalysis reviewed 450 pregnancies in 306 liver transplant recipients. The live birth rate was excellent at 76.9%, which is higher than the US general population (66.7%), but complications also were higher [481]. Outcomes were better if pregnancy was delayed more than 2 years after transplant [481]. Management of immunosuppression during pregnancy is complex and should be directed by an experienced obstetric and transplant team. Antirejection drugs are safe for use in pregnancy except for mycophenolate.

Diagnostic testing and endoscopy during pregnancy

Diagnostic testing should always be placed in the context of risk and benefit to both mother and child. The anatomical changes induced by pregnancy can pose a challenge to interpretation of imaging studies, and ionizing radiation should be limited as increased exposure can be teratogenic, mutagenic, or carcinogenic. Exposure to less than 0.05 Gy has not been associated with fetal abnormalities [482,483]. Initial evaluation should include ultrasonography in most cases. When ultrasound is not adequate, cross-sectional imaging with CT or MR is often considered. Although there are limited safety data on MR during pregnancy, the American College of Radiology considers MRI acceptable during pregnancy when the results would affect clinical management [484]. Use of MR should be limited in the first trimester when organogenesis could potentially be affected. Gadolinium-based intravenous contrast should also be avoided as it can cross the placenta [485].

Box 40.2 BoxGeneral guidelines for endoscopy in pregnancy.

- Obtain a preoperative consultation with an obstetrician, regardless of fetal gestational age.
- Have a strong indication for the procedure, particularly in high-risk pregnancies.
- Defer endoscopy to the second trimester whenever possible.
- Use lowest effective dose of sedative medications.
- Use lowest risk sedation medication when possible.
- Minimize procedure time.
- Position patient in left pelvic tilt or left lateral position to avoid vena cava or aortic compression.
- Decide whether to monitor fetal heart rate. This depends on the gestational age of the fetus and available resources.
  - Before 24 weeks fetal gestation, confirming the presence of the fetal heart rate by Doppler before sedation has begun and after the procedure is complete is sufficient.
  - After 24 weeks of fetal gestation, simultaneous electronic fetal heart and uterine contraction monitoring should be performed before and after the procedure. Ideally, procedures should be done at an institution with neonatal and pediatric services. If possible, the fetal heart rate and uterine contractions should be monitored before, during, and after the procedure by a qualified individual, with obstetric support readily available in case of fetal distress or a pregnancy-related complication.
- Do not perform endoscopy in cases of placental abruption, imminent delivery, ruptured membranes, or uncontrolled eclampsia.

Source: Shergill et al. [491]. Reproduced by permission of Elsevier.

Table 40.13 Medications commonly used for endoscopic sedation in pregnancy.

Drug class	Drug	Recommendations for pregnancy	Recommendations for lactation
Benzodiazepines	Versed	Crosses the placenta. Use lowest dose possible. Limited human data, but animal data suggest low risk	Present in breast milk. Suggest waiting >4 hours after maternal dose to continue breastfeeding
Opioid	Meperidine	No evidence for teratogenicity. Choice of opioid for endoscopy	Caution while breastfeeding risk of CNS and respiratory depression
	Fentanyl	Crosses the placenta. Human data suggest risk. Possible risk of teratogenicity low based on limited conflicting human studies	May use while breastfeeding. Empiric risk of CNS depression in high-risk infant
General anesthetic	Propofol	Crosses the placenta. Weigh risk/benefit in third trimester if prolonged or repeated use. Risk of CNS and respiratory depression	Present in milk. Caution while breastfeeding

CNS, central nervous system.

Magnetic resonance cholangiopancreatography (MRCP) is an excellent and accurate diagnostic tool for biliary diseases [486]. Gallstone complications, especially choledocholithiasis or gallstone pancreatitis, occasionally require intervention during pregnancy. Several case series of endoscopic retrograde cholagiopancreatography (ERCP) have shown that the procedure can be performed safely with few complications during pregnancy. MRCP has been used for stone detection with subsequent extraction by ERCP even without fluoroscopy [487]. Post-ERCP pancreatitis may be more common than in the nonpregnant population [488]. Endoscopic ultrasonography (EUS) is also a sensitive and specific alternative for the evaluation of choledocholithiasis.

Liver biopsy is rarely required, as less invasive testing is normally sufficient for diagnosis. It should be noted that some noninvasive methods such as liver stiffness measurements may be artificially increased in pregnancy due to increased hepatic blood flow and thus cut-offs for fibrosis using nonpregnant standards would not be appropriate [489,490]. In rare instances when the results of a biopsy would impact management, a biopsy can be performed safely through either ultrasound-guided percutaneous or transjugular approaches.

Endoscopy in pregnancy

Endoscopic procedures should only be performed in pregnant patients if failure to perform the procedure places the fetus and/or mother at risk [491]. General guidelines for endoscopy in pregnancy are summarized in Box 40.2. Medications utilized for sedation are summarized in Table 40.13.

References are available at www.yamadagastro.com/textbook7e

Further reading

ASGE Standard of Practice Committee, Shergill A.K., Ben-Menachem T., et al. Guidelines for endoscopy in pregnant and lactating women. Gastrointest Endosc 2012;76:18.

Cappell M.S. Gastric and duodenal ulcers during pregnancy. Gastroenterol Clin North Am 2003;32:263.

Chappell L.C., Bell J.L., Smith A., et al. Ursodeoxycholic acid versus placebo in women with intrahepatic cholestasis of pregnancy (PITCHES): a randomised controlled trial. Lancet 2019;394(10201):849.

Committee on Practice Bulletins – Obstetrics. ACOG Practice Bulletin No. 189: Nausea And Vomiting Of Pregnancy. Obstet Gynecol 2018;131(1):e15.

Gill S.K., O'Brien L., Einarson T.R., et al. The safety of proton pump inhibitors (PPIs) in pregnancy: a meta-analysis. Am J Gastroenterol 2009;104:1541.

Hagstrom H., Hoijer J., Marschall H.U., et al. Outcomes of pregnancy in mothers with cirrhosis: a national population-based cohort study of 1.3 million pregnancies. Hepatol Commun 2018;2(11):1299.

Han L., Zhang H.W., Xie J.X., et al. A meta-analysis of lamivudine for interruption of mother-to-child transmission of hepatitis B virus. World J Gastroenterol 2011;17:4321.

Hashash J.G., Kane S. Pregnancy and inflammatory bowel disease. Gastroenterol Hepatol 2015;11(2):96.

Jourdain G., Ngo-Giang-Huong N., Harrison L., Decker L, et al. Tenofovir versus placebo to prevent perinatal transmission of hepatitis B. N Engl J Med 2018;378(10):911.

Riley LE, Cahill A., Beigi R., et al. Improving safe and effective use of drugs in pregnancy and lactation: workshop summary. Am J Perinatol 2017;34(8):826.

Tran T.T., Ahn J., Reau N.S. ACG Clinical Guideline: Liver Disease and Pregnancy. Am J Gastroenterol 2016;111(2):176.

Westbrook R.H., Dusheiko G., Williamson C. Pregnancy and liver disease. J Hepatol 2016;64(4):933.

CHAPTER 41

Genetic counseling for gastrointestinal patients

Veroushka Ballester and Fay Kastrinos
Columbia University Irving Medical Center, New York, NY, USA

Chapter menu

Genetics is among the most rapidly developing areas of medical science, and this has translated into tremendous opportunities for improved diagnosis, personalized medicine, and new therapeutics in clinical medicine. The Human Genome Project has provided significant insight into the basic structure of our genome, including the number of genes and the importance of the nonprotein encoding portions of the genome, as genomic sequencing on a routine basis is increasingly feasible. As the details of the human genome have been revealed, it has become apparent that there is greater complexity to genomic organization and function than would have been predicted decades ago. Although medical practitioners now have access to genetic information that may explain causation of disease, define disease risk, and impact medical decision making, including the ability to target therapeutic options, they are also confronted by incidental findings and variants of uncertain significance (VUS). This chapter will start with a basic description of the genome, provide an outline for interpreting data that will be presented to the clinician, and review the principles of genetic counseling for patients who are recipients of this information.

Structure and function of nucleic acids

Functional anatomy of the human genome

The human genome consists of 23 pairs of chromosomes, with about 2.85 billion nucleotides (paired), and encodes about 20,000 protein-coding genes, but each may have multiple splice variants [1,2]. The functions of nearly a quarter of all identified genes remain to be determined. Protein-encoding sequences make up only about 1% of the genome. The genome is quite variable among humans and contains at least 5 million single-nucleotide polymorphisms (SNPs; "snips"; with more than 100 million across different populations around the world), 1.4 million short insertion or deletion (in/del) variants, and more than 14,000 larger deletion variants. Some portions of the genome are made up of repetitive elements, which can be so large that they cannot be reliably sequenced. Much or most of the nonprotein-encoding DNA is expressed as noncoding RNAs (ncRNAs), which have a variety of known and yet to be discovered functions. RNA functions include roles as messenger RNAs, transfer RNAs, ribosomal RNAs, and microRNAs, which play an important role in the regulation of gene expression and many other

Yamada's Textbook of Gastroenterology, Seventh Edition. Edited by Timothy C. Wang, Michael Camilleri, Benjamin Lebwohl, Anna S. Lok, William J. Sandborn, Kenneth K. Wang, and Gary D. Wu.

Companion website: www.yamadagastro.com/textbook7e

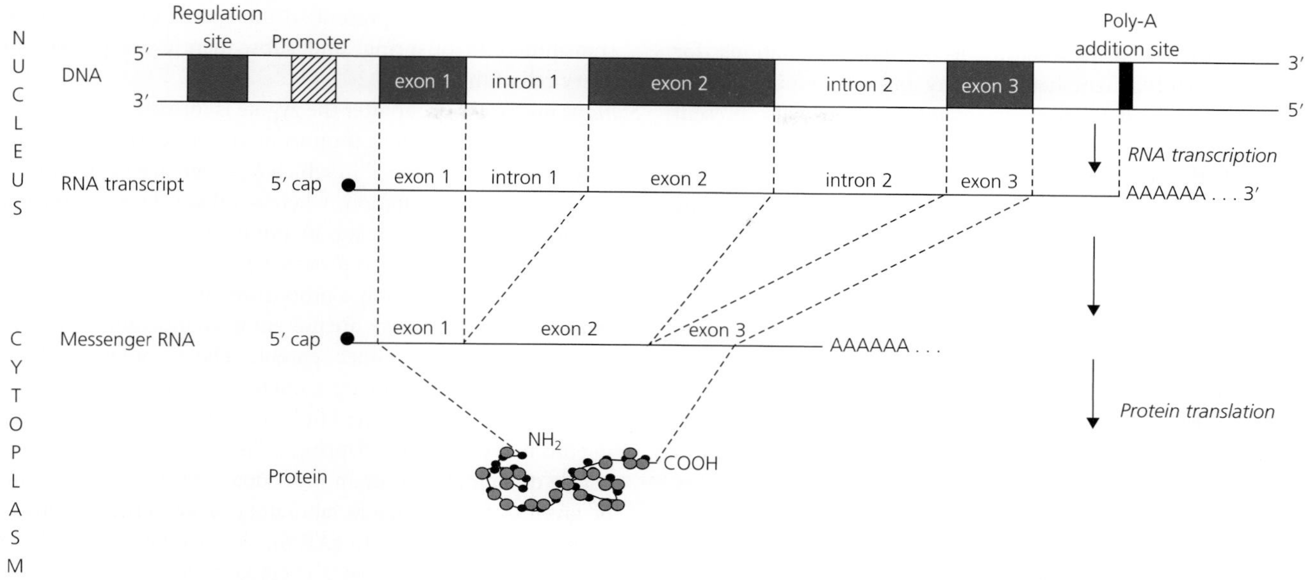

Figure 41.1 Organization of genetic material. DNA is the double-stranded molecule that contains the genetic code and includes coding (exons) and noncoding (introns) segments. In a multistep process, DNA is transcribed into RNA and spliced into messenger RNA (mRNA), which contains regulatory elements and exons, but no introns. The mRNA is translated into a series of amino acids that combine to form a specific protein. Proteins are the molecules that function within cells.

direct enzymatic functions. The size of a gene is variable, but, on average, genes consist of eight exons (each consisting of ~122 base pairs) encoding for 367 amino acids. The genome also harbors a substantial number of pseudogenes, which are inactive copies of protein-coding genes. Currently, approximately 20,000 pseudogenes are estimated, which is comparable with the number of protein-coding genes. It has been recognized that some pseudogenes play essential roles in gene regulation, including regulation of tumor suppressors and oncogenes. The size and variability of DNA sequence among humans and throughout human populations make genetic diagnosis and the interpretation of genetic testing a daunting undertaking [3,4]. The organization of the genome, from DNA to RNA to protein, is illustrated in Figure 41.1.

Methods used to detect mutations

The traditional means to detect germline mutations is to extract DNA from blood and use polymerase chain reaction (PCR)-based techniques to amplify specific genetic targets and sequence them by the traditional Sanger technique. The sequence obtained is compared with a database from which the most common or "wild-type" sequence has been established to determine whether the sequence variation in the patient represents a simple SNP, a rare sequence variation with no functional consequences, or a disease-causing mutation. This is usually accomplished empirically by identifying individuals with the disease phenotype and determining whether the sequence variation is linked to the disease state. Some genotype–phenotype interpretations are relatively straightforward; for example, genetic deletions are unambiguous in their effect. Premature stop codons are also relatively easy to interpret, but the cell may tolerate a truncated protein, or the cell may be able to "ignore" the stop codon in some instances. Missense mutations and sequence variations that change the amino acid encoded are much harder to interpret. In the final analysis, empirical matching of a sequence variation with individuals diagnosed with the disease is the final determinant of interpretation. Population-wide genomic analyses suggest that every individual carries about 250–300 loss-of-function genetic variants, including 50–100 associated with known hereditary diseases, and yet most of these do not result in a disease phenotype. Accordingly, the potential for overinterpretation looms large in every genetic test [4].

There are many different technologies used in genetic/genomic testing; not all provide the same information. One can use a variety of high-throughput "arrays" to determine DNA sequence, quantitate RNA expression, or determine RNA sequences. Analysis of RNA sequences is the most reliable way to determine how the cell has processed or modified the initial RNA transcript and prepared it for protein synthesis (translation). There are several platforms that perform DNA sequencing analysis by massively parallel sequencing of short fragments of DNA and assembling the short "reads" through computer computation using a reference DNA sequence and informatics algorithms. These "next-generation" sequencing (NGS) platforms allow simultaneous testing of multiple susceptibility genes and have the advantage of detecting germline mutations that would not have been discovered based on the patient's clinical phenotype and family history. In addition, NGS can increase the yield of identifying germline mutations for syndromes with genetic heterogeneity and overlapping phenotypes. Although NGS has many advantages, it may also present challenges, including interpretation of VUS with unknown levels of risk, the detection of unexpected high-penetrance susceptibility gene mutations in a patient without a phenotype suggestive of their underlying mutation, and the management of carriers of moderate penetrance mutations for whom the optimal management has not been clearly elucidated. These techniques can also determine DNA copy number, which is another source of human genomic variation.

Genetic tests can, therefore, provide information about DNA sequence, RNA sequence, and copy numbers of either DNA or RNA. Alterations in any of these may be responsible for a genetic disease. Although NGS presents significant challenges, it offers a personalized approach and important opportunities for tailored disease management and prevention strategies for the individual undergoing testing and any at-risk family members.

Key terms in genetics

Genetics has its own terminology, which has evolved as our understanding of genomic structure and function has increased.

DNA repair: Errors in DNA replication are monitored and repaired by a number of protein complexes, including mismatch repair (MMR), base excision repair (BER), nucleotide excision repair, and other DNA glycosylases that can repair spontaneous degradation of DNA. Each system recognizes and repairs specific types of defect in DNA, but the combined effect results in a very low rate of mutation throughout the organism.

Penetrance refers to the likelihood of disease expression if the individual has inherited the disease-causing allele. For example, individuals with familial adenomatous polyposis (FAP) have a nearly 100% chance of developing adenomatous polyps of the colon, one of which will almost certainly develop into colon cancer if prophylactic colectomy is not performed. Therefore, FAP has a 100%, or complete, penetrance, for adenomas. The likelihood of an individual with Lynch syndrome developing colorectal cancer is 60–80%; therefore, Lynch syndrome has incomplete penetrance.

Variable expressivity means that the same genetic disorder is expressed to a different clinical extent in different individuals. In some individuals with hereditary hemochromatosis, cirrhosis of the liver and heart disease may result, where other individuals may have only elevated levels of iron and no organ damage. Gene expression is thought to be modified by intraallelic variation, interactions with other genes, environmental factors, and other unknown factors.

Germline mutations are present in the sperm or egg, may be transmitted to offspring, and subsequently are present in every cell of the body.

Somatic mutations occur after the zygote is formed, and they are therefore found in only a proportion of cells of the body. This may result in a "mosaic," in which a percentage of the body's cells contain the mutation, whereas others do not. Somatic mutations frequently occur in tumor cells (often due to a breakdown in DNA repair processes), in which case the mutation may be found in only a proportion of the tumor cells.

De novo germline mutations are present in an individual but were not inherited from either parent. These mutations have occurred randomly during gamete maturation or early in embryogenesis. The affected individual is now at risk for passing this mutation on to offspring. When interpreting an apparent de novo mutation in an individual, consideration should be given to factors such as laboratory error, germline mosaicism, and nonpaternity. In FAP, the de novo rate is thought to be ~25% (in part because it is a very large gene), whereas individuals with Lynch syndrome rarely have de novo mutations.

Mosaicism occurs when only some of the cells have the mutation. In neurofibromatosis, some individuals have mosaicism, having the mutated allele in certain places of their body (i.e., left arm affected, but right arm unaffected). If the mutation occurs only in the gonads, the parent will be unaffected but will be at risk to pass the disease allele on to offspring ("germline mosaicism").

Pleiotropy: Many genes, such as the mutated *STK11* gene that causes Peutz–Jeghers syndrome (PJS), exhibit pleiotropy, which occurs when a mutated gene has more than one phenotypic effect on the body. Individuals with Peutz–Jeghers may have any combination of colonic polyps; pancreatic cancer; breast cancer; melanin spots on buccal mucosa, vulva, penis, and fingers; and other features.

Genetic heterogeneity is when there are multiple ways of inheriting the same disease. For example, mutations in *BRCA2* and *STK11* both increase the risk for development of breast and pancreatic cancers but result in very different diseases (hereditary breast and ovarian cancer versus PJS).

Locus heterogeneity occurs when a mutation in multiple genes can show the same phenotype. For example, five different genes are associated with Lynch syndrome (*MSH2*, *MSH6*, *PMS2*, *MLH1*, and *EPCAM*).

Allelic heterogeneity refers to the fact that there can be different mutations within the same gene. In FAP, the location of the mutation can predict the polyp burden in an individual. Mutations at either end of the gene (5′ or 3′) are usually associated with an attenuated version of FAP, whereas mutations between codons 1250 and 1464 are associated with profuse carpeting of polyps (>5000).

Compound heterozygosity occurs in a recessive disease when an individual has two different disease-causing mutations; this is distinct from someone who is homozygous for two of the same mutations in that gene. An individual with two copies of

ΔF508 is homozygous, whereas a patient with cystic fibrosis with one copy of ΔF508 and a copy of G542X is a compound heterozygote.

Epigenetics refers to changes in the function of DNA that do not involve a change in the DNA sequence. DNA methylation is the principal mechanism of epigenetic alterations. However, changes in the expression of microRNAs, which can modify the stability of mRNA, are also a source of epigenetic driver changes in function [5].

DNA methylation refers to an epigenetic modification involving the covalent transfer of a methyl group to the C-5 position of the cytosine ring of DNA by DNA methyltransferase. DNA methylation is regarded as a key player in transcriptional silencing in carcinogenesis [6].

Cascade testing refers to a systematic process for the identification of individuals at risk for a hereditary condition. The process begins with the identification of an individual with the condition and/or a pathogenic variant associated with the condition and then extending genetic testing to his/her at-risk biological relatives. This process is repeated as more affected individuals or pathogenic variant carriers are identified.

Inheritance patterns

Patterns of genetic inheritance are somewhat more complicated than suggested by historical Mendelian principles. The classic forms of inheritance are still valid, but more possibilities result from regulatory gene expression.

Autosomal dominant inheritance: This occurs when an alteration in only one of the two alleles is sufficient to cause disease. In this case, one allele has a deleterious mutation, whereas the other copy is "normal" (and is called "wild type"). An individual with an autosomal dominant disease has a 50% chance of transmitting the mutated allele to their offspring. Vertical transmission is typically noted in the pedigree (i.e., the disease is transmitted from grandparent to parent to child and grandchild, etc., with no preference for gender). Males and females are equally at risk, and male-to-male transmission may occur. The mutation does not "skip" generations (although, with variable penetrance, the clinical disease may be missing in a generation). An individual with an autosomal dominant disease, therefore, has a parent with the mutation. In families without a known autosomal dominant disease, the mutation may be a de novo mutation, as described in the previous section. Figure 41.2a shows a typical autosomal dominant pedigree.

Autosomal recessive disorders: These disorders require that an individual inherits two mutant alleles at a given locus – one from each parent. Autosomal recessive conditions, such as *MutYH*-associated polyposis (MAP), express themselves only when both copies of the gene harbor the mutation. Individuals who have only one copy of the mutant allele *typically* do not manifest the symptoms of the disease and are designated carriers. There are exceptions to this rule, because individuals with biallelic (two copies) *ATM* mutations have ataxia telangiectasia. However, carriers of one *ATM* mutation have an increased risk for breast and pancreatic cancer. In other instances, being a carrier may have a survival advantage. Individuals who have one copy of the sickle cell anemia gene have enhanced resistance to malaria. When two carriers have offspring, there is a 25% chance of having an affected child, a 50% chance the child will be a carrier, and a 25% chance that the child will inherit neither of the mutated alleles. This disease may manifest as horizontal transmission, because multiple siblings can be affected, but neither parent will have the disease. As with autosomal dominant inheritance, males and females are equally affected. See Figure 41.2b for a typical autosomal recessive pedigree.

Sex-linked disorders: These disorders involve a mutation on one of the sex-determining chromosomes, X and Y. Y-linked conditions are passed on from father to son but are quite rare. X-linked conditions, such as hemophilia or Duchenne muscular dystrophy, are more commonly observed. Males have only one X chromosome, and thus need only one copy of the mutated allele to show disease. Females usually do not express symptoms of the disease in the carrier state, although there are exceptions (such as in fragile X where carrier mothers may have premature ovarian failure). Female carriers have a 50% chance of passing the mutated allele on to a child. Therefore, 50% of her male children would be affected and 50% will not inherit the mutation. Her female children have a 50% chance of being a carrier and a 50% chance of not inheriting a mutated allele. Males with an X-linked disease will pass the mutation on to all of their daughters and none of their sons. In X-linked conditions, female-to-male transmission is normally noted. In addition, the condition may appear to skip generations, because female carriers typically do not show symptoms of the disease. See Figure 41.2c for a typical X-linked pedigree.

Mitochondrial inheritance: Mitochondria, organelles found in the cytoplasm of a cell, have a 16 569-base pair genome with 13 protein-coding genes, most of which are involved in energy metabolism. Mutations within mitochondrial DNA cause specific genetic conditions, such as mitochondrial encephalomyopathy, lactic acidosis, and stroke-like episodes (MELAS), mitochondrial neurogastrointestinal encephalopathy syndrome (MNGIE), and Pearson syndrome. Mitochondrial genes are maternally inherited through the mitochondria in the cytoplasm of the mother's egg. Sperm have abundant mitochondria (contained in the midpiece), but they are destroyed minutes after fertilization, and thus are not passed on to offspring. A female affected with a mitochondrial disorder will pass the disorder to all her children at variable levels of severity because of heteroplasmy and homoplasmy (see Figure 41.2d). Homoplasmy is when

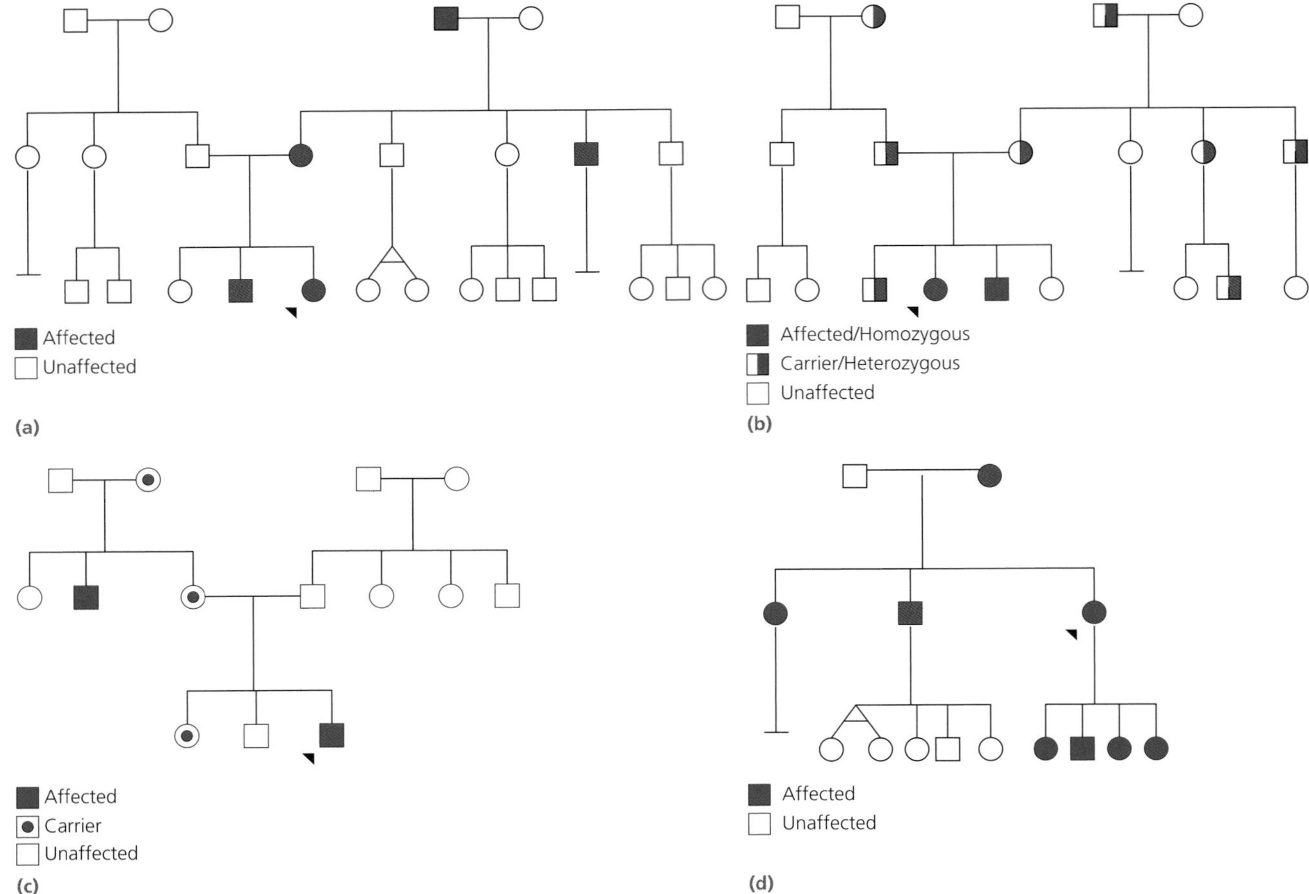

Figure 41.2 Pedigrees showing common patterns of inheritance: **(a)** autosomal dominant, **(b)** autosomal recessive, **(c)** X-linked, and **(d)** mitochondrial. Males are represented by squares and females by circles.

the mitochondria within the eggs are all identical, containing the mutant allele. In homoplasmic cell states, the offspring inherits all mutated alleles. In heteroplasmic cells, there is a mixture of mutated and wild-type alleles. The offspring will show variable expression based on the ratio of mutated versus wild-type alleles that they inherit, which depends on how the cytoplasm of the egg is divided.

Multifactorial inheritance: Although the genetics of the rarer Mendelian diseases are well defined, the genetics of most common diseases are poorly understood; these conditions are probably caused by a combination of gene–gene and gene–environment interactions. Twin studies have been used historically to determine the hereditability of diseases. Many common gastrointestinal conditions, such as Hirschsprung disease, Crohn's disease, and ulcerative colitis, appear to result from a combination of inherited and environmental factors. Even in typical Mendelian disorders, we know that environment can modulate an underlying genetic defect. For example, alcohol and tobacco use in a patient with a *PRSS1* mutation increases the risk for pancreatitis.

Imprinting: Most genes are coexpressed equally from the maternal and paternal alleles. It is a bit more complicated for the sex chromosomes (see earlier discussion on sex-linked disorders in the *Inheritance patterns* section). Every female cell must silence one of the two X chromosomes by methylation of the entire chromosome, to provide dose compensation for genes on the X chromosome. A small number of non-X chromosome genes are expressed from only one allele, as the other allele is silenced by "imprinting," also mediated by methylation of the promoter of the imprinted gene. Imprinting may occur specifically on the paternal or maternal allele. The exact number of imprinted genes is controversial. There are probably a few hundred imprinted genes, although some estimates suggest that there may be a thousand or more [7]. Some diseases are affected by this phenomenon, because a mutation on the nonimprinted gene will act in a dominant fashion, and loss of imprinting will disturb the dose balance of that gene. Diseases caused by perturbations in imprinting include the Beckwith–Wiedemann syndrome, Prader–Willi syndrome, Angelman syndrome, and others.

Genetic mechanisms in disease causation

Many types of genetic change abolish or alter the expression of a protein, or result in a defective protein, thereby causing a genetic disorder. Understanding the basis of the genetic change is crucial in determining the most appropriate test to order. Not every alteration in the DNA sequence causes disease; many alterations are recognized as polymorphisms (benign alterations) or classified as VUS with unknown levels of risk. When a genetic test returns with a VUS, it may be challenging to provide genetic counseling and most often, these results should not be used to guide the clinical management of individuals found to carry them.

Point mutations are single-base-pair changes in the DNA coding sequence. These changes can be silent mutations (making no change in the amino acid sequence of the encoded protein), missense mutations (changing the encoded amino acid to another), and non-sense mutations (which create premature stop codons). Mutations that are silent may be classified as polymorphisms. In some instances, the mutation may not alter the encoded amino acid, but changes a splice site, altering the gene product. In other instances, the change may create a fragile sequence more prone to subsequent mutation. Point mutations are the simplest mutations to detect, and most sequencing approaches can find these.

In/Dels of a small number of nucleotides that are not a multiple of three can result in a frameshift mutation, where the amino acids reading code is shifted downstream of the in/del. In/dels occurring as a multiple of three nucleotides will insert or delete complete codons, altering the composition of the encoded protein. Very small in/dels (several nucleotides) can be detected using standard sequencing techniques; however, larger deletions and duplications require additional testing to be found. One such approach is multiplex ligation-dependent probe amplification, which is a variation on PCR that permits the number of copies of the target DNA to be determined. When there is a large deletion, the DNA sequence appears to be normal, but one copy of the target sequence is being analyzed and the other is missing. Multiplex ligation-dependent probe amplification determines whether the number of copies of that sequence is uniform throughout the DNA under analysis.

Translocations, fusions, and inversions (i.e., rearrangements) can be difficult to detect when there is no deletion of DNA in the rearrangement. A large chromosomal rearrangement requires a karyotype for its detection. One can confirm this by direct sequencing if one identifies the precise "breakpoint" in the gene and sequences through this, demonstrating the inappropriate junction of DNA sequences. Likewise, an inversion of DNA in which all of the genetic material is retained can render the gene nonfunctional, but because DNA sequencing is usually done exon by exon, the rearrangement will not be detected. Again, one must identify the two breakpoints and develop a sequencing strategy for those to demonstrate the rearrangement.

Non-sense-mediated decay refers to a surveillance pathway in the nucleus that eliminates mRNA transcripts that contain premature stop codons. When this pathway is activated, the mutant transcripts are eliminated, sparing the cell the impact of the non-sense mutation. The implication of non-sense-mediated decay is that a diagnostic strategy based on finding an altered mRNA will fail when this pathway is at work.

Pseudogene refers to a DNA sequence that resembles a gene but has been mutated into an inactive form over the course of evolution. It often lacks introns and other essential DNA sequences necessary for function. Although genetically similar to the original functional gene, pseudogenes do not result in functional proteins, although some may have regulatory effects.

Malignant gastrointestinal conditions with genetic testing implications

Inherited colorectal cancer syndromes

Inherited forms of colorectal cancer are estimated to account for approximately 10% of new cases, which involve genes of high and moderate penetrance [8,9]. These syndromes are categorized as polyposis and nonpolyposis syndromes and are identified based on factors such as number and histological features of polyps, molecular features of colorectal tumors, and results of germline testing. Individuals with inherited colorectal cancer syndromes have the highest risk for developing this malignancy. Germline testing is available to identify individuals with these syndromes and determine which family members carry the pathogenic variant. Appropriate colorectal cancer screening and cancer prevention strategies can be personalized for individuals with these syndromes (see Chapter 72).

Lynch syndrome

Lynch syndrome, previously called *hereditary nonpolyposis colorectal cancer syndrome*, is an autosomal dominant cancer predisposition syndrome [10] and the most common cause of inherited colorectal cancer. Individuals with Lynch syndrome also have increased risks for endometrial cancer, cancer of the ureter and renal pelvis, ovarian cancer, stomach cancer, and others [11]. Screening all individuals with colorectal cancer for Lynch syndrome is possible through tumor or germline DNA testing.

Lynch syndrome is caused by a germline pathogenic variant in any of the DNA MMR genes *MLH1*, *MSH2*, *MSH6*, and *PMS2*, or deletions affecting the epithelial cell adhesion molecule (*EPCAM*) gene, which leads to silencing of *MSH2* [10]. Loss of DNA MMR activity results in a hypermutable tumor phenotype called *microsatellite instability* (MSI). Microsatellites are repetitive nucleotide sequences that are highly polymorphic and in microsatellite unstable tumors, the normal (nontumor) DNA has varying alleles than the tumor tissue. About 10–15% of sporadic colon cancers will be microsatellite unstable, and at least 90–95% of patients with Lynch syndrome will have MSI tumors.

In addition, Lynch syndrome-related tumors usually have loss of immunohistochemical (IHC) staining for the associated MMR proteins. When one views pathological tissues microscopically, normal tissue, as well as cancer, is present. The normal tissues will express the four DNA MMR proteins in the nucleus of each cell that is proliferating. Once normal staining is confirmed, one looks for loss of protein expression in the tumor cells. IHC is best done on invasive endometrial or colorectal tumor tissue, although it can also be done on endometrial hyperplasia with complex atypia and large adenomatous polyps. IHC of the cancer tissue will show the absence of expression of specific DNA MMR proteins, revealing which gene has been inactivated.

When MLH1 and PMS2 proteins are both absent, this indicates a defect in the *MLH1* gene. Isolated loss of PMS2 protein indicates a defect in the *PMS2* gene, and MLH1 is stabilized by binding to MLH3 or PMS1. Loss of MLH1 and PMS2 protein expression can also be caused by the nonhereditary, acquired hypermethylation of the *MLH1* gene. This occurs in the context of generalized hypermethylation throughout the tumor DNA, in which *MLH1* is one of many genes silenced by hypermethylation, and the DNA MMR defect occurs secondarily to the primary defect in the control of methylation [5]. This usually occurs in older individuals without a family history of cancer. This confusion can be resolved by quantitative measurement of the methylation of the promoter of *MLH1*. In half or more of these cases, the colon tumor will also have a V600E *BRAF* mutation, which is thought to rarely, if ever, occur in Lynch syndrome.

When MSH2 and MSH6 proteins are both absent, the genetic defect lies in the *MSH2* gene as MSH6 protein binds to MSH2 and requires it for stability. In the case of isolated loss of MSH6 expression, MSH2 protein is stabilized by alternative binding to MSH3; thus, the germline mutation is in the *MSH6* gene. MSH2 can also be inactivated because of a deletion of the stop codon of the next gene upstream of *MSH2*, called *EPCAM*. This results in "read-through" methylation of the *MSH2* gene, which is silenced in any tissue that expresses *EPCAM* (including the colon). Some missense mutations in the MMR genes can abrogate the enzymatic function of the protein, resulting in MSI, but the protein is still expressed, leading to a falsely "normal" IHC result. This can be resolved by performing MSI testing, which will be abnormal. MSI testing is done by extracting DNA from the tumor specimen (easily taken from a paraffin-embedded section on a slide), amplifying five microsatellite sequences by PCR [12], separating these by chromatography, and looking for mutations that alter the length of the PCR products. Alternatively, MSI can be inferred from NGS data by analyzing the percentage of unstable microsatellites as a score from paired tumor-normal genome sequencing data, which allows for comprehensive investigation of MSI sites simultaneously [13]. Such an approach can be more sensitive across various cancers not typically screened for MMR deficiency than the conventional approach using PCR [14].

A cost-effective way to screen for Lynch syndrome in patients with colorectal cancer is through IHC staining for the MMR proteins or MSI testing of the tumor tissue. MSI testing and IHC are each about 90–95% sensitive for defects in the MMR system [5]. Many institutions have adopted universal screening protocols whereby all colorectal cancers are automatically screened with IHC and MSI; in some instances, only tumors that occur before age 70 years are selected for screening [15]. In addition, it is becoming more common to perform IHC or MSI on tumor sites other than the colon (i.e., endometrium, ovary, kidney, breast, etc.). Once the tumor has been determined to have MSI or abnormal IHC, the patient can undergo genetic testing.

Unfortunately, some tumors display abnormal IHC and/or MSI, but the patient with cancer may not have an identifiable pathogenic variant in any of the DNA MMR genes or *MLH1* hypermethylation and are classified as Lynch-like syndrome. Lynch-like syndrome is observed in 2.5–4% of individuals with colorectal cancer [16,17], and many of the MMR-deficient tumors in these individuals have somatic inactivation of MMR genes [18] or are a consequence of inactivating genetic events that have not yet been identified. The incidence of colorectal cancer in patients with Lynch-like syndrome is increased (standard incidence ratio, 2.12; 95% confidence interval, 1.16–3.56) and greater than for families with sporadic colorectal cancer (standard incidence ratio for sporadic CRC, 0.48; 95% confidence interval, 0.27–0.79), although not as high as those with Lynch syndrome (standard incidence ratio, 6.04; 95% confidence interval, 3.58–9.54) [16]. The implications of this recently identified colorectal tumor phenotype on screening and surveillance recommendations are unclear, and colorectal cancer screening may be considered based on family history of colorectal cancer [18]. It is likely that such recommendations will change with time.

Lastly, familial colorectal cancer type X refers to the nearly 50% of individuals suspected of having Lynch syndrome based on family history of colorectal cancer (three affected relatives across two generations), with young-onset colorectal cancer diagnosed before age 50 years, but do not carry pathogenic MMR gene variants and whose colorectal tumors are MMR proficient [19]. The genetic etiology of familial colorectal cancer syndrome X is unknown, and the risk for colorectal cancer in these individuals is twice that of the general population and modest compared with Lynch syndrome with defects in MMR. Therefore, intensive colorectal cancer surveillance recommendations similar to Lynch syndrome are not warranted but are similar to common familial colorectal cancer with colonoscopy every 5 years.

In circumstances where there is no tissue available for MSI or IHC testing, it is reasonable to begin with germline genetic testing [20] in the patient with cancer. Several predictive models are available to estimate the likelihood that an individual will have a pathogenic MMR gene variant [21–23]; PREMM5 and others are freely available online [22,23]. Of the several

Lynch syndrome prediction models, PREMM5 is the one most extensively validated; it includes prediction for all Lynch syndrome MMR genes and is applicable for individuals unaffected by cancer. The models rely on clinical features, such as age, sex, and personal and family history of Lynch-associated malignancies to quantify the likelihood an individual carries a germline pathogenic variant in a related MMR gene. $PREMM_5$ uses a threshold of ≥2.5% to identify individuals suitable for genetic evaluation and testing [23], and the other models generally recommended germline testing when an a priori likelihood exists of 5% or greater.

Because of the increased cancer risks associated with Lynch syndrome, numerous groups have recommended surveillance programs, and there is some variability in what is advised. Frequent colonoscopy is recommended for the prevention or early detection of colorectal cancer and gynecological risk-reducing surgeries for the prevention of endometrial and ovarian cancer. Individuals with Lynch syndrome should undergo intensive screening with frequent colonoscopies at 25 years, or 5 years earlier than the youngest cancer diagnosis in the family, whichever is earlier. Colonoscopy should be repeated every year given the possible accelerated carcinogenesis associated with MMR deficiency. In addition, an esophagogastroduodenoscopy should be performed by age 35 years, treating *Helicobacter pylori* if present. Females are advised to consider prophylactic hysterectomy and oophorectomy at the completion of childbearing and prior to this, should consider annual transvaginal ultrasound and/or endometrial biopsies starting at age 30 years, although these recommendations are debatable. For those who decline surgery, random endometrial biopsy, transvaginal ultrasound, and CA125 may be considered, recognizing these are imperfect, especially for early ovarian cancer detection. Surveillance of other organs, such as small intestine, pancreatic and biliary systems, or brain, is not supported by evidence, although recommendations by expert consensus may vary [15].

Gastrointestinal polyposis syndromes

The gastrointestinal polyposis syndromes are discrete conditions that cause increased colorectal cancer risk [24–27]. The definition and precise characterization of the polyposis conditions have evolved considerably in recent decades. Initial clinical characterizations were made from data in familial registries that demonstrated the inherited and phenotypic details of different polyposis conditions. Pathological characteristics were then integrated to further refine the phenotypes. Finally, identification of relevant causative genes has improved our present understanding of specific polyposis conditions, including phenotypic characteristics and associated cancer risks. The most common feature for when to consider a polyposis diagnosis and germline genetic testing is the finding of 10 or more colonic polyps, polyposis in other parts of the gastrointestinal tract, and polyps in young individuals with a family history of a polyposis diagnosis.

Adenomatous polyposis syndromes

Familial adenomatous polyposis

FAP is an autosomal dominant condition caused by a germline mutation in *APC*. The classic form of FAP causes hundreds to thousands of colon polyps beginning in adolescence. An attenuated version (AFAP), also caused by a mutation in *APC*, typically causes less than 100 polyps. The risk for colorectal cancer in FAP approaches 100% by age 50 years, and the recommended intervention is annual sigmoidoscopies or colonoscopies in adolescence and prophylactic colectomy in young adulthood or when the polyp burden becomes too high [28].

Duodenal polyps occur in up to 90% of patients with FAP, and the risk rate for duodenal cancer is ~6–9% and usually evolves slowly from adenomas. Duodenal polyps can be followed with esophagogastroduodenoscopy on a periodic basis based on the polyp burden. Increased risks also exist for other extracolonic manifestations, such as desmoids, thyroid cancer, congenital hypertrophy of the retinal pigment epithelium, supernumerary teeth, osteomas, and central nervous system tumors, usually medulloblastoma. Children with *APC* mutations have an increased risk for hepatoblastoma up to age 5 years and can be followed with abdominal ultrasonography and α-fetoprotein screening. Genetic testing for FAP can be offered at a young age because of the risks for hepatoblastoma, although some families prefer to wait to test until the child can understand genetic testing at a better level. Families often test for the condition at about 10–12 years, the age when sigmoidoscopies or colonoscopies are first considered to assess polyp burden because it can be variable even among family members with the same causative *APC* gene variant.

Specific mutation locations confer differing risks in FAP. The age of cancer onset can sometimes be estimated based on mutation location; those located at codon 1309 are associated with earlier onset of neoplasia. Mutations in *APC* between codons 1250 and 1464 are associated with a "profuse" polyposis phenotype (i.e., >5000) and those in the first four exons with an "attenuated" phenotype with fewer than 100 adenomatous polyps.

Other non-*APC* gene-related adenomatous polyposis conditions

In recent years, genes other than *APC* have been associated with a colonic adenomatous polyposis phenotype that exhibits both autosomal dominant and recessive patterns of inheritance.

Autosomal dominant adenomatous polyposis conditions

Polymerase proofreading-associated polyposis is associated with pathogenic variants in the *POLE* and *POLD1* genes, which cause an "oligo-polyposis" phenotype in which polyps are often larger but fewer than those in FAP [29]. This disease is rare, where 0.12% to 0.25% of those suspected of having FAP or familial colorectal cancer carry pathogenic variants in one of these two genes. The risk for colorectal cancer is high, although its quantification and mean age of occurrence continue to evolve. In one study, the lifetime risk for colorectal cancer was up to 28% for *POLE* and 82–90% for *POLD1*. With increasing age, the spectrum of associated cancers reported includes endometrial, ovarian, small bowel, and brain cancers [30–32].

The *AXIN2* gene, which regulates β-catenin degradation in the *Wnt* pathway, has been associated with autosomal dominant colonic adenomatous polyposis. The phenotype appears similar to AFAP and may be related to breast and liver cancers.

Autosomal recessive forms of adenomatous polyposis conditions

MAP is an attenuated polyposis condition caused by biallelic germline variants in the BER *MutYH* gene. Carriers typically have a phenotype similar to that of AFAP with 20 and 100 (occasionally more) colonic adenomas and an increased risk for colorectal cancer. MAP is found in 8% to 13% of FAP-like cases, with an estimated mean age of 48 years at time of diagnosis. MAP also confers an increased risk for thyroid and duodenal cancer and other benign extraintestinal findings similar to FAP.

Full gene sequencing of the *MutYH* gene is recommend in individuals with polyposis but without an identified pathogenic *APC* gene variant. Although the majority of Caucasian patients with MAP carry at least one of the two common mutations, p. Tyr179Cys and p.Gly396Asp [33], the prevalence of these variants varies in ethnically and racially diverse populations, and additional pathogenic variants have been reported [34].

Monoallelic pathogenic variants in *MutYH* are commonly detected and do not have much effect on colorectal cancer risk [35] in the absence of family history of colorectal cancer. But even a slight increase in risk might be of consequence because monoallelic variants in *MutYH* are detected in up to 2% of the general population. The risk for colorectal cancer is increased approximately 2-fold in monoallelic *MutYH* carriers with a family history of colorectal cancer [34].

The *NTHL1* gene is associated with an autosomal recessive adenomatous polyposis phenotype and an increased risk for colorectal cancer [36]. Similar to *MutYH*, this gene involves BER and was discovered by whole-exome sequencing in a select cohort of cases with multiple adenomatous polyps occurring at young ages. Carriers of biallelic germline *NTHL1* pathogenic variants have multiple extracolonic malignancies, including breast and endometrial cancers (among others) [37–39], but the cumulative cancer risks are uncertain, as are surveillance guidelines.

Biallelic MMR gene variants express adenomatous polyposis and an elevated colorectal cancer risk at a very young age, often in childhood. This rare condition is called *constitutional mismatch repair deficiency*, where each of the four MMR genes associated with Lynch syndrome can give rise to hematological, central nervous system, small-bowel, ureter, and sarcoma malignancies. In addition, *MSH3*, an MMR gene that does not cause Lynch syndrome, is associated with colonic adenomatous polyposis when both alleles are mutated [40]. The phenotype and cancer risk appear similar to AFAP in both age of occurrence and number of polyps.

Hamartomatous polyposis syndromes

Peutz–Jeghers syndrome

PJS is an autosomal dominant cancer predisposition syndrome caused by a germline mutation in *STK11* (*LBK1*). The condition is characterized by mucocutaneous pigmentation around the mouth, nostrils, and perianal region; hamartomatous polyps in the stomach, small and large intestines, and nasal passages; and increased risks for malignancies in the colon, stomach, pancreas, breast, and ovary. Individuals with PJS often experience bleeding and anemia; they can experience intestinal obstruction or intussusception. Although many children with PJS have hyperpigmented macules in childhood, they may fade in adulthood. Females are at risk for sex cord tumors with annular tubules of the ovaries and adenoma malignum of the cervix; males have increased risks for Sertoli cell tumors of the testes. Patients with PJS need screening for the associated cancer risks. Some individuals would consider prophylactic mastectomies, as well as prophylactic hysterectomies with bilateral salpingo-oophorectomy, after childbearing is complete.

Juvenile polyposis syndrome

Juvenile polyposis syndrome (JPS) is a condition conferring increased risk for hamartomatous polyps in the stomach, small intestine, and colon. The age of the patient is irrelevant; the term *juvenile polyp* refers to the specific histology of the polyp. Polyps develop in early adulthood, and the number ranges greatly between individuals. JPS is suspected when the patient has more than five juvenile polyps in the colon, has multiple juvenile polyps throughout the GI tract, or has juvenile polyps and a positive family history of JPS. Individuals benefit from routine colonoscopy and endoscopy with polypectomy. Both *BMPR1A* and *SMAD4* genes are implicated in JPS; however, they each account for only 20% of patients with JPS, and ~60% of individuals with JPS do not have identifiable germline mutations [41]. Approximately 75% of individuals have an affected parent, suggesting that the de novo rate for this condition is 25%. Some individuals with a *SMAD4* mutation have both JPS and hereditary hemorrhagic telangiectasia. This condition is characterized by arteriovenous malformations, commonly presenting as epistaxis. These lesions occur throughout the body, commonly in the lungs, skin, or mucous membranes. Hereditary hemorrhagic telangiectasia may also be caused by mutations in other genes besides *SMAD4*, including *ENG* and *ACVRL1*.

PTEN hamartoma tumor syndrome

Cowden syndrome is an autosomal dominant genetic disease that predisposes an individual to multiple benign and malignant tumors. The principal gene associated with Cowden syndrome is *PTEN*, although *KILLIN*, *SDHB*, and others also play a role in this disease. Individuals with Cowden syndrome have increased risks for development of cancer of the breast, thyroid, and endometrium. Other risks include kidney cancer and melanoma. Benign growths can include uterine fibroids, lipomas, fibromas, hamartomatous and other polyps, thyroid nodules, and a variety of dermatological lesions, such as trichilemmomas, papillomatous papules, and acral keratoses. Many individuals with Cowden syndrome have a large head circumference, and some have developmental or intellectual delay. A pathognomonic finding is Lhermitte–Duclos disease, a dysplastic cerebellar gangliocytoma.

Other polyposis-related syndromes

Mixed polyposis syndrome is caused by pathogenic variants in the *GREM1* gene, where patients develop oligopolyposis that includes adenomatous, juvenile, and other polyp types [42]. Colorectal cancer risk is high and develops in patients at younger ages. This rare syndrome has been described among Ashkenazi Jews, and the only causal mutation is an ancestral duplication upstream of the *GREM1* gene that was first characterized in Israeli families.

Serrated polyposis syndrome (SPS) is characterized by multiple sessile serrated polyps in the colon with a colorectal cancer risk near 50% by age 63 years [43,44] Fifteen to 25% of cases are due to pathogenic variants of the *RNF43* gene [45] and do not have a clear pattern of inheritance. The estimated prevalence of SPS is less than 0.09% in the general population who have undergone colonoscopy screening programs [46], and surveillance and management of SPS is similar to that of AFAP [47].

Familial gastric cancer

Hereditary diffuse gastric cancer

Hereditary diffuse gastric cancer is a highly penetrant autosomal dominant syndrome that increases the risk for diffuse gastric cancer and lobular breast cancer. Genetic testing can be considered in an individual with diffuse gastric cancer diagnosed at a young age and in individuals with diffuse gastric cancer who have a family history of that and/or lobular breast cancer [48]. This disease has been linked to mutations in the *CDH1* (E-cadherin) gene. Because the penetrance is high for diffuse gastric cancer for individuals with confirmed deleterious germline mutations in *CDH1*, complete gastrectomy is recommended. However, the age at which surgery should occur is unclear and whether it should be pursued in carriers without a gastric cancer phenotype remains controversial [49]. Many physicians make recommendations based on the family history and earliest age of onset, but these clinical factors are not necessarily predictive. Intensive surveillance endoscopy can be attempted, but the sensitivity of this approach is uncertain and thought to be poor for the detection of early disease. In addition, female *CDH1* carriers should begin mammography and breast magnetic resonance imaging (MRI) annually by age 30–35 years and may consider prophylactic mastectomies.

Gastric adenocarcinoma and proximal polyposis

Gastric adenocarcinoma and proximal polyposis (GAPPS) is a rare hereditary gastric polyposis syndrome characterized by proximal gastric polyposis and increased risk for early-onset, intestinal-type adenocarcinoma of the gastric body. It has an autosomal dominant inheritance pattern with incomplete penetrance and has been linked to mutations in the *APC* 1B promoter region. Emerging data have shown that GAPPS is actually a phenotypic variant of FAP, albeit with limited colonic involvement. The lifetime risk for gastric cancer in patients with GAPPS remains undefined. Currently, there are no guidelines on screening, endoscopic surveillance, or timing for prophylactic gastrectomy [50].

Familial intestinal gastric cancer

Familial intestinal gastric cancer is a poorly characterized genetic predisposition for gastric cancer. It is characterized by two or more cases of intestinal-type gastric cancer in first- or second-degree relatives with at least one diagnosed younger than age 50 years, or in families with three or more cases of intestinal-type gastric cancer. There is currently no known pathogenic variant associated with familial intestinal gastric cancer [51].

Inherited pancreatic disorders

Familial pancreatic cancer

Familial pancreatic cancer is a predisposition to cancer in which the majority of cases do not have a known pathogenic variant and in those with known genes, the penetrance is variable and most often low. The best predictor of pancreatic cancer risk relates to the presence of a family history of pancreatic cancer; carriers with a first-degree relative with pancreatic cancer have a 4–6% risk for this disease, as compared with 1–2% for the general population. For those with three close relatives, the likelihood increases to 18–36% [52].

Genes that are typically tested for pancreatic cancer risk include *ATM*, *BRCA1*, *BRCA2*, *CDKN2A*, most Lynch syndrome genes (*MLH1*, *MSH2*, *MSH6*, *EPCAM*), *PALB2*, *STK11*, and *TP53* [53]. Individuals who have hereditary breast and ovarian cancer syndrome, especially those with a germline mutation in *BRCA2*, have increased risk for pancreatic cancer that varies from ~4% to 8%, which is similar to those with pathogenic mutations in *PALB2*, a partner and localizer, that interacts closely with *BRCA2*. Pancreatic and breast cancers are also associated with pathogenic variants in *BRCA1* and *ATM*, where the latter gene is responsible for the neurodegenerative disorder ataxia telangiectasia in biallelic mutation carriers. *ATM* mutation carriage is common, where 1/100 Caucasians are heterozygous carriers with a fourfold to fivefold increased risk for breast cancer. Germline pathogenic variants in the *p16* (*CDKN2A*) gene also confer some increase in risk for pancreatic cancer, as does PJS with a 36% increased risk and Lynch syndrome with a lifetime risk of 3.6% in carriers by age 70 years.

Currently, genetic counseling and germline testing are recommended for all individuals with newly diagnosed exocrine pancreatic cancer [54]. First-degree relatives may be eligible for genetic counseling and germline testing if the individual with pancreatic cancer is unavailable for genetic testing. The goal of testing newly diagnosed patients with pancreatic cancer is for the potential impact on therapeutic decision making based on germline mutation status and for the benefit of cascade testing for the identification of germline mutation carriers among at-risk family members.

Select individuals at high risk for the development of exocrine pancreatic cancer may be considered for pancreatic cancer screening [55]. Currently, individuals who carry the following pathogenic variants and have a family history of pancreatic cancer in first- or second-degree relatives may be eligible: *ATM*, *BRCA1*, *BRCA2*, *CDKN2A*, *MLH1*, *MSH2*, *MSH6*, *EPCAM*, *PALB2*, *STK11*, and *TP53*. In addition, individuals with a high burden of pancreatic cancer in the family may be considered for screening, including those with two or more affected first-degree relatives, one affected first-degree relative and one second-degree relative, or three or more first- and/or second-degree relatives.

Studies continue to evaluate the efficacy of screening with contrast-enhanced MRI/magnetic resonance cholangiopancreatography and/or endoscopic ultrasound in such high-risk individuals, and surveillance recommendations and available modalities will continue to evolve [56].

Multiple endocrine neoplasia type 1

Multiple endocrine neoplasia type 1 (MEN1) is an autosomal dominant disease caused by pathogenic variants in *MEN1*, encoding the protein MENIN [17]. These individuals are at risk for many different types of endocrine neoplasm in the pituitary, parathyroid, foregut, and pancreas. The penetrance is high, and the overall risk for neuroendocrine pancreatic cancer is 40–70%. The most common functional pancreatic tumors are gastrinomas (54%) and insulinomas (15%). Routine surveillance of asymptomatic MEN1 in at-risk individuals by annual biochemical and imaging protocols for early detection is recommended beginning in childhood. Pathogenic variants in the *CDKN1B/p27* gene were recently identified for an MEN1-like condition. *CDKN1B* is a recessive MEN1-like syndrome presenting with variable clinical manifestations typical of both MEN1 and MEN2, such as pheochromocytomas, paragangliomas, thyroid tumors, and parathyroid and pituitary adenomas [57].

Multiple endocrine neoplasia type 2

Multiple endocrine neoplasia type 2 (MEN2) is an autosomal dominant condition associated with increased risks for medullary thyroid cancer (MTC); 25% of individuals with MTC have a germline mutation in the protooncogene *RET*. MEN2 can be subdivided into three clinical entities: MEN2A, MEN2B, and familial medullary thyroid cancer (FMTC), all with lifetime risks for development of MTC that approach 100%. Individuals with MEN2A have increased risks for hyperparathyroidism and pheochromocytomas, whereas the cancer risk in FMTC is limited to MTC. Those with MEN2B have risks for pheochromocytomas, a marfanoid habitus, ganglioneuromatosis, and mucosal neuromas. The specific location of the mutation in the gene determines the extent to which the disease is expressed.

Von Hippel–Lindau syndrome

Von Hippel–Lindau syndrome (VHL) is an autosomal dominant condition that predisposes individuals to the development of cysts, as well as benign and malignant tumors. It is characterized by a pathogenic variant in the *VHL* gene and affects 1/36,000 individuals [58]. Individuals with this condition typically develop symptoms during adolescence, and tumors continue to occur throughout life. Hemangioblastomas commonly occur in the brain and spine, and they can cause pain, ataxia, weakness, and nausea, and when in the retina, affect vision. Cysts may develop in the kidneys, pancreas, and genital tract. The risks for clear cell carcinoma of the kidney and pancreatic neuroendocrine tumors are increased. VHL also increases the risk for pheochromocytomas and endolymphatic sac tumors. VHL mutation carriers are advised to follow surveillance programs, including annual MRI of the abdomen after the age of 15 years, because they are at lifelong risk for development of multiple cysts and tumors [58].

Pheochromocytomas and paragangliomas

Pheochromocytomas and paragangliomas are associated with multiple genes. Four subunits of the mitochondrial enzyme succinate dehydrogenase (SDH) increase risks for pheochromocytomas and paragangliomas: *SDHA*, *SDHB*, *SDHC*, and *SDHD*. *SDHAF2*, another gene that interacts with *SDHA*, can increase risks for pheochromocytomas and paragangliomas when mutated. *TMEM127* and *MAX* are also associated with increased risks for these tumors [59]. These conditions are generally inherited in an autosomal dominant manner; however, *SDHD* and possibly *SDHAF2* and *MAX* exhibit a parent-of-origin affect. With *SDHD* mutations, children of male mutation carriers are much more likely to exhibit the disease phenotype than offspring of female mutation carriers. Phenotype–genotype correlations are apparent for the genes that predispose to these tumors; for example, individuals with germline mutations in *SDHB* are more likely to have malignant transformation, and patients with *SDHD* mutations are more likely to have head and neck paragangliomas than individuals with other mutations or who have sporadic paragangliomas [60,61].

Familial risks for pheochromocytomas and paragangliomas are associated with mutations in *RET* and *VHL*, as well as in *neurofibromin type 1* (*NF1*). In a study of 271 apparently sporadic pheochromocytomas, 66 had mutations in *RET*, *VHL*, *SDHB*, or *SDHD* [62]. Genetic counseling is recommended for any patient with a pheochromocytoma or paraganglioma, regardless of family history.

Nonmalignant gastrointestinal conditions with genetic testing implications

Many gastrointestinal diseases are inherited or have a genetic predisposition involved in disease expression. In clinical practice, gastroenterologists will encounter genetic conditions

Table 41.1 Selected autosomal dominant conditions.

Disease	Gene(s)	Gastrointestinal manifestation(s)
Alagille syndrome	*JAG1, NOTCH2*	Hepatic involvement presenting as cholestasis, jaundice, pruritus, and liver failure
Von Hippel–Lindau syndrome	*VHL*	Pancreatic and kidney cysts, clear cell carcinoma, pheochromocytomas
Hirschsprung disease	*RET, EDN3, ECE-1, EDNRB*	Aganglionic megacolon
Lynch syndrome	*MLH1, MSH2, MSH6, PMS2, EPCAM*	CRC, endometrial cancer, ovarian cancer, small-bowel cancer, biliary tract cancer, renal pelvis and ureter cancer, stomach cancer
Cowden syndrome	*PTEN*	Hamartomatous polyps of the GI tract, CRC
Familial adenomatous polyposis	*APC*	Adenomatous polyposis, CRC, hepatoblastoma, pancreatic cancer, desmoids
Peutz–Jeghers syndrome	*STK11*	Intestinal hamartomatous polyps, CRC and other GI cancers, small-intestinal intussusception, pancreatic cancer
Multiple endocrine neoplasia type 1	*MEN1*	Zollinger–Ellison syndrome, foregut carcinoids
Multiple endocrine neoplasia type 2	*RET*	Pheochromocytoma
Hereditary diffuse gastric cancer	*CDH1*	Diffuse gastric cancer
Hereditary paragangliomas and pheochromocytomas	*SDHA, SDHB, SDHC, SDHD, SDHAF2, TMEM127, MAX*	Paragangliomas and pheochromocytomas, possible GIST
Pancreatitis	*PRSS1*	Chronic and acute pancreatitis
Acute intermittent porphyria	*HMBS*	Neurovisceral attacks, pain, nausea
Erythropoietic protoporphyria	*FECH*	Liver failure (rare)

CRC, colorectal cancer; GI, gastrointestinal; GIST, gastrointestinal stromal tumor.

that may cause congenital malformations, such as Alagille syndrome, or present with particular physical features, such as neurofibromatosis. Other diseases, such as inflammatory bowel disease (IBD), have a complex genetic basis but are usually not linked to a single, clinically actionable pathogenic variant. Some of the common genetically based gastrointestinal disorders are listed in Tables 41.1 and 41.2.

Cystic fibrosis

Cystic fibrosis is an autosomal recessive condition that affects the epithelial lining of the respiratory system, pancreas, male reproductive system, and other organs. Cystic fibrosis is one of the most common autosomal recessive diseases among Caucasians, and 1 in 25 are a carrier of a mutant cystic fibrosis transmembrane conductance (*CFTR*) gene. In other ethnicities, the carrier frequency ranges from 1 in 29 to 1 in 90. Since 2010, all US states include cystic fibrosis in their newborn screening tests.

Pulmonary disease usually dominates the clinical course, but exocrine pancreatic insufficiency is present in 85–90% of patients with cystic fibrosis. The latter causes obstruction of the pancreatic ducts and acinar destruction as a result of inspissated secretion. Cystic fibrosis exhibits wide phenotypic variability; although most individuals have classic pulmonary and pancreatic problems, others have a milder version with retained pancreatic sufficiency.

As more people with cystic fibrosis reach adulthood, they are also at greater risk for development of other diseases, such as colorectal cancer. The risk for colorectal cancer in adults with cystic fibrosis is 5–10 times greater compared with the general population and 25–30 times greater for individuals with cystic fibrosis who receive a lung or solid organ transplant. The Cystic Fibrosis Colorectal Cancer Screening Task Force has published screening recommendations that include initiation of screening at 40 years and subsequently every 5 years. Organ transplant recipients with cystic fibrosis should initiate screening at age 30 years and older and within 2 years of transplantation because of the additional risk for colon cancer associated with immunosuppression [63].

Chronic pancreatitis

Chronic pancreatitis can be inherited in several different ways. Autosomal dominant, gain-of-function mutations in the *PRSS1* gene (a cationic trypsinogen) cause familial pancreatitis, with onset often in childhood. Loss-of-function mutations in *SPINK1* (a secretory trypsin inhibitor) cause an increased risk for pancreatitis by loss of the ability to appropriately inhibit trypsin activity in the pancreas. *SPINK1* mutations are inherited in an autosomal recessive manner.

Table 41.2 Selected autosomal recessive conditions.

Disease	Gene(s)	Gastrointestinal manifestation(s)
Wilson disease	*ATP7B*	Liver disease presenting as recurrent jaundice, acute self-limited hepatitis-like illness, autoimmune-type hepatitis, fulminant hepatic failure, or chronic liver disease
Cystic fibrosis	*CTFR*	Pancreatic insufficiency, meconium ileus in neonates, distal intestinal obstruction syndrome, biliary cirrhosis, rectal prolapse, adenocarcinoma of the ileum
Hereditary hemochromatosis	*HFE TFR2, HJV, HAMP*	Hepatic fibrosis or cirrhosis, inappropriately high iron absorption in gastrointestinal mucosa, liver, and pancreas
α1-Antitrypsin deficiency	*SERPIN1A*	Jaundice, liver cirrhosis, and fibrosis
Ataxia telangiectasia	*ATM*	Carriers have increased pancreatic cancer risks
MutYH-associated polyposis	*MutYH*	Colorectal polyposis, colon cancer
Gilbert syndrome	*UGT1A1* (promoter)	Jaundice, hyperbilirubinemia
Crigler–Najjar syndrome	*UGT1A1* (coding region)	Jaundice, kernicterus, lethargy
Rotor syndrome	*SLCO1B1* and *SLCO1B3*	Hyperbilirubinemia
Dubin–Johnson syndrome	*ABCC2*	Jaundice, weakness, abdominal pain, nausea
Pancreatitis	*SPINK1*	Chronic and acute pancreatitis

Chronis pancreatitis, as well as acute recurrent pancreatitis, may be caused by some mild forms of cystic fibrosis, and some heterozygous carriers of *CFTR* mutations have an increased risk for pancreatitis. The penetrance of these mutations in the heterozygous state is reduced and increases the risk for pancreatitis by twofold to fourfold over the general population. Another pancreatitis-related gene, *CTRC*, which encodes chymotrypsin C, normally functions to prevent premature trypsinogen activation in the pancreas. Mutations in the gene have been shown to reduce chymotrypsin C activity. In addition, pathogenic variants in the *CASR* gene, a calcium-sensing receptor, have been associated with pancreatitis [64,65].

Many patients with pancreatitis have multiple genetic variants or genetic–environmental interactions that are likely contributory; therefore, it is not always possible to find a single gene explanation for the disease. A negative genetic test does not rule out the possibility of a genetic predisposition to pancreatitis. Alternatively, a mutation in the lower penetrant genes (*CASR* and *CTRC*) does not always prove an inherited form of pancreatitis.

Individuals with pathogenic variants in *PRSS1* or other hereditary pancreatitis genes and a clinical phenotype consistent with chronic pancreatitis are at increased risk for pancreatic cancer, and screening can be considered 20 years after onset of pancreatitis or at age 40 years, whichever is earlier [65].

Celiac disease

Celiac disease is an autoimmune disease in which dietary gluten triggers an immune response resulting in a broad range of clinical presentations. The *HLA-DQ2* (*DQA1*0501/DQB1*0201*) haplotype is present in 90% of individuals with celiac disease, but one-third of the general population. Others with celiac disease have the *HLA-DQ8* haplotype (*DQA1*0301/DQB1*0302*), or one of the two genes encoding DQ2. Testing family members at risk for celiac disease for *HLA-DQ2* and *HLA-DQ8* may be helpful because the disease is unlikely to develop in individuals who are negative for both [66]. More than 39 other non-HLA genes have been shown to increase the risk for celiac disease [67]. An increased prevalence of celiac disease has been found in patients with Down syndrome, Turner syndrome, and various autoimmune diseases.

Crohn's disease

Crohn's disease has a strong genetic component. It is most common in Caucasians and Ashkenazi Jewish individuals. Most cases of Crohn's disease are caused by a combination of genetic and environmental factors; however, multiple genes have been implicated in the disease process, including *ATG16L1*, *IL10RA*, *TLR4*, *IL23R*, *IRGM*, and *NOD2* [68], among Caucasians. Other susceptibility genes are being identified in Asian populations. IBD is an excellent example of the complex interactions between genetic and environmental factors in the genesis of disease. At the latest count, 163 loci have been linked to IBD; most, but not all, that link to Crohn's disease are also linked with ulcerative colitis (and vice versa), and many of the implicated genes are involved in the immune response [69].

Liver disorders

HFE hemochromatosis

HFE hemochromatosis (*HFE*-HH) is an autosomal recessive condition that is characterized by excessive iron storage. It is caused by biallelic mutations in the *HFE* gene but can be caused by mutations in other genes as well [70]. This condition exhibits expressive variability, and so the phenotype can differ significantly among individuals with the condition. The diagnosis can be made biochemically or genetically. Biochemically there are elevated transferrin–iron saturation levels and elevated serum ferritin concentrations; however, elevated serum ferritin is not specific for *HFE*-HH. Genetically, two disease-causing mutations in *HFE* are diagnostic; however, the mutation status does not always correlate with the phenotype. Patients are treated with phlebotomy and surveillance for hepatocellular carcinoma.

Mutations in *HFE* are common in Caucasians, and heterozygous mutations occur in one in nine individuals, presumably as an adaptive trait. When two parents are identified with *HFE*-HH, their offspring have a 25% chance of inheriting two mutant alleles and being affected, a 50% chance of inheriting one and being a carrier, and a 25% chance of inheriting neither mutant allele. The parents' adult siblings should be tested for the identified mutations.

Most individuals with *HFE*-HH of European descent have the common mutations, p.Cys282Tyr and p.His63Asp. About 1/200 to 1/400 Caucasians are homozygous for the p.Cys282Tyr variant, which has a more pronounced phenotype than having one copy of each mutation or having two copies of the p.His63Asp mutation. The p.Cys282Tyr allele is especially common in Finland (11.8%) and Ireland (10.2%) and is uncommon in Africa (0.05%).

There are other causes of excess iron storage on a hereditary basis. One is an autosomal recessive condition caused by mutations in *TFR2*. A more severe, rarer form is caused by biallelic mutations in either the *HJV* or *HAMP* genes. Therefore, when a patient clearly has hemochromatosis and no mutations are found in *HFE*, additional genetic testing should be undertaken, especially if the patient is not Caucasian.

Wilson disease

Wilson disease is a rare autosomal recessive disease that results from a defect in copper metabolism. Liver disease, including autoimmune-type hepatitis, fulminant hepatic failure, or chronic liver disease, can result from copper accumulation in the liver. Neuropsychiatric manifestations, hemolytic anemia, and Kayser–Fleischer rings can also result from excess copper storage. The diagnosis can be made by detecting high levels of copper in the liver and urine and low levels of serum ceruloplasmin (and serum copper), although the serum-based tests are not always abnormal. Wilson disease is caused by mutations in the copper transporting ATPase gene, *ATP7B* (also called *WND*). Many of the mutations are missense, and a small number of mutations account for the disease in most affected individuals. H1069Q accounts for 30% of mutations in European-based populations.

Alagille syndrome

Alagille syndrome is an autosomal dominant disorder that involves multiple systems and exhibits marked expressive variability. Many individuals have cholestasis as a result of bile duct paucity. Biliary disease may occur with other birth defects in the heart, pulmonary artery stenosis, butterfly vertebrae, renal defects, or central nervous system defects. There are characteristic facial features with the condition, including a broad prominent forehead, deep-set eyes, and a small pointed chin, as well as embryotoxon in the eye, a ringlike opacity at the edge of the cornea. Mutations in *JAG1* account for about 90% of Alagille syndrome cases; rarely (<1%), a mutation in *NOTCH2* can cause this condition. Many individuals (50–70%) have a de novo form of the disease, whereas 30–50% inherit the mutation from their parents.

Hyperbilirubinemias

Gilbert syndrome is a common physiological variation in the population that is characterized by mild, fluctuating, unconjugated hyperbilirubinemia, caused by a sequence variation in the promoter of the bilirubin uridine diphosphoglucuronate glucuronosyltransferase gene (*BUGT*). The normal *BUGT* promoter contains the sequence $A[TA]_6TAA$, whereas in Gilbert syndrome, the patients have a homozygous sequence variation at this locus, $A[TA]_7TAA$ (designated UGT1A1*28), which reduces expression of the enzyme to 25–40% of normal. The hyperbilirubinemia is modest, and there is usually no jaundice. This condition is typically recognized in adolescence in periods of dehydration, fasting, illness, or physical exertion. Gilbert syndrome is quite common; about 30% of the population of the western hemisphere carry one copy of UGT1A1*28. Consequently, Gilbert syndrome can be detected in 3–7% of the general population.

Crigler–Najjar syndrome is a rare recessive disease caused by mutations in the coding or structural portion of the *BUGT* gene. The disease is arbitrarily classified as type I when the mutations are severely inactivating, there is no BUGT activity in the liver, and affected individuals die in infancy. A milder form of structural gene deficiency, called type II, is compatible with life into adulthood, and the serum bilirubin ranges from 8 to 18 g/dL. There will be a range of disease in compound heterozygotes, depending on the severity of each mutation in *BUGT*.

Dubin–Johnson syndrome is an autosomal recessive disease that is associated with increased levels of conjugated bilirubin, and this is caused by biallelic mutations in the ATP-binding cassette (ABC)-C2 gene known as *MRP2*, which functions as an organic anion transporter. Affected patients may have nonspecific symptoms (such as weakness, abdominal pain, or nausea) but only mild levels of hyperbilirubinemia. The process is generally benign. The liver retains pigment and is black, but it is otherwise histologically normal. This condition is most common among Middle Eastern Jews (1/1300).

Rotor syndrome is a rare autosomal recessive disease, clinically similar to Dubin–Johnson syndrome, except that the liver is not pigmented. The condition is caused by biallelic mutations in the organic anion transporters *OATP1B* and *OATP1B3*. Although this is generally a benign condition with normal liver histology and blood tests, null mutations in these genes alter anion transport and can predispose to unexpected drug toxicity [71].

Porphyrias

The porphyrias can be acquired or inherited conditions caused by a variety of deficiencies of enzymes involved in the synthesis of heme. The accumulation of porphyrins can result in dermatological phototoxicity, or neurological disease [72], and several are essentially caused by abnormal hepatic metabolism of heme. Some porphyrias are caused by null (loss-of-function) mutations that appear to be dominant but may actually be recessive when combined with a partial loss-of-function mutation on the other allele that is silent on its own.

Porphyria cutanea tarda (PCT) is the most common porphyria and is a dermatological disease characterized by blisters and secondary scarring resulting from reduced activity of the *uroporphyrinogen decarboxylase* (*UROD*) gene. In type I PCT, the level of UROD is reduced in the liver because of chronic liver disease (i.e., chronic viral hepatitis, alcoholic liver disease, iron overload, toxic exposure) but not in other tissues; no mutations are found in *UROD*. Type II PCT is a familial disease caused by an autosomal dominant mutation in *UROD* that reduces activity of the enzyme in all tissues to about half of normal. This produces a latent state that can be triggered when the activity of *UROD* is reduced further. Homozygous mutations in *UROD* cause *hepatoerythropoietic porphyria*, a rare but severe form of the disease with blistering often beginning in infancy.

Erythropoietic protoporphyria (EPP) has been presumed to be an autosomal dominant disease of photosensitivity caused by an inactivating mutation in the ferrochelatase (*FECH*) gene. Mutations in the *FECH* gene are typically inherited in an autosomal dominant manner. The levels of FECH enzyme measured in the livers of patients with EPP suggest that one allele is null and the other may be hypomorphic, making this actually an autosomal recessive condition. This situation underscores the complexity of genetic diagnosis and emphasizes that all disorders are not purely dominant or recessive. Liver dysfunction occurs in 20–30% of patients, and 5% may develop liver failure requiring transplantation [73]. Boys who present with EPP without an identifiable mutation in *FECH* may have a gain-of-function mutation in *ALAS2*, which is inherited in an X-linked manner and is associated with liver disease [74].

Acute intermittent porphyria is an autosomal dominant condition resulting from a defect in hydroxymethylbilane (HMB) synthase, coded by the *HMBS* gene. Individuals with acute intermittent porphyria typically have one or a few acute neurovisceral attacks that can be provoked by external stressors, such as medications, psychological stress, infections, hormones, and others. Typically, when an individual with a *HMBS* mutation experiences an acute attack, porphobilinogen will be increased in the urine. Remarkably similar acute neurovisceral attacks can occur in hereditary coproporphyria, variegate porphyria, and 5-ALA dehydratase deficiency porphyria [75]. *Hereditary coproporphyria* is caused by autosomal dominant mutations in COPRO oxidase (*CPOX*). *Variegate porphyria* is found primarily in the white South African population and is caused by autosomal dominant mutations in the PROTO oxidase gene (*PPOX*). *5-ALA dehydratase deficiency porphyria* is a rare, severe, autosomal recessive form of porphyria. Because of codominance of some of the genes involved in the porphyrias, both biochemical studies and genetic studies are required in some instances to determine the correct diagnosis.

Principles of genetic testing and counseling

Genetic testing broadly refers to analysis of DNA, RNA, chromosomes, proteins, or certain metabolites to detect changes related to a genetic disorder. Genetic testing is the standard of care for many gastrointestinal conditions and can identify somatic (noninherited) mutations in specific tissues that may be targets for directed therapies. In colon cancer, genetic testing is commonly performed for *KRAS* and *BRAF* mutations for treatment. Sequencing of tumor DNA can also identify mutation patterns that are characteristic of MMR deficiency or MSI or are suggestive of an underlying germline variant. The ability of NGS to detect pathogenic alterations in tumor samples can subsequently facilitate germline testing of patients.

The inclusion of genetic testing into patient care (notably in oncology) and for risk assessment in healthy populations has been a gradual process. With the advent of NGS technology, there has been a shift from syndrome-specific genetic testing based on phenotypic criteria to multigene panel testing, which allows simultaneous testing of multiple susceptibility genes. In the case of inherited cancer syndromes, these multigene panels have the advantage of detecting germline mutations that would not have been discovered based on the patient's clinical phenotype and family history and increase the yield of identifying germline mutations for syndromes with genetic heterogeneity and overlapping phenotypes. Some panels include gene variants associated with moderate or uncertain risk, with limited or unavailable evidence-based recommendations for management. Such cases require genetic counseling for interpretation of results and individualized recommendations based on personal and family histories [76].

Indications for genetic testing

Genetic testing is useful to confirm a diagnosis of a suspected disorder, or to determine who is at risk for development of disease or at risk for having offspring with a disorder. There are precise screening and treatment recommendations for a wide range of genetic disorders. Genetic test results can significantly alter medical management regimens, such as the recommendation for a total colectomy when the patient has an *APC* mutation, or the recommendation to undergo annual colonoscopies in an individual with Lynch syndrome. Treatment options for oncological care and chemoprevention can also be driven by the results of genetic testing, such as the use of immune checkpoint inhibitor therapy for metastatic solid tumors that display MSI.

Knowledge of a pathogenic germline variant in a family enables geneticists to identify the at-risk individuals, conduct cascade testing, tailor cancer screening strategies for those with the familial variant, and just as importantly, eliminate inappropriate screening and anxiety in those who are not found to be carriers (Table 41.3).

Any patient with a gastrointestinal condition for which a genetic etiology is suspected or known is a candidate for genetic counseling. Although some disorders of the young adolescent and adult population have been linked to genes or genetic loci, most gastrointestinal conditions for which genetic testing is clinically available relate to cancer predisposition. The decision to offer genetic testing can vary based on whether an individual has a personal history of or displays clinical features of the genetic disorder, a personal history of multiple preneoplastic lesions in the case of malignancy (e.g., colorectal polyps), or a family history of disease or cancer but without a personal history of the condition or any associated features.

For the evaluation of gastrointestinal cancers, factors that warrant genetic testing include: (1) early age of GI cancer diagnosis and/or other associated cancers; (2) multiple primary cancers in a single patient; (3) a strong family history of cancer and/or preneoplastic lesions, spanning multiple generations; (4) the existence of other cancers within the kindred consistent with known syndromes and an associated inherited risk for GI malignancy; (5) patients with positive tumor testing (MMR deficiency or abnormal IHC testing); and (6) all patients with a new diagnosis of exocrine pancreatic cancer [77,78].

Genetic risk assessment and genetic counseling

Genetic counseling is the process of communicating information and providing support regarding a genetic disorder (Table 41.4). Given the increasing availability and complexity of genetic testing, healthcare providers need a firm comprehension of the benefits, limitations, and risks of offering specific genetic tests, and they need to recognize the importance of appropriate pretest and posttest counseling. Referral for

Table 41.3 Summary of benefits, risks, and limitations of clinical genetic testing.

Benefits	Risks	Limitations
Better definition of disease risk	Psychological distress	Not all mutations can be detected
Improved and individualized medical screening and management	False sense of security and inappropriate management when results are inaccurately interpreted	Unproven efficacy for some screening protocols
Reduced uncertainty or anxiety; may provide explanation for disease in family	Uncertainty relating to disease penetrance	Results typically indicate probability of disease and not certainty
Aid family in identifying other at-risk individuals; cascade testing	Concerns about discrimination	Uncertain clinical relevance for some mutations (low-penetrance genes, VUS)
Family planning; options for preimplantation genetic testing	Change in family dynamics	Negative results are often uninformative

Table 41.4 Suggested components of genetic counseling.

Family history	Medical history	Patient educational issues
Three-generation pedigree including all individuals' current age or age and cause of death	Demographics	Characteristics of syndrome in question and syndrome management/prevention
Ethnicity of maternal and paternal lineage	Present symptoms	Psychological stability and concerns
Congenital defects, bilaterality of disease, and other pertinent features	Relevant medical history	Possibility of uncertain results/ uninformative results
Diagnosis age of affected relative(s)	Current medications and nontraditional treatments	Concepts of inheritance
Documentation of repeated miscarriages or infertility	Past surgeries and hospitalizations	Risk assessment
Cause of death	Major illnesses and exposures	Financial/insurance information

genetic counseling services provides genetic risk assessment to determine the patient's risk for a genetic disorder. A comprehensive evaluation of the patient's and family's medical history, along with genetic testing results, can outline for healthcare providers how best to incorporate the information into clinical practice. Pretest and posttest counseling should be done in a clear, objective, and nondirective fashion, which allows patients sufficient time to understand information and make informed decisions regarding testing and further evaluation or treatment. If a healthcare provider does not have the necessary knowledge or expertise in genetics to counsel a patient appropriately, referral to a genetic counselor or other genetics specialist should be considered.

Core components of pretest genetic counseling include the evaluation of a patient's risk for a certain genetic disorder based on personal and family histories through pedigree analysis, providing an explanation for the cause of the disorder and relevant inheritance information, discussion of the indications for or against genetic testing based on pretest probability, review of the benefits and limitations of testing, including the performance of genetic testing, and assessment of the patient's personal preferences. In addition, the implications for at-risk family members are also addressed. During pretest counseling, patients should have the option to decline any or all testing.

The primary reasons reported for undergoing genetic testing include a desire to learn about children's risk and to determine whether early detection and screening strategies are needed, as well as to reduce uncertainty. Reasons for declining genetic testing include cost, insurance discrimination concerns, potential adverse emotional effects for oneself or one's family, low anticipated benefit, and lack of time. It is important to be mindful of these factors when offering genetic testing.

Posttest counseling predominantly involves disclosure of genetic testing results. Patients receiving results of susceptibility genetic tests (such as those for cancer susceptibility) or predictive tests (such as those for adult-onset genetic conditions) need counseling on the significance of the results to consider their particular risk status based on their personal and family histories of disease or associated conditions. When a specific diagnosis is made, patient education consists of information about its clinical features, the etiology of the condition, its natural history and prognosis, mode of inheritance, disease risks, recommended preventive measures, screening and treatment options, the availability of research studies, and reproductive options. Patients found to have a pathogenic variant associated with a cancer susceptibility gene are counseled regarding their age-related and lifetime risks of particular types of cancer and the tailored surveillance and management strategies available for risk reduction, as directed by their personal and/or family history. Importantly, in the setting of a high-risk family without a known familial mutation, a patient needs to be counseled that receiving a negative result does not return their risk to baseline general population levels, and the patient can still have an inherited disease.

When disclosing results, it is important to take into consideration feelings of anxiety, cancer worry, and distress. Findings from a study that evaluated psychological distress after disclosure of pathogenic variant status suggested that individuals with Lynch syndrome may experience increased general distress, cancer-specific distress, or cancer worry.

Obtaining a family history and pedigree analysis

Obtaining a family history, typically recorded as a pedigree that demonstrates biological relationships, is an essential component to a genetic risk assessment and most often occurs during pretest counseling. It is pivotal particularly for the unaffected patient because family history may dictate if genetic testing is indicated. A three-generation pedigree illustrates the family structure, documents disease state, and records relevant ages. This tool, when compiled completely and accurately, is an accurate and simple instrument for counseling. Family history is typically collected by a genetic counselor, geneticist, genetics nurse, or other healthcare provider performing genetic counseling. This information is sometimes collected before the clinic visit over the phone or by use of a family history questionnaire; such questionnaires are useful because they allow the patient the opportunity to gather information from family members before the clinic visit.

The pedigree is helpful in identifying single-gene, or Mendelian, disorders because it illustrates inheritance patterns. Inheritance patterns can be determined by examining who has the disease and how the individuals are related to each other (see Figure 41.2). When multiple generations are affected and the pedigree demonstrates male-to-male transmission, the condition is likely being inherited in an autosomal dominant manner. If just one group of siblings is affected, the condition is likely being inherited in an autosomal recessive manner. If only males are affected and the disease does not demonstrate male-to-male transmission, the condition is likely X-linked (or carried on the X chromosome). It is important to keep in mind the concepts of variable expressivity and reduced penetrance, because many conditions will not show an obvious inheritance pattern when some individuals have the genetic mutation but fail to exhibit the phenotype.

The family history can be targeted depending on the indication for genetic counseling. Questions should be asked about specific diagnoses in the family, age at diagnosis, as well as any contributory environmental risk factors, including exposures to alcohol or tobacco. For example, when evaluating a family for pancreatic cancer risk, the patient should be asked about other cancers in the family to determine whether the history suggests hereditary breast and ovarian cancer syndrome (*BRCA* genes), familial atypical mole and melanoma syndrome (*p16*), Peutz–Jeghers syndrome (*STK11*), or others. A history of select benign diseases, such as pancreatitis or endocrine neoplasms, should also be solicited. It is important to ask about physical features that could be clues to a particular condition, such as neurofibromatosis or MEN type 1. Depending on the suspected disorder, a physical examination can be important in determining the likelihood that a specific disorder is present.

In taking a general or targeted family history, several questions should be included, such as questions about birth defects, mental retardation, miscarriages, stillbirths, ancestry, racial background, the presence of any known genetic conditions, and consanguinity. The genetic implications for consanguinity intensify as the degree of relation of the parents increases, most notably in the context of potential autosomal recessive conditions.

A pedigree can also be helpful in predicting risks for common multifactorial diseases and can serve as a risk assessment for likelihood of specific diseases. A positive family history is very helpful in predicting disease risk, but a negative family history can be equally as informative. A negative family history may be present in an autosomal recessive condition because most carriers do not exhibit a phenotype.

Standard nomenclature should be used in collecting a pedigree [79]. The individual who is receiving the genetic counseling is the *consultand*. Oftentimes the consultand is also the proband, the affected individual who brings the family to medical attention. Other times, the consultand is an unaffected individual who is seeking counseling based on the familial risk. The proband or consultand is indicated on the pedigree with an arrow (see Figure 41.2).

The consultand should be centered on the pedigree and should be represented as a circle if female or a square if male. To represent children on the pedigree, a vertical line of descent is drawn from the consultand down to a horizontal sibship line. Individual vertical lines are then drawn from the sibship line to represent each child. If the consultand or the partner is pregnant, the pregnancy is noted by placing a "P" inside the circle or square. If the sex of the fetus is not determined, the most appropriate shape to use is a diamond. The consultand's biological full siblings are connected by use of a horizontal sibship line.

The biological parents are placed above and connected to each other by use of a horizontal relationship line. Another vertical line of descent is drawn from the relationship line to the sibship line. The male parent is oriented to the left, and the female parent is oriented to the right. If the consultand has half siblings, a new relationship line should be made from the mother or father indicating their new partner. Their offspring should be noted directly under that union and not with the consultand's full siblings.

This pattern of indicating parentage and siblings should be continued to the patient's second-degree relatives at a minimum (aunts, uncles, grandparents, nieces, nephews). The pedigree history should extend at least one generation past the diagnosis. For example, if a maternal aunt had hemochromatosis, her children should be included, or if a grandparent died of colon cancer at a young age, great grandparents and great aunts or uncles should be part of the history.

Informed consent

The genetic counselor or clinician should explain the risks, benefits, and limitations of undergoing the test (see Table 41.3). Many clinics, insurance companies, and laboratories require written consent; other times verbal consent is sufficient. Commercial laboratories offer versions of informed consent, although many institutions require use of their own consent form.

Historically, genetic counselors have been trained to be nondirective, allowing the patient to decide how much genetic information they would like to obtain. The benefits of genetic testing should include obtaining an understanding of the cause of disease, the implications for medical management, the possibility of testing in unaffected family members for preventative care, and the utility of this information for reproductive planning. Specimens to be obtained, turnaround time, and cost should be discussed with the patient.

A plan should be developed for the manner in which the individual will receive test results. Some clinics require the patient to return for follow-up counseling regardless of the results. Many base their result disclosure policies on patient preference. Several organizations have guidelines for informed consent when offering genetic testing [80].

The Genetic Information and Nondiscrimination Act (GINA) is a US federal law passed in 2008 and instituted in 2009 to protect unaffected individuals from health insurance and employment discrimination as a result of a genetic mutation or a family history of disease. Unfortunately, the law has some limitations. The law specifies that it is only for unaffected individuals and excludes several populations, including US military, American Indians, and individuals who receive their care through the Department of Veterans Affairs and the Federal Employees Health Benefits Plan. Furthermore, this law does not apply to long-term disability insurance or life insurance. With these limitations, some individuals are reluctant to undergo genetic testing, or they choose to do so without filing through their health insurance.

Implications of genetic evaluation and testing

Cascade testing

Cascade testing refers to predictive testing for at-risk relatives of an index cancer case (proband) in whom a pathogenic germline variant is detected. Review of the pedigree allows the counselor to identify at-risk relatives for whom testing is appropriate. It is the clinician's obligation to warn their patient about the ramifications for their relatives and to document this conversation appropriately. It is ultimately the patient's responsibility, and not the healthcare provider's, to communicate this information to family members, and a genetic counseling program can assist with genetic counseling and testing for at-risk relatives.

When there is a known pathogenic variant, individuals can be offered "site-specific" predictive testing for that specific mutation, instead of sequencing the entire gene; this approach is extremely sensitive, specific, and cost-effective. A positive test result in a presymptomatic family member indicates that the person being tested carries the mutation, has the condition, and provides an estimated risk for development of the manifestations of the disorder. Some genetic conditions show reduced penetrance, and the unaffected carrier may develop the disease later in life or not at all. The patient must be educated about the likelihood of experiencing certain disease features and understand appropriate medical management strategies to prevent or treat the consequences of that condition. A negative site-specific test result means that the individual does not have the known familial mutation or the condition, and medical management is altered to conform to that of the general population or that pertaining to any other relevant family history [81].

Psychosocial issues

Sensitivity to psychosocial issues is important during multiple phases of the genetic risk assessment process. During the assessment of family history, individuals may relive feelings of grief when discussing relatives who have died, or become anxious and fearful when listing their family members who have suffered from the familial condition. There may be incorrect beliefs within the family about the severity of the disease, the cause of the condition, and the inheritance pattern. Issues of guilt are also present in the individual who has the disease and has transmitted it to offspring. The discovery of a familial cancer susceptibility gene variant can have a negative psychological effect on patients, especially those with limited support systems and coping mechanisms [82]. A patient from a high-risk family who receives results indicating that she does not carry a cancer susceptibility mutation may experience "survivor guilt." Providing a patient with additional resources for information and support may help alleviate anxiety by providing examples of how the result can be managed successfully.

In addition, unexpected cases of nonpaternity may be revealed. When the patient misattributes his or her father and tries to assemble a pedigree, the interpretation of disease risk may be incorrect. It has been estimated that as many as 5–10% of individuals may not have the actual biological father on their pedigree, many because of nonpaternity. It is less common to have misattribution of maternity, but it can happen as a result of the actual truth having been kept from the individual.

Family planning

Historically, prenatal testing has been offered to couples at risk for having a child with a condition that is particularly difficult to treat, if not actually untreatable. As our genetic testing capabilities have improved and patient interest has grown, families are opting for prenatal testing opportunities for a myriad of diseases. Carrier screening is performed for autosomal recessive and sex-linked disorders to discover whether an individual is a heterozygous carrier of a gene mutation. Carrier testing may be appropriate for unaffected individuals with a relative who has an autosomal recessive or sex-linked condition. In certain ethnic groups, carrier screening is commonly offered universally based on the increased prevalence of the disease in that population, particularly if marriage within that group is planned or has occurred, such as sickle cell anemia in populations of African descent, Tay–Sachs screening in Ashkenazi Jewish individuals, and cystic fibrosis screening in Caucasians. Larger screening panels have emerged that test couples for a group of conditions that could affect the fetus, regardless of the family history or ethnic background. These tests can help identify couples who are at risk for having a child with an autosomal recessive condition; however, they cannot guarantee a healthy child. Individuals who screen negative still have a residual risk to have a child with an autosomal recessive condition; that is, the possibility exists of having a child with a de novo mutation, chromosomal aneuploidy, or other birth defect.

Chorionic villus sampling and amniocentesis are invasive procedures that can be conducted during the first and second trimester, respectively, for prenatal diagnosis. Theoretically, if a familial mutation is known for any inherited condition, the at-risk fetus could be tested for it with either procedure. These procedures are also commonly used for aneuploidy screening. Chorionic villus sampling or amniocentesis is intended to determine whether the fetus carries the mutation(s) of interest. The proband should have a plan to use the information before having the test, because the implication would be that either the pregnancy would be terminated or some important intervention take place before the birth of the child with the mutation. Some couples solely desire this information for peace of mind and have no actionable plan.

Preimplantation genetic diagnosis (PGD) offers a couple another way to have a child without the known familial condition. If the familial mutation is known, the couple can undergo in vitro fertilization and have a small number of cells removed from the embryo to test for the familial mutation. Embryos without the familial mutation can be implanted.

As a younger generation of healthy at-risk mutation-bearing "previvors" are identified, strategies for counseling this patient population are needed. Some couples opt to do nothing until their child is born, or even grown into adulthood. Others want to consider prenatal testing or PGD. For those who strongly desire a child without the condition, but feel that PGD or prenatal diagnosis compromises their ethical and moral values, they can also consider adoption, sperm donation, or egg donation. While the ethical dilemmas a couple may face are numerous, each state has its own laws surrounding pregnancy termination, with most allowing termination up until the end of the second trimester.

Genetic testing in children

In most jurisdictions, a child is unable to legally provide consent, and therefore lose autonomy in the genetic testing process. The American Academy of Pediatrics and American College of

Medical Genetics issued a joint statement in 2013 suggesting that pediatric diagnostic genetic testing should be considered like any other medical condition, and that consent from the parents or guardians should be obtained. If possible, consent from the child is also desired. Predictive genetic testing is generally discouraged unless the genetic information can help provide medical management and prevention options at the patient's current age. If a parent was diagnosed with pancreatitis, it would be very beneficial for the child to undergo predictive testing as the age of onset is often in childhood. Conversely, testing for Lynch syndrome is generally discouraged in children because the age to begin screening is ~25 years. The American Academy of Pediatrics and American College of Medical Genetics did not endorse carrier screening in children in this instance [83].

Desire not to know

Patients are entitled to make the conscious decision not to know their medical risks based on genetic data. Autonomy is one of the founding principles of genetic counseling, allowing patients to decide what genetic information, if any, they desire to have. In cases where knowing genetic information is helpful for providing medical care, it may become an obstacle for clinicians and their patients to agree not to undergo genetic testing.

Certain diagnostic procedures or tests may disclose genetic information to the patient without specifically obtaining pretest permission. For example, when a patient has a colon cancer resected and immunohistochemistry or MSI testing is performed automatically, the suspected diagnosis of Lynch syndrome may be raised. Although the diagnostic result is not definitive, it raises the possibility of that disease. Certain pathological findings may be pathognomonic of a genetic disease, raising the question of whether there is a legal obligation to inform the patient of the risk. For example, Lhermitte–Duclos disease, a cerebellar dysplastic gangliocytoma, is highly suggestive of Cowden syndrome. The clinician will be in the challenging position of determining whether the patient wants to know more; generally, it is their responsibility to fully inform the patient of risks implied by any finding.

Genomics medicine and challenges

Limitations in the interpretation of genetic testing results

Although genetic testing is a powerful tool to guide the clinical care of the at-risk or affected individual, attention should be given to its current limitations. A negative or indeterminate result in an individual without prior identification of the specific mutation in that family does not indicate the absence of a deleterious mutation for a suspected syndrome or the lack of a genetic etiology. Such misinterpretations are potentially fatal when medical management, particularly surveillance, ceases for an at-risk individual. If a mutation cannot be found in the index case, then all family members should be treated as potentially having the disease. If there are multiple individuals with a history of the same disease, it can be helpful to consider more than one individual as the index case and offer genetic testing to other family members. In some families, there are "phenocopies," where an individual has the at-risk disease (particularly when the disease is common), but it is not due to the family's mutation. This often occurs in a family with Lynch syndrome where one relative without the familial mutation develops a sporadic colon cancer.

Other limitations, particularly as they relate to the increased use of multigene panel testing, include the detection of unexpected high-penetrance cancer susceptibility gene mutations in a patient without a phenotype suggestive of their underlying mutation, detection of variants of moderate penetrance for which the optimal management has not been clearly elucidated, and VUS. Detection of VUS is recognized as a sequence variation, but there is not enough information to know whether this is a simple polymorphism (i.e., a SNP) or a disease-causing pathogenic variant. Detection rates of VUS by clinical laboratories performing germline testing have been reported at nearly 40% and highest among African Americans [84]. A VUS result alone should not be used to guide clinical management of a patient and should not be interpreted as a pathogenic variant. The frequency in detecting VUS will diminish over time as more individuals with disease states are analyzed and sequence variations associated with disease risk become more evident. Until a VUS becomes reclassified, one may attempt to link the VUS in question to additional clinical information (such as a VUS in a DNA MMR gene with the abnormalities found at immunohistochemistry), but caution is needed. Limited knowledge about the risk for cancer associated with VUS is an important challenge, and individuals with these alterations benefit from genetic counseling for interpretation of results and individualized recommendations.

Total genomic sequencing

The cost of sequencing a genome has decreased dramatically. Increasingly, the major factor limiting widespread routine genome sequencing is the ability to accurately interpret the large amount of information, rather than the cost. It will take some time to translate raw DNA sequences into actionable clinical information, because everyone carries a large number of what would historically have been considered disease-causing mutations. A large number of genomes must be correlated with health outcomes to understand how gene–gene interactions and gene–environment interactions result in various states of health and disease. It will take time to develop bioinformatics-driven algorithms that can meaningfully convert an individual's genetic code into a form useful for guiding health maintenance and medical care.

Direct-to-consumer genetic testing

An increasing number of commercial entities are marketing genetic testing directly to consumers. In most instances, this is done without prior counseling. In some, testing is focused on a few SNPs that might provide insight into ethnic background. Others assess commonly identified "founder mutations" for certain genetic diseases. Physicians can expect that some of these individuals will seek explanations of this testing, and each of these panels will present its own challenge. There is concern that these direct-to-consumer tests have not undergone review by the FDA to ensure results are accurate and clinically meaningful. Although numerous associations between common genetic variants and diseases have been established, the quality of the science behind these tests has been questioned. It is likely that exome-wide or genome-wide analyses will soon be available to healthy individuals, who may then seek interpretation from the physician or genetic counselors, or ask the consultant to determine whether the patient carries a disease risk mutation. It will require the development of new software tools to use this information because of the scale of the databases. It is difficult to predict how consumers will use comprehensive sequence data.

Acknowledgments

The authors acknowledge the previous authors of this chapter, Laura E. Panos and C. Richard Boland, on whose work this chapter was based.

References are available at www.yamadagastro.com/textbook7e

Further reading

American Society of Human Genetics. https://www.ashg.org/discover-genetics/genetics-basics/. Accessed January 2020. This website provides links useful for genetic counselors and counseling.

Gene Testing Registry. http://www.ncbi.nlm.nih.gov/sites/GeneTests/. Accessed January 2020. This is a useful website initially supported by the NIH as "Genetests," which provides a central location for voluntary submission of genetic test information by providers. The scope includes the test's purpose, methodology, validity, evidence of the test's usefulness, and laboratory contacts and credentials. The overarching goal of the GTR is to advance the public health and research into the genetic basis of health and disease.

Genetics Home Reference. http://ghr.nlm.nih.gov/. Accessed January 2020. This site provides links for assistance in understanding general and specific genetic conditions.

National Cancer Institute. Publications, PDQ (Physician Data Query) series. https://www.cancer.gov/publications/pdq/information-summaries/genetics. Accessed January 2020. PDQ is the NCI's comprehensive source of cancer information. It contains evidence-based cancer information summaries on a wide range of cancer topics, including genetics, screening, prevention, adult and pediatric cancer treatment, supportive and palliative care, and integrative, alternative, and complementary therapies.

National Center for Advancing Translational Sciences/Office of Rare Diseases Research. http://rarediseases.info.nih.gov/resources/3/genetics-resources. Accessed January 2020. Genetics resources of a collection of links that provide information on genes, genomics, and family history tools.

National Human Genome Research Institute. http://www.genome.gov. Accessed January 2020. This is a website that will provide assistance when there is a question about whether a specific disorder has a genetic basis, and it provides links to clinical research sites.

Pyeritz R.E., Korf B.R., Grody W.W. (eds). Emery and Rimoin's Principles and Practice of Medical Genetics, 7th edn. Philadelphia: Churchill Livingstone/Elsevier; 2019. This is a compendium of clinical descriptions of genetic diseases, with reviews of the genetic bases of the diseases.

Valle D., Antonarakis S., Ballabio A., et al. (eds). The Online Metabolic and Molecular Bases of Inherited Disease, 8th edn. www.OMMBID.com. Accessed January 2020. This is a comprehensive online version of a very complete reference for all inherited diseases.

Vogelstein B., Papadopoulos N., Velculescu V.E., et al. Cancer genome landscapes. Science 2013;339:1546. This is an authoritative review of the somatic genetics of cancer and details the roles of driver mutations in tumor tissues.

PART 3

Gastrointestinal diseases

CHAPTER 42

Motility disorders of the esophagus

John E. Pandolfino[1], David A. Katzka[2], and Peter J. Kahrilas[1]
[1] Department of Medicine, Feinberg School of Medicine, Northwestern University, Chicago, IL, USA
[2] Department of Gastroenterology and Hepatology, Mayo Clinic, Rochester, MN, USA

Chapter menu

Esophageal motility disorders can be categorized based on anatomical localization, neurological control, and muscle type involved. The oropharynx and proximal esophagus are composed of striated muscle and are under central nervous system control. In contrast, the distal esophagus is predominantly composed of smooth muscle and is controlled by the enteric nervous system and vagus nerve via peripheral and central nervous system integration. Recognizing these morphological and functional differences, this chapter on motility disorders of the esophagus will first consider oropharyngeal dysphagia, which includes most physiological aberrations of the upper esophageal sphincter (UES) and proximal esophagus, and then focus on purely esophageal motor disorders that include considerations mainly relevant to the distal esophagus.

Oropharyngeal swallowing disorders

Oropharyngeal dysphagia is associated with high morbidity, mortality, and cost. Estimates of the prevalence rate of dysphagia among individuals older than 50 years range from 16% to 22% [1,2]. Within healthcare institutions, it is estimated that up to 13% of hospitalized patients [3] and 60% of nursing home residents [4] have feeding problems, of which most are attributed to oropharyngeal dysfunction as opposed to esophageal dysfunction. The consequences of oropharyngeal dysphagia are severe: dehydration, malnutrition, aspiration, choking, pneumonia, and death. In fact, mortality of nursing residents with dysphagia and aspiration can be as high as 45% over 1 year [5].

Mechanics of oropharyngeal swallowing

Oropharyngeal swallowing begins with an oral phase that is then followed by a pharyngeal phase. The oral phase of swallowing is largely voluntary and highly variable depending on taste, environment, hunger, motivation, among others. Disorders of the oral phase of swallowing occur with many conditions characterized by global neurological dysfunction, such as head trauma, cerebral tumors, or chorea. Detailed discussion of these conditions can be found in texts on swallow evaluation and therapy [6,7]. The pharyngeal phase of swallowing is the complex integrated oropharyngeal contractile event. Although understood physiologically as the patterned sequential activation of motor neurons and their corresponding motor units, swallowing is clinically evaluated in mechanical terms; specifically, evaluation assesses the effect of this motor activity on the reconfiguration of the oropharyngeal cavity as it transitions from a respiratory to an alimentary conduit. The anatomic complexity of the oropharynx is best evaluated by videofluoroscopic analysis (Figure 42.1).

The pharyngeal swallow consists of several closely coordinated actions: (1) nasopharyngeal closure by elevation and

Yamada's Textbook of Gastroenterology, Seventh Edition. Edited by Timothy C. Wang, Michael Camilleri, Benjamin Lebwohl, Anna S. Lok, William J. Sandborn, Kenneth K. Wang, and Gary D. Wu.

Companion website: www.yamadagastro.com/textbook7e

retraction of the soft palate, (2) UES opening, (3) laryngeal closure, (4) tongue loading (ramping), (5) tongue pulsion, and (6) pharyngeal clearance. Coordination of these actions is imperative, with the most fundamental being the transformation of the oropharynx from a respiratory to a swallow pathway. As shown in Figure 42.1, these events occur in close synchrony as the larynx exhibits substantial axial mobility and the UES is obligated to move in unison with it because the cricopharyngeus attaches to the lateral aspects of the cricoid cartilage. The mechanical determinants of UES opening are laryngeal elevation and anterior traction on the hyoid [8,9]. The mechanical determinants of laryngeal vestibule closure, which is almost exactly synchronized with UES opening, are laryngeal elevation and anterior tilting of the arytenoid cartilages against the base of the epiglottis [6].

The main determinants of bolus transport out of the oropharynx are the action of the tongue and of the pharyngeal constrictors. In the case of the pharyngeal constrictors, the pharyngeal contraction has similar propagation and vigor regardless of bolus volume [10]. However, this is more involved with the process of clearance than the process of bolus propulsion; it strips the last residue from the pharyngeal walls. Tongue motion, in contrast, varies substantially with bolus volume, suggesting that it has a cardinal role in determining differences in bolus propulsion with different swallow volumes [11].

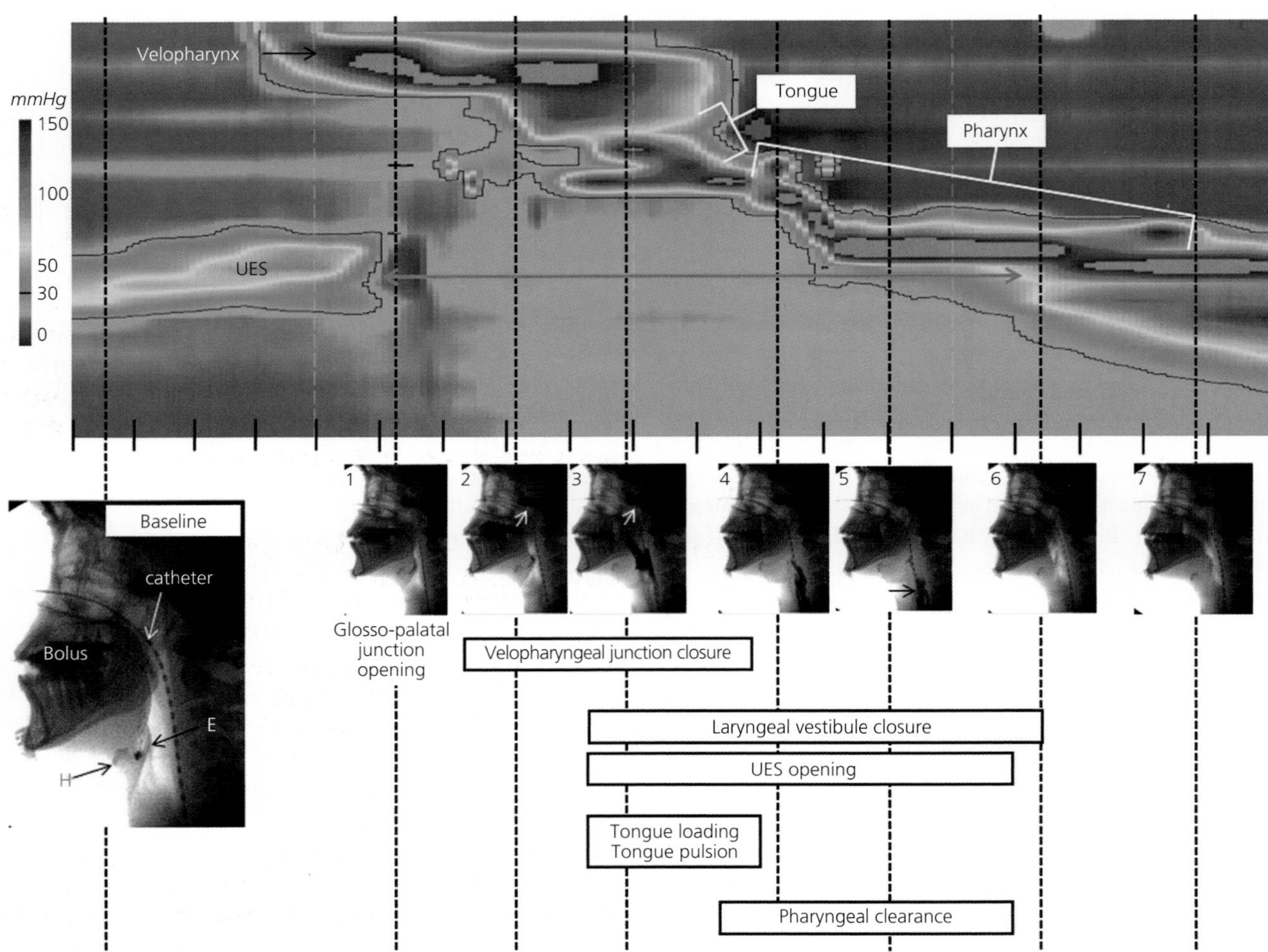

Figure 42.1 High-resolution pharyngoesophageal manometry with combined fluoroscopy. The fluoroscopic images (bottom) are depicted at specific time intervals demarcated on the high-resolution manometry (top). The timeline illustrates the coordination and timing of events within the swallow on fluoroscopy. Each horizontal bar depicts the time period during which the fluoroscopic image is obtained and marks the various stages of the oropharyngeal swallow: 0, baseline anatomy with bolus in the mouth; 1, glossopalatal opening occurring in synchrony with upper esophageal sphincter (UES) relaxation during swallowing, which is typically to less than 10 mmHg; 2, velopharyngeal junction closure sealing off the nasopharynx to prevent regurgitation (note the elevation depicted by the white arrow); 3, laryngeal vestibule closure and UES opening occurring as the epiglottis inverts closing the laryngeal vestibule as the bolus, led by air, is rapidly pushed through the UES; 4, continued bolus transit with onset of the pharyngeal stripping; 5, bolus transfer to the esophagus completed as the pharyngeal stripping traverses the UES and repositions itself to its baseline axial location; 6 and 7, return of the pharynx to the an airway configuration with the laryngeal vestibule opened and the epiglottis back in its upright configuration. The pink arrow depicts the time period of UES relaxation. E, epiglottis; H, hyoid. Source: Courtesy of the Esophageal Center at Northwestern University, Chicago, IL, USA.

UES closure coincides with the arrival of the propagated pharyngeal contraction as evidenced by the fixed time relationship between these events [9]. However, the contractile activity of the sphincter has an added dimension as well, exhibiting increased electromyographic activity during laryngeal descent [12]. The magnitude of this deglutitive UES contraction is further augmented by sphincteric or proximal esophageal distension. The net result is a grabbing effect in which reflexive contraction of the sphincter and laryngeal (UES) descent complement each other to clear residue from the hypopharynx [13]. This clearing function probably acts to minimize the risk for postswallow aspiration by preventing residual material from adhering to the laryngeal inlet when respiration resumes.

Evaluation and classification of oropharyngeal dysphagia

The evaluation of patients with presumed oropharyngeal dysphagia should focus on five fundamental questions:

1. Does the patient describe dysphagia as opposed to globus sensation?
2. Is dysphagia oropharyngeal or esophageal in origin?
3. Is the dysphagia secondary to a structural or functional disorder?
4. Is there an underlying related or causative disorder?
5. Should therapy be directed toward the underlying causative factor or the dysphagia itself?

These questions can usually be answered with a careful history and physical examination. Major objectives of the history are to differentiate oropharyngeal dysphagia from esophageal dysphagia, or globus sensation. Whereas patients almost invariably recognize accurately the locus and consequence of oropharyngeal dysphagia, they mistakenly identify the neck as the locus of bolus hang-up with esophageal dysphagia about 30% of the time. Therefore, elicitation of symptoms such as aspiration, coughing, nasopharyngeal regurgitation, or drooling is of great value in distinguishing oropharyngeal dysphagia from proximally referred esophageal dysphagia.

Distinguishing oropharyngeal dysphagia from globus sensation can be particularly vexing. Globus is defined as a persistent or intermittent, painless sensation of a lump or foreign body in the throat [14]. Unlike dysphagia, which occurs only during swallowing, globus sensation is prominent between meals and swallows. Globus sensation can be associated with anatomic abnormalities, gastroesophageal reflux disease (GERD), or dysmotility [15]. A manometric study suggested that globus patients exhibited a hyperdynamic UES pressure augmentation, independent of the motility findings in the distal esophagus (Figure 42.2) [16]. Another study reported lower thresholds for perception of both electrical and balloon distention in globus patients compared with control subjects [17]. Nonetheless, the clinical history remains the cornerstone for diagnosis.

Physical examination may help to identify features of an underlying systemic or metabolic cause for oropharyngeal dysphagia or localize the anatomic level and severity of a neurological lesion. Examination of the oral cavity, head, and neck for masses, lymph nodes, goiter, and evidence of previous surgery or radiation therapy will help define structural abnormalities associated with dysphagia. Neurological examination may

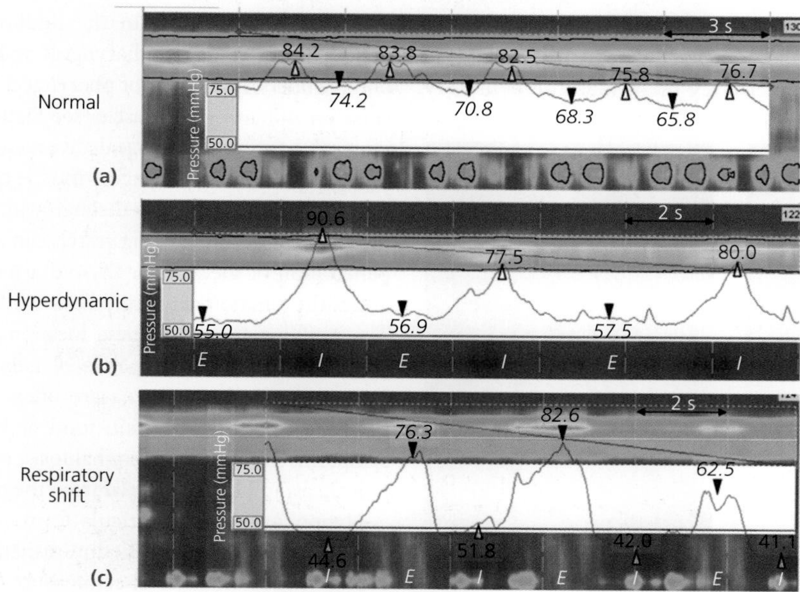

Figure 42.2 Patterns of upper esophageal sphincter (UES) contraction during breathing. (a) The normal pattern is associated with augmentation during inspiration (I) with increases typically less than 27 mmHg. (b) The hyperdynamic pattern suggests a more vigorous change in the inspiratory augmentation during inspiration. (c) A rarer pattern is associated with a shift wherein augmentation occurs during expiration (E). Source: Based on Kwiatek et al. 2009 [16].

indicate cranial nerve dysfunction, neuromuscular disease, cerebellar dysfunction, or an underlying movement disorder. Notably, contrary to popular belief, the gag reflex is not predictive of pharyngeal swallowing efficiency or aspiration risk. The gag reflex is absent in 20–40% of normal adults [18]. Finally, simply observing the patient swallowing water and a solid, such as bread or a marshmallow, can be extremely helpful in determining the most appropriate next step in the evaluation.

If the causative factor of oropharyngeal dysphagia is not readily apparent after initial evaluation, further diagnostic studies are indicated. Because the management implications are so different, *the first task in the evaluation of suspected oropharyngeal dysphagia is to distinguish between structural and functional causative factors*. Structural abnormalities resulting from trauma, surgery, tumors, caustic injury, congenital anomalies, or acquired deformities are identified by endoscopic and/or radiographic examination. Endoscopy may be performed either transorally or transnasally to identify tumors, webs, or hypopharyngeal diverticula. Barium studies may define areas of obstruction and hypopharyngeal diverticula, but they add little structural information to endoscopic examinations (Figure 42.3).

After structural defects have been excluded, videofluoroscopy is used for a functional evaluation of swallowing. Frequently referred to as a modified barium swallow, Logemann [6] has described a protocol composed of a series of swallow tasks. Images are obtained in a lateral projection, framed to include the oropharynx, palate, proximal esophagus, and proximal airway (see Figure 42.1). These images are then evaluated with respect to four major categories of oropharyngeal dysfunction: (1) inability or excessive delay in initiation of pharyngeal swallowing, (2) aspiration, (3) nasopharyngeal regurgitation, and (4) residue of the ingested material within the pharyngeal cavity after swallowing. Furthermore, the procedure allows for evaluation of the efficacy of various compensatory dietary modifications, postures, and swallowing maneuvers in compensating for observed swallowing dysfunction.

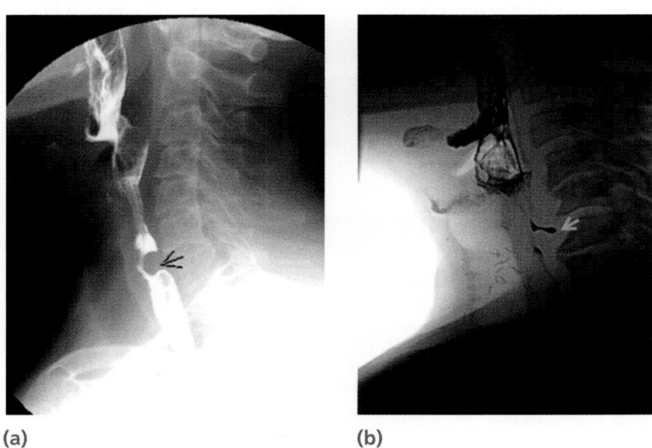

Figure 42.3 Radiographs of obstructive pathology causing oropharyngeal dysphagia. **(a)** Cricopharyngeal bar. **(b)** Zenker's diverticulum. Note the prominent cervical osteophytes below Zenker's diverticulum. Source: Courtesy of the Esophageal center at Northwestern University, Chicago, IL, USA.

Intraluminal manometry can quantify the strength of pharyngeal contraction, the completeness of UES relaxation, and the relative timing of these events. When coupled with concurrent videofluoroscopy, it may provide useful complementary information regarding UES dysfunction. High intrabolus pressures may distinguish impaired UES opening from impaired UES relaxation as a cause of oropharyngeal dysphagia (Figure 42.4).

Structural etiologies of oropharyngeal dysphagia

Implicit in the mechanical description of swallowing summarized earlier is that normal swallowing is associated with minimal outflow resistance from the oropharynx. Identification of obstructing lesions that cause dysphagia will lead to specific management in most cases (see Figure 42.3). For example, cervical webs, pharyngeal or cricopharyngeal strictures, or tumors are indications for surgery, dilation, antineoplastic therapy, or some combination thereof. In the setting of benign strictures or postcricoid webs, simple dilation is safe and effective. Prominent cervical osteophytes also can cause obstructive dysphagia. Because the posterior wall of the pharynx is so closely opposed to the anterior aspect of the cervical vertebrae, cervical osteophytes cause an anterior bulging into the hypopharynx that can impede passage of a normal-size bolus. The most common structural abnormalities of the hypopharynx associated with dysphagia are hypopharyngeal diverticula and cricopharyngeal bars.

Hypopharyngeal diverticula and cricopharyngeal bars

Acquired hypopharyngeal diverticula occur most commonly in men after the age of 60 years. The most common type, Zenker's diverticulum, originates in the midline posteriorly at Killian's dehiscence, a point of pharyngeal wall weakness between the oblique fibers of the inferior pharyngeal constrictor and the transverse cricopharyngeus muscle (see Figure 42.3) [19]. Other locations of acquired pharyngeal diverticula include the lateral slit separating the cricopharyngeus muscle from the fibers of the proximal end of the esophagus through which the recurrent laryngeal nerve and its accompanying vessels run to supply the larynx, at the penetration of the inferior thyroid artery into the hypopharynx, and at the junction of the middle and inferior constrictor muscles. The unifying theme of these locations is that they are sites of potential weakness of the muscular lining of the hypopharynx. Hypopharyngeal diverticula are often asymptomatic until they enlarge sufficiently to retain food or liquid. In most instances, symptoms are of dysphagia, halitosis, postswallow regurgitation, or even aspiration of material from the pharyngeal pouch.

Hypopharyngeal diverticula form as a result of a restrictive myopathy associated with diminished compliance of the cricopharyngeus muscle. Specimens of cricopharyngeus muscle strips from 14 patients with hypopharyngeal diverticula obtained at the time of surgery demonstrated structural changes that would decrease UES compliance and opening [20]. The cricopharyngeus samples from these patients had fibroadipose

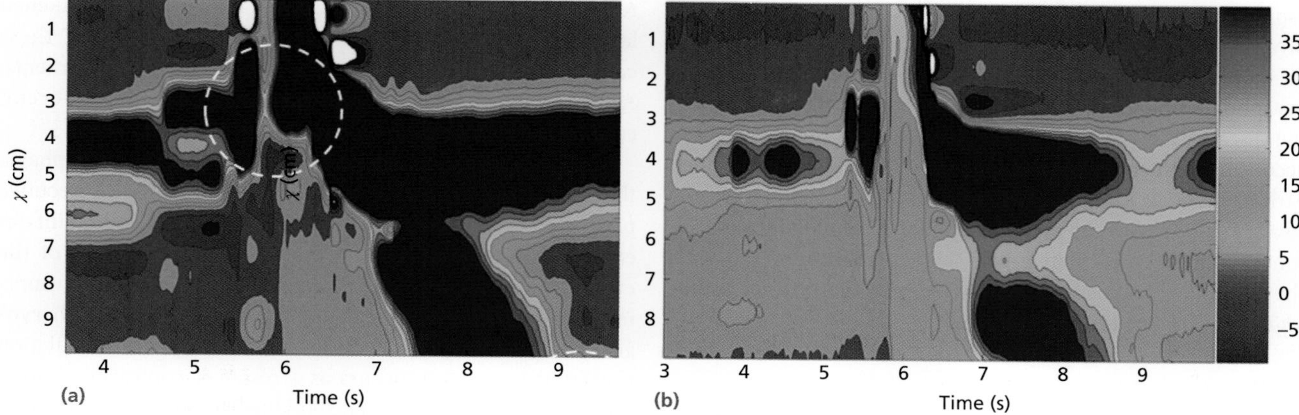

Figure 42.4 Pressure topography plots of high-resolution manometry of the upper esophageal sphincter (UES) before **(a)** and after **(b)** dilation in a subject with a symptomatic cricopharyngeal bar. Typical UES relaxation pressure is less than 10 mmHg. However, **(a)** the mean UES relaxation pressure is >35 mmHg and the relaxation duration is extremely brief. After dilation with an over-the-guidewire polyvinyl dilator, the intrabolus pressure was substantially decreased and relaxation duration prolonged. Source: Courtesy of the Esophageal Center at Northwestern University, Chicago, IL, USA.

tissue replacement and (muscle) fiber degeneration. Thus, although the sphincter relaxes normally during a swallow, it cannot distend normally, resulting in the appearance of a cricopharyngeal indentation, or bar, during a barium swallow (see Figures 42.3 and 42.4). Diminished sphincter compliance necessitates increased hypopharyngeal intrabolus pressure to maintain transsphincteric flow through the smaller UES opening. The increased stress on the hypopharynx from the increased intrabolus pressure may ultimately result in diverticulum formation, that is, pulsion diverticulum.

Management of structural oropharyngeal dysphagia

The treatment of hypopharyngeal diverticula is cricopharyngeal myotomy with or without a diverticulectomy. Resting UES tone is reduced to approximately 50% of baseline, suggesting that the derived benefit is from increased compliance at the UES [20]. Good or excellent results can be expected in 80–100% of patients with Zenker's diverticulum treated by transcervical myotomy combined with diverticulectomy or diverticulopexy wherein the diverticulum is inverted and sutured to the prevertebral fascia [21]. There are instances in which a limited procedure would be adequate, but a definitive approach to the problem of pulsion diverticula should involve both diverticulectomy and myotomy. Diverticulectomy alone risks recurrence because the underlying stenosis at the level of the cricopharyngeus is not remedied. Similarly, myotomy alone risks not solving the problem of food accumulation within the diverticula with attendant regurgitation and aspiration. Small diverticula may, however, disappear spontaneously following myotomy.

Within the past decade, two endoscopic approaches to Zenker's diverticulum have been developed. The principle of the first technique is to divide the common wall between the medial portion of the diverticulum and the hypopharynx [22]. This creates an open communication between the diverticulum and implements a cricopharyngeal myotomy with one cut. Stapling of the margins may also be done to reduce the risk for perforation [23]. Several studies have shown the effectiveness of this procedure both for initial treatment and recurrence [24]. However, endoscopic myotomy is reserved for patients with a diverticulum between 3 and 6 cm in length to assure adequate myotomy of the common wall and drainage of the diverticulum. The second technique is creation of a submucosal tunnel to perform a myotomy similar to that used for achalasia (Zenker's or Z-POEM) [25,26]. This appears to be a promising technique to transect the diverticular septum with submucosal tunneling with minimal risk for perforation. Finally, an endoscopic procedure for repair of Zenker's diverticulum, endoscopic myomectomy [27], has been developed wherein a segment of the cricopharyngeus is excised because of the up to 30% recurrence rate of diverticulum [24]. In this study, 64 patients underwent endoscopic repair for Zenker's diverticulum, 44 with and 20 without cricopharyngeal myectomy. Ten patients (22.7%) had recurrence of Zenker's diverticulum after cricopharyngeal myotomy at a median of 19.1 months, whereas no recurrence was documented in the cricopharyngeal myectomy cohort ($p = .02$), demonstrating promising initial success with the technique.

Whether a cricopharyngeal bar in the absence of a diverticulum requires treatment is less clear. Certainly, if dysphagia exists and combined fluoroscopic/manometric analysis demonstrates reduced sphincter opening in conjunction with elevated upstream intrabolus pressure, there is good rationale for treatment. One uncontrolled series suggested that, in this scenario, dilation with a large-caliber bougie over a guidewire was efficacious in relieving dysphagia, and this is certainly a reasonable treatment option before myotomy [28] (see Figure 42.1).

Functional causative factors of oropharyngeal dysphagia

Primary neurological or muscular diseases involving the oropharynx can be associated with dysphagia. Thus, whereas esophageal dysphagia usually results from esophageal diseases, oropharyngeal dysphagia is frequently the result of neurological or muscular diseases, with oropharyngeal dysfunction being just one pathological manifestation. Although the specifics of the diseases vary, the net effect on swallowing can be analyzed according to the mechanical description of the swallow outlined earlier. Table 42.1 summarizes the mechanical elements of the swallow, along with the manifestation and consequence of dysfunction and representative pathological conditions in which they are likely encountered. Some of the more distinct pathological entities are discussed later.

Neurological causes of oropharyngeal dysphagia

Neurological diseases can damage the neural structures requisite for either the afferent or efferent limbs of the oropharyngeal swallow. Because there is nothing unique to neurons controlling swallowing, their involvement in disease processes is usually random. Furthermore, in most instances, functions mediated by adjacent neuronal structures are concurrently involved. Virtually any disease of the central nervous system can potentially cause dysphagia.

Cerebrovascular accidents

Aspiration pneumonia inflicts an estimated 20% death rate in the first year after a stroke, and 10–15% each year thereafter [29]. It is usually not the first episode of aspiration pneumonia, but the subsequent recurrences over a several-year period that eventually cause death [30]. The ultimate cause of aspiration pneumonia is dysphagia leading to aspiration, which can occur by a number of mechanisms: absence or severe delay in triggering the swallowing reflex (swallow apraxia), reduced lingual control, and unilateral or bilateral weakened laryngopharyngeal musculature [6]. Conceptually, these causes can be divided into motor or sensory impairments. Although sensory and motor impairment frequently co-occur, each will be addressed separately.

Cortical strokes are less likely to result in severe dysphagia than are brainstem strokes [31]. In a report of 100 consecutive patients, 37 of 86 (43%) who sustained an acute cerebral infarct experienced dysphagia when evaluated within 4 days of the event. However, 86% of these patients were able to swallow normally 2 weeks later [31]. Scalp topographic maps of the pharyngeal muscles obtained by transcranial magnetic stimulation suggest that recovery occurs as a result of contralateral areas taking over the lost function [32]. Thus, dysphagia is more prevalent among patients incurring larger strokes and patients who have had prior infarcts.

The sensory cues required for eliciting the pharyngeal swallow are unclear. In pathological circumstances in which the neural substrate of the afferent signal has been damaged, patients may experience a relative inability to initiate a swallow. A study of sensory acuity in the supraglottic and pharyngeal regions revealed either unilateral (n = 9) or bilateral (n = 6) sensory impairment of moderate to severe degree in all 15 patients with stroke studied [33]. Impaired sensation in these critical areas likely results in swallow apraxia. An interesting compensatory strategy for this sensory defect is to accentuate oropharyngeal stimulation during eating to facilitate achieving the threshold for triggering the medullary swallowing center [6]. Preliminary data suggest that sour taste is particularly effective in some patients with swallow apraxia, providing some hope for the treatment of this disabling condition [6].

Table 42.1 Patterns and manifestations of oropharyngeal dysphagia.

Mechanical element	Biomechanical mechanism	Evidence of dysfunction	Typical diseases
Nasopharyngeal closure	Soft palate elevation	Nasopharyngeal regurgitation Nasal voice	Myasthenia gravis
Laryngeal closure	Laryngeal elevation Arytenoid tilt Vocal fold closure	Aspiration during bolus transit	CVA Head trauma
UES opening	UES relaxation Laryngeal elevation Anterior hyoid traction Sphincter distension	Dysphagia Postswallow residue/aspiration Diverticulum formation	Cricopharyngeal bar CVA Parkinson disease
Tongue loading and bolus propulsion	Lingual sensation and control	Sluggish, misdirected bolus	Parkinson disease Surgical defects Cerebral palsy
Pharyngeal clearance	Pharyngeal shortening Pharyngeal contraction Epiglottic flip	Postswallow residue/aspiration	Polio Postpolio Oculopharyngeal dystrophy CVA

CVA, cardiovascular accident; UES, upper esophageal sphincter.

Parkinson disease

Parkinson disease affects swallowing function in 80% of patients over the course of their disease [34,35], often in early phases of the disease [36]. Moreover, this dysfunction is often initially subclinical and diagnosed only with objective testing despite life-threatening manifestations, such as aspiration pneumonia [37]. Because Parkinson disease is a generalized neurodegenerative disorder, it can potentially affect the oral, pharyngeal, and esophageal phases of swallowing [35,38], although the pharyngeal phase is most commonly affected, initially with a brainstem neurodegenerative phase followed by muscle atrophy [35,39]. Videofluoroscopy of swallowing is the most accurate test for assessing swallowing dysfunction in Parkinson [40]. Typical abnormalities include insufficient lip closure, impaired lingual bolus control, lingual pumping, delayed initiation of pharyngeal swallow, and reduced hyolaryngeal excursion [41]. Large liquid bolus volumes are also associated with aspiration [41,42], with delayed initiation of the pharyngeal swallow and reduced hyolaryngeal excursion being predictors for development of pulmonary aspiration [41]. Ultrasound to measure muscle thinning, electromyography, high-resolution manometry (HRM), and fiberoptic endoscopic evaluation of swallowing may aid the evaluation of these patients [35,36,43]. Treatment for dysphagia associated with Parkinson is empirical. It is advised that patients time taking their medications to be maximally active during meals to facilitate swallowing function [44]. Although swallow therapy using maneuvers and dietary changes are often advised, a systematic analysis has not shown clear benefit [45]. Similarly, neither direct electrical stimulation of swallowing nor deep brain stimulation has been proved effective [45,46].

Amyotrophic lateral sclerosis

Amyotrophic lateral sclerosis (ALS) is a progressive neurological disease characterized by degeneration of motor neurons in the brain, brainstem, and spinal cord. Specific symptoms are dependent on the locations of affected motor neurons and the relative severity of involvement. When the degenerative process involves the cranial nerve nuclei, swallowing difficulties ensue. Oropharyngeal dysfunction characteristically begins with the tongue and progresses to involve the pharyngeal and laryngeal musculature. Patients experience choking attacks, become dehydrated or malnourished, and incur aspiration pneumonia. The decline in swallowing function is progressive and predictable, inevitably leading to gastrostomy feeding. A number of patients die as a consequence of their swallowing dysfunction in conjunction with respiratory depression [47].

Tumors

Medullary or vagal tumors are potentially debilitating with respect to swallowing. Astrocytomas are the most common histological type affecting adults, while medulloblastomas are the most common type encountered in children [48]. The relative inaccessibility of the medulla to surgery usually means that substantial morbidity is incurred during attempted resection or palliation.

Unilateral lesions of the vagus can result in hemiparesis of the soft palate and pharyngeal constrictors, as well as of the laryngeal musculature. Surgical manipulation of this region can even result in complete loss of the pharyngeal swallow response [49]. The recurrent laryngeal nerves can be injured as a result of thyroid surgery, polio, aortic aneurysms, pneumonectomy, primary malignancies of the mediastinum, or metastatic lesions to the mediastinum. Owing to its more extensive loop into the chest, the left recurrent laryngeal nerve is more vulnerable to involvement with mediastinal node malignancy. Unilateral recurrent laryngeal nerve injury results in unilateral adductor paralysis of the vocal cords. This defect can result in aspiration during swallowing because of impaired laryngeal closure. Although some reports state the contrary [50], it is probably rare to have any primary pharyngeal dysfunction associated with recurrent laryngeal nerve injury.

Muscular diseases causing oropharyngeal dysphagia

Primary muscular diseases involving the oropharynx are associated with dysphagia reflective of the pattern of involvement. Nasal voice and nasopharyngeal regurgitation indicate either weakness or paresis of the soft palate elevators, and tongue weakness can cause poor control of the bolus within the mouth. Postswallow residue in the valleculae or hypopharynx reflects an ineffective, presumably weakened pharyngeal contraction. Aspiration suggests either weakened laryngeal elevators or postswallow residue that is then aspirated after the swallow sequence is completed. As with neurological disorders, virtually any disorder affecting skeletal muscle can result in dysphagia.

Oculopharyngeal dystrophy

Oculopharyngeal muscular dystrophy (OPMD) is a syndrome characterized by progressive dysphagia and palpebral ptosis first described by Taylor in 1915 [51]. He noted that all of his afflicted patients reaching age 50 years died of starvation resulting from pharyngeal paralysis. The disease is now known to be a form of muscular dystrophy inherited as autosomal dominant with occurrences clustered in families of French-Canadian descent. The underlying cause of OPMD is an expanded GCG repeat in the first exon of the gene encoding poly(A)-binding protein nuclear 1 (PABPN1) localized on chromosome 14. q11.2-q13. The number of GCG expansion ranges from 8 to 13 repeats. PABPN1 is a nuclear multifunctional protein that is involved in transcription regulation and posttranscriptional processes [52,53].

Oculopharyngeal dystrophy affects the striated pharyngeal muscles and the levator palpebrae, which results in ptosis. Other forms of muscular dystrophy occasionally affect the pharyngeal constrictors but rarely, if ever, is this a dominant manifestation. The first symptom of OPMD is usually ptosis that develops slowly and eventually dominates the patient's appearance. Dysphagia may begin before the ptosis but is more often manifest simultaneously or a few years later. The dominant functional abnormalities are weak or absent pharyngeal contraction with hypopharyngeal stasis [54]. Dysphagia progresses slowly but may ultimately lead to starvation, aspiration pneumonia, or asphyxia.

Myasthenia gravis

Myasthenia gravis is a progressive autoimmune disease characterized by high circulating levels of acetylcholine receptor antibody and destruction of acetylcholine receptors at neuromuscular junctions. Musculature controlled by the cranial nerves is almost always involved, particularly the ocular muscles. Dysphagia is prominent in more than a third of myasthenia gravis cases and, in unusual instances, can be the initial manifestation of the disease [6]. In mild cases, dysphagia may not be evident until after 15–20 minutes of eating. Classically manometric studies reveal a progressive deterioration in the amplitude of pharyngeal contractions with repeated swallows. Peristaltic amplitude recovers with rest or following the administration of 10 mg edrophonium chloride. In more advanced cases, the dysphagia can be profound and associated with nasopharyngeal regurgitation and nasality of the voice, even to the extent of being confused with bulbar ALS or brainstem stroke [55].

Management of oropharyngeal dysphagia

Management of oropharyngeal dysphagia begins with definition of the aberrant physiology along the lines summarized in Table 42.1. This is most easily accomplished with a videofluoroscopic swallowing study. Following definition of the patient's swallowing dysfunction, four specific issues pertaining to management of oropharyngeal dysphagia can be addressed:

1. Identification of an underlying systemic disease
2. Characterization of a disorder amenable to surgery or dilation
3. Identification of a specific pattern of dysphagia amenable to swallowing therapy
4. Assessment of aspiration risk.

Identifying underlying disease

A potential outcome of the swallowing evaluation is the identification of an underlying neuromuscular, neoplastic, or metabolic disorder that will dictate specific management. For example, dysphagia can be the presenting symptom in patients with myopathy, myasthenia, thyrotoxicosis, motor neuron disease, or Parkinson disease. In each instance, identification of the underlying disease will result in a specific treatment. Whether identification and treatment of the underlying disorder improves swallowing function depends on both the natural history of the disease and whether an effective treatment exists.

Disorders amenable to surgery

In marked contrast with the high efficacy observed with structural cricopharyngeal disorders, the efficacy of myotomy in neurogenic dysphagia is variable. Furthermore, most series evaluating the efficacy of myotomy in neurogenic dysphagia are uncontrolled without specific outcome measures. Thus, although an overall favorable response rate in excess of 60% is reported, there are currently no validated criteria for preoperative selection. Theoretically, the functional limitation in these circumstances is of pharyngeal propulsion, and the potential benefit of myotomy is less obvious [56].

Specific patterns of dysphagia amenable to swallowing therapy

Following characterization of a patient's swallow dysfunction, the radiographic study should proceed to test selected compensatory or therapeutic treatment strategies. Compensatory treatments include postural changes, modifying food delivery or consistency, or the use of prosthetics. For instance, head turning can eliminate aspiration or pharyngeal residue by favoring the more functional side in patients with hemiparesis [6]. Similarly, diet modifications can reduce the "difficulty" of the swallow [6]. Therapeutic strategies are designed to alter the physiology of the swallow, usually by improving the range of motion of oral or pharyngeal structures using voluntary control of oropharyngeal movement during swallow. Depending on the severity of the impairment, level of motivation, and global neurological intactness, defective elements of the swallow can be selectively rehabilitated. For a detailed description of the techniques and limitations of swallow therapy, the reader is referred to treatises on the topic [6,21].

Detection of severe aspiration

Oropharyngeal dysphagia associated with aspiration is responsible for an estimated 40 000 deaths per year due to aspiration pneumonia [33]. Videofluoroscopy is believed to be the most sensitive test for detecting aspiration, detecting instances not evident by bedside evaluation in 42–60% of patients. However, despite the logical association between aspiration during swallowing and the subsequent development of pneumonia, this sequence is not inevitable. In fact, available data suggest that radiographic aspiration has a positive predictive value of only 19–68% and a negative predictive value of 55–97% for pneumonia [21]. Nonetheless, the balance of evidence suggests that detection of aspiration is a predictor of pneumonia risk, and that its detection dictates that compensatory swallowing strategies, nonoral feeding, or corrective surgery be instituted. Whether nonoral feeding eliminates the risk for aspiration is controversial. A provocative finding by Croghan et al. [5] was that of 22 patients with radiographic aspiration, pneumonia and death were more frequent among patients who received feeding tubes. This finding suggests that aspiration of oral secretions may be important in determining pneumonia risk and has led some to consider procedures such as tracheostomy to protect the airway.

Esophageal motility disorders

Esophageal motility has the consistent objective of emptying the esophagus: primary esophageal peristalsis empties swallowed material from the esophagus; secondary peristalsis eliminates air or fluid refluxed from the stomach; the UES contracts during inspiration to exclude inspired air from the digestive tract; and the crural diaphragm contracts during abrupt increases of intraabdominal pressure, preventing gastroesophageal reflux. A basic characteristic of esophageal motility disorders, in contrast, is failure in preserving esophageal emptiness. Retained material within the esophagus, or the excessive entry of material into the esophagus, is abnormal. Such dysfunction can be categorized as disorders of peristalsis or of sphincter competence. The main dysfunction of sphincter competence occurs with reflux disease, an entity covered in Chapter 43. This discussion will focus on less common causes of sphincter dysfunction and on disorders of peristalsis. For reference, Table 42.2 includes the esophageal motor disorders based on the location and type of impairment in motor function.

Esophageal motor function

The esophagus is a 20- to 22-cm muscular tube with a wall composed of skeletal and smooth muscle. The proportion of each muscle type is species dependent. In the human esophagus, the proximal 5% including the UES is striated, the middle 35–40% is mixed with an increasing proportion of smooth muscle moving distally, and the distal 50–60% is entirely smooth muscle [57]. The bundles of the outer longitudinal muscle arise from the cricoid cartilage, receive slips from the cricopharyngeus, and pass dorsolaterally to fuse posteriorly about 3 cm below the cricoid cartilage. Both the striated and smooth muscle portions of the esophagus contain a nerve network, known as the myenteric or Auerbach's plexus, situated between the longitudinal and circular muscle layers [58]. The inner circular and outer longitudinal muscle layers of the proximal esophagus are composed of striated muscle and are controlled by somatic motor fibers from lower motor neurons in the nucleus retrofacialis and the nucleus ambiguus. Axons of these lower motor neurons course through the vagus nerve by way of the recurrent laryngeal nerve. The thoracic esophagus is composed mainly of smooth muscle that receives innervation from preganglionic neurons in the dorsal motor nucleus of the vagus. Vagal fibers synapse in the myenteric plexus ganglia and are generally considered to be the relay neurons between the vagus and the smooth muscle. A second nerve network, the submucosal or Meissner's plexus, is situated between the muscularis mucosae and the circular muscle layer. The submucosal plexus of the human esophagus is exceedingly sparse [59].

Table 42.2 Patterns of esophageal dysmotility.

Functional impairment	Esophageal region: Body	Esophageal region: LES
Inadequate deglutitive inhibition (or relaxation)	Achalasia DES	Achalasia *Pseudoachalasia*
Impaired retrograde inhibition	—	*Gas bloat (post fundoplication)*
Excess retrograde inhibition	—	GERD (tLESR)
Inadequate peristaltic excitation (or resting tone)	Absent peristalsis Advanced achalasia Weak peristalsis • Transition zone • IEM GERD *Obstruction*	Scleroderma esophagus GERD
Excess peristaltic excitation (or resting tone)	DES Type III achalasia Jackhammer esophagus	Hypercontractile LES Achalasia

Italics indicate structural abnormalities mimicking the findings of primary motor disorders.
DES, diffuse esophageal spasm; GERD, gastroesophageal reflux disease; IEM, ineffective esophageal motility; LES, lower esophageal sphincter; tLESR, transient lower esophageal sphincter relaxation.

The normal esophagus does not exhibit spontaneous contractions, and its resting pressure is an approximate reflection of pleural pressure, becoming negative during inspiration. Analyses of the vigor and propagation of esophageal peristalsis have concluded that progression along the length of the tubular esophagus is not seamless. Rather, there is a distinct transition zone between the first two contractile segments characterized by low peristaltic amplitude, a slight delay in progression, and an increased likelihood of failed transmission [60]. This transition zone becomes quite evident when peristaltic amplitude and progression are plotted topographically (Figure 42.5). The topographic analysis also reveals the segmental characteristic of peristaltic progression through the distal esophagus. Two distinct contractile segments are followed by the lower esophageal sphincter (LES), which contracts with vigor and persistence quite dissimilar to the adjacent esophagus [61].

Esophageal peristalsis commences as the pharyngeal contraction traverses the UES and progresses along the esophagus at 2–4 cm/s. Whereas primary peristalsis is initiated by a swallow, secondary peristalsis can be elicited in response to focal esophageal distention with air, fluid, or a balloon [62]. The mechanical correlate of peristalsis is of a stripping wave that milks the esophagus empty from its proximal to distal end (see Figure 42.5). The efficacy of distal esophageal emptying is inversely related to peristaltic amplitude, such that emptying becomes progressively impaired with peristaltic amplitudes of 30 mmHg or less [63].

Deglutitive inhibition is another cardinal feature of the peristaltic mechanism. A second swallow, initiated while an earlier peristaltic contraction is still progressing in the proximal esophagus, causes rapid and complete inhibition of the contraction induced by the first swallow [64]. If the first peristaltic contraction has reached the distal esophagus, it may proceed distally for

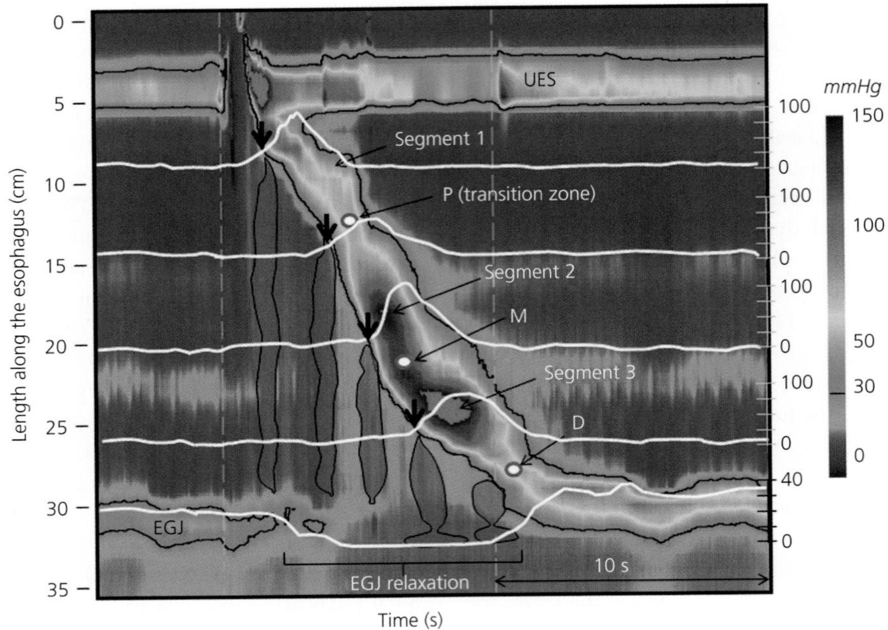

Figure 42.5 Representative physiological data, modified to illustrate the relationship between videofluoroscopic (purple bolus), manometric tracings (white lines), and topographic representations of esophageal peristalsis after a 5-mL water swallow that was completely cleared by the sequence. Tracings of the videofluoroscopic images are overlaid on the esophageal pressure topography (EPT) plot to show the distribution of the bolus. At each recording site, the white line intersecting the pressure scale (mmHg) on the right represents the manometric tracing. Luminal closure, and hence the tail of the barium bolus, coincides at each recording site with the upstroke of the peristaltic contraction (black arrows) and the leading edge of the 30-mmHg isobaric contour (black line). On the isobaric contour plot, four distinct pressure segments separated by three pressure troughs are evident. Physiologically the first trough approximates the transition from striated and smooth muscle, the second is within the smooth muscle segment, and the third separates the peristaltic segment from the lower esophageal sphincter (LES). Note that LES relaxation is reliably recorded using either manometric technique, albeit somewhat differently. From the illustration it is evident that the offset of LES relaxation measured by the sleeve coincides with the peristaltic contraction contacting the proximal portion of the sleeve. In addition to measuring mean residual pressure, topographic analysis allows for more precise measurement of the transsphincteric pressure gradient. D, distal pressure node; EGJ, esophagogastric junction; M, middle pressure node; P: proximal pressure node. Source: Isobaric contour tracing courtesy of the Esophageal Center at Northwestern University, Chicago, IL, USA.

a few seconds after the second swallow, but its amplitude diminishes progressively until it disappears [65]. Deglutitive inhibition results from hyperpolarization of the circular smooth muscle and is mediated by nonadrenergic, noncholinergic neurons in the myenteric plexus.

Esophagogastric junction

The anatomy of the esophagogastric junction (EGJ) is complex. The distal end of the esophagus is anchored to the diaphragm by the phrenoesophageal membrane that inserts circumferentially into the esophageal musculature close to the squamocolumnar junction. The esophagus then traverses the diaphragmatic hiatus and joins the stomach in almost a tangential fashion. Thus, there are several potential contributors to the EGJ high-pressure zone: the LES, the diaphragmatic hiatus, and the muscular architecture of the gastric cardia, which constitutes the distal aspect of this zone.

The LES is a short segment of tonically contracted smooth muscle at the distal extreme of the esophagus (Figure 42.6). Resting LES tone normally varies from 10 to 30 mmHg relative to the intragastric pressure, with considerable temporal fluctuation. Although not fully understood, the mechanism of LES tonic contraction seems to display properties of both the muscle itself and the nerves controlling the sphincter. This conclusion is supported by the observation that pressure within the sphincter is minimally affected after the elimination of neural activity by close intraarterial injection of tetrodotoxin [66].

The neural mediation of LES relaxation has been studied extensively [67–69]. LES relaxation can be triggered by distention on either side of the EGJ or by swallowing [70]. Swallowing induces an initial inhibition of the entire distal esophagus, and LES relaxation is part of this inhibitory response. Deglutitive LES relaxation is mediated by the vagus nerve, which synapses with inhibitory neurons of the myenteric plexus. Current evidence implicates nitric oxide (NO) as the main neurotransmitter in the postganglionic neurons responsible for LES relaxation. NO is produced by neuronal NO synthase, which is a soluble cytosolic enzyme that has been identified in neurons of the myenteric plexus, colocalizing with vasoactive intestinal polypeptide (VIP), which may be a second inhibitory neurotransmitter in the LES, as well as in the esophageal body [71–73].

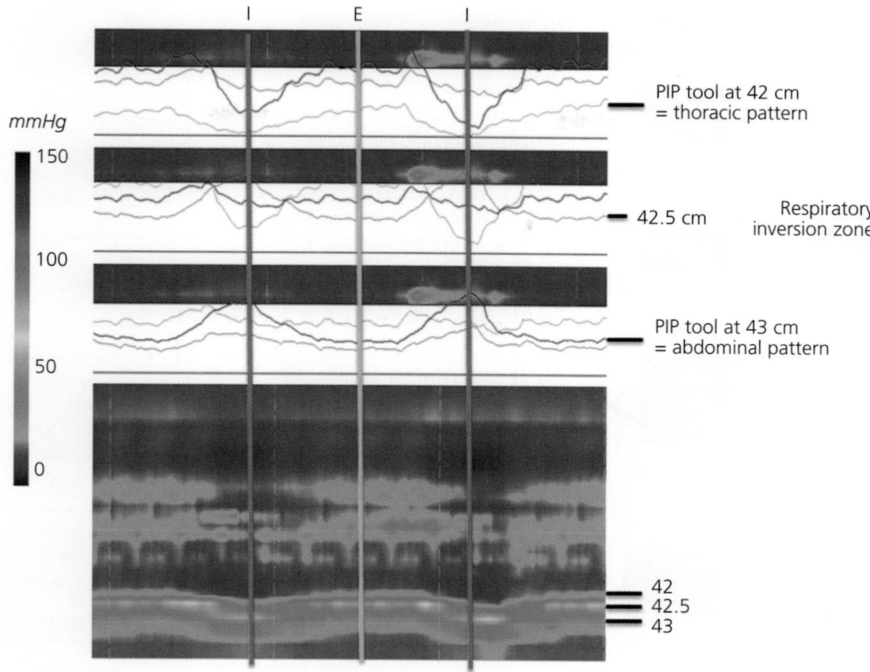

Figure 42.6 Utilization of the pressure inversion point (PIP) tool in a high-resolution manometry study. Peak inspiration is depicted by the pink lines, whereas midexpiratory phase is depicted by the orange line. Scrolling across the esophagogastric junction, the pressure inversion point (PIP) tool subtracts the distal pressure tracing (blue line) from the recording site 1 cm proximal to that (green line) to derive the difference between the two (red line). Note the flattening of the red line occurs at 42.5, indicating the center of the respiratory inversion zone (pink line).

Evaluation and classification of esophageal dysphagia

Dysphagia is a fundamental symptom of esophageal disorders. Esophageal as opposed to oropharyngeal dysphagia is suggested by the absence of associated aspiration, cough, nasopharyngeal regurgitation, dry mouth, pharyngeal residue following swallow, or co-occurring neuromuscular dysfunction. In contrast, the associated conditions of heartburn, regurgitation, chest pain, odynophagia, or intermittent esophageal obstruction suggest esophageal dysphagia. However, an important limitation of the history in patients with esophageal dysphagia is that identification of the location of obstruction is of limited accuracy. Specifically, a distal esophageal obstruction caused by an esophageal ring or achalasia will often be sensed as cervical dysphagia such that patients correctly locate distal dysfunction only 60% of the time [74]. Because of this subjective difficulty in distinguishing proximal from distal lesions within the esophagus, an evaluation for cervical dysphagia should encompass the entire esophagus.

Another important consideration in patient management is that esophageal motility disorders are much less common than mechanical or inflammatory causes of dysphagia: tumors, strictures, rings, and peptic, pill, or infectious esophagitis. Historical points suggestive of a motor disorder are difficulty with both solids and liquids as opposed to only solids, which is more suggestive of mechanical obstruction. However, as will become evident in the ensuing discussion, the functional consequences of mechanical or inflammatory disorders can exactly mimic those of primary motility disorders. Thus, as with oropharyngeal dysphagia, an esophageal motility disorder should be considered *only after exclusion of these more common diagnoses* by endoscopic and/or radiographic examination.

As outlined earlier, the physiological elements of esophageal peristalsis are the coordinated inhibition and excitation of the circular and longitudinal muscle layers of the esophagus. It follows that pathophysiological processes can involve dysfunction of deglutitive inhibition (including sphincter relaxation) and/or of the propagated contraction. Furthermore, because esophageal motor disorders are rarely diagnosed on histopathological grounds, diagnosis depends on defining these functional aberrations using the manometric technique. A relatively new technology, HRM has clearly improved our ability to classify and define relevant clinical phenotypes of abnormal esophageal motor function. This technique has led to the evolution of a new classification of esophageal motor disorders based on esophageal pressure topography (EPT) metrics (Figure 42.7). The Chicago Classification defines esophageal motor disorders using a hierarchal process that distinguishes patients with well-defined motor disorders and those with severe motility aberrations not seen in normal individuals from those that are defined statistically and hence of less certain significance.

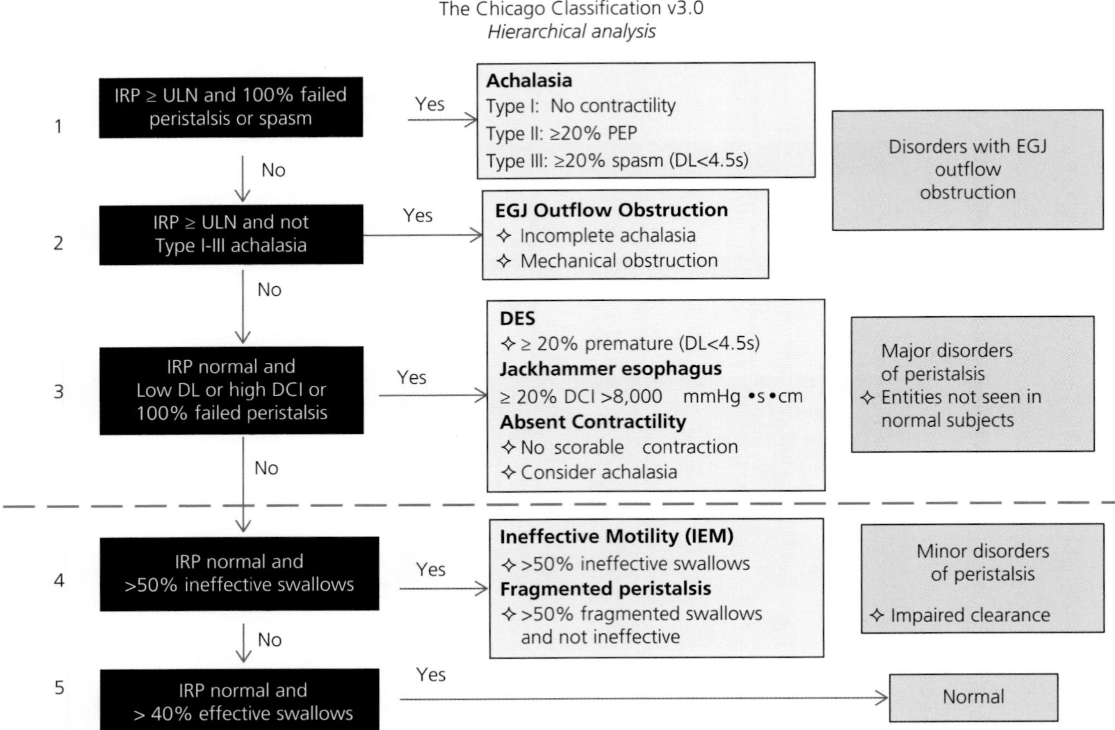

Figure 42.7 Diagnostic algorithm for defining esophageal motor disorders using the Chicago Classification. DCI, distal contractile integral; DL, distal latency; EGJ, esophagogastric junction; IRP, integrated relaxation pressure; PIP, pressure inversion point; ULN, upper limit of normal. Source: Courtesy of the Esophageal Center at Northwestern University, Chicago, IL, USA.

Diagnostic testing in esophageal disease

Endoscopy

Upper endoscopy should be the first test for evaluating new-onset dysphagia when structural causes requiring either dilation or biopsy are being considered. It has excellent specificity for strictures and tumors; however, it has the potential to miss subtle obstructing lesions, such as webs and rings. It also provides only limited information regarding motility disorders.

Radiographic contrast studies

Radiographic contrast studies of the esophagus are useful in assessing dysphagia if upper endoscopy is not readily available. Radiography has the added benefit of providing information regarding the oropharyngeal swallow, UES, peristalsis, and bolus clearance through the EGJ. With good technique and an experienced observer, normal peristalsis can be verified with 91–95% specificity [75,76]. Peristalsis is best evaluated in the prone position so that clearance does not occur by gravity. Abnormalities of peristalsis are inferred by retrograde escape of the bolus through the peristaltic wavefront resulting in delayed esophageal emptying. Spastic contractions are inferred with a corkscrew or “rosary bead” appearance, suggesting that the bolus is trapped in the esophagus during a premature contraction. Normally the EGJ will become widely patent during bolus transit, and impaired relaxation can be inferred with either a smooth tapering noted at the EGJ or esophageal retention.

Manometry

Manometry measures intraluminal pressure at intervals along the length of the esophagus. Conventional manometry devices used either water perfused or solid-state pressure sensors spaced 3–5 cm apart along a transnasally positioned catheter. Pressure recordings were displayed as line tracings, and interpretation relied on assessing the amplitudes and time intervals of events among recording sites to determine propagation velocity. A variety of methods existed to assess EGJ relaxation, but this was not standardized and was often methodologically flawed. Nonetheless, this technology was the foundation for the description of esophageal motility disorders. More recently, the introduction of HRM has vastly improved the characterization of esophageal motility and substantially refined the conventional classification of esophageal motility disorders.

The concept of high-resolution esophageal manometry is to use a sufficient number of pressure sensors within the esophagus such that intraluminal pressure can be monitored as a continuum along the length of the esophagus, much as time is viewed as a continuum in line tracings of conventional manometry (see Figure 42.5). When HRM is coupled with algorithms to display the manometric data as pressure topography plots, pressure differences with time and among pressure sensors are visualized using color gradients on the topography plots. This technology has been leveraged to refine the conventional classification of esophageal motility disorders using clinically relevant criteria to better define subtypes of motility abnormalities. The Chicago Classification of esophageal motor disorders was vetted by a group of international experts over a 5-year period, endorsed by all major national and international motility societies, and published in 2012 [77]. The Chicago Classification was the first classification scheme developed for HRM; it incorporated metrics and physiological concepts not assessed by conventional manometry (distal latency [DL], pressurization events) and refined previous conventional manometry concepts into novel metrics to assess both EGJ relaxation and peristaltic activity (integrated relaxation pressure [IRP], distal contractile integral [DCI], DL). These metrics are detailed and contrasted with conventional manometry in Table 42.3. The Chicago Classification recognizes five categories of motor function: (1) achalasia, (2) EGJ outflow obstruction (EGJOO), (3) major disorders of peristalsis, (4) minor disorders of peristalsis, and (5) normal (see Figure 42.7) [77].

Analysis of an EPT study is done in a stepwise fashion using an algorithmic scheme that first quantifies the adequacy of deglutitive EGJ relaxation and subsequently uses individual swallow patterns defined by EPT metrics to further subclassify the patient into specific categories.

- Step 1: EGJ pressure morphology (see Figure 42.6)
  - EGJ pressure morphology is analyzed to determine whether a hiatus hernia is present and to locate the pressure inversion point. This has significance with respect to reflux disease and as a quality check regarding proper catheter placement.
- Step 2: EGJ relaxation (Figure 42.8)
  - The adequacy of EGJ relaxation is assessed with the IRP. As illustrated in Figure 42.8, the IRP is calculated from the eSleeve recording as the mean eSleeve pressure during the 4 seconds of lowest EGJ pressure in the postdeglutitive period. As such, the IRP is influenced by the completeness of LES relaxation, the persistence of LES relaxation, and intrabolus pressure during transit across the sphincter [78,79].
- Step 3: The integrity of peristalsis (Figure 42.9)
  - Esophageal peristaltic integrity is characterized as intact, failed, or associated with large (>5-cm) breaks in the 20 mmHg isobaric contour spanning from the UES to the EGJ. The subsequent characterization of contractile latency and propagation is dependent on the contraction not being failed (see Figure 42.9). Characterizing peristaltic integrity is similar to using a 30 mmHg threshold at 3 and 8 cm above the proximal border of the LES in conventional manometry to define effective swallows, but provides a more complete assessment of the entire peristaltic sequence [80].
- Step 4: Localizing the contractile deceleration point (CDP) (Figure 42.10)
  - The CDP is the inflection point in contractile wavefront propagation velocity. Conceptually, this is the point at which the peristaltic stripping wave converts to a compartmentalized ampulla to promote emptying of the remaining bolus. This landmark is in close proximity to the proximal border of the LES during maximal shortening and is usually associated with maximal length of concurrent contraction of the esophageal body [81]. The CDP should be localized within the third contractile segment defined by Clouse and Staiano [82], and there is no analogous measure in conventional manometry.
- Step 5: Contractile propagation (see Figure 42.10)
  - Propagation and timing of peristalsis are characterized by the DL to determine whether the contraction is premature in the distal esophagus, indicative of impaired neuronal inhibition. It is measured as the interval between upper esophageal relaxation and the CDP (see Figure 42.10). There is no correlate to this metric in conventional manometry.
- Step 6: Contractile vigor (see Figure 42.9)
  - The contractile activity within the domain of the distal smooth muscle esophagus from the transition zone (typically localized about 6 cm distal to the UES) to the EGJ is quantified as the DCI. The DCI uses the space–time domain of the second and third contractile segments to provide a single number that summarizes the contractile vigor in this region (see Figure 42.9). This is used in place of measuring the mean peristaltic amplitudes at 3 and 8 cm above the proximal aspect of the LES on conventional manometry. The EPT plots also allow a qualitative assessment of the contraction that helps define focal contractile abnormalities and disorders associated with LES after-contraction.
- Step 7: Pressurization patterns (Figure 42.11)
  - Abnormal intrabolus pressure is indicative of abnormal mechanics of bolus transit related to either an outflow obstruction in the distal esophagus/EGJ or a poorly compliant esophageal wall. Intrabolus pressure is characterized using the isobaric contour tool set at 20 mmHg referenced to atmospheric pressure. Abnormal pressurization can be compartmentalized between a propagating contraction and the EGJ or between the two sphincters (panesophageal pressurization) (see Figure 42.11). There is no correlate for this measure in conventional manometry; however, astute clinicians can assess the initial ramp pressure on line tracings or identify isobaric regions among recording sites (see Figure 42.5).

Impedance monitoring

Multichannel intraluminal impedance is a technique described more than two decades ago as a method to assess intraluminal bolus transit without fluoroscopy. The technique uses a catheter with multiple, closely spaced pairs of metal rings. An alternating current is applied across each pair of adjacent rings, and the resultant current flow is dependent on the impedance between the rings. Impedance decreases when the electrodes

Table 42.3 Definitions of esophageal pressure topography (high-resolution manometry) metrics.

EPT metric	Definition	Conventional manometry correlate
IRP (mmHg)	Average minimum EGJ pressure is for 4 contiguous or noncontiguous seconds of relaxation within 10 s of swallow (upper sphincter relaxation). Abnormal value is dependent on contractile and pressure patterns in the esophageal body: • Propagating peristalsis (>15 mmHg) • Absent peristalsis (>10 mmHg) • Premature contractions (>17 mmHg)	LES relaxation is measured with best estimate position through the EGJ • >8 mmHg is abnormal
Peristaltic breaks (cm): peristaltic integrity	Gap in the 20 mmHg isobaric contour of the peristaltic contraction between the UES and EGJ, measured in axial length. • Large break: >5 cm in length	Uses the 30 mmHg amplitude in positions 3 and 8 cm above the LES to distinguish a swallow as ineffective. • Ineffective <30 mmHg at 3 and/or 8 cm recording sites above the LES
DCI (mmHg·s·cm)	Amplitude × duration × length (mmHg·s·cm) of the distal esophageal contraction greater than 20 mmHg measured between the proximal and distal pressure troughs. • Hypertensive: mean DCI of 10 swallows >5000 mmHg·s·cm • Jackhammer: at least two swallows with a DCI >8000 mmHg·s·cm • Weak swallow: DCI <450 mmHg·s·cm • Failed swallow: DCI <100 mmHg·s·cm	Average of 10 swallows at two recording sites positioned 3 and 8 cm above the LES. • Nutcracker >180 mmHg • Revised definitions >220–260 mmHg • Ineffective <30 mmHg at 3 and/or 8 cm recording sites above the LES
CFV (cm/s)	Slope of the tangent to the 30 mmHg isobaric contour between the proximal pressure trough and the CDP • >9 cm/s is abnormal	Peristaltic progression from the UES to the LES at a rate of 2–8 cm/s • >8 cm/s is abnormal
DL (s)	Interval between UES relaxation and the CDP • <4.5 s is abnormal	No correlate in conventional manometry

CDP, contractile deceleration point; CFV, contractile front velocity; DCI, distal contractile integral; DL, distal latency; EGJ, esophagogastric junction; EPT, esophageal pressure topography; IRP, integrated relaxation pressure; LES, lower esophageal sphincter; UES, upper esophageal sphincter.

are bridged by liquid and increases when they are surrounded by air, thereby providing data on the direction, content, and completeness of bolus transit. As illustrated in Figure 42.4, liquid bolus entry is indicated by a 50% decrease in impedance, and return of the impedance tracing to 50% of baseline correlates with the passage of the tail of the bolus on fluoroscopy, also indicated by the contractile upstroke noted during manometry. Validation studies of multichannel intraluminal impedance against videofluoroscopy have shown excellent concordance in ascertaining bolus transit, reporting agreement in 97% (83/86) of swallows analyzed [83].

Multichannel intraluminal impedance has also been combined with HRM to assess the efficacy of esophageal emptying as a function of distal peristaltic amplitude. In a receiver operating characteristic analysis of a large number of swallows, a 30-mmHg cut-off had 85% sensitivity and 66% specificity for identifying incomplete bolus transit [84]. With diminishing peristaltic amplitudes, the sensitivity progressively decreased and the specificity progressively increased. That study illustrated the complementary nature of manometry and impedance testing in assessing esophageal function in the evaluation of dysphagia.

Achalasia

Achalasia is the best-defined motor disorder of the esophagus. First recognized more than 300 years ago, the disorder was initially labeled cardiospasm reflecting the observation that it was caused by a functional obstruction of the esophagus at the cardiac sphincter with no obstructing lesion evident in autopsy specimens. The first reported case was treated by passing a piece of carved whalebone with a sponge affixed to the distal end through the esophagus to facilitate esophageal emptying after meals [85]. That patient apparently sustained himself in this fashion for 15 years. During the next two centuries, there were sporadic reports of cases similarly treated with crude ramrods or dilators. In 1937, Lendrum [86] proposed that the functional esophageal obstruction in this syndrome resulted from incomplete relaxation of the LES and renamed the disease achalasia ("failure to relax"), ushering in our current concept of the disease.

Epidemiology

Achalasia is a rare disease with an estimated incidence of 2–3/100 000 population per year in the United States and Australia [87,88]. The disease affects both sexes equally and

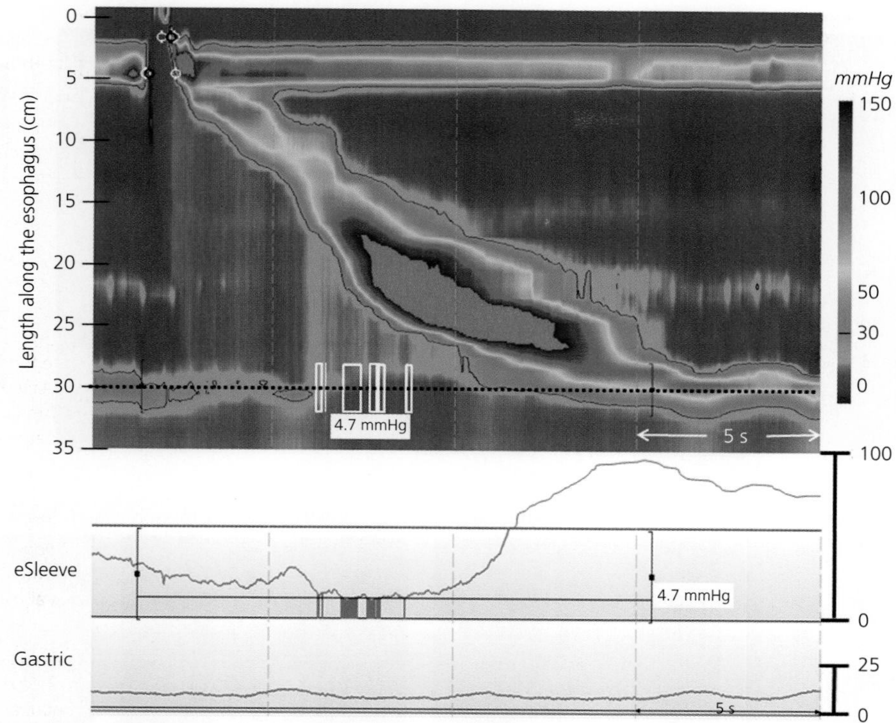

Figure 42.8 Depiction of the integrated relaxation pressure (IRP), which provides a pressure topography metric of esophagogastric junction (EGJ) relaxation after swallowing. The IRP is a complex metric; its computation requires accurately localizing the margins of the EGJ, noting the time window after deglutitive upper sphincter relaxation and then applying an eSleeve measurement (bottom tracings) within that 10-second time box (delineated by the black brackets). The eSleeve is referenced to gastric pressure (red line) and provides a measure of the greatest pressure across the axial domain of the EGJ at each time instant, plotted as a line tracing (orange line). The IRP is the mean value of the 4 seconds during which the eSleeve value is least. These time points are indicated by the white boxes on the esophageal pressure topography (EPT) plot and by the shaded red area under the red line in the eSleeve tracing. In this example, the IRP is 4.7 mmHg, which is normal.

usually presents in adult life, being most common between the ages of 25 and 60 years [89]. Because achalasia is a chronic condition, its prevalence greatly exceeds its incidence. Historic estimates of the prevalence of achalasia in Europe range from 7.1/100 000 in Wales to 13.4/100 000 in Ireland [90], but recent estimates suggest that the prevalence is much greater than this with modern HRM [73].

Reports of familial clustering of achalasia raise the possibility of genetic predisposition; however, the data on this are inconclusive. Achalasia has been reported in monozygotic twins [91], siblings [92], and children of affected parents [93]. However, other reports of the occurrence of achalasia in only one of a pair of monozygotic twins speak against strong genetic determinant [94]. Emphasizing this point, a survey of 1012 first-degree relatives of 159 patients with achalasia identified no affected relatives [95]. A rare genetic achalasia syndrome has also been described; familial adrenal insufficiency with alacrima (absence of tears) is inherited as an autosomal recessive disease that manifests itself with the childhood onset of autonomic nervous system dysfunction, including achalasia, alacrima, sinoatrial dysfunction, abnormal pupillary responses to light, and delayed gastric emptying [96,97]. It is caused by mutations in the *AAAS* gene (achalasia-addisonianism-alacrima syndrome), which encodes a protein known as ALADIN (function not well understood, located in the nuclear envelope). There has been interest in assessing whether polymorphisms in various genes that may have functional significance (e.g., in the expression of NO synthase or vasoactive intestinal peptide receptor 1) are more common in achalasia; however, the data are not conclusive [98].

Neuropathology

Achalasia is characterized by: (1) failure of the LES to relax completely with swallowing, and (2) aperistalsis in the smooth muscle esophagus. The resting LES pressure is elevated in about 60% of achalasia cases. The physiological alterations are thought to result from damage to the innervation of the smooth muscle esophagus (including the LES). Proposed neuroanatomic changes responsible for achalasia include loss of ganglion cells within the myenteric (Auerbach's) plexus, degeneration of the vagus nerve, and degeneration of the dorsal motor nucleus of the vagus. Of these possibilities, the loss of ganglion cells is best substantiated. Several observers report fewer ganglion cells and ganglion cells surrounded by mononuclear inflammatory cells in the smooth muscle esophagus of patients with achalasia [99,100].

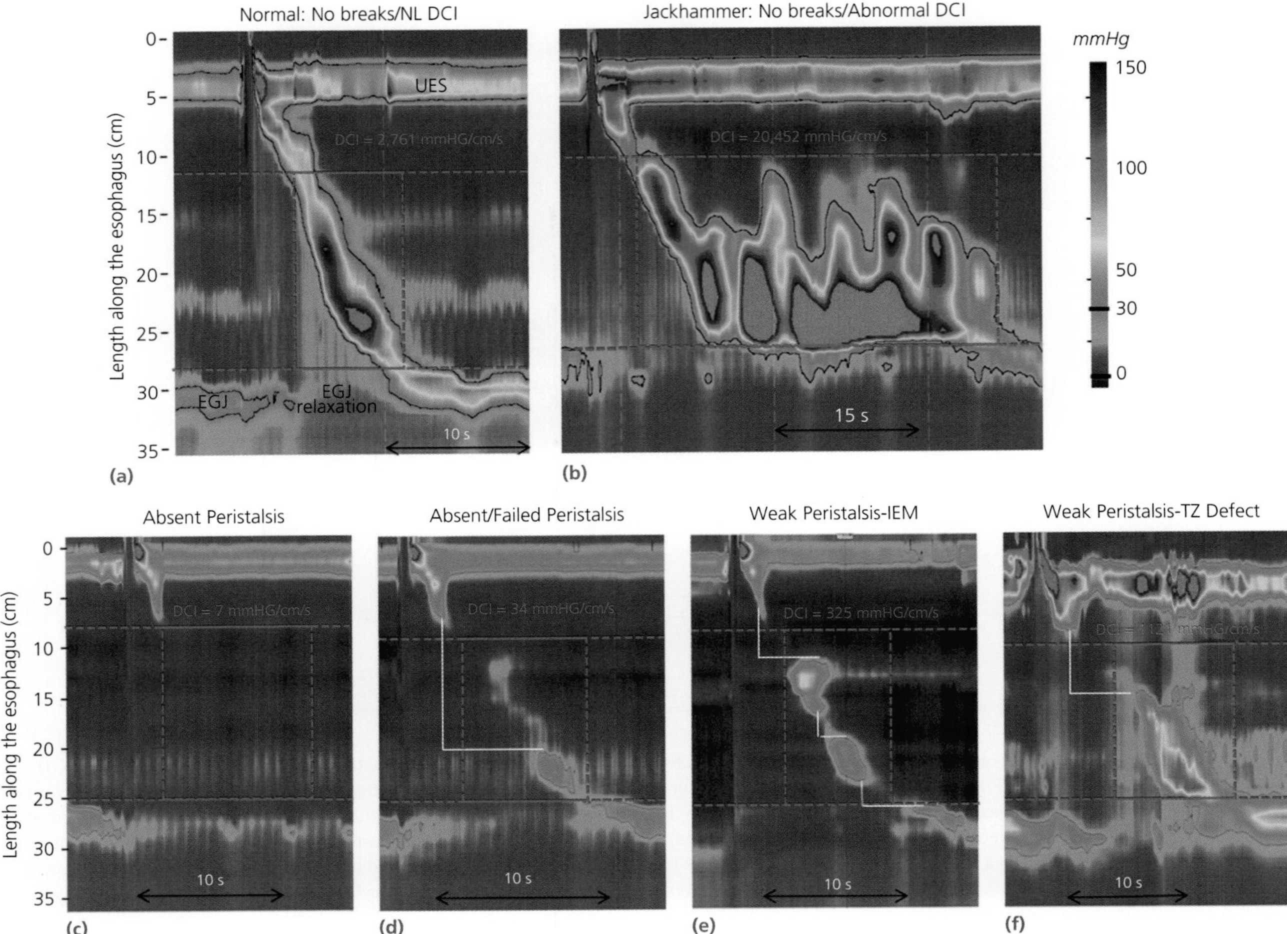

Figure 42.9 The spectrum of postdeglutitive contractile vigor. The distal contractile integral (DCI) space–time box is demarcated by the dashed red lines, with the upper border being the location of the transition zone and the lower border being the upper margin of the esophagogastric junction (EGJ) high-pressure zone. **(a)** A normal swallow with a DCI of 2761 mmHg·s·cm with normal propagation and a single uniform contraction. **(b)** A swallow with a DCI >8000 mmHg·s·cm fulfilling criteria for nutcracker in conventional manometry based on an average peristaltic amplitude >220 mmHg at 3 and 8 cm above the EGJ. This is a hypercontractile pattern classified as "jackhammer" in the Chicago Classification. **(c–e)** Patterns of absent and weak peristalsis in a patient classified as having ineffective esophageal motility (IEM). **(c, d)** Both panels have DCI values <100 mmHg·s·cm indicative of absent or failed peristalsis. **(e)** Panel exhibits a swallow with two defects in the wavefront denoted by the white lines and would qualify as an ineffective swallow with a DCI value <100 mmHg·s·cm. **(f)** A distinct variant of weak peristalsis in which the large isobaric contour break is localized to the transition zone, variably called fragmented peristalsis or a transition zone defect. TZ, transition zone; UES, upper esophageal sphincter. Source: Courtesy of the Esophageal Center at Northwestern University, Chicago, IL, USA.

One report additionally noted ganglion cell degeneration extending into the proximal stomach in half of 34 specimens analyzed [101]. The degree of ganglion cell loss parallels the duration of disease such that ganglion cells are almost absent in patients afflicted for ≥10 years [102]. A morphological study of 42 esophagi resected from patients with advanced achalasia revealed diminished myenteric ganglion cells and inflammation within the myenteric plexus in all cases [103].

The ultimate cause of ganglion cell degeneration in achalasia is unknown; however, there is increasing evidence consistent with an immune-mediated process. Immunohistochemical analysis of the myenteric infiltrate in patients with achalasia revealed that the majority of inflammatory cells are CD3/CD8-positive lymphocytes that express TIA-1 (a 15-kD cytotoxic granule-associated protein expressed in natural killer cells and cytotoxic T lymphocytes), indicating that these cells are either resting or activated cytotoxic T cells [104]. Achalasia may also be associated with degenerative neurological disorders, such as Parkinson disease. Patients with both achalasia and Parkinson disease were noted to have Lewy bodies (intracytoplasmic hyaline or spherical eosinophilic inclusions) in the degenerating ganglion cells of the myenteric plexus [105].

Physiological studies also provide evidence of at least partial postganglionic denervation of esophageal smooth muscle in achalasia. Such damage can potentially affect excitatory (cholinergic) ganglionic neurons, inhibitory (NO with or without VIP)

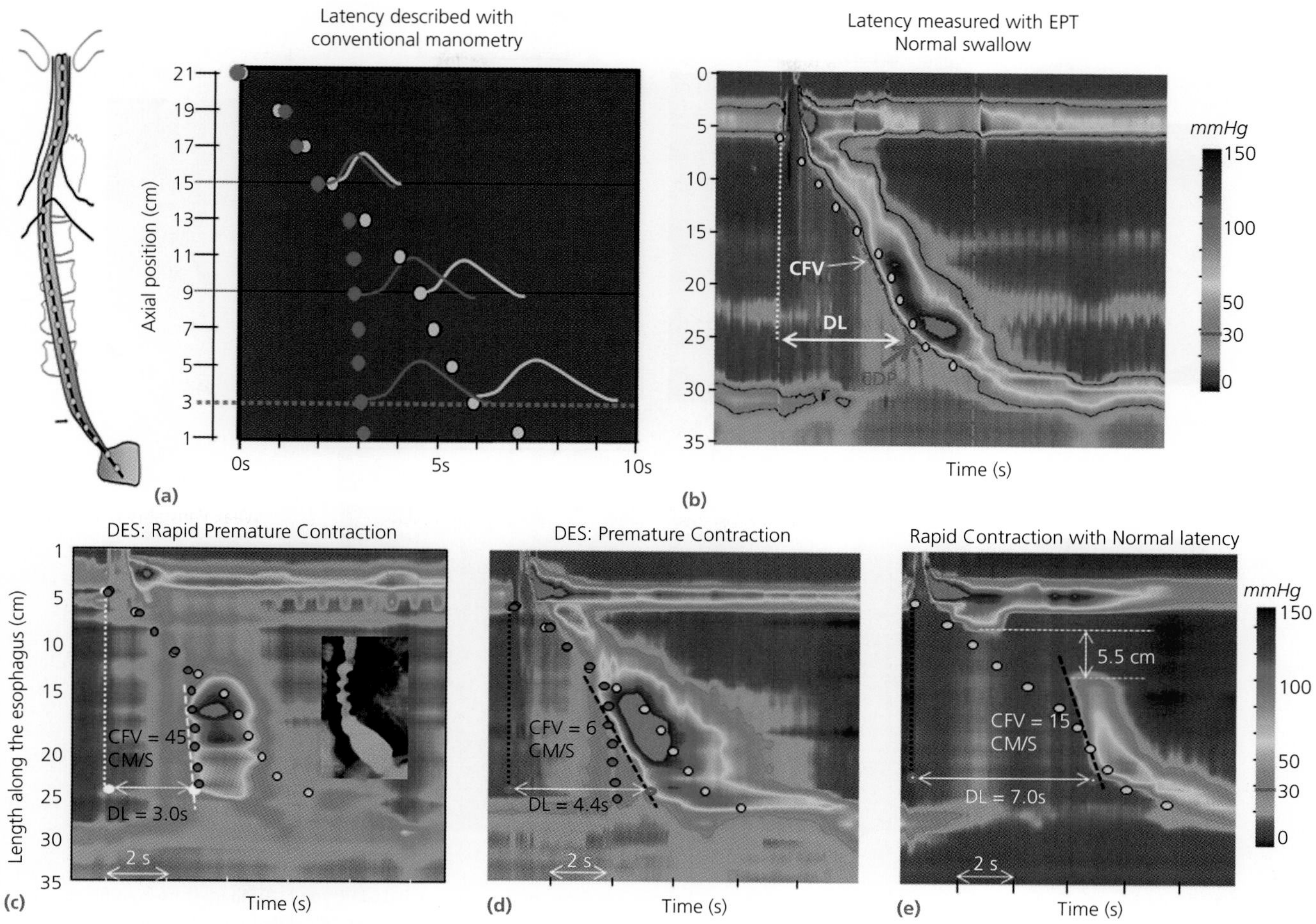

Figure 42.10 The concept of reduced distal latency in spasm as described by Behar and Biancani [196]. **(a)** The latency of propagation for normal subjects (blue circles) and a patient with spasm (red circles). The latency interval was measured as the delay in onset of contraction at sensor 21 relative to sensor 1 suggesting that patients with spasm had an impairment of neural inhibition and premature contraction. **(b)** The latency plots (blue dots) are overlaid on pressure topography of a normal swallow illustrating the metrics used to assess propagation in the Chicago Classification. The contractile front velocity (CFV) is measured along the best tangent extending from the contractile deceleration point (CDP) to the transition zone, thereby focusing on the smooth muscle segments of the esophagus. The distal latency (DL) is a measure of the inhibitory gradient and is measured from the onset of upper esophageal sphincter (UES) relaxation to the CDP. Disorders of propagation are illustrated in **(c)–(e)**. **(c)** Panel represents a patient with diffuse esophageal spasm (DES) with premature contraction characterized by a reduced DL (DL = 3.0 s) and a rapid contraction (45 cm/s). Note that the position of the contractile wavefront closely follows the red dots overlaid from **(a)**. **(d)** Panel represents a patient with reduced latency and a normal contraction velocity. The contractile wavefront approximates the red dots, suggesting that this contraction is premature in the distal esophagus and may be evolving into a spastic pattern. **(e)** Panel represents a patient with normal latency and a rapid propagation velocity. This is an example of weak peristalsis with a large transition zone defect and does not represent impaired neuronal inhibition of the distal esophagus. EPT, esophageal pressure topography. Source: Courtesy of the Esophageal Center at Northwestern University, Chicago, IL, USA.

ganglionic neurons, or both. Consider first the excitatory ganglionic neurons. Muscle strips from the circular layer of the esophageal body of patients with achalasia contract when directly stimulated by acetylcholine but fail to respond to ganglionic stimulation by nicotine, indicating a postganglionic excitatory defect [106]. However, it is likely that loss of excitatory innervation is variable among patients with achalasia. Partial preservation of the postganglionic cholinergic pathway is suggested by the observations that LES pressure in patients with achalasia increases after administration of the acetylcholinesterase inhibitor, edrophonium, and decreases after administration of the muscarinic antagonist, atropine [107]. These observations are crucial to understanding why botulinum toxin may have a therapeutic benefit in achalasia (see later).

Regardless of excitatory ganglionic neuron impairment, it is clear that the inhibitory ganglionic neurons are necessarily impaired as an early manifestation of achalasia. Functionally, these neurons are responsible for deglutitive inhibition (including LES relaxation) and for the timing of propagation of esophageal peristalsis; their absence offers a unifying hypothesis for the key physiological abnormalities of achalasia: impaired LES relaxation and aperistalsis. This is even the case during transient

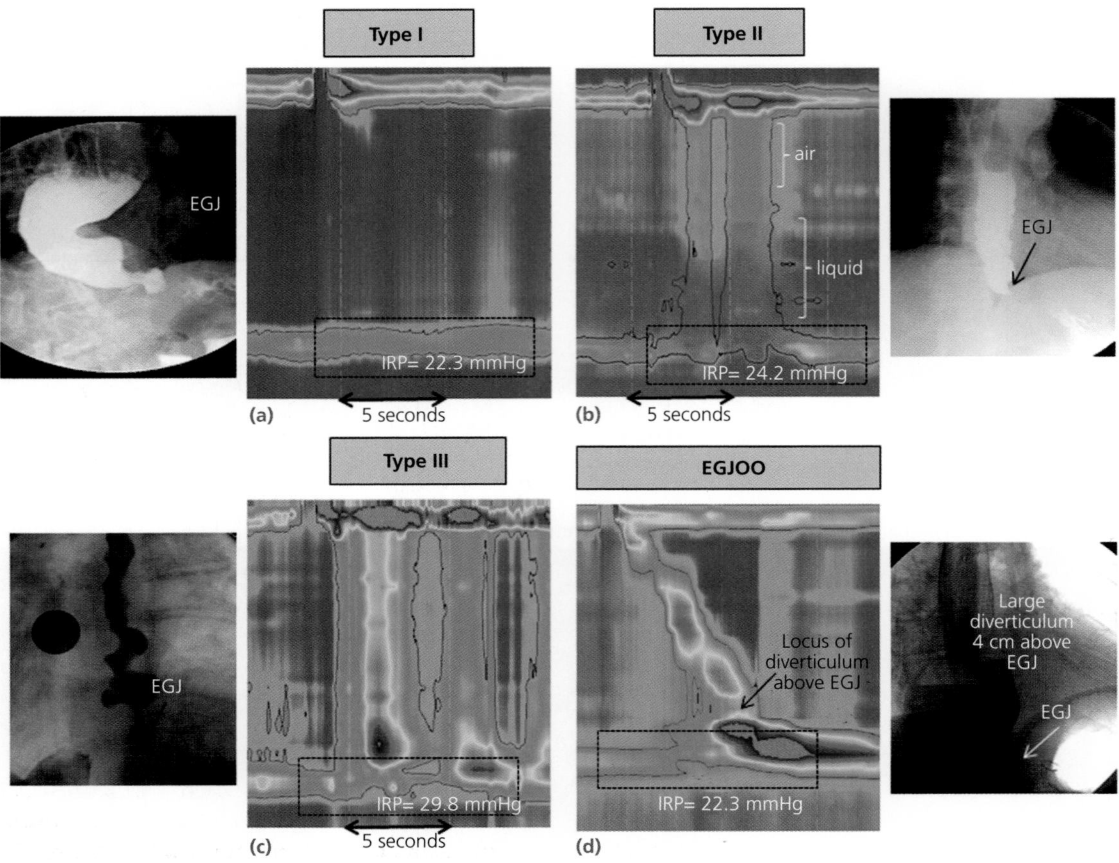

Figure 42.11 Subtypes of achalasia in high-resolution manometry and barium esophagram. In classic achalasia (type I, **a**), there is no significant pressurization within the body of the esophagus and impaired esophagogastric junction (EGJ) relaxation with an integrated relaxation pressure (IRP) of 22.3 mmHg. Patients with type I patterns usually present with esophageal dilatation and poor emptying as evidenced on the esophagram on the left. **(b)** Panel represents a swallow from a patient with type II achalasia exhibiting panesophageal pressurization of the air and fluid column (purple impedance signal = liquid) trapped between the sphincters as the esophagus shortens. The esophagram from this patient is on the right showing only mild esophageal dilatation. **(c)** A pressure topography plot typical of spastic achalasia (type III) achalasia. This is associated with a premature contraction manometrically and abnormal lumen obliterating contractions on the esophagram to the left. **(d)** Panel represents an example of EGJ outflow obstruction wherein the patient exhibits normal propagation of the contractile wavefront with outflow obstruction at the EGJ and a compartmentalized pressurization between the contraction and the wavefront. This patient also had a large diverticulum noted on the esophagram to the right and was eventually treated as an achalasia variant with diverticulectomy and myotomy. Source: Modified from Pandolfino 2008 [129]. Courtesy of the Esophageal Center at Northwestern University, Chicago, IL, USA.

LES relaxations, elegantly demonstrating the selective physiological defect in achalasia. Patients with achalasia can still trigger transient LES relaxations in response to gastric distention and still exhibit the ensuing complex motor pattern of crural diaphragm inhibition, esophageal shortening, and an esophageal after-contraction, but the LES paroxysmally contracts rather than relaxes [108]. Furthermore, patients with achalasia lack NO synthase in the gastroesophageal junction [109], and VIP, which may be a cotransmitter in these neurons, is markedly reduced [110].

Substantial evidence supports impaired function of postganglionic inhibitory innervation in the smooth muscle esophagus of patients with achalasia. Muscle strips from the LES of patients with achalasia do not relax in response to ganglionic stimulation as they do in healthy control subjects [111]. Cholecystokinin octapeptide, which normally stimulates the inhibitory ganglionic neurons, thereby reducing LES pressure, paradoxically increases the LES pressure in patients with achalasia [112]. Impaired inhibitory innervation of the esophagus above the LES is more difficult to demonstrate than within the sphincter itself because of the absence of resting tone in this region. However, Sifrim et al. [113] used an intraesophageal balloon to create a high-pressure zone in the tubular esophagus that then relaxed with the onset of deglutitive inhibition. This deglutitive relaxation in the esophageal body was absent in early, nondilated cases of achalasia.

Clinical presentation

Clinical manifestations of achalasia may include dysphagia, regurgitation, chest pain, weight loss, and aspiration pneumonia. All patients have solid food dysphagia; the majority of patients also have variable degrees of liquid dysphagia. The onset of dysphagia is usually gradual with the duration of symptoms averaging 2 years at presentation [89]. Dysphagia severity fluctuates but eventually plateaus. Predictably, regurgitation occurs when large amounts of food are retained in the dilated esophagus. The regurgitant is often recognized as food that has been eaten hours, or even days, previously. It tends to be nonbilious, nonacid, and mixed with copious amounts of saliva. Chest pain is a frequent complaint early in the course of achalasia occurring in approximately two-thirds of patients [114]. Its etiology is unknown. Treatment of achalasia is less effective in relieving chest pain than it is in relieving dysphagia or regurgitation. However, unlike dysphagia or regurgitation, chest pain may improve or disappear over time [114].

An estimated 10% of patients with achalasia have bronchopulmonary complications from regurgitation [115]. Another interesting, but fortunately rare, symptom of achalasia is airway compromise and stridor as a result of the dilated esophagus compressing the trachea [116]. This is related to dysfunction of the belch reflex either due to neural degeneration or because esophageal dilatation prevents activation of stretch receptors within the esophageal wall [117].

It is paradoxical that many patients with achalasia report heartburn, even after the onset of dysphagia [118]. Although reflux may be a common sequela of the treatments for achalasia, it seems physiologically inconsistent to simultaneously have dysphagia from impaired LES relaxation and reflux from excessive LES relaxation. In support of this skepticism, ambulatory 24-hour esophageal pH studies of patients with achalasia have shown only periods of esophageal acidification caused by the bacterial fermentation of retained food in the esophagus rather than discrete gastroesophageal reflux events [119]. Furthermore, prolonged LES recordings have shown nearly a complete absence of normal transient LES relaxations in patients with achalasia [120]. However, there are occasional exceptions to this, evident from a well-documented case of a patient with achalasia with intact transient LES relaxation despite the absence of deglutitive LES relaxation [121].

Radiography

The characteristic barium swallow x-ray of achalasia is of a dilated intrathoracic esophagus with impaired emptying, an air–fluid level, absence of a gastric air bubble, and an LES that tapers to a point giving the distal esophagus a beaklike appearance (see Figure 42.11). Occasionally, an epiphrenic diverticulum, immediately proximal to the LES, is observed [122]. With longstanding achalasia, the esophagus may assume a sigmoid configuration, and in some instances an air–fluid level, mediastinal widening, and outline of the dilated esophageal wall are even evident on a plain chest film. Note that the characteristic radiographic findings depend on esophageal dilatation. Because dilatation is not always present in achalasia, the sensitivity of the radiographic examination is limited and esophagrams may be unrevealing in up to one-third of patients [123].

Manometry

Manometry is crucial in the diagnosis of achalasia. Because there is no specific serum biomarker or histological correlate for the diagnosis of achalasia, the finding of aperistalsis and incomplete LES relaxation without evidence of a mechanical obstruction solidifies the diagnosis of achalasia [124]. In HRM, the diagnostic criteria are an IRP >15 mmHg and absent peristalsis (see Figure 42.7). Other findings, such as an increased basal LES pressure, an elevated baseline esophageal body pressure, and simultaneous nonpropagating contractions, may also support the diagnosis of achalasia; however, these are not requirements for the diagnosis [125].

Before the introduction of HRM and EPT, there were no data substantiating the prognostic value of conventional manometric measures in achalasia. Although there were qualitative descriptions of variants, such as vigorous achalasia [126], achalasia with preserved peristalsis [121,127], and cases with complete or partial LES relaxation [128], there were no established conventions for making these measurements. However, with the adoption of HRM with EPT, three distinct subtypes of achalasia were quantitatively defined using novel EPT metrics (see Figure 42.11) [129]. Furthermore, there are now five publications supporting the prognostic value of these achalasia subtypes consistently observing that: (1) type II patients have the best prognosis with myotomy or pneumatic dilation; (2) the treatment response of type I patients is less robust (and reduced further as the degree of esophageal dilatation increases); and (3) type III patients have a worse prognosis, likely because the associated spasm is less likely to respond to therapies directed at the LES [129–133]. In addition, patients with impaired EGJ relaxation but some preserved peristalsis (see Figure 42.11) are now recognized as a distinct entity that can be a variant phenotype of achalasia. These findings have led to the demise of the term "vigorous" achalasia because the entity is now subdivided into more discrete subtypes that highlight their unique pathophysiology and the heterogeneity of the previous classification.

Endoscopic findings

Endoscopy is relatively insensitive in the detection of achalasia, with endoscopists prospectively suggesting the correct diagnosis in less than one-third of patients [123]. Typical endoscopic findings include retained food or saliva, dilatation, and atony of the esophageal body. With progressive dilatation and stasis, erythema, friability, and superficial ulcerations may be seen. Whitish plaque covering the epithelial surface may be seen as the result of *Candida* overgrowth; this is usually asymptomatic. The achalasic LES has a constricted, pinpoint appearance and does not open with air insufflation. Nonetheless, the instrument should pass easily through the sphincter into the stomach with minimal pressure. Resistance, or a feeling of stiffness as the endoscope crosses the gastroesophageal junction, should raise the suspicion of a stricture or malignancy (see later *Pseudoachalasia* section). Equivocal mucosal abnormalities of the gastroesophageal junction, evident on forward viewing or retroflexed inspection, should always undergo a biopsy because of the possibility of pseudoachalasia. The motor pattern typical of achalasia may also be encountered in the context of a mechanical obstruction at the EGJ, and endoscopy should be done to rule out stenosis, infiltrative processes, or extrinsic compression.

Differential diagnosis

The differential diagnosis of achalasia includes both other esophageal motility disorders with functional attributes overlapping those of achalasia and diseases of distinct pathophysiology that duplicate the functional consequences of achalasia. With respect to other motility disorders, there are many similarities between esophageal spasm and type III (spastic) achalasia. In fact, the only distinction between these entities is the demonstration of incomplete LES relaxation in achalasia. Thus, it has been speculated that, in some instances, esophageal spasm may represent an early stage of achalasia and may evolve into full-fledged achalasia. Vantrappen et al. [134] first proposed this relationship and reported several cases demonstrating just such an evolution. However, as will become evident later in this chapter, spastic disorders of the esophagus are a heterogeneous lot, and only a small minority, at best, are part of the continuum with achalasia.

Variants of achalasia have also been described. Cases of normal or complete LES relaxation have been described [121,127,128,135], and differentiating these patients from absent peristalsis, as can be seen with reflux disease or collagen vascular disease or distal esophageal spasm, can be difficult. A timed barium esophagram may be extremely useful to help differentiate absent peristalsis from achalasia. Furthermore, there have been descriptions of achalasia variants presenting with propagating contractions, which could represent either early achalasia or a subclinical mechanical obstruction at the EGJ [127,136]. These patients require further evaluation with imaging to rule out mechanical causes for EGJOO because these disorders can present as pseudoachalasia (Figure 42.12).

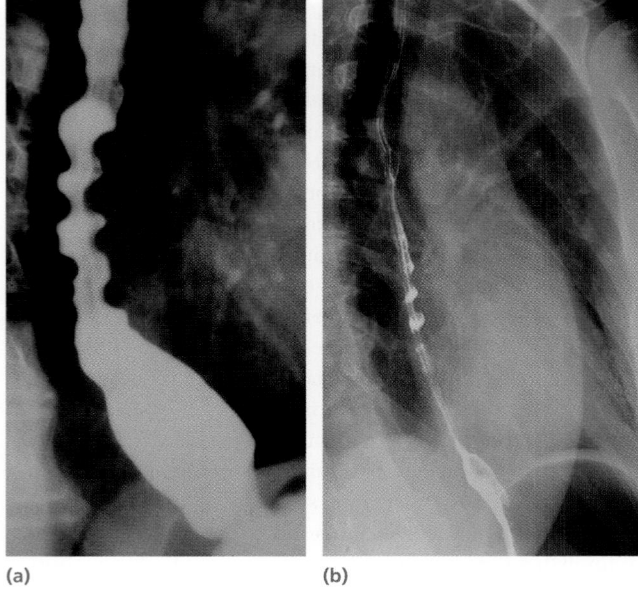

Figure 42.12 Corkscrew esophagus **(a)** and rosary bead esophagus **(b)** on barium x-ray in two patients with symptomatic diffuse esophageal spasm **(a)** and jackhammer esophagus **(b)**. Source: Courtesy John Pandolfino.

Chagas disease

Achalasia can be closely mimicked by esophageal involvement in Chagas disease, which is endemic in areas of central Brazil, Venezuela, and northern Argentina. Chagas disease is spread by the bite of the reduvid (kissing) bug that transmits the culprit protozoan, *Trypanosoma cruzi*. After infection, an acute septicemic phase of the illness develops that varies in severity from being so mild as to go unnoticed to being so severe as to be fatal [137]. The chronic phase of the disease develops many years after infection and results from destruction of autonomic ganglion cells throughout the body, including the heart, gut, urinary tract, and respiratory tract. Chronic cardiomyopathy with conduction system disturbances and arrhythmias is the most common cause of death. The digestive tract organs most often affected are the esophagus, duodenum, and colon. The severity of esophageal dysfunction is directly proportional to the degree of intramural ganglion cell loss; abnormal peristalsis is first detectable after 50% of ganglion cells are destroyed and esophageal dilatation only after 90% are destroyed [137]. Paralleling this, the initial dysfunction is confined to the esophageal body, with LES dysfunction occurring late in the course of the disease [137]. The most useful clinical distinction between idiopathic achalasia and esophageal involvement in Chagas disease is evidence of other tubular organ involvement (megaureter, cardiomyopathy, megaduodenum, megacolon, megarectum) in the latter. Otherwise, patients with Chagas disease have the same clinical, radiographic, and manometric characteristics as idiopathic achalasia. The diagnosis of Chagas disease is confirmed by a serological test using complement fixation or polymerase chain reaction. The treatment of the achalasia syndrome in Chagas disease is similar to that for idiopathic achalasia. Treatment of the infection itself is of limited efficacy in the acute phase of the disease and of no proven efficacy with chronic disease.

Pseudoachalasia

Neither the radiographic nor the manometric features of achalasia are specific for idiopathic achalasia; tumor-related pseudoachalasia accounts for up to 5% of cases with manometrically defined achalasia. Pseudoachalasia is more likely with progressive age (>50 years), abrupt onset of symptoms (<1 year), and early weight loss in excess of 7 kg [89,138]. Tumor infiltration (especially carcinoma in the gastric fundus) can completely mimic the functional impairment seen with idiopathic achalasia [139] (see Table 42.2). It is because of this potential pitfall that a thorough anatomic examination including endoscopy should be done as part of the diagnostic evaluation of every new case of achalasia. A clue to the presence of pseudoachalasia on the endoscopic examination is of more than slight resistance of passage of the endoscope across the gastroesophageal junction. In idiopathic achalasia, the endoscope should pop through with only gentle pressure required. If suspicion of pseudoachalasia persists, endoscopic biopsy, computerized tomography, magnetic resonance imaging, or endoscopic ultrasound should be considered for further evaluation, depending on the special circumstances.

Adenocarcinoma of the gastroesophageal junction accounts for more than half of pseudoachalasia cases, with a myriad of tumors and miscellaneous conditions accounting for the remainder. Within the spectrum of malignancies, pancreatic, oat cell, hepatoma, bronchogenic, esophageal squamous cell, prostate, and lymphoma cases have been reported [89]. These tumors produce an achalasia syndrome by infiltrating the wall of the esophagus at the gastroesophageal junction, in essence causing a malignant obstruction at the LES with proximal esophageal dilatation [139]. Similarly, pseudoachalasia has also been reported to result from esophageal infiltration by amyloid [140], eosinophilic gastroenteritis [141], and sarcoidosis [142]. Although often speculated in the literature, it is less certain, and certainly much less common, that an achalasia-like syndrome occurs as a paraneoplastic syndrome without direct tumor stenosis of the gastroesophageal junction [89]. This syndrome is most commonly associated with small cell lung cancer with production of type I anti-neuronal nuclear (anti-Hu) antibodies [143].

Postfundoplication

Postfundoplication dysphagia is common in the early postoperative period, and patients are often advised to consume soft diets for the first 2–4 weeks. Dysphagia that persists longer than 2–4 weeks should be evaluated with an upper endoscopy or barium esophagram to assess the integrity of the wrap and evaluate for possible paraesophageal hernia. Subjects without an overt mechanical disruption should be evaluated with manometry to assess peristalsis, LES pressure, and LES relaxation to determine whether the wrap is too tight or an underlying motility disorder, such as achalasia, exists. Diagnosing achalasia in the context of fundoplication is difficult because the manometric findings can be quite similar with both entities: aperistalsis and impaired LES relaxation. To distinguish mechanical obstruction as a result of a tight wrap or tight crural repair from a functional obstruction related to achalasia, one can administer amyl nitrite during manometry and observe the effect on the EGJ high-pressure zone. The mechanical effect of a tight fundoplication should be less affected by the smooth muscle relaxing effects of the amyl nitrite than the hypertensive sphincter of a patient with achalasia [144].

Management

Because the underlying neuropathology cannot be corrected, treatment of achalasia is directed at compensating for the functional abnormalities and preventing complications. The main functional abnormality is poor esophageal emptying, and reducing the LES pressure treats this. With a reduced LES pressure, gravity promotes esophageal emptying. LES pressure can be reduced by pharmacological therapy, forceful dilation, or surgical myotomy. Pharmacological treatments, on the whole, are not very effective, perhaps more indicated as temporizing maneuvers than definitive therapies. The definitive treatment of achalasia is still disruption of the LES either surgically (Heller myotomy), endoscopically (per oral endoscopic myotomy), or with a pneumatic dilator. The optimal approach is an issue of debate, and each therapy will be reviewed to highlight its pros and cons.

Pharmacological therapy

Smooth muscle relaxants, such as nitrates or calcium channel blockers, administered sublingually immediately before eating may offer partial relief of the dysphagia accompanying achalasia by reducing the resting sphincter pressure. Amyl nitrite [145], sublingual nitroglycerin [146], theophylline [146], and β_2-adrenergic agonists [146] have also been tried with variable results. The greatest reported experience has been with isosorbide dinitrate and nifedipine [147]. Isosorbide dinitrate, 5–10 mg sublingual before meals, reduces the resting LES pressure by 66% for 90 minutes, with clinical efficacy paralleling the magnitude of LES response [148]. A 19-month trial of this therapy has been reported to provide marked or complete relief of dysphagia [148]. Side-effects, particularly headache, are common. Placebo-controlled trials have not been reported.

Calcium channel blockers (diltiazem, nifedipine, verapamil) reduce the LES pressure by 30–40% for more than an hour with potential benefit in achalasia [148,149]. The greatest clinical experience has been with nifedipine that can be administered 10–30 mg sublingual (capsules are crushed in the mouth) 30–45 minutes before meals. The benefit of nifedipine, 30–40 mg sublingual per day, was assessed in a group of 29 patients with early achalasia (before esophageal dilatation) in a placebo-controlled trial. Nifedipine was significantly better that placebo (which had no significant benefit), yielding good to excellent results in 70% of patients with achalasia followed for 6–18 months [147]. However, subsequent placebo-controlled crossover trials have found only minimal clinical improvement with nifedipine [150]. Limiting side-effects of nifedipine use are flushing, dizziness, headache, peripheral edema, and orthostasis.

Sildenafil is another smooth muscle relaxant that has been shown to decrease the LES pressure and deglutitive relaxation pressure in patients with achalasia by blocking phosphodiesterase type 5, the enzyme that destroys cyclic guanosine monophosphate induced by NO. A double-blind placebo-controlled trial revealed that 50 mg sildenafil caused a significant decrease in LES pressure and relaxation pressure when compared with placebo [151]. The effect peaked at 15–20 minutes after administration and persisted for less than 1 hour. This approach may be reasonable in poor surgical candidates or as a temporizing treatment for those awaiting definitive therapy with pneumatic dilation or surgery.

Botulinum toxin injection

Pasricha et al. [152] first reported the effects of botulinum toxin on the LES in patients with achalasia in 1994. He found that intrasphincteric injection of botulinum toxin decreased LES pressure by 33% and improved dysphagia in 66% of patients for a 6-month period. Botulinum toxin works by irreversibly inhibiting the release of acetylcholine from presynaptic terminals, effectively eliminating the neurogenic component of LES pressure. However, because this effect is eventually reversed by the growth of new axons, the effect of botulinum toxin is not long-lasting. Although most patients initially experience a good response, there is minimal continued efficacy at 1 year [85,153–155]. Doses greater than 100 units have not been shown to be more effective [156]. Studies comparing botulinum toxin with pneumatic dilation suggest that the added expense for repeated injection outweighs the potential economic benefits of the added safety, unless life expectancy is 2 years or less [157]. Thus, this therapeutic option should be mainly reserved for elderly or frail individuals who are poor risks for more definitive treatments.

Pneumatic dilation

Therapeutic dilation for achalasia requires the forceful distension of the LES to a diameter of 3–4 cm to partially disrupt the sphincter and effect lasting reduction of LES pressure. Dilation with an endoscope or with standard bougies (up to 60 F) provides very temporary benefit at best. Only balloon dilators specifically designed to treat achalasia achieve adequate diameter for lasting effectiveness. The basic element of an achalasia dilator is a long, noncompliant, cylindrical balloon that can be positioned fluoroscopically (Rigiflex dilator) or endoscopically (Witzel dilator) across the LES and then inflated in a controlled fashion.

The technique of pneumatic dilation is variable among practitioners in terms of patient preparation, parameters of balloon inflation, and postdilation monitoring. There is general agreement that pneumatic dilation can be done in an outpatient with moderate sedation. In patients with substantial esophageal retention, it is useful to have them on a liquid diet for 1 or more days before the procedure. Reported balloon inflation pressures range from 360 mmHg (7 psi) to 775 mmHg (15 psi), with periods of inflation ranging from several seconds to 5 minutes [158]. Although there is minimal methodological consistency among authors, a cautious approach of beginning with relatively low inflation pressures and/or smaller diameter dilator (3.0 cm) is fairly universal.

The major complication of pneumatic dilation is esophageal perforation; mortality is rare [159]. Although the reported incidence rate of perforation from pneumatic dilation ranges from 0% to 16% [115,158], a systematic review on the topic concluded that the risk was less than 1% when using a modern technique, comparable with the risk for unrecognized perforation during Heller myotomy [160]. Because most perforations are readily evident within a few hours of the procedure, patients should be observed closely for signs of an esophageal leak for 2–6 hours after pneumatic dilation. If a perforation appears small and confined, or intramural, conservative management consisting of close observation, endoscopically clipping the defect closed if feasible, maintaining the patient NPO (nil per os), and administering intravenous antibiotics is appropriate [115]. If any substantial perforation has occurred, or if worsening pain and fever occur during observation of what was thought to be a small perforation, surgical repair should be pursued quickly. Patients with perforation from pneumatic dilation that is recognized and promptly treated surgically (within 6–8 hours) have outcomes that are comparable with those of patients undergoing elective Heller myotomy [161].

Studies using pneumatic dilation as the initial treatment of achalasia have reported excellent long-term symptom control. However, a third of patients will relapse in 4–6 years and may require repeat dilation. Response to therapy may be related to preprocedural clinical parameters, such as age (favorable if age > 45 years), sex (female > male) [162], esophageal diameter (inversely related to response), and achalasia type (type II better than I and III) [129,132]. Although surgical myotomy has a greater response rate than a single pneumatic dilation, it appears that a strategy using a series of dilations with the potential for repeat is comparable with surgery and a reasonable alternative to surgery. A randomized controlled trial compared this type of graded strategy with surgical myotomy and found it to be noninferior in efficacy [163]. It is unclear, however, what additional clinical, radiological, endoscopic, or manometric parameters are predictive of response [164].

Heller myotomy

Surgical series of patients with achalasia treated with myotomy report good to excellent results in 62–100% of patients, with persistent dysphagia troubling fewer than 10% of patients overall [85]. The appeal of myotomy is that it offers a more predictable method of reducing LES pressure than does pneumatic dilatation [165]. Recent studies suggest that laparoscopic and thoracoscopic approaches are associated with similar efficacy and reduced morbidity when compared with myotomy via thoracotomy or laparotomy [85,166–170]. Patti et al. [168] reported the clinical outcomes of 168 patients with achalasia who underwent thoracoscopic myotomy (35 patients) or laparoscopic Heller myotomy accompanied by a partial fundoplication (133 patients). There were no deaths in this series, and only eight patients required reoperation. Relief of dysphagia was obtained in 93% of the patients who underwent the laparoscopic Heller myotomy and 85% of those treated with thoracoscopic myotomy. Not only did the laparoscopic approach more effectively improve dysphagia, it was associated with shorter hospital stay and less postoperative gastroesophageal reflux. Historically, postmyotomy reflux in patients with achalasia could be particularly severe [171]. However, with the availability of proton pump inhibitors, reflux is usually well controlled, making these complications unlikely. Thus, laparoscopic Heller myotomy combined with a partial fundoplication has become the preferred surgical procedure for achalasia.

Occasionally, patients do not respond to dilation and myotomy and require more extensive surgical procedures. In extremely advanced or refractory cases of achalasia, esophageal resection with gastric pull-up or interposition of a segment of transverse colon or small bowel may be the only surgical option [172,173]. Indications for this intervention include unresolvable obstructive symptoms, cancer, development of an esophageal sump, recurrent aspiration, and perforation during dilation. Although excellent long-term functional results can be achieved, the reported mortality rate of this surgery is about 4%, consistent with the mortality rate of esophagectomy done for other indications.

Peroral endoscopic myotomy

In 2010, Inoue et al. [174] published the first series of patients successfully undergoing peroral endoscopic myotomy (POEM). Since this time, more than 300 articles have been published on the use of POEM, and it is accepted as a first-line treatment for achalasia in published guidelines [175]. A metaanalysis of 9 studies with 272 patients with achalasia demonstrated successful performance of POEM in 99.3% and 90.0% after prior myotomy [176]. The principle of POEM technique is creation of a submucosal tunnel in the mid to lower esophagus that is extended on to the gastric cardia. In this third space, the circular (and incidentally, the longitudinal) layers of the muscularis propria are divided, and the mucosal entry point is clipped closed. Although there is some controversy on the ideal length of myotomy to be performed and whether to use an anterior or posterior approach, there is no question of the effectiveness of this procedure. In two randomized multicenter trials comparing POEM with pneumatic dilation [177] and laparoscopic Heller myotomy [178], at 2-year follow-up, POEM demonstrated equal or superior efficacy to both procedures. The main complication of POEM is GERD with reported erosive esophagitis in up to 57% of patients [178]. More severe complications may include complications of mucosal perforation, including pneumomediastinum, but in a large metaanalysis, all complications related to the procedure were managed conservatively using endoscopic clipping, suturing, or hemostasis interventions [179]. What the precise indication for POEM will be in choosing it over pneumatic dilation or laparoscopic myotomy is unclear, but at this time it is offered as an acceptable alternative first-line therapy [179].

Risk for squamous cell cancer

Numerous series report cases of squamous cell carcinoma developing in the achalasic esophagus [180,181], and the relative risk of development of squamous cell cancer has been estimated to be 30-fold relative to the nonachalasia population [182,183]. The pathogenesis of the carcinoma is obscure, but stasis and mucosal inflammation associated with sigmoid deformation of the esophagus [184] may be precipitating factors. The tumors develop many years after the diagnosis of achalasia. Because the tumors often arise in a greatly dilated esophagus, symptoms can be delayed, and the neoplasms are large and advanced at the time of detection. These considerations raise the issue of surveillance endoscopy in patients with achalasia to detect early squamous cell cancer. However, an elegant analysis by Sandler et al. [185] of a database encompassing the entire Swedish population of 1062 patients with achalasia suggests that, after discounting incident carcinomas, the overall squamous cell cancer risk for patients with achalasia compared with age-matched control subjects is 17-fold, resulting in a 0.15% incidence rate of cancer among the patients with achalasia. Consequently, the latest American Society of Gastrointestinal Endoscopy guidelines do not advocate endoscopic surveillance for patients with achalasia [186]. If screening is elected, the use of Lugol's iodine as a vital stain may improve detection [187].

Spastic disorders

The concept of "esophageal spasm" is credited to Hamilton Osgood based on his 1889 description of six patients with episodic chest pain and dysphagia: "sudden and often intense constriction in the epigastrium . . . with an arrest of food at the cardiac orifice." From the time of that report until the present day, further insight into the entity of esophageal spasm has paralleled the development of imaging or measurement technology that might detect it. "Diffuse spasm of the lower part of the esophagus" was first described radiographically in 1934, and the first manometric descriptions of spasm came in the late 1950s. Introduction of the term *diffuse esophageal spasm* (DES) and our present concept of this entity followed Fleshler's 1967 description of a "clinical syndrome characterized by symptoms of substernal distress or dysphagia or both, the roentgenographic appearance of localized, non-progressive waves (tertiary contractions), and an increased incidence of non-peristaltic contractions recorded by intraluminal manometry" [188].

The esophagus of the patient with DES usually retains its ability to propagate normal primary peristaltic waves the majority of the time, suggesting that the responsible neuromuscular pathology must be subtler than with achalasia. Partly because of this fact, the criteria for diagnosing DES (which is the best accepted of proposed disorders of peristalsis) have been variable and confusing [189]. Furthermore, along with the evolution of manometric techniques came the description of minor aberrations of peristalsis (nutcracker esophagus, hypertensive LES, and nonspecific esophageal motor disorders) to which symptomatology, especially chest pain, might be attributed [190]. Despite this proliferation of literature, whether these entities have any clinical significance remains doubtful.

The heterogeneity among patients, the absence of specific pathology, and the absence of well-defined clinical implications caution against considering them akin to achalasia.

Neuromuscular pathology

Patients with spastic disorders of the esophagus rarely undergo esophageal surgery and the diseases are not fatal, making for a paucity of pathological specimens. The most striking reported pathological change is diffuse muscular hypertrophy or hyperplasia, mainly of the distal two-thirds of the esophagus. Little evidence of neuropathology has been reported [191]. Muscular thickening of up to 2 cm has been reported in patients with clinical and manometric evidence of DES [192,193]. However, there are other well-documented cases of spasm in which esophageal muscular thickening was not found at thoracotomy [194] and still other instances of patients with muscular thickening not associated with DES symptoms [195].

Pathophysiology of spastic disorders

Experimental evidence suggests heterogeneity among patients with spastic disorders such that some primarily exhibit a defect of inhibitory myenteric plexus interneuron function, while in others the defect is of excess excitation, now called *hypercontractility*. Two experiments implicate a defect of myenteric plexus inhibitory interneuron function in the genesis of simultaneous contractions in the distal esophagus. Behar and Biancani [196] timed the propagation of a swallow-induced contraction in healthy subjects and in a group of patients whose dominant manometric abnormality was of a simultaneous contraction in the distal 10 cm of esophagus. Figure 42.10 illustrates the key finding of that work. Note that within the proximal (striated muscle) esophagus the two groups exhibited similar contraction propagation, consistent with this timing being the result of the sequenced activation of motor units by vagal efferents programmed within the medullary swallowing center. However, once entering the smooth muscle segment, the patients' contractions diverged from those of the healthy subjects, resulting in a simultaneous contraction in the distal esophagus. The duration and amplitude of contraction at each esophageal locus was normal, but the progressive delay of initiation of that contraction, a function attributable to increasing influence of inhibitory interneurons in the distal esophagus, was absent. Furthermore, if these individuals swallowed twice within a 5-second interval, there was no deglutitive inhibition of the first peristaltic contraction within the smooth muscle esophagus as is observed in healthy individuals. Another experiment demonstrating impaired deglutitive inhibition in DES comes from work using an artificial high-pressure zone within the distal esophagus. Patients with motor disorders characterized by rapidly propagating or simultaneous contractions exhibited only partial relaxation of the artificial high-pressure zone, proportional to the impairment of propagation velocity [113]. Taken together, these findings strongly suggest that one neuropathological process in DES is a selective, intermittent dysfunction of myenteric plexus inhibitory interneurons.

The manometric feature that best equates with impaired deglutitive inhibition, DL, has become the main manometric feature for diagnosing DES in HRM. A recent study assessing patients defined as having spastic peristaltic contractions using conventional definitions focused on peristaltic velocity >8 cm/s suggested that many patients defined with distal esophageal spasm using pressure tracing analysis would be categorized as normal or having weak peristalsis on EPT [197]. When criteria incorporated a surrogate measure of latency defined by the time duration between the onset of UES relaxation and the CDP, it became apparent that most patients labeled with spasm did not have abnormal latency, and that spasm was indeed a rare entity (2.2%).

Epidemiology

No population-based studies exist on the incidence or prevalence of esophageal motility disorders other than achalasia. Thus, the only way to estimate the incidence or prevalence of spastic disorders is to examine data on populations at risk and reference the observed frequency of spastic disorders to the incidence of achalasia, which, as detailed earlier, is 2–3 per 100 000 population. Populations at risk for motility disorders are patients with chest pain and/or dysphagia, so it is among these patients that extensive manometric data have been collected. As detailed in Table 42.4, summarizing representative studies of at least 30 subjects, manometric abnormalities are prevalent among these groups [180,190,198–207]. Asymptomatic volunteers (usually younger than the patients) were evaluated to define normal values in five of these studies [180,206–209]. The manometric pattern of achalasia was not detected in any volunteer. Similarly, although DES is more variably defined than is achalasia [189], simultaneous contractions after ≥30% of swallows were not found in any volunteer [206].

Clinical presentation

Dysphagia for both liquids and solids is reported by 30–60% of patients with spastic disorders [200,210]. Dysphagia is usually intermittent in occurrence, sometimes related to swallowing specific substances or liquids at extreme temperature. Dysphagia is usually not progressive, and weight loss is rare. In some instances, spasm patients experience episodes of esophageal obstruction while eating that persists until relieved by emesis; these instances are probably related to premature prolonged contractions typical of DES. More commonly, the dysphagia reported by patients with spastic disorders does not prevent or prolong eating.

Intermittent substernal chest pain is reported by 80–90% of patients with spastic disorders [200,210]. Esophageal chest pain is very similar to angina; it is usually described as crushing or squeezing in character, often radiating to the neck, jaw, arms, or midline of the back. Pain episodes may last from minutes to hours, but swallowing is usually not impaired during these episodes. Severe

Table 42.4 Manometric abnormalities in patients with chest pain/dysphagia.

Study population	n [reference]	Achalasia	DES	Hypercontractile esophagus
Unselected manometry patients	202 [201]	2%	2%	—[a]
	1013 [206]	6.4%	5%	31%
	429 [207]	13%	4.6%	10%
	1070 [197,231]	—	2.2%	4.1%[b]
Chest pain with a negative cardiac evaluation	112 [180]	12%	10%	12%
	34 [208]	0%	0%	29%
	910 [200]	0.05%	3%	13%
	100 [214]	0%	4%	6%
	100 [205]	0%	2%	21%
	44 [202]	0%	0%	14%
Patients with dysphagia as the principal symptom	251 [200]	19%	7%	5%

[a] Data not provided.
[b] Jackhammer.
DES, diffuse esophageal spasm.

pain episodes may require narcotics or nitroglycerin for relief, further confusing the distinction between esophageal and cardiac pain. The mechanism producing pain is poorly understood; transient ischemia, luminal distension, and altered visceral sensitivity have all been hypothesized [211–213]. More likely, the mechanism responsible for esophageal pain is variable among individuals.

Radiographic and manometric findings

Spastic motor disorders of the esophagus have no pathognomonic endoscopic features. However, endoscopy is useful in the evaluation of patients with dysphagia or suspected esophageal pain to identify either structural lesions or reflux esophagitis. Radiographically, a corkscrew esophagus, rosary bead esophagus, pseudodiverticula, or curling are indicative of DES (see Figure 42.12). It must be emphasized, however, that tertiary contractions (nonperistaltic, simultaneous esophageal contractions) on radiographs are not pathognomonic of esophageal spasm because this may be seen in asymptomatic individuals [190].

The manometric feature universal among proposed classification schemes for DES is the occurrence of simultaneous contractions using normative values of peristaltic velocity as the distinguishing feature of spasm [125,189]. However, the conceptual paradigm of defining a simultaneous contraction based purely on velocity has been challenged and revised to incorporate the measurement of DL with EPT. A recent investigation using a cut-off of 4.5 seconds for DL based on normative data suggests that spastic contractions are rare and when present are more likely to represent type III achalasia. The majority of patients with a classification of rapid contraction based only on velocity are found to have normal peristalsis or weak peristalsis with a focal segment of rapid contraction when analyzed in pressure topography (see Figure 42.10). Hence these findings are characterized as peristaltic abnormalities in the Chicago Classification.

Differential diagnosis

Esophageal dysmotility is not life-threatening as is angina pectoris, the pain of which it can closely mimic. Features suggesting an esophageal causative factor include: (1) pain that is nonexertional and prolonged; (2) pain that interrupts sleep; (3) pain that is meal related; (4) pain relieved with antacids; and (5) the presence of additional esophageal symptoms of heartburn, dysphagia, or regurgitation. However, each of these characteristics still exhibits overlap with cardiac pain in some instances. Thus, an esophageal etiology of chest pain should be considered only after careful consideration and evaluation of potential cardiopulmonary causative factors have been addressed. Furthermore, even within the spectrum of esophageal diseases, neither chest pain nor dysphagia is specific for a spastic disorder because both symptoms are also characteristic of common esophageal disorders, including peptic or infectious esophagitis [214]. Only after these more common diagnostic possibilities have been excluded by appropriate radiographic evaluation, endoscopic evaluation, and in some instances, a therapeutic trial of antisecretory medications should spastic disorders be considered as the cause of the still-unexplained symptoms.

Treatment

There is a paucity of data on the medical treatment of esophageal spasm. Long-term outcome studies of the medical treatment of DES with smooth muscle relaxants are not available. Nitrates [215], calcium channel blockers [216], and hydralazine [217] have all been shown to be beneficial in small trials. In addition, botulinum toxin injected at the EGJ has also been used with some success in patients with nonachalasia esophageal spasm [218]. The only double-blind placebo-controlled trial showing efficacy with medical therapy was in the case of the anxiolytic trazodone, suggesting that reassurance and control of anxiety are important therapeutic goals [219]. Consistent with this conclusion, successful management of symptoms associated with spastic motility disorders has also been reported using behavioral modification programs and biofeedback [220].

Although the rationale is unclear, esophageal dilation with standard bougie dilators has also been suggested as a therapy for dysphagia or chest pain in patients with spastic disorders. However, in the only controlled trial of this therapy, dilation with an 8-mm ("placebo") dilator was as effective as an 18-mm dilator in producing transient symptom relief [221]. Alternatively, pneumatic dilation has been used in patients with DES with severe dysphagia [115,222]. In one practitioner's experience, 45% of patients with DES noted relief, compared with 80% of patients with achalasia [115]. In another series of nine patients with DES and LES dysfunction, dysphagia, but not chest pain, was improved during 37 months of observation [222]. However, it is not clear what distinguishes that group of patients from patients with spastic achalasia, implying that patients likely to derive benefit from pneumatic dilation are those with mixed features of achalasia and DES (type III achalasia) as described by Vantrappen et al. [134]. If dysphagia becomes so severe that weight loss is observed or if pain becomes unbearable, surgical therapy consisting of a Heller myotomy across the LES with proximal extension of the incision to include the involved area of spasm can be considered [223,224]. However, there are no controlled studies of this treatment in patients with well-defined DES, and the indication for this procedure is extremely rare.

In summary, at this point in time the therapy of esophageal spastic disorders is poorly defined. Clearly, most esophageal pain is attributable to reflux, irrespective of the presence or absence of minor motility abnormalities, and antireflux therapy should be extensively pursued before attempting therapy of a spastic disorder. Interestingly, DES most likely responds to specific therapy when it exhibits characteristics indicative of type III achalasia, implying that it is part of a pathophysiological continuum in these cases (see Figure 42.11).

Hypercontractility

Dysfunction of the excitatory ganglionic neurons, or abnormal excitability of the muscle itself, may lead to exaggerated peristaltic contractions. Several lines of evidence suggest instances of excess excitation in response to hormonal or cholinergic stimulation. Representative of such an abnormality is a second group of patients in the analysis of Behar and Biancani [196] whose main manometric abnormality was of frequent spontaneous distal esophageal contractions. These patients had normal propagation latency as defined by the parameters illustrated in Figure 42.10, but a significantly longer and higher amplitude contraction at each locus within the smooth muscle [196]. Examining the categorization of disorders of peristalsis outlined in Table 42.4, these individuals would be labeled hypertensive esophagus or potentially hypercontractile (jackhammer) esophagus if the contractile activity exceeded the level that can be seen in asymptomatic controls. Patients with peristaltic disorders characterized by excess excitation demonstrate heightened sensitivity to stimulation with cholinergic agents [225,226], the cholinesterase inhibitor edrophonium [227], pentagastrin [228], and ergonovine [229]. An additional stimulus for hypercontractility is EGJOO, and this should be carefully considered [230].

Epidemiology

As detailed in Table 42.4, the prevalence of nutcracker esophagus is much greater than that of achalasia or distal esophageal spasm when the primary symptom is chest pain. However, the prevalence of nutcracker esophagus is much less likely in the context of a primary referral for dysphagia when compared with achalasia and DES. A more recent large series found the prevalence rate of hypercontractility (jackhammer) to be 4.1% among 1070 consecutive patients.

Clinical presentation

Symptoms of hypercontractile disorders are chest pain and dysphagia, but there is also a strong overlap with GERD symptoms [231]. Dysphagia is less constant than with achalasia (see Table 42.4) [211]. Similar to DES, the pain with hypercontractile disorders can be described as angina-like, occurring intermittently, and correlating poorly with the occurrence of manometric abnormalities or meals.

Radiographic and manometric findings

Bolus transit is normal with the hypercontractile disorders, and radiographic findings are minimal. Hence hypercontractility is defined manometrically by vigorous peristaltic contractions. High-amplitude peristaltic contractions in the esophagus were first described by Brand et al. [232] in 1977, but the term "nutcracker esophagus" was coined by Benjamin et al. [233] in 1979 in a study linking patients with noncardiac chest pain and high-amplitude peristalsis. Subsequently, Richter et al. [234] suggested a value 2 standard deviations greater than the mean based on a manometric dataset of 95 healthy control subjects and proposed a cut-off of 180 mmHg. However, subsequent analyses have repeatedly demonstrated that poor correlations exist between symptom severity and the degree of manometric abnormality [219,235–237]. Using early versions of the Chicago Classification criteria, hypertensive peristalsis (nutcracker esophagus) was defined as a mean DCI between 5000 and 8000 mmHg·s·cm. This was considered a borderline abnormality, the clinical significance of which is unclear because there is still overlap with control subjects. Consequently, it was abandoned in version 3 of the Chicago Classification. However, if two test swallows exhibit a DCI >8000 mmHg·s·cm, the study qualifies as esophageal hypercontractility (jackhammer esophagus) because this magnitude of contraction is not encountered in healthy subjects.

Treatment

The approach to the patient with a jackhammer pattern is to rule out esophageal obstruction and then to focus on the hypercontractility.

However, data are sparse regarding treatments aimed at attenuating the contractility. A treatment trial in an undifferentiated group of patients with hypertensive peristalsis using nifedipine demonstrated that significant reduction of wave amplitude in patients with nutcracker esophagus was not accompanied by a significant improvement in chest pain [236]. Another controlled trial with diltiazem demonstrated an association of symptomatic and manometric improvement, but the correlation for individual subjects was not reported [205].

Alternatively, treatment for GERD and visceral hypersensitivity may be helpful in patients with noncardiac chest pain. The overlap of nutcracker and GERD supports this concept. A controlled trial of trazodone produced significant symptomatic improvement without a change in manometric findings [219]. In summary, although the extreme phenotype of hypercontractility (jackhammer) is usually indicative of either obstruction or a primary motility disorder, the intermediate phenotype (nutcracker) is of less clear significance, potentially indicative of GERD, hypersensitivity, or even a normal finding.

Esophagogastric junction outflow obstruction

EGJOO is defined in the Chicago Classification by an elevated median IRP with intact or weak peristalsis, thus not meeting the criteria for achalasia [238]. Clinically, this is a heterogenous disorder and often an incidental finding. Studies have shown that patients without dysphagia in whom manometry was performed for another indication can exhibit this pattern [239]. Furthermore, some patients may have resolution of dysphagia without treatment directed at this manometric abnormality [239,240] or have normal findings when tested with functional luminal imaging probe panometry, an investigational alternative to HRM [241]. When EGJOO is pathological, it may be associated with either a mechanical or motility causative factor. For example, esophageal strictures or processes leading to extrinsic compression of the LES, such as fundoplication, may be associated with an EGJOO pattern [242,243]. Pathological findings in EGJOO may include loss of ganglion cells and interstitial cells of Cajal similar to idiopathic achalasia [100,244]. This pattern has also been associated with chronic opioid use [245]. The use of cross-sectional imaging studies to assess for an intramural or extrinsic lesion at the gastroesophageal junction is controversial [240,243,246] and should be used selectively. Treatment is directed at the underlying etiology. When idiopathic EGJOO is suspected to be an early or evolving case of achalasia, a timed barium swallow may be helpful in assessing the need for therapeutic intervention [247]. If the patient's symptoms are determined to result from EGJOO, injection of botulinum toxin [248], pneumatic dilation [249], laparoscopic myotomy [250], and POEM [251] have all been demonstrated to be effective in anecdotal reports or nonrandomized studies.

Hypocontractile motility

At the extreme end of hypocontractility is absent peristalsis. Less extreme is a more common finding, previously defined as ineffective esophageal motility (IEM). The etiology and pathology of these disorders is either idiopathic or secondary to medications, collagen vascular diseases (particularly scleroderma), or infiltrative diseases such as amyloidosis. The entire spectrum of hypocontractility is common with GERD.

The efficacy of peristalsis in terms of bolus clearance is inversely related to peristaltic amplitude such that emptying becomes progressively impaired with amplitudes ≤30 mmHg [63]. However, the description of hypotensive or weak peristalsis has subsequently been refined to incorporate the segmental architecture of peristalsis elegantly revealed by topographic analysis [61,82,252]. As might be predicted from this architecture, hypocontractility becomes most evident at the pressure troughs, which are also the loci of impaired bolus transit. However, the pressure thresholds required for bolus clearance are not uniform along the esophagus and become incrementally greater distally to traverse the EGJ.

Radiographic and manometric findings

Given that the primary abnormality of hypocontractility is poor esophageal clearance and a lack of peristalsis, radiographic and manometric detection hinge on these findings. Spechler and Castell [125] classified a group of hypocontractile disorders as IEM. Criteria for ineffective swallows were any combination of: (1) distal peristaltic wave amplitude ≤30 mmHg; (2) simultaneous contractions with amplitudes ≤30 mmHg; (3) failed peristalsis (the peristaltic wave does not traverse the entire length of the distal esophagus); or (4) absent peristalsis. HRM with EPT allows for a more complete characterization of hypomotility disorders (see Figure 42.9). Studies using EPT and intraluminal impedance have demonstrated that breaks in the 20 mmHg isobaric contour plot that are >2 cm may be associated with impaired bolus clearance, validating this measure as indicative of a weak contraction [253,254]. The Chicago Classification subdivides hypocontractile disorders into "absent peristalsis," "IEM" (>50% of swallows with DCI <450 mmHg·s·cm), and "fragmented peristalsis" (>50% fragmented contractions (large breaks) with DCI >450 mmHg·s·cm) [255]. A comparison of EPT characteristics of 75 healthy subjects and 113 patients with nonobstructive dysphagia demonstrated that weak peristalsis with peristaltic breaks, but not failed peristalsis, were more common in the patients than the control subjects [254]. However, these findings were seen in only about a third of the patients and were also occasionally present in the healthy control subjects.

Treatment

Treatment options for the hypocontractile disorders are limited because promotility drugs have minimal effects on augmenting peristalsis. Hence therapy is directed at reducing or treating secondary causes, such as medications that interfere with peristalsis, or treating underlying disorders including GERD. However, there are no controlled data substantiating that treating GERD will improve peristalsis. Avoiding caustic medications and using liquid formulations may reduce pill esophagitis, and diet modification is paramount.

Esophageal involvement in systemic disease

Esophageal dysmotility occurs as a manifestation of several disease processes with the potential to affect smooth muscle or the autonomic nervous system. The following discussion focuses on esophageal involvement in the collagen vascular diseases and diabetes.

Scleroderma

Scleroderma causes diffuse fibrosis and degenerative changes in the skin and synovium with the potential to involve the heart, kidneys, lungs, intestines, and esophagus. Caucasian women between 30 and 50 years of age are the most commonly afflicted. Two forms of scleroderma are recognized: progressive systemic sclerosis with diffuse scleroderma (the more fulminant form with early involvement of internal organs) and the CREST syndrome (calcinosis, Raynaud phenomenon, esophageal dysfunction, sclerodactyly, telangiectasia). The basic disease process is of smooth muscle atrophy with subsequent fibrosis. With either form of scleroderma, the esophagus is involved in 75–85% of cases [256,257]. Pathological changes are confined to the smooth muscle portion of the esophagus resulting in aperistalsis and atony of the LES [258].

The main clinical manifestations of scleroderma esophagus are dysphagia and heartburn. Symptomatic patients usually have Raynaud phenomenon, but the severity of the esophageal disease does not covary with the disease severity in other organs [259]. The prevalence rate of erosive esophagitis may be as high as 60%, with reported cases of Barrett metaplasia and Barrett adenocarcinoma [260,261]. Dysphagia may be attributable to poor peristalsis or to a stricture complicating the peptic esophagitis (seen in as many as a third of patients) [261]. Radiographic findings typically consist of a slightly dilated aperistaltic esophagus and free reflux. Wide-mouth diverticula of the esophagus, similar to those described in intestines, have also been seen [257]. Manometric abnormalities consist of a hypotensive or absent LES pressure, hypotensive to absent distal esophageal peristalsis, and normal proximal esophageal peristalsis [256]. There is no specific treatment for the esophageal involvement in scleroderma. Gastroesophageal reflux should be identified and treated commensurate with its severity.

Other collagen vascular and connective tissue diseases

Esophageal symptoms are uncommon in systemic lupus erythematosus, although 25–35% of unselected patients have the manometric findings of hypotensive peristalsis and a hypotensive LES [262]. Mixed connective tissue disease exhibits a mixture of clinical features found in scleroderma, polymyositis, and systemic lupus erythematosus and is characterized by high titers of a circulating antibody for a nuclear ribonucleoprotein antigen. More than 60% of patients with mixed connective tissue disease have esophageal involvement defined by cineradiography [263] and up to 82% of patients have manometric findings [262]. Abnormalities of both smooth and skeletal muscle are found. In the largest report to date, 5 of 17 patients had a manometric pattern consistent with scleroderma, and 10 patients had aperistalsis of the entire esophageal body, along with low pressures in both the upper and lower sphincters [262].

Diabetes mellitus

More than 60% of patients with diabetes with peripheral or autonomic neuropathy and an occasional patient without neuropathy have esophageal manometric abnormalities [264]. Reported manometric abnormalities associated with diabetes include hypotensive peristalsis, frequent failed peristalsis, hypotensive LES with impaired deglutitive relaxation, simultaneous contractions, and repetitive contractions [264,265]. The significance of these abnormalities is uncertain because most of these patients are asymptomatic [264]. Histological and pharmacological studies suggest that the esophageal abnormalities are secondary to the degenerative effects of diabetes mellitus on the autonomic nervous system, rather than smooth muscle dysfunction.

References are available at www.yamadagastro.com/textbook7e

Further reading

Boeckxstaens G.E., Annese V., des Varannes S.B., et al. Pneumatic dilation versus laparoscopic Heller's myotomy for idiopathic achalasia. N Engl J Med 2011;364(19):1807.

Cook I.J., Kahrilas P.J. AGA technical review on management of oropharyngeal dysphagia. Gastroenterology 1999;116(2):455.

Crespin O.M., Liu L.W.C., Parmar A., et al. Safety and efficacy of POEM for treatment of achalasia: a systematic review of the literature. Surg Endosc 2017;31(5):2187.

Kahrilas P.J., Bredenoord A.J., Fox M., et al. The Chicago Classification of esophageal motility disorders, v3.0. Neurogastroenterol Motil 2015;27(2):160.

Ponds F.A., Fockens P., Lei A., et al. Effect of peroral endoscopic myotomy vs pneumatic dilation on symptom severity and treatment outcomes among treatment-naive patients with achalasia: a randomized clinical trial. JAMA 2019;322(2):134.

CHAPTER 43

Gastroesophageal reflux disease

Sabine Roman[1], John E. Pandolfino[2], and Peter J. Kahrilas[2]
[1]Digestive Physiology, Lyon I University, Lyon, France
[2]Department of Medicine, Northwestern University Medical School, Chicago, IL, USA

Chapter menu

Definitions and epidemiology

Gastroesophageal reflux is the retrograde movement of gastric content into the esophagus. This physiological phenomenon becomes a disease when it is associated with symptoms of sufficient intensity to impair one's quality of life or with peptic esophagitis. The most typical symptoms of gastroesophageal reflux disease (GERD) are heartburn and regurgitation, but additional esophageal symptoms, such as dysphagia and chest pain, are also common. Finally, extradigestive or atypical symptoms such as cough and laryngitis are often associated with GERD. Typical reflux symptoms are quite prevalent in western countries with 8–28% of individuals having self-reported heartburn [1].

In attempting to be comprehensive in scope, the Montreal Definition of GERD included a number of subgroups within the universe of GERD [2]. Among the "esophageal complications," *reflux esophagitis* is the most common injury, evident by mucosal breaks, or erosions, in the esophageal mucosa. With diminishing frequency, Barrett metaplasia, peptic stricture, and esophageal adenocarcinoma may also complicate GERD. Another disease subgroup in the Montreal Definition, nonerosive reflux disease (NERD), exhibits no esophageal mucosal injury but has GERD defined solely on the basis of typical esophageal symptoms that are of sufficient frequency and/or severity to impair their quality of life.

It has become increasingly clear in recent years that the NERD group is quite heterogeneous. In the Rome IV Classification, three NERD subgroups were proposed: (1) "true NERD" with abnormal esophageal acid exposure on pH-metry and strong correlation between symptoms and gastroesophageal reflux events during reflux monitoring; (2) "reflux hypersensitivity" characterized by normal esophageal acid exposure but strong correlation between symptoms and gastroesophageal reflux events during reflux monitoring; and (3) "functional heartburn" with normal esophageal acid exposure time (AET), absence of symptom-reflux association, and an unsatisfactory response to a proton pump inhibitor (PPI) trial [3]. However, the boundaries between these definitions have varied with time and with iterations of the Rome Classification.

The difficulty of quantifying GERD epidemiology is evident from the Diamond study, conducted in primary care practices in Europe and Canada [4]. A total of 308 patients with upper gastrointestinal (GI) symptoms underwent a comprehensive evaluation with endoscopy, pH-metry, a trial of PPI therapy, structured interviews by physicians, and the Gastroesophageal Reflux Disease Questionnaire to evaluate the diagnostic utility of each for GERD. Not surprisingly, there was substantial disagreement among assessments. Among patients with physiologically defined GERD (116 [38%] with esophagitis and 87 [28%] with abnormal pH-metry), only 49% identified heartburn or regurgitation as their most troublesome symptom. Response to

Yamada's Textbook of Gastroenterology, Seventh Edition. Edited by Timothy C. Wang, Michael Camilleri, Benjamin Lebwohl, Anna S. Lok, William J. Sandborn, Kenneth K. Wang, and Gary D. Wu.

Companion website: www.yamadagastro.com/textbook7e

a 2-week PPI trial was equally ambiguous; a positive response to PPI was observed in 69% of patients with physiologically defined GERD and in 51% of those with negative endoscopy and pH-metry [5]. However, a positive PPI response was significantly more frequent in patients with esophagitis (57%) than in patients with NERD (49%) or patients without physiologically defined GERD (35%, $p = 0.002$). Hence in evaluating the GERD epidemiology data summarized as items a–h in the following list, these pitfalls need to be acknowledged. There has been little consistency in how GERD has been defined among epidemiology studies and over time.

a. Sex: GERD is equally prevalent among male and female individuals [6], but there is a male preponderance of esophagitis (2:1 to 3:1) and of Barrett metaplasia (10:1) [7].
b. Age: The incidence of GERD increases with age; in a systematic review of the UK General Practice Research Database, El-Serag et al. [8] noted that the incidence of GERD was greatest in the 60–69 year range and decreased slightly thereafter.
c. Pregnancy: Pregnancy is associated with the highest incidence of GERD such that half to two-thirds of pregnant women experience typical GERD symptoms [9–11].
d. Geographic variation: GERD prevalence is greater in western countries (10–20%) than in Asia (5–7%) [1]. However, this variation is likely attributable to several factors [12]. The understanding of "heartburn" is not uniform across languages and, in fact, there is no translation for "heartburn" in most Asian languages [13]. There are also substantial differences in diagnostic practices and physician reporting among cultures.
e. Lifestyle, environmental factors, and genetic predisposition: These may influence GERD prevalence among geographic regions.
f. Obesity: In western countries, the increased prevalence of GERD has occurred in parallel with the dramatic increase in obesity [14]. Studies have consistently reported an association between higher body mass index (BMI) and GERD [15–19] such that both obesity (BMI > 30 kg/m^2) and overweight (BMI = 25–30 kg/m^2) are associated with GERD [8,20,21]. Barrett esophagus is also significantly associated with overweight (odds ratio [OR], 1.33; 95% confidence intervals (CIs): 1.07–1.64) and obesity (OR, 1.70; 95% CI: 1.36–2.12) [22].
g. *Helicobacter pylori:* The role of *H. pylori* in GERD merits special attention. As the prevalence of *H. pylori* has decreased, the prevalence of GERD has increased [23]. However, there are conflicting data concerning the influence of *H. pylori* and the effect of eradication of *H. pylori* on GERD. In a metaanalysis of 20 case–control studies, the average prevalence of *H. pylori* infection in patients with GERD was 38.2% (95% CI: 20.0–82.0%) compared with 49.5% (95% CI: 29.0–75.6%) in non-GERD patients (OR, 0.58) [24]. In a systematic review of studies and trials extending up to September 2003, the same author concluded that successful eradication of *H. pylori* in patients with duodenal ulcer disease did not increase the risk for provoking *de novo* esophagitis [25]. The heterogeneous observations regarding the relationship between GERD and *H. pylori* are likely related to the variable effect of *H. pylori* on acid gastric secretion. In patients with *H. pylori*-induced corpus gastritis, acid secretion is reduced, which would tend to reduce GERD symptoms [26], whereas acid secretion is increased in patients with duodenal ulcer disease, which would tend to increase GERD symptoms [27]. *H. pylori* strains and the genetic backgrounds of patients may also influence effects on acid secretion [28].
h. Medications: Several medications (nitrates, calcium channel blockers, anticholinergics, α-adrenergic agonists, theophylline, morphine, benzodiazepines, and sumatriptan) have been reported to promote GERD occurrence [29,30], presumably by reducing lower esophageal sphincter (LES) pressure. Nonsteroidal antiinflammatory drugs are also associated with GERD [15,16,18,31,32], postulated to act by reducing the mucosal protective mechanisms against reflux.

Histopathology of esophagitis

The esophagus is lined with noncornified stratified squamous epithelium. The basal cell layer is predominantly composed of cells with a high nuclear-to-cytoplasm ratio and is the site of cellular proliferation, generally accounting for <15% of the total epithelial thickness. At the squamocolumnar junction (SCJ), the basal cell layer is in continuity with the columnar cells of the stomach [33]. Toward the luminal surface of the squamous epithelium, the basal cell layer ends abruptly in continuity with the stratified squamous cells. The prickle cell layer, adjacent to the basal cell layer, has prominent intercellular bridges. The squamous cells show progressive flattening and nuclear elongation as they migrate toward the surface. Papillae containing thin-walled blood vessels (analogous to the dermal pegs of the skin) indent the overlying squamous mucosa. The length of these papillae is normally less than two-thirds of the overall thickness of the epithelium.

Reflux content (acid, pepsin, and bile acids) is toxic for esophageal mucosa. Mucosal damage identified as distal esophageal mucosal breaks on endoscopy are encountered in 20–40% of patients with GERD symptoms [34–36]. In these cases, histological findings include severe epithelial injury with neutrophilic and eosinophilic infiltration. These changes are confined to the mucosa, lamina propria, and muscularis mucosa. The process of healing esophagitis might lead to complications, such as peptic stricture, Barrett metaplasia, and inflammatory polyps.

Interestingly, a prospective study demonstrated that in patients with severe reflux esophagitis that had been successfully healed with PPI therapy, stopping the PPI medication was associated with T-lymphocyte-predominant esophageal inflammation, along with basal cell and papillary hyperplasia before any loss of surface cells [37]. These data strongly suggest that reflux esophagitis may be cytokine-mediated inflammation beginning at the basal cell layer and progressing to erosion rather than the result of chemical injury working from the surface downward.

Patients with GERD also have microscopic changes in the distal esophageal epithelium without endoscopically evident esophagitis. These changes include elongation of the papillae, proliferation of basal cells, and dilated intercellular spaces within the squamous epithelium [38]. In a review on microscopic esophageal mucosal injury in NERD, Dent [39] emphasized that dilatation of intercellular spaces was the most consistent mucosal change, with the mean intercellular space separation in patients with NERD being at least twice that of controls. Consistent with this, dilated intercellular spaces were observed in 76% of patients with abnormal pH-metry compared with 15% of controls [40]. Based on the literature review of Dent [39], basal hyperplasia and papillary elongation were more frequently encountered in patients with abnormal esophageal acid exposure than in control subjects. These histological changes reversed with acid-suppressive therapy. Importantly, these findings are not encountered more frequently in patients with functional heartburn than in control subjects [41].

Eosinophilic inflammation also can occur in GERD [38,41]. Eosinophils have been demonstrated in the distal esophagus in 69% of patients with esophagitis and 34% of patients with abnormal esophageal acid exposure [38]. Eosinophilic inflammation is important in view of the recent recognition of eosinophilic esophagitis (EoE) as a seemingly distinct disorder. Some authors have suggested that eosinophils in the proximal esophagus are more suggestive of EoE than GERD. However, current consensus recommendations on EoE did not restrict the diagnosis of EoE to proximal eosinophilic inflammation [42]. Clearly an overlap exists between EoE and GERD, and EoE that responds to PPI therapy has also been convincingly demonstrated, even in the absence of physiologically defined GERD [43]. However, the lack of response to PPI therapy is no longer a diagnostic criterion for EoE. Rather, PPIs are now considered an effective treatment for some patients with EoE [44].

In addition to histological examinations of esophageal biopsies, advanced endoscopic techniques have been applied to characterize esophagitis using narrow band imaging, magnification and high-resolution endoscopy, chromoendoscopy, and confocal endomicroscopy. For example, using narrow band imaging, Sharma et al. [45] reported intrapapillary capillary loops and microerosions of the esophagus in patients with GERD with very good intraobserver agreement. Similarly, using confocal laser endomicroscopy, patients with NERD had more intrapapillary capillary loops per image than did controls [46]. Moreover, the diameter of intrapapillary capillary loops and intercellular spaces of squamous cells were greater in patients with GERD than in control subjects.

Pathogenesis

GERD pathogenesis has been studied extensively, primarily with respect to mechanisms promoting esophageal symptoms and injury. The fundamental abnormality is excessive exposure of esophageal mucosa to gastric contents, but this is a multifactorial process. Some degree of gastroesophageal reflux is asymptomatic and "normal," but by definition, GERD occurs when reflux elicits tissue injury or troublesome symptoms. This can occur for a multitude of reasons, including an excessive number of reflux events, prolonged mucosal exposure to reflux, impaired mucosal integrity, or hypersensitivity.

Mechanisms of reflux

The reflux of gastric content into the esophagus is normally prevented by the esophagogastric junction (EGJ), making the anatomical and functional integrity of the EGJ essential. Three dominant, although sometimes overlapping, mechanisms of EGJ incompetence have been observed: (1) anatomic distortion of the EGJ, including hiatal hernia; (2) hypotensive LES; and (3) transient LES relaxations (tLESRs). The latter two mechanisms can occur with or without anatomical abnormalities. Reflux mechanisms can differ from one patient to another. Furthermore, even for a given individual, one mechanism might dominate in specific circumstances. For example, a hypotensive LES or hiatal hernia might be of primary importance during recumbency and tLESR-dominant in the upright position.

The esophagogastric junction, hiatus hernia, and other anatomic variables

Fundamental elements of the EGJ are the LES, the crural diaphragm (CD), and the phrenoesophageal ligament attaching the esophagus to the diaphragmatic hiatus [47]. 3D-high-resolution manometry (HRM) is a new technology that facilitates a detailed analysis of EGJ pressure components (Figure 43.1). Evident in Figure 43.1, EGJ pressure is both radially and axially asymmetrical with the maximal EGJ pressure centered at the apex of the hiatus corresponding to the contact point of the CD and localized 1–2 cm above the SCJ [48]. This pressure asymmetry persists throughout the respiratory cycle, albeit being greatest at inspiration because of diaphragmatic contraction. Using this device, it becomes evident that much of the intraluminal pressure previously attributed to the LES is actually attributable to the CD or local vascular structures (e.g., heart, aorta) such that the length of intrinsic sphincter pressure is only 2.0–2.5 cm [49]. Furthermore, contrary to what has been previously proposed regarding the sphincteric contribution of clasp and sling fibers of the gastric cardia musculature [50], the SCJ closely approximates the distal limit of this circumferential intrinsic sphincter zone.

Supportive of its role as an extrinsic component of the EGJ, independent control of the CD can be demonstrated during esophageal distension, vomiting, and belching when electrical

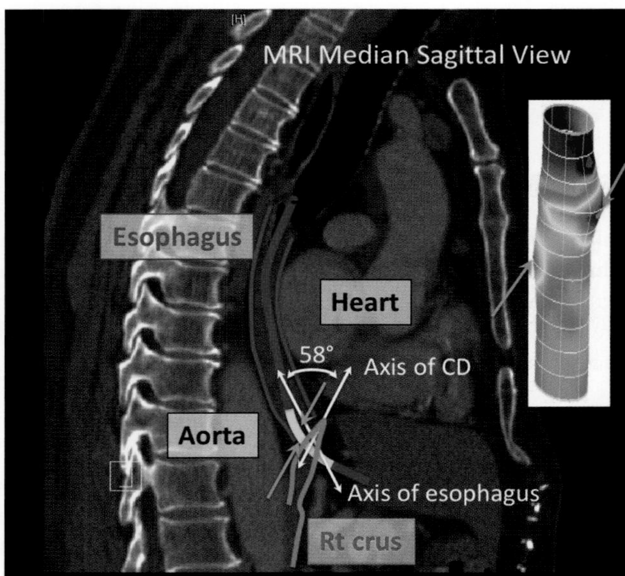

Figure 43.1 Midsagittal magnetic resonance image (MRI) highlighting the esophagogastric junction (EGJ) with the 3D high-resolution manometry device placed within the lumen of the esophagus. Note the characteristic bend imposed on the catheter as it traverses the EGJ. The crural diaphragm (CD) is outlined in orange, while the esophagus is outlined in green. Note that the axis of the crural diaphragm is not perpendicular to the axis of the esophagus and that its 3D pressure signature (cylindrical insert) is reflective of this. The insert, taken at peak inspiration, shows the crural diaphragm apex signal largely restricted to the anterolateral walls of the EGJ. Source: Figure used with permission from the Esophageal Center at Northwestern. Copyright Northwestern University Press.

activity in the CD is selectively inhibited despite continued respiration [51]. This reflex inhibition of CD activity is eliminated with vagotomy. In contrast, CD contraction is augmented during abdominal compression, straining, or coughing [52]. Additional evidence of the sphincteric function of the CD comes from manometric recordings in patients after distal esophagectomy [53]. These patients continued to exhibit an EGJ pressure of about 6 mmHg within the hiatal canal despite having sustained surgical removal of the LES.

The clinical significance of the CD component of the EGJ pertains to a condition potentially associated with its anatomic disruption: hiatus hernia. The impact of hiatus hernia was demonstrated in studies in which the susceptibility to gastroesophageal reflux elicited by straining maneuvers was tested in individuals with and without hiatus hernia. Of several physiological and anatomical variables tested, the size of hiatus hernia had the greatest correlation with the susceptibility to strain-induced reflux [54]. The implication of this observation is that patients with hiatus hernia exhibit progressive impairment of the diaphragmatic component of the EGJ proportional to the extent of upward herniation of the proximal stomach.

Another way to assess the respective roles of LES and CD is with HRM. This technique combines closely spaced pressure sensors and esophageal pressure topography plots, permitting a dynamic representation of EGJ pressure [55]. Hence it is possible to isolate the CD contraction from LES pressure in the inspiratory phase and to differentiate EGJ pressure morphology into three subtypes according to the separation between CD and LES [56]. EGJ type I exhibits no discernible separation between LES and CD, EGJ type II is characterized by a separation of 1–2 cm, and type III by a separation greater than 2 cm (Figure 43.2). Type III EGJ pressure morphology is the manometric criterion for hiatal hernia. Bredenoord et al. [57] reported that the occurrence of acid and weakly acid reflux events was favored by separation between the LES and CD on HRM, and in individuals in whom that separation was intermittent, reflux was more likely during periods of separation. The importance of separation between the CD and LES was also evident in a series of 75 control subjects and 156 patients with suspected GERD wherein Pandolfino et al. [56] showed that the separation was greater in patients with esophagitis compared with control subjects or patients with NERD. Moreover, patients with GERD had significantly less inspiratory augmentation of EGJ pressure (an indicator of CD function) than control subjects or patients without abnormal esophageal pH-metry. Using a multivariate logistic regression model that simultaneously examined expiratory LES pressure, LES-CD separation, and inspiratory EGJ augmentation, while controlling for age and BMI, only inspiration augmentation had a significant independent association with GERD.

Another important physiological variable relevant to reflux is EGJ compliance, the diameter to which the relaxed EGJ opens in response to intraluminal pressure. Although difficult to quantify, this is a measure of laxity within the diaphragmatic hiatus, which determines the diameter to which the EGJ opens following relaxation. The significance of compliance is that the flow rate of refluxed fluid from the stomach into the esophagus is proportional to the EGJ opening diameter to the fourth power. This is consistent with Poiseuille's law for laminar flow. Compliance can be measured by distending the EGJ at controlled pressures and measuring the resultant diameter. Initially this was done using an infinitely compliant balloon kept under constant pressure, called a barostat [58,59]; more recently it has been done with a functional luminal imaging probe [60] to demonstrate that there is a progressive increase in EGJ compliance comparing healthy control subjects with patients with GERD without hiatus hernia and with patients with GERD with hiatus hernia [59]. With all other variables held constant, this change of EGJ compliance results in much greater volumes of reflux during LES relaxation.

A hiatal hernia can also function as a reservoir of potential refluxate. During periods of low sphincter pressure, liquid within the hernia can reflux into the esophagus. When this occurs during swallow-induced LES relaxation, it is a key determinant of prolonged acid clearance, especially with individuals in a supine posture [61,62]. Equally significant, the hernia becomes the site of the acid pocket, a phenomenon in which

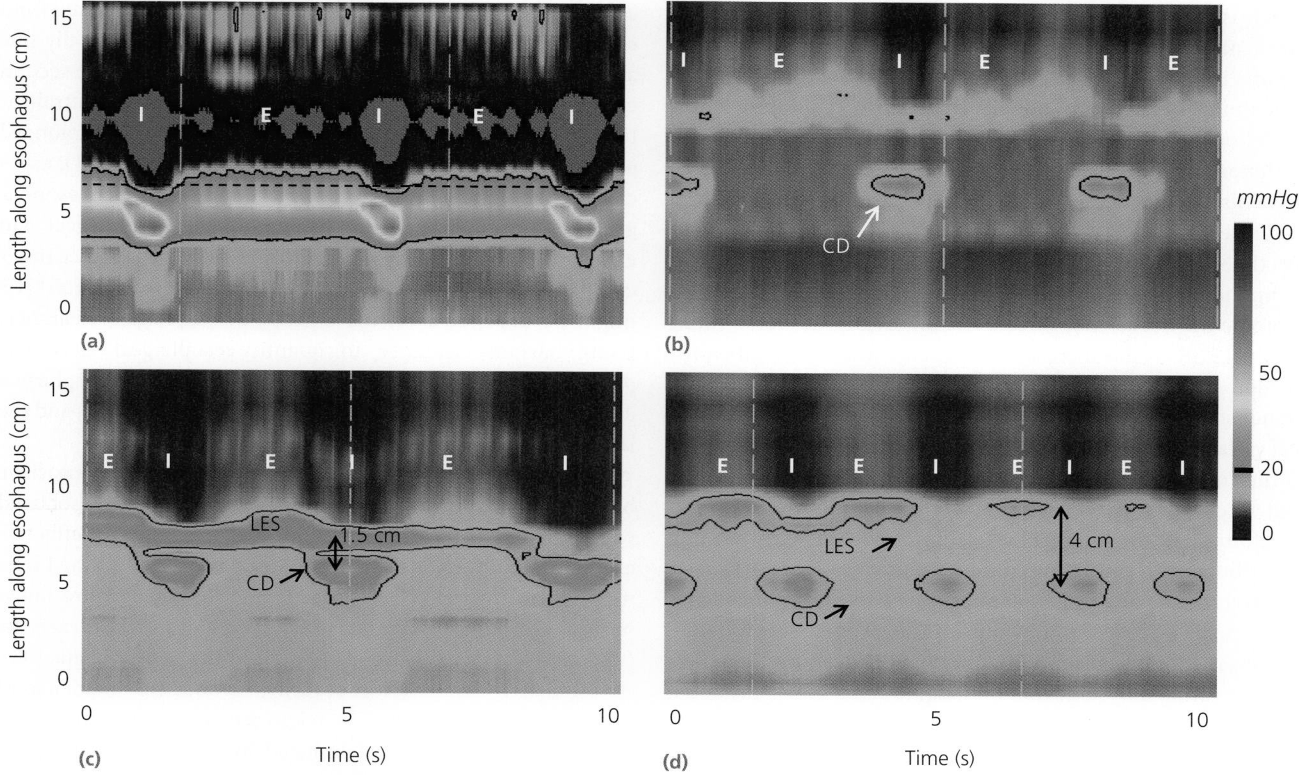

Figure 43.2 Major subtypes of esophagogastric junction (EGJ) morphology demonstrated in high-resolution manometry. The two main EGJ components are lower esophageal sphincter (LES) and crural diaphragm (CD), which cannot be independently quantified when superimposed, classified as type I EGJ **(a)**. During the expiration (E), EGJ pressure decreases, whereas it increases during inspiration (I). In the case of an extremely hypotensive EGJ, only the CD is identified **(b)**. **(c)** Corresponds to type II EGJ defined as LES-CD separation <2 cm. **(d)** Corresponds to type III EGJ defined as LES-CD separation >2 cm. A type III EGJ is the manometric criterion for hiatal hernia.

acid secreted after a meal layers on top of the ingested chyme, serving as a reservoir for acid reflux [63]. The acid pocket is normally located below the EGJ [64]. Beaumont et al. [65] showed that the acid pocket extended continuously above the diaphragm in 40% of patients with large hiatal hernia (>3 cm) and migrated intermittently above the diaphragm in the remainder. At the opposite extreme, the acid pocket was located immediately distal to the SCJ in healthy volunteers and patients with small hiatal hernia. In the same study, acid reflux during a tLESR occurred more often in patients with a hiatal hernia, especially in those with large hiatal hernia, and the risk for having acid reflux was mainly determined by the position of the acid pocket above the diaphragm.

Hypotensive lower esophageal sphincter

Physiologically, the LES is a short segment of tonically contracted smooth muscle at the EGJ [66]. Resting tone of the LES varies among normal individuals from 10 to 30 mmHg relative to intragastric pressure. Continuous LES pressure monitoring reveals considerable temporal variation. Intraabdominal pressure, gastric distention, peptides, hormones, various foods, and many medications (e.g., nitrates, calcium channel blockers, anticholinergics, α-adrenergic agonists, theophylline, morphine, and benzodiazepines) decrease resting LES pressure. The genesis of LES tone is a property of both the muscle itself and of its extrinsic innervation. The myogenic component is calcium dependent [67] and persists after treatment with the neurotoxin tetrodotoxin [68]. Extrinsic neurogenic augmentation of LES tonic contraction is mainly vagal and is cholinergic (atropine sensitive) [69].

A hypotensive LES promotes GERD. Reflux can occur spontaneously when the LES pressure is within 0–4 mmHg of intragastric pressure. A wide-open or patulous hiatus will greatly predispose to reflux as both the LES and CD are compromised. Strain-induced reflux occurs when the LES is overcome and forced open by an abrupt increase of intraabdominal pressure. Manometric data suggest that strain-induced reflux rarely occurred when the LES pressure was greater than 10 mmHg [70].

Transient lower esophageal sphincter relaxation

Transient LES relaxations are prolonged LES relaxations not triggered by swallowing [71] accompanied by CD inhibition and contraction of esophageal longitudinal muscle. The dominant stimulus for tLESR is distension of the proximal stomach, which is not surprising given that tLESR is the physiological mechanism for belching [72,73]. The vagal afferent mechanoreceptors in the gastric cardia project to the nucleus tractus solitarius in the brainstem and subsequently to the dorsal motor nuclei of the vagus. Dorsal motor nucleus neurons project to inhibitory neurons localized within the myenteric plexus of the distal esophagus inducing the tLESR. Gamma aminobutyric acid receptor type B ($GABA_B$) agonists inhibit the vagal pathway for tLESRs both centrally and peripherally [74]. Some food components (fat) or medications (e.g., sumatriptan) may also promote the occurrence of tLESRs. Although the overall number of tLESRs is not increased in patients with GERD, the proportion of tLESRs associated with acid reflux is increased, demonstrating the interplay between anatomical and physiological variables in the pathogenesis of GERD [75,76]. Getting back to the concept of compliance, the increased compliance of the EGJ accounts for the reduced ability to selectively vent gas from the stomach during tLESRs [58]. Ordinarily, elective gas venting is attributable to the 57-fold difference in viscosity between gas and water, allowing large volumes of gas to escape through a very small EGJ aperture while limiting the flow of liquid. However, with increased EGJ compliance, opening diameters become sufficiently large that even liquid refluxes in substantial volumes.

Esophageal HRM, which has supplanted line tracing studies in the assessment of esophageal motility disorders [77], is also superior to conventional manometry in detecting tLESRs [78–80]. CD inhibition [81], upper sphincter relaxation [82,83], and esophageal shortening attributable to longitudinal muscle contraction are easily observed during tLESRs imaged with esophageal pressure topography [84–86]. These observations are consistent with animal studies demonstrating a wide array of musculature involved in tLESRs, including the gastric fundus and even the rectus muscle of the abdomen [87].

Delayed gastric emptying

Delayed gastric emptying may exacerbate GERD by several mechanisms: (1) increasing the gastroesophageal pressure gradient, (2) increasing gastric volume and hence the volume of potential refluxate, (3) increasing tLESR frequency, and (4) increasing gastric acid secretion. However, this is a controversial area [88]. Because there has been little consistency in the methodologies used for quantifying gastric emptying or defining GERD, it is difficult to make generalizations. However, most patients with delayed gastric emptying or meeting the Rome criteria for functional dyspepsia do not have concomitant esophagitis [89], suggesting that although delayed gastric emptying can be a cofactor exacerbating GERD, it is probably not a root cause.

Esophageal acid clearance

After a reflux event, the duration of time that the esophageal mucosa persists at a pH <4 is termed the *esophageal acid clearance time*. Esophageal peristalsis (primary or secondary) is essential for acid clearance because it empties the refluxed fluid containing not only acid but also pepsin (and potentially bile acids and pancreatic enzymes) from the esophagus. The second component of the esophageal acid clearance is the neutralization of the residual acid by swallowed saliva [90]. Prolonged acid clearance occurs in a subset of patients with GERD, especially those with hiatus hernia. For example, using 24-h esophageal pH impedance, patients with pathological esophageal acid exposure exhibited both longer acid and volume clearance times compared with control subjects [91]. The severity of GERD might be dependent on the efficacy of esophageal clearance. Using barium clearance to quantify esophageal clearance, patients with esophagitis had greater impairment of esophageal emptying than patients with GERD without esophagitis, and the latter had greater impairment than control subjects [92].

Two mechanisms of impaired esophageal emptying have been identified: impaired peristalsis and re-reflux associated with larger hiatal hernias. Peristaltic dysfunction or "ineffective esophageal motility" (IEM) in GERD has been described by a number of investigators. Of particular significance are failed peristalsis and hypotensive peristaltic contractions (<30 mmHg), which leave residual fluid in the esophagus [93]. As esophagitis increases in severity, so does the incidence of impaired peristalsis [94]. The relevance of IEM was studied in healthy subjects with IEM induced by the administration of sildenafil [95]. After instillation of an acid bolus, esophageal motility, acid clearance, and volume clearance were evaluated using concurrent manometry, pH, and impedance monitoring. In the upright position, the effect of IEM was minimal. However, in the supine position, severe IEM (>80% of peristaltic sequences) significantly prolonged acid and volume clearance. Recent HRM data suggest that fragmented and failed peristalsis are more relevant than hypotensive contractions in prolonging clearance [96]. In a series of 351 patients with GERD, having >70% fragmented or >50% failed contractions was associated with significantly increased reflux burden. With respect to causative factors, it is unclear whether IEM is the cause or the consequence of GERD [88,97]. However, healing esophagitis does not resolve IEM.

Hiatus hernia also impairs esophageal emptying because of reflux of fluid from the hernia during swallowing as demonstrated radiographically in patients with reducing and nonreducing hiatus hernias compared with control subjects [61]. Emptying was abnormal in both hernia groups but was particularly impaired in the patients with nonreducing hernia who had normal emptying of a swallowed bolus with only one-third of test swallows and exhibited retrograde flow of fluid from the hernia during deglutitive relaxation.

The final phase of esophageal clearance depends on salivation. Just as impaired esophageal emptying prolongs esophageal clearance, diminished salivary neutralizing capacity has the same effect. The role of saliva was demonstrated in a study using radiolabeled hydrochloric acid injected into the esophagus to simulate a reflux event [90]. Concurrent manometry, pH-metry, and radionuclide imaging showed negligible increase in esophageal pH despite nearly complete emptying of labeled acid from the esophagus by secondary peristalsis. Further pH recovery occurred in a series of step increases associated with swallows. Stimulating salivation hastened acid clearance, while aspiration of saliva from the mouth vastly prolonged it. Thus, saliva is essential to neutralize the residual acid in the esophagus. However, saliva is not the only means of reflux neutralization. During sleep, when salivary secretion ceases, some acid clearance is achieved by bicarbonate secretion from esophageal submucosal glands [98]. Nonetheless, acid clearance time is greatly prolonged during sleep because of diminished salivation [99]. Similarly, chronic xerostomia is associated with prolonged esophageal acid exposure and esophagitis [100], and hyposalivation may play a role in promoting reflux disease in cigarette smokers. Even in the absence of GERD symptoms, cigarette smokers exhibited acid clearance times 50% longer than those of nonsmokers, and the salivary titratable alkali content was only 60% that of age-matched nonsmokers [101].

In addition to bicarbonate, saliva contains growth factors that have the potential to enhance mucosal repair. In animal models, epidermal growth factor has been shown to provide cytoprotection against irritants, enhance healing of gastroduodenal ulceration, and decrease the permeability of the esophageal mucosa to hydrogen ions [102]. However, studies have not shown consistent differences in epidermal growth factor concentration in patients with esophagitis or Barrett metaplasia [103,104].

Tissue resistance and injury

The esophageal mucosa possesses several morphological and physiological defenses against cellular acidification; taken together, these are referred to as *tissue resistance*. Conceptually, tissue resistance can be subdivided into preepithelial, epithelial, and postepithelial [105].

The *preepithelial defense* is designed to prevent gastric reflux content from coming into direct contact with squamous esophageal cells. Elsewhere in the GI tract, this consists of a mucous layer, unstirred water layer, and surface bicarbonate ion secretion. Preepithelial defense plays a major role in the protection of gastric and duodenal mucosa but a very minor role in the esophageal epithelium.

Epithelial resistance is the major protective factor against reflux injury in the esophagus. The squamous epithelium is organized into three distinct layers from the lumen to the basal layers: stratum corneum, stratum spinosum, and stratum germinativum. The stratum germinativum produces daughter cells that migrate toward the lumen. During migration, cells undergo morphological and functional transformation. The stratum corneum protects the underlying cells. The combination of cell membranes and intercellular junctional complexes produces a nearly impermeable barrier to hydrogen ions, slowing the rate of hydrogen ion diffusion into the tissue so that they can be effectively neutralized by the cellular buffering system within the esophageal epithelium. Buffers are intracellular (proteins, phosphates, and bicarbonates), as well as extracellular (matrix proteins, bicarbonates). In addition to buffering, epithelial transporters extrude hydrogen ions. The major *postepithelial defense* is an increased vascular perfusion, which provides nutrients and bicarbonate and removes hydrogen ions. This is also essential for tissue resistance and injury.

Luminal acid induces epithelium damage, destroying intercellular junctions, allowing hydrogen ion penetration, and eventually acidifying the intercellular space. Dilated intercellular spaces provide histological evidence of this increased permeability. Eventually, the buffering capacity of the intercellular space is overwhelmed, leading to acidification of the cell cytosol via the basolateral membrane. Acidification of the cytosol is the crucial event leading to cell edema (balloon cells) and death. However, a paradigm-challenging publication added a new twist to this "acid burn" model demonstrating that the earliest histopathological events in the recurrence of esophagitis occurred deep in the epithelium, not at the luminal surface, and "regenerative changes" were initiated before the surface necrosis formerly hypothesized as the stimulus for those changes [37]. Hence although the inciting pathophysiology is unquestionably the reflux of gastric and duodenal secretions into the esophagus, the best current evidence suggests that the effect of that reflux is the initiation of T-lymphocyte-predominant esophageal inflammation and basal cell and papillary hyperplasia without loss of surface cells with cytokine-triggered inflammation rather than the long-held belief of a direct caustic effect of acid, pepsin, and bile on the esophageal epithelium.

Implicit in the model of the pathogenesis of GERD is that the more prolonged the contact of gastric contents with the esophageal mucosa, the more severe is the injury. Acid is the main culprit, and the incidence of GERD is particularly high (around 80%) in patients with acid hypersecretion (with or without Zollinger–Ellison syndrome; see Chapter 50) [106]. Other components of gastric juice (pepsin, bile acids, and pancreatic enzymes), which are not detected with a pH electrode, are also harmful to esophageal epithelium [107–109]. However, their toxicity is dependent on the background pH: Pepsin is activated in an acidic environment; bile acids penetrate through cell membranes only in a weakly acidic medium (pH 3–5) [110]. Using esophageal pH monitoring and an esophageal fiber optic spectrophotometer (Bilitec 2000), which uses the optical properties of bilirubin to document duodenogastroesophageal reflux, Vaezi and Richter [111] demonstrated a graded increase across the GERD spectrum; pathological acid and bile acid exposure was observed in 89% of patients with Barrett esophagus compared with 79% of patients with esophagitis and 50% of patients with NERD.

Ironically, although playing a central role in reflux pathophysiology, abnormalities of gastric secretion are not a major determinant of GERD as determined in a report comparing gastric secretion in 115 patients with esophagitis and in 508 age- and disease-matched control subjects. On a case-by-case basis, neither the occurrence nor severity of esophagitis was related to abnormalities of fasting, basal, or maximal secretion of either acid or pepsin [112].

Genetic factors

Finally, some data suggest that genetic background can be associated with GERD symptoms and susceptibility to complications by interacting with the inflammatory process. Polymorphisms of interleukin-1 gene (*IL-1B*) and *IL-1RN* (gene coding for an interleukin-1 antagonist receptor) are associated with GERD. Thus, the *IL-1B*-511 CC genotype and C allele are associated with higher risk for GERD than the TT genotype (OR, 2.0; 95% CI: 1.12–3.57; $p = 0.01$). In contrast, the *IL-1B*-511*T/*IL-1RN*-*1 haplotype is associated with a lower risk for GERD, particularly among patients with *Hp* infection [113]. This haplotype is associated with higher gastric mucosal IL-1β levels and inflammatory response. This status may decrease the level of acid secretion and explain the protective effect with respect to GERD.

Clinical presentation and natural history

Although widely accepted as one of the most prevalent GI disorders, the clinical detection of GERD can be difficult because of the heterogeneity of potential symptoms. Based on the Montreal definition, GERD can be any condition that develops when the reflux of stomach contents causes troublesome symptoms and/or complications [2]. However, without peptic esophagitis, there can be no gold standard for the diagnosis because of the inherent subjectivity of "troublesome" among individuals. Ambulatory pH-metry or impedance pH-metry are helpful in detecting abnormal esophageal acid exposure and reflux events, but patients differ widely in their sensitivity to reflux, ranging from being extremely symptomatic with minimal acid exposure to being asymptomatic with severe peptic esophagitis or Barrett.

Typical reflux symptoms

The cardinal symptoms of GERD are heartburn and acid regurgitation. Heartburn (pyrosis) is characterized by a discomfort or burning sensation behind the sternum that arises from the epigastrium and may radiate toward the neck. Heartburn is an intermittent symptom, most commonly experienced within 60 minutes of eating, during exercise, and while lying recumbent. The discomfort is relieved with drinking water or antacid, but it can occur frequently and interfere with normal activities. Experiencing heartburn three or more times a week has been shown to impair an individual's perceived quality of life [114]. Although some correlation exists among the frequency of heartburn, the degree of esophageal acid exposure, and the presence or extent of mucosal injury, this correlation is far from perfect [115]. Some patients with severe esophagitis or Barrett metaplasia do not report any heartburn.

In the context of GERD, regurgitation is the effortless return of esophageal or gastric contents into the chest or pharynx without nausea or retching. Patients may note a sour or burning fluid in the throat or mouth that may also contain undigested food particles. Bending, belching, or maneuvers that increase intraabdominal pressure can provoke regurgitation. Although some clinicians restrict the definition of regurgitation to events accompanied by sour taste, others accept the perception of reflux movement into the chest as a sufficient criterion [2].

When heartburn and regurgitations are elicited as dominant symptoms, they have been found to have a high specificity but poor sensitivity for GERD [116]. The poor sensitivity is related to the fact that symptoms are inconsistently characterized by patients, and that the defining symptoms may alternatively be dysphagia, odynophagia, chest pain, water brash, laryngitis, or cough without heartburn or regurgitation.

Some degree of dysphagia is reported by more than 30% of individuals with GERD [117]. It can be caused by peptic stricture, Schatzki ("B") ring, weak peristalsis, or simply by mucosal inflammation. Dysphagia also occurs in the absence of any identifiable abnormality, in which case it is likely the result of abnormal sensitivity to bolus movement within the esophagus during peristalsis.

Less common symptoms of reflux disease include water brash, globus sensation (sensation of food sticking around the level of the throat), and odynophagia (pain on swallowing). Water brash is excessive salivation resulting from a vagal reflex triggered by esophageal acidification. Globus sensation is the perception of a lump or fullness in the throat, which is felt irrespective of swallowing. Odynophagia is more common with pill or infectious esophagitis than with reflux esophagitis and should prompt investigation for these causative factors. When odynophagia does occur in GERD, it is likely related to an esophageal ulcer or deep erosion. The occurrence of exclusive postprandial regurgitation of food is suggestive of rumination syndrome rather than GERD [118]. Rumination is defined as the voluntary, albeit subconscious, return of gastric content to the mouth; it is effortless and usually not associated with heartburn (see Chapter 30). Unlike regurgitation, rumination does not occur during sleep.

Atypical symptoms

Chest pain

Chest pain is sufficiently common in GERD that many consider it a typical symptom. However, given the overlapping characteristics of esophageal and cardiac pain and the potential life-threatening nature of cardiac disease, a cardiac evaluation needs to be prioritized. After a cardiovascular cause has been duly considered, the esophagus is often implicated. Historically, investigators focused on esophageal motor abnormalities, such as achalasia, diffuse esophageal spasm, or hypercontractility (jackhammer esophagus), as potential causes of chest pain. However, the most frequent esophageal causes of chest pain are GERD and hypersensitivity. Abnormal esophageal acid exposure was observed in 21–48% of patients with noncardiac chest pain, and chest pain occurrence was significantly correlated with an acid reflux event in 12–50% [119]. This causal relationship is further supported by the response of unexplained chest pain to PPI therapy in randomized clinical trials [120]. Unexplained chest pain tends to improve with PPIs in patients with endoscopic esophagitis or pathological esophageal acid exposure, whereas GERD-negative patients exhibit minimal PPI response [121].

Cough

Chronic cough has many potential causative factors, of which rhinosinusitis, asthma, and GERD can be the most perplexing [122]. Estimates of the prevalence of GERD-associated cough range from 10% to 40% depending on whether symptoms or pH monitoring is used as the diagnostic criterion for GERD [123]. Because 50–75% of these patients do not report reflux symptoms, the association often goes unrecognized. The pathogenesis of GERD-associated cough is believed to be secondary to acid stimulation of nerve endings in the esophagus, which then activate the cough center. Dual-probe pH studies and esophageal perfusion studies support this hypothesis. Studies using pH monitoring demonstrated a significant correlation between reflux and coughing in patients with chronic cough. Ing et al. [124] examined the response characteristics of distal esophageal afferents in 22 patients with GERD with chronic cough by alternatively challenging them with acid or saline perfusion of the esophagus. Cough frequency was significantly increased with acid infusion compared with saline infusion. Furthermore, lidocaine, acting as a topical anesthetic, blocked acid-induced cough. In contrast, ipratropium, a muscarinic cholinergic blocker, had no effect when instilled in the esophagus but blocked acid-induced cough when inhaled, presumably by preventing activation of the efferent limb of the reflex. These functional studies strongly support the presence of a vagally mediated esophago-tracheo/bronchial reflex activated by stimulation of the esophageal mucosa.

Subsequently, using 24-h pH impedance monitoring for reflux detection and pressure measurement for cough detection, around 30% of cough events were associated with reflux in a series of 22 patients with chronic cough [125]. "Reflux–cough" sequences involved acid (65%) but also weakly acid (29%) and weakly alkaline (6%) reflux events, suggesting that acid was not the only reflux component inducing cough. Equally interesting was the finding that cough preceded reflux in half of the sequences. To further assess the temporal relationship between cough and reflux, acoustic cough recording and esophageal pH impedance were simultaneously monitored in 71 patients with chronic cough [126]. Seventy percent of patients presented temporal association between reflux and cough with a similar proportion of patients having positive association for cough preceded by reflux and for reflux preceded by cough. One-third of patients had both associations. Furthermore, patients with positive reflux–cough association did not exhibit more erosive disease or distinguishing characteristics on impedance pH-metry; the only distinguishing feature relative to reflux patients without cough observed was a more sensitive cough reflex demonstrated by responsiveness to inhaled capsaicin. These findings support a central neuronal sensitization process linking reflux to cough.

Asthma

The relationship between asthma and GERD was first suggested by Osler's observation in 1892 that a distended stomach made wheezing worse. Epidemiological studies subsequently confirmed this association. A systematic review in adults with asthma revealed a 59% prevalence rate of reflux symptom, 51% prevalence rate of abnormal esophageal pH-metry, and 37% prevalence rate of esophagitis [127]. However, despite the association, it is less clear whether GERD causes asthma. Rather, there are several potential mechanisms whereby asthma may provoke reflux [128]. Patients with asthma have autonomic dysregulation with heightened vagal tone. LES pressure may be overcome because of increased negative intrathoracic pressure during labored breathing. Obesity and hiatal hernia are risk factors for both GERD and asthma. Asthma medications (theophylline, α_2-adrenergic receptor agonists) may promote GERD by decreasing LES pressure. Finally, airflow obstruction induces tLESRs.

Both reflex mechanisms and aspiration have been proposed to explain how reflux might exacerbate asthma; both can be demonstrated experimentally. In a unique investigation in which tracheal and esophageal pH were monitored in four patients with severe asthma, peak expiratory flow rates decreased 16 L/min when esophageal and tracheal acid were simultaneously present compared with 4 L/min when only the esophagus was acidified [129]. Another study showed that distal esophageal acid perfusion decreased peak inspiration flow rates and increased airway resistance in patients with asthma with reflux [130].

Finally, a literature review demonstrated that reflux treatment might improve asthma outcomes in selected patients with asthma [128]. Proposed distinguishing factors include the presence of regurgitations at least twice a week, abnormal proximal esophageal acid exposure, high esophageal acid contact time, difficulty to control asthma, and nocturnal asthma.

Ear, nose, and throat symptoms

A variety of ear, nose, and throat (ENT) symptoms have been attributed to laryngopharyngeal reflux. Dysphonia, globus sensation (feeling of a lump in throat), throat clearing, sore throat, and laryngospasm are among the most common [128]. Laryngoscopic findings suggestive of GERD include erythema, posterior commissure hypertrophy, granuloma, pseudosulcus (infraglottic laryngeal edema), vocal cord edema, thick intralaryngeal mucus, ventricular obliteration, hypertrophy, and extralaryngeal signs, such as red mucosa in nasopharynx and lingual tonsil. However, these findings are all nonspecific and also found in asymptomatic individuals when the examinations are interpreted blindly [131].

Diagnostic criteria for ENT-GERD are very controversial. As many as 50% of patients with suspected ENT-GERD may exhibit esophagitis [132], but, alternatively, many ENT practitioners maintain that no esophageal symptoms are required for the diagnosis. Dual-channel esophageal pH-metry, with electrodes in the distal esophagus and just above or below the upper sphincter [133,134], and pharyngeal and esophageal impedance monitoring [135] have shown increased pharyngeal reflux exposure in patients with ENT symptoms, but again, diagnostic thresholds are very controversial. In a study performed in healthy control subjects, more than 88% of pharyngeal acidification episodes corresponded to swallows rather than pharyngeal and/or esophageal reflux [136]. In another study, 24 patients with chronic laryngeal symptoms and suspicion of GERD were studied with pharyngeal and esophageal pH-impedance monitoring [137]. Only 2 of the 24 responded to PPI therapy; both had excessive esophageal reflux but no pharyngeal reflux.

A survey among ENT physicians and gastroenterologists highlighted the different practices in managing suspected ENT-GERD [138]. ENT physicians reported that they diagnosed GERD mainly on symptoms with or without supporting laryngoscopic findings. Half of gastroenterologists proposed endoscopy and pH-metry before treatment. Both groups relied heavily on prolonged periods of PPI therapy for management, although dosing and endpoints were inconsistent. In evaluating treatment response, 70% of gastroenterologists reported a response in <60% of patients treated, whereas 62% of ENT physicians reported a response in >60%.

Dental erosions

Dental erosions, especially on the lingual and palatal tooth surfaces, are increased in patients with GERD. These correlate with both typical GERD symptoms and abnormal esophageal acid exposure measured by pH-metry, and their progression has been shown to slow in a randomized controlled trial of twice-daily PPI therapy [139].

Natural history

Relatively few studies have examined the natural history of GERD. Among the existing reports, some have found progression over time suggesting an evolution from NERD to esophagitis and Barrett esophagus [140,141], whereas other reports suggest regression from erosive disease to NERD. For example, it was reported that there was a decrease of esophagitis prevalence rate (from 40% to 27%) in a cohort of 50 patients assessed 17–22 years after initial referral; improvement of esophagitis did not correlate with the presence of hiatal hernia or symptom severity at the time of referral [35]. Data from a large multicenter study of 6215 patients performed in Germany, Austria, and Switzerland suggest some transition between NERD, esophagitis, and Barrett esophagus [142]. Among 2721 patients who completed the 5-year follow-up, most remained stable or improved under current routine clinical care. Among patients with NERD, 25% had Los Angeles (LA) classification (see later) grade A or B esophagitis and 0.6% had LA grade C or D esophagitis at 5-year follow-up. Among patients with LA grade C or D esophagitis at baseline, 61% had nonerosive disease at 5 years. Progression to Barrett esophagus was observed in 4.2% of patients with NERD, 8.1% of patients with LA grade A or B esophagitis, and 10.3% of patients with LA grade C or D.

Over the past 25 years, the epidemiology of esophageal cancer has dramatically changed in western countries, with an increased incidence of adenocarcinoma and a decreased incidence of squamous cell carcinoma. The former incidence is thought to be related to GERD, while the latter may be attributable to decreased tobacco use, particularly in association with alcohol use and especially in men [143]. The risk for esophageal adenocarcinoma was also shown to be increased in patients with long-standing reflux symptoms in a nationwide study of the Swedish population (OR, 7.7; 95% CI: 5.3–11.4) [144]. Frequent (at least three times a week) and chronic (more than 10–20 years) symptoms increased the adenocarcinoma risk in that study.

Finally, GERD natural history has been modified by the widespread use of PPIs. Esophageal strictures, which are a classic complication of esophagitis, have declined in frequency concurrently with the availability of PPIs [145,146].

Differential diagnosis

Depending on the specific symptom complex, GERD needs to be distinguished from infectious esophagitis, EoE, pill esophagitis, peptic ulcer disease, dyspepsia, biliary colic, coronary artery disease, esophageal motor disorders, and rumination syndrome. It is especially important that coronary artery disease be given early consideration because of its potential lethality. Patients whose symptoms include unexplained chest pain should have a cardiogram and exercise stress test before a GI evaluation. Furthermore, because inferior myocardial ischemia may present with only GI symptoms, patients without chest pain, but with dyspnea, diaphoresis, fatigue, or significant cardiac risk factors, should also first be evaluated for coronary artery disease. Upper endoscopy, esophageal biopsies, barium swallow, esophageal manometry, and biliary tract ultrasonography are useful to address other elements of the different differential diagnosis.

Both infectious and pill esophagitis are accompanied by substantial odynophagia, which is rare in esophagitis. In terms of endoscopic appearance, infectious esophagitis is diffuse and tends to involve the proximal esophagus far more frequently than does reflux esophagitis. In esophageal candidiasis, the esophagus typically has a diffuse, heavy, curdlike exudate, in contrast with the linear streaks emerging from the EGJ typical of peptic esophagitis. The ulcerations seen in peptic esophagitis are usually large, solitary, and distal, whereas infectious ulcerations are punctate and diffuse. Esophageal ulceration from oral medications, such as potassium chloride, quinidine, tetracycline, or nonsteroidal antiinflammatory drugs, are usually singular and deep at points of narrowing, especially near the crossing points of the carina and aortic arch, with sparing of the distal esophagus.

EoE requires special consideration (see Chapter 44). The prevalence of this inflammatory chronic disease is increasing (from 10 per 100 000 inhabitants in western countries in the 1990s to 43–55 per 100 000 in the latest studies) [147]. A wide range of symptoms are associated with EoE, such as dysphagia and food impaction, but also GERD-like symptoms (chest pain, heartburn, regurgitation). EoE should be suspected in cases of GERD resistant to PPIs, although it should also be emphasized that many cases of EoE are responsive to PPIs [148]. Endoscopy might be normal or reveal typical patterns, such as rings, furrows, exudate, edema, and stricture. The diagnosis of EoE is established with esophageal biopsies; 15 eosinophils per high-power field in the most densely inflamed area of the esophageal epithelium is the minimal diagnostic threshold.

Associated conditions

Pregnancy is by far the most common condition predisposing to GERD, with approximately 50–80% of pregnant patients reporting heartburn [149]. As the uterus enlarges, the increased abdominal-to-thoracic pressure gradient promotes reflux. In addition to this anatomical change, LES pressure decreases and gastric emptying is slowed. These motility effects are likely due to increased progesterone levels, explaining why reflux begins early in the first trimester.

Obesity is a major risk factor for GERD based on several mechanisms. First, obesity promotes axial separation between the LES and the CD, causing mechanical disruption of EGJ [150]. The most relevant fat distribution with respect to GERD pathogenesis is abdominal fat, evident by increased abdominal girth [151–153]. LES incompetence and greater esophageal acid exposure have also been observed in obese patients [154–157]. One study even reported an increased tLESR frequency in obese patients [158]. Altered esophageal clearance is also evident in obese patients, with abnormal motility encountered in 25–60% [155,159–161]. Similarly, impaired bolus transit is more frequent in morbidly obese patients with GERD than in patients with GERD with normal weight [162]. Together, these diverse mechanisms help explain the increased incidence of GERD in obese patients.

Scleroderma is associated with impaired esophageal function in at least 80% of patients [163]. Characteristic abnormalities are decreased peristaltic amplitude in the smooth muscle segment of the esophagus and decreased LES pressure. GERD might also contribute to interstitial lung disease in scleroderma [164–166]. Although most frequently found with scleroderma, these esophageal abnormalities are nonspecific and may occur with any of the mixed connective tissue disorders. *Sjögren syndrome*, which disrupts normal salivary secretion and interferes with esophageal acid clearance, also results in an increased risk for reflux esophagitis.

Diabetes mellitus may be associated with GERD [167]; however, there are confounding factors, especially obesity [168]. One Australian study noted that diabetes mellitus and high blood pressure were associated with GERD, but they were not independent risk factors; high cholesterol was, however, independently associated with GERD [169]. GERD prevalence might be greater in patients with diabetes with neuropathy than in those without [170], suggesting a role of delayed gastric emptying or impaired esophageal motility.

Zollinger–Ellison syndrome promotes GERD by increasing the acidity and quantity of refluxate. Thus, an analysis of 122 patients with Zollinger–Ellison syndrome found that 42% had endoscopic esophagitis [171].

Cardiovascular diseases are also associated with GERD. In a case–control study based on a large Norwegian health survey conducted in 1995–1997, a positive association was noted between GERD and angina pectoris (OR, 1.9; 95% CI: 1.6–2.2) [172].

Finally, an interaction exists between *pulmonary disease* and GERD. For example, chronic pulmonary diseases and asthma were associated with a new GERD diagnosis in a study based on the UK General Practice Research Database [8]. *Lung transplantation* is also an important issue that should be addressed. GERD prevalence might be increased in candidates for lung transplantation [173], as well as in lung transplant recipients [174,175]. Patients with cystic fibrosis are at particular risk. This is of clinical importance because GERD is a risk factor for acute rejection [176] and for bronchiolitis obliterans syndrome, which induces chronic rejection [177]. Mechanisms of GERD in lung transplantation are not completely understood. However, impaired esophageal motility and delayed gastric emptying may play a role.

Diagnostic evaluation

It is neither practical nor necessary to embark on a diagnostic evaluation of every patient with classic GERD symptoms. In most cases, a carefully taken history is sufficient to confirm the diagnosis of GERD and begin therapy. However, some patients may present "alarm" signs (dysphagia, bleeding, odynophagia, weight loss), atypical symptoms, or typical symptoms refractory to standard medical therapy. Endoscopy and reflux testing can be useful either to identify esophageal complications as surrogate markers of GERD or to quantify esophageal acid exposure and determine whether symptoms correlate with reflux events. Because these tests are complementary, more than one might be used to optimize management as proposed by the Rome IV consensus [3].

Clinical evaluation and empiric trials

In the case of atypical symptoms, diagnostic studies can confirm that abnormal reflux is occurring and potentially responsible for the syndrome in question. Diagnostic studies are also indicated for a patient with GERD when heartburn is chronic (raising the possibility of Barrett metaplasia), refractory to treatment, or accompanied by the so-called alarm symptoms noted earlier.

Standardized questionnaires to diagnose GERD are far from perfect. For example, the Diamond study evaluated the accuracy of the Reflux Disease Questionnaire in a cohort of 308 patients with troublesome upper GI symptoms [4]. The sensitivity and specificity to diagnose GERD were 62% and 67%, respectively, using pH-metry and endoscopy as the comparator. The advantages of these questionnaires might be to screen patients for GERD in a primary care setting and to use as a standardized symptom evaluation.

Some authors have proposed an empiric PPI trial to diagnose GERD. In the Diamond study [5], a positive response to a 2-week regimen of esomeprazole (40 mg once a day) was observed in 69% of patients with GERD and 51% of those without GERD, again as defined by pH-metry and endoscopy. Response to the PPI trial was greater in patients with esophagitis (57%) than in patients with NERD (49%) or in patients without GERD (35%), but the difference was significant only between patients with esophagitis and those without GERD. Finally, a positive response to a PPI trial may also be indicative of either a placebo effect or response of another peptic disorder, and a negative response may be secondary to persistent acid or weakly acidic reflux despite PPI therapy. PPIs may also mask symptoms of malignancy. Hence it is important that patients be evaluated for warning signs (odynophagia, dysphagia, melena, hematochezia, and weight loss) before this minimalist approach is undertaken. In addition, an empiric trial can lead to inappropriate long-term treatment that may have significant economic and clinical implications. Despite these limitations, its simplicity and low cost make an empiric PPI trial a reasonable option as long as its limitations are understood and appropriate follow-up is arranged.

Endoscopy

Upper endoscopy is the first diagnostic test in the evaluation of GERD. It provides a mean for both detecting and managing complications of GERD, as well as excluding other diseases. Endoscopy is diagnostic of GERD if erosive esophagitis is present, with a specificity of 90–95%; most false-positive results are attributable to either infectious or pill-induced mucosal injury [178,179]. However, esophagitis, defined as distal esophageal mucosal breaks, is encountered in only 20–40% of patients with GERD symptoms [34–36]; thus, endoscopy has poor sensitivity. The majority of patients with GERD do not have esophagitis.

The LA classification system, categorized as grade A, B, C, or D, based on the length and circumferential extent of mucosal breaks, should be used to describe reflux esophagitis severity (Figure 43.3) [180]. This grading scheme has good reproducibility [181] and good correlation with esophageal acid exposure [180]. However, grade A esophagitis might be encountered in 5–7.5% of asymptomatic subjects, and the recent Lyon consensus for GERD diagnosis opined that grade A esophagitis is not sufficient for the diagnosis of GERD [182]. Furthermore, although LA grade B esophagitis might provide enough evidence

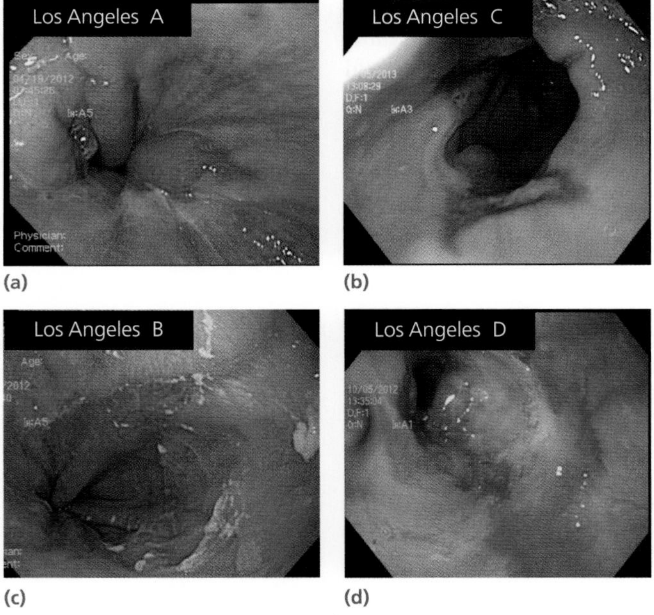

Figure 43.3 Los Angeles classification. Esophagitis is scored into four grades. Grade A is defined as mucosal breaks confined to the mucosal fold, each no longer than 5 mm **(a)**. Grade B corresponds to at least one mucosal break longer than 5 mm confined to the mucosal fold but not continuous between two folds **(b)**. Grade C is characterized by mucosal breaks that are continuous between the tops of mucosal folds but not circumferential **(c)**. Finally, grade D is represented by extensive mucosal breaks engaging at least 75% of the esophageal circumference **(d)**. Source: Courtesy Peter J. Kahrilas.

for the initiation of medical treatment of GERD, the Lyon consensus recommended confirmation of the GERD diagnosis with reflux monitoring if antireflux surgery was being considered. Finally, endoscopically defined minimal changes, such as edema, erythema, and irregular Z line, are not specific for GERD and are poorly reproducible observations; they are not included in the LA classification and should not be taken as definitive evidence of esophagitis [183]. It is important to note that the LA system does not consider strictures, hiatus hernia, or Barrett metaplasia. The endoscopist should describe these entities separately. Endoscopy is also important to obtain esophageal biopsies to rule out EoE in cases of nonresponse to PPI therapy, suggestive associated symptoms, or suggestive endoscopic features [3]. Suspicion of Barrett metaplasia also warrants esophageal biopsies.

In summary, endoscopy is an important test in the evaluation of patients suspected of having complications of GERD or an increased pretest probability of an alternative diagnosis, such as malignancy or peptic ulcer. Thus, endoscopy is reasonable as the first-line evaluation if there is dysphagia, odynophagia, GI bleeding, unintentional weight loss, early satiety, or age at presentation greater than 55 years (to rule out Barrett metaplasia or malignancy). In the absence of warning signs, patients are typically not referred for endoscopy unless they have had an unsuccessful course of PPI therapy. In the case of normal endoscopy and atypical GERD symptoms or refractoriness to empiric PPI therapy, further investigations are required to determine whether abnormal gastroesophageal reflux is present and whether the patient's symptoms are related to gastroesophageal reflux.

Reflux identification: esophageal pH monitoring and pH-impedance monitoring

The principal indications for ambulatory reflux monitoring are to document excessive reflux in patients without endoscopic esophagitis or to evaluate the efficacy of medical or surgical treatment. Quantification of reflux episodes might be achieved using ambulatory 24-h pH monitoring, which may be combined with impedance monitoring. The first technique detects reflux episodes based on the presence of acid in the esophagus and the second on the presence of liquid and/or air in the esophagus.

Catheter-based esophageal pH monitoring

Ambulatory 24-h pH monitoring is the most widely used test to establish the presence of excessive gastroesophageal reflux and to temporally correlate symptoms with reflux. The conventional test is performed by transnasally positioning a thin pH probe 5 cm above the proximal margin of the LES as determined manometrically. The probe is connected to an external data recorder. Ambulatory monitoring allows the patient to conduct normal daily activities while recording symptoms, meals, and sleep in a diary.

Ambulatory pH monitoring provides a marker that acid is present in the esophagus and expresses this as a function of time. Esophageal acid exposure is defined as the percentage of the recording time that the pH is <4, and this is the most useful discriminator between physiological and pathological reflux [184]. Based on studies performed in asymptomatic subjects, the Lyon Consensus defined an esophageal AET >6% of the total time as conclusive diagnosis of GERD [182]. An AET <4% is considered definitively normal (physiological reflux). An AET between 4% and 6% is inconclusive for the diagnosis of GERD, warranting further evaluation.

A composite score, named the DeMeester score, was proposed by Johnson and DeMeester [185] by examining six variables: (1) percent total time the pH is <4, (2) percent upright time the pH is <4, (3) percent supine time the pH is <4, (4) number of reflux events, (5) number of reflux events longer than 5 minutes, and (6) longest reflux event. This composite is considered abnormal if >14.7. Although this score is still used in clinical practice, AET is more reliable than the DeMeester score and should be preferred for the diagnosis of GERD [182].

Although esophageal AET exhibits a graded increase across the GERD spectrum, there is variability among patients, and overlap exists between patients and control subjects [184]. That is one reason why the Lyon Consensus introduced the concept of an inconclusive diagnosis of GERD. Indeed, up to 30% of patients with reflux esophagitis may have normal AET. This lack of sensitivity might be secondary to technical limitations, temporal variability, or that some patients might develop symptoms or erosions at lower threshold values. However, despite this limitation, pH-metry is useful to predict response to reflux therapy [184].

Different indices have been proposed to assess the relationship between reflux events and symptoms. The symptom index (SI) is defined as the percentage of symptom episodes that correlate with documented GERD ([number of reflux-related symptom events/total number of reflux events] × 100) [186]. A SI >50% is considered positive. However, the SI does not take into account the total number of reflux episodes. In patients with frequent reflux episodes, a high SI may be caused by random associations between reflux and symptoms. To circumvent this limitation, the symptom SI was devised to focus on the number of reflux events [187]. This involved dividing the total number of reflux-related symptoms by the total number of reflux episodes. A symptom SI >10% is considered positive. Finally, the best proposed scheme for symptom–reflux correlation is the symptom association probability (SAP). This index uses all relevant data and statistically calculates whether the relationship between symptoms and reflux events can be attributed to chance [188]. This involves constructing a contingency table with four fields: (1) positive symptom, positive reflux; (2) negative symptom, positive reflux; (3) positive symptom, negative reflux; and (4) negative symptom, negative reflux. The Fisher exact test is then applied to calculate the probability that the observed association between reflux and symptoms occurred by chance. A time window of 2 minutes is used to assess the association between reflux and symptom. SAP is significant if greater than 95%. SI and SAP are the most commonly used indices. A strong association between reflux events and symptoms is also a hallmark of hypersensitivity and supports the use of neuromodulators as supplemental therapy.

According to the Lyon consensus, at least three symptom events should be reported by the patient to evaluate the relationship between reflux and symptoms [182]. Further, a combination of positive SI (>50%) and positive SAP (>95%) provides the strongest evidence for a significant association between reflux and symptoms.

Wireless esophageal pH monitoring

Catheter-based pH monitoring has significant methodological limitations. The transnasal probe is uncomfortable and restricts normal daily activities. A wireless device (the Bravo system) composed of a capsule attached to the esophageal mucosa 6 cm above the SCJ offers an alternative method [189] (Figure 43.4). The capsule measures pH and transmits these data to an external receiver worn on the patient's belt. Data are recorded for 48–96 hours. Normative ranges for percentage of time with esophageal pH <4 are 4.4–5.3% for the 48-hour period using this device. The Lyon Consensus proposed to use the same thresholds as for catheter-based pH monitoring that is an AET >6% as conclusive diagnosis of GERD and AET <4% as normal [182]. SI and SAP are calculated as with catheter-based pH monitoring. Several studies have shown the pH capsule to be better tolerated than the conventional pH catheter. Mild-to-moderate chest pain is the main side-effect of the pH capsule; severe chest pain requiring endoscopic capsule removal is rare.

Data demonstrating that wireless pH monitoring is superior to catheter-based studies in diagnosing abnormal reflux are limited; however, there are studies suggesting that extending the duration of pH monitoring from 24 hours to 48–96 hours improves the yield of documenting abnormal reflux. For example, among 38 patients with a negative pH catheter-based study, prolonged (48–96 hours) wireless pH-monitoring revealed pathological acid esophageal exposure in 37% and 47% using average and worst day analysis, respectively [190]. Overall,

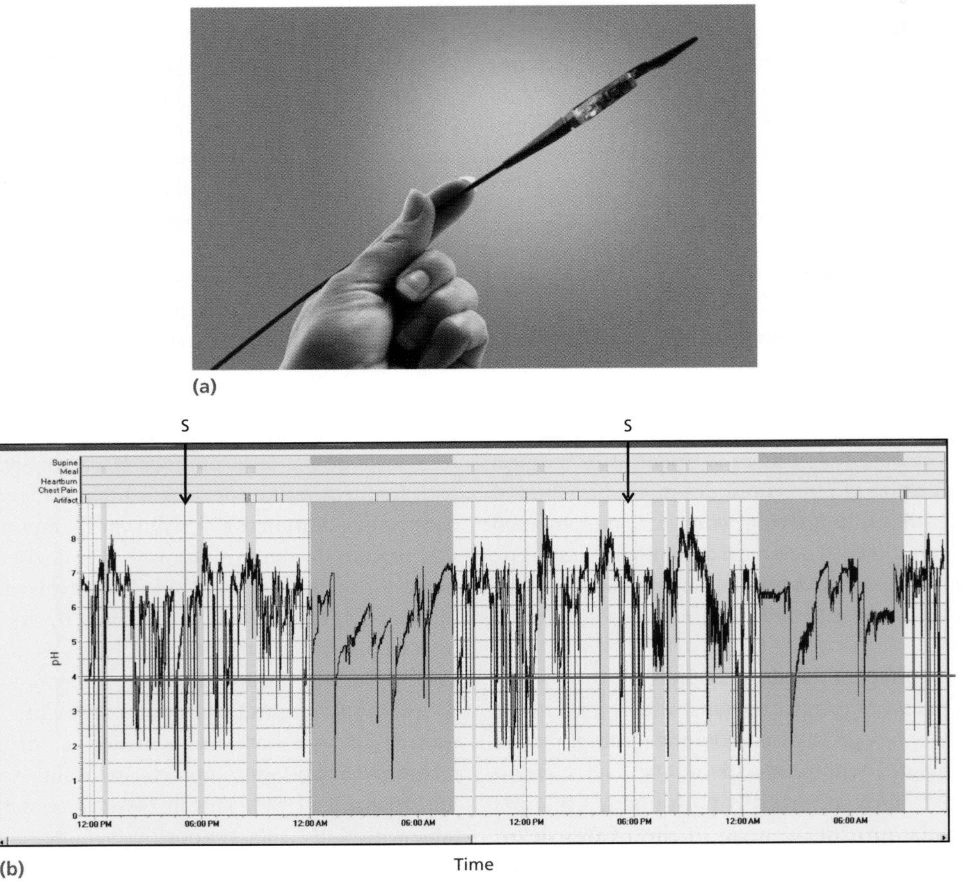

Figure 43.4 Wireless pH monitoring. The Bravo capsule on the delivery system **(a)**. Forty-eight-hour wireless pH monitoring off medication is depicted for a patient with typical GERD symptoms (heartburn) **(b)**. Esophageal pH was recorded 6 cm above the squamocolumnar junction. The horizontal red line corresponds to pH 4. Acid reflux is defined as a pH decline to <4. Meal periods are represented in yellow and the supine position in green. Symptom occurrence (S) is indicated by black arrows. The patient had an esophageal pH <4 during 11.2% of total time on day 1 and during 7.9% on day 2. He had pathological acid reflux off medication on both days. Source: Courtesy Peter J. Kahrilas.

GERD was diagnosed in 61% (average analysis) and 76% (worst day) based on either pathological acid exposure or positive symptom association.

Esophageal pH-impedance monitoring

Standard pH-monitoring detects only acid reflux; that is, reflux with a pH <4. However, weakly acidic or "nonacid" reflux events with pH >4 might still induce symptoms. This is particularly true in patients taking PPIs in whom acid secretion is greatly reduced. Thus, new techniques have evolved to complement pH monitoring for detection and improved characterization (liquid vs gas) of reflux [191]. Intraluminal impedance monitoring detects reflux by determining changes in resistance (impedance) to an electrical current between paired electrodes on the intraesophageal probe. Each reflux episode can be characterized as liquid or gas by their impedance characteristics. When gastric juice bridges electrode pairs, impedance decreases. In contrast, gas venting causes impedance to increase. The sequence of these changes among adjacent electrode pairs defines whether flow is anterograde or retrograde (Figure 43.5). Multichannel intraluminal impedance is usually combined with pH monitoring. Thus, unlike pH monitoring, impedance-pH monitoring can distinguish swallowed acidic foods from gastric reflux. Varying configurations of impedance and pH electrodes on the impedance-pH probes that are passed through the nose are available for use with portable external data recorders. Greater than 73 reflux episodes per 24 hours "off" PPI is considered pathological [184]. "On" PPI treatment, this threshold is 57 per 24 hours [192]. As with pH monitoring, SI and SAP can be calculated. The Lyon Consensus proposed using the same thresholds for studies performed off and on PPI and to consider a total number of reflux episodes >80 per 24 hours as abnormal, but a number <40 physiological [182]. Intermediate values are inconclusive. Because the clinical relevance of an abnormal number of reflux episodes is still debatable, the Lyon Consensus considers the total number of reflux episodes as an adjunctive measurement for the diagnosis of GERD.

One interesting indication for impedance-pH monitoring is in the evaluation of patients who are refractory to PPI therapy. There were distinct phenotypes of PPI nonresponders in a series of 168 patients who underwent impedance-pH monitoring "on" PPI for refractory GERD symptoms [193]. Eleven percent of subjects had persistent pathological esophageal acid exposure despite twice-daily PPI, 31% had a positive association between symptoms and weakly acidic reflux, and 58% had no evidence of pathological reflux and/or positive symptom association. In a series of 200 patients with NERD studied "off" PPI, 27% had normal impedance-pH monitoring and negative SAP, characterizing these patients as functional heartburn rather than GERD [194]. Only 11% of the patients in that series had a positive association between symptoms and weakly acidic reflux without also having a positive association with acid reflux.

Study "off" or "on" PPI

The Lyon Consensus proposed indications for reflux monitoring off and on PPI depending on the strength of evidence supporting a GERD diagnosis [195]. If the patient has no previous evidence of GERD – that is, no previous history of grade C or D

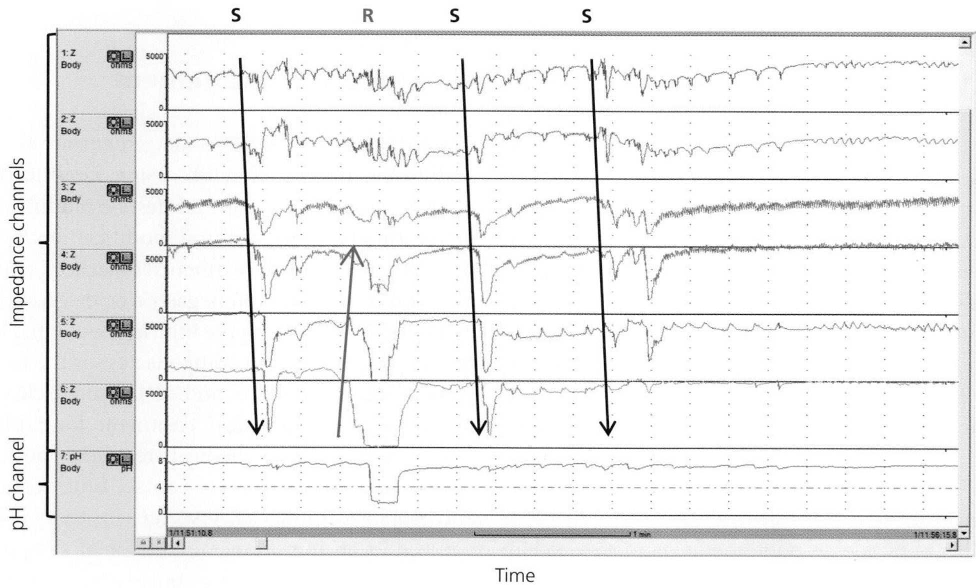

Figure 43.5 Representative 5-minute pH-impedance monitoring. The pH was recorded 5 cm above the proximal border of the lower esophageal sphincter (LES) determined by manometry (channel 7). The impedance was recorded 3, 5, 7, 9, 15, and 17 cm above the LES (channels 1–6). A reflux event (R) is defined by an abrupt retrograde 50% drop of impedance baseline (red arrow). In this example, the pH of this reflux example falls below 4 (dashed horizontal line), thus defining an acid reflux event. Note that swallows (S) are associated with anterograde impedance drops (black arrows).

esophagitis, no Barrett mucosa >1 cm, no peptic stricture, and no abnormal AET on previous reflux monitoring study – the question is whether the reported symptoms can be related to pathological reflux. Hence the patient should be tested "off" PPI to document whether abnormal esophageal acid exposure is present at baseline. This can be accomplished with a standard pH catheter, combined pH-impedance catheter, or a wireless pH capsule. However, if the patient has previous evidence of GERD (grade C or D esophagitis, Barrett mucosa >1 cm, peptic stricture, abnormal AET on reflux monitoring), it is unclear whether the persistent symptoms are related to persistent GERD. In this setting, the patient should be tested on PPI, and pH-impedance monitoring should be used.

An alternative approach to answer the question of whether to test "on" or "off" medication could be prolonged wireless pH monitoring both "off" and "on" PPI in a single examination (2 days off PPI followed by 2 days on PPI) [196]. However, with currently available technologies, this can be achieved only with the wireless pH-monitoring system.

Other investigations

Esophageal manometry

Esophageal manometry has no significant role in the initial diagnostic evaluation of GERD. Even though manometric findings of low LES pressure and tLESRs are key features of the pathophysiology of GERD, their detection seldom alters the clinical management of an individual patient. However, manometry is used routinely for determining the proper placement of pH and pH-impedance probes. It is also used to rule out primary and secondary motility disorders before antireflux surgery, although the utility of this approach is controversial [197].

The Lyon Consensus proposed a classification of esophageal motility disorders frequently encountered in GERD using esophageal HRM [198]. Manometric hiatal hernia and hypotensive EGJ might facilitate the occurrence of GERD. Fragmented peristalsis (at least 50% of esophageal contractions with a break >5 cm), IEM (at least 50% of swallows with a distal contractile integral [DCI] <450 mmHg·s·cm), and absent contractility are in favor of GERD. Finally, the multiple rapid swallow test that consists of five 2-mL swallows less than 2 seconds apart is performed during HRM to evaluate the contraction reserve. If the esophageal contraction after the multiple rapid swallow has a DCI greater than the mean DCI of the single 5-mL swallows performed during HRM, there is contraction reserve. An absence of contraction reserve might be associated with GERD (Figure 43.6).

Esophageal fiber optic spectrophotometer

The esophageal fiber optic spectrophotometer was developed in the 1990s to detect the reflux of bile acids into the esophagus using the optical properties of bilirubin [199]. However, because the detection of bile was based on its color, dietary restriction (white diet) was required to avoid colored food. This technique has been supplanted by pH-impedance monitoring that allows the detection of reflux irrespective of its acidity. The refluxed fluid can be acidic, weakly acidic, or (rarely) weakly alkaline. Bile, per se, is not specifically detected.

Barium esophagogram

Although a barium esophagogram is not needed to diagnose GERD, it can be useful as a preoperative study or in the evaluation of surgical complications. Barium esophagogram offers the ability to assess EGJ anatomy and to classify hiatal hernias. The presence of gastric rugal folds traversing the diaphragm is used as the defining criterion of sliding hiatal hernia. This examination also allows for the identification of paraesophageal hernia. Barium esophagogram is usually performed before antireflux surgery to evaluate the size of hiatal hernia and then predict the difficulty of the surgery. Finally, stricture and segmental narrowing as a result of inflammation can be detected.

Summary of diagnosis of GERD

A diagnosis of GERD usually can be accomplished by a careful medical history and empirical trial of PPIs. Patients with longstanding symptoms or "alarm signs" may benefit from endoscopy. Ambulatory reflux testing is unnecessary in most patients but can be of value in patients refractory to antireflux therapy or to document abnormal acid reflux in an individual undergoing evaluation for antireflux surgery. Patients with atypical symptoms not responding to empiric therapy may also benefit from ambulatory pH or pH-impedance monitoring. Esophageal manometry is of minimal use in managing GERD, with the exceptions of detecting major motor disorders or evaluating peristalsis before antireflux surgery.

Therapeutic management

The principles of GERD management are to minimize reflux and/or the impact of reflux using modifications in lifestyle, pharmaceuticals, or surgery. Lifestyle modifications encompass diet, eating patterns, postural modifications, and weight reduction. Pharmaceutical treatments, especially acid inhibition, play a central role. Even though gastric acid secretion is usually normal in GERD, reducing the injurious potential of gastric juice to the esophageal mucosa compensates for the fundamental problems of excessive reflux and/or impaired clearance. Thus, the dominant pharmaceutical treatment for GERD is inhibiting acid secretion. Other medical treatments aim to inhibit reflux occurrence and to decrease contact time between the refluxate and esophageal mucosa. Visceral sensitivity is increasingly recognized as an important modulator of symptom severity and, when abnormal, should be considered as an adjunct target for GERD treatment. As an alternative to pharmaceutical therapies, surgery and endoscopic techniques aim at restoring the competence of the antireflux barrier. A therapeutic management algorithm is proposed Figure 43.7.

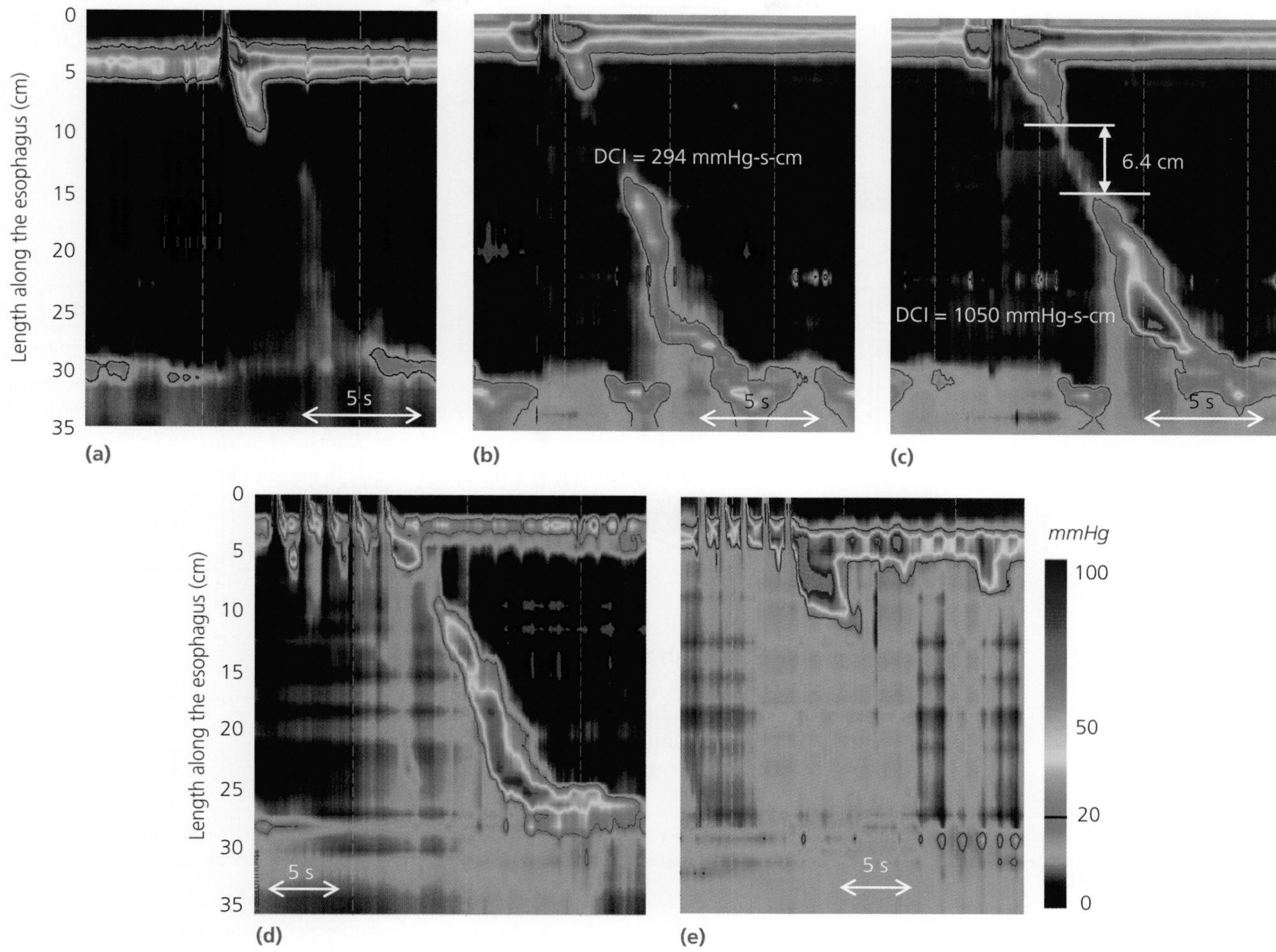

Figure 43.6 Esophageal contractility in gastroesophageal reflux disease (GERD). Absent contraction **(a)**, ineffective contraction **(b)**, and fragmented contraction **(c)** are frequently observed in GERD. Ineffective contraction is defined as a contraction with a distal contractile integral (DCI; metric used to assess the vigor of esophageal contraction) <450 mmHg·s·cm. A fragmented contraction is a contraction with a defect >5 cm in the contractile wavefront. Multiple rapid swallow consists of performing five 2-mL swallows. A contractile reserve is present **(d)** when the vigor of the contraction after the fifth swallow is higher than the vigor of a contraction observed after a single 5-mL water swallow. When there is no contraction after the fifth swallow, there is no contractile reserve **(e)**.

Lifestyle modifications

Recommended lifestyle modifications in GERD fall into three general categories: (1) avoid food that may lead to reflux, presumably by relaxing the LES (coffee, alcohol, chocolate, fatty food); (2) avoid acidic foods that may precipitate heartburn by a direct irritant effect on the esophageal mucosa (citrus, carbonated drinks, spicy foods); and (3) adopt behaviors that may reduce esophageal acid exposure by reducing the occurrence of reflux and/or enhancing the process of acid clearance (weight loss, smoking cessation, raising the head of bed, and avoiding recumbent position for 2–3 hours after meals). Although evidence supporting these recommendations is generally weak [200], they should be encouraged to the extent to which they seem relevant to the individual patient. For instance, patients with regurgitation and heartburn during recumbency should be advised to elevate the head of the bed and to avoid eating for the 2-to 3-hour period before going to bed. Similarly, someone who consistently experiences heartburn after ingestion of alcohol, coffee, or any specific food will benefit from avoidance of these items.

Obesity and weight control merit special attention because accumulating evidence suggests this to be one of the root causes of the GERD epidemic of the past three decades. Epidemiological data suggest a dose-dependent relationship between increasing BMI and frequent reflux symptoms [201]. However, the benefit of weight loss on GERD symptoms has not yet been demonstrated in rigorous clinical trials [202–204]. Nonetheless, if the development of troublesome heartburn paralleled weight gain in a patient, it is very reasonable to propose weight loss as an intervention that may prevent the need for continuous acid-suppressive therapy.

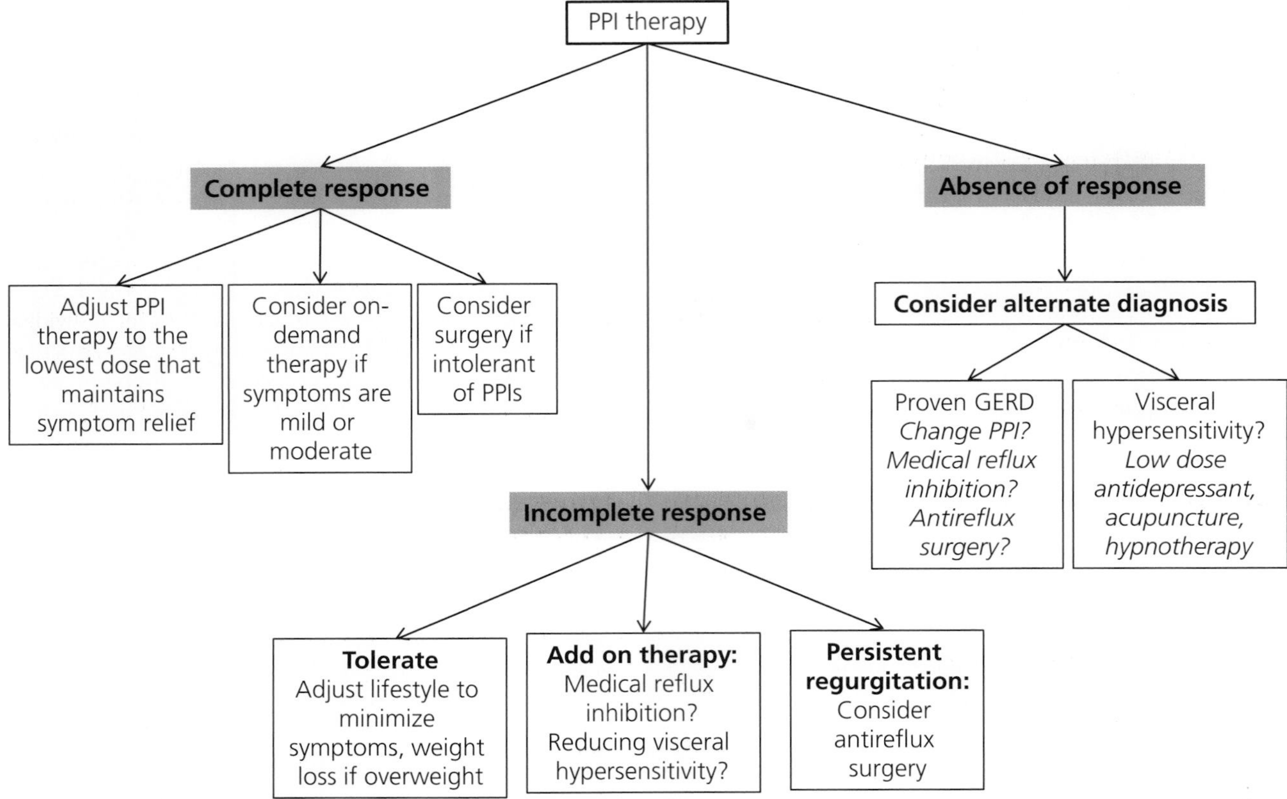

Figure 43.7 Therapeutic management algorithm. Proton pump inhibitors (PPIs) are the first-line therapy. The other alternative should be proposed when PPIs are not well tolerated or in the case of an incomplete and unsatisfactory response. GERD, gastroesophageal reflux disease.

Antacids

Antacids neutralize acid or acidic food without affecting subsequent acid secretion. Until recently they were considered as having limiting effects on GERD symptoms. However, the emerging concept of the acid pocket [64,65] might be a target for antacids combined with alginates. The acid pocket corresponds to the newly secreted acid layer on top of the ingested meal, evident within 20 minutes of eating. Neutralizing this acid layer might be associated with reduction of postprandial GERD symptoms. Alginates are natural polysaccharide polymers isolated from brown seaweed. On contact with gastric acid they precipitate into a low-density viscous gel of near-neutral pH. With the pH change, the sodium bicarbonate contained in the alginate-antacid formulation releases carbon dioxide, which is trapped in the alginate gel and floats on the top of the gastric content [205]. An antacid–alginate formation (Gaviscon) may eliminate or displace the acid pocket in patients with GERD [206]. It may also decrease the number of reflux events that reach the proximal esophagus [207].

A hyaluronic acid–chondroitin sulphate-based bioadhesive formulation (Esoxx) was developed to create a barrier on the esophageal mucosa, and thus reduce the contact between esophageal mucosa and gastric content [208]. A randomized study demonstrated that a combination of mucosal protection and acid suppression could improve symptom relief in patients with NERD compared with acid suppression alone (53% of patients with combined treatment had symptom relief vs 32% receiving only acid suppression; $p < 0.01$).

Acid suppression

Acid neutralization with antacid and pharmacologically inhibiting gastric acid secretion are cornerstones of medical GERD therapy. The most potent drugs are the PPIs, which covalently bind with gastric H^+/K^+-ATPase to block the final common pathway for acid secretion. Histamine-2-receptor antagonists (H_2RAs) competitively block histamine-stimulated acid secretion, making them less potent than PPIs and giving them a duration of action that parallels their serum half-life. Antacids neutralize acid or acidic food without having any effect on subsequent acid secretion.

Proton pump inhibitors

Indications

Evident from the definition, GERD encompasses a diverse set of potential syndromes, and the efficacy of PPI treatment varies substantially among these syndromes. The GERD manifestation most responsive to PPI therapy is esophagitis, in which case, esophageal epithelial injury is directly attributable to gastric acid, and eliminating acid facilitates mucosal healing with close to 100% effectiveness. Furthermore, in the case of esophagitis, higher doses and/or more potent PPIs are more effective than lower doses and/or weaker PPIs; in other words, there is a demonstrable dose–response curve. Similarly, dysphagia without stricture or malignancy, which is reported in about one-third of patients with esophagitis, resolves in 83% of patients with PPI therapy [209].

After esophagitis, heartburn is the second-best case scenario for PPI efficacy. However, the therapeutic gain associated with PPI therapy is sharply reduced from that observed with esophagitis. Furthermore, there is a 10–20% difference in therapeutic gain for heartburn dependent on whether it occurs in the context of erosive esophagitis or NERD. This discrepancy might be because the specificity of heartburn as an acid-induced symptom is less in the absence of esophagitis. This limitation is even more evident in the case of regurgitation wherein the therapeutic gain from PPI therapy is less than 20% [120]. Consequently, persistent regurgitation despite PPI therapy is a major phenotype of treatment-refractory GERD.

Atypical or extraesophageal GERD manifestations remain a controversial topic in disease management. In an analysis based on data from six randomized controlled trials, the therapeutic gain of >50% improvement with PPIs relative to placebo was achieved in 56–85% of patients with chest pain and *abnormal* pH-metry, but only 0–17% of patients with chest pain and *normal* pH-metry [121]. A Cochrane Review explored the efficacy of GERD treatment in patients with chronic cough [210]. Nine adult studies were identified comparing PPI with placebo and were included in a metaanalysis. No significant difference in effect was observed between PPI and placebo in total resolution of cough (OR, 0.46; 95% CI: 0.19–1.15). However, patients receiving PPI did exhibit a slight, but significant, improvement in cough scores after 2–3 months of PPI when data among studies were combined.

Whatever the presentation of GERD, the likelihood of spontaneous, long-term, sustained remission is low, and maintenance therapy is usually required. Although almost all severe esophagitis cases can be healed with PPI therapy, recurrence occurs in approximately 80% of patients within 6 months of discontinuation of therapy [211], and the likelihood of recurrence is directly related to the initial severity of esophagitis. Symptoms also usually relapse after PPI discontinuation. Maintenance therapy should be adjusted to the lowest PPI dose necessary to maintain symptom relief. Regardless of physicians' instructions, most patients do this themselves, adopting on-demand or intermittent PPI dosing as required for symptom control [200].

Dose and pharmacology

Most current practice guidelines endorse empiric treatment with a single US Food and Drug Administration-approved dose PPI therapy for a 4- to 8-week period for a patient with typical GERD symptoms [200]. The appropriate administration of PPI should be 30–60 minutes before breakfast to ensure the best inhibition of proton pumps [212]. However, PPIs exhibit considerable interindividual variation in the degree of acid suppression achieved. This is evident in gastric pH monitoring studies analyzed for the fraction of a 24-hour period that the intragastric pH is maintained >4. In a crossover study, Lind et al. [213] found that 55% of patients taking omeprazole 20 mg/day and 46% of patients taking esomeprazole 20 mg/day failed to maintain intragastric pH >4 for 12 hours or longer, whereas only 8% of patients taking esomeprazole 40 mg/day failed to maintain intragastric pH >4 for 12 hours. The fraction of individuals achieving pH control for 16 hours was proportionately less for all three regimens. The clinical implications of these data are: (1) more potent or higher doses of PPIs are more likely to be effective, and (2) there is a pharmacodynamic rationale for using PPIs in a twice-daily regimen after a once-daily regimen proves ineffective. Consequently, if a patient does not respond successfully to single-dose therapy, it is reasonable to escalate therapy to double dose because there is little risk to this practice and some patients are likely to respond [214]. However, supportive data for dose escalation in patients not responding to single-dose PPI are marginal, and the anticipated gain is likely in the range of 10% to 20% [215]. Becker et al. [216] reported that increasing PPI dosage was more effective in patients with abnormal pH-impedance monitoring while "on" standard PPI therapy (persistent abnormal acid exposure and/or increased number of reflux events) than in patients with normal studies (91% vs 43% symptom relief; $p < 0.001$).

Switching among PPIs is another option when faced with a poor PPI response. Some PPIs have been reformulated to increase or to speed absorption; this is the case with dexlansoprazole and immediate-release omeprazole. Genetic polymorphism of the cytochrome P450 enzyme (CYP2C19), a major metabolic pathway of PPIs, also explains some interindividual variability. Patients of Asian race may have reduced CYP2C19, and they may therefore require lower doses of PPI. Omeprazole and esomeprazole inhibit CYP2C19 [217], and it has been shown that the efficacy of omeprazole and lansoprazole in controlling gastric pH correlated with CYP2C19 status [218,219]. Rabeprazole is not metabolized by CYP2C19, but it is metabolized by CYP3A4. Bioavailability may also differ from among PPIs. In patients with persistent heartburn who are receiving once-daily PPI treatment, Fass et al. [215] compared the strategies of increasing the PPI dosage to twice daily (lansoprazole 30 mg BID) or switching to another PPI (esomeprazole 40 mg). They found that these strategies were equivalent in achieving heartburn control.

Interaction might exist between clopidogrel and PPIs. CYP2C19 is involved with both PPI and clopidogrel metabolism, and in vitro studies suggest that clopidogrel users have decreased CYP2C19 function and less inhibition of platelet aggregation, potentially putting them at risk for increased cardiovascular events. Indeed, initial observational studies suggested that patients receiving PPI and clopidogrel had excess cardiovascular events compared with patients receiving only clopidogrel [220]. However, this was not confirmed in a randomized trial. Nonetheless, despite the lack of evidence, some authors recommend separating the dosing of PPIs and clopidogrel by 12–20 hours to prevent competitive inhibition of CYP and potential diminished efficacy of clopidogrel [220]. A current societal guideline on GERD management concluded that "PPI therapy does not need to be altered in concomitant clopidogrel users" [221].

Safety

For short-term use, PPIs have proved quite safe. Side-effects include headache (<5%) and diarrhea (<5%), both of which are reversible with cessation of therapy. However, several safety concerns related to long-term PPI treatment have been raised. Most proposed adverse consequences are the result of profound inhibition of acid production by parietal cells (hypochlorhydria) or the consequent hypergastrinemia.

Gastric acid-mediated solubilization of dietary calcium salts is believed to be essential for calcium absorption. Thus, it has been suggested that long-term PPI therapy might increase the risk for osteopenia and fracture. In a metaanalysis, the OR for hip fracture was 1.25 (95% CI: 1.14–1.37) in PPI users compared with nonusers or past users [222]. This association was observed with both high-dose and low-dose PPI. Short-duration PPI use was associated with hip fracture risk (OR, 1.24; 95% CI: 1.19–1.28), but long-duration use was not (OR, 1.30; 95% CI: 0.98–1.70); the reason for this discrepancy was not clear. Targownik et al. [223] observed that PPI users had lower bone mineral density than PPI nonusers using the Canadian Multicenter Osteoporosis Study data set. However, there was no significant acceleration of bone mineral density loss after 5 and 10 years of PPI use. Hence although the epidemiological data prompted great concern, prospective studies have yet to demonstrate a significant risk for PPI use with respect to osteopenia or fractures.

PPI use induces hypergastrinemia because gastrin release is modulated by intragastric acidity. Gastrin has growth-promoting effects on a number of epithelial cell types (pancreas, stomach, colonic mucosa) [224]. In transgenic mice that express the mutant form of adenomatous polyposis coli, omeprazole-induced hypergastrinemia increased the proliferation rate of adenoma cells. However, population-based studies have not found an increased risk for colorectal cancer in PPI users [225,226], and long-term PPI use did not influence the frequency, growth, or histology of adenomatous polyps [227]. One study reported that PPI therapy in patients with corpus-predominant *H. pylori* gastritis might promote the development of atrophic gastritis, theoretically increasing the risk for gastric cancer [224], leading them to recommend *H. pylori* screening and treatment for patients beginning long-term PPI therapy. However, that recommendation has not been widely adopted. Finally, long-term PPI therapy can be associated with the development of enterochromaffin-like cells hyperplasia. However, this hyperplasia has not been shown to increase cancer risk in humans [224].

Increased risk for stroke and myocardial infarction has been reported in PPI users. A recent metaanalysis reported an increased risk for any adverse cardiovascular event in patients with PPI treatment as monotherapy (i.e., without antiplatelet treatment) using pooled data from observational studies (risk ratio, 1.25; 95% CI: 1.11–1.42) [228]. However, the risk was not increased using data from randomized controlled trials (risk ratio, 0.89; 95% CI: 0.34–2.33).

Dementia was reported, as well as associated with long-term PPI therapy [229]. The increased risk per patient and per year should be around 0.07–1.5%. Two mechanisms were proposed to explain this increased risk, one related to vitamin B_{12} deficiency and one related to enhanced brain β-amyloid levels. However, there is inconsistency between studies, and the increased risk is debated.

Gastric acid acts as an intraluminal "barrier" preventing bacteria from colonizing the upper GI tract and potentially influencing the composition of normal intestinal flora. A metaanalysis emphasized the association between PPI use and the risk for small-intestinal bacterial overgrowth (OR, 2.282; 95% CI: 1.238–4.205) [230]. However, the significant association was observed only in studies using duodenal or jejunal aspirate culture to diagnose small-intestinal bacterial overgrowth and not in those using hydrogen breath testing. Another limitation of this metaanalysis was the absence of clinical data regarding potential symptoms from small-intestinal bacterial overgrowth. Interestingly, an association between the increase of *C. difficile* infection and PPI use was noted [229]. PPI might reduce the diversity of gut microbiota and thus promote *C. difficile* infection. The absolute excess risk for *C. difficile* infection in chronic PPI users is estimated as 0–0.09% per patient per year.

Finally, reversible severe hypomagnesemia [231], several cases of acute interstitial nephritis [224], and chronic kidney diseases have been reported among PPI users, presumably occurring as sporadic idiosyncratic side-effects [229].

Due to the potential safety issues related to long-term PPI therapy, it is advised to prescribe PPI at the lowest effective dose [229].

Potassium-competitive acid blockers

Potassium-competitive acid blockers (P-CABs) are a new class of acid-suppressant agents that inhibit gastric H^+K^+-ATPase with a faster onset of action than PPIs [232]. The noninferiority of a P-CAB, vonoprazan, compared with PPI to heal esophagitis was demonstrated in randomized studies [233,234]. For example, in a randomized study including 481 patients with erosive esophagitis comparing vonoprazan 20 mg once daily with lansoprazole 30 mg once daily, the 8-week healing rate was 92% in the vonoprazan group compared with 91% in the lansoprazole group (difference 1.1 [95% CI: 3.822–6.087%]) [234]. The yield of vonoprazan was also assessed in patients with refractory GERD. A prospective, single-center, open-label study demonstrated esophagitis healing with vonoprazan 20 mg daily for 4 weeks in 52 out of 60 patients (87%) with persistent erosive esophagitis and symptoms after a PPI treatment for at least 8 weeks [235]. These 52 patients remained symptom free after a 24-week maintenance therapy with vonoprazan 10 mg daily.

It is important to note that a majority of studies evaluating vonoprazan were conducted in Asia, where the prevalence of patients with CYP2C19 polymorphisms is high and consequently PPI metabolism highly variable, ranging from rapid to slow. Contrary to PPIs, the elimination of P-CABs is independent of CYP2C19, and this may partially explain the increased potency of PCABs on acid suppression.

Histamine-2-receptor antagonists

H_2RAs competitively block histamine-stimulated acid secretion. Although they are less potent than PPIs, they are more effective than placebo in healing esophagitis and in relieving GERD heartburn [236,237]. Because they are competitive inhibitors, their duration of action parallels their serum half-life.

Adding a nighttime dose of H_2RAs to a twice-daily PPI has been proposed for patients with GERD with refractory symptoms. The rationale for this strategy was to control histamine-generated "nocturnal acid breakthrough" common with PPI therapy [238]. This strategy was shown to control nocturnal acid breakthrough during intragastric pH studies. However, no clinical correlation with healing or symptom improvement has yet been demonstrated. Furthermore, tachyphylaxis occurs. A study by Fackler et al. [239] showed blunting of the H_2RA effect within 1 week of daily therapy. However, the addition of an H_2RA at night is safe and could potentially be effective in a small proportion of patients with significant nocturnal symptoms, especially if the medication is used intermittently.

Reflux inhibition

Because tLESRs are a dominant mechanism of reflux in most patients with GERD [75], they represent an attractive target for GERD treatment. Conceptually, suppressing tLESRs might be more effective than PPIs in treating regurgitation. Baclofen, a $GABA_B$ agonist, inhibits the vagal pathway for tLESRs both centrally and peripherally [74]. However, because the drug crosses the brain–blood barrier, neurological side-effects (somnolence, dizziness, drowsiness) limit its use for GERD in clinical practice. Therefore, novel $GABA_B$ agonists have been developed in an attempt to limit these side-effects. Experimentally, arbaclofen placarbil, a prodrug of the pharmacologically active *R*-isomer of baclofen, decreases the number of postprandial reflux events [240]. Similarly, lesogaberan, a novel $GABA_B$ agonist, has been shown to decrease postprandial tLESRs [241,242]. However, larger-scale studies failed to show significant additive benefit to PPIs in terms of improvement in heartburn or regurgitation with these investigational drugs. In patients with symptomatic GERD who did not respond successfully to PPI therapy, the proportion of patients who respond to reflux inhibition was modest and not specific for heartburn or regurgitation. In a randomized trial including 244 patients with persistent heartburn and/or regurgitation despite PPI therapy, lesogaberan, used as add-on therapy, increased the number of heartburn-free days by 14% and the number of regurgitation-free days by 13% compared with placebo [243]. Due to the modest effect of these drugs, their development was halted. Another investigational drug, ADX10059, a metabotropic glutamate receptor 5 negative allosteric modulator, reduced reflux events and improved symptoms in patients with GERD [244]. However, the development was stopped because of hepatic side-effects. As a consequence, baclofen is the only reflux inhibitor currently available.

Prokinetic drugs

Patients with GERD can exhibit longer esophageal acid clearance times [91]. Hence limiting the contact time between the refluxate and the esophageal mucosa may reduce symptoms. Ideally, a prokinetic would enhance esophageal clearance by strengthening peristalsis.

Prucalopride, a highly specific 5-HT_4 agonist, has been commercialized for the treatment of constipation. It has been shown to decrease acid esophageal acid exposure and stimulate gastric emptying in healthy volunteers [245]. In patients with GERD, prucalopride might stimulate secondary peristalsis [246]. However, the efficacy of prucalopride on esophageal GERD symptoms has yet to be demonstrated. Another 5-HT4 agonist, mosapride, was tested as an add-on therapy with esomeprazole in patients with erosive esophagitis [247]. The 8-week healing rate was similar in patients receiving PPI alone and in those receiving PPI plus mosapride. However, symptoms tended to improve more rapidly in patients with combined therapy even if the difference did not reach statistical significance.

An alternative approach is to promote gastric emptying, which may have the secondary consequence of reducing the occurrence of tLESR. Metoclopramide, an antidopaminergic agent that also acts as a 5-HT_3 antagonist, 5-HT_4 agonist, and cholinomimetic, may improve gastric emptying [248], leading some to propose its use in GERD, especially if the GERD is accompanied by delayed gastric emptying. However, there are no high-quality data supporting the use of metoclopramide as either monotherapy or adjunctive therapy in esophageal or suspected extraesophageal GERD syndromes. In addition, considering the toxicity profile of the drug (central nervous system side-effects, such as tremor, parkinsonism, depression, or tardive dyskinesia), the current recommendation is against the use of metoclopramide in GERD because the potential risks exceed the potential benefits [200].

Targeting visceral hypersensitivity

Some patients with erosive esophagitis and, especially, NERD exhibit hypersensitivity to esophageal stimuli. This can be demonstrated by balloon distension in the esophagus or acid perfusion (Bernstein test). Hypersensitive patients have a diminished threshold for perceiving these stimuli and a reduced threshold for experiencing pain compared with healthy volunteers [224].

Targeting esophageal sensitivity might be an option for GERD treatment, especially in NERD.

Low-dose antidepressants

Antidepressants may modulate esophageal sensitivity at the central nervous system and/or peripheral level, potentially benefitting symptomatic patients. Low-dose tricyclic antidepressants have been shown to be effective in patients with chest pain after incomplete response to PPI [249]. Trazodone, a serotonin antagonist and reuptake inhibitor, was more effective than placebo in patients with esophageal symptoms (chest pain, dysphagia, heartburn, and/or regurgitation) associated with esophageal contraction abnormalities [250]. Citalopram, another selective serotonin reuptake inhibitor, significantly increased the threshold for perception and discomfort after balloon distension in healthy volunteers [251]. It also prolonged the duration of esophageal acid perfusion required to induce heartburn. Consequently, these medications may be useful to alleviate esophageal discomfort and heartburn in the subset of patients with GERD with hypersensitivity. A placebo-controlled trial of citalopram in patients with pH-impedance findings suggestive of hypersensitivity supports this concept [252].

Acupuncture

Manual acupuncture and electroacupuncture might be an alternative treatment of GERD. A metaanalysis demonstrated superior global symptom improvement with acupuncture compared with traditional GERD treatment (relative risk, 1.17; 95% CI: 1.09–1.26; $p = 0.03$) [253]. An improvement of quality of life was reported in patients who underwent acupuncture.

Hypnotherapy

Response to PPI treatment can be modulated by the level of psychological distress [254]. Consequently, a therapy that reduces psychological distress may be beneficial in some patients who have an inadequate response to PPI. Hypnotherapy has been proposed as such an alternative therapy, especially for patients with atypical GERD symptoms. In a randomized trial including 28 patients with noncardiac chest pain, patients treated with hypnotherapy experienced a global improvement in pain more frequently than did control therapy (80% vs 23%). Similarly, in a case series of patients with globus sensation, hypnotherapy appeared to be a beneficial intervention [255]. It remains to be determined whether this alternative is effective in larger series of patients with GERD-associated functional symptoms.

Surgical fundoplication

Fundoplication attempts to correct the underlying abnormalities associated with GERD. The essential features of fundoplication are to mobilize the lower esophagus, reduce the associated hiatal hernia, and wrap the gastric fundus either partially or totally around the esophagus. The operation reestablishes competence of the antireflux barrier by repairing the hiatus hernia and increasing resting LES pressure [256]. It may also reduce reflux by decreasing the frequency and/or effectiveness of transient LES relaxations [257]. Currently, the two most popular surgical procedures are the laparoscopic Nissen (360°) fundoplication and the Toupet (270°) fundoplication.

High-quality evidence on the efficacy of antireflux surgery exists only for esophagitis and/or excessive distal acid exposure determined without ongoing PPI therapy [200]. Antireflux surgery is at least as effective as PPI therapy in controlling heartburn and acid regurgitation in controlled trials. The LOTUS trial, a large randomized European trial comparing laparoscopic antireflux surgery with esomeprazole treatment for patients with chronic GERD, illustrates the efficacy of antireflux surgery. The diagnosis of GERD was established on the basis of typical symptoms and the presence of esophageal mucosal breaks at endoscopy and/or a pathological esophageal pH-metry study. Only patients with clinical response to esomeprazole during a 3-month run-in period were randomized. Over the first 3 years of follow-up, both laparoscopic fundoplication and PPI therapy were similarly effective in achieving complete symptom remission [258]. The estimated remission rates at 5 years were greater in the esomeprazole group than in the laparoscopic fundoplication group (92% vs 85%, $p = 0.048$) [259]. However, differences were observed between treatments when analyzed by specific symptoms. Specifically, regurgitation was significantly worse in the medical group than in the surgical group (13% vs 2%, respectively; $p < 0.001$), whereas there was no significant difference between the groups in heartburn severity. Dysphagia, bloating, and flatulence were all significantly more common in the fundoplication group than in the PPI group.

Accordingly, the potential benefits of antireflux surgery should be weighed against the potentially deleterious effect of new symptoms consequent from surgery, particularly dysphagia, flatulence, an inability to belch, and postsurgery bowel symptoms (bloating, gas, diarrhea, abdominal pain). Another important requirement for antireflux surgery is the presence of some peristaltic activity in the esophagus. Although the precise cut-off remains uncertain, severe peristaltic dysfunction is a relative contraindication and complete absence of peristalsis an absolute contraindication for antireflux surgery [200]. Given this perspective, esophageal manometry should be done preoperatively to evaluate peristaltic function [197]. It can also exclude major esophageal motility disorders that may masquerade as GERD: achalasia and distal esophageal spasm.

Outcomes of antireflux surgery are highly operator dependent. Efficacy data from community practice [260] are widely divergent from those of the LOTUS trial with reports of as many as 30% of patients resuming PPI therapy within 5 years of antireflux surgery. Revision fundoplication surgery is also common, accounting for up to 50% of operations performed at some referral centers [261]. Hence antireflux surgery should be recommended with caution. Patients with esophagitis who are intolerant of PPIs will likely benefit from antireflux surgery. In contrast, patients with esophagitis who are well maintained on medical therapy may have nothing to gain from antireflux surgery and incur added risk. Patients with esophageal GERD symptoms poorly controlled by PPIs may benefit from surgery, especially in the setting of persistent regurgitation. Even so, the indication must be balanced with the risk for surgery, and patients need to be advised of potential dysphagia, inability to belch, flatulence, and the development of new bowel symptoms. Interestingly, a recent randomized trial conducted in patients with PPI-refractory heartburn demonstrated that highly selected patients, that is, patients with persistent symptoms on PPIs with elevated esophageal acid exposure and/or a positive reflux symptom association on pH-impedance monitoring, might benefit from antireflux surgery [262]. Indeed, these "truly PPI-refractory heartburn patients" responded better to fundoplication than to PPI plus baclofen or PPI alone (treatment success rate at 1 year: 67% vs 28% and 12%; $p = 0.007$ and $p < 0.001$, respectively). It is important to note that the "truly refractory heartburn patients" represented only 21% of the patients screened who were reporting heartburn despite PPI therapy.

Novel antireflux procedures

Recent years have seen many putative endoscopic reflux treatments come and go. Most have ultimately been found to offer minimal efficacy and an unacceptable incidence of adverse events leading to poor acceptance and/or rapid withdrawal from the market. Currently, there are two procedural therapies, both designed to restore competency to the EGJ, that are approved for use, albeit still undergoing evaluation in clinical trials: transoral incisionless fundoplication (TIF) device and magnetic sphincter augmentation.

TIF is done with a device designed to be used in conjunction with an endoscope to create transmural plications in the region of the EGJ. With the TIF procedure, an ω-shaped, full-thickness gastroesophageal valve is created from inside the stomach [263]. In an early open-label study, TIF was compared with laparoscopic fundoplication in patients with persistent heartburn or regurgitation despite PPI therapy [264]. A randomized trial conducted in patients with troublesome regurgitation despite PPI demonstrated that TIF was more effective than PPI to eliminate troublesome regurgitation (67% of patients reported regurgitation elimination in the TIF group at 6 months vs 45% in the PPI group; $p = 0.023$) [265]. A recent metaanalysis confirmed that TIF was a safe and effective procedure with 89% (95% CI: 82–95%; $p < 0.001$) of patients able to stop PPIs after the procedure [266].

Magnetic sphincter augmentation is accomplished with a device (LINX Reflux Management System; Torax Medical, Shoreview, NM, USA) consisting of a miniature band of interlinked titanium beads with magnetic cores that is laparoscopically placed around the EGJ with or without surgical repair of the hiatus [267]. The magnetic attraction between adjacent beads augments sphincter competence by resisting opening and limiting distension. However, the beads do temporarily separate to allow swallowing, belching, or vomiting. A prospective open-label study performed in 100 patients with GERD demonstrated that only 15% were still taking PPIs 5 years after the procedure (vs all of them before LINX) [268]. Bothersome dysphagia was reported in 6% of patients (vs 5% at baseline) and gas bloat in 8% (vs 52% at baseline). In a recent randomized study, magnetic sphincter augmentation controlled regurgitation in 96% of patients at 1 year, whereas only 19% of patients on double-dose PPI reported control of regurgitation [269].

LES electrical stimulation is another minimally invasive surgical procedure under investigation but not yet approved. Electrodes are laparoscopically placed in the LES and connected to an implantable pulse generator [270]. This procedure is associated with reduced esophageal acid exposure and esophageal symptoms in an uncontrolled study [270,271]. These results have not been confirmed in larger controlled trials.

The eventual place of these novel procedures in GERD management remains to be determined, certainly awaiting a more comprehensive understanding of their effectiveness, limitations, and safety. These procedures are designed to be reversible, and it is hoped that they will cause fewer adverse events than laparoscopic fundoplication, potentially representing an intermediate therapy between existing medical and conventional surgical approaches for GERD.

Management of GERD complications: peptic strictures

With the widespread use of PPIs, the incidence of peptic stricture has declined [145,146]. The aims of treatment of peptic strictures are to restore normal lumen diameter, heal esophagitis, and prevent recurrence. PPIs are used to heal esophagitis and prevent recurrences. Endoscopic dilation can be useful to restore esophageal lumen caliber [272]. Different types of dilatators are available: flexible plastic/hard rubber dilators (i.e., Savary) and balloon dilators. The choice between them is a matter of personal preference, cost, availability, and experience; there are no high-quality randomized trials that compare dilators. In cases of refractory stricture despite dilation, intralesion steroid injection can be considered. However, it is extraordinarily rare for peptic strictures as opposed to strictures of other etiologies. Antireflux surgery might also be an option in some cases if more conservative procedures fail.

References are available at www.yamadagastro.com/textbook7e

Further reading

Bredenoord A.J., Pandolfino J.E., Smout A.J. Gastro-oesophageal reflux disease. Lancet 2013;381:1933.

Dunbar K.B., Agoston A.T., Odze R.D., et al. Association of acute gastroesophageal reflux disease with esophageal histologic changes. JAMA 2016;315:2104.

Galmiche J.P., Hatlebakk J., Attwood S., et al. Laparoscopic antireflux surgery vs esomeprazole treatment for chronic GERD. The LOTUS randomized clinical trial. JAMA 2011;305:1969.

Gyawali C.P., Kahrilas P.J., Savarino E., et al. Modern diagnosis of GERD: the Lyon Consensus. Gut 2018;67:1351.

Kahrilas P.J., Boeckxstaens G. Failure of reflux inhibitors in clinical trials: bad drugs or wrong patients? Gut 2012;61:1501.

Katz P.O., Gerson L.B., Vela M.F. Guidelines for the diagnosis and management of gastroesophageal reflux disease. Am J Gastroenterol 2013;108:308.

Lundell L.R., Dent J., Bennett J.R., et al. Endoscopic assessment of oesophagitis: clinical and functional correlates and further validation of the Los Angeles classification. Gut 1999;45:172.

Spechler S.J., Hunter J.G., Jones K.M., et al. Randomized trial of medical versus surgical treatment for refractory heartburn. N Engl J Med 2019;381:1513.

Vakil N., van Zanten S.V., Kahrilas P., et al. The Montreal definition and classification of gastroesophageal reflux disease: a global evidence-based consensus. Am J Gastroenterol 2006;101:1900.

CHAPTER 44
Eosinophilic esophagitis

Nirmala Gonsalves[1] and David A. Katzka[2]

[1] Feinberg School of Medicine, Northwestern University, Rochester, MN, USA

[2] Department of Gastroenterology and Hepatology, Mayo Clinic, Rochester, MN, USA

Chapter menu

Definition

Guideline statements have defined eosinophilic esophagitis (EoE) as a chronic immune-mediated condition of the esophagus consisting of a combination of esophageal symptoms and esophageal tissue eosinophilia [1–4]. Furthermore, whereas previous guidelines may have differed on the level of esophageal eosinophilia used as a definition, more recent guidelines agree on 15 eosinophils per high-power field as a threshold to define the presence of EoE. Prior definitions had also required the use of a proton pump inhibitor for a predefined duration prior to making the diagnosis of EoE, but this too has changed with the recognition that some patients with EoE may have disease that responds entirely to treatment with proton pump inhibition.

While this simple definition has been in place for years, there are aspects that may need to evolve. Reasons for this include: (1) variation in high-power field diameters used by pathologists when counting eosinophils [5]; (2) use of a single highest eosinophil level in a disease with patchy histology; (3) the inability to assess the presence of esophageal degranulation on routine histology [6]; (4) the recognition of other parameters that further assess EoE activity in a complementary fashion. As a result, more recent studies have been using composite scores to diagnose and assess EoE [7] based not only on esophageal eosinophilia but endoscopic activity [8], symptoms [9,10], and measures of histological abnormalities [11] associated with eosinophilic esophagitis. Whether this will become a part of the standard definition of EoE remains to be determined.

Epidemiology

Whereas eosinophilic esophagitis was thought to be a rare disease when first described, more recent data suggest it is becoming more common [12]. This is in part due to increased recognition [13] and also to an increasing incidence of the disease [14,15]. For example, in Denmark, the incidence of EoE increased by 20 times over a 15-year period to 2.6 cases/100 000 when esophageal biopsies were analyzed. The general incidence range is between 1 and 56 patients per 100 000 adult patients [16,17]. The incidence of EoE also varies depending on the time period and population studied. For example, in a study using a military population undergoing clinically indicated endoscopy, the prevalence of EoE was 6.5% [18] whereas patients presenting with food impaction (particularly if under age 40) have up to a 63% chance of having EoE [19,20]. Thus, as symptomatic and demographic features specific to EoE become more evident, the incidence and prevalence increase markedly.

Yamada's Textbook of Gastroenterology, Seventh Edition. Edited by Timothy C. Wang, Michael Camilleri, Benjamin Lebwohl, Anna S. Lok, William J. Sandborn, Kenneth K. Wang, and Gary D. Wu.

Companion website: www.yamadagastro.com/textbook7e

There are clear demographic factors that distinguish EoE. For example, patients are more likely to be white when compared to Hispanic and African American populations [21]. EoE is also approximately 3–4 times more common in men than women [22]. The peak ages for EoE are in the third and fourth decades but patients as young as 1 [22,23] and as old as 89 years [24] have been described. Nevertheless, it is unusual for a patient with EoE to be diagnosed for the first time in their eighth decade and beyond.

Patients with EoE also tend to have additional atopic history. The presence of asthma, atopic dermatitis, seasonal allergies, oral allergy, and other IgE-related syndromes is reported in up to 100% of patients with EoE [25,26] though this is highly variable amongst studies. Family history of EoE may also be an important factor in predisposition to the disease. Indeed, families including multiple members with EoE have been reported [27]. These reports include both parent–child and sibling association [28]. Genetic studies suggest that the estimated risk of EoE in a first-degree relative is 3% [29].

Finally, other diseases have been associated with EoE, including connective tissue disease [30], other autoimmune conditions [31], achalasia [32–34], Barrett esophagus [35] (including after ablation [36]), following esophageal atresia [37–40] and hypertrophic cardiomyopathy [41]. An association with celiac disease has been proposed [42–44] but has not been uniformly demonstrated [45]. Epidemiological studies also suggest that early life exposures can affect the risk of EoE with positive associations with maternal fever, proton pump inhibitor (PPI) therapy, pre- and postnatal antibiotics, and neonatal intensive care unit admission (Table 44.1) [46].

Temporal/secular trends

Almost all studies demonstrate that the incidence of eosinophilic esophagitis is increasing. In a study from the Netherlands analyzing a 20-year period from 1996 to 2015 [47], the incidence increased from 0.01 to 2.07 per 100 000 inhabitants, representing a 200-fold increase. This incidence was higher in males than females, in adults than children, and all despite only a threefold increase in the use of endoscopy. These findings parallel epidemiological data from other countries such as Switzerland [48], Denmark [14], and the United States [49].

Table 44.1 Risk factors for eosinophilic esophagitis (EoE).

Demographic	Environmental	Genetic
White	C-section	First-degree relative with EoE
Male	Bottle fed	
Childhood	Only child	
Early adulthood	Oral immunotherapy	
?Suburban	Other or multiple atopic disorders	
?Northern US	Early proton pump inhibitor or antibiotic exposure	

Geographic factors

There may also be geographic factors that increase the occurrence of EoE. For example, EoE is more common in western countries probably due to the prominence of a white population. Nevertheless, EoE has been described in patients on every continent except Africa. There are also reports of regional differences within countries where EoE is prevalent. For example, EoE appears more common in cold than in tropical and arid zones of the United States [50]. There are also data suggesting that EoE is more likely in suburban than urban populations [51].

Pathogenesis

The pathogenesis of EoE is a complex interaction of genetic predisposition, esophageal mucosal antigenic exposure, initiation of an allergic response, and chronic inflammation leading to fibrosis (Figure 44.1).

Genetics

Several types of data support a genetic contribution to eosinophilic esophagitis. For example, families with multiple members either vertically and/or horizontally related have been described [28]. Twin studies have shown a 36% concordance in dizygotic twins compared to 58% concordance in monozygotic twins in comparison to regular fraternal siblings [28,52]. While many genes have been identified in the EoE transcriptome as playing a role in the development of EoE, the most relevant include a chemokine, eotaxin-3, thymic stromal lymphopoietin (TSLP) gene and CAPN14 gene [53] which is important in barrier function.

Esophageal barrier dysfunction

Several lines of evidence suggest perturbed esophageal epithelial barrier function in patients with EoE. These include histological, morphological, and physiological data. For example, patients with EoE have lower mucosal impedance compared to normal mucosa [54,55]. This presumably represents increased permeability of water and electrolytes through the mucosa that allows greater conductivity of electric current. This is supported by data demonstrating increased permeability of epithelial strips in vitro; from patients with EoE [56]. Histologically, patients with EoE characteristically demonstrate dilation of epithelial intercellular spaces, suggesting increased permeability through these spaces [11]. Morphologically, multiple studies have demonstrated defects in tight junction proteins and desmosomes, structures that help regulate the dynamics of the intercellular space [57–60]. Finally, the presence of food antigens can be identified in the mucosa of patients with active EoE but less so or absent in patients with inactive disease and controls, respectively [61].

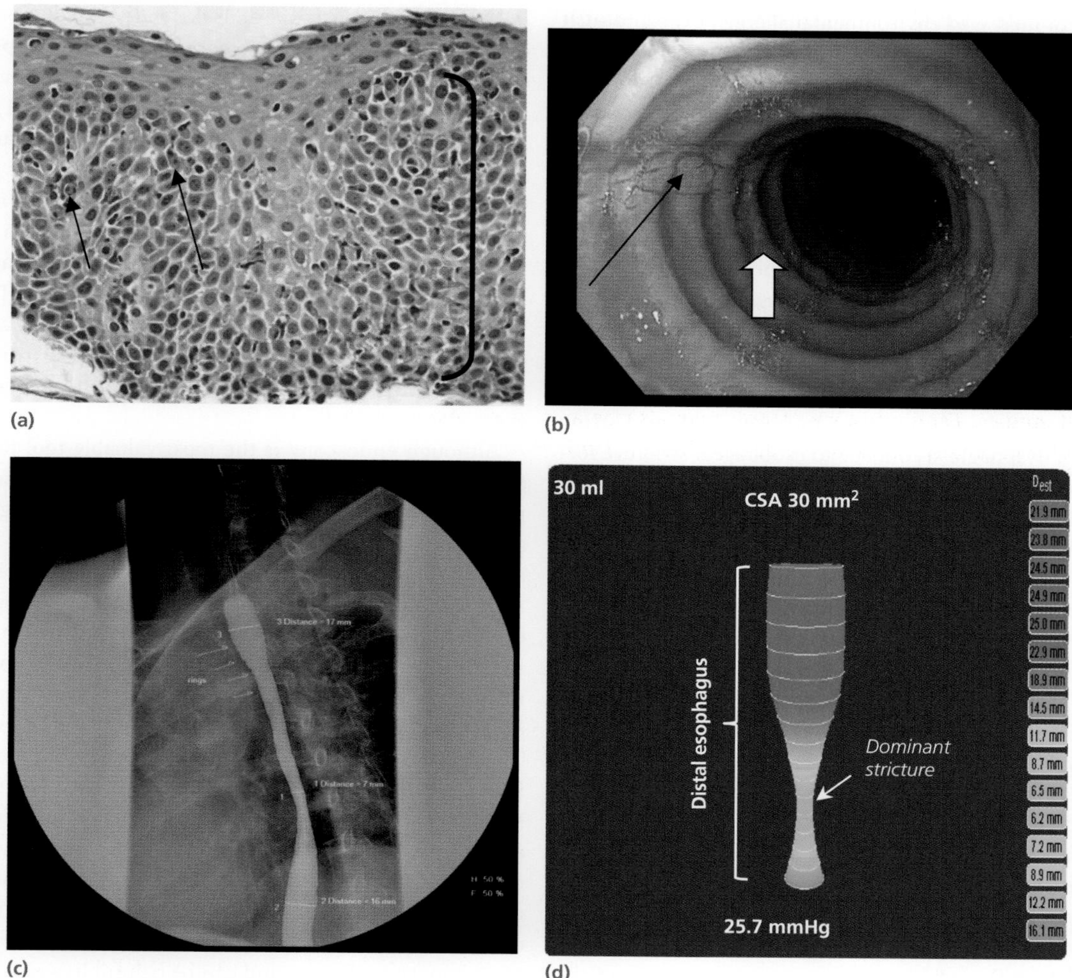

Figure 44.1 Diagnostic testing for eosinophilic esophagitis. **(a)** Histology demonstrating increased eosinophils (black arrow), dilated intercellular spaces (clear spaces surrounding cells), and basal zone hyperplasia (}). **(b)** Endoscopic image demonstrating rings, furrows (black arrow), edema, and exudates (white arrow). **(c)** Barium radiograph of patient with small-caliber esophagus. **(d)** EndoFLIP image of esophagus with marked loss of distensibility in distal esophagus indicating stricture formation.

Inflammatory pathways

Upon antigen exposure in the esophageal epithelium, a cascade of signals and inflammatory events occurs, leading to esophageal inflammation and, in time, fibrosis. This begins with a triggering of a T helper 2 (Th2) cell-mediated response that results in both inflammatory and fibrotic cytokines. Some of these important cytokines include eotaxin-3, interleukin (IL)-5, IL-13, TSLP, transforming growth factor (TGF) β1, and fibroblast growth factor (FGF) 9 [62].

Environmental factors

Predisposition to EoE begins early in life with events that presumably lead to an abnormal gut and perhaps other organ microbiome. Similar to other atopic disorders, patients with EoE are more likely to have been delivered via cesarean section, bottle fed, and have sustained early life antibiotic exposure [46]. They are also more likely to have been born in cold climates [63]. Patients with EoE are also less likely to have *H. pylori* infection [64.65]. This makes intuitive sense as *H. pylori* suppresses the Th2 response. There is also concern that PPI exposure may predispose to EoE [66]. Immunotherapy has also been associated with the development of eosinophilic esophagitis [67–70]. Through childhood, patients who develop EoE also have a series of concordant and perhaps sequential allergic disorders such as atopic dermatitis, asthma, and allergic rhinitis [71]. It is speculated that in this allergic march, patients can start with food-induced anaphylactic allergies but then these disorders may change over time to include asthma, allergic rhinitis, and EoE as patients get older [71]. It is also suggested that activity of other atopic disorders may cause onset of flare of EoE. For example, there is a greater chance of developing EoE in patients undergoing immunotherapy [72] and some patients may report that their symptoms of EoE are worse during times of increased environmental allergen exposure such as in the spring and the fall [73]. Environmental antigens, such as those from dust mites, may also be found in the esophagus mucosa of patients with EoE [74].

Clinical presentation and natural history

The clinical presentation of EoE is age dependent (Table 44.2). This presumably reflects a difference in symptoms that result from esophageal inflammation and fibrosis. In children where inflammation predominates, symptoms can be protean and include failure to thrive, nausea and vomiting at young ages followed by abdominal and chest pain in older children. During teenage years, dysphagia secondary to esophageal stricture formation becomes more prominent and persists into adulthood. A clinical series of adults with EoE suggests that 100% may have dysphagia. A consequence of esophageal stricture and a common presenting symptom may be food impaction. Indeed, EoE is the most common cause of food impaction in patients under the age of 45 and perhaps overall [75]. A rare presentation of EoE resulting from retching with or prolongation of food impaction is Boerhaave syndrome.

Notably, as in many chronic diseases, some of the most prominent symptoms may reflect compensatory maneuvers learned by the patient to avoid dysphagia and food impaction [76]. These include slow eating, careful chewing, avoidance of foods that commonly cause impaction (such as meat and bread), cutting solid food into small pieces, use of gravy or sauces to lubricate the food, and increased fluid consumption during meals. Due to the concern for getting food impaction, some patients may experience a fear of eating at restaurants. Because of the potential complexity of symptoms in EoE patients, several dysphagia scoring systems have been developed for clinical trials and practice as a means of more precisely following symptom response or relapse.

While the diagnosis of EoE is dependent on demonstration of esophageal eosinophilia (>15 eosinophils per high-power field) on esophageal biopsy, several additional techniques are complementary in making this diagnosis (see Figure 44.1). The first and foremost adjunctive test is endoscopy. Key features of EoE seen during endoscopic evaluation include linear furrowing, mucosal edema, mucosal exudates, concentric rings, and fibrotic strictures. These features have been organized into an elegant weighted scoring system termed EREFS (Exudates, Rings, Edema, Furrows, Stricture – see Figure 44.1) [8]. This system has become an essential part of clinical trials and also clinical practice. Other endoscopic signs include crepe paper esophagus (mucosal fragility) and the deep mucosal tears that are seen even after mild dilation.

Although endoscopy is the most valuable tool for assessing gross esophageal changes in EoE, it is limited to evaluating the mucosal surface and not deeper layers of the esophageal wall. As a result, two complementary imaging methods have been applied to EoE. The first is esophagography (see Figure 44.1). Although not accurate for assessing mucosal changes of EoE, esophagography is significantly more sensitive for detecting strictures, particularly in patients with a diffuse esophageal narrowing or narrow-caliber esophagus. In one study, 25% of esophageal strictures <13 mm were missed on endoscopy [77]. The second method is with the endoscopic functional luminal imaging probe (EndoFLIP®) [78]. This is an orally passed long segment balloon-based device that is inflated in a series of steps at known volume and pressure, which measures the resistance or compliance of the esophageal well. Patients with fibrotic change will have lower esophageal wall compliance reflective of a stricture. This test may be used for diagnosis and for monitoring response to therapy and can be helpful in assessing esophageal diameter prior to planned stricture dilation.

Finally, other tools are emerging as important, less invasive measures of EoE activity. These include nonendoscopic esophageal mucosal sampling techniques such as the esophageal string

Table 44.2 Symptoms and conditions that should prompt consideration of eosinophilic esophagitis (EoE).

Symptoms	Compansatory behavior	Demographic factors
Children		
Failure to thrive	Picky eating	Male gender
Nausea and vomiting	Slow eating	Other atopic disorders (allergic rhinitis, eczema, seasonal allergies, asthma, food allergy)
Abdominal pain	Food avoidance	Family history of EoE
Adults		
Dysphagia	Careful chewing	
Intermittent food impaction	Increased fluids with meals	
Refractory heartburn	Avoiding social eating	
Atypical chest pain	Prolonged eating time Avoiding solid foods	

test [79] and the Cytosponge [80], endoscopic tools that obviate the need for endoscopy with biopsy. Other tools being developed include measurement of esophageal mucosal impedance [81] and simpler and less expensive endoscopic devices such as transnasal endoscopy [82].

Although the gold standard for diagnosing EoE has been the level of esophageal eosinophilia, newer tools to better assess histological activity are being devised given the limitations of quantifying a single cell type as a marker of inflammation. These limitations include the patchy nature of the disease in the esophagus and the limited amount of esophagus sampled with a standard biopsy. Therefore, other parameters and markers of histological activity are being investigated, such as a more generalized histological response measured by the EoEHSS (EoE histological scoring system) [11]. For example, in the EoEHSS, other histological findings such as basal zone hyperplasia, dilation of intercellular spaces, esophageal abscesses, surface layering of eosinophils, and lamina propria fibrosis are assessed and scored in severity. Initial studies have suggested that the EoEHSS may correlate better with disease activity than the peak eosinophil score and it has been incorporated into clinical trial design [83,84].

Differential diagnosis

Although most diseases that may cause esophageal eosinophilia are rare (Table 44.3), gastroesophageal reflux disease (GERD) is a common cause of esophageal eosinophilia and difficult to distinguish from EoE. To complicate matters, these disorders are not mutually exclusive and some patients may have an EoE/GERD overlap [85]. As a result, testing such as ambulatory pH monitoring or extent of esophageal eosinophilia does not clearly distinguish the diseases [86,87]. On the other hand, measurement of the location of abnormal mucosal impedance (distal vs whole esophagus) may be helpful [88,89].

At this time, diagnosis is best made by assessing the constellation of findings in an individual patient. For example, esophageal eosinophilia occurring in a 70-year-old white man with central obesity and grade D esophagitis is most likely to be due to gastroesophageal reflux. Conversely, a 20-year-old white man with a 5-year history of solid food dysphagia, a history of asthma and rhinitis and esophageal edema, furrow and rings on endoscopy will have eosinophilic esophagitis. Clinical judgment is required to classify and treat patients with phenotypic characteristics common to both diseases. Finally, achalasia may be associated with EoE and present similarly with dysphagia and heartburn [32–34]. The pathophysiological relationship of these two entities is unclear [34].

Table 44.3 Differential diagnosis and associated conditions.

Differential diagnosis	Associated conditions
Achalasia	Hypermobility syndromes
Allergic vasculitis	Marfan syndrome type II
Crohn's disease of the esophagus	Ehlers–Danlos syndrome
Drug hypersensitivity response	Loeys–Dietz syndrome
Esophageal leiomyomatosis	Eosinophilic gastroenteritis/colitis
Graft-versus-host disease (GVHD)	Collagen vascular disease
Hypereosinophilic syndrome (HES)	Esophageal atresia
Parasitic infection	Celiac disease
Bullous pemphigoid	Inflammatory bowel disease
Gastroesophageal reflux disease	

Complications

The most common complication of eosinophilic esophagitis is esophageal stricture formation which can lead to food bolus impaction. In one study, 85% of patients with greater than 20 years of undiagnosed symptoms had strictures. The severity and locations of strictures in patients with EoE vary widely (see Figure 44.1). These may include localized concentric strictures to diffuse esophageal narrowing termed small-caliber esophagus. Whereas a distal esophageal stricture may occur from either GERD or EoE, proximal esophageal strictures in the absence of Barrett esophagus are typically from EoE. Another complication of EoE is iatrogenic perforation during endoscopic dilation. The incidence of perforation is 1–2% in large experienced medical centers [90,91]. Greater than 50% of these patients will heal with conservative therapy, with the remainder requiring stent placement or surgery. Fortunately, the latter group is relatively rare. Contained esophageal perforation has been seen in patients who have had prolonged food impaction with retching. Spontaneous perforation (Boerhaave syndrome) is significantly more rare but may also occur in patients with EoE due to prolonged bolus impaction and/or retching [92].

Two infections have been associated with eosinophilic esophagitis. *Candida albicans* occurs in up to 5% of patients with eosinophilic esophagitis as a complication of topical steroid therapy [93–97]. It may be difficult to differentiate some symptoms of EoE from *Candida* although the latter is commonly asymptomatic and found incidentally on endoscopy. Additionally, cases of herpes simplex complicating [98] or preceding [99] eosinophilic esophagitis have been reported. Finally, adrenal insufficiency remains a concern with chronic steroid use and biochemical evidence may occur but clinical manifestations are rare [100].

Therapy and management

Endpoints of therapy

Initially, the primary endpoint for therapy of EoE was to reduce esophageal mucosal eosinophils to <15 eosinophils per high-power field. Due to the patchy nature of esophageal

Table 44.4 A step-by-step guide to food elimination diets.

8 Food	6 Food	4 Food	2 Food	Sequences for number of foods to eliminate at a time
Milk	Milk	Milk	Milk	1–3
Wheat	Wheat	Wheat	Wheat	1 – 4–8
Egg	Egg	Egg		Patient preference
Soy	Soy	Soy		
Nuts	Nuts			
Seafood	Seafood			
Corn				
Legume				

eosinophilia, the small fraction of mucosa sampled with standard biopsies and the discordance of eosinophil count to other measures of EoE activity, this single endpoint has been questioned. As a result, a more practical endpoint for successful treatment is not only reduction in eosinophil count but also improvement in endoscopic features and symptom reduction. Similar to inflammatory bowel disease, there is also the concept of deep remission defined by absence of eosinophils, elimination of symptoms, and normalization of endoscopic appearance [101]. Unfortunately, this is achievable in only about 10% of patients with therapy [101]. With this new endpoint in mind, the goals of therapy for eosinophilic esophagitis are to resolve esophageal eosinophilia, reestablish and maintain adequate esophageal caliber and function, and in turn control symptoms.

The three main approaches to treatment of EoE focus on the three Ds: Diet, Drugs and Dilation. Diet therapy is highly effective in EoE by eliminating food antigens that initiate the inflammatory process [102].The most common dietary approaches are the six food elimination diet and the elemental diet (Table 44.4). Allergy testing directed diets are not advised due to lack of predictive value of allergy testing to identify food triggers in EoE. The six food elimination diet (milk, wheat, soy, eggs, nuts, seafood) is 75% effective and as effective as pharmacological therapy [103–106]. In some patients, expansion of dietary restriction to include barley, rye, corn, and legumes is needed [106,107]. The elemental diet may be used in children [108] but, though effective, is rarely needed in adults [109]. The burdens of diet therapy have been the difficulty of avoiding many common foods and the requirement for endoscopy and biopsy between addition and subtraction of tested foods to assess improvement in esophageal eosinophil count as the endpoint of therapy. The convenience of food therapy is improving, with most patients effectively treated with a four food elimination diet or avoidance of milk and/or gluten [110–112] and emerging therapies of nonendoscopic testing such as orally passed minimally invasive esophageal sampling devices.

Pharmacological therapy consists of either PPIs or swallowed topical corticosteroids (Table 44.5). High-dose PPIs given twice daily for 8 weeks are 40–60% effective in achieving histological remission [113,114]. Use of lower doses of PPIs or having the gene for CYP2C19 rapid metabolizers leads to lower efficacy [115]. The mechanism of PPI efficacy appears independent of acid suppression and perhaps due to antiinflammatory effects [116,117] and restoration of esophageal barrier function [56].Topical steroids are 60–95% efficacious [97,118–121]. There is no current medication approved by the FDA for EoE and as a result, steroid therapies have been adapted from steroid asthma inhalers. The two major preparations are fluticasone spray and budesonide liquid. Fluticasone is administered by swallowing the spray or ingesting the powder whereas budesonide is mixed into a viscous solution. Both are administered twice daily and careful instructions must be given to optimize therapy. There are no advantages of using oral steroids such as

Table 44.5 Pharmacological treatments of eosinophilic esophagitis (EoE) in adults.

Initial (8 weeks)	Maintenance[d]
PPIs	
Full dose twice daily[a]	1–2 times daily
Steroids	
Fluticasone 880 μg (4 puffs) twice daily[b]	220–880 μg twice daily 440–880 μg before bed
Budesonide 1 mg twice daily[c]	0.25–1 mg twice daily 1 mg before bed
Montelukast	
No proven efficacy	

[a] Equivalent dose to omeprazole 40 mg twice daily. Efficacy may vary with CYP2C19 genotype.
[b] Careful instructions needed to ensure oral delivery.
[c] Must mix liquid from ampoule in 10 cc viscous fluid such as Splenda packets in water, honey, chocolate syrup. Patient remains NPO for 30 minutes following use. Starting dose 1 mg but some patients may require higher doses.
[d] Maintenance doses unclear and must be assessed individually.

prednisone over topical formulations described above [94]. Trials of biologics that inhibit IL-4 and/or IL-13 show good efficacy but these agents are not available yet for routine use [7,122].

Endoscopic dilation of fibrotic esophageal strictures is a cornerstone of therapy in adults with EoE. One of the early concerns with dilation was the high risk of perforation given the extent of esophageal fibrosis present. Subsequent series from large medical centers, however, have demonstrated that dilation is safe in patients with EoE if done carefully, with a 1–2% rate of perforation [90,91,123]. Most patients who sustain a perforation can be treated with conservative management as most iatragenic perforations are contained esophageal perforations. Safe dilation practices suggest that dilation goals should be modest, at most attempting to increase esophageal diameter by 1–3 mm at a single session. As a result, patients should be aware that multiple sessions may be needed to accomplish adequate dilation. It is also recommended that visualization of the dilated area be obtained to assess for presence of a deep tear. If seen, a tear warrants cessation of further dilation at that time.

There is no clear consensus on what type of dilator is most effective for EoE strictures. Balloon dilation is used for focal concentric strictures whereas for longer or proximal cervical esophageal strictures, Savary dilators may be used. A balloon dilator may also be used for long strictures with a pull-through technique in which an inflated balloon is drawn up the esophagus through the area of stricture formation [124]. It is also unclear what esophageal diameter should be achieved with dilation and this is often symptom dependent. In general, achieving a 15–17 mm diameter throughout the esophagus is adequate. Patients have been reported to experience postprocedure pain 75% of the time [90] and should be counseled that postprocedural chest discomfort may occur after a dilation.

One unresolved question is whether dilation should be performed before or after medical therapy; it is hoped that pharmacological control of inflammation will lead to symptomatic improvement and/or lessen the chance of perforation [125]. In general, this course is suggested unless the patient has severe symptoms such as frequent food impaction, weight loss or limited diet, in which case more urgent dilation is needed.

Maintenance therapy for and monitoring of eosinophilic esophagitis

One of the key questions in eosinophilic esophagitis is the role of maintenance therapy. Whereas earlier recommendations suggested an 8-week course of pharmacological therapy, the almost universal reoccurrence of active disease in adults and the concern over esophageal stricture formation and progression of fibrosis with untreated disease [126] have prompted investigators to recommend long-term treatment. For patients willing to maintain effective diet-based therapy, long-term treatment is easier to apply but for those who require or choose pharmacological therapy, the decision is more circumspect.

At the least, there are certain characteristics of EoE patients that should warrant maintenance therapy. These include patients with rapid relapse off therapy, severe stricture formation, particularly small-caliber esophagus, and those with frequent food impaction. Unfortunately, it is not clear what maintenance dose of either PPIs or steroids should be used. Studies using 0.25 mg of budesonide daily demonstrated superiority to placebo in controlling eosinophilia but not symptoms, with a relapse rate of esophageal eosinophilia of 75% within 12 months [127]. As a result, the use of higher doses has been advocated for chronic treatment [101]. Similarly, for PPI doses effective in inducing remission, the relapse rate is 27% over 12 months [115]. These data are suggesting that the maintenance dose may be the same as or close to the dose required to achieve remission.

Theoretically, diet therapy that is adequate to induce remission should be effective in maintaining long-term remission. Unfortunately, compliance in the long term is challenging, particularly in patients where avoidance of multiple foods is needed. There is also some concern that even with strict avoidance of instigating food antigens, environmental triggers may cause activation of the disease.

Prevention

No interventions have been evaluated to prevent the occurrence of eosinophilic esophagitis. As a result, all that can be done is to modify factors associated with the disease. These are environmental factors and include promoting vaginal delivery and breastfeeding, avoidance of unnecessary antibiotic use in early childhood and perhaps other factors such as growing up with a pet and having siblings. Other than experimental data, no studies have been performed to assess if active means of changing the gut or esophageal microbiome lessen the chances of developing EoE. It is also important to remember that patients who develop EoE likely have a germline genetic predisposition. There is some concern that immunotherapy by either oral or subcutaneous means may cause or lead to a flare of EoE but data are limited in this area [128–130]. Nevertheless, this type of therapy should be implemented cautiously in patients with known EoE.

Conclusions

Eosinophilic esophagitis is a chronic immune-mediated food antigen-driven condition characterized by eosinophilic inflammation of the esophagus resulting in esophageal dysfunction and symptoms. Previously thought to be a rare disorder, this condition is rising in incidence and prevalence. Common symptoms include heartburn, abdominal pain, nausea/vomiting, failure to thrive in children, and dysphagia and food impaction in older adolescents and adults. Pathophysiology includes a combination of food antigen and environmental triggers, genetic predisposition, and barrier dysfunction of the esophagus.

Treatment approaches focus on diet therapy, pharmacological therapy and esophageal dilation, and endpoints of therapy include control of histological inflammation and improvement of endoscopic features and esophageal symptoms. Due to the chronic nature of this disorder, maintenance therapy to prevent complications of esophageal structuring and food impaction is advised.

References are available at www.yamadagastro.com/textbook7e

CHAPTER 45

Esophageal infections and disorders associated with acquired immunodeficiency syndrome

C. Mel Wilcox
University of Alabama-Birmingham, Birmingham, AL, USA

Chapter menu

Introduction

The prevalence of esophageal infections continues to fall with the remarkable efficacy of highly active antiretroviral therapy (HAART) and the selective use and efficacy of antimicrobial prophylaxis for opportunistic infections like cytomegalovirus (CMV) in high-risk transplant patients [1–3]. However, the human immunodeficiency virus (HIV) epidemic continues unabated in developing countries, where gastrointestinal disorders parallel the experience in developed countries more than two decades ago. Despite these advancements, there remain a number of patients at risk for these diseases particularly as the population ages, immunosuppressive therapy becomes more widespread for a variety of indications, the use of organ transplantation expands, and the growth of the AIDS epidemic in developing countries continues. Timely and accurate diagnosis of esophageal infections is critical because treatment is highly effective, results in rapid symptomatic improvement, and often leads to clinical cure. This chapter focuses on the specific causes of esophageal infections, in particular epidemiology, pathology, presentation, diagnosis, and therapy. Esophageal disorders associated with HIV infection and AIDS are also reviewed here.

Epidemiology and predisposing factors

Primary esophageal infection is rare in an otherwise healthy person in whom no permissive factor is present. In this setting, the most common pathogen is *Candida albicans* and, less commonly, herpes simplex virus (HSV) [3,4]. In general, immunocompetent patients who develop esophageal infection have conditions, either local or systemic, that either weaken esophageal defense mechanisms, such as alteration of normal oroesophageal flora (e.g., antibiotics), or reduce esophageal emptying (e.g., achalasia). Infection in adjacent structures may spread into and secondarily involve the esophagus.

More commonly, some form of humoral or cellular immunodeficiency, whether iatrogenic, inherited, or some combination, leads to esophageal infection. Underlying conditions that predispose to infections include diabetes mellitus, alcoholism, malnutrition, malignant diseases, and advanced age. Transplantation predisposes to infections through one of a variety of mechanisms, most of which affect both B-cell and T-cell number and function, including use of immunosuppressive agents, chemotherapy, and neutropenia. Episodes of rejection in solid organ transplant recipients are commonly complicated by infection, because these patients are given more

Yamada's Textbook of Gastroenterology, Seventh Edition. Edited by Timothy C. Wang, Michael Camilleri, Benjamin Lebwohl, Anna S. Lok, William J. Sandborn, Kenneth K. Wang, and Gary D. Wu.

Companion website: www.yamadagastro.com/textbook7e

immunosuppression, including powerful agents such as antithymocyte globulin.

Without antimicrobial prophylaxis, infection after transplantation has a predictable time course. Bacterial and fungal infections are most common during the initial months after transplantation, because it is during this period that granulocyte number or function is most severely compromised. HSV infection also tends to occur early after transplantation related to reactivation of disease, whereas CMV typically presents 2–6 months after transplantation at a time when neutropenia is common and T-cell function is most severely impaired. The development of opportunistic infections in HIV-infected patients reflects severe immunodeficiency; the risk for esophageal infections increases markedly when the CD4 lymphocyte count falls below 200/mm^3 with most infection occurring when the count is less than 100/mm^3 [5].

Fungal infections

Candida species

Epidemiology

Candida species are the most common esophageal pathogens, primarily *C. albicans*, but occasionally *C. tropicalis*, *C. parapsilosis*, *C. glabrata*, and *C. dublinensis*. These organisms are normal components of the oral flora, and their growth is kept in check by bacterial commensals. Conditions predisposing to *Candida* esophagitis in the "normal" host include broad-spectrum antibiotic use, inhaled or ingested corticosteroids, antisecretory therapy (histamine H_2 receptor blockers, proton pump inhibitors) or hypochlorhydric states, diabetes mellitus, alcoholism, malnutrition, old age, head and neck radiotherapy, and esophageal motility disturbances. Alterations in cellular immunity lead to candidal colonization and superficial infection, whereas granulocytes function to prevent invasive disease and dissemination. Chronic mucocutaneous candidiasis, a congenital form of immunodeficiency, may also be complicated by *Candida* esophagitis.

Improvements in immunosuppressive regimens, targeted prophylactic antifungal therapy, and empiric use of fluconazole in symptomatic patients have dramatically reduced the incidence of candidal infections in recipients of solid organ and bone marrow transplants [6]. Candidiasis remains the most common esophageal infection in patients with AIDS; it represents approximately 50% of esophageal infections, and it frequently coexists with other esophageal diseases [7].

Pathology

The gross pathological appearance of esophageal candidiasis can range from a few white or yellow plaques on the mucosal surface to a dense, thick plaque that coats the esophageal mucosa (Figure 45.1a). This plaque material is composed of desquamated squamous epithelial cells, admixed with fungal organisms, inflammatory cells, and bacteria [8] (Figure 45.1b,c). In the absence of granulocytopenia or coinfection, true ulceration is infrequent (Table 45.1).

Clinical manifestations and complications

Although occasionally this infection is detected incidentally in an asymptomatic patient, the usual clinical presentation of esophageal candidiasis is dysphagia, with odynophagia less prominent (Table 45.2). Esophageal symptoms range from mild difficulty with swallowing to severe pain resulting in an inability to eat and secondary dehydration. When odynophagia is very severe, one must consider other causes or coinfections, particularly in patients with AIDS.

Physical examination may be helpful. Approximately two-thirds of patients with AIDS and esophageal candidiasis have oral candidiasis (thrush) [9]. Patients with chronic mucocutaneous candidiasis may have fungal involvement of various mucous membranes, hair, nails, and skin, with a history of adrenal or parathyroid dysfunction. Because the infection is generally superficial, complications of esophageal candidiasis are very rare.

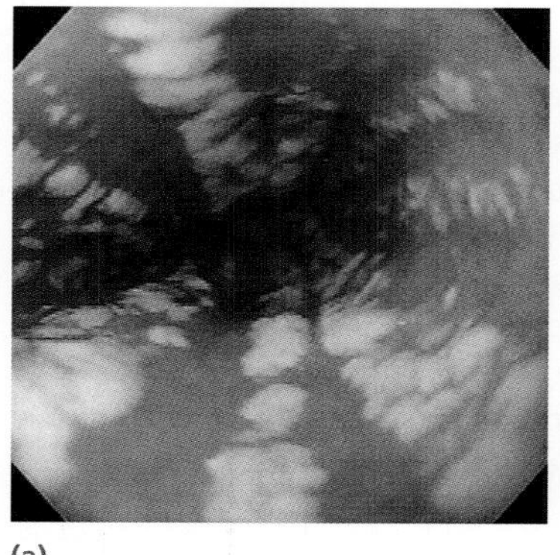
(a)

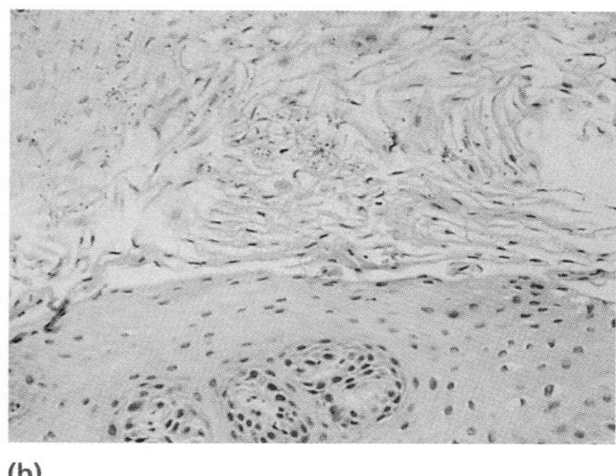
(b)

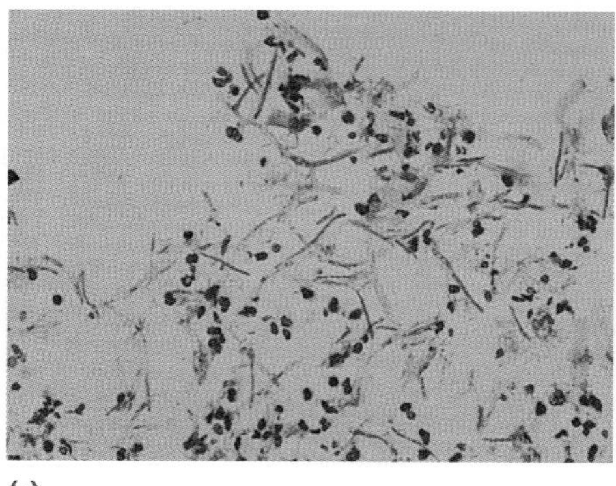
(c)

Figure 45.1 *Candida* esophagitis. **(a)** Endoscopic photograph shows multiple raised plaques involving the esophagus with normal intervening mucosa. **(b)** Desquamated squamous epithelial cells admixed with fungi and inflammatory cells adherent to the mucosa. The underlying squamous epithelium appears normal. **(c)** Close-up view of the plaque material demonstrates mycelia and spores typical of *Candida*.

Table 45.1 Pathological findings of esophageal infections.

	Candida	Other fungi	Viruses	IEU	Bacteria	Mycobacteria	Parasites
Plaque	+ + + +	+	+	0	+ +	+	+ +
Ulcer	+	+ +	+ + + +	+ + + +	+ + +	+ + +	+
Stricture	0	+	+ +	+	0	+ +	0
Fistula	0	+	+	+	0	+ + +	0
Mass	+	+	+	+	0	+ +	0

Not occurring (0), rare (+), occasional (+ +), common (+ + +), uniformly present (+ + + +); IEU, idiopathic esophageal ulcer.

Table 45.2 Symptoms and signs of esophageal infection.

	Candida	Viruses	IEU	Bacteria	Mycobacteria	Parasites
Dysphagia	+ + + +	+	+	+	+ +	+
Odynophagia	+ + +	+ + + +	+ + + +	+ + +	+ +	+ +
Heartburn	+	+	+	+	+	+
Chest pain	+	+ + +	+ + +	+ +	+ +	+
Fever	0	+ +	0	+ + +	+ + + +	0
Bleeding	+	+ +	+ +	+	+	+

Not occurring (0), rare (+), occasional (+ +), common (+ + +), uniformly present (+ + + +); IEU, idiopathic esophageal ulcer.

Diagnosis

Esophageal candidiasis should be suspected in any patient at risk of esophageal infection who complains of dysphagia or odynophagia. The presence of thrush further supports this diagnosis, but the absence of oral involvement does not exclude esophageal disease. On barium esophagram, *Candida* esophagitis is characteristically manifested by multiple plaque-like lesions, often in a linear configuration; when severe, these lesions become confluent to cause a "shaggy" appearance of the esophagus resembling ulcerations (see Figure 45.1) [10]. A large, well-circumscribed ulceration should not be attributed to *Candida*. Importantly, a normal barium esophagram does not exclude esophageal candidiasis. The presence of severe odynophagia may limit the ability of the patient to drink barium and thus hampers the utility of barium studies.

Endoscopic examination of the esophagus is the most accurate method of diagnosing esophageal candidiasis. The gross endoscopic appearance of *Candida* esophagitis is usually diagnostic and may be graded according to published criteria [8]. During endoscopy, mucosal lesions can be brushed and submitted for cytological evaluation or examined by biopsy for histological diagnosis. Multiple biopsies are essential to exclude coexisting disorders when ulceration is identified endoscopically. The use of periodic acid–Schiff or Gomori methenamine silver stain helps to highlight the organisms. Cytological examination of esophageal brushings is more sensitive than histological examination of biopsy specimens because organisms may be washed off tissue surfaces in mild superficial candidiasis (i.e., grades 1 and 2) during processing of biopsy specimens. Rarely, positive cytology but negative histology indicates colonization rather than infection. Skin testing and serological tests for candidiasis play no role in the diagnosis of *Candida* esophagitis.

In patients with AIDS and thrush, the presence of dysphagia or odynophagia usually indicates *Candida* esophagitis [7]. Given the prevalence of *Candida* esophagitis in AIDS, in the symptomatic patient with associated thrush, an empiric trial of antifungal therapy may be instituted, reserving endoscopy for those patients who fail to respond. However, this symptom complex does not exclude coinfection with other pathogens, and one-third of patients with esophageal candidiasis do not have thrush. When patients fail to improve rapidly with empiric antifungal therapy, endoscopy should be performed, given that disorders other than candidiasis are identified in most patients [7,11]. The role of empiric antifungal therapy in symptomatic immunosuppressed patients who do not have AIDS has not been well studied, although this approach is commonly practiced.

Treatment

Both oral and intravenous medications are available that are highly effective for the treatment of *Candida* esophagitis

Table 45.3 Treatment regimens for common esophageal disease in AIDS.

Pathogen	Drug	Dosage	Route	Duration	Efficacy (%)
Candida	Ketoconazole	200–400 mg/day	PO	7–14 days	<80
	Fluconazole	100 mg/day	PO/IV	7–14 days	≈80
	Itraconazole	200 mg/day	PO	7–14 days	≈80
	Amphotericin B	0.5 mg/kg/day	PO/IV	7 days	>95
	Caspofungin	50 mg/day	IV	7 days	>90
Cytomegalovirus	Ganciclovir	5 mg/kg BID	IV	2–4 weeks	≈75
	Foscarnet	90 mg/kg BID	IV	2–4 weeks	≈75
	Cidofovir	5 mg/kg weekly	IV	2–4 weeks	≈75
Herpes simplex virus	Acyclovir	400 mg 5×/day	PO/IV	14 days	>90
	Valaciclovir	1 g TID	PO	14 days	>90
	Famciclovir	500 mg TID	PO	14 days	>90
	Foscarnet	90 mg/kg BID	IV	14 days	>95
	Ganciclovir	5 mg/kg BID	IV	14 days	>95
Idiopathic ulcer	Prednisone	40 mg/day taper	PO	4 weeks	>90
	Thalidomide	200–300 mg/day	PO	4 weeks	>90

BID, twice a day; IV, intravenous; PO, by mouth; TID, three times a day.

(Table 45.3). In general, oral therapies should be initiated first, reserving intravenous treatment for refractory disease or for patients who have contraindications to orally administered medication. Although candidal species other than *C. albicans* may cause esophagitis, speciation is not widely employed because reliable culturing and sensitivity testing are lacking at most centers and the treatment is generally the same. For those patients with mild disease, minimal immunocompromise, or readily reversible immunodeficiency, an abbreviated course of therapy with an orally absorbed, systemically distributed azole (a class of five membered nitrogen heterocyclic ring compounds containing at least one other noncarbon atom of nitrogen, sulfur, or oxygen) should be given, for example clotrimazole, ketoconazole, voriconazole, fluconazole, and itraconazole. Immunocompromised transplant recipients and patients with AIDS with *Candida* esophagitis are best treated with systemically absorbed agents (azoles). In addition, patients with granulocytopenia are at significant risk of disseminated candidal infection, thus warranting the use of systemically acting agents.

Orally administered systemic agents, all of which have efficacy for *Candida* esophagitis, include ketoconazole (Nizoral®), fluconazole (Diflucan®), and itraconazole (Sporanox®). These agents, like other azoles, alter fungal cell membrane permeability by cytochrome P450-dependent interference with ergosterol biosynthesis resulting in fungal cell injury and death. The newer triazoles (itraconazole and fluconazole) have greater affinity than the imidazoles (miconazole and ketoconazole) for fungal cytochrome P450 enzymes [12]. Although other agents such as clotrimazole and nystatin may be effective for oral candidiasis and for prophylaxis against esophageal involvement, these agents are much less effective as primary therapy for esophageal candidiasis.

A number of studies suggest that fluconazole (100 mg/day), the absorption of which does not depend on pH, has significantly greater efficacy for the treatment of *Candida* esophagitis in AIDS than ketoconazole (200 mg/day) [12] and itraconazole [13,14]. Both itraconazole and fluconazole are available in oral forms (both pill and solution) while fluconazole is also available as an intravenous preparation. Fluconazole is minimally metabolized and is excreted unchanged in the urine. Unlike ketoconazole and itraconazole, fluconazole is highly water soluble, is minimally protein bound, and has a half-life of approximately 30 hours if renal function is normal. The adverse effects of ketoconazole, fluconazole, and itraconazole are primarily dose dependent and include nausea, hepatotoxicity, and inhibition of steroid production and cyclosporine metabolism. Finally, because of the effects on hepatic microsomal enzymes, all three azoles (ketoconazole, fluconazole, and itraconazole) inhibit the metabolism of cyclosporine and result in an increase in cyclosporine blood levels. This effect is most pronounced with ketoconazole.

Another major family of antifungal agents consists of the polyene antibiotics, represented by amphotericin and nystatin (see Table 45.3). These agents bind irreversibly to sterols in fungal cell membranes, thereby altering the permeability characteristics of the membrane and causing cell death. Nystatin is effective for treating thrush but much less so for esophageal disease. Although amphotericin B (Fungizone®) is a highly effective treatment for systemic mycoses, it has potential to cause severe side-effects (e.g., renal dysfunction); coupled with the availability of effective alternative agents, amphotericin has limited use for the treatment of esophageal candidiasis.

The newest class of antifungal agents is the echinocandins. These agents have a novel mechanism of action as glucan synthase inhibitors, which inhibit fungal cell wall synthesis [15].

The first agent in this class, caspofungin, has activity against both *Aspergillus* and *Candida* species, including non-*albicans* species. Prospective studies have shown it is as efficacious and as well tolerated as fluconazole for AIDS patients with *Candida* esophagitis and as effective and better tolerated than amphotericin B for azole-resistant esophageal candidiasis [13].

Prophylaxis

The use of nystatin or azoles for the prevention of esophageal candidiasis in patients with cancer and in transplant recipients has yielded mixed results, and it can be problematic, especially for those receiving cyclosporine [16]. Primary prophylaxis has not been recommended in patients with AIDS [13].

Drug resistance

Because of widespread use, azole resistance has become a well-recognized problem in HIV-infected patients. This represents a less common clinical problem today with the widespread use of HAART. Both cumulative exposure and severe immunodeficiency have been shown to be highly associated with the development of resistance [13]. In patients with AIDS, clinical resistance correlates with in vitro; resistance. When resistance occurs, increasing the dose of azole, switching to another azole, or use of oral solution of itraconazole may be tried in higher doses. Because of cross-resistance, higher doses may be needed for efficacy. Echinocandins are efficacious in this setting, as is posaconazole [17]. Improvement in immune function with HAART is also an important component of the treatment of resistant candidiasis.

Other fungi

Epidemiology

Esophageal involvement with other fungal infections is rare [18]. Most instances of histoplasmosis and blastomycosis esophagitis represent secondary esophageal involvement from mediastinal lymph nodes rather than primary esophageal infection associated with dissemination [19,20]. Although no particular geographic distribution within the United States has been reported for aspergillosis or blastomycosis, histoplasmosis is endemic in the Midwestern states and the Mississippi Valley. Mucormycosis and aspergillosis esophagitis have also been described [21,22].

Pathology, clinical manifestations, and complications

Other than the development of fistula to adjacent organs, there are no unique pathological features of these fungal infections (see Table 45.1).

Diagnosis

Histoplasmosis should be considered in endemic areas and if extraesophageal manifestations such as hilar adenopathy, calcification or atelectasis of adjacent pulmonary tissue, or splenic calcification are present. Disseminated disease to multiple organs is well recognized in AIDS. Esophageal blastomycosis should be considered in patients with skin involvement and dysphagia. Barium esophagography or endoscopy may show a focal area of extrinsic compression of the esophagus, usually in the region of the carina, ulcer, or fistula. As with other esophageal infections, the diagnosis is established by the appearance of the abnormality at barium esophagram; the endoscopic appearance at endoscopy; and the use of endoscopic brushings and biopsies with appropriate culture and staining. Serological tests are not useful because of the high prevalence of positive results in endemic areas. However, a urine antigen test is highly specific for the diagnosis of disseminated histoplasmosis [19].

Treatment

Although histoplasmosis may resolve without antifungal therapy in the normal host, therapy should be administered with an induction course of amphotericin B followed by maintenance itraconazole. Blastomycosis responds to itraconazole and amphotericin B. Systemic aspergillosis should be treated with voriconazole [23]. Surgery may be required for drainage of abscesses or excision of fistulas.

Viral infections

As with all esophageal infections, the prevalence of viral esophagitis has also fallen in recent years. In the transplant setting, this reduction has resulted from targeted antiviral prophylaxis for herpesviruses in high-risk transplant recipients, the use of CMV-seronegative organs and blood products for seronegative recipients, and the use of leukocyte-depleted platelets for patients after bone marrow transplantation. An overall reduction in viral esophagitis, attributable to the implementation of HAART, has also been observed in HIV-infected patients [1]. Nevertheless, in patients who fail such therapy or for undiagnosed patients, viral esophagitis continues to be clinically relevant [24].

Herpes simplex virus

Epidemiology

Herpes simplex virus type 1 (HSV-1) is one of three herpesviruses that affect the esophagus, the others being CMV and varicella zoster virus (see sections on Cytomegalovirus and Other viruses). HSV-2 rarely involves the esophagus. After *Candida* species, HSV-1 is the next most frequent agent that causes infectious esophagitis. Although well recognized as an esophageal pathogen in otherwise healthy people, HSV-1 esophagitis has been reported most often in patients with immunosuppression or other predisposing factors. After transplantation, HSV occurs as frequently as CMV as a cause of esophageal disease [18], whereas in patients with AIDS, HSV esophagitis is relatively uncommon and is much less frequent than CMV infection [25].

Pathology

Herpes simplex virus infection is generally limited to squamous mucosa, where the earliest manifestation is a vesicle. As these vesicles enlarge and ulcerate, they may coalesce to form larger lesions. Usually, the intervening mucosa between these lesions is normal. Microscopic examination of the squamous epithelial cells at the edge of the ulcers reveals multinucleation, ground-glass nuclei, and eosinophilic Cowdry type A inclusion bodies that may occupy half of the nuclear volume. These inclusion bodies may be surrounded by haloes and, with time, become more basophilic, filling, enlarging, and deforming the nucleus.

Clinical manifestations and complications

Herpes simplex virus-1 esophageal infection commonly presents with the sudden onset of severe odynophagia, often resulting in an inability to swallow liquids or solids. Herpes labialis (i.e., cold sores) and oropharyngeal ulcers may frequently coexist, antedate, or develop during the esophageal infection, whereas skin infection is rare [5,25]. In untreated immunocompetent persons, spontaneous resolution of HSV-1 esophageal infection occurs 1–2 weeks after the onset of symptoms. Complications are rare and include bleeding, tracheoesophageal fistula, or dissemination [18].

Diagnosis

Esophageal disease caused by HSV-1 usually appears in radiographic studies as focal ulceration on a background of normal mucosa; vesicles are infrequently present (Figure 45.2). These ulcers have been described as stellate or volcanic in appearance, with fewer propensities to form the longitudinal or linear lesions that are commonly seen in CMV infection [26]. Severe, diffuse herpetic esophagitis may result in a cobblestone or "shaggy" mucosal appearance resembling *Candida* esophagitis [26]. Although the radiographic appearance may be suggestive, definitive diagnosis of herpetic esophagitis requires endoscopic mucosal biopsies. The endoscopic appearance of herpetic esophagitis reflects the pathological changes (see Table 45.1) appearing as discrete, usually small (<2 cm) well-circumscribed ulcers [27], diffuse erosive esophagitis, or, rarely, vesicles. Small scattered lesions covered with exudates can mimic esophageal candidiasis. Given the pathophysiological mechanism of disease, deep ulcers, as seen with CMV, are very rare. Cytological or histological brushings or biopsies should be taken from the edge of an ulcer because the viral cytopathic effect with multinucleated giant cells is best identified here, rather than the granulation tissue in the ulcer bed (Figure 45.3).

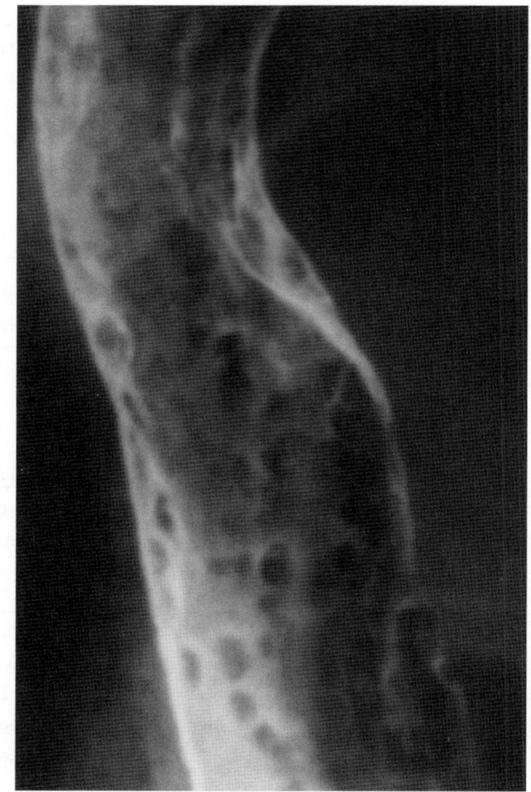

Figure 45.2 Herpes simplex virus esophagitis. Multiple vesicles and ulcers are present throughout the esophagus. Source: Courtesy of Robert Koehler, MD.

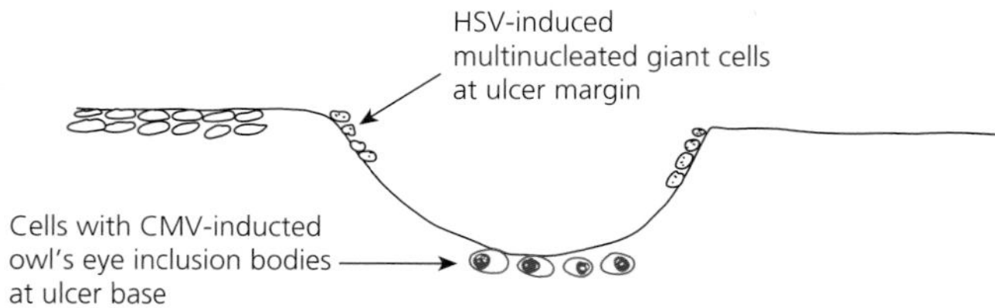

Figure 45.3 Location of viral cytopathic effect in esophageal ulceration.

Immunohistochemistry on biopsy samples using specific monoclonal antibodies to HSV will help to confirm the diagnosis when the viral cytopathic effect is infrequent. Viral culture may also help to establish a definitive diagnosis. As with other causes of infectious esophagitis, serological tests are unhelpful in establishing the diagnosis.

Treatment

Uncontrolled trials and vast clinical experience in both immunocompetent and immunodeficient patients, including those with AIDS [28], suggest efficacy of aciclovir, a nucleoside analog, for the therapy of esophageal viral disease [29]. Valaciclovir, a prodrug of aciclovir, and famciclovir have largely replaced aciclovir as oral therapy given their longer half-life. While not studied for esophagitis, they have shown equivalency for genital HSV disease and, as with aciclovir, minimal toxicity.

Although spontaneous resolution of HSV-1 esophagitis is common in the immunologically normal host, because of its safety and efficacy, therapy is commonly instituted in all patients regardless of immune status. When oral intake is hampered by severe odynophagia or when there is a question of drug absorption, intravenous administration is required. Side-effects of intravenous aciclovir therapy are few and appear limited to irritation of veins (used for drug infusion) and rash. Although rare, drug resistance should be suspected when there is clinical failure of aciclovir; in this setting, foscarnet (see Table 45.3) is the drug of choice and will lead to clinical cure in most patients [30]; cidofovir may also be used. Aciclovir is effective prophylaxis for HSV antibody-positive patients undergoing transplantation. Long-term secondary prophylaxis may be required when immunodeficiency persists because the relapse rate is high.

Cytomegalovirus

Epidemiology

Cytomegalovirus continues to dominate as one of the most common opportunistic infections across all risk groups. This frequency relates to the high background seropositivity rates in the general population, with even higher rates in developing countries and homosexual men. In transplant recipients who receive no antiviral prophylaxis, CMV and HSV are equally common esophageal pathogens [18]. In contrast, CMV is the most frequent cause of esophageal ulcer in patients with AIDS [25].

Pathology

The most prominent histological feature of CMV esophagitis is mucosal ulceration (see Table 45.1). Although there is variability, deep ulcers are very characteristic of disease in AIDS, whereas in immunosuppressed transplant recipients, lesions tend to remain more superficial. In contrast to HSV, the viral cytopathic effect of CMV is present in endothelial and mesenchymal cells in the granulation tissue of the ulcer base and not in the squamous epithelium. Inclusions are large (*cytomegalo*) and often have an eosinophilic appearance that may be present in the nucleus and cytoplasm (Figure 45.4a). Because these inclusions may be atypical in appearance in patients with AIDS [31], immunohistochemical stains are useful in confirming the presence of CMV and often highlight more infected cells than can be appreciated on routine hematoxylin and eosin staining. As with other esophageal infections, CMV may coexist with HSV or *Candida*, especially in patients with AIDS. Whereas HSV leads to disease by a direct cytopathic effect on squamous epithelium, the pathogenesis of disease caused by CMV is not well understood.

Clinical manifestations and complications

In contrast to HSV esophagitis, CMV esophagitis has very rarely been documented in immunocompetent persons [32]. Odynophagia is almost uniformly present and is characteristically severe (see Table 45.2). A prior or coexistent diagnosis of CMV infection in other organs (e.g., retinitis or colitis) is not infrequent. Although rare in transplant recipients, retinitis may be observed in approximately 15% of patients with AIDS and there is a very low CD4 count, usually <50/μL at the time of diagnosis of gastrointestinal disease [33,34]. Complications include gastrointestinal bleeding (~5% of patients) and, rarely, strictures [35] or fistulas to the tracheobronchial tree [36].

Diagnosis

Like HSV-1, the radiological appearance of CMV esophagitis is that of either focal or extensive ulceration and is dependent in large part on the epidemiological setting. Barium esophagography of CMV esophagitis may reveal thickening of mucosal folds or, more typically, ulcers; these ulcers may be vertical, linear with central umbilication, solitary, and deep, or occasionally they may manifest as diffuse superficial ulceration (see Figures 45.3 and 45.4b). In patients with AIDS, these ulcers are often large and deep, may exceed 2 cm in size, or have an appearance suggesting a malignancy. The endoscopic appearance of CMV esophagitis is variable, ranging from multiple shallow ulcers and solitary giant ulcers to diffuse superficial esophagitis (see Figure 45.4c) [37]. Given the high rate of prior exposure to CMV, serological testing is not helpful. In addition, some immunosuppressed transplant recipients fail to develop a brisk antibody response. Blood antigenemia is often present at the time of diagnosis and its presence may predict the subsequent development of end-organ disease [38].

Identification of viral cytopathic effect in mucosal biopsies is the best diagnostic method. Multiple biopsies (up to 10) may be required to establish the diagnosis in patients with AIDS and should be taken from the ulcer base because the viral cytopathic effect is found here [39] (see Figure 45.3). Viral culture of mucosal biopsies is less sensitive and specific than histology and cytological brushings are not helpful [40]. Identification of an isolated inclusion found by immunohistochemical staining should not be considered CMV disease but rather infection, and other causes of mucosal disease should be sought. Because retinitis may coexist with gastrointestinal disease and, when present, alters the duration of antiviral therapy, a diagnosis of CMV gastrointestinal disease in any patient with AIDS warrants ophthalmological examination.

Retinitis as well as GI disease has been described as part of the immune reconstitution inflammatory syndrome (IRIS) [41]. This syndrome is a result of an exuberant inflammatory reaction to foreign antigens following rapid immunological recovery, especially in patients who were most profoundly immunodeficient. Patients may not only develop retinitis or other gastrointestinal problems in association with CMV, but also tuberculosis and Kaposi sarcoma, as well as cryptococcosis [41].

Treatment

The therapies available for the treatment of CMV disease generally require intravenous administration and include ganciclovir, foscarnet, and cidofovir. The most widely used therapy, ganciclovir, is an aciclovir derivative. The time course of the clinical response to ganciclovir is variable; a week of therapy may be required before there is symptomatic improvement in some severely immunosuppressed patients. The total treatment duration should be based on the clinical and endoscopic response; a 2–4-week treatment course is usually adequate. If retinitis is absent and there has been a complete response, the patient may be followed closely without maintenance therapy, especially if

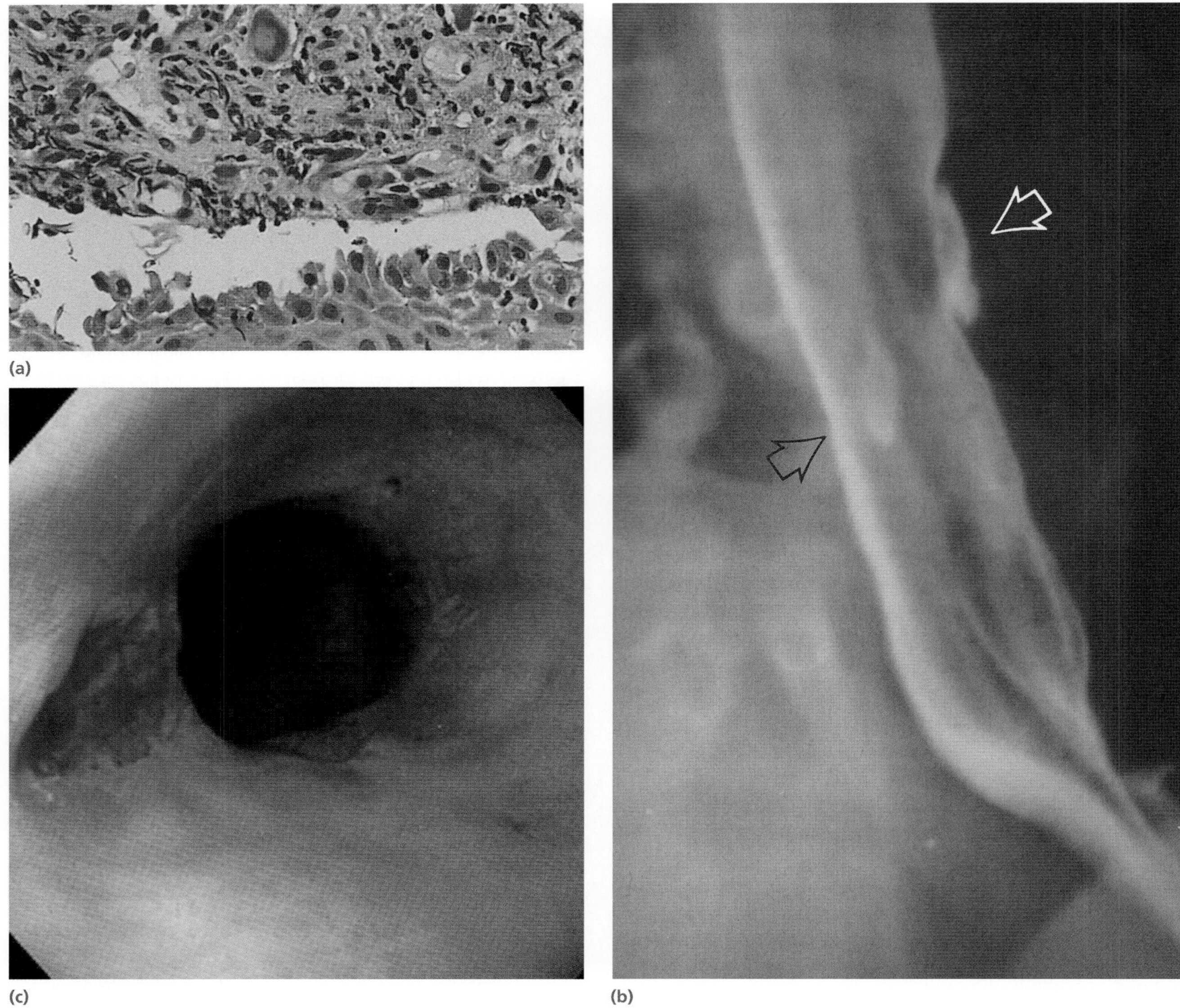

Figure 45.4 Cytomegalovirus esophagitis. **(a)** Biopsies from an ulcer base demonstrate granulation tissue with one large cell with intranuclear and intracytoplasmic inclusions diagnostic for cytomegalovirus. **(b)** Barium swallow demonstrates two well-circumscribed ulcers in the distal esophagus (arrows). **(c)** Endoscopic photograph shows the two ulcers, which are well circumscribed and have some depth, and the surrounding mucosa is normal.

immune function can be optimized with HAART. Because of low bioavailability (<10%), oral ganciclovir is not effective for the treatment of active infections, including those of the gastrointestinal tract.

After acute CMV disease in transplant recipients, treatment with ganciclovir should be given for approximately 1–2 months until the immunosuppressive regimen is either discontinued (bone marrow transplant) or significantly reduced (solid organ transplant). Ganciclovir is well tolerated. Its major side-effect is myelosuppression, which may be severe when other bone marrow suppressive drugs are coadministered. Clinical and virological resistance has been documented, usually in patients receiving prolonged therapy. In this setting, foscarnet is often effective [42].

Valganciclovir, an orally administered prodrug rapidly hydrolyzed to ganciclovir, achieves high blood levels equivalent to intravenous administration of ganciclovir [43]. Given its favorable pharmacokinetics, it has been used successfully for induction therapy for CMV retinitis in AIDS patients as well as for prophylaxis in high-risk solid organ transplant recipients such as those who are donor positive/recipient negative (D+/R−) as well as preemptively for those who develop CMV antigenemia [3,44]. Although potentially effective for treatment of end-organ disease such as esophagitis, trials have not been performed and intravenous ganciclovir remains the treatment of choice. Long-term prophylaxis with this agent following successful therapy is a reasonable option for those in whom severe immunodeficiency persists, although long-term use has been associated with the development of resistance [45].

Foscarnet is a pyrophosphate analog that inhibits viral DNA polymerase and reverse transcriptase. Efficacy is similar to that of ganciclovir. There are fewer data on its use in immunosuppressed patients who do not have AIDS. Because of its recognized toxicity (reversible renal insufficiency and electrolyte disturbances), foscarnet has been most frequently used when there is clinical resistance or intolerance to ganciclovir.

Cidofovir, the newest systemic agent available for the therapy of CMV, has undergone evaluation for the treatment of retinitis in AIDS and less so in other immunocompromised patients. Its long half-life provides the opportunity for once-weekly administration [3].

Newer agents should be available soon which offer the promise of less toxicity and potential for oral administration. All drugs for herpesviruses only inhibit viral replication; thus, relapse is frequent when therapy is discontinued. The relapse rate for transplant recipients also remains high until immunosuppressive therapy is reduced. The relapse rate of CMV esophagitis is approximately 50% and is similar for HSV [28,33]. Initiation of HAART, when associated with significant improvement in CD4 count, may abrogate the need for long-term maintenance therapy.

Prophylaxis

Antiviral prophylaxis will reduce CMV disease and associated mortality, as well as enhance graft survival in transplant patients [3]. As noted previously, at-risk patients should generally receive prophylaxis rather than preemptive therapy based on the appearance of CMV viremia. Oral valganciclovir and intravenous ganciclovir appear to have broadly equivalent efficacy. The duration of therapy is generally dictated by risk and is often extended to approximately 200 days. Oral ganciclovir is recommended to reduce the incidence of CMV disease in patients with solid organ transplant. Oral ganciclovir is also used preemptively in patients who develop CMV viremia. However, in high-risk patients, such as bone marrow transplant patients and solid organ transplant recipients, valganciclovir is the drug of choice [44,46]. Intravenous ganciclovir prophylaxis may be appropriate in very high-risk patients such as D+/R+ transplant recipients. Oral ganciclovir has shown efficacy for prophylaxis for CMV retinitis in AIDS, but HAART represents the ideal choice.

Other viruses

The frequency of esophageal involvement caused by varicella zoster during the course of chickenpox or herpes zoster infections is unknown but clinically uncommon [18]. Papillomavirus may infect the esophagus and may cause small polypoid lesions. Its detection has also been associated with squamous cell carcinoma of the esophagus [47]. Esophageal ulcers have been reportedly caused by papovavirus and Epstein–Barr virus in patients with AIDS [18].

Mycobacterial infections

Epidemiology

Mycobacterial involvement of the esophagus is very rare, even in immunosuppressed patients. In developing countries, the rate of tuberculosis (TB) is much higher, and extrapulmonary manifestations, including esophageal disease, are more common. The combination of the AIDS epidemic with the upsurge in reported cases of systemic TB has increased the incidence of esophageal infection in developed countries. *Mycobacterium avium* complex (MAC) remains primarily a small bowel pathogen with only rare cases of esophageal involvement reported [23].

Pathology

Most commonly, TB affects the middle third of the esophagus at the level of the carina [48]. Esophageal disease is caused by spread of infection from tuberculous-infected mediastinal lymph nodes by way of a draining fistula or obstructed lymphatics, often resulting in tracheoesophageal fistula. TB can also involve the upper third of the esophagus by direct extension from tuberculous pharyngitis or laryngitis. Primary esophageal TB in the absence of extraesophageal disease is exceedingly rare and found in patients from endemic areas.

Clinical manifestations and complications

The symptoms of esophageal TB depend on the degree and type of involvement. Pulmonary complaints often predominate because of the common occurrence of fistula to the trachea, bronchus, or pleural space. Rarely, formation of long strictures or traction diverticula resulting from the fibrotic response causes dysphagia. Upper gastrointestinal hemorrhage from tuberculous esophageal ulcers and tuberculous arterioesophageal fistulas has been reported [49].

Diagnosis

Esophageal TB should be suspected in patients with pulmonary or systemic TB who develop esophageal symptoms. Chest radiography is generally abnormal and CT scan may demonstrate mediastinal adenopathy [50]. Barium esophagram findings, including ulceration and stricture, are nonspecific. A sinus tract or fistulous connection to the bronchial tree or mediastinum is highly suggestive of TB but can also be seen with malignant disease or other infections; in this setting, the diagnosis may often be made by sputum staining and culture, or CT-guided or surgical biopsy [50]. Endoscopic findings include ulcers (which may be solitary and resemble a malignancy), fistula, or strictures [51]. Biopsies from the edge of the lesions may demonstrate granulomata or acid-fast bacilli, and biopsy material may be cultured for further confirmation of the diagnosis and determination of sensitivities to antimycobacterial agents.

Treatment

Regardless of the presence of immunodeficiency, a 9-month course of multidrug therapy (in the absence of drug resistance) will cure esophageal TB and will often close fistulas. If fistulas do not close with medical therapy, surgical or endoscopic intervention will be required. The prevalence of multidrug-resistant TB is an increasingly complex problem; thus, drug sensitivities to antituberculous therapy are essential to guide therapy. The most effective agents for the treatment of MAC are clarithromycin and ethambutol [52]. Although a clinical and bacteriological response is common, long-term therapy for MAC is required in AIDS unless HAART is effective.

Bacterial infections

Epidemiology

Bacterial esophagitis is a rare cause of esophageal disease in immunocompromised patients. It has been described almost exclusively in patients with hematological malignant disease complicated by severe granulocytopenia, occasionally after bone marrow transplantation and diabetic ketoacidosis or those patients receiving radiation and chemotherapy [18,53,54]. Usually, the infecting pathogens are oral flora, particularly gram-positive organisms, including viridans streptococci, staphylococci, and other bacilli. It is likely that these pathogens colonize and then invade mucosa damaged by reflux disease, radiation, or chemotherapy, leading to local infection. Reports in patients with AIDS have broadened the etiological spectrum to include *Bartonella henselae*, the cause of catscratch disease [48], and *Nocardia* [18]. Actinomycosis causes ulcers, sinus tracts, and fistulas [54]. Although esophageal involvement by *Treponema pallidum* was well recognized many years ago, this disease is now only of historical interest [18].

Pathology

The gross pathological appearance of the esophagus in bacterial infection ranges from normal mucosa (colonization) to ulcers associated with erythema, plaques, pseudomembranes, sinus cavities, or hemorrhage [53]. Microscopic examination reveals pseudomembranes and bacterial invasion that may be superficial and invade only the squamous epithelium or may be invasive and transmural with infiltration of blood vessels (i.e., phlegmonous esophagitis). *Bartonella henselae* esophagitis causes multiple nodules of the esophagus resulting from a lobulated proliferation of capillary vessels lined by plump endothelial cells [48].

Clinical manifestations and complications

Bacterial esophagitis is usually found in a neutropenic patient with esophageal complaints who has undergone chemotherapy for a hematogenous malignant disease. Esophageal infection may serve as a focus for bacteremia and seeding of other organs, particularly in patients with granulocytopenia [53]. No unique complications have been reported.

Diagnosis

The diagnosis of bacterial esophagitis should be considered in the clinical setting described above. Radiographic findings are nonspecific, and endoscopic biopsy and culture are necessary to establish this diagnosis. Additional stains, including gram stain, are required to identify the etiological bacteria. Positive blood cultures also pinpoint the bacterial pathogens and direct antimicrobial therapy.

Treatment

Broad-spectrum antibiotics that effectively treat both gram-positive and gram-negative oropharyngeal flora are required for treatment. Treatment of other bacterial infection found in these patients is similar to treatment of disease in other locations.

Protozoal infections

In developed countries, protozoal infections of the esophagus are very rare, occurring almost exclusively in patients with AIDS. In these patients, pathogens include *Pneumocystis carinii*, *Cryptosporidium parvum*, *Leishmania donovani*, and *Trichomonas* [18,55]. In immunologically normal hosts from endemic areas in South America, *Trypanosoma cruzi* may involve the myenteric plexus of the esophagus, resulting in Chagas disease. This disease is indistinguishable clinically, radiographically, endoscopically, and manometrically from idiopathic achalasia. The diagnosis may be established by antibody testing [18]. There is increasing appreciation that Chagas disease is diagnosed in patients who have come from rural areas of Mexico or Central America and who reside in the United States, where 11 species of triatomine bugs have been identified in 29 states. The southwestern states of Texas, Arizona, and New Mexico have the greatest diversity of species, with eight species found in Texas alone, where 50% of collected triatomine specimens tested positive for *T. cruzi* [56,57]. Therefore, gastroenterologists in the United States should be aware that achalasia may result from Chagas disease in the right clinical context.

Specific HIV-related esophageal disorders

In addition to the infections described earlier, certain unique disorders cause esophageal disease in these patients.

Disorders associated with primary HIV infection

Although primary HIV infection is largely asymptomatic, in some patients, a mononucleosis-like illness occurs around the time of infection consisting of fever, sore throat, and myalgias associated with a maculopapular rash, termed a seroconversion illness [58]. Spontaneously resolving oropharyngeal and esophageal ulceration or candidal infection may also be observed during this seroconversion illness. Endoscopically, these esophageal ulcerations are multiple, small, and shallow. The diagnosis can be established at the time of presentation by the detection of HIV RNA in serum [58]. Antibody positivity to HIV occurs within 3–18 months after the illness.

Idiopathic esophageal ulcer

Epidemiology

Early in the AIDS epidemic, large esophageal ulcerations were recognized in which no specific cause could be identified despite extensive histopathological examination of ulcer tissue. These ulcers, termed idiopathic esophageal ulcers (IEU), and aphthous ulcers, are very common and were found in 41% of HIV-infected patients in a large prospective study of patients with esophageal ulcer [25]. They are seen in the later stages of immunodeficiency when the CD4 lymphocyte count is less than 100/μL^3 [25]. Like all opportunistic disorders, their frequency has also fallen markedly in the era of HAART.

Pathology

These ulcers are variable in size, may be large, and are uniformly well circumscribed; diffuse superficial esophagitis has not been described [59]. Ulcer tissue resembles that seen in CMV and HSV infection, except that viral cytopathic effect is absent. The presence of a superficial candidal infection overlying a large well-circumscribed lesion with histopathological findings of granulation tissue without viral cytopathic effect should still lead to the diagnosis of IEU [60]. Although HIV has been suggested as the direct cause of these lesions, there is little histopathological evidence to support a direct cytopathic role for HIV [61].

Clinical manifestations and complications

Idiopathic esophageal ulcer presents in a fashion indistinguishable from CMV esophagitis. Coexistent oropharyngeal aphthous ulcers are infrequent [9], whereas thrush is common, especially if the patient has not been given empiric antifungal therapy. Complications include bleeding and fistula to the stomach, but not to the tracheobronchial tree, and strictures [35].

Diagnosis

The findings of IEU on barium esophagram are typically large, well-circumscribed, and often deep ulcers [62]. Because of the similarity to CMV infection, a definitive diagnosis cannot be based on the radiographic appearance alone. Because IEU is a diagnosis of exclusion, endoscopy and biopsy are the only definitive diagnostic tests. These ulcers are variable in size and appearance, and larger ulcers are endoscopically indistinguishable from CMV infection [37,59]. Distal esophageal ulcer may suggest gastroesophageal reflux disease; the histopathological features alone also cannot distinguish IEU from gastroesophageal reflux disease. Pill-induced esophagitis must be excluded by history because the pathological findings of esophageal biopsies are similar. These ulcers respond rapidly to either prednisone or thalidomide, with clinical and endoscopic cure seen in more than 90% [25,63,64]. HAART therapy alone has also been associated with cure [65]. Relapse may occur.

Neoplasms associated with AIDS

Kaposi sarcoma

With the advent of HAART, Kaposi sarcoma (KS), caused by human herpes virus-8, has shown a sharp fall in frequency. Gastrointestinal KS is common in those with cutaneous disease and clinical experience suggests that gastric or duodenal involvement is more common than esophageal disease, and esophageal lesions, like other areas of the gastrointestinal tract, are most frequently an incidental finding. The endoscopic features of esophageal KS are characteristic and resemble their cutaneous appearance: violaceous macular or plaque-like lesions. These tumors typically involve the submucosa so mucosal biopsy must sample deeper tissue. Bleeding may occur when the tumor becomes large and ulcerated. Effective relatively nontoxic chemotherapy includes Doxil®, a liposomal form of doxorubicin (Adriamycin®). HAART therapy alone has been associated with lesion regression and apparent cure [66]. Radiation therapy is effective to treat local lesions of the head and neck, including the oropharynx.

Non-Hodgkin lymphoma

Despite HAART, lymphoma remains an important opportunistic neoplasm. Although gastrointestinal involvement is common, esophageal disease remains rare [67]. Extraesophageal disease is common at the time of diagnosis [68]. The lesions appear radiographically as large ulcers or mass lesions typical of a carcinoma. The endoscopic appearance of these lesions has been described as an ulcerated polypoid mass, often with a central ulceration, a submucosal lesion or extensive disease resulting in lumenal narrowing resembling an adenocarcinoma, or a solitary ulcer [68]. Complications are rare and include bleeding. Multidrug chemotherapeutic regimens are usually given for non-Hodgkin lymphoma in AIDS, and complete remission may be achieved in approximately 50% or more of patients. Radiation therapy may be a potential option when the disease is localized. Complications are frequent because of chemotherapy-induced neutropenia. The median survival of AIDS-associated non-Hodgkin lymphoma has been enhanced by HAART [69].

Miscellaneous neoplasms

Recent evidence suggests AIDS patients may be at higher risk for esophageal neoplasms, including squamous cell and adenocarcinoma [70].

References are available at www.yamadagastro.com/textbook7e

Further reading

Achenbach C.J., Harrington R.D., Dhanireddy S., et al. Paradoxical immune reconstitution inflammatory syndrome in HIV-infected patients treated with combination antiretroviral therapy after AIDS-defining opportunistic infection. Clin Infect Dis 2012;54:424.

Baehr P.H., McDonald G.B. Esophageal infections: risk factors, presentation, diagnosis, and treatment. Gastroenterology 1994; 106:509.

Fishman J.A. Overview: cytomegalovirus and the herpesviruses in transplantation. Am J Transplant 2013;13:1.

Lortholary O., Petrikkos G., Akova M., et al. ESCMID guideline for the diagnosis and management of Candida diseases 2012: patients with HIV infection or AIDS. Clin Microbiol Infect 2012;18:68.

Monkemuller K.E., Call S.A., Lazenby A.J., et al. Declining prevalence of opportunistic gastrointestinal disease in the era of combination antiretroviral therapy. Am J Gastroenterol 2000;95:457.

Wilcox C.M., Schwartz D.A., Clark W.S. Esophageal ulceration in human immunodeficiency virus infection: causes, diagnosis, and management. Ann Intern Med 1995;123:143.

CHAPTER 46

Barrett esophagus and esophageal adenocarcinoma

Stuart Jon Spechler[1], David H. Wang[2], and Rhonda F. Souza[1]
[1] Baylor University Medical Center and Baylor Scott & White Center for Esophageal Diseases, Dallas, TX, USA
[2] Department of Internal Medicine, The University of Texas Southwestern Medical Center, Dallas, TX, USA

Chapter menu

Barrett esophagus is the condition in which a metaplastic columnar mucosa that is predisposed to malignancy replaces a portion of the squamous mucosa that normally lines the distal esophagus (Figure 46.1) [1,2]. The condition is a consequence of gastroesophageal reflux disease (GERD), which both injures the esophageal squamous mucosa and provides the abnormal intraluminal milieu that leads to mucosal healing through columnar metaplasia rather than through regeneration of more squamous cells. For reasons that remain incompletely understood, the metaplastic columnar mucosa predisposes to the development of esophageal adenocarcinoma. Indeed, GERD and Barrett esophagus are the major risk factors for esophageal adenocarcinoma, a tumor whose frequency has increased more than sevenfold over the past several decades [2–4].

Diagnostic criteria for Barrett esophagus

Endoscopic examination is required to diagnose Barrett esophagus, and two diagnostic criteria must be fulfilled: (1) the endoscopist must document that columnar epithelium extends proximal to the gastroesophageal junction (GEJ) to line ≥1 cm of the distal esophagus, and (2) biopsy specimens of the esophageal columnar epithelium must reveal the specialized intestinal metaplasia with goblet cells (also called specialized columnar epithelium or just intestinal metaplasia) that is characteristic of Barrett esophagus (Figure 46.2).

To document that columnar epithelium lines the esophagus, the endoscopist must identify both the squamocolumnar junction (SCJ) and the GEJ (Figure 46.3). Columnar epithelium has a reddish color and coarse texture on endoscopic examination, whereas squamous epithelium has a pale, glossy appearance. The juxtaposition of those epithelia at the SCJ forms a visible, typically zigzag line called the Z line. The GEJ, the conceptual level at which the esophagus ends and the stomach begins, is not so readily identified with precision.

In western countries, the GEJ is recognized endoscopically as the level of the most proximal extent of the gastric folds [5]. However, the most proximal extent of the gastric folds is not a static marker, and its location can vary considerably with the level of air distention

Yamada's Textbook of Gastroenterology, Seventh Edition. Edited by Timothy C. Wang, Michael Camilleri, Benjamin Lebwohl, Anna S. Lok, William J. Sandborn, Kenneth K. Wang, and Gary D. Wu.

Companion website: www.yamadagastro.com/textbook7e

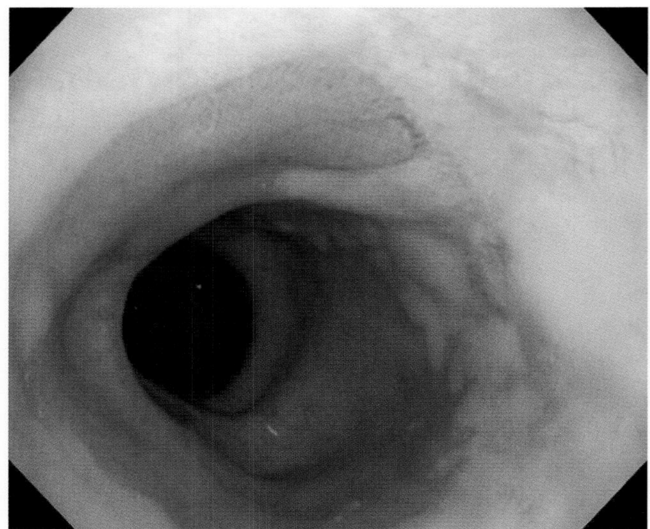

Figure 46.1 Endoscopic photograph of Barrett esophagus. Note the contrast between the pale, glossy squamous epithelium of the proximal esophagus and the red Barrett epithelium of the distal esophagus. Source: Courtesy Stuart Jon Spechler.

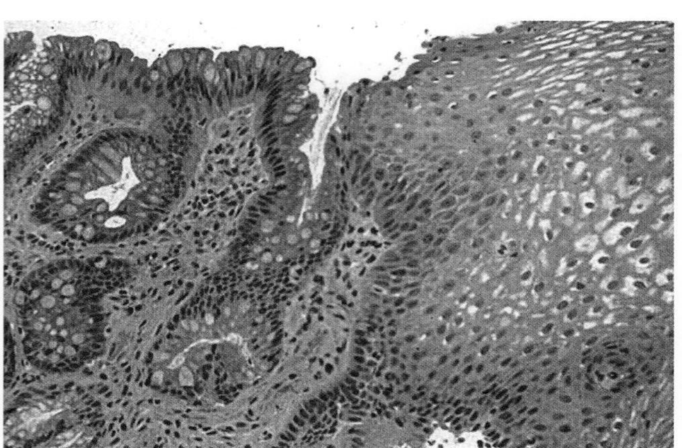

Figure 46.2 Photomicrograph showing the junction between stratified squamous epithelium (right) and specialized intestinal metaplasia (left). Note the numerous goblet cells characteristic of the intestinal-type epithelium. Source: Courtesy Stuart Jon Spechler.

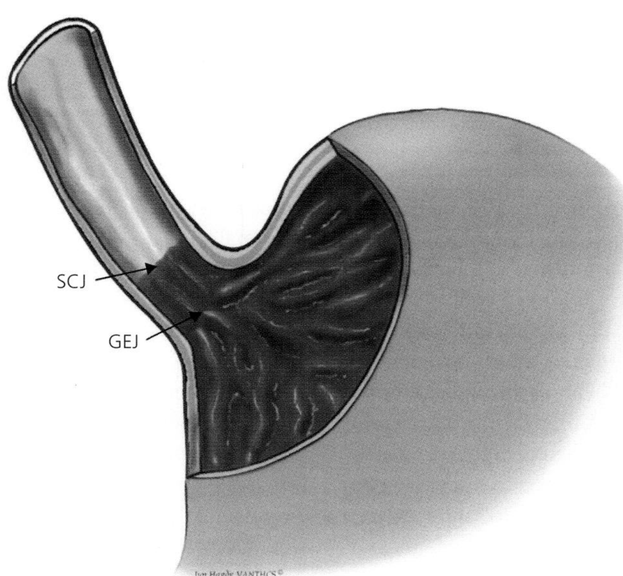

Figure 46.3 Landmarks at the gastroesophageal junction (GEJ) region. The squamocolumnar junction (SCJ, also called the Z line) is the visible line formed by the juxtaposition of squamous and columnar epithelia. The GEJ is the conceptual line at which the esophagus ends and the stomach begins. The GEJ corresponds to the most proximal extent of the gastric folds. When the SCJ is located proximal to the GEJ, as it is in this figure, then the region between the two landmarks is a columnar-lined segment of esophagus.

of the esophagus and stomach, as well as with respiration. Noting these shortcomings of the gastric folds as a landmark for the GEJ, endoscopists in some Asian countries instead identify the GEJ as the distal extent of the esophageal palisade vessels, which are fine, longitudinal veins located in the lamina propria of the distal esophagus [6,7]. Palisade vessels can be difficult to visualize in the presence of reflux esophagitis, and their distal extent is often located ≥1 cm below the proximal extent of the gastric folds [8]. Controversy regarding which is the best endoscopic landmark for the GEJ remains unresolved. Both landmarks have shortcomings, neither has a compelling conceptual basis for its use, and the two frequently disagree by a centimeter or more in location. The use of different endoscopic landmarks for the GEJ might explain some differences between Asian and western studies on Barrett esophagus.

In this chapter, we use the proximal extent of the gastric folds as the endoscopic landmark for the GEJ. When the SCJ is located proximal to the GEJ, there is a columnar-lined segment of esophagus. When the SCJ and GEJ coincide (Figure 46.4), the entire esophagus is lined by squamous epithelium. If biopsy specimens from a columnar-lined segment of esophagus ≥1 cm in length show specialized intestinal metaplasia, then the patient has Barrett esophagus.

Before 1994, endoscopists generally diagnosed Barrett esophagus only when they saw long segments of esophageal columnar mucosa extending >3 cm above the GEJ. In 1994, Spechler and colleagues [9] reported the results of a study in which consecutive patients undergoing elective endoscopic examinations in a general endoscopy unit had biopsy specimens taken at the SCJ in the distal esophagus, irrespective of its appearance and location. Among 142 patients who had columnar epithelium involving <3 cm of the distal esophagus, 26 (18%) were found to have specialized intestinal metaplasia typical of Barrett esophagus in the biopsy specimens. A number of subsequent studies confirmed this observation that intestinal metaplasia is present frequently in short segments of columnar epithelium in the distal esophagus, even in patients without symptoms or endoscopic signs of GERD [10]. Since the description by Spechler and colleagues [9], Barrett esophagus has been categorized as "long-segment" if the distance between the Z line and the GEJ is ≥3 cm and "short-segment" if that distance is <3 cm [11] (Figure 46.5).

The "Prague C and M criteria" is a system used to describe the endoscopic appearance of Barrett esophagus by evaluating both the circumferential (C) and the maximum (M) extent of Barrett metaplasia above the GEJ [12]. The Prague C and M system has

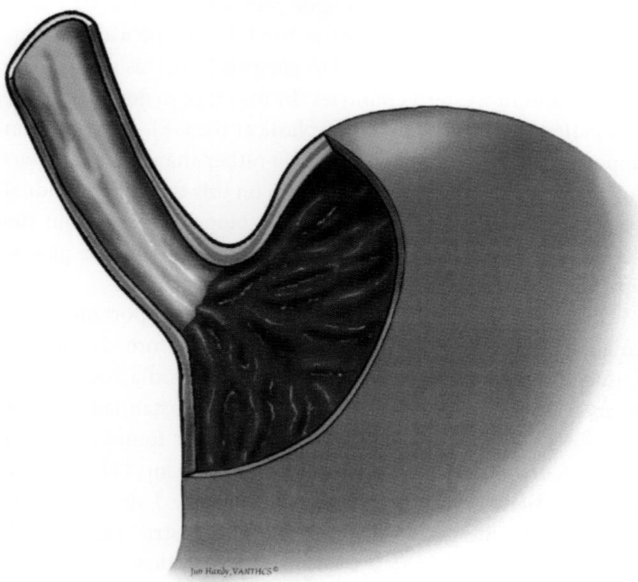

Figure 46.4 The squamocolumnar junction (SEJ) and gastroesophageal junction (GEJ) coincide. In this situation, there is no columnar-lined esophagus (i.e., the entire esophagus is lined by squamous epithelium).

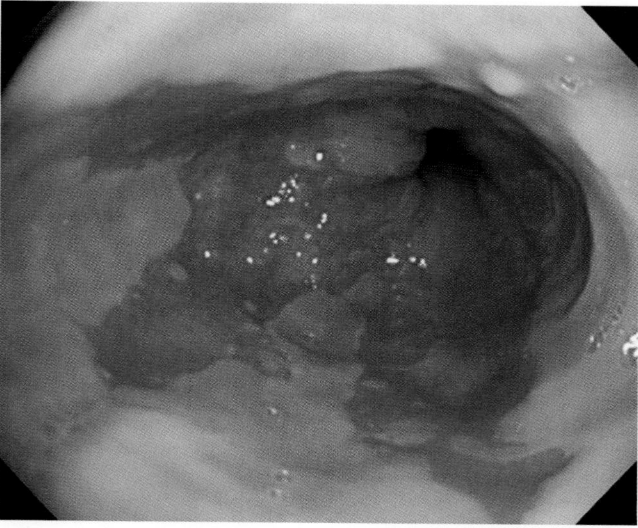

Figure 46.5 Endoscopic photograph of short-segment Barrett esophagus. Columnar epithelium extends <3 cm above the gastroesophageal junction (GEJ). Source: Courtesy Stuart Jon Spechler.

been found to have excellent reproducibility among endoscopists for a number of features of Barrett esophagus, with the notable exception of columnar metaplasia that extends <1 cm above the GEJ, for which interobserver agreement is poor. Based on this and other observations, modern diagnostic criteria for Barrett esophagus require that intestinal metaplasia line at least 1 cm of the distal esophagus.

To optimize the identification of specialized intestinal metaplasia when Barrett esophagus is suspected, at least eight biopsy specimens should be taken from the columnar-lined esophagus [13]. For patients with short segments (1–2 cm) of columnar-lined esophagus in whom it may not be possible to obtain eight biopsies, at least four should be taken from the circumferential portion.

Cardiac mucosa in the esophagus

As discussed earlier, the presence of ≥1 cm of specialized intestinal metaplasia in the esophagus establishes the diagnosis of Barrett esophagus. However, two other columnar mucosal types also have been described in Barrett esophagus [14]: (1) cardiac mucosa (also called junctional-type or nongoblet columnar mucosa) comprised exclusively of mucous-secreting glands lined by gastric foveolar-type columnar cells without goblet cells or oxyntic cells, and (2) an atrophic gastric fundic-type mucosa (also called oxyntocardiac) that contains some acid-secreting parietal cells. Biopsy specimens of Barrett esophagus often reveal a mosaic of these three mucosal types with an admixture of cardiac glands, oxyntocardiac glands, and intestinal metaplasia with variable densities of goblet cells. Traditionally, cardiac mucosa has been considered the normal lining of the most proximal portion of the stomach (the gastric cardia). In the late 1990s, Chandrasoma [15] suggested that cardiac mucosa is not normal, but rather a metaplastic mucosa acquired as a consequence of reflux esophagitis. According to this unproved and controversial hypothesis, the normal epithelial junction at the end of the esophagus is one between esophageal squamous and gastric oxyntic (acid-producing) mucosae, and the finding of squamous abutting cardiac mucosa defines the presence of GERD [16]. In support of the concept that cardiac mucosa is metaplastic, it has been shown to express molecular markers of intestinal differentiation (e.g., villin, CDX2) and to exhibit genetic abnormalities similar to those found in specialized intestinal metaplasia [17,18].

Some clinical studies have suggested that cardiac mucosa, like specialized intestinal metaplasia, has a malignant predisposition. One study of 141 patients who had endoscopic mucosal resections (EMRs) of small esophageal adenocarcinomas found that 71% had cardiac mucosa, not intestinal metaplasia, adjacent to the cancer [19]. Another retrospective study of 688 patients in one hospital who had endoscopic biopsy specimens taken from esophageal columnar epithelium found no significant difference in the rate of esophageal adenocarcinoma development between patients with and without intestinal metaplasia (4.5% vs 3.6% rate of cancer development, respectively) during a median follow-up interval of 12 years [20]. Interestingly, although cardiac mucosa is distinguished from specialized intestinal metaplasia largely by the presence of goblet cells, high goblet cell counts in intestinal metaplasia are associated with a decreased risk for esophageal adenocarcinoma [21] Noting these observations, some authorities have proposed that cardiac mucosa in the esophagus should be considered a form of Barrett esophagus [22]. In 2005, the British Society of Gastroenterology (BSG) defined Barrett esophagus as one "in which any portion of the normal squamous lining has been replaced by a metaplastic columnar epithelium which is visible macroscopically" [23]. This definition includes patients with cardiac mucosa in the esophagus. Although the BSG's most recent definition of Barrett esophagus requires ≥1 cm of visible esophageal columnar epithelium (rather than "any portion"), the BSG still does not require intestinal metaplasia and still accepts cardiac mucosa as a diagnostic criterion [24].

The debate about whether patients who have only cardiac epithelium lining the distal esophagus have "Barrett esophagus" is largely a semantic issue. Norman Barrett [25], the Australian surgeon who described the condition that now bears his name, did not mention either intestinal metaplasia or cardiac epithelium in his original report on the condition in 1950. The columnar-lined esophagus has clinical importance only because it predisposes to the development of esophageal cancer. The great majority of studies on the risk for cancer in Barrett esophagus have included patients with specialized intestinal metaplasia either primarily or exclusively [1]. Although the data mentioned earlier suggest that cardiac mucosa might also predispose to malignancy, the magnitude of that risk is not clear. Furthermore, more recent reports suggest that the risk for cancer in cardiac mucosa is minimal [26]. For all these reasons, the authors of the American Gastroenterological Association's (AGA's) 2011 medical position statement [27] on Barrett esophagus made a distinction between the conceptual definition of Barrett esophagus and its diagnostic criteria. They defined Barrett esophagus conceptually as "the condition in which any extent of metaplastic columnar epithelium that predisposes to cancer development replaces the stratified squamous epithelium that normally lines the distal esophagus." The authors also wrote, "Presently, intestinal metaplasia [with goblet cells] is required for the diagnosis of Barrett esophagus because intestinal metaplasia is the only type of esophageal columnar epithelium that clearly predisposes to malignancy" [27]. That statement remains valid today.

Intestinal metaplasia at the GEJ

Chronic reflux esophagitis leads to the development of intestinal metaplasia in the esophagus. Intestinal metaplasia also occurs commonly in the stomach as a consequence of chronic gastritis caused by infection with *Helicobacter pylori* [28]. On histological examination, intestinal metaplasia in the stomach cannot be distinguished reliably from intestinal metaplasia in the esophagus. Because the GEJ cannot be identified with great precision, it can be difficult to determine whether short segments of intestinal metaplasia found in the GEJ region are lining the esophagus (i.e., short-segment Barrett esophagus) or the proximal stomach (i.e., intestinal metaplasia of the gastric cardia). The term "intestinal metaplasia at the GEJ" has been used to describe the condition in which intestinal metaplasia is found at a Z line that appears to coincide precisely with the GEJ [29]. Although intestinal metaplasia at the GEJ can be a manifestation of a diffuse, chronic *H. pylori* gastritis [30], this seems to be uncommon in western countries. In the large majority of western patients with intestinal metaplasia at the GEJ, the condition appears to be associated with GERD rather than with *H. pylori* infection [31]. Any clinical confusion on this issue in individual patients can be resolved by obtaining biopsies throughout the stomach to look for *H. pylori* associated with diffuse gastric atrophy and gastric intestinal metaplasia [30].

Until relatively recently, it was thought to be important to distinguish short-segment Barrett esophagus from *H. pylori*-induced intestinal metaplasia of the gastric cardia because the former condition was believed to have a substantially higher risk for malignancy. For example, one study found dysplasia (the precursor of malignancy) in 20 of 177 patients (11.3%) with short-segment Barrett esophagus, but in only 1 of 76 patients (1.3%) with intestinal metaplasia in the gastric cardia [32]. Consequently, authorities recommended endoscopic cancer surveillance routinely for patients with Barrett esophagus, but not for patients with intestinal metaplasia in the stomach [33,34]. A number of histochemical and immunological biomarkers were proposed to differentiate gastric intestinal metaplasia from short-segment Barrett esophagus, including cytokeratin staining patterns [35–38], immunoreactivity for Das-1 (a monoclonal antibody raised against colonic epithelial cells) [39], and mucosal expression of colonic-type sulfomucins [29]. However, the utility of biomarkers in distinguishing short-segment Barrett esophagus from intestinal metaplasia of the gastric cardia was never established, and it was recommended that clinical decisions should not be based on the presence of those biomarkers [40]. Furthermore, more recent studies have clarified that diffuse gastric intestinal metaplasia has a similar, if not greater risk for malignancy than short-segment Barrett esophagus [41]. Societal guidelines currently discourage the practice of obtaining biopsies at a normal-appearing Z line. However, if such biopsies are taken and intestinal metaplasia at the GEJ is identified, any confusion regarding the presence of diffuse gastric atrophy can be resolved by obtaining systematic biopsies throughout the stomach [42].

Intestinal metaplasia at the GEJ might cause an adenocarcinoma that straddles the GEJ. For patients with such tumors, therefore, it might be difficult to determine whether they developed as a complication of *H. pylori*-induced intestinal metaplasia of the stomach or from short-segment Barrett esophagus. The fact that the epidemiology of adenocarcinoma at the GEJ in western countries resembles that of esophageal adenocarcinoma more than that of distal gastric cancers suggests that most such tumors arise from esophageal intestinal metaplasia [43].

Epidemiology of Barrett esophagus

Long-segment Barrett esophagus is strongly associated with chronic heartburn, hiatal hernia, and severe reflux esophagitis [44]. Barrett esophagus typically is discovered in middle-aged and older adults, usually during endoscopic examinations performed for the evaluation of chronic GERD symptoms, such as heartburn, regurgitation, and dysphagia. Barrett esophagus is rare in children of any age and virtually nonexistent in children younger than 5 years [45]. In a retrospective study of 6731 children who had upper gastrointestinal (GI) endoscopy in 12 pediatric facilities, only 17 (0.25%) had suspected Barrett esophagus, and only 9 of those had intestinal metaplasia confirmed by esophageal biopsy [46]. Barrett esophagus is two to three times more common in men than in women. The condition has a predilection for white individuals and appears to be uncommon in Black and Asian individuals [47,48], although recent data suggest that the prevalence is increasing in Asian countries [49]. Obesity is associated with Barrett esophagus, especially obesity with a predominantly intraabdominal distribution of fat [50]. Cigarette smoking is also a risk factor [51].

Barrett esophagus is common in the general adult population, but the precise prevalence is not clear. In one study of 961 patients scheduled for elective colonoscopy who agreed to have an upper GI endoscopy performed for research purposes, Barrett esophagus (predominantly short-segment) was found in 6.8% [52]. In another study in which individuals in the general population of Sweden were invited to have endoscopic examinations, the prevalence rate of Barrett esophagus was found to be 1.6% [53].

A familial form of Barrett esophagus has been described and can be recognized in patients who have a first- or second-degree relative with Barrett esophagus, esophageal adenocarcinoma, or adenocarcinoma of the GEJ [54]. In the United States, the familial form accounts for less than 12% of all cases of Barrett esophagus [54,55].

Screening for Barrett esophagus

Currently, endoscopy is considered the method of choice for screening high-risk populations to identify patients with Barrett esophagus. Before performing such screening, the physician should ensure that the patient understands the implications of finding Barrett esophagus, including the need for regular endoscopic surveillance and the need for therapy if dysplasia is detected (see later). Current societal guidelines suggest that patients to be considered for screening are those with chronic GERD symptoms who have other risk factors for Barrett esophagus, including male sex, age ≥50 years, white race, central obesity, a history of cigarette smoking, or a family of a first-degree relative with Barrett esophagus or esophageal adenocarcinoma [24,27,56]. The risk for esophageal adenocarcinoma in women is so low that screening for Barrett esophagus generally is not recommended, although screening can be considered for women who have multiple risk factors. When considering these guidelines, the clinician should appreciate that two systematic reviews and one overview recently produced for the Canadian Task Force on Preventive Health Care concluded that there is little evidence that supports the effectiveness of screening for Barrett esophagus [57].

Screening methods for Barrett esophagus other than standard endoscopy have been explored. For example, transnasal endoscopy can be performed without sedation in an office setting, although transnasal endoscopy is inferior to standard endoscopy for the identification of subtle mucosal abnormalities and for acquiring adequate biopsy specimens [58,59]. Capsule endoscopy also has been evaluated as a screening tool, with sensitivity rates of 60–79% and specificity rates of 75–100% for identifying Barrett esophagus [60–63]. A number of nonendoscopic, minimally invasive screening tests also are in development. Cytosponge is a gelatin capsule that contains a mesh sponge attached to a string. The capsule is swallowed and dissolves in the stomach where the sponge expands. When the sponge is pulled out of the mouth by the string, attached esophageal cells can be analyzed for trefoil factor 3 (TFF3), a molecular marker of Barrett metaplasia [64–66]. Even less invasive screening tests for Barrett esophagus include "liquid biopsy" blood tests that can detect circulating abnormal cells, their DNA or their microRNA, and "electronic nose" breath testing that detects volatile organic compounds indicative of Barrett esophagus that are exhaled in the breath [59].

Epidemiology of esophageal adenocarcinoma

There are two major histological types of esophageal cancer: squamous cell carcinoma and adenocarcinoma. In the 1960s, squamous cell cancers comprised well more than 90% of all esophageal tumors in the United States, whereas adenocarcinoma of the esophagus was considered so uncommon that some authorities questioned its very existence. Since then, the frequency of adenocarcinoma of the esophagus has increased dramatically, to the point that adenocarcinoma surpassed squamous cell carcinoma in frequency in the 1990s (see later) [67,68]. The cause of this dramatic increase in the frequency of adenocarcinoma is not clear. GERD and Barrett metaplasia esophagus are the major risk factor for this tumor [69], and all of the risk factors for Barrett esophagus discussed previously also are risk factors for adenocarcinoma [70]. Changes in the frequency of some of those risk factors (e.g., GERD, obesity) might underlie the rising incidence of esophageal adenocarcinoma.

The prevalence of obesity has increased substantially over the past several decades, paralleling the increase in the frequency of esophageal adenocarcinoma [71]. The association with obesity might be related to the fact that obesity predisposes to the development of GERD and Barrett esophagus [72–75]. In addition, obesity (especially central obesity) is associated with insulin resistance that results in high serum levels of insulin-like growth factors, which might increase proliferation in Barrett epithelial cells [76]. Obesity also is associated with increased serum levels of leptin [77], a hormone that stimulates cellular proliferation, and decreased levels of adiponectin, a hormone that has antiproliferative effects [78].

In contrast with the increasing frequency of obesity, the frequency of infection with *H. pylori* has declined dramatically over the last century in the United States [79]. *H. pylori* is a well-established carcinogen for adenocarcinoma of the stomach, but this infection has not been identified as a positive risk factor for esophageal adenocarcinoma. Indeed, most studies on this issue suggest just the opposite – infection with *H. pylori*, particularly with the more virulent cagA^{+} strains, may protect against the development and neoplastic progression of Barrett esophagus [80–83]. The mechanism of this alleged protective effect is not clear, but it has been suggested that *H. pylori* infections that cause pangastritis can decrease gastric acid secretion, thereby protecting against the development of GERD. It has been proposed that the declining prevalence of *H. pylori* infection may be contributing to the increasing frequency of esophageal adenocarcinoma. It also has been proposed that other modern alterations of the gut microbiome that have resulted from the widespread use of antibiotics, dietary changes, and numerous other factors might combine with known risk factors to promote the development and neoplastic progression of Barrett esophagus [84].

Other factors that appear to protect against the development of esophageal adenocarcinoma include the use of aspirin and other nonsteroidal antiinflammatory drugs (NSAIDs) [85,86] and the consumption of a diet high in fruits and vegetables [87]. Although cigarette smoking and excessive alcohol consumption are very strong risk factors for squamous cell carcinoma of the esophagus, cigarette smoking only modestly increases the risk for esophageal adenocarcinoma, and alcohol does not appear to affect that risk at all [88].

Cancer risk in Barrett esophagus

Published estimates on the annual incidence of cancer in patients with long-segment Barrett esophagus have ranged from 0.2% to 2.9% [89]. In the 1990s, investigators pooled data from those reports to derive composite estimates of cancer risk in Barrett esophagus, which appeared to be approximately 1% per year [90]. In 2000, however, Shaheen [89] presented compelling evidence that the cancer risk had been overestimated because of publication bias, and estimated that risk at approximately 0.5% per year. For the next decade, many authorities estimated the risk for cancer in Barrett esophagus at approximately 0.5% per year. More recent estimates place the risk at 0.12–0.33% per year [91–94]. In addition, one study suggests that the cancer risk is not static but decreases over time [95]. This study included 1401 patients with nondysplastic Barrett who were followed for a mean of 5.6 years. When those patients had their first endoscopy showing nondysplastic Barrett, their annual rate of cancer development was 0.32%. However, the cancer risk decreased with every subsequent endoscopy. For patients who had five endoscopies showing nondysplastic Barrett mucosa, the annual cancer risk was only 0.11%. However, a more recent study has challenged this contention, finding that the annual risk for esophageal adenocarcinoma does not decrease over time [96].

The large majority of observational studies on this issue of cancer risk in Barrett esophagus suggest that the cancer risk varies directly with the length of the metaplastic segment [97–104]. Patients with longer segments of metaplasia have more progenitor cells undergoing cell division (when they are vulnerable to DNA damage) and, therefore, should be more likely to acquire the critical mutations that cause malignancy. However, in one older report of 235 patients with Barrett esophagus, the cancer risk was not found to vary significantly with the extent of metaplasia [105]. Despite all the evidence suggesting that patients with long-segment Barrett have a greater cancer risk than those with short-segment disease, American GI society guidelines currently do not distinguish between short- and long-segment Barrett esophagus in management recommendations.

Pathogenesis of metaplasia in the esophagus

Metaplasia, the process in which one adult cell type replaces another, is a response to chronic inflammation in a number of organs [29,106]. Because the metaplastic cells may be more resistant to the factors inducing the inflammation than the native cells, metaplasia can be viewed teleologically as a protective mechanism. Unfortunately, for reasons that are not clear, metaplasia also can predispose to malignancy. In the esophagus, chronic inflammation caused by GERD results in columnar metaplasia in which the acid-sensitive squamous epithelium is replaced by a columnar epithelium that may be more resistant to peptic injury.

Physiological perturbations

A number of physiological abnormalities that predispose to severe GERD have been described in patients with long-segment Barrett esophagus. For example, gastric acid hypersecretion and duodenogastric reflux have been described in some patients [107–109], and extreme hypotension of the lower esophageal sphincter is common [110]. Manometric studies also often reveal ineffective esophageal motility, an abnormality that may delay the clearance of refluxed material from the esophagus [111]. Some patients have diminished esophageal pain sensitivity, and thus may not sense the effects of reflux of damaging gastric contents [112]. Some patients have decreased salivary secretion of epidermal growth factor, a peptide thought to enhance the healing of peptic ulceration [113]. Individual patients may exhibit any, all, or none of these abnormalities, and the frequency of the potential GERD-predisposing factors in Barrett esophagus is disputed. For example, there may be normal gastric acid secretion in patients with long-segment Barrett esophagus [114]. Furthermore, many patients with short-segment Barrett esophagus have no GERD symptoms and no endoscopic signs of esophagitis whatsoever [10].

Exposure to noxious agents at the GEJ

The distal esophagus frequently is exposed to noxious agents that might play a role in the development of Barrett esophagus. Even in healthy individuals, the intraluminal environment of the GEJ appears to be especially hostile to the lining mucosa. After meals, there is a pocket of acid at the GEJ that escapes the buffering effects of ingested food [115]. This postprandial acid pocket often extends above the SCJ to affect the distal esophagus. Studies have shown that the very distal esophagus (5–10 mm above the SCJ) of healthy volunteers can be exposed to acid for more than 10% of the day [116,117]. This can result in acid-peptic injury of the distal esophagus and also in exposure to high concentrations of nitric oxide (NO) generated from dietary nitrate (NO_3^-). Most dietary nitrate comes from green leafy vegetables. The ingested nitrate is absorbed by the small intestine, concentrated by the salivary glands, and secreted into the mouth, where bacteria on the tongue reduce the recycled nitrate to nitrite (NO_2^-). When swallowed nitrite encounters acidic gastric juice at the GEJ, the nitrite is converted rapidly to NO. After nitrate ingestion, high levels of NO can be found at the GEJ [118]. Those high concentrations of NO can damage DNA and are potentially carcinogenic. Thus, the GEJ is exposed repeatedly to acid, pepsin, NO, and other noxious agents in gastric juice. Chronic exposure to those agents may induce the injury and inflammation that results in the intestinal metaplasia of Barrett esophagus [119].

Cells of origin for Barrett metaplasia

The process of Barrett metaplasia is thought to start with reflux-induced injury to the esophageal squamous mucosa, followed by replacement of the damaged squamous cells with metaplastic columnar cells. However, it is not known which cells give rise to the specialized intestinal metaplasia of Barrett esophagus [106,120–123]. Barrett metaplasia conceivably could result from the process of transdifferentiation, in which mature esophageal squamous cells change into columnar cells through reflux-induced alterations in the expression of key developmental transcription factors. More likely, metaplasia might result from transcommitment, in which esophageal stem cells (in the basal layer of the squamous epithelium or in the ducts of esophageal submucosal glands) that normally differentiate into squamous cells instead differentiate into columnar cells. Biopsy specimens at the SCJ can reveal a "multilayered epithelium" with features of both squamous and columnar epithelia [124], and scanning electron microscopy of such specimens has demonstrated a distinctive, hybrid cell that has morphological features of both squamous and columnar cells [125,126]. These observations could support either a transdifferentiation or transcommitment origin for Barrett metaplasia. In a rat model of reflux esophagitis, Barrett metaplasia appears to develop from circulating bone marrow stem cells [127]. Finally, recent research using mouse models has suggested that Barrett metaplasia might result from the proximal migration of stem cells from the gastric cardia [128], or from the expansion of nests of residual embryonic cells or transitional basal cells at the GEJ [129,130].

Although the identity of the Barrett progenitor cell remains unclear, metaplasia must arise from changes in the progenitor cell's expression of key developmental transcription factors. Cells from any of the locations described in the previous paragraph might contribute to reepithelization of the reflux-damaged esophagus initially via a wound healing process, with GERD-induced reprogramming resulting in metaplasia [131]. Most investigations on molecular events underlying the intestinal metaplasia of Barrett esophagus have focused primarily on the upregulation of genes involved in intestinal differentiation, such as *SOX9* and *CDX*. However, it is likely that this metaplasia also involves the downregulation of transcription factors involved in squamous differentiation such as *SOX-2* and *p63*. In mice, high levels of Sox-2 in the embryonic esophagus promote the development of stratified squamous epithelium [132] and after birth, strong expression of p63 is found in basal cells of the mouse stratified squamous esophagus [133]. In humans and in a rat model of Barrett esophagus, *SOX-2* and *p63* are expressed in esophageal squamous epithelium, but not in Barrett metaplasia [133–135]. These and other data suggest that gastroesophageal reflux may induce the expression of *CDX* and *SOX9* while suppressing *SOX-2* and *p63* expression in esophageal progenitor cells, thereby mediating their differentiation into the intestinal-type cells characteristic of Barrett esophagus.

Bone morphogenetic protein (BMP)-4 also may be involved in the squamous-to-columnar metaplasia of Barrett esophagus [136]. In a rat model of Barrett esophagus and in patients with Barrett esophagus, BMP-4 has been found in stromal tissues of inflamed esophageal squamous mucosa and in specialized intestinal metaplasia, but not in normal esophageal squamous mucosa [137]. When cultures of human esophageal squamous cells are exposed to BMP-4, they express *SOX9* and cytokeratins typical of columnar cells, and their gene expression patterns change to resemble those of Barrett epithelial cells [137,138]. These data suggest that reflux esophagitis may induce the esophageal stroma to express BMP-4, which mediates the change from esophageal squamous cells to the columnar cell types of Barrett esophagus.

BMP-4 is a target of the hedgehog signaling pathway that is active during the embryonic development of the gut [138]. Sonic hedgehog (Shh), the most ubiquitous hedgehog ligand, is expressed by the embryonic columnar-lined esophagus, which later becomes squamous lined as hedgehog signaling is downregulated [139]. Recently, Shh expression has been observed in Barrett metaplasia, but not in normal adult esophageal squamous epithelium [138]. In a mouse model of reflux esophagitis and Barrett esophagus, Shh expression is found in Barrett metaplasia, as well as in esophageal squamous cells, just before the development of that metaplasia [138].

In an in vivo; transplant culture system, overexpression of Shh by mouse esophageal squamous cells induces esophageal fibroblasts to express BMP, which causes the epithelial cells to express SOX9 and columnar cell cytokeratins and to assume an intestinal-like morphology [138]. Thus, hedgehog signaling appears to play an important role in the pathogenesis of Barrett esophagus. Data suggest that the gastroesophageal reflux of acid and bile causes esophageal epithelial cells to express Shh, which induces esophageal stromal cells to express BMP-4, which signals back to the epithelium to induce squamous cells to produce SOX9 and FOXA2, columnar transcription factors that might mediate the squamous-to-columnar metaplasia of Barrett esophagus [140]. In support of the importance of hedgehog signaling, inhibition of the hedgehog pathway in a rat model of reflux esophagitis decreased the development of Barrett esophagus and esophageal adenocarcinoma by approximately 36% [141].

Notch is another developmental signaling pathways that has been implicated in Barrett pathogenesis. The Notch pathway participates in maintaining the normal intestinal crypt progenitor cell pool [142]. As intestinal cells begin to differentiate, persistent Notch signaling leads to the development of absorptive cells, whereas cessation of Notch signaling leads to a secretory phenotype with the appearance of enteroendocrine, goblet, and Paneth cells [143,144]. In HET-1A human esophageal squamous cells, the expression of CDX2 downregulates Hes1, a downstream target of Notch. This suggests that inhibition of Notch signaling by CDX2 might contribute to goblet cell metaplasia. Bile salt exposure also decreases the expression of Notch pathway components by HET-1A cells and human esophageal adenocarcinoma cells [145,146]. Although Notch inhibition appears to be linked to the development of the goblet cell metaplasia that characterizes Barrett esophagus, Notch signaling is increased in esophageal adenocarcinoma, perhaps because this signaling drives a cancer stem cell phenotype by regulating genes that establish stemness [147].

Genetic susceptibility to develop Barrett esophagus and esophageal adenocarcinoma

Recent advances in genomic techniques have provided considerable insights into genetic factors that determine the risk for development of Barrett esophagus and its progression to esophageal adenocarcinoma. Genome-wide association studies (GWAS) can compare genetic variations throughout the genome of patients who have Barrett esophagus (with or without neoplasia) with individuals who do not. The most common types of genetic variations studied are single-nucleotide polymorphisms (SNPs). Each SNP represents a difference in a nucleotide at a specific location in the individual's DNA that can then be mapped to a specific gene, thus enabling the association of specific genes with a disease. GWASs are usually performed on whole blood DNA to identify germline (i.e., inherited) alterations.

Most GWASs on Barrett esophagus and esophageal adenocarcinoma have used the Barrett and Esophageal Adenocarcinoma Consortium (BEACON) dataset, which contains clinical information and blood samples from subjects enrolled in 14 epidemiological studies from Australia, Europe, and North America [148]. With this dataset, Ek et al. [149] analyzed GWAS data on a subset of subjects with white European ancestry (including 1509 patients with esophageal adenocarcinoma, 2383 with Barrett esophagus, and 2170 control subjects). Using complex bioinformatic analyses, they estimated that 25% of patients with esophageal adenocarcinoma and 35% of those with Barrett esophagus have a polygenic component underlying disease risk, meaning that many common SNP variants (any one of which alone might not increase risk for disease) together accounted for the increased risk for Barrett esophagus and esophageal adenocarcinoma [149]. Moreover, unrelated subjects with Barrett esophagus and esophageal adenocarcinoma were found to have substantial overlapping of SNPs, suggesting a shared genetic susceptibility for the two disorders. Another study that combined DNA samples from the BEACON cohort with those from the Aspirin Esomeprazole Chemoprevention trial, the Chemoprevention of Premalignant Intestinal Neoplasia genetic study, and the Esophageal Adenocarcinoma Genetics consortium estimated that the genetic risk for Barrett esophagus was only 9.99% [150], considerably less than the 35% reported by Ek et al. [149].

Many of the SNPs identified by GWASs as risk factors for Barrett esophagus and esophageal adenocarcinoma are located in or around genes that regulate esophageal development (i.e., FOXF1, FOXP1, BARX1), the cystic fibrosis transmembrane conductance regulator (CFTR) gene, and the major histocompatibility complex (MHC) locus that regulates activation of the immune system [148,151–153]. In contrast, SNPs that genetically result in low vitamin D levels have not been associated with risk for these diseases [154]. Noting the male predominance for Barrett esophagus and esophageal adenocarcinoma, GWASs have looked for differences in genes that regulate sex hormones. Higher genetically predicted levels of follicle-stimulating hormone have been associated with an increased risk for Barrett esophagus and esophageal adenocarcinoma in both men and women, whereas genetically predicted greater levels of luteinizing hormone are associated with a reduced risk for both disorders in women and a reduced risk only for esophageal adenocarcinoma in men [155].

Barrett esophagus and esophageal adenocarcinoma are far more prevalent in white individuals (of European ancestry) than in African Americans despite the fact that Barrett risk factors, such as GERD and obesity, are at least as common in African American as in white individuals. This suggests a genetic susceptibility to Barrett esophagus in individuals of European ancestry [156]. In a study in which DNA was extracted from paraffin-embedded tissue samples from 54 African American patients with Barrett esophagus or esophageal adenocarcinoma, SNPs identified by genotyping were compared with genotype data from a European and an African ancestry population in the 1000 Genome Project [156]. In the African American patients with Barrett esophagus and esophageal adenocarcinoma, the investigators identified two broad chromosomal regions (one on chromosome 11p15 and the other on chromosome 8q22–24) containing SNPs suggestive of excess European ancestry. Moreover, transcriptional profiling of esophageal squamous mucosa from African Americans and European Americans with and without GERD, Barrett esophagus, or esophageal adenocarcinoma has demonstrated increased messenger RNA (mRNA) expression of glutathione *S*-transferase θ 2, GSTT2/GSTT2B, a gene that protects against oxidant-induced DNA damage, in the squamous mucosa of African Americans [157]. In contrast, European Americans had a duplication within the promoter region of GSTT2/GSTT2B that is associated with lower promoter activity and lower mRNA expression. Thus, esophageal squamous mucosa of African Americans might have greater innate protection against the GERD-induced injury that leads to Barrett esophagus and esophageal adenocarcinoma than white individuals.

Finally, there is a familial form of Barrett esophagus that appears to account for 7–11% of all cases [158–161]. It is unclear whether this familial clustering is due to common environmental exposures, such as smoking and diet, and/or to an inherited predisposition. Germline mutations in the macrophage scavenger receptor 1 (MSR1), activating signal cointegrator 1 complex subunit 1 (ASCC1), and collagen triple-helix repeat containing 1 (CTHRC1) genes, which are involved in macrophage function and inflammatory pathways, have been associated with the presence of Barrett esophagus and esophageal adenocarcinoma [162]. Cases of familial Barrett esophagus have a significantly younger age of onset of heartburn symptoms and of esophageal adenocarcinoma diagnoses, as well as more frequent reports of reflux symptoms in their first-degree relatives than nonfamilial cases [159–161].

Genetic susceptibility and epidemiological risk factors for Barrett esophagus and esophageal adenocarcinoma

A number of studies have analyzed genetic interactions between Barrett esophagus and/or esophageal adenocarcinoma and their epidemiological risk factors, including GERD, cigarette smoking, and body mass index (BMI). A genome-wide gene–environment interaction study found several significant interactions between SNPs associated with Barrett esophagus and esophageal adenocarcinoma and these risk factors [163]. Conversely, individuals with increased genetic risk for high BMI (determined by a genetic risk score involving 29 BMI-associated SNPs) were found to have high rates of Barrett esophagus and esophageal adenocarcinoma [164]. On a genome-wide level, there is a high degree of correlation between genetic risk for obesity and genetic risk for Barrett esophagus and esophageal adenocarcinoma [165].

Combining epidemiological risk with genetic risk has been explored as a strategy to improve risk prediction for the development of Barrett esophagus and esophageal adenocarcinoma. For example, Dai et al. [166] used a candidate-based SNP approach involving SNPs located in or near seven genes that GWASs had identified as associated with risk for Barrett esophagus (i.e., FOXF1, TBX5, GDF7, MHC, CRTC1, BARX1, and FOXP1) [148,150,151,166]. They found that patients with GERD symptoms who had no SNPs in their FOXP1 gene had the highest odds ratio (OR) for development of Barrett esophagus (OR, 6). The combination of GERD symptoms and a SNP in the FOXP1 gene significantly decreased the risk for Barrett esophagus from an OR of 6.0 to 5.44, whereas a SNP in the FOXP1 gene in patients without GERD symptoms had an OR for Barrett esophagus of 1.5. No significant associations were found between any of the seven candidates' SNPs, BMI, or cigarette smoking and the risk for development of Barrett esophagus, or between any of these SNPs and any of the epidemiological risk factors for esophageal adenocarcinoma [166].

More recently, a polygenetic risk score (PRS) was developed using 23 SNPs associated with Barrett esophagus or esophageal adenocarcinoma [167]. An increased PRS was found to be associated with a significant increase in risk for Barrett esophagus and esophageal adenocarcinoma, such that individuals in the highest PRS quartile had >2-fold greater risk for Barrett esophagus and esophageal adenocarcinoma than those in the lowest quartile. When the PRS score was combined with demographic and lifestyle factors (age, sex, smoking, BMI, and NSAID use) and GERD symptoms, the area under the receiver operating characteristic curve (AUC) increased only slightly above that for the clinical variable alone in distinguishing individuals with Barrett esophagus or esophageal adenocarcinoma from those without either condition. In a similar study, Kunzmann et al. [168] found that combining 18 SNPs associated with esophageal adenocarcinoma with a clinical risk score (age, sex, BMI, smoking status, and esophageal conditions) did not change the AUC for predicting the 5-year risk for development of esophageal adenocarcinoma.

Because GERD causes chronic esophageal inflammation that contributes to the development of Barrett esophagus and esophageal adenocarcinoma, it is not surprising that genetic susceptibility within inflammatory pathways has been linked to risk for these conditions. Investigators have analyzed selected SNPs within five different inflammation-related pathways linked with Barrett esophagus and esophageal adenocarcinoma, including cyclooxygenase (COX), proinflammatory and antiinflammatory cytokines, oxidative stress, human leukocyte antigen, and nuclear factor κ-light-chain-enhancer of activated B cells (NF-κB) [169]. Significant associations with risk for Barrett esophagus alone and in combination with adenocarcinoma were found only for germline variations in the COX pathway (specifically in the antioxidant microsomal glutathione *S*-transferase 1 [MGST1] gene). Interestingly, none of these pathways were associated with risk for esophageal adenocarcinoma alone. In esophageal squamous and Barrett epithelial cells, refluxed acid and bile salts induce oxidative stress via the production of reactive oxygen species. Glutathione *S*-transferase genes such as MGST1 encode proteins that respond to oxidative stress [170]. Huo et al. [171] have shown that the intensity of activation of the inflammation-related NF-κB pathway caused by acid and bile salt-induced reactive oxygen species is substantially greater in esophageal squamous cells from patients with Barrett esophagus than from patients with GERD without Barrett esophagus. In the esophageal squamous cells from the former but not the latter patients, the intensity of this NF-κB pathway activation was sufficient to induce expression of caudal-related homeobox transcription factor 2 (CDX2), a key developmental transcription factor that determines the formation of intestinal epithelium. It is intriguing to speculate that perhaps germline mutations in genes that modify inflammatory responses to oxidative stress (such as MGST1) might help to explain the reported differences in intensity of NF-κB activation and CDX2 expression in esophageal squamous cells from patients with GERD with and without Barrett esophagus, and why Barrett esophagus develops in only some patients with GERD.

Conceptual framework for the progression of Barrett metaplasia to dysplasia and adenocarcinoma

The exact sequence and precise molecular changes necessary to produce dysplasia and adenocarcinoma in Barrett metaplasia remain incompletely understood. However, the notion that several distinct physiological properties distinguish the behavior of cancer cells from normal cells, and that genetic alterations within several key molecular pathways allow normal cells to acquire these essential cancer properties has been the underlying conceptual framework for cancer development since the year 2000 [172]. These acquired cancer properties include limitless proliferative ability (generally acquired through oncogene activation), the ability to evade growth suppressors (generally through inactivation of tumor suppressor genes), avoidance of apoptosis, replicative immortalization, angiogenesis induction, the ability to invade adjacent structures and to metastasize to distant structures, reprogramming of energy metabolism to support enhanced proliferation, and the ability to evade cancer-destroying immune cells (Figure 46.6) [172,173]. Features that facilitate the acquisition of these cancer properties include genomic instability (often reflected by aneuploidy or whole-genome doubling) and mutation, and a cancer-promoting, inflammatory microenvironment (see Figure 46.6) [172–174].

Processes involved in communication between cells appear to play key roles in delivering messages that can regulate cancer properties. In the past few years, exosomes, a subtype of extracellular vesicles that are between 50 and 150 nm in diameter, have gained attention as an important means of cell-to-cell communication [175]. Membrane-bound exosomes that contain molecular cargo, such as proteins, mRNAs, and microRNAs, are released by cells, including benign Barrett cells and esophageal adenocarcinoma cells [176–178].

Cell-to-cell communication occurs by the transfer of this molecular cargo from the releasing cell to a recipient cell, resulting in modification of the physiological state of the recipient cell. Through such cargo transfer, cancer-derived exosomes can initiate molecular pathways that regulate the acquisition of cancer properties in benign cells or in other neoplastic cells (see Figure 46.6) [179]. Studies by Ke et al. [180] have shown that gastric organoids co-cultured with esophageal adenocarcinoma cell-derived extracellular vesicles for 6 weeks exhibit changes in morphology, proliferation, and growth rates. Moreover, exposure to esophageal adenocarcinoma cell-derived extracellular vesicles causes gastric organoids to become crowded, compact, and multilayered through the uptake of extracellular vesicle-derived microRNAs that increase cell proliferation, suggesting a role for such molecular cargo transfer in the neoplastic progression of stem/progenitor Barrett cells.

As we are entering an era of precision medicine, the conceptual framework provided earlier can be useful in aiding the clinician to classify data stemming from studies involving next

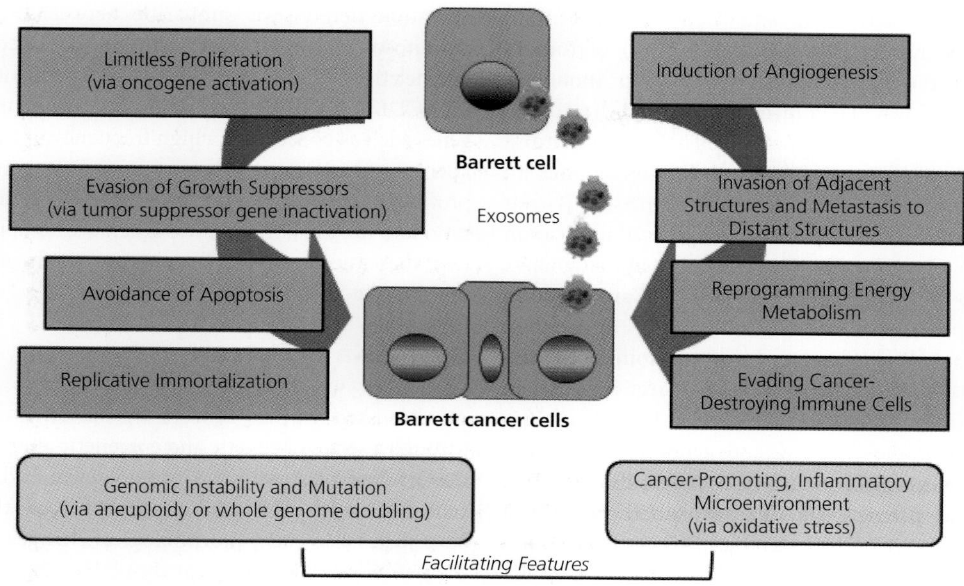

Figure 46.6 Conceptual framework for the progression of Barrett metaplasia to dysplasia and adenocarcinoma. The essential properties of cancer cells are shown in the blue boxes. In general, activation of oncogenes, such as ERBB2, is the way in which a stem/progenitor Barrett cell can attain limitless proliferation, and inactivation of tumor suppressor genes, such as p53 and p16, is a common way in which stem/progenitor Barrett cells evade growth suppressors. The rounded boxes in orange are the facilitating features, such as genomic instability and mutation and a cancer-promoting inflammatory microenvironment rich in oxidative stress as a result of chronic gastroesophageal reflux disease, that allow stem/progenitor Barrett cells faster acquisition of these cancer properties. Cell-to-cell communications by exosomes released from Barrett cancer cells can initiate molecular pathways that regulate the acquisition of these essential cancer properties by metaplastic stem/progenitor Barrett cells. Sources: Hanahan and Weinberg 2000 [172]; Hanahan and Weinberg 2011 [173]; and Fouad and Aanei 2017 [174].

generation sequencing (alterations in gene sequence), metabolomics (alterations in cellular functions), and proteomics (alterations in protein products). Such studies can identify alterations in the entire biologic phenotype as Barrett cells progress toward malignancy [181]. It is also important to realize that a single alteration may have multiple disparate effects and may endow more than one essential cancer property. For example, inactivation of the tumor suppressor gene *TP53* not only enables cells to evade growth suppressors but also enables them to avoid apoptosis [182].

Molecular pathways of neoplastic progression in Barrett esophagus

Advances in genomic techniques, such as whole-genome sequencing and whole-exome sequencing (i.e., sequencing limited only to coding regions of genes) have revolutionized our understanding of how premalignant Barrett cells are transformed into tumor cells. Unlike GWASs, these sequencing techniques are performed on tissue specimens of Barrett metaplasia, dysplasia, and esophageal adenocarcinoma to identify somatic (i.e., acquired, not inherited) alterations involved in neoplastic progression. For example, whole-exome sequencing of DNA extracted from specimens of benign Barrett metaplasia and esophageal adenocarcinoma from the same patient has revealed that nondysplastic Barrett esophagus has a high frequency of somatic mutations ranging from 1.3 to 5.4 mutations per megabase of DNA [183]. These rates of mutation in benign Barrett metaplasia are even greater than those found in cancers of the prostate and breast. Furthermore, the mutational signature in nondysplastic Barrett tissues is commonly a transversion (i.e., a shift from an adenine–adenine pair to an adenine–cytosine pair), a mutational pattern typical of genotoxic damage from oxidative stress presumably because of GERD. Dysplastic Barrett esophagus and esophageal adenocarcinoma share similar somatic mutational frequencies, which are higher than those found in nondysplastic Barrett esophagus. Most esophageal adenocarcinomas harbor a p53 mutation, and that same somatic p53 mutation can be detected in the nondysplastic Barrett metaplasia of patients who have cancer, often preceding inactivation of p16 [183]. The growth advantage endowed to a cell by p53 mutation would enable the clonal expansion of that cell. A high degree of diversity in clones within Barrett's metaplasia has been associated with an increased risk for neoplastic progression [184]. In contrast with inactivation of the p53 and p16 tumor suppressor genes found early in nondysplastic Barrett tissues, activation of oncogenes such as ERBB2 appear later in the dysplastic stages of carcinogenesis [183]. Surprisingly, however, this recent study found that only a minority of Barrett's tumors progress along this "traditional pathway" that involves the stepwise accumulation of alterations in tumor suppressor genes, followed by oncogene activation, and then development of genomic instability. Rather, the majority (62.5%) of tumors arising in Barrett esophagus appear to develop though a "genome-doubled pathway" (Figure 46.7) [183].

In the genome-doubled pathway, cells first acquire a p53 mutation, followed by doubling of the whole genome, an alteration primarily detected in areas of dysplastic Barrett esophagus. Genomic instability and oncogene amplification develop after whole-genome doubling, resulting in malignancy (see Figure 46.2). Cells with p53 mutations also are prone to genomic catastrophes, which have been reported to occur in about 30% of esophageal adenocarcinoma genomes, causing structural genomic rearrangements leading to large increases in oncogene amplification (see Figure 46.2) [185,186]. Thus, it is possible that the genome-doubling and genomic catastrophe pathways may be more rapid pathways to cancer development than the traditional pathway and may explain the failure of endoscopic surveillance to detect such rapid cancer progression in some patients with Barrett esophagus.

Advances in genomic techniques also have revealed a strong molecular resemblance between Barrett-associated esophageal adenocarcinomas and gastric adenocarcinomas of the chromosomal instability subtype. For example, analyses of mRNA expression, DNA methylation, and somatic copy-number alterations demonstrate similarities between these two tumors in chromosomal aberrations, including amplified oncogenic loci and deletions in genes such as cyclin-dependent kinase inhibitor 2A (CDKN2/p16^{INK4a}), in mutations within tumor suppressor genes such as p53, and in a high frequency of transversions from adenine–adenine to adenine–cytosine base pairs [187,188]. Such profound similarity at the genetic level provides a molecular rationale for the similar chemotherapeutic approaches used to treat these tumors arising from opposite sides of the GEJ.

Dysplasia in Barrett esophagus

As discussed earlier, cancers in Barrett esophagus develop through a series of genetic and epigenetic alterations that endow the affected cells with the physiological hallmarks of cancer cells. Some of the DNA changes that give cells these proliferative advantages also cause morphological changes in the tissue that the pathologist recognizes as dysplasia. Thus, dysplasia can be viewed as the histological expression of genetic and epigenetic alterations that favor cell growth and neoplasia [189].

Dysplasia is categorized as low-grade or high-grade depending on the degree of histological abnormalities. Histological changes similar to those of low-grade dysplasia can be seen in

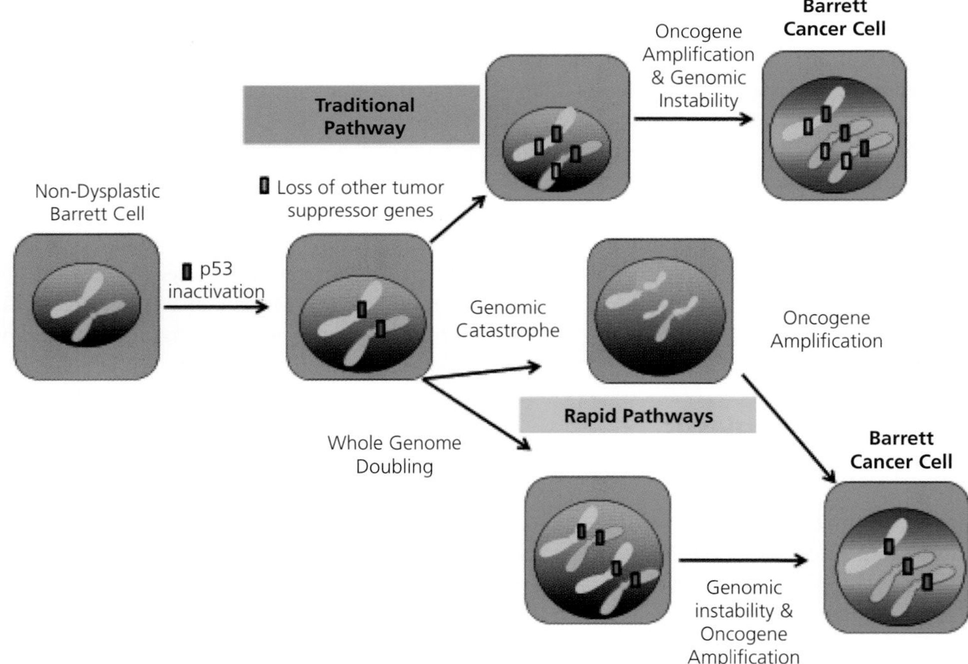

Figure 46.7 Molecular pathways of neoplastic progression in Barrett esophagus. Metaplastic Barrett cells first acquire a mutation leading to inactivation of p53. The traditional pathway involves the stepwise accumulation of alterations in tumor suppressor genes, such as p16, followed by oncogene activation and genomic instability, finally resulting in cancer formation. In the genome-doubled pathway, the p53-mutant Barrett cells undergo whole-genome doubling, followed by genomic instability and oncogene amplification, resulting in cancer formation. Cells with inactivation of p53 are also prone to genomic catastrophes with structural genomic rearrangements leading to large increases in oncogene amplification, resulting in cancer formation. Both the genome-doubled and genomic catastrophe pathways have been proposed to be more rapid pathways to cancer development and may possibly explain the failure of endoscopic surveillance to detect early cancer progression in Barrett esophagus. *Source:* Based on Stachler MD, Taylor-Weiner A, Peng S, et al. Paired exome analysis of Barrett's esophagus and adenocarcinoma. *Nat Genet.* 2015;47(9):1047–1055.

nonneoplastic tissue that is regenerating in response to injury from reflux esophagitis, and it can be difficult for pathologists to distinguish low-grade dysplasia in Barrett esophagus from reactive changes caused by reflux esophagitis. Consequently, interobserver agreement among experienced pathologists for the diagnosis of low-grade dysplasia is poor (<50%) [190–193]. One study conducted in the Netherlands found that when community pathologists rendered a diagnosis of low-grade dysplasia in Barrett esophagus, expert pathologists confirmed that diagnosis in only 15% of cases [194]. Interobserver agreement is better (approximately 85%) for high-grade dysplasia, but far from perfect. There is also substantial disagreement among pathologists when distinguishing high-grade dysplasia from intramucosal carcinoma [195] and for recognizing dysplasia confined to the crypts of the Barrett mucosa [196].

Endoscopic perspectives

On high-resolution, white-light endoscopy, dysplasia in Barrett esophagus is frequently, but not always, associated with visible abnormalities (e.g., ulcerations, nodules, mucosal and vascular irregularities), although those abnormalities can be subtle and easily overlooked [197]. In addition, dysplasia can be patchy both in extent and severity, factors contributing to the substantial problem of biopsy sampling error for dysplasia in Barrett esophagus [198,199]. Endoscopists traditionally have used a system of random, four-quadrant biopsy sampling of every 1–2 cm of columnar-lined esophagus (the Seattle biopsy protocol) in an attempt to maximize the chance of finding an endoscopically inconspicuous lesion, but it is clear that this system can miss dysplastic areas [198,200]. For patients found to have dysplasia, furthermore, foci of invasive cancer can be missed because of sampling error. In older series of patients who had esophagectomy for high-grade dysplasia in Barrett esophagus, a number of studies suggested that invasive cancer was present in as many as 30–40% of the resected specimens [201]. More recently, a critical review of those reports suggested that 13% is a more accurate estimate of the frequency of invasive cancer in this situation and, when a careful endoscopic examination excludes all visible lesions, the frequency of finding invasive cancer at esophagectomy is only approximately 3% [202].

A number of advanced imaging techniques have been used to enhance the endoscopic detection of dysplasia in Barrett esophagus. In chromoendoscopy, dyes (e.g., methylene blue, indigo carmine) or other agents (e.g., acetic acid) are sprayed on the esophageal mucosa to highlight dysplastic mucosal irregularities [203–206]. "Virtual chromoendoscopy" includes techniques such as Narrow Band Imaging (NBI; Olympus), Fujinon intelligent color enhancement (FICE; Fujinon), and i-Scan (Pentax) that use optical filters to highlight mucosal and vascular patterns associated with dysplasia [207]. A randomized trial comparing standard white-light endoscopy with Seattle protocol biopsies with NBI-directed targeted biopsies found that NBI detected a higher proportion of areas with dysplasia (30% vs 21%; $p = 0.01$) [208]. Confocal laser endomicroscopy provides real-time magnification of the esophageal mucosa to target areas suspicious for dysplasia [209–214], and there are several forms of spectroscopy (laser induced, elastic scattering, and infrared spectroscopy) that identify epithelial abnormalities by changes in fluorescence or in the reflection and scattering of light. Volumetric laser endomicroscopy (VLE) uses optical coherence tomography (OCT) technology to evaluate long segments of the esophageal mucosa to depths of 3 mm to detect neoplasia in Barrett esophagus [215,216]. Despite all the recent progress with advanced endoscopic imaging techniques, high-resolution white-light endoscopy with careful inspection and Seattle biopsy protocol sampling for dysplasia remains the clinical standard for managing patients with Barrett esophagus. However, the most recent guideline from the American Society for Gastrointestinal Endoscopy (ASGE) recommends the use of chromoendoscopy or virtual chromoendoscopy as an adjunct to Seattle protocol biopsy sampling during endoscopic evaluation of Barrett esophagus [217].

Wide-area transepithelial sampling (WATS) with computer-assisted three-dimensional (3D) analysis is another test that can be used to enhance the identification of dysplasia in Barrett esophagus. WATS uses an abrasive cytology brush that is passed through the channel of an endoscope, and the endoscopist uses the brush to scrape cells from the entire segment of Barrett metaplasia. The brush sample is smeared on a microscope slide, yielding a tissue specimen that is up to 150 μm in thickness. This slide is analyzed by a neural network computer system that captures up to 50 "optical slices" (each 3 μm in thickness) of the specimen, creating 3D images of the Barrett glands sampled. The computer then scans these images and flags areas it deems suspicious for dysplasia for final interpretation by a human pathologist. In one recent study, 12 899 patients undergoing screening or surveillance endoscopies for Barrett esophagus had both standard forceps biopsies and WATS samples taken by community endoscopists [218]. Forceps biopsies identified dysplasia in 88 patients, while WATS identified an additional 213 patients with dysplasia, increasing the dysplasia detection rate from 0.68% to 2.33%. The most recent guideline on screening and surveillance of Barrett esophagus from the ASGE suggests using WATS-3D in addition to Seattle protocol biopsy sampling for patients with known or suspected Barrett esophagus [217].

Histopathological perspectives

Although cancers in Barrett esophagus are thought to evolve from nonneoplastic metaplasia to low-grade dysplasia to high-grade dysplasia and to adenocarcinoma, this orderly sequence of progression is documented only infrequently. For patients with verified dysplasia, subsequent endoscopies often reveal no dysplastic epithelium, or patchy areas of dysplasia with varying severities [193,219,220]. Furthermore, adenocarcinomas have been found in patients whose previous surveillance biopsy specimens revealed only low-grade or even no dysplasia [192,220,221]. It is not clear whether these findings are the result of biopsy sampling error, of true regression or rapid progression of dysplasia between surveillance endoscopies, or of cancers developing directly from metaplastic epithelium that does not manifest dysplastic changes. One study suggests that patients who have Barrett esophagus experience low-grade dysplasia at the rate of 4.3% per year and high-grade dysplasia at the rate of 0.9% per year [222].

Reports on the natural history of low-grade dysplasia in Barrett esophagus yield contradictory data, perhaps because of poor agreement among pathologists regarding the diagnosis. In a series of 48 patients with low-grade dysplasia followed for a mean duration of 41 months, 5 (10%) progressed to high-grade dysplasia (4 patients) or adenocarcinoma (1 patient) [223]. Another group described a 12% cumulative incidence rate of adenocarcinoma at 5 years for 43 patients with low-grade dysplasia on baseline endoscopy [217]. Skacel and colleagues [192] followed 25 patients with low-grade dysplasia for a mean duration of 26 months, during which 7 (28%) progressed to high-grade dysplasia (5 patients) or adenocarcinoma (2 patients). In this series, agreement among pathologists in the diagnosis of low-grade dysplasia was associated with neoplastic progression. Seven of the 17 patients (41%) in whom at least two of the three study pathologists agreed on the diagnosis of low-grade dysplasia exhibited progression, while progression was seen in four of the five patients (80%) for whom there was unanimous agreement among the study pathologists. One study that included 156 patients with low-grade dysplasia described a cancer incidence rate of 0.6% per year [222]. In a Dutch study in which pathology slides for 147 patients who had low-grade dysplasia diagnosed at community hospitals were reviewed by two expert pathologists, the experts confirmed the diagnosis in only 15% of cases [194]. When the diagnosis was downgraded to "no dysplasia" or "indefinite for dysplasia," neoplastic development was unusual. In contrast, when low-grade dysplasia was confirmed by the experts, the cumulative risk rate of neoplastic progression was 85% at 109 months. Finally, in an American study of 210 patients with low-grade dysplasia followed for a mean of 6.2 years, the annual rate of progression was only 0.4% and a consensus diagnosis among the pathologists of low-grade dysplasia was not associated with neoplastic progression [92].

Relatively few studies provide meaningful data on the rate at which high-grade dysplasia in Barrett esophagus progresses to cancer, and reported estimates vary considerably. Hameeteman and colleagues [224] described eight patients with high-grade dysplasia in Barrett esophagus, five (63%) of whom were found to have adenocarcinomas on repeat endoscopic examinations performed within 1 year. Reid and colleagues [219] reported a 59% 5-year cumulative cancer incidence among 76 patients with high-grade dysplasia in Barrett esophagus. However, Schnell and colleagues [220] observed a much lower cancer incidence in 75 patients with high-grade dysplasia in Barrett esophagus, only 12 of whom (16%) developed adenocarcinoma during a mean follow-up period of 7.3 years. The reasons underlying the large disparities in the results of these three studies are not clear. In Schnell et al.'s series [220], it is possible that "over-reading" of dysplastic changes contributed to the low incidence of adenocarcinoma [225]. In addition, Schnell et al.'s analysis excluded patients who were found to have cancer within 1 year of the diagnosis of high-grade dysplasia, because the investigators considered those cancers to be prevalent (present at the first endoscopy but missed because of sampling error) rather than incident malignancies (developing during the period of follow-up). This exclusion criterion would have disqualified all five patients with cancer described by Hameeteman et al. [224] and would have reduced the 5-year cumulative cancer incidence rate in Reid's series from 59% to 31% [219].

Buttar [226] found that the extent of high-grade dysplasia in Barrett esophagus correlated with the risk for adenocarcinoma. In that report, high-grade dysplasia was defined as "focal" if the histological abnormalities were confined to a single focus involving up to five crypts, and as "diffuse" when those features were seen in more than five crypts or in multiple biopsy specimens. The cumulative cancer incidence rate at 3 years was 56% for the 67 patients with diffuse high-grade dysplasia, compared with only 14% for the 33 patients initially found to have focal high-grade dysplasia. However, the histological criteria for focal or diffuse dysplasia used in this study were arbitrary; there is no clear consensus on this classification among GI pathologists, and these observations require confirmation [227]. Indeed, other investigators have not confirmed the observation that focal high-grade dysplasia is associated with such a low cancer risk [228,229].

The category of "indefinite for dysplasia" has been especially problematic because there are no well-established diagnostic criteria for this diagnosis. A recent systematic review and metaanalysis on the risk for neoplastic progression in Barrett esophagus indefinite for dysplasia found that the pooled incidence of progression to high-grade dysplasia or adenocarcinoma was 1.5 per 100 person-years (95% confidence interval [CI]: 1.0–2.0). The most recent guideline on Barrett esophagus from the American College of Gastroenterology (ACG) recommends that when patients are given a diagnosis of indefinite for dysplasia, repeat endoscopy after optimization of acid suppression for 3–6 months should be performed [56]. If the diagnosis of indefinite for dysplasia is confirmed on this repeat endoscopy, then yearly surveillance is recommended.

In summary, it appears that patients with nondysplastic Barrett esophagus experience low-grade dysplasia at the rate of approximately 4.0% per year and high-grade dysplasia at the rate of 0.9% per year [222]. The overall rate of cancer development in patients with nondysplastic Barrett esophagus is approximately 0.1–0.3% per year. For patients with high-grade dysplasia, the rate of demonstrable cancer development is approximately 6% per year [1,230]. For patients with low-grade dysplasia in Barrett esophagus, the incidence of cancer is so poorly defined that it is not possible to provide a precise, meaningful estimate. Presumably, that incidence is greater than that of the general population of patients with Barrett esophagus (0.1–0.3% per year) and less than that of patients with high-grade dysplasia (6% per year).

Biomarkers for assessing risk for neoplastic progression

Noting the shortcomings of the histological demonstration of dysplasia for predicting the risk for neoplastic progression in Barrett esophagus, investigators have sought molecular markers that might be used to predict that risk with greater precision [231]. Although a myriad array of such biomarkers has been studied over the past four decades, American GI societies currently do not endorse the routine use of any biomarker in the management of Barrett esophagus. However, the British Society of Gastroenterology suggests that "The addition of p53 immunostaining to the histopathological assessment may improve the diagnostic reproducibility of a diagnosis of dysplasia in BE and should be considered as an adjunct to routine clinical diagnosis" [24]. As discussed earlier, inactivation of the p53 tumor suppressor gene appears to be a key event that occurs early and often during Barrett's carcinogenesis. A recent systematic review and metaanalysis has concluded that case–control and cohort studies of Barrett patients have shown consistent, strong, and significant associations between aberrant p53 immunostaining in Barrett biopsies and subsequent progression to high-grade dysplasia or esophageal adenocarcinoma [232]. Although these findings support the use of p53 immunostaining as an adjunct to routine histology, such immunostaining is performed uncommonly for clinical purposes in the United States.

Because the development of Barrett cancers involves numerous genetic and epigenetic derangements, perhaps it is not surprising that no single biomarker has been able to predict neoplastic progression with precision. Recently, however, new tests that evaluate panels of biomarkers, along with histological features, have shown promise for risk stratification. As discussed earlier, Barrett's cancers often exhibit genomic instability (an increased tendency for genome alterations during cell division) manifested both by small structural alterations (e.g., base pair mutations, microsatellite instability [MSI]) and large structural alterations (e.g., changes in chromosome number, loss of heterozygosity). Mutational load is an index of genomic instability, and one new test (BarreGEN; Interpace Diagnostics) measures mutational load in Barrett biopsy specimens from which a pathologist microdissects the most worrisome-looking areas. Using those microdissected targets, loss of heterozygosity mutations and MSI are assessed at 10 loci for tumor suppressor genes using polymerase chain reaction and quantitative capillary electrophoresis of DNA to determine the mutational load, which is quantitated on a scale of 0–10. In one case–control study, mutational load in baseline Barrett biopsies from 23 patients (cases) who subsequently experienced high-grade dysplasia or esophageal adenocarcinoma were compared with baseline Barrett biopsies from 46 similar control subjects who did not exhibit neoplastic progression [233]. At a mutational load of ≥1, the receiver operating curve for prediction of neoplastic progression exhibited excellent sensitivity and specificity, with an area under the curve of 0.95. The authors concluded that mutational load in baseline Barrett biopsies could be used to predict progression to high-grade dysplasia or esophageal adenocarcinoma. However, a subsequent study of similar design found an AUC of only 0.50, indicating poor discrimination of mutational load in predicting neoplastic progression [234]. Unlike the positive former study that used purified DNA for analysis, the latter study used crude lysates prepared from archived tissue specimens, and the authors proposed this as a possible explanation for the disparities between the two studies.

TissueCypher (Cernostics) is another promising test for predicting Barrett neoplastic progression [235]. In this test, formalin-fixed, paraffin-embedded Barrett biopsy specimens are immunofluorescence labeled with a panel of 14 biomarkers associated with Barrett neoplasia. The labeled slides are analyzed by computer to calculate an array of fluorescence intensity features in epithelial and stromal tissue compartments and within subcellular compartments, and these analyses are displayed and quantitated using computer algorithms. In a case–control study, TissueCypher results in baseline Barrett biopsies from 79 patients (cases) who subsequently had high-grade dysplasia or esophageal adenocarcinoma were compared with baseline Barrett biopsies from 287 similar control subjects who did not exhibit neoplastic progression [236]. Biopsy specimens were randomly assigned to either training or validation sets. The top-performing training set classifier used 15 biopsy features to predict neoplastic progression and to classify patients as low, intermediate, or high risk for progression. When this classifier was used in the validation set, it was found to predict the probability of progression with a high degree of accuracy that outperformed histology. These good results were confirmed in a follow-up case–control study [237]. Promising as these results are, American GI societies have not yet endorsed the use of biomarkers for routine management of patients with Barrett esophagus.

Proton pump inhibitors, NSAIDs, and antireflux surgery for cancer prevention in Barrett esophagus

The general approach to the treatment of GERD for patients with Barrett esophagus is very similar to that recommended for patients who have GERD without Barrett esophagus [238]. However, acid control might be especially important for patients with Barrett esophagus, and a number of studies have shown that patients with Barrett esophagus may be rendered asymptomatic by proton pump inhibitors (PPIs) given in dosages that fail to normalize esophageal acid exposure [239–241]. For example, in one study of 48 patients with Barrett esophagus, 50% had persistently abnormal acid exposure documented by esophageal pH monitoring while they were receiving dosages of PPIs that abolished GERD symptoms [241]. In patients with GERD who are treated with PPIs, lower healing rates of reflux esophagitis have been reported for those with Barrett esophagus than for those who have esophagitis of similar severity but without columnar metaplasia [242], and it has been suggested that patients with Barrett esophagus are unusually resistant to PPI treatment [241]. One study has suggested that this problem is not due to gastric resistance to the antisecretory effects of PPIs, because patients with Barrett esophagus treated with high doses of esomeprazole exhibited gastric acid suppression to levels similar to those reported for normal individuals [243]. However, despite the significant decrease in gastric acidity with the high dose of PPIs, up to 23% of patients with Barrett esophagus still had abnormal esophageal acid exposure. This suggests that the "PPI resistance" in patients with Barrett esophagus is a consequence of their profound reflux diathesis. In other words, PPIs may reduce gastric acid secretion appropriately, but the little acid that remains in the stomach refluxes into the esophagus because of the strong reflux diathesis, and so pathological levels of acid reflux persist despite effective gastric acid suppression.

For patients with Barrett esophagus, many authorities advocate maintenance therapy with a PPI for chemoprevention, irrespective of the severity of the underlying GERD and irrespective of the presence or absence of GERD symptoms. This practice is based primarily on indirect evidence suggesting that acid reflux promotes carcinogenesis in Barrett metaplasia, and that aggressive control of acid reflux may interfere with carcinogenesis. Acid causes DNA double-strand breaks in Barrett epithelial cells in vitro and in Barrett esophagus in vivo [244], and any agent that induces such double-strand breaks can be considered a potential carcinogen. Thus, effective acid suppression with PPIs would limit exposure to this carcinogen. Brief esophageal acid exposure in vivo also activates the mitogen-activated protein kinase pathways in Barrett esophagus [245]. In a clinical study in which esophageal biopsy specimens were taken from patients with Barrett esophagus at baseline and after 6 months of antireflux therapy, the expression of proliferating cell nuclear antigen (a proliferation marker) decreased significantly in biopsy specimens from 24 patients in whom treatment had normalized esophageal acid exposure, but not in the 15 with persistently abnormal acid reflux [230]. Another group found no significant change in the proliferative activity of Barrett esophagus in 22 patients treated with a PPI for 2 years, whereas proliferative activity increased significantly in 23 patients treated for the same time with a histamine H_2-receptor antagonist, which is far less effective at reducing gastric acid secretion [246]. During PPI therapy, most patients with Barrett esophagus experience partial regression of Barrett epithelium, which takes the form of islands of squamous epithelium that appear within their metaplastic columnar lining [247]. All this is indirect evidence that PPIs might prevent carcinogenesis in Barrett esophagus.

Observational studies on the efficacy of PPIs for reducing the neoplastic progression of Barrett esophagus have yielded confusing, contradictory results. In 2014, a metaanalysis of seven such studies found that the use of PPIs was associated with a 71% reduction in the risk for development of advanced neoplasia in Barrett esophagus [248]. Following the publication of this metaanalysis, a large case–control study on the same issue from Denmark found that the relative risk for development of high-grade dysplasia or adenocarcinoma in long-term users of PPIs was 2.2 for low-adherence PPI users and 3.4 for high-adherence PPI users, suggesting that PPIs *increase* the risk for neoplasia in Barrett esophagus [249]. A similar study in Sweden also found that the chronic use of PPIs was associated with a significantly increased risk for esophageal adenocarcinoma, even in patients who took PPIs for non-GERD indications [250]. In contrast, a nested case–control study of 29 536 male veteran patients with Barrett esophagus found that PPI use was associated with a 41% lower risk for cancer [251]. Unfortunately, all of these observational studies suffer from a number of biases that limit the conclusions that can be drawn.

It has been proposed that aspirin and NSAIDs that inhibit COX also might have a chemopreventive role for patients with Barrett esophagus. The rationale for this contention is that the specialized intestinal metaplasia of Barrett esophagus exhibits increased expression of COX-2 [252], and inhibition of COX-2 has antiproliferative and proapoptotic effects in Barrett-associated esophageal adenocarcinoma cell lines [253]. Furthermore, COX-2 inhibitors have been found to prevent the development of esophageal adenocarcinoma in an animal model of Barrett esophagus [254]. However, like the observational studies on PPIs discussed earlier, observational studies on the efficacy of NSAIDs for preventing the neoplastic progression of Barrett esophagus also have yielded contradictory results. One metaanalysis found that the use of aspirin and other NSAIDs decreased that risk by approximately 40% [85], whereas a recent large, population-based, case–control study concluded that neither NSAIDs (including aspirin) nor PPIs were associated with a significant reduction in the risk for cancer and high-grade dysplasia in Barrett esophagus [255].

The Aspirin and Esomeprazole Chemoprevention in Barrett's Metaplasia Trial (AspECT) was a large, prospective, randomized trial designed to establish the safety and efficacy of aspirin and esomeprazole for patients with Barrett esophagus [256]. In this study, 2557 patients with Barrett esophagus were randomized to receive high-dose PPI (esomeprazole 40 mg BID) with no aspirin, low-dose PPI (esomeprazole 20 mg daily) with no aspirin, high-dose PPI plus aspirin 300 mg daily, or low-dose PPI plus aspirin 300 mg daily, and endoscopy was performed at years 2, 4, 6, 8, and 10. In total, there were 20 095 patient-years of follow-up, with a median follow-up of 8.9 years. The primary endpoint was time to a composite of events including all-cause mortality, high-grade dysplasia, or esophageal adenocarcinoma, whichever came first, and the analyses used accelerated failure time modeling to determine whether the treatments accelerated or decelerated progression to the composite endpoint. Of patients receiving low-dose PPI, 13.8% had a primary endpoint event, compared with 10.9% of patients in the high-dose PPI group, with a time ratio of 1.27 (95% CI: 1.01–1.58; $p = 0.038$), meaning that high-dose PPI therapy significantly increased the time to death, high-grade dysplasia, or esophageal adenocarcinoma by

27%. For the comparison of aspirin with no aspirin, the time ratio for a primary endpoint event was 1.24 (95% CI: 0.98–1.57; $p = 0.068$), which was not statistically significant. However, when patients taking other NSAIDs together with aspirin were censored from the analysis, then aspirin was significantly better than no aspirin with a time ratio of 1.29 (95% CI: 1.01–1.66; $p = 0.043$). When high-dose PPI plus aspirin (with its 9.1% rate of primary endpoint events) was compared with low-dose PPI alone (with its 14.2% rate of primary endpoint events), the effects of PPI and aspirin appeared to be additive, with a time ratio of 1.59 (95% CI: 1.14–2.23; $p = 0.007$). Although high-dose PPIs and aspirin had significant beneficial effects for the composite endpoint that included all-cause mortality or high-grade dysplasia or esophageal adenocarcinoma, secondary analyses revealed that the only significant effect was for all-cause mortality. In other words, the study found no significant benefit of high-dose PPIs and aspirin for preventing high-grade dysplasia, esophageal adenocarcinoma, or death from esophageal adenocarcinoma. Furthermore, there was no placebo-treated control group, and thus the study cannot establish that PPIs are better than placebo for protecting against these endpoints. Clearly, AspECT was a monumental effort and a high-quality trial. Unfortunately, the results are not robust, and the proper roles for high-dose PPIs and aspirin as chemopreventive agents for patients with Barrett esophagus remain disputed.

Medical therapy for GERD in Barrett esophagus focuses almost exclusively on acid suppression with PPIs, which do not eliminate the reflux of other noxious gastric material, such as bile acids. Some have proposed that surgical antireflux therapy, which controls the reflux of all potentially damaging gastric material, might be more effective than antisecretory therapy for preventing cancer in Barrett esophagus [257]. Although some observational studies have found fewer cases of dysplasia and cancer among patients with Barrett esophagus who had fundoplication than among those who had received medical treatment [258,259], high-quality studies have found no significant difference in cancer incidence between medically and surgically treated patients with GERD. For example, during a 10- to 13-year follow-up of patients who had participated in a randomized trial of medical and surgical therapies for complicated GERD, 4 of 165 patients (2.4%) in the medical group and 1 of 82 (1.2%) in the surgical group developed an esophageal adenocarcinoma [260]. The difference between the treatment groups in the incidence of this tumor was not statistically significant, but with such a low observed rate of cancer development, the study did not have sufficient statistical power to detect small differences in the incidence of esophageal cancer. Much larger studies using patient databases [261–265] and metaanalyses [265,265] also have found no superior cancer-preventive effects for antireflux surgery compared with medical GERD therapy. A recent metaanalysis of 10 studies comparing cancer risk for patients who had fundoplication or medical treatment for GERD found that medical and surgical GERD treatments were very similar in their effects on cancer risk [266]. However, a subanalysis limited to only the four most modern studies in that metaanalysis suggested that surgery might decrease the risk for cancer in Barrett esophagus by 74% compared with medical therapy. Nevertheless, it is not at all clear that this potential advantage justifies the risks for antireflux surgery. We do not feel that antireflux surgery should not be advised with the expectation that the procedure will prevent esophageal cancer better than medical treatment.

Endoscopic surveillance for dysplasia

Although a number of medical societies recommend endoscopic surveillance for patients with Barrett esophagus, there is no proof (in the form of a randomized control trial) that surveillance is beneficial. The rationale for endoscopic surveillance for patients with Barrett esophagus includes the following questionable assumptions: (1) without interventions based on surveillance, patients with Barrett esophagus have decreased survival because of deaths from esophageal adenocarcinoma, (2) surveillance will reliably detect neoplasia in Barrett esophagus at a curable stage, and (3) treatment of the neoplasia found by surveillance will prolong survival and improve quality of life by preventing death and morbidity from esophageal cancer.

In several small series, survival for patients with Barrett esophagus did not differ significantly from that for control subjects in the general population [267–269]. Such small studies might not have the statistical power to demonstrate a small decrement in survival. However, in a large, population-based study comprising 7413 person-years of follow-up in 2373 patients with Barrett esophagus, Anderson and colleagues [270] found that overall mortality in the patients with Barrett esophagus was not increased above that of the general population of Northern Ireland. In contrast, Solaymani-Dodaran et al. [271] found that 1677 patients with Barrett esophagus had a 37% increase in mortality compared with a standard reference cohort of 13 416 individuals representing the general population of the United Kingdom. Approximately 45% of the excess mortality in the patients with Barrett esophagus was due to esophageal cancer, with the remainder due to other causes, mostly cardiovascular disease.

Available data suggest that the incidence of esophageal adenocarcinoma and the frequency of deaths as a result of esophageal cancer for patients with Barrett esophagus are increased significantly above the general population. Nevertheless, esophageal cancer is an uncommon cause of death in patients with Barrett esophagus. Older patients with Barrett esophagus succumb far more often to common illnesses like coronary artery disease than to esophageal adenocarcinoma. Thus, overall mortality in patients with Barrett esophagus appears to be affected only slightly by their higher frequency of esophageal cancer.

Observational studies have shown that some patients with Barrett esophagus have had curable neoplasms detected by endoscopic surveillance, and that asymptomatic cancers discovered in surveillance programs are less advanced than those found when patients present to the hospital with cancer symptoms such as dysphagia and weight loss [272–275]. For example, Corley and colleagues [276] reviewed the records of 589 patients who had adenocarcinomas at the GEJ, only 23 of whom were known to have had Barrett esophagus before the cancer was discovered [274]. Fifteen of those 23 patients had the cancer discovered during endoscopic surveillance for Barrett esophagus, and 11 of those (73%) survived, whereas there were no survivors among 8 patients who were not in surveillance and whose cancers were discovered when they presented with symptoms of dysphagia and weight loss. However, a more recent case–control study by Corley and colleagues [277] did not find a benefit for surveillance. In that study of 8272 patients known to have Barrett esophagus, 70 had an esophageal adenocarcinoma. Thirty-eight of those died of esophageal cancer and were included as the cases in the case–control study. For control subjects, the investigators identified 101 living patients with Barrett esophagus who were matched with the cases for age, sex, and duration of follow-up. Fifty-five percent of the cases had a surveillance endoscopy performed within 3 years of their cancer diagnosis, as did 60% of the control subjects, and the difference in the frequency of surveillance endoscopy between the groups was not statistically significant. If surveillance had been effective at preventing deaths from esophageal cancer, then it would be expected that the control subjects would have a higher frequency of surveillance than the cases. The authors concluded that surveillance endoscopy was not associated with a decreased risk for death from esophageal cancer. In contrast, a more recent study identified 29,536 veteran patients with Barrett esophagus, 424 of whom had esophageal adenocarcinoma during a mean follow-up of 5 years [228]. In 209 of those cases, the cancer was diagnosed during an endoscopy performed for surveillance of Barrett esophagus, while in 215, the cancer was diagnosed during an endoscopy performed for reasons other than surveillance. The patients whose cancers were diagnosed by surveillance endoscopy had earlier stage tumors, longer median survival, and less cancer-related mortality, and the authors concluded that surveillance endoscopy was associated with a significantly decreased risk for death from esophageal cancer.

Observational studies, such as those described earlier, cannot be considered definitive because they are subject to numerous biases (e.g., healthy volunteer bias, lead-time bias, length-time bias) that might inflate the benefits of surveillance programs [229]. A recent systematic review and metaanalysis on this topic concluded that surveillance as currently performed is associated with detection of earlier-stage esophageal adenocarcinoma and may provide a small survival benefit [278]. However, the authors added that the effects of confounding biases on these estimates are not fully defined and may completely or partially explain the observed differences between surveyed and unsurveyed patients. Although observational studies have documented the feasibility of endoscopic surveillance for detecting curable neoplasia, no study has established the reliability of surveillance in that regard. Indeed, a number of reports have documented the development of incurable esophageal malignancies in patients participating in endoscopic surveillance programs [279,280].

Surveillance programs seek to detect curable neoplasms in the form of dysplasia and early cancers, but the mere detection of these lesions cannot prolong survival. To prolong survival, there must be an effective treatment that prevents the progression of curable neoplasms to incurable cancers. Traditionally, the only treatment available for dysplasia and early cancer in Barrett esophagus was esophagectomy, a procedure associated with considerable morbidity and mortality. For older patients with comorbidities, the risks for esophagectomy often far exceeded the potential benefits [281]. When the only treatment for dysplasia was esophagectomy, it made little sense to recommend endoscopic surveillance for any patient who was not fit enough for that major operation. Today, however, dysplasia can be treated with endoscopic eradication therapy that is far less invasive and better tolerated than esophagectomy. Although studies have not yet proved that endoscopic eradication therapy prolongs life for patients found to have dysplasia during surveillance programs, the availability of endoscopic treatment has substantially expanded the population of patients who might benefit from surveillance. In other words, patients no longer need to be fit enough to undergo esophagectomy to justify endoscopic surveillance.

A number of modeling studies have supported the practice of endoscopic screening and surveillance for Barrett esophagus [57,282–290]. Cost-efficacy studies often use a benchmark value between $50 000 and $100 000 per life-year saved as something that society deems to be worthwhile, and all of these studies estimate that the costs of endoscopic screening and surveillance for patients with Barrett esophagus are within that range. Unfortunately, the computer models are not definitive because they rely on soft data and make many questionable assumptions. Furthermore, the internal programs of the models are largely "black boxes," with no external means to validate their accuracy.

The major points of the arguments for and against endoscopic surveillance for Barrett esophagus are summarized in Table 46.1. There have been numerous debates at medical meetings and in medical journals regarding the wisdom of surveillance for Barrett esophagus, with no clear winners. Current, most gastroenterology societies recommend endoscopic surveillance for patients with Barrett esophagus [24,27,56].

Treatment of dysplasia in Barrett esophagus

When evaluating reports on treatments for dysplasia in Barrett esophagus, it is important to consider the issue of what constitutes adequate follow-up. Specifically, when can the patient treated for dysplasia be considered "cured"? Patients treated for carcinomas traditionally are deemed cured if there is no evidence of recurrence at 5 years, because it is assumed that any cancer cells that survived the treatment would have become

Table 46.1 Arguments for and against endoscopic surveillance for patients with Barrett esophagus.

Against	For
No randomized controlled trial has established efficacy in preventing deaths from esophageal cancer	No randomized controlled trial establishing efficacy will be available in the foreseeable future
Some observational and computer model studies show no reasonable benefit for patients in surveillance programs [315,321–323]	Some observational and computer model studies show reasonable benefit for patients in surveillance programs [274,312,314,317]
Endoscopy has medical risks	The medical risks of elective endoscopy are minimal, and no study has found decreased survival for patients in surveillance programs [324]
A diagnosis of Barrett esophagus has adverse consequences (anxiety, decreased quality of life, higher life insurance costs) [325,326]	The adverse consequences of diagnosing Barrett esophagus are far less serious than missing the opportunity to cure esophageal cancer
Endoscopy is expensive	Some computer models show reasonable cost–benefit for surveillance in extending life-years [312,314,317]
The large majority of patients derive no benefit from surveillance	For some patients, surveillance can be lifesaving

Source: Spechler and Souza [2].

clinically manifest within that period. As discussed earlier, however, it often takes considerably longer than 5 years for dysplasia to progress to invasive cancer. Consequently, it is not appropriate to conclude that the cancer risk has been eliminated for a patient who has survived 5 years after treatment of dysplasia. Unfortunately, the follow-up duration in most reported studies on treatments for dysplasia in Barrett esophagus is considerably less than 5 years, and this factor severely limits the conclusions that can be drawn regarding the long-term efficacy of therapy.

Three management options have been studied for patients with high-grade dysplasia in Barrett esophagus: (1) intensive endoscopic surveillance in which invasive therapies are withheld until biopsy specimens reveal adenocarcinoma, (2) esophagectomy, and (3) endoscopic eradication therapy. Today, endoscopic eradication therapy is considered the procedure of choice for the treatment of dysplasia. Esophagectomy for dysplasia is required only in unusual circumstances, and intensive endoscopic surveillance is no longer recommended.

Intensive endoscopic surveillance

Before 2011, a program of expectant management with intensive endoscopic surveillance (endoscopy every 3–6 months) was considered a valid management option for patients with high-grade dysplasia in Barrett esophagus [33]. This approach was based on the findings of several observational studies. Schnell and colleagues [220] described 12 patients who developed adenocarcinoma during intensive endoscopic surveillance for high-grade dysplasia in Barrett esophagus. The cancers were deemed potentially curable at the time of detection in all 11 patients who were compliant with the surveillance program, but 1 patient who was lost to follow-up returned 10 years later with an unresectable tumor. In Reid et al.'s [291] series of 32 patients with high-grade dysplasia who developed adenocarcinoma during intensive endoscopic surveillance, only 1 patient (3%) had incurable disease (metastases) when the cancer was first detected on surveillance endoscopy. Weston and colleagues [292] performed intensive endoscopic surveillance in 15 patients with high-grade dysplasia for a mean duration of 36.8 months, during which 4 experienced development of adenocarcinoma. One of those four had metastatic disease, and the authors concluded that an observational approach to the management of high-grade dysplasia should be discouraged. These studies showed that intensive endoscopic surveillance generally was safe, but even patients who were compliant with the programs occasionally developed incurable cancers. With the widespread availability of endoscopic eradication therapy, the AGA, BSG, ACG, and ASGE no longer recommend intensive endoscopic surveillance for patients with high-grade dysplasia who are deemed fit enough for endoscopic treatment [24,27,56,217,293].

Esophagectomy

Esophagectomy, which removes both the abnormal esophagus and adjacent lymph nodes that might harbor metastases, is the most definitive but riskiest (in terms of procedure-related morbidity and mortality) of the treatments for dysplasia in Barrett esophagus. During hospitalization for esophagectomy, 30–50% of patients have at least one serious postoperative complication (e.g., pneumonia, arrhythmia, myocardial infarction, heart failure, wound infection, anastomotic leaks) [294–296]. Reported mortality rates for esophagectomy are high, and they vary with the frequency with which the operation is performed at any given medical center. In a study of data from the Dutch National Medical Registry, for example, the mortality rates for esophagectomy were 12.1%, 7.5%, and 4.9% at centers performing 1–10, 11–20, and >50 esophagectomies per year, respectively [297]. However, estimated mortality rates for esophagectomy have been based largely on series of patients with symptomatic esophageal cancer, many of whom are elderly and debilitated. Substantially lower mortality rates (generally <3%) are described in reports on esophagectomy performed to treat younger and otherwise healthy patients with dysplasia in Barrett esophagus (reviewed by Spechler et al. [1]).

Esophagectomy can have substantial long-term morbidity, with symptoms such as dysphagia, early satiety, loss of appetite, and fatigue that seriously impair the quality of life. However, most studies that have addressed the issue of quality of life after esophagectomy have included primarily patients with advanced esophageal cancer, and the results of those studies may not be applicable to patients with early neoplasia in Barrett esophagus. Several studies that focused on quality of life primarily in patients who had esophagectomy for high-grade dysplasia or early cancer in Barrett esophagus suggest that these patients generally have a good, long-term quality of life after the operation. One study of 34 such patients found that short form (SF)-36 results obtained at a mean of 46 months after esophagectomy were equal to or better than those of a healthy control population [298]. Another study included 36 patients who had esophagectomy for high-grade dysplasia or intramucosal carcinoma and who were followed for a mean duration of 4.9 years. Similar to the previous study, SF-36 scores for the patients were similar to those of age- and sex-matched control subjects [299]. One study compared SF-36 scores 12–60 months after treatment in 27 patients who had esophagectomy and 64 patients who had endoscopic treatment for early Barrett neoplasia [300]. No statistically significant differences between endoscopy and surgery patients were found in the mean scores of the eight subscales of the SF-36. Surgery patients reported significantly more reflux and eating problems than endoscopy patients, while endoscopy patients reported significantly higher fear of cancer recurrence than surgery patients.

In summary, esophagectomy for early neoplasia in Barrett esophagus definitively removes all of the esophagus at increased risk for malignancy, provides a specimen that can be examined for evidence of invasion (unlike endoscopic ablation procedures), and obviates the concern that local lymph nodes might contain metastases (unlike endoscopic therapy). When performed in otherwise healthy individuals, the mortality rate for the operation is generally less than 3%, and the long-term quality of life is good in most cases. Thus, even though endoscopic eradication therapy is the procedure of choice for the large majority of patients with dysplasia in Barrett esophagus, esophagectomy still warrants consideration in special circumstances, for example, in younger patients who have extensive Barrett metaplasia with multiple areas of dysplastic foci that are resistant to endoscopic eradication [301].

Endoscopic eradication therapy

Endoscopic eradication therapy can be performed using the techniques of endoscopic ablation, EMR, endoscopic submucosal dissection (ESD), or any combination of these modalities. Endoscopic ablation is the use of endoscopic techniques that deliver damaging energy to the esophagus with the intent of destroying the Barrett metaplasia. Because the intent is to destroy tissue, ablation does not provide a specimen for histological analysis. EMR and ESD are techniques that remove large segments of the esophageal mucosa and submucosa, providing specimens that are submitted for histological examination. The term "endoscopic eradication therapy" is used to describe the use of one or any combination of these endoscopic modalities with the specific goal of completely eradicating all of the Barrett metaplasia, both dysplastic and nondysplastic [302].

Endoscopic eradication therapy can cure neoplasms confined to the Barrett mucosa but cannot cure cancers that have metastasized to lymph nodes. Because the frequency of lymph node metastases varies with the depth of neoplasia, careful T staging of esophageal neoplasia is critical when considering endoscopic eradication therapy. Endoscopic ultrasonography (EUS), the best of the noninvasive techniques available for T staging esophageal tumors, accurately identifies the T stage for early esophageal cancers in only 50–60% of cases [303]. In contrast, studies have found excellent T-stage agreement between preoperative EMR findings and histological examination of esophagectomy specimens for patients with neoplasia in Barrett esophagus [304]. Therefore, in addition to its role as an eradication procedure, EMR is an invaluable T staging procedure.

Mucosal neoplasia (dysplasia) in Barrett esophagus can be categorized as T1am1 (high-grade dysplasia confined to the epithelium), T1am2 (intramucosal carcinoma with invasion into the lamina propria but not involving the muscularis mucosae), and T1am3 (intramucosal carcinoma with invasion into the lamina propria involving but not penetrating the muscularis mucosae). For patients with T1am1 and T1am2 neoplasms, the risk for lymph node metastases is <2% [305]. For T1am3 lesions, that risk increases to 4% [306]. The risk for lymph node metastases is considerably greater for T1b neoplasms, which penetrate the muscularis mucosae to invade the submucosa. The submucosa can be divided into a superficial third (sm1), a middle third (sm2), and a deep third (sm3). The risk rate for lymph node metastases is approximately 13% for sm1 lesions, 26% for sm2 lesions, and up to 67% for sm3 lesions [306–308]. Thus, when EMR or ESD specimens show submucosal invasion, endoscopic eradication therapy generally is not recommended, although patients with sm1 lesions have been treated successfully by endoscopy in some highly specialized endoscopy units [309]. EMR or ESD of visible mucosal irregularities (e.g., nodularity) in Barrett esophagus often reveal submucosal invasion that is not apparent in forceps biopsy specimens, and it is strongly recommended that endoscopists evaluate all such visible lesions by EMR before initiating eradication therapy [272,273]. The most recent ACG guideline states specifically that the inability to perform EMR in the setting of Barrett esophagus with nodularity should lead to consideration for referral to a tertiary care center [56].

Endoscopic ablation

Endoscopic ablative therapies (e.g., potassium titanyl phosphate, argon, Nd:YAG laser; multipolar electrocoagulation; argon plasma coagulation; photodynamic therapy (PDT); cryoablation; radiofrequency ablation [RFA]) have used thermal, photochemical, and radiofrequency energy to ablate the abnormal epithelium in Barrett esophagus [274,275,302,310]. After the epithelium is ablated, patients are given potent antireflux therapy (usually PPIs) so that the injured mucosa heals with the growth of new squamous epithelium. Early reports on ablative therapies for dysplasia in Barrett esophagus were not randomized or controlled, involved small numbers of patients, and had short durations of follow-up. Consequently, the conclusions that could be drawn from those studies were very limited. Now, randomized controlled trials are available for two of the ablative modalities: PDT and RFA.

Photodynamic therapy

For PDT, patients are given a systemic dose of a light-activated chemical (usually a porphyrin or porphyrin precursor) that is taken up by the esophageal cells. The esophagus is then irradiated using a low-power laser that activates the chemical, which transfers the energy acquired from laser light to oxygen. This results in the formation of singlet oxygen, a toxic molecule that destroys the abnormal cells and their vasculature. In a multicenter, randomized trial of PDT using porfimer sodium for ablation of high-grade dysplasia in Barrett esophagus, 138 patients were treated with PDT plus omeprazole 20 mg BID, and 70 received omeprazole 20 mg BID alone (without PDT) [311,312]. No dysplasia was seen on repeat endoscopy in 77% of the patients treated with PDT and in 39% of the patients who received omeprazole alone ($p < 0.0001$). During up to 5 years of follow-up, 15% of the PDT patients developed cancer, compared with 29% of those treated with omeprazole alone ($p = 0.027$). There was no procedure-related mortality, but 69% of the patients who received PDT developed photosensitivity reactions and 36% developed esophageal strictures that required one or more sessions of dilation therapy. Although these results show that PDT is clearly superior to omeprazole alone for eradicating dysplasia and preventing cancer in Barrett esophagus, the frequency of serious complications is disconcerting, as is the fact that cancer developed in 15% of the patients who received PDT. For these reasons, PDT has largely been replaced by RFA.

Radiofrequency ablation

RFA uses endoscopic guidance to position a balloon with a circumferential array of electrodes to deliver radiofrequency energy to the Barrett esophagus [313,314]. Using a generator to control the power, density, and duration of the radiofrequency energy applied, RFA was designed to inflict a uniform, circumferential thermal injury of limited depth. There are also smaller, endoscope-mounted, paddle-shaped RFA devices that are used to destroy localized segments of metaplasia. In a multicenter, randomized, sham-controlled trial of RFA, 127 patients with dysplasia in Barrett esophagus (64 low grade, 63 high grade) were randomized to receive either RFA (ablation group) or a sham endoscopic procedure (control group) [315]. At 1 year, intention-to-treat analyses revealed complete eradication of low-grade dysplasia in 90.5% of patients in the ablation group, compared with 22.7% of those in the control group ($p < 0.001$). Similarly, complete eradication of high-grade dysplasia was found in 81.0% of patients in the ablation group, compared with 19.0% of those in the control group ($p < 0.001$). Complete eradication of intestinal metaplasia was found in 77.4% of all patients in the ablation groups, compared with 2.3% of those in the control group ($p < 0.001$). In addition, patients in the ablation group had less progression in their degree of neoplasia (3.6% vs 16.3%; $p = 0.03$) and fewer cancers noted 1 year later (1.2% vs 9.3%; $p = 0.045$). Serious complications occurred in 6 (7%) of the 84 patients who received ablation, including one upper GI hemorrhage and five esophageal strictures.

The Surveillance vs Radiofrequency Ablation (SURF) study, a European randomized trial, has established the superiority of RFA over endoscopic surveillance for patients with low-grade dysplasia in Barrett's esophagus [316]. In this study, 136 patients with low-grade dysplasia confirmed by expert pathologists were randomized to receive either RFA or endoscopic surveillance. Progression to high-grade dysplasia or cancer was found at 3 years in 1.5% of the RFA group and in 26.5% of the surveillance group, indicating that RFA had decreased the risk for neoplastic progression by 25% (95% CI: 14.1–35.9%; $p < 0.001$). Progression to cancer was seen at 3 years in 1.5% of the RFA group and in 8.8% of the surveillance group, indicating that RFA decreased the risk for cancer by 7.4% (95% CI: 0–14.7%; $p = 0.03$). Esophageal strictures that required dilation developed in 12% of ablated patients.

The safety record of RFA is far superior to that of esophagectomy or PDT, although serious side-effects of RFA are not rare. A recent systematic review and metaanalysis of 37 articles, including a total of 9200 patients treated with RFA, found an 8.8% (95% CI: 6.5–11.9%) pooled rate of all adverse events, with the most common being strictures (5.6%; 95% CI: 4.2–7.4%) followed by bleeding (1.0%; 95% CI: 0.8–1.3%) and perforation (0.6%; 95% CI: 0.4–0.9%) [317].

Cryotherapy

Cryotherapy for Barrett esophagus involves the endoscopic application of a very cold cryogen, typically liquid nitrogen or liquid nitrous oxide, to the Barrett mucosa, thereby inducing freeze–thaw events that destroy tissue by disrupting cell membranes, inducing apoptosis, and thrombosing blood vessels [318]. There are two types of delivery systems: a spray delivery device and a closed-balloon system device. With spray delivery, the liquid nitrogen sprayed on the mucosa expands rapidly into nitrogen gas, and so a concomitant system for decompression of the gas is required. In the closed-balloon system, cold nitrous oxide is sprayed within a closed balloon that contacts the mucosa, so there is no need for a separate decompression system. Unlike RFA, cryotherapy appears to preserve extracellular collagen matrix architecture, which theoretically might limit stricture formation [319]. However, the clinical advantage of cryotherapy over RFA in this regard is not established and, in one recent study of 41 patients treated with cryotherapy, esophageal strictures developed in 4 (9.7%) [320]. As initial therapy for dysplasia in Barrett esophagus, observational studies suggest that the efficacy and safety of cryotherapy are very similar to RFA [320,321]. Cryotherapy has been used to treat bulky lesions that might not be amenable to RFA, and as a second-line therapy for patients with persistent dysplasia or metaplasia after RFA treatment [322]. A recent systematic review and metaanalysis of such patients found that cryotherapy was successful in achieving complete eradication of dysplasia in three-fourths and complete eradication of metaplasia in half of patients with Barrett esophagus who did not respond to RFA [323]. Compared with RFA, however, available studies on cryotherapy are small and limited, and there are as yet no randomized trials. Thus, RFA remains the first-line ablation technique for Barrett esophagus, and cryotherapy remains a second-line therapy.

Endoscopic mucosal resection and endoscopic submucosal dissection

In EMR, a diathermy snare or endoscopic knife is used to remove a large segment of esophageal mucosa, including a portion of the submucosa [324,325]. EMR can be performed using a "suck and cut" method in which the endoscopist elevates the dysplastic area by injecting fluid into the submucosa, and the elevated mucosa is suctioned into a cap that fits over the tip of the endoscope. A polypectomy snare is then deployed around the suctioned area to remove it. EMR also can be performed without submucosal fluid injection using a ligating device, similar to that used for endoscopic variceal ligation, that deploys elastic bands around the suctioned mucosal segment [326]. ESD uses specially designed needle knives to achieve en bloc dissection of large esophageal lesions, often much larger than those that can be removed en bloc by EMR. The advantage of en bloc removal of mucosal Barrett tumors by ESD rather than EMR must be weighed against ESD's considerable disadvantages of longer procedure times and greater risk for serious complications such as perforation. For endoscopic eradication therapy in Barrett esophagus, EMR generally is preferred over ESD except in special circumstances [327].

EMR and ESD provide large tissue specimens that can be examined by the pathologist to determine the character and extent of the lesion and the adequacy of resection. As mentioned earlier, these specimens allow histological examination to determine whether there is submucosal invasion, which is a contraindication to endoscopic eradication therapy. Therefore, EMR and ESD can be both diagnostic (revealing submucosal invasion that might not be apparent by less invasive techniques, which would require esophagectomy or other modalities for cure) and therapeutic (if there is no submucosal extension and no tumor in the margins of the specimen) [328]. Considering the depth and size of the mucosal specimens obtained by EMR, there have been surprisingly few reports of serious complications (bleeding, perforation) and virtually no procedure-related mortality [329]. However, circumferential EMR frequently is complicated by esophageal stricture formation [330].

Limited data are available on long-term survival for patients with dysplasia and early cancers in Barrett esophagus treated by EMR alone. Ell and colleagues [331] performed EMR on 100 patients with early adenocarcinomas in Barrett esophagus. The mean age of the patients was 62 years, and 69 of the 100 had short-segment Barrett esophagus. The cancers were early, meaning that the tumor diameter was <20 mm, the histology was well differentiated, there was no invasion of lymphatics or blood vessels, and there were no metastases, submucosal invasion, or lymph node involvement. EMR resulted in no serious complications, and the calculated 5-year survival rate was an extraordinary 98%. However, recurrent or metachronous cancers were found in 11% of the patients during a mean follow-up period of 37 months. The recurrent tumors were treated successfully with more endoscopic therapy, but this high rate of recurrence shows that EMR alone (without ablation of the remaining Barrett metaplasia) often leaves behind cells with neoplastic potential.

Endoscopic ablation and EMR combined

Investigators from the Mayo Clinic retrospectively reviewed long-term survivals in patients with high-grade dysplasia in Barrett esophagus who were treated with either esophagectomy or a combination of EMR and PDT [332]. There was no statistically significant difference in overall long-term survival for patients treated with either of the therapies, although 6.2% of the patients treated endoscopically had esophageal cancer during the follow-up period.

A report of the largest experience with endoscopic therapy for mucosal neoplasms in Barrett esophagus published to date describes the long-term results of endoscopic therapies in 349 patients who had high-grade dysplasia or mucosal adenocarcinoma in Barrett esophagus [333]. Endoscopic treatments included EMR alone for 279 patients, PDT alone for 55, EMR and PDT combined for 13, and argon plasma coagulation alone for 2. A complete remission (complete elimination of the neoplastic lesion and at least one follow-up endoscopy showing no neoplasia) was achieved in 97%. However, during a mean follow-up of 64 months, metachronous neoplasms were discovered in 21%. The investigators noted that a major risk factor for these metachronous lesions was failure to eradicate the residual Barrett epithelium. Metachronous neoplasms occurred in 17% of 200 patients who had their Barrett epithelium ablated after the primary neoplasm was removed, but in 30% of the 137 patients whose Barrett epithelium was not ablated. Based largely on this experience, experts now recommend that endoscopic eradication therapy for mucosal neoplasms in Barrett esophagus should include an attempt to eradicate all of the Barrett mucosa, not just the apparent foci of neoplasia. A recent systematic review of nine studies (774 patients) treated with the combination of EMR for focal lesions followed by RFA (which is now the standard procedure for endoscopic eradication therapy) found that this combination achieved complete eradication of dysplasia in 93% and complete eradication of metaplasia in 73% of cases [334].

Recurrence of dysplasia and metaplasia after endoscopic eradication

Early reports suggested that RFA results were extremely durable, with very low rates of metaplasia recurrence identified in patients who achieved complete eradication of intestinal metaplasia [335–337]. Subsequent studies have refuted these early findings, and it now is clear that there is a substantial rate of recurrence of metaplasia and neoplasia after complete eradication of Barrett metaplasia by RFA [338].

Two major problems confound attempts to provide precise estimates on the rate of recurrence after complete eradication of metaplasia in Barrett esophagus. First, there is no clear consensus on how to define complete eradication. Studies agree that there is complete eradication if follow-up endoscopies reveal no visible or histological evidence of metaplasia in the ablated segment of esophagus. However, studies have differed regarding whether one or two such negative endoscopies are required, and biopsy protocols have differed substantially among studies, with some taking biopsy samples only from the ablated tubular esophagus and others including samples from the GEJ and gastric cardia, where persistent or recurrent metaplasia is found far more frequently. The second problem relates to the biopsy protocol used to identify recurrences. Studies agree that there is recurrence if intestinal metaplasia, dysplasia, or adenocarcinoma is found in any biopsy specimen obtained in any endoscopy performed after complete eradication, and that recurrence can be classified as visible if seen by the endoscopist or nonvisible if detected only in biopsy specimens. However, biopsy protocols have differed substantially among studies on recurrence, and recurrence rates are higher in studies that included biopsy samples of the GEJ and cardia than in those that took samples only from the tubular esophagus. With these caveats, modern studies suggest that intestinal metaplasia recurs at the rate of 8–10% per patient-year of surveillance, and that the annual rate of dysplasia recurrence is 2–3% [339].

Risk factors for recurrence identified in observational studies have included longer segments of Barrett metaplasia, high-grade dysplasia, or intramucosal carcinoma at baseline, erosive esophagitis, older age, male sex, nonwhite race, smoking, obesity, and poor control of underlying GERD [339,340]. A number of studies have suggested that the highest rates of recurrence are found in the first 12–18 months after successful eradication [341,342]. However, a large recent study has refuted that contention [343]. In this study of 594 patients who achieved complete eradication of intestinal metaplasia, 151 experienced recurrence during a median follow-up of 2.8 years. There was a 19% cumulative recurrence risk rate within 2 years and an additional 49% risk rate over the next 8.6 years, with no evidence of a meaningful change in recurrence rates over time. The reasons underlying the disparate findings of these studies are not clear.

Fortunately, most recurrences of intestinal metaplasia are nondysplastic, and most recurrences can be managed successfully with endoscopic therapy. Among the minority of recurrences that are dysplastic, most are at or below the grade of dysplasia found at baseline [342,344]. In one study, the histological grade of recurrence was worse than the baseline grade in only 20 of 334 cases (6%) [344]. Nevertheless, there are well-documented cases of adenocarcinomas developing after apparent complete eradication of intestinal metaplasia [338]. The large majority of recurrences are located at or very close to the GEJ [345,346]. In a study of 198 patients who achieved endoscopic eradication of Barrett esophagus and who had four-quadrant biopsies taken at 1-cm intervals throughout the ablated segment and at the GEJ on follow-up endoscopies, 32 (16%) had a recurrence during a mean follow-up of 3 years [346]. Twenty-nine of the 32 total recurrences were either at the GEJ or 1 cm above it, and all of the three recurrences found in the more proximal esophagus were visible endoscopically. Other studies have confirmed that most recurrences in the tubular esophagus are visible, whereas most at the GEJ are not, and that the yield of biopsies of normal-appearing neosquamous mucosa to identify recurrence is extremely small [343]. The reason for the high rate of recurrence is not entirely clear, but it might be related to failure to extend RFA adequately into the gastric cardia to eliminate intestinal metaplasia in this area. To minimize this problem, recent guidelines recommend that ablation should be extended into the cardia, 5–10 mm distal to the GEJ [347].

Because of the substantial rates of recurrence of metaplasia and dysplasia after endoscopic eradication, regular surveillance endoscopy is recommended. After complete eradication of metaplasia has been achieved, the present ACG guidelines recommend that patients who had high-grade dysplasia or intramucosal carcinoma at baseline should have surveillance endoscopy every 3 months for the first year, every 6 months for the following year, and annually thereafter [56]. For patients with low-grade dysplasia at baseline, surveillance is recommended every 6 months for the first year and annually thereafter. These guidelines are based solely on expert opinion, and a statistical model based on data from the US RFA Registry has suggested that it would be preferable to perform surveillance at intervals of 3 months, 6 months, 1 year, and then annually after complete eradication of high-grade dysplasia or intramucosal carcinoma, and at 1 year and 3 years after complete eradication of low-grade dysplasia [348]. However, this model has not been validated. During surveillance endoscopy, current ACG guidelines recommend taking four-quadrant biopsies every 1 cm throughout the ablated segment and at the GEJ. Based on data discussed in the previous paragraph on the low yield of biopsies of normal-appearing neosquamous mucosa, it has been suggested that posteradication surveillance endoscopies should include careful inspection and targeted biopsies of any visible esophageal abnormalities, followed by four-quadrant biopsies taken from the top of the gastric folds (i.e., the GEJ), four-quadrant biopsies taken from 1 and 2 cm proximal to the GEJ, and a set of random biopsies in the region 3–5 cm above the GEJ [340].

Subsquamous intestinal metaplasia

After endoscopic eradication of Barrett esophagus, biopsy specimens of what appears to be normal neosquamous epithelium can reveal metaplastic glands "buried" under squamous epithelium in the lamina propria [349]. A review of reports of 18 studies in which endoscopic biopsies of neosquamous epithelium were taken from 1004 patients who had RFA of Barrett esophagus found such buried metaplastic glands in nine cases (0.9%). These structures have been called buried glands, buried Barrett, and subsquamous intestinal metaplasia (SSIM). We prefer the latter term. SSIM are located in the subepithelial lamina propria, and most forceps biopsies of esophageal squamous mucosa do not reach the lamina propria. For example, in one study in which the investigators evaluated the adequacy of 1692 forceps biopsies of squamous-lined esophagus, fewer than 11% contained subepithelial lamina propria [350]. Because esophageal biopsies sample only a tiny fraction of the esophageal mucosal surface, and because the large majority of those biopsy samples are not of sufficient depth to be informative for the presence of SSIM, the frequency of SSIM after RFA remains unclear.

SSIM originally was thought to be a consequence of incomplete ablation procedures that destroyed only the superficial layer of Barrett metaplasia, leaving behind a viable layer of Barrett glands to be "buried" by subsequent overgrowth of squamous epithelium. Subsequent studies demonstrated that SSIM often could be found in patients who had not had ablation procedures, especially in areas where Barrett metaplasia abuts squamous epithelium (e.g., at the Z line and in islands of squamous epithelium within the Barrett segment) [349]. It was suggested that those areas of SSIM developed as a consequence of extensive biopsy sampling of metaplastic epithelium during endoscopic surveillance, with the esophageal biopsy sites healing via growth of squamous epithelium that buries metaplastic glands [351]. Even more recent studies suggest that SSIM is very common in the region of the SCJ in Barrett esophagus, even without ablation or extensive biopsy sampling. Zhou and colleagues [352] used 3D-OCT to determine the frequency of buried glands in patients with short-segment Barrett esophagus before and after treatment with RFA. OCT uses light reflected from tissues to construct images of the bowel wall with a resolution close to that provided by a low-power microscope, and each 3D-OCT dataset can cover an area some 60-fold larger than that sampled by standard biopsy forceps. The investigators identified "buried glands" by 3D-OCT in 13 (72%) of 18 patients before complete eradication and in 10 (63%) of 16 patients after complete eradication of visible Barrett metaplasia by RFA. The buried glands were found within 5 mm of the squamocolumnar mucosal junction in approximately two-thirds of cases. A subsequent study using VLE (a more modern OCT technology) disputed these findings, noting that although VLE detected subsquamous glandular structures in 13 of 17 patients with Barrett neoplasia, EMR of those areas revealed that most were not Barrett glands but rather normal histological structures (e.g., dilated glands and blood vessels). However, in a study of 110 patients with neoplasia in Barrett esophagus, Anders and colleagues [353] analyzed 138 EMR specimens that crossed the SCJ and found SSIM extending a mean distance of 3.3 mm in 108 of the 110 patients (98.2%).

Zhang et al. [354] have demonstrated that Barrett epithelial cells exposed to acid and bile salts undergo the process of epithelial–mesenchymal transition (EMT) in which the cells acquire mesenchymal cell features, including the ability to migrate. They propose that GERD triggers EMT in Barrett epithelial cells, enabling them to migrate into the lamina propria under adjacent squamous epithelium to become SSIM. An EMT-mediated mechanism for the development of SSIM also is supported by findings in a rat model of reflux esophagitis and Barrett esophagus [131]. Irrespective of how SSIM forms, it appears to be a common condition both before and after endoscopic eradication of Barrett metaplasia, and the clinical importance of SSIM is unclear and disputed. Some contend that it is generally a benign lesion of little importance [340]. However, there are well-documented cases of cancers found in SSIM [349]. Furthermore, it has been proposed that SSIM hidden from endoscopists is a potential cause of Barrett cancers that develop despite endoscopic surveillance and of recurrences of Barrett metaplasia after apparent complete eradication by RFA [354]. Because SSIM in the lamina propria might be shielded from RFA destruction by the overlying squamous epithelium, SSIM might persist after RFA to become a source for recurrent metaplasia, dysplasia, or cancer.

Endoscopic eradication for nondysplastic Barrett esophagus

Noting the technical simplicity, relative safety, and efficacy of endoscopic eradication for patients with dysplasia, some authorities have proposed that even nondysplastic Barrett metaplasia should be ablated routinely to prevent the development of esophageal cancer [355]. Some even have argued that RFA for nondysplastic Barrett esophagus is, in principle, equivalent to the widely accepted practice of routinely removing all colonic polyps found during colonoscopy [356]. To restrict RFA only to Barrett esophagus with neoplasia, they contend, would be like limiting colonoscopic polypectomy only to polyps that are very large or clearly malignant. Although these are interesting arguments, there are a number of unresolved issues that must temper enthusiasm for using RFA to treat the millions of patients with nondysplastic Barrett esophagus, most of whom will never develop esophageal cancer even without ablation. No study has established the efficacy of RFA for cancer prevention in patients with nondysplastic Barrett esophagus. Rather, that efficacy is inferred from studies showing that RFA can eliminate visible evidence of Barrett metaplasia for a number of years in most patients. Those studies do not establish that the cancer risk has been eliminated, especially considering the problems of recurrence and SSIM described earlier. RFA generally requires several endoscopic procedures to achieve complete eradication, and its complication rate is low but not trivial. Furthermore, data from the US RFA Registry indicate that when RFA is used to ablate nondysplastic Barrett metaplasia, that metaplasia recurs at the rate of approximately 7% per year [344], suggesting that patients will still require endoscopic surveillance after endoscopic eradication. Thus, endoscopic eradication for nondysplastic Barrett esophagus would entail considerable expense, inconvenience, and risk in the absence of data establishing its efficacy. To date, no GI society has recommended endoscopic eradication for the general population of patients with nondysplastic Barrett esophagus.

General management recommendations

No management strategy for patients with Barrett esophagus has been verified to prolong life. The bulk of the indirect evidence available suggests that acid suppression with PPIs may reduce the cancer risk in Barrett esophagus. With that proviso, patients with Barrett esophagus should be treated with a PPI using whatever dose is needed to control GERD symptoms and to maintain the healing of esophagitis. Antireflux surgery should not be prescribed solely as a cancer preventive strategy, although there well may be other valid reasons to recommend this operation for patients with Barrett esophagus with poorly controlled GERD.

The authors endorse the following management policy, which is in general agreement with the recommendations of the AGA, ACG, and ASGE:

- PPIs are the medical therapy of choice for GERD in patients with Barrett esophagus. PPIs should be used in conventional doses unless higher doses are needed to control GERD symptoms or to heal the endoscopic signs of reflux esophagitis.
- Patients with Barrett esophagus should be screened to identify cardiovascular risk factors for which aspirin therapy is indicated.
- Patients with Barrett esophagus should have regular surveillance endoscopy, during which the esophageal mucosa should be examined carefully using high-resolution endoscopy. For patients without suspicious lesions or known dysplasia, four-quadrant esophageal biopsy specimens should be obtained every 2 cm throughout the Barrett metaplasia (Seattle biopsy protocol). WATS and chromoendoscopy/virtual chromoendoscopy can be used as adjuncts to Seattle protocol biopsy sampling during endoscopic evaluation of Barrett esophagus. EMR is recommended to sample any visible mucosal irregularities.
- For patients who have no dysplasia, surveillance endoscopy is recommended at an interval of every 3–5 years.
- When dysplasia is first noted, another endoscopy should be performed with extensive biopsy sampling to look for invasive cancer if there is any question regarding the adequacy of the initial examination. The histology slides should be interpreted by at least two expert pathologists.
- In patients known to have dysplasia, four-quadrant biopsy specimens should be taken at intervals of every 1 cm throughout the length of the Barrett metaplasia. EMR is recommended to sample any visible mucosal irregularities.
- For patients with verified low-grade dysplasia, high-grade dysplasia, or intramucosal carcinoma after extensive biopsy sampling (including EMR of visible irregularities showing no submucosal invasion), endoscopic eradication therapy using RFA to ablate all remaining Barrett metaplasia generally is the treatment of choice.
- After endoscopic eradication therapy, patients should have regular endoscopic surveillance to identify and treat recurrences of metaplasia.

Adenocarcinoma of the esophagus

See Chapter 47 for discussion of squamous cell cancer of the esophagus.

Clinical suspicion for esophageal cancer

Patients with an esophageal malignancy typically present with progressive dysphagia, sometimes with odynophagia, and often with weight loss. Less frequent presenting symptoms, such as nonspecific chest or abdominal pain, fatigue, upper GI bleeding, hoarseness, recurrent pneumonia, cough, hiccups, or dyspnea, that are not attributable to other causes should prompt diagnostic evaluation for an esophageal cancer. This can be done initially with either a double-contrast barium esophagram or an endoscopy, although an endoscopy generally is preferred because it allows tissue sampling to establish a histological diagnosis [357,358].

Natural history

The two most frequent histological types of esophageal cancer are squamous cell carcinoma and adenocarcinoma, and for most of the 20th century, squamous cell carcinoma was by far the most common type in the United States. Data from 93 167 patients with primary carcinoma of the esophagus or gastric cardia from the National Cancer Institute's Surveillance, Epidemiology, and End Results (SEER) program between 1973 and 2009 demonstrate that adenocarcinoma recently has become the predominant histology in this country [359]. The percentage of esophageal cancers in the SEER database that are adenocarcinomas has increased from 35% in the 1970s to 61% in the 2000s. This is despite the percentage of distal esophageal tumors remaining relatively stable at around 40%. Advances in esophageal cancer diagnosis and treatment are likely responsible for a meaningful improvement in median survival in patients with local or regional disease, but not in those with metastatic disease, over the last three decades. Patients with local or organ-confined esophageal cancers in the 2000s have a median survival of 30 months as compared with 10 months in the 1970s, while patients with regional disease (direct tumor extension into adjacent organs or lymph node involvement) have a median survival of 13 months in the 2000s compared with 6 months in the 1970s [359]. Median survival for patients with metastatic disease has increased marginally from 4 months in the 1970s to 6 months in the 2000s. Additional survival data specific to esophageal adenocarcinoma are derived from a surgical series in which patients did not receive any other therapy [360]. In patients with organ-confined cancer, the 5-year overall survival rate ranged from 50% to 80% depending on depth of tumor invasion [360,361]. Patients with regional disease had a 5-year overall survival rate of 15–40%, depending on the number of lymph nodes involved [361].

Staging systems

The Worldwide Esophageal Cancer Collaboration was formed in 2009 to recommend esophageal staging criteria for the seventh edition of the *American Joint Committee on Cancer (AJCC)'s Staging Manual*, which was published a year later [360,362]. In the seventh edition, separate staging systems for esophageal squamous cell carcinoma and esophageal adenocarcinoma were established, and the category of grade (G, i.e., differentiation) was added to the tumor (T), node (N), metastasis (M) classification system [363]. In addition, tumor location within the esophagus was incorporated into the staging system for squamous cell carcinoma. Although these changes might seem to complicate the staging process, they were added to align staging groups with all-cause, time-related mortality [360]. Other changes included expanding the T1 classification to distinguish mucosal (T1a) and submucosal tumors (T1b), a crucial distinction for deciding whether endoscopic eradication therapy is appropriate, and expanding the T4 classification to distinguish resectable tumors (T4a) from unresectable tumors (T4b); adjusting the N classification to quantify the number of involved periesophageal lymph nodes; and removing cervical or celiac lymph node involvement from the M1 category. Because the Worldwide Esophageal Cancer Collaboration data were generated from patients who underwent surgical resection, pathological TNM staging could be accurately matched to patient outcome [364]. Overall, patients with resected early-stage adenocarcinoma fared better than those with resected early-stage squamous cell carcinoma [360].

An update in 2016 occurred with the publication of the AJCC's eighth edition [365], which went into effect in the United States in 2018. Unlike the seventh edition, in which the staging was based on 4627 esophagectomy patients from 13 institutions worldwide, the AJCC's eight edition used survival data from 22 654 patients from 33 institutions who had been treated with neoadjuvant and/or adjuvant therapy [366]. Other major changes included differentiating clinical (cTNM, before any treatment), pathological (pTNM, after surgery), and post-neoadjuvant treatment (ypTNM, after neoadjuvant therapy and surgery) staging; redefining Siewert type III tumors, which is discussed later; and reclassifying lymph node groups or stations. As in AJCC's seventh edition, supraclavicular and celiac lymph nodes were classified as regional lymph nodes. Minor changes included adding grade to the staging for adenocarcinoma, removing location from T2 squamous cell carcinoma, and moving peritoneal invasion into the T4a resectable category. Given the much larger number of patients combined with real-world treatment (i.e., after neoadjuvant and adjuvant therapy and surgery) survival data, prognostic information from AJCC's eighth edition is considered more accurate.

Because GEJ tumors have a worse prognosis than more distal gastric cancers, GEJ tumors are included with esophageal adenocarcinoma for AJCC staging purposes [367]. Siewert and colleagues [368] define GEJ tumors as those centered within 5 cm of the GEJ: Siewert type I tumors are distal esophageal tumors that cross the GEJ from above, type II tumors are centered at the GEJ, and type III tumors are proximal gastric tumors that cross the GEJ from below. In AJCC's eighth edition, Siewert type III tumors that have an epicenter greater than 2 cm from the GEJ are now staged as gastric carcinomas even if they involve the GEJ [366]. Although distal esophageal, GEJ, and proximal gastric adenocarcinomas are molecularly similar [369], the Siewert classification for GEJ tumors is used by surgeons to determine the surgical approach and by medical and radiation oncologists to recommend neoadjuvant chemoradiation versus perioperative chemotherapy to patients (discussed further later).

An additional classification system has been developed for T1 tumors, driven by the shift toward endoscopic management of these superficial tumors, with mucosal (M) and submucosal (SM) designations [370]. In this system, intraepithelial neoplasms (high-grade dysplasia) are designated as M1, neoplasms that invade the lamina propria are designated M2, and tumors that invade or are in contact with the muscularis mucosae are designated M3. Tumors that breach the muscularis mucosae to invade the superficial one-third of the submucosa are designated SM1, while those that invade the middle and deepest third of the submucosa are designated SM2 and SM3, respectively. M2 and M3 neoplasms are equivalent to T1a tumors and are sometimes called intramucosal carcinomas. SM tumors are equivalent to T1b tumors in the AJCC classification system.

Staging studies

Once a patient has been diagnosed histopathologically with esophageal adenocarcinoma and undergone a history and physical examination, staging studies should be performed to determine the appropriate treatment. In general, staging procedures should include EUS and, where available, whole-body ^{18}F-fluorodeoxyglucose (^{18}F-FDG) positron emission tomography (PET), along with a dedicated chest and abdominal computed tomography (CT) scan, or with a combined PET/CT study. These tests are used to estimate the depth of tumor invasion, assess for tumor involvement of periesophageal lymph nodes, and search for distant metastases [371–374]. Recent metaanalyses have documented the accuracy of EUS staging of esophageal cancer [375–377]. The pooled sensitivity and specificity of diagnosing T1 tumors by EUS were 82% and 99%, for T2 tumors sensitivity and specificity were 81% and 96%, for T3 tumors 91% and 94%, and for T4 tumors 92% and 97% [375]. Discrimination between T1a and T1b tumors by EUS was also possible with a pooled sensitivity of 85–86% and a pooled specificity of 86–87% [376]. Nevertheless, EMR is recommended for areas of nodularity within lesions judged to be T1a by EUS, because EMR often reveals submucosal invasion (T1b) in these nodules.

Detection of regional lymph node involvement by EUS has a sensitivity of 80% and specificity of 70% [377]. With the addition of fine needle aspiration, EUS sensitivity for detecting regional lymph node involvement increases to 97% [375]. By comparison, the sensitivity and specificity of detecting involved regional lymph nodes by CT scan are 50% and 83%, while those of PET scan are 57% and 85%, respectively [377]. For identifying distant esophageal cancer metastases, PET is more accurate than combined use of CT and EUS, with a sensitivity of 74% and a specificity of 90% as compared with 47% and 78% for combined CT and EUS [372]. Sequencing a PET/CT study before EUS has two advantages: (1) it allows foregoing EUS if distant metastases are found, and (2) it may identify hypermetabolic periesophageal lymph nodes to target for biopsy sampling by fine needle aspiration [371].

If the esophageal tumor is located at the level of the tracheal bifurcation or higher, then bronchoscopy with biopsies and brush and washing cytologies should be performed to assess for airway invasion [367,378]. Invasion into the trachea renders the tumor unresectable [379]. Magnetic resonance imaging has not been used routinely for staging because of lack of demonstrated superiority to EUS and PET/CT in determining T and N staging, although advances in technique may make magnetic resonance imaging more useful in the future [380]. Staging laparoscopy should be considered in distal esophageal and GEJ cancers because this procedure is more accurate than either EUS or CT in detecting peritoneal metastases and has been shown to prevent unnecessary esophagectomies in patients with previously undetected stage IV disease in the abdomen [381]. Staging laparoscopy can be performed at the time of planned resection or during the initial staging workup. This can facilitate placement of a jejunostomy feeding tube for nutritional support during neoadjuvant chemoradiation and ischemic conditioning of the gastric conduit favored by some surgeons [382,383].

Treatment summary

All patients with esophageal adenocarcinoma are best evaluated by a multidisciplinary team composed of gastroenterologists and surgical, radiation, and medical oncologists. Treatment of esophageal adenocarcinoma has evolved from the results of disparate clinical trials that often included patients with esophageal squamous cell carcinoma, GEJ carcinoma, and gastric carcinoma in addition to esophageal adenocarcinoma [379]. The patient population should be considered in interpreting individual trial results. In general, all patients with resectable disease (stage 0 to stage IIIC) should be considered for esophagectomy. In patients with Tis, endoscopic eradication therapy is a reasonable alternative to esophagectomy. Endoscopic eradication therapy is also an option for patients with T1a disease without lymph node involvement. In patients with T1b disease, occult lymph node metastases have been found in more than 10% of cases [384,385], and these patients generally are advised to undergo esophagectomy. The added benefit of neoadjuvant chemoradiation before esophagectomy is unclear in stage I patients [386]. For patients who are surgical candidates with T2 disease or higher or lymph node involvement, neoadjuvant chemoradiation followed by esophagectomy is preferred [379]. Perioperative chemotherapy and esophagectomy (in distal adenocarcinomas) or definitive chemoradiation (in squamous cell carcinomas or nonsurgical candidates) are also acceptable alternatives. In patients with stage IV disease or T4b tumors, a palliative approach should be taken. Guidelines support using gastric cancer chemotherapy regimens in the treatment of metastatic esophageal or GEJ adenocarcinomas [379]. This is justified by The Cancer Genome Atlas consortium study showing that distal esophageal, GEJ, and proximal gastric adenocarcinomas resemble each other molecularly [369].

Types of esophagectomy

Because esophagectomy is often required for cure, an understanding of the various surgical techniques is helpful. Open approaches include transhiatal esophagectomy (THE), transthoracic esophagectomy (TTE) such as the Ivor–Lewis procedure, esophagectomy with three-field lymph node dissection, and the left thoracoabdominal esophagectomy [361,387]. THE consists of a laparotomy and a left-sided cervical incision with a cervical anastomosis, whereas TTE consists of a laparotomy and a right-sided thoracotomy with an intrathoracic anastomosis. THE and TTE are performed on midesophageal, distal esophageal, and GEJ cancers. A three-field lymph node dissection is usually performed for esophageal cancers at the level of the carina or higher and consists of thoracotomy, laparotomy, and cervical anastomosis (McKeown procedure). Advantages of a THE include lower surgical morbidity, a statistically similar survival rate to TTE despite higher recurrence rates, and less catastrophic anastomotic leaks [387,388]. Disadvantages of THE include a higher frequency of anastomotic leaks and recurrent laryngeal nerve injury. Advantages of TTE include improved access to the tumor, more thorough mediastinal lymph node dissection, and fewer anastomotic leaks, although such leaks that occur within the chest are often fatal [387,389]. Disadvantages of TTE include greater surgical morbidity and longer recovery.

Multiple studies have demonstrated that institutional esophagectomy volume is inversely related to mortality rate, although the definitions of "high-volume" centers vary [390,391]. It is recommended that patients undergo esophagectomy at a center with experience in surgical treatment of esophageal cancer. Minimally invasive esophagectomy (MIE) has been gaining increased interest and is performed in specialized centers. The MIE surgical flow is similar to a TTE but consists of laparoscopy and thoracoscopy [361]. A series from the University of Pittsburgh of 222 patients who underwent a MIE reported a median intensive care unit stay of 1 day and median hospitalization of 7 days with a 30-day all-cause mortality rate of 1.4% [392]. Eastern Cooperative Oncology Group (ECOG) Study E2202, a prospective phase II trial evaluating mortality after MIE in 16 institutions, had a 30-day mortality rate of 2%, confirming the benefit of MIE [393].

Esophagectomies are classified by surgeons using the residual (R) tumor category of the AJCC, where R0 denotes no residual tumor, R1 denotes microscopic residual tumor, and R2 denotes macroscopically visible residual tumor [363]. Tumor response to neoadjuvant treatment can be classified by pathologists as a complete response (pathological CR) if there is no residual tumor, near-complete response, partial response, or no response. The various currently used tumor response grading systems and their criteria are reviewed by Donohoe et al. [394].

Radiation therapy

Radiation can be delivered to the esophagus using external beam radiation therapy (EBRT) or brachytherapy, while metastases may sometimes be treated with stereotactic body radiation therapy. Definitive EBRT, which has fallen out of favor, is usually delivered at a dose between 60 and 66 Gy using divided 1.8–2.0 Gy fractions to minimize toxicity [395,396]. EBRT given concurrently with chemotherapy ranges from a total dose of 41.4–50.4 Gy [397]. Palliative EBRT is usually delivered as 30–40 Gy with fractions of 2.5–3 Gy. Brachytherapy can be used as an alternative to stenting for dysphagia or tumor bleeding [396]. A catheter is placed into the esophagus, and then a radioactive source is placed within the catheter to treat the luminal component of the tumor. Doses of 16–18 Gy in two or three divided fractions are used.

Treatment of stage IA cancer

Stage IA cancers generally are treated with endoscopic eradication therapy, which is discussed in a previous section of this chapter. Esophagectomy sometimes is recommended for patients with stage IA cancers in long-segment Barrett esophagus containing multiple foci of dysplasia or intramucosal carcinoma, which can be difficult to eradicate endoscopically. Esophagectomy also is used when endoscopic eradication therapy fails to eradicate the neoplasia, or when submucosal invasion or lymph node metastases occur despite endoscopic eradication. Another important factor to consider when choosing between endoscopic therapy and esophagectomy for stage IA cancer is the patient's willingness and reliability to adhere to a rigorous follow-up process. Endoscopic therapy usually requires multiple treatment sessions to achieve complete eradication and frequent, regular surveillance for recurrences. Patients unwilling or unable to comply with the frequent follow-up required for successful endoscopic eradication might be better advised to have surgery.

Surgical candidates with stage IB–IIIC cancer

Multiple studies have demonstrated the added survival benefit of adding chemotherapy or chemoradiation to surgical resection in patients with esophageal cancer. The following discussion reviews the clinical trials that support definitive chemoradiation, neoadjuvant chemotherapy and chemoradiation, perioperative chemotherapy, and adjuvant chemotherapy and chemoradiation. The current, preferred multimodality therapy for resectable esophageal adenocarcinoma is either neoadjuvant chemoradiation, based on the RTOG 8501 [395] and CROSS trials [398], or perioperative chemotherapy, based on the MAGIC [399] and FLOT4-AIO [400] trials. Which approach is superior is being investigated in two ongoing clinical trials, ESOPEC and ICORG 10-14: Neo-AEGIS. Induction chemotherapy and the use of imaging studies to assess response during treatment are also reviewed further on.

Definitive chemoradiation

RTOG 8501 was a phase III trial that enrolled 121 patients with resectable esophageal cancer [395]. Any gastric involvement was an exclusion criterion; 88% of patients had squamous cell carcinoma and 12% had adenocarcinoma. Patients were randomized to either radiation alone with a total dose of 64 Gy or to chemoradiation with a total radiation dose of 50 Gy. The chemotherapy consisted of 5-fluorouracil (5-FU) 1000 mg/m^2/day administered via continuous infusion over 96 hours and cisplatin 75 mg/m^2 both given on day 1. This was repeated every 4 weeks for four total cycles, with the first two cycles given concurrently with radiation therapy. Median overall survival was 12.5 months in the chemoradiation arm, compared with 8.9 months in the radiation therapy arm, which was a statistically significant difference. Long-term follow-up demonstrated that 5-year overall survival was 26% for patients who received chemoradiation and 0% for patients who received radiation alone [401].

The INT 0123 clinical trial sought to determine the optimal radiation dose to be used concurrently with chemotherapy [402]. Using the 5-FU/cisplatin chemotherapy regimen from RTOG 8501, 218 patients with resectable esophageal cancer were randomized to a total radiation dose of either 64.8 or 50.4 Gy. The proportion of patients with squamous cell and adenocarcinoma was 86% and 14%, respectively, similar to the RTOG 8501 trial. Median overall survival was not significantly different between the two arms: 13 months in the high-dose 64.8-Gy arm compared with 18.1 months in the standard dose of the 50.4-Gy arm. No significant difference was seen in local/regional or distant failure. There were 11 treatment-related deaths in the high-dose arm and two treatment-related deaths in the standard-dose arm. INT 0123 established 50.4 Gy as the radiation dose to be given with concurrent chemotherapy at that time.

FFCD 9102 was a randomized controlled trial of 444 patients with T1-3, N0-1 resectable esophageal cancer [403]. All patients were treated with chemoradiation using conventional (total dose of 46 Gy) or split-course radiation (total dose of 30 Gy) and chemotherapy consisting of 5-FU 800 mg/m^2/day via continuous infusion over days 1–5 and cisplatin 15 mg/m^2 given daily on days 1–5. Of the 444 patients, 259 demonstrated a treatment response and were then randomized to esophagectomy or continued chemoradiation (three cycles of 5-FU and cisplatin with either conventional radiation of 20 Gy or split-course radiation of 15 Gy). Median overall survival was 17.7 months in the surgical arm versus 19.3 months in the chemoradiation arm, demonstrating equivalence. Because 88% of randomized patients had squamous cell carcinoma and 11% had adenocarcinoma, chemoradiation as an acceptable alternative to esophagectomy is more accepted in patients with squamous cell carcinoma.

A randomized controlled trial was performed in 172 German patients, all with locally advanced esophageal squamous cell carcinoma, T3-4, N0-1 [404]. Patients received chemotherapy consisting of three cycles of 5-FU 500 mg/m^2, leucovorin 300 mg/m^2, etoposide 100 mg/m^2, and cisplatin 30 mg/m^2 on days 1–3 every 3 weeks. Patients were then randomized to either low-dose chemoradiation with a total radiation dose of 40 Gy followed by surgical resection or chemoradiation alone with a total radiation dose of 65 Gy. The concurrent chemotherapy regimen used was cisplatin 50 mg/m^2 given on days 2–8 and etoposide 80 mg/m^2 given on days 3–5. Median overall survival for the low-dose chemoradiation and surgical arm was 16.4 months and for the chemoradiation arm 14.9 months, which was not statistically different.

The ACCORD 17 randomized phase III trial examined whether six cycles of biweekly FOLFOX chemotherapy (oxaliplatin 85 mg/m^2, leucovorin 200 mg/m^2, 5-FU bolus of 400 mg/m^2 followed by a 46-hour continuous infusion of 1600 mg/m^2) with three cycles given concurrently with radiation was as effective as the RTOG 8501 chemoradiation regimen [405]. Two hundred sixty-seven patients with esophageal cancer, of which 85% had squamous cell histology, were randomized to the two treatment arms. Median progression-free survival was similar, 9.7 months for the patients receiving FOLFOX and 9.4 months for those patients receiving 5-FU and cisplatin. This demonstrated the safety and efficacy of using FOLFOX, a more tolerable chemotherapy regimen, during concurrent radiotherapy to treat esophageal cancer.

Several conclusions can be drawn from these five clinical trials. First, definitive chemoradiation is superior to definitive radiation therapy alone. Second, the optimal radiation dose is less than 64 Gy. Third, definitive chemoradiation appears to be equivalent to surgical resection in patients with esophageal squamous cell carcinoma. In patients with esophageal adenocarcinoma, surgical resection is still preferred [362], but definitive chemoradiation based on RTOG 8501 can be considered in nonsurgical candidates. In such patients, all four cycles of chemotherapy should be given.

Neoadjuvant radiation therapy

Five prospective randomized trials have examined the effects of neoadjuvant radiation therapy followed by surgery versus surgery alone in esophageal cancer, and all but one limited enrollment to patients with squamous cell carcinoma [406]. A metaanalysis of a total of 1147 patients demonstrated a 43% survival difference at 5 years, which was not statistically significant. The authors of this metaanalysis concluded that neoadjuvant radiation should not be considered outside of a clinical trial.

Neoadjuvant chemotherapy

The next question was whether neoadjuvant chemotherapy could improve on surgical resection alone. The INT 0113 was a multiinstitutional randomized controlled trial that enrolled 440 patients in the United States with stage I–III esophageal cancer [407]. Histology was divided as 46% squamous cell carcinoma and 54% adenocarcinoma of the distal esophagus or GEJ. Patients were randomized to receive either surgery alone or three cycles of 5-FU/cisplatin administered every 4 weeks followed by surgery. Chemotherapy was given as continuous infusion 5-FU 1000 mg/m^2/day over days 1–5 and cisplatin 100 mg/m^2 on day 1. At the time of resection, a determination of treatment response was made in patients who received neoadjuvant chemotherapy. For those patients who had a treatment response and were able to tolerate it, two additional cycles of chemotherapy were given postoperatively using the same 5-FU dose and cisplatin in a dose reduced to 75 mg/m^2. Median overall survival was 14.9 months in the chemotherapy and surgery arm and 16.1 months in the surgery-only arm, which was not statistically different.

A trial in the United Kingdom also investigated the potential benefit of adding neoadjuvant chemotherapy to surgery in esophageal cancer. The OEO-2 trial was a randomized controlled trial that enrolled 802 patients, 31% with squamous cell carcinoma, 63% with esophageal adenocarcinoma, and 10% with GEJ adenocarcinoma [408]. Patients were randomized to immediate surgery or two cycles of 5-FU/cisplatin chemotherapy followed by surgery. Chemotherapy consisted of 5-FU 1000 mg/day administered continuously on days 1–4 and cisplatin 80 mg/m^2 on day 1; both drugs were given again 3 weeks later. OEO-2 demonstrated a significant survival benefit with a median overall survival of 16.8 months in the chemotherapy and surgery arm as compared with 13.3 months in the surgery-only arm. More importantly, 5-year overall survival between the two arms was significantly different, with 17.1% of the patients in the chemotherapy and surgery arm alive compared with 5.1% in the surgery-only arm.

Several reasons for the negative result seen in INT 0113 and the positive effect to neoadjuvant chemotherapy seen in OEO-2 have been considered [408]. First, OEO-2 had almost twice as many patients, which may have enabled detection of a small, but significant, survival difference. Second, a higher proportion of patients had adenocarcinomas in OEO-2 than in INT 0113 (73% vs 54%). Third, the time to surgery was longer in INT 113 compared with OEO-2 because of the chemotherapy regimen, possibly allowing more time for micrometastases to develop.

The goal of the OEO-5 trial was to improve on the OEO-2 trial results through intensifying chemotherapy by adding epirubicin and increasing the number of cycles to four [409]. This open-label, randomized phase III trial enrolled 897 patients with esophageal adenocarcinoma. Patients either received two cycles of 5-FU and cisplatin, per the OEO-2 protocol, or four cycles of ECX (epirubicin 50 mg/m^2 on day 1, cisplatin 60 mg/m^2 on day 1, and capecitabine 1250 mg/m^2 daily) repeated every 3 weeks. Of 451 patients randomized to 5-FU and cisplatin, 96% completed chemotherapy and 91% went on to surgical resection. Of the 446 patients randomized to ECX, 81% completed chemotherapy and 87% underwent surgical resection. Median overall survival was 23.4 months with 5-FU and cisplatin and 26.1 months with ECX, which was not significantly different. Although ECX was more toxic, it did result in better pathological responses; however, this did not translate to improved survival.

Neoadjuvant chemoradiation

The CROSS trial enrolled 368 patients (366 available in the final analysis) with esophageal cancer or GEJ cancer that were considered resectable, T2-3 and N0-1 [398]. Patients were randomized to neoadjuvant chemoradiation followed by surgery or surgery alone. Chemotherapy was administered weekly for 5 weeks using paclitaxel 50 mg/m^2 and carboplatin dosed to achieve an area under the curve of 2 mg/mL/min. This regimen has the advantage of being given peripherally without use of an infusion pump. The total radiation dose was 41.4 Gy given in 23 divided fractions. Of the patients enrolled, 75% had esophageal or GEJ adenocarcinoma (Siewert type II) and 23% had squamous cell carcinoma. Median survival was significantly improved in the chemotherapy and surgery arm (49.4 months) as compared with the surgery-alone arm (24 months). Importantly, the R0 resection rate improved significantly from 69% in the surgery-alone arm to 92% in the chemoradiation and surgery arm. A pathological CR was found in 29% of patients who received neoadjuvant therapy. The chemotherapy regimen in this trial was well tolerated with a single grade 4 toxicity of leukopenia. This study provided data that a lower dose of radiation could be used, and that a well-tolerated carboplatin and paclitaxel regimen is an acceptable alternative to cisplatin and infusional 5-FU. Long-term follow-up for the CROSS trial has now been published [397], confirming the survival benefit. When broken out by histology, median overall survival was 43.2 months with chemoradiotherapy plus surgery and 27.1 months with surgery alone in those patients with adenocarcinoma.

Perioperative chemotherapy

The Medical Research Council of the United Kingdom undertook the MAGIC trial to investigate the role of perioperative chemotherapy in gastric cancer [399]. The 503 patients with stage II or higher resectable adenocarcinoma (15% with lower esophageal, 12% with Siewert type II GEJ, and 74% with gastric) were randomized to surgery alone or to three cycles of epirubicin, cisplatin, and 5-FU (ECF) followed by surgery, followed by another three cycles of ECF. ECF consisted of epirubicin 50 mg/m^2 and cisplatin 60 mg/m^2 each given on day 1 and continuous infusion of 5-FU 200 mg/m^2/day for days 1–21. This three-drug chemotherapy regimen was repeated every 3 weeks. There was a statistically significant 5-year overall survival difference: 36% in the chemotherapy plus surgery arm compared with 23% in the surgery-alone arm. Only 42% of the patients randomized to chemotherapy and surgery were able to complete all six cycles of chemotherapy because of toxicity. Given the inclusion of patients with lower esophageal and GEJ adenocarcinoma in the MAGIC trial, these results are used to treat patients with esophageal adenocarcinoma where radiation therapy is unavailable or where addition of radiation therapy could lead to treatment delay.

The results of the MAGIC trial were strengthened by the results of the ACCORD-07/FFCD 9703 trial [410]. In this phase III trial, 204 patients with resectable adenocarcinoma of the lower esophagus (11%), Siewert type II GEJ (64%), and stomach (25%) were randomized to surgery alone or to six cycles of perioperative chemotherapy with surgery. The chemotherapy used was 5-FU 800 mg/m^2/day given on days 1–5 and cisplatin 100 mg/m^2 given on day 1. This was repeated every 4 weeks. The trial mandated a minimum of two cycles or a maximum of three cycles of chemotherapy be given preoperatively, with the remainder given postoperatively. Five-year overall survival rate was significantly in favor of chemotherapy added to surgery, with 38% of patients alive as compared with 24% of patients in the surgery-alone group. Chemotherapy also improved the R0 resection rate. Importantly, the majority of patients in this trial had esophageal or GEJ cancer.

More recently, the FLOT-4 trial improved on the results seen with the MAGIC trial by using a different chemotherapy regimen [359]. In this phase II/III trial, 716 patients with locally advanced (T2 and above or node positive), resectable gastric or GEJ adenocarcinoma were randomized to either three cycles of preoperative and three cycles of postoperative ECX/ECF or four cycles of preoperative and four cycles of postoperative FLOT (biweekly docetaxel 50 mg/m^2, oxaliplatin 85 mg/m^2, leucovorin 200 mg/m^2, and 5-FU 2600 mg/m^2 continuous infusion given over 24 hours). By tumor location, 24% were Siewert type I, 32% Siewert types II or III, and 44% gastric. Median overall survival was 50 months with FLOT and 35 months with ECX/ECF, which was statistically significant, with estimated 5-year survival rates of 45% and 36%, respectively. Not only was FLOT superior in terms of survival, but the chemotherapy was also better tolerated such that more patients were able to receive postsurgical chemotherapy. Notably, FLOT was associated with a greater rate of neutropenia, infections, diarrhea, and neuropathy. In 2020, FLOT was the preferred perioperative chemotherapy regimen.

Adjuvant therapy

Currently, the majority of patients with esophageal adenocarcinoma who present to a multidisciplinary esophageal cancer center before surgical resection are treated with neoadjuvant chemoradiation or perioperative chemotherapy. For those patients with distal esophageal or GEJ adenocarcinoma who undergo surgical resection before evaluation for neoadjuvant therapy, adjuvant chemoradiation or chemotherapy still should be considered. Chemoradiation for these patients is based on findings from the INT 0116 trial, which randomized 556 patients with resected GEJ (20%) and gastric (80%) adenocarcinoma, nonmetastatic stage IB–IV, to either observation or adjuvant chemoradiation [411]. Adjuvant therapy was given as a single 4-week cycle of daily 5-FU 425 mg/m^2 and leucovorin 20 mg/m^2 both given on days 1–5, followed by radiation to a total dose of 45 Gy in divided fractions over 5 weeks concurrently with 5-FU 400 mg/m^2 and leucovorin 20 mg/m^2 given on the first 4 days and the last 3 days of radiation therapy, followed by two additional 4-week cycles of 5-FU and leucovorin given in the same fashion as the first cycle. Median overall survival was significantly improved in the adjuvant chemoradiation arm (36 months) compared with patients who were observed without chemoradiation (27 months).

In patients with gastric cancer, the ARTIST trial suggested that the addition of radiation to adjuvant chemotherapy gives improved survival in patients who have lymph node-positive disease at the time of resection [412]. Final results from the CALGB 80101 clinical trial suggest that intensifying chemotherapy by using ECF before and after 5-FU/cisplatin-based chemoradiation in resected GEJ or gastric cancers is not superior to the INT 0116 regimen [413].

A phase II trial (ECOG 8296) of 59 patients with resected adenocarcinoma of the distal esophagus, GEJ, or gastric cardia with R0 resection and T2N1M0 to T4N1M0 disease found a benefit to adjuvant treatment with paclitaxel 175 mg/m^2 and cisplatin 75 mg/m^2 given on day 1 every 3 weeks for a total of four cycles [414]. Despite 89% of patients having nodal disease, 60% were alive at 2 years, which was significantly different from a 38% expected survival rate for historic controls with R0 resections. This regimen was fairly well tolerated with the median number of cycles administered being 3.7. Main toxicities were cytopenias, nausea/vomiting, metabolic, and neuropathy. These results suggest that adjuvant chemotherapy is beneficial in patients who did not receive neoadjuvant therapy.

Induction chemotherapy

Given that systemic therapy is more easily tolerated before esophagectomy, there has been interest in adding chemotherapy before neoadjuvant chemoradiation, which has been termed *induction chemotherapy*. This concept was explored in the POET study [415]. In this randomized controlled study of 126 patients with locally advanced adenocarcinoma of the lower esophagus or GEJ, patients were randomized to one of two arms. Patients in arm 1 received two 6-week cycles plus one 3-week cycle of induction PLF chemotherapy consisting of weekly 5-FU 2000 mg/m^2, leucovorin 500 mg/m^2, and biweekly cisplatin 50 mg/m^2, followed by surgery. Patients in arm 2 received two 6-week cycles of PLF chemotherapy followed by chemoradiation with PE chemotherapy (cisplatin 50 mg/m^2 on days 1 and 8 and etoposide 80 mg/m^2 on days 3–5) with concurrent radiation given to a total dose of 30 Gy, followed by surgery. Three-year overall survival differences did not reach statistical significance but favored chemoradiation therapy (47.4% in arm 2) over chemotherapy (27.7% in arm 1). Improvements in R0 resection, pathological CR, and tumor-free nodes trended toward favoring the patients who received chemoradiation.

Assessing response to treatment

As discussed earlier, PET scans are effective in detecting metastatic disease. There has also been interest in using PET scans to define treatment response and to select additional therapy. In a prospective trial of 65 patients with T3NX distal esophageal or GEJ (Siewert type I or II) adenocarcinoma treated with neoadjuvant chemotherapy, PET findings were able to predict overall survival [416]. Metabolic responders, defined as a decrease of FDG uptake greater than 35% on a day 14 scan compared with one done before treatment, had a 3-year overall survival rate of 70% compared with 35% in nonresponders. In the MUNICON clinical trial, PET was used to select further therapy for 119 patients with GEJ adenocarcinomas treated with 5-FU and cisplatin [417]. After 2 weeks of chemotherapy, a repeat PET was performed; if patients had a decrease in FDG avidity, they continued with additional chemotherapy, but if not, they went on to immediate surgical resection. Two-thirds of the patients (68%) had type I distal esophageal tumors. In a median follow-up of 2.3 years, nonresponders had a median overall survival of 25.8 months, while median overall survival was not yet reached in responders. Progression-free survival was 29.7 months in metabolic responders and 14.1 months in nonresponders.

Treatment of metastatic disease

The goal of treatment for patients with metastatic disease is palliation, treating symptoms and prolonging survival while optimizing quality of life. Palliative radiation therapy can be used to control GI bleeding or improve dysphagia. Covered stents can be placed endoscopically in the airway and esophagus to treat tracheoesophageal or bronchoesophageal fistulas. Palliative chemotherapy can extend survival and improve quality of life. A metaanalysis of chemotherapy in metastatic gastric cancer demonstrates that overall survival is improved with chemotherapy, and that response rates increase with more than one chemotherapeutic agent [418]. Typically, two- or three-agent regimens are used and individualized based on the patient's performance status, preferences, and medication side-effect profile [419,420]. Patients with metastatic esophageal adenocarcinoma should have their tumor tested for expression of HER2/Neu because of the results of the ToGA trial, which explored the use of trastuzumab, a monoclonal antibody that interferes with the HER2/neu receptor [421]. Other testing that should be considered includes MSI/mismatch repair status, expression of programmed death ligand 1 (PD-L1), and next generation sequencing to identify actionable mutations [369,422].

Phase III trials in metastatic disease

A common multidrug chemotherapy regimen to treat metastatic esophageal cancer is ECF [379,423]. Given the development of newer platinum agents and capecitabine, an orally bioavailable fluoropyrimidine prodrug, the Medical Research Council of the United Kingdom conducted the REAL-2 trial [424]. This was a noninferiority study designed to demonstrate the equivalence of infusional 5-FU to capecitabine and cisplatin to oxaliplatin. A total of 1002 patients were randomized in a 2 × 2 format to epirubicin 50 mg/m^2 on day 1, cisplatin 60 mg/m^2 on day 1, 5-FU 200 mg/m^2/day continuous infusion for days 1–21 (ECF); epirubicin, oxaliplatin 130 mg/m^2 day 1, and 5-FU (EOF); epirubicin, cisplatin, and capecitabine 625 mg/m^2 orally twice daily (ECX); or epirubicin, oxaliplatin, and capecitabine (EOX). All regimens were repeated every 3 weeks. Patients were previously untreated and were required to have inoperable or metastatic esophageal, GEJ, or gastric cancer; 90% of patients had adenocarcinoma, and the number of patients was evenly divided among esophageal, GEJ, and gastric cancers. Median overall survival was 9.9 months for ECF, 9.9 months for ECX, 9.3 months for EOF, and 11.2 months for EOX. This has led to capecitabine-containing regimens being commonly used in metastatic esophageal cancer. Quality-of-life measures were not significantly different between the treatment groups.

Given the frequent overexpression of epidermal growth factor receptor (EGFR) and other HER family members in esophagogastric cancers, the phase III ToGA trial randomized 594 patients with inoperable or metastatic GEJ (20%) or gastric (80%) adenocarcinoma that overexpressed HER2/Neu to receive a fluoropyrimidine with cisplatin, with or without trastuzumab [421]. Patients could have recurrent disease, but they could not have received prior treatment for metastatic disease. Chemotherapy consisted of 5-FU 800 mg/m^2/day given days 1–5 or capecitabine 1000 mg/m^2 orally twice daily for 14 days given with cisplatin 80 mg/m^2 on day 1, repeated every 3 weeks. Patients randomized to receive trastuzumab were given a loading dose of 8 mg/kg on day 1, which was then followed by 6 mg/kg every 3 weeks indefinitely until progression, or unacceptable toxicity. Median overall survival was significantly improved in patients who received trastuzumab (13.8 months) compared with those who did not (11.1 months). Trastuzumab increased diarrhea, nausea, and neutropenia associated with the prescribed chemotherapy. The trial established criteria for determining HER2/Neu expression positivity in esophagogastric tumors, which differed from those used in breast cancer. Although not US Food and Drug Administration (FDA)-approved as second-line therapy, the ToGA regimen with trastuzumab is commonly given to patients who progress on a conventional multiagent chemotherapy regimen.

Molecularly targeted therapy

Given the success of trastuzumab, there has been great interest in targeting HER2 in other settings or with other agents. Other pathways of interest for molecularly targeted therapies include EGFR and vascular endothelial growth factor (VEGF), although data on agents that target EGFR have been disappointing. The SCOPE-1 phase II/III trial randomized 258 patients with stage I–III esophageal carcinoma to receive definitive chemoradiation with or without cetuximab (an antibody directed against the EGFR receptor) [425]. Cetuximab was given as a loading dose of 400 mg/m^2 on day 1, followed by 250 mg/m^2 weekly. Chemoradiation consisted of four cycles of cisplatin 60 mg/m^2 on day 1, with oral capecitabine 625 mg/m^2 given twice daily on days 1–21, with the third and fourth cycle given concurrently with radiation to a total dose of 50 Gy. The trial was halted in the phase II stage because the addition of cetuximab led to worse outcomes with higher toxicity. The EXPAND phase III trial, which assessed the addition of cetuximab to cisplatin and capecitabine in 904 patients with previously untreated, unresectable, or metastatic gastric adenocarcinoma [426], also failed to show a significant difference in progression-free survival in those receiving cetuximab.

Finally, in patients receiving another antibody directed against EGFR, panitumumab actually showed reduced survival in the phase III REAL-3 trial [427]. Results from targeting the VEGF pathway have been more encouraging. The AVAGAST trial combined bevacizumab (an antibody directed against the VEGF ligand) with cisplatin and capecitabine as first-line therapy in patients with unresectable or metastatic GEJ or gastric cancer [428]. A total of 774 patients were randomized to receive cisplatin 80 mg/m^2 on day 1 and capecitabine 1000 mg/m^2 twice daily on days 1–14 every 3 weeks, with or without bevacizumab 7.5 mg/kg on day 1. Median overall survival was not significantly different but favored patients who received bevacizumab (12.1 months) versus those who did not (10.1 months). Progression-free survival (6.7 months) and tumor response (46%) were significantly improved in patients who received bevacizumab compared with those who did not (5.3 months and 37%, respectively).

Clearer results have been seen with ramucirumab, an antibody against the VEGFR2 receptor, in three published trials. Side-effects of ramucirumab included hypertension, anemia, abdominal pain, ascites, fatigue, anorexia, and hyponatremia. In the randomized, double-blind, placebo-controlled phase III REGARD trial, patients with advanced gastric or GEJ adenocarcinoma who had progressed on a first-line chemotherapy regimen containing a platinum or fluoropyrimidine were randomized 2 : 1 to receive either ramucirumab 8 mg/kg given every 2 weeks or placebo [429]. A total of 238 patients received ramucirumab, and 117 patients received placebo; 25% in each arm had GEJ adenocarcinoma. Ramucirumab statistically improved survival from 3.8 to 5.2 months compared with placebo. The randomized, double-blind, placebo-controlled phase III RAINBOW trial enrolled 665 patients with advanced gastric or GEJ adenocarcinoma who had progressed within 4 months of receiving a first-line platinum- and fluoropyrimidine-containing regimen [430]. Patients were randomized equally to ramucirumab 8 mg/kg or placebo given on days 1 and 15 with paclitaxel 80 mg/m^2 given on days 1, 8, and 15 of a 28-day cycle. Twenty percent of the patients had GEJ adenocarcinoma. Median overall survival was 9.6 months with ramucirumab and paclitaxel versus 7.4 months with paclitaxel alone, which was statistically significant. Finally, the randomized, double-blind, placebo-controlled phase III RAINFALL trial enrolled 645 untreated patients with metastatic gastric or GEJ adenocarcinoma that were HER2/Neu negative [431]. Patients were randomized to ramucirumab 8 mg/kg or placebo on day 1, along with cisplatin 80 mg/m^2 on day 1 and capecitabine 1000 mg/m^2 twice daily. In this trial that included 25% GEJ adenocarcinomas, no statistically significant overall or progression-free survival difference was noted. Based on these results, ramucirumab was approved for use in the second-line setting either as a monotherapy or in combination with paclitaxel for GEJ and gastric adenocarcinomas.

Refractory disease

Recent data show that second-line chemotherapy is superior to best supportive care in patients with metastatic esophageal cancer, although multiple prediction factors have been proposed using clinical factors to identify patients who would benefit from chemotherapy [432]. In COUGAR-02, a randomized phase III trial, docetaxel 75 mg/m^2 given every 3 weeks significantly improved overall survival versus active symptom control in patients with locally advanced or metastatic gastroesophageal cancer who had progressed within 6 months of initial chemotherapy [433]. Median overall survival was 5.2 months with docetaxel as compared with 3.6 months with active symptom control alone. As or more important, quality-of-life measures were better in patients receiving docetaxel.

Immunotherapy

In 2018, the Nobel Prize in Physiology or Medicine was awarded for the discovery of cancer therapy by inhibition of negative immune regulation, in particular work done characterizing the immune checkpoint proteins cytotoxic T-lymphocyte-associated protein 4 (CTLA-4) and programmed cell death protein 1 (PD-1) (https://www.nobelprize.org/prizes/medicine/2018/summary/). Activation of T cells occurs when antigen bound to an MHC molecule on the surface of an antigen-presenting cell interacts with the appropriate T-cell receptor on the T lymphocyte [434]. This primary signal also requires costimulatory signals, typically a B7 ligand (CD80 or CD86) on the antigen-presenting cell binding to CD28 on the T cell in the presence of secreted cytokines, such as IL-2 [435]. Conversely, to maintain self-tolerance and avoid autoimmunity, immune checkpoint proteins act as inhibitory signals. Two such protein receptors found on the surface of the T cell are CTLA-4 and PD-1 (Figure 46.8). CTLA-4 is upregulated in activated T cells and has a higher affinity for B7 ligand, outcompeting CD28 for ligand binding and decreasing the costimulatory signal. Tumor cells can induce tolerance and escape immune surveillance by expressing PD-L1. This leads to PD-L1/PD-1 signaling and downregulation of stimulatory cytokine secretion.

To reactivate recognition of tumor cells by the immune system, antibodies have been developed against CTLA-4 (e.g., ipilimumab, tremelimumab), PD-1 (nivolumab, pembrolizumab), and PD-L1 (atezolizumab, avelumab, durvalumab) and have been approved for use in or are currently being investigated in

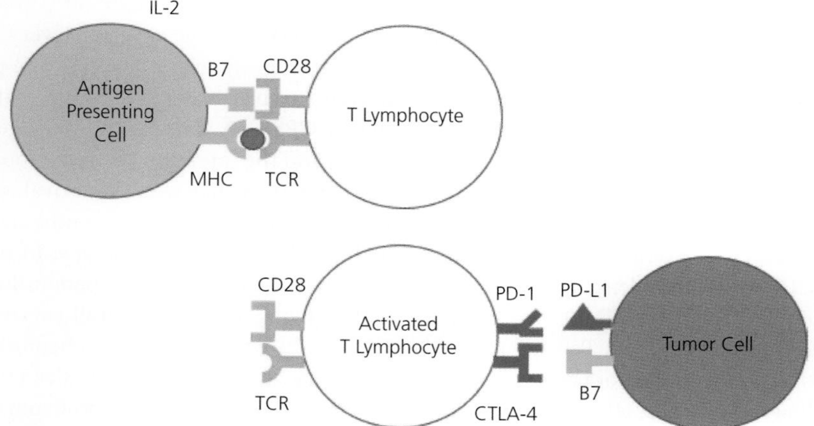

Figure 46.8 When antigen (represented by blue circle) is presented by a major histocompatibility complex (MHC) molecule of an antigen-presenting cell, this complex interacts with the T-cell receptor (TCR) of a resting T lymphocyte. In the context of costimulatory cytokines (e.g., interleukin-2 [IL-2]) and a cosignal induced by binding of B7 ligand to the T lymphocyte's CD28 molecules, the T lymphocyte can become activated. Activated T lymphocytes then transiently express the immune checkpoint proteins programmed cell death protein 1 (PD-1) and cytotoxic T-lymphocyte-associated protein 4 (CTLA-4). CTLA-4 outcompetes the T lymphocyte's CD28 molecules for B7 ligand to diminish the costimulatory signal. Tumor cells can express programmed death ligand 1 (PD-L1), which binds PD-1, leading to decreased stimulatory cytokine production.

clinical trials for gastroesophageal cancers. Clinicians who use these immune checkpoint inhibitor drugs have become familiar with their efficacy in treatment-refractory patients, especially in biomarker-identified subsets, and their unique spectrum of side-effects. Subsets of patients who have an improved response to immune checkpoint inhibitors are those with tumors that express neoantigens because of defects in mismatch repair or after radiation therapy and those who have high tissue expression of PD-L1. The most common PD-L1 expression assay uses immunohistochemical staining with the proprietary 22C3 antibody [436]. Results can be reported as the combined positive score (CPS) where PD-L1-positive tumor and infiltrating immune cells are counted and then divided by the total number of tumor cells, or tumor proportion score where PD-L1-positive tumor cells are divided by the total number of tumor cells. Because immune checkpoint inhibitors break tolerance, autoimmune side-effects can occur and are classified as immune-related adverse events [437]. These can range from life-threatening requiring hospitalization, cessation of therapy, and use of steroids and other immunosuppressants to less serious events permitting outpatient management.

Although many immune checkpoint inhibitor trials have been reported in gastroesophageal cancers, the ones that have impacted treatment guidelines will be highlighted. The phase II KEYNOTE-059 trial was a single treatment arm of pembrolizumab 200 mg given every 3 weeks to patients who had previously received at least two lines of treatment for recurrent, locally advanced or metastatic GEJ and gastric adenocarcinoma [413]. Of the 259 patients treated, 51% had GEJ adenocarcinoma, 57% were PD-L1 positive with CPS ≥1, and 4% were MSI-high. Primary endpoints were safety and tolerability and overall response rate as measured radiographically every 6 weeks during the first year. The drug was fairly well tolerated with 17.8% of patients experiencing at least one immune-related adverse event. The overall response rate was 11.6% in all patients and 15.5% in the subset of PD-L1-positive patients. Median duration of response was 16.3 months in the PD-L1-positive patients and 6.9 months in the PD-L1-negative patients. Based on these results, pembrolizumab was FDA approved for use in GEJ and patients with gastric adenocarcinoma with PD-L1 CPS ≥1 tumors third line or later.

KEYNOTE-061 was a randomized, controlled phase III trial comparing pembrolizumab with paclitaxel as second-line therapy in patients with metastatic GEJ or gastric adenocarcinoma [438]. Of the 592 patients randomized, 395 were PD-L1 CPS ≥1, and roughly one-third had GEJ adenocarcinoma. Patients received either pembrolizumab 200 mg every 3 weeks or paclitaxel 80 mg/m^2 weekly for 3 weeks followed by 1 week off until progression, intolerable toxicity, or patient withdrawal. Primary endpoints were overall survival and progression-free survival. At a median follow-up of 8.5 months in the PD-L1 CPS ≥1 patient population, no patients continued to receive paclitaxel, while 13 patients continued to receive pembrolizumab. Pembrolizumab did not significantly prolong median overall survival at 9.1 months compared with 8.3 months in the paclitaxel arm. Median progression-free survival was not significantly different either, at 1.5 months with pembrolizumab and 4.1 months with paclitaxel. Post hoc analysis demonstrated that in patients with PD-L1 CPS ≥10, the treatment effect was greater with pembrolizumab having a median overall survival of 10.4 months compared with 8.0 months with paclitaxel. In patients who were MSI-high, median overall survival in patients treated with pembrolizumab was not reached versus 8.1 months for those treated with paclitaxel.

The benefit seen in metastatic MSI-high GEJ and gastric tumors is in line with results from five early-stage trials (KEYNOTE-012, -028, -016, -158, and -164) in other tumors [439]. A total of 149 patients with MSI-high tumors (90 with metastatic colorectal cancer and 59 with other metastatic types of cancer) received pembrolizumab in these trials. The median number of prior lines of therapy was two. Overall, there were 59 responders (39.6%), with 7% having a complete response. Based on this, in May 2017, the FDA granted its first tissue agnostic approval for use of pembrolizumab in MSI-high metastatic solid tumors after progression on a single prior line of therapy. Based on this, metastatic esophageal and GEJ cancers that are MSI-high could be treated with pembrolizumab second line no matter the PD-L1 expression level.

Based on the negative results of KEYNOTE-061 and the positive results of the phase II KEYNOTE-180 trial examining the clinical benefit of pembrolizumab third line in metastatic esophageal and GEJ adenocarcinoma [440], KEYNOTE-181 was initiated. Results were presented at ASCO GI 2019 in abstract form but have yet to be published [441]. This was a phase III trial in which 628 patients with advanced or metastatic esophageal or GEJ adenocarcinoma (Siewert type I only) that had progressed on or after one prior line of therapy were randomized 1 : 1 to either pembrolizumab 200 mg given every 3 weeks or investigators' choice of paclitaxel 80–100 mg/m^2 given weekly for 3 weeks followed by 1 week off, docetaxel 75 mg/m^2 given every 3 weeks, or irinotecan 180 mg/m^2 given every 2 weeks. The primary endpoints were overall survival in three separate patient subsets: those with PD-L1 CPS ≥10, those with esophageal squamous cell carcinoma, and the intention-to-treat groups. In patients with PD-L1 CPS ≥10, median overall survival was significantly different with pembrolizumab at 9.3 months compared with 6.7 months with single-agent chemotherapy. In patients with esophageal squamous cell carcinoma, pembrolizumab was statistically better, giving a median overall survival of 8.2 months versus 7.1 months with single-agent chemotherapy. Using intention-to-treat analysis, no difference was seen with pembrolizumab. Based on these results, pembrolizumab was approved for use in esophageal squamous cell carcinoma in the second-line setting in tumors with PD-L1 CPS ≥10.

Two other studies that inform on use of immune checkpoint inhibitors in gastroesophageal cancer were presented at ESMO 2019, although final results have not yet been published. The phase III ATTRACTION-3 trial randomized 419 patients with recurrent unresectable or metastatic esophageal squamous cell carcinoma to nivolumab or chemotherapy [442]. Median overall survival was significantly different at 10.9 months with nivolumab versus 8.4 months with chemotherapy. Importantly, the survival benefit with nivolumab did not depend on PD-L1 expression level. Also, nivolumab had an improved toxicity profile compared with chemotherapy. In the phase III KEYNOTE-062 trial, untreated patients with metastatic GEJ or gastric adenocarcinoma were randomized to pembrolizumab 200 mg given every 3 weeks; pembrolizumab 200 mg given with cisplatin 80 mg/m^2 and continuous infusion 5-FU for 5 days or daily oral capecitabine repeated every 3 weeks; or placebo with chemotherapy [443]. In patients with PD-L1 CPS ≥1, pembrolizumab was noninferior to chemotherapy with median overall survival of 10.6 months with pembrolizumab and 11.1 months with chemotherapy. What was striking was that in an exploratory analysis of 50 MSI-high patients, median overall survival was not reached in both pembrolizumab arms but was 8.5 months in patients who received placebo with chemotherapy. Some clinicians now advocate for pembrolizumab monotherapy as first-line therapy in patients with MSI-high GEJ and gastric tumors, although this may still be premature.

Recommendations for the current use of immune checkpoint inhibitors in esophageal adenocarcinoma, especially in those that involve the GEJ, are as follows: In tumors that are PD-L1 CPS ≥1, pembrolizumab monotherapy can be given third line or later. In MSI-high tumors, pembrolizumab monotherapy can be given second line, without consideration of PD-L1 expression levels. In tumors that are PD-L1 CPS ≥10, clinical guidelines suggest considering pembrolizumab monotherapy in the second-line setting. Ongoing clinical trials are examining combining PD-1/PD-L1 antibodies with CTLA-4 antibodies along with chemotherapy first line in metastatic tumors, targeting other immune checkpoints, such as LAG-3, and using PD-1/PD-L1 antibodies in patients with localized cancers in combination with neoadjuvant chemoradiation and/or adjuvantly in patients found to have residual tumor at the time of esophagectomy.

Treatment recommendations

Treatment recommendations for esophageal adenocarcinoma include:

1. Once diagnosed with esophageal adenocarcinoma, patients should undergo staging with a PET/CT scan and EUS. Bronchoscopy should be performed for tumors at the level of the carina or higher. Staging laparoscopy should be done as part of the initial staging evaluation or at the time of planned esophageal resection.
2. For patients with stage IA disease, endoscopic eradiation therapy generally is preferred to esophagectomy.
3. For patients with stage IB–III disease, neoadjuvant chemoradiation (CROSS trial) followed by esophagectomy is preferred. Acceptable alternatives are perioperative chemotherapy (FLOT4 preferred over MAGIC regimen) and esophagectomy, *or* definitive chemoradiation (RTOG 8501 regimen) for nonsurgical candidates.
4. Esophagectomy should be performed in a specialized, high-volume center by a surgeon experienced in esophageal cancer surgery.
5. For patients who have surgery without prior neoadjuvant therapy, adjuvant chemotherapy or chemoradiation (INT 0116 regimen) should be offered.
6. For patients with metastatic disease, the tumor should be tested for HER2/Neu amplification, MSI status, and PD-L1 expression with consideration of next generation sequencing. If HER2/Neu positive and the patient is a chemotherapy candidate, a trastuzumab-containing regimen should be used (ToGA regimen). If HER2/Neu negative and the patient is a chemotherapy candidate, a multiagent chemotherapy regimen (REAL-2 regimen) should be chosen based on the patient's performance status. Three-drug regimens may be reserved for patients with an excellent performance status.
7. Second-line therapy options for metastatic disease include single-agent chemotherapy, ramucirumab with or without paclitaxel, and pembrolizumab in MSI-high tumors or PD-L1 CPS ≥10 tumors.
8. Third-line therapy or later options for metastatic disease include single-agent chemotherapy or pembrolizumab in MSI-high tumors or PD-L1 CPS ≥1 tumors.
9. Palliative adjuncts, such as radiation therapy or stent placement, should be considered by members of a multidisciplinary team.
10. Enrollment in clinical trials should be prioritized.

References are available at www.yamadagastro.com/textbook7e

Further reading

Hvid-Jensen F., Pedersen L., Drewes A.M., et al. Incidence of adenocarcinoma among patients with Barrett's esophagus. N Engl J Med 2011;365:1375.

Ku G.Y. The current status of immunotherapies in esophagogastric cancer. Hematol Oncol Clin N Am 2019;33(2):323.

Phoa K.N., van Vilsteren F.G., Weusten B.L., et al. Radiofrequency ablation vs endoscopic surveillance for patients with Barrett esophagus and low-grade dysplasia: a randomized clinical trial. JAMA 2014;311(12):1209.

Que J., Garman K.S., Souza R.F., Spechler S.J. Pathogenesis and cells of origin of Barrett's esophagus. Gastroenterology 2019;157:349.

Shaheen N.J., Sharma P., Overholt B.F., et al. Radiofrequency ablation in Barrett's esophagus with dysplasia. N Engl J Med 2009;360:2277.

Spechler S.J., Souza R.F. Barrett's esophagus. N Engl J Med 2014;371:836.

CHAPTER 47

Esophageal squamous cell carcinomas and other neoplasms

Adam J. Bass[1] and Anil K. Rustgi[2]

[1]Dana-Farber Cancer Institute and Harvard Medical School, Boston, MA, USA

[2]Herbert Irving Comprehensive Cancer Center, Columbia University Irving Medical Center, New York, NY, USA

Chapter menu

Definition

Squamous cell carcinoma (SCC) is the most common malignancy of the esophagus. It typically occurs in the proximal and midesophagus. Although worldwide SCC is the most common esophageal cancer, in the western world esophageal adenocarcinoma is increasingly prevalent. Esophageal adenocarcinomas, which typically occur in the setting of Barrett esophagus and are more commonly found in the distal esophagus and gastroesophageal junction, are discussed in Chapter 46.

Epidemiology and risk factors

Esophageal SCC is the most common form of esophageal malignancy worldwide and is one of the leading causes of cancer mortality in men, especially African American men.

Tobacco and alcohol

Tobacco and alcohol constitute the largest risk factors for the development of esophageal SCC. Because tobacco and alcohol are commonly consumed together, their individual contribution may be difficult to ascertain, and their effects may be synergistic [1]. In one study, the relative risk was 2.0 for those who smoked fewer than 15 cigarettes per day and 6.2 for those who smoked more than 25 cigarettes per day [2]. Not surprisingly, there is a substantial increase in risk in patients who consume both tobacco and alcohol; the risk correlates with the amount and duration of use [1]. Thus, smokers who have a large intake of beer and whiskey incur a 10- to 25-fold increased risk for esophageal SCC compared with smokers who do not drink alcohol [3]. In addition, the risk may be greater for pipe and cigar smokers than for cigarette smokers [3].

Risk for esophageal SCC is decreased 10 years after cessation of smoking. Although cigarette smoking is a key risk factor in North America and Western Europe, chewing tobacco, betel, or combinations of these with lime may account for the high incidence of esophageal SCC in southern and Southeast Asia [4]. Tobacco tars and cigarette smoke contain various chemical carcinogens, such as aromatic amines, lactones, peroxy compounds, halo ethers, *N*-nitroso compounds, and polycyclic aromatic hydrocarbons [5,6], which individually or in combination likely lead to esophageal epithelial hyperproliferation and eventual malignant transformation.

Yamada's Textbook of Gastroenterology, Seventh Edition. Edited by Timothy C. Wang, Michael Camilleri, Benjamin Lebwohl, Anna S. Lok, William J. Sandborn, Kenneth K. Wang, and Gary D. Wu.

Companion website: www.yamadagastro.com/textbook7e

The type of alcohol (beer, spirits), duration, and quantity of use are risk factors for esophageal SCC. Groups of people who do not consume alcohol have a substantially lower risk than those who do. Alcoholic beverages may contribute to the pathogenesis of esophageal cancer, as well as other cancers, through a variety of mechanisms [7]. Some alcoholic beverages contain congeners or other ingredients, such as *N*-nitroso compounds, urethane, mycotoxins (toxins from fungi), tannins, pesticide residues, and asbestos products, which are directly or indirectly carcinogenic. Because it is a solvent for fat-soluble compounds, ethanol itself may facilitate the absorption of other carcinogens. Carcinogens that are oxidants may increase the risk for DNA damage. Acetaldehyde, a metabolite of ethanol, can inhibit DNA methyltransferase activity [8], and methyl deficiency may potentiate the carcinogenic effect of a methyl-deficient diet.

Diet and nutrition

Vitamin deficiencies, especially of vitamins A, C, folic acid, E, B_{12}, and B_2 (riboflavin), are crucial risk factors [9]. Diets with greater red meat or processed meat are associated with increased risk for esophageal SCC [10]. Lower plasma levels of folic acid have been documented in patients with esophageal SCC [11]. Riboflavin deficiency manifested by cheilosis and glossitis is common in the Linxian province of China, where esophageal cancer is endemic [11]. It is likely that vitamins A, C, and E exert antioxidant effects; vitamins C and E are known to influence the formation of nitrosamines. Conversely, diets that contain high amounts of green and yellow vegetables (which are rich in β-carotene) and citrus fruits (which are high in vitamin C) are associated with a decreased risk for esophageal SCC [12,13].

Tissue and blood levels of certain trace elements, such as selenium, molybdenum, and zinc, show an inverse association with mortality from esophageal cancer in high-incidence areas of the world [14]. Furthermore, *N*-nitrosomethylbenzylamine in combination with a zinc-deficient diet induces a significance increase in SCC in rats [15]. Mechanistically, zinc deficiency enhances the microsomal activation of *N*-nitrosomethylbenzylamine to a methylating agent that yields *O*-6-methylguanine adducts in esophageal DNA [15]. As a component of superoxide dismutase, zinc also protects against oxygen-derived radical damage and free radical formation [16]. Similarly, selenium has protective effects, in part mediated through the inhibition of lipid peroxidation of cell membranes through the actions of selenium-dependent glutathione peroxidase [17]. Molybdenum deficiency could conceivably lead to the accumulation of nitrates that are precursors of nitrosamines because this trace element is a key constituent of nitrate reductase [18].

Achalasia

The average interval from onset of dysphagia, weight loss, and chest pain attributable to achalasia to the development of esophageal SCC is approximately 15–20 years [19]. In a study of 195 consecutive patients with achalasia, the incidence of esophageal SCC was 3.4 per 1000 patients per year, representing a 33-fold increase when compared with age- and sex-matched controls [20]. A follow-up study of 146 of 147 patients with achalasia treated with myotomy revealed that 10 patients progressed to esophageal SCC, with a mean interval of 16.7 years [21]. Thus, the condition of achalasia eventually may lead to cancer, but the exact risk and mechanism remain to be determined [22]. Some have advocated endoscopic surveillance of patients with achalasia; however, the frequency of examinations remains the subject of debate. Management of achalasia with conventional botulinum toxin, Heller myotomy, and more recently, peroral endoscopic myotomy is discussed in Chapter 42.

Head and neck squamous cell carcinoma

Patients with head and neck SCC are at an increased risk for development of esophageal SCC, presumably reflecting the known risk of tobacco and/or alcohol use that is common to all these conditions. Either synchronous (coexisting) or metachronous (sequential) esophageal SCC can develop, although the rate of esophageal SCC development is highly variable [23,24]. As a result, endoscopic surveillance of the esophagus has been advocated in patients with head and neck SCC, although the optimal frequency has not been established. Toluidine blue staining enhances the detection of indolent esophageal SCC in patients with head and neck cancer SCC. Not surprisingly, survival of patients with head and neck SCC is adversely affected by the coexistence of esophageal SCC. A reduction in the incidence of second primary tumors from 24% to 4% in patients with head and neck cancers has been observed with the use of isotretinoin, a chemopreventive agent that induces epithelial differentiation [25].

Tylosis

Although some studies from China have suggested familial aggregation of esophageal SCC, it is difficult to discriminate between a common environmental exposure and an actual genetic basis for these observations. However, a genetic predisposition to esophageal SCC is clear in tylosis palmaris et plantaris, an autosomal dominant disorder manifested by hyperkeratosis of the palms and soles. There is an association between esophageal SCC and oropharyngeal leukoplakia in this condition. In endoscopic surveillance studies over a 5-year period, 4 of 29 patients were found to have dysplasia, and one patient had carcinoma in situ [26]. The locus responsible for tylosis palmaris et plantaris was linked originally to chromosome 17q11-q23 [27,28] and subsequently to a smaller genomic locus in chromosome 17q25. Of note, this locus is commonly deleted in sporadic esophageal SCC [29,30]. Missense mutations have been found in *RHBDF2*, a gene that encodes an inactive rhomboid protease, in tylosis palmaris et plantaris-related esophageal SCC [31].

Other factors

Lye ingestion, which results in stricture formation, has been postulated as a risk factor for esophageal SCC, mostly appearing at the level of the tracheal bifurcation. Lye strictures constitute only a very small proportion of esophageal SCC cases, and the progression to cancer after initial exposure may require four to five decades.

Other factors implicated in the pathogenesis of esophageal SCC include high-dose mediastinal ionizing radiation [32], celiac sprue, human papillomavirus (HPV), Plummer-Vinson syndrome (also referred to as Paterson-Brown-Kelly syndrome, involving postcricoid dysphagia from esophageal webs, atrophic glossitis, and iron-deficiency anemia), lichen planus, and consumption of high-temperature beverages [33]. HPV, especially HPV-16, which has been increasingly associated with head and neck SCC in the western world, has been reported in up to 20–25% of esophageal SCCs from a metaanalysis [34]. HPVs infect squamous epithelial cells, replicate, and produce oncogenic proteins that contribute to hyperproliferation and malignant transformation.

Temporal/secular trends

In the western world, where alcohol and tobacco are the primary risk factors for esophageal SCC, rates have been decreasing, presumably because of decreasing tobacco and alcohol usage. In Asia, however, trends remain different from in the west. As in the west, esophageal adenocarcinoma rates have also been increasing in the Middle East (Iran), while the incidence of esophageal SCC remains unchanged. In the same period that a dramatic increase in esophageal adenocarcinoma in the west was observed, there was no change in incidence rates in Taiwan. However, during the period from 1979 to 2003, the age-standardized rate of esophageal SCC increased from 2.63 to 4.37 per 100 000 years. Studies in the Japanese population have observed some increases in esophageal SCC rates, especially in men, since the late 1970s. This study also noted a decreasing rate of esophageal SCC in China during this period, consistent with other reports [35].

Geographic variation

The incidence of esophageal SCC varies according to geographical location, with a global range from 2.5 to 5.0 for men and from 1.5 to 2.5 for women per 100 000 population. High-incidence regions, where rates may exceed 100 per 100 000 population, include northern China, India, northern Iran, areas north and east of the Caspian Sea, and the Transkei area of South Africa [36]. Indeed, esophageal SCC comprises nearly 50% of all cancers in southeastern South Africa [35]. In the United States, African Americans have a fourfold to fivefold increased risk compared with whites, especially African American men, in whom the risk is 15.1 per 100 000 compared with 2.9 per 100 000 in whites [37].

The geographical variation in esophageal SCC is presumed to reflect a significant impact of environmental factors. The incidence of esophageal SCC is very low in those younger than 40 years, but it increases with each succeeding decade of life [37]. It is more common in men than in women, with a twofold to threefold higher risk, regardless of ethnicity and age. However, there are some exceptions to this general finding. In northern Iran, the rate is 263 per 100 000 for women and 206 per 100 000 for men [38], and esophageal SCC occurring in association with Plummer–Vinson syndrome is found primarily in women.

There are likely biological differences superimposed on environmental factors in the high-incidence areas compared with western countries, which may account for the apparently lengthy period from dysplasia to cancer in China and the good prognosis there after resection of early esophageal SCC, with a 5-year survival rate approaching 90%. It is not entirely clear whether the same early esophageal SCC is prevalent in North America and Western Europe. Several nonbiological explanations can be invoked: the use and accuracy of balloon cytology in China, the definition of early esophageal SCC, and proper staging with aggressive therapy [39]. Some genomic studies also have identified differences in the types of mutation found in esophageal SCCs between Asian and western cohorts [40].

Pathogenesis

It is believed that the development of esophageal SCC results from the accumulation of alterations in oncogenes and tumor suppressor genes. It is likely that environmental, dietary, and lifestyle factors cooperate or interact with genetically determined processes to increase cancer risk. For example, environmental factors injure the esophageal epithelium, which results in changes in key genes through point mutations or augmented gene expression.

Perhaps the most critical oncogene product in esophageal SCC pathogenesis is cyclin D1. Mammalian cyclins are a large family of cell-cycle regulatory proteins that associate, in turn, with catalytic subunit partners, designated cyclin-dependent kinases (CDKs). The activity of cyclin D1 is restricted to the G1 phase, and it preferentially associates with CDK4 or CDK6. The complex of cyclin D1 and CDK4 or CDK6 phosphorylates the retinoblastoma tumor suppressor gene product (pRb). This relieves the negative regulation of pRb in the G1 phase through the release of key transcriptional factors, such as E2F. It has been shown that cyclin D1 is overexpressed in more than 50% of esophageal SCCs and is associated with a poor prognosis [41,42]. Cyclin D1 may be altered through additional mechanisms, including point mutation [43] or mutation in its E3 ligase, Fbx4 [44]. Knowledge of the association of cyclin D1 and esophageal cancer has enabled the development of a transgenic mouse model. Targeting cyclin D1 to the esophageal squamous epithelium with an Epstein–Barr virus promoter results in dysplasia and cell-cycle abnormalities [45,46]. A subset of esophageal SCC also shows c-*myc* and epidermal growth factor receptor overexpression as a result of gene amplification. SOX2, a transcriptional factor important in esophageal development during embryogenesis, plays a role in esophageal SCC pathogenesis by virtue of amplification [47]. In addition, mutations in *KEAP1* or *NFE2L2*, both of which are believed to lead to stabilization of the NFR2 transcription factor, have been noted in esophageal SCC [48].

The key tumor suppressor gene *p53* has many functions, including cell-cycle regulation, induction of apoptosis in response to environmental insults, transcriptional regulation of genes, and DNA replication. *p53* is mutated in >50% of esophageal cancers [49,50]. One of the functional consequences of *p53* mutation is the transcriptional downregulation of *p21*, a general CDK inhibitor. In addition, *p16*, also referred to as *INK4a* (designated $p16^{INK4a}$), is an inhibitor of CDK4. Located on chromosome 9p22–23, $p16^{INK4a}$ can be deleted, mutated, or hypermethylated, resulting in loss of its inhibitory function in esophageal SCC [49,51]. It appears that either cyclin D1 is overexpressed or $p16^{INK4a}$ is altered to accelerate the cell-cycle progression through G1 phase in esophageal SCC. Loss of E-cadherin and transforming growth factor-β type II receptor has been observed in esophageal SCC [52]. Similarly, loss of p120-catenin, which stabilizes E-cadherin at the cell membrane, in a mouse model has been demonstrated to lead to development of esophageal SCC and is accompanied by the development of an infiltrate with immature myeloid cells, as well as desmoplasia [53]. More recent studies have identified loss-of-function mutations in *Notch1* in esophageal SCC [40]. With the advent of new technologies for comprehensive genomic sequencing, new large-scale analysis of the esophageal SCC genome has been performed, finding additional mutations in *RB1* and epigenetic regulatory factors such as *MLL2*, *ASH1L*, *MLL3*, *SETD1B*, and *EP300* [48].

Clinical presentation and natural history

Early esophageal SCC may be asymptomatic, associated with only mild specific symptoms. Dysphagia is present in nearly 90% of patients and odynophagia in 50% of patients at the time of diagnosis. This is usually a reflection of partial or total luminal obstruction. Anorexia and weight loss from malnutrition may be observed in about 75% of patients. Retrosternal pain or radiation of pain to the back suggests mediastinal involvement by the cancer. Nausea, vomiting, and hematemesis may occur. Cough may reflect aspiration pneumonia or, rarely, tracheoesophageal fistula. Recurrent laryngeal nerve involvement as a result of extraesophageal extension can result in hoarseness. Skeletal metastases can cause bone pain. Physical examination may reveal cachexia, lymphadenopathy, hepatomegaly (if distant metastatic disease is present), and the presence of occult blood in stool. Evaluation of dysphagia is imperative. The differential diagnosis may include peptic acid esophagitis with stricture, caustic ingestion resulting in stricture, malignant disease (either squamous or adenocarcinoma), and motility disorders such as achalasia or scleroderma.

Esophageal SCC in western countries usually presents at an advanced stage; consequently, nearly 75% of untreated patients succumb to the disease within 1 year [54]. Biologically, esophageal SCC is not a rapidly growing tumor, and there is a prolonged period between the development of dysplasia and progression to advanced cancer. In China and Iran, the early stages of esophageal SCC have been shown to persist for more than two decades. Indeed, serial balloon cytological examinations, used to monitor the natural history of esophageal squamous dysplasia in China, indicate that dysplasia progresses to cancer in 26.6% of patients, but it regresses to mild dysplasia or a normal state in 40.5% of patients. Of those with mild dysplasia, nearly 15% progressed to severe dysplasia and about 45% regressed [55]. Other studies in China indicate that superficial esophageal SCCs remain in this state in 58% of cases for a follow-up period of 19–78 months [56]. Patients with untreated early esophageal SCC in China have a median survival time of 75 months [56].

Differential diagnosis

The differential diagnosis of esophageal SCC includes a variety of mass lesions of the esophagus. Esophageal adenocarcinoma is discussed in Chapter 46. Pathological evaluation of tissue obtained from esophageal mass lesions remains the mainstay of guiding diagnosis.

Benign epithelial tumors (squamous cell papilloma)

Squamous cell papillomas are usually discovered incidentally at endoscopy or during barium radiography. Generally, they are small, sessile, polypoid growths of normal or hyperplastic squamous epithelium covering a core of connective tissue. They are more common in Japan and central Asian countries [57]. They typically do not recur after removal. Most are solitary and located in the distal third of the esophagus. Papillomas may result from chronic irritation from reflux esophagitis. Morphological features suggest that papillomas result from HPV infection, and HPV DNA has been found in a subset of papillomas [58]. Development of cancer is rare in these papillomas [59], which may reflect the fact that esophageal papillomas are associated with the nononcogenic genotypes of HPV.

Other malignant epithelial tumors

Squamous cell carcinoma with a spindle cell component

SCC with a spindle cell component is also referred to as carcinosarcoma, pseudosarcoma, spindle cell carcinoma, and polypoid carcinoma [60]. Originally, carcinosarcoma was believed to be malignant, whereas pseudosarcoma was designated benign without metastatic potential. Local and distant metastases of spindle cells, however, have been reported.

Spindle cell carcinomas are either solitary or multiple and are large and polypoid. Histologically, the squamous component at the surface is associated with dysplasia or carcinoma in situ. One may also observe adenocarcinoma, or undifferentiated epithelial components can occur. The spindle cell component ranges from mild proliferation to marked proliferation with pleomorphism, giant cells, and mitoses. Differentiation into smooth or skeletal muscle, bone, or cartilage is rarely observed. Immunohistochemical and electron microscopic analyses indicate that the spindle cells derive from mesenchymal metaplasia of malignant squamous cells. Although there are reports that spindle cells contain epithelial cell markers such as cytokeratins, suggesting multiclonality, most pathologists believe that spindle cell carcinomas arise from SCCs that produce a spindle cell component [61].

Men are affected more often than women, and most patients are middle aged or elderly. Located in the middle to distal esophagus, these cancers can produce obstruction and dysphagia by virtue of their large size. Most patients present with esophageal wall invasion and lymph node involvement. There is little prospective information on the treatment of these cancers. Surgical resection, when feasible, is the mainstay of therapy.

Verrucous squamous cell carcinoma

Classically, verrucous SCC of the esophagus is a slow-growing malignant tumor that is often limited to local invasion without distant metastasis [62]. However, some do metastasize to other organs, with resulting poor prognosis.

Adenoacanthoma and adenosquamous carcinoma

These rare tumors feature adenocarcinoma with either squamous metaplasia (adenoacanthoma) or squamous carcinoma (adenosquamous carcinoma) [63]. These lesions can arise in the setting of Barrett esophagus or occur de novo. It is likely that these tumors arise in the squamous epithelium, which has the ability to achieve squamous and glandular differentiation. Alternatively, squamous metaplasia or transformation within an adenocarcinoma may have occurred. Clinically, these tumors behave like adenocarcinomas.

Adenoid cystic carcinoma

This rare tumor, usually found in elderly men, resembles salivary adenoid cystic carcinoma. These tumors are multilobulated or ulcerated and are located in the midesophagus [64]. Histologically, adenoid cystic carcinomas contain many cystic spaces and are primarily submucosal.

Mucoepidermoid carcinoma

This cancer consists of glandular and squamous elements; however, the mixture is more pronounced than in adenosquamous carcinoma [64]. Mucoepidermoid carcinomas develop in the middle to distal esophagus and probably arise from submucosal glands or their ducts. Prognosis is poor.

Melanoma

Melanoma is a rare esophageal cancer that can be primary or metastatic, although the esophagus is less commonly a site of metastatic melanoma than the stomach, small intestine, or colon [65]. The mean age of patients is 60 years, and there are more cases in Japan than in other countries. Melanomas are polypoid and may be multiple, with a propensity for lateral spread. Primary esophageal melanomas arise from melanocytes in the basal layer. Amelanotic melanomas may require confirmation with immunohistochemical demonstration of S100 protein; alternatively, electron microscopy may reveal premelanosomes. Overall, the prognosis of malignant melanoma is dismal; most patients succumb to the disease within 2 years [66].

Neuroendocrine tumors

Small cell carcinoma of the esophagus includes a small cell variant of SCC, as well as oat cell carcinoma. Oat cell carcinoma of the esophagus can be primary or secondary from the lung, and both are rare. A disease of the elderly, who present with dysphagia, primary small cell carcinoma of the esophagus (typically distal and sometimes multiple) carries an especially dismal prognosis, with an average survival of 5 months [67]. These tumors occasionally secrete ectopic antidiuretic hormone or may be associated with hypercalcemia. Microscopically, this tumor is an anaplastic small cell carcinoma resembling those found in the lung, with solid sheets of small anaplastic cells and frequent mitoses. There can be evidence of squamous or glandular differentiation. Neuroendocrine markers used are chromogranin and synaptophysin, as well as electron microscopic evidence of neurosecretory granules.

Esophageal carcinoid tumors are rare, with most occurring at the gastroesophageal junction [68]. Carcinoid syndrome has not been reported in association with esophageal carcinoid tumors. There is little or no malignant potential; consequently, prognosis is good.

Choriocarcinoma of the esophagus is an exceedingly rare tumor that may be primary or an adenocarcinoma with trophoblastic differentiation [69]. Secretion of human chorionic gonadotropin has been reported.

Benign nonepithelial tumors

Leiomyoma

Leiomyomas are the most common benign esophageal tumor [70]. Men are affected twice as frequently as women. These tumors are typically solitary. Most occur in the distal esophagus and arise in the inner circular layer of the muscularis propria. Most leiomyomas are asymptomatic and are found incidentally. Symptoms, if present, include dysphagia and chest pain; gastrointestinal bleeding is rare.

The diagnosis is usually suggested by barium esophagography, which shows a smooth, round defect with sharp margins (Figure 47.1), or endoscopy, in which a well-circumscribed, rounded mass with normal overlying mucosa is seen. Biopsy is usually not helpful because the tumor lies deep in the mucosa. Endoscopic ultrasonography (EUS) is helpful for diagnosis.

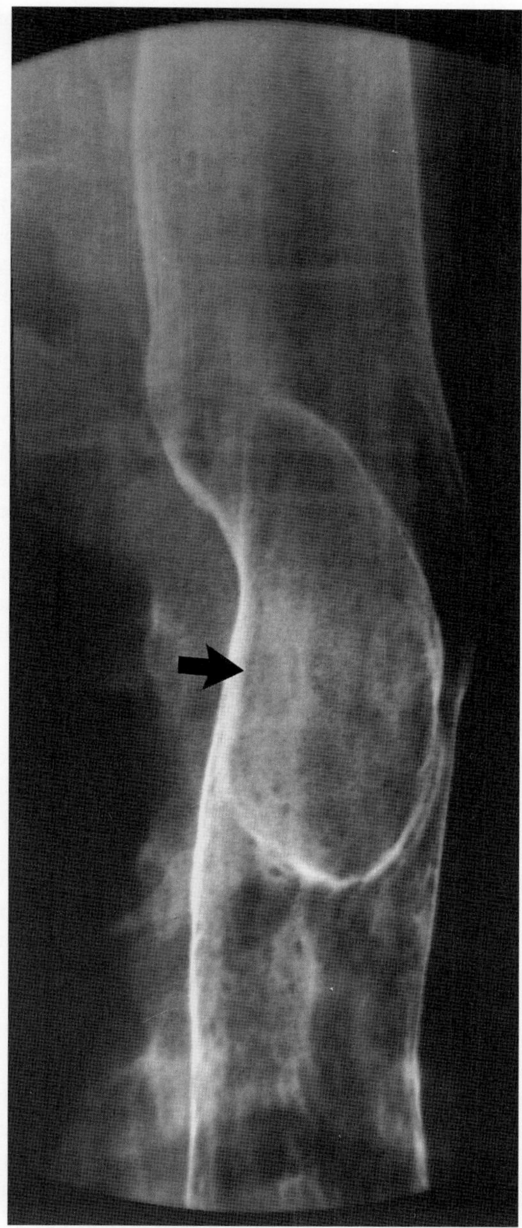

Figure 47.1 Leiomyoma of the esophagus represented by a smooth intramural mass (arrow) outlined with air-contrast barium. Source: Courtesy of Deborah Hall, MD.

Granular cell tumor

Granular cell tumors are derived from neural or Schwann cell elements, as evidenced by positive staining for S100 protein and neuron-specific enolase [71]. Endoscopically, granular cell tumor is characterized as a small, smooth, sessile polyp with overlying normal mucosa and intramural nodules or plaques [71]. Most tumors occur in the distal esophagus and may be single or multiple. Patients are usually asymptomatic. Malignant transformation is rare. Microscopically, there are sheets of monomorphic histiocyte-like cells.

Fibrovascular polyp

Intraluminal fibrovascular polyps of the esophagus are rare tumors that may prolapse into the larynx [72]. Other symptoms include dysphagia, nausea, vomiting, and occasionally, gastrointestinal bleeding from ulceration. The polyps are covered by a smooth mucosa and are composed of fibrous and vascular tissue, although adipose tissue occasionally predominates, prompting the designation of a fibrolipoma or pedunculated lipoma. Fibrovascular polyps do not have any malignant potential.

Hemangioma

Hemangiomas are small, asymptomatic lesions found incidentally on endoscopy [73].

Lymphangioma

Lymphangiomas are rare and have the appearance of a translucent, easily compressed mass on endoscopy [74], differentiating them from leiomyomas, which are nontranslucent and firmer but also well circumscribed. Histologically, they contain dilated endothelial spaces.

Lipoma and fibroma

Sessile submucosal nodules composed of adipose or fibrous tissue are called lipomas and fibromas, respectively. Together, they constitute fewer than 5% of all benign esophageal tumors.

Malignant nonepithelial tumors

Leiomyosarcoma and other sarcomas

Leiomyosarcoma in the esophagus is uncommon [75,76]. These tumors may be polypoid or infiltrative and can arise throughout the esophagus. Other esophageal sarcomas include soft tissue sarcoma, rhabdomyosarcoma, neurogenic sarcoma, and Kaposi sarcoma.

Metastatic carcinoma

Metastatic carcinoma of the esophagus is unusual. The most common primary tumor serving as a source of metastatic spread to the esophagus is melanoma, followed by breast cancer and, less commonly, gastric, renal, liver, prostate, testicular, bone, skin, lung, and head and neck cancer. Primary esophageal and head and neck squamous cancers may coexist or may develop as metachronous lesions. In this context, an esophageal stricture is usually extrinsic, without mucosal involvement.

Lymphoma

Both Hodgkin and non-Hodgkin lymphoma can originate primarily in the esophagus, although this is much less common than primary lymphomas in the stomach or small intestine. Symptomatic esophageal lymphoma may be present in immunocompromised patients, as in those with acquired immunodeficiency syndrome. Lymphoma of the esophagus also occurs as a result of disseminated disease or infiltration from adjacent lymph nodes.

Management and therapy

Diagnostic evaluation

A complete history and physical examination are the cornerstones of the diagnostic evaluation. A laboratory profile may reveal anemia, hypoalbuminemia, elevated prothrombin time reflecting vitamin K deficiency, and possibly elevated liver function tests if metastatic disease is present. Serological markers of cancer, such as CEA and CA19-9, have not proved to be of high sensitivity and specificity in esophageal SCC. Evaluation is dependent on tissue diagnosis through biopsy and cytology, followed by staging for prognosis and therapeutic planning.

Endoscopy

The diagnosis of esophageal cancer requires endoscopy with biopsy and cytology. Because endoscopy may prove too costly in some regions of the world, some advocate barium esophagography alone, especially in patients with dysphagia. Advantages include reduction in cost, noninvasiveness, and reduced complication rate. In addition, a barium study allows information to be obtained about motility, as well as challenge with a solid bolus, such as a tablet of known size. Ultimately, endoscopy is a better diagnostic test for patients in whom one suspects esophageal cancer because of the ability to obtain tissue in one test and the greater positive predictive value of upper endoscopy.

The endoscopic appearance of early esophageal SCC includes a superficial erosive ulcer(s), a raised plaque, a "congestive" lesion marked by red spots on the mucosa, and a small polypoid lesion. Vital staining dyes, such as toluidine blue, aniline blue, or Lugol's iodine, can enhance detection and simultaneously discriminate early cancers from normal adjacent mucosa. In a study of 178 patients who underwent endoscopy and vital staining, nine esophageal cancers were found, of which seven were early cancers [77]. By contrast, endoscopy without vital staining detected only four of nine cancers. Limiting the usefulness of vital staining is its inability or failure to distinguish inflammation from dysplasia. Molecular imaging using fluorescent lectins has been helpful in the diagnosis of dysplasia in Barrett esophagus and might be applicable to squamous dysplasia in the future [78]. In recent years, the development and greater use of chromoendoscopy and narrow band imaging, both of which facilitate the evaluation of mucosal morphology, have played an important role in the detection of early esophageal SCC [79].

Advanced esophageal SCCs are typically exophytic, ulcerated, and even circumferential. Submucosal invasion produces friable nodules or strictures. When feasible without risking perforation, the endoscope should be advanced through the stricture to determine the proximal–distal extent of tumor and any distal abnormalities. The majority of SCCs are found in the proximal esophagus to the midesophagus.

Barium esophagography

Radiologically, early esophageal SCC may have a granular mucosal appearance with single or multiple small ulcerations observed as small filling defects. Polypoid lesions are characterized by small intraluminal filling defects affecting one wall of the esophagus with ulcerations. Advanced esophageal cancer can appear as an infiltrative or an ulcerative lesion, but the most common presentation of advanced esophageal carcinoma is that of a polypoid mass within the lumen produced by an exophytic cancer. The mass may have the characteristic appearance of an "apple-core" lesion with circumferential involvement by the cancer (Figure 47.2). Infiltrating carcinomas often result in diminished esophageal motility with or without stricture. Such a stricture may be symmetric or asymmetric and can sometimes be difficult to distinguish from a benign stricture. The primary ulcerative type of esophageal cancer is rare, although ulceration can be a component of either polypoid or infiltrating cancer. Ulcerative cancers are well-demarcated lesions with a thin rim of lucency.

Staging and staging systems

After the diagnosis of cancer is established, staging is necessary to optimize management and to establish prognosis. This should ideally include computed tomography (CT) scanning of the chest and abdomen supplemented with EUS to assess depth of esophageal wall involvement and local lymph node involvement. In addition, where available, positron emission tomography (PET) scanning is often performed in conjunction with CT given its better sensitivity in detecting metastatic spread compared with CT alone.

Endoscopic ultrasound

The critical determinants of survival are depth of invasion, the presence or absence of lymph node metastases, and the presence or absence of distant metastases. Although several staging systems have been recommended for esophageal cancer, surgical pathological staging has increasingly been replaced by EUS for preclinical staging as detection for both depth of invasion and nodal involvement has improved (Figure 47.3). The staging system for esophageal SCC is listed in Table 47.1.

EUS has been shown to have an 81% sensitivity for T1–2 disease but a 91–92% sensitivity for detection of T3–4 disease. EUS is superior to CT scan in the determination of the primary tumor (T) and regional lymph node (N) status [80]. The EUS accuracy rate in staging the depth of tumor invasion varies from 87% to 92%, making it more accurate than CT [81]. The overall accuracy rate of EUS in detecting nodal involvement (N staging) is about 90%. In these studies, EUS sensitivity varied from 92% to 95%, and specificity varied from 50% to 54%, whereas CT accuracy rate ranged from 51% to 74%, with a sensitivity of 34% and specificity of 88% [82]. EUS-fine needle aspiration has

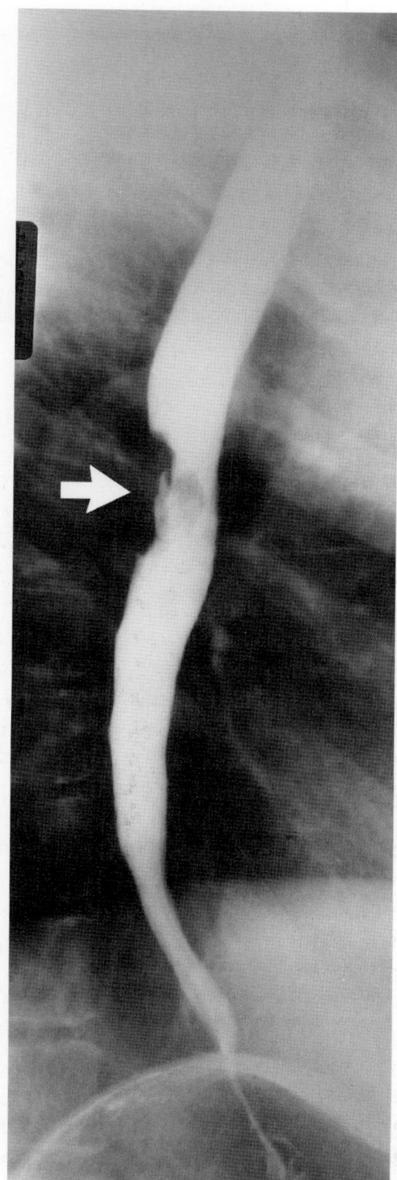

Figure 47.2 Advanced squamous cell carcinoma represented by an ulcerated mass (arrow) in the midesophagus. Source: Courtesy of Deborah Hall, MD.

improved the accuracy of EUS for N staging. EUS-fine needle aspiration has a more than 90% accuracy rate in confirming celiac axis lymph node metastases but only a limited role for staging distant metastases [81]. Therefore, it is generally recommended that CT or MRI be performed before EUS for detection of distant metastases.

EUS is useful in the assessment of resectability of cancer. Although EUS is superior to CT scan for staging after preoperative chemotherapy and radiation, EUS may not be able to distinguish inflammation and fibrosis from residual cancer. However, a decrease of 50% or more in tumor cross-sectional area or diameter correlates with treatment response. Because of its potential to reduce unnecessary surgery, EUS has been deemed to be cost-effective in the evaluation of nonmetastatic esophageal cancer.

Positron emission tomography

PET is a whole-body, metabolic-based imaging modality using fluorine 18-labeled deoxyglucose (18-FDG). There is an increased accumulation of the radiotracer in malignant tissues, which is believed to be the result of increased glucose transport into tumor cells together with increased activity of the enzymes in the first steps of the glycolytic pathway. The degree of FDG accumulation in a lesion can be assessed semi-quantitatively and expressed as a standard uptake value [83]. The results of a prospective study comparing the staging accuracy of FDG-PET with the standard combined use of CT and EUS showed that FDP-PET significantly improved the detection of stage IV disease [84]. Thus, FDG-PET has been documented as a highly accurate modality for the primary preoperative staging of patients with esophageal cancer, and its greater capacity to identify occult metastatic disease can help avoid unnecessary surgery in patients for whom curative surgical therapy is not possible.

Beyond its use in staging, FDG-PET is a promising noninvasive tool for the assessment of preoperative (neoadjuvant) therapy. There is a good correlation between clinical response demonstrated through serial PET scans and pathological response and survival. PET with the nucleoside analog 3′deoxy-3′-^{18}F-fluorothymidine (FLT) may be more accurate than FDG-PET in visualizing early changes in tumor proliferation [85]. Using an experimental model of esophageal cancer (human xenografts), FLT-PET was more accurate than FDG-PET in detecting early changes in proliferation after docetaxel and radiation therapy, with a much stronger correlation with histological findings. Clinical studies are needed to determine whether FLT-PET can distinguish between degrees of response to neoadjuvant chemoradiation in patients with esophageal cancer [85].

Laparoscopy/bronchoscopy

Abdominal metastases are more common from distal esophageal tumors, and these subdiaphragmatic metastases can be confirmed by laparoscopy. Nonetheless, laparoscopy is not routinely needed for the staging of esophageal cancer. Preoperative bronchoscopy may be considered to exclude potential airway invasion.

Therapy for esophageal SCC

Presentation of esophageal SCC at advanced stages often precludes curative surgical resection. However, with better understanding of the disease and the development of new anticancer agents, the overall survival of patients with esophageal SCC has been improving. Based on Surveillance, Epidemiology, and End Results information, the 5-year overall survival rate in the

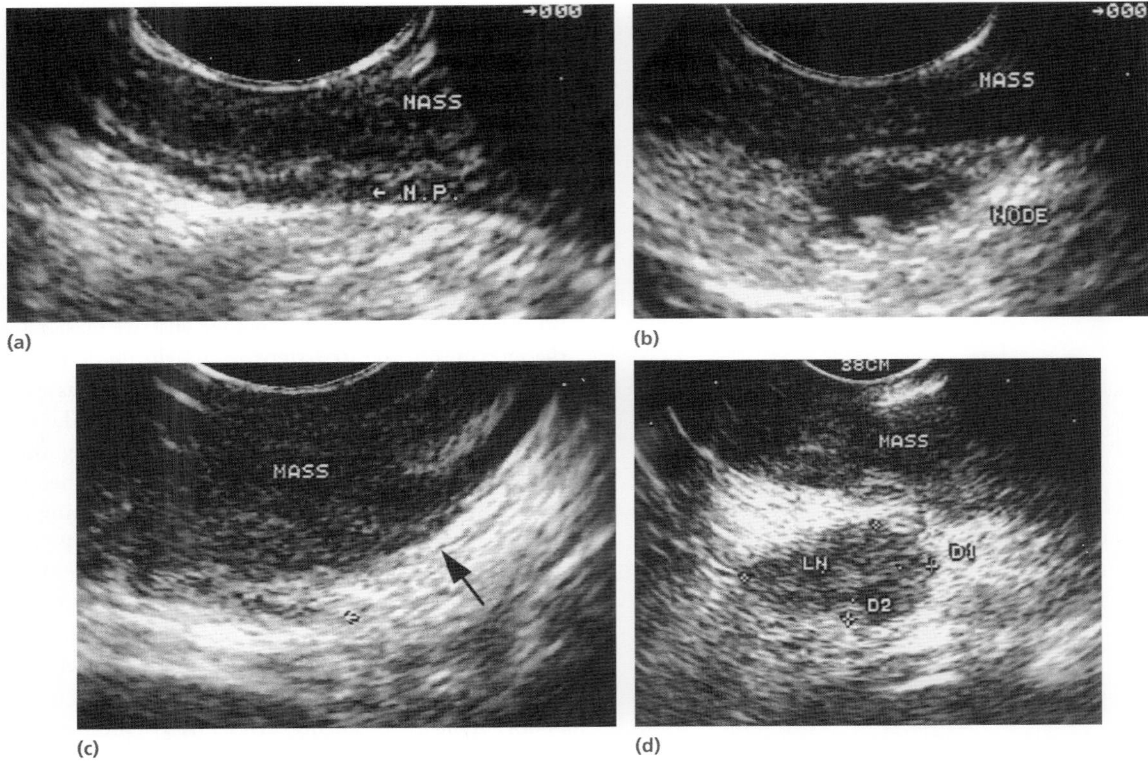

Figure 47.3 Endoscopic ultrasound images of different stages of esophageal cancer. **(a)** T2N0 stage. Note the prominent muscularis propria (M.P.). **(b)** T2N1 stage. The mass is directly adjacent to the muscularis propria. **(c)** T3N0 stage. Note invasion into the muscularis propria (arrow). **(d)** T3N1 stage. A mass with a large lymph node (LN) in mediastinal fat. Source: Courtesy of William Brugge, MD.

United States increased from 4.7% in 1976 to 20% in 2009 [86]. The following discussion is divided into categories of potential curative modalities, as well as palliative measures.

Surgery

Where feasible, surgery remains a cornerstone of treatment of esophageal SCC, especially cancers of the noncervical esophagus, with curative intent for resectable, local, and locoregional disease. Surgical therapy alone, without neoadjuvant chemoradiation therapy, is generally recommended in those with T1N0 tumors with endoscopic therapies feasible with pT1a disease per National Comprehensive Cancer Network guidelines. There is greater controversy in those with T2N0 disease regarding the need for multimodality therapy before surgical resection, especially in patients with well-differentiated tumors. National Comprehensive Cancer Network guidelines recommend consideration of esophagectomy for noncervical esophageal tumors that are T2/N0 if deemed low risk with size <2 cm and well differentiated. Advances in surgical therapy, staging techniques, patient selection, and supportive care in recent years have resulted in a marked improvement in surgery-related mortality and morbidity. Surgery is rarely used in the setting of incurable disease as a palliative measure as a means to control dysphagia or esophageal obstruction, because radiation therapy or esophageal stenting is generally more suitable for this indication.

There are various surgical approaches for esophageal cancer, including transthoracic, transhiatal, and radical en bloc resections. Despite the different advantages and disadvantages of each, and the controversies surrounding them, there is no evidence to suggest improved survival with any particular one [87]. Factors that influence the choice of technique include tumor location, depth of tumor invasion, status of lymph node involvement, overall performance status and body habitus of the patient, previous treatment (e.g., radiation or chemoradiation therapy), and the preferences and biases of the surgeon and institution. A feeding tube is typically placed at the time of surgery to facilitate nutritional support during recovery.

In the past, midesophageal tumors were approached through the left side of the chest. The benefits of a right-sided approach (Ivor Lewis) have been advocated since then and include enhanced accessibility to the upper two-thirds of the esophagus, location of the aorta as a barrier to the left pleural space, and visualization of the entire esophagus after division of the azygos vein. This approach has been applied as well for distal esophageal cancers, thus allowing for a longer segment of esophageal resection with a higher anastomosis.

Table 47.1 TNM staging system for cancer of the esophagus.

Primary tumor (T)	
TX	Primary tumor cannot be assessed
T0	No evidence of primary tumor
Tis	High-grade dysplasia
T1	Tumor invades lamina propria or muscularis mucosae (T1a) or invades submucosa (T1b)
T2	Tumor invades muscularis propria
T3	Tumor invades adventitia
T4	Tumor invades adjacent structures that are resectable (T4a) or unresectable (T4b)
Regional lymph nodes (N)	
NX	Regional lymph nodes cannot be assessed
N0	No regional lymph node metastasis
N1	Metastasis in 1–2 regional nodes
N2	Metastasis in 3–6 regional nodes
N3	Metastasis in ≥7 regional lymph nodes
Distant metastasis (M)	
MX	Distant metastasis cannot be assessed
M0	No distant metastasis
M1	Distant metastasis
Histological grade	
Gx	Grade cannot be assessed
G1	Well differentiated
G2	Moderately differentiated
G3	Poorly differentiated
G4	Undifferentiated

Location category	
Lx	Location unknown
Upper	Cervical esophagus to lower border of azygos vein
Middle	Lower border of azygos vein to lower border of IVC
Lower	Lower border of IVC to stomach

Stage grouping					
Stage 00	Tis (HGD)	N0	M0	G1	Any location
Stage IA	T1a	N0	M0	G1, X	Any location
Stage IB	T1b	N0	M0	G1, X	Any location
	T1	N0	M0	G2–3	Any location
	T2	N0	M0	G1	Any location
Stage IIA	T2	N0	M0	G2–3, X	Any location
	T3	N0	M0	Any	Lower
	T3	N0	M0	G1	Upper/Middle
Stage IIB	T3	N0	M0	G2–3	Upper/Middle
	T3	N0	M0	X	Any location
	T3	N0	M0	Any	X
	T1	N1	M0	Any	Any location
Stage IIIA	T1	N2	M0	Any	Any location
	T2	N1	M0	Any	Any location
	T3	N2	M0	Any	Any location
Stage IIIB	T4a	N0–1	M0	Any	Any location
	T3	N1	M0	Any	Any location
	T2–3	N2	M0	Any	Any location
Stage IVA	T4a	N2	M0	Any	Any location
	T4b	N0–2	M0	Any	Any location
	T1–4	N3	M0	Any	Any location
Stage IV	Any	Any	M1	Any	Any location

IVC, inferior vena cava.
Source: Based on data from the American Joint Committee on Cancer (AJCC). Esophagus. In: AJCC Cancer Staging Manual, 8th edn. New York: Springer; 2017.

Potential early complications after transthoracic esophagectomy include anastomotic leak (0–13%); pulmonary problems, such as pneumonia, retained secretions, and pulmonary emboli (6–50%); recurrent laryngeal nerve injury (1–13%); and cardiac problems, such as myocardial infarction, arrhythmia, and congestive heart failure (2–27%) [88]. The mortality rate may range from 1% to 13% [89].

Because of the morbidity and mortality linked to the thoracotomy associated with transthoracic esophagectomy, the transhiatal approach has also been advocated, although this has not been shown to reduce operative mortality. The mortality rate ranges between 2% and 13%, and the 5-year survival rate ranges from 12% to 27% [90]. Transhiatal esophagectomy reduces the extent of thoracic lymph node dissection that is feasible. Transhiatal esophagectomy is often used in the resection of benign and malignant disease. Potential advantages over transthoracic esophagectomy include a significant reduction in respiratory complications and mediastinitis because of the avoidance of thoracotomy and intrathoracic anastomosis [90]. New approaches include the triincisional approach, which borrows from both the transhiatal and transthoracic approaches and brings the advantage of enabling lymphadenectomy for both mediastinum and upper abdomen. The en bloc resection of cancers of the distal esophagus and the cardia involves removal of 10 cm of the esophagus on either side of the tumor, along with contiguous tissues, vascular supply, and lymph nodes. The extent of lymphadenectomy has been linked to survival; removal of as many nodes as possible is generally advocated.

An important consideration during surgery is the choice of esophageal replacement. The stomach, by virtue of its rich blood supply, length, and muscular wall, is preferred, whereas the left colon, because of its similarity to the esophagus in caliber, can be used to replace the esophagus when the stomach cannot be used. Jejunal interposition may be used for reconstitution of the hypopharynx and the cervical esophagus. Subsequent complications of esophageal replacement include anastomotic leaks (2–5%), anastomotic stricture (9–29%), and gastric dysfunction.

As a result of modern surgical management, mortality associated with anastomotic leak has been markedly reduced and has no impact on long-term survival. As a result, clinical decisions regarding the use of intrathoracic anastomoses should not be affected by concerns of increased mortality from leak.

Minimally invasive laparoscopic esophagectomy has been investigated in highly selected patients with esophageal cancer, typically in those with early disease. Advantages include less intraoperative blood loss, a smaller incision, and potentially faster postoperative recovery. However, no definitive benefits in terms of mortality and morbidity with the minimally invasive approaches have emerged [91]. A concern with minimally invasive approaches, however, lies in the limited extent of lymph node dissection that is feasible and the ability to get wide cancer-free margins. Some surgeons are now also performing hybrid approaches that combine open and minimally invasive approaches.

Occasionally, a bypass procedure using a portion of the stomach, jejunum, or colon as a conduit may be warranted in a patient with unresectable esophageal cancer. However, bypass surgery is fraught with high morbidity and mortality rates, and it should be reserved for patients with a tracheoesophageal fistula or those in whom conservative medical measures have failed. Effective palliative resection of the cervical esophagus usually requires total laryngectomy and esophagectomy.

When occurring in the cervical esophagus, SCCs of the esophagus pose greater clinical challenges because surgical procedures typically require radical neck dissections and removal of portions of the larynx and pharynx. Given the greater morbidity, treatments are often adapted from those from the head and neck field, where combined chemoradiation is used in a definitive form.

Radiation therapy

Radiation (external beam) alone

Radiation is seldom used as a single modality in either definitive or adjuvant therapy. It is limited to patients who are not candidates for surgical resection because of unresectable disease or because they are medically unable to tolerate either a surgical procedure or multimodality treatment with chemoradiation. Randomized trials have shown that radiation alone is inferior to combination concurrent chemoradiotherapy [92]. However, radiation alone may lead to amelioration of dysphagia, with 50% of patients receiving relief for 2 months or more and 15% of patients for more than 1 year. In the acute setting, radiation-induced esophagitis may lead to dysphagia and can result in fibrotic strictures. Unusual complications of radiation therapy include pulmonary fibrosis, myelitis, and cutaneous burns.

Brachytherapy

Intraluminal radiation (brachytherapy) can ameliorate symptoms resulting from obstructing cancers. Compared with external beam treatment, higher doses of radiation can be delivered with this technique without inducing injury to pulmonary, cardiac, and mediastinal structures. Complications of brachytherapy include ulcers, strictures, and tracheoesophageal fistulas in up to 25% of patients [93]. Brachytherapy is commonly used for palliation of esophageal obstruction due to inoperable cancer. Brachytherapy may deliver better long-term relief of dysphagia than metal stent placement and is also associated with fewer complications than stent placement [93].

Preoperative (neoadjuvant) and postoperative (adjuvant) radiation therapy

The potential advantages of neoadjuvant radiation therapy include increased resectability, decreased tumor seeding at the time of surgery, and that enhanced blood flow to the tumor may enhance radiosensitivity by increasing free radical formation. Neoadjuvant radiation therapy has not been shown to improve the overall survival of patients with resectable disease. However, the use of neoadjuvant radiation has largely been supplanted with the use of neoadjuvant concurrent chemoradiotherapy, as discussed later.

Postoperative adjuvant radiation therapy provides the advantages of accurate pathological staging and the direction of treatment to areas with a high risk for disease recurrence. Postoperative radiation therapy is often given when the surgical margins are positive or the resection is incomplete. A slightly higher total dose range (4500–5500 cGy) than that administered in the neoadjuvant randomized trials has not yielded a survival advantage [94]. Adjuvant chemoradiation strategies are discussed later in this chapter.

Chemotherapy

Because approximately 30% of patients present with metastatic disease and at least 50% of others present with stage II and III disease, chemotherapy holds promise for the local control of disease, the prevention of distant metastasis, and increased survival. Cisplatin and 5-fluorouracil (5-FU) have been used as a standard regimen, and they have produced response rates of 35–40% in advanced disease with a median survival of 33 weeks and a 1-year survival rate of 38% [95]. Other active agents are mitomycin, bleomycin, taxanes (paclitaxel and docetaxel), irinotecan, gemcitabine, oxaliplatin, and anthracyclines such as doxorubicin and epirubicin.

Neoadjuvant (preoperative) chemotherapy

The rationale of neoadjuvant chemotherapy is to eradicate occult metastases before surgery and also to enhance the resectability of the primary tumor. Data from a large (802 patients), randomized, well-controlled study of neoadjuvant chemotherapy in esophageal SCC conducted by the UK Medical Research Council (MRC) upper gastrointestinal tract cancer group demonstrated that preoperative chemotherapy with 5-FU and cisplatin improved relapse rates, overall survival, and cure rate [96]. Patients with esophageal cancer, 67% of whom had adenocarcinoma and 33% of whom had SCC, were randomized to neoadjuvant chemotherapy before surgery or to surgery alone. Resectability was significantly higher in the treatment arm (78% vs 70%; $p < 0.001$), as was overall survival ($p = 0.003$). Two-year survival rates were 43% in the neoadjuvant chemotherapy arm compared with 34% in the surgery-alone arm. Overall survival was superior in patients who received preoperative chemotherapy (hazard ratio, 0.79; $p = 0.0004$). There was no increase in postoperative complications in patients receiving preoperative chemotherapy (40–41%). These findings have established preoperative chemotherapy as a standard treatment in the United Kingdom and in much of Europe. New data from neoadjuvant chemoradiotherapy from the Dutch CROSS trial (see later *Neoadjuvant chemoradiation therapy* section) are leading to increased adoption of chemoradiotherapy before surgical resection, especially in patients with SCC given greater responses of neoadjuvant chemoradiation in SCC compared with adenocarcinoma in the CROSS study.

Adjuvant (postoperative) chemotherapy

A trial to evaluate the efficacy of postoperative chemotherapy in resectable lesions showed an advantage in disease-free survival in the treatment arm ($p = 0.05$), but there was no overall survival benefit [97]. The MRC Adjuvant Gastric Infusional Chemotherapy (MAGIC) trial was designed to determine whether perioperative chemotherapy (given both before and after surgery) could improve outcomes in patients with resectable gastric and distal esophageal adenocarcinomas. In total, 503 patients with operable disease were randomized to receive either three cycles of epirubicin, cisplatin, and 5-FU before and after surgery or surgery alone [98]. The resected tumors were significantly smaller and less advanced in patients who received perioperative chemotherapy. The perioperative chemotherapy patients also had higher overall survival, with a 5-year survival rate of 36.3% versus 23.0% ($p = 0.009$), and a statistically significant improved progression-free survival ($p < 0.001$). Postoperative complications and mortality were similar between the two groups. The applicability of these results to esophageal SCC is unknown. A metaanalysis of patients treated with adjuvant chemotherapy or surgery alone for esophageal SCC revealed disease-free survival benefits at 1 year across patients, but by 3 years these benefits were limited to those with more advanced disease [99]. The field of adjuvant chemotherapy is now being furthered by the use of emerging tests of tumor-derived circulating DNA, the finding of which has been demonstrated to be a marker of risk for recurrence when seen postoperatively in esophageal cancer [100]. The combination of markers such as circulating DNA to identify patients with greatest risk for recurrence and the greater potential tolerability of adjuvant therapy with better surgical managements opens new opportunities to study introduction of adjuvant therapy to improve on survival rates. Moreover, ongoing studies are also exploring the potential for adjuvant immune checkpoint inhibitors to be integrated into therapy to minimize risk for recurrence postoperatively.

Primary chemoradiation therapy

Cisplatin and 5-FU combined with radiation therapy can substantially improve 5-year survival in patients with esophageal cancer compared with radiation alone. Cisplatin and 5-FU are radiosensitizers and improve the response to radiation therapy. Definitive primary chemoradiation therapy for locoregional esophageal carcinoma is increasingly considered an alternative to neoadjuvant therapy followed by surgical resection, especially in patients with an endoscopic complete response to preoperative therapy and those whose age or comorbidities add greater risk to surgical resection. The largest single-institution trial of primary chemoradiation was conducted in 57 patients with stage T1 and T2 esophageal cancer [99]. These patients were treated with 6000 Gy radiation and two cycles of 5-FU delivered as a continuous 4-day infusion during the first and fifth week of radiation therapy, and a single bolus of mitomycin C on day 2. The median survival was 18 months, and 3-year and 5-year survival rates were 29% and 18%, respectively [101]. One study from France, FFCD 9102, randomized patients with esophageal cancer to neoadjuvant chemoradiation, with those patients with at least partial response to therapy then randomized to surgery or additional chemoradiation. Survival was not significantly improved with surgery, but there was a reduction in locoregional recurrence and complications due to local disease progression with surgery [102]. Although definitive chemoradiation is increasingly viewed as an option, trimodality therapy with surgery in optimal candidates is typically preferred given reduced rates of local control after attempted definitive treatment with dual-modality chemoradiotherapy. Notably, PET scans performed after chemoradiation have not been clearly shown to mark those with response to therapy, indicating the importance of endoscopic evaluation [103] for those being considered for potential definitive therapy.

A phase III multiple-institution randomized trial (RTOG 85-01) compared combination therapy with radiation therapy alone [90]. Patients randomized to combination therapy received a total dose of 5000 cGy radiation and 5-FU for 4 consecutive days and cisplatin on day 1 in weeks 1, 5, 8, and 11. Patients in the radiation-alone group were given a total dose of 6400 cGy. This trial was stopped early after an interim analysis demonstrated a survival advantage for patients in the combination therapy group. The 5-year survival rate for patients who had chemoradiation was 26% versus 0% for those receiving radiation only ($p < 0.001$), with a median survival of 14.1 versus 9.3 months, respectively. There was no statistical difference in survival related to histology of the cancer (adenocarcinoma vs SCC). The support for avoiding surgery based on this regimen was tempered by the observation of 46% incidence rate of locally recurrent disease after chemoradiation. No further benefit but more treatment-related death was shown in a later study (RTOG 94-05) using a higher dose of radiation (6480 cGy) and the same chemotherapy regimen [104].

Neoadjuvant chemoradiation therapy

Data from several nonrandomized studies suggest that neoadjuvant therapy with chemotherapy (5-FU and cisplatin) plus radiation before surgery yielded complete response rates of 24–42%, with a median survival of 12–23 months [94,95]. The Dutch CROSS trials randomized patients with esophageal cancer (mostly adenocarcinoma) to preoperative paclitaxel/carboplatin in conjunction with external beam radiation (41.4 Gy) followed by surgery or to radiation alone [105]. The combined treatment group had a higher rate of R0 resection, 92% versus 69%, and also was observed to have an improved overall survival, with median survival of 49.4 versus 24 months. An US study, CALGB 9781, also conducted to address the question of trimodality therapy versus surgery alone, was limited by low accrual [106]. However, the results were consistent with that of the CROSS trial with a trend toward increased survival with the multimodality therapy. Some newer studies are investigating the potential to enhance neoadjuvant chemoradiation with a phase of higher-dose induction chemotherapy. However, definitive data supporting this approach are still lacking.

Another trial, in a Chinese population of resectable thoracic esophageal SCC, demonstrated superiority of radiation concurrent with vinorelbine and cisplatin compared with surgery alone [107]. This regimen has not been compared directly with the CROSS regimen, which has become adopted largely in the western world. Pending potential improvements to neoadjuvant chemoradiation include the integration of novel immune checkpoint inhibitors. Ongoing clinical studies are investigating the addition of these agents.

Adjuvant chemoradiation therapy

Medical and radiation oncologists also have administered combined modality chemoradiation therapy postoperatively to patients with esophageal cancer, based on the proven benefit observed in other gastrointestinal malignancies, such as rectal cancer. However, chemoradiation is more commonly given before surgery; when neoadjuvant chemoradiotherapy with cisplatin and 5-FU was compared with postoperative treatment in a Japanese study of patients with advanced stages of esophageal SCC, improved survival was observed with the neoadjuvant approach [108].

Palliative treatment

Local disease

Because fewer than 50% of patients are candidates for a curative approach after careful staging and preoperative assessment of comorbid disease, palliative approaches are essential [109]. Total esophagectomy is fraught with high mortality rates in palliative situations, and thus endoscopic stents should be considered for those patients with a limited expected survival. External beam radiation therapy (with or without chemotherapy) may be suitable for annular or nearly obstructive lesions, but radiation-induced esophagitis may be problematic. Lower doses may be an option. Brachytherapy should be considered for relief of symptoms (see earlier *Brachytherapy* section).

Endoscopic esophageal interventions with various techniques, including endoscopic dilation, self-expanding metal stents, and ablative methods, such as laser therapy, can be used to relieve malignant strictures, which are mostly associated with low serious complication rates. Endoscopic dilation is not usually done alone because of the transience of the relief of dysphagia and need for repeated procedures, but rather in combination with other endoscopic palliations, including laser therapy. The insertion of self-expandable metal stents has largely replaced conventional plastic stents as a more definitive option to maintain patency with sustained symptomatic improvement. A covered metal stent is also considered to be an effective nonsurgical tool in the management of malignant tracheoesophageal fistulas. Potential stent-related complications include retrosternal pain, recurrent dysphagia, and esophagopulmonary fistulas. Among endoscopic ablative approaches, laser therapy, mainly Nd:YAG laser, and brachytherapy are available as alternative or complementary modalities to palliative stent therapy with comparable efficacy and safety to expandable metal stenting.

Metastatic disease

For distant metastatic disease, systemic chemotherapy is the main modality for palliative care. Although there is no standard first-line therapy, the combination of 5-FU and cisplatin has long been accepted but is now often being replaced by combinations of a fluoropyrimidine with oxaliplatin given the greater tolerability relative to cisplatin. With additional agents, such as paclitaxel, docetaxel, gemcitabine, irinotecan, and oxaliplatin, response rates have improved to 50–60% and median survival has increased to 10–14 months, with gains in quality of life [110,111]. The combination of epirubicin, cisplatin, and 5-FU has been considered a standard treatment for esophageal and gastric adenocarcinoma in Europe. Other fluoropyrimidines are often used in place of 5-FU, including the oral agent capecitabine. As mentioned earlier, oxaliplatin is used instead of cisplatin as a component of combination therapy; a regimen of oxaliplatin with epirubicin and capecitabine is at least equivalent to cisplatin with epirubicin and capecitabine [110]. An emerging understanding of the molecular characteristics of cell growth, the cell cycle, apoptosis, angiogenesis, and signaling pathways has provided novel targets in cancer therapy, including for esophageal cancer. Genomic biomarkers will likely be used to select the most appropriate therapy in individual patients in the future.

Beyond chemotherapy and targeted therapies, immune checkpoint inhibitors have now entered routine use in the care of patients with metastatic esophageal SCC. Pembrolizumab, a PD-1 directed antibody, was approved in 2019 by the US Food and Drug Administration for treatment in locally advanced or metastatic esophageal SCC with positive expression of the marker PD-L1 (as defined by a combined positive score of ≥10) after progression to one or more lines of prior systemic therapy. This approval followed the Keynote-181 study, where patients were randomized to pembrolizumab or empiric chemotherapy on progression [112]. Among 167 patients with PD-L1$^+$ SCC, response rates were 22% with Keytruda compared with 7% with cytotoxic therapy.

Prognostic factors

The chances of curative surgical resection are optimal for lesions less than 5 cm, confined to the mucosa, and without lymph node involvement. For those patients who achieve a pathological complete response to neoadjuvant chemotherapy, long-term survival is significantly improved.

Molecular markers may have prognostic value. Increased cyclin D1 expression and reduced E-cadherin expression portend a less favorable outcome [113]. A high serum vascular endothelial growth factor concentration has been associated with tumor progression, poor treatment response, and poor survival in patients with SCC [114]. Patients with higher serum levels of C-reactive protein have a poorer response to chemoradiotherapy and worse overall disease-free survival rates [115]. It has also been suggested that high expression of BAX and p16INK4a are associated with a favorable prognosis, and that loss of the RB protein is correlated with poor prognosis [116]. Clinically, patients should abstain from tobacco and alcohol consumption during treatment for better outcomes.

The extent of disease is an important prognostic factor. After resection, negative surgical margins are important for improving prognosis; conversely, the development of distant metastasis during treatment portends a poor prognosis. The type of operation is not an independent prognostic factor. Identification of micrometastatic disease in lymph nodes of patients with esophageal cancer may permit stratification to better or worse survival. Moreover, emerging applications of circulating tumor DNA will likely increasingly guide assessment of risk for recurrence and inform use of adjuvant therapies in the coming years.

Complications

The average survival of untreated patients with advanced, symptomatic cancer is less than 1 year. Patients may experience aspiration pneumonia or other complications, including extension into the tracheobronchial tree and other mediastinal structures. Fistulas most often communicate with the trachea, the main stem bronchi, and the lung parenchyma and carry a poor prognosis. They are manifest as cough, chest pain, dyspnea, hoarseness, and hemoptysis. Direct extension of the esophageal cancer, as opposed to fistula formation, may involve the lung and tracheobronchial tree, aorta, pericardium, and upper abdomen. Hoarseness suggests recurrent laryngeal nerve involvement. Apart from direct extension or fistula formation, esophageal cancer can metastasize to lymph nodes, lung, and liver as frequent sites.

Prevention

Screening

Screening of the general population may have merit in high-incidence areas, such as northern China. Although balloon cytology has achieved success in China, its application in US veterans has not proved successful [117]. The reasons were the low prevalence of esophageal cancer and the low specificity of dysplasia because of confounding factors such as inflammation resulting from reflux esophagitis. Follow-up measures included biannual endoscopy with vital staining and biopsy, balloon cytology, laryngoscopy, and chest radiography. However, most positive results found in screened patients proved to be "false positives." Institution of screening and surveillance endoscopic programs may be applied to certain clinical situations, such as in patients with head and neck SCC.

Ingestible esophageal capsule endoscopy and transnasal endoscopy

An office-based noninvasive diagnostic approach has been developed as an alternative to conventional endoscopy or other screening techniques to evaluate patients with esophageal abnormalities, especially those with Barrett esophagus, gastroesophageal reflux disease, and esophageal varices. A small plastic capsule with a tiny video camera glides down the esophageal tract taking video images and transmitting these to a recording device. The disposable capsule passes through the gastrointestinal tract, usually within 24 hours. This approach is not as effective as direct endoscopy for evolving or advanced esophageal SCC [118]. Other approaches to less invasive endoscopy have included the use of unsedated transnasal endoscopy.

References are available at www.yamadagastro.com/textbook7e

Further reading

Chaber-Ciopinska A., Kirprian D., Kawecki A., Kaminski A. Surveillance of patients at high-risk of squamous cell esophageal cancer. Best Pract Res Clin Gastroenterol 2016;30:893e900.

Chow T.L., Lee D.T., Choi C.Y., et al. Prediction of simultaneous esophageal lesions in head and neck squamous cell carcinoma: a multivariate analysis. Arch Otolaryngol Head Neck Surg 2009;135:882.

Cunningham D., Allum W.H., Stenning S.P., et al. Perioperative chemotherapy versus surgery alone for resectable gastroesophageal cancer. N Engl J Med 2006;355:11.

Hardefeldt H.A., Cox M.R., Eslick G.D. Association between human papillomavirus (HPV) and oesophageal squamous cell carcinoma: a meta-analysis. Epidemiol Infect 2014;142:1119.

Heresbach D., Leray E., D'Halluin P.N., et al. Diagnostic accuracy of esophageal capsule endoscopy versus conventional upper digestive endoscopy for suspected esophageal squamous cell carcinoma. Endoscopy 2010;42:93.

Liu X., Wang X., Lin S., et al. Dietary patterns and oesophageal squamous cell carcinoma: a systematic review and meta-analysis. Br J Cancer 2014;110:2785.

Napier K.J., Scheerer M., Misra S. Esophageal cancer: a review of epidemiology, pathogenesis, staging workup and treatment modalities. World J Gastrointest Oncol 2014;6:112.

Karthik Ravi K., Chamil Codipilly D., Sunjaya D., et al. Esophageal lichen planus is associated with a significant increase in risk of squamous cell carcinoma. Clin Gastroenterol Hepatol 2019;17:1902.

Kijima T., Nakagawa H., Shimonosono M., et al. Three-dimensional organoids reveal therapy resistance of esophageal and oropharyngeal squamous cell carcinoma cells. Cell Mol Gastroenterol Hepatol 2018;7:73.

Song Y., Li L., Ou Y., et al. Identification of genomic alterations in oesophageal squamous cell cancer. Nature 2014;509:91.

Stairs D.B., Bayne L.J., Rhoades B., et al. Deletion of p120-catenin results in a tumor microenvironment with inflammation and cancer that establishes it as a tumor suppressor gene. Cancer Cell 2011;19:470.

Tepper J., Krasna M.J., Niedzwiecki D., et al. Phase III trial of trimodality therapy with cisplatin, fluorouracil, radiotherapy, and surgery compared with surgery alone for esophageal cancer: CALGB 9781. J Clin Oncol 2008;26:1086.

Van Hagen P., Hulshof M.C., Van Lanschot J.J., et al. Preoperative chemoradiotherapy for esophageal or junctional cancer. N Engl J Med 2012;366:2074.

CHAPTER 48

Miscellaneous diseases of the esophagus: foreign bodies, physical injury, and systemic and dermatological diseases

Craig C. Reed, Evan S. Dellon, and Nicholas J. Shaheen
Department of Medicine, Division of Gastroenterology and Hepatology, School of Medicine, University of North Carolina, Chapel Hill, NC, USA

Chapter menu

Introduction

The esophagus is susceptible to a variety of environmental exposures and the effects of systemic and dermatological diseases. This chapter discusses causes of esophageal pathology not addressed elsewhere in the textbook. Although some of these diseases and disorders are rare, their timely recognition, in many cases, improves patients' outcomes.

Esophageal trauma

Mallory–Weiss syndrome (see Chapter 38)

In 1929, Mallory and Weiss described a syndrome in alcoholics of retching and emesis preceding massive, and sometimes fatal, upper gastrointestinal (GI) hemorrhage caused by linear lacerations at the gastroesophageal junction [1]. In subsequent retrospective series, Mallory–Weiss syndrome accounts for 5–15% of cases of upper GI bleeding [2,3]. These mucosal lacerations are generally 3–20 mm long, 2–3 mm wide, and parallel to the long axis of the esophagus (Figure 48.1) [4].

Vomiting, retching, and coughing abruptly raise intraabdominal pressure, which likely represents the major pathogenic mechanism of a Mallory–Weiss tear. Accordingly, tears have been putatively ascribed to ingestion of ipecac syrup or administration of chemotherapeutic agents, diabetic ketoacidosis, seizures, hiccups, blunt trauma, straining at defecation, asthma exacerbations, heavy lifting, cardiopulmonary resuscitation, primal scream therapy, after abrupt changes in air pressure, and as a complication of carbon monoxide poisoning [2,5–8]. Rarely, tears have been reported during upper endoscopy in patients with excessive retching during the procedure (less than 0.5% of all endoscopies) [9–12]. Hiatal hernia is an established risk factor for Mallory–Weiss syndrome [4,13–15], though some authors have disputed this association [16].

The "classic" presentation of a Mallory–Weiss tear is repeated, violent retching, vomiting, or coughing preceding hematemesis. However, the presentation is often atypical, with 40% of patients exhibiting no antecedent explanation for the tear, and 50% of patients having hematemesis with the first episode of emesis [2,4]. The mean age at presentation is in the fifth decade, but the syndrome can occur at any age [4,17]. Male patients are affected more frequently than females (4:1) [2,4]. Twenty-seven percent of patients have multiple lacerations, and up to 77% have other associated upper GI lesions [2,3]. Though bleeding stops spontaneously in up to 90% of patients, blood transfusion may be needed

Yamada's Textbook of Gastroenterology, Seventh Edition. Edited by Timothy C. Wang, Michael Camilleri, Benjamin Lebwohl, Anna S. Lok, William J. Sandborn, Kenneth K. Wang, and Gary D. Wu.

Companion website: www.yamadagastro.com/textbook7e

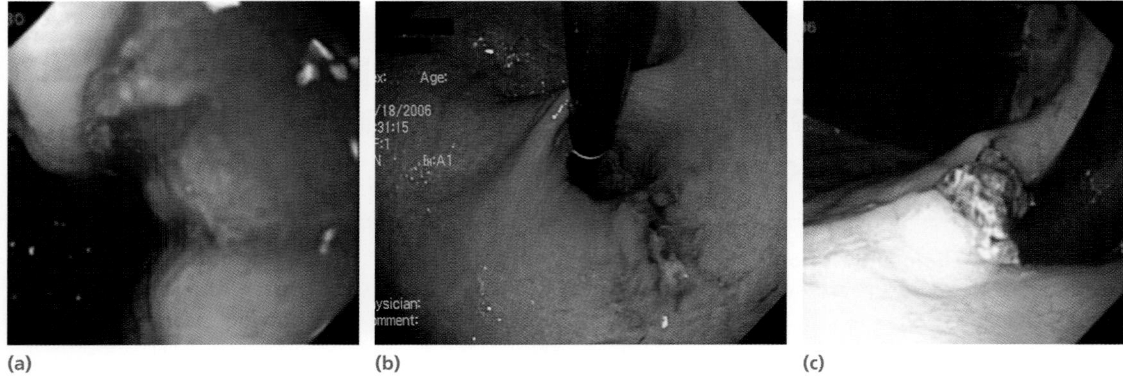

Figure 48.1 Examples of different morphologies of Mallory–Weiss tears in three different patients, seen in antegrade (a) and retroflexed (b, c) views in the proximity of the gastroesophageal junction.

and mortality may be as high as 12% [2,3]. Patients with portal hypertension and coagulation defects are at increased risk of bleeding from Mallory–Weiss tears [3,18]. Presentation with shock or ongoing active bleeding predicts recurrent bleeding episodes, and advanced age, low hemoglobin, elevated aspartate aminotransferase (AST), and melena have been independently associated with increased mortality [19,20].

Treatment is recommended only for lesions with active bleeding or stigmata of bleeding [21]. Scoring systems can stratify patients into high- and low-risk groups to determine the need for urgent endoscopic evaluation [22]. The injection of anhydrous ethanol, polidocanol, or 1:10 000 epinephrine, cautery with multipolar coagulation or heater probe, endoscopic band ligation, and application of hemoclips can achieve endoscopic hemostasis [2,23–32]. Endoscopic injection of epinephrine and polidocanol may reduce recurrent bleeding and decrease length of hospital stay [33]. Angiographic embolization may treat Mallory–Weiss tears though typically following inadequate hemostasis with endoscopic methods [34,35]. Surgery may be required in rare instances when bleeding cannot be controlled by the aforementioned means [2].

Esophageal perforation and rupture

Injury to the esophagus resulting in perforation or rupture is life threatening, and successful management depends on early diagnosis and prompt intervention [36]. The most common cause of esophageal perforation, accounting for about half of cases, is medical instrumentation, including rigid and flexible endoscopy [37–39]. Therapeutic endoscopic stricture dilation by bougie or balloon carries a perforation risk, and in the treatment of achalasia with pneumatic dilation the perforation rate can be as high as 3–4% [40–47]. Perforation has also been reported following nasogastric tube placement, inflation of a gastric variceal tamponade balloon in the esophagus, sclerotherapy, insertion of an intragastric balloon for weight loss, transesophageal echocardiography, and atrial fibrillation ablation procedures most commonly by radiofrequency energy catheter ablation [39,48–53]. In addition to medical instrumentation, penetrating injury from knife and gunshot wounds or sword swallowing, as well as blunt trauma to the neck, chest, and upper abdomen, may cause esophageal perforation [54–56]. The degree of blunt trauma may vary from grave, as in blast and crush injuries, to less severe, as in assault or the Heimlich maneuver [57–62]. Esophageal perforation may also be attributed to foreign body ingestion [63,64], and in rare instances, may manifest following esophageal infection [65].

In 1724, Herman Boerhaave described the spontaneous transmural rupture of the esophagus in a patient, Baron von Wassenauer, who died suddenly after severe retching [66]. Ninety percent of spontaneous ruptures, or Boerhaave syndrome, occur in the distal esophagus, with more than two-thirds on the left side. This is likely due to an anatomical weakness of the left posterolateral aspect of the esophagus just above the diaphragm [67,68]. The typical description involves a bout of vomiting after a copious meal, sometimes by an alcoholic patient [69]. Most patients have antecedent retching and vomiting, although any maneuver that suddenly increases the intraabdominal pressure may result in rupture [67,70]. Interestingly, some patients with Boerhaave syndrome lack a muscularis mucosae, which may predispose them to rupture [71]. Boerhaave syndrome is also an unusual but severe initial presentation for eosinophilic esophagitis [72–74].

Chest pain, dysphagia, odynophagia, nausea, vomiting, hoarseness, or aphonia can be seen in an upper esophageal perforation, whereas lower esophageal perforations manifest with abdominal pain, pneumothorax or hydropneumothorax, or pneumomediastinum. Hematemesis is rarely severe, but occurs in 55% of patients [39,67,70,71,75,76]. Of note, iatrogenic perforations often may remain asymptomatic for up to 8 h [39].

Physical examination reveals tachypnea, tachycardia, and sometimes fever. Subcutaneous emphysema is present in at least 30% of patients [77]. If present, Hamman's sign (a mediastinal "crunch" appreciated with each heartbeat with patients in the left lateral decubitus position) suggests pneumomediastinum. With pleural involvement, there may be reduced or absent breath sounds on the side of the perforation. Signs of tension pneumothorax, hypotension, or shock are indicative of sudden massive esophageal rupture [78–80].

Early diagnosis and treatment are mandatory to avoid the high mortality rate (25–75%) associated with presentation beyond 24 h from the rupture [76,79,81,82]. Misdiagnosis or treatment delay occurs in more than 50% of patients [80,83]. After obtaining a history and performing the physical examination, radiographs of the chest and abdomen should be acquired. There is a range of findings, including subcutaneous emphysema, pneumomediastinum, mediastinal widening, pleural effusion, among others [67,70]. A completely normal chest radiograph is present in fewer than 5% of patients [81].

The next step in evaluation is to perform an esophagram with water-soluble contrast; multidirectional views are diagnostic in most cases, and barium should be avoided on the initial study as it can contaminate the mediastinum if there is a perforation [39,67,70]. If this cannot be obtained, a noncontrast computed tomography (CT) scan may identify small quantities of air or oral contrast in the pleural space, and provides views of the mediastinum, pleura, and aorta [70,84]. Unfortunately, it does not always allow for localization of the perforation [85]. Flexible upper endoscopy is highly accurate and has been advocated with suspected blunt or penetrating esophageal trauma, but does present the risk of extending the perforation [86].

Until the patient develops fever, mediastinitis, pleural effusion, empyema, or sepsis, the diagnosis may be obscure. If examined, the pleural fluid is exudative, and due to leakage of gastric acid, esophageal rupture is one of the few conditions that can be associated with a pleural fluid pH as low as 6.0 [87]. Because the pleural fluid is salivary in origin, the pleural fluid amylase may be elevated [88]. A wide range of community and nosocomial organisms can cause empyema in this setting [89,90].

No gold standard management paradigm exists, and as such, management relies upon individualizing therapy. Factors influencing treatment decisions include the location, timing, and etiology of the perforation in addition to the hemodynamic status of the patient and associated contamination of normally sterile spaces [91,92]. Historically, open surgical repair was thought mandatory for both spontaneous rupture and traumatic perforation [82,93]. However, advances in stent and endoscopic closure devices have made nonoperative management a more tenable approach, particularly in iatrogenic settings [94–98].

Initially, all patients should take nothing by mouth (NPO), and broad-spectrum antibiotics should be administered. Small perforations of the cervical esophagus can be treated conservatively with antibiotics and without surgery, or with localized drainage of the neck without esophageal repair [99,100]. Intrathoracic perforations, especially when associated with hemodynamic instability, noncontained leaks, and respiratory compromise [91,92], must be treated aggressively with debridement and irrigation of the mediastinum, followed by primary closure of the defect [101]. With early intervention, the mortality is less than 10%, but this rate triples if surgery is delayed for more than 24 h [37,82,102]. Yet even in patients with a delayed diagnosis, primary esophageal repair remains the treatment of choice [37,101,103–105]. Esophagectomy is typically performed only when the diagnosis has been significantly delayed such that severe infection has developed [45,106]. Patients with perforation caused by endoscopy with dilation tend to have a good prognosis due to prompt diagnosis and treatment [107].

In carefully selected patients, minimally invasive interventions are increasingly utilized. This includes thoracoscopic and endoscopic repair. Novel endoscopic techniques such as through-the-scope hemoclips [108–112], removable, self-expanding plastic or fully covered metal stents [94–98], over-the-scope clips [113,114], and endoscopic suturing devices have all been advocated for the closure of esophageal perforations in the right clinical setting [115,116].

Esophageal intramural hematomas

Esophageal intramural hematomas are rare and usually produced by local trauma [117–119]. They occur in the setting of vomiting or retching, although spontaneous [117–124] and iatrogenic hematomas [125–133] occur.

Patients typically present with an abrupt onset of substernal or epigastric pain followed by hematemesis. Hemorrhage is usually of small volume, though up to 10% of patients require blood transfusion [117,134]. Dysphagia and odynophagia are common, and in some cases the esophagus can be completely obstructed [123,125,134–136].

Chest radiographs to rule out perforations should be obtained in patients presenting with hematemesis and substernal chest pain. If negative, an esophagram with a water-soluble contrast agent should follow [135]; the most common abnormality is a filling defect [137]. On endoscopy, a bluish or violet esophageal mass protruding into the lumen may be found, sometimes associated with a mucosal tear [118,138,139]. CT with contrast or magnetic resonance imaging (MRI) can reveal a nonenhancing esophageal mass with the density of blood [120,122,139,140]. Endoscopic ultrasound shows an intramural submucosal hypoechoic mass [139].

Most patients respond to conservative management with complete resolution in 2–3 weeks [124,129,134]. However, the development of fever or a pleural effusion may indicate an esophageal perforation not detected during initial evaluation [129,137]. Endoscopic incision and drainage of esophageal hematomas has been described [141,142], as has treatment with angiography and embolization [143]. Surgery, whether open or through a thoracoscopic approach [144], is needed in 19% of cases to control bleeding or to repair perforations [134].

Esophageal foreign bodies

Epidemiology

Multiple objects can become lodged in the esophagus, and this varies by age group [145]. Adults at particularly high risk for EFBI include denture wearers and edentulous individuals, prisoners, the mentally impaired, substance abusers, and psychiatric patients [145–151]. The annual incidence of food impaction in adults is approximately 13 episodes/100 000 people [152–154].

Food, particularly meat and bones, is the most common source of esophageal foreign body impactions (EFBI) in adults. In children, most cases occur between the ages of 6 months and 6 years, and small objects such as coins, toys, crayons, buttons, and batteries are commonly ingested [145–148,150,155,156].

Pathogenesis

Foreign body impaction can occur in areas of anatomical esophageal narrowing, such as the cervical esophagus, aortic arch, and gastroesophageal junction [150]. However, adults with food impaction often have an underlying esophageal anatomical, structural, or motility disorder such as a peptic stricture or Schatzki ring, web, hiatal hernia, esophageal cancer, or achalasia (Figure 48.2) [147,157]. Moreover, a sizeable proportion may have eosinophilic esophagitis, and this condition is now the most common cause of EFBI in patients presenting to the emergency room (see Chapter 44) [154,158].

Presentation

Dysphagia is the most common symptom. If the esophagus is obstructed, odynophagia, choking, or drooling can be present [159]. The latter symptoms may be the only clue in young children or adults who cannot communicate. In children with foreign objects lodged proximally, 5–15% may present with respiratory symptoms [146].

Complications depend on the type of impacted object, and more frequently occur with large, irregularly shaped, or sharp objects [150]. If a foreign body perforates the esophagus, mediastinitis can result in abscess formation, requiring drainage [63,64]. Fistulization to surrounding vasculature such as the aorta or innominate artery may lead to life-threatening hemorrhage [160–162]. Equally serious consequences can also occur with fistulization to the airway or pericardium [163,164]. Disk batteries pose a unique threat as leakage of alkali causes direct tissue damage, potentially leading to perforation or fistulization [165,166].

Diagnosis

Neck swelling, erythema, tenderness, or crepitus from subcutaneous emphysema suggests proximal perforation. Imaging can confirm the diagnosis prior to an invasive procedure. Neck and chest radiographs show radiopaque foreign objects, and, in the case of esophageal perforation, subcutaneous air [149,167,168]. Both anteroposterior and lateral views are indicated to properly identify and locate radiopaque objects potentially obscured by orientation or shadowing from the vertebral column [169]. Contrast esophagrams should be avoided when obstruction is suspected due to the risk of aspiration. Moreover, barium may coat both the foreign body and esophagus, hampering localization, endoscopy, and removal. Gastrografin is a transparent contrast agent but may cause severe pneumonitis if aspirated [150]. Metal detectors can detect metallic foreign bodies [162,170]. Point-of-care ultrasound may be a viable option for detecting EFBI in children [171,172].

Treatment

Flexible endoscopy represents the mainstay of therapy with a success rate up to 98% with low morbidity [145,150,157,173–176]. Rigid laryngoscopy may be required for EFBI in the high cervical esophagus or pharynx [147]. Blind bougienage carries a significant perforation risk and is not recommended [149]. The risks of aspiration and airway obstruction should be minimized, and elective endotracheal intubation prior to endoscopic intervention should be considered.

Disk batteries, sharp objects, and objects lodged in the proximal esophagus require immediate intervention [150,177]. Cases of complete esophageal obstruction where patients have difficulty handling secretions should also be dealt with urgently [145,149,177]. It is safe to observe coins in the distal esophagus for up to 24 h. [178]. If such an object moves into the stomach, it typically progresses through the remainder of the GI tract without incident [179]. Because of the increased risk of progressive mucosal damage, aspiration, and prolonged odynophagia, frankly impacted objects should not be allowed to remain in the esophagus for more than 24 h even if they are nonobstructing [149,153].

Nonendoscopic medical treatments are generally of limited value in EFBI. Glucagon, given in a 1 mg intravenous bolus, can relax the esophagus to allow spontaneous passage of a food

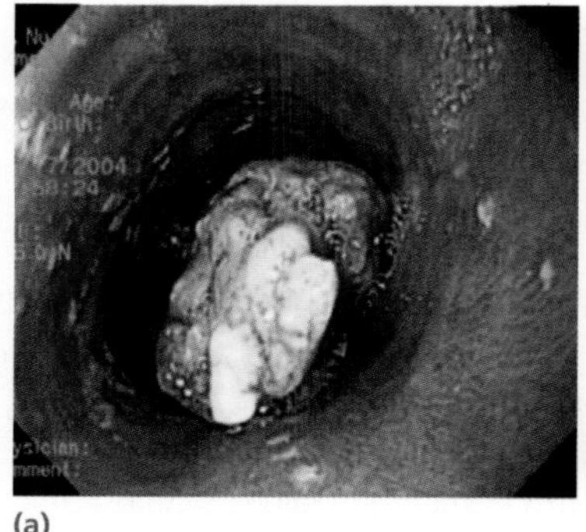
(a)

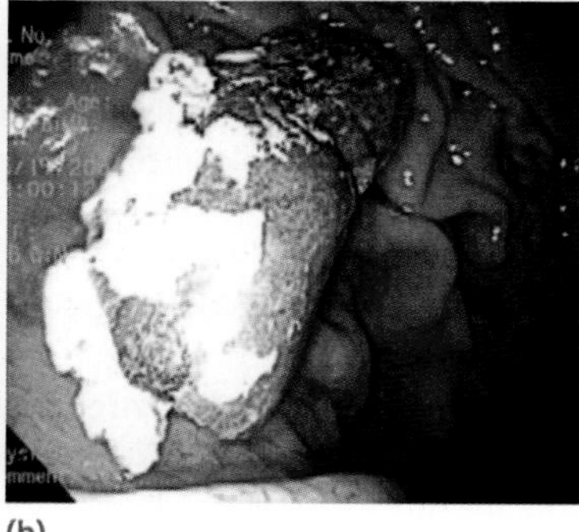
(b)

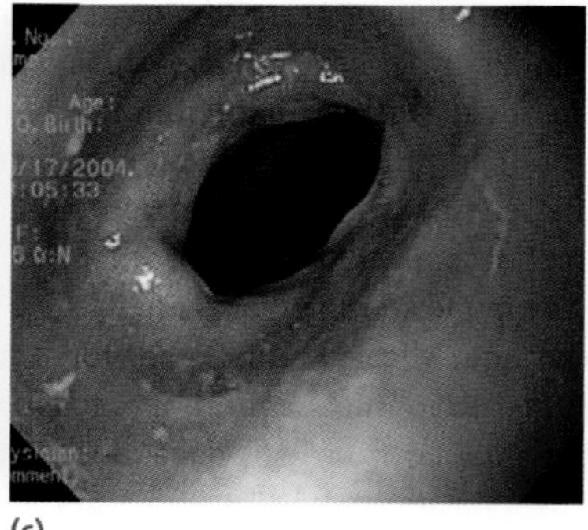
(c)

Figure 48.2 Food impaction in the distal esophagus **(a)** which is cleared by gently advancing the bolus under direct endoscopic vision into the stomach **(b)**. A reexamination of the esophagus reveals a Schatzki ring as the underlying cause **(c)**.

bolus or foreign body, though is often not successful [157,180–182]. Recent systematic reviews and metaanalyses suggest that glucagon may be no more effective than placebo [183,184]. Effervescent agents are also of limited efficacy, carry a perforation risk, interfere with subsequent endoscopy, and are therefore not recommended [185]. The use of enzymatic digestion of a meat bolus (with papain or other meat tenderizer) is also not recommended; both perforation and death have been reported [186,187]. Even if a patient experiences medication-assisted passage of an object, subsequent esophageal examination is recommended to determine whether an underlying cause of mechanical obstruction exists.

A number of endoscopic instruments, including snares, nets, and multiple varieties of grasping forceps, are available to facilitate removal of an esophageal foreign body (Figure 48.3) [188,189]. Prior to the procedure, a practice session with a similar object can identify the appropriate endoscopic tool(s) for the removal and increase proficiency [177]. An esophageal overtube can potentially protect the airway [190], though this increases the risk of perforation, and therefore it should be used cautiously [191].

Coins can be removed with a grasping forceps, net, or retrieval basket, depending on the coin's size and shape [178,192]. Special care should be taken when traversing the upper esophageal sphincter with a coin to prevent loss into the trachea. Round objects, including disk batteries, are also amenable to retrieval in a net [188]. If a small (<2.0 cm), smooth object cannot be securely grasped in the esophagus under direct visualization, advancement into the stomach where there is more room to maneuver may facilitate removal. Sharp objects, however, are best removed where they lie with retrieval forceps or a polypectomy snare [188]. Orienting a sharp object with its point trailing during extraction can minimize mucosal injury, as does fitting a protector hood to the end of the endoscope [149,193,194].

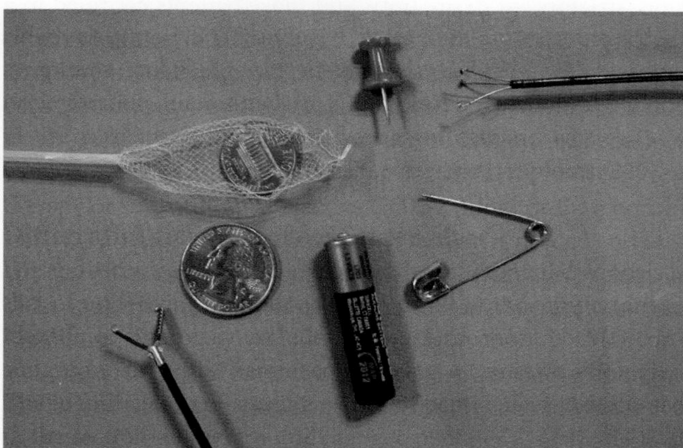

Figure 48.3 An example of the array of devices available for foreign body removal. From top left and proceeding clockwise, a Roth net (with a captured penny), a three-pronged grasping forceps, and a rat-tooth forceps are pictured. Objects that can potentially be impacted in the esophagus are shown for size comparison.

Techniques for clearing a food impaction are similar. A bolus can often be gently advanced into the stomach under direct visualization with the tip of the endoscope, which is safe in most cases [152,195]. Alternatively, the food bolus can be removed (or debulked) with snares, baskets, or forceps. An esophageal overtube can be helpful to facilitate repeated passage of the endoscope during piecemeal removal of a food bolus, and to prevent stray food particles from dropping into the airway [149,177]. A friction-fit adaptor, such as a cap, can be placed on the end of the endoscope as a suction device [196].

After clearing an esophageal foreign body, the endoscopist must still assess for underlying structural abnormalities. If an esophageal stricture is found, it can be biopsied or dilated, provided severe esophagitis is not present [145,152,158,195]. Eosinophilic esophagitis is an important cause of EFBI, and esophageal biopsies at the time of the therapeutic procedure should be considered to diagnose this disorder [197].

Surgery is rarely needed to remove an impacted object or food bolus, and should be reserved for instances when endoscopic management has failed. Other potential indications for surgery include when an object is embedded in the esophageal wall, extraction carries a high risk of perforation, if a perforation has already occurred, or if endoscopic removal of the object poses additional risk of systemic effects, such as in the case of ingested packets of illicit drugs [145,149,161,177].

Pill esophagitis

Epidemiology

Pill esophagitis, also known as drug-related esophageal injury, is widely reported in the literature. Though many medications have been implicated in hundreds of cases (Box 48.1), the majority are caused by tetracycline-class antibiotics, potassium chloride, nonsteroidal antiinflammatory drugs (NSAIDs), and quinidine [198–200]. The overall incidence of pill esophagitis has been estimated at 0.004% per year, but ranges from 0.04% for alendronate to as high as 20% for NSAIDs [200–203].

Elderly patients are at increased risk for pill esophagitis due to frequent use of high-risk medications, decreased salivation, and a higher prevalence of esophageal dysmotility [199,200]. Similarly, women are more likely to be treated with high-risk medications and are twice as likely as men to have pill esophagitis [199,200,204].

Pathogenesis

Prolonged direct contact of a caustic medication with the esophageal mucosa may cause pill esophagitis [200,205,206]. This is particularly typical of quinidine, potassium, and bisphosphonates [202]. Tetracycline and ferrous sulfate, in contrast, injure the esophageal epithelium as a result of local pH changes or hyperosmolarity [207]. NSAIDs appear to be absorbed by the esophageal mucosa and cause injury from within, potentially due to prostaglandin inhibition [203].

Box 48.1 Selected medications implicated in pill esophagitis.

Antibiotics

- Tetracycline
- Tetracycline derivatives (doxycycline, erythromycin)
- Penicillin
- Penicillin derivatives (amoxicillin, ampicillin)
- Trimethoprim
- Clindamycin
- Rifampin
- Zidovudine
- Zalcitabine
- Telithromycin

Nonsteroidal antiinflammatory drugs

- Aspirin
- Ibuprofen
- Naproxen
- Many others in class (indomethacin, diclofenac, etc.)

Other drugs

- Bisphosphonates (alendronate, pamidronate, etidronate)
- Potassium chloride and potassium citrate
- Quinidine
- Emepronium
- Ascorbic acid
- Papain
- Isotretinoin
- Theophyllines
- Oxybutynin
- Iron preparations (ferrous sulfate)
- Captopril
- Nifedipine
- Diltiazem
- Warfarin
- Valproic acid
- Phenytoin
- Phenobarbital
- Cromolyn sodium
- Chloral hydrate
- Alprenolol
- Corticosteroids
- Kayexalate

Data from [198,200,208].

The middle and distal regions of the esophagus are at highest risk for injury. Extrinsic compression by the left atrium or aortic arch may slow transit and increase contact time with the medication in the middle region of the esophagus. In the distal esophagus, concomitant acid reflux may worsen pill esophagitis [209].

Presentation

Pain and odynophagia are the hallmarks of pill esophagitis, which may be severe enough to inhibit adequate oral intake [207]. Retrosternal chest pain is also a frequent complaint. Dysphagia is less common and usually related to edema and ulceration rather than stricture. Rarely, patients may present with hematemesis or perforation [199].

Diagnosis

Upper endoscopy typically demonstrates erosions or ulcers, usually in the middle or distal third of the esophagus, which are often circular or oval in nature. Rarely, the culprit medication is still in place (Figure 48.4). Focal epithelial damage, which spares the majority of the distal esophagus, is nearly pathognomonic of pill esophagitis, and effectively excludes reflux esophagitis. "Kissing" ulcers, or ulcers at the same level of the esophagus but on adjacent walls, can also be seen [210]. If a stricture is found, it more likely is the cause, rather than a result, of the esophagitis, and may be responsible for delayed transit of a pill. Finally, though nonspecific, barium esophagram can show discrete ulcers in the middle or distal esophagus [211,212]. Histological findings are inadequately sensitive or specific to establish the diagnosis [213].

Treatment

Pill esophagitis may be prevented with patient education. Patients should ingest medications in an upright position with at least 100 mL of fluid, and remain upright for 30 min after ingestion. If possible, patients with known esophageal compression, stricture, or dysmotility, and those patients confined to a bed should avoid medications frequently associated with esophageal injury [199].

Most mucosal lesions heal within days to weeks of withdrawal of the offending agent [198,200]. Occasionally, patients may have such severe symptoms that intravenous fluids or dietary modifications are needed. Antisecretory therapy is usually prescribed to protect the esophageal mucosa from further injury related to reflux of gastric contents [200]. Similarly, agents that provide a protective coating over the esophagus, such as sucralfate, may be of benefit.

Corrosive esophagitis

Epidemiology

Corrosive esophagitis is caused by ingestion of caustic agents, in particular those with a pH higher than 12 or less than 2. More

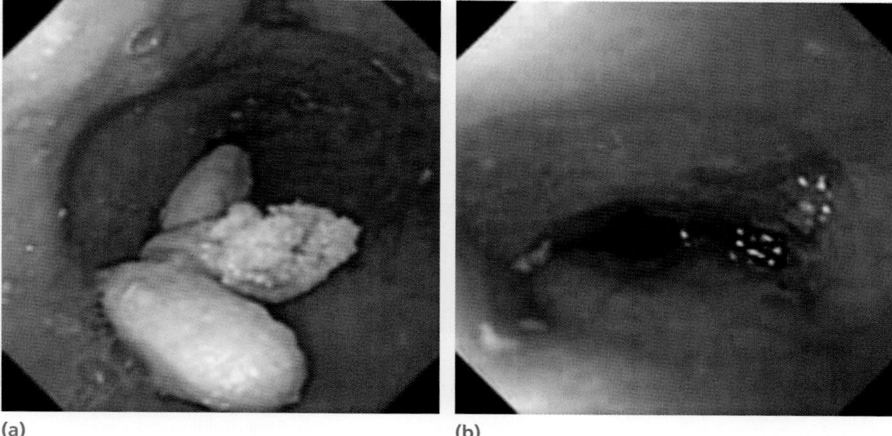

Figure 48.4 Three pills (one partially dissolved) lodged in the midesophagus with nearby erosions **(a)**. After removal of the tablets, pill esophagitis and an underlying esophageal stricture are evident **(b)**.

than 26 000 patients ingest corrosive substances in the United States each year, approximately 17 000 of whom are children (half are less than 4 years of age) [214]. Most corrosive esophagitis in children occurs between 1 and 3 years of age [215,216]. The majority of caustic ingestions involve alkaline agents such as drain cleaners, but strong acids and chlorine bleach are also common [215,217]. Long-term esophageal complications occur in one quarter to one half of caustic ingestions, and ingestion of corrosive substances remains a leading cause of pediatric death [214,215,218].

Caustic esophageal injury dramatically increases the risk factor for esophageal squamous cell carcinoma. One study found that this malignancy may be a thousand times more common in patients after caustic injury than in the general population [219,220], even though the mean time between ingestion and cancer is 50 years [214,221]. This association has prompted the recommendation for yearly endoscopic surveillance beginning 15–20 years after caustic esophageal injury [222].

Pathogenesis

The ingestion of corrosive substances directly injures the esophagus. The liquefactive necrosis of alkaline caustic injury produces a deeper depth of injury than acidic substances [214,223]. The pH required for esophageal damage is 12.5, but the severity is dependent on both concentration and mucosal contact time [214].

The formulation of corrosive agents is also important. Granular corrosives may cause less esophageal injury than liquids, because the granules adhere to the mucous membranes of the mouth rather than being carried into the esophagus [224,225].

Presentation

Presentation partly depends on the time preceding ingestion and evaluation. Symptoms include abdominal pain, retrosternal chest pain, dysphagia, nausea, vomiting, and odynophagia and may last days to weeks [226]. Children may present with feeding refusal or increased salivation.

The most common long-term consequences of severe or circumferential caustic ingestion injuries are esophageal strictures [216,226]. These strictures are long and narrow, adversely affect distal esophageal peristalsis, and cause dysphagia or food impaction [227]. Strictures and subsequent dysmotility may also lead to decreased clearance of refluxate, esophagitis, and peptic stricture.

Diagnosis

An accurate history usually suggests the diagnosis but upper endoscopy is often utilized to confirm the diagnosis and grade the severity of the injury (Figure 48.5) [214,223,224]. A grading system for the endoscopic classification of caustic esophageal injury has been developed, which helps to determine the prognosis and optimal management (Table 48.1) [228]. While the majority of patients with grade 2b and 3 corrosive injury develop strictures and complications, those with grade 0–2a injuries generally do not [228,229]. Imaging modalities may also be helpful in the diagnostic evaluation; plain abdominal or chest radiographs can show evidence of pleural fluid, mediastinitis, or frank perforation. If an esophageal perforation is found, upper endoscopy is relatively contraindicated. Barium swallow may demonstrate esophagitis, gastric abnormalities, or poor distension of the esophagus [230–232].

Treatment

Once a corrosive injury has occurred, there is no role for inducing emesis, lavaging the esophagus, or using a "neutralizing" agent because these modalities have the potential to cause further mucosal damage [214]. If there is any sign of severe oral or pharyngeal injury, there may be a need for urgent endotracheal intubation.

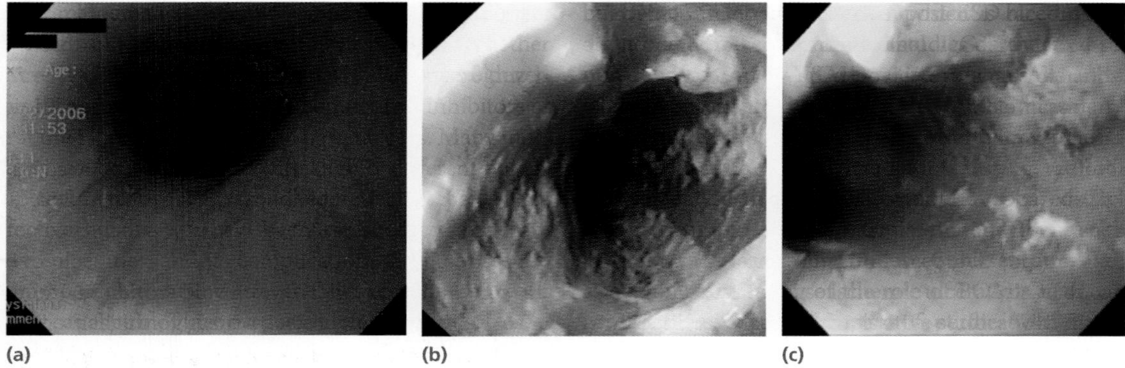

Figure 48.5 Examples of caustic esophageal injury in three pediatric patients after ingestion of a household alkali cleaning agent. Grade 1 injury is manifest by mucosal erythema **(a)** while grade 2 injury results in sloughing of the mucosa with ulceration **(b, c)**.

Table 48.1 Grading system for endoscopic classification of corrosive esophagitis.

Grade	Description
0	Normal
1	Superficial mucosal edema and erythema
2	Mucosal and submucosal ulcerations
2a	Superficial ulcerations, erosions, exudates
2b	Deep discrete or circumferential ulcerations
3	Transmural ulcerations with necrosis
3b	Focal necrosis
3c	Extensive necrosis
4	Perforations

Source: Data from Zargar et al. 1991 [228].

Though frequently recommended, the use of corticosteroids is controversial [233,234]. While some retrospective studies suggest lower stricture rates in patients treated with steroids [233], systematic reviews have shown no benefit in patients with grade 2 or 3 burns [235–237]. Routine steroid treatment for corrosive esophagitis is not currently recommended.

The timing of resumption of oral feeding is not well established, but some recommend keeping patients NPO for at least 1 week in cases of severe esophageal burns [238,239]. Finally, given that concomitant reflux may also contribute to stricture formation, it is reasonable to prescribe antisecretory agents such as proton pump inhibitors [240,241]. A nasogastric tube, placed carefully during initial endoscopic evaluation, can allow for "esophageal rest" and early enteral feeding, prevent complete stricturing, and may facilitate future dilation procedures [242,243]. However, some authors argue that nasogastric tubes may worsen gastroesophageal reflux and interfere with mucosal healing. Moreover, nasogastric tubes should not be inserted blindly due to the risk of further esophageal injury or perforation [244].

When strictures secondary to caustic esophagitis occur, endoscopic dilation is effective more than 50% of the time [245,246]. Topical mitomycin-C (an antifibrotic agent) has also been used for recalcitrant caustic strictures with some success [247–252]. Additionally, the use of fully covered, self-expandable metal and plastic stents has been described for the treatment of refractory caustic strictures [253,254]. Patients with severe corrosive injury complicated by perforation or those with dilation-refractory strictures require esophagectomy. If the stomach is uninvolved, a gastric conduit can be used (e.g., Ivor Lewis procedure) [255]. Alternatively, colonic interposition grafts have been utilized in this situation [256–258].

Acute esophageal necrosis

Epidemiology

Acute esophageal necrosis (AEN) or "black esophagus" is a rare disorder characterized by acute circumferential necrosis of the esophagus in the absence of antecedent corrosive ingestion [259]. The epidemiology of this disorder is poorly understood due to its rarity [260], though endoscopic series report a prevalence of 0.0–0.2% [259–262]. The condition is typically found in the elderly, though cases in younger patients are seen, with a male predominance [260,262]. The majority of patients with AEN have suspected predisposing comorbidities and/or a concurrent critical illness [259,260,262].

Pathogenesis

The pathogenesis of AEN is incompletely understood. Ischemia likely plays a central role, as evidenced by histological findings and that cases of AEN have been reported with concurrent shock and ischemic conditions [263,264]. In most reports, a clear predisposing factor or associated condition has been reported with AEN: antibiotic exposure, gastric outlet obstruction, gastric volvulus, esophageal varices, stroke, major surgery, malignancy, infections, hyperglycemia and diabetic ketoacidosis, acute hepatitis, and alcohol and cocaine abuse [260,265–271].

Presentation

Patients with AEN report an abrupt onset of symptoms and may evidence signs of GI bleeding and fever [272,273]. Symptoms of chest pain, epigastric or abdominal pain, dysphagia, and nausea and vomiting may be present [274].

Diagnosis

Endoscopically, the esophagus appears black and friable with exudates (Figure 48.6) [262] erosions, and hemorrhage [275]. The distal esophagus is typically involved, though the discoloration and necrosis do not typically extend beyond the gastroesophageal junction [259,276]. Histology shows diffuse necrosis involving the mucosa and submucosa, and frequently the muscularis propria [259,276].

Treatment

Treatment for AEN primarily consists of supportive care and treatment of the suspected underlying disorder. Patients should be kept NPO, and intravenous proton pump inhibitor therapy is advocated to facilitate mucosal healing [274]. While there are numerous reports of patients recovering from AEN [264,277], there remains a high mortality rate in excess of 30%, which is likely related to the high prevalence of comorbid diseases in affected persons [274,278]. For patients who do survive the initial episode of AEN, there is a risk of stricture formation and dysphagia [279].

Lymphocytic esophagitis

Epidemiology

The increased recognition of eosinophilic esophagitis (see Chapter 44) prompted GI practitioners to obtain esophageal biopsies in patients with unexplained dysphagia and refractory reflux [280–282]. With this, a new clinicopathological entity, entitled lymphocytic esophagitis, emerged [283]. Lymphocytic esophagitis is characterized clinically by esophageal symptoms (e.g., dysphagia, heartburn, or chest pain), and histologically by lymphocyte-predominant esophageal mucosal inflammation in the absence of granulocytes following the exclusion of alternative etiologies of esophageal lymphocytosis (e.g., reflux, esophageal motility disorders, Crohn's disease, candidiasis) [283–287].

The condition is uncommon. In large US and Australian pathology databases, it was seen in less than 0.1% and 0.3% of esophageal biopsies, respectively [285,288]. Moreover, subanalysis of a population-based study of Barrett esophagus found no cases histopathologically consistent with lymphocytic esophagitis in the 1000 subjects enrolled in the study [289]. There is some evidence that the diagnosis is becoming more prevalent [284]. Lymphocytic esophagitis is described more commonly in women (53% in a systematic review) [290], and typically affects patients in the 5th–8th decades of life, although there are reports in children [283–286,290]. Lymphocytic esophagitis may be more common in nonwhite patients, patients who use tobacco, and those with additional lymphocytic disorders of the GI tract [291,292]. The natural history of the disease is unknown. In one study where patients with lymphocytic esophagitis were contacted a median of 3.3 years after diagnosis, nearly all reported persistent GI symptoms, and almost half had visited an emergency room for their GI symptoms in the past 5 years [284]. There is also one case report of lymphocytic esophagitis presenting with an esophageal perforation [293].

Pathogenesis

Few investigations exist into the pathogenesis of lymphocytic esophagitis. The lymphocytic infiltrate has been characterized as containing CD3+ T cells, split between CD4 and CD8 subtypes [283], or as a CD8 predominant infiltrate [285]. The triggers of this immune response have not been identified. Some speculated that lymphocytic esophagitis represents an unusual pathological manifestation of gastroesophageal reflux disease

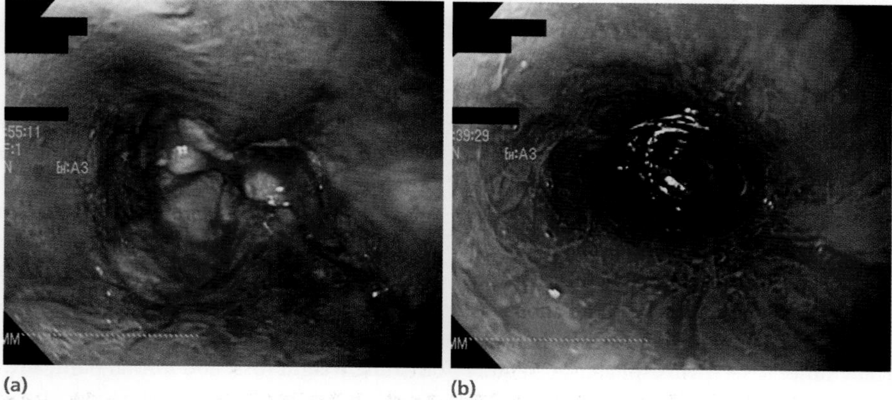

Figure 48.6 Endoscopic appearance of acute esophageal necrosis, with characteristic circumferential blackened **(a)** and friable mucosa with underlying hemorrhagic tissue **(b)** involving the distal esophagus.

(GERD), and not a separate clinical entity [289]. Additionally, a relatively consistent association between Crohn's disease and lymphocytic esophagitis exists [283,284,286,294]. Between 11% and 40% of patients with lymphocytic esophagitis have an inflammatory bowel disease [283,284,286]. In one study of children with Crohn's disease, the converse was also seen: 28% of children with Crohn's disease had evidence of lymphocytic esophagitis on upper endoscopy and biopsy [294]. In a subgroup of these patients, granulomas were also present, suggesting that lymphocytic esophagitis was a manifestation of esophageal Crohn's disease.

At the current time, it remains unclear if the observed association between lymphocytic esophagitis and Crohn's disease is coincidental or whether the two conditions share a common pathogenesis. Similarly, up to 10% of patients with lymphocytic esophagitis have concurrent celiac disease, but the significance of this association is also unclear [283,285].

Presentation

In the four largest case series [283–286], up to 67% of patients reported dysphagia, 18–47% had symptoms related to GERD, approximately half had abdominal pain, and almost one-third had nausea and vomiting. On endoscopy, a range of findings have been reported [283–286]. Though not necessarily always present simultaneously, these include esophageal rings, strictures, furrows, plaques, erosive esophagitis, erythema, and nodularity (Figure 48.7) [285,295]. In a recent systematic review, the most common symptom was dysphagia (49%), and the esophagus was endoscopically normal in a minority (31%) [290].

Diagnosis

No consensus diagnostic criteria for lymphocytic esophagitis exist, but it is felt that similar to eosinophilic esophagitis, lymphocytic esophagitis is a clinicopathological condition requiring clinical symptoms and histological findings for diagnosis following the exclusion of alternative etiologies for lymphocytic inflammation of the esophagus. Haque and Genta found that patients with lymphocytic esophagitis had at least 30 intraepithelial lymphocytes (IELs)/hpf (hpf = 0.237 mm^2, equivalent to a density of 125 IELs/mm^2). They also proposed three pathological features as criteria for diagnosis: (1) dense peripapillary lymphocytic infiltrates; (2) peripapillary spongiosis involving the lower two-thirds of the epithelium; and (3) the absence of significant neutrophil or eosinophilic infiltrates [285]. Determination of a threshold number of lymphocytes for diagnosis has been challenged by the patchy distribution of the disease. As such, the presence of spongiosis and pattern of distribution of lymphocytes may be more important. A recent study suggested that esophageal lymphocytosis may be more common in the middle and proximal esophagus [287]. At the current time, it seems reasonable to require clinical symptoms and the above pathological findings as minimum criteria for the diagnosis of lymphocytic esophagitis, but most likely the diagnostic algorithm will evolve in the future.

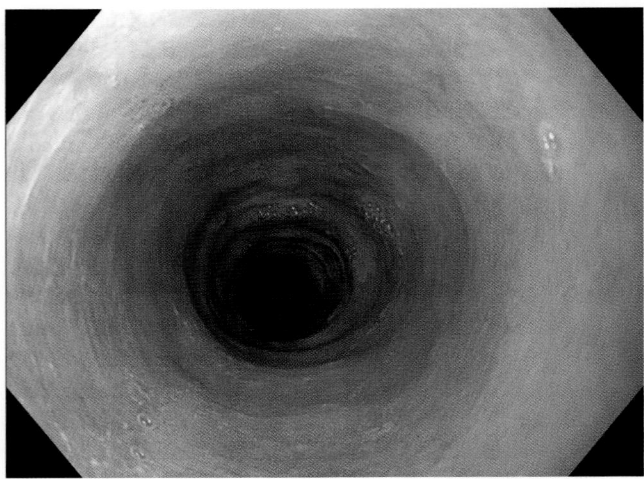

Figure 48.7 Endoscopic image of the proximal esophagus in a patient with lymphocytic esophagitis. Subtle mucosal edema with loss of normal vasculature is present, along with narrowing and mild rings. With these findings, the appearance may be confused with eosinophilic esophagitis. Source: Evan S. Dellon, MD MPH.

Treatment

There are no clinical trial data on treatments for lymphocytic esophagitis, no pharmaceutical agents approved by the United States Food and Drug Administration, and all information comes from retrospective case series. Because lymphocytic inflammation can be seen in reflux and many patients with lymphocytic esophagitis also have GERD-related symptoms, a trial of a proton pump inhibitor or other antireflux therapy is reasonable, and there have been reports of patients responding to these measures [284]. As with eosinophilic esophagitis, topical steroid therapy may be of benefit in this patient population. However, this has been poorly studied and is limited to heterogeneous and small case series and case reports [295–300]. If there is concomitant inflammatory bowel disease, then treatment of the underlying condition can be effective [284]. If esophageal strictures are present, endoscopic dilation can improve the symptoms of obstructive dysphagia [284]. Treatment approaches are expected to change as more is learned about this new condition.

Systemic diseases

Sarcoidosis

Approximately 10% of patients with known sarcoidosis, a systemic granulomatous disease, may have granulomas in the submucosa of their GI tracts, but associated symptoms are rare [301–303]. Dysphagia is the most common clinical manifestation of esophageal sarcoidosis. Less common symptoms include weight loss, abdominal pain, and odynophagia [304]. Perforation and aortoesophageal fistula have also been reported [305,306]. Causes of dysphagia in sarcoidosis include extrinsic compression from enlarged lymph nodes, an achalasia-like dysmotility syndrome, neurosarcoidosis with cranial nerve involvement, and granulomatous stricture formation [304,307–310]. Because granulomas are present in both diseases, esophageal sarcoidosis may be difficult to differentiate from Crohn's disease [310]. Transbronchial ultrasound-guided fine-needle aspirate of enlarged mediastinal lymph nodes often demonstrates granulomas [311].

Medical therapy primarily targets the underlying systemic disease. Dysphagia may respond to steroid treatment, though endoscopic dilation of strictures may be required [308,309]. Esophageal surgery is very rarely needed [309].

Crohn's disease

Esophageal involvement in Crohn's disease is rare. The prevalence of esophageal disease in several series ranges from 0.002% to 2% [312–314]. Moreover, many patients with esophageal involvement are asymptomatic. Of 75 patients with esophageal Crohn's disease in one study, only 55% presented with esophageal symptoms [315]. The prevalence may also be higher in children, though this may be a detection bias, as children undergo upper endoscopy more frequently during the evaluation of Crohn's disease [313,316–318].

Patients with Crohn's esophagitis usually have active disease elsewhere in the GI tract, and the degree of inflammation typically parallels the activity in the other involved segments [319,320]. Rarely, dysphagia alone can be the presenting symptom of Crohn's disease, and isolated esophageal involvement has been reported [319,321–323]. Other symptoms include odynophagia, pyrosis, and substernal chest pain [312,319].

On upper endoscopy, aphthous ulceration can be seen early in the course of the disease, while cobblestoning and deep linear ulcerations may be present later, leading to decreased motility and distensibility (Figure 48.8). Esophageal stricturing and the formation of sinus tracts, fistulas, or mucosal bridges have been reported [319,320,324]. In severe cases, there is perforation and fistulization to the bronchi, mediastinum, pleura, or stomach [313,323,325–327]. For diagnostic purposes, endoscopic mucosal biopsies can evaluate the degree of inflammation, but cannot demonstrate transmural inflammation; granulomas are rarely found [312,319,320]. The transmural nature of the inflammatory process may be better illustrated with endoscopic ultrasound, though this is not routinely used [328,329]. Barium studies may demonstrate aphthous ulcers, radiographically demonstrated as minute pools of retained barium [330].

The tenets of treating Crohn's disease of the esophagus are the same as for the small or large intestine (see Chapter 64), with a focus on controlling systemic inflammation and local complications [313]. Altogether, the literature on medical therapy of Crohn's disease isolated to the esophagus is too scant to allow firm recommendations, and therapy is usually dictated by the involvement of other GI organs. Treatment of the inflammatory component of esophageal Crohn's disease may include topical corticosteroids, systemic corticosteroids, and/or biologic medications [314]. Of patients who respond to corticosteroids or other immunosuppressants, more than half will remain free of both esophageal lesions and upper GI symptoms, while the remainder will have either refractory lesions or recurrence [312,319,320]. Tumor necrosis factor (TNF) antagonists may have value for treating fistulizing disease of the esophagus [331].

Strictures may respond to both medical management and dilation; extensive mucosal bridges may be endoscopically excised with a papillotomy needle knife [324]. In some patients, placement of a percutaneous endoscopic gastrostomy may be needed for malnutrition [332,333]. Surgical resection is reserved for medically refractory fistulas, endoscopically refractory strictures, or when malignancy cannot be excluded [322].

Graft-versus-host disease

Uncommonly, acute graft-versus-host disease (GVHD) involves the esophagus. Esophageal GVHD typically occurs in the

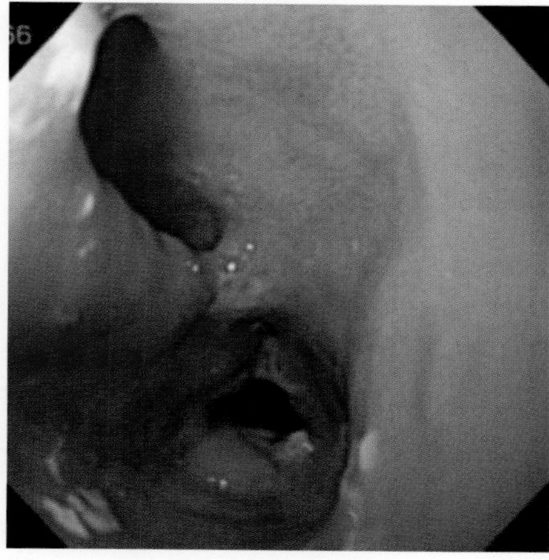
(a)

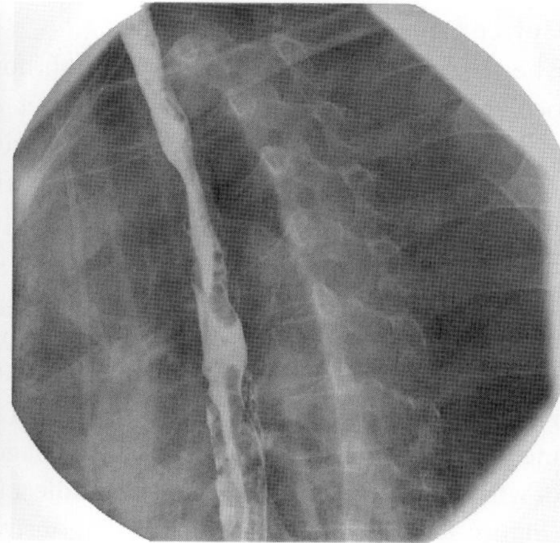
(b)

Figure 48.8 An endoscopic view of Crohn's disease of the esophagus with diffuse esophageal narrowing, a prominent sinus tract, and exudative plaques **(a)**. A barium swallow from the same patient showing esophageal narrowing, mucosal irregularity, ulceration, and nodularity, and sinus tracts parallel to the esophagus **(b)**.

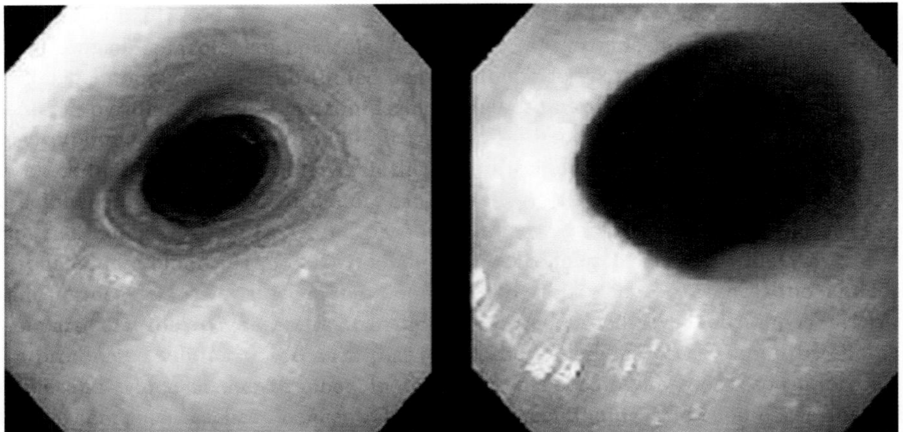

Figure 48.9 An endoscopic view of graft-versus-host disease showing multiple fine mucosal webs in the esophagus.

context of severe multisystem disease involving the upper and lower GI tracts [334–337]. Symptoms of GVHD esophagitis include odynophagia, dysphagia, pyrosis, and retrosternal chest pain.

Upper endoscopy with biopsy and culture is the most sensitive way to differentiate GVHD esophagitis from opportunistic infections such as herpes simplex virus, cytomegalovirus, or *Candida* [338,339]. The esophageal mucosa may appear erythematous and friable, and strictures, webs, bullae, or esophageal casts may be found (Figure 48.9) [334,335,340]. Biopsies to rule out GVHD should be taken regardless of endoscopic appearance, as a sizeable minority of those with GVHD have normal endoscopic appearances [341,342].

Therapy guided by hematologists specializing in bone marrow transplantation utilizes immunosuppressants such as prednisone, azathioprine, cyclosporine, mycophenolate mofetil, and infliximab [333,343,344]. Esophageal symptoms can respond to antireflux medications and to dilation of webs and strictures, although the risk of iatrogenic perforation may be increased in these patients [336].

Behçet syndrome

The constellation of oral and genital aphthous ulceration with ocular inflammation characterizes Behçet syndrome. Behçet syndrome rarely involves the esophagus, with less than 5% of cases demonstrating esophageal abnormalities [345,346]. It is most common in eastern Mediterranean, Middle Eastern, and East Asian populations, primarily affecting young adults [347].

As with other esophageal processes, symptoms can include dysphagia, odynophagia, chest pain, and hematemesis [346]. An association with downhill esophageal varices has been reported [348]. Upper endoscopy can reveal a range of findings including erosions, esophagitis, and esophageal strictures, most of which have been reported in the middle and distal esophagus (Figure 48.10) [349–352]. Biopsies demonstrate ulceration with nonspecific inflammation and neutrophilic infiltration [345].

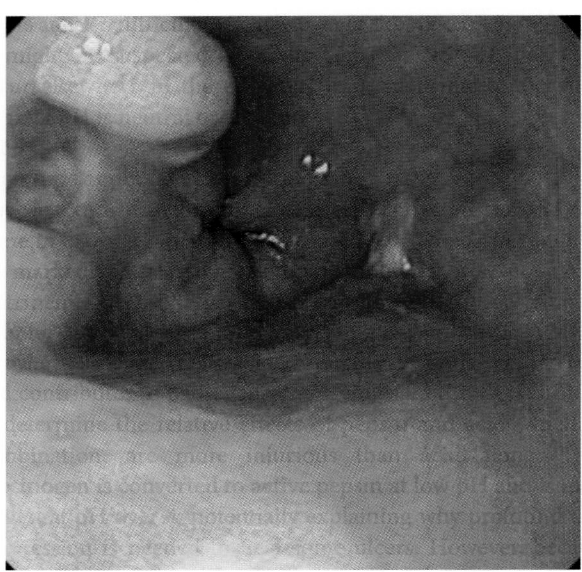

Figure 48.10 Endoscopic view of esophageal Behçet disease, with a small punched-out active ulceration in the distal esophagus. From Yi et al. 2009 [346]. Reproduced with permission from the Journal of Korean Medical Science.

The clinical course is one of unpredictable remissions and exacerbations. While dysphagia caused by esophageal ulcers may resolve spontaneously, corticosteroids have been reported to improve symptoms, and intestinal and esophageal ulcers have also responded to sulfasalazine, antitumor necrosis factor agents, and low-dose cyclosporine [345,347,349,350,353–355].

Miscellaneous autoimmune diseases

More than one-half of patients with *Sjögren syndrome* complain of difficulty swallowing, though the severity of dysphagia does not appear to correlate with the degree of xerostomia [356,357].

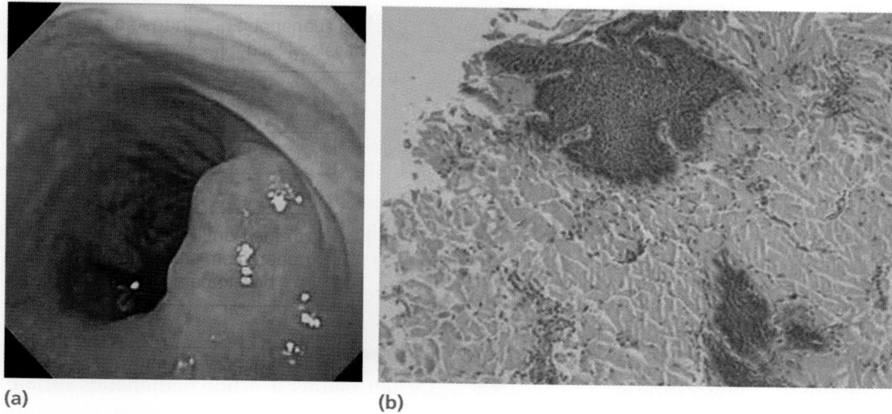

Figure 48.11 Endoscopic view of an amyloidoma in the distal esophagus **(a)** and corresponding histopathology, showing focal eosinophilic amyloid deposition in the esophageal submucsa **(b)**. Source: Kahi et al. 2007 [363]. Reproduced by permission of Nature Publishing Group.

Esophageal webs are responsible for dysphagia in approximately 10% of patients [358]. Several potential etiologies of dysphagia may be diagnosed via esophageal manometry, and heartburn and its severity may be measured by pH probe [359–362].

Primary or secondary *amyloidosis* may cause dysphagia due to amyloid deposition in the esophageal muscle or nerves (Figure 48.11) [363]. The resulting motility abnormalities can mimic achalasia [364–366]. In rare cases, amyloid deposition may predispose to spontaneous esophageal rupture [367].

The *antiphospholipid antibody syndrome* may present with esophageal vascular thrombosis and ischemic esophageal perforation or esophageal varices secondary to portal vein thrombosis [368–370].

Esophageal intramural pseudodiverticulosis is a rare condition first described in 1960 (Figure 48.12) [371,372]. It is benign, more common in men than woman, and may be asymptomatic, though more frequently presents with dysphagia from stricture formation [371,373,374]. Associated diseases seen with esophageal intramural pseudodiverticulosis include HIV, esophageal candidiasis, esophageal motility disorders, and EoE [373–376]. Treatment should include management of associated disorders. Patients may benefit further from treatment aimed at esophageal strictures [373–376].

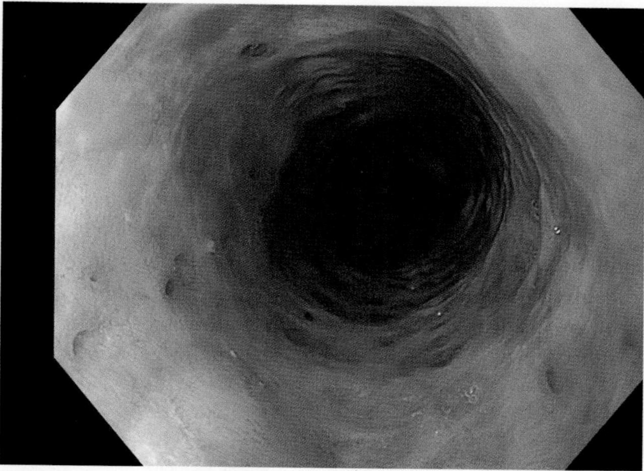

Figure 48.12 Endoscopic image of the proximal esophagus showing esophageal intramural pseudodiverticulosis. Multiple small pseudodiverticuli are noted throughout this segment, which also has a chronic scarred appearance, with mild narrowing and congestion/decrease in vascularity. Source: Evan S. Dellon, MD MPH.

Dermatological diseases

Pemphigus vulgaris

The esophageal mucosa can be affected by diseases of the squamous epithelium of the skin. One example is pemphigus vulgaris, a chronic autoimmune blistering disease of older adults in which flaccid intraepidermal blisters and oral erosions are caused by IgG autoantibodies against desmoglein-3 in keratinocytes [377–379]. Patients may be asymptomatic, but the 50% who have esophageal involvement usually present with dysphagia or food impaction [380–382]. Isolated esophageal involvement without significant skin manifestations has rarely been reported [383–385]. Certain medications are associated with this condition, such as thiol compounds (e.g., penicillamine), angiotensin converting enzyme inhibitors, and antibiotics (e.g., penicillins, rifampin, cephalosporins) [384].

Diagnosis requires upper endoscopy with biopsy [386]. Advances in forceps design may allow for deeper, more diagnostic biopsies in esophageal pemphigus [386]. Immunohistochemistry cannot distinguish idiopathic pemphigus vulgaris from drug-induced or paraneoplastic pemphigus [379,387,388]. Therefore, serological testing for pemphigus antibodies and antidesmoglein-3 antibodies is needed [389]. Corticosteroids are the primary treatment modality in pemphigus vulgaris, though other immunosuppressive drugs may be required to induce a complete remission or withdraw steroids [379,390]. In severe cases, plasmapheresis has been successful [379].

Bullous pemphigoid

In contrast to pemphigus vulgaris, bullous pemphigoid is characterized by tense bullae on the flexor surfaces of the skin [379,391]. The disease is caused by immunoglobulin G (IgG) autoantibodies directed against the basement membrane of squamous epithelium [379,392]. Though 20% of patients have involvement of the oropharynx, the prevalence of esophageal bullous pemphigoid is unknown and may be underestimated given infrequent symptoms [393,394]. Rarely, patients complain of dysphagia and odynophagia. Upper GI hemorrhage, scarring, mucosal sloughing, and hemorrhage are also rare [395]. Treatment with prednisone is highly effective, but azathioprine, cyclophosphamide, cyclosporine, and methotrexate have also been used [379].

Benign mucous membrane pemphigoid

Benign mucous membrane pemphigoid (BMMP), or cicatricial pemphigoid, is a chronic blistering disease of the conjunctivae, oral and genital mucosa, and adjacent areas of skin. In this disease, IgG or immunoglobulin A (IgA) autoantibodies are deposited in the basement membrane zone [379,396–399]. BMMP usually occurs after the sixth decade of life, producing tense blisters with scarring and strictures of the esophagus, trachea, anus, or vagina [400]. Between 2% and 13% of affected patients have esophageal involvement, which can present up to 10 years into the course of disease as dysphagia, odynophagia, or chronic cough due to aspiration [401]. Rarely, patients have isolated esophageal BMMP with no other disease manifestations [402]. On endoscopy, esophageal webs or strictures may be seen (Figure 48.13) [403]. Persistent dysphagia can be treated with dilation, although these patients may be at increased risk of esophageal injury [403,404]. In severe cases, BMMP requires prednisone, whereas milder cases often respond to dapsone [379,405,406]. Surgical treatment of strictures is rarely required [407].

Lichen planus

Lichen planus is a mucocutaneous inflammatory condition of unknown etiology [408]. Most frequently, the skin and oral mucosa are affected though other mucus membranes, including the esophagus, may be involved, and in certain cases, esophageal involvement may be the presenting finding [408–410]. Most afflicted patients are female and diagnosed in their 7th decade of life after presenting for dysphagia [409,411,412]. Endoscopic findings include a friable mucosa, white plaques, webs, and strictures, most commonly within the proximal esophagus [409,411–413]. Histological findings compatible with esophageal lichen planus include a band-like esophageal infiltrate of the superficial lamina propria and basal epithelium as well as Civatte bodies [414,415]. Limited data support the use

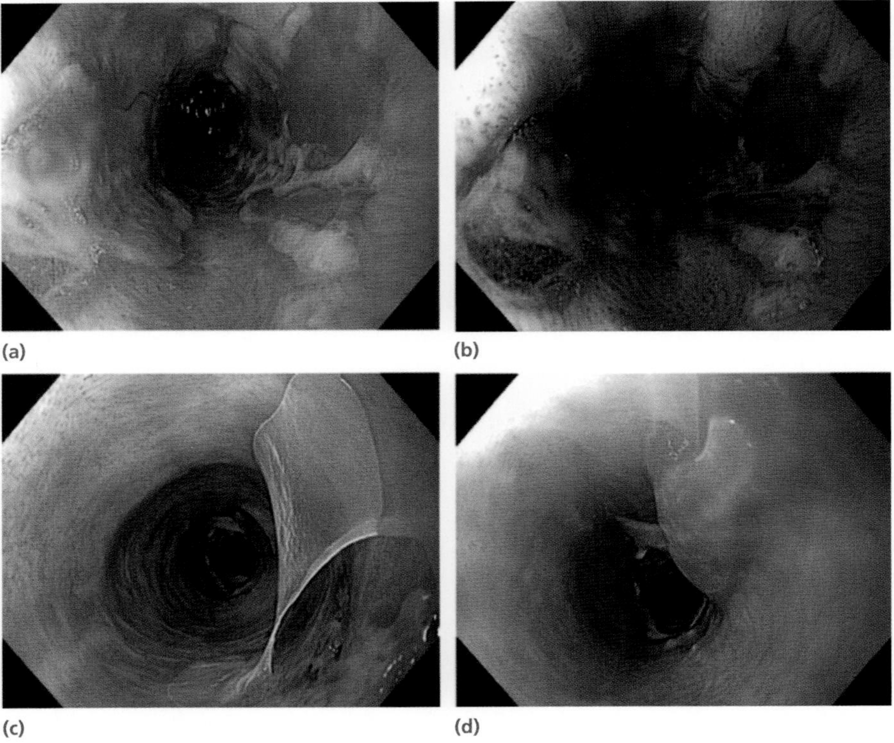

Figure 48.13 Endoscopic view of esophageal involvement of benign mucous membrane pemphigoid, showing erosions and scarring under white light endoscopy **(a)** and narrow band imaging **(b)**, and blister formation after trauma from balloon dilation **(c, d)**. From Tang 2009 [429]. Reproduced by permission of Elsevier.

of systemic corticosteroids, topical corticosteroids, cyclosporine, and tacrolimus [416–418]. Dilation may be required for associated strictures [412,419].

Epidermolysis bullosa dystrophica

A final, and also rare, esophageal manifestation of dermatological disease is epidermolysis bullosa dystrophica (EBD), a blistering disease of the squamous epithelium caused by mutations in the collagen type VII gene (*COL7A1*) [420,421]. Histopathologically, the basal lamina separates from the dermis due to a reduction in or absence of the fibrils normally attaching these two layers [422]. Cutaneous bullae are evident beginning in early childhood and form at sites of minor trauma, especially in the hands and extremities. Over time, the cycle of chronic scarring and healing leads to contractures and syndactyly, a process termed mummification. Both dominant and recessive forms of this inherited disease exist, but esophageal involvement is only clinically important in the recessive form [423,424]. There is also an acquired form of the disease (epidermolysis bullosa acquisita) which causes nonscarring bullous lesions of the esophagus [425,426].

In the esophagus of patients with EBD, trauma from routine swallowing begins a cycle of bullae formation, healing, and scarring, leading to the development of strictures, esophageal shortening, and dysmotility [427,428]. Clinically, these cause symptoms of dysphagia, odynophagia, and food impaction [427,428]. In younger patients, malnourishment is common and parenteral nutrition may be required. The constellation of esophageal symptoms and the prominent cutaneous manifestations suggest the diagnosis of EBD. In uncomplicated cases, the risk of traumatic bullae formation due to endoscopy outweighs the incremental diagnostic yield. If a diagnostic test is needed, barium esophagram can reveal strictures or webs [427,428]. Complications include esophageal perforation and occlusion due to scarring [427,428].

Treatments for EBD are limited, and when the esophagus is involved, the prognosis tends to be poor [428]. From a dietary standpoint, patients should avoid coarse or hot foods and use nutritional supplements to avoid malnutrition. Medical therapies lack efficacy [427,428,430,431]. For endoscopic therapy of strictures, balloon dilators may be preferable to bougienage to avoid damage to friable mucosa, and a preprocedural barium swallow may help plan the procedure by assessing angulation within the stricture [432]. Because dilation carries an increased risk of esophageal trauma and perforation, fluoroscopy may be a valuable adjunct [428,433,434]. In patients with esophageal perforation or malnutrition from refractory esophageal stenosis, esophagectomy and conduit reconstruction may be necessary [428,430,435].

References are available at www.yamadagastro.com/textbook7e

Further reading

Abid S., Mumtaz K., Jafri W.., et al. Pill-induced esophageal injury: endoscopic features and clinical outcomes. Endoscopy 2005;37:740.

ASGE Standards of Practice Committee, Ikenberry S.O., Jue T.L.., et al. Management of ingested foreign bodies and food impactions. Gastrointest Endosc 2011;73:1085.

Aslanian H., Chander B., Robert M.., et al. Prospective evaluation of acute graft-versus-host disease. Dig Dis Sci 2012;57:720.

Contini S., Scarpignato C. Caustic injury of the upper gastrointestinal tract: a comprehensive review. World J Gastroenterol 2013;19:3918.

de Wijkerslooth L.R., Vleggaar F.P., Siersema P.D. Endoscopic management of difficult or recurrent esophageal strictures. Am J Gastroenterol 2011;106:2080.

Dua K.S. Expandable stents for benign esophageal disease. Gastrointest Endosc Clin North Am 2011;21:359.

Gurvits G.E. Black esophagus: acute esophageal necrosis syndrome. World J Gastroenterol 2010;16:3219.

Haque S., Genta R.M. Lymphocytic oesophagitis: clinicopathological aspects of an emerging condition. Gut 2012;61:1108.

Le Cleach L., Chosidow O. Clinical practice. Lichen planus. N Engl J Med 2012;23:723.

Pasricha S., Gupta A., Reed C.C.., et al. Lymphocytic esophagitis: an emerging clinicopathologic disease associated with dysphagia. Dig Dis Sci 2016;61:2935.

Schmidt E., Zillikens D. Pemphigoid diseases. Lancet 2013;381:320.

Sperry S.L., Crockett S.D., Miller C.B.., et al. Esophageal foreign-body impactions: epidemiology, time trends, and the impact of the increasing prevalence of eosinophilic esophagitis. Gastrointest Endosc 2011;74:985.

CHAPTER 49

Peptic ulcer disease

Mohammad Yaghoobi and David Armstrong
Department of Medicine, McMaster University, Hamilton, Ontario, Canada

Chapter menu

Introduction

Peptic ulcers are localized defects of the gastrointestinal (GI) mucosa, most commonly found in the duodenum or stomach (Figure 49.1). Before the discovery of *Helicobacter pylori*, ulcers were attributed to stress, hyperacidity and a variety of host, genetic, and environmental factors; *H. pylori* infection and nonsteroidal antiinflammatory drugs (NSAIDs) are now known to be the major etiologies. Alongside pharmacological acid suppression for immediate ulcer healing [1], the identification and treatment of these underlying causes are the basis of rational management. Interestingly, there has been a steady increase in reports of non-*H. pylori*, non-NSAID ulcers, particularly in developed countries, and although they are still relatively uncommon, their recognition and management are important [2–8]. Worldwide, peptic ulcer disease (PUD) and its complications remain the cause of much suffering and significant mortality. PUD is also a major drain on national resources; in the United States, the annual cost through medication, physician visits, hospitalization, and missed work days has been estimated at nearly US$ 6 billion [9].

Definition

Peptic ulcers are localized defects of the GI mucosa, extending at least to the depth of the muscularis mucosa and affecting one or more sites, simultaneously. Superficial lesions are less likely to result in bleeding or perforation since blood vessels are located deep to the muscularis. An ulcer is identifiable endoscopically as a mucosal break with depth. Ulcers smaller than 5 mm are arbitrarily called erosions although they represent the same underlying disease and the utility of this distinction is therefore debatable.

Ulcer locations

Peptic ulcers are traditionally categorized as gastric ulcers (GU) and duodenal ulcers (DU) (see Figure 49.1) but GUs and DUs can occur concurrently and peptic ulcers can occur elsewhere in the GI tract. Mechanistically, DUs and pyloric and prepyloric GUs are distinct from other GUs (see "Pathogenesis"); however, there are only minor differences in their management. Ulcers may occur at other sites including the distal esophagus, the gastroesophageal junction, sites of GI anastomosis and in ectopic

Yamada's Textbook of Gastroenterology, Seventh Edition. Edited by Timothy C. Wang, Michael Camilleri, Benjamin Lebwohl, Anna S. Lok, William J. Sandborn, Kenneth K. Wang, and Gary D. Wu.

Companion website: www.yamadagastro.com/textbook7e

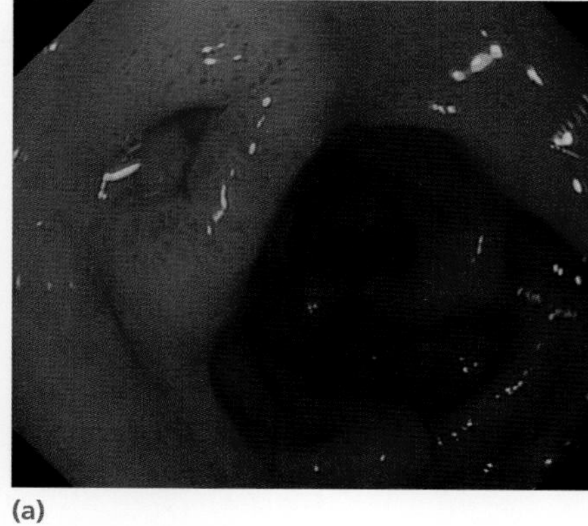

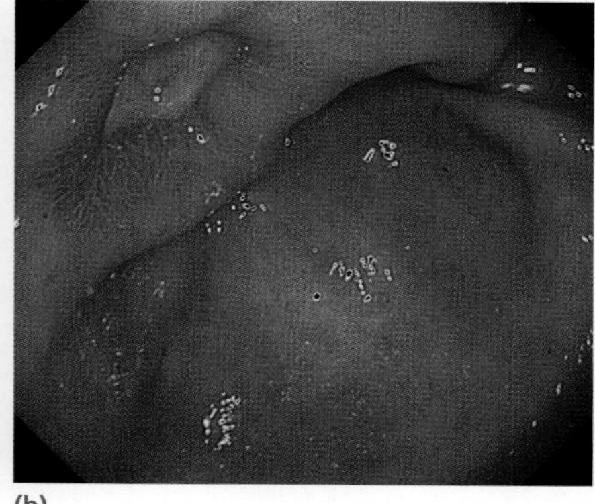

(a) (b)

Figure 49.1 Endoscopic views of duodenal ulcer **(a)** and gastric ulcer **(b)**.

gastric mucosa, most frequently within a Meckel diverticulum or in esophageal inlet patches. These less common ulcers are discussed elsewhere while this chapter concentrates on duodenal and gastric ulceration.

Duodenal ulcers typically occur in the duodenal bulb and are usually attributable to *H. pylori*; if more distal DUs are found, other etiologies, such as NSAIDs or gastrinoma, should be considered. NSAIDs can cause ulceration along the whole GI tract. GUs can occur anywhere in the stomach but are found most frequently in the distal rather than the proximal stomach.

Epidemiology (risk factors)

The epidemiology of PUD has changed markedly over the last century due to changes in the epidemiology of its environmental risk factors, including *H. pylori* and NSAID/aspirin use. The current epidemiology of PUD is directly affected by the different trends in prevalence of these risk factors and, thus it varies between different communities. The incidence and prevalence of PUD are lower in high and very high Human Development Index (HDI) countries but there are marked geographical and regional variations. Age is also important, particularly in relation to hospitalization and mortality. Therefore, to understand the epidemiology of PUD, temporal, demographic, and geographic trends, the relationship with *H. pylori* and NSAID use, and the growing significance of non-*H. pylori*, non-NSAID ulcers will be discussed.

Epidemiology of *H. pylori*-related ulcers

The global prevalence of gastric *H. pylori* infection is about 50% and, once acquired, it persists lifelong if left untreated. The prevalence varies widely by country, age, socioeconomic status, and living conditions (Table 49.1) (10). In many low and medium HDI countries, over 80% of people are infected by early adulthood, most acquiring infection in childhood before 10 years of age. In contrast, *H. pylori* infection in high and very high HDI countries is uncommon in childhood but increases in prevalence with increasing age. In the US, *H. pylori* is now rare before 10 years of age, rising to 10–20% of individuals between 18 and 30 years and to 50–60% in those older than 60 years [11]. A similar relationship between *H. pylori* prevalence and age exists in Japan, with infection in 70–80% born before 1950, 45% born between 1950 and 1960, and 25% born between 1960 and 1970 [12]. These age associations are not due to continuing acquisition of *H. pylori* with aging but rather to a birth cohort effect in which successive cohorts have had a lower risk of childhood infection. For example, in Japan before 1950, 70–80% of children acquired *H. pylori*, which explains why so many elderly Japanese have the infection. In contrast, only 25% of Japanese born between 1960 and 1970 acquired the infection, explaining why it is much less common amongst those aged 40–50 years old.

Helicobacter pylori is most likely spread by fecal–oral or oral–oral transmission although the precise mechanisms and their relative importance require further investigation [13]. There is indirect evidence for a fecal–oral route by finding *H. pylori* in the stool of children with diarrhea as well as in the swimming water in endemic areas. Those who swim in these waters might acquire the infection by ingestion [14–18]. Transmission between family members has been reported and mostly happens between younger children in endemic areas; the importance of this mode of transmission is supported by isolating genetically similar species of *H. pylori* in family members [19]. The evidence for direct oral–oral transmission is lacking apart from the rare isolation of *H. pylori* in dental plaque [20] but in a domestic environment and also in school or kindergarten, *H. pylori* may be transmitted by the vomito-oral route. Transmission through exposure to gastric secretions by healthcare professionals has also been reported and should be considered when disinfecting equipment exposed to human gastric secretions to prevent transmission [21].

Local differences in prevalence exist where there has been substantial immigration from countries with a higher prevalence of infection. Some reports suggest that certain ethnic and racial groups are at increased risk not fully explained by socioeconomic difference, such as Hispanics and African

Table 49.1 *Helicobacter pylori* infection globally.

Region/country	Age group (years)	*H. pylori* prevalence (%)	Region/country	Age group (years)	*H. pylori* prevalence (%)
Africa			South Korea	16	56
Ethiopia	2 to 4	48		≥16	40.6
	6	80	Sri Lanka	6 to 19	67
	Adults	>95		Adults	72
Nigeria	5 to 9	82	Taiwan	9 to 12	11
	Adults	91		13 to 15	12.3
	Adults	70 to 90		≥25	45.1
Central America				Adults	50 to 80
Guatemala	5 to 10	51	*Australasia*		
	Adults	65	Australia	1 to 59	15.4
Mexico	5 to 9	43		Adults	20
	Adults	70 to 90	*Europe*		
North America			(Eastern)	Adults	70
Canada	5 to 18	7.1	(Western)	Adults	30 to 50
	50 to 80	23.1	Albania	16 to 64	70.7
USA and Canada	Adults	30	Bulgaria	1 to 17	61.7
South America			Czech Republic	5 to 100	42.1
Bolivia	5	54	Estonia	25 to 50	60
Brazil	6 to 8	30	Germany	50 to 74	48.8
	10 to 19	78	Iceland	25 to 50	36
	Adults	82	Netherlands	2 to 4	1.2
Chile	3 to 9	36	Serbia	7 to 18	36.4
	Adults	72	Sweden	25 to 50	11
	Adults	70 to 90	Switzerland	18 to 85	11.9, 26.6
Asia			*Middle East*		
Bangladesh	0 to 2	50 to 60	Egypt	3	50
	0 to 4	58		Adults	90
	8 to 9	82	Libya	1 to 9	50
	Adults	>90		10 to 19	84
Hong Kong	6 to 19	13.1		Adults	94
India	0 to 4	22	Saudi Arabia	5 to 9	40
	10 to 19	87	Arabia	Adults	80
	Adults	88	Turkey	6 to 17	64
India, south	30 to 79	80			
Japan, 3 areas	20 to >70	55.4		Adults	80
Japan, western	Adults	70.1			
Siberia	5	30			
	15 to 20	63			
	Adults	85			

Source: Reproduced from Hunt et al. 2011 [10], with permission from Wolters Kluwer Health.

Americans when compared with Caucasians. Twin studies support a role for genetic susceptibility, but also reinforce the importance of childhood environment. In addition, the increased availability and use of antibiotics, particularly in childhood for intercurrent illness, may also have contributed to the continued decline in *H. pylori* prevalence in high and very high HDI countries.

Relationship with peptic ulcer disease

Helicobacter pylori is a major cause of PUD so the variations and changes in *H. pylori* infection are key to understanding PUD epidemiology. About 15–20% of people infected with *H. pylori* will develop peptic ulceration or gastric cancer as a long-term consequence of infection. The risk of these diseases is determined by bacterial virulence, host genetic susceptibility, and immune response (see "Pathogenesis"), and by environmental and other cofactors (see "Risk factors"). The annual incidence and the 1-year point prevalence of PUD in the *H. pylori*-positive group are around 1% and 2% respectively, with an estimated 500 000 new cases annually in the US [22, 23]. The incidence and prevalence of ulcer disease are up to 10-fold higher in *H. pylori*-infected than uninfected individuals [24].

Epidemiology of NSAID-related ulcers

Both NSAIDs and aspirin can cause adverse GI effects including endoscopic erosions and ulcers throughout the digestive tract, including the duodenum and stomach. In the US, 1.2% of the population use nonaspirin NSAIDs on a daily basis [25]. In 2010, about one-fifth of American adults were reported to be taking aspirin regularly and about one-eighth were taking NSAIDs regularly, increases of 57% and 41% respectively compared with 2005, the use of both increasing with age [26]. The estimated point prevalence of gastric erosions is 50–90% in patients taking NSAIDs or low-dose aspirin [27,28] although erosions do not necessarily cause significant clinical consequences. Symptomatic or complicated ulceration occurs in 5% of NSAID users, and is approximately three times more frequent in elderly individuals [29]; duodenal or gastric ulceration has been reported in 12–30% of NSAID users in some other studies [30], with complications developing in 1–2 per 100 patient-years [31]. NSAIDs are responsible for 30% of hospitalizations and deaths from PUD, with older people most at risk [32].

Fortunately, the overall risk of serious GI complications due to NSAIDs is declining, attributed to the use of lower doses, less toxic agents, and co-prescription of antisecretory therapy [33] even though the use of potentially ulcerogenic drugs is increasing.

Selective COX-2 inhibitors cause less gastroduodenal injury than nonselective agents, but despite their initial promise of better outcomes, it became clear that they did not abolish gastroduodenal injury and, furthermore, concerns about cardiovascular safety have resulted in the withdrawal of several COX-2 selective drugs, and those still available are used sparingly (see "Prevention"). Over recent years, NSAID prescriptions have continued to decline due to greater physician awareness regarding the potential adverse events and the need to limit the indications, for example, to use for joint inflammation rather than pain.

Important NSAID-related risk factors for peptic ulcer disease include duration of therapy, with increased complication risk from within the first week, peaking within the first month and then remaining constant to around 3 months [34]; the dose and degree of suppression of prostaglandin synthesis, with greatest risk with drugs of high potency at high doses or with simultaneous use of multiple NSAIDs; and cotherapy with low-dose aspirin, which increases the risk of complications. Although there has been controversy as to whether *H. pylori* infection has an additive effect with NSAIDs in producing ulcers, the most recent evidence suggests a significant and synergistic increase in the risk of uncomplicated PUD [35]. This has resulted in recommending "test and treat" for *H. pylori* before prescribing long-term NSAID therapy. Other risk factors for complications of NSAID-induced PUD are considered later in the chapter but the most important are age greater than 60 years, previous history of ulcer or bleeding, concomitant drug therapies (including glucocorticoids and anticoagulants), and comorbidity [36].

Epidemiology of non-*H. pylori*, non-NSAID idiopathic ulcers

Data on the epidemiology of idiopathic ulcers vary according to how rigorously *H. pylori* infection and exposure to NSAIDs/ aspirin have been excluded but over the last three decades, there has been a steady rise in the relative incidence of *H. pylori*-negative and NSAID/aspirin-negative PUD [37,38]. This is seen particularly in countries where *H. pylori* infection rates are low or declining, though studies do not necessarily support a perfect inverse relationship between the decline in prevalence of *H. pylori* infection and idiopathic ulcers (Table 49.2) (2,5–8,38–47). Cohorts from the same countries and between different ethnic groups have not provided consistent results on point prevalence of idiopathic PUD, partly due to methodological differences in defining these cohorts, with retrospective study designs and suboptimal exclusion of *H. pylori* infection, along with unidentified exposures to NSAIDs including over-the-counter or herbal medications. Some non-*H. pylori*, non-NSAID ulcers may be due to rare established etiologies (Box 49.1), but truly idiopathic ulcers are rare.

Pragmatically, the rising prevalence of non-*H. pylori*, non-NSAID ulcers means that the investigation and management of these patients (at both the individual and population level) are increasingly important considerations.

Risk factors

There are several important risk factors for PUD with various influences depending on the primary underlying etiology: *H. pylori* infection or NSAID use. Cotherapy with other drugs is particularly important in the context of NSAID-related ulcers (see "Prevention"). The roles of emotional stress and psychological factors are controversial. Peptic ulceration is more common in the context of comorbidity and in association with specific diseases.

Table 49.2 Epidemiology of non-*H. pylori*, non-NSAID peptic ulceration.

Prevalence (%)	Country	Source
Broadly low H. pylori prevalence		
1	Spain	Gisbert et al. (1999) [41]
6	Spain	Arroyo et al. (2004) [42]
22	Sweden	Aro et al. (2006) [43]
12	UK	Musumba et al. (2012) [5]
39	USA	Jyotheeswaran et al. (1998) [44]
27	USA	Ciociola et al. (1999) [45]
Broadly high H. pylori prevalence		
17	Hong Kong	Xia et al. (2001) [7]
4 (bleeding PUD)	Hong Kong	Chan et al. (2001) [2]
2	Japan	Tsuji et al. (1999) [46]
1	Japan	Nishikawa et al. (2000) [6]
3	Japan	Aoyama et al. (2000) [47]
22	Korea	Jang et al. (2008) [38]
29	Pakistan	Yakoob et al. (2005) [8]

NSAID, nonsteroidal antiinflammatory drug (including aspirin); PUD, peptic ulcer disease.
Source: Data from [39] and [40].

Box 49.1 Peptic ulcer disease etiologies.

Common causes of peptic ulcer
Helicobacter pylori
NSAIDs including aspirin

Other causes
Peptic
Acid hypersecretion, with hormone- or mediator-induced ulcers
Gastrin
Gastrinoma in Zollinger–Ellison syndrome and MEN1
Antral G-cell hyperfunction (controversial independent of *H. pylori*)
Histamine
Systemic mastocytosis
Basophilia associated with myeloproliferative diseases
Rebound acid secretion after withdrawal of PPI therapy
Nonpeptic
Other infectious agents
Non-*pylori Helicobacters* including *H. heilmannii*
HSV
CMV
EBV
Other rare infectious causes, e.g., streptococcus, tuberculosis, syphilis
Other potentially ulcerogenic drugs
Possibly high doses of acetaminophen (paracetamol) with NSAIDs
Bisphosphonates (especially alendronate)
Colchicine
Clopidogrel and other antiplatelet agents
Glucocorticoids with NSAIDs
Iron tablets
Mycophenolate mofetil
Nicorandil
Potassium chloride
Sirolimus
Spironolactone
SSRIs and venlafaxine
Immunosuppressives including chemotherapy, e.g., hepatic infusion of 5-fluorouracil, some tyrosine kinase inhibitors
Malignancy
Adenocarcinoma
Lymphoma
Other neoplastic conditions, e.g., malignant melanoma, breast cancer, renal cell carcinoma
Inflammatory and infiltrative disease
Crohn's disease
Eosinophilic gastroenteritis
IgG4-positive inflammatory and autoimmune disease
Other uncommon forms, e.g., sarcoidosis, Wegener granulomatosis, Behçet disease
Radiation therapy
Ischemic mechanisms
Critical celiac axis vascular disease
Crack cocaine use
Methamphetamine use
Other uncommon forms of vascular insufficiency, e.g., enterocolic Lymphocytic phlebitis
Mechanical duodenal obstruction, e.g., duodenal webs, pyloric stenosis, annular pancreas, preduodenal portal vein
Ingestion of batteries or magnets
Iatrogenic
Following EMR or ESD, particularly for early gastric cancer postsurgical and postprocedural, e.g., gastroenterostomy, anastomotic ulcer after subtotal gastric resection, laparoscopic fundoplication, migration of surgical clips or embolization microcoils, nonabsorbable suture material

Other forms of peptic ulceration
Idiopathic peptic ulcer, including idiopathic hypersecretory *Hp*-negative duodenal ulcer
Ulceration in the context of comorbidity[a]
Esophageal ulcers related to GERD, e.g., in Barrett esophagus
Region of hiatus hernia where this passes through diaphragmatic hiatus; termed Cameron ulcer
Meckel diverticulum
Other ectopic gastric mucosa, e.g., inlet patch, in gallbladder

Note

[a] Ulceration in the context of comorbidities such as acute multisystem failure, decompensated chronic disease, and specific scenarios (e.g., Cushing ulcer with head injury, Curling ulcer with burns) are considered under "Risk factors."

CMV, cytomegalovirus; EBV, Epstein–Barr virus; EMR, endoscopic mucosal resection; ESD, endoscopic submucosal dissection; GERD, gastroesophageal reflux disease; ***Hp*, *Helicobacter pylori***; HSV, herpes simplex virus; MEN1, multiple endocrine neoplasia type 1; NSAID, nonsteroidal antiinflammatory drug; PPI, proton pump inhibitor; SSRI, serotonin-selective reuptake inhibitor.

Proven risk factors

Patient age is an important risk factor for both major etiologies, with an increased risk of occurrence and complications with age over 75. Cigarette smoking also enhances the risk of both DU and GU in proportion to the amount smoked and is an independent risk factor for development of PUD and more complicated PUD [48–52]. PUD is also harder to treat in smokers [53]. A metaanalysis showed that the attributable risk of smoking for PUD is 23% [54]. This is particularly true for patients with *H. pylori* infection, in whom the risk is considerably increased, though the risk of recurrent DU is not significantly different between smokers and nonsmokers following eradication of *H. pylori* [52,55,56]. A history of PUD or ulcer complications, whether due to *H. pylori* infection or NSAID use, is an important risk factor for further PUD [57]. The influence of family history on risk probably mainly reflects shared *H. pylori* infection within the family unit; whether shared genetic risk also contributes is unclear.

Unproven risk factors

Although ethanol stimulates the secretion of gastrin and gastric acid, it is unlikely that alcohol intake is an important risk factor in the absence of cirrhosis (see "Disease associations") [58–60], though alcohol misuse may impair patient compliance with management [61]. Indeed, alcohol consumption in moderation has been linked with improved ulcer healing [62,63]. Specific diets play no clear role and historical dietary advice to avoid spicy or rich foods is not evidence based – chilli may actually be protective for DU [64]! Similarly, caffeine is not a true risk factor for PUD [59].

Context-dependent risk factors – glucocorticoids and cotherapy with other drugs

Glucocorticoids or other steroids alone impart no significant ulcer risk but there is a synergistic effect leading to an increased ulcer risk if they are used concurrently with NSAIDs, particularly for PUD complicated by bleeding. The relative risk for concomitant therapy is four- to 11-fold above that with NSAIDs alone [36,65]. In this context, there are no data on the benefit of ulcer prevention strategies, such as prophylactic antisecretory therapy or substituting a selective COX-2 inhibitor for a nonselective NSAID. Therefore, the utmost caution is needed and ideally this combination of drugs should not be used, especially in older patients or individuals with other risk factors (see "Prevention").

Concurrent use of other drugs with NSAIDs can also increase the risk of ulcer complications. Aspirin, even at low dose for cardio- and cerebrovascular prophylaxis, increases the risk of NSAID ulcers. Other drugs which increase risk include clopidogrel and other antiplatelet agents, bisphosphonates (especially alendronate), serotonin selective reuptake inhibitors, and anticoagulants (with relative risk of concomitant therapy as much as 13-fold above NSAIDs alone) [36].

Unclear risk factors – psychological factors and stress

There is controversy as to whether psychological risk factors (including stress) are clinically relevant in causing peptic ulceration in the majority of patients. Associations have been explained by other confounding risk factors. Initial efforts to develop a useful biopsychosocial model of PUD [66] have been hampered by the multiplicity of proposed risk factors in the literature, particularly from poorly designed studies that do not account for now well-established pathophysiological factors, nor clearly define psychological stressors and their temporal relationship with ulcer identification.

Recently, some compelling evidence has been presented. Ulcer complications are increased during catastrophic events, first demonstrated during the bombing of London during the Blitz in 1940 and 1941 [67]. The incidence of GUs, particularly bleeding ulcers in older patients, was increased relative to DUs after the Hanshin-Awaji earthquake in Japan in 1995 [68]. More recent prospective studies have shown that the risk of subsequent ulcer occurrence or recurrence is increased compared to controls in cohorts with psychosocial stressors including adverse life events, stress, anxious and depressive symptoms, social problems, and posttraumatic stress disorder [69]. In two more recent observational studies, including a prospective study of a population-based Danish cohort and a population-based, cross-sectional US study, multivariate analysis showed that mental health issues such as severe stress, depressed mood, suicidal ideation, and psychological counseling were associated with a higher prevalence of PUD [70,71]. Overall, the quality of evidence in this area is not high due to the nature of the risk factor and ethical and logistic limitations regarding study design and it is therefore difficult to establish causality; however, it does appear that there is an independent relationship between psychological factors and the risk of developing PUD.

Disease associations and comorbid ulcers

It has long been recognized that comorbidities such as acute multisystem failure and decompensated chronic disease or specific scenarios including organ transplantation may predispose to PUD. However, for chronic diseases associated with lifestyle or social class, disease associations do not prove that there is a mechanistic role in causation; referral, selection, and ascertainment biases may have overstated the importance of the putative causative factors.

Acute multisystem failure and intensive care stress ulcers

Stress-related mucosal disease (ulceration, mucosal erosions) occurs in around three-quarters of patients within a few days of acute major illness (particularly burns or head injury). It is usually found in the proximal stomach, although it can develop at any site. These early ulcers tend to be superficial; in contrast, late stress ulceration that occurs around 2 weeks after admission is typically deeper, and distal or duodenal. Complications are less common for stress ulcers than for other ulcers; overt bleeding, occurring in 1.5–10% of patients in intensive care, is less prevalent than subclinical bleeding confirmed during endoscopy and perforation is rare. The most important risk factors for complications, particularly hemorrhage, are invasive ventilation for over 48 hours (odds ratio [OR] 16) and coagulopathy (OR 4) [72]. Other risk factors largely relate to the severity of the acute illness or multisystem failure. Importantly, bleeding from stress ulcers is associated with increased mortality although this is probably mostly due to comorbid conditions [73].

Prophylactic ulcer prevention therapy with proton pump inhibitors (PPIs) is often prescribed for critically ill patients in intensive care as part of a defined management protocol although the most important aspect of ongoing management is to treat the underlying condition. However, this practice has been challenged because of more recent evidence [74]. Various guidelines on ulcer prophylaxis in intensive care have been developed that seek to balance the baseline and incremental risks, potential harms and efficacy, including the choice of antisecretory agent, availability of the enteral route for nutrition and medication, and cost. A metaanalysis of eight studies showed that coagulopathy (relative effect [RE] 4.76), shock (RE 2.60), and chronic liver disease (RE 7.64) were predictors of clinically significant GI bleeding in ICU patients [75]. The Stress Ulcer Prophylaxis in the Intensive Care Unit (SUP-ICU) trial, a large randomized controlled trial in 1140 ICU patients who had a Simplified Acute Physiology Score (SAPS) II >53, showed a higher mortality in patients receiving prophylactic pantoprazole compared to placebo [76]. The 1-year mortality rate was comparable [(77)]. Therefore, routine prophylactic PPI treatment in ICU patients is not recommended.

Outside the intensive care setting, prophylaxis should be restricted to high-risk patients (see "Prevention" and "Mucosal protection – coprescription of prophylactic agents"). Standardized prescribing guidelines may help to limit overuse of PPIs [74,78] and clear direction to primary care colleagues on the indication for and intended duration of any therapy is advisable [79].

Chronic disease, including COPD and cirrhosis

Chronic lung disease, principally chronic obstructive pulmonary disease (COPD), is associated with both GUs and DUs, which occur in up to 30% of such patients. Chronic lung disease is also 2–3 times as frequent in PUD patients as in the general population [49,80,81]. It is likely that these observed associations are confounded, at least in part, by cigarette smoking. Ulcer risk is also increased in coal miners.

Cirrhosis of any etiology is associated with PUD, with an annual ulcer incidence of 4–5% and prevalence of 10–50% [82–84]. The risk is greatest in those with more severe cirrhosis by Child–Pugh score. Some of the increased ulcer risk may be due to shared risk factors. The major concerns for clinicians are the high rate of complicated PUD in these patients, recurrence (up to 50%), and the fact that complications may precipitate a decompensation in other aspects of their health. There should be a low threshold for maintenance antisecretory therapy. The incidence of PUD in cirrhosis was independent of the high prevalence of *H. pylori* in this population [85]. Peptic ulcer is also more commonly described in patients with renal failure and coronary artery disease, though data are conflicting and shared risk factors are likely important.

Other specific scenarios – organ transplantation, head injuries, and burns

The important risk factors for PUD in the transplant setting are pretransplant history of PUD, glucocorticoids (particularly pulsed methylprednisolone), immunosuppression (less frequent with cyclosporine), CMV infection (ameliorated by antivirals), other comorbidities, and stress ulcers. Most centers routinely offer antacid prophylaxis, particularly early after transplant when the risk is highest [86,87]. Given the observation that active PUD may be exacerbated after transplantation, such patients should be treated and resolution should be confirmed by endoscopy before transplantation.

Cushing ulcers and Curling ulcers are peptic ulcers that occur in the settings of head injuries, with elevated intracranial pressure (ICP) and severe burns, respectively. These lesions probably reflect subtypes of ulceration seen in the wider context of acute multisystem failure, although raised ICP may contribute to vagally mediated hyperchlorhydria and the hypovolemia associated with severe burns may lead to ischemic necrosis of the gastroduodenal mucosa. These ulcers are much less frequent with modern intensive care management protocols that specify ulcer prophylaxis and early enteral nutrition.

Etiology

In the overwhelming majority of patients, PUD is caused by *H. pylori* infection or NSAIDs, including aspirin. Although there are many other causes of ulcers (see Box 49.1), these are all uncommon or rare. Thus, before making a diagnosis of non-*H. pylori*, non-NSAID or idiopathic ulcer, it is crucial to rule out false-negative results for *H. pylori* and to obtain a detailed medication history to exclude unrecognized, inadvertent or surreptitious use of NSAIDs. Decreasing prevalence of *H. pylori* and greater awareness of the importance of NSAIDs may be responsible, at least in part, for the relative increase in the proportion of patients diagnosed with non-*H. pylori*, non-NSAID PUD. PUD in the context of comorbidity (acute multisystem failure or chronic disease) and specific disease associations is considered in the section on risk factors.

Helicobacter pylori

Identification of *H. pylori* as the major etiological agent for PUD after its discovery in 1982 by Warren and Marshall has revolutionized the management of PUD [88] (Figure 49.2). As a result, the prevalence of *H. pylori* infection is decreasing worldwide; despite this, about one in two of the global human population is still believed to be infected (see Table 49.1). In general, *H. pylori*

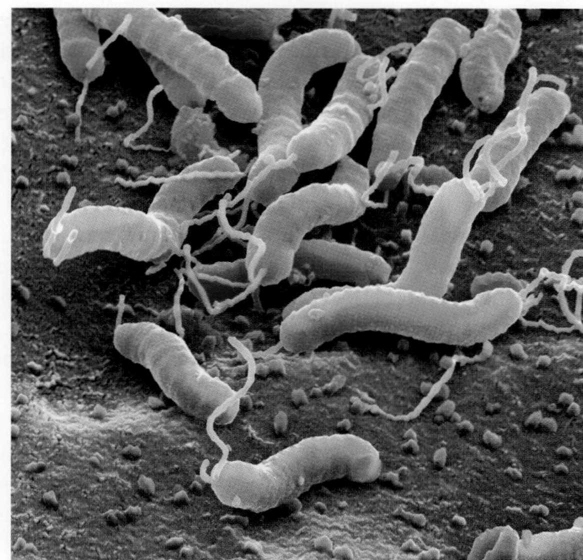

Figure 49.2 *Helicobacter pylori*. False colored scanning electron micrograph showing *H. pylori* bacteria (red) on the surface of gastric epithelial cells. Source: Reproduced with permission of Juergen Berger (Max-Planck Institute) and Science Photo Library.

prevalence is decreasing more rapidly in high or very high HDI countries than in low or medium HDI countries but the decrease is not uniform and prevalence rates remain high, even in some very high HDI countries, particularly in marginalized, indigenous or immigrant communities and in individuals with mental or physical disabilities. The rate of reinfection after complete eradication is also higher in low and medium HDI countries.

Amongst infected individuals, development of *H. pylori*-associated disease depends on several factors including bacterial virulence, host susceptibility, and environmental factors (see "Pathogenesis"). The average lifetime risk of PUD in people with *H. pylori* is around 10–20%. Accordingly, although worldwide *H. pylori* is commonly described as being the cause of about 90% of DUs and up to 80% of GUs, this no longer applies in most high or very high HDI countries. For DU, *H. pylori* is usually still the most common cause and is found in about 75% of cases. However, for GU, although *H. pylori* remains a common cause, NSAIDs and aspirin have become the most common causes in many industrialized nations.

Nonsteroidal antiinflammatory drugs

Nonsteroidal antiinflammatory drugs and aspirin (including low-dose aspirin) inhibit the synthesis of protective gastroduodenal prostaglandins, which are critical for mucosal defense, leading to GI toxicity and the development of gastroduodenopathy (discussed further in Chapter 51) and ulceration. In some high and very high HDI countries, NSAIDs have become the most common cause of GU, and their increased use, associated with a decreased rate of *H. pylori* infection, is held responsible for the relative rise in complicated ulcer disease. NSAID-induced PUD depends on multiple factors including the type of NSAID (e.g., COX-2 nonselective more than selective NSAIDs), the dose of NSAID (directly proportional to risk), concurrent use of multiple NSAIDs, concurrent use of other medicaitons (e.g., glucocorticoids, bisphosphonates), patient age (more common in older patients), history of PUD, and smoking (see "Risk factors").

Non-*H. pylori*, non-NSAID causes

The less common causes of ulcers continue to increase in relative importance in high or very high HDI countries, as *H. pylori* prevalence declines and risks with NSAID and aspirin use are better managed by PPI prophylaxis and *H. pylori* eradication in susceptible individuals. There are several important, less common specific causes of PUD (see Box 49.1) which require specific management. Presentations that should increase suspicion of these forms are discussed under "Clinical features – scenario two." Truly idiopathic ulcers remain uncommon but are increasingly reported (see "Epidemiology of non-*H. pylori*, non-NSAID ulcers").

Other infectious agents

Several non-*H. pylori* species, such as *H. heilmannii*, *H. felis*, *H. suis*, and *H. pullorum*, have been identified in human gastroduodenal mucosa and at other sites [89]. They have been isolated from patients with PUD in whom no other cause is found and, in some cases, ulcers have remitted and not recurred following treatment, implying causality. Non-*pylori Helicobacter* species are most commonly described as being associated with a chronic mild gastritis and occasionally in association with disease, most usually GU or gastric MALT lymphoma (a rare lymphoma associated with *H. pylori*, see Chapter 52). Management is with standard *H. pylori* eradication regimens [89,90].

In addition, even in healthy individuals, there are multiple, non-*Helicobacter* species that reside in the stomach; the most common are Actinobacteria (*Rothia*, *Actinomyces*, *Micrococcus*), Bacteroidetes (*Prevotella*), Firmicutes (*Streptococcus*, *Bacillus*), and Proteobacteria (which include *H. pylori* as well as *Haemophilus*, *Actinobacillus*, and *Neisseria*). The predominant genus is *Streptococcus* which may originate from the oral or nasal cavities and has been associated with PUD in one study from Malaysia [91].

Viruses are an important consideration in immunocompromised patients, and occasionally in patients without systemic disease or immunosuppression. They should be considered in patients with renal or other organ transplants, and in those with acquired immunodeficiency and low CD4 counts. Viruses which are well described as causing ulcers in the GI tract include herpes simplex virus types I and II (HSV-1 and -2) [92–94], cytomegalovirus (CMV, which often causes large and multiple ulcers) [95–97], and Epstein–Barr virus (EBV) [98,99]. Viruses should be sought and treated if the ulcer is unusual in appearance and particularly if other etiologies are absent. HSV has been shown to be present in the margin of the ulcers in nonimmunocompromised individuals and was absent in the center or the tissue distant from the ulcer [94] while CMV and EBV are mostly isolated from immunocompromised patients. Whether they also have a role as cofactors in ulcers with better recognized etiologies is disputed.

Other drug exposures

Although NSAIDs and aspirin are the most important drug exposures to consider in cases of PUD, several other drugs may contribute to ulceration and its complications. Some drugs are especially more problematic when used in combination with NSAIDs, such as aspirin, glucocorticoids, clopidogrel, selective serotonin uptake inhibitors (SSRIs) and bisphosphonates, particularly alendronate, although they can cause GI bleeding even when used separately. High doses of acetaminophen (paracetamol) also increase the risk of bleeding when taken with NSAIDs [100,101].

Hormone- or mediator-induced ulcers

Gastrinoma and its associated syndromes cause high gastrin levels and hypersecretion of acid and pepsin, leading to severe PUD and GI bleeding; these are covered in Chapter 50 (Zollinger–Ellison syndrome). Systemic mastocytosis is a very rare type of myeloproliferative neoplasm with mast cell infiltration in tissues. Patients may be asymptomatic but gastrointestinal symptoms, including abdominal pain, reflux, diarrhea, nausea and vomiting, may be accompanied by systemic manifestations of pruritus, flushing, rash, organomegaly, and lymphadenopathy [102]. Histamine release from mast cell degranulation is believed to drive acid hypersecretion, leading to severe duodenal inflammation and DU in 30–50% of patients. Antisecretory drugs are effective for these ulcers. Myeloproliferative disorders such as basophilic leukemia and chronic myelogenous leukemia, characterized by severe basophilia, have been linked with PUD mediated by histamine release. Other disorders such as polycythemia vera may contribute to PUD through increased blood viscosity leading to altered mucosal blood flow.

Malignancy

Gastric ulcers may be caused directly by underlying primary gastric adenocarcinoma or lymphoma (see Chapter 52) and they can sometimes be difficult to distinguish from benign ulcers, although their context, appearance or site usually gives a strong clue. Malignancy is reported in about 3% of GUs but is extremely rarely in DUs. Malignant melanomas can rarely arise as gastric primary tumors. Occasionally, metastatic carcinoma is found in the stomach, most commonly from melanoma or from breast or renal cell carcinoma. Gastric neuroendocrine tumors (carcinoids) can also be associated with PUD, likely due to histamine release [103,104].

Other rare etiologies

Gastroduodenal ulceration can occur in Crohn's disease, with gastroduodenal manifestations in 0.5–4% of cases [105,106], or in eosinophilic gastroenteritis, which is rare but increasingly described [107]. Gastrointestinal IgG4-related disorders can cause infiltration by IgG4-positive plasma cells and ulceration of the stomach and duodenum [108]. Ulceration can also rarely occur with sarcoidosis, Wegener granulomatosis, and Behçet disease. Gastroduodenal irradiation during radiotherapy can lead to acute or chronic PUD. Critical celiac axis vascular disease can cause PUD at atypical sites, often with intense pain, and will respond to revascularization. Crack cocaine and methamphetamine misuse cause ischemic ulceration secondary to vasoconstriction with a high risk of perforation. Rare causes of duodenal obstruction, including duodenal webs, pyloric stenosis, annular pancreas, and preduodenal portal vein, can lead to secondary DU. Ingested foreign bodies, such as sharp objects, magnets and button batteries, have also been reported to cause ulceration [109].

Iatrogenic

Ulceration can be expected as a consequence of interventions which breach the mucosa and clinicians should therefore be aware that procedures such as mucosal biopsy, polypectomy, endoscopic mucosal resection (EMR), and endoscopic submucosal dissection (ESD) may cause ulceration. Bariatric surgeries such as antral exclusion, Roux-en-Y procedures or sleeve gastrectomy can lead to PUD or anastomotic ulcers. Simultaneous presence of ischemia, *H.pylori*, and NSAIDs can also increase the risk of PUD after surgery [110,111]. Metallic or even plastic stents used for a variety of procedures such as biliary stenosis and obstruction, pseudocyst drainage or cholecystogastrostomy may cause traumatic injury and ulceration.

Idiopathic

Idiopathic hypersecretory DU, the cause of up to 10% of DUs, is typified by basal acid output >15 mmol/h, the absence of hypergastrinemia, and the absence of *H. pylori* infection. The mechanism is undefined but the condition responds to long-term antisecretory therapy.

Pathogenesis

For much of the last century, research into the pathogenesis and treatment of peptic ulcer disease was grounded in the dictum "No acid, no ulcer" enunciated in 1910 by Dragutin (Carl) Schwarz, a surgeon in Zagreb [112]. It was already known that the normal human stomach produces acid and pepsin; in the early 19th century, William Prout (1785–1850) demonstrated that gastric juice contains hydrochloric acid and subsequently, in 1836, Theodor Schwann (1810–1882) reported the discovery of pepsin. The recognition in the following decades that acid is necessary for the formation of peptic ulcers [113,114] led to the development of a range of surgical techniques and medical therapies to reduce acid secretion and produce peptic ulcer healing.

Gastric acid secretion

Secretion of acid by the stomach is widely conserved across many animal species, ranging from fish to mammals, and the maintenance of appropriate acid secretion and gastric acidity is closely regulated by multiple physiological mechanisms to achieve a successful balance between the beneficial effects of luminal acid and the potential for acid and pepsin to injure the gastroduodenal mucosa. In health, gastric acid serves to reduce the load of ingested organisms and protect the gastrointestinal tract and, indeed, the whole body from infections and injury, to increase the absorption of iron, calcium, and other dietary nutrients, and to activate pepsinogen and protein digestion [115].

The anatomy of the stomach and the functions of the different parts of the stomach are uniquely adapted to its role which consists of holding ingested food temporarily so that it can be mixed with acid and pepsin and ground down physically into a particulate suspension that can then be passed on, in a controlled manner, to the proximal small intestine.

Ingested food is held, initially, in the gastric body, where it is suspended in gastric secretions, including hydrochloric acid and pepsin, that are products, respectively, of the parietal and chief cells, located in the oxyntic glands of the gastric corpus and fundus. Portions of the food then pass on from the gastric corpus to the antropyloric region where they are ground down in the process of trituration and mixed thoroughly with gastric secretions, the acidity of which is monitored by "G" and "D" cells, located in the pyloric glands of the gastric antrum.

The control of acid secretion and hence of gastric luminal acidity is regulated by the coordinated actions of a number of neural, endocrine, and paracrine processes which respond to central stimuli, such as taste and smell, to local mechanical and chemical stimuli such as distension, nutrients and acid and to neurohormonal stimuli such as gastrin, somatostatin, and histamine.

Neural stimulation of acid secretion is mediated by efferent fibers of the vagus nerve which synapse with intramural enteric neurons which release acetylcholine (ACh) that binds to muscarinic type 3 (M_3) receptors on the parietal cell. Hormonal stimulation of acid secretion is mediated by gastrin which is secreted by antral G cells and binds to CCK subtype 3 receptors (CCK-2) on the parietal cell, whilst paracrine stimulation is mediated primarily by histamine which is secreted by enterochromaffin-like (ECL) cells and binds to histamine type 2 (H_2) receptors on the parietal cell. Histamine release by ECL cells is stimulated by gastrin which binds to CCK-2 receptors and is inhibited by somatostatin which binds to somatostatin subtype 2 (SSTR2) receptors, both located on the ECL cell. Somatostatin, released by oxyntic gland D cells, also inhibits acid secretion, directly, acting via SSTR2 receptors on the parietal cell. Increases in intracellular calcium, resulting from activation of M_3 and CCK-2 receptors by acetylcholine and gastrin respectively, and generation of adenosine 3',5'-cyclic monophosphate (cAMP) resulting from activation of H_2 receptors, lead to protein kinase activation and activation of H^+,K^+-ATPase proton pumps that secrete hydrochloric acid into the gastric lumen.

In addition to its stimulatory effects on acid secretion, mediated by cholinergic intramural enteric neurons, the vagus nerve also acts via cholinergic enteric neurons on D cells in the gastric corpus and gastric antrum and on G cells in the gastric antrum and via peptidergic enteric neurons, mediated by vasoactive intestinal peptide (VIP) on D cells and by gastrin-releasing peptide (GRP) on G cells in the gastric antrum. In the antrum, gastrin from G cells stimulates D cells to secrete somatostatin which in turn inhibits G cell secretin of gastrin. Somatostatin release is also modulated by increased luminal acidity which stimulates the release of calcitonin gene-related peptide (CGRP) from extrinsic sensory neurons which then stimulates somatostatin secretion by D cells in both the antrum and corpus. These core neural, endocrine, and paracrine mechanisms are also subject to modulation by numerous other factors acting at multiple points along these pathways.

Acetylcholine stimulates acid secretion directly via the M_3 receptor on the parietal cell, activating phospholipase C to generate inositol triphosphate and release intracellular calcium. Acetylcholine also stimulates acid secretion indirectly via M_2 and M_4 receptors on D cells which inhibit somatostatin release and thereby decrease the inhibition of acid secretion. Acetylcholine release occurs in response to activation of the cholinergic enteric neurons by the vagus nerve, largely in response to central activity in the vagal dorsal motor nucleus (DMN), the nucleus tractus solitarius (NTS), and hypothalamus. Central neuronal activity in these areas is triggered by the thought, sight, smell, and taste of food and this is responsible for about half of the acid secretion that occurs after eating. The presence of food in the stomach then leads to mechanical and chemical activation of the same cholinergic enteric neurons, triggering further acid secretion, and the acid-neutralizing effect of food decreases gastric acidity which also increases the drive to acid secretion.

Gastrin is produced predominantly by G cells in the gastric antrum but also in the small intestine, the large intestine, and pancreas; it is the main mediator of meal-stimulated gastric acid secretion. The precursor to gastrin is converted from a 101-amino acid molecule to progastrin, an 80-amino acid molecule that is further processed and amidated to generate the active forms: gastrin 34 (G34amide) and gastrin 17 (G17amide). The larger form, G34, is less abundant (5–10% of amidated gastrins) but has a longer half-life (30 minutes) than G17 (3–7 minutes); as a result, G34 is the main form in circulation during fasting whereas G17 predominates after meals.

Gastrin secretion is stimulated by ACh, GRP, secretin, 5-hydroxytryptamine (5-HT), b-adrenergic agonists, calcium, and a variety of dietary factors, including amines, amino acids, protein, capsaicin, and fermented alcoholic drinks, while it is inhibited by somatostatin, adenosine, bradykinins, galanin, and menin. Through its actions on the ECL cell progenitors, gastrin is trophic for ECL cells and when stimulating ECL cells it causes both the release of stored histamine and the production of more histamine from L-histidine by increasing histidine decarboxylase (HDC) activity.

Histamine release from the ECL cell occurs primarily in response to gastrin but its release is also stimulated by VIP, pituitary adenylate cyclase-activating peptide (PACAP) – a VIP-like protein – and ghrelin. Conversely, histamine release from the ECL cell is inhibited not only by somatostatin but also by prostaglandins, galanin, peptide YY (PYY), and CGRP. Histamine stimulates acid secretion directly via H_2 receptors on the parietal cell, activating adenylate cyclase to generate cAMP, and indirectly via the H_3 receptors on oxyntic D cells which inhibit somatostatin release.

Somatostatin is produced mainly by D cells in the gastric antrum and corpus but also in the pancreas and small intestine. The precursor to somatostatin is a 91-amino acid molecule (pre-prosomatostatin) that is processed to generate somatostatin-14 (half-life 1–3 minutes), which predominates in the stomach, pancreas, and enteric neurons, and somatostatin-28 (half-life 15 minutes), which predominates in the small intestine. Somatostatin acts via SSTR2 receptors on its targets, G cells in the gastric antrum and ECL and parietal cells in the gastric corpus; the SSTR2 receptor is a member of the G-protein binding receptor family which leads to inhibition of adenylyl cyclase and calcium channels. The D cells are located in very close proximity to their target cells, acting indirectly via the local circulation or directly via cytoplasmic processes to provide tonic inhibition of gastrin secretion, histamine secretion, and acid secretion. Somatostatin secretion is stimulated by gastric luminal acidity, gastrin, CGRP, GRP, PACAP, VIP, secretin, atrial natriuretic peptide (ANP), adenosine, b-adrenergic agonists, adrenomedullin, amylin, phenylalanine, and tyrosine whereas somatostatin secretion is inhibited by ACh, glucose, glutamine, and interferon (IFN)-g.

Several other peptides modulate gastric acid secretion. Ghrelin, orexin-A, and, under some circumstances, PACAP have been reported to increase acid secretion by various mechanisms including vagal and histamine-mediated mechanisms for ghrelin, gastrin-mediated mechanisms for orexin-A and a balance of ECL cell- and D cell-mediated effects for PACAP. Many other peptides, some encompassed by the term enterogastrone, including ANP, CCK, glucagon-like peptide 1 (GLP-1), adrenomedullin, amylin, epidermal growth factor (EGF), glicentin, leptin, oxyntomodulin, neurotensin, PYY, and secretin, appear to act by stimulating somatostatin release although interleukin (IL)-1b appears to act via a different pathway.

All of these control mechanisms, which allow gastric acidity to be regulated very tightly in response to a huge number of external and internal stimuli, lead to the final common pathway of acid secretion, the H^+,K^+-ATPase proton pumps in the gastric parietal cells. Parietal cells secrete hydrochloric acid at a pH of about 0.8 (160 mM); the concentration of the secreted acid is constant and the normal pH of the gastric lumen (1.5–3.5) is therefore determined by the volume of gastric acid secreted and the volume and acidity of other gastric contents, including other gastric secretions, ingested food, and refluxed duodenal contents.

Parietal cells are located in the neck and pits of the oxyntic glands which are found throughout the gastric corpus and fundus (Figure 49.3) [116]. In humans, there are about 1 billion parietal cells, each of which is able to secrete hydrochloric acid in addition to producing intrinsic factor, amphiregulin, heparin-binding EGF, hepcidin, leptin, sonic hedgehog, and transforming

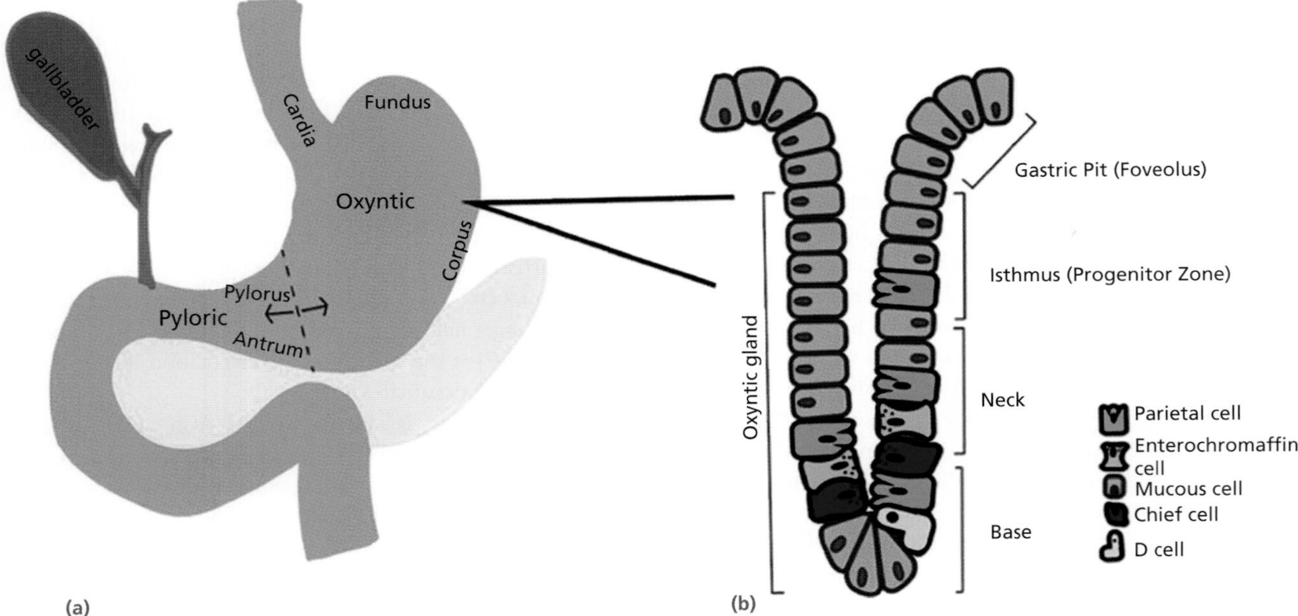

Figure 49.3 Schematic representations of the stomach **(a)** and oxyntic gland **(b)**. **(a)** The stomach is divided into two functional regions, the oxyntic region (composed of the cardia, fundus, and corpus) and the pyloric region (composed of the antrum and pylorus). **(b)** A representative oxyntic gland from the oxyntic region of the stomach features a gastric pit, isthmus, neck, and base. A variety of stomach cell types exist, including parietal cells, enterochromaffin cells, and mucous cells. Source: Reproduced with permission from Baratta et al. [116].

growth factor (TGF)-a. Parietal cells are formed in the isthmus region of the oxyntic gland and migrate down to the base of the gland, becoming progressively less active as they go; in the neck and base of the oxyntic gland, the parietal cells are in close proximity to chief cells (pepsinogen), D cells (somatostatin), ECL cells (histamine or ANP), and mucous neck cells.

The secretion of hydrochloric acid by parietal cells is achieved by the transport of hydronium ions via the H^+,K^+-ATPase pump (Figure 49.4a) [(116)]; when activated, the proton pump secretes intracellular protons in exchange for extracellular potassium, leading to electroneutral ion exchange [117]. The H^+,K^+-ATPase has a and b subunits that are assembled in the endoplasmic reticulum and trafficked to the plasma membrane as a heterodimeric oligomer. In the resting state, the H^+,K^+-ATPase is located in cytoplasmic tubulovesicles which undergo morphological change when acid secretion is stimulated and the parietal cell is activated. Activation leads to translocation of the tubulovesicles which fuse with the apical secretory canaliculi to form an extensive canalicular secretory system which is 6–10 times larger in surface area than in the resting cell. The H^+,K^+-ATPase is then activated by translocation into the canalicular membrane in the presence of potassium ions in the lumen so that it can secrete hydronium ions against a huge concentration gradient. In order to achieve this, the parietal cell also requires apical potassium and chloride channels to provide luminal potassium that can be exchanged for the hydronium ions and chloride for hydrochloric acid formation, as well as basolateral bicarbonate and chloride exchangers that can export one bicarbonate ion for every hydronium ion secreted by the H^+,K^+-ATPase and import chloride for export at the apical membrane (Figure 49.4b) [116,118].

Once secreted, the gastric acid must then traverse the overlying mucus layer to enter the gastric lumen, probably via channels created by the relatively high pressure generated in the oxyntic gland during acid secretion [119] (see also Chapter 17).

Pharmacological inhibition of gastric acid secretion

The multitude of mechanisms involved in the control of acid secretion would suggest that there should be many therapeutic targets for pharmacological invention but in general, attempts to inhibit the neural, endocrine, and paracrine pathways have had only limited success because of the degree of redundancy in the control mechanisms. The development of anticholinergic agents and gastrin inhibitors to reduce acid secretion is only of historical interest now and although histamine H_2 receptor antagonists (H_2-RAs) such as cimetidine, ranitidine, famotidine, and nizatidine have been hugely successful commercially, their therapeutic potential is limited as they block only one of the pathways leading to acid secretion and CCK-2 receptor upregulation leads to tachyphylaxis and loss of effect with time. Furthermore, in April 2020, all formulations of ranitidine were withdrawn from the market due to the risk of contamination by the probable human carcinogen N-nitrosodimethylamine (NDMA), concentrations of which may increase with time and exposure to higher than room temperatures [120,121].

The most effective and successful pharmacological agents have therefore been those which target the H^+,K^+-ATPase or proton pump as the final common pathway of acid secretion. The most widely used and studied agents are the PPIs but they have been joined in recent years by the potassium competitive acid blockers (PCABs).

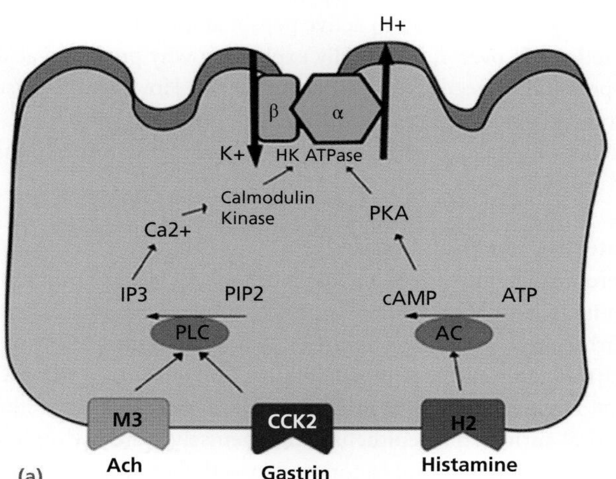

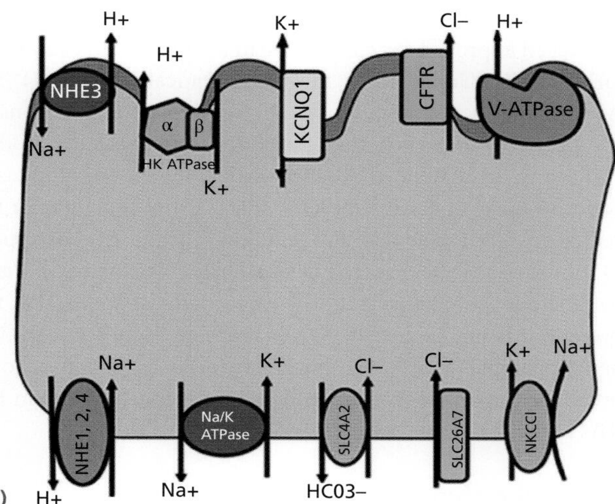

Figure 49.4 Schematic representations of the parietal cell **(a)** and gastric acid stimulants **(b)** exchangers, transporters, channels. **(a)** The H,K,ATPase is stimulated through three primary inputs: acetylcholine (ACh), gastrin, and histamine. ACh and gastrin bind to their receptors and trigger activation of phospholipase C (PLC), which converts PIP2 to IP3 and triggers release of Ca2Cfrom the sarcoplasmic reticulum. This leads to downstream activation of the H,K,ATPase. Histamine binds to the H_2 receptor, triggering activation of adenylyl cyclase and PKA. **(b)** Multiple apical and basolateral anion and cation movements occur to maintain the gradient and electroneutral transport of hydrogen. Source: Reproduced with permission from Baratta et al. Figure 4 [116].

Proton pump inhibitors

Current PPIs (omeprazole, esomeprazole, lansoprazole, dexlansoprazole, rabeprazole, pantoprazole) are substituted benzimidazoles composed of a pyridine ring and benzimidazole ring, joined by a methylsulphinyl group. They are all prodrugs when taken and they block the proton pump only when they have converted to the sulphenamide form in the secretory canaliculus of the parietal cell. Being weak bases, with a pKa of 4–5, PPIs are nonprotonated at a blood pH of 7.35–7.45 and are therefore membrane permeable. However, when they enter the parietal cell, and in particular the active secretory canaliculus, they change to a protonated sulphenamide form that is membrane impermeable and which is then trapped in the secretory canaliculus where it reaches concentrations 100 000–1 000 000 greater than in the blood. Serendipitously, it is this protonated form that then binds covalently with the proton pump to inhibit acid secretion completely. Resumption of acid secretion occurs only when the inhibited proton pumps are replaced by new proton pumps inserted into the canalicular membranes.

Proton pump inihibitors have proven to be very effective for the treatment of acid-related disorders and are generally very safe although there are continuing concerns, more than 30 years after their introduction, that the chronic hypergastrinemia caused by decreased gastric acidity may be harmful or that the long-term reduction in gastric acidity may have multiple deleterious effects related to reduced clearance of ingested organisms or reduced absorption of nutrients or medications whose uptake is facilitated by gastric acid [122].

Potassium competitive acid blockers

Potassium competitive acid blockers have been developed more recently than PPIs and, to date, only revaprazan and vonaprazan have been approved for clinical use in a very limited number of jurisdictions. Unlike PPIs, they bind ionically to the H^+,K^+-ATPase and in doing so, block the access of potassium ions to the proton pump such that they cannot activate the H^+,K^+-ATPase. Like the PPIs, PCABs are weak bases and they too reach concentrations that are 100 000–1 000 000 times greater in the secretory canaliculus than in the blood. Current PCABs appear to inhibit gastric acid secretion to an extent that is comparable to PPIs but they do have a more rapid onset of action. For the present, it is not clear that PCABs offer any significant clinical benefit compared with PPIs but the two classes do appear to be broadly comparable in effect and demonstrably better than H_2-RAs for acid-related disorders.

Mucosal defense

Acid and pepsin, produced by the normal stomach, are potentially injurious agents; as a result, the stomach and duodenum have a number of mucosal defense systems to protect themselves from peptic digestion (Figure 49.5). Damage to the mucosa allows acid access to already damaged mucosa, thereby causing an ulcer. For some ulcers, increased acidity may also contribute. The two main agents which disrupt these systems are *H. pylori* infection and NSAIDs, and these cause ulcers in different ways. Acid is needed for peptic ulcers to form [113,114], giving rise to Schwarz's 1910 dictum of "No acid, no ulcer" [112]. However, this concept is more useful in directing treatment than in understanding pathogenesis: most peptic ulcers heal with acid-suppressive therapy, but acid is only rarely the sole underlying cause of an ulcer, and acid production is actually reduced in many patients with GU.

To stop ulcer recurrence, the underlying cause must be removed, usually by eradicating *H. pylori* or stopping NSAIDs. If the underlying cause cannot be eliminated, for example in patients needing low-dose aspirin for vascular disease prophylaxis, continuing acid-suppressive therapy is required and is often successful. If ulcers do not heal with strong acid-suppressive therapy, unusual (i.e., nonpeptic) causes should be suspected and testing for these is indicated, including malignancy, viruses or Crohn's disease (see Box 49.1). Some NSAID ulcers are also difficult to heal with acid suppression alone [123], as might be suspected from the fact that NSAID ulcers can occur elsewhere in the GI tract (e.g., small intestine), where luminal pH is neutral or alkaline.

Injurious agents – acid and pepsin

It is well known that luminal acid can damage tissue and acid alone in extreme situations can cause DUs. The best example is the markedly increased acid output stimulated by severe hypergastrinemia in Zollinger–Ellison syndrome (or gastrinoma, Chapter 50) or by histamine in systemic mastocytosis [124]. In *H. pylori*-associated DUs, acid production is modestly increased and contributes to pathogenesis. Having said this, it is difficult to determine the relative effects of pepsin and acid which, in combination, are more injurious than acid alone [125]. Pepsinogen is converted to active pepsin at low pH and is inactivated at pH over 4, potentially explaining why profound acid suppression is needed to heal some ulcers. However, because therapeutic interventions to reduce acid production also inactivate pepsin, one cannot be certain of the relative contributions of these two agents.

Protective mucosal defense

There are several mucosal defense mechanisms (see Figure 49.5). Luminally, initial protection is provided by gastric mucus and bicarbonate produced by epithelial cells. The mucus forms an unstirred layer and bicarbonate buffers acid, creating a pH gradient ranging from 1–2 in the gastric lumen to 6–8 at the mucosal surface. The epithelial cells themselves are hydrophobic. Production of trefoil factors and growth factors helps maintain this barrier and allows epithelial restitution – movement of cells to fill gaps – following immediate damage. Larger gaps can be filled more slowly by cellular proliferation. Finally, local blood flow is important in eliminating backdiffusion of acid and supporting healing; angiogenesis is increased at the healing margins of ulcers.

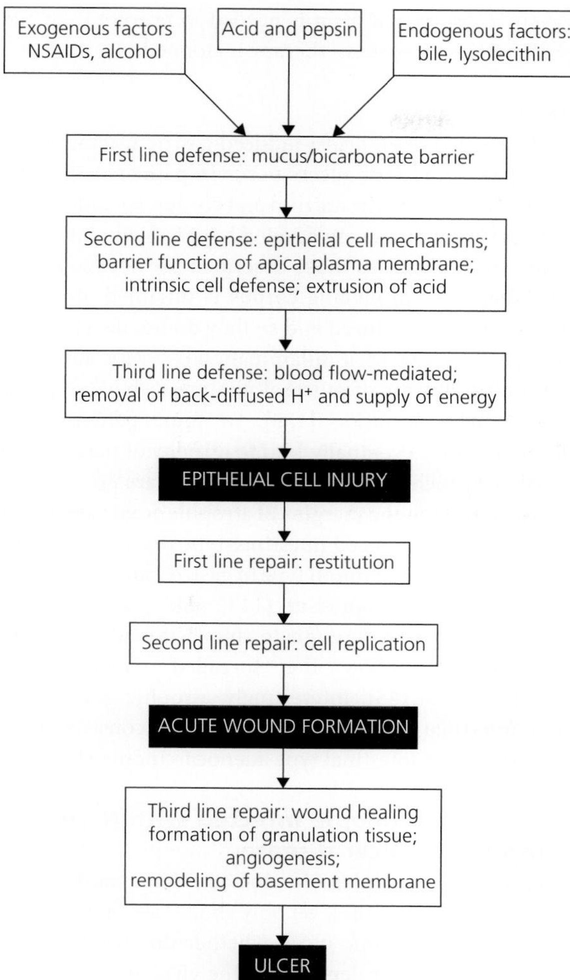

Figure 49.5 Cascade of mucosal defense and repair mechanisms. Damaging effects on epithelial cells of exogenous and endogenous factors are amplified by acid-peptic activity. If the three lines of defense mechanisms fail, epithelial cell injury occurs, which will be repaired by restitution and cell replication. If these repair mechanisms fail, an acute wound forms. Ulcers form when these normal defense and repair mechanisms fail or are overwhelmed. NSAIDs, nonsteroidal antiinflammatory drugs.

These mucosal defensive mechanisms are mediated through constitutively expressed prostaglandins and nitric oxide, and the key mechanism underlying NSAID-associated ulceration is prostaglandin inhibition. *H. pylori*-associated ulcers are related to mucosal inflammation, which directly disrupts host defense. Stress ulcers arise largely through impaired mucosal defense, including reduced mucosal blood flow. Cameron ulcers in the neck of a hiatus hernia are thought to have an ischemic etiology and may be associated with iron deficiency anemia [126]. Impaired mucosal defense may also contribute to the observation that ulcers often recur at the site of the original lesion: underlying damage and fibrosis may impair local blood flow, inducing tissue ischemia and retarding local repair mechanisms.

Duodenal ulcers

Duodenal, pyloric, and immediately prepyloric ulcers share a common pathogenesis and are generally classified together (Figure 49.6). The vast majority of ulcers are due to *H. pylori* infection. DUs are usually associated with increased acid, most obviously in Zollinger–Ellison syndrome where DUs often extend distal to the duodenal bulb. However, *H. pylori*-induced DUs are also in part caused by increased acid, usually in association with elevated fasting serum gastrin levels. Patients have increased parietal cell mass, increased acid response to stimulation (for example, by food), and prolonged acid secretion after a meal, due to a combination of increased production and reduced inhibition [127–129]. Suppression of mucosal defense is also a factor in DU pathogenesis and bicarbonate secretion is reduced [130]. As explained later, *H. pylori* inhabits areas of gastric metaplasia in the duodenum, leading to local inflammation and damage [131]. NSAIDs can cause DUs but much less commonly than they cause GUs.

Gastric ulcers

Helicobacter pylori is still a major cause of GUs worldwide, but in many high and very high HDI countries, NSAIDs, including low-dose aspirin, have overtaken *H. pylori* as the primary cause. GU patients usually have normal or reduced acid secretion [132]. Ulcers occur in areas of heavy inflammation, transitional zones between different parts of the stomach, or other areas of mucosal fragility [133]. For example, they frequently occur in the transitional zone on the lesser gastric curve where oxyntic and antral mucosa meet, and in *H. pylori*-induced

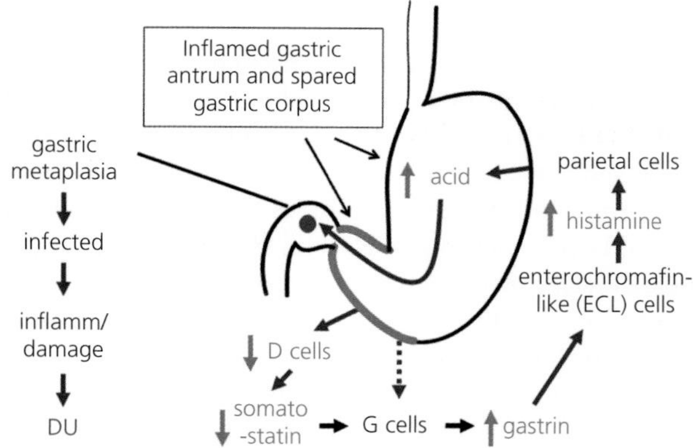

Figure 49.6 How gastric infection with *Helicobacter pylori* causes duodenal ulceration. Inflammation in the gastric antrum causes reduced somatostatin production from D cells and increased gastrin production from G cells, leading to increased meal-stimulated acid output from the healthy gastric corpus. The increased acid load in the duodenum encourages the formation of gastric metaplasia which can become infected by *H. pylori*. This then becomes inflamed and may ulcerate, leading to duodenal ulcer (DU). If *H. pylori* colonizes and causes inflammation in the whole stomach, acid production is usually reduced from the inflamed and damaged gastric corpus. These patients do not develop DUs but are prone to gastric ulceration and gastric adenocarcinoma.

pangastritis this transitional zone is often heavily inflamed. They may also occur where atrophic mucosa from long-standing *H. pylori* infection abuts normal oxyntic mucosa. Some drug-induced ulcers or erosions occur in the dependent stomach where tablets cause local damage (pill ulcers). Recurrent GUs are often found at the same site as the original ulcer, emphasizing the important role of local mucosal defense in ulcer localization and pathogenesis.

The pathogenesis of *H. pylori*-induced peptic ulcer disease

Helicobacter pylori is a gram-negative bacillus measuring roughly 3.5 microns in length and 0.5 microns in width with a spiral shape that enables it to corkscrew through gastric mucus [134]. Approximately 4.4 billion people worldwide are infected with *H. pylori* [135]. It lives only on gastric-type mucosa, deep to the mucus layer. It is well adapted to this niche, possessing several acid-protective mechanisms, most notably a powerful urease enzyme which hydrolyzes urea to release bicarbonate and ammonia, allowing it to maintain its periplasm at neutral pH when exposed to acid [136]. This enzyme is the basis of two of the important clinical tests for *H. pylori*: the biopsy urease test and the urea breath test. All *H. pylori* infections are associated with histological gastritis – infiltration of lymphocytes and neutrophils into the gastric mucosa [133,137]. The pattern of this gastritis influences whether a patient is prone to duodenal or gastric ulceration, and the severity of the gastritis is a major determinant of overall ulcer risk (see Chapter 51).

Mechanisms of *H. pylori*-induced duodenal and gastric ulceration

Duodenal ulceration

The mechanism whereby a gastric infection causes DUs is now reasonably well understood. Duodenal ulceration occurs in individuals how have an *antral-predominant* pattern of *H. pylori* colonization and gastritis, with sparing of the acid-producing gastric corpus. Antral inflammation suppresses somatostatin production by antral D cells and as somatostatin normally exerts negative feedback on gastrin, this results in hypergastrinemia [138–140].

Gastrin is a growth factor that increases parietal cell mass and consequently increases meal-stimulated acid secretion from the healthy and largely uninflamed gastric corpus [140]. Gastrin also acts on ECL cells in the corpus to stimulate histamine production, and both histamine and gastrin stimulate parietal cells to produce acid (see Chapter 17). The increased acid load emptying from the stomach contributes to gastric metaplasia of the duodenum, possibly as a protective response [141,142]. *H. pylori* can only colonize gastric-type mucosa but gastric metaplasia of the duodenum enables colonization of the duodenum, causing inflammation, damage, and ulceration. The increased acid load in the duodenum may also contribute directly to ulceration and certainly, the acid, possibly associated with pepsin, is necessary for this ulceration, as evidenced by the fact that *H. pylori*-induced ulcers heal with acid suppression. However, *H. pylori* treatment is needed to prevent their recurrence after acid-suppressive therapy is stopped.

Gastric ulceration

The pathogenesis of *H. pylori*-induced gastric ulceration is less well understood. Gastric ulcers occur in patients with inflammation involving both the antrum and corpus, so-called *pangastritis*. These individuals may develop hypergastrinemia through the same mechanisms as those described previously. However, because their acid-producing corpus is inflamed, gastric acid production is often reduced and so they do not develop duodenal ulcers [132]. Instead, if inflammation is severe, and particularly if it crosses areas of mucosal weakness, they are prone to develop gastric ulceration [133]. In some patients, corpus inflammation may eventually lead to atrophy of parietal glands and further hypochlorhydria. These patients are prone to ulceration, particularly at the margins of atrophic areas. They are also at risk of *H. pylori*-induced intestinal-type distal gastric adenocarcinoma, the most common type of gastric cancer. Continuing hypergastrinemia is important [143], and progression from atrophy to metaplasia through to dysplasia and carcinoma is hypothesized to follow the so-called Correa pathway (Figure 49.7) [144,145]. Interestingly, atrophic gastritis, compared to intestinal metaplasia, has been more consistently associated with gastric intestinal type adenocarcinoma [146].

Why only some people infected with *H. pylori* develop peptic ulcer disease

Helicobacter pylori colonizes the stomach from childhood to old age unless it is treated [147], yet only about 15% of infected people ever develop a peptic ulcer, whether duodenal or gastric. Who develops an ulcer depends on the virulence of the infecting *H. pylori* strain, host genetic susceptibility, host immune response, and environmental cofactors [148]. These factors usually affect the risk of both duodenal and gastric ulceration as they tend to affect the severity of damage and inflammation rather than its pattern or site.

Bacterial virulence

Helicobacter pylori is a mobile organism and uses its flagella to swim or swarm in a liquid or semiliquid environment [149]. Several mutations in genes that encode specific flagellar proteins such as fliD, FlaA, and FlaB are reported to reduce or even abolish its capacity to colonize the gastric mucosal layer by impairing the proper motility of *H. pylori* [150].

The best characterized *H. pylori* virulence factor is the *cag* pathogenicity island (*cag* PAI, Figure 49.8). Pathogenicity islands are collections of genes acquired distantly in the evolution of a bacterium, which render the bacterium pathogenic. Strains of *H. pylori* that possess the *cag* PAI (*cag*-positive strains) induce more local inflammation and are more likely to cause peptic ulceration and gastric adenocarcinoma than are *cag*-negative strains [148,151]. Genes in the *cag* PAI encode proteins that make up a bacterial type IV secretion system, a sort of

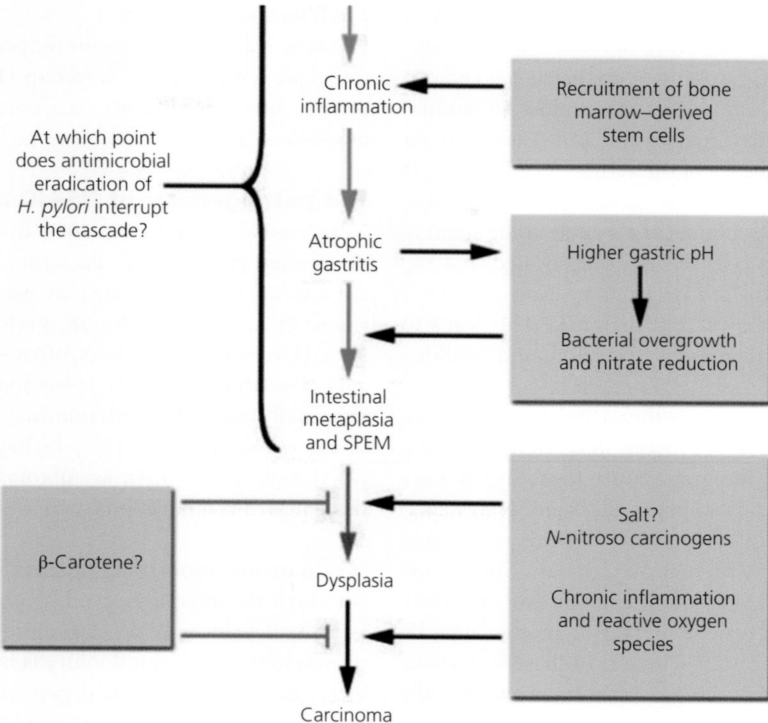

Figure 49.7 Proposed cascade of pathological events in gastric adenocarcinoma. Source: Reproduced with permission from Fox and Wang [145].

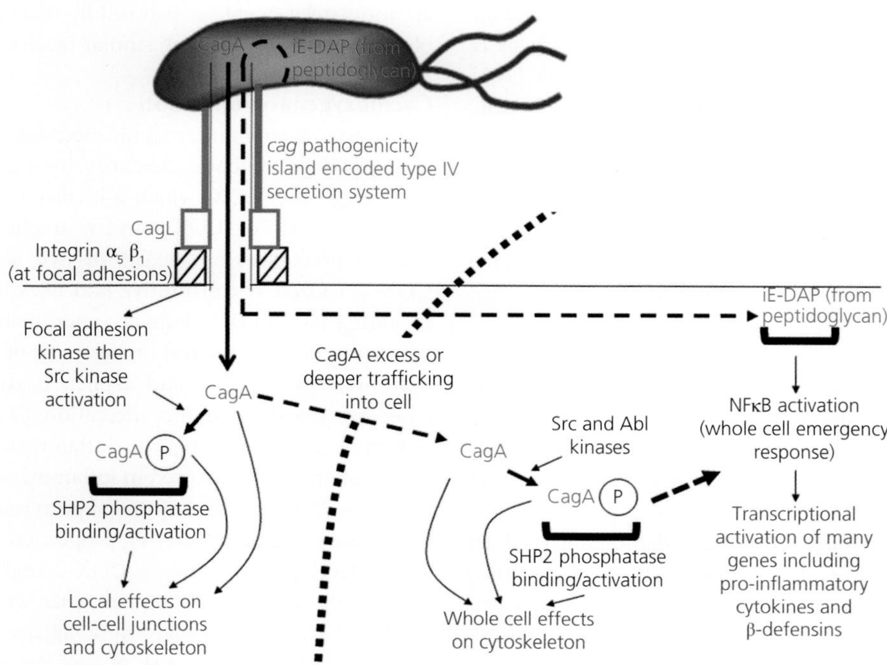

Figure 49.8 Mechanisms and effects on epithelial cells of the Cag virulence system of *Helicobacter pylori*. Bacterial factors are shown in red, host epithelial cell factors are in black, and effects on the cell are in blue.

molecular syringe through which an effector protein, CagA, is translocated into epithelial cells [152)]. Several signaling pathways are activated by CagA, resulting in epithelial cell changes and proinflammatory cytokine release that induce inflammation [153]. The *cag* PAI also induces inflammation in other ways. The protein coating the tip of the syringe, CagL, interacts with an integrin on the host cell to stimulate specific signaling pathways [154]. Also, small amounts of a soluble component of the bacterial peptidoglycan cell wall are translocated in a *cag* PAI-dependent manner, and are detected by Nod1, a major pathogen recognition protein in epithelial cells. This leads to activation of further proinflammatory signaling and cytokine release by the cell [155].

A second major virulence factor is the vacuolating cytotoxin, VacA, a pore-forming toxin which inserts into cell membranes. Strains of *H. pylori* that produce more active forms of VacA are more closely associated with both peptic ulcer and gastric cancer, independently of *cag* status [151,156,157]. Other recognized virulence factors associated with increased disease risk include an adhesin, BabA [158,159], an outer membrane inflammatory protein, OipA [160], and a genetic marker of another type IV secretion system, *dupA* [161,162]. The last of these is particularly interesting, as some studies suggest that it may specifically increase the risk of duodenal ulceration (hence its name, duodenal ulcer promoting gene A, *dupA*) but in some populations reduce the risk of gastric cancer [163].

Host genetic susceptibility

Specific polymorphisms in some cytokine genes, such as the gene encoding IL-1β, increase the level of inflammation induced by *H. pylori* [164], predispose to pangastritis, and, in some populations, are associated with a modestly increased risk of *H. pylori*-associated gastric atrophy and adenocarcinoma [165]. Such polymorphisms appear to be less important in determining peptic ulcer risk, although it is likely that those same patients would be more susceptible to GU. The increased risk of peptic ulceration seen in first-degree relatives of patients is likely to be mostly due to the increased risk of *H. pylori*, which can be passed from primary caregiver to child or between children. It is unclear whether there is a further small genetic risk.

Immune response

Helicobacter pylori infection induces both innate [166] and acquired immune responses [167]. The acquired response is orchestrated by proinflammatory T-helper (Th)-1 and Th-17 cells and is modulated by an antiinflammatory regulatory T cell response [168]. Patients who mount a weak regulatory T cell response develop more intense gastric inflammation and are more likely to have a peptic ulcer than those mounting a strong regulatory T cell response [169]. Strains of *H. pylori* that are better equipped to interact with their human host, for example those that possess the *cag* PAI, appear to exert a stronger influence on the immune response. NF-κB and c-jun N-terminal kinase activation are the known signaling pathways [170].

Environmental factors

Smoking is a strong risk factor for peptic ulceration, particularly in people with *H. pylori* infection [171]. Its mechanism is not known, but it may affect bicarbonate secretion and/or local blood flow [130].

The pathogenesis of NSAID/aspirin-induced PUD

Nonsteroidal antiinflammatory drugs and low-dose aspirin more often cause gastric ulceration or erosions, although they are also an important cause of duodenal ulceration and erosions. Erosions are common, perhaps almost ubiquitous, in NSAID users but deep ulcers, often with a punched-out appearance, also occur. Unlike *H. pylori*-induced ulcers, NSAID ulcers are usually associated with minimal inflammatory cell infiltrate in surrounding tissue [137]. Perhaps in part because of this, NSAID ulcers are often asymptomatic and so more prone to present with complications such as bleeding or perforation.

Mechanisms underlying mucosal damage

Although the most important mechanism underlying NSAID/aspirin ulceration is prostaglandin inhibition, other mechanisms contribute. Topical injury is important, and erosions and ulcers are common in the dependent stomach. Many NSAIDs and aspirin are weakly acidic and become trapped in epithelial cells where they have concentrated effects. However, enteric-coated NSAIDs and aspirin can still cause ulcers and ulcer complications, illustrating that topical injury is not necessary. The antiplatelet action of aspirin is also important. As well as increasing the risk of significant bleeding, it may affect ulcer healing through inhibition of angiogenesis [172]. Clopidogrel, an antiplatelet agent, is also mildly ulcerogenic and increases bleeding, probably through similar mechanisms [172].

Cyclooxygenase inhibition

The most important ulcerogenic mechanism of NSAIDs/aspirin is to damage mucosal defences by inhibiting the enzyme cyclooxygenase (COX) which is involved in local prostaglandin synthesis [173,174]. COX converts arachidonic acid to prostaglandin precursors and exists in two isoforms: COX-1 and COX-2. COX-1 is constitutive and is expressed in many sites including the stomach, kidneys, endothelium, and platelets. In the stomach, it is a central orchestrator of mucosal defense. Its inhibition by NSAIDs and aspirin is the main mechanism whereby these drugs induce ulceration. COX-2 is inducible and is expressed most strongly in inflammatory cells, fibroblasts, and synovium. It is involved in inflammation and pain; its inhibition by NSAIDs is the key mechanism underlying their antiinflammatory and pain-relieving properties.

The development of specific COX-2 inhibitory drugs appeared to offer the possibility for pain relief without GI side-effects (29,175–177]. Unfortunately these agents were also associated with a slightly increased risk of vascular events and have now either been withdrawn or are used with caution [178]. However, it is now becoming clear that many nonselective NSAIDs have similar vascular effects [179,180] and physicians are beginning to use COX-2 inhibitors again if an NSAID is indicated, ulcer risk is high, and vascular risk is low [181] (see "Prevention").

Effects of prostaglandin inhibition

Following COX-1 inhibition, the precise mechanism of ulceration is unclear as many protective processes are inhibited. Mucin suppression allows backdiffusion of acid and pepsin. Bicarbonate, surface active phospholipid, epithelial restitution, and epithelial cell proliferation are all suppressed. There is also relative stasis in the microvasculature. In animal models, neutrophils adhere to the microvasculature before migrating into the mucosa, although in chronic ulceration in humans, inflammatory cells are usually scarce. Profound acid suppression is sometimes needed to heal NSAID ulcers [182]. This may imply a role for pepsin in their pathogenesis or may reflect the fact that acid is less important in their pathogenesis than it is in *H. pylori* ulcers; NSAID damage can occur elsewhere in the GI tract where there is no acid.

Differential risk in NSAID users

The ulcer risk conferred by aspirin and NSAIDs differs depending on the precise agents used and how they are employed (Figure 49.9) [(183)]. The risk depends on the extent of COX-1 inhibition, but also on dose, solubility, duration of action, coprescription with other drugs such as steroids, age of the patient, and whether there is a history of previous ulceration [65,177].

The pathogenesis of idiopathic, non-*H. pylori*, non-NSAID ulcers

The scenario of non-*H. pylori*, non-NSAID PUD has been increasingly recognized in recent years. Except for certain rare etiologies with defined disease mechanisms (see "Etiology"), the pathogenesis of non-*H. pylori*, non-NSAID ulcers is largely unknown [3]. Systemic reviews have emphasized the importance in this group of false-negative results for *H. pylori* diagnosis, NSAID use, and smoking [184]. When these have been excluded, the remaining group of DUs includes those associated with gastric hypersecretion, isolated duodenal *H. pylori* colonization, and other diseases of the duodenal mucosa, and non-*pylori Helicobacter* infection.

One interesting hypothesis is that genetic and epigenetic changes in mucin expression may be responsible for otherwise idiopathic ulcers [39]. Mucins are essential components of the mucus layer that protects the underlying mucosa from luminal low pH contents and enzymatic damage. This theory is supported by more reasonably well-established pathogenic mechanisms – mucin secretion is reduced by COX pathway inhibition, and different mucin subtypes are relevant for *H. pylori* adhesion and invasion. The clinical impact of non-*H. pylori*, non-NSAID ulcers, and potential opportunities for targeted management in these patients, await further research.

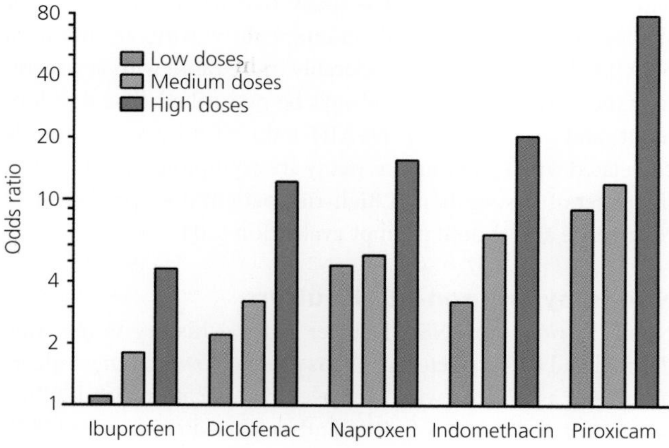

Figure 49.9 Odds ratios for peptic ulcer bleeding for different NSAIDs and drug doses. All odds ratios are adjusted and relative to nonuse of NSAIDs or aspirin. Note that confidence intervals were wide. NSAIDs, nonsteroidal antiinflammatory drugs. Source: Adapted from Lewis et al. 2002 [183], with permission from Wiley Blackwell.

Genetics of peptic ulcer disease

The importance of genetic influences is unclear but they probably moderate the overall susceptibility to PUD. Early twin and family studies suggested a genetic component to peptic ulcer as a *H. pylori*-related disease. Monozygotic twin pairs showed greater similarities in the acquisition of *H. pylori* infection although, unsurprisingly, a shared rearing environment also contributes to shared risk [185]. The ABO blood group is one determinant of *H. pylori* infectivity [186]. Individuals with blood group O appear to be at higher risk of peptic ulcers, with significantly lower relative risks for blood groups A, B, and AB, ranging from 0.75 to 0.91 [187]. Risk profiles were similar for GU and DU, and for ulcer complications. The mechanisms are not completely clear, but *H. pylori* does express adhesins that can bind to blood group antigens and so are likely responsible in part [188]. In addition, correlations between blood group O and the development of gastric cancer under the age of 50 have been shown in previous observational studies, which might be explained based on this elevated risk for *H. pylori* infection [189].

Genetic influences in PUD go beyond the acquisition of *H. pylori* infection. A cross-sectional study used the Swedish twin registry for a total of 691 twin pairs overall, reared together or separately [190]. The greatest influence on PUD risk was observed for monozygotic twins reared apart, with estimates for genetic effects (heritability) of approximately 65%, and for nongenetic (environmental) effects of approximately 35%. Moreover, twins reared together were not more similar than twins reared apart, which may suggest that shared environment is not an important source of familial similarity for PUD (though age at separation varied widely). Interestingly, genetic influences for PUD were largely independent of genetic effects important for acquiring *H. pylori* infection (*H. pylori* status was determined by serology).

Host genetic factors are important determinants of disease risk, particularly cytokine and innate immune response gene polymorphisms, though as previously discussed these are less convincing for PUD risk than for gastric cancer and precursors to cancer [191]. Polymorphisms can influence the expression of inflammatory mediators in the gastric mucosa, influencing mucosal inflammation in response to *H. pylori* infection and acid secretion. However, they are mostly linked to hypochlorhydria and atrophy, potentially explaining the much closer associations with gastric cancer than with DU. Most of these reports concern polymorphisms in genes for IL-1β, the antagonist for its receptor (IL-1RA, *IL1RN*), and for tumor necrosis factor (TNF)-α, though others including IL-2, IL-4, IL-6, and IL-8 have been identified. There appear to be quite major population differences in their influence on disease expression [192]. Genetic and pharmacogenetic factors have also been identified that predispose to NSAID-induced peptic ulcers [193]. Polymorphisms in the genes for COX-1 and IL-1β are examples thought to increase the risk of ulcer in NSAID and aspirin users, whereas polymorphisms associated with hypoacidity and corpus gastritis seem to reduce this risk [194].

Other genetic differences, including HLA-DQA1 genotype, have been reported for *H. pylori*-negative ulcer disease [195]. A syndromic form of cytosolic phospholipase A2 a deficiency has been reported, which is associated with recurrent GI ulcers and bleeding diathesis, as well as mild inherited deficiency of factor XI and extremely low levels of platelet thromboxane A2 biosynthesis [196].

Natural history

The natural history of PUD depends on the underlying cause, but essentially ulcers may remit (even without antisecretory treatment), persist, or develop complications such as bleeding or perforation. *H. pylori*-related ulcers follow these classic scenarios but NSAID ulcers are more likely to persist if the NSAID is not stopped. Following antisecretory treatment, most ulcers heal, although DUs generally heal more quickly than GUs, and small ulcers heal more quickly than large ones. After healing, ulcers will usually relapse when antisecretory therapy is stopped, unless the underlying cause – typically *H. pylori* infection or NSAID use – is removed. Persistent ulceration, particularly during antisecretory therapy, should prompt a search for another underlying cause. For GUs, repeat endoscopy after antisecretory therapy should be performed to confirm healing and exclude underlying malignancy. Ulcer complications are relatively more common for NSAID than *H. pylori* ulcers. This may be because NSAID ulcers are more often asymptomatic and so, presumably, persist longer without treatment. Indeed, they more commonly present for the first time with a complication such as bleeding or perforation than *H. pylori* ulcers.

Helicobacter pylori ulcers

Helicobacter pylori-associated ulcers have been observed to relapse without eradication or medical treatment; over a 12-month period, 26% of patients did not experience further symptoms after documented DU healing, whereas 33% experienced one recurrence, 24% had two episodes, and 17% had three or more episodes [197]. Treatment of *H. pylori* infection markedly reduces recurrences and alters natural history. The symptomatic benefit is greatest for DU [198]. Duodenal erosions may occur after treatment [199,200], and this may be responsible in part for occasional reports of an unexpectedly high DU recurrence rate of up to 20% despite successful eradication [201]. However, duodenal erosions often heal spontaneously and their clinical relevance is questionable. Alternative explanations for DU recurrence after *H. pylori* eradication are a persistent predisposition to mucosal injury or that the ulcer was falsely attributed to *H. pylori*. Eradication of *H. pylori* is more effective at preventing recurrent bleeding from peptic ulcer than antisecretory therapy alone – less than 3% following *H. pylori* eradication, compared with 6% during long-term antisecretory therapy and 20% in the absence of maintenance antisecretory therapy (see "Complications").

In the modern management of dyspepsia, antisecretory therapy is recommended for symptomatic patients under the age of 60 rather than performing an endoscopy if *H. pylori* infection is ruled out, and this is a more cost-effective approach where community prevalence of *H. pylori* is less than 20% [202]. In these cases, the natural history determines that the ulcer (and so symptoms) will often relapse, usually within weeks of stopping treatment.

Nonsteroidal antiinflammatory drug ulcers

Upper GI events, including symptomatic and complicated ulcers, occur in 1 in 20 NSAID users and in 1 in 7 older adults using NSAIDs (203]. The natural history of NSAID ulcers has not been established for patients who continue on NSAIDs without ulcer treatment. It is likely that particularly small or shallow ulcers would heal spontaneously with cessation of NSAIDs, but healing is considerably more rapid with antisecretory therapy, which should always be prescribed. The development and resolution of NSAID-induced ulcers are poorly correlated with symptoms, as many are asymptomatic. However, the onset of dyspepsia in a high-risk patient does predict ulcer recurrence and should prompt evaluation [203–206].

Non-*H. pylori*, non-NSAID ulcers

Non-*H. pylori*, non-NSAID ulcer natural history is less well defined and this is a heterogeneous group. However, these ulcers have been associated with increased complication risk [207], a longer initial duration of ulcer, and increased recurrence [184]. These patients are treated with the highest PPI dose for 40–60 days [208]. Follow-up endoscopy showed a cure rate of 97.6%; age (OR 3.5), male sex (OR 3.1), hospitalization (OR 3.0), number of medications (OR 2.8), and a clinical history positive for PUD (OR 3.7) are the major risk factors.

Relationship between natural history and symptoms

The natural history of PUD means that the most usual course is one of recurrent episodes of upper abdominal pain. In trials of antisecretory therapy, before *H. pylori* eradication and PPI therapy, ulcer recurrence rates of 50–80% were observed in the placebo-treated control groups in the 6–12 months following initial ulcer healing [209–211]. The predictive value of symptoms remains poor in this context: the disappearance of symptoms does not correlate with ulcer healing (15–44% have endoscopic ulceration despite being asymptomatic) and ongoing symptoms do not correlate with ulceration (40% have persistent symptoms despite endoscopic healing) [212,213]. These observations may relate to the relapsing and remitting nature of PUD, or the coexistence and symptomatic overlap with functional dyspepsia.

Clinical presentation and differential diagnosis

Uncomplicated ulcers may present with a variety of symptoms, usually collectively termed "dyspepsia." Dyspepsia is difficult to define. The International Rome III consensus group described it as "a symptom or set of symptoms that most physicians consider to originate from the gastroduodenal area," including postprandial heaviness, early satiety, and epigastric pain or burning [214].

Clinical features are of limited value in identifying or excluding uncomplicated ulcers – patients with ulcers may report dyspepsia (with or without the classic ulcer symptoms), other upper GI complaints, or be asymptomatic (Table 49.3). Therefore, the aims of the initial clinical evaluation are to exclude symptoms arising from outside the GI tract; to identify risk factors for peptic ulceration; and to determine the presence of red flags (Box 49.2), which would prompt urgent investigation to exclude malignancy.

Presentation with dyspepsia

The Rome IV criteria divide dyspepsia into epigastric pain syndrome, postprandial distress syndrome, and overlap of these two entities [217,218], either of which can indicate peptic ulceration. Approximately 10% of adults in high or very high HDI countries suffer from functional dyspepsia which is associated with significant health impairment [219]. Pain is the hallmark symptom of uncomplicated peptic ulceration, typically burning epigastric pain. Peptic ulceration is also frequently asymptomatic. Traditionally, patients with PUD, and in particular duodenal ulceration, were considered to have stereotypical presentations – the classic ulcer symptoms (see further on). However, several conditions commonly present with pain or discomfort centered predominantly in the upper abdomen, with or without associated features.

PUD may also be accompanied by other symptoms, including postprandial fullness or bloating, early satiety, belching, nausea, or vomiting; reflux-like symptoms including heartburn, water and acid brash; or other features including reversible anorexia, weight loss, constipation, and symptoms typical of irritable bowel syndrome. There is considerable overlap between these patterns.

Only 5–10% of patients presenting with simple dyspepsia in high or very high HDI countries will have a peptic ulcer. Population endoscopy studies suggest that three-quarters of patients with dyspepsia have a normal upper GI tract [220]. Therefore, the role of the clinical assessment in this setting is to discriminate upper GI symptoms from those arising from other systems, and to identify red flags (see Box 49.2) that will usually mandate endoscopy. The approach to the patient with dyspepsia is discussed in the section on therapy and management and is the subject of Chapter 31.

Differential diagnosis of dyspepsia

The differential diagnosis of dyspepsia is presented in detail in Chapter 31 and that of abdominal pain in general in Chapter 34. In patients with uninvestigated dyspepsia in whom etiologies outside the GI tract have first been identified through clinical assessment (in particular cholelithiasis with biliary pain, pancreatitis, medications, and extraabdominal causes), the differential diagnosis of PUD includes any cause of dyspepsia [215,216]. The most common diagnosis in this group is functional dyspepsia (in up to 60–75%). Other important causes of nonulcer dyspepsia include gastroesophageal reflux disease (GERD) and malignancy, though early-stage gastric cancer is often asymptomatic.

Clinical features of uncomplicated peptic ulcer disease

Nowadays, it is well recognized that it is not possible to reliably diagnose peptic ulceration by the history alone or to distinguish DU, GU, or nonulcer dyspepsia based on symptoms (see Table 49.3). The prevalence of dyspeptic symptoms is broadly similar in patients with and without ulcers. Although some specific symptoms such as food relief have some positive predictive value for PUD and others such as postprandial pain, food intolerance, and nausea have some negative predictive value [221], they provide no certainty as to the diagnosis.

Physical examination is also rarely helpful. The most predictive sign is the "pointing sign": when asked to indicate the location of pain, the patient points to a discrete epigastric site. This is moderately predictive of DU but again gives little certainty. One systematic review reported that the clinical diagnosis of PUD, or its absence, had a positive likelihood ratio of 2.2 (95% confidence interval (CI) 1.9–2.9) and a negative likelihood ratio of 0.45 (95% CI 0.38–0.53) respectively [222]. These figures were similar whether the diagnosis was made by a primary care physician, a specialist, or a computer model. Thus, overall clinical assessment has poor predictive value for peptic ulceration in the scenario of uninvestigated dyspepsia.

Table 49.3 Symptoms of gastric and duodenal ulcers and functional dyspepsia.

Symptom	Gastric ulcer (%)	Duodenal ulcer (%)	Functional dyspepsia (%)
Pain/discomfort	100	100	100
Features of the pain:			
Primary pain			
Epigastric	67	61–86	52–73
Right hypochondrium	6	7–17	4
Left hypochondrium	6	3–5	5
Frequently severe	68	53	37
Within 30 minutes of food	20	5	32
Gnawing pain	13	16	6
Increased by food	24	10–40	45
Clusters (episodic)	16	56	35
Relieved by alkali	36–87	39–86	26–75
Food relief	2–48	20–63	4–32
Occurs at night	32–43	50–88	24–32
Not related to food or variable	22–53	21–49	22–65
Radiation to back	34	20–31	24–28
Increased appetite		19	
Anorexia	46–57	25–36	26–36
Weight loss	24–61	19–45	18–32
Nausea	54–70	49–59	43–60
Vomiting	38–73	25–57	26–34
Heartburn	19	27–59	28
Nondyspeptic symptoms	2	8	18
Fatty food intolerance		41–72	53
Bloating	55	49	52
Belching	48	59	60

Note: Asymptomatic and silent ulcers are also common – see text.

Patients are either managed with a diagnosis of uninvestigated dyspepsia (the cause being recognized as uncertain) or investigated with endoscopy. Whether to perform endoscopy depends on the presence of red flag symptoms (see Box 49.2), age, and whether symptoms recur.

Classic ulcer symptoms – duodenal ulcer

Despite the overall poor predictive value of symptoms and the lack of utility in management algorithms, some ulcers do present with classic symptoms of epigastric pain or discomfort that occurs in the fasted state, typically at night or 2–3 hours after meals, with food relief. These classic symptoms may occur in up to half of patients (see Table 49.3), but they also occur in patients with other diagnoses. Pain may wake the patient from sleep but is absent by morning; this pattern is thought to follow the circadian stimulation of acid secretion that is maximal between 11 pm and 2 am. Postprandial pain occurs in the presence of ongoing acid secretion following emptying of food from the upper GI tract. Discomfort may localize to the left or right hypochondrium but mainly occurs in the epigastrium and may radiate to the back. Qualitative descriptions of pain are not very helpful in diagnosis, but the pain is typically reported as burning, aching, gnawing, or as a "hunger pain" or discomfort. Relief may be provided by food, such that most patients maintain or increase weight, or by antacids and antisecretory agents. Because of their clinical course and chronicity, characteristically ulcers cause clusters of pain lasting for 1–3 months with intervening asymptomatic periods of weeks or months.

Box 49.2 Red flags (or alarm symptoms) in dyspepsia.

Age older than 55 years with new-onset dyspepsia[a]

- Family history of upper gastrointestinal cancer
- Unintended weight loss
- Gastrointestinal bleeding
- Progressive dysphagia
- Odynophagia
- Unexplained iron deficiency anemia
- Persistent vomiting
- Palpable mass or lymphadenopathy
- Jaundice

Note

[a] Some national guidelines do not recommend an age cut-off or use an alternative such as 45 years. See text for further discussion (under Therapy and management). Source: Reproduced from Talley [215] and Talley et al. [216], with permission from Elsevier.

Patients may also present with acute or chronic complications of PUD, including hemorrhage, perforation or penetration, and gastric outlet obstruction.

Classic ulcer symptoms – gastric ulcer

In GU, the classic symptom is epigastric pain shortly after meals (within 30 minutes of food); however, the presentation is usually less stereotypical. Symptoms are less often relieved by eating or antacids, and more likely to be provoked. Associated symptoms are more prominent, including anorexia or weight loss in around 50% (see Table 49.3). If the ulcer is near the pylorus then poor gastric emptying may result, leading to reflux symptoms, vomiting, and early satiety. Clusters of pain are less common.

Asymptomatic or silent ulcers

Upper GI endoscopy or other tests are sometimes performed in patients without dyspepsia, and chronic asymptomatic ulcers are identified surprisingly frequently [223–225]. In particular, in elderly patients, NSAID-induced ulcers often cause no antecedent symptoms until manifesting as complicated disease with bleeding or perforation. Interestingly, in a European population, about one in five participants with ulcers were asymptomatic, whereas in a Chinese study, 72% of individuals reported no symptoms [226].

Differential diagnosis of confirmed ulcer

For endoscopically confirmed ulcer, the differential diagnosis is that of underlying conditions (see Box 49.1). It is important to identify or rigorously exclude *H. pylori* infection, NSAID consumption, or both, before considering alternative etiologies. The identification of specific causes of peptic ulcer is discussed in the section on therapy and management.

Clinical features of complicated peptic ulcer disease

This scenario is considered separately in the section on complications. The cardinal features that suggest acute complicated PUD include upper GI bleeding (hemorrhage), severe pain (perforation or penetration), and vomiting (gastric outlet obstruction). Patients may present with a change in symptoms or without antecedent ulcer symptoms, and many present late having ignored or underestimated their significance. Chronic complications include iron deficiency anemia and chronic gastric outlet obstruction secondary to scarring.

Differential diagnosis of complicated PUD

In the context of presentation with clinical features suggestive of ulcer complications, other causes of vomiting (see Chapter 33), of an acute abdomen (see Chapter 37), and of upper GI bleeding and anemia (see Chapter 38) enter into the differential diagnosis.

Special scenarios – other clinical or endoscopic findings

Peptic ulcer in association with gastroesophageal reflux

Gastroesophageal reflux disease (see Chapter 43) and peptic ulceration can occur simultaneously, particularly in the pathophysiological settings of increased acid secretion or reduced gastric emptying. Risk factors for GERD in an ulcer patient include acid hypersecretory states (basal acid output >15 mmol/h), decreased lower esophageal sphincter pressure, frequent vomiting, and obesity. The relationship is complex, as patients with severe duodenal or pyloric ulceration and impaired gastric emptying frequently also have reflux esophagitis, and this may cooccur with *H. pylori* or NSAID ulcers. Symptomatic improvement after *H. pylori* eradication therapy is less frequent overall in patients with coexisting GERD, presumably because the GERD is likely to persist and in many patients is the predominant cause of symptoms [227]. However, strong evidence from systematic review and metaanalysis shows that the overall incidence of GERD with or without erosive esophagitis does not increase after *H. pylori* eradication [228].

Giant ulcers

Giant ulcers are larger than 2–3 cm in diameter and typically occur in the gastric body, although giant duodenal (typically on the posterior wall) and prepyloric ulcers have been reported. They are commonly related to NSAID consumption but have also been reported in end-stage renal failure, Crohn's disease, transplantation, and amphetamine misuse. Weight loss is more common with giant ulcers and may increase the suspicion of malignancy, which should be considered and excluded in all cases as the risk is increased fourfold for giant GU. However, giant benign-appearing ulcers rarely turn out to be malignant.

Giant ulcers heal slowly, necessitating sustained medical treatment, and this is to be expected as healing progresses at around 3 mm per week for all GUs [229]. Giant ulcers are also more prone to complications, including more frequent relapses (particularly in the presence of dense scarring and resulting deformity), severe hemorrhage (twofold relative risk), and penetration (four- to fivefold relative risk). While giant DUs no longer routinely require surgery, they still have a higher rate of complications and mortality, and early surgical consultation is advisable [230].

Pyloric channel ulcers

Pyloric channel ulcers are a type of GU sited within 3 cm of the pylorus. The edema and scarring associated with larger ulcers can affect gastric emptying such that patients may present with features of gastric outlet obstruction.

Postbulbar ulcers

Duodenal ulcers are typically located in the duodenal bulb within a few centimeters of the pylorus. Postbulbar ulcers are uncommon and suggest hormonally mediated acid hypersecretion although alternative diagnoses such as duodenal diverticula or adhesive bands, local or locally invasive neoplasia, and annular pancreas should be considered. Unusual endoscopic appearances are rare even in the presence of alternative etiologies such as carcinoma of the duodenum or pancreas, although additional clinical features, a mass at endoscopy, or refractory ulceration may raise suspicion.

In gastrinoma, not only are DUs often located atypically but they are often also multiple and refractory to therapy. Additional clues to gastrinoma include a positive family history, hypoglycemic episodes, weight loss or gain, diarrhea and steatorrhea (islet cell tumors), hypercalcemia and renal stones (hyperparathyroidism), and visual disturbance, headache, and hormonal abnormalities (pituitary tumors). See Chapter 50 on Zollinger–Ellison syndrome.

Multiple ulcers

Multiple simultaneous ulcers occur in up to one in five patients with PUD and are often clustered around the same site; they are more common in male smokers, NSAID users, and in gastrinoma. DU and GU can also occur simultaneously but this is less common; coexisting DU and GU heal more slowly and follow a more complicated course.

Childhood peptic ulcer disease

Duodenal ulcer in the first two decades usually presents with nocturnal pain, but presentation with hemorrhage is reported in up to one in three. Infection with *H. pylori* and NSAID use (typically short term for febrile illness) account for the majority of cases of childhood PUD, though non-*H. pylori*, non-NSAID ulcers were diagnosed in around one-third of patients in one series from Taiwan [4], albeit in older children with a family history of PUD. Severe general illness is an important cause of secondary ulcer, particularly in children younger than 10 years [231].

Therapy and management

There are three major therapeutic scenarios in the approach to PUD. First, uninvestigated dyspepsia, a common scenario for a large number of patients, often in a primary care setting; second, an uncomplicated ulcer that has been identified at endoscopy; and third, a complicated PUD. The approach to ulceration is twofold: first, management of ulceration and second, the identification and treatment of specific causes/risk factors (*H. pylori* infection, NSAID use, others). The management of recurrent and refractory ulcers is an important consideration for physicians in secondary and tertiary care settings.

Uninvestigated dyspepsia

The approach to the patient with dyspepsia is covered in Chapter 31 and several guidelines have been published [232]. Dyspepsia is common and only a minority of patients with uninvestigated dyspepsia have PUD [233]. Clinical evaluation is largely directed at excluding causes outside the GI tract and determining whether there are any red flags (or alarm symptoms) that could indicate underlying malignancy (see Box 49.2). Taking a comprehensive drug history is important to identify potentially ulcerogenic drugs (including unreported, occasional, or surreptitious use of NSAIDs), or drugs associated with dyspepsia such as iron supplements or narcotics. Collateral histories from family members can be helpful. The history should also determine any personal history of peptic ulceration and risk factors for *H. pylori* infection (for example, family history, recent migration, or certain ethnic backgrounds).

Following this initial evaluation, the aims of management are prompt, effective, and cost-effective treatment, without exposing patients to unwarranted investigations or prolonged empirical treatments that prove ineffective [234]. A definitive diagnosis is not always required but the most recent North American guidelines suggest a trial of PPI in the absence of alarm features and *H. pylori* and do not recommend endoscopy to investigate dyspepsia in patients under the age of 60 [202]. This is despite a metaanalysis showing that patient satisfaction and symptomatic relief were better achieved by endoscope-and-treat compared to test-and-treat strategies since the test-and-treat strategy proved to be more cost-effective [235].

Population approaches

In areas of high *H. pylori* prevalence (>20% in general population) and in the absence of red flags (see Box 49.2), screening for and eradication of infection is usually the next step (the test and treat approach). This will treat some cases of PUD without a definitive diagnosis being made and is an effective and cost-effective strategy.

In regions of low *H. pylori* prevalence (less than 10%) and in the absence of red flags, treatment with empirical antisecretory agents (mainly PPIs) is widely used (the empirical therapy approach) as mentioned above.

An investigative approach to dyspepsia, with urgent upper GI endoscopy, is indicated in patients over the age of 60 or, more controversially, those under the age of 60 but with red flags. This approach aims to establish a definitive diagnosis in these patients, as the selected population has a higher risk of gastric malignancy and also of PUD. A cut-off at age 60 years is most common, though different nationally determined thresholds are used (such as 45 years), depending on the population risk of gastric cancer. Earlier thresholds may be appropriate for certain populations at higher risk, such as patients from Asian, Hispanic, and Afro-Caribbean ethnic backgrounds. Some national guidelines do not use an age cut-off for two reasons. In some countries, most dyspeptic patients undergo endoscopy, despite the cost, in an attempt to make a definitive diagnosis and guide management. At the other extreme, some guidelines argue that early gastric cancer is unlikely to cause symptoms, and do not advise endoscopy at all in simple dyspepsia (as excluding cancer is the main indication). We advise an age cut-off of 60 years at first presentation with simple dyspepsia for arranging endoscopy in accordance with the most recent North American guidelines [202].

Individualized approach, including test and treat

A more individualized or personalized approach is increasingly being advocated for the management of dyspepsia, particularly for identifying and treating *H. pylori* infection (see "Treating *H. pylori* – Recommended therapeutic paradigm"). The goal is to estimate the pretest probability of *H. pylori* infection. This should be informed by the local prevalence of *H. pylori* and the patient's age, country of origin, ethnic background, and socioeconomic status in early life. Other considerations are a prior history of ulcer; previous investigations and treatment for *H. pylori*; smoking status; and comorbidity. Patient preference should also be considered. Taken together, these factors inform decisions on the optimal management strategy and, in particular, whether to test for (and to treat) *H. pylori* infection. If *H. pylori* testing is indicated, urea breath testing or the stool antigen test is usually most appropriate (refer to "Testing for *H. pylori*"). Eradication therapy for *H. pylori* is discussed later.

Empirical antisecretory therapy, including for NSAID users

An empirical trial of treatment with a PPI for 4 weeks is recommended when *H. pylori* prevalence is low, and for patients following a test and treat strategy who are uninfected [236,237]. Some guidelines recommend a trial for up to 8 weeks but, even with an early change in drug class and optimized dosing, only around one in 5–7 patients with uninvestigated dyspepsia respond to empirical PPI (and one in 15 with functional dyspepsia) [238]. Prolonged PPI use can cause rebound acid hypersecretion on withdrawal [239], promoting dependency, and therefore it is important to taper or discontinue the PPI if there is no significant early improvement in symptoms. A metaanalysis of 15 RCTs comparing PPI and placebo showed a 30.4% response in the PPI group compared to 24.8% in the control group ($p < 0.00001$) with a number needed to treat (NNT) of 10 [202].

Many experts use test and treat and empirical therapy strategies together; they test for *H. pylori* and at the same time start a PPI while waiting for results. Such strategies may not be cost-effective but are suitable for some healthcare systems. Suspected NSAID-associated dyspepsia should receive immediate treatment with a PPI if there are no red flags (with relief of symptoms expected within 2–4 weeks) [240], along with testing for *H. pylori* if not already performed, and discontinuation of the offending drug whenever possible (see "Prevention"). The test and treat strategy has been more cost-effective than an endoscopy-first strategy in patients under the age of 60 [202]. We recommend waiting for at least 4 weeks to assess the effect of eradication on dyspepsia.

Ongoing symptoms

Persistent or recurrent dyspepsia is common regardless of the treatment approach and, particularly where empirical therapy has been employed initially, it is important to reconsider whether to test for *H. pylori* infection. Most patients following a test and treat strategy who are infected with *H. pylori* will have ongoing symptoms despite successful treatment – only one in 14 *H. pylori*-infected patients with dyspepsia will completely respond to eradication therapy. Such patients should be treated with a trial of PPI. We recommend endoscopy for any individual developing red flags and also, on occasion, for individuals with persistent troublesome symptoms despite therapy. For further discussion and management considerations, see Chapter 31.

Identification of ulcer

Definitive diagnosis of ulceration requires a diagnostic test, and endoscopy is the test of choice. Endoscopy provides a sensitive, specific, and safe method for identifying peptic ulcers, allowing direct inspection, tests to determine *H. pylori* status, and tissue sampling via biopsy where necessary. In the past, barium contrast studies were routinely used to investigate persistent dyspepsia, and these are still occasionally employed in patients who cannot tolerate endoscopy or who have failed intubation. Demonstration of barium within an ulcer crater is diagnostic, though secondary changes may be present from edema, scarring, or other deformity. Computed tomography (CT) scans are much less sensitive but can occasionally demonstrate a gastric or duodenal ulcer but are not the test of choice. In case of findings in the stomach suggestive of GU, supplementary gastroscopy with biopsy is still recommended to increase the diagnostic specificity and rule out malignancy.

Treatment of peptic ulcer disease

Regardless of etiology of the ulcer, antisecretory agents relieve ulcer-associated dyspeptic symptoms and effectively heal most peptic ulcers. Continued use greatly reduces ulcer recurrence and the risk of complications.

Antisecretory and antiulcer agents

There are several classes of drugs licensed for use in PUD that have an antisecretory and/or antiulcer mechanism of action (Table 49.4). Drugs that inhibit acid secretion are the most effective for management of peptic ulcer – both for healing of active ulcer and for maintenance therapy – and are by far the most commonly used.

Histamine type 2 receptor antagonists (H_2-RAs) were developed in the 1970s and 1980s. They are competitive inhibitors of histamine at the H_2 receptors found on parietal cells. Many individual drugs have been developed with slightly different potencies, pharmacokinetic properties, and side-effect profiles. They are all effective but have largely been replaced by the more potent PPIs.

Proton pump inhibitors bind irreversibly to proton pumps in the secretory canaliculi of gastric parietal cells and block acid secretion more durably and more effectively than H_2-RAs (see Chapter 17). PPIs heal a greater proportion of ulcers more rapidly than H_2-RAs. Available PPIs differ to some extent with respect to potencies, pharmacokinetic properties, and side effect profiles, but all are effective and the least expensive is usually selected. In general, they are very safe drugs and there are minimal safety concerns with long-term use (see Table 49.4) based on RCT data [202,241]. PPIs may reduce the sensitivity of *H. pylori* tests and slightly reduce the sensitivity of endoscopy for diagnosing malignancy (see "Identification of specific causes of ulcer"). They have minor drug interactions, the most potentially important, though still controversial, being interference with the efficacy of clopidogrel (see "Prevention"). A randomized crossover study suggested that the effect of PPIs in attenuating the efficacy of clopidogrel was less with dexlansoprazole or lansoprazole than esomeprazole or omeprazole [242], although a more recent study of the effect of six different PPIs (rabeprazole, pantoprazole, omeprazole, lansoprazole, esomeprazole, dexlansoprazole) in healthy volunteers reported no significant difference in platelet aggregation between the clopidogrel monotherapy arm and any of the clopidogrel-PPI arms [243].

Potassium competitive acid blockers, like PPIs, enter the parietal cell secretory canaliculus and act on the proton pump but they have a different mechanism of action, binding ionically to the H+,K+-APTase enzyme to prevent activation by the K+ cation [244]. This class of drugs, which includes linaprazan, revaprazan, soraprazan, and vonaprazan, offers rapid onset with reversible and very effective acid suppression. PCABs have been in development for over two decades but revaprazan, the first PCAB to market, is available only in India and South Korea and vonoprazan is available only in Japan. Initial randomized, controlled clinical studies have reported that revaprazan 200 mg daily is similar in efficacy to omeprazole 20 mg daily for the treatment of DU over 4 weeks [245] and GU over 4–8 weeks [246]. More recent studies have reported comparable healing rates with vonaprazan 20 mg daily and lansoprazole 30 mg daily for DU over 6 weeks and GU over 8 weeks [247]. Similarly, 24-week maintenance studies have reported comparable efficacy for vonoprazan 10 mg daily, vonoprazan 20 mg daily, and lansoprazole 15 mg daily in preventing recurrent ulceration in patients taking NSAIDs [248] or low-dose aspirin [249]. A recent metaanalysis concluded that vonoprazan was superior to PPI therapy for ulcer shrinkage rate and healing of post-ESD ulcers but there were no differences in post-ESD bleeding [250]. There are no randomized, controlled studies on the use of PCABs for non-*H. pylori*, non-NSAID ulcers but a small observational study in 33 patients concluded that, with a healing rate of 81% after 6–8 weeks, vonoprazan was insufficient to heal idiopathic ulcers [251].

Metaanalyses indicate that vonoprazan-based triple therapy is superior to PPI-based triple therapy for clarithromycin-resistant and clarithromycin-susceptible *H. pylori* strains but a clearer understanding of the role of PCABs in *H. pylori* treatment requires further comparative studies with different PCAB dosing and antibiotic regimens in different geographic regions [252].

In summary, PCABs appear to be comparable to PPIs for the management of acid-related disorders, including PUD, but there are not yet any conditions for which PCABs are clearly superior.

Misoprostol and sucralfate have minor roles in modern ulcer management (see Table 49.4). Misoprostol may occasionally be useful to prevent NSAID ulcers but PPIs are preferable in most situations (see "Prevention"). Misoprostol may also have a role in *H. pylori*-negative GU [253]. Sucralfate is sometimes used in the setting of stress ulcer (see "Disease associations and comorbid ulcers") and is occasionally used with PPIs in severe refractory non-*H. pylori*, non-NSAID ulceration.

Other drugs are rarely used for PUD. Antacids offer rapid symptom relief in other acid-related disorders and are often used by patients with dyspepsia; at high dose they can heal ulcers although they are much less effective than antisecretory drugs. Bismuth was a traditional remedy that is now used predominantly in *H. pylori* eradication regimens; combination convenience pills, containing bismuth and antibiotics, may provide suboptimal antibiotic dosing in some situations [254]. Anticholinergic medications are of historical interest only.

Medical therapy

Proton pump inhibitors are most often used, given that they are most effective. The approach taken to heal an ulcer is determined by location, *H. pylori* status, ulcer complications or an expectation of slow healing. Standard doses of PPI are adequate, with higher dose treatment reserved for those with complications.

Active ulcers

For patients with an uncomplicated, *H. pylori*-positive shallow DU, *H. pylori* eradication therapy without further antisecretory treatment is usually adequate. Otherwise, DUs should be treated with standard-dose PPI for 4 weeks (to achieve a healing rate of 80–100%), though the majority will have healed by 2 weeks (60–90%). H_2-RAs can be used for 4 weeks (70–80%) but 8 weeks of treatment is more effective (90–95%). Longer initial therapy with PPI can be considered for complicated ulcers and those that may take longer to heal (such as those associated with severe scarring or the rare giant DU and smokers).

Table 49.4 Antisecretory and antiulcer drugs licensed in the USA for use in peptic ulcer disease in adults.

Generic name	Brand names	Total daily dosages	Dosing intervals	Pregnancy
Proton pump inhibitors (PPIs)				
Potently inhibit acid secretion: irreversibly bind and inhibit H⁺,K⁺-ATPase pumps on parietal cell luminal surface membrane Side-effects: headache, diarrhea, constipation, abdominal discomfort, nausea, rash Potential safety concerns in some patients during long-term use: ***Clostridium difficile***-associated diarrhea (not a statistically significant difference) [241]				
Esomeprazole	Nexium®	20 to 40 mg	Once or twice daily when used as part of ***H. pylori*** treatment	B/C
Lansoprazole	Prevacid®	15 to 30 mg[a]		B
Omeprazole	Prilosec®, Zegerid®	20 to 40 mg[a]		C
Pantoprazole	Protonix®	20 to 40 mg		B
Rabeprazole	Aciphex®	20 mg		B
Dexlansoprazole	Dexilant®	30 or 60 mg	Once daily	
H_2-receptor antagonists (H_2-RAs)				
Inhibit acid secretion: reversibly and competitively inhibit histamine H_2 receptors on parietal cell Side-effects: generally well tolerated; although minor side-effects occur, major side-effects are rare; cimetidine more frequently causes side-effects and drug interactions. Potential concerns: tachyphylaxis				
Cimetidine	Tagamet®	400, 800, 1600 mg[a]	qhs ***or*** twice daily (***or*** four times daily for cimetidine)	B
Famotidine	Pepcid®	20 to 40 mg[a]		B
Nizatidine	Axid®	150 to 300 mg[a]		B
Ranitidine	Taladine®, Zantac®	150 to 300 mg[a]		B
Prostaglandin analogs				
Inhibit acid secretion: reduce secondary messenger signaling from histamine H_2 receptors Enhance mucosal defense: by prostaglandin-mediated effects on epithelial cells Side-effects: diarrhea, abdominal discomfort, cramps, abortifacient (contraindicated in women of childbearing potential not on contraception)				
Misoprostol (PG-E2 analog)	Cytotec®	800 micrograms	Note 1	X
Sucralfate				
Mucosal protection: coating of ulcer sites (various other actions proposed) Side-effects: potential aluminum toxicity				
Sucralfate	Carafate®	2 to 4 g (Note 2)	Twice daily ***or*** four times daily	B
Bismuth salts				
Antibacterial effects against ***H. pylori*** and promote ulcer healing: various mechanisms proposed Side-effects: blackened stool, potential bismuth intoxication and nervous system toxicity (with prolonged use at high dosage), potential salicylate toxicity (with BSS, platelet function unaffected)				
BSS	Pepto-Bismol®	2096 mg	Four times daily	Not assigned
	Helidac®			
CBS	Pylera® (Note 3)	1680 mg		Note 3
TPDCB	De-Noltab® (Note 4)	480 mg		Note 4

Drug classes are given along with mechanism of action and certain side-effects highlighted. ***Brand names*** are for example only and are not exhaustive. ***Total daily dosages*** are the maximum doses in 24 hours that are licensed in adults by the FDA for indications related to peptic ulcer disease. ***Dosing intervals*** are the licensed dosing patterns; therefore, individual doses will vary and relate to the ***Total daily dosage***. Double doses of PPI are used as part of ***H. pylori*** eradication therapy. ***Pregnancy*** is the FDA pregnancy category.

All information correct at November 2020. Consult other sources for current and complete prescribing information in different regions.

[a] Indicates that over-the-counter preparations of different dosage are available for other indications.

[1]Misoprostol: Although licensed for ulcer healing (at twice daily or four times daily dosing interval), its main current use is for prevention of NSAID ulcer (alternative dosing to improve tolerability is discussed under "Prevention").

[2]Sucralfate: Daily dosages of up to 6 g total (1 g every 4 hours) are licensed for stress ulcer prophylaxis.

[3]Pylera: Each Pylera capsule contains CBS (140 mg), metronidazole (125 mg), and tetracycline (125 mg) in combination; recommended dosage is three capsules per dose with four doses daily alongside PPI as one form of ***H. pylori*** eradication therapy. This and other combination convenience pills such as Helidac could provide suboptimal dosing of some antibiotics in some situations [254].

[4]TPDCB. This bismuth salt is not currently available in the USA but is available in the UK and elsewhere. It is contraindicated in pregnancy on theoretical grounds, according to the UK licensing agency. Note that bismuth subcitrate (120–240 mg four times daily) has largely been superseded by other bismuth salts because of potential toxicity concerns. BSS, bismuth subsalicylate; CBS, colloidal bismuth subcitrate; FDA, US Food and Drug Administration; H,K-ATPase, hydrogen-potassium adenosine triphosphatase; ***H. pylori***, ***Helicobacter pylori***; PG, prostaglandin; qhs, every night at bedtime (quaque hora somni); TPDCB, tri-potassium di-citratobismuthate.

For patients with GU, healing is less rapid and longer courses of up to 8 weeks of PPI are licensed. This treatment should continue alongside any cause-specific management (e.g., *H. pylori* eradication regimen). The length is determined by anticipated healing rate and any plan for follow-up endoscopy (see "Endoscopy and exclusion of malignancy"). Four to 6 weeks is adequate for low-risk patients where the underlying cause has been treated. Six to 8 weeks is more standard, with at least 8 weeks for complicated ulcers and up to 12 weeks for giant GU.

Maintenance

Patients with uncomplicated DU do not need further treatment once *H. pylori* has been eradicated or any other cause removed. Continuing acid suppression unnecessarily can delay testing to confirm *H. pylori* eradication. Persistence or relapse of symptoms should prompt further evaluation (see "Recurrent and refractory ulcers").

Similarly, for patients with uncomplicated GU, providing *H. pylori* has been treated or NSAIDs have been discontinued, no maintenance therapy is required. In other cases, maintenance therapy will reduce the risk of ulcer relapse.

Special scenarios – ulcer management

Treatment during pregnancy

Eradication therapy for *H. pylori* is typically delayed in this setting, and antisecretory therapy is the focus of treatment.

None of the antisecretory drugs are licensed for use in pregnancy. Most have animal but not human reproduction data and are in FDA Category B (see Table 49.4), although misoprostol is absolutely contraindicated and there is less experience with some drugs than others. Ranitidine, which is now off the market, was often used initially as it had been used in several pregnancy-associated conditions for many years. PPIs are generally considered safe though most experience is derived from studies of patients in their third trimester [255,256]. A large Danish cohort study of 5082 exposures to PPIs between 4 weeks before conception and the end of the first trimester of pregnancy in over 840 000 live births showed no significant increase in adverse events [257].

Some obstetricians confine the treatment of pregnant ulcer patients to antacids, particularly in uninvestigated dyspepsia, and high-dose regular antacids do have ulcer healing properties, albeit weaker than the more usual antisecretory drugs. We recommend that antisecretory drugs be used if ulcer suspicion is moderate or high as ulcer complications can be disastrous in pregnancy. Discussion with the patient and obstetrician is required. In patients with confirmed or suspected *H. pylori* ulceration, follow-up arrangements should be made for *H. pylori* eradication after parturition. Note that tetracyclines and bismuth cannot be used in pregnancy, or during breastfeeding.

The approach is broadly similar for breastfeeding. Although some commonly used drugs (including ranitidine and omeprazole) are excreted in breast milk [258], they are unlikely to affect the baby. Caution and patient discussion are advised [255, 256].

Renal and hepatic impairment

Dose adjustment of PPI is typically necessary for patients with moderate hepatic impairment and advised for some agents in renal impairment. The physician should consult national formularies and other sources for complete prescribing information.

Peptic ulcer in association with gastroesophageal reflux

Symptoms are often attributable predominantly to coexisting GERD [227] and, following treatment of the peptic ulcer, this should guide the management (see Chapter 43).

Giant ulcers

These ulcers take longer to resolve so a longer course of antiulcer therapy at a higher dose is needed. For giant GUs, and probably for giant DUs especially with nodular edges [230], multiple biopsies to exclude malignancy are required at index and interval endoscopy. Further decisions on healing and maintenance therapy are made after follow-up endoscopy. Often 12 weeks of treatment is necessary and for ulcers that do not resolve, early consultation with surgeons is helpful.

Pyloric channel

Longer duration maintenance antisecretory therapy may ameliorate the greater risk of obstructive complications in this group. Treatment can be stopped after the underlying cause has been removed, and edema and deformity have resolved.

Postbulbar and multiple ulcers

These ulcers require high-dose PPI until a definitive diagnosis is reached.

Endoscopic therapy

Endoscopic therapy is of benefit to patients with active bleeding ulcers only [259]. This is discussed in the section on complications and in further detail in Chapters 38 and 123.

Interventional radiology

Interventional radiology may play a role in the management of refractory bleeding from gastric or duodenal ulcer (see "Complications").

Surgical therapy

Over recent decades, the development of potent antisecretory agents (especially PPIs) and the discovery of *H. pylori* have essentially eliminated the need for elective surgery [260]. Once the most common indication for gastric surgery, PUD now only infrequently requires operative intervention. Elective surgical management of recurrent or refractory ulcers is discussed with that topic. Emergent surgery is also indicated for early life-threatening complications of an ulcer, particularly for perforation or penetration, or for rare instances of hemorrhage when medical, endoscopic, and/or radiological interventions have failed [259,261]. Late complications such as chronic gastric outlet obstruction may also necessitate surgery.

Other therapies

There are some reports evaluating nondrug complementary therapies for PUD, including acupuncture and moxibustion (a traditional Chinese medicine therapy). Although not recommended, Chapter 116 discusses the role of complementary alternative medicine and CBT in gastroenterology. There is no evidence that addressing stress and psychological comorbidity is beneficial for ulcer healing. No firm dietary recommendations are necessary.

Identification of specific causes of PUD

Most peptic ulcers are caused by *H. pylori* infection or NSAID use, although there are other important etiologies to consider in the case of non-*H. pylori*, non-NSAID ulcers (see "Etiology"). In routine cases, diagnosing and excluding the various causes of ulcer can occur concomitantly with ulcer treatment. In complicated PUD, diagnosis can be delayed but must not be forgotten or ignored. Usually investigations should be initiated in secondary care with a clear plan for follow-up agreed upon with the primary care physician.

Testing for *H. pylori*

There are several tests for *H. pylori* infection [262], some based on endoscopy with biopsy and others which do not require endoscopy; the choice of test will be influenced by the clinical scenario, the pretest probability of infection, local availability, and cost considerations. More than one test may be required in some situations.

Endoscopic biopsy-based tests are most convenient if an endoscopy is being performed anyway in the investigation of symptoms. Three major types are available: biopsy urease tests (convenient and rapid); histology (other information can be gleaned); and bacterial culture (less sensitive, but useful where antibiotic susceptibilities are needed). These all rely on a sufficient *H. pylori* bacterial load or colonization density (Box 49.3). The choice of test will usually depend on whether additional information is required. If the test is done merely to determine *H. pylori* status, the biopsy urease test is sensitive, convenient, and inexpensive.

Box 49.3 Optimal conditions for all tests for ***H. pylori*** except serological antibody detection.

Patients should be asked to:

avoid antibiotics and bismuth compounds for at least 4 weeks
avoid proton pump inhibitors (PPIs) for at least 2 weeks[a]

False-negative results are increased for ***H. pylori*** tests that depend on bacterial load. Positive results may still be diagnostic

PPIs may also alter the appearance of malignant GU (see "Endoscopy and exclusion of malignancy")

PPIs may also heal peptic ulcers or other acid-related conditions, potentially resulting in a falsely negative endoscopy

Longer periods before testing of 2 or 3 months may occasionally be preferred (see "Recurrent and refractory ulcers")

[a] Histamine type 2 receptor antagonists (H_2-RAs) do not reduce bacterial load as severely as PPIs and are often used when it is necessary to test for ***H. pylori*** treatment success and acid suppression cannot safely be stopped. However, the sensitivity of tests that depend on bacterial load is slightly reduced.

The major types of nonendoscopic investigations are urea breath testing, stool antigen tests, and serology. Urea breath testing and stool antigen tests also depend on bacterial load and so require optimal conditions (see Box 49.3). Serological tests depend on detection of antibodies against ***H. pylori***. A Cochrane diagnostic test accuracy metaanalysis using histological examination as reference standard showed that urea breath tests have high diagnostic accuracy followed by serology and stool antigen tests based on an indirect test comparison [263].

Biopsy urease tests

Biopsy urease tests are inexpensive if endoscopy with biopsy is already indicated. The test relies on the *H. pylori* urease in endoscopic biopsy specimens to hydrolyze urea which is present, along with a pH indicator, in a gel in the test kit well. The gastric biopsy specimen is embedded in the gel and if *H. pylori* urease is present, urea hydrolysis releases ammonia which increases the pH, leading to a change in indicator color.

Typically, one large or two regular gastric antral biopsies are tested using a commercial kit. Some positive results may be available within 1 hour, though usually results are read at 24 hours. False-positive results are rare but can occur when other urease-producing organisms are present (non-*pylori Helicobacter* species typically give a weakly positive result). False-negative results are more likely with recent upper GI bleeding and medications that reduce bacterial load (see Box 49.3). Rapid urease tests have sensitivities of 80–100% with specificities of 97–99% [264]. Sensitivity is greater when two samples are used, one each from the antrum and the corpus. The corpus sample is particularly important if the patient is taking an antisecretory drug (particularly a PPI) which reduces *H. pylori* density in the antrum and increases it in the corpus. Biopsies from both antrum and corpus should also be used when assessing the success of *H. pylori* eradication therapy.

Several rapid urease tests are available commercially and they can also be prepared in local laboratories. They enable a diagnosis to be made within a few minutes based on the actions of *H. pylori* urease. However, locally made tests may be less accurate and should not be used in isolation without validation.

Histology

Optimal histological evaluation of gastric biopsies is performed in accordance with the updated Sydney system [137] (see Chapter 51). The clinical utility and cost-effectiveness of routine upper gastrointestinal histopathology have been questioned [265], though staging using a system established by an international group of pathologists – the Operative Link for Gastritis Assessment (OLGA) – may inform gastric cancer risk [266]. Histology can accurately identify *H. pylori* organisms, typically appearing as curved rod or short spiral organisms associated with or sometimes crossing the epithelium; however, it is sensitive only if special stains are used, most usually a modified Giemsa stain, a silver-based stain, or toluidine blue, although immunostaining is increasingly used. For non-*pylori Helicobacter* species, the appearance is diagnostic (long tight spirals). Providing sufficient biopsies are taken by the endoscopist (two from each of the antrum and corpus, with or without one from the incisura [137]), the pathologists can report on the distribution and severity of gastric inflammation, and the pattern and presence of any atrophy and/or intestinal metaplasia. Chronic active gastritis is invariably seen with *H. pylori* infection, although the number of neutrophils is variable and may be very low.

Some authorities suggest that, in an effort to manage costs, biopsies for histology are taken but not sent to pathology for analysis until the results of biopsy urease testing are available. This strategy assumes that the additional information that can be gleaned from histology is not needed in the patient under investigation. Brush cytology may be useful for identifying *H. pylori* if endoscopic mucosal biopsies cannot be obtained.

Bacterial culture

Microbiological culture for identification of *H. pylori* is not routinely recommended and is not available in most centers although it is useful to guide eradication therapy in cases of treatment failure. For *H. pylori* this requires microaerobic culture on complex media; small translucent colonies are seen after 3–5 days. Organisms are identified as gram-negative spiral or curved bacilli with multiple flagella, which test positive for urease, oxidase, and catalase activities.

In principle, culture is not difficult but *H. pylori* is very slow-growing and overgrowth of culture plates with other bacteria is common, sometimes requiring selective antibiotic-containing plates. In practice, few centers culture *H. pylori* successfully in more than 80% of cases so although culture is the most specific test, it is generally performed only for antibiotic susceptibility testing [267].

If culture is not possible, there are now molecular, PCR-based tests for antibiotic resistance, most notably clarithromycin and fluoroquinolones, which can be performed on gastric biopsy specimens directly without prior culture of *H. pylori* [267]. There is also increasing interest in simple, nonendoscopic tests for antibiotic susceptibility based on stool testing but their role in clinical practice is not yet established.

Other tests based on endoscopic biopsy specimens

Methods for detection and strain characterization are of great interest, with many reports of molecular tests on gastric biopsies, fixed tissue, and other samples such as gastric juice, typically employing DNA hybridization and/or based on PCR. These tests are not currently used in standard clinical practice, in part because the biopsy urease test and histology are so reliable.

Urea breath testing

Urea breath tests are simple and noninvasive, and involve the patient drinking a solution of urea labeled with the nonradioactive 13C carbon isotope or a very small dose of radioactive 14C. Urease from *H. pylori* catalyzes the hydrolysis of urea to ammonia, liberating labeled carbon dioxide that can be detected in breath samples. This test is dependent on the presence of a sufficient number of organisms. However, because the urea solution comes into contact with much of the stomach, urea breath testing is not prone to the sampling error of many biopsy-based tests.

Its sensitivity and specificity are consistently among the highest of all tests for *H. pylori*, perhaps for this reason. The estimated sensitivity at a fixed specificity of 0.90 is 0.94 (95% CI 0.89–0.97) for the 13C urea breath test and 0.92 (95% CI 0.89–0.94) for the 14C urea breath test which implies that on average, given a prevalence of 53.7%, out of 1000 people tested for *H. pylori* infection, there will be 46 false positives. In addition, the 13C and 14C urea breath tests will give 30 (95% CI 15–58) and 42 (95% CI 30–58) false negatives respectively [263].

Serology

Serological tests, which detect IgG antibodies against *H. pylori*, are convenient and relatively cheap. The best tests are very accurate although some, including near-patient or point-of-care tests, are not. Antibodies against *H. pylori* may persist for several years after eradication and sometimes for life, so serology cannot be used to reliably determine treatment success. If a patient is found to be seronegative several years after treatment, this likely reflects previous treatment success. However, seropositivity in this scenario is uninformative. Paired serological tests that show a decreased antibody titer 6 months after eradication accurately reflect success, but this is too slow and inconvenient to be of practical use in most situations. Even before treatment, the positive and negative predictive values of serology are inadequate in populations where *H. pylori* prevalence is low, and in this scenario further testing is required. Serology has a role in patients who cannot stop medications that reduce the sensitivity of other preferred tests of active infection and it is also useful in the context of acute GI bleeding when other tests have reduced sensitivity.

The sensitivity of serology based on a fixed specificity of 0.90 was estimated at 0.84 (95% CI 0.74–0.91) in a recent Cochrane review, corresponding to 86 (95% CI 50–140) false negatives in 1000 patients tested [263]. Serology should not be used as a test to confirm eradication.

Stool antigen testing

Fecal tests are widely available and simple to perform, though some patients dislike stool testing. Stool antigen tests consist of fixed polyclonal or monoclonal antibodies that bind and detect *H. pylori* antigens and are therefore dependent on the presence of sufficient organisms. The monoclonal antibody tests are more accurate and laboratory tests are more reliable than near-patient tests. Validated tests are accurate and cost-effective. Most recent studies show accuracy comparable with urea breath testing even for posteradication testing. Their accuracy may be reduced after GI bleeding. The sensitivity of stool antigen testing, at a fixed specificity of 0.90, is estimated at 0.83 (95% CI 0.73–0.90), which means that in a population with a prevalence of 53.7%, out of 1000 people tested for *H. pylori* infection, there will be 89 (95% CI 52–146) false negatives [263]. It is often the test of choice in children as it is accurate, noninvasive and does not require significant patient cooperation for sample collection.

Other nonendoscopy-based tests

Tests on saliva, urine, and a 13C urea blood test have been developed but are not used in clinical practice.

Approach to *H. pylori* testing in different scenarios and clinical settings

Test and treat strategy for uninvestigated dyspepsia

Accurate, convenient, nonendoscopic tests – urea breath testing and stool antigen testing – are recommended in the absence of other indications for endoscopy; serology may be recommended if *H. pylori* prevalence is moderate or high. The pretest probability of *H. pylori* infection is low in most populations in high or very high HDI countries and in this setting a positive result from serology requires validation by another test.

Testing in a patient with an uncomplicated ulcer

Upper GI endoscopy, where already indicated, is the most convenient time to establish *H. pylori* status, provided that the patient has not recently taken antibiotics, bismuth, or PPI (see Box 49.3). The pretest probability of *H. pylori* is high when an ulcer is identified at endoscopy, particularly where NSAID use has been excluded and/or when a DU is found, so a single positive test result is highly likely to reflect *H. pylori* infection. Conversely, the impact of false-negative results is greater, and a negative test for *H. pylori* should be confirmed by a second test. Typically, this involves initial biopsy urease testing and saving/sending samples for histology. Breath and stool tests are appropriate nonendoscopic alternatives, and a good serological test is also reasonably reliable in this setting. In some countries with more limited resources and a very high prevalence of *H. pylori*, empirical *H. pylori* eradication without testing may be a cost-effective approach. However, particularly due to the complexity and adverse effects of currently available treatments, it is now recommended that evidence of infection be sought before attempting *H. pylori* eradication.

Complicated ulcer – testing in the presence of upper gastrointestinal bleeding

Unfortunately, many patients hospitalized with bleeding peptic ulcer are not tested for *H. pylori*, and appropriate treatment is delayed. Prompt diagnosis is important and *H. pylori* treatment can be commenced as soon as the acute episode has been treated and a normal diet restarted. However, it is also safe and acceptable to delay investigations for *H. pylori* for several weeks until they can be performed under optimal conditions.

Endoscopic tests have high specificity but lower sensitivity in the presence of acute bleeding [268], and other more pressing concerns often dominate at the time of index endoscopy. Stool antigen tests lack specificity when blood is present in stool. Early urea breath testing during hospitalization is accurate although there is a limited window of opportunity given the central role for PPIs in the management of upper GI bleeding. Pragmatically, serological testing is most often used in the acute phase but results should be interpreted in light of the past medical history and its lesser sensitivity. Follow-up in primary or secondary care should be planned, and the patient informed of the benefits of accurate testing to determine the need for eradication therapy.

NSAIDs

Diagnosis of NSAID ulcer depends on the patient history although this is not always reliable. NSAIDs are widely available over the counter and present in various commonly used analgesic remedies. Unidentified, sporadic, or even surreptitious NSAID use are important considerations. Specific tests to identify NSAID use are not clinically available, though measurements of prostaglandin metabolites and COX activity in platelets are technically feasible. Urine and serum salicylate measurements are available but their main utility is in the setting of suspected overdose.

Endoscopy and exclusion of malignancy

Upper GI endoscopy allows direct inspection and biopsy for tissue sampling. Benign and malignant ulcers can usually, but not always, be distinguished by inspection. Benign ulcers are characterized by smooth and regular edges, an ulcer base that is flat and smooth, and an ulcer crater filled by exudate. Malignant lesions are often associated with an irregular ulcerated mass that protrudes into the lumen with wall deformity, and abnormal folds surrounding the ulcer crater with overhanging or irregular margins. Larger ulcers are more likely to be malignant. The Paris endoscopic classification of superficial neoplastic lesions describes this in more detail [269,270]. Site is also an important consideration: the lesser curve and pylorus are common sites for noncardia malignancy.

The reference standard for determining whether an ulcer is benign or malignant is biopsy. Biopsy should be performed even if gastric lesions appear benign endoscopically, or small (less than 1 cm diameter) as such lesions may still harbor malignancy. In contrast to GU, most DUs do not require biopsy but these should be considered in cases of giant DU with abnormal edges [230].

The number of biopsies to be obtained has been debated, but seven or more specimens taken using regular-sized biopsy forceps have a diagnostic yield over 98% in suspected malignancy, with at least four biopsies required for a yield over 95% [271]. Biopsies should be taken from the ulcer crater, ulcer edge, and surrounding mucosa. Brush cytology may increase the yield, and the combination of multiple biopsies and cytology has been shown to detect nearly all cancers although this approach is not routinely employed. The role of advanced endoscopic modalities, mainly endoscopic ultrasound [272], and the endoscopic approach to early gastric cancer are discussed elsewhere (see Chapters 52, 118, 126, and 128).

One point of current controversy is whether or not the index endoscopy should be performed with the patient on PPI therapy. Inflammation can confound the diagnosis of dysplasia so acid suppression ought to be beneficial. However, treatment with a PPI may potentially mask endoscopic findings, delay diagnosis, or result in a misdiagnosis on the first endoscopy [273]. In particular, PPIs can cause apparent healing or otherwise alter the appearance of malignant ulcers [274]. To avoid this ambiguity, and because PPIs render endoscopic tests for *H. pylori* infection unreliable [275], it is advisable to perform the index endoscopy having advised the patient not to take any antiulcer healing medication for at least 2 weeks before the endoscopy. However, because of considerations of urgency and difficulties of communication between primary and secondary care, index endoscopies are often performed with the patient on a PPI.

A second point of controversy concerns indications for follow-up endoscopy for GU and whether this confers a survival benefit [276, 277]. Repeat endoscopy with further biopsies is often recommended to confirm successful healing, after a course of antiulcer medication and treatment of any underlying causes. This is strongly recommended when histology from the index endoscopy was inadequate, the ulcer's appearance suggests malignancy, the ulcer etiology remains undefined, or where there are other risk factors for gastric cancer (see Chapter 52). It may be safe not to repeat endoscopy when all of the following apply: index endoscopy identifies one (or multiple) small and benign-appearing GU; the ulcer is due to NSAIDs; *H. pylori* infection is absent; the patient is young (e.g., <50 years, though patients from some ethnic backgrounds are at increased risk from a younger age); there is no family history of gastric cancer; and no premalignant conditions such as gastric atrophy are present. Retrospective data suggest that no new diagnoses of malignancy are made at surveillance endoscopy in patients after antiulcer therapy [278,279]. However, most guidelines are more cautious and advise follow-up endoscopy in all cases of GU [277].

The optimal strategy for taking biopsies at follow-up endoscopy has not been defined but a similar strategy to that for index endoscopy is reasonable, and samples should be taken from the ulcer edges and the ulcer bed even if the ulcer has healed, given the possibility of apparent healing of malignant ulcers with PPI.

Laboratory evaluation of acid secretion

Acid hypersecretory states should be considered in patients with multiple peptic ulcers, which are typically postbulbar and refractory to conventional treatment (see "Other clinical scenarios or endoscopic findings"). The additional clinical features of gastrinoma and Zollinger–Ellison syndrome, and the diagnosis and work-up of hypergastrinemia, are covered in Chapter 50.

Laboratory measurement of pepsinogen I and the pepsinogen I:II ratio has been used to infer, noninvasively, the pattern and severity of gastric inflammation (serological biopsy) [280,281]. The main potential application is in screening for atrophic gastritis, when both are reduced, allowing identification of a group of patients at increased risk of gastric adenocarcinoma who may benefit from endoscopic surveillance [282,283]. Measurement of serum pepsinogens does not have a defined role in PUD management.

Other investigations

Upper GI radiography using barium contrast was used before modern endoscopy became widely available. These studies may be more useful in special circumstances as described in the section "Identification of ulcer." Definitive diagnosis requires endoscopy and biopsy. CT is indicated if an ulcer complicated by perforation or penetration is suspected. If this is not immediately available, then upright chest and abdominal radiographs may detect free air.

Treatment of specific causes of PUD

Treating *H. pylori*

In the context of established *H. pylori*-associated PUD, the aims of therapy are to heal the ulcer and prevent recurrence. *H. pylori* eradication is extremely successful in achieving these aims, particularly for DU and, when used with antiulcer therapy, for GU and complicated ulcers. Multiple metaanalyses have also shown significant improvement in gastric atrophy after eradication of *H. pylori* and thus the overall value of eradication is well established [284–286], although it has not been shown to improve gastric intestinal metaplasia.

Systemic review and metaanalysis of 34 trials in a total of 3910 patients demonstrated that eradication is superior to antiulcer therapy in initial healing of DU (relative risk [RR] of persisting ulcer 0.66, 95% CI 0.58–0.76), but not in initial healing of GU in 13 trials [287]. However, the main aim of treating *H. pylori* is to prevent ulcer recurrence. Eradication therapy was superior to no treatment in preventing DU recurrence (RR of recurrent ulcer 0.20, 95% CI 0.15–0.26, analysis of 27 trials in 2509 patients), and in preventing GU recurrence (RR of recurrent ulcer 0.28, 95% CI 0.18–0.43, analysis of 10 trials in 1029 patients) [287]. The number needed to treat to prevent one ulcer recurrence was only two for DU and three for GU. In a 1995 study of cost-effectiveness modeled over the course of 15 years, the cost of treating *H. pylori* infection ($995) was over 10-fold less than antisecretory therapy and other strategies [288].

The challenge for treating *H. pylori*-associated PUD and other *H. pylori*-associated diseases comes in selecting the optimal eradication strategies, both at a population level and, increasingly, at an individual patient level.

Here, we first consider the current therapeutic approach, types of eradication therapy, and the patient and bacterial predictors of treatment outcome. The choice of treatment is discussed in light of national and international guidelines that exist to inform these decisions, and their limitations in the face of increasing antimicrobial resistance and eradication failure. The importance of patient education and confirmation of eradication is emphasized. Finally, we consider the optimal modern therapeutic paradigm.

Current therapeutic paradigm

The current approach is to begin with the most effective and cost-effective eradication regimen, usually referred to as first-line therapy, followed, if this is unsuccessful, by empirical second-line therapy. If this in turn is unsuccessful, one recommended approach is to perform endoscopy and culture biopsy specimens for *H. pylori* antibiotic sensitivity testing, so that further treatment can be based on known sensitivities. However, because *H. pylori* culture and sensitivity testing is not widely available, empiric rescue therapies (also termed salvage or third-line therapy) are often employed. Relevant guidelines include several different regimens at each level that are considered acceptable based on population-level evidence and consensus (see "Guidelines for *H. pylori* eradication therapy").

The definition of acceptability has varied but an initial cure rate over 90% has been used. However, perhaps due to changing antibiotic resistance patterns, some of the regimens which performed well in initial trials now have reported cure rates of 80% or less in everyday practice, and recently optimal regimens for first-line therapy have been reexamined.

Unfortunately, most treatment regimens are complex and difficult for some patients to comply with fully. Lack of compliance is the major cause of treatment failure, which in turn leads to acquired antibiotic resistance, making further treatment more difficult. Therefore, treatment of this serious infection needs to be precise and optimal.

Types of *H. pylori* eradication therapy

Triple therapy

Failure of monotherapy and dual therapy for treatment of *H. pylori* infection prompted the development of triple therapy and other multidrug regimens. Triple therapy is classically a 7-day regimen with twice-daily PPI and two antibiotics (Table 49.5), though there are other permutations and a 10–14-day course is usually suggested (particularly in North America). Acid suppression with PPI has synergistic bactericidal effects and stabilizes antibiotics, so increasing their half-life. Empirical triple therapy emerged as the dominant treatment strategy worldwide and was initially widely successful, with clarithromycin-containing regimens most often used. However, with the rise in clarithromycin resistance in *H. pylori* due to the increasing use of macrolides for respiratory infections, these regimens have become less effective in most countries [289–291].

Using triple therapy as first-line treatment, cure rates of less than 80% (and even below 50%) are now widely reported across countries on different continents [292], including in Greece [293], India [294], Italy [295], Japan [296,297], Mexico [298], and Spain [299,300]. However, evidence suggests that an acceptable cure is still achievable in some regions, for example Korea [301,302], Singapore [303], and Thailand [304].

Table 49.5 Types of conventional triple therapy for eradication of *Helicobacter pylori*.

Regimen	Drug	Dosage
PAC	PPI[a]	Standard dose; twice daily
	Amoxicillin	1 g twice daily
	Clarithromycin	500 mg twice daily
PCM	PPI[a]	Standard dose; twice daily
	Clarithromycin	250–500 mg twice daily
	Metronidazole	400 mg twice daily
PAM	PPI[a]	Standard dose; twice daily
	Amoxicillin	1 g twice daily
	Metronidazole	400 mg twice daily

[a] A proton pump inhibitor (PPI) is given every 12 hours (esomeprazole 40 mg, lansoprazole 30 mg, omeprazole 20 mg, pantoprazole 40 mg, or rabeprazole 20 mg) or 24 hours (dexlansoprazole 60 mg).
PAC and PCM are equivalent, though PCM is used in penicillin-allergic individuals.
The nonclarithromycin regimen (PAM) is not usually recommended for first-line therapy as it is less effective in most studies.
Other imidazole antibiotics have been used in place of metronidazole.

Clarithromycin resistance is a major determinant of the success of triple therapy and primary resistance is rising in many countries (see "Bacterial resistance to antimicrobial drugs"). One strategy to account for the increasing prevalence of clarithromycin-resistant strains of *H. pylori* was proposed in the Maastricht IV/Florence consensus guidelines [305]. This was further emphasized in the more recent Maastricht V/Florence consensus guidelines [306]. The expert consensus recommended that different regions be classified into high-resistance areas (>15%) and low resistance areas (<15%). Clarithromycin-containing triple therapy was considered acceptable first-line therapy only in low-resistance areas, and even then quadruple therapy was considered an acceptable alternative. Triple therapy should not be used as the first-line treatment in areas with high clarithromycin resistance rates. The Maastricht V/Florence consensus report recommends the decision in areas with high clarithromycin resistance based on the rate of metronidazole and dual clarithromycin and metronidazole resistance (Figure 49.10) [306].

If triple therapy is used, various approaches to improve effectiveness have been suggested [306], including longer courses (14 days rather than 7 or 10 days improves eradication success by about 5% without adding to the adverse effects [307]); PPI at high doses (increases cure rate by 6–10%) or more potent PPI (increases cure rate by 8–12%) [308]); possibly using PCM instead of PAC (see Table 49.5) [309]; or possibly adding an adjuvant treatment (see "Adjuvant therapies"). The crucial importance of patient factors and patient education is discussed later in this chapter. Esomeprazole and rabeprazole may have a better effect in Europe and North America

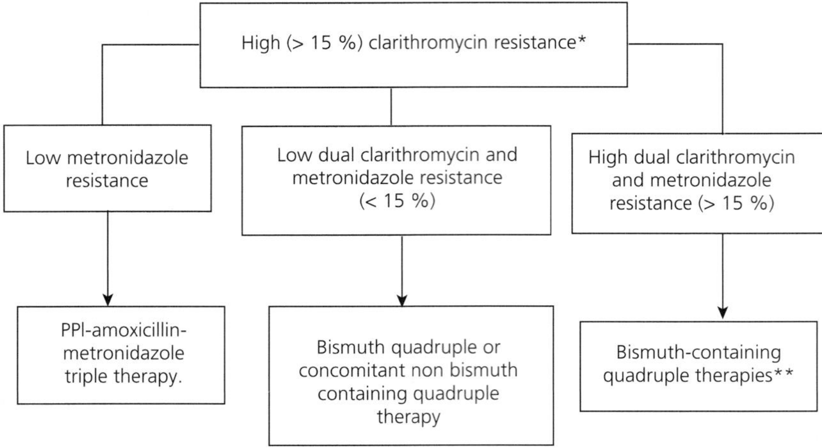

Figure 49.10 Recommended approach to eradication therapy for *Helicobacter pylori* in regions with high clarithromycin resistance rates, with or without metronidazole resistance. Source: Maastricht V/Florence Consensus Report [306].

where the majority of the population have a CYP2C19 polymorphism leading to a phenotype of extensive metabolism of PPI [306]. *H. pylori* is more likely in a nonreplicative state in low gastric pH but is more replicative and therefore susceptible to amoxicillin and clarithromycin when the pH rises, which explains the role of high-dose PPI in achieving a higher eradication rate [310].

Even in countries where clarithromycin resistance in *H. pylori* is thought to be low, clarithromycin-based triple therapies should only be used after proper consideration. It is likely that clarithromycin resistance patterns in these countries will differ in different locales and populations, and primary antibiotic resistance monitoring in different regions is often inadequate. The chance of a patient's *H. pylori* strain being clarithromycin resistant is high if they have a personal exposure to clarithromycin or repeated exposure to other macrolide antibiotics [311]. In these scenarios, quadruple therapy is recommended by many guidelines, though other effective regimens are available that may be more appropriate for some patients. Overall, there are probably a declining number of settings where empirical triple therapy should be used [289,311,312]. Bismuth-based quadruple therapy or a fluoroquinolone-containing triple or quadruple therapy should be considered as a second-line treatment if PPI-clarithromycin-amoxicillin triple therapy or a nonbismuth quadruple therapy fails or as a first line in patients with previous exposure to macrolides or penicillin allergy [306,313,314].

Rifabutin triple regimen (PPI, amoxicillin, rifabutin) or high-dose dual therapy (PPI and amoxicillin) can also be considered as second-line treatment after failure of initial therapy [313].

Bismuth-based quadruple therapy In the Maastricht V/Florence, American College of Gastroenterology and Toronto guidelines [306,313,314], bismuth quadruple therapy is recommended for first-line empirical treatment in areas of high clarithromycin resistance, as second-line or alternative first-line empirical treatment in areas of low clarithromycin resistance, and for patients with recent or repeated exposure to clarithromycin or metronidazole [311]. We therefore recommend it as a first-line therapy in all patients.

Bismuth quadruple therapy [315] is a 14-day regimen with twice-daily PPI, a bismuth salt usually given four times daily (see Table 49.4), and two further antibiotics (usually metronidazole at various dosages, e.g., 400 mg three times daily, in the proprietary combination capsule Pylera® at 375 mg four times daily or the proprietary combination capsule Helidac® at 250 mg four times daily, and tetracycline hydrochloride at various dosages, e.g., Helidac 500 mg four times daily, Pylera 375 mg four times daily). Eradication rates of 90% or higher are achievable for first-line therapy [316–319]. A lower rate of 78% reported in a metaanalysis is more difficult to interpret, as heterogeneous dosing regimens were included [320]. Successful cure is achieved in 79–88% in studies when it is used as second-line therapy [321–323].

A major drawback of bismuth quadruple therapy regimens is that they comprise around 17–34 pills per day, which can be impractical for many patients. The combination capsule Pylera (see Table 49.4) has a much simpler dosing regimen of 14 pills per day. However, combination medications may contain suboptimal antibiotic doses for some settings [254]. Pylera was evaluated as a 7-day regimen against triple therapy in a trial that also included patients with *H. pylori* infection but without PUD and reported an eradication rate of 80% [324]. One advantage of quadruple therapy is that it contains metronidazole rather than clarithromycin; resistance to metronidazole has much less impact in clinical practice than does clarithromycin resistance. Metronidazole resistance is only partial, and the efficacy of quadruple therapy containing metronidazole is only slightly reduced in patients with metronidazole-resistant strains [291,311,317,320,325].

Levofloxacin-based triple therapy The most common fluoroquinolone-based regimen is levofloxacin-based triple therapy which is a 10–14-day regimen with twice-daily PPI, levofloxacin at various dosages (mostly 500 mg twice daily), and amoxicillin 1 g twice daily. In current guidelines, it is proposed for second-line or rescue therapy. Eradication rates of 78–93% as first-line therapy have been reported [292], including in China [326], India [327], Italy [328], and Spain [329]. Higher rates were observed with 10–14-day regimens than with 7-day regimens. Eradication rates of 74–86% as second-line therapy have been reported [292], including in China [330], Italy [331], Spain [332], and Taiwan [333].

Other levofloxacin-based therapies have been reported that include clarithromycin in place of or in addition to amoxicillin [334], and other fluoroquinolone-based therapies have been proposed with moxifloxacin, gemifloxacin or sitafloxacin [292].

Fluoroquinolone resistance in *H. pylori* varies between countries (see "Bacterial resistance to antimicrobial drugs"), is increasing, and could potentially increase further if used widely in first-line *H. pylori* treatment regimens. This is an important consideration in identifying optimum second-line therapy options in different settings [331], and for this reason we do not recommend fluoroquinolone-based regimens as first-line therapy or in areas with high fluoroquinolone resistance rates.

Sequential therapy Sequential therapy is usually a 10–14-day regimen that is split into two consecutive 5–7-day treatments. Split regimens comprising two sets of 7-day treatment periods (a 14-day regimen) have also been used. Standard sequential therapy is with twice-daily PPI and amoxicillin 1 g twice daily for days 1–5 (or 1–7), then with twice-daily PPI and two further antibiotics (usually clarithromycin 500 mg twice daily and nitroimidazole 500 mg twice daily) for days 6–10 (or 8–14). Other imidazole antibiotics have been used.

Sequential therapy performs better than standard triple therapy in some [335] but not all [336] randomized trials, but overall sequential therapy is superior in systematic reviews [337,338]. Sequential therapy and concomitant therapy (see further on) are both effective in certain settings. Various eradication rates have been reported, though differences between these did not reach statistical significance (over 90% for both in Italy [338] and Taiwan [339]; 81% and 87% respectively in Spain [340], where clarithromycin resistance is increased; and 80% and 88% respectively in China [341]. Lower success rates have also been reported for sequential therapy [292]: 82–84% in Korea and Morocco and only 76–78% for sequential therapy in trials from China, India, Iran, and Korea [342].

Antimicrobial resistance patterns have been proposed as the most important determinant of differences between studies. Other considerations include the role of dual resistance (when concomitant therapy may be more suitable), potential for higher cure rates with 14 rather than 10 days of sequential therapy [335], and differences in cost (shorter courses of concomitant therapy can be as effective but less expensive than sequential therapy). Overall, recent guidelines have recommended against the use of sequential therapy [314].

Concomitant therapy Concomitant therapy regimens refer to nonbismuth quadruple therapies. This is usually a 10–14-day regimen with PPI and three antibiotics (most often amoxicillin 1 g, clarithromycin 500 mg and a nitroimidazole 500 mg) twice daily [313,314]. Eradication rates of 81–96% have been reported in different settings [292], with a mean of 88% cure and superior performance to triple therapy in a systematic review [343]. Concomitant therapy is contrasted with sequential therapy above; the regimens are typically less complex and so more practical.

Other eradication therapies Various other regimens have been reported [292,312], including hybrid therapy (a combination of sequential and concomitant therapies), amoxicillin-PPI dual therapy (PPI double dose and amoxicillin 750 mg 4 times/day) [344], and regimens that contain rifabutin, the nitrofurantoin antibacterial furazolidone, the antiprotozoal nitazoxanide, or ecabet sodium. These require further evaluation but are sometimes used by specialists for patients with multiple antibiotic-resistant strains. Interestingly, clarithromycin-based triple therapy is the only FDA-approved regimen for the treatment of *H. pylori* [313].

Adjuvant therapies Probiotics and prebiotics may reduce or prevent side-effects (particularly diarrhea) during *H. pylori* eradication and they may therefore improve treatment tolerability. The prebiotic lactoferrin may be beneficial [345,346] but is not recommended due to insufficient evidence [305]. Butyric acid and inulin have also been used in combination [347].

Several probiotics have been studied, including *Lactobacillus* species [348] and *Saccharomyces boulardii* [349–351]. Early studies comparing different probiotics reported similar protection from side-effects independent of the species used, though without an associated improvement in compliance [352]. Some studies of *S. boulardii* have reported increased eradication rates with standard triple therapy for *H. pylori*, likely through better compliance [350], though others report fewer side-effects but no difference in eradication [351]. In one metaanalysis, *S. boulardii* reduced the absolute risk of therapy-related adverse effects by 11% (95% CI 7–16%) and increased the absolute eradication rate by 9% (95% CI 4–14%) [349]. In a recent double-blind randomized placebo-controlled trial in Thailand, 100 *H. pylori*-infected patients received either 7- or 14-day high-dose PPI-bismuth-containing quadruple therapy with or without

Lactobacillus reuteri 37.5 mg twice daily [353]. The 14-day regimen with probiotics was effective in 96% of all patients and 100% of patients with clarithromycin, metronidazole or dual clarithromycin and metronidazole resistance. In addition, adverse effects were significantly less with probiotics compared to placebo (6% versus 26%, $p = 0.002$). Therefore, probiotics may have a role as therapeutic adjuvants but should not be used instead of standard *H. pylori* treatments since they have proved ineffective in multiple trials [347,353–355]. These data notwithstanding, the Toronto Consensus recommended against the routine addition of probiotics to reduce adverse events or improve outcomes for *H. pylori* eradication therapy [314].

Simvastatin as an adjuvant to *H. pylori* triple therapy has been reported in one study to increase the absolute eradication rate by 17% (95% CI 2–32%), despite demonstrating no differences in side-effects or compliance [356]. Larger confirmatory trials and mechanistic clarification are needed.

Experimental and possible future therapies The in vitro antimicrobial effects of photodynamic therapy on *H. pylori* were first reported in 1990 [357]. More recently, a ruthenium-based photosensitizer activated by visible blue light was observed to cause a 7-log reduction in colony number in vitro across several strains [358]. Successful targeting of *H. pylori* in its niche in vivo has not yet been determined.

Further concerted efforts to develop a therapeutic vaccine against *H. pylori* have been recommended to enable individual patient or population-based eradication for many years [305]. Although the main aim of any vaccine would be primary prevention of gastric cancer, prophylactic or therapeutic *H. pylori* vaccines could be useful tools in the prevention or management of PUD [359]. A recent double-blind, placebo-controlled, phase III trial in China randomized 4464 healthy children aged 6–15 years to receive the *H. pylori* vaccine or placebo and showed an efficacy of 71.8% (95% CI 48.2–85.6) with comparable adverse events [360].

Predictors of treatment outcome

Patient factors The most important factors in determining outcome are the previous use of antimicrobial agents and compliance with eradication treatment. A thorough antibiotic history should be obtained, focusing on recent and recurrent treatments, including any previous *H. pylori* eradication therapies used. Regimens are complex and at least mild side-effects are common. Inadequate therapy through noncompliance can quickly result in acquired resistance. Careful explanation and written information may be helpful (see "Patient education, including potential side-effects of therapy").

Smoking is another important factor and current smokers are more likely to fail eradication therapy (eradication rate 8% lower, OR 1.95, 95% CI 1.55–2.45) [361].

Intragastric pH during treatment is affected by PPI pharmacokinetics; *MDR1* and cytochrome P450 *2C19* polymorphisms modulate metabolism [305]. The latter can identify subpopulations of extensive metabolizers and slow metabolizers of PPIs. Significantly lower eradication rates have been identified with some PPIs in extensive metabolizers, but studies in slow metabolizers have found that even amoxicillin-PPI dual therapy was able to cure over 90% of *H. pylori* infections [362–365]. This is the rationale for recommending esomeprazole and rabeprazole and more potent PPIs in populations with high rates of fast metabolizers [366].

Bacterial resistance to antimicrobial drugs Antimicrobial resistance in *H. pylori* varies widely between and within different countries and regions but is increasingly common overall [289–291,367–369]. The most important resistances are to clarithromycin, metronidazole, and levofloxacin and, hence, to other macrolides, imidazoles, and fluoroquinolones. Resistance is very rare for other commonly used antimicrobials, though when it occurs for amoxicillin, it can be a cause for treatment failure. Resistance has also been demonstrated for rifampins such as rifabutin, which is included in some other eradication therapies. The rise in *H. pylori* antibiotic resistance is mainly due to antibiotics being used for other infections. The most clear-cut example is the increasing use of clarithromycin or other highly absorbed macrolides for chest infections in many countries; the proportion of *H. pylori* resistant to macrolides correlates reasonably with the use of these drugs in the local community [289].

Data on local primary antibiotic resistance patterns are helpful for deciding on strategies for first-line treatment of *H. pylori*, but often are not available. Surveillance of primary antibiotic resistance in *H. pylori* is useful [370], but local microbiology laboratories may not perform *H. pylori* culture despite the availability of relatively straightforward, standard protocols [267] and there is no national *H. pylori* reference laboratory in many countries. Available data may not be relevant for migrant populations. At the level of the individual patient, a thorough history of recent and recurrent antibiotic usage, and previous eradication therapies attempted (with indication of compliance) can be a useful guide to optimal treatment.

Resistance can be acquired rapidly during treatment and increases as further empirical therapies are attempted: this is termed secondary resistance. The majority of patients who fail second-line therapy will have single and usually double resistance to clarithromycin and/or metronidazole. Resistance to clarithromycin or levofloxacin renders these agents useless for further treatment. However, metronidazole resistance is only partial, and metronidazole is still a useful component of treatment regimens for metronidazole-resistant strains. The efficacy of most regimens containing metronidazole is reduced by only about 10% if the strain is metronidazole resistant.

Patient education, including potential side-effects of therapy

Patient education may improve concordance with treatment, and therefore its success [371,372]. Discussion should include information about *H. pylori* and the indication for treatment; the benefits of successful treatment; the benefits of stopping smoking on long-term ulcer healing; the intended regimen (many are complex with multiple drugs and dosing schedules); the likelihood of side-effects (in up to 50%) even if often mild and transient; the symptomatic management of mild adverse effects; clear advice on when to stop treatment for severe adverse events such as allergic reaction; the importance of compliance with the full course for successful eradication and to guard against increasing antibiotic resistance that can make future treatments ineffective; and the need for further testing to confirm treatment success. Written instructions about how to take the pills are helpful.

Patients should be informed of minor side-effects such as bowel disturbance and mild diarrhea (most) or constipation (bismuth); metallic taste (metronidazole, clarithromycin); disulfiram/Antabuse-like reaction with alcohol (metronidazole); photosensitivity (tetracyclines, especially in sunny climates); blackening of stools (bismuth); and transient headache (PPIs at very high doses). Patients should be told to continue treatment without missing doses even if they develop mild side-effects. They should stop if they develop severe watery diarrhea (*Clostridium difficile* colitis can occur but is rare) or a clear allergic reaction. Extra time taken for explanation and discussion, even during a busy clinic, may improve adherence, minimize repeat consultations and further interventions and, even more importantly, increase the treatment success rate and decrease acquired antibiotic resistance.

Guidelines for H. pylori eradication therapy

Currently available guidelines for the management of *H. pylori* infection [10,306,313,314,373–376] are summarized in Table 49.6.

Confirmation of eradication and follow-up

Confirmation of *H. pylori* eradication is suggested for all *H. pylori*-associated ulcers, given increasing antibiotic resistance and effective nonendoscopic tests, and has been explicitly recommended by expert consensus particularly for PUD complicated by bleeding [305,376]. Its role in uninvestigated dyspepsia managed with a test and treat approach is debated. Either a urea breath test or a validated stool antigen test should be used, taking note of the prerequisites for reliable negative results (see Box 49.3). Tests should be performed at least 4–6 weeks after eradication therapy has been completed. Delay is necessary in cases when the patient needs a longer course of PPI for ulcer healing. As already noted, serological tests have no role in confirming *H. pylori* eradication in clinical practice.

Endoscopy-based tests are appropriate alternatives if an endoscopy is planned and the conditions are optimal (see Box 49.3). The majority of patients undergoing follow-up endoscopy for GU will still be taking PPIs (see "Endoscopy and exclusion of malignancy"), so in these cases testing for *H. pylori* at endoscopy is unhelpful, and urea breath testing or a stool test should be performed at an appropriate interval following cessation of PPIs.

If eradication is successful, further follow-up is not required except for recurrent ulcers (see "Refractory and recurrent ulcers"). Reinfection is rare (less than 1%) in high and very high HDI regions but increases in inverse proportion to socioeconomic development [377]. Very high reinfection rates have been described in some low and medium HDI countries, but it is often unclear from reports whether this represents true reinfection or failed initial treatment.

Management of treatment failures

Potential explanations for treatment failure should be considered. Patient compliance is particularly important, as this can potentially be improved in the subsequent treatment round. Determining the likely antibiotic resistance profile of the infecting strain is also vital [267].

One should assume that the strain is resistant to clarithromycin or levofloxacin if these agents have been used previously in specific *H. pylori* treatment regimens. Exposure to these antibiotics if used for other purposes is also likely to have induced resistance. Data on primary *H. pylori* resistance patterns in the community will also be helpful.

Rational treatment is most straightforward if the *H. pylori* strain is cultured and actual sensitivities are determined. The increasing availability of molecular tests makes this possible even where local laboratories find culture difficult. These tests still require endoscopy and gastric biopsy specimens. DNA sequencing and molecular analysis for *H. pylori* antibiotic resistance are rapidly expanding and will likely be the main option in the future [267,378]; the accuracy of this is at present unknown and so not currently recommended [378]. The concordance of gastric and stool *H. pylori* DNA tests in detection of clarithromycin and fluoroquinolone resistance was 53% and 35% respectively in one study and 86% with eradication success in another study [379,380]. Regardless, determination of *H. pylori* antibiotic resistance is logical and underused. We recommend testing for sensitivity as third line for all patients and second line where individual patient history means resistance to all the commonly used antibiotics is possible.

Assuming that second-line treatment is being given without direct determination of antibiotic resistance and that the treatment will not include antibiotics that have been used previously, other than metronidazole, additional considerations may help treatment success. Full length, 14-day courses of treatment should be used [314]. Meticulous attention to optimizing patient understanding and compliance is vital. Local guidelines and advice should be followed [292,381,382]. Adjuvant therapy for treatment failure may be beneficial but evidence is limited. Smoking cessation should be encouraged. Not treating and delayed treatment are also options for some patients, particularly if personal factors mean careful compliance is unlikely. In this scenario treatment is likely to do more harm than good; the *H. pylori* strain is likely to acquire further antibiotic resistance, making future efforts to treat even more difficult. Eradication should be pursued in patients with complicated PUD and those at increased risk of malignancy based on gastric histology or personal risk, though evidence to support this approach is limited. Multiple treatments in the setting of nonulcer dyspepsia are probably less important for future outcomes.

Table 49.6 Summary of the most recent international guidelines for the management of ***Helicobacter pylori***. This summary is based on the most recently available guidelines for Europe, Developing Countries, Asia-Pacific, Japan, the US, and Canada. Recently, an English-language version of the Chinese guidelines has been published [376]. Several other national guidelines are available.

Regimen	Europe 2017 [306]	Developing Countries 2011 [10]	Asia-Pacific 2009 [373]	Japan 2019 [374]	USA 2017 [313]	Toronto 2016 [314]
Triple therapy PCA	*LC*: first-line (14 days) *HC*: do not use	First-line Rescue (7 to 14 days)	First-line Second-line Salvage (7 to 14 days)	First-line (7 days)	LC: First-line (14 days)	LC: Restricted First-line (14 days)
Triple therapy PCM	*LC/PA*: first-line (14 days) *HC*: do not use	First-line Rescue (7 to 14 days)	Alt. first-line Second-line Salvage *PA*: first-line (7 to 14 days)		LC: First-line (14 days)	LC: Restricted First-line (14 days)
Triple therapy PAM		First-line Rescue (7 to 14 days)	Alt. first-line Second-line Salvage (7 to 14 days)	Second-line (5 to 10 days)		HC: Restricted First-line(14 days)
Bismuth quadruple therapy	*LC*: alt. first-line *LC*: second-line *HC*: first-line or third-line if not used	First-line Rescue (10 days)	Alt. first-line (10 days) Second-line Salvage (7 to 14 days)		First-line (10 to 14 days) Salvage (14 days)	First-line (14 days) Rescue(14 days)
Sequential therapy	*HC*: alt. first-line (not stated)		[a]	[a]	First-line (5 to 7 plus 5 to 7 days)	Not recommended
Concomitant therapy	*HC*: alt. first-line			First-line (7 days)	First-line 10 to 14 days Salvage (10 to 14 days)	First-line (14 days)
Levofloxacin PAL	*LC*: second-line *HC*: first-line	Rescue (10 days)	Second-line Salvage (10 days)	Third-line (not stated)	First-line (10 to 14 days) Salvage (14 days)	HC: Rescue(14 days)
Levofloxacin PCL	*LC/PA*: alt. second-line					LC: Rescue(14 days)
Other eradication therapies / approaches	[b]	PPI, bismuth, amoxicillin, clarithromycin: first-line	PPI, rifabutin, amoxicillin: second-line salvage (7 to 10 days)	High-dose PPI, amoxicillin: can consider (14 days)		PPI, amoxicillin, rifabutin(14 days)

[a] Insufficient local data to recommend.

[b] Guided by antimicrobial susceptibility testing whenever possible.

The different terms for levels of therapy for each guideline are used: first-line, second-line, third-line, salvage, and rescue therapies. Treatment durations recommended by the guidelines for their respective indications are provided where reported (in the table, these apply to all preceding indications in that box). Please see text for further discussion of current recommendations.

Alt., alternative; ***LC***, areas of low clarithromycin resistance; ***HC***, areas of high clarithromycin resistance; ***PA***, recommendation for patients with penicillin allergy; PCA/PCM/PAM, different types of triple therapy (see Table 49.5); PAL/PCL, levofloxacin-based therapies containing amoxicillin and clarithromycin respectively.

Recommended therapeutic paradigm

Several experts have challenged established treatment paradigms [292,311,312,325,383–387]. *H. pylori* resistance has increased markedly in recent years and even an 80% cure rate may be out of reach of standard eradication therapies in some settings. Each empirical trial of ineffective therapy can exacerbate antimicrobial resistance, further decreasing the prospects of treatment success at both patient and population levels.

Helicobacter pylori should be recognized as a serious and potentially life-threatening infection, and time and effort should be devoted to selecting the best eradication therapy for the individual patient. This selection should be based on known primary resistance patterns in the local population and on suspected resistance patterns in the individual patient, based on their personal history of antibiotic exposure and country where they spent their early childhood. An important facet of any approach to first-line treatment is that the patient is educated and empowered to be fully compliant with therapy.

Therefore, overall, in most cases 14-day courses of bismuth-based or nonbismuth-based quadruple therapy (i.e., concomitant therapy) will be appropriate for first-line use. Triple therapy will be an acceptable first-line option in some countries where clarithromycin resistance rates are low in local populations, for example in most parts of the United Kingdom. The most recent national resistance data currently available for the United States were collected nearly two decades ago [388], with subsequent smaller studies suggesting that rates of clarithromycin resistance have risen. In the absence of specific local or further national resistance data, triple therapy should not be used [383].

In the case of treatment failure, empirical second-line treatments should be selected from unused first-line options in a similar fashion, but include the option of fluoroquinolone-based therapies, avoiding clarithromycin if that was used first line. *H. pylori* antibiotic sensitivity testing should be the norm for third-line treatment and deserves more use for second-line therapy where resistance to multiple antibiotics is suspected.

Treating NSAID ulcers

Treatment of NSAID- and aspirin-associated ulcers should include discontinuation of the drug if possible in conjunction with a PPI to promote healing. Concurrent *H. pylori* infection should also be sought and, if present, treated as above. PPIs accelerate ulcer healing in this setting and are preferred to H_2-RAs [389,390]. Misoprostol [391] and sucralfate [392] are inferior to PPI, particularly if NSAIDs are continued, and the utility of misoprostol is limited by its GI side-effects. Management should then be directed at assessment and modification of risk factors, with secondary preventive strategies. Maintenance therapy with a PPI is particularly important for patients who continue or resume NSAID treatment [393].

Discontinuation of NSAID or low-dose aspirin will be informed by drug indication, the balance of risk factors (primarily GI, cardiovascular, and cerebrovascular risks), and patient preference. Consultation with colleagues in cardiology or stroke medicine may be sensible to guide both patient and gastroenterologist in the immediate and longer term.

Helicobacter pylori eradication alone is inadequate to prevent relapse if the NSAID or ASA is continued, and in this situation gastroprotective prophylaxis will usually be required [30,305,393,394].

Risk management, patient education, and monitoring

If it is not possible to stop the NSAID or aspirin, the least ulcerogenic agent should be used at the lowest effective dose [393]. Secondary ulcer prevention in patients with ongoing NSAID and/or aspirin use is addressed under "Prevention." Gastrointestinal complications should be suspected in patients who develop severe dyspepsia or iron deficiency anemia while taking NSAIDs or aspirin, and these patients should be investigated by upper GI endoscopy [204–206]. Unfortunately, many of these patients will present with complications such as overt GI bleeding or perforation (see "Complications").

Treating suspected non-*H. pylori*, non-NSAID ulcers

The approach to non-*H. pylori*, non-NSAID ulcers is based on treating the underlying etiological factors (Table 49.7) after rigorous exclusion of *H. pylori* infection and NSAID use [184,395]. Management is specific to the underlying cause. In truly idiopathic ulcers where no cause is identified, maintenance antisecretory therapy in higher doses is often needed.

Diagnostic approach

Tests for *H. pylori* may be falsely negative. Before concluding that a patient is truly *H. pylori* negative, we suggest that at least two tests for *H. pylori* are used – including a nonendoscopic test – which will increase their combined negative predictive value. Apparently isolated duodenal colonization by *H. pylori* is too infrequent for routine clinical evaluation [396], though duodenal biopsy can be considered in this subpopulation.

Ulcerogenic drug use may be difficult to identify, requiring a meticulous drug history and a collateral history to identify over-the-counter and herbal remedies and illicit drugs that can cause vascular insufficiency. Where available, serum, urine, and platelet function testing may help to identify the use of NSAIDs and, in particular, illicit drugs. However, it should be recognized that that many other drugs, apart from ASA and NSAIDs, can injure the gastroduodenal mucosa (see Box 49.1) so the patient's entire medication list should be scrutinized for potential ulcerogens.

Once *H. pylori* and ulcerogenic drugs have been excluded, multiple endoscopic biopsies should be obtained from the ulcer edges and bed or crater, the surrounding mucosa, and the "normal" gastric antrum and corpus. Malignancy is uncommon in DUs [184] but 3% of GUs harbor malignancy (usually carcinoma or lymphoma). Biopsies can also be evaluated for other infectious agents such as non-*pylori Helicobacter* species (long tight spirals are seen on histology with the special stains usually used to detect *H. pylori*), cytomegalovirus, or herpes simplex viruses. Colonization with other bacterial and fungal species can occur in advanced gastric atrophy, though these are unlikely to cause disease in an immune-competent host. An experienced GI pathologist may identify evidence suggestive of inflammatory or infiltrative disease such as Crohn's disease, eosinophilic gastroenteritis, etc. (see Box 49.1), which require specific evaluation.

Investigations for acid hypersecretion may be indicated, particularly to exclude hypergastrinemia in Zollinger–Ellison or other syndromes (see Chapter 50). Usually additional clinical features, family history, and the endoscopic appearances are clues to gastrinoma. However, PPI therapy may mitigate the classic features. Diagnosis of mastocytosis and myelodysplasia with basophilia requires special tests, including blood film, bone marrow and other organ biopsies, serum tryptase, and molecular tests. In nongastrinoma acid hypersecretion and in the absence of these syndromes, measurements of stimulated acid output are sometimes used to guide PPI treatment and dosing decisions. However, it is more common to use high-dose PPI empirically in such ulcers. Finally, smoking and comorbidities are important considerations for patient management.

Management

Proton pump inhibitors are less effective for acid suppression and ulcer healing in true idiopathic non-*H. pylori*, non-NSAID ulcers than in *H. pylori*-infected patients [397,398]. Ulcers in uninfected patients are more prone to complications [37], with patients at greater risk of recurrent bleeding and death [207]. Therefore, higher doses of PPI and maintenance therapy are recommended. Patients who smoke should be encouraged to stop; this is sometimes the key therapeutic intervention.

In the case of malignancy (see Chapters 52 and 61), inflammatory and infiltrative disease (see Chapters 51 and 64), and acid hypersecretion, management is that of the underlying cause. Acid suppression, almost always with a PPI, is also given. For the management of gastrinoma in Zollinger–Ellison syndrome, refer to Chapter 50. Non-*pylori Helicobacter* species are managed with similar eradication therapy to *H. pylori*. However, many of these organisms are only weakly urease positive, so follow-up breath testing is unreliable and stool antigen tests are unhelpful. In the very rare situation where clearance needs to be assessed, repeat endoscopy and biopsy for histology is needed. Other infectious etiologies need specific discussion with clinical microbiology or virology colleagues. Patients using illicit drugs, such as crack cocaine or methamphetamine, should be managed in collaboration with drug rehabilitation services. Iatrogenic ulcers following bariatric surgery or endoscopic interventions for early gastric cancer such as EMR or ESD require high-dose PPI and removal of other causes (see Chapters 126 and 128). For truly idiopathic ulcers, management is usually with maintenance high-dose PPI to control acid secretion and prevent ulcer relapse [184].

Recurrent and refractory ulcers

Ulcers may recur or be refractory to standard treatment. Before the discovery of *H. pylori* and the development of effective antisecretory agents, PUD was a relapsing condition characterized by ulcer recurrence (see "Relationship between natural history and symptoms") [209–213] but most PUD now responds to medical therapy. Recurrent and refractory PUD has declined, actually, slightly in advance of PPI availability and declining *H. pylori* prevalence [399]. In the era of H_2-RAs, ulcers were defined as refractory if unhealed after 8–12 weeks of therapy, allowing for ulcer size [400]. Ulcers can now be considered refractory if unhealed after 8 weeks of PPI therapy. Most ulcers heal more rapidly than this on PPIs, with DUs healing more rapidly than GUs and smaller ulcers healing more rapidly than larger ulcers. Gastric ulcer healing may be slowed if NSAID or aspirin use needs to be continued, but with modern PPI therapy is still expected before 8 weeks [401]. For GUs, healing can be confirmed as endoscopy is usually repeated after 6–8 weeks of treatment (for discussion see "Endoscopy and exclusion of malignancy"). For both DUs and GUs, refractory or recurrent ulceration should be considered in patients with ongoing symptoms or evidence of complications.

In patients with refractory or recurrent symptoms, key considerations include whether persisting symptoms are due to PUD and, if so, whether the major etiological factors of *H. pylori* infection and NSAID/or aspirin have been addressed before considering other perpetuating factors that may impair healing or lessen the response to antisecretory therapy (such as continued smoking, dense fibrosis, or giant ulcer). Antisecretory therapy may fail because of PPI resistance or H_2-RA tolerance, hypersecretory states, or nonpeptic causes of PUD.

Etiology

The etiology of recurrent and refractory ulcers is broadly similar to PUD in general – *H. pylori* infection, NSAID use, and the causes of non-*H. pylori*, non-NSAID ulcers. Prevalence of truly idiopathic ulcers is increasing (see Tables 49.2 and 49.7), and these patients are at greater risk of recurrent bleeding and death than those with ulcers from *H. pylori* infection [207].

For *H. pylori*-associated ulcers, persisting infection may relate to a failure to recognize infection through inadequate or false-negative testing, or a failure to cure a diagnosed infection as a result of poor patient compliance, inadequate eradication therapy, or *H. pylori* antibiotic resistance.

Continued NSAID or aspirin use (or resumption of use) should be considered in all patients, as these are the most frequent causes of nonhealing ulcer [402]. It is surprisingly common for patients to deny NSAID use. This is usually because of an inadequate drug history, unidentified use of over-the-counter therapies, or sporadic use that is not recalled, but surreptitious misuse does occur. Denial may persist even in the face of objective laboratory evidence or in the context of multiple recurrences or surgery [403,404]. Patients with coronary artery disease are a particular at-risk group, given their use of multiple antiplatelet agents and older age.

The most important etiologies to consider for non-*H. pylori*, non-NSAID ulcer recurrence are malignancy, acid hypersecretory states, unusual infections and inflammatory conditions, though there are many other rare causes (see Box 49.1 and Table 49.7).

Table 49.7 Approach to idiopathic non-*H. pylori*, non-NSAID ulcers.

Etiological factor	Diagnoses	Evaluation
Malignant disease	Gastric adenocarcinoma Gastric MALT lymphoma Metastatic disease Gastrointestinal stromal tumors (GIST)	Endoscopic biopsy of ulcer and adjacent mucosa
Inflammatory and infiltrative disease	Crohn's disease Behçet disease Mastocytosis Eosinophilic gastroenteritis Sarcoidosis Wegener granulomatosis Celiac disease	Endoscopic biopsy of ulcer, adjacent and distant mucosa Colonoscopy, ileoscopy and biopsy
Infectious agents	Non-*pylori Helicobacter* spp. *Streptococcus* spp. *Mycobacterium tuberculosis* *Treponema pallidum* Herpes simplex virus Epstein–Barr virus Cytomegalovirus	Endoscopic biopsy of ulcer and related mucosa Special stains for infectious organisms
Acid hypersecretion	Hypergastrinemia (Zollinger–Ellison syndrome) Carcinoid syndrome Neuroendocine tumors (NET)	Serum gastrin levels (off PPI therapy) Chromogranin A levels Secretin stimulation test NET work-up
Ischemia	Profound hypertension (shock) Recreational drugs (cocaine, methamphetamine) Radiation gastritis Mesenteric atherosclerosis	Detailed history Blood and urine testing Angiography
Iatrogenic	Gastric surgery (ulcer, bariatric) Endoscopic mucosal resection Endoscopic submucosal dissection Nasogastric, orogastric, and nasoenteral (feeding) tubes	Detailed history
Concurrent disease	Stress-related mucosal disease (ICU)	Detailed history and clinical evaluation
Mucosal abnormality	Smoking Site of prior ulcer	Detailed history Endoscopic biopsy of ulcer and related mucosa
Medications	5-Fluorouracil Bisphosphonates Clopidogrel Colchicine Mycophenolate mofetil Potassium chloride Selective serotonin reuptake inhibitors Sirolimus	Detailed history
Foreign bodies	Bezoars Magnets or batteries Intentional foreign body ingestion	Detailed history Radiological imaging Upper endoscopy

ICU, intensive care unit; MALT, mucosa-associated lymphoid tissue; NSAID, nonsteroidal antiinflammatory drug; PPI, proton pump inhibitor.
Source: Adapted based on Table 56.1, Gisbert and Calvet 2009 [184], and Kavitt et al. 2019 [395].

Impaired healing

Ulcers can be refractory because of impaired healing. Restitution and repair may be delayed in the face of an intense inflammatory response, impaired mucosal blood flow or severe local scarring. These same factors promote rapid recurrence if healing was inadequate, mucosal architecture was not restored, or the underlying etiology perpetuates.

Large or giant ulcers: these take longer to heal completely since the rate of healing is approximately 3 mm per week for GU [229], and are often associated with scarring. Ulcers up to 2–2.5 cm in diameter should resolve within 8 weeks [229].

In complicated ulcers: mucosal injury is often deeper and more extensive, again with associated scarring or deformity.

Smoking: cigarette smoke impairs ulcer healing and the deleterious effects increase for heavy smokers. This can delay healing and is associated with ulcer relapse despite adequate antisecretory therapy. However, most studies were performed before *H. pylori* was discovered and this effect may be less when *H. pylori* has been eradicated from infected patients; as a result, the authors do not believe that smoking is an independent factor for impaired healing [405].

Comorbidity: many comorbid diseases linked with chronic catabolism can precipitate or perpetuate ulcers.

Concurrent therapy: glucocorticoids, cytotoxics, and vasoconstrictors may delay healing.

Inadequate control of acid secretion

Gastrinoma: will occasionally be the cause of refractory duodenal ulceration (see Chapter 50).

Nongastrinoma acid hypersecretion: increased basal and stimulated acid secretion has been described in patients with nonhealing ulcers. However, this is much less problematic with standard doses of PPI than with H_2-RAs, and the dose of PPI can easily be increased.

Rapid drug metabolism: pharmacokinetic differences between drugs used for treatment and class-specific differences between individuals can affect acid control, particularly for cytochrome P450-mediated metabolism of PPIs (via *CYP2C19*). Occasionally this may translate into poorer clinical outcomes [362]. In practice, PPI dose is usually empirically increased in patients responding poorly to PPIs, but in a future era of personalized prescribing based on known genetic polymorphisms, this may change.

Clinical features

Refractory or recurrent symptoms require clinical evaluation. Although many patients attribute the recurrence of symptoms to the "return of their ulcer," as for dyspepsia in general, the differential diagnosis is broad (see "Clinical features") and recurrent symptoms do not necessarily indicate ulcer recurrence. Symptoms can return even with ulcer healing [406] and functional GI syndromes are common in these patients. Conversely, 25–40% of ulcer recurrences are asymptomatic [212,213,407].

Diagnostic approach

Endoscopy is required to identify patients with refractory or recurrent ulceration, particularly for overt bleeding, anemia, or symptoms of gastric outlet obstruction. In patients with uncomplicated ulcer and refractory or recurrent symptoms, the history should identify ulcerogenic drugs and treatment compliance. Nonendoscopic testing for *H. pylori* by urea breath or stool antigen test is reasonable to identify eradication failure (though around 10% of treatment failures may be missed). Endoscopy will identify the ulcer and, if the patient is off PPI, antibiotics or bismuth, will provide the opportunity for urease testing, histological evaluation (particularly in urease-negative cases, to detect *H. pylori* organisms, or the presence of chronic active gastritis, or other rare etiologies) and *H. pylori* culture with antibiotic susceptibility testing. All refractory or recurrent ulcers should be inspected carefully with a low threshold for biopsy to identify unusual etiological factors.

The ulcer location is important. Persistent GU in any form mandates meticulous exclusion of malignancy whereas the cancer risk for DU is very low (but not zero). Multiple ulcers and postbulbar DU may reflect acid hypersecretion and gastrinoma (see "Other clinical scenarios or endoscopic findings"). However, in all cases, persisting *H. pylori* infection and NSAID use must be considered. The approach is identical to that for non-*H. pylori*, non-NSAID ulcers (see "Treating suspected non-*H. pylori*, non-NSAID ulcers").

Treatment

Treatment of *H. pylori* infection after failed eradication therapy, the prevention of NSAID and aspirin ulcers, and the management of non-*H. pylori*, non-NSAID ulcers are considered above. Refractory ulcers are more likely to recur if the underlying cause is not identified and managed.

Antisecretory therapy

The mainstay of treatment remains an adequate PPI regimen, adapted to clinical response. Patients initially treated with H_2-RA should be switched to a PPI. Standard doses of PPI are effective though higher doses are more effective, and we recommend full-dose PPI in all cases, for maximal acid inhibition.

Antisecretory therapy should be continued at least until healing is confirmed and, if possible, until the underlying cause has been addressed. However, in all cases of refractory ulcer, and particularly where impaired healing is anticipated or in cases with complications, maintenance full-dose PPI is reasonable for a sustained period of 6 months to several years. Therapy may be required indefinitely if the underlying cause cannot be identified and treated successfully.

Maintenance therapy is also indicated to prevent recurrent ulcers, particularly in high-risk groups defined by previous ulcer complications, previously refractory or recurrent ulcers, and risk factors for impaired healing.

If high-dose PPI is not effective, there is no evidence to guide subsequent medical therapy. One can try empirical switching to an alternative PPI, or addition of bedtime H_2-RA to control acid breakthrough. Direct measurement of acid output may be useful in these patients, with therapy adjusted if pH remains low. Addition of sucralfate or even misoprostol may also be effective although there are no prospective studies of combination therapy for this indication. Very occasionally, PUD persists despite full medical therapy and this is an appropriate indication for elective surgery.

Surgery

Elective surgery for refractory or recurrent PUD still has a very occasional role. Surgery is rarely advisable for erosions or shallow ulcers and is performed very rarely in the absence of previous complications, such as recurrent bleeding. We advise particular caution in performing surgery primarily for symptom relief; it is extremely difficult to be sure that resistant symptoms arise from resistant ulcers.

Ulcer surgery usually involves one or more of the following operations: vagotomy, pyloroplasty, gastrojejunostomy, or rarely partial gastrectomy. Some operations are linked to subsequent postgastrectomy syndromes including early and late dumping syndromes [408]. Nowadays, a laparoscopic approach is increasingly used [409]. Recent advances in endoscopic techniques, such as over-the-scope clips, permit endoscopic treatment of perforated or treatment-resistant bleeding ulcers and there may be a diminishing role for surgery in managing complicated ulcers in the near future [410] although some conditions, such as clinically significant Cameron's lesions [126], may still merit surgical intervention.

Complications

Complications of PUD include hemorrhage (either overt or chronic, the latter causing chronic iron deficiency anemia), perforation and penetration, and gastric outlet obstruction (acute or chronic). The relative frequency, epidemiology, and management of complications differ between regions and have changed markedly in recent years related, in part, to the changing epidemiology of *H. pylori* [411] (see "Epidemiology"). All patients presenting with complications require appropriate identification of and intervention for *H. pylori* infection and NSAID use, with successful *H. pylori* eradication confirmed after treatment. Non-*H. pylori*, non-NSAID ulcers are associated with increased complications [207]. Early multidisciplinary coordination between emergency room and medical teams, gastroenterology and endoscopy teams, surgeons, radiologists, and intensivists/ICU specialists is recommended.

Hemorrhage

The most common presentation of complicated PUD is with upper GI bleeding, accounting for over 70% of acute complications in high and very high HDI countries [412]. The incidence of bleeding in these countries has declined over the last 20 years, from around 50–170 per 100 000 to an estimated 19–57 per 100 000 [413], with the highest risk in people over 60 years of age and a significant minority aged over 80 years, reflecting increased NSAID use. However, bleeding accounted for only 10% of complications in a Nigerian center, where obstruction and perforation were more frequent [414].

Clinical features and diagnosis

Patients typically present with nausea, hematemesis and/or melena, and may have symptoms or signs of hemodynamic instability, including dizziness or syncope. Around 10% of patients presenting with hematochezia and apparent acute lower GI bleeding will have a source in their upper GI tract, most commonly duodenal ulceration. A subset of patients with PUD will present with complications without preceding symptoms (silent ulcers). Peptic ulceration is usually diagnosed at endoscopy.

Nonsteroidal antiinflammatory drugs, including aspirin, are the most important risk factor for bleeding. Drug-specific factors influence the relative risk (see "Prevention"). Therefore, an accurate drug history is essential.

Helicobacter pylori is also an important risk factor. There are some specific considerations for the diagnosis of *H. pylori* infection in bleeding patients: higher rates of false-negative results for *H. pylori* status using urease and stool antigen tests; difficulty in diagnosing *H. pylori* due to suppression with PPIs or antibiotics; and that endoscopists are disinclined to take biopsies during the acute bleeding episode. Diagnosis can be safely delayed until after the acute episode or even after the ulcer has healed, though procedures should be in place within primary or secondary care to follow up this cohort. Typically, serological testing will be performed during the acute episode, particularly when other tests are not available early in the hospitalization. In the setting of complicated PUD, though a single negative test has some negative predictive value, interval testing is indicated to confidently exclude *H. pylori* infection, especially in high-prevalence populations and in high-risk patients. This is usually in the form of urea breath testing, a stool antigen test, or even repeat endoscopy for biopsy-based tests.

Management

The management of upper GI bleeding is addressed in detail in Chapter 38. Key elements in management are resuscitation and stabilization with fluids and/or blood products in proportion to severity; multidisciplinary input including risk assessment based on clinical, laboratory, and endoscopic parameters; intravenous acid suppressive therapy (to promote ulcer healing and reduce rebleeding); management of hemorrhage by endoscopic modalities (and sometimes timely angiography or surgical intervention if indicated); and identification of the etiology so that definitive treatment can be arranged. Without definitive treatment, the risk of recurrent bleeding is 10–36% per patient-year [415–417]. Appropriate eradication of *H. pylori* and/or discontinuation of NSAIDs will significantly reduce this risk, and typically the treatment effect size is greater than for long-term maintenance antisecretory therapy alone. Management strategies where it is not possible to stop NSAIDs or aspirin use are discussed under "Prevention."

At endoscopy, the appearance of the ulcer as per the modified Forrest classification can predict the risk of rebleeding, the need for intervention, and death. Ulcers with high-risk features of active spurting (IA), active oozing (IB), or a nonbleeding visible vessel (IIA) have a high risk of further bleeding and warrant endoscopic therapy. A metaanalysis of endoscopic therapy shows a significant decrease in further bleeding for both actively bleeding ulcers and ulcers with nonbleeding visible vessels [418]. For ulcers with adherent clot (IIB), endoscopic therapy may be performed by targeting the underlying lesion after clot removal. This has been shown to reduce recurrent bleeding compared to medical therapy alone, although significant heterogeneity exists among the studies [419]. Endoscopic therapy is generally not recommended for ulcers with a flat pigmented spot (IIC) or a clean base (III).

Perforation and penetration

Perforation results in leakage of air and intraluminal contents into the peritoneal cavity. It is less frequent than ulcer bleeding in developed countries, occurring in up to 10% of cases and with an estimated annual incidence of 4–14 per 100 000. In Nigeria, perforation accounts for 30% of surgical procedures for complicated PUD [414]. Duodenal ulcers are the most common site for perforation (60%) with the remaining cases evenly split between the gastric antrum and corpus.

Presentation is typically with sudden onset of severe generalized abdominal pain, features of peritonitis and shock. The clinical picture will often gradually improve over the first few hours but this should not necessarily be taken as reassurance – prompt assessment and management decisions are essential. Following initial fluid resuscitation, cross-sectional imaging has largely replaced plain radiographs in establishing the diagnosis. Patients are managed nil per os with a nasogastric tube, intravenous fluids, empirical broad-spectrum antibiotics guided by local policies, and often high-dose intravenous PPI therapy (extrapolated from studies on peptic ulcer hemorrhage).

The decision on whether to operate and, if so, when, should consider patient comorbidity and functional status, whether the patient is stable or improving, evidence that the perforation has spontaneously sealed, and the availability of percutaneous peritoneal drainage. Detailed discussion of the different surgical approaches to perforated ulcers is beyond the scope of this chapter. The prognosis is very good with mortality of 1–5%, though poor outcomes are more likely in older patients, those with comorbid disease including diabetes mellitus, in the context of more severe illness (initial hypotension, metabolic acidosis, and organ failure), and with delayed presentation past 12 hours.

The management of apparently sealed-off perforations is an increasingly frequent issue for medical gastroenterologists, where perigastric or periduodenal pockets of air have been identified on the CT scan. Patients may have presented along the spectrum of symptoms outlined above but then improved. Management should be in close collaboration with the surgical team, but endoscopy may be the most appropriate step rather than operative intervention. Parenteral, then maintenance anti-ulcer therapy, and an evaluation for reversible underlying causes are also central aspects of management.

Ulcers may also penetrate into retroperitoneal organs without free perforation into the peritoneal cavity. Penetration is characterized by constant severe pain and usually a sudden change in symptoms. However, penetration often remains subclinical. Penetration may result in pancreatic damage with raised serum amylase but usually without overt pancreatitis (antral GUs and DUs); abscess formation; erosion into the biliary tree or liver (DUs); gastroduodenal fistulas (pyloric or prepyloric ulcers); gastrocolic fistulas (GUs on greater curve; may present with feculent vomiting, postprandial diarrhea, dyspepsia, and halitosis); or aortoenteric fistulas or erosion into other vascular structures (may present with herald bleed or catastrophic hemorrhage). Management is usually surgical.

Gastric outlet obstruction

Gastric outlet obstruction (GOO) occurs in PUD because of local fibrosis, scarring, and edema as well as gastric atony; historically, PUD accounted for about 90% of GOO cases but it is now responsible for only about 5% of GOO cases and it is the least frequent ulcer complication in most populations, likely affecting less than the quoted 2–3% of PUD patients. However, in low and medium HDI countries, it is still the most common reason for surgical intervention (in 50–60% of cases) in complicated PUD. However, other causes of GOO have increased in relative importance in the differential diagnosis of gastric retention, including neoplasia (50–80%) and upper GI tract webs, other obstructing lesions and inflammatory conditions (Table 49.8). GOO is more frequent in Zollinger–Ellison syndrome (in around 10%, see Chapter 50), with DU and pyloric channel ulcers, and with long-standing or NSAID-associated ulcers.

Clinical features and diagnosis

Upper abdominal pain, vomiting after a meal, bloating and distension, early satiety, and weight loss are suggestive of GOO. Physical examination may reveal a succussion splash caused by food or drink retained in the stomach. The spectrum of associated clinical features of the underlying etiology is broad.

Diagnostic work-up includes both imaging and endoscopy although diagnostic efforts are usually preceded by initial management steps, at least in acute presentations. Radiological investigations are often the first step, typically cross-sectional imaging, though ultrasound, contrast studies, and plain films are often informative. Endoscopic evaluation facilitates definitive diagnosis and therapeutic intervention, although prolonged fasting or aspiration of stomach contents using a nasogastric tube (NGT) may be necessary first. The traditional saline load test (where 750 mL of sodium chloride solution is administered via NGT, with mechanical obstruction suggested when more than 400 mL can be aspirated after 30 minutes) has declined in importance, though serial assessment to gauge response to medical management may be useful (aspirated residual volume below 200 mL after 30 minutes suggests resolution). At endoscopy, the stomach is cleansed and decompressed, then inspected for evidence of an intrinsic obstructing lesion, with targeted endoscopic biopsies to identify or exclude malignancy. Sometimes additional tissue evaluation by endoscopic ultrasound, deeper biopsies, or full-thickness surgical biopsies is required, particularly if there is a strong suspicion of malignancy or tuberculosis.

Management

The management of GOO is multidisciplinary. Priorities include initial stabilization, administration of antisecretory agents, optimization of nutritional status and fluid balance, endoscopic intervention if indicated, and specific management according to the definitive diagnosis.

In most cases, the first step is aspiration of retained stomach contents via a large-bore NGT to reduce the risk of aspiration.

Table 49.8 Differential diagnosis of gastric outlet obstruction.

Etiology	Notes on management
Peptic ulcers (5%)	See text
Duodenal ulcers	
Pyloric channel ulcers	
Gastric ulcers	
Malignancy (50–80%)	
Local extension of pancreatic cancer	Usually palliation including endoscopic enteral stent or surgical bypass by gastrojejunostomy
Gastric carcinoma	As for pancreatic cancer
Gastric lymphoma	Usually chemotherapy
Other causes of malignant obstruction, e.g., proximal duodenal and ampullary neoplasms, local extension of gallbladder or biliary tree neoplasms, gastric carcinoid	
Inflammatory and infiltrating disease	
Crohn's disease (5%)	Antiinflammatory therapy to target nonfibrotic disease, multiple endoscopic balloon dilations, 40% require surgery (including gastrojejunostomy, gastroduodenostomy, stricturoplasty)
Chronic and acute severe pancreatitis (1–5%)	Usually surgical, limited long-term outcome data with endoscopic dilation
Large pancreatic pseudocyst	Drainage: percutaneous, endoscopic by transpapillary route or via gastrostomy or duodenostomy, or surgical
Other causes, e.g., cholecystitis, eosinophilic gastroenteritis, infiltration with amyloid or granulomata, including gastric tuberculosis	
Miscellaneous	
Caustic injury	Balloon dilation, various temporary and definitive surgeries
Migration of PEG tube	Usually endoscopic
Postsurgical complications	Usually surgical
Large pedunculated gastric polyp	Usually endoscopic
Bouveret syndrome[a]	Extracorporeal lithotripsy and endoscopic removal or surgery
Gastric bezoars	See Chapter 61
Other causes, e.g., adult hypertrophic pyloric stenosis, upper gastrointestinal tract webs and bands, annular or ectopic pancreas, gastric volvulus	

[a] Impaction of gallstone in pyloric channel or duodenum, following migration through gastrocholecystic or enterocholecystic fistula.
PEG, percutaneous endoscopic gastrostomy.

The patient is managed nil per os, and fluid and electrolyte abnormalities are corrected. These steps are usually necessary prior to endoscopy or contrast studies. Parenteral PPIs, often given intravenously, are also indicated to reduce gastric secretion. Nutritional support, sometimes intravenous, is essential. Endoscopic therapy with balloon dilation or stent insertion may aid initial recovery, though this is rarely definitive and repeated interventions may be needed (see Chapter 122).

Once the underlying cause has been identified, the patient is rehydrated, and electrolyte derangement and malnutrition addressed, specific treatment should be instigated (see Table 49.8). If the cause is PUD, then the usual work-up is again to identify *H. pylori* infection and/or NSAID use. Most of these patients will respond (at least initially) to acid suppression and, if indicated, *H. pylori* eradication and NSAID cessation. This is particularly the case for NSAID-induced PUD, though there is a risk of recurrent obstruction if patients continue NSAIDs even following interventional therapy. In the absence of evidence for maintenance antisecretory therapy, full-dose oral medication should be started after the obstruction has resolved and continued long term. However, it may ultimately be possible to discontinue this if NSAIDs are stopped or, in the case of *H. pylori* infection, when eradication is confirmed and deformities in the antrum and/or duodenum have resolved.

Prevention

The primary and secondary prevention of PUD are key aspects of management, aiming to assess and modify risk. The primary prevention of ulcers is focused on users of NSAIDs and aspirin. Broader primary prevention of PUD through targeted screening and eradication of *H. pylori* in asymptomatic individuals is not currently recommended, except in certain patients receiving long-term NSAID or aspirin treatment in whom there is strong evidence of benefit. Effective secondary prevention of NSAID and aspirin ulcers is also important. Secondary prevention of non-NSAID ulcers by an adequate search for, and eradication of, *H. pylori* infection should also be reemphasized because it is far too frequently overlooked in some healthcare settings.

Ulcer healing and long-term antisecretory treatment for non-NSAID ulcers are considered with maintenance medical therapy (see "Treatment of peptic ulcer disease"). Modulation of other important factors (see "Risk factors") such as smoking, in particular, is also possible and likely to be of benefit.

A recent metaanalysis of more than 1200 trials quantified the relative treatment effects of available gastroprotective agents in the settings of ulcer prevention, ulcer healing, and treatment of acute upper gastrointestinal bleeding and showed benefits in all three clinical contexts, with PPIs showing superiority to other available agents [420]. In prevention trials, protective agents reduced development of endoscopic ulcers, symptomatic ulcers, and upper gastrointestinal bleeding, but did not significantly reduce mortality (OR 0.85, 95% CI 0.69–1.04, $p = 0.11$). PPIs were superior to all other agents in preventing PUD, preventing bleeding irrespective of the use of NSAIDs, and ulcer healing. In trials among patients with acute bleeding, gastric protective agents prevented further bleeding (OR 0.68, 95% CI 0.60–0.78, $p < 0.0001$), blood transfusion (OR 0.75, 95% CI 0.65–0.88, $p = 0.0003$), further endoscopic intervention (OR 0.56, 95% CI 0.45–0.70, $p < 0.0001$) and surgery (OR 0.72, 95% CI 0.61–0.84, $p < 0.0001$) but did not reduce mortality significantly (OR 0.90, 95% CI 0.72–1.11, $p = 0.31$). PPIs were superior to H_2-RAs for preventing further bleeding ($p = 0.01$) and blood transfusion ($p = 0.01$).

Prevention of NSAID and aspirin ulcers

Nonsteroidal antiinflammatory drugs and aspirin are widely used and cause considerable GI morbidity and mortality (see "Epidemiology"). Low-dose aspirin (<325 mg daily) is associated with a 2–4-fold increased risk [421]. It is frequently not possible to avoid or discontinue these agents so both primary and secondary prevention of NSAID-associated ulcers are important issues in clinical practice.

Earlier studies on prevention were largely based on endpoints of questionable clinical significance (endoscopic ulceration defined by arbitrary size criteria, rather than symptomatic or complicated ulcers), and undertaken in less relevant populations (healthy volunteers, often young and without comorbidities or a history of PUD). The management strategy includes assessment of risk factors for GI toxicity (and cardio- and cerebrovascular risks) and patient stratification, consideration of *H. pylori* status and other modifiable risk factors (e.g., smoking), drug-specific factors, and consideration of coprescription of prophylactic agents to protect the mucosa.

Risk stratification

Assessment of risk factors for GI toxicity is central when considering which strategy to follow to prevent NSAID- and aspirin-associated ulcers and their complications. Many individuals are not at significantly increased clinical risk, particularly healthy individuals using NSAIDs at low doses in the short term. No special preventive strategy is needed and the majority of patients can be reassured. However, as NSAIDs carry an FDA black box warning for both GI (increased risk of serious GI bleeding, ulceration, perforation) and cardiovascular risk (cardiovascular thrombotic events, myocardial infarction, stroke), these should always be discussed with patients and documented.

Several guidelines and consensus statements have been published (Table 49.9), with more recent guidelines recommending that patients be stratified into high-, medium-, and low-risk groups (Table 49.10) [32,394,422]. We recommend prophylaxis primarily for GI high-risk groups [393]. Although a large number of trials have been undertaken, direct comparisons of different strategies for GI protection are limited and many trials are at risk of bias [423]. Therefore, guidelines and cost-effectiveness analyses are not necessarily informed by high-grade evidence. New NSAIDs releasing vasoactive gaseous mediators such as nitric oxide (COX-inhibiting nitric oxide donators) or hydrogen sulfide (H_2S) have been associated with fewer GI adverse effects and hold promise as safer alternatives with regard to gastric protection [424]. Interestingly, these agents may also provide a better cardiovascular safety profile [425].

Key considerations in risk stratification include a history of complicated or uncomplicated PUD, patient age (with older patients at higher risk), and concurrent drugs, of which the most important are aspirin, clopidogrel or other antiplatelet agents, anticoagulants, and glucocorticoids. Drug combinations such as dual antiplatelet therapy or the combination of NSAIDs with selective serotonin reuptake inhibitors or bisphosphonates are associated with increased risks of bleeding and other complications.

Cardiovascular and cerebrovascular risk stratification

The need to consider cardiovascular and cerebrovascular risk was affirmed in a randomized trial of 156 adults in Hong Kong who developed peptic ulcer bleeding while taking low-dose aspirin [426]. After endoscopic and PPI therapy, patients were assigned to continue aspirin (80 mg daily) or placebo for 8 weeks. There were significantly fewer deaths in the aspirin arm at 8 weeks: lower all-cause mortality (1.3% vs 12.9%, difference 11.6%, 95% CI 3.7–19.5%) and lower mortality attributed to cardiovascular, cerebrovascular or GI complications (1.3% vs 10.3%, difference 9.0%, 95% CI 1.7–16.3%). Recurrent ulcer bleeding within 30 days was nonsignificantly increased in patients taking aspirin (10.3% vs 5.4%, difference 4.9%, 95% CI −3.6% to 13.4%). The mortality benefit with aspirin was much greater than expected from larger secondary prevention trials. This underlines an important message in clinical practice: the management of cardiovascular and cerebrovascular risk should be considered alongside the immediate priority to control hemorrhage and prevent rebleeding.

Table 49.9 Risk factors for gastrointestinal toxicity from nonsteroidal antiinflammatory drugs.

ACCF/ACG/AHA 2008 consensus statement	ACG 2009 guidelines	ACCF/ACG/AHA 2010 focused update
High risk		
Previous history of a complicated ulcer	Previous history of a complicated ulcer, especially recent	Prior GI bleeding
Previous history of ulcer disease (nonbleeding)	≥3 other risk factors	Advanced age
Dual antiplatelet therapy or anticoagulants		Concurrent use of anticoagulants, steroids, or NSAIDs including aspirin
≥2 other risk factors		***Helicobacter pylori*** infection
Moderate risk		
Classification level not used	1 or 2 other risk factors	
Low risk		
1 or no other risk factors	No other risk factors	
Other risk factors		
Age ≥60 years	Age >65 years	
Concurrent use of glucocorticoids	Concurrent use of aspirin (including low-dose), glucocorticoids, or anticoagulants	
Dyspepsia or GERD symptoms	Previous history of an uncomplicated ulcer	
	High-dose NSAID therapy	

Helicobacter pylori is an independent and additive risk factor and needs to be addressed separately, along with consideration of cardiovascular and cerebrovascular risks (see text).
GERD, gastroesophageal reflux disease; NSAID, nonsteroidal antiinflammatory drug.
Source: Adapted from the American College of Cardiology Foundation (ACCF)/American College of Gastroenterology (ACG)/American Heart Association (AHA) 2008 consensus statement [32] and ACCF/ACG/AHA 2010 focused update [422], with permission from Elsevier. Reproduced from the American College of Gastroenterology 2009 guidelines [394], with permission from Nature Publishing Group.

Table 49.10 A proposed strategy to prevent NSAID-related ulcer complications.

	Low GI risk	Moderate GI risk	High GI risk
Low CV risk	NSAID alone – the least ulcerogenic at the lowest effective dose	NSAID plus PPI or misoprostol	Alternative therapy if possible, or COX-2 inhibitor plus PPI or misoprostol
High CV risk	Naproxen plus PPI or misoprostol	Naproxen plus PPI or misoprostol	Avoid NSAID or COX-2 inhibitors, use alternative therapy

Choice between different strategies based on clinical and cost-effectiveness analysis, and any cardioprotective benefits of naproxen over other agents remains controversial (see text).
GI risk: This is stratified into low, moderate, and high (see Table 49.9 and text). We recommend prophylaxis primarily for patients in high GI risk groups on the basis of currently available evidence (see text).
CV risk: High CV risk is arbitrarily defined by the ACG 2009 guidelines as the requirement for low-dose aspirin for prevention of serious CV events. There are other approaches to assessing CV risk that can provide more gradation and account for vascular risk factors in individual patients (see text).
All patients with a history of ulcers who require NSAIDs should be tested for ***H. pylori*** and if the infection is present, eradication therapy should be given.
COX-2, cyclooxygenase 2; CV, cardiovascular; GI, gastrointestinal; NSAID, nonsteroidal antiinflammatory drug; PPI, proton pump inhibitor.
Source: Lanza et al. 2009 [394]. Reproduced from the American College of Gastroenterology 2009 guidelines, with permission from Nature Publishing Group.

The effect of age should not be underestimated. A recent large prospective population-based study showed that the severity, case fatality, and poor functional outcome of bleeds increase significantly in patients older than 75 on long-term antiplatelet treatment for secondary prevention [427]. Most major upper gastrointestinal bleeds were disabling or fatal in this age group. Interestingly, the number needed to treat with PPIs to prevent one disabling or fatal upper gastrointestinal bleed at 5-year follow-up decreased, from 338 for patients younger than 65 years [428] to 25 for patients over the age of 85 [427].

Close collaboration between the gastroenterology team and cardiology or stroke medicine is advised, particularly for high-risk patients with coronary artery stents or a recent history of significant myocardial or cerebral ischemia.

Guidelines, including those from the American College of Gastroenterology in 2009 [394], updated in 2010 [422], have also addressed cardiovascular risk, with patients at high risk arbitrarily defined as those taking low-dose aspirin. These guidelines recommend different management strategies depending upon the combined GI and cardiovascular risk profile. Some authors recommend further caution in the prescription of NSAIDs in patients with cardiovascular disease [429], citing inadequate long-term randomized outcome data. Other useful tools for clinical practice have become available such as the ASA Risk Calculator (www.asariskcalculator.com) [430]. This assesses the baseline risk and expected benefit of aspirin on the 10-year risk of cardiovascular events using Framingham estimations. Gastrointestinal risk calculations are based on large European primary care databases and systematic review.

As is often stated, guidelines and evidence may not directly relate to the individual patient under consideration, but tools such as this can be useful in informing collaborative discussions between physician and patient.

Vascular risk – clopidogrel and omeprazole

There have been concerns regarding a pharmacokinetic interaction between clopidogrel and PPIs, particularly omeprazole. in vitro studies have highlighted this interaction, with further work suggesting that other factors than *CYP2C19* metabolism can also determine clopidogrel efficacy. Studies including an observational self-controlled cohort study of 24 471 patients in the United Kingdom [431] concluded that this interaction is not clinically important. Other observational studies have reached different conclusions.

The only randomized evidence comes from the COGENT trial [432], which compared clopidogrel alone with a clopidogrel/omeprazole combination pill, with the properties of this omeprazole formulation being slightly different than other generic forms. The two primary endpoints were composites of significant GI and cardiovascular events at 180 days. The authors did not find a significant difference in cardiovascular events but they highlighted a 66% reduction in GI events and an 87% reduction in overt upper GI bleeding. Unfortunately, the study was underpowered, recruiting only around 75% of its target of 5000 patients. In another post hoc analysis, 2676 patients enrolled in COGENT undergoing percutaneous coronary intervention (PCI) within 14 days of randomization and 1573 patients presenting with acute coronary syndrome (ACS) managed with or without PCI were included [433]; omeprazole significantly reduced rates of composite GI events at 180 days for both PCI (1.2% versus 2.7%, $p = 0.02$) and non-PCI (1.1% versus 2.7%, $p = 0.05$) patients without increasing composite cardiovascular events. Another post hoc analysis of this RCT showed that the effect of PPI in preventing GI adverse events is independent of the dose of aspirin (1.2% versus 3.1% in low-dose ASA group and 0.9% versus 2.6% for high-dose ASA [>100 mg])] [434]. Based on this evidence, we recommend patients with cardiovascular and GI risk factors requiring dual antiplatelet therapy receive prophylactic daily PPI therapy.

Helicobacter pylori

Helicobacter pylori infection significantly and synergistically increases the risk of uncomplicated and complicated ulcers in NSAID users [35]. Screening for and eradication of infection is widely recommended to avoid this risk [32,305,394]. We recommend that all patients be tested for *H. pylori* and treated if positive before initiating long-term NSAID therapy. There are benefits whether or not patients have a personal history of peptic ulceration, but those who have such a history benefit most. However, this strategy alone does not reduce ulcer risk in patients already receiving long-term NSAID treatment. Aspirin users with a history of PUD, whether complicated or not, should also be tested and treated, with a lower long-term incidence of ulcer bleeding after eradication even in the absence of gastroprotective treatment. The HEAT trial is an RCT started in 2012 with an expected completion date in early 2021 [435], that is designed to test whether peptic ulcer bleeding is reduced by *H. pylori* eradication, compared to no eradication, in an estimated 6600 regular aspirin users (≤325 mg daily) over 60 years of age.

Primary prevention of ulcer disease through population screening is not practiced, although may be a beneficial outcome of other *H. pylori* screening programs such as those aimed to reduce gastric cancer in East Asian countries. Other potential tools such as *H. pylori* vaccines are not available despite much research [359].

NSAID factors – duration, choice and dose of agent, and formulation

Several important NSAID- or aspirin-specific factors influence the risk of GI complications, namely the duration of treatment, the class of NSAID (nonselective or COX-2 selective), toxicity of particular drugs, the dose used, cotherapy with aspirin, and the formulation. Strategies that target these factors may be used to reduce the risk of ulcer development [393].

The risk of GI complications is related to the duration of treatment, with increasing risk for longer exposures. This risk is most significant after 1–3 months of treatment [34], though is present within 1 week for some higher-risk agents such as indomethacin or piroxicam. Therefore, short-term treatment courses of NSAIDs with the lowest GI toxicity, and infrequent or occasional use such as for relief of temporary pain, are unlikely to cause significant problems in the majority. In particularly high-risk individuals, such as older patients with a history of complicated ulcer, NSAID prescriptions for analgesia should be avoided and alternative agents used. Although it is advisable to use the shortest possible course of therapy, this strategy is usually not an option for those taking prophylactic aspirin or

NSAIDs for inflammatory conditions. Patient risk and the prevention of GI complications should be considered regardless of the duration of therapy [436].

Some drugs or drug classes are potentially more ulcerogenic (see Figure 49.9). Compared to no NSAIDs, indomethacin has a higher risk of GI complications (RR 2.3), with moderate risk for naproxen, diclofenac, and piroxicam (RR 1.7–1.8), and lower but still increased risk for tenoxicam and ibuprofen (RR 1.4) and meloxicam (RR 1.2) [437]. Other drugs with higher ulcer risk include tolmetin, ketoprofen, and azapropazone [438]. As previously highlighted, concurrent use of NSAIDs and aspirin (even at low doses) will further increase the risk.

Selective COX-2 inhibitors, developed to reduce or avoid the gastroduodenal toxicity of nonselective NSAIDs [439], have been shown in large clinical studies and systematic reviews to be less ulcerogenic than other NSAIDs with similar cardiovascular adverse effects [178]. However, switching from nonselective to selective NSAIDs for secondary prevention in high-risk patients is generally, but not always, less effective than a PPI for prophylactic mucosal protection (see further on), although concomitant use of a selective COX-2 inhibitor and a PPI does appear to further reduce ulcer risk. Concomitant use of aspirin with COX-2 inhibitors negates any benefit from reduced ulcer risk, by effectively reestablishing nonselective COX inhibition [439].

Longer-term outcome data have linked COX-2 inhibitors with an increased risk of cardio- and cerebrovascular events. Some drugs, including rofecoxib, lumiracoxib, and valdecoxib, were withdrawn from the market in some regions because they were associated with more myocardial infarctions and/or strokes. However, several drugs have kept their licensing approvals, including celecoxib, and are widely available although used less since the safety data received widespread public attention. COX-2 inhibitors are effective antiinflammatory agents and analgesics.

The choice of agent is influenced by the assessment of GI risk, but generally the least ulcerogenic NSAID is recommended (which may be a COX-2 inhibitor) with or without mucosal protection [394]. However, treatment decisions must be individualized for patients with high cardiovascular or cerebrovascular risk, in whom COX-2 inhibitors and most nonselective NSAIDs may further increase the vascular risk and reduce the effectiveness of antiplatelet agents. The impact of naproxen on the antiplatelet effect is believed to be less, such that this NSAID is putatively mildly cardioprotective, though this remains controversial and in January 2014 an FDA panel voted 16 against and nine in favor of a lower cardiovascular risk for naproxen. Management decisions that balance these complex risks should be informed by the latest evidence, guidelines, and regulatory agency advice, rather than blanket recommendations.

The PRECISION Trial enrolled over 24 000 patients to compare celecoxib with ibuprofen and naproxen in a double-blind, parallel-group study of cardiovascular, GI and renal safety in patients with osteoarthritis or rheumatoid arthritis and a high risk of cardiovascular disease. Overall, celecoxib was noninferior to ibuprofen and naproxen for a composite cardiovascular outcome endpoint (cardiovascular death, nonfatal myocardial infarct, nonfatal stroke) which was reported in 2.3%, 2.5%, and 2.7% of patients in the celecoxib, naproxen, and ibuprofen arms, respectively [440]. Evaluation of other outcomes in subsidiary analyses led to the conclusion that celecoxib was associated with similar or lower risks of adverse cardiovascular, GI and renal events than ibuprofen or naproxen in patients with osteoarthritis or rheumatoid arthritis [441]. When given without aspirin, celecoxib was associated with lower risk than naproxen (hazard ratio [HR] 1.52, 95% CI 1.22–1.90) or ibuprofen (HR1.81, 95% CI 1.46–2.26) for the primary composite adverse event endpoint which comprised noncardiovascular death and major cardiovascular, GI and renal events. The addition of aspirin reduced the safety benefit associated with celecoxib and, although there was still benefit compared with ibuprofen, this was not seen in comparison with naproxen [442].

The dosage used is also relevant – ulcer risk from NSAIDs is closely associated with dose (see Figure 49.9 and Table 49.9). This increased risk with higher doses of NSAIDs has been observed for many agents, both selective and nonselective, leading to the recommendation that the lowest effective dose be used. This is perhaps more complicated for aspirin at low dose (50–325 mg daily) with the GI risk increasing proportionately, but the degree of vascular protection is considered by some to be greater with doses at the higher end of this range for some indications. Additional care is needed to adequately address ulcer risk in these cases.

Alternative formulations of aspirin, including enteric-coated and buffered forms, can reduce endoscopic ulceration (which can be in part a topical effect) but not clinically important upper GI bleeding (where systemic effects and other risk factors are important).

Safe prescription of NSAIDs

There is a variety of mitigation strategies to reduce the risk of NSAID-induced gastroduodenopathy and peptic ulceration, based on avoidance of NSAIDs, selection of less injurious agents, dose minimization, and pharmacological prophylaxis (Box 49.4) [393].

Using alternative therapy

Pharmacological alternatives to NSAID therapy include acetaminophen (paracetamol) which is less effective but safer when taken within the recommended dose range [443]. Nonpharmacological methods include cognitive behavioral therapy, acupuncture, alternative medicine, and transepithelial electrical nerve stimulation which activates native opioid receptors but these approaches are generally less accessible and more expensive and their efficacy is unpredictable.

Mucosal protection – coprescription of prophylactic agents

Primary and secondary prevention strategies in patients requiring NSAIDS include coprescription of a PPI or misoprostol; H_2-RAs are not as effective [389,391,444] with several cost-effectiveness

Box 49.4 Prevention strategies for safe prescription of NSAIDs [393].

Use alternative management
- Nonpharmacologcal
- Pharmacological

Choose NSAID with lowest gastrointestinal adverse events
- Nonselective NSAIDs
- Selective COX-2 inhibitors
- Other newer NSAIDs

Use lowest effective dose of NSAIDs
Avoid combination NSAID therapy
Be aware of self-medication
Patient education
Test and treat *H. pylori*
Pharmacological prevention
- PPI
- H_2-RA
- Misoprostol
- Rebamipide
- DA-9601 (Stillen)
- β-D-glucuronidase inhibitors

analyses reaching different conclusions [423,445,446]. Nowadays, where prophylaxis is indicated, PPIs are used in almost all situations. Therapy should continue for as long as the NSAID or low-dose aspirin is used and risk factors remain. Physicians should note that although there is strong evidence that PPIs decrease the rate of adverse events from NSAIDs in the upper GI tract, there is no evidence for benefit more distally in the GI tract [393].

When combined with risk assessment and other factors previously discussed, several strategies are possible, including those proposed by the American College of Gastroenterology guidelines (see Table 49.9) [394]. Management should be tailored to each individual – no strategy is universally effective or safe, evidence remains limited, and health economic evaluations are incomplete. We recommend prophylaxis in patients at high risk, consideration in those at medium risk informed by up-to-date evidence, and clear communication between primary and secondary care physicians [79].

Proton pump inhibitors

Proton pump inhibitors are useful in both the primary and secondary prevention of NSAID ulcers [447–449]. There is no compelling evidence that a particular PPI is more or less effective. PPIs are also the most effective agents for preventing ulcers in patients taking low-dose aspirin [450–452]. In these patients, clopidogrel is not an effective alternative to aspirin plus PPI if the goal is to prevent recurrent ulcer bleeding or complications [453,454].

Proton pump inhibitors are more effective at preventing ulcers than other drugs although comparative data with misoprostol are conflicting. However, PPIs are also usually the most attractive choice because they are more convenient for patients, once-daily dosing is typical, and less costly generic versions are available. Particular considerations may be relevant to some patients, for example in the context of breastfeeding or pregnancy.

Misoprostol

Misoprostol is a prostaglandin E analog that can protect the gastroduodenal mucosa against the deleterious effects of COX-1 inhibition from a wide range of NSAIDs. It is approved for prevention of NSAID-associated gastric and duodenal ulceration. The relative risk of ulcer is reduced by over 90% (absolute risk reduction [ARR] 1.4–21.7%) regardless of ulcer size [455], and the relative risk of ulcer complications is reduced by 40% (ARR 0.38–0.95%) [456].

The use of misoprostol is limited by lower GI side-effects of abdominal discomfort and diarrhea in about one in five patients. However, the background prevalence of these symptoms is itself high, with up to 15% treatment withdrawals in the placebo arm of randomized trials. The licensed dose of misoprostol, 200 micrograms four times daily, is needed for maximum efficacy, but lower doses are better tolerated and can be titrated to reduce side-effects; the manufacturer advises caution in patients with cardiovascular disease, in the elderly and in women of child-bearing age as it is an abortifacient.

Comparative data on relative effectiveness of misoprostol and PPIs are conflicting. One study showed that lansoprazole (15 or 30 mg/day) and misoprostol (800 mg) were more effective than placebo at preventing duodenal ulcers [457]. Most other studies have reported that omeprazole is superior to misoprostol in secondary prevention [389,391], with no additive benefit of dual therapy [458].

H_2 receptor antagonists

There is evidence that H_2-RAs may prevent NSAID DUs [444] although this is of questionable importance as GUs are much more frequent in NSAID users. H_2-RAs also prevent endoscopic ulcers when used at very high doses [459]. Overall, however, other agents are much more effective [444,460].

Selective COX-2 inhibitors

There are conflicting reports of the relative merits of using a combination therapy of a nonselective NSAID and a prophylactic agent (PPI or misoprostol) versus using a COX-2 inhibitor (with or without PPI) [461,462]. All these strategies significantly reduce the risk of complications but the former strategy is used more often in clinical practice because of concerns that COX-2 selective NSAIDs increased vascular events. Despite this, it is still appropriate to consider a selective COX-2 inhibitor, with or without a PPI, for some patients and the combination of a COX-2 inhibitor and a PPI is logical in those at greatest risk.

Other newer agents

Several newer agents have been developed specifically to protect the GI tract against the adverse effect of NSAIDs. Rebamipide, a cytoprotective antiulcer agent that increases gastric mucus and stimulates endogenous prostaglandin production, was shown to decrease the rate of diclofenac-induced small intestinal mucosal injury compared with placebo in a prospective RCT [463].

Eupatilin (DA-9601; Stillen®) prevents the formation of reactive oxygen species and is under investigation to prevent NSAID-induced GI complications [464]. DA-9601 was noninferior to misoprostol in preventing endoscopic gastroduodenal adverse events in healthy volunteers in a randomized, double-blinded, multicenter noninferiority study [465]. However, the adverse event rate (diarrhea, abdominal pain, bloating, nausea) with DA-9601 was higher than with misoprostol. In another multicenter, double-blind, stratified randomized noninferiority study, 520 patients taking NSAID (aceclofenac, 100 mg twice daily) over a 4-week period were randomly assigned to receive DA-9601 (60 mg three times daily) or misoprostol (200 g three times daily) [466]. At week 4, the gastric protection rates with DA-9601 was 81.4% and not inferior to misoprostol (89.3%). Adverse event rates were similar.

β-D-glucuronidase inhibitors have also been shown to significantly reduce the small intestinal damage due to diclofenac, indomethacin or ketoprofen in rats if given before introduction of NSAIDs but did not show clinical benefit when given after the administration of NSAIDs [467].

Further studies are needed before any of these newer agents can be recommended in routine practice.

Temporal/secular trends

In westernized societies, the prevalence of DU initially increased during the first half of the 20th century but has declined since the 1960s. By contrast, humans and *H. pylori* have coevolved for tens of thousands of years and until the second half of the last century, most humans in all countries were likely infected with *H. pylori* [147]. Thus, the rise of DU must be explained by an environmental change increasing ulcer risk in infected people.

One major contributor is likely to be the widespread increase in smoking in the early 20th century which could explain the time trend and might also contribute to the 2:1 male predominance of DU. Other contributors may be dietary changes (with more fresh fruits, vegetables, and fortified foods), and improved childhood health, which may have resulted in a healthier stomach and so gastric inflammation that spares the function of the corpus. This antral-predominant pattern of gastritis is associated with raised acid secretion and duodenal ulceration (see "Pathogenesis"). The subsequent decrease in DU incidence in the latter third of the 20th century is usually attributed to preceding improvements in standards of living, sanitation, and hygiene, which contributed to reduced transmission of many infectious diseases including *H. pylori*. However, it is likely that the widespread use of antibiotics has also contributed, particularly in childhood, when *H. pylori* is first acquired.

Although gastric ulceration was described before duodenal ulceration, for most of the 20th century DUs have been more common, particularly in men [468]. By the 1970s, four times as many DUs as GUs were diagnosed in the United States [469]. The accelerating decline in *H. pylori* in North America and western Europe then coincided with an increase in the use of NSAIDs and aspirin. Probably because of these changes in underlying causes, the relative incidences of GU and DU are now more equal in these regions, particularly for uncomplicated disease, though DU usually still dominates. Both morbidity and mortality are generally more common with gastric ulceration, particularly in NSAID users; 3% of GUs harbor malignancy. The same trend has been observed in high and very high HDI Asian countries, suggesting similar trends in the epidemiology of risk factors [470].

Demographic trends

Duodenal and gastric ulcers differ in their incidence by age and gender. The incidence of PUD increases with age but the peak for DU is two decades earlier than for GU (at around 30–40 years). Historically, PUD has a male predominance, driven by the male preponderance in DUs. However, the gender distribution of PUD is now more balanced in high or very high HDI countries partly due to the decreased incidence of DU and the increased incidence of GU. These PUD trends are reflected in important differences and distinct trends in hospitalization, mortality and complications based on age and gender (see further on). The changing age demographics are largely due to the declining incidence of *H. pylori* in children and, hence, PUD in adults, to increased use of NSAIDs, aspirin and other medications, and to additional age-related comorbidities.

Ulcer incidence and prevalence

There are large geographic variations in ulcer incidence and prevalence with estimates of the annual PUD incidence ranging from 0.1% to 0.19% based on physician-centered diagnosis and 0.03% to 0.17% according to hospitalization data and estimates of the point prevalence in asymptomatic adults ranging from 0.12% to 1.5% [471]. The incidences of bleeding and perforation in PUD have been reported, respectively, to be 0.57 and 0.1 per 1000 patient-years [472].

Geographic variation

The rates of PUD are generally higher in Asia than in the West, although there are marked variations in prevalence between regions. In the US, the 1-year point prevalence of PUD is around 1.8% (reports range from 1% to 6%) with an estimated 500 000 new cases annually [22]. Two large European population studies showed a 4–6% prevalence of PUD (DU: 2.1–3.9%, GU: 2.0–2.3%) [43, 220] consistent with findings of DU in 2.8% and GI in 3.0% of a Canadian primary care population with uninvestigated dyspepsia [233]. In a large study from Shanghai,

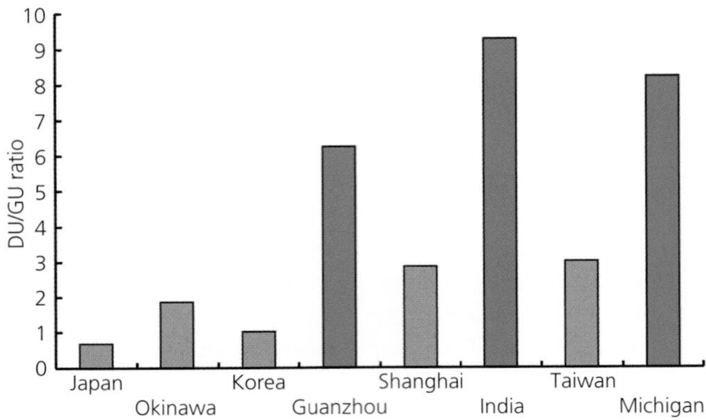

Figure 49.11 The duodenal ulcer (DU) to gastric ulcer (GU) ratio between and within different countries. Blue bars show relatively lower DU:GU ratios (particularly for Japan where the ratio is less than 1.0) and green bars show relatively more DU than GU (Guangzhou is in southern China). Source: Adapted from Chiba et al. 2006 [473]. Reproduced by permission of Springer Science and Business Media. Data were collected at the International Conference during Japanese Digestive Disease Week, Japan, in 1999.

China, the prevalence of PUD was 17% (DU: 13%, GU: 6%) but this may be an overestimate as subjects were invited to volunteer for endoscopy and the one in three who accepted were, perhaps, more likely to have ulcers than those who declined [226].

The relative frequency of DU and GU (DU:GU ratio) varies between and within countries (Figure 49.11) [473]. Duodenal and gastric ulcers occur around twice as frequently in southern compared to northern China, with this pattern reversed for gastric cancer (despite similar *H. pylori* prevalence), emphasizing the role of cofactors in determining differential disease risk in infected people [474]. In Japan and other regions where gastric cancer is common, GU is more frequent and the DU:GU ratio is lower (see Figure 49.11). In consecutive asymptomatic Taiwanese individuals, 9% had PUD [223]. In a single urban Indian center, there was a substantial reduction in PUD prevalence in dyspeptic patients from 17% in 1988 to 6% in 2008 [475]. The decline in DU was more marked than for GU (DU: from 12% to 4.5%, GU: from 2.9% to 2.7%). In India, as in China, DU is more common in the south than in the north. As *H. pylori* prevalence, smoking and, presumably, NSAID use are similar in north and south, it may be that this difference is explained by diet: southern India is predominantly rice-eating whereas northern India is mainly wheat-eating [476].

Ethnicity may be an important risk factor. In Singapore, individuals of Chinese ethnicity have an increased risk of PUD but a lower prevalence of *H. pylori* infection than those of Indian ethnicity [477] although it is also possible that Chinese individuals carry more pathogenic strains of *H. pylori*.

Not all geographical trends hold up to careful examination. The so-called African enigma – that *H. pylori*-associated diseases were believed to be uncommon in Africa despite the near ubiquity of *H. pylori* infection – has been shown not to hold true for much of Africa [478,479]. The low reported rate of PUD was largely due to underreporting and difficulties in accessing healthcare, and *H. pylori*-related diseases actually appear to be common in this region (DU: 21%, GU: 3%, gastric cancer: 2%).

Worldwide, *H. pylori* infection remains the major cause of PUD, but geographical and regional trends in ulcer risk and predominant site (and the risks of other *H. pylori*-associated diseases) are not explained by colonization rates alone. Other factors likely to be important include *H. pylori* strain virulence, NSAID use, smoking, diet, and genetic differences.

Trends in hospitalization, mortality, and complications

Trends in hospitalizations, deaths, and complications from PUD in developed nations are complicated by differing patterns in different subgroups. Hospital admission rates fluctuated but changed little overall in England during the three decades before the millennium although rates declined in younger patients but increased in those older than 65 years [480,481]. Mortality and hospitalization for complicated PUD also declined over this period in England and Scotland although, again, for older people, hospitalizations increased for hemorrhage [482,483]. This parallels a modest decline in prescriptions for NSAIDs but marked increases in consumption of low-dose aspirin, oral anticoagulants, and selective serotonin reuptake inhibitors. In Denmark, trends in uncomplicated and complicated PUD were similar, although the incidence of bleeding peptic ulcer remained stable [484]. This study reported standardized all-cause mortality rates, 1 month after PUD diagnosis of 37 per 1000 for complicated and 12 per 1000 for uncomplicated PUD, falling to 5.1 and 4.0 respectively

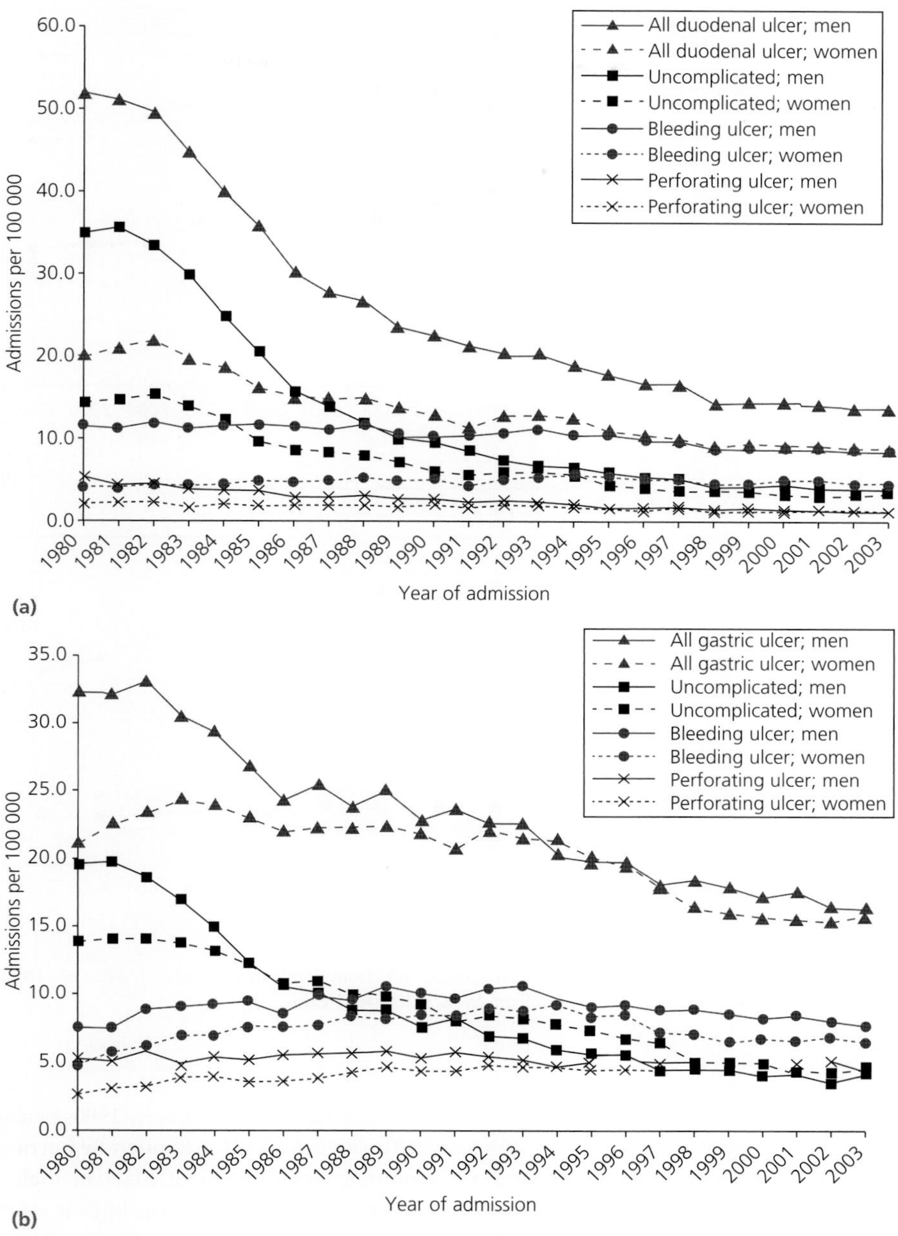

Figure 49.12 Trends in peptic ulcer hospitalization; admission rates with duodenal ulcer **(a)** and gastric ulcer **(b)** in The Netherlands. Source: Post et al. 2006 [485]. Reproduced with permission from John Wiley & Sons.

at 1 year, and 2.6 and 2.5 respectively in subsequent years. Early all-cause mortality is high in most studies following a diagnosis of PUD and may reflect further complications and comorbidities that are more frequent in older patients with complicated PUD (see "Disease associations and comorbid ulcers").

In The Netherlands, hospitalization for uncomplicated PUD declined by more than half, although rates for complicated ulcers remained stable or increased slightly (Figure 49.12) [485]. In the US, data from 1995 to 2005 from five large studies show that the rates of diagnosis of PUD and its complications were stable [486]. However, another US study using nationwide data

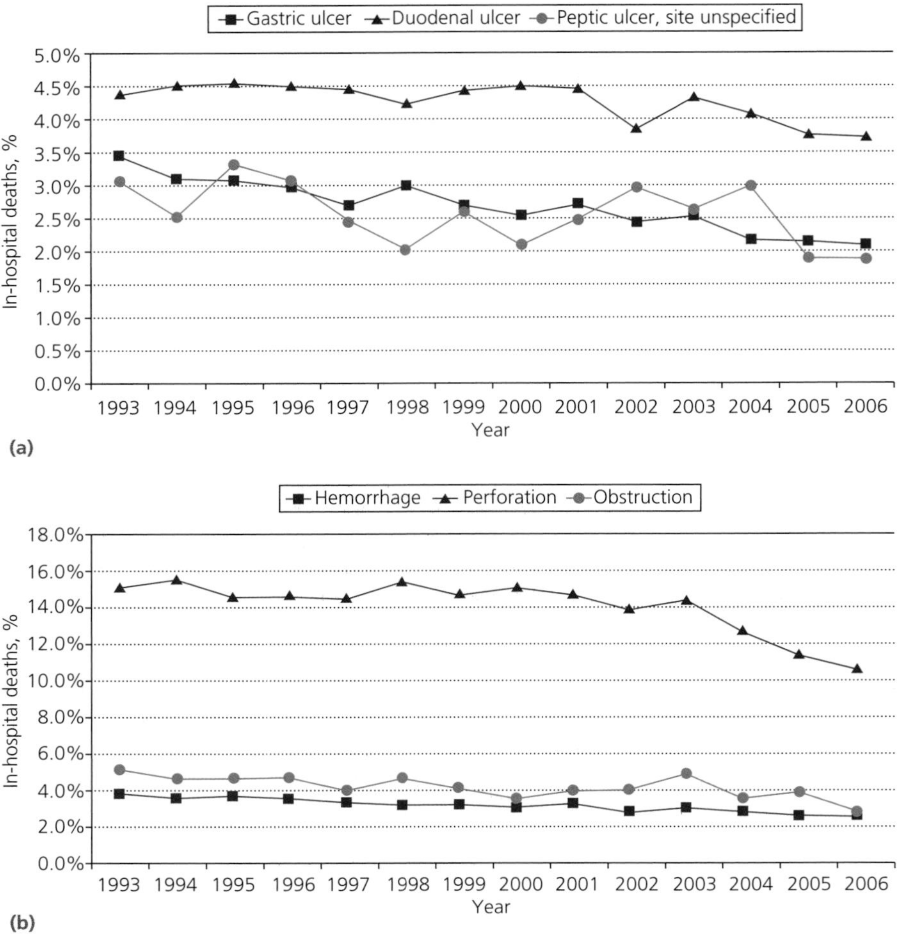

Figure 49.13 Trends in peptic ulcer mortality and complications; in-hospital deaths from peptic ulcer disease by ulcer site **(a)** and complication **(b)** in the United States. Source: Wang et al. 2010 [260], with permission from Wolters Kluwer Health.

on hospitalizations with PUD as the primary diagnosis reported a 30% decrease between 1993 and 2006 (DU: 37%, GU: 20%), and a similar decrease in PUD complications [260]. In Sweden, ulcers complicated by hemorrhage decreased in men (DU: 64%, GU: 54%) and, to a lesser extent, in women (DU: 37%, GU: 35%) between 1987 and 2004 [412]. In-hospital mortality rates in these two studies remained stable or perhaps declined slightly, from around 3–5% in the early 1990s to about 1–4% in the mid-2000s (Figure 49.13). Although hemorrhage remains the most common complication of PUD in high and very high HDI countries, perforation has the highest mortality at 10–15% (see Figure 49.13) [260].

References are available at www.yamadagastro.com/textbook7e

CHAPTER 50

Zollinger–Ellison syndrome

David C. Metz[1] **and Robert T. Jensen**[2]

[1] Perelman School of Medicine, University of Pennsylvania, Philadelphia, PA, USA

[2] National Institute of Diabetes and Digestive and Kidney Diseases, National Institutes of Health, Bethesda, MD, USA

Chapter menu

Introduction

Zollinger–Ellison syndrome (ZES) is a clinical syndrome characterized by excess gastric acid secretion leading to abdominal pain, severe peptic ulcer disease (PUD), diarrhea, and gastroesophageal reflux disease (GERD), entirely due to the autonomous release of gastrin from a particular neuroendocrine tumor (NET) also called a gastrinoma, islet cell tumor, or non-β islet cell tumor [1–3]. NETs are a heterogeneous group of tumors that can occur anywhere in the body but predominantly in the lung, alimentary tract or pancreas (pNETs) [4,5]. Gastrinomas are generally included in the pNET group, which includes functional or nonfunctional pNETs, though most gastrinomas are now known to occur in the duodenum [5–8]. The syndrome is named after two surgeons at Ohio State University who described two patients in 1955 with severe refractory PUD, controlled only by total gastrectomy, who had extreme gastric acid hypersecretion and pancreatic non-β islet cell tumors [1]. There had been previous reports of this syndrome [9] but Zollinger and Ellison were the first to propose it was due to the release of a biologically active substance by an islet cell tumor [1]. Within 5 years, Gregory and colleagues [10] demonstrated a gastrin-like secretagog in the tumoral extracts of ZES patients that subsequently was shown to be identical to antral gastrin [11,12]. Later, specific gastrin radioimmunoassays were developed, which demonstrated elevated serum levels in ZES patients and its presence in their tumors [7,13–15].

Many clinicians use the terms gastrinoma and ZES synonymously, and some pathologists use the term gastrinoma to describe any tumor containing gastrin identified by immunohistochemistry [4,5,8] but neither of these are correct. In fact, immunoreactive gastrin is present in a number of tumors not associated with ZES or even hypergastrinemia (e.g., colorectal cancers, pheochromocytomas, acoustic neuromas, bronchogenic carcinomas, and other pNET syndromes) [4,15]. The diagnosis of ZES requires the presence of typical clinical features (i.e., the syndrome) together with biochemical confirmation of inappropriate hypergastrinemia [2,5,6,16–19]. The term "gastrinoma" implies a NET that produces gastrin as opposed to other pNETs that produce other products. Please see Chapter 80 for a broader discussion on pancreatic NETs (pNETs) in general.

Yamada's Textbook of Gastroenterology, Seventh Edition. Edited by Timothy C. Wang, Michael Camilleri, Benjamin Lebwohl, Anna S. Lok, William J. Sandborn, Kenneth K. Wang, and Gary D. Wu.

Companion website: www.yamadagastro.com/textbook7e

Epidemiology

Pancreatic neuroendocrine tumors including gastrinomas, other functional pNETs (insulinomas, vasoactive intestinal polypeptide-secreting tumors, etc.) and nonfunctional pNETs account for 1–10% of all pancreatic tumors and 1.3% of pancreatic tumors in the Surveillance, Epidemiology, and End Results (SEER) database of malignant tumors [20–23]. Autopsy studies have shown that 0.5–1.5% of individuals harbor a pNET but <1/1000 cause symptoms during life, so that the overall prevalence and incidence of pNETs are low, approximately 10/million [23–25] and 1–5 cases/million/year [26], respectively (see also Chapter 80). The overall incidence of ZES specifically is 0.5–3/million/year [7,24]. Gastrinomas are the most common functional malignant pNETs and comprise up to 30% of the pNETs in various series [7,8,24]. Duodenal tumors were originally thought to be uncommon (i.e., <20%) but now make up 50–88% of gastrinomas in sporadic ZES patients and 70–100% in MEN1/ZES patients [2,3,7,8]. In rare instances, gastrinomas occur in other nonpancreatic nonduodenal abdominal (stomach, liver, bile duct, ovary) (5–15%) and extraabdominal (heart, small cell lung cancer) locations [27–30]. The incidence of pNETs, like all gastrointestinal NETs, has increased in a number of studies, which may be due to better detection, and it is unclear whether the incidence of ZES itself has actually changed [22,23].

Zollinger–Ellison syndrome can occur without an accompanying inherited syndrome (i.e., sporadic ZES) or as part of the multiple endocrine neoplasia type 1 syndrome (MEN1) (20–25%) [19,31,32]. The distinction between ZES patients with or without MEN1 is particularly important because their management differs significantly and MEN1-associated cases also require evaluation for other associated conditions and genetic counseling [24,33,34]. ZES also rarely occurs in neurofibromatosis type 1 [32,35], or tuberous sclerosis [32,36]. Approximately 10–17% of patients with von Hippel–Lindau disease (VHL) develop pNETs; however, these are almost invariably nonfunctional and not gastrinomas [32].

Zollinger–Ellison syndrome occurs with a slight male predominance (55–65%) [2,19,31,37,38] and has been found in patients varying from age 5 to 85 years [2,7,19,37]. The mean age at onset is 41 years, with the onset of ZES in patients with MEN1/ZES occurring 10 years earlier than those without MEN1 (sporadic ZES) (33.7 vs 43.3 years) [19].

Pathophysiology

The presenting symptoms of ZES are all due to gastric acid hypersecretion [18,19,39–41]. Symptoms of tumor progression (e.g., pain, anorexia, weight loss) only occur late in the disease course [8,18,19,39–41]. Accordingly, in a typical patient, presenting symptoms (including PUD, pain, diarrhea, GERD symptoms, and weight loss) resolve once the gastric acid hypersecretion is adequately controlled [7,8,39,42–45].

The gastric acid hypersecretion is due to uncontrolled and inappropriate ectopic release of gastrin by the gastrinoma [46]. This results in a markedly increased basal acid output (BAO), approximately fourfold (42 mEq/h) [47], but in some patients as high as >10-fold [7,39,41,47–51] (Figure 50.1a). Chronic hypergastrinemia also has trophic effects on the gastric mucosa, which increase the number of gastric parietal and enterochromaffin-like (ECL) cells [45,52–55], with the result that the parietal cell mass can be 4–6 times normal [7,56,57], elevating maximal acid output (MAO) (Figure 50.1a) and BAO to MAO ratio (>0.7) as well [7,47,51,58]. On average, gastric ECL cells are increased twofold in ZES [51,59–61]. With time, ZES patients can develop advanced ECL-proliferative responses, similar to those seen in animal models of chronic hypergastrinemia, which can, in some cases, undergo neoplastic change [45,52,62–65]. It has been proposed that ECL cells undergo a hyperplasia–neoplasia sequence of events progressing from simple hyperplasia to linear hyperplasia, micronodular hyperplasia, adenomatoid hyperplasia, dysplasia (a precarcinoid state), and finally the development of gastric ECL cell carcinoids [45,63,64,66]. Greater than 98% of ZES patients develop ECL hyperplasia [64,65], with about 50% of sporadic and MEN1/ZES patients having advanced changes (with 7% and 2% having dysplasia, respectively) [64,65]. In ZES, there is a close correlation between the degree of ECL hyperplasia and the fasting serum gastrin level [64,65]. Even though advanced ECL proliferative changes are seen in both sporadic and MEN1/ZES patients, there is a marked difference in the rate of occurrence of macroscopic gastric carcinoids. Gastric carcinoids occur in 0–33% of MEN1/ZES patients (Figure 50.1b); a single prospective study found a rate of 23% [31,60,65,67–69]. However, gastric carcinoids occur only rarely (<1%) in sporadic ZES patients [51,64,70,71], and it has been estimated they occur at least with 70-fold greater frequency in MEN1/ZES patients [65].

Pathology and classification

Gastrinomas were originally reported to be non-β islet cell tumors [1] and thus were originally thought to be pancreatic in origin with a distribution ratio of 4:1:4 in the head, body, and tail [1,7,8,40,72–76]. Later studies proposed that a small percentage were duodenal [77,78]. Today, duodenal gastrinomas are found 2–4 times more frequently than pancreatic gastrinomas (Table 50.1) [34,79–86]. This change likely occurred because duodenal tumors were being missed on preoperative localization studies or with standard laparotomy because of their small size (see Table 50.1) [7,34,79–81,85]. When careful attention was paid to the duodenum at surgery, more duodenal tumors were found [34,80–84]. Primary gastrinomas also occur in other intraabdominal sites (e.g., ovary, liver, bile duct, pylorus, spleen, mesentery, stomach, or kidney), and very rarely (<0.5%) in extraabdominal locations, including the heart and lung (see

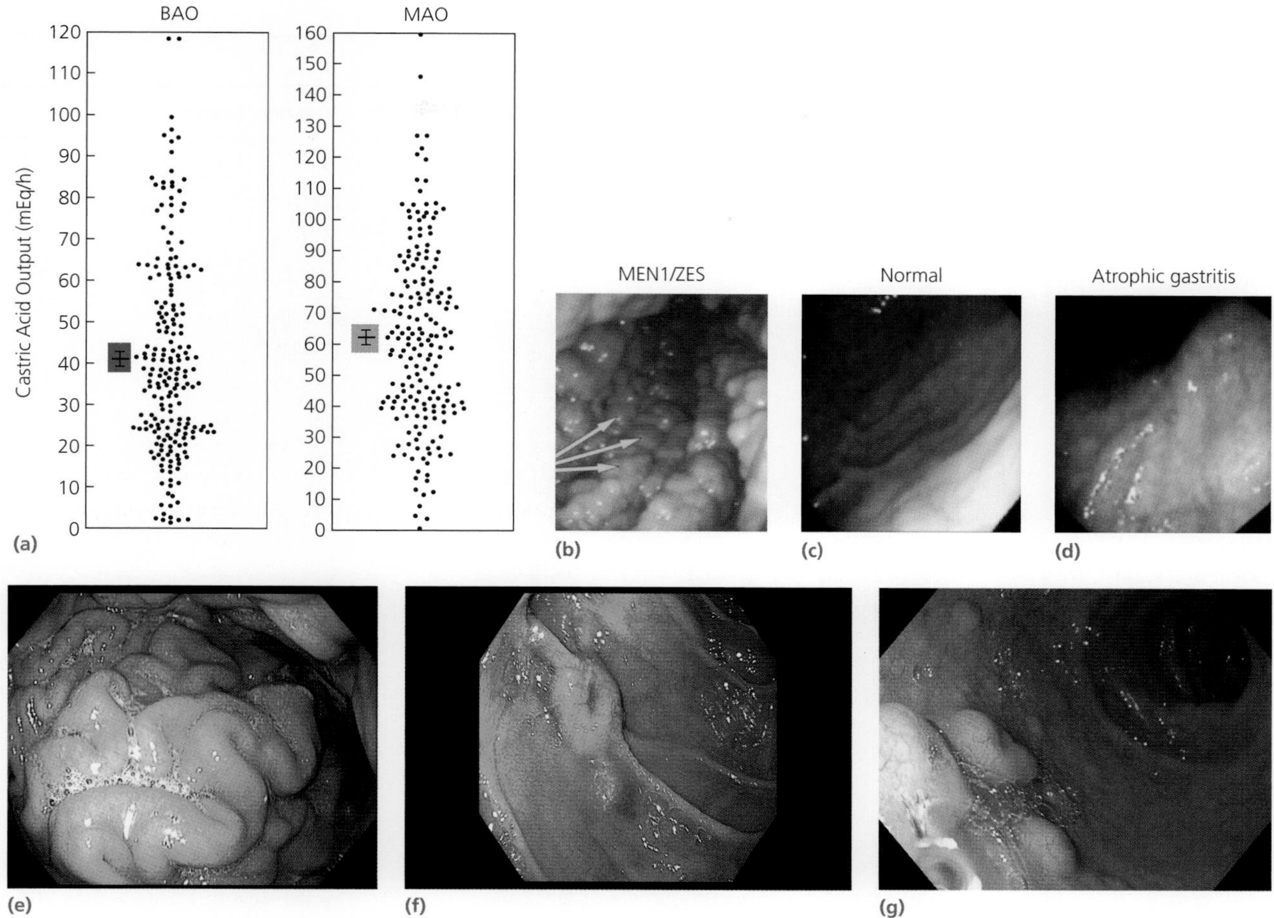

Figure 50.1 Endoscopic and acid secretory findings in Zollinger–Ellison syndrome (ZES). **(a)** Markedly elevated gastric basal acid secretion (BAO) (upper limit of normal [ULN] <15 mEq/h) and maximal acid secretion (MAO) (ULN 48 mEq/h) in 235 patients with ZES. Source: Data from Roy et al. 2001 [47]. **(b)** Multiple gastric carcinoids (type 2) (arrows) that frequently occur in patients with multiple endocrine neoplasia type 1 syndrome (MEN1)/ZES (23%) [65,294]. **(c–e)** Typical gastric endoscopic findings in normal patients, patients with atrophic gastritis (loss of folds, thin mucosa), or ZES (prominent folds, present in >94%), respectively see [19]. **(f)** A typical isolated duodenal primary gastrinoma in a patient with sporadic ZES. **(g)** Multiple duodenal primary tumors in a patient with MEN1/ZES.

Table 50.1) [8,27,28,30,73,87–93]. It is controversial whether gastrinomas can arise in lymph nodes or whether those cases reported represent metastases from occult primaries [7,8,79,91,92,94–96]. Long-term biochemical cures have occurred after resection of only a lymph node gastrinoma [8,91,92,95]. In addition, 3–25% of patients without pNETs have chromogranin-positive rests in abdominal lymph nodes [94,97]. The National Institutes of Health (NIH) prospective series, classified 11% of ZES patients as having primary lymph node gastrinomas (see Table 50.1). With improved more modern imaging (see below), this figure is likely to diminish.

Histologically, gastrinomas show the typical features of any NET, with cuboidal cells with few mitoses and fine granular eosinophilic cytoplasm [73,98]. They can demonstrate trabecular, gyriform, or glandular morphology but no specific pattern is predictive of biological behavior [7,72,98]. Duodenal gastrinomas occur in the submucosa, frequently infiltrate the mucosa, and, in the case of tumors >1 cm, the muscular layer as well [73]. Duodenal gastrinomas usually have proliferative rates <10%, whereas pancreatic gastrinomas frequently have higher proliferative rates [73]. Both duodenal and pancreatic gastrinomas may demonstrate blood vessel invasion [73,98]. Gastrinomas are usually identified as a NET by their histological appearance and positivity with immunohistochemistry for NET markers (chromogranin A [CgA], synaptophysin, etc.) [4,7,17,73,98]. Gastrin immunoreactivity can be detected in most gastrinomas [7,73,99,100] and approximately one-half produce multiple hormones [7,73,99,100].

At surgery, 60–90% of gastrinomas are found within the "gastrinoma triangle" bound by the junction of the cystic/common bile ducts, the junction of the second/third parts of the duodenum, and the junction of the pancreatic neck/body [8,81,82,85,101]. Duodenal gastrinomas demonstrate a decreasing frequency distally, with almost 90% occurring in the first or second part of the duodenum (see Table 50.1) [29,34,102].

Table 50.1 Characteristics of gastrinomas (NIH prospective studies and literature).

Characteristic	%	
	NIH data (n = 221) Mean [range]	Literature [range]
Primary location		
Pancreas	24%	[21–70%]
Duodenum	49%	[6–32%]
Lymph node	11%	<1%
Other[a]	9%	[0–18%]
Unknown	16%	[7–48%]
Duodenal location		
D1	57%	ND
D2	32%	ND
D3	5%	ND
D4	4	ND
Extent of disease		
No tumor found	13%	[7–48%]
Localized disease	70%	[23–51%]
Metastatic disease to liver	17	[13–53%]
Extent of metastases		
Primary only	36%	[23–51%]
Primary + lymph nodes	29%	[8–61%]
Primary + liver metastases	23%	[15–38%]
Liver metastases only	3%	[4–14%]
Lymph node metastases only	16%	[4–23]
Gastrinoma size (cm)		
Mean (largest)	1.9 ± 0.2 [0.1–4.8]	[1–6]
Duodenal	0.89 ± 0.05 [0.1–5]	[0.2–5.5]
Pancreatic	3.8 ± 0.3 [0.5–7]	[0.5–10]
Metastases: duodenal vs pancreatic		
Lymph node metastases (%)		
Duodenal	47%	[20%–80%]
Pancreas	48%	[Up to 48% of patients had no primary 0–60%]
Liver metastases (%)		
Duodenal	5%	10
Pancreas	52%	[15%–45%]

D1–4, duodenal regions 1, 2, 3, and 4; ND, no data; NIH, National Institutes of Health.
[a] Other tumor locations include additional intraabdominal sites (liver, bile duct, spleen, pylorus, mesentery, ovary, lymph nodes) and very rarely extraabdominal sites (heart, nonsmall cell lung cancer).
Source: Data are from [8,27–30,87–93,110].

In older studies, 60–90% of gastrinomas were associated with metastases (primarily to lymph nodes or liver) and therefore they should all be considered potentially malignant [2,30,40,73,103,104]. The presence of metastases or gross invasion of normal tissue remains the only generally accepted, reliable criterion for the diagnosis of malignancy [7,8,98]. Gastrinomas metastasize first to regional lymph nodes and then the liver [7,27,73]. More widespread metastases to lungs, bone, brain, skin, etc. are generally late findings [105–109]. Bone metastases occur in 31% of patients with advanced disease, but are rarely seen in ZES patients who do not have liver metastases [105,106,109] and occur primarily in the axial skeleton initially.

Duodenal gastrinomas are typically small (see Table 50.1) and frequently <1 cm in diameter but nevertheless are associated with lymph node metastases in 47% of the cases in the NIH prospective studies (20–80% in the literature). This percentage is similar for the larger pancreatic gastrinomas (mean size 3.8 cm) (see Table 50.1). However, in the NIH series, liver metastases occurred in only 5% of duodenal gastrinomas (10% in the literature) but 52% of pancreatic gastrinomas (15–45% in the literature) (see Table 50.1) [27,28,110]. These data suggest that both gastrinoma primary sites are equally malignant but not equally aggressive. Unfortunately, the NIH database does not include information on tumor grade.

In the last decade, it has been proposed that all NETs, including gastrinomas, other pNETs (see also Chapter 80) and gastrointestinal NETs (carcinoid tumors), should have a common classification [111]. A number of classification systems have been proposed, including those of the World Health Organization (WHO), the European Neuroendocrine Tumor Society (ENETS), and in the USA the American Joint Cancer Committee/International Union for Cancer Control (UJCC/IUCC) [4,111]. The WHO originally classified these tumors into poorly differentiated neuroendocrine (G3) carcinomas or well-differentiated neuroendocrine tumors/neoplasms, with the well-differentiated group further divided into two grades (G1 or G2) with different behavior depending on proliferative indices (Ki67 value and/or mitoses per high-power field) in addition to a tumor/node/metastasis (TNM) classification as with other solid malignancies [111]. Recently, the WHO revised its classification, dividing the G3 pNETs into two groups based on differentiation, with G3-NETs being well differentiated and G3-NECs (neuroendocrine carcinomas) being poorly differentiated [112]. This division is important because these two G3 groups differ in pathogenesis, prognosis and treatments, as will be discussed below [112]. Other possible prognostic factors are size, functionality, location, necrosis, and invasiveness [111]. Proper classification of gastrinomas is essential, because recent studies demonstrate this has prognostic value and may affect the type of treatment recommended [111,113]. Most gastrinomas are well-differentiated grade 1 or grade 2 pNETs [73].

Tumor biology

Gastrinomas frequently synthesize and secrete multiple gastrointestinal peptides, as well as chromogranins and neuron-specific enolase [7,98,100]. Plasma levels of hormones other than gastrin are elevated in 62% of ZES patients, with one additional hormone elevated in 44% and two in 18% [100]. Motilin is the most common plasma hormone also elevated (30%), followed by human pancreatic polypeptide (27%), neurotensin (20%), and gastrin-releasing peptide (10%) [100].

The gastrin gene spans a 4 kb area and consists of three exons and two introns, with the coding region translating into a 101-amino acid peptide, preprogastrin [15,45,114,115]. In normal G cells, preprogastrin undergoes a series of posttranslational processing steps including dibasic cleavages, removal of the glycine extended COOH terminal amino acids and sulfation, leading to the formation of progastrin, then COOH terminal glycine-extended forms, and finally the biologically active forms consisting of two COOH-amidated gastrins, gastrin-17 (G-17) and gastrin-34 (G-34), existing in sulfated and nonsulfated forms [15,45,114,115]. Normally, >90% of antral gastrin is G-17, while in the duodenum only 40–50% is G-17 [15,45,114,115]. In the circulation, normal G-34 is the predominant form (>60%) and sulfated/nonsulfated forms occur equally [15,45,114,115]. In contrast, in patients with gastrinomas, the relative concentrations of G-17 are higher (74–80%), and increased concentrations of partially processed forms are found (progastrin, NH_2 and COOH terminal fragments, COOH glycine extended fragments, incompletely amidated fragments) [7,15,45,114–117]. Alterations in posttranslational processing have been correlated with the presence of metastatic disease [7,45,114,116,117]; however, no prospective studies have established their usefulness in an individual case [45] and they are currently rarely measured.

Chromogranin A is a 48 kD protein stored in the secretory granules of neuroendocrine cells and is widely used as an immunohistochemical marker of NETs [4,7,73,102,118,119]. CgA is released simultaneously with the release of polypeptides and thus can be used as a general plasma tumor marker too [118–125]. CgA is elevated in 80–100% of ZES patients, as it is in patients with other pNETs or carcinoids [120–124]. Changes in plasma CgA levels are reported to be useful for assessing changes in tumor mass in some studies; however, in other studies, including in patients with gastrinomas, it has been found to be a relatively insensitive marker for tumor progression [120–124]. One problem with using plasma CgA as a tumor marker in ZES patients is that chronic hypergastrinemia causes gastric ECL cell proliferation which increases plasma CgA [18,123,119,125]. Thus, in ZES, elevated plasma CgA can come from the gastrinoma or from hyperplastic ECL cells [18,126–128]. Unfortunately, plasma CgA is also increased by inflammatory disorders, other endocrine diseases, gastrointestinal disorders, cardiovascular disorders, and altered renal function, and therefore mild or moderately elevated plasma CgA levels in the range frequently seen with small gastrinomas/pNETs overlap with values found in these other disorders [118,119,123]. Finally, proton pump inhibitor (PPI) therapy, commonly employed in ZES patients, interferes with the normal feedback control of gastrin release which also contributes to CgA elevation [119].

In patients with ZES, secretin [129–134], glucagon [135], calcium [131–134,136], and a standard meal [133,134,137] all stimulate increased serum gastrin levels; in addition, native and synthetic somatostatin analogs (octreotide, lanreotide) can decrease serum gastrin [43,45,138,139]. These findings have been used clinically with the development of secretin, calcium, glucagon, and standard meal provocative tests for ZES diagnosis [17,43,45]. The exact mechanism by which secretin, calcium, glucagon, or a meal increase, and somatostatin analogs decrease, serum gastrin in ZES patients is not completely understood [7,133]. The most likely explanation is a direct effect on gastrin release from the gastrinoma, although others have proposed (in the case of the secretin test) that it is an exaggerated physiological response [140–142]. The evidence for a direct effect is that secretin [141,143] and somatostatin receptors [144,145] as well as the calcium-sensing receptor, which regulates cellular hormone release [146,147], are all present on gastrinomas. Furthermore, calcium and secretin stimulate gastrin release, and secretin activates adenylate cyclase from dispersed/cultured gastrinoma cells [141,147–153] whereas somatostatin inhibits it [151,152]. Finally, a direct relationship exists between the magnitude of expression of secretin receptors on gastrinomas and the magnitude of the secretin-stimulated response in ZES patients [141]. Normally, native antral G cells exist in close association with inhibitory D cells that also respond to secretin, thereby dampening the secretin stimulation response in normal individuals.

The cell of origin of gastrinomas remains unclear too. Although gastrinomas and other pNETs are frequently called islet cell tumors, it is not proven that they actually arise from pancreatic islets [154]. Gastrin is found in the fetal/developing pancreas in islet cells but it is not present in the adult pancreas [114,155,156]. Duodenal and pancreatic gastrinomas differ in biological behavior [28,110,157–159], and gastrin-producing G cells are found in the adult duodenum but not in the adult pancreas; therefore, a different cell of origin has been proposed for duodenal and pancreatic gastrinomas [7,8,157–159]. It has been suggested that gastrinomas in the gastrinoma triangle area (duodenum/pancreatic head) originate from the ventral pancreatic bud, and those from the pancreatic body/tail from the dorsal pancreatic bud [156]. Others have proposed that gastrinomas originate from multipotential, endocrine programmed stem cells that undergo inappropriate and incomplete differentiation toward the G cell [7,155,157]. In MEN1/ZES patients, duodenal gastrinomas may arise from the G cells by a process of hyperplasia similar to that proposed for the response of ECL cells to gastrin in the stomach [160]. In MEN1/ ZES patients, the pivotal event in the development of the multifocal gastrin neoplasms is likely the allelic deletion of the second MEN1 allele [160,160]. However, this sequence was not seen in sporadic gastrinomas [160,161]. For pancreatic pNETs in MEN1 patients, two studies have come to different conclusions, with one concluding that PETs arise from duct cells [154] and the other concluding that they arise from islet cells [160,162]. Although some recent studies propose that cancer stem cells, which have been described in a number of solid tumors, could also be important in the pathogenesis of pNETs or gastrointestinal NETs, at present they have not been convincingly identified and isolated in gastroenteropancreatic NET pathological samples [163].

Studies of the natural history of ZES patients have provided some important insights [27,28,164,165] regarding outcome. In patients with sporadic ZES, 25% of the gastrinomas show a pattern of aggressive growth behavior [27,28]. Aggressive growth is associated with a decreased 10-year survival (30%) compared to the excellent survival in those with nonaggressive disease (10-year survival 96%) [28]. A similar pattern has been described in patients with MEN1/ZES but the percentages are different, with only 14% demonstrating aggressive growth [164], although it is unclear whether this difference is due to a lag time bias or not. In the sporadic ZES patients, those with aggressive growth are characterized by more frequently having liver metastases, a pancreatic primary, a large primary (>3 cm), a short disease history, higher gastrin levels, female gender, and sporadic ZES [27,28]. In general, patients with MEN1/ZES have a better prognosis than patients with sporadic ZES [28]. Finally, follow-up studies demonstrate that even in patients with liver metastases, their rate of growth varies markedly: 42% demonstrate rapid growth, 26% show no growth, and 32% slow growth over a 3-year period [166]. Deaths only occurred in the group with rapid growth (62% died during follow-up) [166]. This result has important implications for treatment; the growth slope prior to treatment is rarely considered in most treatment studies, but it can clearly have a marked effect on patient outcome and survival.

Molecular pathogenesis (see also Chapter 80)

In contrast to many common malignances, the pathogenesis of gastrinomas, as well as other NETs, was relatively unstudied until recently [24,167,168]. In contrast to many adenocarcinomas, mutations of common tumor suppressor genes (*p53*, retinoblastoma [*RB*], etc.) and oncogenes (*Ras*, *myc*, *jun*, *Src*, etc.), are infrequent in gastrinomas and other pNETs [24,167,169–171]. However, recent studies show that both the p53 pathway and the RB pathway are altered in pNETs [172,173]. The Rb pathway is inactivated in most pNETs (including gastrinomas) [173] by amplification of genes encoding the cyclin-dependent kinases Cdk4/Cdk6. A second study [172] found a low rate of *p53* mutations in pNETs (<3%); however, the p53 pathway was altered in 70% of pNETs through aberrant activation of its negative regulators – mouse double minute 2

Table 50.2 Clinical features of patients with Zollinger–Ellison syndrome (NIH prospective studies and literature).

Feature	NIH (*n* = 261)	Literature [range]
Gender (% male)	56%	[44–70]
Mean age onset (years)	41	[41–53]
MEN1 present (%)	22%	[10%–48%]
Initial symptom (%)		
Abdominal pain	75%	[26–98%]
Diarrhea	73%	[17–73%]
Heartburn/reflux symptoms	44%	[0–56%]
Weight loss	17%	
Nausea	30%	[0–37%]
Vomiting	25%	[0–51%]
Bleeding	24%	[8–75%]
Pain + bleeding	19%	[19–44%]
Pain + diarrhea	55%	[28–56%]
Mean duration of symptoms (years)	5.2	[3.2–8.7]
Previous gastric acid-reducing surgery (%)	32%	[0–45%]
History-confirmed peptic ulcer	71%	[71–93%]
Peptic acid complication		
Perforation	4%	[4–6%]
Esophageal stricture	5%	[5–18%]
Pyloric/duodenal scarring	10%	ND
Prominent gastric folds	94%	[13–30%]

MEN1, multiple endocrine neoplasia type 1; ND, no data; NIH, National Institutes of Health.
Source: Data from [7,19,31,81,189] and from 11 series with 12–359 patients (see Table 9 in [19]).

homolog (MDM2) (22%), mouse double minute 4 homolog (MDDM4) (30%), and wild-type p53-induced phosphatase-1 (WIPI) (51%).

Since gastrinomas and other pNETs occur as part of inherited syndromes, including MEN1, tuberous sclerosis, neurofibromatosis, von Recklinghausen disease [32], and VHL, studies of the genes altered in these diseases have provided insights into the molecular pathogenesis of pNETs [32,168,170]. Approximately 20–25% of patients with ZES (Table 50.2) [7,31,32,174,175] have MEN1 (Wermer syndrome) (MEN1/ ZES). MEN1 is an autosomal dominant disorder due to mutations in the *MEN1* gene on the long arm of chromosome 11 (11q13). The *MEN1* gene has 10 exons encoding for a 610 amino acid protein, MENIN [31,32,176,177]. The exact molecular alteration that occurs with MENIN mutations that results in pNETs, including gastrinomas, is not clear. However, it is known that MENIN is a nuclear protein that interacts with a large number of other proteins [32,175,177,178]. MENIN interacts with SMAD3, RPA2 (a DNA-processing factor), the AP1 transcription factor, JunD, nuclear factor-κB, Pem, FANCD2 (a DNA-repair factor), nucleoside diphosphate kinase, NM23β, cytoskeletal-associated proteins, and various histone-modifying enzymes [32,175,177,178]. Mutations in the *MEN1* gene occur in one-third of sporadic gastrinomas [32,167,170,171,179]. A recent study [169] reported results of exomic sequencing of 10 sporadic pNETs, and found the *MEN1* gene was the most frequently altered gene. *MEN1* gene mutations occurred in 44% [169], followed in frequency by mutations in 43% in genes encoding for two subunits of a transcription/chromatin-remodeling complex consisting of DAXX (death domain associated protein) and ATRX (α-thalassemia/mental retardation syndrome X linked), followed by mutations in mTor pathway genes (15%). The VHL locus occurs at 3p25, and chromosome 3 alterations are reported in 21–50% of sporadic pNETs [170,180]. However, these chromosome 3 alterations are rarely associated with a mutation at the VHL locus, suggesting that it is not involved in pNET development, although a locus telomeric to the VHL locus may be involved. At present there are no specific data from complete exomic or next-generation sequencing specifically in gastrinomas, although in the near future this likely will be available and may provide some important molecular insights for the differences between duodenal and pancreatic gastrinomas.

Recent studies provide evidence for the importance in pNETs/gastrinomas of alterations in the *DPC4/Smad* gene (20% in pNETs), the *p16/MTS1* tumor suppressor gene (50– 90%), mTor/Akt/PI3K pathway, amplification of the *HER-2/neu* protooncogene, as well as increased expression of a number of growth factors and/or their receptors (platelet-derived growth factor [PDGF], hepatocyte growth factor, epidermal growth factor [EGF], insulin-like growth factor 1) [167,168,170,171,181,182]. Numerous recent studies provide evidence that the mTor/Akt/PI3K pathway is particularly important for mediating the growth of pNETs [181,182]. This evidence includes the success of the mTOR inhibitor, everolimus, in extending disease-free survival in patients with advanced pNETs [183], but studies also show that the mTor/Akt/PI3K signaling cascade plays a central role in pNET cell growth and proliferation [168,181,182,184]. Additional evidence for the importance of the mTor/Akt/PI3K pathway comes from a study [185] reporting the effects of a single nucleotide polymorphism. Replacing arginine by glycine in codon 388 (R388) of the fibroblast growth factor receptor 4 (FGF4) diminishes the responsiveness to mTor inhibitors in pNETs, and its presence in pNETs is associated with advanced tumor stage and liver metastases.

Comparative genomic hybridization (CGH) and genomic-wide allelotyping studies report that chromosomal gains/losses occur frequently in pNETs, including in gastrinomas, and that the distribution of these changes differs between gastrointestinal NETs (carcinoids) and pNETs, supporting the conclusion that they have a different pathogenesis [24,170,171]. In pNETs, allelic losses occur most frequently at chromosomal locus 1p (25–75%), 1q (20–90%), 3p (40–95%), 11p (30–50%), 11q (30–70%), and 22q (40–95%) [167,170,171,181]. With pNETs, chromosomal gains occur most frequently at 17q (10–55%), 7q (15–70%), and 4 q (33%) [167,170,171,181]. A number of these alterations are associated with malignant behavior including deletions at chromosome 1, 3p, 6, 11q, 17p, and 22p, and gains on chromosome 4, 7, 14q, and Xp [1677, 170,171,181].

Results have been reported from a number of studies in which pNETs were studied using microarrays to perform gene expression profiling [170,171,181]. Results from eight studies in pNETs have been summarized [184] and they demonstrate a wide variation in the number of genes upregulated (45–668) or downregulated (25–323). It is not clear presently which gene changes are important in the molecular pathogenesis of pNETs.

Clinical presentation and features

General clinical features

The initial clinical features of ZES are entirely due to gastric acid hypersecretion (see Table 50.2 and Figure 50.1a) [19,39,72,186]. Abdominal pain, clinically indistinguishable from that seen in typical patients with idiopathic PUD, occurs in >90% of ZES patients (see Table 50.2) [39,72,186]. The pain is typically due to duodenal ulceration, traditionally described as multiple and/or occurring in unusual locations. More recent data, however, suggest most ZES patients present with typical duodenal ulcers [7,19,186]. Pain occurs alone or associated with diarrhea in up to 55% of patients (see Table 50.2) which, in part, explains the long delay in diagnosis commonly seen with this disease [7,17,19,24].

Diarrhea is an important presenting feature occurring in 73% of the patients in the NIH prospective studies, in 28–73% in the literature (see Table 50.2), and in up to 20% as the sole presenting symptom [19,186]. The diarrhea is typically not large volume (<1 L/day), but on occasion can be significant [187]. It is characterized by increased frequency with a watery consistency, and may be associated with mild steatorrhea (<15 g/day) [187,188]. In the past, up to 40–50% of patients had diarrhea >1 L/day, compared to <10% today [19]; therefore, unless a careful history is taken, its presence may be missed. The diarrhea is a direct result of gastric acid hypersecretion because any method of control (e.g., nasogastric suction, medical therapy, or surgical treatment) results in its cessation [39,72,186]. The diarrhea is due to multiple effects of acid hypersecretion, including inactivation of lipase and other pancreatic enzymes, structural effects on the intestinal mucosa, precipitation of bile acids, and altered motility [7,39,187,188].

Gastroesophageal reflux disease symptoms (e.g., heartburn, regurgitation, chest pain) are increasingly recognized in ZES patients, with 44% having GERD symptoms at presentation in the prospective NIH series, and 49–61% in the recent literature (see Table 50.2) [19,186,189]. In early studies, GERD symptoms were uncommon or not reported, with the result that in seven series of ZES patients prior to 1986, the frequency was listed at 0–2% [19].

Other upper gastrointestinal symptoms such as nausea (30%), vomiting (25%), and weight loss (17%) are not infrequent in ZES patients at presentation (see Table 50.2). The cause of the weight loss is multifactorial but mainly due to maldigestion and malabsorption. Control of acid hypersecretion commonly leads to weight gain [190].

Before effective medical control of acid hypersecretion was available, many patients with ZES developed severe complications of gastric acid hypersecretion [1,39,40,72]. These included PUD (with penetration or perforation, with or without fistula formation), bleeding, strictures with gastric outlet obstruction (up to 20%), or GERD complications (esophageal strictures, ulcers, bleeding, rarely perforation) (up to 20%) [1,19–40,72,191]. At present, because of widespread off-label antisecretory drug use, it is uncommon to have patients present with symptoms due to complications from advanced PUD/GERD [19,186]. In the NIH prospective study, only 4% of ZES patients had a perforation due to PUD and 5% had esophageal strictures, although 10% had duodenal scarring due to chronic PUD (see Table 50.2). Features of the presentation of ZES patients related to its modern diagnosis are discussed in more detail in the section on diagnosis later in the chapter.

Specific clinical features in MEN1/ZES

For the 20–25% of patients with ZES who also have MEN1 syndrome (MEN1/ZES) (see Table 50.2) [7,31,32,175,176], ZES may be suspected because of the presence of other MEN1 features [19,31,65,192–194]. MEN1 causes NETs and hyperplasia in multiple endocrine organs that classically includes: (1) hyperparathyroidism due to four-gland parathyroid hyperplasia, (2) pancreatic NETs (nonfunctional pNETs > gastrinoma > insulinoma >> other), and (3) pituitary adenomas (prolactinomas > adrenocorticotrophic hormone secreting > growth hormone secreting) (Table 50.3) [31,32,175,195,196]. Each may cause functional syndromes. The most frequent pNET is a nonfunctional pNET (NF-pNET) with 80–100% developing microscopic NF-pNETs; however, NF-pNETs cause symptoms in only 0–13% [23,32]. Gastrinomas are the most frequent functional pNET (mean 54%, range 20–61%) [19,31,175,196,197] (see Table 50.3). Adrenal tumors (rarely functional) and thyroid disease can also occur in <50% of MEN1 patients and there also is an increased incidence of carcinoid tumors of the stomach (see Figure 50.1b), lung and thymus (see Table 50.3). Other non-NET tumors associated with MEN1 include smooth muscle tumors (leiomyomas, leiomyosarcomas), central nervous system (CNS) tumors (meningiomas, schwannomas, ependymomas), and skin tumors (angiofibromas > collagenomas > lipomas > melanoma) (see Table 50.3).

Zollinger–Ellison syndrome in MEN1 patients presents at a younger age (10 years earlier) than in patients with sporadic ZES [19,31,197]. The initial clinical manifestation of MEN1 is usually renal colic due to nephrolithiasis from hyperparathyroidism, and therefore it was generally thought that MEN1 and sporadic ZES could be easily distinguished by the presence or absence of hyperparathyroidism [31,32,39,194,198]. However, this is not always the case, and recent studies suggest that up to one-third of ZES/MEN1 patients present initially with features of ZES [31,32,194]. Almost all MEN1/ZES patients have hyperparathyroidism when they present with ZES symptoms but it is often mild [31,194]. Moreover, hyperparathyroidism can be difficult to diagnose with routine laboratory studies because the total serum calcium levels may be normal and the changes in plasma parathyroid hormone (PTH) levels minimal [31,194]. In general, the clinical manifestations of ZES are largely similar in patients with sporadic and MEN1/ZES, although patients with MEN1/ZES tend to have diarrhea less frequently at presentation (26% vs 53%). A detailed clinical, personal, and family history of endocrinopathies can be particularly important because up to 75% of MEN1/ZES patients have a family history of MEN1 (see Table 50.3) and 24–42% have a personal history compatible with renal colic [31,32,174].

Diagnosis and differential diagnosis

Unfortunately, recent studies report that the diagnosis of ZES is not being made any more quickly, with a persistent mean delay in diagnosis of 4–7 years [7,17,19,24,199–201]. Moreover, this diagnosis is also becoming more difficult to make [17,200,202–207]. The diagnosis of ZES has historically been delayed because ZES is an uncommon cause of PUD (1–3 new cases/million population/year), whereas idiopathic PUD is 1000-fold more frequent (2300 cases/year/million) and their clinical manifestations closely mimic each other so that physicians often fail to consider ZES [7,8,17,199,206]. Furthermore, most patients present with a typical appearing duodenal ulcer as seen in patients with idiopathic PUD [18,38,199]. In addition, the diagnosis is now becoming more difficult primarily for two additional reasons: first, the widespread use of PPIs which can both mask the diagnosis and lead to a false-positive diagnosis of ZES [17,18,203–208]; and second, the increasing unreliability of serum gastrin assays which are essential for the diagnosis of ZES [17,202,206,209]. Each of these points is discussed in detail later in this section.

A number of clinical/laboratory findings should suggest the diagnosis of ZES. Particularly important is the clinical association of diarrhea with GERD/PUD, because >60% of ZES patients have diarrhea, and it is now uncommon in idiopathic PUD because high doses of antacids are no longer used (see Table 50.2). Similarly, in any patient with unexplained chronic diarrhea, ZES should be suspected (see Table 50.2) because up to a third of the time diarrhea is the only presenting symptom [19,32,186–188]. ZES should be suspected in patients with PUD (generally duodenal) without *H. pylori* infection or a history of nonsteroidal antiinflammatory drug (NSAID)/aspirin use, because they are frequently not present in ZES patients with a duodenal ulcer (approximately 50%); in contrast, either *H. pylori* or NSAID/aspirin use is present in >80% of patients with idiopathic PUD [210–212]. In any patient with severe PUD or with a PUD complication (e.g., stricture, obstruction, perforation, bleeding, penetration), ZES should be considered (see Table 50.2). Because of the occurrence of MEN1 in 20–25% of ZES patients, a personal/family history of an endocrinopathy or a laboratory finding suggesting an endocrinopathy should lead to suspicion of ZES (see Table 50.2). Prominent gastric folds on upper gastrointestinal endoscopy are an important sign of ZES present in 94% of patients [19] (see Figure 50.1c–e and Table 50.2) but it is important to recognize that other causes of hypertrophic folds exist as well [24].

When ZES is suspected, the initial study is usually a fasting serum gastrin level (FSG) [2,6,17,24,200, 201,206]. FSG levels are elevated in >98% of ZES patients, except in some unusual circumstances, such as after noncurative gastrinoma resection or postparathyroidectomy in MEN1/ZES [3,13,186,199,213–217]. Because of its high sensitivity, the assessment of FSG is an excellent screening test [8,17,186]. However, an elevation of FSG alone, no matter how high the value, is not sufficient for a ZES diagnosis [8,17,24,186,200,201,206] (Table 50.4). Many physicians assume that a very high level of FSG (>10–100-fold elevated) is indicative of ZES; however, comparable levels can occur in patients with chronic atrophic gastritis (CAG)/pernicious anemia, renal failure, or even in those taking PPIs [17,24,206].

Table 50.3 Features of patients with multiple endocrine neoplasia type 1 syndrome (MEN1) and Zollinger–Ellison syndrome (ZES).

	Number/%	
Feature	**NIH data (*n* = 106) Mean [range]**	**Literature [range]**
MEN1 tumor/hyperplasia		
Hyperparathyroidism	101 (94%)	88.3% [78–100%]
Pituitary disease	60%	31.4% [28–60%]
Adrenal abnormality[a]	45%	13.1% [13–35%]
Carcinoid	29%	6.4%[c]
Gastric	20%	3.5%[c]
Bronchial	8%	1.5%[c]
Thymic	6%	2.3%[c]
Other functional pNET[b]	6%	15.7%[c]
Smooth muscle tumor	7%	0.2%[c]
Thyroid disease	6%	4.6% [3–25%]
CNS tumor (meningioma, etc.)	8%	<1%
Skin tumor		
Lipoma	5%	3%[c]
Melanoma	2%	<1%
Collagenoma	72%	<1%
Angiofibroma	88%	<1%
Age/duration		
Age (years)		
Age at study	51.2 ± 1.2 [23.8–79.6]	43.5 ± 0.5 [43–51]
Age at onset ZES	29.7 ± 1.1 [10.2–60.6]	36.6 ± 0.6[c]
Age onset MEN1	34.6 ± 1.0 [12.1–60.6]	34.1 ± 0.5[c]
Duration (years)		
Of ZES	16.6 ± 0.9 [1.4–43.1]	ND
Of MEN1	21.5 ± 1.1 [1.4–57.8]	ND
Other MEN1 features		
First MEN1 symptom		
Asymptomatic (screening)	11%	1.3%[c]
HPT	38%	38.4%[c]
ZES	44%	41.5%[c]
Pituitary	8%	11.6%[c]
Other	2%	7.6%[c]
Family history of MEN1	72%	76%[c]

CNS, central nervous system; HPT, hyperparathyroidism; MEN1, multiple endocrine neoplasia type 1; ND, no data; pNET, pancreatic neuroendocrine tumor; ZES, Zollinger–Ellison syndrome.

[a] "Adrenal abnormality" refers to the presence of an abnormality detected on imaging studies (*n* = 45) and/or clinically (pheochromocytoma [*n* = 1], adrenal Cushing syndrome [*n* = 2]) (*n* = 3).

[b] "Other functional PET" includes insulinoma (*n* = 6), glucagonoma (*n* = 1), or carcinoid syndrome (*n* = 1). One patient had an insulinoma and carcinoid syndrome.

[c] Data from [31] literature review of MEN1/ZES patients (*n* = 1009).

National Institutes of Health (NIH) data from [7,19,31,65,421–423].

Table 50.4 Causes of chronic hypergastrinemia (frequency).

Associated with gastric acid hyposecretion/achlorhydria
Chronic atrophic gastritis/pernicious anemia (common)
Treatment with potent gastric acid antisecretory agents (especially PPIs) (common)
Chronic renal failure (uncommon)
H. pylori infections (common)
Post acid-reducing surgery/vagotomy (uncommon)
Associated with gastric acid hypersecretion
H. pylori infections (common)
Gastric outlet obstruction
Antral G-cell hyperfunction/hyperplasia (uncommon)
Chronic renal failure (uncommon)
Short bowel syndrome (rare)
Retained gastric antrum syndrome (rare)
Zollinger–Ellison syndrome

PPIs, proton pump inhibitors

Table 50.5 Criteria to make the diagnosis of Zollinger–Ellison syndrome (ZES).

FSG and gastric fluid pH ≤2
If FSG >10 times elevated (over ULN) and gastric pH ≤2, the diagnosis of ZES is established (can exclude retained antrum almost always by history) (40%)
If FSG is <10-fold elevated and gastric pH ≤2, need to perform additional testing to exclude other causes of increased FSG/ hyperchlorhydria (60%) • Secretin test positive (≥120 pg/mL increase) • Elevated basal acid output (>15 mEq/h)

CAG, chronic atrophic gastritis; FSG, fasting serum gastrin level; ULN, upper limit of normal.
Source: Data are from [133,206, 217, 218].

Hypergastrinemia can either be physiological/appropriate (caused by hypo-/achlorhydria) or pathological/inappropriate (occurs in the presence of normal/elevated gastric acid secretion) (see Table 50.4). Unfortunately, physiological hypergastrinemia (especially due to CAG/pernicious anemia, use of PPIs, or to *H. pylori* infections) is much more frequent than ZES, and needs to be excluded as the cause of hypergastrinemia. Therefore, if fasting hypergastrinemia is detected, the next study generally recommended is an assessment of gastric pH [2,7,16,17,24,200,206]. If the patient has hypergastrinemia with a concomitant gastric pH ≤2, ZES should be strongly suspected [200,217,218] (Table 50.5); an NIH ZES study found that fasting pH was ≤2 in all ZES patients off antisecretory drug [218].

Use of PPIs makes the diagnosis of ZES challenging. PPIs are potent gastric acid suppressants and because of their long durations of action (up to 1 week), they induce hypergastrinemia in 80–100% of normals [17,200, 201,206]. The hypergastrinemia with PPIs develops rapidly (within 5 days), and is common since these agents are widely prescribed and are also now available as over-the-counter medications. The degree of hypergastrinemia is variable among PPI users, with 20–25% developing FSG levels >4-fold elevated and occasionally >10-fold [17,206]. Furthermore, in contrast to H_2 receptor (H2R) antagonists (e.g., cimetidine, ranitidine, nizatidine, famotidine), PPIs control symptoms in most ZES patients at conventional doses used in the treatment of idiopathic PUD [43,219–223], whereas with H2R antagonists, higher doses and/or more frequent dosing are usually needed [8,223,224]. In the past, ZES patients treated with conventional doses of H2R antagonists continued to have symptoms suggesting the diagnosis, whereas this is not the case with PPIs [17,207]. Therefore, PPIs mask and delay the diagnosis of ZES because of their effective symptom control at conventional doses and their ability to cause a false suspicion for ZES by inducing hypergastrinemia in normals [17,206,207].

When the gastric pH is >2 in the context of PPI use, it may be difficult to determine whether hypergastrinemia is physiological or pathological. To accomplish this distinction, both the North American Neuroendocrine Tumor Society (NANETS) and the European Neuroendocrine Tumor Society (ENETS) guidelines recommend stopping the PPI for up to 1 week and then determining gastric pH and FSG [2,6,16,43,225,226]. This approach must be undertaken with extreme caution [17,200,203,209,225,226]. In each set of guidelines, it is pointed out that this must be performed with a careful history about the prior effects of stopping PPIs, that high-dose H2R antagonists should be substituted for the PPI (equivalent to ranitidine 300–600 mg every 4–6 h), and this should only be performed after it is has been established that all acute PUD/GERD lesions are healed with careful follow-up during this time of PPI avoidance [17,200,203,209,225,226]. After 5–7 days, the H2R can be stopped for 30 h because they have a shorter serum half-life, and antacids can be used instead until midnight the night before repeat testing is performed. A recent study [203] reported two patients with ZES who developed severe PUD/ GERD complications when PPIs were suddenly stopped, and recommended the diagnosis of ZES should be established by not stopping the PPI. Two subsequent papers [17,200] have pointed out that it may be possible in some patients to decrease the dose/frequency of PPI to obtain gastric pH ≤2, or use other findings (e.g., the presence of gastrinoma on imaging) to establish the diagnosis; however, in most cases this will not be possible. The only established criteria, which usually require discontinuation of PPIs, are listed in Table 50.5. Because of the potential risk in a patient who does have ZES, repeat testing off PPIs is best performed at experienced centers. This highly controversial issue is described in some detail in a recent manuscript [206].

Previously, gastric acid secretory studies were widely performed and used for ZES diagnosis. Most ZES patients without previous gastric acid-reducing surgery have elevated basal acid outputs (BAO) and MAO with a mean BAO of 42 mEq/h (normal <10 mEq/h) and mean MAO of 62.7 mEq/h (normal 48 mEq/h [men]/30 mEq/h [women]) [47] (see Figure 50.1a). Various levels of BAO, MAO, BAO/MAO ratios as well as basal gastric fluid volume and basal/maximal acid concentration or pH were proposed to identify ZES patients [47]. A study of gastric acid secretory results in 234 NIH ZES patients and 984 ZES patients from the literature found a number of these secretory criteria had high sensitivity for identifying ZES patients, with the commonly used BAO criteria of ≥15 mEq/h (no previous gastric acid-reducing surgery) or ≥5 mEq/h (with previous gastric surgery) having a sensitivity of 87–90% and 81–100%, respectively [47] (see Figure 50.1a). However, gastric acid secretion studies are now performed by only a few centers and are thus not generally available, so that these secretory criteria are no longer used regularly. Nonetheless, the aforementioned NIH study [47] demonstrated that >99% of ZES had a fasting gastric pH ≤2 off antisecretory drugs, indicating that this is a useful criterion that can potentially be applied more widely than formal gastric analysis. Furthermore, another study [227] described the validity of measuring gastric pH at the time of gastrointestinal endoscopy in ZES patients, further supporting that this criterion can be generally applied [47].

A FSG level >10-fold elevated with a gastric pH ≤2 occurs in 40% of ZES patients, which firmly establishes the diagnosis (see Table 50.5), as long as the possibility of a retained antrum syndrome, which can mimic ZES (see Table 50.4), has been ruled out by previous history/records [7,228]. Unfortunately, 60% of ZES patients have FSG <10-fold elevated [7,51,132,217] with a gastric pH ≤2 (Table 50.6), which overlaps with a number of other disorders (see Table 50.4). *H. pylori* infection can result in both gastric acid hypersecretion and hyposecretion [229–231], and may thus be particularly confusing. To exclude these other disorders (see Table 50.4), patients may be referred to a center where BAO and/or secretin testing are performed (see Table 50.5). Previously, secretin- [7,129,132–134,232], calcium- [8,132–134,136,232], and meal-stimulated [7,133,134,137] gastrin provocative tests were used to diagnose ZES. The secretin/calcium tests were based

Table 50.6 Tumor imaging results in patients with Zollinger–Ellison syndrome (ZES).

	Sensitivity (%)		Specificity (%)
	NIH studies Mean [range]	Literature Mean [range]	Literature Mean [range]
Extrahepatic lesions			
Ultrasound	13 [9–16]	24 [0–28]	92 [92–93]
CT scan	38 [31–51]	38 [0–59]	90 [83–100]
MRI	40 [30–57]	22 [20–25]	100 [99–100]
Angiography	48 [28–57]	68 [35–68]	89 [84–94]
EUS	ND	70 [28–86]	85 [80–93]
SRS (Octreoscan)	69 [58–78]	72 [57–77]	86 [86–100]
SRI (^{68}Ga PET)	80	80[68–100]	97 [95–100]
PVS	71	68 [60–94]	ND
Intraarterial secretin test	86	89 [55–100]	ND
IOUS	ND	83 [75–100]	
Liver metastases			
Ultrasound	46	40 [15–77]	100 [99–100]
CT scan	42	48 [37–56]	99 [99–100]
MRI	71	63 [60–75]	92 [88–100]
Angiography	65	62 [33–86]	98 [96–100]
SRS (Octreoscan)	92	97 [92–100]	97 [95–100]
SRI(^{68}Ga PET)	95	95[90–100]	97 [95–100]
Intraarterial secretin test	40	ND	ND

CT, computed tomography; EUS, endoscopic ultrasound; MRI, magnetic resonance imaging; ND, no data; NIH, National Institutes of Health; IOUS, intraoperative ultrasound; PVS, portal venous sampling for gastrin; SRS, somatostatin receptor scintigraphy with ^{111}In-labeled somatostatin analogs with SPECT imaging (Octreoscan); SRI, ^{68}Ga-labeled somatostatin analogs with PET scanning.
Source: Data from [2,7,8,107,247–249,253,257,259].

on the finding that these stimuli caused a marked increase in serum gastrin in ZES patients compared to normal individuals [129,136]. With the meal test, ZES patients generally show <100% increase in serum gastrin [133,134,137], whereas patients with antral G-cell hyperfunction/hyperplasia have an augmented and much larger response [133,134,137,233].

At present, only the secretin test is widely used because of its convenience, sensitivity, specificity, and lack of side-effects [133]. This is a reasonable approach to diagnosis in locations that do not have access to gastric analysis but it is potentially confounded by achlorhydria. An NIH study of 293 ZES patients (NIH) and 537 ZES cases (in the literature) [133] demonstrated that a value of 120 pg/mL increase with secretin had a sensitivity of 94% and specificity of 100% for ZES [136], and was more sensitive than previously proposed criteria of increases of 200 pg/mL, 50% over basal or 110 pg/mL [130,132,134,232], and therefore the former criterion is now the recommended diagnostic threshold [6,16,30,206]. It is recommended that secretin testing be performed in patients with fasting gastrin levels <10-fold increased and gastric pH ≤2 in order to confirm the diagnosis. In some countries, secretin is not available and a glucagon stimulation test has been proposed as an alternative [226,234]; however, there is much less experience with this test. Unfortunately, it is important to recognize that secretin test results can be affected by PPI-induced hypo-/achlorhydria or by the presence of hypo-/achlorhydria for other reasons; therefore, it cannot be reliably performed while the patient is taking PPIs or is hypo- or achlorhydric [235,236]. This too has contributed to the great difficulty with which ZES is diagnosed in the modern era as atrophy is so much more common than ZES [206].

Finally, the availability of a reliable serum or plasma gastrin assay is critical in all the diagnostic approaches for ZES. However, a recent study [202] of the 12 commercial assays for gastrin assessment widely used by different laboratories in both the USA and Europe demonstrated that only five assays reliably measured gastrin concentrations, while the others either over- or underestimated the true value. Therefore, the results of seven of these commercially used assays gave gastrin values that could lead to false or missed diagnoses [17,202,206]. The inaccuracy occurred because inadequately characterized antibodies were used that either recognized precursor/inactive fragments or did not interact with all biologically active, circulating gastrin forms [202]. Lack of a reliable gastrin assay affects both the assessment of FSG levels and the secretin test results. This is obviously a potentially major problem, and the best approach is to determine whether the laboratory uses one of the five reliable gastrin assays listed in this paper [202] or to obtain advice from a center that routinely performs these studies.

Given all these issues, diagnosing ZES in the current era is quite challenging and if any doubt exists or there is any concern about withdrawal of therapy to try and make a diagnosis we recommend referral to a center with experience in managing and diagnosing these patients. The interested reader is also referred to the manuscript mentioned above which examines this issue in more detail, including a discussion of the potential value of functional imaging (see below) which, if positive, supports the presence of a NET and even ZES in the correct setting [206].

Tumor localization

Tumor localization, which involves assessment of both the primary site and tumor extent, is essential to the management of all ZES patients [2,7,16,24,237–240]. It is needed to determine whether surgery should be considered; to plan the extent of surgery; to define the location, extent, and in some cases the rate of growth of metastatic disease; to restage patients post resection; or to determine changes in tumor load with antitumor therapies or with time [2,7,16, 24,237–240]. A combination of imaging modalities is usually needed for each patient.

A large number of imaging modalities have been used in the evaluation of ZES patients (see Table 50.6) [2,238,241]. These include cross-sectional imaging (computed tomography [CT] scanning, magnetic resonance imaging [MRI], ultrasound); selective angiography; somatostatin receptor scintigraphy (SRS) using ^{111}indium-labeled somatostatin analogs with single photon emission computed tomographic (SPECT) imaging or, more recently, somatostatin receptor imaging (SRI) using ^{68}gallium-labeled somatostatin analogs with positron emission tomographic (PET) scanning; endoscopic ultrasound (EUS); and the assessment of serum gastrin gradients determined in either the portal venous drainage through transhepatic venous sampling or in hepatic veins after selective, intraarterial secretin injections [2,7,16,27,239–246]. These modalities vary in sensitivities for the detection of the primary/metastatic tumor (see Table 50.6). It is important to note that ^{68}gallium-labeled somatostatin scintigraphy (discussed in more detail below) represents a significant advance over indium-labeled imaging (octreoscan) as well as all other modalities, which has had a major impact on diagnosis, staging, and therapy of ZES patients, including potentially for diagnosis in the absence of diagnostic biochemistries [206].

Patients usually undergo a cross-sectional imaging study followed by SRS imaging to initially define whether surgical resection should be considered [2,6,16] as the former studies provide important anatomical detail and the latter the best in formation regarding tumor extent. Gastrinomas are hypervascular tumors and are often best detected with the administration of contrast; therefore, the recommended study is a triphasic CT with contrast or an MRI with contrast (gadolinium), with the contrast material given by intravenous infusions [238,240,241]. With each of the cross-sectional imaging studies, the detection of the primary tumor is influenced by its size [8,240,247,248]. In general, with gastrinomas <1 cm in diameter, <15–20% are detected, with tumors 1–3 cm in diameter 15–40% are detected, and with tumors >3 cm >90% are detected [8,240,247,248]. Thus, cross-sectional imaging studies miss most primary duodenal gastrinomas, which are characteristically <1 cm in diameter; however, they detect most pancreatic primaries which are frequently >3 cm in diameter by the time a diagnosis is made [28,34,79,81,210]. The sensitivity of cross-sectional imaging for the detection of primary gastrinomas varies markedly among different series (see Table 50.6). In general, they detect <50% of the primaries, with lower yields in series with a high percentage of duodenal gastrinomas. For the detection of a patient with liver metastases, cross-sectional CT/ultrasound identifies approximately one-half of the patients, whereas MRI detects nearly three-quarters (see Table 50.6).

Selective angiography is a sensitive method for localizing gastrinomas, and was previously widely used [7,247–249]. Angiography was generally more sensitive than cross-sectional imaging studies for localizing primary gastrinomas, but still missed approximately half of primary gastrinomas, particularly in patients with duodenal gastrinomas [8,34,79,247,248] (Table 50.7). Because of its invasive nature and because of increasing sensitivity of cross-sectional imaging, as well as the high sensitivity of modern SRS, angiography is no longer commonly used. Functional gastrin localization at angiography to identify selective vessel hormonal gradients after secretin stimulation as a localization test [249–251] is now generally reserved for rare patients in whom all imaging procedures are negative prior to surgery, and in whom an additional localization approach is considered necessary, but this is not commonly required in the modern era. It should be noted that inappropriate hypergastrinemia is pathognomonic of ZES (especially in patients who have not undergone prior gastric surgery, in whom retained antrum is not possible). Consequently, negative imaging, even with highly sensitive SRI using ^{68}gallium-labeled somatostatin analogs, should not preclude a careful exploration, including a duodenotomy by an experienced ZES surgeon, as tumor is identified under such circumstances in about 95% of cases and long-term biochemical cure is achievable in about 30–40% of cases [88,252,253].

Gastrinomas, like other NETs/pNETs (see also Chapter 80), overexpress somatostatin receptors in >90% of cases, with the result that SRS using radiolabeled somatostatin analogs is a particularly sensitive method to identify both the primary and metastatic gastrinoma tumors [16,145,238,248,253–255]. There are five classes of somatostatin receptors (sst1–5), and all can be detected in gastrinomas; however, sst2 (80–100%) and sst5 (30–600%) are most often overexpressed [256]. Somatostatin interacts with all five receptor subtypes with high affinity; however, it is rapidly degraded and therefore is not useful therapeutically or for radioimaging studies [254,256]. Two synthetic analogs of somatostatin, octreotide and lanreotide, have high affinity for sst2 and sst5 specifically, are metabolically more stable, and formulations of these two analogs or related compounds are now generally used for SRI and for the treatment of pNETs including gastrinomas [254,256]. In the NIH ZES prospective studies (see Table 50.6), SRS using ^{111}In-labeled somatostatin analogs (Octreoscan®) and SPECT imaging detected primaries in 69% of patients and in one prospective study of 80 consecutive ZES patients [257], SRS was more sensitive than any single cross-sectional imaging study or angiography, and was equal in sensitivity to the combination of all three cross-sectional imaging studies (ultrasound, CT, MRI) and angiography together (58% vs 48%) [257]. SPECT detection is particularly important in ZES patients for SRS to have maximal sensitivity [248,257]. The sensitivity of SRS, similar to cross-sectional imaging, is influenced by the size of the gastrinoma, with SRS using ^{111}In-labeled somatostatin analogs (Octreoscan) visualizing only 20% of gastrinomas <0.5 cm in diameter and 30–40% <1 cm in diameter [258]. Because the mean size of duodenal gastrinomas is <1 cm, SRS detects only 32% of duodenal gastrinomas [34,258]. However, the use of ^{68}Ga-labeled somatostatin analogs with PET scanning, which has far greater resolution with increased sensitivity, is an important recent advance. SRI using ^{68}Ga-labeled somatostatin analogs with PET imaging detects 60–80% of lesions <1.5 cm and 70–100% of lesions >2.5 cm [259] (see Table 50.6).

Figure 50.2 illustrates ^{68}Ga-labeled imaging in two patients with ZES. Figure 50.2a shows imaging findings in a patient with a small sporadic duodenal primary that is not well visualized on routine cross-sectional imaging but is easily identified on SRS. Figure 50.2b shows a patient with widely metastatic disease which is also not well visualized on routine noncontrast CT. ^{68}Ga-labeled somatostatin analogs with PET scanning were approved in the USA in early 2018 and this has now become the imaging modality of choice for identification of primary gastrinomas and determination of disease extent in the USA and wherever it is available elsewhere [238,260,261]. The reader is directed to a recent consensus manuscript for appropriate use of somatostatin receptor imaging in NET patients [262].

Somatostatin receptor imaging is particularly valuable for detecting distant metastases, with a detection rate of 97% for patients with metastatic disease in the liver (see Table 50.6). Studies demonstrate that bone metastases are relatively common in patients with gastrinomas, occurring in up to 31% of those with liver metastases [105,106,263]. Their identification has clinical importance, because they may not only require specific treatment, they also have important prognostic significance [27,106]. In one prospective study from the NIH, SRS had greater sensitivity than bone scanning for detecting bone metastases, and for imaging metastases in the spine it was equal in sensitivity to MRI [105]. Because 15–25% of the initial metastases occur outside the axial skeleton, SRS was recommended as the initial study over MRI to detect bone metastases [105]. SRI using ^{68}Ga-labeled somatostatin analogs with PET imaging is more sensitive than SRS for detecting small bone metastases, so in the future it is likely the rate of detection of small bone metastases will be higher than the numbers found using SRS with ^{111}In-labeled somatostatin analogs with SPECT imaging in the prospective NIH studies.

Table 50.7 Prognostic factors in patients with gastrinomas (survival or associated with increased development of liver metastases).

Prognostic factor for decreased survival	References
Gastrinomas only	
Diagnosis before 1980 ($p = 0.010$)	[424]
Poorly controlled acid hypersecretion	[1,7,40,270,310]
Female gender ($p = 0.024$)	[237,28]
Older age at diagnosis ($p = 0.001$)	[424]
Short disease history prior to diagnosis (<3 years) ($p < 0.001$)	[27,28]
MEN1 absent (sporadic ZES) ($p < 0.03$) (see Figure 50.4d)	[27,28,425,426]
Extent/presence of liver metastases ($p < 0.0001$)	[7,27,28,165,310,426]
Diffuse > localized ($p < 0.0001$)	
Diffuse > both lobes > single lobe > none (see Figure 50.4a)	
Lymph node metastases ($p < 0.004$)	[27,311,426]
Time to diagnosis of liver metastases	
Present initially > develop on follow-up ($p = 0.02$)	[27]
Develop bone or extrahepatic metastases ($p < 0.0001$) (see Figure 50.4c)	[27,105,258,310]
Develop ectopic Cushing syndrome ($p = 0.0049$) (see Figure 50.4c)	[27,312]
Rate of growth of liver metastases	
Rapid > slow, none	[166]
Increased tumor markers	
High gastrin ($p = 0.022$)	[27,28,305]
Large primary tumor size (>3 cm)	[27,28,310,424]
Primary gastrinoma location	
Pancreatic > duodenal ($p < 0.004$) (see Figure 50.4b)	[27,28,110,424,426]
Left SMA > right of SMA (gastrinoma triangle)	[158]
Tumor features	
Flow cytometric results	
• High S phase, low % nontetraploid aneuploid, multiple stem line aneuploid frequent	[427]
Molecular changes	
• Chromosome 1qLOH ($p = 0.019$)	[428]
• Chromosome XLOH ($p = 0.042$)	[429]
Additional features shared with other pNETs	
Histological features	
Poorly differentiation	[239,430]
High Ki-67 > low Ki-67 proliferative index	[239,431–433]
Cytokeratin 19-IR positivity	[434–436]
Vascular, neural invasion	[21,437]
Classification	
Advanced TNM classification (ENETS, UICC/AJCC/WHO)	[239,432,434,438]

AJCC, American Joint Committee on Cancer; ENETS, European Neuroendocrine Tumor Society; IR, immunoreactivity; LOH, loss of heterozygosity; MEN1, multiple endocrine neoplasia type 1; pNET, pancreatic neuroendocrine tumor; SMA, superior mesenteric artery; UICC, Union for International Cancer Control; WHO, World Health Organization; ZES, Zollinger–Ellison syndrome.

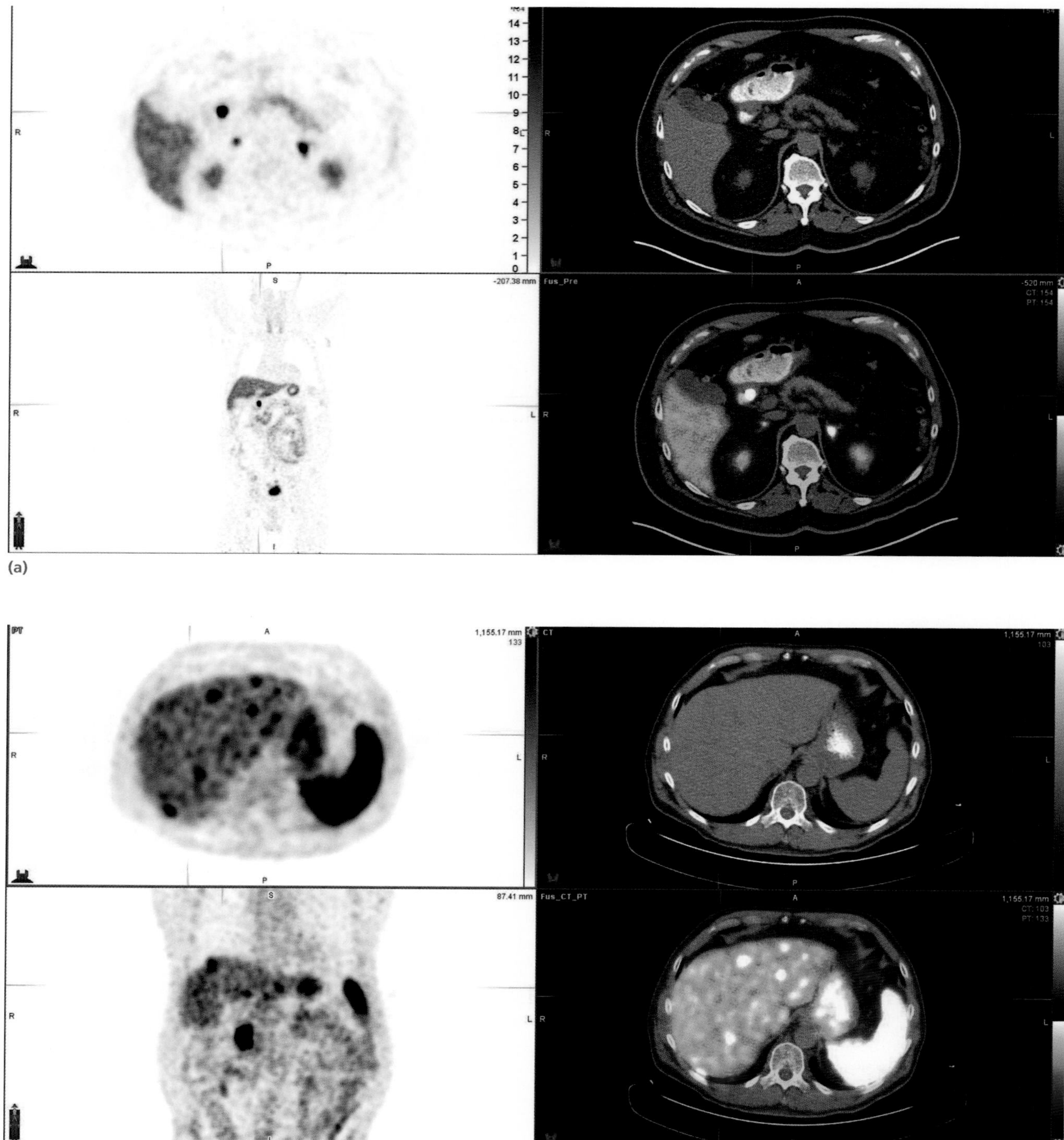

Figure 50.2 [68]Gallium dotatate PET scanning in two patients with ZES. **(a)** Imaging findings in a patient with a sporadic duodenal primary whereas **(b)** shows findings in a patient with widely metastatic disease. Both figures are arranged as follows: bottom L is a coronal PET scan image, top L is a cross-sectional PET scan image, top R is a cross-sectional noncontrast CAT scan image, and bottom R is a fused PET/CAT scan image. Source: Photographs courtesy of Daniel Pryma, MD.

Endoscopic ultrasound is reported to be sensitive for localizing gastrinomas [7,86,253,264–267]. EUS detected a mean of 83% of gastrinomas in different studies (see Table 50.6) and has the advantage of allowing histological verification of the presence of a NET; however, its result is operator dependent and false positives can occur [86,253,257,266]. An important issue in patients with ZES is the sensitivity of EUS for detecting gastrinomas in different locations. In one review, EUS detected pancreatic gastrinomas in 83% of cases, whereas it detected duodenal gastrinomas in only 43% [253]. This is a major problem for EUS in patients with ZES because in recent studies 3–10 times more gastrinomas are found to be duodenal rather than pancreatic [2,6,16]. Because of this, many experts do not recommend EUS as a routine preoperative imaging study in patients with ZES, especially in the 75–85% of patients with sporadic ZES [253]. As discussed below, serial EUS studies may be used in patients with MEN1/ZES to evaluate growth rates of pNETs in patients who do not undergo routine exploration [268,269] and specifically for the identification of insulinomas (which often are ^{68}Ga-scan negative). At present, it is recommended that a cross-sectional imaging study and a ^{68}Ga SRI with PET imaging be performed in all patients to evaluate tumor location/extent [2,6,16]. However, even if all imaging is negative, many experts still favor exploration as long as the diagnosis of ZES has otherwise been confirmed, MEN1/ZES is not present and the patient is likely to live for a decade or more [88,253]. This issue is discussed further under the section on surgical management.

Treatment of gastric acid hypersecretion

General

When initially described, patients with ZES succumbed to the ravages of uncontrolled gastric acid hypersecretion (see Figure 50.1a). However, with the development of effective therapy for acid hypersecretion, it soon became clear that additional therapy would be required for the gastrinoma itself. Long-term curative resection would solve both problems; unfortunately, it is only possible in about 30% of sporadic patients (Figure 50.3a,b) and rarely, if at all, in patients with MEN1/ZES [225,226]. In general, antitumor therapy for controlled ZES patients should not differ significantly from that for other pNETs. Patients with MEN1/ZES also require treatment directed at their other endocrinopathies as well as genetic counseling [32,175,196].

Control of gastric acid hypersecretion

Control of gastric acid hypersecretion acutely and in the long term is essential in ZES patients [2,16,43,201]. Prior to the availability of effective acid antisecretory drugs, most patients who did not have a total gastrectomy developed complications of gastric acid secretion, and the majority died from these complications rather than from tumor progression [1,7,39,40,43,72,174,201,270]. This occurred because mean basal acid secretion is typically four times normal and can reach 12 times normal [8,47] (see Figure 50.1a). Therefore, it is essential to acutely control acid hypersecretion as soon as ZES is suspected and as the initial step in management [2,6,16,17].

Surgical treatment of gastric acid hypersecretion

Initially, the only effective means of controlling gastric acid hypersecretion was by total gastrectomy [1,39,44,75,270,271]. Lesser operations were almost invariably inadequate [1,39,75,270,271]. Total gastrectomy often had to be performed as an emergency procedure and was associated with considerable morbidity and mortality [1,8,40,270]. However, with the ability to preoperatively control acid hypersecretion medically, total gastrectomy can now be performed electively and is relatively safe, with an overall mortality of 5.8% in 248 cases since 1980, and 2.4% for elective cases [44]. However, long-term morbidity is not insignificant, and in some studies up to 50% of patients have moderate or severe side-effects, including weight loss, pain, stenosis of the anastomoses, vomiting, and early satiety [7,8,272]. At present, because of the effectiveness of medical therapy, total gastrectomy is rarely performed and reserved for patients (<0.3%) [2,7,273] who cannot or will not regularly take oral antisecretory drugs.

Vagotomy, as well as anticholinergic agents, reduces gastric acid secretion in ZES patients and potentiates H2R antagonists [7,8,274,275]. Because most ZES patients are not cured at surgery, and because many continued to require frequent high-dose H2R antagonists, it was previously proposed that parietal cell vagotomy could be performed at the time of surgery to limit the risks of acid hypersecretion. In patients who underwent selective vagotomy [274,275], BAO decreased by 50%, H2R antagonist dosage was reduced by 40%, and in 36% of patients all antisecretory drugs could be stopped postoperatively. Today, because of the effectiveness of PPIs, vagotomy is rarely performed.

In patients with hyperparathyroidism and MEN1/ZES, parathyroidectomy can have a dramatic effect on fasting gastrin levels, BAO, and sensitivity to gastric antisecretory drugs [213–215,276], with a mean decrease in BAO of 56% and in FSG of 55% [8,213–215]. Furthermore, in some patients, the fasting gastrin levels can revert to normal and positive secretin testing can normalize too [8,213–215]. Because MEN1 patients, with or without ZES, have parathyroid hyperplasia which involves all four parathyroid glands, if recurrent hyperparathyroidism is to be avoided, a 3.5-gland resection or a four-gland resection with a parathyroid implant is needed [32,175,213,214].

Long-term curative gastrinoma resection is possible in up to 40% of patients with sporadic ZES undergoing surgery [34,79] (see Figure 50.3a); unfortunately, it does not completely correct gastric acid hypersecretion in all patients [277,278]. In NIH prospective studies of acid hypersecretion postcurative resection, MAO decreased 50%, BAO decreased 75% within 6–12 months and then remained unchanged for up to 4 years, and the H2R antagonist dose could be reduced by >60% [277,278]. However, even though BAO decreased by 75%

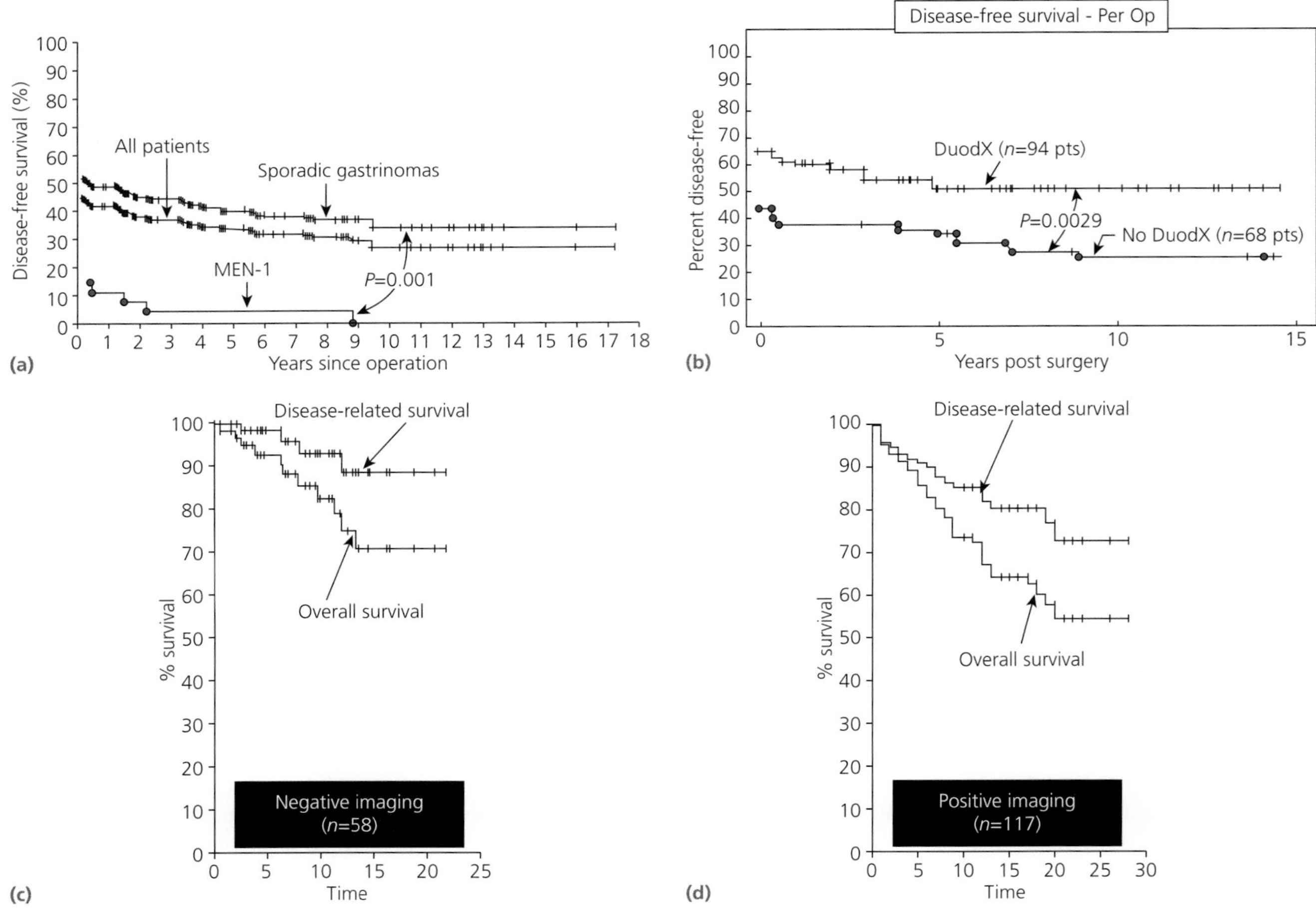

Figure 50.3 Surgical results in patients with Zollinger–Ellison syndrome (ZES) from prospective studies. **(a)** Disease-free survival in 151 patients with ZES (sporadic = 123 patients with multiple endocrine neoplasia type 1 syndrome [MEN1]; ZES = 28 patients) after attempted surgical cure (without Whipple resection). Data show that 34% of sporadic ZES patients have a long-term cure (10 years), but none of the MEN1/ZES patients do. Data from [79]. **(b)** The importance of performing a duodenotomy in 162 ZES patients. Duodenotomy results in more duodenal gastrinomas being found, in a higher cure rate, and a better ZES-related survival. Data from [34]. **(c, d)** Survival (disease-related and total survival) in patients with negative preoperative imaging (n = 58) or positive preoperative imaging (n = 117). Data from [88]. These results demonstrate that the survival rates are as good in patients with negative preoperative imaging as those with positive imaging, and thus the lack of positive preoperative imaging should not be used to postpone surgery in patients with sporadic ZES [88].

after curative resection for up to 4 years, 56–62% of the patients remained acid hypersecretors [277,278]. The 56–62% of the postcurative hypersecretors included 34% who were mild hypersecretors (BAO 15–24.9 mEq/h) and 28% who had marked to extreme hypersecretion (≥25 mEq/h; range 25–69 mEq/h) [278]. The mechanism of this continued hypersecretion postcurative resection is unclear [278]. Practically, it means that all ZES patients should continue to be followed carefully postcurative resection and many will continue to need low doses of antisecretory drugs [278].

Medical treatment of gastric acid hypersecretion

Oral gastric acid hypersecretory drugs are required to control gastric acid hypersecretion acutely and in the long term in ZES patients. PPIs (e.g., omeprazole, esomeprazole, lansoprazole, dexlansoprazole, pantoprazole, rabeprazole) are the drugs of choice because of their long durations of action and potency [2,8,6,16,43]. Most ZES patients without complicated disease are manageable with once-daily dosing and many are controlled on doses equivalent to those used in idiopathic PUD disease (i.e., equivalent to 20 mg/day omeprazole) [201,219,220,222]. However, because loss of acid control and severe morbidity can occur rapidly if drugs are withdrawn, we favor BID dosing in all patients and recommend that patients obtain a Medicalert bracelet stating "gastrinoma; PPI dependent.. In patients with complicated disease (i.e., with MEN1/ZES, moderate-to-severe GERD, or post Billroth II surgery), higher doses and/or frequency are usually needed [201,219,220,222,279]. In general, increasing the dose frequency is more effective than increasing the dosage once per day [219,222]. Most long-term studies were performed with omeprazole or lansoprazole but other PPIs (e.g., pantoprazole, rabeprazole, esomeprazole, dexlansoprazole) are also effective in ZES, and it is not apparent that any one agent has an advantage over the others [43,201,280].

There is no complete agreement on the recommended starting dose of PPI. This becomes an important point in patients with ZES because many of the PPI formulations are acid labile and thus starting a patient on a low PPI dose could delay its action, and in acutely ill ZES patients with PUD this could result in complications [281]. One study attempted to address this question [281] by starting patients on a low dose of omeprazole (20 mg/day), and found that in 32%, acid secretion was not controlled and higher doses were needed. This study proposed that ZES patients with uncomplicated ZES (no MEN1/ZES, moderate-to-severe GERD, post Billroth II surgery) be started on higher PPI doses (equivalent to omeprazole 60 mg/day) and then the doses can be reduced during follow-up. Both the American NANETS guidelines [6,225] and the European ENETS guidelines [16,226] recommend that ZES patients with uncomplicated disease (no MEN1/ZES, moderate-to-severe GERD, post Billroth II surgery) be started on the equivalent of 60 mg/day of omeprazole and that patients with complicated disease be started on PPI doses equivalent to omeprazole 40–60 mg BID and then, with time, dose reduction can be considered. It is ideal to titrate the PPI dose to control the acid output (<10 mEq/h for patients with no prior gastric surgery, <5 mEq/h for those with previous gastric surgery) [7,8,42,189,201,280], but few physicians now have access to this modality.

Symptom control (particularly diarrhea, pain, heartburn) can be used to guide management, and if mucosal disease is present, repeat upper gastrointestinal endoscopy should be performed after 6–8 weeks to confirm healing has occurred. Because of their potency, dose titration is less important with PPIs; however, it is essential with H2R antagonists.

Studies report continued long-term efficacy of PPIs in ZES patients for 9–15 years [220,222,282]. Tachyphylaxis does not develop with long-term PPI treatment in ZES patients, and on average <20% of patients require a PPI dose increase/year (rate 0.13/patient), whereas with long-term H2R antagonist treatment, on average at least one dose increase/year was required [7,221,222,224,283,284].

Long-term PPI use has proven safe; fewer than 0.1% of patients will stop because of a side-effect [43]. A potential concern of long-term PPI treatment is the drug-induced hypo-/achlorhydria, which may lead to effects on nutrient absorption (vitamin B_{12}, iron, calcium) as well as enhanced hypergastrinemia resulting in an increased risk of gastric carcinoid tumors [285–289]. Low vitamin B_{12} levels are frequent in ZES patients [287,288,290,291] and are more frequent in ZES patients treated with PPIs, and correlate with the PPI-induced hypo-/achlorhydria [290]. In another study of ZES patients [292], deficiencies in body iron stores were not found with long-term PPI treatment. Epidemiological and various correlative studies in the general population have suggested that long-term PPI use may result in an increased incidence of bone fractures, particularly in the spine/hip, but there are no specific studies in ZES patients [287,288,293] and the findings may well be confounded. On the basis of these studies, it has been proposed [16, 29,226] that vitamin B_{12} levels be periodically assessed in ZES patients on long-term PPI treatment, especially the group of patients who might have low vitamin B_{12} level initially or a poorer nutritional status (for instance, elderly patients with a long history of malabsorption). The 2016 ENETS minimum consensus update on the medical treatment of ZES also stressed the need to monitor B_{12} levels and to be aware of the possibility of hypomagnesemia with any of the PPIs [226].

Prolonged hypergastrinemia in humans and animals stimulates gastric ECL cell proliferation and in animal models, gastric carcinoid tumors (ECLomas) can develop, some of which are malignant [64,286,287,289]. In patients with ZES, ECL cell proliferative changes develop in >90% [64]. However, patients with sporadic ZES rarely develop gastric carcinoids [43,64,289], whereas MEN1/ZES patients have a >70-fold greater risk of developing gastric carcinoids [65] (see Figure 50.1b). In one prospective study [65], 23% of MEN1/ZES patients had gastric carcinoids (see Figure 50.1b), and other studies have indicated that these can be malignant in 10–30% of patients [65,192,287,289,294]. There is no evidence that the long-term use of PPIs accelerates gastric carcinoid development either with sporadic ZES or MEN1/ZES [43,289]. However, because of the association of hypergastrinemia with gastric carcinoids, all patients with ZES should undergo an initial upper gastrointestinal endoscopy; those with MEN1/ZES should have a repeat upper gastrointestinal endoscopy yearly, while in those with sporadic ZES, if there are no upper gastrointestinal symptoms, follow-up upper gastrointestinal endoscopy can be less frequent.

For brief periods (e.g., after surgery, during chemotherapy or gastroenteritis) when ZES patients are unable to take oral medications, a parenterally administered gastric antisecretory drug may be necessary. Parental H2R antagonists can be used, but continuous infusions of high doses are required [7,43,245,295], whereas with parenteral PPIs (e.g., omeprazole, pantoprazole, lansoprazole), because of their long durations of action, intermittent parenteral administration (every 8–12 h) can be used [43,296–298]. IV PPIs should be administered three times daily in the absence of correlative acid secretory testing as this dose will control acid hypersecretion in *all* patients [296].

Antitumor therapy

Surgical

Previously, the role of routine surgery for ZES cure was controversial, with some recommending that surgery should not be routinely performed because gastrinomas were frequently not found at surgery and cure was uncommon. In addition, many patients had negative preoperative imaging, and most patients with nonimaged or small gastrinomas had a good prognosis without surgery [299,300]. The situation changed with both the ENETS (2012) [16] and NANETS (2013) guidelines [6] as well as more recent expert reviews/series [2,3,95,225,252,301] and an upcoming NANETS pNET consensus (in press) recommending that sporadic ZES patients should routinely be considered for surgery unless they have some accompanying illness limiting life expectancy, inoperable disease, or their medical condition increases surgery risk. This recommendation is supported by results from a number of studies.

In an NIH prospective surgical study [79] of sporadic ZES patients (n = 123), the immediate postoperative cure rate was 51% and after 10 years 34% (see Figure 50.3a). Three other prospective studies [88,302,303] from NIH provided additional support for routine surgery, with one study [302] demonstrating that patients who underwent routine exploration had a lower incidence of developing liver metastases post resection (3% vs 23%, $p < 0.003$). A subsequent NIH study [303] with more patients (n = 160) and a longer follow-up (mean 12 years post resection) demonstrated that patients undergoing surgery had a better overall survival (15 years, 98% vs 74%, $p = 0.0002$); the survival advantage was disease related ($p = 0.0012$), due to less tumor progression, and fewer patients developed liver metastases (5% vs 29%, $p = 0.0002$).

Two studies have demonstrated that the development of liver metastases is the most important prognostic marker of long-term survival in ZES patients [27,28]. Neither of these studies was randomized, but in each case the comparative groups were well matched [83,301]. A third NIH study [88] specifically investigated the value of surgery in patients with preoperative negative imaging. In ZES patients (n = 58) with negative preoperative imaging (40% negative SRS), a gastrinoma was found in almost every patient (98%), and nearly 50% were cured (see Figure 50.3c,d). Improvement in the surgical success of finding and curing gastrinomas in sporadic ZES patients has occurred because of a number of factors. Particularly important is the appreciation that the majority of gastrinomas are small duodenal tumors that can only be found using procedures such as duodenotomy and duodenal transillumination [34,81,82,] (see Figure 50.3b); improved imaging; routine resection of lymph nodes because of the possibility of lymph node primaries [91,92]; and an understanding that patients with sporadic ZES have a different surgical outcome from those with MEN1/ZES [2,32,79,301] (see Figure 57.3a).

The surgical management of MEN1/ZES patients remains controversial. This has occurred because most studies demonstrate that these patients are rarely cured by the standard ZES operation involving local tumor resection/enucleation, and that cure is only potentially possible if a Whipple resection is performed, which is not routinely recommended [2,6,16,79,304] (see Figure 50.3a). This poorer outcome stems from the fact that MEN1/ZES patients almost invariably have multiple duodenal gastrinomas which are small (many <0.5 cm) and thus difficult to find at surgery, and >50% have metastatic lymph nodes at surgery [79,305–308]. The pancreatic NETs frequently visualized on preoperative imaging studies in MEN1/ZES patients are usually not gastrinomas (<15%) (mostly nonfunctional pNETs), and studies show that if preoperative imaging studies identify a tumor <2 cm, these patients have an excellent long-term prognosis; in fact, survival is not different from MEN1 patients without a pNET seen [2,7,305,309] (Figure 50.4d–f). For these reasons, the ENETS [6,13,225] and NANETS [16,226] guidelines for the treatment of pNETs in MEN1 patients recommend that MEN1/ZES patients with preoperative imaging studies demonstrating pNETs <2 cm in diameter should not undergo routine surgical exploration. These guidelines also recommend that when surgical exploration is performed, Whipple resections not be routinely undertaken [13,16].

Advanced metastatic disease

General

With increasingly effective medical control of gastric acid hypersecretion, the natural history of the gastrinoma itself is becoming the major determinant of long-term survival in ZES patients [3,27,28,171,174,310]. In older studies, gastrinomas were malignant in 60–90% and currently approximately one-third of patients present with metastatic disease, frequently in the liver, and because most are not cured surgically, an increasing proportion develop advanced metastatic disease over time [3,8,21,27,28,165,174,310]. Overall, 25% of sporadic ZES and 15% of MEN1/ZES patients have aggressive disease [27,28,164], and in 40% of patients with hepatic metastases, aggressive growth occurs [166]. As a result, currently one-half of ZES patients have tumor-related deaths [27].

A number of clinical, laboratory, and tumoral features in ZES patients are associated with a poor prognosis (see Table 50.7). Most important is the presence of any liver metastases (initially or their development) (see Figure 50.4a and Table 50.7). The 10-year survival of ZES patients with no liver metastases initially is 96%, with liver metastases limited to one hepatic lobe is 78%, and with diffuse liver metastases 16% (see Figure 50.4a) [327,28]. If liver metastases develop for the first time during follow-up, 10-year survival is decreased to 85% (see Figure 50.4a) [34]. However, the presence of lymph node metastases alone is only a weak predictor of poor prognosis, and was not predictive in a number of early studies (see Table 50.7) [27,28,165,311]. Other particularly important prognostic factors include the need for control of acid hypersecretion. The fact that duodenal and pancreatic gastrinomas are equally malignant (40–70% lymph node metastases) but not equally aggressive, with liver metastases present in 25–40% of pancreatic gastrinomas but in only 2% of duodenal gastrinomas, results in pancreatic gastrinomas having a worse prognosis

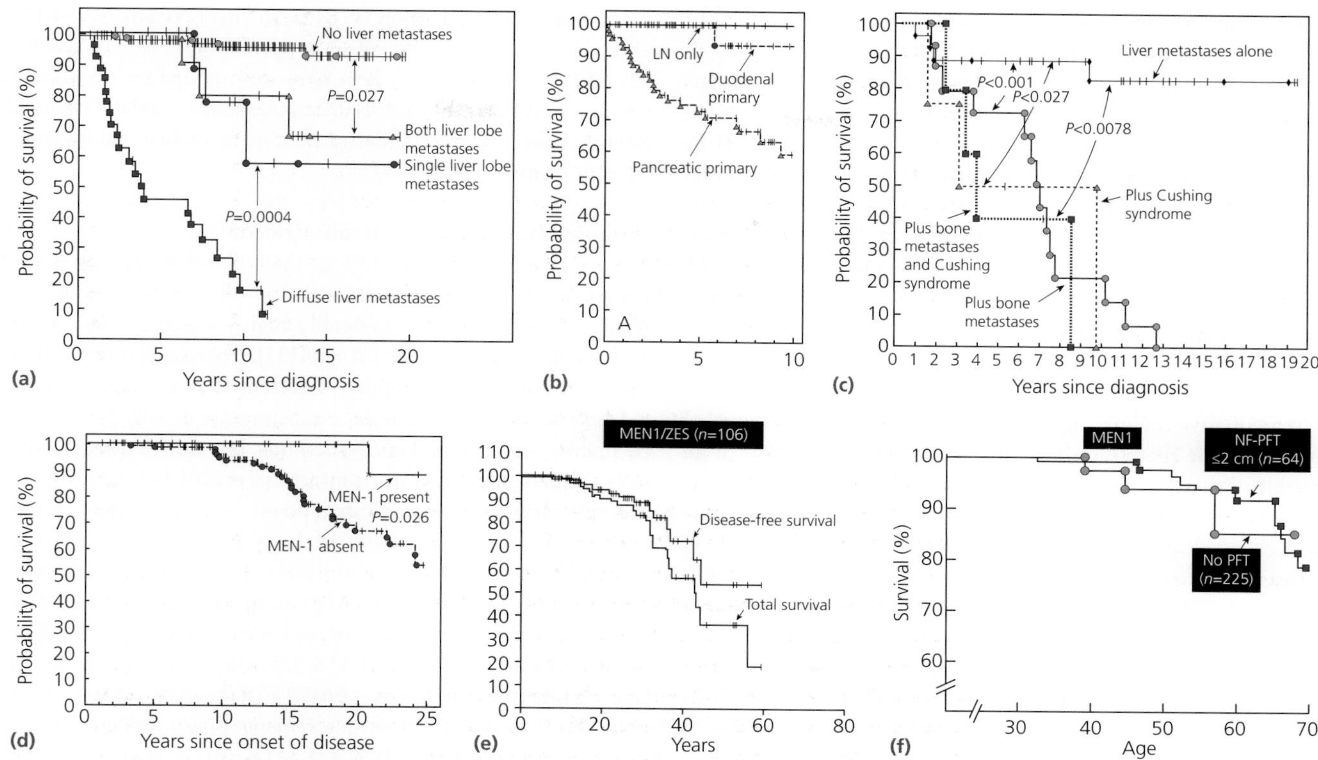

Figure 50.4 Effect on survival of disease extent, primary location, ectopic Cushing syndrome, bone metastases, or presence of multiple endocrine neoplasia type 1 syndrome (MEN1) in Zollinger–Ellison syndrome (ZES) patients. **(a)** The effect of increasing the extent of liver metastases on survival in 212 ZES patients. Data from [27]. **(b)** The difference in survival for ZES patients with a pancreatic primary (n = 20), duodenal primary gastrinoma (n = 42), or gastrinoma only in the lymph nodes (LN) (n = 24). Data from [28]. **(c)** The poor prognosis in ZES patients (n = 27) with liver metastases who develop Cushing syndrome (n = 4), bone metastases (n = 15), or both (n = 5). Data from [27]. **(d)** The difference in survival for ZES patients with (n = 34) or without MEN1 (n = 151). Data from [28]. **(e)** The long-term survival in 106 MEN1/ZES patients followed at the National Institutes of Health (NIH). Data from [174]. This survival is much better than that reported in 182 MEN1/ZES patients in the literature [174]. **(f)** The effect on survival of a nonfunctional pancreatic endocrine tumor (NF-PET) ≤2 cm (n = 64) in patients with MEN1 compared to MEN1 patients (n = 225) with no pancreatic neuroendocrine tumor (No-pNET). Data from [309]. This result, in addition to other studies showing very low cure rate and excellent long-term survival, lead to the North American Neuroendocrine Tumor Society (NANETS)/European Neuroendocrine Tumor Society (ENETS) recommendations not to routinely operate on MEN1 patients with or without ZES with small pNETs ≤2 cm [6,16,225,226,305].

(see Table 50.7 and Figure 50.4b) [7,27,28,165,310]. The development of ectopic Cushing syndrome (see Figure 50.4c) or bone metastases (see Figure 50.4c) has a particularly poor prognosis, with survival averaging only 1 year [27,106,263,312]. Other features of gastrinomas associated with a poor prognosis include advanced ENETS/WHO classification, higher ENETS/WHO grade, poor differentiation, other histological features, and rapid growth (see Table 50.7) [4,5,239]. It is important to recognize that these data are all relatively dated and with more modern systemic therapies, including PRRT (see below), all these results are likely to improve.

At present, depending on the extent of metastatic disease, rate of growth, and various histological features, a number of different treatments may be considered [2,6,16,313]. However, there is as yet no recognized algorithm for the approach to widely metastatic gastrinomas (or pNETs in general). Most authorities favor somatostatin analogs (SSAs) for first-line antitumor therapy and follow this when necessary with systemic agents (usually peptide receptor radiotherapy [PRRT], chemotherapy or small molecule therapy), without any specific approach being dominant. Liver-directed therapy is also frequently considered for patients with liver-dominant disease as liver failure is a common cause of patient demise even with widespread disease throughout the body.

The available modalities include cytoreductive surgery [2,8,239,305,313–319]; hepatic-directed therapies including embolization or chemoembolization [2,6,16,239,318,320–325], radioembolization [2,6,16,239,318,320,322,326–334], radiofrequency ablation (RFA), and other locally ablative techniques [2,6,16,239,317,318,320,335–341]; chemotherapy [2,6,16,239,318,320,332–346]; biotherapy with somatostatin analogs [2,6,16,239,256,318,320,347–349] or interferon [2,6,16,239,318,320,350–353]; liver transplantation [2,6,16,239,318,320,354–356]; targeted molecular therapies [2,6,16,239,318,320,357–360] including using mTOR inhibitors (everolimus) [2,6,16,182,183,239,318,320,360] or tyrosine kinase (TK) inhibitors (sunitinib) [2,6,16,239,318,320,360–364] and PRRT using radiolabeled somatostatin analogs [2,6,16,239,318,320,365–368]. In general, there are few specific studies that include only patients with advanced gastrinomas, and most studies have included patients with all pNETs, because of the low frequency of the individual pNET syndromes (see also Chapter 80). Whether all pNETs respond similarly is not clear and, as was mentioned above, the natural history of duodenal and pancreatic gastrinomas appears different. Below, gastrinoma-specific studies are mentioned in addition to the results of series containing pNETs with some gastrinomas.

Cytoreductive surgery

Cytoreductive (debulking) surgery or the systematic removal of all resectable metastatic disease is recommend if >90% of all visible disease is resectable and the patient is an adequate candidate [2,8,239,319,305,313–318]. Unfortunately, only 5–15% of all gastrinoma/pNET patients with metastatic liver disease fit into this category, as most have diffuse nonresectable metastases. Five-year survival rates after cytoreductive surgery are 70–80% and in many studies, the resected patients have increased survival [8,238,313–318,363–365]. Although this approach is generally recommended and included in the ENETS/NANETS [6,313,318] and other guidelines [320,322], there are no prospective studies that have proven its value, and almost all the retrospective studies contain some bias. However, recent data, not confined to gastrinomas, indicate that removal of as little as 70% of measurable disease may also lead to an improved outcome.

Liver-directed therapies

General

These therapies are reserved for patients with advanced metastatic disease in the liver who either have metastases limited to the liver or have liver-predominant disease, particularly in patients with functional syndromes that are not controlled by other means [313,318,321,322,325,326,337]. Liver-directed therapies can be considered as alternative methods of debulking and analogous to cytoreductive surgery. This approach has value as liver failure is the most common cause for demise in patients with widespread disease [313,318,369,370].

Radiofrequency ablation and other ablative therapies

Radiofrequency ablation and other ablative techniques (e.g., cryotherapy, ethanol injections) are administered either at surgery to ablate isolated metastases or by radiological techniques under guidance [239,317,335–341]. RFA involves using a probe that converts radiofrequency waves into heat, causing tissue destruction at temperature >60 °C [239,335,338]. Patient selection criteria differ between studies but general contraindications include too many lesions (>5–15), large lesions (>3.5–5.5 cm), or metastases near vital structures [318,320,321,336,338–341]. Response rates are 80–95% with durations of 2–3 years. Even though no prospective studies have established the value of RFA, in the ENETS, NANETS, and other recent guidelines [6,16,225, 226,239,313,318,322,337], RFA is recommended for antitumor therapy and can be used as a supplement to ablate isolated lesions at surgery or as palliative therapy to avoid a major surgical procedure.

Embolization and chemoembolization

Normal livers receive 20–25% of their blood supply from the hepatic artery and 75–80% from the portal vein, whereas metastatic pNETs, which are generally highly vascular, receive an arterial blood supply [239,321,325,335]. Therefore, interrupting the tumoral arterial supply preferentially affects metastases [239,321,325,335]. Arterial occlusions are usually performed by interventional radiological methods, but can be done at surgery and can be done alone (transarterial embolization [TAE]) or accompanied with chemotherapeutic agents (transarterial chemoembolization [TACE]) such as doxorubicin, cisplatin, 5-fluorouracil (5-FU), mitomycin C, or streptozotocin (STZ) [239,321,325,335]. TAE/TACE are most frequently accomplished by administering polyvinyl alcohol particles or gel-foam powder [239,321,323–325,335]. Contraindications include metastases involving >50–75% of the liver, portal venous occlusion, liver failure, poor performance status, and postsurgical biliary reconstruction [239,321,324,325,371]. A symptomatic response occurs in 60–100%, objective response in 25–85%, and the mean duration of response is 6–45 months [239,323–325,339]. Five-year survival rates for TAE/TACE are 20%–35% and the progression-free survival is 1.5 years [239,325,371]. TAE/TACE has a complication rate of 10%–85% in different studies, including most frequently a postembolization syndrome (pain, fever, nausea) [239,321,323,325,335,342]. The mortality is <6%; however, serious side-effects can occur including hepatic failure, abscess formation, gallbladder necrosis, and renal failure [321,323–325,335,372]. In general, liver-directed therapies are not recommended after Whipple operations because of these infection risks.

There are no prospective studies that have established the value of TAE/TACE; however, both NANETS and ENETS guidelines recommend TAE/ TACE be considered for palliative treatment in an experienced center if the patient has hepatic-only or hepatic-predominant disease that is not surgically resectable [6,225,313,319,373]. It is currently unknown whether adding chemotherapy to the embolotherapy is beneficial or not but the RETNET trial which is comparing TACE to TAE is currently accruing (a third arm of drug-eluting bead TACE [Deb TACE] was abandoned in this trial for lack of efficacy) [373].

Radioembolization or selective internal radiation therapy

Radioembolization (selective internal radiation therapy [SIRT]) is an alternative technique for the treatment of hepatic metastases from pNETs/NETs using ^{90}yttrium (^{90}Y)-labeled microspheres for radioembolization [2,6,16,239,318,320,322,326–334].

Initially, <600 patients had been treated using radioembolization [239,326–332,334,374,375] and because of this limited experience, it was considered experimental in the ENETS 2012 guidelines [313,318] but its use has increased in the last decade.

Two different types of ^{90}Y-microspheres are avaialable: ^{90}Y-glass microspheres (TheraSpheres®, Nodion, Canada) have a 20–30 µm diameter and a radioactive content of 2500 Bq/sphere, and ^{90}Y-resin microspheres (SIR® spheres, Sirtex Medical, Australia) are 20–60 µm in diameter and have 50 Bq/sphere [239,335,376,377]. Prior to their administration, the position of the catheter tip needs to be properly established so that microsphere administration does not enter the cystic or duodenal arteries, which can result in cholecystitis or ulceration, and the amount of lung shunting must be determined to avoid radiation pneumonitis [239,374,377]. Contraindications include the presence of excessive shunting to the lung/gastrointestinal tract, inadequate liver reserve and the inability to isolate the liver arterial tree from the gastric/small intestinal branches [239,374,376,378]. The main side-effects include postembolization syndrome (fever, nausea, vomiting, abdominal pain) (25–45%) and radiation-induced liver disease (<1%) [239,326,335,374,377]. Side-effects from radioembolization are reported to be milder than those from embolization/chemoembolization [239] but the delayed effects can be severe. The objective response rate varies from 12% to 90% with a mean rate of 55%, and stable disease is seen in 10–60% (mean 32%) [239,326,377]. The mean survival is 30 months and 50% of patients have symptomatic improvement in quality of life indices [238,328–330,377].

With the advent of PRRT (see below), many authorities are avoiding radioembolization so as not to end up with dose-limiting toxicity in the future if PRRT is required.

Medical treatment (see also Chapter 80)

Biotherapy

Somatostatin analogs

In addition to its ability to inhibit hormonal secretion, somatostatin inhibits the growth of pNETs and gastrointestinal NETs, both in vitro; and in vivo; in animal models, as well as in nonrandomized studies in patients, supporting a possible role for the treatment of advanced NETs (pNETs, gastrointestinal carcinoids) [239,256,318,347–350,379]. The exact molecular basis for this antiproliferative effect is not entirely clear, but SSAs inhibit the release of growth factors from NETs, have antiproliferative effects on neighboring cells (stromal, immune, vascular, etc.), and activate intracellular cascades that have antiproliferative effects (phosphatases, inhibition of adenylate cyclase, etc.) [256,348,349,380,381].

The utility of SSAs as antiproliferative agents in patients with pNETs/NETs was first demonstrated in a double-blind, randomized prospective study called the PROMID study (*P*lacebo-controlled, double-blind, *R*andomized study of the effect of *O*ctreotide LAR in control of tumor growth in patients with metastatic *MID*gut carcinoid tumors) [382]. In this study of 85 patients with advanced metastatic midgut carcinoids (none with ZES), the long-acting somatostatin analog octreotide LAR increased progression-free survival (PFS) (14.3 vs 6 months, $p < 0.000072$) [382]. The effect was only seen in patients with low hepatic tumor burden (<10%) and there was no change in overall survival, perhaps because of the study's low death rate [382]. A similar randomized, double-blind, prospective study with the long-acting somatostatin analog lanreotide-autogel, CLARINET, showed a similar positive effect. The CLARINET study (*C*ontrolled study of *L*anreotide *A*ntiproliferative-*R*esponse in *NET*s) involved 204 patients with metastatic, inoperative pNETs [383] (45% pNETs) with well/moderately differentiated nonfunctional GI-NETs (pNET, carcinoids) with <10% Ki67. At the end of the study after 2 years following the initiation of treatment, PFS was not reached with lanreotide compared to 18 months with placebo (hazard ratio 0.47, $p = 0.0002$). Furthermore, neither disease progression nor death occurred in 62% of lanreotide-treated patients compared to 22% for placebo.

The results of the PROMID [382] and CLARINET studies [383] are consistent with those of numerous uncontrolled studies in which SSAs were used to treat NETs/pNETs (including gastrinomas), where primarily a tumoristatic effect with growth stabilization was seen (only 10–15% show decreased tumor size) [256,318,347,349,350,380,381,384].

At present, treatment with SSAs has not been proven to extend survival in these patients but it is commonly used first line because it is generally well tolerated. Although 50% of patients develop some side-effects, they rarely lead to cessation of therapy [24,239,313,318, 347,349,350]. The most frequent mild side-effects include pain at the injection site and various gastrointestinal side-effects (<20%). More important but less frequent side-effects include elevation of blood sugar with the development or exacerbation of diabetes, steatorrhea, and the development of gallbladder sludge or stones (mean 29%), although only 1% develop symptomatic gallbladder disease [24,239,318,347,349,350]. It is for this reason that we generally recommend prophylactic cholecystectomy in all patients undergoing exploration. The US National Comprehensive Cancer Network (NCCN) guidelines [322,385] recommend that the use of somatostatin analogs be considered (level 2B evidence) in patients with locoregional unresectable pNETs.

Interferon

Interferons (primarily α-interferon) have effects similar to somatostatin analogs in controlling the symptoms of the hormone excess state in pNETs (gastrinomas)/gastrointestinal NETs (carcinoids), and have a predominantly tumoristatic effect on tumor size, causing primarily growth stabilization (30–85%) and only uncommonly a decrease in tumor size (<10–15%) [239,318,350–353,386]. In the only study of interferon limited to gastrinoma patients (13 patients with advanced metastatic progressive disease) [386], 46% of patients showed disease stabilization, and in 23% it lasted almost 2 years. The antiproliferative effect on pNETs/NETs of interferon is putatively mediated by blocking cell cycle progression in G1, inhibiting DNA synthesis, stimulating an increase in Bcl-2, inhibiting protein synthesis, inhibiting angiogenesis, and induction of apoptosis [350–353]. Interferon causes frequent side-effects (>70%) including flu-like symptoms (40– 80%), weight loss/anorexia (60%), and fatigue (51%), which frequently abate with continued treatment [318,350,352,353,386]. More serious side-effects include hyperlipidemia (31%), hepatotoxicity (31%), bone marrow toxicity, autoimmune disorders, particularly thyroid abnormalities, and uncommonly CNS toxicity [350,352,353,386].

The ENETS guidelines conclude that interferon treatment should be considered if the pNET is well differentiated, slowly proliferative, and somatostatin receptor negative; should be avoided if the pNET/NET is associated with a large tumor burden [313,318]; and the dose should be titrated to reduce the leukocyte count to <3000 [239,313,318,351–353]. This recommendation is made because treatment with SSAs is associated with fewer side-effects and thus should be considered first [318]. In the recent NANETS guidelines [225], while octreotide is ranked as a second-line therapy after everolimus/sunitinib, interferon is not even ranked as a possible therapy. The US NCCN guidelines [322,385] classify interferon use for antiproliferative activity as category 3 for metastatic pNETS/NETs, and recommend its use after SSAs or if a patient had hepatic-predominant metastases, and then only after embolization/radioembolization. Interferon has been used in combination with SSAs, frequently after patients with advanced metastatic disease failed other individual treatments; however, this use is controversial because a number of studies, including some randomized studies, do not show enhanced efficacy with the combination [239,350,352,387].

Chemotherapy

In contrast to gastrointestinal NETs (carcinoid), chemotherapy continues to play an important role in the treatment of patients with advanced metastatic gastrinomas and other pNETs [2,6,16,239,313,318,320,342–346,388]. The recommended chemotherapeutic regimens for the treatment of advanced pNET that are well differentiated (grade 1, 2) differ from those recommended for poorly differentiated tumors (grade 3) [239,313,342,343,346,388,389]. The previously recommended regimen for well-differentiated advanced pNET/gastrinomas is STZ/ doxorubicin with or without 5-FU [2,6,16,239,322,342,344–346,388,390]. STZ is a glycosamine-nitrourea derivative which was found to have cytotoxic effects on pancreatic islets [39], and since 1968 has been used for the treatment of patients with metastatic pNETs/gastrinomas [2,6,16,239,322,342,344–346,390]. The combination of STZ/doxorubicin (±5-FU) has an objective response rate of 20–45%, but complete responses are rare and the median response duration is only 5–20 months [2,6,16,239,322,342,344–346,388,390]. In patients with advanced gastrinomas only, the response rate varied from 5% to 40% [391,392]. Treatment with STZ/doxorubicin (±5-FU) is associated with significant toxicity, with 70–100% developing some side-effect [2,6,16,239,322,342,344–346,388,390–392]. The main side-effects are nausea/vomiting (70–100%), leukopenia, thrombocytopenia, hepatic functional abnormalities, and renal dysfunction (15–50%) including proteinuria (40–50%), decreased creatinine clearance, and occasionally renal failure [239,342,344,345,392].

Recently, the combination of temozolomide (TMZ)/capecitabine has shown promising results for the treatment of patients with advanced pNETs [238,346,388,393–396]. In a study of 30 patients with advanced pNETs [384], TMZ/capecitabine achieved a partial response rate of 70%, a 2-year survival of 92%, and a median PFS of 18 months. This high response rate is supported by results from other studies [388,393,395,396] and also by a study of the possible cellular basis of the enhanced responsiveness of pNETs over alimentary tract carcinoids to treatment with TMZ/capecitabine [396]. This study found a frequent deficiency of the DNA repair enzyme O^6-methyl-guanine DNA methyl transferase (MGMT) in many pNETs, in contrast to carcinoids, and MGMT deficiency correlated with sensitivity to the alkylating agent, TMZ [396]. Prospective trials are needed to confirm this high response rate but the regimen is well tolerated and is currently favored by most authorities after progression on SSA therapy (with PRRT, see below, as an alternative).

Poorly differentiated pNETs make up only 2–6.5% of all pNETs and are not typically seen with ZES; however, it is important that they be identified because they have an aggressive course, poor prognoses, and respond to different chemotherapeutic agents than the well-differentiated pNETs [239,313,337,346,389,397,398]. Poorly differentiated gastrinomas (WHO/ENETS, grade G3), like other pNETS with this grading/classification, are treated by a combination of etoposide either alone or in combination with other agents (vincristine, paclitaxel) [239,318,346,378,389,397–399]. The initial response rate to this chemotherapeutic regimen varies markedly in different series (14–80%) and the duration of response is usually <1 year [239,346,389,397,398]. This cisplatin-based regimen is associated with significant toxicity, particularly related to the gastrointestinal tract; this includes frequent vomiting and nausea, as well as renal toxicity and myelosuppression [239,389,397–400]. Even with chemotherapeutic treatment, the survival is only 3–16 months with 5-year survival <15% [239,346,389,397,398].

Molecular targeted therapies

mTor inhibitors (everolimus)

Numerous in vitro; and in vivo; studies of isolated pNET/NET cells have shown that the mTor cellular signaling cascade plays an important role in mediating cell growth [182,239,335,343,349,359,401–403]. mTor is a serine-threonine kinase critically involved in a variety of cellular functions including apoptosis, cell growth, and cell proliferation [357,359,401–403].

Two mTOR inhibitors have progressed in clinical development. Temsirolimus has been evaluated in phase II studies, and everolimus has been approved for treatment of advanced metastatic pNETs in the USA, Japan, and Europe after completing phase III trials [183,239,357,403,404]. The latter study [183] was a prospective randomized double-blind placebo-controlled study (RADIANT-1: *RAD*001 [everolimus] *i*n *a*dvanced *n*euroendocrine *t*umors) involving 410 patients with progressive metastatic pNETs. Everolimus treatment increased the number of patients with PFS at 18 months 3.7-fold (37% vs 9%), and yielded a significant overall improvement in PFS (11 vs 4.6 months, $p < 0.0001$) [183]. Everolimus treatment was associated with a twofold increase in adverse events, the majority being grade 1 or 2; however, grade 3 or 4 toxicity did occur in 2–7%, primarily hematological, gastrointestinal (diarrhea), stomatitis, or hyperglycemia [183]. Most side-effects were controlled by dose reduction or drug interruption [183].

Although approved for use in metastatic pNETs, at present there is no general agreement on when everolimus should be used in relation to the other treatments available for advanced metastatic pNETs. The NANETS US guidelines [370,225] list everolimus, similar to the TK inhibitor sunitinib, as a first-line treatment for well-differentiated advanced metastatic pNETs, whereas the ENETS European guidelines conclude that everolimus, similar to the TK inhibitor sunitinib, should be considered as first-line treatment in only selected cases [313,316]. The US NCCN guidelines [322,385] rank both everolimus and sunitinib as possible first-line treatments (category 2A), on the same level as cytotoxic chemotherapy for patients with progressive well-differentiated metastatic pNETs. At present, it is not established whether everolimus' ability to increase PFS will result in an increase in overall survival [239,404].

Tyrosine kinase receptor inhibitors (sunitinib)

Pancreatic neuroendocrine tumors usually possess multiple TK receptors [362,402,405,406] which have important effects on the growth of pNETS/NETs [239,318,326,349,362,363,407]. TK receptors comprise >20 families of transmembrane receptors that mediate the actions of a number of different growth factors that include the receptors for insulin-like growth factor 1 receptor (IGF1R), EGF receptor family (EGFRs), hepatocyte growth factor (c-Met), PDGF receptor family (PDGFRs), vascular endothial growth factor receptor family (VEGFRs), stem cell factor (c-Kit); and a number of others [239,363,402]. In various cells, including pNETS/carcinoids, activation of TK receptors is important in mediating angiogenesis, cell growth, cell differentiation, and apoptosis [239,362,363,402].

A number of different TK inhibitors have antigrowth effects on pNETs/NETs in both in vitro; and in vivo; studies [239,362,363,402,408]; however, only sunitinib is approved (in the USA, Japan, and Europe) for use in patients with advanced pNETs [239,361,404,408]. Sunitinib (Sutent®, SU11248) is an orally active inhibitor of a number of TK receptors, including VEGFR-1, PDGFRs, VEGFR-2, FLT-3, and c-Kit [360–362]. Sunitinib was shown to have antiproliferative activity against pNETS in both phase II [364,407,408] and phase III studies [361]. In a phase III double-blind randomized placebo-controlled prospective study of 171 patients with progressive metastatic pNETs [358], sunitinib treatment increased PFS 2.5-fold (11.4 vs 4.5 months, $p < 0.001$), objective tumor response (9% vs 0%, $p = 0.007$), and overall survival [361]. Sunitinib treatment was associated with a threefold increase in side-effects, with most being grade 1 or 2, although some grade 3 and 4 toxicity occurred [361]. The most frequent, severe side-effects were neutropenia (12%) and hypertension (9.6%) [361]. A quality of life analysis [361] showed sunitinib did not have a significant effect, with most side-effects able to be managed by dose reduction and/or temporary cessation of treatment.

The ENETS guidelines [313,318] conclude that sunitinib, similar to everolimus, represents a novel therapeutic option but it should not be used as first-line therapy. The recent NANETS guidelines [225] recommend sunitinib and everolimus as primary options for the treatment of patients with progressive metastatic pNETs, ahead of cytotoxic chemotherapy and embolization/chemoembolization/octreotide LAR. Similarly, the US NCCN [322,385] guidelines, and a recent review of treatment of patients with metastatic well-differentiated pNETs [335], list sunitinib, as well as everolimus, as first-line treatment options.

Peptide receptor radiotherapy using radiolabeled somatostatin analogs

The fact that >90% of gastrinomas/other pNETs (excluding insulinomas) overexpress or ectopically express at least one of the five classes of somatostatin receptors (sst1–5) led to the development of peptide receptor radiotherapy (PRRT) using radiolabeled somatostatin analogs to deliver receptor-directed cytotoxicity [239,256,365–368,409]. Two different isotopes have been used in most studies: ^{90}yttrium (^{90}Y)- and ^{177}lutetium (^{177}Lu)-labeled SSAs [239,365–368,409]. ^{177}Lu emits β-particles and γ-rays, has a maximum tissue penetration of 2 mm, and a half-life of 6.7 days, whereas ^{90}Y strongly emits β-particles, has a maximal tissue penetration of 12 mm, and a half-life of 2.7 days [365–368,409].

A number of different synthetic SSAs have been used, with the most frequent being octreotide or octreotate coupled to the radiolabel by different chelators, including diethylene triamine pentaacetic acid (DTPA) and 1,4,7,10-tetraazaacyclododecane-1,4,7,10-tetraacetic acid (DOTA) [239,365,366,368]. Of 440 patients (10 studies) with various malignant NETs, including gastrinomas, treated with ^{90}Y-labeled SSAs, complete tumor remission was rare (0– 6%), partial remission occurred in 7–37%, and tumor stabilization in 40–86% [24,239,365,366,368]. Of 510 patients with malignant NETs treated with ^{177}Lu-[DOTA^0, Tyr^3] octreotate, a complete response occurred in 2%, partial response in 28%, and tumor stabilization in 35% [367,410]. With ^{177}Lu-[DOTA^0, Tyr^3] octreotate, a number of prognostic factors were identified which predicted a poor outcome after PRRT, which included the presence of progressive metastatic disease prior to treatment, Karnofsky performance score of ≤70, no tumor response to PRRT, weight loss at the time of treatment, presence of bone metastases, extensive liver involvement, poor uptake of the radiolabeled analog by the tumor and the presence of malignant gastrinoma, vasoactive intestinal polypeptide-secreting tumor, or insulinoma [239,365–368,410,411]. Gastrinomas are one of the malignant pNET/NETs that were most responsive to PRRT (42% at 3 months); however, they also had one of the highest recurrence rates, leading to a poorer overall prognosis in comparison with other primary sites [239,365–368,410,411]. In one detailed study of 11 patients with metastatic ZES [412] treated with either ^{90}Y- and/or ^{177}Lu-labeled somatostatin analogs, the mean serum gastrin decreased by 81%, complete response occurred in 9%, partial tumor response in 45%, tumor stabilization in 45%, and in 64% the antitumor effect persisted for a median period of 14 months.

Peptide receptor radiotherapy with ^{177}Lu-[DOTA^{0}, Tyr^{3}] octreotate has now been approved for routine use in both Europe and the USA. FDA approval in 2018 was based on a single, double-blind, randomized, controlled trial of Lu-177 dotatate versus high-dose cold octreotide in patients with progressive metastatic well-differentiated small bowel NETs, the NETTER-1 trial [413], and a systematic review of selected retrospective data in a subset of 1214 patients (360 for efficacy and 811 for safety, deemed eligible for inclusion by the FDA) who were treated at a single center in Europe (Erasmus Medical Center, Rotterdam, The Netherlands). The latter cohort included primary tumors other than the small bowel including some gastrinomas. The NETTER-1 trial demonstrated an improvement of PFS for ^{177}Lu-DOTATATE compared to the control arm (8.4 months for the control arm vs not reached for ^{177}Lu-DOTATATE; hazard ratio [HR] 0.21, 95% confidence interval [CI] 0.13–0.33), which was a significant improvement over any other form of systemic therapy. Objective response rate with ^{177}Lu-DOTATATE was 18%, versus 3% with high-dose octreotide [413]. Preliminary analysis of overall survival (OS) demonstrated a HR of 0.4 ($p = 0.004$) favoring ^{177}Lu-DOTATATE; final OS is still pending. Analysis of health-related quality of life demonstrated that ^{177}Lu-DOTATATE significantly delayed decline in clinically relevant endpoints such as global health, physical functioning, role functioning, and in symptoms such as pain, fatigue, and diarrhea [413].

While older guidelines such as ENETS 2012, NANETS 2010 and 2013, and ESMO all previously considered PRRT an investigational treatment [6,225,226,313,370,414], most authorities now consider PRRT as second-line therapy in patients with SSA-avid metastatic disease (together with chemotherapy – see above). This approach has been termed "theranostics," indicating utilization of the same ligand, somatostatin, for diagnosis (SRS) and treatment (PRRT). NANETS and the Society for Nuclear Medicine and Molecular Imaging (SNMMI) have collaborated on two guidelines for PRRT, a "how to do it" manuscript [415] and a "who to do it in" manuscript, which is still in press.

Most PRRT side-effects are mild and do not require treatment to be stopped [239,365,366,368,409]. The most frequent acute side-effects are vomiting, pain, and nausea (30%) and the most serious side-effects include liver toxicity (0.6%), hematological toxicity (0.8% develop a myelodysplastic disorder, 15% acute toxicity), and renal toxicity, with the latter occurring primarily in patients receiving ^{90}Y-labeled SSAs [239,365,366,368,409–411].

Liver transplantation

In contrast to the situation with most other neoplasms, liver transplantation continues to be used in management of some patients with metastatic, unresectable, hepatic metastases [239,313,354–356,378,416–419]. In a summary [356] of 213 cases of NET/pNETs (94 pNETs) who underwent liver transplantation in Europe, the 5-year survival was 52% and the disease-free survival was 32%. These results are similar to those from 150 liver transplants performed in patients with metastatic NETs in the USA reported from the United Network for Organ Sharing Database [354], where the 1-, 3-, and 5-year survival rates were 81%, 65%, and 49%, respectively, with a similar survival for pNETs and gastrointestinal NETs (carcinoids). In the European study [356], the most important prognostic factors for a poor outcome were poorly differentiated tumor, hepatomegaly, and the occurrence of a major resection in addition to the liver transplantation. When these three factors were taken into consideration in the selection of patients, the overall survival at 5 years increased to 59% [356]. In other studies, additional risk factors associated with a poor outcome have been reported to include primary NET in the duodenum or a pNET, the presence of extrahepatic metastases at the time of the transplant, an accompanying upper abdominal exenteration, extensive liver involvement (>50%), and certain histological features such as a Ki-67 proliferative index >10% or abnormal E-cadherin staining [239,354,417,418,420].

The ENETS guidelines [313,318] conclude that liver transplantation should be considered only for providing palliative care, and thus be reserved for patients suffering life-threatening hormonal effects refractory to other treatments or for selected patients with unresectable nonfunctional NETs/pNETs refractory to all other treatments. If liver transplantation is considered, important selection criteria include the presence of a well-differentiated NET/pNET; patient age <45–50 years; a Ki-67 index of <10%; the absence of extrahepatic metastases as determined using the most sensitive methodology (^{68}Ga-labeled somatostatin analogs and PET imaging); the absence of other resections at the time of liver transplantation; and some groups consider various histological features such as E-cadherin tumor staining characteristics [239,313,318,337,417,418].

References are available at www.yamadagastro.com/textbook7e

Further reading

Batukbhai B.D.O., de Jesus-Acosta A. The molecular and clinical landscape of pancreatic neuroendocrine tumors. Pancreas 2019;48:9.

Desai H., Borges-Neto S., Wong T.Z. Molecular imaging and therapy for neuroendocrine tumors. Curr Treat Options Oncol 2019;20:78.

Falconi M., Eriksson B., Kaltsas G., et al., Vienna Consensus Conference Participants. ENETS consensus guidelines update for the management of patients with functional pancreatic neuroendocrine tumors and non-functional pancreatic neuroendocrine tumors. Neuroendocrinology 2016;103:153.

Hope T.A., Abbott A., Colucci K., et al. NANETS/SNMMI procedure standard for somatostatin receptor-based peptide receptor radionuclide therapy with (177)Lu-DOTATATE. J Nucl Med 2019;60:937.

Inzani F., Petrone G., Rindi G. The new World Health Organization classification for pancreatic neuroendocrine neoplasia. Endocrinol Metab Clin North Am 2018;47(3):463.

Jensen R.T., Cadiot G., Brandi M.L., et al. ENETS consensus guidelines for the management of patients with digestive neuroendocrine neoplasms: functional pancreatic endocrine tumor syndromes. Neuroendocrinology 2012;95:98.

Kunz P.L., Reidy-Lagunes D., Anthony L.B., et al. North American Neuroendocrine Tumor Society consensus guidelines for the management and treatment of neuroendocrine tumors. Pancreas 2013;42:557.

Metz D.C., Cadiot G., Poitras P., etal. Diagnosis of Zollinger–Ellison syndrome in the era of PPIs, faulty gastrin assays, sensitive imaging and limited access to acid secretory testing. Int J Endocr Oncol 2017;4:167.

Pavel M., Baudin E., Couvelard A., et al. ENETS consensus guidelines for the management of patients with liver and other distant metastases from neuroendocrine neoplasms of foregut, midgut, hindgut, and unknown primary. Neuroendocrinology 2012;95:157.

Raj N., Fazio N., Strosberg J. Biology and systemic treatment of advanced gastroenteropancreatic neuroendocrine tumors. Am Soc Clin Oncol Educ Book 2018;38:292.

CHAPTER 51

Gastritis and gastropathy

Mary Kay Washington and Richard M. Peek Jr
Vanderbilt University Medical Center, Nashville, TN, USA

Chapter menu

Definition

Gastritis is defined as microscopic inflammation of the stomach and represents a histological, not a clinical entity; of interest, the majority of persons harboring gastric inflammation are completely asymptomatic. Many etiological agents can induce gastritis, but the most common cause is infection by *Helicobacter pylori*, a bacterium that resides in the mucus gel layer overlaying the gastric mucosa [1]. Barry Marshall and Robin Warren were awarded the Nobel Prize in Medicine in 2005 as the first investigators to identify and culture these spiral bacilli from gastric tissue of patients with chronic gastritis [1,2]. Since that time, a strong link has been established between *H. pylori* and a diverse spectrum of gastroduodenal diseases, including gastric and duodenal ulceration, gastric adenocarcinoma, mucosa-associated lymphoid tumor (MALToma), and non-Hodgkin lymphoma of the stomach (Figure 51.1) [1]. *H. pylori* colonizes the stomach for years or decades, not days or weeks as is usually the case for other bacterial pathogens, and this organism virtually always induces chronic gastritis; however, only a fraction of *H.pylori*-colonized individuals ever develop disease. Identification of mechanisms that regulate *H. pylori*–host interactions will not only improve diagnostic and therapeutic modalities, but also provide insights into other diseases that arise within the context of pathogen-initiated inflammatory states, such as chronic viral hepatitis and hepatocellular carcinoma. In addition to *H. pylori*, other pathogens and exogenous agents that induce gastric inflammation and gastropathy will be discussed in this chapter.

Classification of gastritis using the Sydney system

The most widely used method for classification of gastritis and reporting of nonneoplastic gastric biopsies in the research setting is the updated Sydney system [3], which classifies chronic gastritis based on topography, morphology, and etiology

Yamada's Textbook of Gastroenterology, Seventh Edition. Edited by Timothy C. Wang, Michael Camilleri, Benjamin Lebwohl, Anna S. Lok, William J. Sandborn, Kenneth K. Wang, and Gary D. Wu.

Companion website: www.yamadagastro.com/textbook7e

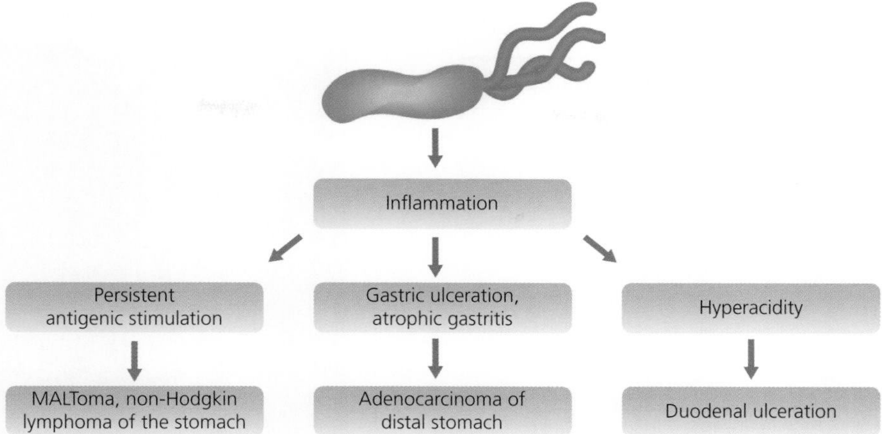

Figure 51.1 Disease outcomes that develop within the context of *H. pylori*-induced gastric inflammation. Source: Based on Amieva, M., and Peek, R. M. (2016). Pathobiology of Helicobacter pylori–Induced Gastric Cancer. Gastroenterology, 150(1), 64–78.

(Table 51.1). More recently, a system of staging gastritis, the Operative Link for Gastritis Assessment (OLGA), has been proposed. The OLGA system incorporates the updated Sydney system biopsy mapping protocol but includes more detailed assessment of glandular atrophy, with the goal of providing increased information about gastric cancer risk [4].

Biopsy protocol

The Sydney system requires histological sampling with separate submission of biopsies from five locations in the stomach: the greater and lesser curvature in the antrum, the greater and lesser curvature of the corpus, and the incisura. The incisura is a typical site for atrophy, intestinal metaplasia, and dysplasia [3], although some data suggest that biopsies from endoscopically normal incisura add little additional clinical information [5]. Histological features assessed on a 0 to 4+ scale include *H. pylori* density, neutrophil infiltration, mononuclear cell infiltration, atrophy, and intestinal metaplasia. A series of diagrams illustrating the scoring is available to assist in standardizing histopathological grading [3]. Additional features assessed as present or absent but not otherwise graded are surface epithelial damage, lymphoid follicles, and foveolar hyperplasia. Other findings such as granulomas are noted when present. The final diagnosis represents a synthesis of individual histological findings, topographical location, and available clinical information.

While the Sydney and OLGA systems are useful for research purposes, in clinical practice, failure to obtain the specified numbers of biopsies from the various regions of the stomach and the complexity of the scoring systems limit their widespread use.

Histological features of chronic gastritis

Three patterns of chronic nonspecific gastritis are recognized: (1) diffuse antral gastritis (nonatrophic gastritis in the Sydney system), which is associated with *H. pylori* infection; (2) multifocal atrophic gastritis, which is also highly associated with *H. pylori*; and (3) diffuse corporal atrophic gastritis (autoimmune gastritis).

Nonatrophic chronic gastritis

In the nonatrophic chronic gastritis associated with *H. pylori* infection, a diffuse chronic inflammatory infiltrate, composed of lymphocytes, plasma cells, and scattered eosinophils and mast cells, is present in the lamina propria. The density of this infiltrate is variable and tends to be sparser in atrophic gastritis. The presence of lymphoid aggregates (Figure 51.2), especially with germinal centers, is highly associated with *H. pylori* colonization and may persist after eradication of infection. The presence of neutrophils indicates an "active" gastritis and is often associated with *H. pylori* organisms in the nearby superficial epithelium. Neutrophils infiltrate gastric glandular epithelium, typically in the neck area of the gland, and may form "pit abscesses" (Figure 51.3). The foveolar epithelium often shows degenerative changes, and superficial erosions may be seen. Mucosal edema and hyperemia are common but nonspecific findings, and there is poor correlation between endoscopic and histological findings [6]. *H. pylori* organisms are generally readily identifiable on routine hematoxylin and eosin-stained slides in the superficial mucus layer and extend into the lumen of the gastric pits (Figure 51.4).

Multifocal atrophic gastritis

In atrophic gastritis, specialized glands are lost, such as chief and parietal cells in the gastric corpus and deep mucinous glands in the antrum, and are replaced by metaplastic epithelium or by fibrous tissue. Multifocal atrophic gastritis (MAG) involves both the gastric antrum and corpus and, while patchy in distribution, often begins at the incisura, which notably represents a hotspot for gastric cancer occurrence. However, atrophic gastritis may be extensive instead of patchy, forming continuous sheets in stomachs containing intestinal-type gastric adenocarcinoma. Intestinal metaplasia, in which the

Table 51.1 Classification of chronic gastritis based on topography, morphology, and etiology (updated Sydney system).

Type of gastritis	Etiology	Synonymous terms
Nonatrophic chronic gastritis	*H. pylori*	Chronic superficial gastritis
	? Other factors	Diffuse antral gastritis Chronic antral gastritis Type B gastritis
Atrophic gastritis		
Autoimmune gastritis	Autoimmunity ? *H. pylori*	Type A gastritis Diffuse corporal gastritis
		Pernicious anemia-associated gastritis
Multifocal atrophic gastritis	*H. pylori*	Type B or type AB gastritis
	Environmental factors	Atrophic pangastritis
Special forms of gastritis		
Reactive gastropathy	NSAIDs Bile reflux Other chemical irritation	Chemical gastropathy Reflux gastropathy
Radiation	Radiation injury	
Lymphocytic	? Gluten	Celiac disease associated
	? Autoimmune mechanisms	Varioliform
	Drugs	
	? *H. pylori*	
	? Idiopathic	
Noninfectious granulomatous gastritis	Crohn's disease Sarcoidosis	Isolated granulomatous gastritis
	Foreign substances	
	? Idiopathic	
Eosinophilic gastritis	Food sensitivity ? Other allergies	Allergic
Collagenous gastritis	Unknown ? Autoimmune	
Other infectious gastritides	Bacteria, other than *H. pylori*	Phlegmonous gastritis Emphysematous gastritis
	Viruses	Cytomegalovirus
	Fungi	
	Parasites	Anisakiasis

NSAIDs, nonsteroidal antiinflammatory drugs.
Source: Data from Dixon et al. 1996 [3].

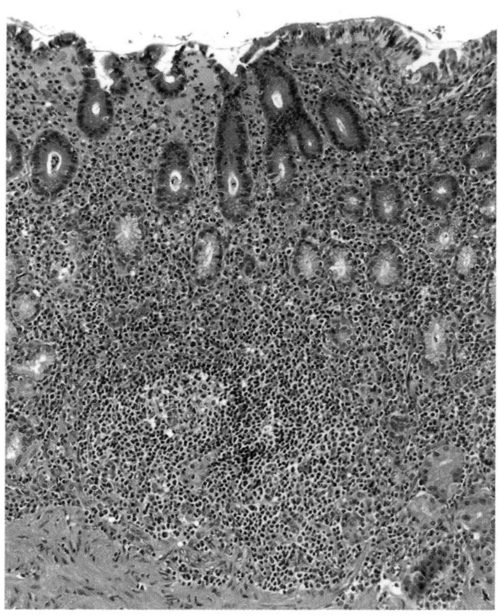

Figure 51.2 Lymphoid aggregates are common findings in *H. pylori*-induced gastritis. The lamina propria contains a mixed inflammatory infiltrate of plasma cells, lymphocytes, neutrophils, and eosinophils.

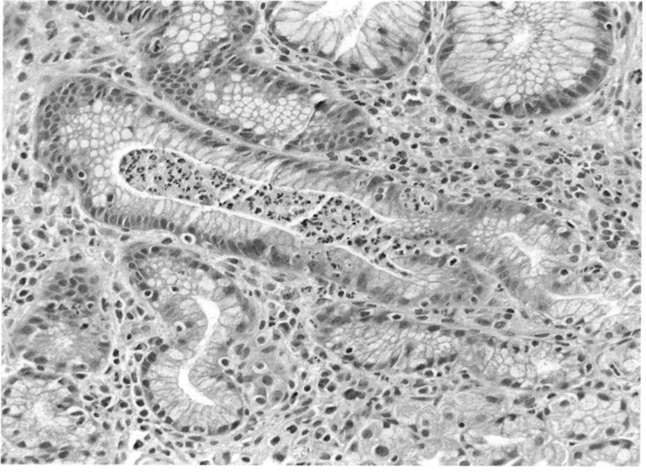

Figure 51.3 Neutrophils infiltrating in the lamina propria and foveolar epithelium and forming pit abscesses are characteristic of *H. pylori*-induced gastritis.

gastric mucosa is replaced by mucosa resembling the small or large intestine, is common in MAG (Figure 51.5). The oxyntic glands of the corpus are replaced by mucinous glands resembling antral mucosa, a change known as pseudopyloric metaplasia, antralization, or spasmolytic peptide-expressing metaplasia (SPEM) [7], making it difficult to distinguish corpus from gastric antrum. Endocrine cell hyperplasia secondary to hypergastrinemia is common, although partial loss of

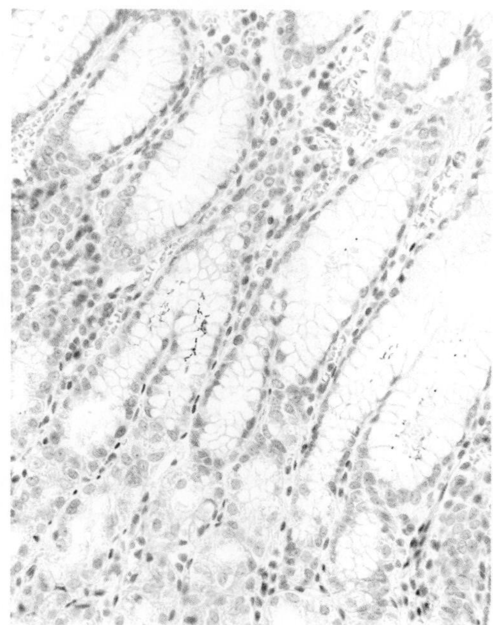

Figure 51.4 *H. pylori* organisms are found in the surface mucous layer and extending into the lumen of the gastric pits (immunohistochemistry).

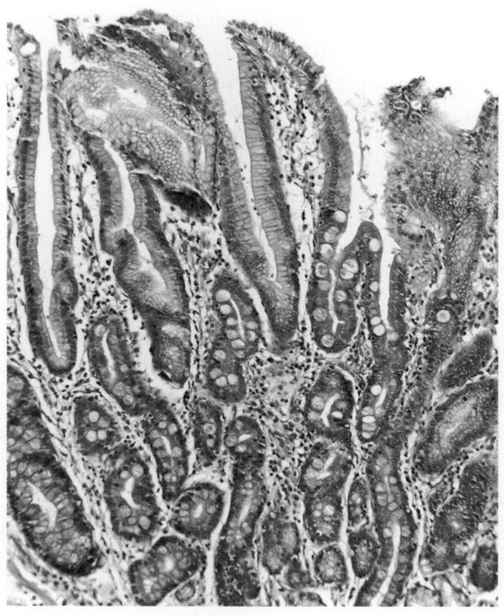

Figure 51.5 Multifocal atrophic gastritis and intestinal metaplasia involving the gastric corpus, showing patchy loss of oxyntic glands and intestinal metaplasia.

antral G cells may prevent significant gastrin elevations in many patients. As gastric acid production falls in atrophic gastritis, *H. pylori* organisms colonize more sparsely and are more difficult to detect.

Diffuse corporal atrophic gastritis (autoimmune gastritis)

The hallmark of this pattern of gastritis is the destruction of oxyntic glands. Atrophic gastritis is confined to the corpus and involves the antrum only minimally (see section on Autoimmune gastritis).

Epidemiology of *Helicobacter pylori*-induced gastritis

Helicobacter pylori colonizes the stomachs of at least half of the world's population and people in all geographic regions have been shown to carry the bacteria [8]. Infection is usually acquired in childhood and, when left untreated, persists for the lifetime of the host. The prevalence of *H. pylori* is higher in developing than developed countries. In the United States, *H. pylori* is present in 10–15% of children under 12 years of age compared with 50–60% of people older than 60 years [9]. The rate of acquisition of new *H. pylori* infections among adults in developed countries is less than 1% per year, and most carriers in the US acquired *H. pylori* during childhood. Over the past half-century, however, progressively fewer children have been shown to carry *H. pylori* [10].

Risk factors for *H. pylori* acquisition include lower socioeconomic status and household crowding, and colonization rates reflect country of origin and ethnicity [10]. Colonization is related to intrafamilial clustering but not to the presence of nonprimate reservoirs, favoring person-to-person transmission as the mode of initial infection. Experimental induction of regurgitation and catharsis increases *H. pylori* culture positivity rates from vomitus and diarrheal specimens [11], suggesting that *H. pylori* transmission rates may increase during childhood episodes of gastroenteritis and occurs via a fecal–oral route.

Gastric colonization

Helicobacter pylori has evolved several mechanisms to elude primary host defenses such as gastric acidity and peristalsis, in order to establish persistent infection within the stomach. *H. pylori* resides within the gastric mucus, which contains a pH gradient ranging from 7.2 to 2. *H. pylori* is considered to be a neutralophile and can replicate at a pH of 5 and survive at a pH of 4. One pH-manipulating mechanism utilized by *H. pylori* is production of urease, and isolates that cannot produce urease fail to colonize animal models of infection or survive at pH levels less than 4 [12,13], indicating that urease is a necessary factor for establishment of infection. *H. pylori* cytoplasmic urease produces ammonia via hydrolysis of urea, thereby increasing the pH of the environment. Urease activity is tightly linked to cytoplasmic urea uptake, which is mediated by a pH-dependent urea channel encoded by *ureI* [14].

To facilitate locomotion within gastric mucus and to counteract peristalsis, *H. pylori* possesses between one and five polar flagella. As is the case for urease production, bacterial motility is required for persistent infection [15]. Approximately 20% of the *H. pylori* population in the stomach bind to gastric epithelial cells, and adhesion is important for acquisition of nutrients, such as iron, from the host and for resistance to shedding of the mucus gel layer. Several cognate *H. pylori* and host ligands have been identified, including three outer membrane proteins (BabA, SabA, HopQ) that bind Lewis^b, sialyl-Lewis^x, and CEACAM proteins, respectively [16–19].

Histopathological studies in human subjects have shown that *H. pylori* binds to specific regions of gastric epithelium, and that bacterial density is greatest in the upper portion of the gastric glands. However, using state-of-the-art microscopy techniques, Sigal et al. identified foci of replicating *H. pylori* adjacent to progenitor and stem cell niches within gastric glandular units [20,21]. Thus, the host seems to have evolved mechanisms to restrict *H. pylori* to certain microniches within the gastric mucosa.

Helicobacter pylori can also limit the bactericidal effects of proinflammatory molecules, such as nitric oxide. *H. pylori* expresses an enzyme, arginase, which siphons the nitric oxide substrate L-arginine away from inducible nitric oxide synthase (iNOS), limiting the production of iNOS-generated nitric oxide [22]. Another level of host defense circumvented by *H. pylori* is innate immunity. Toll-like receptors (TLRs) are a conserved family of host receptors that function in innate immunity via recognition of invariant regions in bacterial molecules termed pathogen-associated molecular patterns. *H. pylori* avoids global activation of this system as *H. pylori* lipopolysaccharide (LPS) and flagellin are relatively anergic compared with LPS and flagellins of other enteric bacteria [23–25]. *H. pylori* can also actively suppress the adaptive immune response [26] and survive within epithelial cells and macrophages [27,28]. However, despite these strategies that facilitate persistence, substantial immune activation still occurs as evidenced by proinflammatory cytokine release, infiltration of the mucosa by inflammatory cells, and cellular and humoral recognition of *H. pylori* antigens.

Development of *H. pylori*-induced gastric inflammation

The gastric inflammatory response induced by *H. pylori* consists of neutrophils, dendritic cells, lymphocytes, plasma cells, and macrophages, along with varying degrees of epithelial cell degeneration and injury (see Figures 51.2 and 51.3), and the most distinctive feature of *H. pylori*-induced gastritis is infiltration of the gastric epithelium by neutrophils. Within the lamina propria, polymorphonuclear cells are admixed with lymphocytes, lymphoid follicles, plasma cells, and eosinophils, and the severity of gastritis is greatest in the superficial portions of the lamina propria. *H. pylori* colonization also induces an exuberant systemic and mucosal humoral response directed at multiple antigens; however, antibody production does not result in eradication.

Dendritic cells (DCs) are strategically positioned within the gastric mucosa to sample both self and *H. pylori* antigens, are primary responders to *H. pylori* products, and can subsequently differentiate into antigen-presenting cells (APCs) [29]. An alternate mechanism of DC activation was reported by Nagai et al., who demonstrated that *H. pylori* in a coccoid form could become phagocytosed by DCs present within Peyer's patches in the small intestine of mice, which mediated the proximal gastric inflammatory response [30]. Following activation, DCs activate T cells in different ways, being capable of inducing either a Th1 or Th2/regulatory T cell (Treg) response; thus the nature of DC interactions with other immune cells is a major determinant of the characteristics of the adaptive immune response [29].

Gastric lymphocyte populations from *H. pylori*-infected patients contain an increased number of γ-interferon (IFN)-producing T cells, consistent with a Th1 cytokine response [31], and *H. pylori*-specific T-cell clones derived from gastric mucosa have a Th1 profile in patients with peptic ulcer disease. Because of the consistent identification that, similar to Crohn's disease, *H. pylori* infection induces a Th1-skewed response, this reaction is considered to be a cause of pathological inflammation, and is atypical for a pathogen that is predominantly noninvasive. However, evidence suggests that Th1-mediated responses are of value to the host in regulating infection, and that the actual defect is that the response is not vigorous enough to eliminate the pathogen. Murine studies have demonstrated that an insufficient Th1 response is associated with increased bacterial colonization, suggesting that the development of a strong Th1 response can attenuate *H. pylori* colonization. However, there is also evidence that adoptive transfer of $CD4^+$ T cells from mice that lack IFN-γ production and Th1 differentiation into immunodeficient SCID mice still results in gastritis. These findings indicate that other T-cell populations are important in pathogenesis and persistence of inflammation.

Interleukin (IL)-17 has been linked to neutrophil infiltration and IL-17 levels are increased in *H. pylori*-infected human and mouse gastritis tissues. Immunization of mice with *H. pylori* lysates enhances IL-17 expression in the gastric mucosa and in $CD4^+$ T cells isolated from spleens and cocultured with *H. pylori*-pulsed DCs or macrophages, and these findings are associated with increased gastric inflammation but decreased colonization, suggesting that the IL-17/Th17 response may be defective in a normal host, thereby contributing to chronic persistence of the bacterium [32].

Along with IL-17-producing T cells, Tregs have been implicated in the pathogenesis of *H. pylori* infection. *H. pylori*-infected individuals have increased gastric mucosal levels of $CD4^+CD25^{high}$ T cells that express *FOXP3*, a gene involved in the development of Tregs. There are also a higher number of $CD4^+CD25^{high}$ T cells in *H. pylori*-associated gastric adenocarcinoma tissues than in adjacent tissue. *H. pylori*-infected persons with peptic ulceration have significantly fewer gastric Tregs but increased Th1 and Th2 responses compared to infected subjects without ulcers [33], suggesting that imbalances within the Treg cellular network may predispose to diseases that develop within the context of *H. pylori* infection. Collectively, these data are consistent with a model in which an inappropriate host T-cell response towards an extracellular pathogen, *H. pylori*, facilitates the development and chronicity of gastric inflammation.

Clinical presentation and natural history

Patterns of *H. pylori*-induced gastritis and disease outcome

There is a distinct dichotomy between *H. pylori*-induced duodenal ulceration and gastric cancer, and this is dependent on the topography of inflammation within the stomach. In the majority of infected persons residing in developed countries, *H. pylori*-induced gastritis is more severe in the gastric antrum, with only minimal involvement of the corpus, a pattern termed "diffuse antral gastritis" or "nonatrophic chronic gastritis." Gastric atrophy and intestinal metaplasia are typically absent in this type of gastritis. Persons with such corpus-sparing inflammation are at increased risk for duodenal ulcer disease, and gastric acid production in this population is either normal or increased. In contrast, those who progress to gastric ulcer disease and distal gastric adenocarcinoma have a different pattern of gastritis – involvement not only of the antrum but also the acid-secreting corpus – and, as predicted, patients with pangastritis tend to have reduced acid outputs. Corpus gastritis is often accompanied by gastric atrophy and intestinal metaplasia, in both the antrum and the corpus. This pattern of gastric inflammation is most common among infected people residing in Southeast Asia, South America, and certain regions of central, eastern, and southern Europe [34].

Helicobacter pylori virulence factors and gastric injury

Helicobacter pylori strains from different individuals are extremely diverse and genetically unique derivatives of a single strain are present simultaneously within an individual human host [35]. The *cag* pathogenicity island (*cag* PAI) is a well-characterized and intensively studied strain-specific *H. pylori* virulence determinant (Figure 51.6), and strains that harbor the *cag* PAI augment the risk for peptic ulcer disease and distal gastric cancer compared to strains that lack the *cag* island [1]. Genes within the *cag* island encode proteins that form a bacterial type IV secretion system (T4SS), which translocates effector molecules across the bacterial membrane into host gastric epithelial cells. The terminal gene product of the *cag* island is CagA, and this effector is one of the substrates translocated into host cells by the T4SS [36]. CagA can also be delivered into host epithelial cells by T4SS-induced externalization of phosphatidylserine from the inner leaflet of the cell membrane [37].

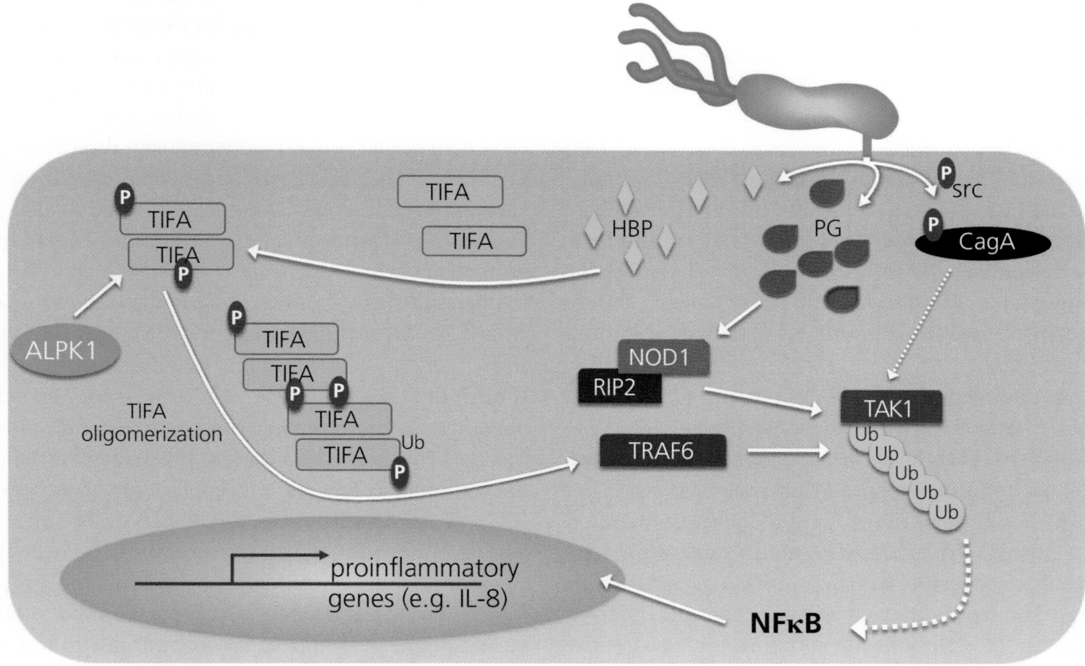

Figure 51.6 *H. pylori* affects multiple pathways in gastric epithelial cells that induce proinflammatory gene expression. CagA is translocated into host cells where it becomes phosphorylated by Src kinases and activates NF-κB. Translocation of components of peptidoglycan (PG) by the *cag* secretion system triggers NOD1 activation and activation of NF-κB. The metabolite HBP is also translocated into host cells by the *H. pylori cag* secretion system leading to increased NF-κB activation and IL-8 expression. ALPK, α-kinase 1; HBP, heptose bisphosphate; IL, interleukin; NOD1, nucleotide-binding oligomerization domain-containing protein 1; P, phosphate; RIP2, receptor-interacting protein 2; TAK1, TGF-β-activated kinase 1; TIFA, TRAF-interacting protein with forkhead-associated domain; TRAF6, TNF receptor-associated factor 6; Ub, ubiquitin.

Once inside host cells, CagA is tyrosine phosphorylated by Src and Abl kinases and phospho-CagA targets and interacts with numerous intracellular effectors to lower the threshold for carcinogenesis. For example, phospho-CagA activates a eukaryotic tyrosine phosphatase (SHP-2), leading to morphological transformations similar to those induced by growth factor stimulation [38]. Nonphosphorylated CagA also exerts effects within host cells that contribute to pathogenesis. CagA in an unmodified form interacts with the cell adhesion protein E-cadherin and the hepatocyte growth factor receptor c-Met, and activates β-catenin [39–42], which culminate in proinflammatory and mitogenic responses, disruption of cell–cell junctions, and loss of cell polarity, all of which promote neoplastic progression. CagA can increase the risk for gastric cancer by increasing spermine oxidase (SMO) production in gastric epithelial cells. Induction of SMO generates oxidative damage and selects for a subpopulation of cells with damaged DNA, which are resistant to apoptosis [43]. *H. pylori* also targets the tumor suppressor protein p53 to regulate apoptosis in a CagA-dependent manner [44].

CagA is not the only bacterial product delivered into host cells via the T4SS, as components of *H. pylori* peptidoglycan are also delivered into host cells and trigger signaling pathways that lower the threshold for carcinogenesis [45]. Peptidoglycan interacts with the host intracellular pattern recognition molecule Nod1, which leads to activation of NF-κB-dependent proinflammatory responses such as secretion of IL-8 [46] or β-defensin-2, as well as production of type I IFN [47,48]. Translocated peptidoglycan can also activate PI3K-AKT signaling, leading to decreased apoptosis, increased proliferation, and increased cell migration [49].

Additional effectors shown to be translocated by the *cag* T4SS include the metabolite heptose bisphosphate (HBP), a component of bacterial LPS synthesis. This molecule activates NF-κB signaling via the host adaptor molecule TIFA, resulting in inflammatory cytokine production [50–52]. *H. pylori* DNA has also been shown to be translocated into host epithelial cells by the T4SS, where it activates the intracellular innate immune receptor TLR9 [53,54].

Vacuolating cytotoxin A (VacA) is a toxin produced by *H. pylori* that is associated with increased disease risk. VacA exerts a multitude of effects on epithelial cells, including vacuolation, as well as inducing apoptosis and suppressing T-cell responses, which may contribute to the longevity of infection [26,55]. The majority of *H. pylori* strains possess the *vacA* gene but there is considerable variation in *vacA* gene structures within the signal (s) region, the middle (m) region, and the intermediate (i) region [56]. The s region and m region are stratified into s1 or s2 and m1 or m2 alleles, respectively. *vacA* s1/m1 strains induce greater vacuolation than s1/m2 strains, and there is typically no vacuolating activity in s2/m2 strains [57]. The *vacA* s1/m1 allele is strongly associated with ulcer disease and gastric cancer [57]. There are two i region subtypes, i1 and i2, and the i region plays a functional role in vacuolating activity [56]. Colonization with *vacA* i1 strains is strongly associated with the presence of CagA, *vacA* s1 alleles, and gastric cancer [56].

In order for *H. pylori* to colonize, deploy virulence factors, and persist within the gastric niche, adherence of *H. pylori* to gastric epithelium is required. Sequence analyses have revealed that an unusually high proportion of the *H. pylori* genome is committed to encoding outer membrane proteins (OMPs), and OMP expression is associated with gastroduodenal ulceration and may heighten the risk for developing gastric cancer. Blood group antigen binding adhesin (BabA) is an OMP encoded by the *babA2* gene and binds to fucosylated Lewis^b antigen (Le^b) on the surface of gastric epithelial cells [16]. Le^b-mediated colonization may increase the pathogenic potential of *H. pylori* [58], and *H. pylori babA2*$^+$ strains are associated with an increased risk of developing gastric cancer, especially when *babA2* is found in conjunction with *cagA* and *vacA* s1 alleles [59]. Another *H. pylori* adhesin is sialic acid-binding adhesin (SabA). SabA binds to the carbohydrate structure sialyl-Lewis^x antigen expressed on gastric epithelium, and is associated with increased gastric cancer risk. Sialyl-Lewis^x expression is induced during chronic gastric inflammation, suggesting that *H. pylori* modulates host cell glycosylation patterns to enhance attachment and colonization [17]. Finally, the OMP HopQ has recently been shown to bind to host cell surface molecules within the CEACAM family [18,19].

Human genetic polymorphisms and development of disease among *H. pylori*-infected persons

Most people colonized with disease-associated *H. pylori* strains remain asymptomatic. *H. pylori cag*$^+$ toxigenic strains are related to both duodenal ulcer disease and distal gastric cancer, considered to be two mutually exclusive disease outcomes. The inability of bacterial virulence components to completely account for pathological outcomes has highlighted the need to explore host factors that may influence disease, particularly gastric cancer.

Interleukin 1β is a Th1 cytokine that inhibits acid secretion and is increased within gastric mucosa of *H. pylori*-infected persons (Table 51.2). Polymorphisms within the *IL-1β* gene cluster, specifically *IL*-1β-31 and *IL*-1β-511, are associated with increased IL-1β production, and with a significantly increased risk for hypochlorhydria, gastric atrophy, and distal gastric adenocarcinoma compared to people with genotypes that limit IL-1β expression. However, these relationships are only present among those infected with *H. pylori* [60,61]. Given that IL-1β is a potent inhibitor of acid secretion, is profoundly proinflammatory, and is upregulated by *H. pylori*, colonized individuals harboring high-expression IL-1β polymorphisms are at increased risk for the development of gastric cancer.

Another cytokine that may increase the risk for gastric cancer is tumor necrosis factor (TNF) α. TNF-α is a proinflammatory, acid-suppressive cytokine that is increased within *H. pylori*-colonized human gastric mucosa. Polymorphisms that increase TNF-α production are associated with an increased risk of

Table 51.2 Human genetic polymorphisms that influence the development of distal gastric cancer.

Genetic locus	Function of expressed protein	Genotype associated with enhanced risk
IL-1β	Induces expression of inflammatory cytokines, potently inhibits acid secretion from parietal cells	31 C/C 511 T/T
IL-1RN	Receptor for IL-1β	Pentaallelic 86 bp tandem repeat in intron 2
TNF-α	Activates intracellular signaling pathways related to inflammation and apoptosis; inhibits acid secretion from parietal cells	308 A/A
IL-10	Inhibits production of proinflammatory cytokines	592 ATA/ATA 819 ATA/ATA 1082 ATA/ATA

IL, interleukin; TNF, tumor necrosis factor.

gastric cancer and its precursors (see Table 51.2) [62]. In contrast to *IL-1β* and *TNF-α* polymorphisms that increase cytokine production and are associated with increased gastric cancer risk, polymorphisms that decrease the production of the anti-inflammatory cytokine IL-10 reciprocally increase the risk for distal gastric cancer [62]. Investigations into the combinatorial effects of *IL-1β, TNF-α*, and *IL-10* polymorphisms on the development of cancer have revealed that the risk of cancer increases progressively with increasing number of proinflammatory polymorphisms, and three high-risk polymorphisms increased the risk of cancer 27-fold over baseline [62].

Diagnosis of *H. pylori* infection

The presence of *H. pylori* should only be determined if such results will affect clinical management decisions. Persons in whom an indication for *H. pylori* testing exists are those with peptic ulcer disease, MALToma, premalignant lesions such as atrophic gastritis or intestinal metaplasia, prolonged nonsteroidal anti-inflammatory drug (NSAID) or aspirin use, uninvestigated dyspepsia without alarm symptoms (e.g., weight loss, gastrointestinal bleeding, age >55) in populations where the prevalence of *H. pylori* is high, those with a strong family history of distal gastric cancer and those who reside in communities with a high prevalence of gastric cancer, prolonged usage of proton pump inhibitors (PPIs), unexplained iron deficiency anemia, or idiopathic thrombocytopenic purpura (ITP). Techniques to diagnose *H. pylori* can be classified as either invasive (requiring endoscopy) or noninvasive, which require breath samples, body fluid, or stool (Table 51.3). Invasive methods utilize gastric tissue and include histology, rapid urease tests,

Table 51.3 Diagnostic tests for *Helicobacter pylori*.

Test	Clinical utility for		
	Primary diagnosis	Confirmation of cure	Detects viable bacteria
Invasive			
Histology	+	+	-
Rapid urease testing	+	+	+
Culture	+/-	+/-	+
Polymerase chain reaction	-	-	-
Noninvasive			
Urea breath testing	+	+	+
Serology	+	-	-
Stool antigen tests	+	+	-

culture, or, rarely, polymerase chain reaction. Although none of the currently available diagnostic tests are completely reliable due to heterogeneity in colonization density, most are sufficiently accurate so as to permit their widespread use, either for initial diagnosis and/or confirmation of cure (see Table 51.3).

Histological detection of *H. pylori*

The presence of *H. pylori* within biopsy specimens can be determined histologically with or without the use of special stains that enhance bacterial visibility. Commonly used special histological studies include Warthin–Starry, Giemsa, Diff-Quik, stains and immunohistochemistry and these enhance detection rates. Advantages of histological diagnosis include direct visualization of the organism, assessment of the severity of gastritis, identification of more severe gastric lesions such as atrophic gastritis, intestinal metaplasia, adenocarcinoma or lymphoproliferative disease, and accuracy for both initial diagnosis and confirmation of cure. Although histology is considered by many to be the gold standard, its reliability is dependent upon the number and sites of biopsy harvest, staining technique, and the experience of the histopathologist. Evaluation of between three and five biopsy specimens obtained from the greater and/or lesser curvature of the antrum and corpus respectively, as well as the angularis, reliably distinguishes infected from uninfected mucosa [63]. Gastric biopsies taken after *H. pylori* is no longer detectable frequently show a mild residual infiltrate of lymphocytes with scattered plasma cells.

Rapid urease tests

Rapid urease tests take advantage of the robust production of urease by *H. pylori*, and the most widely used form consists of a gel tablet containing urea and a pH indicator. When an infected biopsy is placed into the gel, urea is converted to ammonia by urease, the pH within the tablet increases, and the pH indicator undergoes a color change (typically from yellow to red), often within 30 minutes. Additional forms of rapid urease tests have been developed and include paper and tablet tests, but their superiority to gel forms has not been established.

Advantages of rapid urease testing include ease of use, cost-effectiveness, and rapid acquisition of results, and they can be utilized for both initial diagnosis and follow-up of therapy. Sensitivities of rapid urease tests range from 93% to 97% with specificities of approximately 98%; however, biological conditions can affect their accuracy. Achlorhydria that develops as a consequence of atrophy or medication use (i.e., PPIs) can lead to both false-positive (bacterial overgrowth with urease-producing organisms such as *Proteus*) and false-negative (decreased *H. pylori* colonization density) results. False-positive results may also occur when non-*H. pylori Helicobacter* species, such as *H. heilmanni*, colonize the stomach. Heterogeneity in sites of colonization can alter the accuracy of biopsy-based rapid urease tests. For these reasons, it is recommended to wait at least 4–6 weeks following completion of anti-*H. pylori* therapy and at least 1 week after discontinuing PPIs before performing a rapid urease test.

Helicobacter pylori culture

Helicobacter pylori can be grown directly from gastric tissue either by gently rubbing a biopsy specimen onto selective or nonselective media or by homogenizing gastric tissue in sterile saline and plating serial dilutions of homogenate. Samples are then incubated for up to 10 days at 37 °C in an environment containing 5% CO_2. Similar to rapid urease testing, medications such as antibiotics or acid-suppressive drugs that alter bacterial colonization patterns in vivo; may affect culture sensitivity. Despite significant advances over the past two decades, microbiological culture has not been widely accepted as a practical means to diagnose *H. pylori* primarily due to cost, the special conditions required for growth, and the long interval between specimen harvest and test results, which delays treatment decisions. *H. pylori* culture is advantageous, however, if antimicrobial susceptibility patterns for specific isolates need to be determined.

Detection of *H. pylori*-specific DNA sequences in vivo

Helicobacter pylori DNA can be successfully detected in gastric tissue by polymerase chain reaction (PCR). Using specific primers, PCR amplifies DNA sequences specific for *H. pylori* and can yield high levels of sensitivity (93%) and specificity (100%) by detecting as few as 10 *H. pylori* colony-forming units (CFU). *H. pylori* DNA has also been amplified from gastric juice, saliva, dental plaque, and stool. Disadvantages of this technique include a high rate of false-positive results due to contamination within either the clinical (i.e., contaminated or improperly cleaned endoscopes) or the laboratory setting. Since PCR is only detecting DNA, a positive result cannot be equated with the presence of viable organisms. False-negative results can occur due to the presence of PCR inhibitors within gastric tissue, extremely low numbers of organisms, or DNA damage that occurs during specimen processing. For these reasons, as well as the availability of other diagnostic techniques with comparable levels of sensitivity and specificity, PCR is still considered a research technique.

Urea breath tests

A noninvasive technique that also capitalizes on urease production is urea breath testing. When urea labeled with either ^{13}C or ^{14}C is ingested by a patient with active *H. pylori* infection, gastric urease hydrolyzes labeled urea to ammonia and labeled CO_2, which is quickly absorbed into the bloodstream and can be detected in expired breath samples. Urea breath tests accurately ascertain the presence of active infection, unlike PCR or serological methods, and allow a more global assessment of *H. pylori* within the stomach than can be provided by biopsy-based techniques. Breath tests also are effective for detection of *H. pylori* post therapy, and due to their noninvasive nature and high levels of sensitivity and specificity, they represent the gold standard for confirmation of cure.

Serological testing for *H. pylori*

Antibody production against *H. pylori* antigens does not result in eradication; however, quantitating levels of anti-*H. pylori* immunoglobulins is an effective technique for primary diagnosis. A variety of serological methods have been developed, which include bacterial agglutination, complement fixation, hemagglutination, enzyme-linked immunosorbent assay (ELISA), immunofluorescence, radioimmunoassay, and latex agglutination. Patient samples range from blood obtained by venipuncture and/or finger-stick, to saliva. As a rule, whole-blood tests are less accurate than serum-based tests due to the presence of chylomicrons within whole blood, and finger-stick tests have reduced sensitivity and specificity compared to venipuncture tests. Levels of anti-*H. pylori* antibodies in saliva are much more variable than in blood, and thus saliva-based tests are less optimal than serum-based tests. Commercially available serology kits provide an extremely accurate way to diagnose *H. pylori* in patients who have not been previously treated, and levels of sensitivity are comparable to those obtained by histology, culture, or urea breath testing. Additionally, there are clinical situations in which serology may be preferable to other techniques, such as patients who present with an actively bleeding ulcer. Other tests for detecting antibodies directed against *H. pylori* include urine assays, and sensitivities range from 82% to 94% with specificities of 68–92%, depending on the population under study, but these are less useful clinically.

The most significant limitation of serological testing is its inability to reliably confirm cure. Following treatment, anti-*H. pylori* antibody levels decrease slowly and unpredictably, and often 6 months or more elapse before serum antibody concentrations decrease below the cut-off value for positivity. In addition, serology is not cost-effective for confirming eradication in clinical practice due to the potential for multiple patient return visits and tests, and the requirement for storing pretherapy samples as a standard to which posttherapy antibody levels must be compared. The availability, accuracy, and simplicity of urea breath tests also preclude using serology as a practical means to confirm cure.

Helicobacter pylori stool antigen tests

An enzymatic immunoassay (HpSA®, Meridian Diagnostics) that detects the presence of bacterial antigens in feces was developed as a noninvasive diagnostic technique for *H. pylori*. This test was originally formulated as a sandwich ELISA in which polyclonal anti-*H. pylori* antibody is bound to microtiter wells. Stool samples are then added and *H. pylori* antigens (if present) are "captured" by the bound antibody. A secondary antibody is then added followed by the addition of substrate, and bound *H. pylori* antigens are detected by a color change. This assay has also been modified into an immunocard.

The *H. pylori* stool antigen test is both sensitive and specific, and the United States Food and Drug Administration approved HpSA for initial diagnosis and for monitoring posttherapy responses in *H. pylori*-infected adults. Several trials have reported the sensitivity and specificity of HpSA to range from 91% to 96%. Concomitant use of PPIs does not affect the accuracy of detecting *H. pylori* antigens in stool, in contrast to urea breath tests or biopsy-based techniques. Following successful treatment of *H. pylori*, stool antigen levels rapidly decline and, in the majority of patients, are undetectable by 5 days post treatment. Stool samples can be stored for prolonged periods of time and multiple samples can be assayed at once. HpSA testing is safe and accurate in pediatric patients infected with *H. pylori*. Finally, testing stool for *H. pylori* antigens is cost-effective. Thus, the *H. pylori* stool antigen test is a highly accurate technique that can identify the presence of *H. pylori* prior to and shortly following initiation of antimicrobial therapy.

Therapy and management of *H. pylori* infection

The goal of *H. pylori* therapy is to eliminate the organism from the stomach and successful eradication is defined as a negative test for the bacterium ≥4 weeks after the completion of therapy. Treatment regimens should be straightforward, well tolerated, and cost-effective. There are several different options for treating *H. pylori* infections, and selection of a particular therapy is dependent on many factors, including drug availability, antimicrobial resistance patterns, and cost.

Proton pump inhibitor triple therapy consists of a PPI plus clarithromycin and either amoxicillin or metronidazole, each ingested twice daily. There are no consistent advantages to using a particular PPI for *H. pylori* eradication so any agent in this class can be used as a component of triple therapy. Bismuth-based quadruple therapy consists of a PPI dosed twice daily plus bismuth, metronidazole, and tetracycline for 14 days. Nonbismuth quadruple therapy, known as concomitant therapy (PPI with clarithromycin, metronidazole, and amoxicillin), is highly effective for the initial treatment of *H. pylori* when taken for 14 days. Anti-*H. pylori* therapies are also available as prepackaged formulations such as Prevpac® (lansoprazole 30 mg, clarithromycin 500 mg, amoxicillin 500 mg; each taken twice a day for 7 days) and Helidac® (bismuth subsalicylate 262.4 mg, metronidazole 250 mg, tetracycline 500 mg; each taken four times a day for 14 days). Although these may be more convenient, they are not cost-effective and the shorter duration (7 days) and lower dosage of amoxicillin (500 mg) in Prevpac as well as the need for combination therapy with a PPI (Helidac) preclude recommending these formulations as optimal first-line anti-*H. pylori* therapies. A concern with all of these regimens is that they fail to eradicate *H. pylori* in up to 15–25% of patients, likely due to an increased global prevalence of antibiotic-resistant *H. pylori* strains [64]. This has necessitated the development of several guidelines for initial management of *H. pylori* infection and recommendations for regimens to be used when initial attempts at eradication fail [64].

The three guidelines, all published in 2017, include the Maastricht V/Florence Consensus, the Toronto Consensus, and the American College of Gastroenterology recommendations [65–67]. The primary determinant for selection of a specific regimen was the level of *H. pylori* resistance to clarithromycin in a particular community. In general, in areas with known low rates of *H. pylori* clarithromycin resistance (below 15%), PPI-clarithromycin-containing triple regimens are recommended as first-line treatment. In areas of known high clarithromycin resistance (>15%), bismuth-containing or nonbismuth-containing quadruple regimens are recommended as first-line empirical treatment [64]. One practical issue is that in many countries outside Europe, local or community *H. pylori* resistance rates are not available. In these cases, empiric approaches must be used and a collective recommendation from the three guidelines was that bismuth quadruple therapy should be first-line therapy with concomitant therapy as an alternative, especially when bismuth is not available [64]. A summary of the three collective recommendations is shown in Figure 51.7.

In patients who fail initial eradication, the most common reason is *H. pylori* resistance to clarithromycin and/or metronidazole and therefore, these drugs, if used in the initial eradication regimen, should be avoided. Second-line therapies should be either bismuth quadruple therapy or levofloxicin triple therapy, depending on suspected resistance patterns [64]. Salvage therapies should include rifabutin-based triple or high-dose dual amoxicillin/PPI therapy [64]. Recently, a new FDA-approved anti-*H. pylori* treatment regimen containing rifabutin, omeprazole, and amoxicillin has become available, which increases the therapeutic options for *H. pylori* eradication.

Eradication rates in clinical practice are frequently below 90%, primarily due to differences in patient populations, genetic

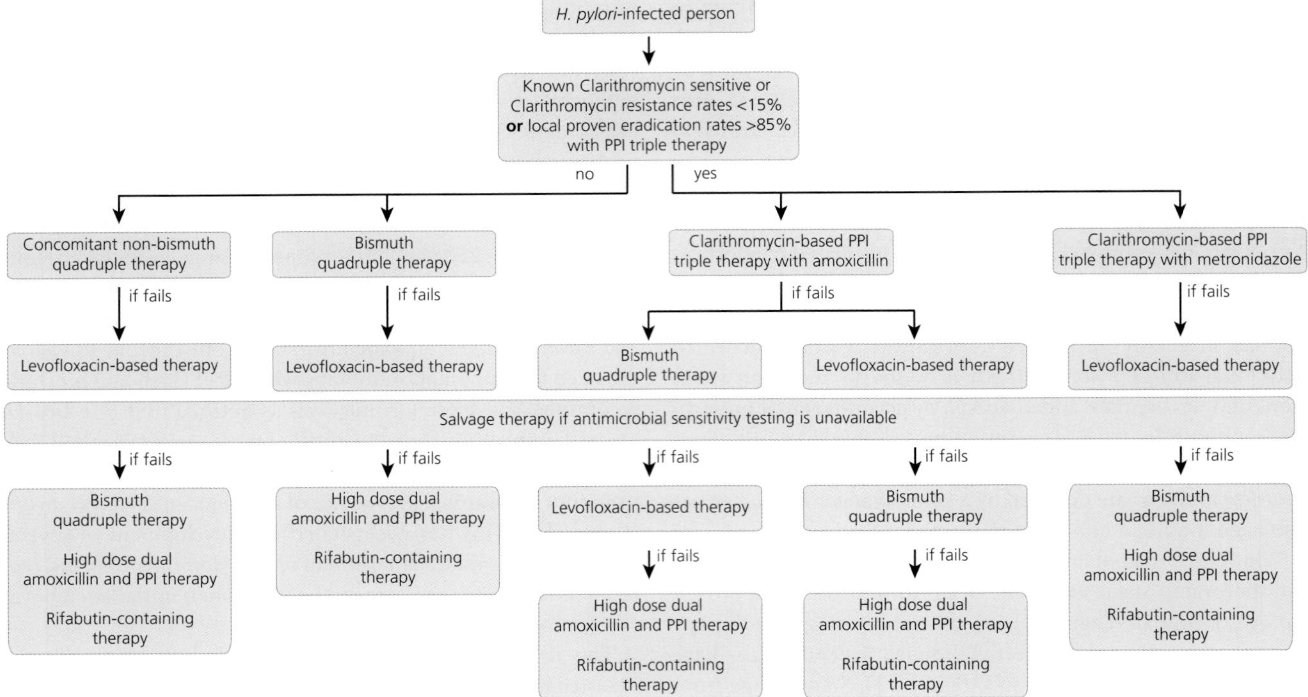

Figure 51.7 Therapeutic recommendations for eradication of *H. pylori* infections. PPI, proton pump inhibitor.

diversity of infecting *H. pylori* isolates, and bacterial antibiotic resistance patterns. It is therefore recommended that urea breath testing or stool antigen tests be performed post intervention to confirm successful cure. Follow-up testing should be performed at least 4 weeks after the completion of therapy.

Infectious gastritis (excluding *Helicobacter pylori*)

Bacteria

Bacterial colonization of the achlorhydric [68] or dysmotile stomach does not elicit a marked inflammatory response (although scattered mononuclear inflammatory cells may be found on biopsy) and is generally asymptomatic. True bacterial infections of the stomach, excluding *H. pylori* gastritis, are exceedingly rare. Acute suppurative gastritis, or *phlegmonous gastritis*, is a life-threatening condition caused by infection of the submucosa and muscularis propria of the stomach by pyogenic bacteria, most often α-hemolytic streptococci [69]. Immunocompromised patients, the elderly, and alcoholics are at greatest risk [70], and iatrogenic causes include endoscopic mucosal resection [71] and polypectomy [72]. Patients typically present with acute abdominal pain, peritonitis, fever, and hypotension. When gas-forming bacteria such as *Clostridium* species invade the stomach wall, the term *emphysematous gastritis* is used [72].

This form of gastritis has been associated with *Sarcina* infection [73], intake of large amounts of alcohol, AIDS, infected peritoneal–jugular venous shunts, and biopsy procedures [74]. Surgical intervention with gastrectomy may be necessary [75,76], and mortality is high for both conditions. *Helicobacter heilmanii*-like organisms, which are easily identified by their larger size and multiple spirals [77], cause an active gastritis that may mimic mild *H. pylori* gastritis. Other rare causes of gastric bacterial infections include syphilis, which may cause ulcerated lesions [78] and nodular masses [79], and *Mycobacterium tuberculosis* [80], which may present as gastric outlet obstruction. In gastric tuberculosis, biopsies show necrotizing granulomas, with acid-fast bacilli demonstrated on appropriate stains. Gastric infection by *Mycobacterium avium* complex is rarely seen, even in AIDS patients, even though the organism is resistant to low pH environments [81].

In contrast to pathogens, the gut microbiota is essential to maintain host physiology through its integral role in cellular metabolism, nutrient absorption, and immune defense against invading pathogens. Research has previously focused on a single organism causing disease in the stomach, (e.g., *H. pylori*); however, a rapid increase in molecular technologies such as next-generation sequencing in combination with computational analysis has transformed our understanding of how the gastric microbiota is associated with disease states such as gastritis. Using such refined techniques, a diverse bacterial community has been found within the stomach, with colonization densities reported to range from between 10^1 and 10^3 colony-forming units/g [82]. The gastric microbiota in *H. pylori*-negative individuals is highly diverse. Through one sequencing study, 128 phylotypes were identified within eight bacterial phyla; the five most abundant phyla were Proteobacteria, Firmicutes, Bacteroidetes, Fusobacteria, and Actinobacteria [83,84]. In an independent study using tagged 454 pyrosequencing analysis, 262 phylotypes representing 13 phyla were identified in gastric biopsies from *H. pylori*-negative persons [85]. In stark contrast, in *H. pylori*-infected individuals, *H. pylori* is the single most abundant phylotype present in the stomach and accounts for between 72% and 97% of all sequence reads [83,85,86].

Currently, there are very few studies that have examined differences in microbial composition and outcomes stratified by disease. The hypochlorhydric environment found in atrophic gastritis permits colonization of other bacteria that may enter the stomach and may further promote the progression towards gastric cancer. One study using pyrosequencing found distinct differences when the gastric microbiota was compared in different disease stages from chronic gastritis, to intestinal metaplasia and gastric cancer. In gastric cancer, the Bacilli class and Streptococcaceae family were significantly increased compared to what was found in chronic gastritis and intestinal metaplasia, where the Epsilonproteobacteria class and Helicobacteraceae family were both decreased [87]. In a recent large study, the gastric microbiota was compared in chronic gastritis and gastric cancer and significant differences were identified between the two groups. Specifically, the microbiota in gastric cancer had decreased diversity, reduced *Helicobacter* abundance and overabundance of *Citrobacter*, *Clostridium*, *Lactobacillus*, *Achromobacter*, and *Rhodococcus*, which are usually found in the intestinal microbiota [88].

These studies are intriguing and demonstrate associations between the human gastric microbiota and *H. pylori* with gastric disease; however, they are not able to differentiate between cause and effect. To begin to address whether changes in the gastric microbiota play a direct role in the development of gastric cancer, or are secondary to the changing gastric environment, further detailed molecular studies to define the composition of the gastric microbiota in well-characterized human populations, with and without gastric cancer, will need to be conducted. As of now, infection with *H. pylori* is the strongest known risk factor for developing gastritis and gastric cancer; however, a large longitudinal human study suggests that other components of the gastric microbiota may influence gastric disease progression. In a 15-year follow-up study of 3365 subjects, antibiotic treatment of *H. pylori* infection significantly reduced the incidence of gastric cancer despite less than half of the treated individuals remaining free of *H. pylori* infection. The incidence of gastric cancer was decreased to a similar level in individuals who remained free of *H. pylori* over 15 years versus those where eradication was not successful, suggesting that treatment with antibiotics may modify the microbiota in such a way that the development of gastric cancer is attenuated despite the presence of *H. pylori* [89]. Along similar lines, computational analysis of bacterial DNA within known cancer genomes determined that gastric adenocarcinoma contained the second highest number of bacterial DNA sequences. Interestingly, this bacterial DNA was not *H. pylori* but was, instead, *Pseudomonas* [90].

Viruses

While enteric viruses cause a clinical picture of acute gastritis, biopsy is rarely performed in such cases and no distinctive findings have been reported. The most common viral infection identified in gastric biopsies is cytomegalovirus (CMV), usually seen in immunocompromised patients as part of disseminated infection, although it is occasionally found in elderly apparently immunocompetent patients [91]. Clinically, gastric involvement by CMV may be manifested by nausea and upper abdominal pain or occasionally by gastric outlet obstruction [92] or hemorrhage. Endoscopically, erosions, ulcers, hypertrophic folds, and edema are identified. In children, cytomegalovirus gastritis causes massive foveolar hyperplasia [93] that is indistinguishable from Ménétrier disease. Nuclear cytomegalovirus inclusions may be found in enlarged epithelial, endothelial, smooth muscle, and stromal cells and range in number from numerous to impossible to detect on routine histology. The inflammatory response is variable; in some cases, patchy acute inflammatory infiltrates often centered about small vessels in the lamina propria and submucosa may be seen. Diagnosis is established by demonstration of the characteristic viral inclusions (Figure 51.8), highlighted by immunohistochemical or in situ hybridization techniques. Treatment is with ganciclovir.

A few cases of Epstein–Barr virus (EBV) as a cause of gastritis and gastric ulcers [94] have been reported. The dense infiltrate of atypical lymphocytes may mimic lymphoma. Detection of EBV RNA by in situ hybridization is helpful in making the diagnosis.

Fungi

Fungal colonization of gastric ulcers by *Candida* species is relatively common [95] but is of little clinical consequence.

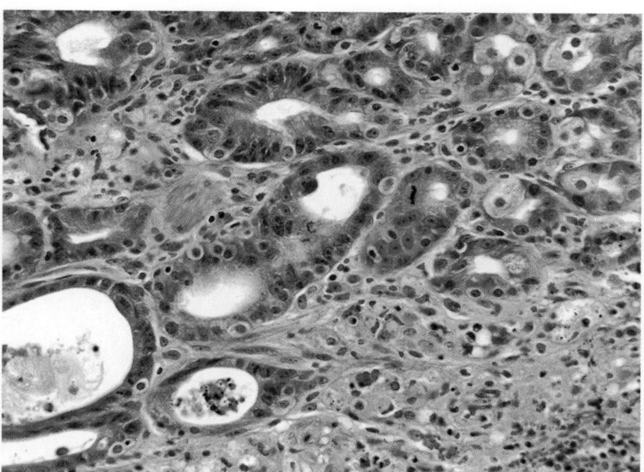

Figure 51.8 In cytomegalovirus gastritis, the inflammatory infiltrate is variable; characteristic nuclear viral inclusions may be seen in endothelial cells, stromal cells, epithelium, and smooth muscle.

Invasive or disseminated fungal infections with *Histoplasma capsulatum* [96], *Crytococcus neoformans* [97], and *Zygomycetes* species [98] (among others) involving the stomach have been reported in immunocompromised patients.

Parasites

Although involvement of the stomach by parasites is rare in western countries, many cases of invasive anisakiasis have been reported in Japan, where raw marine fish is commonly consumed. Nematode larvae of the genus *Anisakis* may migrate into the gastric wall and cause sporadic epigastric pain. Multiple gastric erosions are typical on endoscopy, and microscopically an eosinophilic granulomatous inflammatory infiltrate with abscess formation and granulation tissue is seen [99]. A small worm may be identified in some cases. Other parasites occasionally found in gastric mucosa, primary in immunocompromised patients, include *Cryptosporidium* species [100], *Giardia intestinalis* [101], and *Strongyloides stercoralis* [102].

Eosinophilic gastritis

Small numbers of eosinophils (up to 38 per mm^2) [103] are normally found in the gastric lamina propria, and eosinophils are a typical component of the inflammatory infiltrate in a wide range of inflammatory diseases involving the stomach, including parasitic infection. Eosinophilic gastritis, the gastric component of eosinophilic gastroenteritis, should only be diagnosed when numerous eosinophils out of proportion to the other components of the inflammatory infiltrate are present (Figure 51.9). The stomach is less commonly involved than duodenum, ileum, and colon [104]. Eosinophilic gastroenteritis is considered a polygenic allergic disorder; in the majority of cases, serum IgE is elevated and peripheral eosinophilia is present [105]. Endoscopic findings are nonspecific and include friability, erythema, erosions, and enlarged gastric folds, particularly in the antrum; the endoscopic appearance may be normal even when the gastric mucosa is heavily infiltrated by eosinophils. Biopsy diagnosis may be difficult, as selective involvement of the deeper layers of the gastric wall may be seen, with minimal or only patchy mucosal collections of eosinophils [106]. Eosinophilic gastritis has also been described in the setting of collagen vascular disease [107]. In noninfectious cases, the disease often responds to corticosteroid therapy [108], although flares following steroid withdrawal may occur [105].

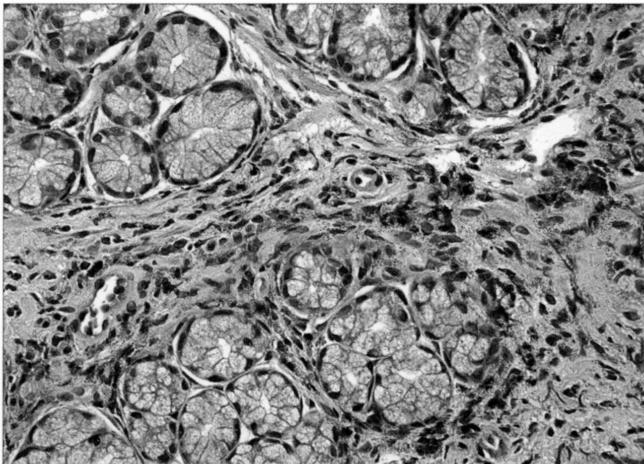

Figure 51.9 Eosinophilic gastritis is characterized by a dense but irregularly distributed infiltrate of eosinophils in the lamina propria or deeper layers of the stomach.

Granulomatous gastritis

Granulomas are found in less than 1% of gastric mucosal biopsies [74] in adults and up to 1.7% in children [109], but occur in a wide variety of infectious and noninfectious inflammatory disorders. Clinical and endoscopic findings generally reflect the underlying disease. Small erosions and ulcers are common [110], but the gastric mucosa may also be entirely normal on endoscopy. While in most cases of granulomatous gastritis, a specific diagnosis can be made by integrating histological findings with clinical data, in a small number of cases, termed idiopathic, no etiology can be identified. Etiology of granulomatous gastritis varies with the patient population, and is more likely to represent Crohn's disease in children, whereas adults in one case series from a single institution were more likely to have sarcoidosis or idiopathic granulomatous gastritis [109].

Infectious causes of granulomatous gastritis include acid-fast bacilli (*Mycobacterium tuberculosis*), fungi (*Histoplasma capsulatum*), and parasites (*Anisakis simplex*). *H. pylori* is not considered to cause granulomatous gastritis, although occasionally granulomas are found in the superficial mucosa in the antrum in close proximity to injured gastric glands and probably represent reaction to ruptured glands. Foreign bodies such as sutures may also give rise to a granulomatous reaction. Rarely, a granulomatous response to tumor antigens may be seen in non-neoplastic mucosa or perigastric lymph nodes in patients with gastric adenocarcinomas or gastric lymphomas.

In most series, Crohn's disease, followed by sarcoidosis, is the most common disorder associated with granulomatous gastritis [111], with over half of all cases identified in retrospective series attributed to upper GI involvement by Crohn's disease. A prevalence of 10–15% for gastric granulomas (Figure 51.10) and up to 70% of "focally enhanced gastritis," characterized by focal periglandular mononuclear inflammatory infiltrates composed of T cells and $CD68^+$ histiocytes, has been reported in these patients [112]. It should be noted that focally enhanced gastritis has also been reported in children [113] and adults with ulcerative colitis. In unselected gastric biopsies, this pattern of gastric inflammation is relatively rare, and has a low positive predictive value for inflammatory bowel disease [114]. In many cases, involvement of the stomach by Crohn's disease is an incidental finding; however, severe involvement with strictures and fistulas refractory to medical management also occurs.

Gastrointestinal involvement by sarcoidosis is generally an incidental finding and rarely has clinical importance. In severe

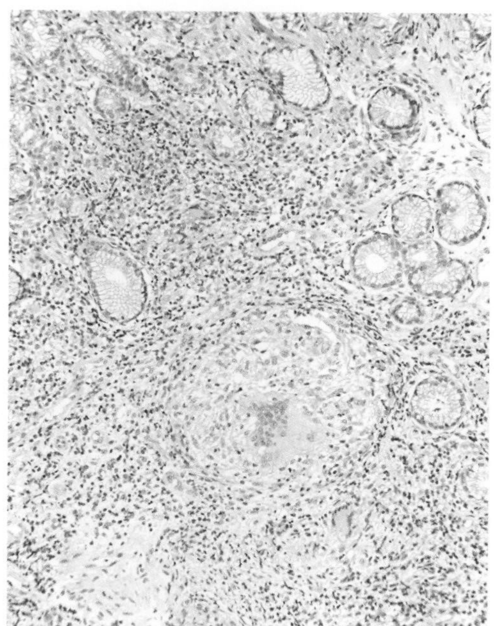

Figure 51.10 Nonnecrotizing granulomas composed of epithelioid histiocytes with occasional giant cells are found in up to 15% of gastric biopsies from patients with Crohn's disease.

cases, scarring and ulcers are seen, which may mimic gastric carcinoma or cause gastric outlet obstruction.

Autoimmune gastritis

Autoimmune gastritis is a chronic atrophic gastritis restricted to the body of the stomach and associated with circulating antiparietal cell and anti-intrinsic factor antibodies with resulting intrinsic factor deficiency. Only a small subset of patients with autoimmune gastritis will have classic pernicious anemia.

Pangastritis can develop in the setting of other autoimmune diseases, such as autoimmune enteropathy, systemic lupus erythematosus, and autoimmune hemolytic anemia, and is often not associated with antiparietal cell and anti-intrinsic factor antibodies. This form of gastritis is not limited to the gastric body but involves the entire mucosa. In contrast to classic autoimmune gastritis, neuroendocrine cell hyperplasia is not seen [115]. Chronic atrophic pangastritis may also be seen in the setting of congenital or acquired immunodeficiency [116].

Clinical features and pathogenesis

Patients with autoimmune gastritis may be clinically asymptomatic for many years, until parietal cell mass has decreased to the point that hypo- or achlorhydria results. Achlorhydric patients have hypergastrinemia, and injury to the chief cells results in reduced pepsin activity. Achlorhydria results in iron deficiency anemia in over 20% of patients [117] due to lack of absorption of nonheme iron. Patients who present with pernicious anemia may complain of anorexia, weight loss, sore tongue, and neurological disturbances including numbness and paresthesias in the extremities, weakness, and ataxia.

Patients with autoimmune gastritis may have other autoimmune diseases such as Graves disease, idiopathic adrenocortical insufficiency, and vitiligo. It has been hypothesized that *H. pylori* infection may trigger autoimmune gastritis in a genetically susceptible individual due to molecular mimicry between *H. pylori* and gastric mucosal antigens, supported by evidence that up to 80% of patients with *H. pylori* may have autoantibodies with H^+/K^+ ATPase specificity directed against the canalicular membranes of parietal cells, the same target autoantigen in autoimmune gastritis [118]. However, additional evidence is needed before it can be concluded that *H. pylori* is the causative agent for autoimmune gastritis [119].

Endoscopic appearance

Progressive thinning of the mucosa in atrophic gastritis results in loss of gastric folds and increased visibility of fine submucosal vessels. The antrum is endoscopically normal in most cases of autoimmune gastritis. Multiple hyperplastic polyps may develop in advanced stages of the disease.

Pathological features

The corpus of the stomach is most severely affected in autoimmune gastritis. Characteristic histological findings include a diffuse chronic atrophic gastritis with variable degrees of intestinal metaplasia (Figure 51.11). Early in the disease, deep, midzonal [120] or diffuse lymphoplasmacytic infiltrates

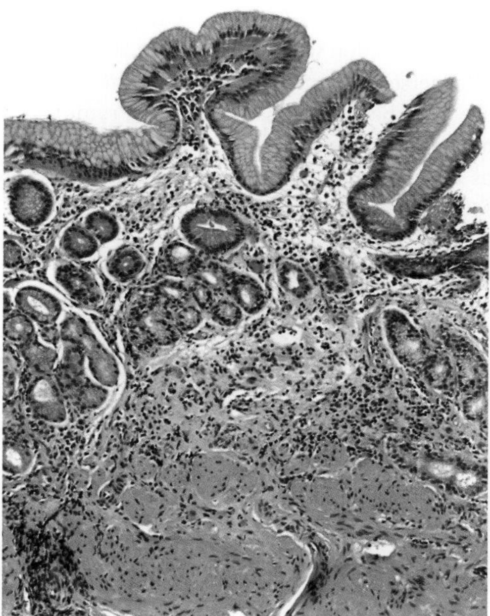

Figure 51.11 In autoimmune gastritis, loss of oxyntic glands results in atrophic gastritis primarily affecting the gastric corpus. A diffuse lymphoplasmacytic infiltrate is common.

in the lamina propria with foci of epithelial infiltration and damage, intestinal or pyloric metaplasia, and linear enterochromaffin-like (ECL) cell hyperplasia are typical features [121]. Pyloric metaplasia tends to predominate over intestinal metaplasia in early stages. In late-stage disease, the oxyntic mucosa is largely destroyed, with replacement of chief and parietal cells by metaplastic cells; at this stage, the inflammatory infiltrate is minimal. Extreme degrees of ECL cell hyperplasia often lead to the formation of multiple microcarcinoids secondary to hypergastrinemia. The antrum may show mild chronic inflammation with intestinal metaplasia, and hyperplasia of gastrin cells may be seen.

Management

The mucosal changes in autoimmune gastritis are irreversible. While patients with multiple hyperplastic polyps and extensive metaplasia may be at increased risk for gastric adenocarcinoma, there are no standards for frequency of endoscopic surveillance. Most abnormalities resulting from cobalamin deficiency are reversible with replacement therapy, except for neurological manifestations.

Lymphocytic gastritis

Lymphocytic gastritis is characterized by large numbers of mature lymphocytes infiltrating the surface and foveolar epithelium (i.e., intraepithelial lymphocytes in contrast to lamina propria lymphocytes). It occurs most commonly in patients with celiac disease [122], with up to 45% of celiac disease patients [123] having evidence of lymphocytic gastritis on biopsy. The pathogenesis of lymphocytic gastritis is unknown but given its association with celiac disease, it likely represents a response to persistent antigens; *Propionibacterium acnes* overabundance has been implicated [124]. Prominent foveolar hyperplasia may also be seen in lymphocytic gastritis, a pattern known as hypertrophic lymphocytic gastritis, and protein loss may be found in about 20% of patients [125].

Clinical and endoscopic features

Patients with lymphocytic gastritis may be asymptomatic, and the condition is discovered by random biopsy of endoscopically normal mucosa. In more severe disease, there may be scattered erosions and enlarged mucosal folds resembling Ménétrier disease and accompanied by anemia and hypoalbuminemia (hypertrophic lymphocytic gastritis).

Pathological features

The minimum number of lymphocytes considered diagnostic for lymphocytic gastritis is 25 per 100 epithelial cells [126]; counts of up to 65 lymphocytes per 100 epithelial cells are not uncommon. Virtually all of the lymphocytes are of T-cell origin. Lymphocytes are distributed singly (Figure 51.12), but rarely small clusters resembling lymphoepithelial lesions may be seen. The antrum is more severely involved in patients with celiac disease compared to patients with *H. pylori* gastritis [126], in which the lymphocytic gastritis pattern is more likely to be corpus predominant and to show concomitant infiltration of the mucosa by neutrophils. The intraepithelial lymphocytes are more numerous in hypertrophic forms of lymphocytic gastritis.

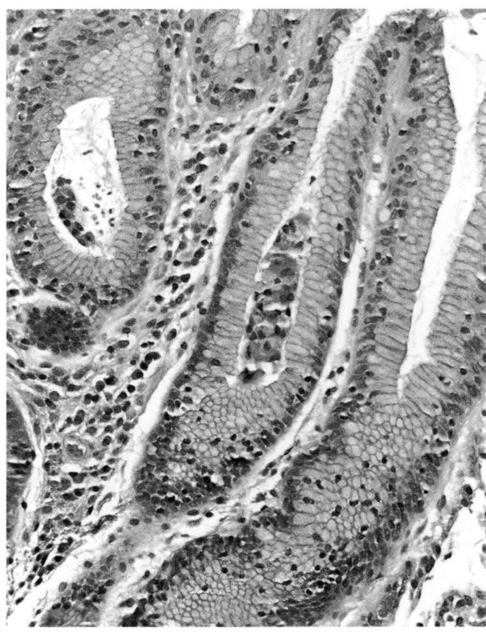

Figure 51.12 Numerous intraepithelial lymphocytes are found in the mucosa in lymphocytic gastritis.

Management

Treatment of lymphocytic gastritis is aimed at the underlying *H. pylori* gastritis or celiac disease; for patients with lymphocytic gastritis not associated with these diseases, therapy has largely consisted of PPIs [127]. Children with celiac disease and lymphocytic gastritis may have more severe celiac disease at the time of diagnosis by clinical and laboratory measures [128] than those without concomitant lymphocytic gastritis.

Collagenous gastritis

Collagenous gastritis is a rare but histologically distinctive disorder characterized by thickening of the subepithelial collagen layer in the gastric mucosa (Figure 51.13). It occurs in association with collagenous colitis in older adults and with celiac disease, although it may also be limited to the stomach. Collagenous gastritis may show a nodular pattern on endoscopy [129]. On biopsy, in addition to the markedly thickened and irregular subepithelial collagen band, the mucosa contains a variable chronic inflammation infiltrate, and the surface epithelium shows degenerative changes and infiltration by

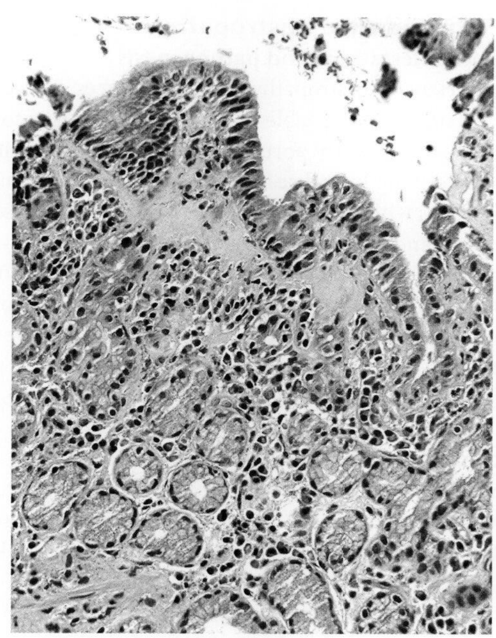

Figure 51.13 The histological hallmark of collagenous gastritis is irregular thickening of the subepithelial collagen band, with degenerative changes and inflammation in the surface epithelium.

lymphocytes and eosinophils. Three histological patterns have been described: a lymphocytic gastritis-like pattern, an eosinophil-rich pattern, and an atrophic pattern [130].

Reactive (chemical) gastropathy (NSAID and bile reflux)

Reactive gastropathy, also referred to as chemical gastropathy or gastritis, is a distinctive constellation of endoscopic and microscopic findings first described in the setting of bile reflux in stomachs subjected to gastric surgery, most commonly Billroth II gastrojejunostomy. More recently, it has been recognized that bile reflux in the intact stomach may lead to reactive gastropathy. Most cases, however, are associated with use of NSAIDs, with an estimated prevalence of reactive gastropathy of up to 45% in this group [131]. The prevalence of reactive gastropathy is age dependent [132], ranging from 2% in children under 10 years of age to over 20% in adults over age 80 [133], perhaps reflecting increasing use of NSAIDs in older patients.

Clinical manifestations and pathogenesis

Reactive gastropathy may be seen in three clinical settings: postgastrectomy alkaline reflux, bile reflux secondary to gastroduodenal dysmotility, and aspirin or NSAID ingestion. Other medications that may cause this pattern of injury include bisphosphonates, tetracyclines, iron, and selective serotonin reuptake inhibitors [134]. Patients with bile reflux complain of burning midepigastric pain unresponsive to antacids; bilious vomiting may occur. In persons ingesting aspirin or NSAIDs on a regular basis, epigastric pain is common, but no relationship has been established between the mucosal appearance and the presence or severity of symptoms. Unless complicating erosions or ulcers are present, reactive gastropathy may be an asymptomatic lesion.

Disruption of the mucus barrier of the antrum and direct damage to surface epithelium, from either reflux of alkaline duodenal contents or reduced prostaglandin synthesis secondary to NSAID use, is a major factor in the pathogenesis of reactive gastropathy. Cyclooxygenase- and prostaglandin-independent mechanisms may also be involved in NSAID-induced gastric injury, perhaps through production of additional proinflammatory mediators [135]. The gastric injury induced by NSAIDs is exacerbated by acid, and use of potent acid suppression therapy is a common approach to reducing NSAID-related complications.

Endoscopic appearance

In patients with nonoperated stomachs, the mucosa in reactive gastropathy may show edema, vascular congestion and erythema, and erosions. In the operated stomach, the mucosa shows similar features, often primarily involving the anastomotic site. Superficial erosions may be seen in this setting but are not specific for reactive gastropathy.

Histological features

The characteristic histopathological features of reactive gastropathy are best seen in the antrum and include foveolar hyperplasia imparting a corkscrew appearance to the superficial mucosa, reactive epithelial changes (nuclear enlargement and loss of cytoplasmic mucin), increased lamina propria smooth muscle fibers, and edema of the lamina propria [136] (Figure 51.14). Acute and chronic inflammatory cells are typically sparse. In children with reactive gastropathy, the degree of foveolar hyperplasia has been reported to correlate with the severity of bile reflux [137].

Hemorrhagic gastropathy

Hemorrhagic gastropathies are a multifactorial group of conditions characterized by mucosal hemorrhages and erosions. The major etiological factors are NSAID use, major physical stress, and ingestion of large quantities of alcohol. Hemorrhagic gastropathy has also been reported in the setting of crack cocaine use [138]. The most severe examples of hemorrhagic gastropathy are *stress ulcers*, originally described by Dr. Thomas Curling in 1842 [139] and therefore sometimes referred to as Curling ulcers, seen in patients who suffer major physical or thermal trauma, shock, sepsis, or head injury. Respiratory failure requiring mechanical ventilation for more than 48 hours and coagulopathy are independent risk factors for the development of bleeding from hemorrhagic gastropathy [140]. The pathogenesis of hemorrhagic gastropathy is related to disruption of the mucosal

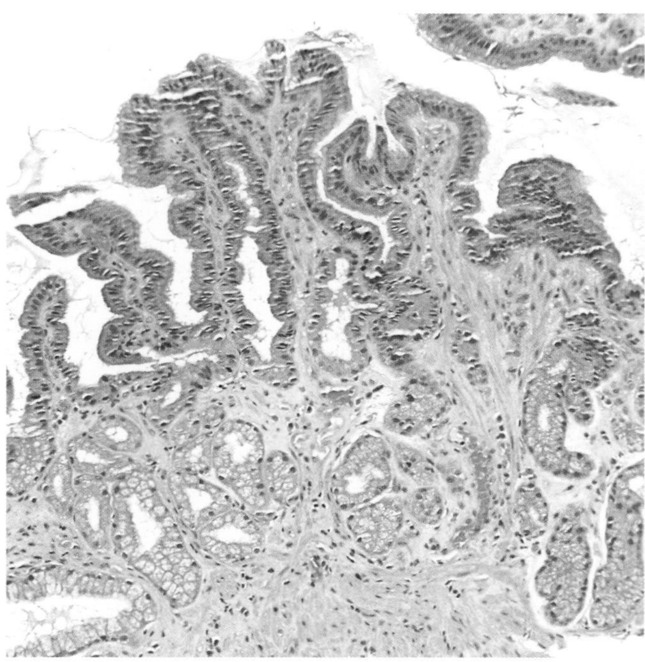

Figure 51.14 Chemical gastropathy is characterized by reactive epithelial changes out of proportion to the sparse inflammatory infiltrate, foveolar hyperplasia with corkscrew appearance to the superficial mucosa, and increased lamina propria smooth muscle fibers.

protective mechanisms secondary to compromise of gastric mucosa microcirculation in some cases; gastric acid secretion likely contributes to the injury [140] and *H. pylori* infection has been implicated as a contributing factor in some cases [141].

In hemorrhagic gastropathy, the mucosal lesions are multiple, superficial, and nontransmural. Microscopically, the superficial mucosa is eroded and edematous; a neutrophilic inflammatory response may be seen, but mononuclear inflammation is not present unless there is concomitant chronic mucosal injury as in *H. pylori* infection. Hemorrhagic gastropathy usually produces no symptoms and blood loss is minor. However, because of the increased mortality associated with gastrointestinal bleeding in critically ill patients, prophylactic treatment with PPIs is advocated by some investigators [140].

Vascular gastropathy

Vascular gastropathies are due to alterations in gastric circulation; the most common are gastric antral vascular ectasia ("watermelon stomach") (see Chapter 113) and portal hypertensive gastropathy (see also Chapter 124). Congestive heart failure may also cause a congestive gastropathy [142] endoscopically resembling portal hypertensive gastropathy. Frank ischemic necrosis of gastric mucosa is rarely seen, but occasionally occurs in patients with severe atherosclerotic disease, and gastric ulcers have been reported in chronic mesenteric ischemia [143].

Portal hypertensive gastropathy

Clinical manifestations and pathogenesis

Portal hypertensive gastropathy (PHG) produces characteristic mucosal changes recognizable at endoscopy, and is a common finding in patients with portal hypertension, both with and without underlying liver disease. Although the development of PHG correlates with duration and severity of liver disease [144] and presence and size of gastroesophageal varices, the severity and presence of portal hypertensive gastropathy do not correlate in a linear fashion with severity of portal hypertension, and measurements of gastric blood flow to the stomach have shown variable results [145]. Although blood loss from PHG is usually chronic and mild, it may also cause acute bleeding [146].

Endoscopic appearance

Portal hypertensive gastropathy is more prominent in the body and fundus of the stomach and is rare in the gastric antrum. Characteristic patterns on endoscopy are a mosaic or snake-skin pattern, scarlatina rash, cherry red spots, and/or black-brown spots. Endoscopic two-category classification systems (mild and severe) are recommended because of better reproducibility; bulging red marks and active bleeding are considered indicative of severe changes [146].

Histopathology

Small veins in the mucosa and submucosa show dilation, tortuosity, and thickened walls (Figure 51.15). The mucosa is otherwise generally normal in appearance, with no erosions, significant inflammation, or thrombi. Correlation of histological findings with endoscopic impression of PHG is poor, because

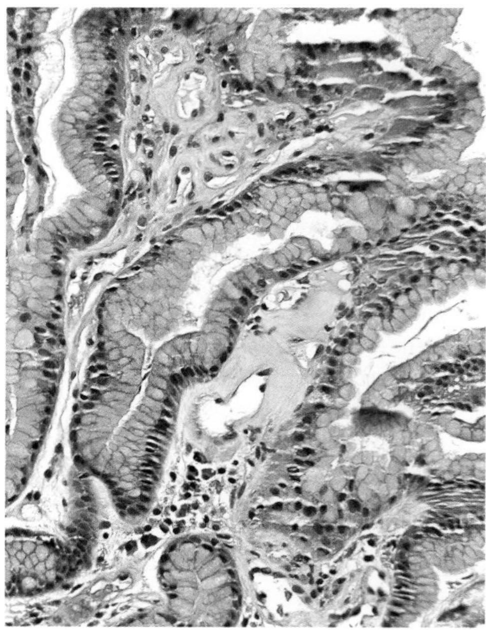

Figure 51.15 In portal hypertensive gastropathy, dilated small veins are found in the submucosa and lamina propria.

the vascular changes are more pronounced in submucosal vessels, and small mucosal biopsies may not show diagnostic changes.

Management

Because clinically significant bleeding is rare, most patients require no specific treatment for PHG. Nonselective β-blockers such as propranolol or nadalol may be used to lower portal pressure and gastric mucosal blood flow. Endoscopic intervention is of limited value because of the mild and diffuse nature of the bleeding in most cases. Transjugular intrahepatic portosystemic shunt (TIPS) and shunt surgery have been used to treat PHG hemorrhage in refractory cases [146].

Hypertrophic gastropathy

Hypertrophic gastropathy is characterized by diffuse macroscopic enlargement of the gastric folds, primarily in the body of the stomach. These markedly enlarged folds follow the normal rugal pattern of the stomach, and may resemble cerebral convolutions at endoscopy. Three main types are recognized, on the basis of which mucosal compartment is hyperplastic:

- foveolar hyperplasia (Ménétrier disease), usually accompanied by atrophy of oxyntic glands
- hyperplasia of oxyntic glands, without foveolar hyperplasia (Zollinger–Ellison syndrome, see Chapter 50)
- mixed foveolar/oxyntic hyperplasia, seen in a diverse group of conditions (see above), including *H. pylori* infection, cytomegalovirus gastritis in children, lymphocytic gastritis, sarcoidosis, and Cronkhite–Canada syndrome (see Chapter 71).

Ménétrier disease

While enlarged gastric folds may be associated with a wide variety of inflammatory conditions, classic Ménétrier disease is very rare, affecting primarily men in their 50s and 60s. Patients may present with weight loss, abdominal pain, nausea, and vomiting. Histologically, the enlarged folds in Ménétrier disease show massive expansion of the foveolar compartment, with normal or reduced numbers of chief and parietal cells (Figure 51.16). The foveolae are tortuous and dilated, and cystic glands may be seen. Inflammation is not typically a feature, although the enlarged folds are subject to erosion, and may thus show secondary inflammatory changes in the superficial mucosa. In well-developed Ménétrier disease, severe protein loss from the abnormal gastric mucosa leads to hypoalbuminemia; low acid secretion is due to loss of parietal cell mass.

Transient forms of hypertrophic gastropathy resembling Ménétrier disease are seen in children and are almost always associated with cytomegalovirus gastritis [147], although cow's milk protein allergy [148] and other inflammatory disorders have also been implicated. CMV-associated Ménétrier disease has also been reported in adults [149]. The pathogenesis of the classic form of the disorder is unknown, although overexpression of transforming growth factor (TGF)-α, which stimulates epithelial cell proliferation and inhibits gastric acid secretion, among other functions, has been implicated [150]. Medical treatments for Ménétrier disease include antacids, corticosteroids, and PPIs, but thee have been inconsistently effective; treatment with a monoclonal antibody directed against the epidermal growth factor receptor has proven effective in a few patients treated on an experimental basis [151].

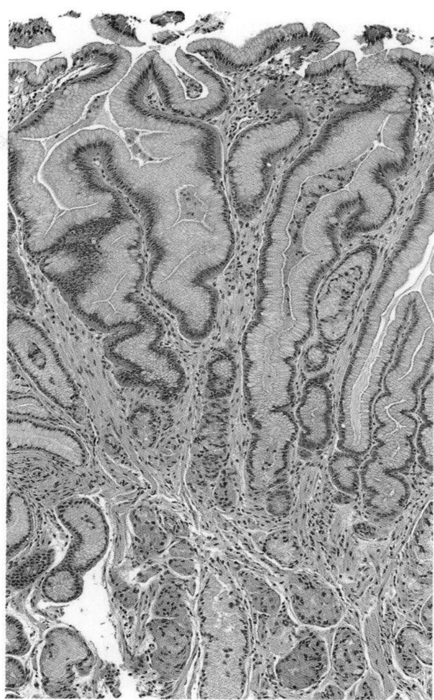

Figure 51.16 The enlarged folds in Ménétrier disease are composed of massively expanded foveolar epithelium, leading to protein loss and hypoalbuminemia.

Gastritis of the cardia

The cardia is an ill-defined anatomical zone of the stomach extending 10–20 mm distal to the lower end of the esophagus. Histologically, cardiac mucosa resembles antral mucosa in that it lacks oxyntic glands. Inflammation of the cardia ("carditis") may be seen in the setting of pangastritis due to *H. pylori* infection; its intensity parallels that of antral inflammation. Similarly, the presence of intestinal metaplasia in the cardia is associated with multifocal atrophic gastritis in the remainder of the stomach. Recent studies suggest that cardiac mucosa at the gastroesophageal junction is associated with gastroesophageal reflux disease in Asian as well as in western populations [152,153]. Intestinal metaplasia of the cardia is present in roughly 3% of *H. pylori*-negative patients with reflux esophagitis and without significant inflammation elsewhere in the stomach [154], raising the issue of whether this finding represents short-segment

Barrett esophagus. Gene expression profiling of microdissected samples suggests that cardiac intestinal metaplasia is more closely related to Barrett's esophagus than gastric antral or corpus intestinal metaplasia in its pattern of gene expression [155].

References are available at www.yamadagastro.com/textbook7e

Further reading

Carr N.J., Leadbetter H., Marriott A. Correlation between the endoscopic and histologic diagnosis of gastritis. Ann Diagn Pathol 2012;16:13.

El-Zimaity H., Choi W.T., Lauwers G.Y., Riddell R. The differential diagnosis of *Helicobacter pylori* negative gastritis. Virchows Archiv 2018;473(5):533.

Fallone C.A., Chiba N., van Zanten S.V., et al. The Toronto consensus for the treatment of Helicobacter pylori infection in adults. Gastroenterology 2016;151(1):51.

Fallone C.A., Moss S.F., Malfertheiner. P. Reconciliation of recent Helicobacter pylori treatment guidelines in a time of increasing resistance to antibiotics. Gastroenterology 2019;157(1):44

Greenberg E.R., Anderson G.L., Morgan D.R., et al. 14-day triple, 5-day concomitant, and 10-day sequential therapies for *Helicobacter pylori* infection in seven Latin American sites: a randomised trial. Lancet 2011;378:507.

Langner C., Schneider N.I., Plieschnegger W., et al. Cardiac mucosa at the gastro-oesophageal junction: indicator of gastro-oesophageal reflux disease? Data from a prospective central European multicentre study on histological and endoscopic diagnosis of oesophagitis (histoGERD trial). Histopathology 2014;65(1):81.

Malfertheiner P., Megraud F., O'Morain C.A., et al. Management of Helicobacter pylori infection-the Maastricht V/Florence Consensus Report. Gut 2017;66(1):6.

Massironi S., Zilli A., Elvevi A., Invernizzi P. The changing face of chronic autoimmune atrophic gastritis: an updated comprehensive perspective. Autoimmunity Rev 2019;18(3):215.

Meyer A.R., Goldenring J.R. Injury, repair, inflammation and metaplasia in the stomach. J Physiol 2018;596(17):3861.

Sato H., Honma T., Owaki T., et al. Clinical and pathological profile of eosinophilic gastroenteritis. Eur J Gastroenterol Hepatol 2019;31(2):157.

Suarez G., Romero-Gallo J., Piazuelo M.B., et al. Nod1 imprints inflammatory and carcinogenic responses toward the gastric pathogen *Helicobacter pylori*. Cancer Res 2019;79(7):1600.

Tan S., Noto J.M., Romero-Gallo J., et al. *Helicobacter pylori* perturbs iron trafficking in the epithelium to grow on the cell surface. PLoS Pathog 2011;7:e1002050.

Wroblewski L.E., Peek R.M. Jr. *Helicobacter pylori*, cancer, and the gastric microbiota. Adv Exp Med Biol 2016;908:393.

CHAPTER 52

Tumors of the stomach

Emad M. El-Omar and Howard Yim
Microbiome Research Center, St George and Sutherland Clinical School, University of New South Wales, Sydney, Australia

Chapter menu

Gastric neoplasia

The earliest descriptions of gastric cancer can be found in ancient Egyptian medical papyri such as the Ebers papyrus dating to around 1550 BC. Gastric tumors are mass lesions arising from any part of the stomach (cardia, corpus or antrum). Ninety percent of gastric malignancy is adenocarcinoma, which is traditionally classified according to the Lauren scheme [1]. This is a simple and still widely used three-tiered system comprising the intestinal type (well differentiated and accounting for approximately half the cases), diffuse type (poorly differentiated and accounting for one-third of cases), and a mixed or unclassified type. In the intestinal type, the malignant cells form glandular-like structures of different degrees of differentiation (Figure 52.1). In the diffuse type, the cells infiltrate through the wall of the stomach, giving rise to a rigid "leather bottle" stomach (Figure 52.2). The 2019 WHO classification of tumors of the digestive system has recently updated the histological classification of gastric cancer [2]. Newer classification systems based on molecular features have also been introduced in the past 5 years.

In this chapter, we primarily discuss gastric adenocarcinoma; other less common gastric malignancies such as lymphoma, GIST, and endocrine tumors will be discussed only briefly.

Gastrointestinal stromal tumors

Gastrointestinal stromal tumors (GISTs) are rare mesenchymal tumors arising from connective tissue [3,4] (Box 52.1). They are mostly located in the stomach (>60%) [5] and most are benign (>70%). Malignant GISTs metastasize into the peritoneal cavity and the liver [3]. Gastric GISTs can present with gastrointestinal bleeding or anemia if ulceration occurs. Otherwise, symptoms depend on location; distal gastric GISTs can cause gastric outlet obstruction and proximal lesions cause dysphagia. Around 20% are identified incidentally on endoscopy or radiological imaging. Patients with GISTs have an increased risk of synchronous and metachronous tumors, including both solid and hematological cancers.

The diagnosis is aided by positive cKit expression in >95% of cases, assessed by positive immunohistochemical staining of CD117. Other immunohistochemical markers can also be positive (CD34, vimentin, smooth muscle actin) [2–4]. The molecular basis is most commonly an activating mutation in the receptor tyrosine kinase, KIT, driving downstream ligand-independent constitutive activation of the MAPK pathway [6]. An alternative mutually exclusive mutation in platelet-derived growth factor receptor α (PDGFRA) has been identified in a minority [7]. GISTs can also be "wild type"

Yamada's Textbook of Gastroenterology, Seventh Edition. Edited by Timothy C. Wang, Michael Camilleri, Benjamin Lebwohl, Anna S. Lok, William J. Sandborn, Kenneth K. Wang, and Gary D. Wu.

Companion website: www.yamadagastro.com/textbook7e

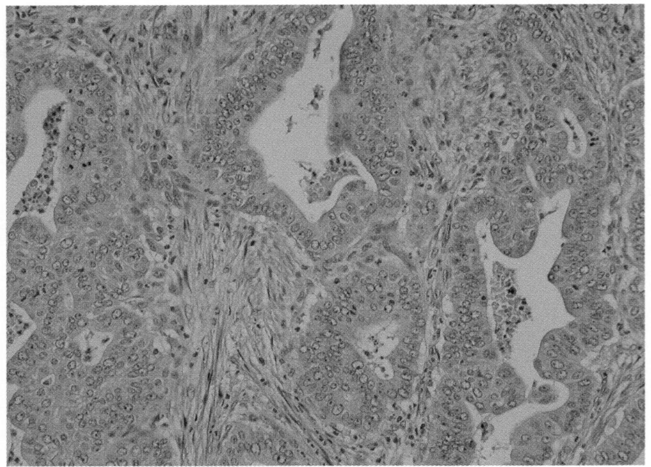

Figure 52.1 Intestinal type gastric adenocarcinoma. Source: Courtesy of Professor Graeme Murray, Aberdeen University.

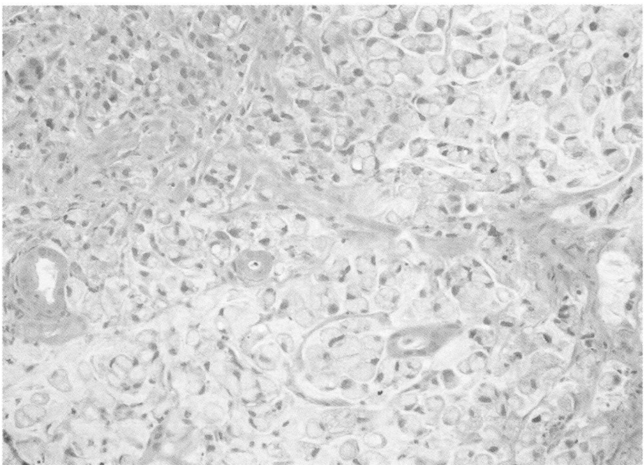

Figure 52.2 Diffuse type gastric cancer. This is characterized by lack of cellular cohesion, invasion throughout the stroma, and poor cellular differentiation. The pathognomonic feature is the presence of signet ring cell morphology. Source: Courtesy of Professor Graeme Murray, Aberdeen University.

Box 52.1 Key facts.

- Gastric cancer remains a common malignancy in many parts of the world, but the incidence shows great geographic variation
- Symptomatic presentation is usually a sign of advanced disease.
- The 5-year survival is less than 20% and depends on stage
- Known predisposing conditions include:
  - *H. pylori*
  - Autoimmune gastritis
  - Previous gastric surgery
- Diagnosis is usually made by endoscopy
- Surgery is the mainstay of treatment

with no demonstrable kinase activation; therefore, CD117 negativity does not exclude the diagnosis.

Surgical resection with curative intent is the primary treatment. The discovery of the oncogenic driver KIT/PDGFRA mutations has led to successful use of the tyrosine kinase inhibitors imatinib or sunitinib for unresectable, metastatic or recurrent GIST [8]. These agents are being assessed in an adjuvant and neoadjuvant capacity and several clinicopathological parameters are used in a risk assessment capacity to aid treatment strategies [8,9]. Several prognostic algorithms are proposed and include tumor size, location, mitotic index, and presence of rupture [8–10]. However, resistance to these chemotherapeutic agents develops due to kinase mutations and disease progresses.

Neuroendocrine tumors

Neuroendocrine neoplasms (NENs) of the stomach are gastric epithelial neoplasms with neuroendocrine differentiation, including well-differentiated neuroendocrine tumors (NETs), poorly differentiated neuroendocrine carcinomas (NECs), and mixed neuroendocrine–nonneuroendocrine neoplasms (MiNENs)– an umbrella category including mixed adenoneuroendocrine carcinoma (MANEC) [2].

Neuroendocrine tumors are a heterogeneous group of neoplasms, thought to arise mainly from enterochromaffin-like (ECL) cells or their progenitors. While many have assumed that gastric carcinoids arise from ECL cells, there is no lineage tracing data to support this, and some have proposed stem or progenitor cells as the source of these tumors [11]. NETs are divided into subgroups 1, 2, and 3 based on histological features [12,13], namely Ki67 score and mitotic index. It has been long recognized that different types exhibit differing characteristic biochemical features. Type 1 NETs are associated with achlorhydria arising as a consequence of varying etiologies, such as previous surgery with vagotomy, pharmacological reduction of acid secretion, or *H. pylori*-induced chronic atrophic gastritis, and hypergastrinemia [14]. Fraenkel and colleagues reported a systematic review of the epidemiology of these tumors over the last four decades and noted an increasing incidence worldwide [15]. The majority of gastric NETs are type 1. Each type is associated with a different prognostic outcome. Type 3, described as neuroendocrine carcinoma and mixed adenoneuroendocrine carcinoma, often has evidence of metastases at diagnosis and is associated with a poor prognosis.

The WHO classification criteria have supported the emergence of a prognostic and treatment algorithm, based on clinicopathological parameters. Surgery or endoscopic resection is prominent in the treatment algorithm, although regular endoscopic surveillance of type 1 gastric NETs <1 cm is recommended as first-line management [16]. Given the poorer prognosis, type 3 NETs are treated more aggressively with gastrectomy and lymph node dissection. Chemotherapy is suitable for a cohort of patients, including those with "functioning," hormone-secreting tumors. Chemotherapeutic options include somatostatin analogs or α-interferon [17].

Lymphomas

The stomach is the most common extranodal site of lymphomas [18,19]. These are almost exclusively B cell in origin. Two main subtypes present in this location: marginal zone lymphoma of mucosa-associated lymphoid tissue (MALT lymphoma) and diffuse large B-cell lymphomas. The former accounts for >50% of gastric lymphomas and although incidence has been increasing, it remains rare, representing <2% of gastric malignancies. MALT lymphoma is low grade and behaves in an indolent fashion, although metastases to lymph node, liver, lung, and bone marrow can occur. Typical lymphoma B symptoms are rare, and most patients present with nonspecific upper gastrointestinal symptoms.

Macroscopically, MALT lymphomas manifest as a wide range of lesions, from overt ulcerated mass to single erosions or gastric fold thickening. The etiological factor that drives this malignancy is *H. pylori* infection [18,19]. However, given the high incidence of this infection worldwide and the rare occurrence of MALT lymphoma, other factors must be crucial in the pathophysiology of this disease. It is known that the pathogenesis of MALT lymphoma involves interplay between B cells and T cells, cytokine signaling via *H. pylori*-induced macrophage-derived a proliferation-inducing ligand (APRIL), and also genetic factors, including translocations and polymorphisms of innate immune genes [20]. By far the most common translocation, which occurs in approximately 25% of gastric MALT lymphomas, is t(11;18). This causes reciprocal fusion of the API2 and MALT1 genes and generates an API2-MALT1 fusion product, which is a potent NFκB activator. in vitro studies show that the API2-MALT1 fusion product protects cells from both p53- and FAS-induced apoptosis and this protective effect depends on its ability to activate NFκB. *H. pylori* eradication is first-line treatment for low-grade, nonmetastatic MALT lymphoma and this results in remission in >75% patients [21]. Persistent, recurrent or progressive disease is treated successfully with radiotherapy, followed by chemotherapy or surgical options.

Gastric adenocarcinoma

Definition and classification

Gastric adenocarcinoma is a malignant epithelial neoplasm of the gastric mucosa, with glandular differentiation [2]. The tumor arises in any of the three compartments of the stomach (cardia, corpus or antrum) and has the potential for invasive growth and metastasis to regional lymph glands and distant organs. According to the Eighth Edition of the Union for International Cancer Control (UICC) TNM classification, any cancer whose epicentre lies >2 cm distal to the esophagogastric junction is regarded as gastric [22].

Macroscopic classification

According to the Japanese Classification of Gastric Cancers Third Edition [23], early gastric adenocarcinomas are classified as follows.

- Type 0-I (protruding): polyploid lesions, protruding >3 mm
- Type 0-IIa (superficial elevated): slightly elevated lesions protruding <3 mm
- Type 0-IIb (superficial flat): tumors without elevation or depression
- Type 0-IIc (superficial depressed): slightly depressed lesions
- Type 0-III (excavated): lesions with a deep depression
- Type 0 denotes the early superficial nature of the lesions

Advanced gastric cancers, more prevalent in the west, are usually described using the Borrmann classification. This system was first proposed in 1926 and relies on assessment of gross appearance during surgery or after resection or preoperatively by endoscopy. The scheme classifies advanced gastric cancers into four types.

- Type I: polypoid fungating
- Type II: ulcerative with elevated distinct borders
- Type III: ulcerative with indistinct borders
- Type IV: diffuse, indistinct borders

Types I and II are localized, while types III and IV are infiltrative. The type IV diffusely infiltrating growth is also referred to as linitis plastica where most of the gastric wall is involved by infiltrating tumor cells (signet ring cells). Recently, Song et al. showed that the clinicopathological characteristics and prognosis of patients with Borrmann types of gastric cancer are different and can be used as a valuable factor to predict survival in advanced gastric cancer patients, especially in those TNM stage III undergoing curative resection [24].

Histopathology

Histologically, gastric cancer is traditionally classified according to Laurén into intestinal, diffuse, mixed, indeterminate, and undefined types [1]. Other classification schemes include the Japanese Gastric Cancer Association classification and the WHO scheme. In the latest (2019) WHO classification of tumors of the digestive system, gastric cancer is classified into five main subtypes [2].

1. Tubular adenocarcinoma: this is the most common subtype ranging in frequency between 45% in Europe and 64% in Japan.
2. Papillary adenocarcinoma: this subtype is relatively rare (2.7–9.9% of cases) and is most commonly well differentiated yet is associated with a higher frequency of liver metastasis and poor survival.
3. Poorly cohesive adenocarcinoma, including signet ring cell carcinoma and other subtypes: this subtype accounts for 20–54% of cases, with higher frequencies in Japan. Poorly cohesive adenocarcinomas can be of either signet ring or

nonsignet ring cell type. Some evidence suggests that signet ring cell carcinomas have a lower sensitivity to chemo(radio) therapy [25,26].

4. Mucinous adenocarcinoma: this subtype is relatively rare (2.1–8.1% of cases) and has two main growth patterns – a glandular structure with interstitial mucin and a form characterized by nests or single tumor cells (including signet ring cells) surrounded by mucin.
5. Mixed-pattern adenocarcinoma: this subtype accounts for 6–22% of cases and may contain two histological components – glandular and signet ring cell type. Mixed cancers have a poorer prognosis than those with a single component.

In addition to the five main subtypes, there are other rare subtypes including adenocarcinoma with lymphoid stroma (medullary carcinoma); hepatoid adenocarcinoma; micropapillary adenocarcinoma; adenocarcinoma of fundic gland type; and other rare subtypes (mucoepidermoid carcinoma, Paneth cell carcinoma, parietal cell carcinoma). Some histological variants have a poor prognosis (e.g., adenocarcinoma with enteroblastic differentiation), while others have a good (e.g., gastric carcinoma with lymphoid stroma = EBV-positive gastric cancer) or very good prognosis (e.g., gastric adenocarcinoma of fundic gland type).

Gastric cancers are also classified on the basis of their location in the stomach into cardia cancers (arising from the narrow rim of cardiac mucosa around the esophago-gastric junction), proximal cancers (involving the proximal third of the stomach), or distal cancers (involving the distal third of the stomach). Interestingly, location of gastric cancer shows a geographic pattern that matches the incidence. Thus, in high-incidence areas such as Asia, Central and South America and eastern Europe, 80% of gastric cancers are classified as distal whereas in low-incidence areas such as North America and the UK, 50–60% of gastric cancers are located in the cardia or fundus [27].

Finally, gastric cancers are classified on the basis of stage into early gastric cancer (EGC) and advanced gastric cancer. Early gastric cancer is very common in the Far East, particularly in Japan, and carries an excellent prognosis (>90% 5-year survival), while advanced gastric cancer is the more common presentation in the west and carries a dismal prognosis (<20% 5-year survival). Gastric cancers are also classified on the basis of molecular features. Lei et al. classified cancers into three subtypes based on gene expression profiling: proliferative, metabolic, and mesenchymal [28]. The three subtypes differed on the basis of molecular and genetic features and also in their response to therapy. More recently, the Cancer Genome Atlas (TCGA) has proposed a molecular classification dividing gastric cancer into four subtypes [29]; this classification system will be discussed in more detail below.

Epidemiology

Incidence and mortality

Gastric cancer remains a global health burden, being a leading cause of death worldwide. There is great geographic variation in the incidence of gastric cancer. According to the latest GLOBOCAN estimates, 1 089 103 new cases (5.6% of the total) of stomach cancer were estimated to have occurred in 2020, making it the fifth most common malignancy in the world, after cancers of the breast, lung, colorectum, and prostate [30]. This represents a substantive change since the very first estimates in 1975 when stomach cancer was the most common neoplasm. Gastric cancers are diagnosed more frequently in developed nations with an average incidence rate among high-middle Human Development Index (HDI) nations of 20 per 100 000 for males, compared to 6.6 per 100 000 among low-middle HDI nations. Two-thirds of the world total occurs in eastern Asia, mainly in China. Age-standardized (world) incidence rates range from 4.5 in middle Africa to 32.5 in eastern Asia for men, and from 2.4 in southern Africa to 13.2 in eastern Asia for women [30].

Stomach cancer is the fourth leading cause of cancer death in both sexes worldwide (768 793 deaths, 7.7% of the total). The highest age-standardized (world) mortality rates for both genders combined are in East Asia (22.4 per 100 000). High mortality rates are also present in both sexes in central and eastern Europe, and in Central and South America [30]. Gastric cancer is twice as common in males than females [30]. In recent years, there has been an observed increase in the incidence in younger people (<50 years) in both low-incidence and high-incidence countries such as the USA and the UK, Chile and Belarus, suggesting a change in the disease risk and epidemiology of gastric cancer [31]. In the USA, gastric cancer in those aged younger than 50 years is more common in females and Hispanics, is more likely to be of diffuse and poorly differentiated histology and is generally more aggressive with a propensity for metastasis [32]. Cho et al. reported that early-onset diffuse gastric cancers contained somatic mutations in CDH1 or TGFBR1 compared with late-onset counterparts [33]. Interestingly, early-onset diffuse gastric cancers in women contained significantly more mutations in CDH1 or TGFBR1 than similar cancers in men [33]. Attention to ongoing transitions in gastric cancer epidemiology is therefore relevant to future cancer control and clinical practice. Gastric cancer exerts a major global burden and it is estimated that over 19 million disability-adjusted life-years (DALYs) are currently lost due to the disease [34].

Geographic and regional variations in incidence are thought to reflect differences in environmental factors, which could include differences in dietary habits and the prevalence of *H. pylori* infection. There have been substantial reductions in the incidence rates of gastric cancer across the globe. The reasons for this reduction include improved hygiene and the widespread use of refrigeration, ensuring year-round availability of fresh fruits and vegetables, less reliance on salted/preserved foods, and reduction of bacterial content of foods. Another important reason is the reduction in the incidence of *H. pylori* infection in many parts of the world. In terms of mortality, this remains very high in most countries except Japan, which instituted a mass screening program based on fluoroscopy which has allowed recognition and treatment of early gastric cancer.

According to data from the Surveillance, Epidemiology, and End Results Program (SEER), approximately 0.8% of men and women will be diagnosed with gastric cancer at some point during their lifetime. The median age at diagnosis is 68 years and 71 at death. The estimated new cases of gastric cancers in the US in 2020 are 27 600 and deaths 11 010 [35]. The median age at diagnosis is 68 years and the median age at death is 71 years, although in some parts of the US there has been an unusual increase in the gastric cancer incidence in patients under 30 years of age. Almost twice as many men as women are diagnosed with gastric cancer and the same applies for the death rate, independent of ethnic background. All races have a higher rate of diagnosis compared to whites. The overall 5-year relative survival rate in the US is 32.0%. The survival rate is dramatically different depending on the stage of the disease: 70% for stage IA and 5.5% for stage IV [35].

Risk factors

Hereditary factors

Approximately 10–15% of gastric cancers arise in individuals with a significant family history of the condition [36]. An increased risk of gastric cancer is associated with several of the recognized dominantly inherited cancer predisposition syndromes, such as familial adenomatous polyposis, hereditary nonpolyposis colon cancer (HNPCC), and Peutz–Jeghers syndrome. Hereditary diffuse gastric cancer (HDGC) is an autosomal dominant cancer syndrome characterized by a high prevalence of diffuse gastric cancer and lobular breast cancer [37]. HDGC is highly penetrant and the average age at diagnosis is 38 years. The worldwide population incidence is around 5–10 per 100 000 births. It is largely caused by inactivating germline mutations in the tumor suppressor gene CDH1, which encodes the epithelial cell adhesion protein E-cadherin. A minority of families harbor pathogenic variants in CTNNA1. The updated 2020 HDGC genetic testing criteria and clinical practice recommendations have recently been published [37].

H. pylori infection

By far the most important etiological risk factor is *H. pylori* infection, which is the most common single chronic bacterial infection that affects half the world's population. The discovery of *H. pylori* by Warren and Marshall in 1983 proved to be pivotal in the understanding of the etiology of gastric cancer. In 1994 the WHO and the International Agency for Research on Cancer consensus group concluded that there was sufficient evidence to classify *H. pylori* as a Class I (i.e., definite) human carcinogen [38]. The evidence as it stood at that time comprised epidemiological studies only, many of which were poorly controlled for confounding risk factors for gastric cancer. Over the subsequent decade, numerous cohort and case–control studies were published demonstrating an association between serological evidence of *H. pylori* infection and increased risk of gastric cancer. Many of these data have been subjected to metaanalysis with the conclusion that *H. pylori* infection carries at least a twofold increased risk for the development of gastric cancer [39].

Some of these metaanalyses addressed the question of cardia versus noncardia cancer and also the histological subtype. For example, the metaanalysis of Huang et al. [40] found an odds ratio (OR) of 3.08 (95% confidence interval [CI] 1.78–5.31) for noncardia cancer compared to an OR of 1.23 (95% CI 0.56–2.71) for cardia cancer. The same study found the association between *H. pylori* infection and gastric cancer was equally strong for intestinal and diffuse type cancer (OR 2.49, 95% CI 1.41–4.43, and OR 2.58, 95% CI 1.47–4.53, respectively). The study by the Helicobacter and Cancer Collaborative Group, headed by Forman, analyzed the data from 12 case–control studies nested within prospective cohorts [41]. They reported an overall OR for gastric cancer in those who were *H. pylori* positive of 2.36 (95% CI 1.98–2.81). The risk was confined to noncardia cancer (OR 2.97, 95% CI 2.34–3.77) and not to cardia cancer (OR 0.99, 95% CI 0.72–1.35). Furthermore, they found that the OR for noncardia gastric cancer was stronger when blood samples for *H. pylori* serology were collected more than 10 years before cancer diagnosis (OR 5.9, 95% CI 3.4–10.3) and they argued that this higher estimate is a more accurate reflection of the risk. Finally, the authors found that *H. pylori* infection was associated with an equally increased risk of intestinal and diffuse noncardia cancer (OR 4.45, 95% CI 2.74–7.24, and OR 3.39, 95% CI 1.70–6.76, respectively).

Another remarkable study that was published since the above metaanalyses were carried out is the study of Uemura et al. [42]. The authors prospectively studied 1526 Japanese patients who had duodenal ulcers, gastric ulcers, gastric hyperplasia, or nonulcer dyspepsia at the time of enrollment; 1246 of these patients had *H. pylori* infection and 280 were negative. The mean follow-up was 7.8 years, and the patients underwent endoscopy with biopsy at baseline and then between 1 and 3 years after enrollment. Gastric cancers developed in 36 (2.9%) of the infected and none of the uninfected patients. The authors identified corpus-predominant gastritis as the most serious gastric phenotype giving a relative risk for cancer of 34.5 (95% CI 7.1–166.7). Presence of severe gastric atrophy and intestinal metaplasia were also distinct risk factors. Interestingly, none of the 275 patients with duodenal ulcers (DU) developed gastric cancer, confirming previous studies that DU disease protects from this malignancy.

As *H. pylori* may disappear in advanced gastric cancer, it is informative to compare the risk of the disease in early versus advanced cases. Wang et al. performed a metaanalysis to systematically review the relationship between *H. pylori* infection and early gastric cancer [43]. Their findings indicated that *H. pylori* infection is strongly associated with early gastric cancer when compared with nonneoplasm controls or advanced gastric cancer.

Thus, *H. pylori* infection increases the risk of gastric cancer, but are all strains of the bacterium equally harmful? It is well established that strains possessing the cytotoxin-associated gene A (CagA) cause more severe tissue damage and are associated with increased risk of DU disease and gastric cancer. Huang et al. carried out a metaanalysis of the relationship between

CagA seropositivity and risk of gastric cancer [44]. They identified 16 qualified studies with 2284 cases and 2770 controls. *H. pylori* and CagA seropositivity significantly increased the risk for gastric cancer by 2.28-fold and 2.87-fold, respectively. Furthermore, among *H. pylori*-infected populations, CagA seropositivity further increased the risk for gastric cancer by 1.64-fold (95% CI 1.21–2.24) overall and by 2.01-fold (95% CI 1.21–3.32) for noncardia gastric cancer. Interestingly, not all CagA strains are equal and studies suggest that the C-terminal variable region of *H. pylori* CagA containing Glu-Pro-Ile-Tyr-Ala (EPIYA) motifs can influence virulence of the strains. EPIYA motifs are classified as A, B, C, and D. CagA from western strains contains EPIYA A and B motifs followed by 0–3 repeats of EPIYA C motifs. East Asian-type CagA contains the EPIYA A and B motifs, followed by one EPIYA D motif. East Asian-type CagA has been found to be more carcinogenic than the western-type CagA [45,46].

In addition to CagA, there are other bacterial virulence factors that have been associated with increased risk of gastric cancer. These include the vacuolating cytotoxin VacA and some outer membrane proteins such as OipA and BabA [47].

In summary, the epidemiological evidence strongly suggests that *H. pylori* infection increases the risk of noncardia gastric cancer of both histological subtypes while the risk of cardia cancer is dependent on geography, being higher in the east [48] but not increased in the west. Virulent strains, such as CagA-positive strains, further increase the risk of cancer. While this epidemiological evidence is impressive, it is not sufficient to ascribe causality unless clear evidence is provided by suitable animal models. Several such models have been developed (e.g., INS-GAS mice, Mongolian gerbil models, and CagA transgenic mice) and the evidence is now incontrovertible ([49]. Perhaps the most impressive evidence for the critical role of *H. pylori* in gastric cancer has come from studies showing that successful eradication of the infection reduces the incidence of this cancer [50–52], as will be discussed later in this chapter.

Other risk factors

Pernicious anemia, with its hallmark of autoimmune gastritis leading to atrophy, has long been known to confer an increased risk of gastric cancer [53], but this risk is very small compared to *H. pylori*-induced multifocal atrophic gastritis. Song et al. carried out a systematic review and metaanalysis to examine the association between autoimmune conditions and gastric cancer risk. In addition to pernicious anemia, they identified eight other conditions with increased risk, including dermatomyositis, Addison disease, diabetes mellitus type 1 and dermatitis herpetiformis [54]. The authors concluded that these associations may reflect unreported links between these conditions and autoimmune gastritis [54].

Similarly, it is well established that benign ulcer surgery, such as partial gastrectomy, is also associated with increased risk of gastric cancer [55]. Following gastric surgery, inflammation of the gastric remnant is common and usually associated with bile reflux. In addition, most of these patients harbor *H. pylori* infection and thus have chronic gastritis. Rendering the stomach achlorhydric by the surgery itself increases the chances of neoplastic transformation. Indeed, both pernicious anemia and the postsurgical stomach share this common pathophysiological abnormality, namely hypochlorhydria. This abnormal physiological state leads to bacterial overgrowth and it is likely that this altered microbiota sustains and drives chronic inflammation and subsequent carcinogenesis, with or without *H. pylori*.

There has been concern that inducing hypochlorhydria pharmacologically might increase the risk of gastric cancer. Recent observational studies have questioned whether proton pump inhibitors increase the risk of gastric cancer by 2.4-fold in subjects who have had successful eradication of *H. pylori* infection [56]. However, the findings from such observational studies have been criticized for inadequate adjustment for confounders, surveillance bias, a lack of dose response or duration response, and other critically important flaws in study design [57,58]. Finally, patients who have developed gastric cancer are also at increased risk of developing further lesions (either synchronous or recurrent). This is particularly seen in Japanese patients in whom early gastric cancers were removed endoscopically. It is mandatory in such patients to eradicate *H. pylori* infection if present at the time of the first resection of cancer.

Although *H. pylori* plays a crucial role in the pathogenesis of sporadic gastric cancer, it cannot be considered as the sole causative agent in this malignancy. There are other factors that clearly contribute, including diet and smoking.

Diet

The marked geographic variation in gastric cancer incidence suggests that environmental influences play an important etiological role, and much attention in the past focused on the possible association between diet and gastric cancer risk. It has been postulated that the downward trend in gastric cancer incidence may in part be due to the advent of widespread refrigeration of food, hence increased intake of fresh produce, and less reliance on food preservation.

Numerous retrospective studies have suggested a protective effect from diets rich in fresh fruit and vegetables; however, when one considers case–control and prospective data only, the evidence is less robust (59). Data from a large European prospective study (EPIC-EURGAST) analyzed in 2006 failed to show an overall association between fruit or vegetable consumption and gastric cancer risk but showed a statistically significant association between total dietary vegetable content (and onion and garlic intake) and the intestinal histological subtype [60]. Additionally, a nonsignificant negative association was observed between cardia cancer risk and citrus fruit consumption. Interestingly, the effect of fruit and vegetable intake appeared to be independent of *H. pylori* status. However, a more up-to-date reanalysis of the EPIC-EUROGAST data in 2012 based on a longer follow-up and twice the number of gastric cancer cases showed no association between total or specific vegetable intake and gastric cancer risk [61]. The inverse association between fresh fruit and citrus fruits and risk of gastric cancer was restricted to smokers and the northern European countries. Overall, the authors concluded that fresh fruit and citrus fruit consumption may protect against diffuse and cardia GC, respectively [61].

In summary, prospective and interventional studies have not confirmed a large role for diet in gastric cancer pathogenesis and this may be due to the complex interaction between diet, host genetics, and the microbiome. The importance of the latter is just beginning to be appreciated.

Vitamin C and other antioxidant nutrients have attracted a lot of attention as the potential mediators of any dietary influence on gastric cancer risk. Vitamin C seems a promising candidate since its levels are reduced in the serum of *H. pylori*-infected individuals, and, as well as being a free radical scavenger, it reduces the formation of potentially carcinogenic N-nitroso compounds [62]. Data from the prospective EPIC cohort show a negative association between gastric cancer risk and serum vitamin C, but not dietary vitamin C intake, and this was unaffected by *H. pylori* status [63].

A review by the Cochrane Collaboration, which included a number of high-quality randomized trials, concluded that there is no evidence that dietary supplementation with antioxidants, including vitamin C, reduces gastric cancer risk [64].

Salt and nitrite are other dietary components that have been implicated in gastric cancer risk. Both are frequently used in food preservation. Pickled and smoked foods may also contain potential carcinogens such as N-nitroso compounds and benzp(a)yrene. Of note is the fact that the Japanese diet is particularly rich in salted fish and pickled vegetables. Dietary nitrate, of which a significant portion may come from water depending on the source, can be converted to nitrite by nitrate reductase-synthesizing bacteria. *H. pylori* infection and hypochlorhydria facilitate the growth of such bacteria.

Dietary salt and nitroso compounds appear to exert a synergistic effect with *H. pylori* in animal models of gastric carcinogenesis. Several case–control studies in humans have shown a positive association between gastric cancer risk and both salt and dietary nitrate/nitrite intake although data from prospective studies are conflicting [65–67].

Iron is another factor that is emerging as a link between *H. pylori* infection and pathogenesis of *H. pylori*-induced gastric cancer. Noto et al. showed that iron deficiency enhances *H. pylori* virulence and represents a measurable biomarker to identify populations of infected persons at high risk for gastric cancer [68]. Experimentally, iron-deficient Mongolian gerbils infected with CagA+ *H. pylori* develop more severe inflammation and accelerated premalignant and malignant lesions compared with infected animals fed an iron-replete diet [68].

In summary, it is very likely that dietary constituents directly influence the pathogenic potential of *H. pylori* by augmenting the expression and function of cancer-associated microbial virulence determinants [69].

Smoking

Smoking is an independent risk factor for gastric intestinal metaplasia and gastric cancer. Thrift et al. recently showed that ever smokers had a twofold increased risk of gastric intestinal metaplasia compared to never smokers while risk in former smokers remained significantly elevated until 15 years post cessation [70]. Prospective studies have demonstrated a significant dose-dependent association between tobacco smoke and gastric cancer risk [71,72]. In the EPIC cohort, it was estimated that 17.6% of gastric cancers in this European population were attributable to cigarette smoking [73].

Pathogenesis

Gastric cancer is a paradigm for inflammation-induced and microbially driven cancer. The etiology in most cases is *H. pylori* infection and the pathogenesis is strongly influenced by host genetic factors and environmental exposures (Box 52.2). The molecular pathway of cancer progression in the stomach is well understood. Most sporadic gastric cancers are considered inflammation driven, and their etiology is characteristically environmental, usually triggered by *H. pylori* infection [74]. The infectious etiology explains why gastric cancer may be viewed as a potentially preventable malignancy, though it remains lethal. Chronic gastric inflammation leads to glandular loss and atrophy with inevitable reduction, and eventually total loss, of gastric acid secretory capacity. The loss of gastric acid leads to

Box 52.2 Causes and risk factors.

Significant risk factors

Conditions associated with hypochlorhydria

H. pylori-associated gastritis
Autoimmune gastritis
Post gastric surgery (>20 years)
Chronic atrophic gastritis

Chronic mucosal changes

High-grade dysplasia
Barrett esophagus (adenocarcinoma of cardia and distal esophagus)
Gastric adenoma
Intestinal metaplasia

Genetic risk factors

Gastric cancer families
Familial adenomatous polyposis coli (FAP)
Hereditary nonpolyposis coli
Germline E-cadherin (CDH1) mutations
Proinflammatory cytokine gene polymorphisms
Novel polymorphisms identified by genome-wide association studies (e.g., PSCA, MUC1)

Possible risk factors

Peutz–Jeghers syndrome
Ménétrier disease
Smoking
Diets low in fresh fruit and vegetables
Diets high in preserved, pickled or smoked items
Alcohol

changes in the gastric microbiome and colonization by proinflammatory and nitrosamine-generating bacteria that exert genotoxic pressure on the stem cell compartment [75]. The mucosal atrophy and metaplasia may then progress to neoplasia after further molecular alterations. Metaplastic changes in the upper gastrointestinal tract are well recognized as early cancer precursors, but their precise molecular mechanisms and the exact role of progenitor cells play in the oncogenic cascade remain a subject of intense investigation [74].

In the section below, we discuss the contribution of genetic factors to the pathogenesis of gastric cancer. We also outline the most widely accepted model of gastric cancer pathogenesis.

Genetic factors contributing to gastric cancer

The vast majority of gastric cancers arise sporadically with no demonstrable inherited component. Less than 15% of cases are thought to have familial clustering and most of these are not associated with a definitive germline mutation. Less than 3% of gastric cancer cases are linked to hereditary cancer syndromes [76].

The most frequent hereditary gastric cancer syndrome is HDGC [37,76]. This autosomal dominant condition is associated most frequently with a CDH1 germline mutation, the gene encoding E-cadherin. E-cadherin protein exerts an essential role in cell–cell adhesion. Indeed, acquired somatic mutation of this gene resulting in an impaired protein function is widely associated with cancers at many different sites. The molecular mechanism of HDGC most frequently involves a heterozygous germline mutation of CDH1 that can take many forms such as deletion, frameshift mutation, splice site mutation, or missense mutation, involving a variety of gene sites and not only restricted to coding regions but possibly including the untranslated regions. Loss of function mutation in the remaining allele can be caused by a number of mechanisms such a loss of heterozygosity or promoter hypermethylation and lead to clinical phenotype [77].

Recently, an additional hereditary gastric cancer syndrome has been reported, named Gastric Adenocarcinoma and Proximal Polyposis of the Stomach (GAPPS) [78,79]. It has an autosomal dominant pattern of inheritance and is characterized by >100 gastric polyps carpeting the proximal stomach in the absence of colorectal and duodenal polyposis and other hereditary polyposis syndromes. Histology is predominantly that of fundic gland polyps with regions of dysplasia, some of which undergo malignant progression to intestinal type gastric adenocarcinoma. It is important to note that fundic gland polyps are frequently seen in patients on long-term proton pump inhibitor therapy but are almost always benign and require no further follow-up. The underlying genetic abnormality in GAPPS was described by Li et al. who identified point mutations in APC promoter 1B that cosegregated with disease in all families studied [79]. These mutations reduced binding of the YY1 transcription factor and impaired activity of the APC promoter 1B in luciferase assays. Analysis of blood and saliva from carriers showed allelic imbalance of APC, suggesting that these mutations lead to decreased allele-specific expression in vivo [79].

Hereditary nonpolyposis colon cancer (HNPCC), also known as Lynch syndrome, carries an increased risk of intestinal type gastric cancer, arising through disordered DNA repair mediated by mutation in the DNA mismatch repair genes such as MLH1, MLH2, PMS2, and MSH6. This in turn increases mutation rate in oncogene and tumor suppressor genes, leading to cancer initiation and progression; instability of repeat nucleotide sequences or microsatellites is a key characteristic of this phenotype, termed microsatellite instability. Gastric cancer appears to be a common extracolonic manifestation of this syndrome. A study of cancer registries in northern Europe and the USA by the Lynch group and collaborators reported that the lifetime gastric cancer risk in HNPCC families is around 7%, occurring primarily over the age of 50 years [80]. In an analysis of data from 3828 carriers of Lynch syndrome-associated mutations, Kim et al. found history of gastric cancer to be independently associated with male sex, older age, mutations in MLH1 or MSH2, and number of first-degree relatives with gastric cancer [81].

There are other rarer hereditary syndromes (associated with malignancies in a vast array of organs) that carry an increased risk of gastric cancer, such as Li–Fraumeni syndrome (germline mutation in TP53 gene) and Peutz–Jeghers syndrome (mutation within STK11 (serine/threonine-protein kinase 11) [76]. Familial adenomatous polyposis (FAP), an autosomal dominant condition with mutation of the APC gene, predominantly manifests with colonic adenomatous lesions that exert a high risk of malignant transformation. This condition is associated with polyp lesions throughout the gastrointestinal tract, including the proximal stomach. Martin et al. observed gastric adenomas in 14% of patients with FAP; of these, 5% contained high-grade dysplasia [82]. The risk of high-grade dysplasia correlated with adenoma size. Endoscopic resection was feasible but did not completely eliminate the cancer risk. There are several reported cases of gastric cancer in patients with FAP and therefore current surveillance guidelines suggest regular endoscopies to assess for this and also to detect the more common duodenal adenoma phenotype that carries a high risk of malignant transformation [83].

Acquired genetic factors contributing to sporadic gastric cancer

Acquired genetic abnormalities can be a result of chromosomal insufficiency, microsatellite instability, changes in the epigenetic landscape or microRNA profile that profoundly affect downstream gene expression, somatic gene mutations or single nucleotide polymorphisms (SNPs) within key candidate genes. All these mechanisms can lead to dysregulated signaling pathways, altered interaction between host and environment such as response to intraluminal pathogens/dietary components, disruption of the cell cycle, growth proliferation or cell death characteristics that favor the hallmarks of cancer [84]. These molecular aberrations do not occur in isolation and an individual tumor may exhibit many simultaneous changes in molecular profile compared to a nonmalignant cell, leading to documented intra- and interpatient heterogeneity.

A comprehensive molecular characterization of gastric adenocarcinoma has been undertaken by the Cancer Genome Atlas Research Network [85]. The authors propose a molecular classification dividing gastric cancer into four subtypes:

1. tumors positive for Epstein–Barr virus, which display recurrent PIK3CA mutations, extreme DNA hypermethylation, and amplification of JAK2, CD274, and PDCD1LG2
2. microsatellite unstable tumors, which show elevated mutation rates, including mutations of genes encoding targetable oncogenic signaling proteins
3. genomically stable tumors, which are enriched for the diffuse histological variant and mutations of RHOA or fusions involving RHO-family GTPase-activating proteins
4. tumors with chromosomal instability, which show marked aneuploidy and focal amplification of receptor tyrosine kinases.

Around 9% of gastric cancers are associated with Epstein–Barr virus (EBV) and around 80 000 patients are estimated to develop EBV-associated gastric cancer annually. This subtype of gastric cancer is characterized by male predominance, younger age, predisposition to the proximal stomach, low prevalence of *H. pylori* infection, a high proportion in diffuse-type gastric carcinomas, and a relatively favorable prognosis. The characteristic molecular abnormality is global and nonrandom CpG island methylation of the promoter region of many cancer-related genes, which causes downregulation of their expression [85].

Chromosomal instability

Gastric cancers with chromosomal instability (CIN) account for 50% of cases. CIN is a hallmark of malignancy that can occur as an early or late event in disease progression and may also be transient. In gastric cancer, chromosomal aberrations are numerous [86]. These have been linked to histological type; for example, intestinal and diffuse gastric cancer is associated with copy number gains at 8q, 17q, 20q, 12q, and 13q chromosomal locations, respectively, with similar unique patterns of loss of chromosomal material in each histological type, with particular patterns of CIN linked to patient outcome and other clinicopathological parameters [87,88]. Genomic instability has also been shown to differ according to geographical location, highlighting the importance of gene–environment interactions in disease pathogenesis [89].

Creation of fusion genes via translocations is common in hematological cancers but less so in solid tumors. In gastric cancer, Tao et al. identified a SLC1A2 gene breakpoint mutation with detectable SLC1A2-CD44 fusion protein due to chromosomal inversion. This led to physiological alteration of cell growth properties, likely due to aberration in metabolic pathways [90]. Similarly, a novel fusion protein involving the ROS1 gene has been identified as a consequence of genetic rearrangement in gastric cancer, although occurring at a lower frequency [91]. The ROS1 gene encodes a transmembrane receptor tyrosine kinase. Notably, genetic rearrangements leading to constitutive expression of this gene within a fusion protein confer transforming potential [92]. The identification of this particular genetic rearrangement is important given that a potential therapeutic option is available for this patient subgroup using small molecule kinase inhibitor drugs. These studies highlight a novel mechanism of CIN in gastric cancer and have uncovered a potential novel therapeutic target, although it should be noted that these occur at low frequency.

The literature on chromosomal aberrations, such as amplification, deletion or loss of heterozygosity (LOH) in gastric cancer is vast and involves a multitude of genes. LOH affects many chromosomal sites in gastric cancer, with 18 loci on 17 chromosomes implicated [86]; the degree of LOH (LOH-high or LOH-low) appears important in disease progression and the most common genes involved are APC, TP53 and nm23, all occurring at greater than 30% frequency. Amplification of the HER2 gene offers an example of this particular molecular mechanism in gastric cancer [93,94]. This amplification leads to overexpression of the HER2 protein in a subset of gastric cancer patients, estimated to occur at approximately 15% frequency. HER receptors belong to the tyrosine kinase/EGFR family, signaling via MAPK pathways, and activation mutations confer characteristics conducive to transformation of cells. Despite many studies over the last decade, it is still unclear how overexpression of HER2 impacts on prognosis. HER2-positive patients have the potential to benefit from monoclonal antibodies blocking this receptor, and thus this may represent an example of successful translational molecular profiling in this malignancy [93,94].

The humanized monoclonal antibody against HER2 (trastuzumab) has been FDA approved in the USA for treatment of patients with HER2-overexpressing metastatic gastric adenocarcinoma for several years, based on results from an international randomized controlled trial (ToGA) of this agent [95]. At the second interim analysis, the authors reported a median overall survival of 13.8 months in patients receiving HER2-directed therapy along with standard chemotherapy, reflecting a 2.5-month improvement in survival compared to the control group. Particular improvement was seen in patients who highly expressed HRT2 in their gastric tumor (3+ by immunohistochemistry). However, this treatment strategy is only suitable for a minority of patients with benefits that are relatively short-lived.

Microsatellite instability

In addition to exerting a pivotal role in the development of HNPCC clinical phenotype, microsatellite instability is also found in up to 50% of sporadic gastric cancers and is largely caused by epigenetic changes of the mismatch repair genes, particularly MLH1 [96]. This commonly is a consequence of hypermethylation of the promoter region, impairing DNA mismatch repair, resulting in multiple mutations within simple nucleotide repeats, impacting on expression levels of many downstream genes and exerting profound functional consequences on a number of cell functions, such as the cell cycle, cell signaling, and tumor suppression. Gastric tumors can be categorized into high (MSI-H), low (MSI-L) or stable (MSS) MSI tumors, dependent on frequency of mutations within microsatellite markers. It is not clear from the literature whether MSI status impacts on clinicopathological parameters and prognosis of gastric cancer. Reports suggest that MSI-H gastric cancers are associated with antral location, intestinal subtype, and overall better survival in several populations [96,97].

In summary, the clinical relevance (e.g., prognosis and response to therapy) of molecular classifications is currently only strongly supported for the MSI or EBV+ gastric cancer subtypes [98–101]. In routine clinical practice, mismatch repair deficiency and HER2 are routinely tested as these are strongly predictive biomarkers for drug therapy, while additional molecular subgroup testing is not yet carried out as clinical decisions are currently not based on molecular subtypes [98].

Pathogenesis of *H. pylori*-induced gastric cancer

Chronic inflammation, caused by *H. pylori* colonization over decades, is the driving force for neoplastic transformation in the stomach. Correa proposed a multistage model of carcinogenesis in the 1970s that detailed the gradual transformation of the normal gastric mucosa through stages of chronic gastritis, gastric atrophy, intestinal metaplasia, dysplasia, and finally cancer [102]. This cascade applies mainly to noncardia gastric cancer, particularly the intestinal type, while in the diffuse type there is rapid progression from *H. pylori*-induced gastritis to cancer. In both types, more than 90% of patients are achlorhydric and this physiological abnormality precedes the onset of malignancy by decades. It is now known that the increased proliferation induced by chronic inflammation creates a genetically unstable gastric mucosa, which is further compromised by the presence of genotoxic substances generated by inflammatory and bacterial products. The hypochlorhydria contributes to bacterial overgrowth and the generation of an aberrant gastric microbiome characterized by bacteria that further exacerbate the inflammation and leads to the generation of carcinogenic nitrogenous products.

These changes have become far better understood in the past few years due to the massive technical improvements in high-throughput sequencing and advanced bioinformatics. Coker et al. identified differences in microbial diversity and richness between gastric cancer and superficial gastritis, atrophic gastritis and intestinal metaplasia, indicating the presence of microbial dysbiosis along the gastric carcinogenesis continuum [103]. Ferreira et al. reported that gastric carcinoma microbiota is dysbiotic and characterized by reduced microbial diversity, reduced *H. pylori* abundance and overrepresentation of bacterial genera that include intestinal commensals [75]. Most crucially, they found that the microbial community that characterizes gastric cancer has increased nitrosating functions consistent with increased genotoxic potential. This provides great support for Correa's original hypothesis on gastric carcinogenesis.

Sung et al. examined the gastric microbiome 1 year after eradication of *H. pylori* infection. They found that a distinct cluster of oral bacteria comprising *Peptostreptococcus*, *Streptococcus*, *Parvimonas*, *Prevotella*, *Rothia*, and *Granulicatella* were associated with emergence and persistence of atrophy and intestinal metaplasia, while probiotic *Faecalibacterium prausznii* was depleted in subjects who developed atrophy 1 year after *H. pylori* eradication [104]. This study demonstrated the contribution of gastric microbes in the development and perpetuation of precancerous gastric lesions after *H. pylori* eradication. The identified microbes associated with progression of gastric inflammation, atrophy or intestinal metaplasia are potential therapeutic targets in gastric cancer prevention.

In the 1990s, the etiology of the first stage, namely chronic gastritis, was finally confirmed with the discovery of *H. pylori* infection [74]. With a better understanding of the gastric microbiome in the past 10 years, we now have a more complete picture of the pathogenesis of gastric cancer. Microbially induced inflammation (*H. pylori* and other microbiota) will impact on the gastric stem cell compartment and initiate a cascade that may, in some genetically predisposed individuals, lead to cancer formation. For an excellent review on the topic, see Hayakawa et al. [105].

In addition to the role of *H. pylori*-induced inflammation, there is strong evidence that *H. pylori* may also exert a direct carcinogenic effect on the gastric mucosa. *H. pylori*'s CagA protein is now regarded as having direct oncogenic potential (for an excellent review see [46]). CagA, a product of the cagA gene, is delivered into gastric epithelial cells by the bacterial type IV secretion system, an apparatus very much akin to a molecular syringe. Once injected, CagA undergoes tyrosine phosphorylation by SRC family kinases at the Glu-Pro-Ile-Tyr-Ala (EPIYA) motifs in its C-terminal region. Phosphorylated CagA specifically binds and activates SHP2, a phosphatase that acts as a human oncoprotein. SHP2 transmits positive signals for cell growth and motility and deregulation of SHP2 by CagA is thought to be an important mechanism by which cagA-positive *H. pylori* strains may promote gastric carcinogenesis [106]. Furthermore, the in vivo oncogenic activity of CagA is further potentiated in the presence of chronic inflammation, which is clearly the hallmark of *H. pylori* infection, and this feedforward stimulation loop augments the oncogenic actions of CagA [46]. Through CagA and other proteins, *H. pylori* is capable of subverting cell physiology towards several preneoplastic processes, e.g., activation of growth factor receptors, increased proliferation, activation of β-catenin, evasion of apoptosis, sustained angiogenesis and cell dissociation and tissue invasion.

There is, however, a clinical paradox. The clinical outcomes of *H. pylori* infection are varied and include neoplastic (gastric cancer) and nonneoplastic (peptic ulcer, nonulcer dyspepsia and simple asymptomatic gastritis) conditions. Furthermore, it is known that duodenal ulcer disease is actually protective against risk of gastric cancer. What then determines who gets cancer, ulcer or simple gastritis? This paradox highlights the role of host genetic factors in the pathogenesis of gastric cancer, in addition to the role of environmental exposures that likely modulate this risk. In the next section we discuss the main determinants of the divergent outcomes of *H. pylori* infection, including gastric cancer.

What determines the clinical outcome of *H. pylori* infection?

Helicobacter pylori is responsible for three separate phenotypes in the infected host. The first is corpus-predominant gastritis leading to atrophic gastritis, hypochlorhydria, and the development of gastric cancer. The second is the benign phenotype where *H. pylori* infection results in a mild mixed gastritis that has minimal effect on the physiology of gastric acid production. The third phenotype is the duodenal ulcer phenotype where an antrum-predominant gastritis leads to increased gastric acid secretion and duodenal ulceration [107]. Individual differences in the host response to *H. pylori* infection, determined by host genetic polymorphisms, might, in part, explain why some individuals are more likely to develop the gastric cancer phenotype than others. Evidence for the importance of host genetic factors initially came from the finding of an increased incidence of atrophic gastritis and hypochlorhydria in *H. pylori*-infected relatives of gastric cancer patients when compared to matched controls [108].

Interleukin (IL)-1β is a proinflammatory cytokine and also a potent inhibitor of gastric acid secretion. The IL1 gene was therefore a potential candidate for host genetic polymorphisms that may influence gastric cancer risk. Individuals with proinflammatory IL1 gene cluster polymorphisms were found to be at increased risk of developing mucosal atrophy and hypochlorhydria in response to *H. pylori* infection, and this is reflected in a 2–3-fold increase in the risk of noncardia cancer [109,110].

The association between gastric cancer susceptibility and inflammation-related gene polymorphisms was examined in a Human Genome Epidemiology (HuGE) systematic review and metaanalysis [111]. Persson and colleagues conducted a series of metaanalyses using a predefined protocol and looked at the most studied polymorphisms in inflammatory genes, including IL1B, IL1RN, IL8, IL10, and tumor necrosis factor (TNF)-α. They stratified gastric cancers on the basis of histological subtype and anatomical subsite, *H. pylori* infection status, geographic location (Asian or non-Asian study population), and by a quantitative index of study quality. The analysis spanned the period 1990–2006. There was a consistent positive association between carriage of IL1RN*2 and increased risk of gastric cancer. This risk was specific to non-Asian populations and was seen for intestinal and diffuse cancers, and particularly for distal cancers. In Asian populations, reduced risk was observed in association with IL1B-31C carrier status.

When considering all the conflicting associations in the literature, it is essential to recognize the importance of the tumor factors mentioned above in addition to *H. pylori* infection status and ethnic origin of the population under study. Many of these discrepant studies could be explained by variations in study design, including power, and laboratory techniques.

It is interesting to note that experimental work in murine models lends strong support for the role of IL-1β in gastric carcinogenesis. In a seminal study, Tu et al. used transgenic mice engineered to exclusively overexpress IL-1β in the stomach. IL-1β in such mice leads to spontaneous gastric inflammation and cancer that correlate with early recruitment of myeloid-derived suppressor cells to the stomach [112]. IL-1β transgenic mice infected with *H. felis* developed more severe gastric inflammation and histological alterations 5 months post infection. Antagonism of IL-1 receptor signaling inhibited the development of gastric preneoplasia and suppressed MDSC mobilization [112].

Genome-wide association studies

Over the past decade, the focused candidate gene-based approach has been overtaken by technological advancements allowing the use of hypothesis-free genome-wide association studies (GWAS). GWAS have identified variation in novel susceptibility loci, offering new molecular insights into gastric cancer pathogenesis.

Sakamoto et al. were the first to report a GWAS on gastric cancer in 2008. They identified a significant association between diffuse gastric cancer and polymorphic genetic variation (rs2294008 and rs2976392) within exon 1 of the PSCA (prostate stem cell antigen) gene, in a large Japanese population [113]. Allelic differences at this site, G>A and C>T at rs2976392 and rs2294008, respectively, interfered with transcription initiation and conferred risk of diffuse gastric cancer with an adjusted odds ratio of 4.18 (95% CI 2.88–6.21, $p = 1.5X10^{17}$). This effect was subsequently confirmed within a Korean population of over 450 diffuse type gastric cancer patients. Interestingly, the same polymorphism had a much weaker effect in intestinal type gastric cancer, though still significant (OR 1.59, 95% CI 1.15–2.21, $p = 0.0041$). Functional analysis revealed that the PSCA protein is expressed in areas of the glandular crypts along with stem cell progenitors, the proposed initiator cell for this particular histological subtype of gastric cancer. In a cohort of gastric cancer tissue specimens, PSCA was downregulated at both the gene and protein level.

To unravel the biological consequence of this, in vitro transfection studies revealed a role for PSCA in the inhibition of epithelial cell proliferation. This unexpected molecular association has been subsequently validated in several Asian population-based case–control studies, albeit with variable frequency and with risk of both intestinal and diffuse histological subtypes [114–117]. This risk association was also reported in a Caucasian population, with carriage of the rs2294008 T allele conferring risk of chronic atrophic gastritis (OR 1.5, 95% CI 1.1–1.9) in addition to overt noncardia gastric malignancy (OR 1.9, 95% CI 1.3–2.8) [118]. Similarly, analysis of the EPIC cohort (European Prospective Investigation into Cancer and nutrition) confirmed positive association of similar strength (OR 1.42,

95% CI 1.23–1.66) with carriage of the T allele and both intestinal and diffuse histological subtypes of gastric cancer [119]. Given the numerous published reports of the risk of this particular genetic susceptibility on development of gastric cancer, several metaanalyses have been performed, and even allowing for study selection potential bias, the relationship between gastric cancer risk and polymorphic alleles in the PSCA gene remains significant [120].

Gastric mucins have long been targets of study in the context of gastric cancer. These heavily glycosylated proteins play a role in epithelial barrier protection between host and environment that includes creating the protein scaffold for the intestinal glycocalyx mucus layer. Phosphorylation of the cytoplasmic tail of membrane-bound MUC1 can profoundly influence many important cell functions through its multifaceted functional repertoire, such as stimulation of the β-catenin/Wnt pathway with subsequent influence on cyclin-D1 transcription and cell growth, inhibition of apoptosis via mitochondrial influences, influences on cell–cell adhesion, stimulation of kinase-driven cell signaling pathways and interaction with several transcription factors, such as the STATs and NF-κB. As such, MUC1 has been termed an oncoprotein and has been implicated in a number of cancers [121]. Notably, MUC-1 interaction with other proteins such as β-catenin, I-CAM, and EGFR has been targeted pharmacologically, as well as the development of anti-muc1 anticancer immunotherapy, and these strategies are currently being explored as a cancer therapeutic [122].

Hence, given the potential therapeutic implication of MUC-1 in gastric cancer, it has been widely investigated, with several studies reporting the aberrant expression of this protein in malignant gastric tissue. From a genetic perspective, several studies have investigated MUC1 as an important gene associated with gastric cancer risk in different geographical and ethnic populations, using a candidate gene approach and GWAS studies [123–125]. Overall, the consensus appears to be that rs4072037 (G>A) polymorphism in exon 2 confers risk, with carriage of the G allele protective in this setting. This association was confirmed within a metaanalysis that found G allele carriage to be associated with a 28% reduced risk of GC overall, across 10 studies that included over 6000 gastric cancer cases and 10 000 controls across several geographical and ethnic populations [126]. The mucins, including MUC-1, expressed on the surface of gastric epithelial cells, interact with *H. pylori* during infection, and this interaction blocks effective binding of the bacteria directly to the epithelial cells, ultimately interrupting and attenuating the host inflammatory response [127].

Investigations with gastric cancer cell lines and muc1 knockout mice have shown that muc1 regulates host inflammatory response through inhibition of IL-8 and NF-κB in response to *H. pylori* infection [128]. Overall, functionally, the inference is that carriage of the A allele reduces protein expression of MUC1, allowing *H. pylori* to directly interact with the gastric epithelium, thus creating a chronic and persistent, unchecked inflammatory response in the host that could exert genotoxic pressure and favor transformation. This would imply that MUC1 has a central role in gastric cancer initiation and progression. However, this is not fully understood as a study revealed that genetic variation in this and other MUC family member genes did not impact on clinical outcome and progression to overt gastric malignancy in individuals with premalignant phenotype followed up over at least a 12-year period [129]. In addition, it has been noted that carriage of more than one of these susceptibility-associated SNPs confers a cumulative risk effect, with greater than eightfold increased risk of gastric cancer with carriage of both MUC1 and PSCA risk alleles [125]. This may account for the high incidence of gastric cancer in the Japanese population, despite relatively low *H. pylori* colonization, where more than 60% of the population is believed to carry one or both susceptibility SNPs [130].

Mocellin et al. conducted a systematic review and metaanalysis of the evidence on the association between DNA variation and risk of developing stomach cancer [131]. The authors graded the credibility of summary evidence using the Venice criteria and calculated the false-positive report probability (FPRP) to validate the result worthiness. The metaanalysis was conducted for subgroups defined by ethnicity (Asian vs Caucasian), tumor histology (intestinal vs diffuse), tumor site (cardia vs noncardia) and *H. pylori* infection status (positive vs negative). Eleven variants were found to be significantly associated with disease risk and assessed to have a high level of summary evidence: MUC1 rs2070803 at 1q22 (diffuse carcinoma subgroup), MTX1 rs2075570 at 1q22 (diffuse), PSCA rs2294008 at 8q24.2 (noncardia), PRKAA1 rs13361707 5p13 (noncardia), PLCE1 rs2274223 10q23 (cardia), TGFBR2 rs3087465 3p22 (Asian), PKLR rs3762272 1q22 (diffuse), PSCA rs2976392 (intestinal), GSTP1 rs1695 11q13 (Asian), CASP8 rs3834129 2q33 (mixed), and TNF rs1799724 6p21.3 (mixed), with the first nine variants characterized by a low FPRP; 110 polymorphisms were identified with lower quality significant associations. These data are updated annually and may contribute to future screening programs [131].

The recent advent of large GWAS studies has also allowed the construction of polygenic risk scores.

Polygenic risk scores

Jin et al. employed polygenic risk scores recently to look at genetic risk, incident gastric cancer and a healthy lifestyle [132]. They first conducted a fixed-effects metaanalysis of the association between genetic polymorphisms and gastric cancer in six independent GWAS studies that had a case–control design. Collectively, these studies included 21 168 Han Chinese individuals (10 254 had gastric cancer and 10 914 were geographically matched controls without cancer). They then constructed five polygenic risk scores for gastric cancer in a range of five thresholds from $p = 5 \times 10^{-4}$ to $p = 5 \times 10^{-8}$. These scores were then applied to an independent, prospective, nationwide cohort of 100 220 individuals from the China Kadoorie Biobank (CKB), with more than 10 years of follow-up. They calculated the relative and absolute risk of incident gastric cancer associated with four healthy lifestyle factors (smoking, never consuming alcohol, low consumption of preserved foods, and frequent intake of fresh fruits and vegetables), and stratified by genetic risk based on the five quintiles of the polygenic risk score: low (quintile 1), intermediate (quintiles 2–4) and high (quintile 5). A favorable lifestyle was defined as adoption of all four healthy lifestyle factors, an intermediate lifestyle adoption of two or three factors, and an unfavorable lifestyle adoption of none or one factor.

The polygenic risk score derived from 112 single nucleotide polymorphisms ($p < 5 \times 10^{-5}$) showed the strongest association with gastric cancer risk ($p = 7.56 \times 10^{-10}$). When this polygenic risk score was applied to the prospective CKB cohort, there was a significant increase in the relative risk of incident gastric cancer across the quintiles of the polygenic risk score (ptrend <0.0001). A similar increase in the relative risk of incident gastric cancer was observed across the lifestyle categories (ptrend <0.0001). The remarkable take-home message from this study is that individuals at an increased risk of incident gastric cancer could be identified by use of this newly developed polygenic risk score. More importantly, compared with individuals at a high genetic risk who adopt an unhealthy lifestyle, those who adopt a healthy lifestyle could substantially reduce their risk of incident gastric cancer [132].

Helicobacter pylori and cancer of the gastric cardia

The association between *H. pylori* infection, atrophic gastritis, and cancer of the cardia region of the stomach is less clear than it is for distal cancers. In western countries there appears to be a negative association between *H. pylori* infection and cardia cancer, whereas there is a trend toward positive association in eastern Asia [133].

A nested case–control study based in Norway has helped elucidate the etiology of cardia cancer [134]. The study set out to compare the premorbid state of the gastric mucosa between individuals with cardia and noncardia gastric cancer. Out of an original cohort of 101 601 individuals, 129 noncardia and 44 cardia cancers were included and matched with three controls each. Serum samples had been collected a median of 11.9 years before the diagnosis of cancer. The serum samples were analyzed for *H. pylori* serology and the ratio of pepsinogen I:II, which is a marker of *H. pylori*-induced atrophic gastritis. As expected, there was a strong association between *H. pylori* seropositivity and noncardia cancer; however, there was a negative association between *H. pylori* infection and cardia cancer. The predominant histological subtype of cardia cancer was intestinal and was not associated with gastric atrophy. In persons with cardia cancer plus serological evidence of atrophic gastritis, however, there was a strong association with *H. pylori* infection, and the intestinal:diffuse ratio was 1:1, similar to noncardia cancer.

These findings indicate that there are two etiologically distinct types of cardia cancer: a less common type (<20%) associated with *H. pylori*-induced atrophic gastritis, similar to noncardia cancer, and a more common type (>80%) associated with nonatrophic gastric mucosa, resembling esophageal adenocarcinoma [134].

In summary, therefore, the pathogenesis of gastric cancer appears to be multifactorial with hypochlorhydria being the common phenotypic trait predisposing to the onset of carcinogenesis in the distal type. The route to hypochlorhydria and gastric atrophy varies from patient to patient and is influenced by host genetic, bacterial, and environmental factors. Cardia cancer remains poorly understood and probably has a different pathogenesis from distal cancer.

Clinical presentation and natural history (Boxes 52.3 and 52.4)

Early gastric carcinoma is asymptomatic in 80% of patients. Ten percent of patients may have peptic ulcer symptoms or nonspecific features such as nausea, anorexia or early satiety. The majority of cases of early gastric carcinoma outwith Japan are usually found by chance whilst investigating nonspecific upper intestinal symptoms.

In advanced gastric carcinoma, the most common symptoms are weight loss, anorexia, abdominal pain, nausea and vomiting, early satiety, a sense of fullness in the upper abdomen after eating, and dysphagia. The latter is particularly common with proximal gastric and junctional cancers. Patients may present

Box 52.3 Clinical presentation.

- Early gastric cancer is often asymptomatic
- Upper abdominal discomfort or pain
- New-onset dyspepsia
- Anorexia and early satiety
- Weight loss
- Vomiting (may be unaltered food in gastric outlet obstruction)
- Iron deficiency anemia
- Distant lymphadenopathy (Virchow's node, etc.)
- Metastatic spread: hepatomegaly, malignant ascites, bone pain, pulmonary metastases

Box 52.4 Clinical tips.

- Gastric cancer is increasingly a disease of the elderly
- It often presents with vague upper abdominal symptoms or iron deficiency anemia.
- The diffuse form of gastric cancer is less common but can be difficult to diagnose at endoscopy
- The presence of concomitant disease is often a crucial determining factor in the decision process for treatment
- Early gastric cancer has a better prognosis but is frequently asymptomatic and is often a chance endoscopic finding
- Surgery remains the treatment of choice when curative treatment is attempted
- Radical surgery is a major undertaking, and the patient must be fit enough to survive. A careful assessment of any concomitant disease and the anesthetic risks is required

with anemia and signs of chronic GI blood loss, but acute gastrointestinal hemorrhage is relatively uncommon. Because the symptoms are nonspecific, patients often present late. Forty percent of patients will have had symptoms of less than 3 months' duration, 60% will have been symptomatic for 3 months or longer, and up to 20% may have had symptoms for 1 year.

The clinical manifestations also depend on the location of the tumor. Tumors in the antrum interfere with gastric emptying or may directly infiltrate the pylorus and present with gastric outlet obstruction, sometimes manifesting as a succussion splash. Tumors of the fundus and body may reach a very large size with no symptoms other than chronic blood loss. Involvement of the gastroesophageal junction can produce dysphagia.

Physical examination in most cases, particularly early ones, is normal. For advanced cases, the signs of gastric cancer include a palpable epigastric mass, anemia, supraclavicular or axillary lymphadenopathy, hepatomegaly, malignant ascites and evidence of weight loss and cachexia. None of these features is specific to gastric cancer and investigations are usually required.

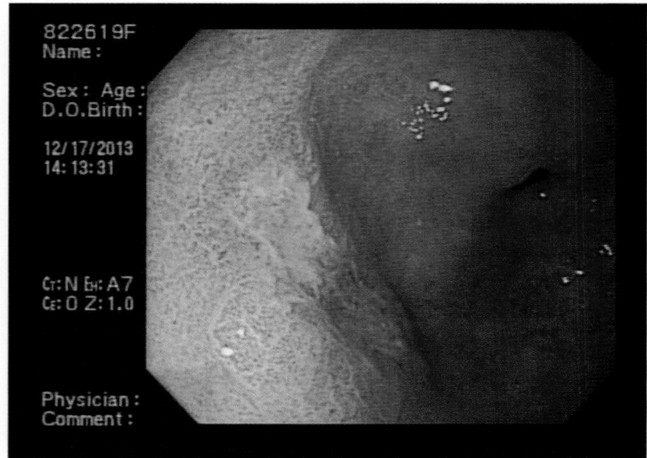

Figure 52.3 Early gastric cancer in the antrum. The patient was a 73-year-old female. Endoscopy showed a 2 cm ulcer in the prepyloric region. Histology confirmed poorly differentiated adenocarcinoma with signet ring cell features. The same lesion was seen with greater precision and clarity in narrow band imaging mode.

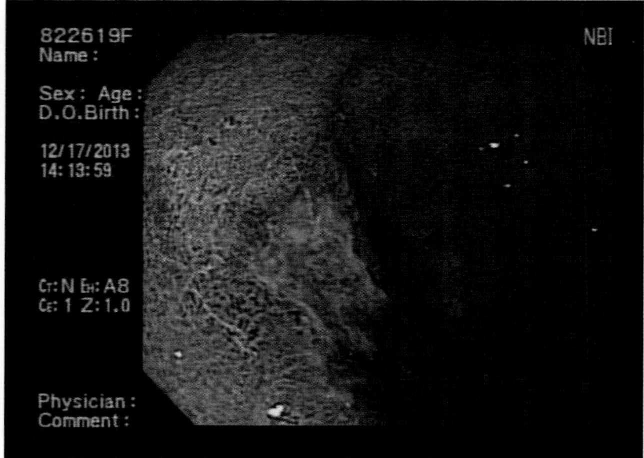

Figure 52.4 Narrow band imaging view of the lesion in Figure 52.3.

Natural history

Early gastric cancer

Early lesions are typically asymptomatic and in the west are usually found by chance. By contrast, in Japan, where the frequency of the disease is sufficiently high to warrant screening, true early gastric carcinoma is seen more frequently and is usually classified according to the Japanese Research Society for Gastric Cancer (JRSCG) scheme [23]. By definition, early gastric cancer involves only the mucosa and submucosa. Type I lesions are polypoid, type II lesions are superficial and are divided into elevated, flat and depressed forms, whilst type III lesions are excavated and usually penetrate through the mucosa into the submucosa but not through the muscularis propria. Type I and IIa lesions have a tendency to be better differentiated than type III. The mucosal appearance of early gastric carcinoma is often extremely subtle and requires very careful inspection of the stomach (Figures 52.3–52.5). As gastric carcinoma is less common in western Europe, Australia and the USA, endoscopists are probably less familiar with its detection and this may explain the lower diagnostic rates.

Advanced gastric cancer

Unfortunately, most gastric carcinoma is advanced and will have penetrated through the submucosa by the time of presentation (Figure 52.6). The histopathology is usually that of an adenocarcinoma that may vary from well-differentiated to poorly differentiated forms. Tumor cells may contain mucus, giving rise to the so-called "signet ring" appearance. Macroscopically, tumors may present as raised nodular areas, often with extensive infiltration of the gastric wall. Presentation with ulceration, however, is also common and macroscopic appearances can be indistinguishable from a benign gastric ulcer. For this reason, gastric ulcers should always be biopsied. Typically, malignant ulcers tend to be more asymmetrical, producing distortion of the rugae and often altering the surrounding mucosal appearance as infiltration occurs. Malignant areas often appear nodular and the tissue is frequently more friable. Endoscopic biopsy of such areas often lacks the characteristic elastic "tug" of normal gastric tissue. In diffuse forms, the anatomy of the stomach may be distorted, making retroflexion and inflation more difficult. At surgery, advanced gastric carcinoma is often palpable and unfortunately local spread and metastatic dissemination are common.

Local and distant spread

Gastric cancer will commonly spread to the esophagogastric junction and to local and regional lymph nodes. Spread into the antrum may distort the pylorus and lead to gastric outlet

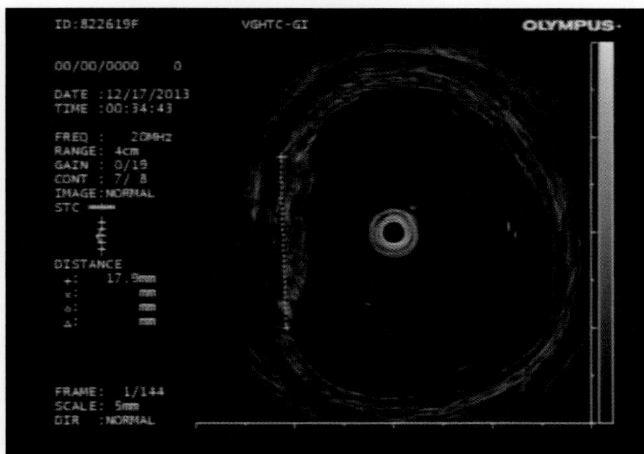

Figure 52.5 Endoscopic ultrasound appearance of the lesion in Figure 52.3. The submucosa was invaded but the muscularis propria layer is intact.

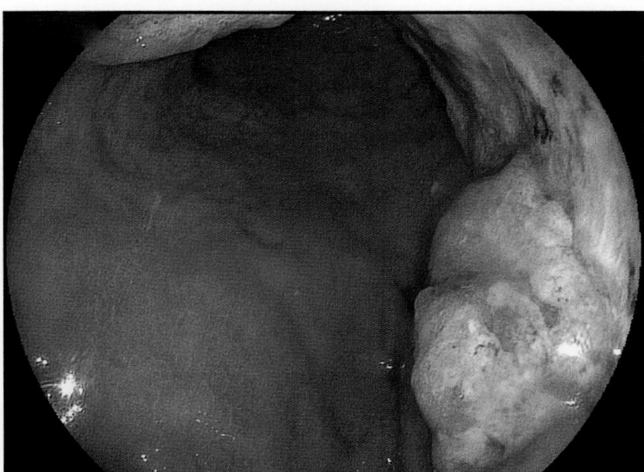

Figure 52.6 Advanced gastric cancer. Endoscopy shows a large lesion (>4 cm) at the posterior wall of the lower corpus and angularis, consistent with Borrmann type II. Histology showed moderately to poorly differentiated adenocarcinoma of the intestinal type. The tumor penetrated the serosa and metastasized to perigastric lymph nodes (2/6). Pathological TNM stage: pT4aN3aMx (according to the American Joint Committee on Cancer Staging. Guidelines for Tumors, 7th edn, 2010/ CAP Guideline, 2010).

obstruction. The omentum and spleen can be involved as well as organs in close proximity such as the transverse colon, occasionally giving rise to gastrocolic fistula.

Distant spread is most frequently to the liver and lungs (approximately 40%) and the peritoneum and bone marrow in 10%. Spread to supraclavicular nodes (Virchow's node), left axillary nodes, and even umbilical nodes (Sister Mary Joseph's node) have all been documented. Peritoneal spread may result in malignant ascites, and ovarian involvement in the form of Krukenberg tumors is recognized.

At presentation, many patients will have distant metastases, with liver being the most common site followed by lung, peritoneum, and bone marrow. Other organs include bone, brain, bladder, kidney, heart, thyroid, adrenal glands, and ovaries.

Differential diagnosis (Box 52.5)

Benign peptic ulcer

The most important differential diagnosis is benign peptic ulceration of the stomach. Whilst large gastric ulcers may inherently appear suspicious, they can sometimes occur in the context of nonsteroidal antiinflammatory drug (NSAID) use. Similarly, a gastric cancer may be indistinguishable from a "benign" ulcer, and "healing" of malignant ulcers, particularly with proton pump inhibitors, is well recognized. Needless to say, the healing process is temporary and malignant ulcers will always reappear eventually. For this reason, it is essential to biopsy gastric ulcers irrespective of whether they appear benign or malignant. Ulcers should be followed to complete healing and rebiopsy undertaken whilst any mucosal break remains. However, surveillance in the majority of cases has a low yield [135] and some have questioned the value of doing so [136]. As such, it is appropriate to base the decision on the individual circumstances of patients; young patients on NSAIDs whose symptoms resolve after treatment do not require follow-up whereas older patients with suspicious-looking ulcer on index endoscopy or whose symptoms persist after treatment clearly require follow-up endoscopy.

Lymphoma

Lymphoma accounts for 5% of all malignant gastric tumors and can appear identical to gastric carcinoma. Typically, patients with MALTomas (gastric B cell lymphoma) may appear less ill than would be expected for the size of the tumor, but again it is important to stress that biopsy is essential.

Box 52.5 Differential diagnosis.

Benign gastric (peptic) ulcer
Gastric lymphoma
Benign polyps and pseudo-polyps
+ Gastric adenomas and polyps
Hyperplastic polyps (cystic fundal hyperplasia)
Gastrointestinal stromal tumors (leiomyoma, and leiomyosarcoma)
Carcinoid tumors
Causes of large gastric folds:
  Helicobacter gastritis
  Ménétrier disease

Other infiltrating conditions of the stomach
  Crohn's disease
  Amyloid
  Sarcoid
  Kaposi sarcoma

Benign polyps and pseudo-polyps

True gastric adenomas are relatively rare but gastric polyps and pseudo-polyps are common.

Hyperplastic polyps (cystic fundal hyperplasia)

Hyperplastic polyps are usually distinguished by being small and by their biopsy appearance. Cystic fundal hyperplasia with multiple small "polyps" in the fundus and body is also common and usually easily recognized at endoscopy.

Diagnostic methods (Box 52.6)

Whilst the diagnosis of gastric cancer may be straightforward in advanced cases, none of the symptoms or signs is unique. For this reason, a high index of suspicion is often required in association with a careful history and physical examination. Physical examination is unfortunately often unrewarding even in advanced gastric cancer. Hematology and chemical pathology results may be supportive, but none are diagnostic. A hypochromic, microcytic anemia is a common finding, and the fecal occult blood test may be positive, but this does not localize the source of blood loss and is therefore rarely diagnostic on its own. Liver function tests may be deranged in advanced disease and both the C-reactive protein (CRP) and erythrocyte sedimentation rate (ESR) may be elevated but all of these findings can occur in other conditions and are particularly common in elderly patients. For these reasons, if gastric cancer is suspected, some form of visualization of the upper GI tract is indicated.

Endoscopy

Endoscopic identification of early gastric cancer

As experience grew in the endoscopic detection of EGC in Japan, it was felt necessary to devise a new macroscopic classification for gastric cancers [137]. This system was subsequently adopted internationally and updated in 2005 [138].

A lesion that is felt endoscopically to represent an EGC is denoted as 0 rather than T1, as would be used in pathological staging. Lesions are then subclassified as being protruding (greater than 2.5 mm), flat, or excavated. Flat lesions are further subdivided according to whether they are completely flat or slightly elevated or depressed. In the west, most EGCs are identified because of the presence of an obvious mass or ulcer seen at endoscopy; flat lesions are likely to be easily overlooked. Indeed, there are data from the UK demonstrating that a significant proportion of patients presenting with gastric or esophageal cancer have had an endoscopy within the preceding 3 years, at which time the diagnosis had been missed [139]. Endoscopist error may be partly explained by the use of acid-suppressing medications that may cause reepithelialization and masking of an underlying malignancy. Another explanation is that our approach to diagnostic endoscopy in a patient with dyspeptic symptoms is to exclude peptic ulcer disease and not to examine the whole of the gastric mucosa in detail for subtle alterations in appearance.

> **Box 52.6** Diagnostic methods.
>
> **Establishing a diagnosis**
> Upper gastrointestinal endoscopy and biopsy
> Barium meal
>
> **Methods mainly for staging**
> Computed tomography scanning
> Ultrasound scanning
> Endoscopic ultrasound
> Positron emission tomography scanning

The vast majority of diagnostic upper GI procedures performed in the west use standard white-light endoscopy (WLE). Standard WLE has its limitations when carrying out surveillance endoscopy for dysplastic premalignant lesions. This is clear from our experience of screening in Barrett esophagus where repeated WLE with systematic biopsy is time-consuming both for the endoscopist and pathologist, and results in poor diagnostic yield.

The Japanese have led the way in the adoption of technologies whereby the detection of EGC can be enhanced. There are numerous established and emerging diagnostic modalities including high-resolution and magnification endoscopy, chromoendoscopy, point spectroscopy, fluorescence imaging, and confocal endoscopy. Chromoendoscopy is being increasingly employed in endoscopy units in the west. The technique involves the topical application of stains to aid the endoscopic visualization of lesions. The nature and mechanism of action of the stains vary. Methylene blue, for example, stains intestinal-type epithelium but not normal gastric mucosa. Indigo carmine accentuates mucosal patterns, helping to identify distorted surface topography. Techniques such as point spectroscopy and confocal endoscopy allow the mucosa to be assessed in vivo for spectroscopic or microscopic evidence of dysplasia or malignancy. Although these techniques do not replace conventional biopsy for histology, they allow biopsies to be targeted, thus increasing diagnostic yield.

Upper GI endoscopy has long superseded barium radiology in the diagnosis of gastric cancer. The procedure is generally well tolerated even in elderly patients, although complications can occur in patients with comorbid disease. Results from retrospective studies typically indicate that upper GI endoscopy carries a significant complication rate of 1:1000 procedures but the mortality is much less, at 1:10 000. The principal advantage of endoscopy is its ability to closely inspect the gastric mucosa and this is really the only circumstance under which early gastric carcinoma is found. Equally important is the ability to obtain endoscopic biopsies from which a firm histological diagnosis can be made.

While advanced gastric carcinoma is usually obvious at endoscopy, certain presentations are difficult. As previously discussed, gastric cancer can present as a typical gastric ulcer. Nonsteroidal antiinflammatory drugs can produce large malignant -ooking ulcers which are, however, benign. Perhaps the most difficult presentation at endoscopy is diffuse gastric carcinoma because the mucosa itself may appear normal. An experienced endoscopist may note a different "feel" to the stomach and it may be more difficult to produce adequate air insufflation of the fundus and body, making retroflexion more difficult. However, the changes are often subtle and mucosal biopsies may not be diagnostic because the carcinoma can infiltrate through the submucosal tissues, giving rise to the "leather bottle" appearance. Under these circumstances, a double contrast barium meal demonstrating abnormal motility or CT scanning to confirm the thickened wall may be helpful.

It is also recognized that the examination of the postoperative stomach can present particular difficulties. Malignancy in the postoperative stomach often presents in the seventh and eighth decades. While rarely performed now, a variety of operative procedures were common in the past, including antrectomy and gastroenterostomy (Polya gastrectomy), antrectomy and primary anastomosis (Billroth I partial gastrectomy), vagotomy and pyloroplasty, and vagotomy and gastroenterostomy. It may be very difficult in the presence of a gastroenterostomy to achieve adequate inflation of the stomach and in addition, bile reflux gastritis is almost invariable and may produce a fragile and mottled mucosa. The appearance of gastric cancer around the margins of a gastroenterostomy can therefore be difficult to find. Multiple biopsies are usually essential for diagnosis, particularly as gastric atrophy and intestinal metaplasia are common findings in older patients. The presence of high-grade dysplasia is always suspicious because it is known to indicate a high risk of malignant transformation or may occur in areas of the mucosa adjacent to established malignancy.

With the advent of artificial intelligence and machine learning, endoscopic diagnosis of gastrointestinal malignancy has been at the translational forefront of this revolution. Luo et al. recently developed the Gastrointestinal Artificial Intelligence Diagnostic System (GRAIDS), which is a deep learning semantic segmentation model capable of providing real-time automated detection of upper gastrointestinal cancers from suspicious lesions during endoscopic examinations [140]. The system was based on >1 million endoscopy images obtained from 84424 individuals from different tier hospitals across China and was shown to be capable of detecting upper gastrointestinal cancer at a latency of less than 40 ms in real-time imaging analysis, with high diagnostic accuracy.

In addition to endoscopy, deep residual learning has been successfully employed in histopathology. Using routinely available hematoxylin and eosin slide images, Kather et al. used deep learning methodology to predict microsatellite instability in gastric tumors with high sensitivity and specificity. Such an approach has the potential to provide immunotherapy to a much broader subset of patients with gastrointestinal cancer and could be implemented in routine histopathology labs in tertiary centers at low cost and without any additional laboratory tissue testing [141,142].

Imaging studies

Double contrast barium meal was for many years the main diagnostic method in gastric cancer. Barium is swallowed with a gassing agent to produce distension of the stomach and is usually well tolerated, making it useful for older or frailer patients. Frail patients can find it difficult to retain gas and double contrast barium meals are more difficult to interpret if the stomach is not fully distended. A noninvasive alternative is CT scan, which has the advantage of offering some staging information in case malignancy is detected. If an abnormality is detected on barium examination, endoscopy is usually required to confirm the diagnosis and obtain biopsies. For these reasons, if gastric carcinoma is suspected, endoscopy should be the primary investigation and barium meal should be seen as second line.

Techniques for staging and preoperative assessment

Staging in the USA is based on the TNM system proposed by the American Joint Commission on Cancer (AJCC) [143]. The latest classification is provided below and modified from [144].

T: Tumor

TX: The main (primary) tumor cannot be assessed.
T0: No evidence of a primary tumor.
Tis: Carcinoma in situ.
T1: The cancer has grown from the top layer of cells of the mucosa into the next layers below such as the lamina propria, muscularis mucosa, or submucosa.
T1a: The tumor is growing into the lamina propria or muscularis mucosa.
T1b: The tumor has grown through the lamina propria and muscularis mucosa and into the submucosa.
T2: The tumor is growing into the muscularis propria layer.
T3: The tumor is growing into the subserosa layer.
T4: The tumor has grown into the serosa and may be growing into a nearby organ.
T4a: The tumor has grown through the stomach wall into the serosa, but the cancer has not grown into any of the nearby organs or structures.
T4b: The tumor has grown through the stomach wall and into nearby organs or structures.

N: Nodes

NX: Nearby (regional) lymph nodes cannot be assessed.
N0: No spread to nearby lymph nodes.
N1: The cancer has spread to 1–2 nearby lymph nodes.
N2: The cancer has spread to 3–6 nearby lymph nodes.
N3: The cancer has spread to 7 or more nearby lymph nodes.
N3a: The cancer has spread to 7–15 nearby lymph nodes.
N3b: The cancer has spread to 16 or more nearby lymph nodes.

M: Metastasis

M0: No distant metastasis.
M1: Distant metastasis to organs such as liver, lungs, brain, or peritoneum.

According to this classification, gastric cancers are staged from 0 to IV. Stage 0 is defined as Tis (carcinoma in situ) N0M0; Stage IA (T1N0M0); Stage IB (T1N1M0) or (T2N0M0); Stage IIA (T1N2M0) or (T2N1M0) or (T3N0M0); Stage IIB (T1N3aM0) or (T2N2M0) or (T3N1M0) or (T4aN0M0); Stage

IIIA (T2N3aM0) or (T3N2M0) or (T4aN1M0) or (T4aN2M0) or (T4bN0M0); Stage IIIB (T1N3bM0) or (T2N3bM0) or (T3N3aM0) or (T4aN3aM0) or (T4bN2M0); Stage IIIC (T3N3bM0) or (T4aN3bM0) or (T4bN3aM0) or (T4bN3bM0); Stage IV (Any T, Any N, M1).

Methods of staging

Ultrasonography is useful as part of the staging of a gastric cancer. It may detect lymphadenopathy but is particularly valuable in assessing liver metastases. Endoscopic ultrasound (EUS) provides good definition of the gastric wall and will also detect lymph nodes adjacent to the stomach but is less useful for imaging distant lymph nodes, liver or lungs. It has particular value, however, in determining the depth of invasion and defining early gastric carcinoma with its better prognosis. Similarly, with its ability to determine gastric wall thickness, it can be useful in detecting diffuse gastric carcinoma. EUS is particularly helpful for identifying superficial lesions that do not penetrate further than the submucosa (T1) or muscularis propria (T2) from advanced cancers (T3–T4). Early T-stage, along with tumor size, differentiation, and the presence of ulceration, might be helpful to identify patients suitable for endoscopic resection [98]. See Figures 52.7 and 52.8 for endoscopic and EUS views of early and advanced gastric cancer.

A chest x-ray may detect pulmonary metastases but for more detailed staging and detection of metastatic disease, CT scanning is the mainstay. Chest CT scans are useful for detecting pulmonary metastases whilst abdominal CT scanning will detect hepatic metastases and may define perigastric involvement. Lesions <5 mm in diameter may not be detected by CT scanning or may be difficult to define. The primary role of CT is to detect the size of lymph nodes so nodes that are involved but not enlarged will not be detected on scanning. It may detect peritoneal or omental disease and has been reported to have an accuracy of up to 90% in detecting distant metastases. However, some studies suggest that up to 50% of tumors are understaged and more importantly, 15% are overstaged. In other words, a percentage of patients who appear to have inoperable disease may actually be operable at the time of surgery. As a result, some surgeons may perform intraoperative ultrasound scanning or laparoscopy before deciding on surgery. The most important point, however, is that in the absence of distant metastases, a patient who is otherwise fit and capable of undergoing surgery should not be refused surgery on the basis of a single screening modality.

In locally advanced gastric cancer, FDG-PET/CT identifies occult metastatic lesions in approximately 10% of patients and is worth considering in this situation as it may avoid futile and expensive surgery [145]. According to the European Society for Medical Oncology guidelines, for patients with gastric cancer at stage 1B or higher, and in whom surgical resection is planned, laparoscopy is recommended to detect peritoneal metastases as patients with positive cytology on peritoneal lavage have high rates of disease recurrence following surgery [146].

Therapy and management (Box 52.7)

The treatment of gastric cancer is dependent on:

- making an accurate diagnosis
- careful assessment and staging of the disease
- consideration of the patient's overall condition, including age, nutritional state and particularly whether they have concomitant disease. The latter is probably more important than age per se.

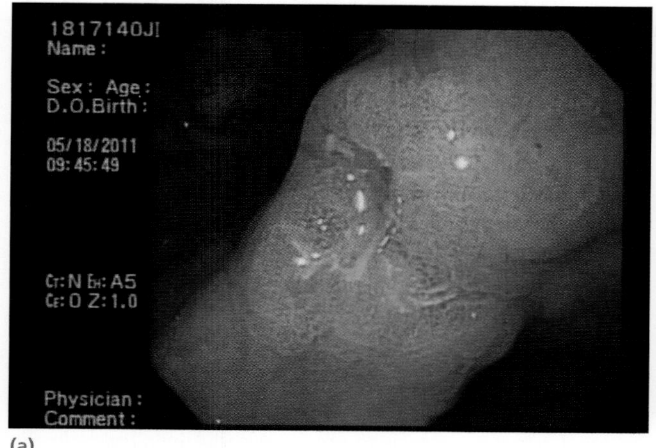

(a)

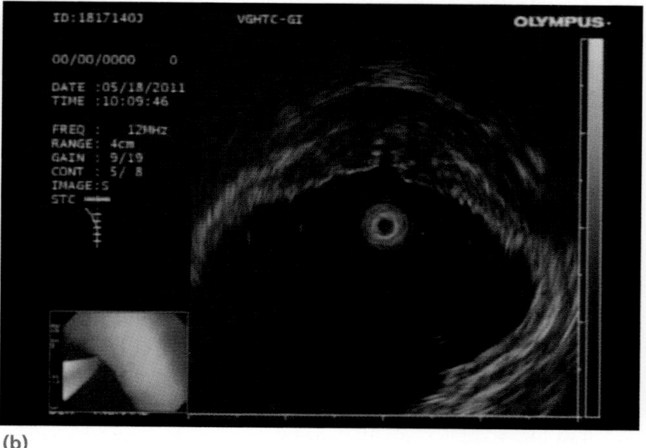

(b)

Figure 52.7 Early gastric cancer. **(a)** Endoscopic findings: uneven elevated mucosal patch over angularis, with some healing ulcers. Possible adenocarcinoma in situ. Invasive carcinoma cannot be ruled out. **(b)** EUS findings: prominent thickening of focal gastric wall over angularis with predominantly mucosal and submucosal infiltration. The focal muscularis propria layer was also thickened and blurred. Serosal interruption was not prominent with UM3R probe. Operative report: adenocarcinoma, intestinal type, moderately differentiated. Tumor invaded to muscularis propria. Pathological TNM stage: pT2N2Mx (according to the American Joint Committee on Cancer. Staging Guidelines for Tumors, 7th edn, 2010/CAP Guideline, 2010).

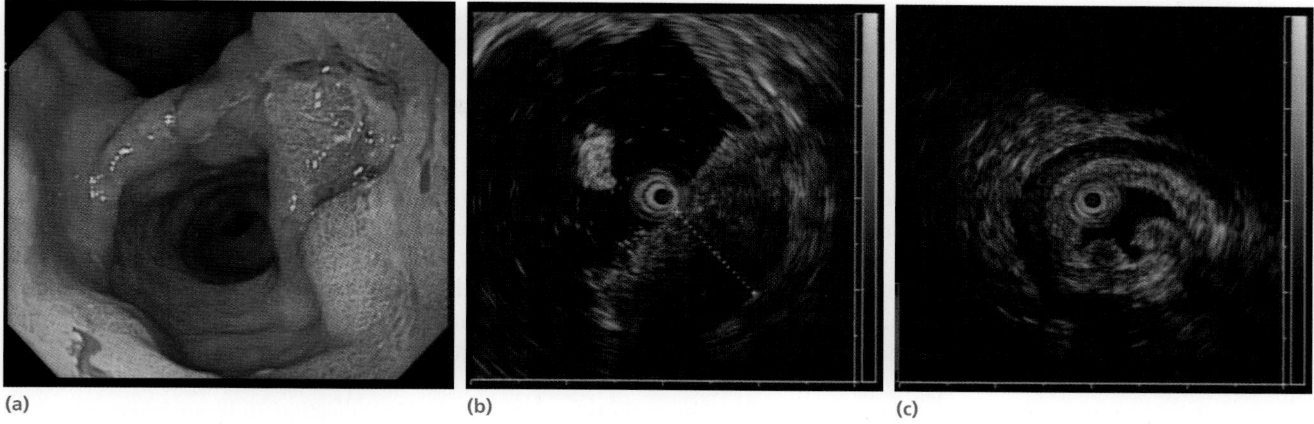

Figure 52.8 **(a)** Endoscopic findings: prominent mucosal elevation with multiple ulcerations over antrum to low body, chiefly the lower curvature and posterior wall. **(b, c)** EUS findings: marked thickening of the gastric wall over antrum and low body was noted with transmural infiltration. Prominent serosal invasion and penetration was also noted. Pathological findings: adenocarcinoma, moderately differentiated. Operative report: adenocarcinoma, intestinal type, poorly differentiated, of posterior wall of antrum. Tumor invaded to perigastric soft tissue and metastasized to perigastric lymph node (greater curvature: 0/0, lesser curvature: 1/3). Pathological TNM stage: pT3N2Mx (according to the American Joint Committee on Cancer. Staging Guidelines for Tumors, 7th edn, 2010/CAP Guideline, 2010).

Box 52.7 Treatment and prevention.

Early gastric cancer
Surgical resection
Endoscopic mucosal resection (nonulcerated lesions)

Advanced gastric cancer
Curative
Radical surgery: D1 or D2 lymph node resection
Possibly combined with: adjuvant, neo-adjuvant, and chemoradiotherapy chemotherapy (still subject to trials)

Palliative
Debulking surgery
Bypass procedures for gastric outlet obstruction
Endoscopic laser therapy, or injection with absolute alcohol to debulk
Stenting of the gastroesophageal junction for dysphagia

Early gastric cancer

The outlook with true EGC is good and if treated appropriately, many patients will be cured. The only proven method of producing long-term survival in patients with gastric cancer is surgery with complete resection of both macro- and microscopic disease. In EGC that is not suitable for endoscopic resection, proximal or distal partial resection is appropriate with limited lymphadenectomy. The approach to cardia, subcardia and some type II esophagogastric junctional cancers can be extended total gastrectomy or esophagogastrectomy. There has been increasing interest in the potential for laparoscopic resection of gastric cancer, with the procedures being either totally laparoscopic or more usually laparoscopic assisted. Evidence thus far suggests that laparoscopic-assisted distal gastrectomy takes longer and yields fewer lymph nodes while there is a trend towards faster recovery postoperatively.

Surgery is a major undertaking, and for this reason alternatives to full resection have been explored for early tumors. Laser ablation, photodynamic therapy, and in particular endoscopic mucosal resection (EMR) have all been proposed for tumor confined to the gastric mucosa and where lymphatic spread appears to be minimal. As soon as tumors encroach into the submucosa, the incidence of lymphatic spread rises and mucosal ablation techniques are unlikely to achieve clearance of the disease. More recently, endoscopic submucosal dissection (ESD) has been used to treat EGC, especially in older patients with comorbid disease. Currently in Japan and Korea, endoscopic resection (EMR and ESD) is considered a standard treatment for EGC that meets the absolute indications defined in the Japanese gastric cancer treatment guidelines for endoscopic resection [147]. For EGC within expanded indications [147], ESD could potentially be comparable to surgery. Ahn et al. recently carried out a nationwide multicenter study in South Korea and compared ESD and surgery for the curative resection of undifferentiated type early gastric cancer. They concluded that ESD produced comparable outcomes to surgery for this type of EGC within expanded indications but cautioned that appropriate patient selection was needed for ESD due to the possibility of lymph node metastasis [148]. The risk of lymph node metastasis is increased by presence of lymphovascular invasion, submucosal invasion, poor differentiation, ulceration, and large tumor size [98]. ESD has become a standard of treatment for EGC in Asia and Europe but long-term follow-up studies are still needed.

Unfortunately, no imaging technique is entirely reliable in assessing the depth of tumor invasion. For this reason, it is essential that if a mucosal resection technique is undertaken, excessive diathermy should be avoided, and the resected mucosa (carefully oriented) should be sent for detailed histological examination. If histological examination shows that the lateral margins of the resected specimen are clear of tumor and that the malignancy has not spread into the submucosa, the chance of a cure is likely to be good. Tumors that are ulcerated, however, are thought to pose particular problems with infiltration and there are some suggestions that metastases to regional lymph glands occur early. Accordingly, EMR should probably not be undertaken in these forms of EGC unless the patient is so unfit that no other treatment would be possible. If histological examination suggests any of the criteria have not been fulfilled and that there is a possibility that the tumor has breached the submucosa or spread beyond the resection then laparotomy and full surgical resection should be performed if the patient is fit. In addition, patients who undergo EMR or ESD need to be monitored for the presence of synchronous lesions and/or recurrence of gastric cancer.

Advanced gastric cancer

Patients with evidence of distant metastases, or where spread has occurred outwith the regional lymph glands, have a very poor prognosis. A radical surgical approach is usually not indicated, although palliative procedures to relieve specific complications such as gastric outlet obstruction or hemorrhage may be required. In patients who are thought to have a potentially resectable cancer, a partial or more usually total gastrectomy is the operation of choice. Procedures that preserve pylorus function, e.g., pylorus-preserving gastrectomy or proximal gastrectomy with double tract reconstruction, show promising results with acceptable oncological outcomes and less dumping symptoms and less weight loss [149,150].

Whilst there is no controversy about removing the primary tumor, there has been some debate about the extent of lymphadenectomy that is required. There are three types of lymph node dissection (D1, D2, D3). A D1 dissection clears perigastric and left gastric artery lymph nodes, which have the highest risk involvement. A D2 dissection involves clearance of all D1 lymph nodes and those along the common hepatic, proper hepatic, and splenic arteries, excluding the splenic hilar nodes as well as those along the coeliac axis [147]. Finally, a D3 dissection clears all D2 lymph node stations and well-defined abdominal paraaortic and hepatoduodenal lymph nodes [147]. Extended lymph node dissection is thought to produce better control of local disease and a more accurate determination of tumor stage but appears to have a higher morbidity because of the greater technical difficulty of the operation and the length of surgery.

Work in Japan involving meticulous mapping of lymph nodes has suggested that systematic lymphadenectomy may improve the outcome of patients when compared with historical controls. In Europe, however, two randomized controlled trials comparing systematic lymph node dissection (D2) with localized lymph node dissection (D1) suggested that D2 operations were associated with increased mortality and morbidity and did not improve long-term outcome [151,152]. In both trials, however, distal splenectomy and pancreatectomy were performed as part of the systematic lymphadenectomy and this contributed to the morbidity. In the Dutch trial, after a median follow-up of 15 years, D2 lymphadenectomy was associated with lower locoregional recurrence and gastric cancer-related death rates than D1 surgery [153]. Other centers have demonstrated that D2 dissections can be performed without the need for splenectomy and pancreatectomy, providing a more acceptable morbidity.

Prospective audit of D2 gastrectomy has suggested an advantage in patients with stage II and IIIa tumors, but the majority of patients from Europe and the United States present with more advanced tumors and therefore probably do not receive benefit from the more detailed D2 resection. In Japan, where organized screening is able to identify early gastric carcinomas, the benefits of D2 resection may be higher. Finally, a Japanese randomized trial compared D2 with the more extensive D3 lymphadenectomy and found no improvement in the survival rate in curable gastric cancer [154].

Advanced gastric cancer is associated with a poor survival even after surgery, with 5-year survival rates as low as 10% in some studies. This has led to the development of postoperative (adjuvant) chemotherapy and preoperative (neo-adjuvant) therapy. Early trials using chemotherapy or single-dose radiotherapy suggested that there might be some survival advantage.

In neo-adjuvant chemotherapy, treatment is given before surgical resection. In theory, less toxic regimes could be used, and it might allow tumors to be downstaged from the inoperable to potentially resectable. Numerous small studies have been reported, none having more than 59 patients. The large UK Medical Research Council (MRC) MAGIC trial reported its final results in 2006 [155] and the French FFCD 9703 trial reported its final results in 2007 [156,157]. These two studies, both with substantial amounts of evidence, support the efficacy of perioperative (preoperative and postoperative) chemotherapy in terms of survival rate (36% vs 23%, estimated at 5 years for MAGIC; 38% vs 24% estimated at 5 years for FFCD 9703) [158]. Even in these large well-organized studies, however, the improved survival was very modest, but the results overall imply that perioperative chemotherapy may have a role.

Smalley et al. performed a randomized phase III trial of postoperative radiochemotherapy in those at moderate risk of locoregional failure (LRF) following surgery [159]. They reported the 10-year median follow-up and presented data on failure patterns and second malignancies. They found that there was persistent benefit from adjuvant radiochemotherapy, while toxicities, including second malignancies, appeared acceptable. They concluded that adjuvant radiochemotherapy remains a rational standard therapy for curatively resected gastric cancer with primaries T3 or greater and/or positive nodes [159].

At present, treatment should be carried out by oncologists with an interest in GI malignancies and patients should be part of organized clinical trials or looked after in units that audit their results. Chemoradiotherapy is used more frequently in North America than Europe, and further clinical trials will be necessary to define its role more clearly. Furthermore, a number of newer chemotherapeutic agents and drug combinations are under trial and it seems likely that the results of chemotherapy will improve in the future. Curative surgery is not always possible and in patients with complications, palliative treatment may be required.

The standard treatment for advanced gastric cancer is chemotherapy since it has been shown to provide a survival benefit and improved quality of life compared with best supportive care alone [160]. Five classes of cytotoxic agents are currently used in gastric cancer (fluoropyrimidines, platinums, taxanes, topoisomerase inhibitors, and anthracyclines). The optimal combination is not well defined, but choice of treatment has to take into account several factors including comorbidities, performance status, and organ function. Generally speaking, most guidelines advocate the use of combination regimens incorporating a platinum agent and a fluoropyrimidine. Capecitabine is preferred by some to 5-FU. Other first-line options include irinotecan plus 5-FU and taxane-based regimens.

For HER2+ patients with advanced gastric cancer, trastuzumab combined with a fluoropyrimidine (5-FU or capecitabine) plus cisplatin is widely used. Trastuzumab has allowed major progress in the treatment of advanced HER2-overexpressing gastric adenocarcinoma but all other HER2-targeting molecules (e.g., lapatinib and pertuzumab) have regrettably failed to provide benefit in first- or second-line treatment in large randomized phase III studies, and the value of continuing trastuzumab after disease progression remains uncertain [94]. Improved understanding of the mechanisms leading to resistance to HER2-targeting treatments may lead to better therapeutic options.

The field of chemotherapy is developing fast with new therapeutic approaches being tested or approved, recently including targeted therapies, such as BRAF and MEK inhibitors, and novel immunotherapies, such as anti-CTLA4 or anti-PD1 therapies. Emerging methods for detection of circulating tumor DNA and new treatments, such as combination with immunotherapy, have shown interesting results and could become an integral part of the strategy of care of this disease [94]. The EORTC-1707 VESTIGE trial [161] is investigating the role of adjuvant immunotherapy with nivolumab and ipilimumab in patients with a high risk for relapse, such as tumors that have cancer cells found in lymph nodes at resection following neo-adjuvant chemotherapy or patients who have a margin-positive (R1) resection (NCT03443856). Advanced gastric cancer is set to benefit from these novel approaches and the results of trials are awaited with great anticipation. Some of these novel approaches include claudin-18.2 (more commonly expressed in diffuse type gastric cancer), inhibitors of the fibroblast growth receptor 2 pathway, and combinations of antiangiogenic therapies and immune checkpoint blockade [98].

Complications and palliative treatment (Box 52.8)

Gastric outlet obstruction

Antral tumors frequently affect gastric emptying. This may be related to direct infiltration of the pylorus by the tumor-producing stenosis but the antrum itself plays an important role in gastric emptying and an infiltrated section with loss of peristalsis may greatly impede emptying of the stomach.

Diagnosis

Delayed gastric emptying produces early satiety, nausea and vomiting that may be severe and projectile and often contains undigested food. Weight loss is almost invariable. Patients are often anorexic and thin with a poor nutritional status. Physical examination may reveal a succussion splash.

A plain abdominal x-ray will sometimes show an enlarged fluid-filled stomach. At endoscopy, the stomach is often filled with fluid despite fasting overnight. A patient with a distended stomach due to outlet obstruction may be at considerable risk of aspirating during endoscopy, particularly as the scope enters the stomach. If there is any doubt, it is often prudent to empty the stomach first with a nasogastric tube to minimize this risk. Similarly, barium should be given with caution to patients with outlet obstruction.

Treatment

Treatment of malignant outlet obstruction is often difficult. Some patients may respond to balloon dilation of the pylorus, but the effects are usually transient. Stenting of the pylorus and duodenum is difficult. Even if the pylorus is patent, patients may still have delayed gastric emptying because of antral involvement and stenting will usually not help. Prokinetics such as domperidone or metoclopramide may offer some benefit but are likely to become less effective as the disease progresses. Surgical bypass will often be required, typically with a gastroenterostomy or sometimes with resection of the tumor and anastomosis if technically possible. If a major surgical procedure

Box 52.8 Complications and their management.

Complication	Management
Gastric outlet obstruction	Surgery Balloon dilation and stenting
Hemorrhage	Endoscopic therapy,laser, heater probe, adrenaline injection Surgery
Dysphagia and involvement of the cardia	Esophageal stenting Surgery Endoscopic laser therapy
Liver metastases	Rarely resected
Malignant ascites	Paracentesis, instillation of doxorubicin
Poor nutritional state	Oral sip feeds and supplements Intravenous feeding in carefully selected patients

cannot be contemplated, a drainage percutaneous endoscopic gastrostomy (PEG) can be considered and in this technique the gastrostomy is used to drain the stomach rather than to feed. Whilst the insertion of a drainage PEG is often an attractive proposition, it can be technically challenging as it may be difficult to find an area of transillumination if the stomach is very thickened.

Hemorrhage

Severe hemorrhage from gastric cancer is unusual but can occasionally occur if the tumor ulcerates and invades a large blood vessel. The effects are usually obvious, with hematemesis or melena, but endoscopy is usually required to confirm the site of bleeding. Sometimes a localized bleeding point may be amenable to laser or heater probe therapy, or the injection of 1:10 000 adrenaline. Often bleeding gastric ulcers are very large and it can be very difficult to stop bleeding.

Chronic blood loss from gastric cancer is common and patients will often require transfusion. When chronic blood loss becomes excessive and the need for transfusion frequent, palliative treatment may be required. Treatment options include laser to shrink the tumor but in the authors' experience this is often difficult in advanced large tumors and very often does not result in decreased blood loss. Similarly, argon plasma coagulation can be tried whilst the injection of absolute alcohol may also produce necrosis and shrinkage of the tumor. In many patients where blood loss is a problem, the tumor is often large and at best only temporary relief is obtained.

Dysphagia and involvement of the gastric cardia

Tumors of the fundus and body may involve the lower esophagus and cardia of the stomach, producing dysphagia.

Diagnosis

Usually made at endoscopy or sometimes a barium swallow can be used.

Treatment

Laser coagulation can be successful in reestablishing a lumen and opening a malignant stricture. Balloon dilation will often produce short-term relief but if a definitive procedure is not possible then esophageal stenting through the stricture and into the stomach may restore swallowing.

Metastatic spread to the liver

The appearance of liver metastases is usually a very bad prognostic sign and most patients have very limited survival under these circumstances. The presence of a single metastasis is unusual, and resection is rarely undertaken. Occasionally spread to involve the common bile duct can occur and may require stenting.

Malignant ascites

Omental spread may result in malignant ascites.

Diagnosis

Usually confirmed at ultrasound scanning and by paracentesis and cytological examination.

Treatment

Treatment is usually by paracentesis. Sometimes a chemotherapeutic agent such as doxorubicin can be given intraperitoneally.

Poor nutritional status

Advanced gastric cancer often has profound effects on appetite and the ability to take normal-sized meals. Most patients with advanced stomach cancer lose weight and their nutritional status may deteriorate rapidly. Some gastroenterologists, particularly in Europe and the United States, advocate total parenteral nutrition (TPN) to try and maintain nutritional status. This is controversial as there is no evidence that TPN prolongs life and effects on the quality of life are difficult to ascertain. TPN is, however, associated with some potentially dangerous complications such as infection or thrombosis. Training a patient to go home on TPN may take several weeks and they will often require support from community nurses. It is suggested that the pros and cons of parenteral nutrition are discussed carefully with the patient on an individual basis and routine use cannot be recommended in gastric cancer.

General palliative measures

As gastric cancer spreads, patients can experience pain and alteration in bowel habit, particularly constipation. Involvement of the palliative care team can be extremely useful, and it is recommended that this be considered early rather than late in the course of treatment.

Prognosis with and without treatment

At present, surgery is the only treatment that offers the possibility of cure. Patients with potentially curative lesions should be offered surgery. A partial or total gastrectomy is, however, a major undertaking and may involve several weeks in hospital. Patients with more advanced disease who undergo noncurative surgery may therefore lose some of their best quality time recovering from surgery and may not receive a survival advantage as a result of their operation. In advanced tumors, therefore, where surgery is unlikely to alter the prognosis, palliative measures and supportive treatment of the patient may offer a longer period of good-quality life. As in all aspects of treatment, it is very important to discuss these issues with the patient and determine what suits them as an individual.

Prevention

Screening for early gastric cancer is not feasible in most populations, and prevention therefore represents the most promising approach to reducing gastric cancer mortality on a global scale. There is no doubt that the gradual and spontaneous disappearance of *H. pylori* infection will, in due course, lead to a reduction in the incidence of gastric cancer. Although the exact mechanisms by which *H. pylori* promotes gastric carcinogenesis remain unclear, it is the single most important etiological agent in gastric cancer and therefore the target of preventive strategies. *H. pylori* is believed to be acquired in infancy or childhood. There is therefore a long latency period before the development of malignancy during which *H. pylori* eradication may be effective in preventing gastric carcinogenesis. Despite what appears to be a logical assumption – that *H. pylori* eradication in infected individuals will prevent the development of gastric cancer – there was, until recently, minimal supporting clinical evidence from controlled trials. This is partly due to the difficulty of recruiting infected individuals who may be randomized to placebo, and the consequent ethical issues this generates. In addition, the follow-up period required for such studies is often prohibitively lengthy.

The largest randomized controlled trial, conducted in a high-risk region of China, was published by Wong et al. in 2004 [162]. In this study, 1630 healthy *H. pylori* carriers were randomized to receive either eradication therapy or placebo. There was no overall difference in the incidence of gastric cancer between the two groups over a follow-up period of 7.5 years. Within the subgroup of patients who had no endoscopic evidence of atrophy or intestinal metaplasia at recruitment, there was, however, a significant reduction in the risk of gastric cancer in the active treatment group. This suggests that there is likely to be a "point of no return" in gastric carcinogenesis, beyond which *H. pylori* eradication is ineffective in preventing the progression to carcinoma.

In the Shandong Interventional Trial, You et al. recruited most of the adults aged 35–64 years in 13 randomly selected villages in Linqu County, Shandong Province, China. Subjects were identified and given baseline endoscopies in 1994 [163]. In 1995, 3365 eligible subjects were randomly assigned in a factorial design to three interventions or placebos: amoxicillin and omeprazole for 2 weeks in 1995 (*H. pylori* treatment); vitamin C, vitamin E, and selenium for 7.3 years (vitamin supplement); and aged garlic extract and steam-distilled garlic oil for 7.3 years (garlic supplement). Subjects underwent endoscopies with biopsies in 1999 and 2003, and the prevalence of precancerous gastric lesions was determined by histopathological examination of seven standard biopsy sites. *H. pylori* treatment significantly decreased the combined prevalence of severe chronic atrophic gastritis, intestinal metaplasia, dysplasia, or gastric cancer in 1999 (OR 0.77, 95% CI 0.62–0.95) and in 2003 (OR 0.60, 95% CI 0.47–0.75) and had favorable effects on the average histopathological severity and on progression and regression of precancerous gastric lesions in 2003. *H. pylori* treatment did not reduce the combined prevalence of dysplasia or gastric cancer. However, fewer subjects receiving *H. pylori* treatment (19/1130; 1.7%) than receiving placebo (27/1128; 2.4%) developed gastric cancer (adjusted $p = 0.14$).

In 2012, Ma et al. reported the 15-year follow-up of these subjects [50]. Gastric cancer was diagnosed in 3.0% of subjects who received *H. pylori* treatment and in 4.6% of those who received placebo (OR 0.61, 95% CI 0.38–0.96, $p = 0.032$). For the first time ever, the results showed a significant reduction in the incidence of gastric cancer in those who lost *H. pylori* infection [50]. In their latest analysis from this landmark study, Li et al. reported the 15-year effect of treatment on gastric cancer incidence and mortality in subgroups defined by age, baseline gastric histopathology, and posttreatment infection status [164]. Treatment was associated with a statistically significant decrease in gastric cancer incidence (OR 0.36, 95% CI 0.17–0.79) and mortality (hazard ratio 0.26, 95% CI 0.09–0.79) at age 55 years and older and a statistically significant decrease in incidence among those with intestinal metaplasia or dysplasia at baseline (OR 0.56, 95% CI 0.34–0.91). These exciting results suggest that antibiotic treatment (with or without *H. pylori* eradication) can benefit an entire population, not just the young or those with mild histopathology [164]. This perhaps suggests that eradication of non-*pylori* microbiota can also be protective.

Two very recent studies add further support to the concept that *H. pylori* eradication leads to prevention of gastric cancer development. Choi et al. carried out a prospective, double-blind, placebo-controlled, randomized trial where they assigned 470 patients who had undergone endoscopic resection of early gastric cancer or high-grade adenoma to receive either *H. pylori* eradication therapy with antibiotics or placebo [52]. During a median follow-up of 5.9 years, metachronous gastric cancer developed in 14 patients (7.2%) in the treatment group and in 27 patients (13.4%) in the placebo group (hazard ratio in the treatment group, 0.50; 95% CI 0.26–0.94, $p = 0.03$) [52]. In addition to the reduction in the incidence of gastric cancer, eradication therapy also led to improvement from baseline in the atrophy grade at the gastric corpus lesser curvature in 48.4% of the patients in the treatment group compared to 15.0% in the placebo group ($p < 0.001$) [52]. Choi et al. also examined the protective effect of *H. pylori* eradication therapy on the development of gastric cancer in subjects with a family history of gastric cancer in a first-degree relative [51]. Such relatives are known to have a 2–3-fold increased risk of gastric cancer and a high prevalence of *H. pylori*-induced precancerous changes in the stomach [108]. Choi et al. conducted a double-blind, placebo-controlled trial where they randomly assigned 1838 participants with *H. pylori* infection to receive either eradication therapy or placebo. The primary outcome was development of gastric cancer and the median follow-up was 9.2 years. Gastric cancer developed in 0.8% of participants (5 of 608) in whom *H. pylori* infection was eradicated and in 2.9% of participants (28 of 979) who had persistent infection (hazard ratio, 0.27; 95% CI 0.10–0.70) [51].

A global consensus meeting, employing Delphi methodology, was held in Taipei in late 2019 to review current evidence and knowledge gaps and propose collaborative studies on population-wide screening and eradication of *H. pylori* for prevention of gastric cancer [165]. The Taipei Global Consensus concluded that evidence supports the proposal that mass screening and eradication of *H. pylori* should be considered in populations at higher risk of gastric cancer [165].

Overall, these studies have finally offered hope that *H. pylori* eradication could act as a form of primary prevention against gastric cancer. As mentioned earlier, it is likely that not all gastric cancers will be prevented by *H. pylori* eradication since some individuals will already have developed premalignant mucosal changes that may no longer be dependent on *H. pylori* for driving the progression to carcinoma. For those unfortunate patients, other forms of chemoprevention (e.g., NSAIDs) or enhanced surveillance (serologically or through endoscopy) are required.

Conclusions

Our understanding of the mechanisms by which gastric cancer arises is more advanced than for the majority of other solid tumors. *H. pylori* is the single most important environmental risk factor for the development of noncardia gastric cancer as well as for at least a proportion of cardia cancers. Prevention of gastric cancer will only be achievable through prevention of acquisition of *H. pylori* or eradication of the infection before an as yet undetermined critical committal stage in the gastric carcinogenesis. Further studies are required to determine the efficacy of *H. pylori* eradication as a preventive strategy in gastric cancer. The evidence implicating dietary factors, and the potential for dietary modification to reduce gastric cancer risk, is conflicting and merits further investigation.

Screening for EGC in high-risk populations reduces gastric cancer mortality and facilitates endoscopic therapy, thus reducing the morbidity associated with the condition. It may eventually be possible to target screening to those individuals most at risk of developing gastric cancer within nonhigh-risk populations. Risk estimation is likely to incorporate factors such as age, family history, and *H. pylori* status combined with serological testing for gastric atrophy, and possibly molecular genetic analysis for predisposing polymorphisms and bacterial virulence factors.

References are available at www.yamadagastro.com/textbook7e

CHAPTER 53

Miscellaneous diseases of the stomach

Tamas A. Gonda[1] **and Abraham Krikhely**[2]

[1] Department of Medicine, Tisch Hospital, and Pancreas Disease Program, New York University, New York, NY, USA

[2] Columbia University Irving Medical Center, New York, NY, USA

Chapter menu

Hiatal hernias

Definition and etiology

Hiatal hernias are abnormal protrusions of abdominal organs into the thoracic cavity via the esophageal hiatus through the diaphragm. Under normal circumstances, the phrenoesophageal membrane anchors the esophagus to the diaphragm and maintains the anatomic position of the esophagogastric junction throughout the "physiological" movement of the gastric cardia during the swallowing mechanism. The gastrophrenic, gastrohepatic, gastroduodenal, and gastrosplenic ligaments, in turn, hold the stomach in its intraabdominal position [1,2]. Structural defects in these anatomic structures and disruption at the crux enlarge the hiatus contributing to the formation of hiatal hernias.

Conditions that magnify the positive pressure gradient between the intraperitoneal and intrapleural cavity and increase the laxity in the phrenoesophageal ligament, such as pregnancy, obesity, vomiting, and gastroesophageal reflux disease (GERD), are risk factors for hiatal hernia formation [3]. Hiatal hernias may also be associated with shortening of the esophagus in longstanding GERD. One retrospective study found that 45% of patients with GERD had hiatal hernias [4]. Hiatal hernias have been found in association with 96% of patients with long-segment Barrett esophagus, 72% of patients with short-segment Barrett esophagus, and 71% of those with esophagitis [5,6].

Hiatal hernias are classified into four types. Type I hernias are called *sliding hiatal hernias* and are differentiated from type II–IV hernias, which are referred to as *paraesophageal hernias* (PEHs) as a group.

Sliding hiatal hernias

Type I hernias account for more than 95% of all hiatal hernias. In a type I hiatal hernia, the gastroesophageal junction (GEJ) migrates longitudinally cephalad from its normal anatomic position within the abdominal cavity into the mediastinum. The fundus of the stomach remains below the GEJ. The herniation is often associated with an attenuated and stretched phrenoesophageal ligament. Type I hernia is a commonly acquired condition with the prevalence rate of 10–80%, peaking in the fifth decade of life [7].

The clinical presentation of type I hernias goes in hand with the presentation of reflux disease. Symptoms include dysphagia, heartburn, cough, and regurgitation. Severe symptoms and complications related to sliding hernias, such as dysphagia or gastric ulcers, are rare [8]. Most patients with GERD in the

Yamada's Textbook of Gastroenterology, Seventh Edition. Edited by Timothy C. Wang, Michael Camilleri, Benjamin Lebwohl, Anna S. Lok, William J. Sandborn, Kenneth K. Wang, and Gary D. Wu.

Companion website: www.yamadagastro.com/textbook7e

setting of hiatal hernias are often treated with standard medical therapy (e.g., proton pump inhibitors [PPIs]) (Figures 53.1 and 53.2). The 2013 Society of American Gastrointestinal and Endoscopic Surgeons recommended surgical repair of type I hiatal hernias when they are associated with gastroesophageal reflux disease [9].

Paraesophageal hernias

Type II hernias, also known as *true* PEHs, are the least common of the hiatal hernias. PEHs are characterized by the GEJ in its normal anatomic position, with a portion of the gastric fundus acting as the lead point herniating through an enlarged diaphragmatic hiatus. A true hiatal hernia is due to a weakness in the phrenoesophageal ligament and a widened hiatus (Figures 53.3–53.7).

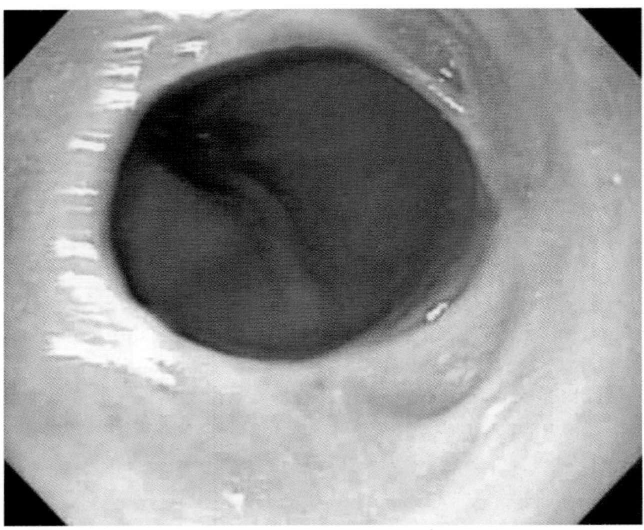

Figure 53.1 Endoscopic appearance of large hiatal hernia with Schatzki ring.

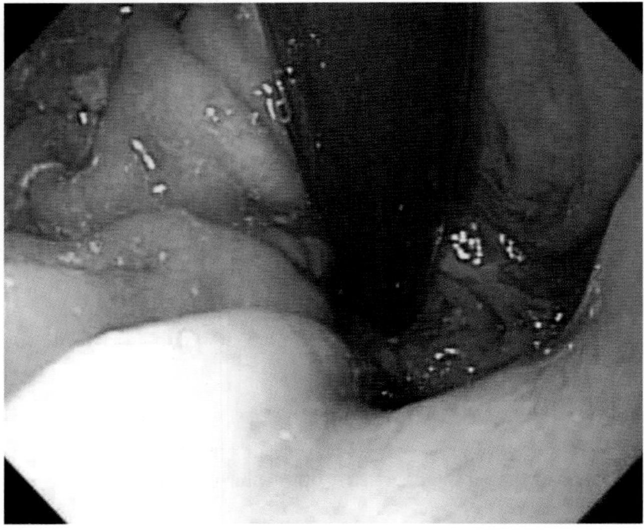

Figure 53.2 Retroflexion view of hiatal hernia.

Type III hernias are a combination of both type I and II hernias and make up more than 90% of the PEHs group [10]. Both the GEJ and the gastric fundus herniate through the hiatus, with the gastric fundus migrating above the GEJ. Type IV hiatal hernias are defined by the presence of other intraabdominal organs in the hernia sac, such as the colon, small bowel, or spleen protruding into the thorax along with the stomach.

PEHs can also be complications arising from surgical procedures that disrupt the region of the esophageal hiatus, such as Nissen fundoplication and gastrectomy. PEHs develop as postoperative complications in 1–6% of cases after laparoscopic Nissen fundoplications [11–14]. Although most PEHs are acquired, a limited number of familial cases have been reported [15]. No genetic predisposition has been identified.

Patients with PEHs present with a wide range of symptoms, with the most common being nausea, epigastric or substernal pain, dysphagia, postprandial fullness, and dry retching [16]. Reflux and regurgitation may be present. Regurgitation and coughing while in bed may be particularly troublesome to patients. Initially, symptoms may be intermittent, vague, and nonspecific. Gradually, the hernia sac around the esophagus enlarges with more stomach migrating into the mediastinum. This can be associated with progressive symptoms from compression of the esophagus, gastric volvulus, gastric outlet obstruction, and gastric ischemia. Postprandial nausea, pain, and fullness are described to be epigastric and substernal and are often relieved by vomiting. Patients may also present with fatigue from anemia as a result of chronic and occult bleeding from the herniated stomach or Cameron ulcer. Pulmonary compression and recurrent aspirations can lead to respiratory symptoms, such as difficulty breathing, shortness of breath, and aspiration pneumonias [17,18].

Untreated PEHs are thought to progressively enlarge until the entire stomach flips on its longitudinal axis into the thorax, resulting in an organoaxial gastric volvulus. Rarely, the stomach rotates vertically on a line parallel to the gastrohepatic ligament, a condition known as *mesenteroaxial rotation*.

The risk for progression from asymptomatic to symptomatic PEH has been estimated to be 14% per year [19]. In chronic cases where vascular compromise of the stomach has occurred because of gastric distention and engorgement of the gastric veins at the hiatus, gastric mucosal ischemia, erosions, ulcerations, bleeding, and anemia have been reported [20,21]. Iron-deficiency anemia can be seen in up to 50% of patients with a paraesophageal hiatal hernia [22]. In fact, a recent study showed that performing a PEH repair in patients with anemia, PEH, an otherwise unremarkable esophagogastroduodenoscopy, and no other identifiable causes of gastrointestinal (GI) bleeding resulted in resolution of the anemia 72% of the time [23].

The most severe and life-threatening complication of a PEH can occur when the stomach in volvulus obstructs, strangulates, and ruptures with profuse bleeding. Some report up to 20% of

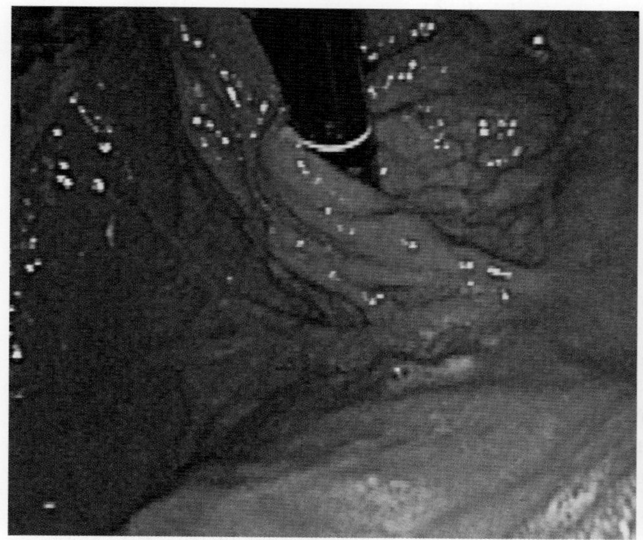
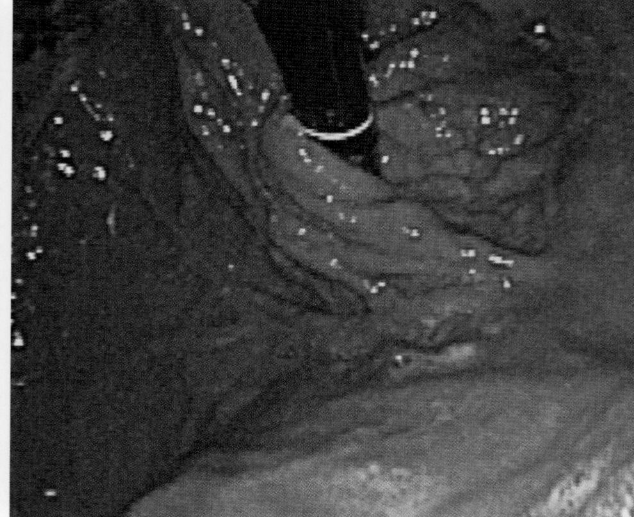

Figure 53.3 Endoscopic views of paraesophageal hernia.

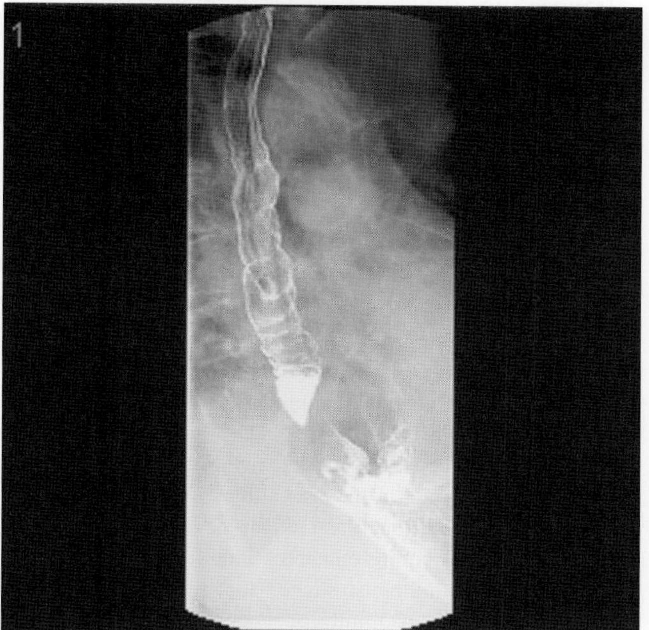

Figure 53.4 Barium esophagogram of a paraesophageal hernia.

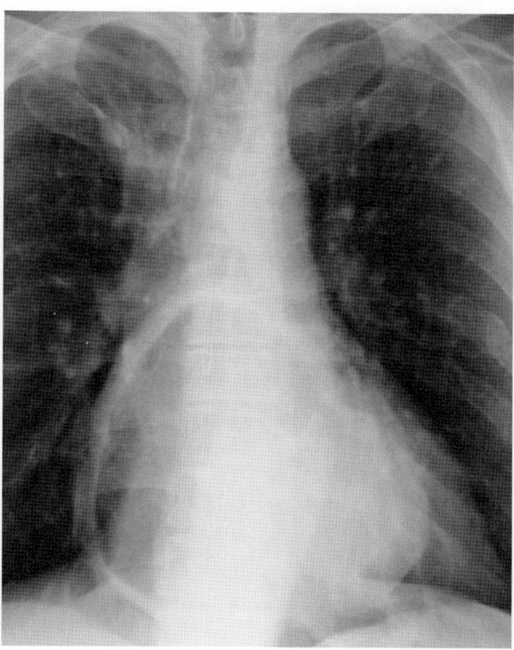

Figure 53.5 Large gastric bubble, seen on chest x-ray, suggestive of paraesophageal hernia.

patients with PEHs presenting with acute gastric strangulation or perforation, resulting in mortality rates as high as 50% [24–26]. In another analysis of the National Inpatient Survey database, Stylopoulos, Gazelle, and Rattner [27] found a lower but still substantial mortality rate associated with emergency surgery for PEHs of 5.4%.

Diagnosis

Hiatal hernias are commonly found during workup of GERD, respiratory symptoms, dysphagia, or anemia. Various diagnostic modalities can play a role in the evaluation of patients suspected of having a hiatal hernia [16,28]. Common studies include contrast swallow radiograph, upper endoscopy, pH study (Bravo vs impedance), and high-resolution esophageal manometry. A contrast swallow study and endoscopy are often performed before elective surgical intervention (see Figure 53.4). The swallow study provides important anatomical information about the size of the hernia, the relative displacement of the GEJ, and flow of contrast through the esophagus.

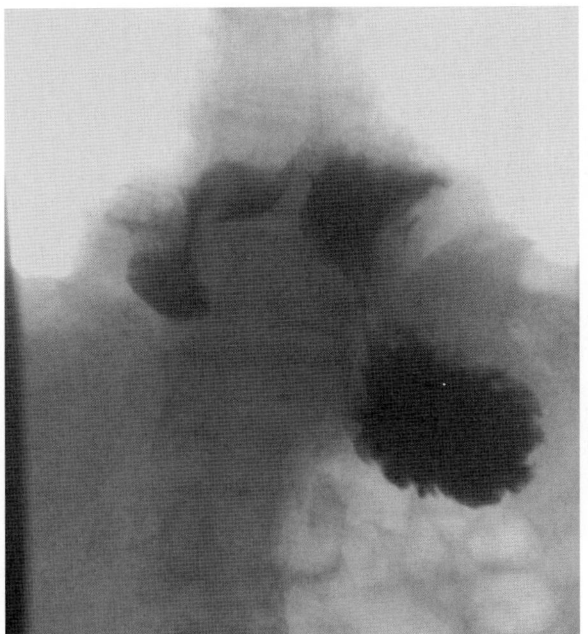

Figure 53.6 Upper gastrointestinal series showing paraesophageal hernia with a large portion of the fundus in the chest.

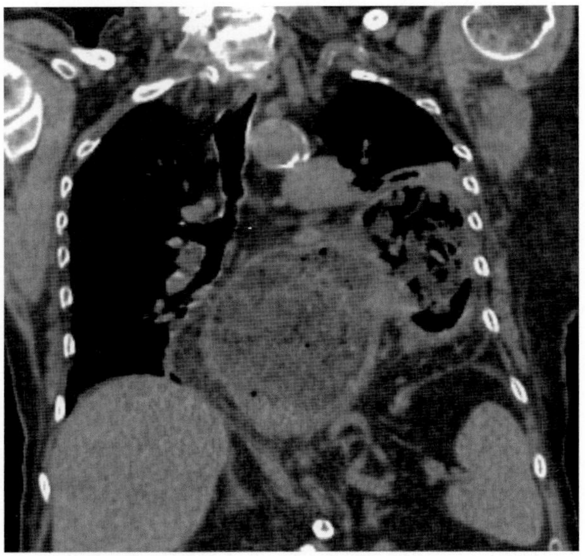

Figure 53.7 Large paraesophageal hernia complicated by a large food bezoar.

Upper endoscopy supplements these data, along with the visualization of the mucosal surfaces of the esophagus, stomach, and duodenum, which allows for evaluation of changes, such as Barrett esophagus, erosions, ulcerations, and other lesions. If a hiatal hernia is small and the workup otherwise shows no evidence of reflux, a pH study can be helpful to confirm GERD. Manometry is also helpful in assisting to evaluate esophageal motility, which may be contributing to the presenting symptoms, as well as help guide the type of surgical repair. If GERD presents in conjunction with upper abdominal cramps and bloating, one might also consider a gastric emptying study. Computed tomography (CT) abdomen might be considered if there are also significant abdominal symptoms not clearly explained by the hiatal hernia. Sometimes, a PEH can be noted on a chest radiograph with a classic retrocardiac air–fluid level. In cases presenting as an emergency, studies should be limited to those needed to confirm the diagnosis without delaying surgical intervention. If there are significant chest pain or respiratory symptoms, evaluation for cardiac or pulmonary disease should be considered.

Therapy and management

Treatment for sliding hiatal hernias depends on the presence of GERD. If GERD is present, the patient can be trialed on acid suppression and lifestyle optimization. If that acid suppression and behavior optimization does not adequately treat the symptoms or if acid suppression is not desired, surgery becomes the treatment of choice.

Treatment for symptomatic PEH is surgical repair. Mild symptoms can be managed with acid suppression and diet and behavior modification. However, symptoms and sequelae can often be more significant and require surgery. Also, elective surgical repair can avoid emergent operative interventions for potentially life-threatening complications of PEH. Another indication for repair of PEH is the presence of PEH in a patient who has recently received a fundoplication [12–14,29,30]. However, surgical repair of PEHs in asymptomatic patients has been debated [31,32]. This is due in part to reports that have demonstrated a marked decrease in the mortality rate of patients undergoing emergency surgical repair in the setting of acute complications from PEH. Therefore, in asymptomatic older patients (>65 years of age), an approach without surgical intervention is reasonable.

Mortality rates for emergency repair have declined, in contrast with the high rates in the last century [27,31–33]. In addition, studies indicate that the risk for development of acute complications that require emergent intervention is less than 2% per year [34]. Studies also suggest that elective repair in the absence of significant symptoms or sequelae may even decrease the quality of life for patients older than 64 years [27,35–37]. However, in practice, truly asymptomatic patients with PEH are uncommon. Therefore, the evaluation of a patient diagnosed with PEH must be thorough, and the decision for surgical intervention individualized to the patient's risks and benefits analysis.

A successful hiatal hernia repair reduces the contents of the hernia sac, repositions the stomach and lower esophageal sphincter (LES) back into the abdomen without tension, mobilizes and ensures the length of the intraabdominal esophagus, closes the defect in the crura to prevent reherniation of abdominal contents into the mediastinum, and commonly creates a fundoplication as an antireflux measure.

In the past, open transabdominal (TA) and open transthoracic (TT) approaches were attempted for PEH repair. Following the increasing adoption of minimally invasive techniques, laparoscopic TA approach has become the standard of care for the elective treatment of PEHs, especially in the hands of those experienced with minimally invasive surgery. A NSQIP (National Surgical Quality Improvement Program) analysis of more than 8,000 cases from 2005 to 2011 showed that 78% of all cases were done laparoscopically, 19% open TA, and 2% open TT. Laparoscopic PEH repair had significantly lower mortality (0.5% laparoscopically vs 2.6% TA vs 1.5% TT) and morbidity. The laparoscopic approach also had a shorter length of stay (3.3 days laparoscopically vs 7.8 days TA vs 6.5 days TT) [38]. Studies demonstrate that laparoscopic hiatal hernia repair is as effective as open TA or open TT repair, with a reduced rate of intraoperative blood loss, less postoperative pain, decreased pulmonary complications, quicker recovery of bowel function, and shorter hospital stays. The smaller incisions of minimally invasive surgery are less likely to be complicated by incisional hernias and wound infection [39]. Quality of life has also been shown to be improved [40]. Furthermore, being able to advance the laparoscope into the mediastinum can make it easier to see relative to the open TA approach. Robot-assisted surgery using the DaVinci platform is the latest advance in the surgeon's armamentarium. It is increasingly being applied to hiatal hernia repairs with good reported results in both primary and revisional settings [41,42]. In our practice, laparoscopic and robot-assisted approaches are the standard, and many of our patients are discharged home on postoperative day 1 after elective repair.

Gastroesophageal fundoplication is commonly performed at the same time as a hiatal hernia repair. Although long-term surgical data are limited, Robinson and Swanstrom et al. [43] have reported long-term sustained results after laparoscopic fundoplication. Ninety-four percent of patients reported only occasional or less reflux at 20-year follow-up; however, 18% required surgical revision to maintain those results. Complete and partial fundoplications in the setting of a PEH have both been described with good results [39,44]. Trepanier et al. [44] compared PEH repair with Nissen fundoplication versus Dor fundoplication. The authors demonstrated a significantly higher rate of severe dysphagia with Nissen fundoplication at 1 month, but there was no longer a significant difference at 6 months. One study documented that preoperative high-resolution manometry done on 200 patients with a large PEH revealed abnormal motility in 53% of patients [45]. In another study, Roman et al. [46] described significant alterations in the measurements obtained in the manometry as a result of abnormalities in the anatomy in the setting of a large PEH [47]. Because of the incidence of abnormal motility and impacted reliability of the high-resolution manometry in the setting of a PEH, some authors advocate a partial fundoplication [39,48]. Collis gastroplasty has also been described as an important option in the setting of a PEH with a foreshortened esophagus [49].

The necessity of a fundoplication during a PEH repair has also been examined. Muller-Stich et al. [50] suggest that fundoplication should be combined with a PEH repair to decrease reflux. Patients were randomized to PEH repair with fundoplication versus PEH repair with gastropexy. At 12 months, there were greater rates of esophagitis in the gastropexy group, 53% versus 17%. There were no significant differences in dysphagia, gas bloating, and quality of life [49]. However, Daigle et al. [51] suggest that one can consider PEH repair without fundoplication with the majority of patients not experiencing significant GERD. The study reported experience on 101 patients with laparoscopic PEH repair, without fundoplication and with anterior gastropexy. Seventy percent of patients had no symptoms of reflux. Despite not having an antireflux procedure, only 22% required PPIs postoperatively. Hiatal hernia recurrence rates were 16.8% with a median follow-up of 10.8 months [51].

Magnetic sphincter augmentation of the LES using the LINX device at the same time as a PEH repair is a novel approach with limited but promising data. Buckley et al. [52] reported on a laparoscopic experience in 200 patients. Seventy-eight percent of patients had a hiatal hernia >5 cm or a large paraesophageal component. The repairs were reinforced with nonpermanent mesh in 83% of patients. There were two readmissions for dehydration, two patients with PE, and one patient with cardiac ischemia. Nineteen patients required endoscopic dilation. Ninety-four percent of patients were completely off PPIs. Three of 51 patients had a recurrent hiatal hernia at a median of 11 months [52].

Use of mesh to augment a crural repair during PEH repair is an often-debated topic. It is more likely to be considered in the setting of a wide defect or poor quality of fascia overlying the crura. In 2002, Frantzides et al. [53] demonstrated a reduction in hiatal hernia recurrence when using PTFE nonabsorbable mesh to augment the crural repair (0% recurrence in PTFE group vs 22% in mesh-free group) [52]. However, erosions of mesh into the esophagus have been reported [54], and alternatives to the use of permanent mesh have been investigated. Oelschlager et al. [55,56] randomized 108 patients to primary sutured diaphragm repair and to primary repair buttressed with a biologic absorbable prosthesis. At 6 months, the radiological hiatal hernia recurrence was lower in the biologic mesh group at 9% versus 24% in the primary repair group [55]. However, in a follow-up analysis, at a median follow-up of 58 months, hiatal hernia recurrence was high in both groups (54% in the biologic mesh group vs 59% in the primary repair group, without statistical significance). There were also no statistically significant differences in associated symptoms or quality of life [56]. Watson et al. [57] randomized 126 patients in four academic centers in Australia to sutured repair, repair augmented with absorbable mesh, and repair augmented with nonabsorbable mesh. The authors assessed results from endoscopy and barium swallow studies 3–4 years out from surgery and found recurrence rates of 39.3% in the sutured group, 56.7% in the absorbable mesh group, and 42.9% in the permanent mesh group (not statistically significant). It should be noted that most recurrences were less than 2 cm. Whether to use mesh, when to use mesh, and what type of mesh to use continues to be debated.

Obesity continues to have a high prevalence throughout the world. Some authors have investigated its impact on GERD and antireflux surgery. Perez et al. [58] reported a higher failure rate of antireflux surgery in obese patients of 31% versus 4.5% in patients with normal body mass index. Winslow et al. [59] did not find a significant difference when comparing obese patients with nonobese patients. Anvari et al. [60] reported significant improvement in GERD in both obese and nonobese groups, but a higher reflux symptom score in the obese group. Although the data are mixed, it makes sense that obesity would impact hiatal hernia repair.

There is concern that obesity can increase the gastroesophageal pressure gradient, as well as add pressure to the crural repair. Performing bariatric surgery together with PEH repair (for those who qualify) instead of fundoplication has been proposed as an option that addresses the PEH, the morbid obesity, and the risk for hernia recurrence that obesity poses [61]. Repairing the hiatal hernia, restoring the LES below the diaphragm, and weight loss are factors that contribute to treating GERD. Sleeve gastrectomy and gastric bypass have both been reported to have success in the short term when performed in conjunction with a PEH repair [61–64]. However, long-term data are lacking. Although the sleeve gastrectomy was the most common bariatric surgery performed in the United States in 2018, GERD is one of its drawbacks. New-onset GERD has also been reported in many patients who did not have symptomatic GERD before the surgery. Furthermore, gastric bypass has been shown to be more effective at treating GERD [65]. It is thus often reasoned that the gastric bypass should be the bariatric surgery of choice in the setting of significant GERD. Patients sometimes have strong preferences on which bariatric surgery is desired despite the GERD; the surgical choice will need to individually weigh the benefits and the risks.

Complications

The postoperative complications associated with PEH repair include bleeding, pneumothorax, vagal injury, esophageal or gastric perforations, gastric volvulus, and recurrences. Up to 20% of patients will have dysphagia initially, and 6% will have chronic dysphagia [48,66].

Gastric volvulus

Definitions

Gastric volvulus is a rare but potentially life-threatening structural disorder in which a portion of the stomach abnormally rotates more than 180° on its own axis. The pathological rotation can lead to obstruction of the stomach, strangulation, and infarction, either in the abdomen or the thorax. Berti first described this clinical entity in 1866 and was the first to treat it successfully with surgery in 1897. There have been only a few hundred reported cases since [67]. Primary gastric volvuli do not have a known etiology; secondary gastric volvuli are the result of preexisting conditions, such as PEHs, conditions that result in the abnormal attachment of the stomach (i.e., prior surgery, neoplasia, connective tissue disorders, possibly severe gastric inflammation), and anterior abdominal wall defects [68].

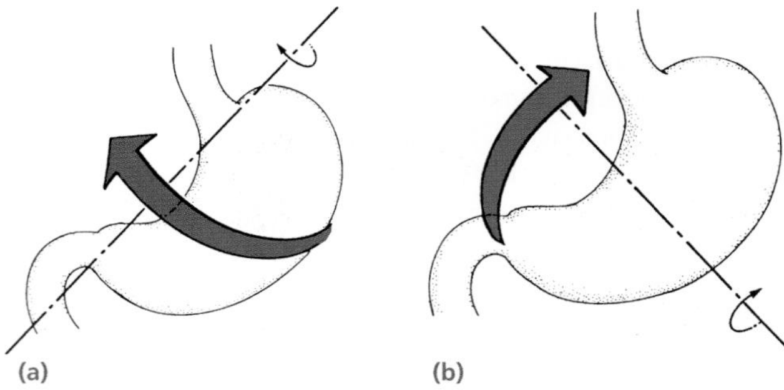

Figure 53.8 Schematic representation of organoaxial volvulus **(a)** and mesenteroaxial volvulus **(b)**.

Due to the transient nature of most chronic gastric volvuli, the exact incidence and prevalence of gastric volvulus is unknown. In the adult population, the peak occurrence is in the sixth decade, affecting men and women equally. Congenital diaphragmatic defects are the cause of gastric volvuli in children before 1 year of age, accounting for about 10–20% of cases [69,70].

Singleton [71] proposed the most commonly used classification of gastric volvulus according to the axis of rotation of the stomach: organoaxial, mesenteroaxial, and combined-unclassified (Figures 53.8 and 53.9) The organoaxial gastric volvulus (type I gastric volvulus) comprises 59% of the cases, mesenteroaxial volvulus 29% (type II), and combined-unclassified 12% (type III) [72]. In the organoaxial type, the stomach excessively rotates anteriorly on its longitudinal axis, with the pylorus and the GEJ as the points of rotation. In such cases, a closed-loop obstruction occurs and can lead to strangulation of the stomach, which has been reported in as many as 28% of the cases [73]. Mesenteroaxial gastric volvulus occurs when the stomach rotates anteroposteriorly about the short transgastric axis to fold on itself toward the right of the abdomen (see Figure 53.6). This axis is defined by the bisection of the lesser and greater curvature of the stomach. Unlike the organoaxial gastric volvulus, infarction of the stomach is uncommon because most cases of mesenteroaxial gastric volvuli are incomplete and intermittent. In the combined-unclassified type, the stomach twists along both axes and is usually seen in chronic cases.

Pathophysiology

Consistent with its function in storing and mechanically breaking down food, the stomach is a relatively mobile organ loosely anchored in the intraabdominal cavity by its ligaments.

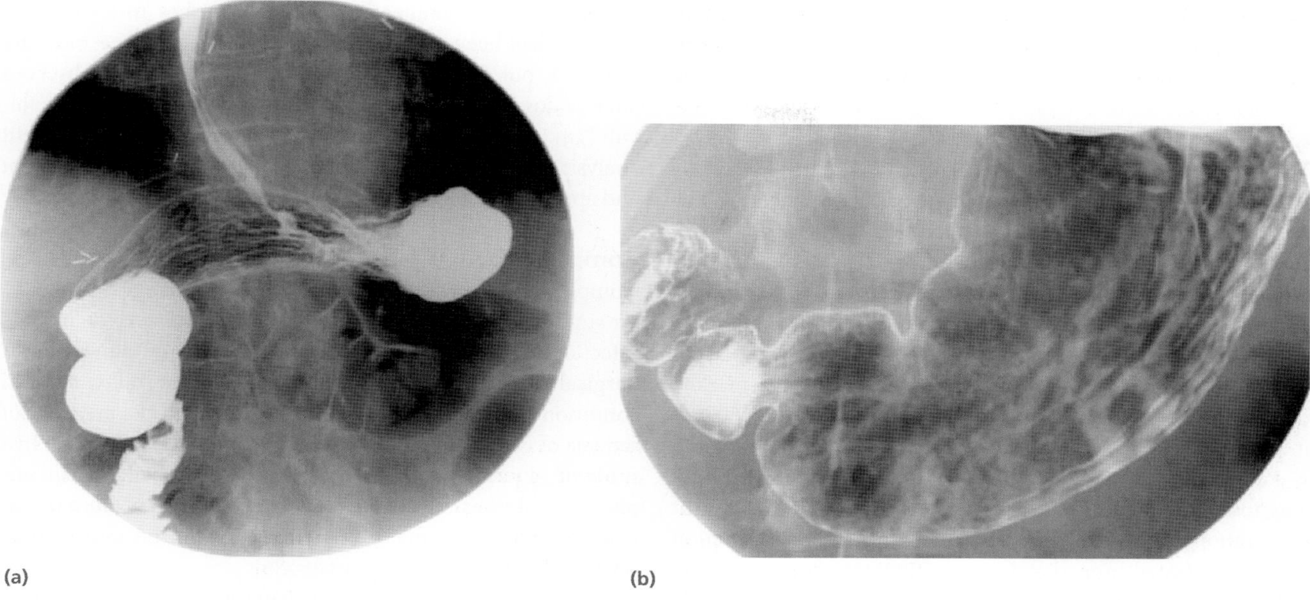

Figure 53.9 (a) Barium radiograph of an organoaxial volvulus associated with a large hiatal hernia. (b) Barium radiograph after resolution of organoaxial volvulus (same patient as in a).

However, the laxity in the gastric ligaments permits excessive rotation of the stomach along its axes leading to a volvulus. Defect or enlargement of the diaphragmatic esophageal hiatus is another permissive factor. In the pediatric population, diaphragmatic and gastric ligament defects are associated with the majority of gastric volvuli (43% and 32%, respectively) [74]. It is not surprising that gastric volvulus is most commonly found in adults with underlying hiatal hernias. Surgical interventions, including Nissen fundoplications and gastrectomies, which can predispose patients to hiatal hernias, are also implicated in the cause of gastric volvulus [74]. Phrenic nerve paralysis and large gastric lesions also place patients at risk for development of gastric volvulus [75].

Clinical presentation

Acute gastric volvulus

Clinical presentation of gastric volvulus can be acute or chronic in nature with signs and symptoms associated with the timing of onset, the severity of rotation of the stomach, and the presence of complications. Patients with acute gastric volvuli report sudden onset of severe epigastric or substernal pain, which radiates to the neck and shoulders. Thus, acute gastric volvulus should be in the differential diagnosis of patients who present with symptoms of myocardial infarction. This is usually accompanied by intractable dry heaving. Borchardt's triad encompasses the three diagnostic elements of the classic presentation of acute gastric volvulus occurring in 70% of cases: (1) acute-onset abdominal pain, (2) violent retching, and (3) inability to pass a nasogastric tube into the stomach [76].

On physical examination, the patients with acute gastric volvulus are often found in acute distress with upper abdominal distention and tenderness. The inability to pass a nasogastric tube is concerning for a complete volvulus and closed-loop obstruction. Plain radiographs and contrast studies evaluating the chest and abdomen are essential initial diagnostic tools. X-ray findings that may aid in early diagnosis include a completely intrathoracic stomach in the retrocardiac position and a gas-filled viscus in the lower chest or upper abdomen with paucity of air in the rest of the GI tract seen on chest and abdominal radiographs [77]. The stomach appears spherical in supine films obtained in patients with mesenteroaxial volvulus. Because plain films may be falsely negative, when gastric volvulus is highly suspected or when diagnosis is uncertain, a CT scan can offer immediate diagnosis by defining the volvulus and providing additional information, such as pockets of free air, abscesses, and the ability to exclude other processes. Some recommend a CT scan with oral and intravenous contrast as the study of choice [78].

Chronic gastric volvulus

Most adult patients with gastric volvulus have a chronic form of the disorder, which is less likely to become symptomatic or lead to severe complications than the acute type. Moreover, chronic gastric volvulus is more likely to involve the mesenteroaxial rotation. Usually, the chronic form is found incidentally on imaging done for other reasons, and at the time of presentation the patient may describe only intermittent vague upper abdominal symptoms. Other primary symptoms include pyrosis, early satiety, bloating, shortness of breath, and episodes of burping. Patients report that these symptoms can be exacerbated with large meals, and vomiting may alleviate the discomfort [79]. Because of the nonspecific and remitting nature of the symptoms, patients can be undiagnosed for years and often are discovered to have chronic gastric volvulus only after workup for other conditions, such as peptic ulcer disease, myocardial infarction, or cholecystitis. The mortality rate of chronic gastric volvulus is less than 13% [80].

Therapy and management

In approximately 5–25% of cases, acute gastric volvulus is complicated by gastric strangulation, infarction, or perforation [8]. Hematemesis is an ominous sign of mucosal ischemia and can rapidly progress to hypovolemic shock. In addition, patients may manifest signs of other complications, such as GI bleeding and multisystem organ failure. Improvements in diagnosis and management of acute gastric volvulus have led to a marked decrease in the historical mortality rates of 30–50% to 15–20% in recent years [17,68,81–83].

Acute gastric volvulus is a surgical emergency, and prompt diagnosis and appropriate management can be lifesaving. In preparation for operative intervention, volume resuscitation should be started immediately, the patient's medical condition optimized, and a careful attempt made at placement of a nasogastric tube to decompress the stomach. Analgesics and antiemetics are also helpful. In line with the goal of therapy of relieving the symptoms, correcting the anatomic abnormality, and preventing recurrence, the surgical strategy to treat acute gastric volvulus must include reduction of volvulus, decompression of the stomach, evaluation of the viability of the stomach, repair of predisposing conditions, and prevention of recurrence by fixing the stomach [80]. Several options for surgical repair were described by Tanner in 1968 [80]. These include simple gastropexy, gastropexy with division of the gastrocolic omentum, partial gastrectomy, gastrogastrostomy, diaphragmatic hernia repair, and repair of diaphragmatic eventration. In patients without gastric necrosis, anterior gastropexy has become the procedure of choice [84]. However, subtotal or total gastrectomy may be mandated in cases where gastric necrosis or perforation has occurred. Laparoscopic and open approaches can both be considered depending on the skillset of the surgeon, the stability of the patient, the quality of tissue, and whether there is sufficient intraperitoneal space in which to work in the setting of distended viscera.

Although surgery is the standard of care in the treatment of acute gastric volvulus, endoscopic options may be considered in a select group of patients without evidence of gastric necrosis. With advancements in endoscopic equipment and skills, successful intubation of the stomach with the endoscope beyond the point of volvulus to rotate it back to its normal anatomic position, temporarily reducing the volvulus, has been reported [18,85–88]. Emergent endoscopic reduction may be especially useful to allow for preoperative optimization of the patient; if this is not feasible due to availability of endoscopy or patient's clinical status, emergent surgery is recommended [79].

The benefit of electively repairing an asymptomatic chronic gastric volvulus is uncertain. Although the standard treatment is surgical, endoscopic reduction of chronic gastric volvulus and placement of percutaneous gastrostomy tubes to anchor the stomach has been reported [87]. Higher recurrence rates are expected, but few serious complications have been observed after endoscopic interventions to correct chronic gastric volvuli [18]. As in all surgically correctable disorders, risk–benefit analysis should be considered and discussed with the patient and appropriate family members.

Complications

Complications after surgical treatment of acute gastric volvulus are similar to other major abdominal operations and can include infections, bleeding, and injury to surrounding anatomy. Surgical complication rates can depend on the frailty, medical condition, and optimization of the patient, and the presence of sequela of volvulus, such as gastric ischemia or perforation. In a study of 44 patients treated for acute gastric volvulus, the complication rate was 38% [89]; in contrast, two other more recent studies reported no major complications and no mortality in series of 29 and 14 patients [18,85–88].

Gastric rupture

Definitions

Spontaneous gastric rupture is an extremely rare clinical entity. The first case of gastric rupture was recorded in 1818, and the literature principally consists of case reports and small series [89]. Gastric ruptures affect both children and adults, with more incidences reported in female than male patients [90]. Several factors contribute to gastric rupture, including massive gastric distension (usually >4 L), increased intragastric pressure with or without associated outlet obstruction, and conditions, whether acquired or congenital, that weaken the stomach wall. In all cases, the rupture originates with a tear in the mucosal layer and dissects through the serosa. Sixty percent of the ruptures that occur in the presence of gastric dilation are located along the lesser curve near the cardia or at the fundus [89]. However, ruptures induced by vomiting are associated with herniation of the stomach into the thorax and are typically found on the greater curve. The latter type of gastric rupture is similar in pathogenesis and management to Boerhaave syndrome (esophageal rupture) [91].

Gastric rupture has been reported in patients with a history of anorexia nervosa, bulimia, and binge eating. In addition, gastric necrosis and rupture were the cause of death in 3–6% of 152 reported deaths in patients with Prader–Willi syndrome, suggesting that these patients are at risk [92]. Finally, neonates may be at increased risk for gastric perforation for unknown reasons; in a series of 13 newborns with gastric rupture, 45% were preterm, and the mortality rate was 54% [93].

Clinical presentation

Gastric rupture typically presents with acute onset of severe abdominal pain, marked abdominal distention, and dyspnea [89]. Patients usually have examination findings consistent with peritonitis and shock [94]. In some cases, subcutaneous emphysema in the chest and neck has also been reported. These symptoms and findings can mimic other intraabdominal catastrophes, such as ulcer perforation, pancreatitis, appendicitis, neoplastic perforation, and splenic rupture.

Therapy and management

Without surgical intervention, uncontained gastric rupture can have a 100% mortality rate as patients succumb to shock and multisystem organ failure [90]. Once the diagnosis is suspected from the clinical presentation and history, a plain radiograph is typically all that is required to confirm the diagnosis and plan for immediate surgical intervention.

Even with immediate surgical treatment, mortality rates can exceed 60%. Gastric ruptures are usually greater than 5 cm, with larger size of rupture associated with greater peritoneal contamination and higher mortality rates [95]. The operation begins with an intraabdominal exploration, evacuation of the gastric spillage, adequate intraperitoneal lavage, complete resection of nonviable gastric tissue (sometimes requiring a subtotal or total gastrectomy), and correction of any other underlying anatomic condition if the hemodynamic stability of the patient permits.

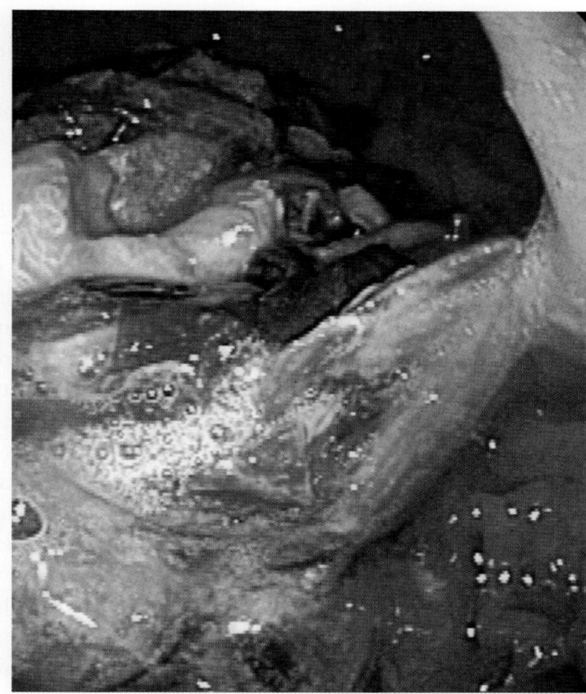

Figure 53.10 Endoscopic view of a gastric bezoar.

Foreign bodies

Definitions and epidemiology

In the United States, 1500 persons die each year from either swallowing or aspirating foreign bodies [95]. The majority of foreign object ingestions occur in children and are most commonly small toys or coins [96]. In adults, items may be accidentally swallowed as a result of carelessness, cognitive impairment, poor vision, or alcohol intoxication [97,98]. Such items may be articles that are frequently placed in the mouth, such as toothbrushes, dental prostheses, or nails. Patients with dementia or psychological disease are most likely to intentionally ingest a foreign body, but patients with bulimia may inadvertently swallow objects while trying to induce emesis [99,100]. Multiple or repeated ingestion is most common in the psychiatric population [99]. Incarcerated criminals may swallow objects for secondary gain (hospitalization), whereas drug traffickers may be "body-packers," who intentionally ingest small packets of illicit drugs [97,101] (Figures 53.7 and 53.10).

Clinical presentation and natural history

Unlike esophageal impaction, where underlying pathology is quite common (especially with food bolus), in gastric foreign body ingestion cases, management greatly depends on knowing the contents, shape, and size of the ingested material. Most foreign bodies will traverse the stomach without causing gastric symptoms; symptoms induced by a gastric foreign body suggest mucosal penetration or perforation, peritonitis, or obstruction [97,99]. Mucosal tears, ulceration, perforation, abscess formation, hemorrhage, and fistula formation may all develop as a result of a retained foreign object [97,98]. Sharp objects, such as splinters or animal bones, are more likely to induce a perforation. Whether and when to remove foreign bodies from the stomach are clinical uncertainties. Serious consideration should be given for removal of objects more than 2 cm in diameter or 5 cm in length because such items may lead to duodenal obstruction or perforation [102]. Due to the risk for perforation, sharp objects regardless of size also should be removed promptly. If a sharp object is too large to be reasonably retrieved endoscopically, a laparoscopic gastrostomy or other surgical methods may be necessary [103]. Blunt objects that are less than 2 cm in diameter or 5 cm in length may be followed with serial radiographs. If the object remains in the stomach for 3 weeks or if the patient experiences symptoms of mucosal irritation, endoscopic retrieval of the foreign body should be pursued. However, batteries that do not pass from the stomach should be removed within 48 hours, and if they have passed into the small intestine, the patient needs to be managed closely to ensure progression through the GI tract.

Therapy and management

Endoscopy should be performed in the left lateral position. Glucagon may be administered to limit motility (although this is more likely to be beneficial for objects in the duodenum than those in the stomach). The efficacy of glucagon has not been established, but side-effects are minimal. Although removal of foreign bodies usually can be managed without endotracheal intubation, this should be strongly considered in difficult-to-sedate individuals or in cases when removal may be challenging or lengthy. Similarly, a protective overtube should almost always be placed when esophageal injury is a concern. If available, longer overtubes (>45 cm) should be used for gastric ingestions. These may allow both safer removals and/or can be removed in one motion with the foreign body if that cannot pass through the rigid overtube [104,105]. Standard biopsy forceps or snares may be used, although these are typically low yield. Oval or round objects may be trapped within a basket or net. Depending on the circumstances, the endoscopist may also consider use of other instruments, such as the grasping forceps, endoscopic scissors, loop cutters, three-armed grasping devices, or tools used during pancreatobiliary manipulation. With the use of commercially available forceps, snares, baskets, nets, and at times a creative combination of devices, as well as with safe anesthesia for the procedure, endoscopic retrieval of foreign bodies is successful in 94–98% of cases [106,107]. Surgery should be considered before endoscopy for large, jagged objects and for "body-packers," where there is a significant risk for death from rupture during endoscopic removal.

Button batteries are especially concerning; therefore, a thorough history should be taken to elicit their ingestion and abdominal films carefully scrutinized for this finding. These batteries contain alkaline compounds, such as sodium or potassium hydroxide. Damage to the stomach may occur as a result of low-voltage burns, pressure necrosis, or direct corrosion [18]. Batteries lodged within the esophagus should be removed immediately by endoscopy. If the plain radiograph demonstrates the battery within the stomach and the patient is asymptomatic, the patient can be followed with serial radiographs. Endoscopic removal is warranted if the battery remains in the stomach at 48 hours, if it is greater than 15 mm in diameter, if it is a mercury-based battery, or if the patient is symptomatic with localized abdominal pain, hematemesis, or melena [108]. If the battery passes beyond the stomach into the duodenum, the vast majority will pass through the GI tract and need to be followed by occasional (every 3–4 days) radiographs. Ipecac syrup should never be administered in cases of battery ingestion because it has not been shown to be effective and may result in esophageal impaction of the battery [98]. If there is battery disruption, heavy metal levels (dependent on the type of battery) in the blood and urine should be measured.

Caustic ingestion injury

Definitions and epidemiology

Ingestion of caustic materials is often more dangerous and damaging than foreign bodies. Common sources of alkaline products (containing sodium or potassium hydroxide, ammonium hydroxide, sodium or potassium hydroxide, and potassium permanganate) include drain openers, automatic dishwasher detergents, alkaline batteries, and toilet, swimming pool, and radiator cleaning agents. Any compound with a pH >11 is capable of inducing alkali injury. Products that contain acids include anti-rust compounds, etching compounds, car batteries, and pool sanitizers. The discomfort caused by acids is likely to lead to immediate vomiting and limited ingestion. In contrast, alkali compounds are often odorless and tasteless and are therefore more likely to be consumed in dangerous quantities. Furthermore, alkali agents penetrate tissue more rapidly than acidic agents because of their solvent action on lipoproteins [109].

Clinical presentation

Acute manifestations of a caustic ingestion include persistent salivation, odynophagia or even a complete inability to swallow, and the development of palatal or pharyngeal ulcers and white plaques [110,111]. Hoarseness, stridor, and hematemesis may also develop. In a series of 378 patients with acid ingestions, 3% experienced massive upper GI bleeding between 9 and 21 days after the ingestion [112]. The majority of these hemorrhages arose from the stomach rather than the duodenum, and 90% of gastric bleeds required surgical intervention. The presence of peritonitis or mediastinitis suggests a perforation. Acute and chronic manifestations of a caustic ingestion are more commonly seen in the oropharynx and esophagus, but gastric damage may result in late manifestations, such as early satiety, weight loss, and vomiting (symptoms of a possible outlet obstruction).

Therapy and management

The first goal in the evaluation of the patient with caustic injury is to assess for evidence of perforation. This can be done with abdominal and chest radiographs. If no free air is seen but perforation is still suspected, a CT scan should be pursued. The patient may be sent home if there is no free air on plain films, if there are no symptoms, and if the ingestion was accidental. Admission and surgical consultation are warranted if there is evidence of perforation. If the patient has respiratory or GI symptoms, or if the ingestion was intentional, the patient should be admitted to the hospital. The patient should ingest nothing by mouth initially, and psychiatric consultation should be considered. If the patient has significant respiratory complaints, laryngoscopy should be considered to determine the need for intubation or tracheostomy. Endoscopy is warranted in all cases, but the timing of an endoscopic examination is unclear. Although some authors recommend immediate endoscopy, waiting 24–36 hours may allow for better assessment for the extent of injury [110,111].

A grading system based on endoscopic appearance has been developed to guide postingestion management:

1. Grade I: erythema and edema
2. Grade II: hemorrhage, erosions, blisters, and superficial ulcers (IIA, linear; IIB, circumferential)
3. Grade III: multiple, deep, brown-black or gray ulcers
4. Grade IV: full perforation.

For grade I–IIA damage, liquids can be started with dietary advancement as tolerated. Grade IIB or III patients should have a nasogastric tube placed for gastric decompression, and acid suppression should be employed. Oral liquids may be started approximately 48 hours after endoscopy if the patient is swallowing well. Immediate surgery is warranted in patients with grade IV damage.

Acid neutralizers have been used to limit caustic damage in the past, but these are no longer recommended because heat production from the neutralization process has been shown to worsen tissue injury [113]. Owing to the risk for esophageal strictures and antral stenosis, some investigators have proposed administering oral corticosteroids, based on animal and anecdotal data. The only randomized controlled trial performed suggested that steroids did little to prevent or limit esophageal strictures, and routine steroid use is not recommended by all clinicians [114].

Complications

In the long term, caustic gastric injury may lead to antral stenosis within 3–6 weeks of the ingestion, or it may be delayed for many years. It is not unreasonable to perform an upper GI series at 3–6 weeks to look for this complication. Some cases of antral or pyloric stenosis may respond well to endoscopic balloon dilation, but most patients will eventually require a surgical pyloroplasty or distal gastrectomy. In patients with prior caustic injury who are undergoing endoscopy for other reasons, antral hyalinization has been reported and may mimic gastric Crohn's disease or cancer [115]. Corrosive damage may increase the risk for subsequent gastric cancer, but such reports are isolated. Unlike in the case of esophageal corrosive injury, where an increased risk for squamous cancer warrants surveillance, such a recommendation cannot be made for gastric cancer risk [116].

Gastric bezoars

Definition

Bezoars are concretions of foreign material that are retained, most frequently within the stomach (see Figure 53.10), but have also been found in the esophagus and rectum [117]. Such matter may include plant and vegetable debris (phytobezoar), hair (trichobezoar), medications (pharmacobezoar), inspissated milk (lactobezoar), and persimmons (diospyrobezoar). Rapunzel syndrome is a form of trichobezoar when the hair extends to the small intestine (at times to the ileocecal valve) and causes obstruction.

Epidemiology

The true prevalence of bezoars is uncertain because many patients are asymptomatic, but bezoars are uncommon in the intact stomach, with a reported prevalence rate of 0.4%. However, 10–25% of patients with prior antrectomies have been found to have symptomatic bezoars, and in one study, more than 50% of all patients presenting with a bezoar have had prior gastric surgery [118,119].

Pathogenesis

The formation of bezoars is likely multifactorial. Altered gastric motility and emptying are the primary causes, but size and digestibility of swallowed material are factors as well. Inadequate mastication, missing teeth, and poorly fitting dentures may also contribute to bezoar formation [120,121]. Prior gastric surgery, whether it be a pyloroplasty, antrectomy, Roux-en-Y gastric bypass, or partial gastrectomy, clearly places patients at risk for phytobezoar or fungus ball formation [122,123]. Surgery can induce gastric atony and dysmotility, but outlet obstruction from stenosis and decreased secretion of acid and pepsin also play a role in bezoar formation. Furthermore, many postsurgical patients experience chronic gastropathy that leads to increased mucous production, and this mucus may act like cement for developing concretions [124]. In an era of bariatric surgery, Roux-en-Y gastric bypass and laparoscopic adjustable gastric banding have been associated with bezoar formation [122,125]. In addition to surgery, gastric stasis and bezoars have been linked to PEHs (see Figure 53.7), diabetic gastroparesis, mixed connective tissue disease, hypothyroidism, and myotonic dystrophy [126–129].

Phytobezoars commonly comprise apples, grapes, oranges, pomegranates, cherries, raisins, bran, oats, cabbage, potato peels, peanuts, and celery [120,130]. Bezoars may also be composed of nonfood items, such as plastic, paper, string, or Styrofoam. Diospyrobezoars develop when unripe persimmon material comes into contact with gastric acid; tannin in the fruit forms a coagulum that acts as a base for bezoar formation. Trichobezoars may be large, depending on the amount of hair consumed. Medications have reportedly been trapped within hair fibers, and drug toxicity has been attributed to altered drug metabolism [131]. Trichobezoars may also contain food material and fat. Fungus balls, also termed yeast bezoars, are associated with prior gastric surgery and frequently resolve without therapy. For symptomatic fungus balls, gastric lavage, antimycotics, and gastric outlet reconstruction have all been used [132,133].

Concretions are typically hard bezoars. Shellac, furniture polish, and concrete are classic components of such bezoars, and surgery may be necessary to remove concretions because other therapies are generally ineffective. Pharmacobezoars may develop in patients with normal or abnormal gastric physiology. Aluminum hydroxide antacids have caused bezoars in patients with renal failure, and the cellulose-based coating of enteric-coated aspirin has been problematic in other patients [134,135]. In patients with achlorhydria, calcium and magnesium carbonate preparations may not dissolve normally. Sucralfate will occasionally form concretions at normal doses and in patients with gastric outlet obstruction, so this agent should be avoided in patients with outlet obstruction or significant dysmotility [136]. Other drugs with capsules that do not digest (such as certain nifedipine or mesalamine preparations) should also be avoided in patients with gastric outlet narrowing [137].

Clinical presentation

Many patients with bezoars are asymptomatic, but epigastric pain, early satiety, nausea, and vomiting are common manifestations of a bezoar [111,120]. Bloating, malaise, and weight loss may also be reported. In some patients, these symptoms persist despite bezoar resolution; in such cases, the nonspecific symptoms may be more reflective of the gastric dysmotility than of the actual presence of a bezoar. In patients at risk for bezoar formation, symptoms of small-bowel obstruction may reflect the passage of a bezoar into the small bowel, although this is rare [138]. Gastric outlet obstruction and gastric bleeding (hematemesis or melena) can also be complications of bezoars. Given the nonspecific nature of the symptoms, the patient's history may suggest other causes, such as peptic ulcer disease, gastric cancer, or many other intraabdominal processes. On physical examination, potential findings include abdominal tenderness, a palpable mass, and a succussion splash [111]. Plain radiographs may demonstrate an air shadow or a mottled-appearing mass in the stomach. Barium studies are much more likely to demonstrate a bezoar; trichobezoars "absorb" barium and have a mottled appearance, whereas phytobezoars and concretions are typically impermeable to barium (see Figure 53.7). Radiographic studies may miss a bezoar, and endoscopy remains the test of choice. Although other studies such as ultrasound or CT may demonstrate a bezoar, endoscopy is best for determining the type of bezoar, for excluding cancer, and for evaluating the mucosa for associated ulceration or outlet obstruction.

Therapy and management

Endoscopic therapy aimed at resolution is warranted for symptomatic bezoars. Incidentally found bezoars do not require immediate endoscopic treatment; however, evaluation of delayed gastric emptying should be undertaken, and treatment should probably be proteolytic therapy or prokinetic agents.

Enzyme therapy

Because many bezoars contain cellulose, protein, and mucus, enzymatic degradation of phytobezoars may be possible. For bezoars that contain fibrous material, papain can be a useful proteolytic enzyme. Although this enzyme can be individually purchased, papain can be obtained more cheaply by using Adolph's Meat Tenderizer (1 teaspoon in 115 mL [4 ounces] of water before each meal) [111,139]. Some caution should be used with the latter salt-containing preparation (1800 mg per tablespoon) because hypernatremia is a potential problem. An important caveat that limits the use of papain in practice is that the safe amount to be ingested has not been established.

Phytobezoars can be treated with cellulase. Cellulase tablets are frequently crushed and given after each meal, or 2 L of cellulase solution may be consumed over the course of 2 days (20 g cellulase in 2 L of water) [139,140]. Biochemical supply companies can provide papain and cellulase preparations. Because many phytobezoars contain mucus as well, the mucolytic agent acetylcysteine may also be used. This agent has been reported to be effective at a dose of 15 mL in 50 mL of saline administered through a nasogastric tube two times per day for 2 days; although not specifically stated in this case report, presumably a commercially available 20% acetylcysteine preparation was used and diluted to a 5% solution as recommended by the manufacturer for other indications [139].

Several case series have reported significant benefit from Coca-Cola lysis [141], with a nearly 50% complete resolution. The average amount of Coca-Cola consumed was close to 3–4 L [141] (typically administered via nasogastric tube and over 12 hours). If there is ulceration associated with the bezoar, some investigators have suggested that mucolytic and cellulolytic agents are safer than the proteolytic regimens provided.

Mechanical therapy

Many bezoars contain insoluble agents that are not amenable to enzyme therapy, and some patients are sufficiently symptomatic that more urgent therapy is warranted. Small bezoars may be retrieved like other foreign bodies with endoscopic baskets, snares, or forceps. An esophageal overtube is frequently used to prevent inadvertent aspiration of the bezoar [142]. Similarly, many bezoars can be mechanically disrupted into small pieces with forceps such that the pieces are retrieved by suction or allowed to pass through the pylorus. For soft and permeable bezoars, a large-bore orogastric lavage tube can be placed for aggressive water lavage with subsequent aspiration of the fragmented bezoar. Frequently, a combination of endoscopic fragmentation and subsequent orogastric lavage is used, with immediate relief for the patient.

Other modes of mechanical disruption have been proposed. Plastic tubing has been placed through an endoscope channel and attached externally to a Teledyne Water Pik system. Water or an enzymatic solution can be pulsated against the bezoar to allow fragmentation and subsequent gastric lavage [131,143]. Neodymium : yttrium–aluminum–garnet (Nd : YAG) laser may be useful for refractory bezoars, although multiple sessions may be necessary [144]. Electrohydraulic lithotripsy, laser lithotripsy, and mechanical lithotripsy – with an endoscopic retrograde cholangiopancreatography lithotriptor for hard bezoars – have also been successful [145,146]. In patients who have undergone gastroplasty and in whom the surgical stoma may be too small (predisposing to bezoar formation and not allowing passage of bezoar fragments), the stoma may require balloon dilation or even an endoscopic incision with a papillotome [147,148].

Medical therapy

Prokinetic agents such as metoclopramide may be used on a long-term basis to aid in the prevention and recurrence of bezoars. Metoclopramide has been used alone and with concomitant endoscopic therapy in the acute setting (40 mg intravenously over 24 hours) with some success for the management of symptomatic bezoars, but patients should also be placed on a clear liquid diet under such circumstances [149]. In the absence of a documented underlying gastroparesis, this is not a US Food and Drug Administration-approved indication, and patients should be counseled about potential serious side-effects. Although liquid diets may have some benefit in bezoar dissolution, this is a slow process that is not practical as a sole therapy. Domperidone, which is not available within the United States, may be another option, with fewer side-effects but similar gastric effects compared with metoclopramide. Erythromycin is another agent that can be used to promote gastric motility and to decrease the risk for bezoar formation, although this should be used for a limited period to aid in resolution [150].

For patients with or at risk for the development of bezoars, prokinetic agents should be considered, based on the patient's symptom severity. Conversely, all such patients should follow basic dietary guidelines to limit bezoar formation. Specifically, smaller but more frequent meals are advisable to promote gastric emptying. Patients should chew their food adequately into small pieces. Foods that easily coalesce into a bezoar, such as persimmons, raw fruits, and stringy vegetables, should be avoided [121].

Surgical therapy

Surgery is rarely required for bezoars but may be necessary in the setting of bezoar complications, such as perforation, gastric or small-bowel obstruction, and uncontrollable hemorrhage. Symptomatic trichobezoars require surgery more often than other bezoar types because they are resistant to standard management techniques. Other types of bezoars may also require surgery if they cannot be treated by the methods outlined earlier. Because surgery is unlikely to correct the underlying cause of bezoar formation and may worsen gastric motility and emptying, careful consideration is warranted before proceeding.

Heterotopic pancreas

Heterotopic pancreas is defined as the presence of pancreatic tissue in a location without direct anatomical or vascular continuity with the pancreas. Heterotopic pancreatic tissue, also termed a "pancreatic rest," has been identified in 0.5–14% of persons at autopsy [151]. The stomach is the most common site, although heterotopic pancreas can also be found in the duodenum, jejunum, and much less frequently, the esophagus, gallbladder, colon, and spleen. Histologically, it is classified based on its similarity to the pancreas (type I, consists of all components of pancreas tissue; type II, acini and ducts but no islets; type III, ducts only; type IV, islets only). In the stomach, the typical location is the greater curvature, and more than half of the lesions have a central umbilication (Figure 53.11). Typically, these rests are asymptomatic, but abdominal pain, nausea, vomiting, and rarely bleeding have been attributed to rests located in the stomach. However, identical complications to pancreatic disease (i.e., neoplasia, inflammation) have been described. Typically, lesions greater than 1.5 cm can cause pain, and this is possibly due to secretion of pancreatic juice; in most of these, symptomatic improvement after resection has been described [140]. However, given that the majority of lesions are smaller and likely asymptomatic, the role of resection is limited [152].

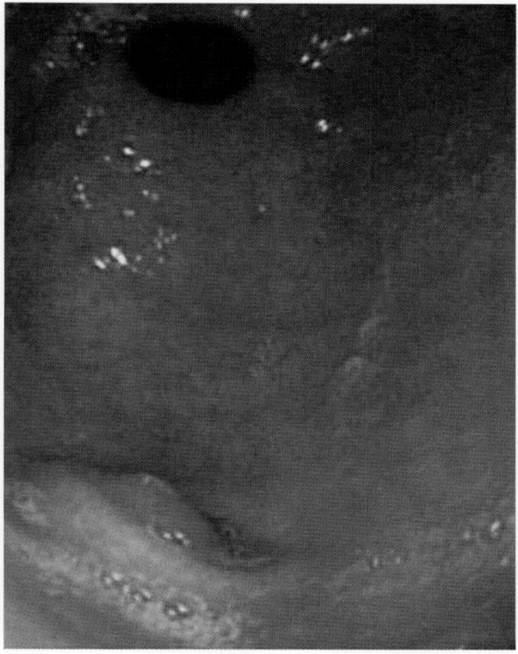

(a)

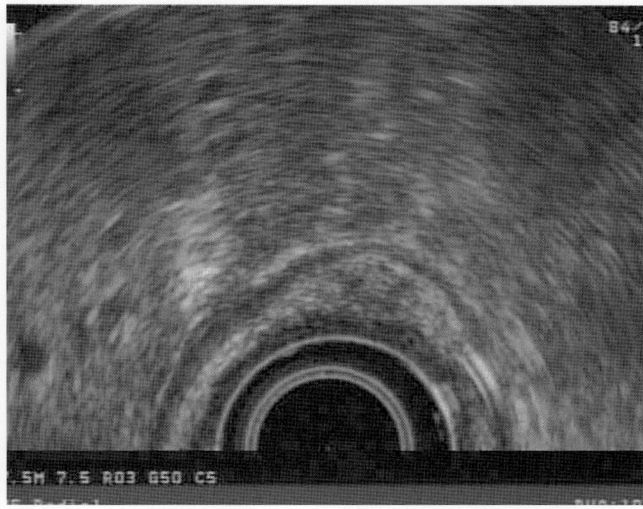

(b)

Figure 53.11 Pancreatic rest: **(a)** endoscopic view; **(b)** radial endosonographic image.

The characteristic endoscopic appearance is a smooth raised lesion with a central dimpling or umbilication. Most of the lesions are found in the antrum of the stomach. If the endoscopic appearance is not diagnostic, endoscopic ultrasound (EUS) may be helpful in the evaluation, especially when deep biopsies or surgical resection are being considered [153]. Either radial EUS or miniprobe EUS can be used to characterize these lesions. The typical appearance is that of a hypoechoic or intermediate echogenic lesion arising most often from the third (submucosa) or fourth (muscularis propria) layer.

Endoscopic resection using techniques of mucosal resection (band EMR, snare polypectomy) are generally effective, but in cases where the lesion is larger than 1.5 cm, endoscopic submucosal dissection may be considered. Surgery is rarely necessary.

Squamous cardiac epithelium

Squamous epithelial extension into the proximal stomach has been reported. In the earliest report, 16 patients (all male and nearly all Caucasian), were described [154]. Most of the patients had pyrosis (75%) and hiatal hernias (100%), and many had Barrett esophagus (38%). None of the patients had a history of caustic ingestion or prior gastric surgery. Most had solitary tongues of this squamous epithelium in the proximal stomach, but multiple tongues and islands were also identified. Squamous metaplasia of the stomach has also been described on the lesser curvature of the stomach, near the cardia [144]. Prior gastric injury, such as that from gastric ulcers or electrocautery, has been proposed as an underlying factor [142,154–156]. For example, 12 patients with previous ablation of Barrett esophagus using multipolar electrocautery have been reported to develop squamous epithelium in the gastric cardia (mean length, 1.7 cm). Although some investigators have proposed that squamous epithelium in the stomach represents metaplasia from prior injury, others believe this phenomenon is a normal variant [156]. The true incidence and clinical significance of this finding are unknown.

References are available at www.yamadagastro.com/textbook7e

Further reading

Byrne W.F. Foreign bodies, bezoars, and caustic ingestion. Gastroenterol Clin North Am 1994;4:99.

Fullum T.M., Oyetunji T.A., Ortega G., et al. Open versus laparoscopic hiatal hernia repair. JSLS 2013;17:23.

Kahrilas P.J., Kim H.C., Pandolfino J.E. Approaches to the diagnosis of hiatal hernia. Best Pract Res Clin Gastroenterol 2008;22:601.

Katsinelos P., Kountouras J., Paroutoglou G., et al. Endoscopic techniques and management of foreign body ingestion and food bolus impaction in the upper gastrointestinal tract: a retrospective analysis of 139 cases. J Clin Gastroenterol 2006;40:784.

Oelschalager B.K., Pellegrini C.A., Hunter J., et al. Biologic prosthesis reduces recurrence after laparoscopic paraesophageal hernia repair: a multicenter, prospective, randomized trial. Ann Surg 2006;244:481.

Watson D.I. Evolution and development of surgery for large paresophageal hiatus hernia. World J Surg 2011;35:1436.